QUICK LOOK DRUG BOOK

2007

Leonard L. Lance, RPh, BSPharm
Senior Editor
Pharmacist
Lexi-Comp, Inc.
Hudson, Ohio

Charles F. Lacy, PharmD, FCSHP
Editor
Vice President, Information Technologies
Professor, Pharmacy Practice
Professor, Business Leadership
University of Southern Nevada
Las Vegas, Nevada

Morton P. Goldman, PharmD, BCPS, FCCP
Associate Editor
Assistant Director, Pharmacotherapy Services
Department of Pharmacy
Cleveland Clinic Foundation
Cleveland, Ohio

Lora L. Armstrong, PharmD, BCPS
Associate Editor
Vice President, Clinical Affairs
Pharmacy & Therapeutics Formulary Process
Clinical Program Oversight
CaremarkRx
Northbrook, Illinois

Wolters Kluwer Health | Lippincott Williams & Wilkins

Philadelphia • Baltimore • New York • London
Buenos Aires • Hong Kong • Sydney • Tokyo

QUICK LOOK DRUG BOOK

2007

Leonard L. Lance, RPh, BSPharm
Senior Editor
Pharmacist
Lexi-Comp, Inc.
Hudson, Ohio

Charles F. Lacy, PharmD, FCSHP
Editor
Vice President, Information Technologies
Professor, Pharmacy Practice
Professor, Business Leadership
University of Southern Nevada
Las Vegas, Nevada

Morton P. Goldman, PharmD, BCPS, FCCP
Associate Editor
Assistant Director, Pharmacotherapy Services
Department of Pharmacy
Cleveland Clinic Foundation
Cleveland, Ohio

Lora L. Armstrong, PharmD, BCPS
Associate Editor
Vice President, Clinical Affairs
Pharmacy & Therapeutics Formulary Process
Clinical Program Oversight
CaremarkRx
Northbrook, Illinois

NOTICE

This handbook is intended to serve the user as a handy quick reference and not as a complete drug information resource. It does not include information on every therapeutic agent available. The publication covers 1600 commonly used drugs and is specifically designed to present certain important aspects of drug data in a more concise format than is generally found in medical literature or product material supplied by manufacturers.

Although great care was taken to ensure the accuracy of the handbook's content when it went to press, the editors, contributors, and publisher cannot be responsible for the continued accuracy of the supplied information due to ongoing research and new developments in the field. Further, the *Quick Look Drug Book* is not offered as a guide to dosing. The reader, herewith, is advised that information shown under the heading **Usual Dosage** is provided only as an indication of the amount of the drug typically given or taken during therapy. Actual dosing amount for any specific drug should be based on an in-depth evaluation of the individual patient's therapy requirement and strong consideration given to such issues as contraindications, warnings, precautions, adverse reactions, along with the interaction of other drugs. The manufacturers' most current product information or other standard recognized references should always be consulted for such detailed information prior to drug use.

The editors and contributors have written this book in their private capacities. No official support or endorsement by any federal agency or pharmaceutical company is intended or inferred.

This manual was produced using Lexi-Comp's Information Management System™ (LIMS) — a complete publishing service of Lexi-Comp Inc.

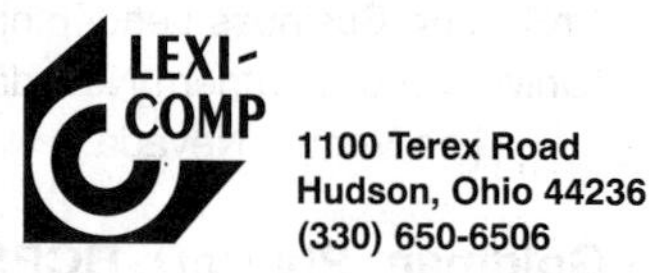

1100 Terex Road
Hudson, Ohio 44236
(330) 650-6506

TABLE OF CONTENTS

ABOUT THE AUTHORS

Leonard L. Lance, RPh, BSPharm

Leonard L. (Bud) Lance has been directly involved in the pharmaceutical industry since receiving his bachelor's degree in pharmacy from Ohio Northern University in 1970. Upon graduation from ONU, Mr Lance spent four years as a navy pharmacist in various military assignments and was instrumental in the development and operation of the first whole hospital I.V. admixture program in a military (Portsmouth Naval Hospital) facility. His last 15 months in the Navy were spent on the USS Independence CV-62.

After completing his military service, he entered the retail pharmacy field and has managed both an independent and a home I.V. franchise pharmacy operation. Since the late 1970s, Mr Lance has focused much of his interest on using computers to improve pharmacy service. The independent pharmacy he worked for was one of the first retail pharmacies in the State of Ohio to computerize (1977).

His love for computers and pharmacy led him to Lexi-Comp, Inc. in 1988. He was the first pharmacist at Lexi-Comp and helped develop Lexi-Comp's first drug database in 1989 and was involved in the editing and publishing of Lexi-Comp's first *Drug Information Handbook* in 1990.

As a result of his strong publishing interest, he presently serves in the capacity of pharmacy editor and technical advisor as well as pharmacy (information) database coordinator for Lexi-Comp. Along with the *Quick Look Drug Book*, he provides technical support to Lexi-Comp's *Drug Information Handbook for the Allied Health Professional* and Lexi-Comp's reference publications. Mr Lance also assists approximately 300 major hospitals in producing their own formulary (pharmacy) publications through Lexi-Comp's custom publishing service. Mr Lance is also Manager of the Dosage Forms database in the Medical Sciences Division at Lexi-Comp.

Mr Lance is a member and past president (1984) of the Summit Pharmaceutical Association (SPA). He is also a member of the Ohio Pharmacists Association (OPA), the American Pharmaceutical Association (APhA), and the American Society of Health-System Pharmacists (ASHP).

Charles F. Lacy, PharmD, FCSHP

Dr Lacy is the Vice President for Information Technologies, Professor of Pharmacy Practice, and Professor of Business Leadership at the University of Southern Nevada. In his capacity at the university, Dr Lacy oversees the directors of the Library and Learning Resources Center and the University Information Systems. Additionally, Dr Lacy is a co-founder of the University. Currently, Dr Lacy is also the Director of International Programs for the university, which includes the College of Pharmacy, the College of Business Administration, and the College of Nursing. Previously, Dr Lacy was the Facilitative Officer for Clinical Programs for the College of Pharmacy where he managed the clinical curriculum, clinical faculty activities, student experiential programs, pharmacy residency programs, and the college's continuing education programs.

Prior to co-founding the Nevada College of Pharmacy, Dr Lacy was the Clinical Coordinator for the Department of Pharmacy at Cedars-Sinai Medical Center. With 20 years of clinical experience, he has developed a reputation as an acknowledged expert in drug information, pharmacy practice, and critical care drug therapy.

Dr Lacy received his doctorate from the University of Southern California School of Pharmacy. Presently, Dr Lacy holds teaching affiliations with the University of Southern Nevada, the University of Southern California, the University of the Pacific School of Pharmacy, Western University of Health Sciences School of Pharmacy, Hokkaido College of Pharmacy in Otaru, Japan, and the University of Alberta at Edmonton, School of Pharmacy and Health Sciences.

Dr Lacy is an active member of numerous professional associations including the American Society of Health-System Pharmacists (ASHP), the American College of Clinical Pharmacy (ACCP), the American Society of Consultant Pharmacists (ASCP), the American Association of Colleges of Pharmacy (AACP), American Pharmacists Association (APhA), and the California Society of Hospital Pharmacists (CSHP), through which he has chaired many committees and subcommittees.

Morton P. Goldman, PharmD, BCPS, FCCP

Dr Goldman received his bachelor's degree in pharmacy from the University of Pittsburgh, College of Pharmacy and his Doctor of Pharmacy degree from the University of Cincinnati, Division of Graduate Studies and Research. He completed his concurrent 2-year hospital pharmacy residency at the VA Medical Center in Cincinnati. Dr Goldman is presently the Assistant Director of Pharmacotherapy Services for the Department of Pharmacy at the Cleveland Clinic Foundation (CCF) after having spent over 4 years at CCF as an Infectious Disease pharmacist and 4 years as Clinical Manager. He holds faculty appointments from The University of Toledo, College of Pharmacy and Case Western Reserve University, College of Medicine and is the Pharmacology Curriculum Coordinator for the new Cleveland Clinic Lerner College of Medicine. Dr Goldman is a Board-Certified Pharmacotherapy Specialist (BCPS) with added qualifications in infectious diseases.

In his capacity as Assistant Director of Pharmacotherapy Services at CCF, Dr Goldman remains actively involved in patient care and clinical research with the Department of Infectious Disease, as well as the continuing education of the medical and pharmacy staff. He is an editor of CCF's *Guidelines for Antibiotic Use* and participates in their annual Antimicrobial Review retreat. He is a member of the Pharmacy and Therapeutics Committee and many of its subcommittees. Dr Goldman has authored numerous journal articles and lectures locally and nationally on infectious diseases topics and current drug therapies. He is currently a reviewer for the *Annals of Pharmacotherapy* and the *Journal of the American Medical Association*, an editorial board member of the *Journal of Infectious Disease Pharmacotherapy*, and coauthor of the *Infectious Diseases Handbook*, the *Drug Information Handbook*, and the *Drug Information Handbook for the Allied Health Professional* produced by Lexi-Comp, Inc. He also provides technical support to Lexi-Comp's Clinical Reference Library™ publications.

Dr Goldman is an active member of the Ohio College of Clinical Pharmacy, the Society of Infectious Disease Pharmacists, the American College of Clinical Pharmacy (and is a Fellow of the College), and the American Society of Health-Systems Pharmacists.

Lora Armstrong, PharmD, BCPS

Dr Armstrong received her bachelor's degree in pharmacy from Ferris State University and her Doctor of Pharmacy degree from Midwestern University. Dr Armstrong is a Board-Certified Pharmacotherapy Specialist (BCPS).

In her current position, Dr Armstrong serves as Vice President of Clinical Affairs with responsibility for the National Pharmacy & Therapeutics Committee process, Clinical Program Oversight process, and Pharmaceutical Pipeline Services at Caremark. Caremark is a prescription benefit management company (PBM). Dr Armstrong is also responsible for monitoring drug surveillance and communicating Pharmacy & Therapeutics Committee Formulary information to Caremark's internal and external customers.

Prior to joining Caremark, Inc, Dr Armstrong served as the Director of Drug Information Services at the University of Chicago Hospitals. She obtained 17 years of experience in a variety of clinical settings including critical care, hematology, oncology, infectious diseases, and clinical pharmacokinetics. Dr Armstrong played an active role in the education and training of medical, pharmacy, and nursing staff. She coordinated the Drug Information Center, the medical center's Adverse Drug Reaction Monitoring Program, and the continuing Education Program for pharmacists. She also maintained the hospital's strict formulary program and was the editor of the University of Chicago Hospitals' *Formulary of Accepted Drugs* and the drug information center's monthly newsletter *Topics in Drug Therapy*.

Dr Armstrong is an active member of the Academy of Managed Care Pharmacy (AMCP), the American Society of Health-Systems Pharmacists (ASHP), the American Pharmaceutical Association (APhA), the American College of Clinical Pharmacy (ACCP), and the Pharmacy & Therapeutics Society (P & T Society). Dr Armstrong wrote the chapter entitled "Drugs and Hormones Used in Endocrinology" in the 4th edition of the textbook *Endocrinology*. She is an Adjunct Clinical Instructor of Pharmacy Practice at Midwestern University. Dr Armstrong currently serves on the Drug Information Advisory Board for pharmacist.com and on the American Pharmaceutical Association Scientific Review Panel for Evaluations of Drug Interactions (EDI).

EDITORIAL ADVISORY PANEL

David S. Jacobs, MD
President, Pathologists Chartered
Consultant in Pathology and Laboratory Medicine
Overland Park, Kansas

Polly E. Kintzel, PharmD, BCPS, BCOP
Clinical Pharmacy Specialist - Oncology
Spectrum Health
Grand Rapids, Michigan

Jill M. Kolesar, PharmD, FCCP, BCPS
Associate Professor of Pharmacy
University of Wisconsin
Madison, Wisconsin

Donna M. Kraus, PharmD, FAPhA
Associate Professor of Pharmacy Practice
Departments of Pharmacy Practice and Pediatrics
Pediatric Clinical Pharmacist
University of Illinois
Chicago, Illinois

Daniel L. Krinsky, RPh, MS
Director, Pharmacotherapy Sales & Marketing
Lexi-Comp, Inc
Hudson, Ohio

Kay Kyllonen, PharmD
Clinical Specialist
The Cleveland Clinic Children's Hospital
Cleveland, Ohio

Charles Lacy, RPh, PharmD, FCSHP
Vice President, Information Technologies
Professor, Pharmacy Practice
Professor, Business Leadership
University of Southern Nevada
Las Vegas, Nevada

Brenda R. Lance, RN, MSN
Program Development Director
Northcoast HealthCare Management Company
Northcoast Infusion Therapies
Oakwood Village, Ohio

Leonard L. Lance, RPh, BSPharm
Clinical Pharmacist
Lexi-Comp, Inc
Hudson, Ohio

Jerrold B. Leikin, MD, FACP, FACEP, FACMT, FAACT
Director, Medical Toxicology
Evanston Northwestern Healthcare-OMEGA
Glenbrook Hospital
Glenview, Illinois
Associate Director
Toxikon Consortium at Cook County Hospital
Chicago, Illinois
Professor of Medicine
Pharmacology and Health Systems Management
Rush Medical College
Chicago, Illinois
Professor of Medicine
Feinberg School of Medicine
Northwestern University
Chicago, Illinois

EDITORIAL ADVISORY PANEL

Amy VanOrman, PharmD
Pharmacotherapy Specialist
Lexi-Comp, Inc
Hudson, Ohio

David M. Weinstein, PhD
Pharmacotherapy Specialist
Lexi-Comp, Inc.
Hudson, Ohio

Anne Marie Whelan, PharmD
College of Pharmacy
Dalhouise University
Halifax, Nova Scotia

Richard L. Wynn, PhD
Professor of Pharmacology
Baltimore College of Dental Surgery
Dental School
University of Maryland Baltimore
Baltimore, Maryland

PREFACE

Working with clinical pharmacists, hospital pharmacy and therapeutics committees, and hospital drug information centers, the editors of this handbook have directly assisted in the development and production of hospital-specific formulary documentation for several hundred major medical institutions in the United States and Canada. The resultant documentation provides pertinent detail concerning use of medications within the hospital and other clinical settings. The most current information on medications has been extracted, reviewed, coalesced, and cross-referenced by the editors to create this *Quick Look Drug Book*.

Thus, this handbook gives the user quick access to data on 1600 medications with cross-referencing to 5709 U.S. and Canadian brand or trade names. Selection of the included medications was based on the analysis of those medications offered in a wide range of hospital formularies. The concise standardized format for data used in this handbook was developed to ensure a consistent presentation of information for all medications.

All generic drug names and synonyms appear in lower case, whereas brand or trade names appear in upper/lower case with the proper trademark information. These three items appear as individual entries in the alphabetical listing of drugs and, thus, there is no requirement for an alphabetical index of drugs.

Mailing and WEB site addresses for Pharmaceutical Manufacturers' and Drug Distributors are provided in the appendix section of this book.

The Indication/Therapeutic Category Index is an expedient mechanism for locating the medication of choice along with its classification. This index will help the user, with knowledge of the disease state, to identify medications which are most commonly used in treatment. All disease states are cross-referenced to a varying number of medications with the most frequently used medication(s) noted.

— L.L. Lance

ACKNOWLEDGMENTS

The *Quick Look Drug Book* exists in its present form as the result of the concerted efforts of the following individuals: Robert D. Kerscher, publisher and chief executive officer of Lexi-Comp, Inc; Steven Kerscher, president and chief operating officer; Mark F. Bonfiglio, BS, PharmD, RPh, chief content officer; Stacy S. Robinson, editorial manager; Cynthia Forney, drug identification database manager; Daniel L. Krinsky, director, pharmacotherapy sales and marketing; Ginger S. Stein, project manager; David C. Marcus, chief information officer; Leslie Jo Hoppes, pharmacology database manager; and Alexandra Hart, composition specialist.

Special acknowledgment goes to all Lexi-Comp staff for their contributions to this handbook.

USE OF THE HANDBOOK

The *Quick Look Drug Book* is organized into a drug information section, an appendix, and an indication/therapeutic category index.

The drug information section of the handbook, wherein all drugs are listed alphabetically, details information pertinent to each drug. Extensive cross-referencing is provided by brand name and synonyms.

Drug information is presented in a consistent format and for quick reference will provide the following:

Generic Name	U.S. Adopted Name (USAN) or International Nonproprietary Name (INN) If a drug product is only available in Canada, a ***(Canada only)*** will be attached to that product and will appear with every occurrence of that drug throughout the book
Pronunciation Guide	Subjective aid for pronouncing drug names
Sound-Alike/Look-Alike Issues	Lists drugs with similar sounding names or names that look alike
Synonyms	Official names and some slang
Tall-Man	"Tall-Man" lettering revisions recommended by the FDA
U.S./Canadian Brand Names	Common trade names used in the United States and Canada
Therapeutic Category	Lexi-Comp's own system of logical medication classification
Controlled Substance	Drug Enforcement Agency (DEA) classification for federally scheduled controlled substances
Use	Information pertaining to appropriate use of the drug
Usual Dosage	The amount of the drug to be typically given or taken during therapy
Dosage Forms	Information with regard to form, strength and availability of the drug

Appendix

The appendix offers a compilation of tables, guidelines, and conversion information that can often be helpful when considering patient care.

Indication/Therapeutic Category Index

This index provides a listing of accepted drugs for various disease states thus focusing attention on selection of medications most frequently prescribed in relation to a clinical diagnosis. Diseases may have other nonofficial drugs for their treatment and this indication/therapeutic category index should not be used by itself to determine the appropriateness of a particular therapy. The listed indications may encompass varying degrees of severity and, since certain medications may not be appropriate for a given degree of severity, it should not be assumed that the agents listed for specific indications are interchangeable. Also included as a valuable reference is each medication's therapeutic category.

TALL-MAN LETTERS

Confusion between similar drug names is an important cause of medication errors. For years, The Institute for Safe Medication Practices (ISMP), has urged generic manufacturers use a combination of large and small letters as well as bolding (ie, chlorpro**MAZINE** and chlorpro**PAMIDE**) to help distinguish drugs with look-alike names, especially when they share similar strengths. Recently the FDA's Division of Generic Drugs began to issue recommendation letters to manufacturers suggesting this novel way to label their products to help reduce this drug name confusion. Although this project has had marginal success, the method has successfully eliminated problems with products such as diphenhydr**AMINE** and dimenhy**DRINATE**. Hospitals should also follow suit by making similar changes in their own labels, preprinted order forms, computer screens and printouts, and drug storage location labels.

In order for all involved to become more familiar with the FDA's recent suggestion, in this edition of the *Quick Look Drug Book* the "Tall-Man" lettering revisions will be listed in a field called **Tall-Man**.

The following is a list of product names and recommended FDA revisions.

Drug Product	Recommended Revision
acetazolamide	aceta**ZOLAMIDE**
acetohexamide	aceto**HEXAMIDE**
bupropion	bu**PROP**ion
buspirone	bus**PIR**one
chlorpromazine	chlorpro**MAZINE**
chlorpropamide	chlorpro**PAMIDE**
clomiphene	clomi**PHENE**
clomipramine	clomi**PRAMINE**
cycloserine	cyclo**SERINE**
cyclosporine	cyclo**SPORINE**
daunorubicin	**DAUNO**rubicin
dimenhydrinate	dimenhy**DRINATE**
diphenhydramine	diphenhydr**AMINE**
dobutamine	**DOBUT**amine
dopamine	**DOP**amine
doxorubicin	**DOXO**rubicin
glipizide	glipi**ZIDE**
glyburide	gly**BURIDE**
hydralazine	hydr**ALAZINE**
hydroxyzine	hydr**OXY**zine
medroxyprogesterone	medroxy**PROGESTER**one
methylprednisolone	methyl**PREDNIS**olone
methyltestosterone	methyl**TESTOSTER**one
nicardipine	ni**CAR**dipine
nifedipine	**NIFE**dipine
prednisolone	predniso**LONE**
prednisone	predni**SONE**

sulfadiazine	sulfa**DIAZINE**
sulfisoxazole	sulfi**SOXAZOLE**
tolazamide	**TOLAZ**amide
tolbutamide	**TOLBUT**amide
vinblastine	vin**BLAS**tine
vincristine	vin**CRIS**tine

Institute for Safe Medication Practices. "New Tall-Man Lettering Will Reduce Mix-Ups Due to Generic Drug Name Confusion," *ISMP Medication Safety Alert*, September 19, 2001. Available at: http://www.ismp.org.

Institute for Safe Medication Practices. "Prescription Mapping, Can Improve Efficiency While Minimizing Errors With Look-Alike Products," *ISMP Medication Safety Alert*, October 6, 1999. Available at: http://www.ismp.org.

U.S. Pharmacopeia, "USP Quality Review: Use Caution-Avoid Confusion," March 2001, No. 76. Available at: http://www.usp.org.

SAFE WRITING

Health professionals and their support personnel frequently produce handwritten copies of information they see in print; therefore, such information is subjected to even greater possibilities for error or misinterpretation on the part of others. Thus, particular care must be given to how drug names and strengths are expressed when creating written health care documents.

The following are a few examples of safe writing rules suggested by the Institute for Safe Medication Practices, Inc.*

1. There should be a space between a number and its units as it is easier to read. There should be no periods after the abbreviations mg or mL.

Correct	**Incorrect**
10 mg	10mg
100 mg	100mg

2. Never place a decimal and a zero after a whole number (2 mg is correct and 2.0 mg is incorrect). If the decimal point is not seen because it falls on a line or because individuals are working from copies where the decimal point is not seen, this causes a tenfold overdose.
3. Just the opposite is true for numbers less than one. Always place a zero before a naked decimal (0.5 mL is correct, .5 mL is **in**correct).
4. Never abbreviate the word "unit." The handwritten U or u, looks like a 0 (zero), and may cause a tenfold overdose error to be made.
5. IU is not a safe abbreviation for international units. The handwritten IU looks like IV. Write out international units or use int. units.
6. Q.D. is not a safe abbreviation for once daily, as when the Q is followed by a sloppy dot, it looks like QID which means four times daily.
7. O.D. is not a safe abbreviation for once daily, as it is properly interpreted as meaning "right eye" and has caused liquid medications such as saturated solution of potassium iodide and Lugol's solution to be administered incorrectly. There is no safe abbreviation for once daily. It must be written out in full.
8. Do not use chemical names such as 6-mercaptopurine or 6-thioguanine, as 6-fold overdoses have been given when these were not recognized as chemical names. The proper names of these drugs are mercaptopurine or thioguanine.
9. Do not abbreviate drug names (5FC, 6MP, 5-ASA, MTX, HCTZ CPZ, PBZ, etc) as they are misinterpreted and cause error.
10. Do not use the apothecary system or symbols.
11. Do not abbreviate microgram as µg; instead use mcg as there is less likelihood of misinterpretation.
12. When writing an outpatient prescription, write a complete prescription. A complete prescription can prevent the prescriber, the pharmacist, and/or the patient from making a mistake and can eliminate the need for further clarification. The legible prescriptions should contain:
    a. patient's full name
    b. for pediatric or geriatric patients: their age (or weight where applicable)

*From "Safe Writing" by Davis NM, PharmD and Cohen MR, MS, Lecturers and Consultants for Safe Medication Practices, 1143 Wright Drive, Huntingdon Valley, PA 19006. Phone: (215) 947-7566.

c. drug name, dosage form and strength; if a drug is new or rarely prescribed, print this information

d. number or amount to be dispensed

e. complete instructions for the patient, including the purpose of the medication

f. when there are recognized contraindications for a prescribed drug, indicate to the pharmacist that you are aware of this fact (ie, when prescribing a potassium salt for a patient receiving an ACE inhibitor, write "K serum leveling being monitored")

ALPHABETICAL LISTING OF DRUGS

1370-999-397 *see* anagrelide *on page 55*

A_1-PI *see* alpha$_1$-proteinase inhibitor *on page 31*

A200® Lice [US-OTC] *see* permethrin *on page 655*

A-200® Maximum Strength [US-OTC] *see* pyrethrins and piperonyl butoxide *on page 720*

A and D® Original [US-OTC] *see* vitamin A and vitamin D *on page 876*

abacavir (a BAK a veer)

Synonyms abacavir sulfate; ABC

U.S./Canadian Brand Names Ziagen® [US/Can]

Therapeutic Category Nucleoside Reverse Transcriptase Inhibitor (NRTI)

Use Treatment of HIV infections in combination with other antiretroviral agents

Usual Dosage Oral:

Children: 3 months to 16 years: 8 mg/kg body weight twice daily (maximum: 300 mg twice daily) in combination with other antiretroviral agents

Adults: 300 mg twice daily or 600 mg once daily in combination with other antiretroviral agents

Dosage Forms

Solution, oral:

Ziagen®: 20 mg/mL (240 mL) [strawberry-banana flavor]

Tablet:

300 mg

abacavir and lamivudine (a BAK a veer & la MI vyoo deen)

Synonyms abacavir sulfate and lamivudine; lamivudine and abacavir

U.S./Canadian Brand Names Epzicom™ [US]; Kivexa™ [Can]

Therapeutic Category Antiretroviral Agent, Reverse Transcriptase Inhibitor (Nucleoside)

Use Treatment of HIV infections in combination with other antiretroviral agents

Usual Dosage Oral: Adults: HIV: One tablet (abacavir 600 mg and lamivudine 300 mg) once daily

Dosage Forms

Tablet:

Epzicom™: Abacavir 600 mg and lamivudine 300 mg

abacavir, lamivudine, and zidovudine

(a BAK a veer, la MI vyoo deen, & zye DOE vyoo deen)

Synonyms azidothymidine, abacavir, and lamivudine; AZT, abacavir, and lamivudine; compound S, abacavir, and lamivudine; lamivudine, abacavir, and zidovudine; 3TC, abacavir, and zidovudine; ZDV, abacavir, and lamivudine; zidovudine, abacavir, and lamivudine

U.S./Canadian Brand Names Trizivir® [US]

Therapeutic Category Antiretroviral Agent, Nucleoside Reverse Transcriptase Inhibitor (NRTI)

Use Treatment of HIV infection (either alone or in combination with other antiretroviral agents) in patients whose regimen would otherwise contain the components of Trizivir®

Usual Dosage Oral: Adolescents and Adults: 1 tablet twice daily; **Note:** Not recommended for patients <40 kg

Dosage Forms

Tablet:

Trizivir®: Abacavir 300 mg, lamivudine 150 mg, and zidovudine 300 mg

abacavir sulfate *see* abacavir *on this page*

abacavir sulfate and lamivudine *see* abacavir and lamivudine *on this page*

abarelix (a ba REL iks)

Synonyms PPI-149; R-3827

Therapeutic Category Gonadotropin Releasing Hormone Antagonist

Use Palliative treatment of advanced symptomatic prostate cancer; treatment is limited to men who are not candidates for LHRH therapy, refuse surgical castration, and have one or more of the following complications due to metastases or local encroachment: 1) risk of neurological compromise, 2) ureteral or bladder outlet obstruction, or 3) severe bone pain (persisting despite narcotic analgesia)

Usual Dosage I.M.: Male prostate cancer: 100 mg administered on days 1, 15, 29 (week 4), then every 4 weeks

Dosage Forms [DSC] = Discontinued product
Injection, powder for reconstitution [preservative free]: 113 mg [provides 100 mg/2 mL depot suspension when reconstituted; packaged with diluent and syringe] [DSC]

abatacept (ab a TA sept)

Synonyms CTLA-4Ig
U.S./Canadian Brand Names Orencia® [US]
Therapeutic Category Antirheumatic, Disease Modifying
Use Treatment of rheumatoid arthritis not responsive to other disease-modifying antirheumatic drugs (DMARD); may be used as monotherapy or in combination with other DMARDs (**not** in combination with TNF-blocking agents)
Usual Dosage I.V.: Adults: Dosing is according to body weight: Repeat dose at 2 weeks and 4 weeks after initial dose, and every 4 weeks thereafter:
<60 kg: 500 mg
60-100 kg: 750 mg
>100 kg: 1000 mg
Dosage Forms Injection, powder for reconstitution [preservative free]: 250 mg

Abbokinase® *(Discontinued)*

abbott-43818 *see* leuprolide *on page 486*

ABC *see* abacavir *on previous page*

ABCD *see* amphotericin B cholesteryl sulfate complex *on page 50*

abciximab (ab SIK si mab)

Synonyms C7E3; 7E3
U.S./Canadian Brand Names ReoPro® [US/Can]
Therapeutic Category Platelet Aggregation Inhibitor
Use Prevention of acute cardiac ischemic complications in patients at high risk for abrupt closure of the treated coronary vessel and patients at risk of restenosis; an adjunct with heparin to prevent cardiac ischemic complications in patients with unstable angina not responding to conventional therapy when a percutaneous coronary intervention (PCI) is scheduled within 24 hours
Usual Dosage
Acute coronary syndromes: PCI: I.V.: 0.25 mg/kg bolus administered 10-60 minutes before the start of intervention followed by an infusion of 0.125 mcg/kg/minute (to a maximum of 10 mcg/minute) for 12 hours
Patients with unstable angina not responding to conventional medical therapy and who are planning to undergo percutaneous coronary intervention within 24 hours may be treated with abciximab 0.25 mg/kg intravenous bolus followed by an 18- to 24-hour intravenous infusion of 10 mcg/minute, concluding 1 hour after the percutaneous coronary intervention.
Dosage Forms Injection, solution: 2 mg/mL (5 mL)

Abelcet® [US/Can] *see* amphotericin B lipid complex *on page 52*

Abenol® [Can] *see* acetaminophen *on page 5*

Abilify® [US] *see* aripiprazole *on page 73*

ABLC *see* amphotericin B lipid complex *on page 52*

A/B Otic [US] *see* antipyrine and benzocaine *on page 62*

Abraxane™ [US] *see* paclitaxel (protein bound) *on page 631*

Abreva® [US-OTC] *see* docosanol *on page 270*

absorbable cotton *see* cellulose, oxidized regenerated *on page 165*

absorbable gelatin sponge *see* gelatin (absorbable) *on page 377*

Absorbine® Antifungal *(Discontinued)* *see* tolnaftate *on page 834*

Absorbine® Jock Itch *(Discontinued)* *see* tolnaftate *on page 834*

AC 2993 *see* exenatide *on page 332*

acamprosate (a kam PROE sate)

Synonyms acamprosate calcium; calcium acetylhomotaurinate
U.S./Canadian Brand Names Campral® [US]
Therapeutic Category GABA Agonist/Glutamate Antagonist
Use Maintenance of alcohol abstinence
(Continued)

acamprosate *(Continued)*

Usual Dosage Oral: Adults: Alcohol abstinence: 666 mg 3 times/day (a lower dose may be effective in some patients)

Dosage Forms Tablet, enteric coated, delayed release, as calcium: 333 mg [contains calcium 33 mg and sulfites]

acamprosate calcium *see* acamprosate *on previous page*

acarbose (AY car bose)

Sound-Alike/Look-Alike Issues

Precose® may be confused with PreCare®

U.S./Canadian Brand Names Prandase® [Can]; Precose® [US]

Therapeutic Category Antidiabetic Agent, Oral

Use

Monotherapy, as indicated as an adjunct to diet to lower blood glucose in patients with type 2 diabetes mellitus (noninsulin dependent, NIDDM) whose hyperglycemia cannot be managed on diet alone

Combination with a sulfonylurea, metformin, or insulin in patients with type 2 diabetes mellitus (noninsulin dependent, NIDDM) when diet plus acarbose do not result in adequate glycemic control. The effect of acarbose to enhance glycemic control is additive to that of other hypoglycemic agents when used in combination.

Usual Dosage Oral:

Adults: Dosage must be individualized on the basis of effectiveness and tolerance while not exceeding the maximum recommended dose

Initial dose: 25 mg 3 times/day with the first bite of each main meal

Maintenance dose: Should be adjusted at 4- to 8-week intervals based on 1-hour postprandial glucose levels and tolerance. Dosage may be increased from 25 mg 3 times/day to 50 mg 3 times/day. Some patients may benefit from increasing the dose to 100 mg 3 times/day.

Maintenance dose ranges: 50-100 mg 3 times/day.

Maximum dose:

≤60 kg: 50 mg 3 times/day

>60 kg: 100 mg 3 times/day

Patients receiving sulfonylureas: Acarbose given in combination with a sulfonylurea will cause a further lowering of blood glucose and may increase the hypoglycemic potential of the sulfonylurea. If hypoglycemia occurs, appropriate adjustments in the dosage of these agents should be made.

Dosage Forms Tablet: 25 mg, 50 mg, 100 mg

A-Caro-25® [US] *see* beta-carotene *on page 106*

Accolate® [US/Can] *see* zafirlukast *on page 883*

AccuHist® PDX Drops [US] *see* brompheniramine, pseudoephedrine, and dextromethorphan *on page 120*

AccuHist® Pediatric *(Discontinued)* *see* brompheniramine and pseudoephedrine *on page 118*

AccuNeb® [US] *see* albuterol *on page 23*

Accupril® [US/Can] *see* quinapril *on page 725*

Accuretic® [US/Can] *see* quinapril and hydrochlorothiazide *on page 725*

Accutane® [US/Can] *see* isotretinoin *on page 466*

Accuzyme® [US] *see* papain and urea *on page 637*

ACE *see* captopril *on page 143*

acebutolol (a se BYOO toe lole)

Sound-Alike/Look-Alike Issues

Sectral® may be confused with Factrel®, Seconal®, Septra®

Synonyms acebutolol hydrochloride

U.S./Canadian Brand Names Apo-Acebutolol® [Can]; Gen-Acebutolol [Can]; Monitan® [Can]; Novo-Acebutolol [Can]; Nu-Acebutolol [Can]; Rhotral [Can]; Rhoxal-acebutolol [Can]; Sandoz-Acebutolol [Can]; Sectral® [US/Can]

Therapeutic Category Antiarrhythmic Agent, Class II; Beta-Adrenergic Blocker

Use Treatment of hypertension, ventricular arrhythmias, angina

Usual Dosage Oral: Adults:

Hypertension: 400-800 mg/day (larger doses may be divided); maximum: 1200 mg/day; usual dose range (JNC 7): 200-800 mg/day in 2 divided doses

Ventricular arrhythmias: Initial: 400 mg/day in divided doses; maintenance: 600-1200 mg/day in divided doses

Dosage Forms Capsule, as hydrochloride: 200 mg, 400 mg

acebutolol hydrochloride *see* acebutolol *on previous page*

Aceon® [US] *see* perindopril erbumine *on page 655*

Acephen™ [US-OTC] *see* acetaminophen *on this page*

Acetadote® [US] *see* acetylcysteine *on page 15*

Aceta-Gesic [US-OTC] *see* acetaminophen and phenyltoloxamine *on page 8*

acetaminophen (a seet a MIN oh fen)

Sound-Alike/Look-Alike Issues

Acephen® may be confused with AcipHex®

FeverAll® may be confused with Fiberall®

Tylenol® may be confused with atenolol, timolol, Tuinal®, Tylox®

Synonyms APAP; n-acetyl-p-aminophenol; paracetamol

U.S./Canadian Brand Names Abenol® [Can]; Acephen™ [US-OTC]; Apo-Acetaminophen® [Can]; Apra Children's [US-OTC]; Aspirin Free Anacin® Maximum Strength [US-OTC]; Atasol® [Can]; Cetafen Extra® [US-OTC]; Cetafen® [US-OTC]; Comtrex® Sore Throat Maximum Strength [US-OTC]; FeverAll® [US-OTC]; Genapap™ Children [US-OTC]; Genapap™ Extra Strength [US-OTC]; Genapap™ Infant [US-OTC]; Genapap™ [US-OTC]; Genebs Extra Strength [US-OTC]; Genebs [US-OTC]; Infantaire [US-OTC]; Mapap Children's [US-OTC]; Mapap Extra Strength [US-OTC]; Mapap Infants [US-OTC]; Mapap [US-OTC]; Nortemp Children's [US-OTC]; Novo-Gesic [Can]; Pain-Eze [US-OTC]; Pediatrix [Can]; Silapap® Children's [US-OTC]; Silapap® Infants [US-OTC]; Tempra® [Can]; Tycolene Maximum Strength [US-OTC]; Tycolene [US-OTC]; Tylenol® 8 Hour [US-OTC]; Tylenol® Arthritis Pain [US-OTC]; Tylenol® Children's with Flavor Creator [US-OTC]; Tylenol® Children's [US-OTC]; Tylenol® Extra Strength [US-OTC]; Tylenol® Infants [US-OTC]; Tylenol® Junior [US-OTC]; Tylenol® [US-OTC/Can]; Valorin Extra [US-OTC]; Valorin [US-OTC]

Therapeutic Category Analgesic, Nonnarcotic; Antipyretic

Use Treatment of mild-to-moderate pain and fever (antipyretic/analgesic); does not have antirheumatic or anti-inflammatory effects

Usual Dosage Oral, rectal:

Children <12 years: 10-15 mg/kg/dose every 4-6 hours as needed; do **not** exceed 5 doses (2.6 g) in 24 hours; alternatively, the following age-based doses may be used:

0-3 months: 40 mg

4-11 months: 80 mg

1-2 years: 120 mg

2-3 years: 160 mg

4-5 years: 240 mg

6-8 years: 320 mg

9-10 years: 400 mg

11 years: 480 mg

Note: Higher rectal doses have been studied for use in preoperative pain control in children. However, specific guidelines are not available and dosing may be product dependent. The safety and efficacy of alternating acetaminophen and ibuprofen dosing has not been established.

Adults: 325-650 mg every 4-6 hours or 1000 mg 3-4 times/day; do **not** exceed 4 g/day

Dosage Forms [DSC] = Discontinued product

Caplet: 500 mg

Cetafen Extra® Strength, Genapap™ Extra Strength, Genebs Extra Strength, Mapap Extra Strength, Tycolene Maximum Strength, Tylenol® Extra Strength: 500 mg

Caplet, extended release:

Tylenol® 8 Hour, Tylenol® Arthritis Pain: 650 mg

Capsule: 500 mg

Elixir: 160 mg/5 mL (120 mL, 480 mL, 3780 mL)

Apra Children's: 160 mg/5 mL (120 mL, 480 mL, 3780 mL) [alcohol free; contains benzoic acid; cherry and grape flavors]

Mapap Children's: 160 mg/5 mL (120 mL) [alcohol free; contains benzoic acid and sodium benzoate; cherry flavor]

Gelcap:

Mapap Extra Strength, Tylenol® Extra Strength: 500 mg

Geltab:

Tylenol® Extra Strength: 500 mg

(Continued)

acetaminophen *(Continued)*

Geltab, extended release:
Tylenol® 8 Hour: 650 mg
Liquid, oral: 500 mg/15 mL (240 mL)
Comtrex® Sore Throat Maximum Strength: 500 mg/15 mL (240 mL) [contains sodium benzoate; honey lemon flavor]
Genapap™ Children: 160 mg/5 mL (120 mL) [contains sodium benzoate; cherry and grape flavors]
Silapap®: 160 mg/5 mL (120 mL, 240 mL, 480 mL) [sugar free; contains sodium benzoate; cherry flavor]
Tylenol® Extra Strength: 500 mg/15 mL (240 mL) [contains sodium benzoate; cherry flavor]
Solution, oral: 160 mg/5 mL (120 mL, 480 mL)
Solution, oral drops: 80 mg/0.8 mL (15 mL) [droppers are marked at 0.4 mL (40 mg) and at 0.8 mL (80 mg)]
Genapap™ Infant: 80 mg/0.8 mL (15 mL) [fruit flavor]
Infantaire: 80 mg/0.8mL (15 mL, 30 mL)
Silapap® Infant's: 80 mg/0.8 mL (15 mL, 30 mL) [contains sodium benzoate; cherry flavor]
Suppository, rectal: 120 mg, 325 mg, 650 mg
Acephen™: 120 mg, 325 mg, 650 mg
FeverAll®: 80 mg, 120 mg, 325 mg, 650 mg
Mapap: 125 mg, 650 mg
Suspension, oral:
Mapap Children's: 160 mg/5 mL (120 mL) [contains sodium benzoate; cherry flavor]
Nortemp Children's: 160 mg/5 mL (120 mL) [alcohol free; contains sodium benzoate; cotton candy flavor]
Tylenol® Children's: 160 mg/5 mL (120 mL, 240 mL) [contains sodium benzoate; bubble gum yum, cherry blast, dye free cherry, grape splash, and very berry strawberry flavors]
Tylenol® Children's with Flavor Creator: 160 mg/5 mL (120 mL) [contains sodium 2 mg/5 mL and sodium benzoate; cherry blast flavor; packaged with apple (4), bubblegum (8), chocolate (4), & strawberry (4) sugar free flavor packets]
Suspension, oral drops:
Mapap Infants: 80 mg/0.8 mL (15 mL, 30 mL) [contains sodium benzoate; cherry flavor]
Tylenol® Infants: 80 mg/0.8 mL (15 mL, 30 mL) [contains sodium benzoate; cherry, dye free cherry, and grape flavors]
Syrup, oral:
ElixSure™ Fever/Pain: 160 mg/5 mL (120 mL) [bubble gum, cherry, and grape flavors] [DSC]
Tablet: 325 mg, 500 mg
Aspirin Free Anacin® Extra Strength, Genapap™ Extra Strength, Genebs Extra Strength, Mapap Extra Strength, Pain Eze, Tylenol® Extra Strength, Valorin Extra: 500 mg
Cetafen®, Genapap™, Genebs, Mapap, Tycolene, Tylenol®, Valorin: 325 mg
Tablet, chewable: 80 mg
Genapap™ Children: 80 mg [contains phenylalanine 6 mg/tablet; fruit and grape flavors]
Mapap Children's: 80 mg [contains phenylalanine 3 mg/tablet; bubble gum, fruit, and grape flavors]
Mapap Junior Strength: 160 mg [contains phenylalanine 12 mg/tablet; grape flavor]
Tylenol® Children's: 80 mg [fruit and grape flavors contain phenylalanine 3 mg/tablet; bubble gum flavor contains phenylalanine 6 mg/tablet] [DSC]
Tylenol® Junior: 160 mg [contains phenylalanine 6 mg/tablet; fruit and grape flavors] [DSC]
Tablet, orally disintegrating: 80 mg, 160 mg
Tylenol® Children's Meltaways: 80 mg [bubble gum, grape, and watermelon flavors]
Tylenol® Junior Meltaways: 160 mg [bubble gum and grape flavors]

acetaminophen and chlorpheniramine *see* chlorpheniramine and acetaminophen *on page 176*

acetaminophen and codeine (a seet a MIN oh fen & KOE deen)

Sound-Alike/Look-Alike Issues
Capital® may be confused with Capitrol®
Tylenol® may be confused with atenolol, timolol, Tuinal®, Tylox®

Synonyms codeine and acetaminophen

U.S./Canadian Brand Names Capital® and Codeine [US]; ratio-Emtec [Can]; ratio-Lenoltec [Can]; Triatec-30 [Can]; Triatec-8 Strong [Can]; Triatec-8 [Can]; Tylenol® No. 1 Forte [Can]; Tylenol® Elixir with Codeine [Can]; Tylenol® No. 1 [Can]; Tylenol® No. 2 with Codeine [Can]; Tylenol® No. 3 with Codeine [Can]; Tylenol® No. 4 with Codeine [Can]; Tylenol® With Codeine [US]

Therapeutic Category Analgesic, Narcotic

Controlled Substance C-III; C-V

Use Relief of mild-to-moderate pain

Usual Dosage Doses should be adjusted according to severity of pain and response of the patient. Adult doses ≥60 mg codeine fail to give commensurate relief of pain but merely prolong analgesia and are associated with an appreciably increased incidence of side effects. Oral:

Children: Analgesic:

Codeine: 0.5-1 mg codeine/kg/dose every 4-6 hours

Acetaminophen: 10-15 mg/kg/dose every 4 hours up to a maximum of 2.6 g/24 hours for children <12 years; **alternatively, the following can be used:**

3-6 years: 5 mL 3-4 times/day as needed of elixir

7-12 years: 10 mL 3-4 times/day as needed of elixir

>12 years: 15 mL every 4 hours as needed of elixir

Adults:

Antitussive: Based on codeine (15-30 mg/dose) every 4-6 hours (maximum: 360 mg/24 hours based on codeine component)

Analgesic: Based on codeine (30-60 mg/dose) every 4-6 hours (maximum: 4000 mg/24 hours based on acetaminophen component)

Dosage Forms [DSC] = Discontinued product; [CAN] = Canadian brand name

Caplet:

ratio-Lenoltec No. 1 [CAN], Tylenol No. 1 [CAN]: Acetaminophen 300 mg, codeine phosphate, 8 mg and caffeine 15 mg [not available in the U.S.]

Tylenol No. 1 Forte [CAN]: Acetaminophen 500 mg, codeine phosphate 8 mg, and caffeine 15 mg [not available in the U.S.]

Elixir, oral [C-V]: Acetaminophen 120 mg and codeine phosphate 12 mg per 5 mL (5 mL, 10 mL, 12.5 mL, 15 mL, 120 mL, 480 mL) [contains alcohol 7%]

Tylenol® with Codeine [DSC]: Acetaminophen 120 mg and codeine phosphate 12 mg per 5 mL (480 mL) [contains alcohol 7%; cherry flavor]

Tylenol Elixir with Codeine [CAN]: Acetaminophen 160 mg and codeine phosphate 8 mg per 5 mL (500 mL) [contains alcohol 7%, sucrose 31%; cherry flavor; not available in the U.S.]

Suspension, oral [C-V] (Capital® and Codeine): Acetaminophen 120 mg and codeine phosphate 12 mg per 5 mL (480 mL) [alcohol free; fruit punch flavor]

Tablet [C-III]: Acetaminophen 300 mg and codeine phosphate 15 mg; acetaminophen 300 mg and codeine phosphate 30 mg; acetaminophen 300 mg and codeine phosphate 60 mg

ratio-Emtec [CAN], Triatec-30 [CAN]: Acetaminophen 300 mg and codeine phosphate 30 mg [not available in the U.S.]

ratio-Lenoltec No. 1 [CAN]: Acetaminophen 300 mg, codeine phosphate 8 mg, and caffeine 15 mg [not available in the U.S.]

ratio-Lenoltec No. 2 [CAN], Tylenol No. 2 with Codeine [CAN]: Acetaminophen 300 mg, codeine phosphate 15 mg, and caffeine 15 mg [not available in the U.S.]

ratio-Lenoltec No. 3 [CAN], Tylenol No. 3 with Codeine [CAN]: Acetaminophen 300 mg, codeine phosphate 30 mg, and caffeine 15 mg [not available in the U.S.]

ratio-Lenoltec No. 4 [CAN], Tylenol No. 4 with Codeine [CAN]: Acetaminophen 300 mg and codeine phosphate 60 mg [not available in the U.S.]

Triatec-8 [CAN]: Acetaminophen 325 mg, codeine phosphate 8 mg, and caffeine 30 mg [not available in the U.S.]

Triatec-8 Strong [CAN]: Acetaminophen 500 mg, codeine phosphate 8 mg, and caffeine 30 mg [not available in the U.S.]

Tylenol® with Codeine No. 3: Acetaminophen 300 mg and codeine phosphate 30 mg [contains sodium metabisulfite]

Tylenol® with Codeine No. 4: Acetaminophen 300 mg and codeine phosphate 60 mg [contains sodium metabisulfite]

acetaminophen and diphenhydramine (a seet a MIN oh fen & dye fen HYE dra meen)

Sound-Alike/Look-Alike Issues

Excedrin® may be confused with Dexatrim®, Dexedrine®

Percogesic® may be confused with paregoric, Percodan®

Tylenol® may be confused with atenolol, timolol, Tuinal®, Tylox®

Synonyms diphenhydramine and acetaminophen

U.S./Canadian Brand Names Excedrin® P.M. [US-OTC]; Goody's PM® [US-OTC]; Legatrin PM® [US-OTC]; Percogesic® Extra Strength [US-OTC]; Tylenol® PM [US-OTC]; Tylenol® Severe Allergy [US-OTC]

Therapeutic Category Analgesic, Nonnarcotic

Use Aid in the relief of insomnia accompanied by minor pain

Usual Dosage Oral: Adults: 50 mg of diphenhydramine HCl (76 mg diphenhydramine citrate) at bedtime or as directed by physician; do not exceed recommended dosage; not for use in children <12 years of age

(Continued)

acetaminophen and diphenhydramine *(Continued)*

Dosage Forms

Caplet: Acetaminophen 500 mg and diphenhydramine hydrochloride 25 mg
- Excedrin® P.M.: Acetaminophen 500 mg and diphenhydramine citrate 38 mg
- Legatrin PM®: Acetaminophen 500 mg and diphenhydramine hydrochloride 50 mg
- Percogesic® Extra Strength: Acetaminophen 500 mg and diphenhydramine hydrochloride 25 mg
- Tylenol® PM: Acetaminophen 500 mg and diphenhydramine hydrochloride 25 mg [also available in vanilla caplets]
- Tylenol® Severe Allergy: Acetaminophen 500 mg and diphenhydramine hydrochloride 12.5 mg

Gelcap:
- Tylenol® PM: Acetaminophen 500 mg and diphenhydramine hydrochloride 25 mg

Geltab: Acetaminophen 500 mg and diphenhydramine hydrochloride 25 mg
- Excedrin® P.M.: Acetaminophen 500 mg and diphenhydramine citrate 38 mg
- Tylenol® PM: Acetaminophen 500 mg and diphenhydramine hydrochloride 25 mg

Liquid:
- Tylenol® PM: Acetaminophen 500 mg and diphenhydramine hydrochloride 25 mg per 15 mL (240 mL) [contains sodium benzoate; vanilla flavor]

Powder for oral solution:
- Goody's PM®: Acetaminophen 500 mg and diphenhydramine citrate 38 mg [contains potassium 41.9 mg and sodium 3.15 mg per powder]

Tablet: Acetaminophen 500 mg and diphenhydramine hydrochloride 25 mg
- Excedrin® P.M.: Acetaminophen 500 mg and diphenhydramine citrate 38 mg

acetaminophen and hydrocodone *see* hydrocodone and acetaminophen *on page 420*

acetaminophen and oxycodone *see* oxycodone and acetaminophen *on page 627*

acetaminophen and pentazocine *see* pentazocine and acetaminophen *on page 651*

acetaminophen and phenyltoloxamine (a seet a MIN oh fen & fen il to LOKS a meen)

Sound-Alike/Look-Alike Issues
Percogesic® may be confused with paregoric, Percodan®

Synonyms phenyltoloxamine citrate and acetaminophen

U.S./Canadian Brand Names Aceta-Gesic [US-OTC]; Dologesic® [US]; Flextra 650 [US]; Flextra-DS [US]; Genesec™ [US-OTC]; Hyflex-DS® [US]; Percogesic® [US-OTC]; Phenagesic [US-OTC]; Phenylgesic [US-OTC]; RhinoFlex 650 [US]; RhinoFlex™ [US]; Staflex [US]

Therapeutic Category Analgesic, Nonnarcotic

Use Relief of mild pain

Usual Dosage Oral:

Analgesic: Based on acetaminophen component:
- Children: 10-15 mg/kg/dose every 4-6 hours as needed (maximum: 5 doses/24 hours
- Adults: 325-650 mg every 4-6 hours as needed (maximum: 4 g/day)

Product-specific labeling:

Flextra-650:
- Children 6 to <12 years: 1/2 tablet every 6 hours (maximum: 2 tablets/day)
- Children ≥12 years and Adults: 1/2-1 tablet every 6 hours (maximum: 4 tablets/day)

Flextra-DS, Hyflex-DS®, RhinoFlex™, RhinoFlex™-650:
- Children 6 to <12 years: 1/2 tablet every 4 hours (maximum: 2.5 tablets/day)
- Children ≥12 years and Adults: 1/2-1 tablet every 4 hours (maximum: 5 tablets/day)

Percogesic®:
- Children 6-12 years: 1 tablet every 4 hours (maximum: 4 tablets/24 hours)
- Adults: 1-2 tablets every 4 hours (maximum: 8 tablets/24 hours)

Dosage Forms

Caplet:
- Dologesic®: Acetaminophen 500 mg and phenyltoloxamine citrate 30 mg
- Staflex: Acetaminophen 500 mg and phenyltoloxamine citrate 55 mg

Capsule:
- Dologesic®: Acetaminophen 500 mg and phenyltoloxamine citrate 30 mg

Liquid:
- Dologesic®: Acetaminophen 500 mg and phenyltoloxamine citrate 30 mg per 15 mL (180 mL)

Tablet: Acetaminophen 325 mg and phenyltoloxamine citrate 30 mg
- Aceta-Gesic, Genasec™, Percogesic®, Phenagesic, Phenylgesic: Acetaminophen 325 mg and phenyltoloxamine citrate 30 mg
- Flextra-650: Acetaminophen 650 mg and phenyltoloxamine citrate 60 mg

Flextra-DS, Hyflex-DS®, RhinoFlex™: Acetaminophen 500 mg and phenyltoloxamine citrate 50 mg
RhinoFlex™-650: Acetaminophen 650 mg and phenyltoloxamine citrate 50 mg

acetaminophen and propoxyphene *see* propoxyphene and acetaminophen *on page 708*

acetaminophen and pseudoephedrine (a seet a MIN oh fen & soo doe e FED rin)

Sound-Alike/Look-Alike Issues

Ornex® may be confused with Orexin®, Orinase®
Sudafed® may be confused with Sufenta®
Tylenol® may be confused with atenolol, timolol, Tuinal®, Tylox®

Synonyms pseudoephedrine and acetaminophen

U.S./Canadian Brand Names Alka-Seltzer® Plus® Cold and Sinus Liqui-Gels [US-OTC]; Cetafen Cold® [US-OTC]; Contac® Cold and Sore Throat, Non Drowsy, Extra Strength [Can]; Dristan® N.D. [Can]; Dristan® N.D., Extra Strength [Can]; Genapap® Sinus Maximum Strength [US-OTC]; Mapap Sinus Maximum Strength [US-OTC]; Medi-Synal [US-OTC]; Ornex® Maximum Strength [US-OTC]; Ornex® [US-OTC]; Sinus-Relief® [US-OTC]; Sinutab® Non Drowsy [Can]; Sinutab® Sinus [US-OTC]; Sudafed® Head Cold and Sinus Extra Strength [Can]; Sudafed® Sinus and Cold [US-OTC]; Sudafed® Sinus Headache [US-OTC]; SudoGest Sinus [US-OTC]; Tylenol® Cold, Infants [US-OTC]; Tylenol® Decongestant [Can]; Tylenol® Sinus Day Non-Drowsy [US-OTC]; Tylenol® Sinus [Can]; Tylenol® Sinus, Children's [US-OTC]

Therapeutic Category Decongestant/Analgesic

Use Relief of mild-to-moderate pain; relief of congestion

Usual Dosage Oral:

Analgesic: Based on acetaminophen component:
Children: 10-15 mg/kg/dose every 4-6 hours as needed; do **not** exceed 5 doses in 24 hours
Adults: 325-650 mg every 4-6 hours as needed; do **not** exceed 4 g/day
Decongestant: Based on pseudoephedrine component:
Children:
2-6 years: 15 mg every 4 hours; do **not** exceed 90 mg/day
6-12 years: 30 mg every 4 hours; do **not** exceed 180 mg/day
Children >12 years and Adults: 60 mg every 4 hours; do **not** exceed 360 mg/day

Product labeling:

Alka-Seltzer Plus® Cold and Sinus:
Children 6-12 years: 1 dose with water every 4 hours (maximum: 4 doses/24 hours)
Adults: 2 doses with water every 4 hours (maximum: 4 doses/24 hours)
Children's Tylenol® Sinus: Children:
Liquid:
2-5 years (24-47 lb): 1 teaspoonful every 4-6 hours (maximum: 4 doses/24 hours)
6-11 years (48-95 lb): 2 teaspoonfuls every 4-6 hours (maximum: 4 doses/24 hours)
Tablet, chewable:
2-5 years (24-47 lb): 2 tablets every 4-6 hours (maximum: 4 doses/24 hours)
6-11 years (48-95 lb): 4 tablets every 4-6 hours (maximum: 4 doses/24 hours)
Sinutab® Sinus: Children >12 years and Adults: 2 doses every 6 hours (maximum: 8 doses/24 hours)

Dosage Forms

Caplet:
Allerest® Allergy and Sinus Relief, Ornex®: Acetaminophen 325 mg and pseudoephedrine hydrochloride 30 mg
Genapap™ Sinus Maximum Strength, Mapap Sinus Maximum Strength, Ornex® Maximum Strength, Tylenol® Sinus Daytime: Acetaminophen 500 mg and pseudoephedrine hydrochloride 30 mg
Capsule, liquid:
Sudafed® Multi-Symptom Sinus and Cold: Acetaminophen 325 mg and pseudoephedrine hydrochloride 30 mg [contains sodium 16 mg]
Gelcap:
Tylenol® Sinus Daytime: Acetaminophen 500 mg and pseudoephedrine hydrochloride 30 mg
Liquid:
Childrens Tylenol® Cold Daytime: Acetaminophen 160 mg and pseudoephedrine hydrochloride 15 mg per 5 mL (120 mL) [contains sodium benzoate; fruit flavor[
Liquid, oral [drops]:
Infants Tylenol® Cold: Acetaminophen 80 mg and pseudoephedrine 7.5 mg per 0.8 mL [contains sodium benzoate; bubble gum flavor]
Tablet:
Medi-Synal, Sinus-Relief: Acetaminophen 325 mg and pseudoephedrine hydrochloride 30 mg
Oranyl Plus: Acetaminophen 500 mg and pseudoephedrine hydrochloride 30 mg

acetaminophen and tramadol (a seet a MIN oh fen & TRA ma dole)

Synonyms APAP and tramadol; tramadol hydrochloride and acetaminophen

U.S./Canadian Brand Names Tramacet [Can]; Ultracet™ [US]

Therapeutic Category Analgesic, Miscellaneous; Analgesic, Nonnarcotic

Use Short-term (≤5 days) management of acute pain

Usual Dosage Oral: Adults: Acute pain: Two tablets every 4-6 hours as needed for pain relief (maximum: 8 tablets/day); treatment should not exceed 5 days

Dosage Forms Tablet: Acetaminophen 325 mg and tramadol hydrochloride 37.5 mg

acetaminophen, aspirin, and caffeine (a seet a MIN oh fen, AS pir in, & KAF een)

Sound-Alike/Look-Alike Issues

Excedrin® may be confused with Dexatrim®, Dexedrine®

Synonyms aspirin, acetaminophen, and caffeine; aspirin, caffeine, and acetaminophen; caffeine, acetaminophen, and aspirin; caffeine, aspirin, and acetaminophen

U.S./Canadian Brand Names Excedrin® Extra Strength [US-OTC]; Excedrin® Migraine [US-OTC]; Fem-Prin® [US-OTC]; Genaced™ [US-OTC]; Goody's® Extra Strength Headache Powder [US-OTC]; Goody's® Extra Strength Pain Relief [US-OTC]; Pain-Off [US-OTC]; Vanquish® Extra Strength Pain Reliever [US-OTC]

Therapeutic Category Analgesic, Nonnarcotic

Use Relief of mild-to-moderate pain; mild-to-moderate pain associated with migraine headache

Usual Dosage Oral: Adults:

Analgesic:

Based on **acetaminophen** component:

Mild-to-moderate pain: 325-650 mg every 4-6 hours as needed; do **not** exceed 4 g/day

Mild-to-moderate pain associated with migraine headache: 500 mg/dose (in combination with 500 mg aspirin and 130 mg caffeine) every 6 hours while symptoms persist; do not use for longer than 48 hours

Based on **aspirin** component:

Mild-to-moderate pain: 325-650 mg every 4-6 hours as needed; do **not** exceed 4 g/day

Mild-to-moderate pain associated with migraine headache: 500 mg/dose (in combination with 500 mg acetaminophen and 130 mg caffeine) every 6 hours; do not use for longer than 48 hours

Product labeling:

Excedrin® Extra Strength, Excedrin® Migraine: Children >12 years and Adults: 2 doses every 6 hours (maximum: 8 doses/24 hours)

Note: When used for migraine, do not use for longer than 48 hours

Goody's® Extra Strength Headache Powder: Children >12 years and Adults: 1 powder, placed on tongue or dissolved in water, every 4-6 hours (maximum: 4 powders/24 hours)

Goody's® Extra Strength Pain Relief Tablets: Children >12 years and Adults: 2 tablets every 4-6 hours (maximum: 8 tablets/24 hours)

Vanquish® Extra Strength Pain Reliever: Children >12 years and Adults: 2 tablets every 4 hours (maximum: 12 tablets/24 hours)

Dosage Forms

Caplet:

Excedrin® Extra Strength, Excedrin® Migraine: Acetaminophen 250 mg, aspirin 250 mg, and caffeine 65 mg

Vanquish® Extra Strength Pain Reliever: Acetaminophen 194 mg, aspirin 227 mg, and caffeine 33 mg

Geltab (Excedrin® Extra Strength, Excedrin® Migraine): Acetaminophen 250 mg, aspirin 250 mg, and caffeine 65 mg

Powder (Goody's® Extra Strength Headache Powder): Acetaminophen 260 mg, aspirin 520 mg, and caffeine 32.5 mg [contains lactose]

Tablet:

Excedrin® Extra Strength, Excedrin® Migraine, Genaced™, Pain-Off: Acetaminophen 250 mg, aspirin 250 mg, and caffeine 65 mg

Fem-Prin®: Acetaminophen 194.4 mg, aspirin 226.8 mg, and caffeine 32.4 mg

Goody's® Extra Strength Pain Relief: Acetaminophen 130 mg, aspirin 260 mg, and caffeine 16.25 mg

acetaminophen, butalbital, and caffeine *see* butalbital, acetaminophen, and caffeine *on page 129*

acetaminophen, caffeine, and dihydrocodeine

(a seet a MIN oh fen, KAF een, & dye hye droe KOE deen)

Synonyms caffeine, dihydrocodeine, and acetaminophen; dihydrocodeine bitartrate, acetaminophen, and caffeine

U.S./Canadian Brand Names Panlor® DC [US]; Panlor® SS [US]; ZerLor™ [US]
Therapeutic Category Analgesic Combination (Opioid)
Controlled Substance C-III
Use Relief of moderate to moderately-severe pain
Usual Dosage Oral: Adults: Relief of pain:
Panlor® DC: 2 capsules every 4 hours as needed; adjust dose based on severity of pain (maximum dose: 10 capsules/24 hours)
Panlor® SS, ZerLor™: 1 tablet every 4 hours as needed; adjust dose based on severity of pain (maximum dose: 5 tablets/24 hours)
Dosage Forms
Capsule:
Panlor® DC: Acetaminophen 356.4 mg, caffeine 30 mg, and dihydrocodeine bitartrate 16 mg
Tablet:
Panlor® SS, ZerLor™: Acetaminophen 712.8 mg, caffeine 60 mg, and dihydrocodeine bitartrate 32 mg

acetaminophen, caffeine, hydrocodone, chlorpheniramine, and phenylephrine *see* hydrocodone, chlorpheniramine, phenylephrine, acetaminophen, and caffeine *on page 424*

acetaminophen, chlorpheniramine, and pseudoephedrine

(a seet a MIN oh fen, klor fen IR a meen, & soo doe e FED rin)
Sound-Alike/Look-Alike Issues
Thera-Flu® may be confused with Tamiflu®, Thera-Flur-N®
Tylenol® may be confused with atenolol, timolol, Tuinal®, Tylox®
Synonyms acetaminophen, pseudoephedrine, and chlorpheniramine; chlorpheniramine, acetaminophen, and pseudoephedrine; chlorpheniramine, pseudoephedrine, and acetaminophen; pseudoephedrine, acetaminophen, and chlorpheniramine; pseudoephedrine, chlorpheniramine, and acetaminophen
U.S./Canadian Brand Names Actifed® Cold and Sinus [US-OTC]; Alka-Seltzer® Plus® Cold Liqui-Gels® [US-OTC]; Comtrex® Flu Therapy Day/Night [US-OTC]; Comtrex® Flu Therapy Nighttime [US-OTC]; Kolephrin® [US-OTC]; Sinutab® Sinus & Allergy [Can]; Sinutab® Sinus Allergy Maximum Strength [US-OTC]; Thera-Flu® Cold and Sore Throat Night Time [US-OTC]; Tylenol® Allergy Complete [US-OTC]; Tylenol® Allergy Sinus [Can]; Tylenol® Children's Plus Cold Nighttime [US-OTC]
Therapeutic Category Antihistamine/Decongestant/Analgesic
Use Temporary relief of sinus symptoms
Usual Dosage Oral:
Analgesic: Based on **acetaminophen** component:
Children: 10-15 mg/kg/dose every 4-6 hours as needed; do **not** exceed 5 doses in 24 hours
Adults: 325-650 mg every 4-6 hours as needed; do **not** exceed 4 g/day
Antihistamine: Based on **chlorpheniramine maleate** component:
Children:
2-6 years: 1 mg every 4-6 hours (maximum: 6 mg/24 hours)
6-12 years: 2 mg every 4-6 hours (maximum: 12 mg/24 hours)
Children >12 years and Adults: 4 mg every 4-6 hours (maximum: 24 mg/24 hours)
Decongestant: Based on **pseudoephedrine** component:
Children:
2-6 years: 15 mg every 4 hours (maximum: 90 mg/24 hours)
6-12 years: 30 mg every 4 hours (maximum: 180 mg/24 hours)
Children >12 years and Adults: 60 mg every 4 hours (maximum: 360 mg/24 hours)

Product labeling:
Alka-Seltzer Plus® Cold Medicine Liqui-Gels®:
Children 6-12 years: 1 softgel every 4 hours with water (maximum: 4 doses/24 hours)
Children >12 years and Adults: 2 softgels every 4 hours with water (maximum: 4 doses/24 hours)
Sinutab® Sinus Allergy Maximum Strength: Children >12 years and Adults: 2 tablets/caplets every 6 hours (maximum: 8 doses/24 hours)
Thera-Flu® Cold and Sore Throat Night Time: Children >12 years and Adults: 1 packet dissolved in hot water every 6 hours (maximum: 4 packets/24 hours)
Dosage Forms [DSC] = Discontinued product
Caplet: Acetaminophen 325 mg, chlorpheniramine maleate 2 mg, and pseudoephedrine hydrochloride 30 mg
Actifed® Cold and Sinus, Sinutab® Sinus Allergy Maximum Strength, Tylenol® Allergy Complete [DSC]: Acetaminophen 500 mg, chlorpheniramine maleate 2 mg, and pseudoephedrine hydrochloride 30 mg
Kolephrin®: Acetaminophen 325 mg, chlorpheniramine maleate 2 mg, and pseudoephedrine hydrochloride 30 mg
(Continued)

acetaminophen, chlorpheniramine, and pseudoephedrine *(Continued)*

Capsule, softgel:

Alka-Seltzer® Plus Cold Liqui-Gels®: Acetaminophen 325 mg, chlorpheniramine maleate 2 mg, and pseudoephedrine hydrochloride 30 mg [contains potassium 25 mg]

Combination package: (Comtrex® Flu Therapy Day/Night):

Caplet [Daytime]: Acetaminophen 500 mg and pseudoephedrine hydrochloride 30 mg

Caplet [Nighttime]: Acetaminophen 500 mg, chlorpheniramine maleate 2 mg, and pseudoephedrine hydrochloride 30 mg

Liquid:

Comtrex® Flu Therapy Nighttime: Acetaminophen 100 mg, chlorpheniramine maleate 4 mg, and pseudoephedrine hydrochloride 60 mg per 30 mL (240 mL) [contains alcohol; cherry flavor]

Tylenol® Children's Plus Cold Nighttime: Acetaminophen 160 mg, chlorpheniramine maleate 1 mg, and pseudoephedrine hydrochloride 15 mg per 5 mL (120 mL) [contains sodium benzoate; grape flavor]

Tablet:

Drinex: Acetaminophen 650 mg, chlorpheniramine maleate 4 mg, and pseudoephedrine hydrochloride 60 mg

acetaminophen, codeine, and doxylamine *(Canada only)*

(a seet a MIN oh fen, KOE deen, & dox IL a meen)

Synonyms codeine, doxylamine, and acetaminophen; doxylamine succinate, codeine phosphate, and acetaminophen

U.S./Canadian Brand Names Mersyndol® With Codeine [Can]

Therapeutic Category Analgesic, Opioid; Antihistamine

Controlled Substance CDSA-1

Use Relief of headache, cold symptoms, neuralgia, and muscular aches/pain

Usual Dosage Oral: Children >12 years and Adults: 1-2 tablets every 4 hours as needed; total dose should not exceed 12 tablets in a 24-hour period

Dosage Forms [CAN] = Canadian brand name

Tablet:

Mersyndol® With Codeine [CAN]: Acetaminophen 325 mg, codeine 8 mg, and doxylamine 5 mg [not available in the U.S.]

acetaminophen, dextromethorphan, and pseudoephedrine

(a seet a MIN oh fen, deks troe meth OR fan, & soo doe e FED rin)

Sound-Alike/Look-Alike Issues

Sudafed® may be confused with Sufenta®

Thera-Flu® may be confused with Tamiflu®, Thera-Flur-N®

Tylenol® may be confused with atenolol, timolol, Tuinal®, Tylox®

Synonyms dextromethorphan, acetaminophen, and pseudoephedrine; pseudoephedrine, acetaminophen, and dextromethorphan; pseudoephedrine, dextromethorphan, and acetaminophen

U.S./Canadian Brand Names Alka-Seltzer® Plus® Flu Liqui-Gels [US-OTC]; Comtrex® Non-Drowsy Cold and Cough Relief [US-OTC]; Contac® Complete [Can]; Contac® Cough, Cold and Flu Day & Night™ [Can]; Contac® Severe Cold and Flu/Non-Drowsy [US-OTC]; Infants' Tylenol® Cold Plus Cough Concentrated Drops [US-OTC]; Sudafed® Cold & Cough Extra Strength [Can]; Sudafed® Severe Cold [US-OTC]; Triaminic® Cough and Sore Throat Formula [US-OTC]; Tylenol® Cold Day Non-Drowsy [US-OTC]; Tylenol® Cold Daytime [Can]; Tylenol® Flu Non-Drowsy Maximum Strength [US-OTC]; Vicks® DayQuil® Multi-Symptom Cold and Flu [US-OTC]

Therapeutic Category Cold Preparation

Use Treatment of mild-to-moderate pain and fever; symptomatic relief of cough and congestion

Usual Dosage Oral:

Analgesic: Based on acetaminophen component:

Children: 10-15 mg/kg/dose every 4-6 hours as needed; do **not** exceed 5 doses/24 hours

Adults: 325-650 mg every 4-7 hours as needed; do **not** exceed 4 g/day

Cough suppressant: Based on dextromethorphan component:

Children 6-12 years: 15 mg every 6-8 hours; do **not** exceed 60 mg/24 hours

Children >12 years and Adults: 10-20 mg every 4-8 hours **or** 30 mg every 8 hours; do **not** exceed 120 mg/24 hours

Decongestant: Based on pseudoephedrine component:

Children:

2-6 years: 15 mg every 4 hours (maximum: 90 mg/24 hours)

6-12 years: 30 mg every 4 hours (maximum: 180 mg/24 hours)

Children >12 years and Adults: 60 mg every 4 hours (maximum: 360 mg/24 hours)

Product labeling:

Alka-Seltzer Plus® Cold and Flu Liqui-Gels®:

Children 6-12 years: 1 dose every 4 hours (maximum: 4 doses/24 hours)

Children >12 years and Adults: 2 dose every 4 hours (maximum: 4 doses/24 hours)

Infants' Tylenol® Cold Plus Cough Concentrated Drops: Children 2-3 years (24-55 lb): 2 dropperfuls every 4-6 hours (maximum: 4 doses/24 hours)

Sudafed® Severe Cold, Tylenol® Flu Non-Drowsy Maximum Strength: Children >12 years and Adults: 2 doses every 6 hours (maximum: 8 doses/24 hours)

Tylenol® Cold Non-Drowsy:

Children 6-11 years: 1 dose every 6 hours (maximum: 4 doses/24 hours)

Children ≥12 years and Adults: 2 doses every 6 hours (maximum: 8 doses/24 hours)

Dosage Forms [DSC] = Discontinued product

Caplet:

Contac® Severe Cold and Flu/Non-Drowsy, Sudafed® Severe Cold, Tylenol® Cold Non-Drowsy: Acetaminophen 325 mg, dextromethorphan hydrobromide 15 mg, and pseudoephedrine hydrochloride 30 mg

Comtrex® Non-Drowsy Cold and Cough Relief: Acetaminophen 500 mg, dextromethorphan hydrobromide 15 mg, and pseudoephedrine hydrochloride 30 mg [contains benzoic acid]

Tylenol® Cold Day Non-Drowsy: Acetaminophen 325 mg dextromethorphan hydrobromide 15 mg, and pseudoephedrine hydrochloride 30 mg

Capsule, liquid:

Alka-Seltzer Plus® Flu Liqui-Gels®: Acetaminophen 325 mg, dextromethorphan hydrobromide 10 mg, and pseudoephedrine hydrochloride 30 mg

Vicks® DayQuil® Multi-Symptom Cold and Flu: Acetaminophen 250 mg, dextromethorphan hydrobromide 10 mg, and pseudoephedrine hydrochloride 30 mg

Gelcap:

Tylenol® Cold Day Non-Drowsy: Acetaminophen 325 mg, dextromethorphan hydrobromide 15 mg, and pseudoephedrine hydrochloride 30 mg [contains benzyl alcohol]

Tylenol® Flu Non-Drowsy Maximum Strength: Acetaminophen 500 mg, dextromethorphan hydrobromide 15 mg, and pseudoephedrine hydrochloride 30 mg

Liquid:

Triaminic® Cough and Sore Throat Formula: Acetaminophen 160 mg, dextromethorphan hydrobromide 7.5 mg, and pseudoephedrine hydrochloride 15 mg per 5 mL (120 mL, 240 mL) [contains benzoic acid; grape flavor]

Vicks® DayQuil® Multi-Symptom Cold and Flu: Acetaminophen 325 mg, dextromethorphan hydrobromide 10 mg, and pseudoephedrine hydrochloride 30 mg per 15 mL (175 mL)

Suspension, oral drops (Infants' Tylenol® Cold Plus Cough Concentrated Drops): Acetaminophen 160 mg, dextromethorphan hydrobromide 5 mg, and pseudoephedrine hydrochloride 15 mg per 1.6 mL (15 mL) [1.6 mL = 2 dropperfuls] [cherry flavor] [DSC]

acetaminophen, dichloralphenazone, and isometheptene *see* acetaminophen, isometheptene, and dichloralphenazone *on this page*

acetaminophen, isometheptene, and dichloralphenazone

(a seet a MIN oh fen, eye soe me THEP teen, & dye KLOR al FEN a zone)

Sound-Alike/Look-Alike Issues

Midrin® may be confused with Mydfrin®

Synonyms acetaminophen, dichloralphenazone, and isometheptene; dichloralphenazone, acetaminophen, and isometheptene; dichloralphenazone, isometheptene, and acetaminophen; isometheptene, acetaminophen, and dichloralphenazone; isometheptene, dichloralphenazone, and acetaminophen

U.S./Canadian Brand Names Amidrine [US]; Duradrin® [US]; Midrin® [US]; Migquin [US]; Migratine [US]; Migrazone® [US]; Migrin-A [US]

Therapeutic Category Analgesic, Nonnarcotic

Controlled Substance C-IV

Use Relief of migraine and tension headache

Usual Dosage Oral: Adults:

Migraine headache: 2 capsules to start, followed by 1 capsule every hour until relief is obtained (maximum: 5 capsules/12 hours)

Tension headache: 1-2 capsules every 4 hours (maximum: 8 capsules/24 hours)

Dosage Forms

Capsule: Acetaminophen 325 mg, isometheptene mucate 65 mg, dichloralphenazone 100 mg

Amidrine, Duradrin®, Midrin®, Migquin, Migrazone®, Migratine, Migrin-A: Acetaminophen 325 mg, isometheptene mucate 65 mg, and dichloralphenazone 100 mg

acetaminophen, pseudoephedrine, and chlorpheniramine *see* acetaminophen, chlorpheniramine, and pseudoephedrine *on page 11*

Acetasol® HC [US] *see* acetic acid, propylene glycol diacetate, and hydrocortisone *on next page*

acetazolamide (a set a ZOLE a mide)

Sound-Alike/Look-Alike Issues

acetaZOLAMIDE may be confused with acetoHEXAMIDE

Diamox® Sequels® may be confused with Dobutrex®, Trimox®

Tall-Man aceta**ZOLAMIDE**

U.S./Canadian Brand Names Apo-Acetazolamide® [Can]; Diamox® Sequels® [US]; Diamox® [Can]

Therapeutic Category Anticonvulsant; Carbonic Anhydrase Inhibitor

Use Treatment of glaucoma (chronic simple open-angle, secondary glaucoma, preoperatively in acute angle-closure); drug-induced edema or edema due to congestive heart failure (adjunctive therapy); centrencephalic epilepsies (immediate release dosage form); prevention or amelioration of symptoms associated with acute mountain sickness

Usual Dosage Note: I.M. administration is not recommended because of pain secondary to the alkaline pH

Children:

Glaucoma:

Oral: 8-30 mg/kg/day or 300-900 mg/m^2/day divided every 8 hours

I.V.: 20-40 mg/kg/24 hours divided every 6 hours, not to exceed 1 g/day

Edema: Oral, I.V.: 5 mg/kg or 150 mg/m^2 once every day

Epilepsy: Oral: 8-30 mg/kg/day in 1-4 divided doses, not to exceed 1 g/day; extended release capsule is not recommended for treatment of epilepsy

Adults:

Glaucoma:

Chronic simple (open-angle): Oral: 250 mg 1-4 times/day or 500 mg extended release capsule twice daily

Secondary, acute (closed-angle): I.V.: 250-500 mg, may repeat in 2-4 hours to a maximum of 1 g/day

Edema: Oral, I.V.: 250-375 mg once daily

Epilepsy: Oral: 8-30 mg/kg/day in 1-4 divided doses; **extended release capsule is not recommended for treatment of epilepsy**

Mountain sickness: Oral: 250 mg every 8-12 hours (or 500 mg extended release capsules every 12-24 hours)

Therapy should begin 24-48 hours before and continue during ascent and for at least 48 hours after arrival at the high altitude

Note: In situations of rapid ascent (such as rescue or military operations), 1000 mg/day is recommended.

Dosage Forms

Capsule, extended release:

Diamox® Sequels®: 500 mg

Injection, powder for reconstitution: 500 mg

Tablet: 125 mg, 250 mg

acetic acid (a SEE tik AS id)

Sound-Alike/Look-Alike Issues

VoSol® may be confused with Vexol®

Synonyms ethanoic acid

Therapeutic Category Antibacterial, Otic; Antibacterial, Topical

Use Irrigation of the bladder; treatment of superficial bacterial infections of the external auditory canal

Usual Dosage

Irrigation (**Note:** Dosage of an irrigating solution depends on the capacity or surface area of the structure being irrigated):

For continuous irrigation of the urinary bladder with 0.25% acetic acid irrigation, the rate of administration will approximate the rate of urine flow; usually 500-1500 mL/24 hours

For periodic irrigation of an indwelling urinary catheter to maintain patency, about 50 mL of 0.25% acetic acid irrigation is required

Otic: Insert saturated wick; keep moist 24 hours; remove wick and instill 5 drops 3-4 times/day

Dosage Forms [DSC] = Discontinued product

Solution for irrigation: 0.25% (250 mL, 500 mL, 1000 mL)

Solution, otic (VoSol® [DSC]): 2% (15 mL)

acetic acid, hydrocortisone, and propylene glycol diacetate *see* acetic acid, propylene glycol diacetate, and hydrocortisone *on next page*

acetic acid, propylene glycol diacetate, and hydrocortisone

(a SEE tik AS id, PRO pa leen GLY kole dye AS e tate, & hye droe KOR ti sone)

Synonyms acetic acid, hydrocortisone, and propylene glycol diacetate; hydrocortisone, acetic acid, and propylene glycol diacetate; propylene glycol diacetate, acetic acid, and hydrocortisone

U.S./Canadian Brand Names Acetasol® HC [US]; VoSol® HC [US]

Therapeutic Category Antibiotic/Corticosteroid, Otic

Use Treatment of superficial infections of the external auditory canal caused by organisms susceptible to the action of the antimicrobial, complicated by swelling

Usual Dosage Children ≥3 years and Adults: Otic: Instill 3-5 drops in ear(s) every 4-6 hours

Dosage Forms Solution, otic drops: Acetic acid 2%, propylene glycol diacetate 3%, and hydrocortisone 1% (10 mL)

acetohydroxamic acid (a SEE toe hye droks am ik AS id)

Sound-Alike/Look-Alike Issues

Lithostat® may be confused with Lithobid®

Synonyms AHA

U.S./Canadian Brand Names Lithostat® [US/Can]

Therapeutic Category Urinary Tract Product

Use Adjunctive therapy in chronic urea-splitting urinary infection

Usual Dosage Oral:

Children: Initial: 10 mg/kg/day

Adults: 250 mg 3-4 times/day for a total daily dose of 10-15 mg/kg/day

Dosage Forms Tablet: 250 mg

Acetoxyl® [Can] *see* benzoyl peroxide *on page 102*

acetoxymethylprogesterone *see* medroxyprogesterone *on page 524*

acetylcholine (a se teel KOE leen)

Sound-Alike/Look-Alike Issues

acetylcholine may be confused with acetylcysteine

Synonyms acetylcholine chloride

U.S./Canadian Brand Names Miochol-E® [US/Can]

Therapeutic Category Cholinergic Agent

Use Produces complete miosis in cataract surgery, keratoplasty, iridectomy, and other anterior segment surgery where rapid miosis is required

Usual Dosage Adults: Intraocular: 0.5-2 mL of 1% injection (5-20 mg) instilled into anterior chamber before or after securing one or more sutures

Dosage Forms

Powder for solution, intraocular, as chloride:

Miochol®-E: 1:100 [20 mg; packaged with diluent (2 mL)]

acetylcholine chloride *see* acetylcholine *on this page*

acetylcysteine (a se teel SIS teen)

Sound-Alike/Look-Alike Issues

acetylcysteine may be confused with acetylcholine

Mucomyst® may be confused with Mucinex®

Synonyms acetylcysteine sodium; mercapturic acid; NAC; *n*-acetylcysteine; *n*-acetyl-L-cysteine

U.S./Canadian Brand Names Acetadote® [US]; Acetylcysteine Solution [Can]; Mucomyst® [Can]; Parvolex® [Can]

Therapeutic Category Mucolytic Agent

Use Adjunctive mucolytic therapy in patients with abnormal or viscid mucous secretions in acute and chronic bronchopulmonary diseases; pulmonary complications of surgery and cystic fibrosis; diagnostic bronchial studies; antidote for acute acetaminophen toxicity

Usual Dosage

Acetaminophen poisoning: Children and Adults:

Oral: 140 mg/kg; followed by 17 doses of 70 mg/kg every 4 hours; repeat dose if emesis occurs within 1 hour of administration; therapy should continue until acetaminophen levels are undetectable and there is no evidence of hepatotoxicity.

I.V. (Acetadote®): Loading dose: 150 mg/kg over 60 minutes. Loading dose is followed by 2 additional infusions: Initial maintenance dose of 50 mg/kg infused over 4 hours, followed by a second maintenance dose of 100 mg/kg infused over 16 hours. To avoid fluid overload in patients <40 kg and those requiring

(Continued)

acetylcysteine *(Continued)*

fluid restriction, decrease volume of D_5W proportionally. Total dosage: 300 mg/kg administered over 21 hours.

Experts suggest that the duration of acetylcysteine administration may vary depending upon serial acetaminophen levels and liver function tests obtained during treatment. In general, patients without measurable acetaminophen levels and without significant LFT elevations (>3 times the ULN) can safely stop acetylcysteine after ≤24 hours of treatment. The patients who still have detectable levels of acetaminophen, and/or LFT elevations (>1000 units/L) continue to benefit from addition acetylcysteine administration

Adjuvant therapy in respiratory conditions: **Note:** Patients should receive an aerosolized bronchodilator 10-15 minutes prior to acetylcysteine.

Inhalation, nebulization (face mask, mouth piece, tracheostomy): Acetylcysteine 10% and 20% solution (dilute 20% solution with sodium chloride or sterile water for inhalation); 10% solution may be used undiluted

Infants: 1-2 mL of 20% solution or 2-4 mL of 10% solution until nebulized given 3-4 times/day

Children and Adults: 3-5 mL of 20% solution or 6-10 mL of 10% solution until nebulized given 3-4 times/day; dosing range: 1-10 mL of 20% solution or 2-20 mL of 10% solution every 2-6 hours

Inhalation, nebulization (tent, croupette): Children and Adults: Dose must be individualized; may require up to 300 mL solution/treatment

Direct instillation: Adults:

Into tracheostomy: 1-2 mL of 10% to 20% solution every 1-4 hours

Through percutaneous intratracheal catheter: 1-2 mL of 20% or 2-4 mL of 10% solution every 1-4 hours via syringe attached to catheter

Diagnostic bronchogram: Nebulization or intratracheal: Adults: 1-2 mL of 20% solution or 2-4 mL of 10% solution administered 2-3 times prior to procedure

Dosage Forms

Injection, solution:

Acetadote®: 20% [200 mg/mL] (30 mL) [contains disodium edetate]

Solution, inhalation/oral: 10% [100 mg/mL] (4 mL, 10 mL, 30 mL); 20% [200 mg/mL] (4 mL, 10 mL, 30 mL)

acetylcysteine sodium *see* acetylcysteine *on previous page*

Acetylcysteine Solution [Can] *see* acetylcysteine *on previous page*

acetylsalicylic acid *see* aspirin *on page 77*

Aches-N-Pain® *(Discontinued)* *see* ibuprofen *on page 437*

achromycin *see* tetracycline *on page 816*

aciclovir *see* acyclovir *on page 18*

acidulated phosphate fluoride *see* fluoride *on page 354*

Aci-jel® *(Discontinued)* *see* acetic acid *on page 14*

Acilac [Can] *see* lactulose *on page 478*

AcipHex® [US/Can] *see* rabeprazole *on page 727*

acitretin (a si TRE tin)

Sound-Alike/Look-Alike Issues

Soriatane® may be confused with Loxitane®

U.S./Canadian Brand Names Soriatane® [US/Can]

Therapeutic Category Retinoid-like Compound

Use Treatment of severe psoriasis

Usual Dosage Oral: Adults: Individualization of dosage is required to achieve maximum therapeutic response while minimizing side effects

Initial therapy: Therapy should be initiated at 25-50 mg/day, given as a single dose with the main meal

Maintenance doses of 25-50 mg/day may be given after initial response to treatment; the maintenance dose should be based on clinical efficacy and tolerability

Dosage Forms Capsule: 10 mg, 25 mg

Aclasta® [Can] *see* zoledronic acid *on page 889*

Aclovate® [US] *see* alclometasone *on page 24*

acrivastine and pseudoephedrine (AK ri vas teen & soo doe e FED rin)

Synonyms pseudoephedrine hydrochloride and acrivastine

U.S./Canadian Brand Names Semprex®-D [US]

Therapeutic Category Antihistamine/Decongestant Combination

Use Temporary relief of nasal congestion, decongest sinus openings, running nose, itching of nose or throat, and itchy, watery eyes due to hay fever or other upper respiratory allergies

Usual Dosage Oral: Adults: 1 capsule 3-4 times/day

Dosage Forms Capsule: Acrivastine 8 mg and pseudoephedrine hydrochloride 60 mg

ACT *see* dactinomycin *on page 227*

ACT® [US-OTC] *see* fluoride *on page 354*

Act-D *see* dactinomycin *on page 227*

Actagen® Syrup *(Discontinued)* *see* triprolidine and pseudoephedrine *on page 853*

Actagen® Tablet *(Discontinued)* *see* triprolidine and pseudoephedrine *on page 853*

Act-A-Med® *(Discontinued)* *see* triprolidine and pseudoephedrine *on page 853*

ACTH *see* corticotropin *on page 215*

ActHIB® [US/Can] *see* *Haemophilus* B conjugate vaccine *on page 405*

Acticin® [US] *see* permethrin *on page 655*

Actidose-Aqua® [US-OTC] *see* charcoal *on page 169*

Actidose® with Sorbitol [US-OTC] *see* charcoal *on page 169*

Actifed® [Can] *see* triprolidine and pseudoephedrine *on page 853*

Actifed® Allergy Tablet (Night) *(Discontinued)* *see* diphenhydramine and pseudoephedrine *on page 263*

Actifed® Cold and Allergy [US-OTC] *see* triprolidine and pseudoephedrine *on page 853*

Actifed® Cold and Sinus [US-OTC] *see* acetaminophen, chlorpheniramine, and pseudoephedrine *on page 11*

Actigall® [US] *see* ursodiol *on page 862*

Actimmune® [US/Can] *see* interferon gamma-1b *on page 457*

actinomycin *see* dactinomycin *on page 227*

actinomycin D *see* dactinomycin *on page 227*

actinomycin CI *see* dactinomycin *on page 227*

Actiq® [US/Can] *see* fentanyl *on page 340*

Activase® [US] *see* alteplase *on page 34*

Activase® rt-PA [Can] *see* alteplase *on page 34*

activated carbon *see* charcoal *on page 169*

activated charcoal *see* charcoal *on page 169*

activated dimethicone *see* simethicone *on page 772*

activated ergosterol *see* ergocalciferol *on page 301*

activated methylpolysiloxane *see* simethicone *on page 772*

activated protein C, human, recombinant *see* drotrecogin alfa *on page 282*

Activella® [US] *see* estradiol and norethindrone *on page 310*

Actonel® [US/Can] *see* risedronate *on page 747*

Actonel® and Calcium [US] *see* risedronate and calcium *on page 747*

Actos® [US/Can] *see* pioglitazone *on page 669*

ACT® Plus [US-OTC] *see* fluoride *on page 354*

ACT® x2™ [US-OTC] *see* fluoride *on page 354*

Acular® [US/Can] *see* ketorolac *on page 472*

Acular LS™ [US/Can] *see* ketorolac *on page 472*

Acular® PF [US] *see* ketorolac *on page 472*

ACV *see* acyclovir *on next page*

acycloguanosine *see* acyclovir *on this page*

acyclovir (ay SYE kloe veer)

Sound-Alike/Look-Alike Issues
Zovirax® may be confused with Zostrix®, Zyvox™

Synonyms aciclovir; ACV; acycloguanosine

U.S./Canadian Brand Names Apo-Acyclovir® [Can]; Gen-Acyclovir [Can]; Nu-Acyclovir [Can]; ratio-Acyclovir [Can]; Zovirax® [US/Can]

Therapeutic Category Antiviral Agent

Use Treatment of genital herpes simplex virus (HSV), herpes labialis (cold sores), herpes zoster (shingles), HSV encephalitis, neonatal HSV, mucocutaneous HSV in immunocompromised patients, varicella-zoster (chickenpox)

Usual Dosage Note: Obese patients should be dosed using ideal body weight

Genital HSV:

I.V.: Children ≥12 years and Adults (immunocompetent): Initial episode, severe: 5 mg/kg every 8 hours for 5-7 days

Oral: Adults:

Initial episode: 200 mg every 4 hours while awake (5 times/day) for 10 days (per manufacturer's labeling); 400 mg 3 times/day for 5-10 days has also been reported

Recurrence: 200 mg every 4 hours while awake (5 times/day) for 5 days (per manufacturer's labeling; begin at earliest signs of disease); 400 mg 3 times/day for 5 days has also been reported

Chronic suppression: 400 mg twice daily or 200 mg 3-5 times/day, for up to 12 months followed by re-evaluation (per manufacturer's labeling); 400-1200 mg/day in 2-3 divided doses has also been reported

Topical: Adults (immunocompromised): Ointment: Initial episode: ½" ribbon of ointment for a 4" square surface area every 3 hours (6 times/day) for 7 days

Herpes labialis (cold sores): Topical: Children ≥12 years and Adults: Cream: Apply 5 times/day for 4 days

Herpes zoster (shingles):

Oral: Adults (immunocompetent): 800 mg every 4 hours (5 times/day) for 7-10 days

I.V.:

Children <12 years (immunocompromised): 20 mg/kg/dose every 8 hours for 7 days

Children ≥12 years and Adults (immunocompromised): 10 mg/kg/dose or 500 mg/m²/dose every 8 hours for 7 days

HSV encephalitis: I.V.:

Children 3 months to 12 years: 20 mg/kg/dose every 8 hours for 10 days (per manufacturer's labeling); dosing for 14-21 days also reported

Children ≥12 years and Adults: 10 mg/kg/dose every 8 hours for 10 days (per manufacturer's labeling); 10-15 mg/kg/dose every 8 hours for 14-21 days also reported

Mucocutaneous HSV:

I.V.:

Children <12 years (immunocompromised): 10 mg/kg/dose every 8 hours for 7 days

Children ≥12 years and Adults (immunocompromised): 5 mg/kg/dose every 8 hours for 7 days (per manufacturer's labeling); dosing for up to 14 days also reported

Topical: Ointment: Adults (nonlife-threatening, immunocompromised): ½" ribbon of ointment for a 4" square surface area every 3 hours (6 times/day) for 7 days

Neonatal HSV: I.V.: Neonate: Birth to 3 months: 10 mg/kg/dose every 8 hours for 10 days (manufacturer's labeling); 15 mg/kg/dose or 20 mg/kg/dose every 8 hours for 14-21 days has also been reported

Varicella-zoster (chickenpox): Begin treatment within the first 24 hours of rash onset:

Oral:

Children ≥2 years and ≤40 kg (immunocompetent): 20 mg/kg/dose (up to 800 mg/dose) 4 times/day for 5 days

Children >40 kg and Adults (immunocompetent): 800 mg/dose 4 times a day for 5 days

Dosage Forms [DSC] = Discontinued product

Capsule: 200 mg

Zovirax®: 200 mg

Cream, topical:

Zovirax®: 5% (2 g, 5 g)

Injection, powder for reconstitution, as sodium: 500 mg, 1000 mg

Zovirax®: 500 mg [DSC]

Injection, solution, as sodium [preservative free]: 25 mg/mL (20 mL, 40 mL); 50 mg/mL (10 mL, 20 mL)

Ointment, topical:
Zovirax®: 5% (15 g)
Suspension, oral: 200 mg/5 mL (480 mL)
Zovirax®: 200 mg/5 mL (480 mL) [banana flavor]
Tablet: 400 mg, 800 mg
Zovirax®: 400 mg, 800 mg

Aczone™ [US] *see* dapsone *on page 229*

Adacel™ [US/Can] *see* diphtheria, tetanus toxoids, and acellular pertussis vaccine *on page 265*

Adagen® [US/Can] *see* pegademase (bovine) *on page 642*

Adalat® XL® [Can] *see* nifedipine *on page 592*

Adalat® CC [US] *see* nifedipine *on page 592*

Adalat® *(Discontinued)* *see* nifedipine *on page 592*

adalimumab (a da LIM yoo mab)

Sound-Alike/Look-Alike Issues
Humira® may be confused with Humulin®

Synonyms antitumor necrosis factor apha (human); D2E7; human antitumor necrosis factor alpha

U.S./Canadian Brand Names Humira® [US/Can]

Therapeutic Category Antirheumatic, Disease Modifying; Monoclonal Antibody

Use Treatment of active rheumatoid arthritis, active psoriatic arthritis (moderate to severe), or ankylosing spondylitis

Note: May be used alone or in combination with disease-modifying antirheumatic drugs (DMARDs).

Usual Dosage SubQ: Adults:
Rheumatoid arthritis: 40 mg every other week; may be administered with other DMARDs; patients not taking methotrexate may increase dose to 40 mg/week
Ankylosing spondylitis, psoriatic arthritis: 40 mg every other week

Dosage Forms
Injection, solution [preservative free]:
Humira®: 40 mg/0.8 mL (1 mL) [prefilled glass syringe or Humira® pen; packaged with alcohol preps; needle cover contains latex]

adamantanamine hydrochloride *see* amantadine *on page 38*

adapalene (a DAP a leen)

U.S./Canadian Brand Names Differin® XP [Can]; Differin® [US/Can]

Therapeutic Category Acne Products

Use Treatment of acne vulgaris

Usual Dosage Topical: Children >12 years and Adults: Apply once daily at bedtime; therapeutic results should be noticed after 8-12 weeks of treatment

Dosage Forms [DSC] = Discontinued product
Cream, topical: 0.1% (15 g, 45 g)
Gel, topical: 0.1% (15 g, 45 g) [alcohol free]
Pledget, topical: 0.1% (60s) [DSC]
Solution, topical: 0.1% (30 mL) [DSC]

Adderall® [US] *see* dextroamphetamine and amphetamine *on page 244*

Adderall XR® [US/Can] *see* dextroamphetamine and amphetamine *on page 244*

adefovir (a DEF o veer)

Synonyms adefovir dipivoxil

U.S./Canadian Brand Names Hepsera™ [US]

Therapeutic Category Antiretroviral Agent, Non-nucleoside Reverse Transcriptase Inhibitor (NNRTI)

Use Treatment of chronic hepatitis B with evidence of active viral replication (based on persistent elevation of ALT/AST or histologic evidence), including patients with lamivudine-resistant hepatitis B

Usual Dosage Oral: Adults: 10 mg once daily

Dosage Forms Tablet, as dipivoxil: 10 mg

adefovir dipivoxil *see* adefovir *on this page*

ADEKs [US-OTC] *see* vitamins (multiple/pediatric) *on page 878*

ADH *see* vasopressin *on page 868*
Adipex-P® [US] *see* phentermine *on page 659*
Adlone® Injection *(Discontinued)* *see* methylprednisolone *on page 547*
Adoxa™ [US] *see* doxycycline *on page 278*
Adrenalin® [US/Can] *see* epinephrine *on page 295*
adrenaline *see* epinephrine *on page 295*
adrenocorticotropic hormone *see* corticotropin *on page 215*
adria *see* doxorubicin *on page 277*
Adriamycin® [Can] *see* doxorubicin *on page 277*
Adriamycin PFS® [US] *see* doxorubicin *on page 277*
Adriamycin RDF® [US] *see* doxorubicin *on page 277*
Adrucil® [US] *see* fluorouracil *on page 356*
adsorbent charcoal *see* charcoal *on page 169*
Adsorbocarpine® Ophthalmic *(Discontinued)* *see* pilocarpine *on page 668*
Adsorbonac® *(Discontinued)* *see* sodium chloride *on page 777*
Adsorbotear® Ophthalmic Solution *(Discontinued)* *see* artificial tears *on page 75*
Advair Diskus® [US/Can] *see* fluticasone and salmeterol *on page 360*
Advanced Formula Oxy® Sensitive Gel *(Discontinued)* *see* benzoyl peroxide *on page 102*
Advanced NatalCare® [US] *see* vitamins (multiple/prenatal) *on page 879*
Advantage-S™ [US-OTC] *see* nonoxynol 9 *on page 597*
Advate [US] *see* antihemophilic factor (recombinant) *on page 59*
Advicor® [US/Can] *see* niacin and lovastatin *on page 589*
Advil® [US-OTC/Can] *see* ibuprofen *on page 437*
Advil® Allergy Sinus [US] *see* ibuprofen, pseudoephedrine, and chlorpheniramine *on page 439*
Advil® Children's [US-OTC] *see* ibuprofen *on page 437*
Advil® Cold and Sinus Plus [Can] *see* ibuprofen, pseudoephedrine, and chlorpheniramine *on page 439*
Advil® Cold, Children's [US-OTC] *see* pseudoephedrine and ibuprofen *on page 715*
Advil® Cold & Sinus [US-OTC/Can] *see* pseudoephedrine and ibuprofen *on page 715*
Advil® Infants' [US-OTC] *see* ibuprofen *on page 437*
Advil® Junior [US-OTC] *see* ibuprofen *on page 437*
Advil® Migraine [US-OTC] *see* ibuprofen *on page 437*
Advil® Multi-Symptom Cold [US] *see* ibuprofen, pseudoephedrine, and chlorpheniramine *on page 439*
Aerius® [Can] *see* desloratadine *on page 237*
Aeroaid® *(Discontinued)* *see* thimerosal *on page 822*
AeroBid® [US] *see* flunisolide *on page 352*
AeroBid®-M [US] *see* flunisolide *on page 352*
Aerodine® *(Discontinued)* *see* povidone-iodine *on page 689*
aeroKid™ [US] *see* chlorpheniramine, phenylephrine, and methscopolamine *on page 180*
Aerospan™ [US] *see* flunisolide *on page 352*
Afeditab™ CR [US] *see* nifedipine *on page 592*
A-Free Prenatal [US] *see* vitamins (multiple/prenatal) *on page 879*
Afrin® Children's Nose Drops *(Discontinued)* *see* oxymetazoline *on page 628*
Afrin® Extra Moisturizing [US-OTC] *see* oxymetazoline *on page 628*
Afrinol® *(Discontinued)* *see* pseudoephedrine *on page 712*
Afrin® Original [US-OTC] *see* oxymetazoline *on page 628*
Afrin® Saline Mist *(Discontinued)* *see* sodium chloride *on page 777*

Afrin® Severe Congestion [US-OTC] *see* oxymetazoline *on page 628*

Afrin® Sinus [US-OTC] *see* oxymetazoline *on page 628*

Aftate® Antifungal *(Discontinued)* *see* tolnaftate *on page 834*

AG *see* aminoglutethimide *on page 42*

agalsidase beta (aye GAL si days BAY ta)

Sound-Alike/Look-Alike Issues

agalsidase beta may be confused with alglucerase, alglucosidase alfa

Synonyms alpha-galactosidase-A (human, recombinant); r-h α-GAL

U.S./Canadian Brand Names Fabrazyme® [US/Can]

Therapeutic Category Enzyme

Use Replacement therapy for Fabry disease

Usual Dosage I.V.: Adults: 1 mg/kg every 2 weeks

Dosage Forms Injection, powder for reconstitution: 5 mg [contains mannitol 33 mg; derived from Chinese hamster cells]; 35 mg [contains mannitol 222 mg/vial; derived from Chinese hamster cells]

Agenerase® [US/Can] *see* amprenavir *on page 55*

Aggrastat® [US/Can] *see* tirofiban *on page 830*

Aggrenox® [US/Can] *see* aspirin and dipyridamole *on page 79*

AGN 1135 *see* rasagiline *on page 733*

$AgNO_3$ *see* silver nitrate *on page 772*

Agrylin® [US/Can] *see* anagrelide *on page 55*

AGT *see* aminoglutethimide *on page 42*

AHA *see* acetohydroxamic acid *on page 15*

AH-Chew® [US] *see* chlorpheniramine, phenylephrine, and methscopolamine *on page 180*

AH-Chew II [US] *see* chlorpheniramine, phenylephrine, and methscopolamine *on page 180*

AH-chew® D *(Discontinued)* *see* phenylephrine *on page 660*

AHF (human) *see* antihemophilic factor (human) *on page 59*

AHF (recombinant) *see* antihemophilic factor (recombinant) *on page 59*

AICC *see* anti-inhibitor coagulant complex *on page 61*

Airet® *(Discontinued)* *see* albuterol *on page 23*

Airomir [Can] *see* albuterol *on page 23*

AKBeta® *(Discontinued)* *see* levobunolol *on page 488*

Ak-Chlor® Ophthalmic *(Discontinued)* *see* chloramphenicol *on page 172*

AK-Con™ [US] *see* naphazoline *on page 577*

AK-Dilate® [US] *see* phenylephrine *on page 660*

AK-Fluor [US] *see* fluorescein sodium *on page 354*

Ak-Homatropine® Ophthalmic *(Discontinued)* *see* homatropine *on page 415*

Akineton® [US/Can] *see* biperiden *on page 111*

AK-Nefrin *(Discontinued)* *see* phenylephrine *on page 660*

Akne-Mycin® [US] *see* erythromycin *on page 303*

AK-Pentolate® *(Discontinued)* *see* cyclopentolate *on page 220*

AK-Poly-Bac® [US] *see* bacitracin and polymyxin B *on page 90*

AK-Pred® [US] *see* prednisolone (ophthalmic) *on page 694*

AK-Spore® H.C. Ophthalmic *(Discontinued)* *see* bacitracin, neomycin, polymyxin B, and hydrocortisone *on page 91*

AK-Spore® H.C. Otic *(Discontinued)* *see* neomycin, polymyxin B, and hydrocortisone *on page 584*

AK-Spore® Ophthalmic Ointment *(Discontinued)* *see* bacitracin, neomycin, and polymyxin B *on page 91*

AK-Taine® *(Discontinued)* *see* proparacaine *on page 706*

AKTob® [US] *see* tobramycin *on page 831*

AK-Tracin® *(Discontinued)* *see* bacitracin *on page 90*

AK-Trol® Ophthalmic Ointment *(Discontinued)* *see* neomycin, polymyxin B, and dexamethasone *on page 584*

AK-Trol® Ophthalmic Suspension *(Discontinued)* *see* neomycin, polymyxin B, and dexamethasone *on page 584*

Akwa Tears® [US-OTC] *see* artificial tears *on page 75*

Alamag [US-OTC] *see* aluminum hydroxide and magnesium hydroxide *on page 36*

Alamag Plus [US-OTC] *see* aluminum hydroxide, magnesium hydroxide, and simethicone *on page 37*

Alamast® [US/Can] *see* pemirolast *on page 645*

Alavert® [US-OTC] *see* loratadine *on page 505*

Alavert™ Allergy and Sinus [US-OTC] *see* loratadine and pseudoephedrine *on page 505*

Alazide® *(Discontinued)* *see* hydrochlorothiazide and spironolactone *on page 420*

Albalon® [US] *see* naphazoline *on page 577*

Albalon-A® Ophthalmic *(Discontinued)*

albendazole (al BEN da zole)

U.S./Canadian Brand Names Albenza® [US]

Therapeutic Category Anthelmintic

Use Treatment of parenchymal neurocysticercosis caused by *Taenia solium* and cystic hydatid disease of the liver, lung, and peritoneum caused by *Echinococcus granulosus*

Usual Dosage Oral: Children and Adults:

Neurocysticercosis:

<60 kg: 15 mg/kg/day in 2 divided doses (maximum: 800 mg/day) for 8-30 days

≥60 kg: 400 mg twice daily for 8-30 days

Note: Give concurrent anticonvulsant and steroid therapy during first week.

Hydatid:

<60 kg: 15 mg/kg/day in 2 divided doses (maximum: 800 mg/day)

≥60 kg: 400 mg twice daily

Note: Administer dose for three 28-day cycles with a 14-day drug-free interval in between.

Dosage Forms Tablet: 200 mg

Albenza® [US] *see* albendazole *on this page*

Albert® Glyburide [Can] *see* glyburide *on page 387*

Albert® Pentoxifylline [Can] *see* pentoxifylline *on page 653*

Albert® Tiafen [Can] *see* tiaprofenic acid *(Canada only)* *on page 826*

Albumarc® [US] *see* albumin *on this page*

albumin (al BYOO min)

Sound-Alike/Look-Alike Issues

Albutein® may be confused with albuterol

Buminate® may be confused with bumetanide

Synonyms albumin (human); normal human serum albumin; normal serum albumin (human); salt poor albumin; SPA

U.S./Canadian Brand Names Albumarc® [US]; Albuminar® [US]; Albutein® [US]; Buminate® [US]; Flexbumin [US]; Plasbumin® [US]; Plasbumin®-25 [Can]; Plasbumin®-5 [Can]

Therapeutic Category Blood Product Derivative

Use Plasma volume expansion and maintenance of cardiac output in the treatment of certain types of shock or impending shock; may be useful for burn patients, ARDS, and cardiopulmonary bypass; other uses considered by some investigators (but not proven) are retroperitoneal surgery, peritonitis, and ascites; unless the condition responsible for hypoproteinemia can be corrected, albumin can provide only symptomatic relief or supportive treatment

Usual Dosage I.V.:

5% should be used in hypovolemic patients or intravascularly-depleted patients

25% should be used in patients in whom fluid and sodium intake must be minimized

Dose depends on condition of patient:

Children: Hypovolemia: 0.5-1 g/kg/dose (10-20 mL/kg/dose of albumin 5%); maximum dose: 6 g/kg/day

Adults: Usual dose: 25 g; initial dose may be repeated in 15-30 minutes if response is inadequate; no more than 250 g should be administered within 48 hours

Hypoproteinemia: 0.5-1 g/kg/dose; repeat every 1-2 days as calculated to replace ongoing losses

Hypovolemia: 0.5-1 g/kg/dose; repeat as needed; maximum dose: 6 g/kg/day

Hypovolemia: 5% albumin: 0.5-1 g/kg/dose; repeat as needed. **Note:** May be considered after inadequate response to crystalloid therapy and when nonprotein colloids are contraindicated. The volume administered and the speed of infusion should be adapted to individual response.

Dosage Forms

Injection, solution [preservative free; human]:

Albuminar®: 5% [50 mg/mL] (50 mL, 250 mL, 500 mL) [contains sodium 130-160 mEq/L and potassium ≤1 mEq/L; packaging contains dry natural rubber]; 25% [250 mg/mL] (20 mL, 50 mL, 100 mL) [contains sodium 130-160 mEq/L and potassium ≤1 mEq/L; packaging contains dry natural rubber]

AlbuRx™: 5% [50 mg/mL] (250 mL, 500 mL) [contains sodium 130-160 mEq/L and potassium ≤2 mEq/L]; 25% [250 mg/mL] (50 mL, 100 mL) [contains sodium 130-160 mEq/L and potassium ≤2 mEq/L]

Albutein®: 5% [50 mg/mL] (250 mL, 500 mL) [contains sodium 130-160 mEq/L and potassium ≤2 mEq/L]; 25% [250 mg/mL] (50 mL, 100 mL) [contains sodium 130-160 mEq/L and potassium ≤2 mEq/L]

Buminate®: 5% [50 mg/mL] (250 mL, 500 mL) [contains sodium 130-160 mEq/L and potassium ≤2 mEq/L]; 25% [250 mg/mL] (20 mL, 50 mL, 100 mL) [contains sodium 130-160 mEq/L and potassium ≤2 mEq/L]

Flexbumin: 25% [250 mg/mL] (50 mL, 100 mL) [contains sodium 130-160 and potassium ≤2 mEq/L]

Human Albumin Grifols®: 25% [250 mg/mL] (50 mL, 100 mL) [contains sodium 130-160 mEq/L and potassium ≤2 mEq/L]

Plasbumin®: 5% [50 mg/mL] (50 mL, 250 mL) [contains sodium ~145 mEq/L and potassium ≤2 mEq/L]; 25% [250 mg/mL] (20 mL, 50 mL, 100 mL) [contains sodium ~145 mEq/L and potassium ≤2 mEq/L]

Albuminar® [US] *see* albumin *on previous page*

albumin (human) *see* albumin *on previous page*

Albumisol® ***(Discontinued)*** *see* albumin *on previous page*

Albunex® ***(Discontinued)*** *see* albumin *on previous page*

Albutein® [US] *see* albumin *on previous page*

albuterol (al BYOO ter ole)

Sound-Alike/Look-Alike Issues

albuterol may be confused with Albutein®, atenolol

Proventil® may be confused with Bentyl®, Prilosec® Prinivil®

salbutamol may be confused with salmeterol

Ventolin® may be confused with phentolamine, Benylin®, Vantin®

Volmax® may be confused with Flomax®

Synonyms albuterol sulfate; salbutamol

U.S./Canadian Brand Names AccuNeb® [US]; Airomir [Can]; Alti-Salbutamol [Can]; Apo-Salvent® CFC Free [Can]; Apo-Salvent® Respirator Solution [Can]; Apo-Salvent® Sterules [Can]; Apo-Salvent® [Can]; Gen-Salbutamol [Can]; PMS-Salbutamol [Can]; ProAir™ HFA [US]; Proventil® HFA [US]; Proventil® [US]; ratio-Inspra-Sal [Can]; ratio-Salbutamol [Can]; Rhoxal-salbutamol [Can]; Salbu-2 [Can]; Salbu-4 [Can]; Ventolin® Diskus [Can]; Ventolin® HFA [US/Can]; Ventolin® [Can]; Ventrodisk [Can]; VoSpire ER® [US]

Therapeutic Category Adrenergic Agonist Agent

Use Bronchodilator in reversible airway obstruction due to asthma or COPD; prevention of exercise-induced bronchospasm

Usual Dosage

Oral:

Children: Bronchospasm (treatment):

2-6 years: 0.1-0.2 mg/kg/dose 3 times/day; maximum dose not to exceed 12 mg/day (divided doses)

6-12 years: 2 mg/dose 3-4 times/day; maximum dose not to exceed 24 mg/day (divided doses)

Extended release: 4 mg every 12 hours; maximum dose not to exceed 24 mg/day (divided doses)

Children >12 years and Adults: Bronchospasm (treatment): 2-4 mg/dose 3-4 times/day; maximum dose not to exceed 32 mg/day (divided doses)

Extended release: 8 mg every 12 hours; maximum dose not to exceed 32 mg/day (divided doses). A 4 mg dose every 12 hours may be sufficient in some patients, such as adults of low body weight.

Inhalation: MDI 90 mcg/puff:

Children ≤12 years:

Bronchospasm (acute): 4-8 puffs every 20 minutes for 3 doses, then every 1-4 hours; spacer/holding-chamber device should be used

Exercise-induced bronchospasm (prophylaxis): 1-2 puffs 5 minutes prior to exercise

(Continued)

albuterol *(Continued)*

Children >12 years and Adults:
Bronchospasm (acute): 4-8 puffs every 20 minutes for up to 4 hours, then every 1-4 hours as needed
Exercise-induced bronchospasm (prophylaxis): 2 puffs 5-30 minutes prior to exercise
Children ≥4 years and Adults: Bronchospasm (chronic treatment): 1-2 inhalations every 4-6 hours; maximum: 12 inhalations/day
NIH guidelines: 2 puffs 3-4 times a day as needed; may double dose for mild exacerbations
Nebulization:
Children ≤12 years:
Bronchospasm (treatment): 0.05 mg/kg every 4-6 hours; minimum dose: 1.25 mg, maximum dose: 2.5 mg
2-12 years: AccuNeb®: 0.63 mg or 1.25 mg 3-4 times/day, as needed, delivered over 5-15 minutes
Children >40 kg, patients with more severe asthma, or children 11-12 years: May respond better with a 1.25 mg dose
Bronchospasm (acute): Solution 0.5%: 0.15 mg/kg (minimum dose: 2.5 mg) every 20 minutes for 3 doses, then 0.15-0.3 mg/kg (up to 10 mg) every 1-4 hours as needed; may also use 0.5 mg/kg/hour by continuous infusion. Continuous nebulized albuterol at 0.3 mg/kg/hour has been used safely in the treatment of severe status asthmaticus in children; continuous nebulized doses of 3 mg/kg/hour ± 2.2 mg/kg/hour in children whose mean age was 20.7 months resulted in no cardiac toxicity; the optimal dosage for continuous nebulization remains to be determined.
Note: Use of the 0.5% solution should be used for bronchospasm (acute or treatment) in children <15 kg. AccuNeb® has not been studied for the treatment of acute bronchospasm; use of the 0.5% concentrated solution may be more appropriate.
Children >12 years and Adults:
Bronchospasm (treatment): 2.5 mg, diluted to a total of 3 mL, 3-4 times/day over 5-15 minutes
NIH guidelines: 1.25-5 mg every 4-8 hours
Bronchospasm (acute) in intensive care patients: 2.5-5 mg every 20 minutes for 3 doses, then 2.5-10 mg every 1-4 hours as needed, **or** 10-15 mg/hour continuously

Dosage Forms
Aerosol, for oral inhalation: 90 mcg/metered inhalation (17 g) [200 metered inhalations; contains chlorofluorocarbons]
Proventil®: 90 mcg/metered inhalation (17 g) [200 metered inhalations; contains chlorofluorocarbons]
Aerosol, for oral inhalation:
ProAir™ HFA: 90 mcg/metered inhalation (8.5 g) [200 metered inhalations; chlorofluorocarbon free]
Proventil® HFA: 90 mcg/metered inhalation (6.7 g) [200 metered inhalations; chlorofluorocarbon free]
Ventolin® HFA: 90 mcg/metered inhalation (18 g) [200 metered inhalations; chlorofluorocarbon free]
Solution for nebulization: 0.042% (3 mL); 0.083% (3 mL); 0.5% (0.5 mL, 20 mL)
AccuNeb® [preservative free]: 0.63 mg/3 mL (3 mL) [0.021%]; 1.25 mg/3 mL (3 mL) [0.042%]
Proventil®: 0.083% (3 mL) [preservative free]; 0.5% (20 mL) [contains benzalkonium chloride]
Syrup, as sulfate: 2 mg/5 mL (480 mL)
Tablet: 2 mg, 4 mg
Tablet, extended release:
VoSpire ER®: 4 mg, 8 mg

albuterol and ipratropium *see* ipratropium and albuterol *on page 460*

albuterol sulfate *see* albuterol *on previous page*

Alcaine® [US/Can] *see* proparacaine *on page 706*

Alcalak [US-OTC] *see* calcium carbonate *on page 135*

alclometasone (al kloe MET a sone)

Sound-Alike/Look-Alike Issues
Aclovate® may be confused with Accolate®

Synonyms alclometasone dipropionate

U.S./Canadian Brand Names Aclovate® [US]

Therapeutic Category Corticosteroid, Topical

Use Treatment of inflammation of corticosteroid-responsive dermatosis (low potency topical corticosteroid)

Usual Dosage Topical: Apply a thin film to the affected area 2-3 times/day. Therapy should be discontinued when control is achieved; if no improvement is seen, reassessment of diagnosis may be necessary.

Dosage Forms
Cream, as dipropionate: 0.05% (15 g, 45 g, 60 g)
Ointment, as dipropionate: 0.05% (15 g, 45 g, 60 g)

alclometasone dipropionate *see* alclometasone *on previous page*

alcohol, absolute *see* alcohol (ethyl) *on this page*

alcohol, dehydrated *see* alcohol (ethyl) *on this page*

alcohol (ethyl) (AL koe hol, ETH il)

Sound-Alike/Look-Alike Issues

ethanol may be confused with Ethyol®, Ethamolin®

Synonyms alcohol, absolute; alcohol, dehydrated; ethanol; ethyl alcohol; EtOH

U.S./Canadian Brand Names Biobase-G™ [Can]; Biobase™ [Can]; EpiClenz™ [US-OTC]; Gel-Stat™ [US-OTC]; GelRite [US-OTC]; Isagel® [US-OTC]; Lavacol® [US-OTC]; Prevacare® [US-OTC]; Protection Plus® [US-OTC]; Purell® 2 in 1 [US-OTC]; Purell® with Aloe [US-OTC]; Purell® [US-OTC]

Therapeutic Category Intravenous Nutritional Therapy; Pharmaceutical Aid

Use Topical anti-infective; pharmaceutical aid; therapeutic neurolysis (nerve or ganglion block); replenishment of fluid and carbohydrate calories

Usual Dosage

Oral: **Note:** Oral dosing is not recommended outside of a hospital setting: Initial dose: 600 mg/kg [equivalent to 1.8 mL/kg using a 43% solution]

Maintenance dose:

Nondrinker: 66 mg/kg/hour [equivalent to 0.2 mL/kg/hour using a 43% solution]

Chronic drinker: 154 mg/kg/hour [equivalent to 0.46 mL/kg/hour using a 43% solution]

I.V.: Initial: 600 mg/kg [equivalent to 7.6 mL/kg using a 10% solution]

Maintenance dose:

Nondrinker: 66 mg/kg/hour [equivalent to 0.83 mL/kg/hour using a 10% solution]

Chronic drinker: 154 mg/kg/hour [equivalent to 1.96 mL/kg/hour using a 10% solution]

Antiseptic: Children and Adults: Liquid denatured alcohol: Topical: Apply 1-3 times/day as needed

Therapeutic neurolysis (nerve or ganglion block): Adults: Dehydrated alcohol injection: Intraneural: Dosage variable depending upon the site of injection (eg, trigeminal neuralgia: 0.05-0.5 mL as a single injection per interspace vs subarachnoid injection: 0.5-1 mL as a single injection per interspace); single doses >1.5 mL are seldom required

Replenishment of fluid and carbohydrate calories: Adults: Dehydrated alcohol infusion: Alcohol 5% and dextrose 5%: 1-2 L/day by slow infusion

Dosage Forms [DSC] = Discontinued product

Foam, topical:

Epi-Clenz™: 62% (240 mL, 480 mL) [instant hand sanitizer; contains aloe vera and vitamin E]

Gel, topical:

Epi-Clenz™: 70% (45 mL, 120 mL, 480 mL) [instant hand sanitizer; contains aloe vera and vitamin E]

GelRite: 67% (120 mL, 480 mL, 800 mL) [instant hand sanitizer; contains vitamin E)

Gel-Stat™: 62% (120 mL, 480 mL) [instant hand sanitizer]

Isagel®: 60% (59 mL, 118 mL, 621 mL, 800 mL) [instant hand sanitizer]

Prevacare®: 60% (120 mL, 240 mL, 960 mL, 1200 mL, 1500 mL) [instant hand sanitizer]

Protection Plus®: 62% (800 mL) [instant hand sanitizer]

Purell®: 62% (15 mL, 30 mL, 59 mL, 120 mL, 236 mL, 250 mL, 360 mL, 500 mL, 800 mL, 1000 mL, 2000 mL) [instant hand sanitizer; contains moisturizers and vitamin E]

Purell® Moisture Therapy: 62% (75 mL) [instant hand sanitizer]

Purell® with Aloe: 62% (15 mL, 59 mL, 236 mL, 360 mL, 800 mL, 1000 mL, 2000 mL) [instant hand sanitizer; contains aloe and tartrazine]

Infusion [in D_5W, dehydrated]: Alcohol 5% (1000 mL)

Injection, solution [dehydrated]: 98% (1 mL, 5 mL)

Liquid, topical [denatured]: 70% (3840 mL)

Lavacol®: 70% (473 mL)

Lotion, topical:

Purell® 2 in 1: 62% (60 mL, 360 mL, 1000 mL) [instant hand sanitizer]

Towelettes, topical:

Isagel®: 60% (50s, 300s) [instant hand sanitizer]

Purell®: 62% (35s, 175s) [instant hand sanitizer]

Alcomicin® [Can] *see* gentamicin *on page 381*

Alconefrin® Nasal Solution *(Discontinued)* *see* phenylephrine *on page 660*

Aldactazide® [US] *see* hydrochlorothiazide and spironolactone *on page 420*

Aldactazide 25® [Can] *see* hydrochlorothiazide and spironolactone *on page 420*

Aldactazide 50® [Can] *see* hydrochlorothiazide and spironolactone *on page 420*

Aldactone® [US/Can] *see* spironolactone *on page 789*

Aldara™ [US/Can] *see* imiquimod *on page 443*

aldesleukin (al des LOO kin)

Sound-Alike/Look-Alike Issues

aldesleukin may be confused with oprelvekin

Proleukin® may be confused with oprelvekin

Synonyms epidermal thymocyte activating factor; ETAF; IL-2; interleukin-2; lymphocyte mitogenic factor; NSC-373364; T-cell growth factor; TCGF; thymocyte stimulating factor

U.S./Canadian Brand Names Proleukin® [US/Can]

Therapeutic Category Biological Response Modulator

Use Treatment of metastatic renal cell cancer, melanoma

Usual Dosage Refer to individual protocols.

I.V.:

Renal cell carcinoma: 600,000 int. units/kg every 8 hours for a maximum of 14 doses; repeat after 9 days for a total of 28 doses per course. Retreat if needed 7 weeks after previous course.

Melanoma:

Single-agent use: 600,000 int. units/kg every 8 hours for a maximum of 14 doses; repeat after 9 days for a total of 28 doses per course. Retreat if needed 7 weeks after previous course.

In combination with cytotoxic agents: 24 million int. units/m^2 days 12-16 and 19-23

SubQ:

Single-agent doses: 3-18 million int. units/day for 5 days each week, up to 6 weeks

In combination with interferon:

5 million int. units/m^2 3 times/week

1.8 million int. units/m^2 twice daily 5 days/week for 6 weeks

Dosage Forms Injection, powder for reconstitution: 22 x 10^6 int. units [18 million int. units/mL = 1.1 mg/mL when reconstituted]

Aldex™ [US] *see* guaifenesin and phenylephrine *on page 396*

Aldomet® *(Discontinued)* *see* methyldopa *on page 544*

Aldoril® [US] *see* methyldopa and hydrochlorothiazide *on page 545*

Aldoril® D50 *(Discontinued)* *see* methyldopa and hydrochlorothiazide *on page 545*

Aldroxicon I [US-OTC] *see* aluminum hydroxide, magnesium hydroxide, and simethicone *on page 37*

Aldroxicon II [US-OTC] *see* aluminum hydroxide, magnesium hydroxide, and simethicone *on page 37*

Aldurazyme® [US/Can] *see* laronidase *on page 483*

alefacept (a LE fa sept)

Synonyms B 9273; BG 9273; human LFA-3/IgG(1) fusion protein; LFA-3/IgG(1) fusion protein, human

U.S./Canadian Brand Names Amevive® [US/Can]

Therapeutic Category Monoclonal Antibody

Use Treatment of moderate to severe chronic plaque psoriasis in adults who are candidates for systemic therapy or phototherapy

Usual Dosage Adults:

I.M.: 15 mg once weekly; usual duration of treatment: 12 weeks

A second course of treatment may be initiated at least 12 weeks after completion of the initial course of treatment, provided CD4$^+$ T-lymphocyte counts are within the normal range.

Note: CD4$^+$ T-lymphocyte counts should be monitored before initiation of treatment and every 2 weeks during therapy. Dosing should be withheld if CD4$^+$ counts are <250 cells/µL, and dosing should be permanently discontinued if CD4$^+$ lymphocyte counts remain at <250 cell/µL for longer than 1 month.

Dosage Forms

Injection, powder for reconstitution:

Amevive®: 15 mg [for I.M. administration; contains sucrose 12.5 mg; supplied with SWFI]

alemtuzumab (ay lem TU zoo mab)

Synonyms C1H; campath-1H; DNA-derived humanized monoclonal antibody; humanized IgG1 anti-CD52 monoclonal antibody

U.S./Canadian Brand Names Campath® [US]
Therapeutic Category Antineoplastic Agent, Monoclonal Antibody
Use Treatment of B-cell chronic lymphocytic leukemia (B-CLL)
Usual Dosage **Note: Dose escalation is required;** usually accomplished in 3-7 days. Do not exceed single doses >30 mg or cumulative doses >90 mg/week.
I.V. infusion, SubQ (unlabeled route): Adults: B-CLL:
Initial: 3 mg/day; increase to 10 mg/day, then to 30 mg/day as tolerated
Maintenance: 30 mg/day 3 times/week on alternate days for up to 12 weeks
Dosage Forms [DSC] = Discontinued product
Injection, solution [ampul]: 10 mg/mL (3 mL) [DSC]
Injection, solution [vial]: 30 mg/mL (1 mL)

alendronate (a LEN droe nate)

Sound-Alike/Look-Alike Issues
Fosamax® may be confused with Flomax®
Synonyms alendronate sodium
U.S./Canadian Brand Names Apo-Alendronate® [Can]; CO Alendronate [Can]; Fosamax® [US/Can]; Gen-Alendronate [Can]; Novo-Alendronate [Can]; PMS-Alendronate [Can]; ratio-Alendronate [Can]; Riva-Alendronate [Can]
Therapeutic Category Bisphosphonate Derivative
Use Treatment and prevention of osteoporosis in postmenopausal females; treatment of osteoporosis in males; Paget disease of the bone in patients who are symptomatic, at risk for future complications, or with alkaline phosphatase ≥2 times the upper limit of normal; treatment of glucocorticoid-induced osteoporosis in males and females with low bone mineral density who are receiving a daily dosage ≥7.5 mg of prednisone (or equivalent)
Usual Dosage Oral: Adults: **Note:** Patients treated with glucocorticoids and those with Paget disease should receive adequate amounts of calcium and vitamin D.
Osteoporosis in postmenopausal females:
Prophylaxis: 5 mg once daily **or** 35 mg once weekly
Treatment: 10 mg once daily **or** 70 mg once weekly
Osteoporosis in males: 10 mg once daily **or** 70 mg once weekly
Osteoporosis secondary to glucocorticoids in males and females: Treatment: 5 mg once daily; a dose of 10 mg once daily should be used in postmenopausal females who are not receiving estrogen.
Paget disease of bone in males and females: 40 mg once daily for 6 months
Retreatment: Relapses during the 12 months following therapy occurred in 9% of patients who responded to treatment. Specific retreatment data are not available. Following a 6-month post-treatment evaluation period, retreatment with alendronate may be considered in patients who have relapsed based on increases in serum alkaline phosphatase, which should be measured periodically. Retreatment may also be considered in those who failed to normalize their serum alkaline phosphatase.
Dosage Forms **Note:** Strength expressed as free acid
Solution, oral, as monosodium trihydrate:
Fosamax™: 70 mg/75 mL [contains parabens; raspberry flavor]
Tablet, as sodium:
Fosamax™: 5 mg, 10 mg, 35 mg, 40 mg, 70 mg

alendronate and cholecalciferol (a LEN droe nate & kole e kal SI fer ole)

Synonyms alendronate sodium and cholecalciferol; cholecalciferol and alendronate; vitamin D_3
U.S./Canadian Brand Names Fosamax Plus D™ [US]; Fosavance [Can]
Therapeutic Category Bisphosphonate Derivative; Vitamin D Analog
Use Treatment of osteoporosis in postmenopausal females; increase bone mass in males with osteoporosis
Usual Dosage Oral: Adults: One tablet once weekly
Dosage Forms
Tablet:
Fosamax Plus D™: 70/2800: Alendronate 70 mg and cholecalciferol 2800 int. units

alendronate sodium *see* alendronate *on this page*

alendronate sodium and cholecalciferol *see* alendronate and cholecalciferol *on this page*

Alenic Alka Tablet [US-OTC] *see* aluminum hydroxide and magnesium trisilicate *on page 36*

Aler-Cap [US-OTC] *see* diphenhydramine *on page 261*

Aler-Dryl [US-OTC] *see* diphenhydramine *on page 261*

Aler-Tab [US-OTC] *see* diphenhydramine *on page 261*

Alertec® [Can] *see* modafinil *on page 562*

Alesse® [US/Can] *see* ethinyl estradiol and levonorgestrel *on page 320*

Aleve® [US-OTC] *see* naproxen *on page 578*

Alfenta® [US/Can] *see* alfentanil *on this page*

alfentanil (al FEN ta nil)

Sound-Alike/Look-Alike Issues

alfentanil may be confused with Anafranil®, fentanyl, remifentanil, sufentanil

Alfenta® may be confused with Sufenta®

Synonyms alfentanil hydrochloride

U.S./Canadian Brand Names Alfentanil Injection, USP [Can]; Alfenta® [US/Can]

Therapeutic Category Analgesic, Narcotic; General Anesthetic

Controlled Substance C-II

Use Analgesic adjunct given by continuous infusion or in incremental doses in maintenance of anesthesia with barbiturate or N_2O or a primary anesthetic agent for the induction of anesthesia in patients undergoing general surgery in which endotracheal intubation and mechanical ventilation are required

Usual Dosage Doses should be titrated to appropriate effects; wide range of doses is dependent upon desired degree of analgesia/anesthesia

Children <12 years: Dose not established

Adults: Dose should be based on ideal body weight.

Dosage Forms

Injection, solution [preservative free]: 500 mcg/mL (2 mL, 5 mL, 10 mL)

Alfenta®: 500 mcg/mL (2 mL, 5 mL, 10 mL, 20 mL)

alfentanil hydrochloride *see* alfentanil *on this page*

Alfentanil Injection, USP [Can] *see* alfentanil *on this page*

Alferon® N [US/Can] *see* interferon alfa-n3 *on page 457*

alfuzosin (al FYOO zoe sin)

Synonyms alfuzosin hydrochloride

U.S./Canadian Brand Names Uroxatral™ [US]; Xatral [Can]

Therapeutic Category Alpha-Adrenergic Blocking Agent

Use Treatment of the functional symptoms of benign prostatic hyperplasia (BPH)

Usual Dosage Oral: Adults: 10 mg once daily

Dosage Forms Tablet, extended release, as hydrochloride: 10 mg

alfuzosin hydrochloride *see* alfuzosin *on this page*

alglucerase (al GLOO ser ase)

Sound-Alike/Look-Alike Issues

Ceredase® may be confused with Cerezyme®

Synonyms glucocerebrosidase

U.S./Canadian Brand Names Ceredase® [US]

Therapeutic Category Enzyme

Use Replacement therapy for Gaucher disease (type 1)

Usual Dosage I.V.: Children and Adults: Initial: 30-60 units/kg every 2 weeks; dosing is individualized based on disease severity; average dose: 60 units/kg every 2 weeks. Range: 2.5 units/kg 3 times/week to 60 units/kg 1-4 times/week. Once patient response is well established, dose may be reduced every 3-6 months to determine maintenance therapy.

Dosage Forms [DSC] = Discontinued product

Injection, solution [preservative free]: 10 units/mL (5 mL) [DSC]; 80 units/mL (5 mL) [contains human albumin 1%]

alglucosidase *see* alglucosidase alfa *on this page*

alglucosidase alfa (al gloo KOSE i dase AL fa)

Sound-Alike/Look-Alike Issues

alglucosidase alfa may be confused with agalsidase beta, alglucerase

Synonyms alglucosidase; GAA; rhGAA
U.S./Canadian Brand Names Myozyme® [US]
Therapeutic Category Enzyme
Use Replacement therapy for Pompe disease (infantile onset)
Usual Dosage I.V.: Children 1 month to 3.5 years (at first infusion): 20 mg/kg over ~4 hours every 2 weeks
Dosage Forms
Injection, powder for reconstitution [preservative free]:
Myozyme®: 50 mg [contains mannitol 210 mg; polysorbate 80; derived from Chinese hamster ovary cells]

Alimta® [US/Can] *see* pemetrexed *on page 645*

Alinia® [US] *see* nitazoxanide *on page 593*

alitretinoin (a li TRET i noyn)

Sound-Alike/Look-Alike Issues
Panretin® may be confused with pancreatin
U.S./Canadian Brand Names Panretin® [US/Can]
Therapeutic Category Antineoplastic Agent, Miscellaneous; Retinoic Acid Derivative
Use Orphan drug: Topical treatment of cutaneous lesions in AIDS-related Kaposi sarcoma
Usual Dosage Topical: Apply gel twice daily to cutaneous lesions
Dosage Forms Gel: 0.1% (60 g tube)

Alka-Mints® [US-OTC] *see* calcium carbonate *on page 135*

Alka-Seltzer® Plus® Cold and Cough [US-OTC] *see* chlorpheniramine, phenylephrine, and dextromethorphan *on page 179*

Alka-Seltzer® Plus® Cold and Sinus Liqui-Gels [US-OTC] *see* acetaminophen and pseudoephedrine *on page 9*

Alka-Seltzer® Plus® Cold Liqui-Gels® [US-OTC] *see* acetaminophen, chlorpheniramine, and pseudoephedrine *on page 11*

Alka-Seltzer® Plus® Flu Liqui-Gels [US-OTC] *see* acetaminophen, dextromethorphan, and pseudoephedrine *on page 12*

Alkeran® [US/Can] *see* melphalan *on page 526*

AllanFol RX [US] *see* folic acid, cyanocobalamin, and pyridoxine *on page 365*

AllanHist PDX [US] *see* brompheniramine, pseudoephedrine, and dextromethorphan *on page 120*

AllanTan Pediatric [US] *see* chlorpheniramine and phenylephrine *on page 176*

AllanVan-DM [US] *see* phenylephrine, pyrilamine, and dextromethorphan *on page 664*

AllanVan-S [US] *see* phenylephrine and pyrilamine *on page 662*

Allanzyme [US] *see* papain and urea *on page 637*

Allanzyme 650 [US] *see* papain and urea *on page 637*

Allbee® C-800 [US-OTC] *see* vitamin B complex combinations *on page 876*

Allbee® C-800 + Iron [US-OTC] *see* vitamin B complex combinations *on page 876*

Allbee® with C [US-OTC] *see* vitamin B complex combinations *on page 876*

Allegra® [US/Can] *see* fexofenadine *on page 344*

Allegra® 60 mg Capsule *(Discontinued)* *see* fexofenadine *on page 344*

Allegra-D® [Can] *see* fexofenadine and pseudoephedrine *on page 344*

Allegra-D® 12 Hour [US] *see* fexofenadine and pseudoephedrine *on page 344*

Allegra-D® 24 Hour [US] *see* fexofenadine and pseudoephedrine *on page 344*

Aller-Chlor® [US-OTC] *see* chlorpheniramine *on page 175*

Allercon® Tablet *(Discontinued)* *see* triprolidine and pseudoephedrine *on page 853*

Allerdryl® [Can] *see* diphenhydramine *on page 261*

Allerest® 12 Hour Nasal Solution *(Discontinued)* *see* oxymetazoline *on page 628*

Allerest® Eye Drops *(Discontinued)* *see* naphazoline *on page 577*

Allerest® Maximum Strength Allergy and Hay Fever [US-OTC] *see* chlorpheniramine and pseudoephedrine *on page 177*

Allerfrim® [US-OTC] *see* triprolidine and pseudoephedrine *on page 853*

Allerfrin® Syrup *(Discontinued)* *see* triprolidine and pseudoephedrine *on page 853*

Allerfrin® Tablet *(Discontinued)* *see* triprolidine and pseudoephedrine *on page 853*

Allerfrin® with Codeine *(Discontinued)* *see* triprolidine, pseudoephedrine, and codeine *(Canada only) on page 853*

Allergen® [US] *see* antipyrine and benzocaine *on page 62*

AllerMax® [US-OTC] *see* diphenhydramine *on page 261*

Allernix [Can] *see* diphenhydramine *on page 261*

Allersol® [US] *see* naphazoline *on page 577*

Allerx™ [US] *see* chlorpheniramine and phenylephrine *on page 176*

Allfen-DM [US] *see* guaifenesin and dextromethorphan *on page 394*

Allfen Jr [US] *see* guaifenesin *on page 392*

allopurinol (al oh PURE i nole)

Sound-Alike/Look-Alike Issues

allopurinol may be confused with Apresoline

Zyloprim® may be confused with Xylo-Pfan®, ZORprin®

Synonyms allopurinol sodium

U.S./Canadian Brand Names Aloprim™ [US]; Apo-Allopurinol® [Can]; Novo-Purol [Can]; Zyloprim® [US/Can]

Therapeutic Category Xanthine Oxidase Inhibitor

Use

Oral: Prevention of attack of gouty arthritis and nephropathy; treatment of secondary hyperuricemia which may occur during treatment of tumors or leukemia; prevention of recurrent calcium oxalate calculi

I.V.: Treatment of elevated serum and urinary uric acid levels when oral therapy is not tolerated in patients with leukemia, lymphoma, and solid tumor malignancies who are receiving cancer chemotherapy

Usual Dosage

Oral: Doses >300 mg should be given in divided doses.

Children ≤10 years: Secondary hyperuricemia associated with chemotherapy: 10 mg/kg/day in 2-3 divided doses **or** 200-300 mg/m^2/day in 2-4 divided doses, maximum: 800 mg/24 hours

Alternative (manufacturer labeling): <6 years: 150 mg/day in 3 divided doses; 6-10 years: 300 mg/day in 2-3 divided doses

Children >10 years and Adults:

Secondary hyperuricemia associated with chemotherapy: 600-800 mg/day in 2-3 divided doses for prevention of acute uric acid nephropathy for 2-3 days starting 1-2 days before chemotherapy

Gout: Mild: 200-300 mg/day; Severe: 400-600 mg/day; to reduce the possibility of acute gouty attacks, initiate dose at 100 mg/day and increase weekly to recommended dosage.

Recurrent calcium oxalate stones: 200-300 mg/day in single or divided doses

I.V.: Hyperuricemia secondary to chemotherapy: Intravenous daily dose can be given as a single infusion or in equally divided doses at 6-, 8-, or 12-hour intervals. A fluid intake sufficient to yield a daily urinary output of at least 2 L in adults and the maintenance of a neutral or, preferably, slightly alkaline urine are desirable.

Children ≤10 years: Starting dose: 200 mg/m^2/day

Children >10 years and Adults: 200-400 mg/m^2/day (maximum: 600 mg/day)

Dosage Forms

Injection, powder for reconstitution, as sodium (Aloprim™): 500 mg

Tablet (Zyloprim®): 100 mg, 300 mg

allopurinol sodium *see* allopurinol *on this page*

all-*trans*-retinoic acid *see* tretinoin (oral) *on page 844*

Almacone® [US-OTC] *see* aluminum hydroxide, magnesium hydroxide, and simethicone *on page 37*

Almacone Double Strength® [US-OTC] *see* aluminum hydroxide, magnesium hydroxide, and simethicone *on page 37*

Almora® [US-OTC] *see* magnesium gluconate *on page 513*

almotriptan (al moh TRIP tan)

Sound-Alike/Look-Alike Issues

Axert™ may be confused with Antivert®

Synonyms almotriptan malate
U.S./Canadian Brand Names Axert™ [US/Can]
Therapeutic Category Serotonin 5-HT_{1D} Receptor Agonist
Use Acute treatment of migraine with or without aura
Usual Dosage Oral: Adults: Migraine: Initial: 6.25-12.5 mg in a single dose; if the headache returns, repeat the dose after 2 hours; no more than 2 doses in 24-hour period
Note: If the first dose is ineffective, diagnosis needs to be re-evaluated. Safety of treating more than 4 migraines/month has not been established.
Dosage Forms Tablet, as malate: 6.25 mg, 12.5 mg

almotriptan malate *see* almotriptan *on previous page*

Alocril® [US/Can] *see* nedocromil (ophthalmic) *on page 581*

Aloe Vesta® 2-n-1 Antifungal [US-OTC] *see* miconazole *on page 553*

Alomide® [US/Can] *see* lodoxamide *on page 502*

Alophen® [US-OTC] *see* bisacodyl *on page 111*

Aloprim™ [US] *see* allopurinol *on previous page*

Alor® 5/500 *(Discontinued)* *see* hydrocodone and aspirin *on page 422*

Alora® [US] *see* estradiol *on page 308*

alosetron (a LOE se tron)

Sound-Alike/Look-Alike Issues
Lotronex® may be confused with Lovenox®, Protonix®
U.S./Canadian Brand Names Lotronex® [US]
Therapeutic Category 5-HT_3 Receptor Antagonist
Use Treatment of women with severe diarrhea-predominant irritable bowel syndrome (IBS) who have failed to respond to conventional therapy
Usual Dosage Oral:
Children: Safety and efficacy have not been established.
Adults: Female: Initial: 0.5 mg twice daily for 4 weeks, with or without food; if tolerated, but response is inadequate, may be increased after 4 weeks to 1 mg twice daily. If response is inadequate after 4 weeks of 1 mg twice-daily dosing, discontinue treatment.
Note: Discontinue immediately if constipation or signs/symptoms of ischemic colitis occur. Do not reinitiate in patients who develop ischemic colitis.
Dosage Forms Tablet: 0.5 mg, 1 mg

Aloxi® [US] *see* palonosetron *on page 632*

alpha$_1$-antitrypsin *see* alpha$_1$-proteinase inhibitor *on this page*

alpha$_1$-PI *see* alpha$_1$-proteinase inhibitor *on this page*

alpha$_1$-proteinase inhibitor, human *see* alpha$_1$-proteinase inhibitor *on this page*

alpha$_1$-proteinase inhibitor (al fa won PRO tee in ase in HI bi tor)

Synonyms alpha$_1$-antitrypsin; α_1-PI; alpha$_1$-proteinase inhibitor, human; A_1-PI
U.S./Canadian Brand Names Aralast [US]; Prolastin® [US/Can]; Zemaira® [US]
Therapeutic Category Antitrypsin Deficiency Agent
Use Replacement therapy in congenital alpha$_1$-antitrypsin deficiency with clinical emphysema
Usual Dosage I.V.: Adults: 60 mg/kg once weekly
Dosage Forms Injection, powder for reconstitution [preservative free]:
Aralast, Prolastin®: 500 mg, 1000 mg [packaged with diluent]
Zemaira®: 1000 mg [packaged with diluent]

alpha-galactosidase-A (human, recombinant) *see* agalsidase beta *on page 21*

Alphagan® [Can] *see* brimonidine *on page 116*

Alphagan® *(Discontinued)* *see* brimonidine *on page 116*

Alphagan® P [US] *see* brimonidine *on page 116*

Alphamul® *(Discontinued)* *see* castor oil *on page 155*

Alphanate® [US] *see* antihemophilic factor (human) *on page 59*

AlphaNine® SD [US] *see* factor IX *on page 333*

Alphaquin HP [US] *see* hydroquinone *on page 430*

Alph-E [US-OTC] *see* vitamin E *on page 876*

Alph-E-Mixed [US-OTC] *see* vitamin E *on page 876*

alprazolam (al PRAY zoe lam)

Sound-Alike/Look-Alike Issues

alprazolam may be confused with alprostadil, lorazepam, triazolam

Xanax® may be confused with Lanoxin®, Tenex®, Tylox®, Xopenex®, Zantac®, Zyrtec®

U.S./Canadian Brand Names Alprazolam Intensol® [US]; Alti-Alprazolam [Can]; Apo-Alpraz® [Can]; Gen-Alprazolam [Can]; Niravam™ [US]; Novo-Alprazol [Can]; Nu-Alprax [Can]; Xanax TS™ [Can]; Xanax XR® [US]; Xanax® [US/Can]

Therapeutic Category Benzodiazepine

Controlled Substance C-IV

Use Treatment of anxiety disorder (GAD); panic disorder, with or without agoraphobia; anxiety associated with depression

Usual Dosage Oral: **Note:** Treatment >4 months should be re-evaluated to determine the patient's continued need for the drug

Adults:

Anxiety: Immediate release: Effective doses are 0.5-4 mg/day in divided doses; the manufacturer recommends starting at 0.25-0.5 mg 3 times/day; titrate dose upward; maximum: 4 mg/day. Patients requiring doses >4 mg/day should be increased cautiously. Periodic reassessment and consideration of dosage reduction is recommended.

Anxiety associated with depression: Immediate release: Average dose required: 2.5-3 mg/day in divided doses

Panic disorder:

Immediate release: Initial: 0.5 mg 3 times/day; dose may be increased every 3-4 days in increments ≤1 mg/day. Mean effective dosage: 5-6 mg/day; many patients obtain relief at 2 mg/day, as much as 10 mg/day may be required

Extended release: 0.5-1 mg once daily; may increase dose every 3-4 days in increments ≤1 mg/day (range: 3-6 mg/day)

Switching from immediate release to extended release: Patients may be switched to extended release tablets by taking the total daily dose of the immediate release tablets and giving it once daily using the extended release preparation.

Preoperative sedation: 0.5 mg in evening at bedtime and 0.5 mg 1 hour before procedure

Dose reduction: Abrupt discontinuation should be avoided. Daily dose may be decreased by 0.5 mg every 3 days, however, some patients may require a slower reduction. If withdrawal symptoms occur, resume previous dose and discontinue on a less rapid schedule.

Dosage Forms

Solution, oral [concentrate]:

Alprazolam Intensol®: 1 mg/mL (30 mL)

Tablet: 0.25 mg, 0.5 mg, 1 mg, 2 mg

Xanax®: 0.25 mg, 0.5 mg, 1 mg, 2 mg

Tablet, extended release: 0.5 mg, 1 mg, 2 mg, 3 mg

Xanax XR®: 0.5 mg, 1 mg, 2 mg, 3 mg

Tablet, orally disintegrating [scored]:

Niravam™: 0.25 mg, 0.5 mg, 1 mg, 2 mg [orange flavor]

Alprazolam Intensol® [US] *see* alprazolam *on this page*

alprostadil (al PROS ta dill)

Sound-Alike/Look-Alike Issues

alprostadil may be confused with alprazolam

Synonyms PGE_1; prostaglandin E_1

U.S./Canadian Brand Names Caverject Impulse® [US]; Caverject® [US/Can]; Edex® [US]; Muse® Pellet [Can]; Muse® [US]; Prostin VR Pediatric® [US]; Prostin® VR [Can]

Therapeutic Category Prostaglandin

Use

Prostin VR Pediatric®: Temporary maintenance of patency of ductus arteriosus in neonates with ductal-dependent congenital heart disease until surgery can be performed. These defects include cyanotic (eg, pulmonary atresia, pulmonary stenosis, tricuspid atresia, Fallot tetralogy, transposition of the great vessels) and acyanotic (eg, interruption of aortic arch, coarctation of aorta, hypoplastic left ventricle) heart disease.

Caverject®: Treatment of erectile dysfunction of vasculogenic, psychogenic, or neurogenic etiology; adjunct in the diagnosis of erectile dysfunction

Edex®, Muse®: Treatment of erectile dysfunction of vasculogenic, psychogenic, or neurogenic etiology

Usual Dosage

Patent ductus arteriosus (Prostin VR Pediatric®):

I.V. continuous infusion into a large vein, or alternatively through an umbilical artery catheter placed at the ductal opening: 0.05-0.1 mcg/kg/minute with therapeutic response, rate is reduced to lowest effective dosage; with unsatisfactory response, rate is increased gradually; maintenance: 0.01-0.4 mcg/kg/minute

PGE_1 is usually given at an infusion rate of 0.1 mcg/kg/minute, but it is often possible to reduce the dosage to 1/2 or even 1/10 without losing the therapeutic effect. The mixing schedule is as follows. Infusion rates deliver 0.1 mcg/kg/minute. **Note:** 500 mcg equals 1 ampul.

For a concentration of 2 mcg/mL, add 500 mcg to 250 mL; infuse at 0.05 mL/kg/minute (72 mL/kg/24 hours)

For a concentration of 5 mcg/mL, add 500 mcg to 100 mL; infuse at 0.02 mL/kg/minute (28.8 mL/kg/24 hours)

For a concentration of 10 mcg/mL, add 500 mcg to 50 mL; infuse at 0.01 mL/kg/minute (14.4 mL/kg/24 hours)

For a concentration of 20 mcg/mL, add 500 mcg to 25 mL; infuse at 0.005 mL/kg/minute (7.2 mL/kg/24 hours)

Therapeutic response is indicated by increased pH in those with acidosis or by an increase in oxygenation (PO_2) usually evident within 30 minutes

Erectile dysfunction:

Caverject®, Edex®: Intracavernous: Individualize dose by careful titration; doses >40 mcg (Edex®) or >60 mcg (Caverject®) are not recommended: Initial dose must be titrated in physicians office. Patient must stay in the physician's office until complete detumescence occurs; if there is no response, then the next higher dose may be given within 1 hour; if there is still no response, a 1-day interval before giving the next dose is recommended; increasing the dose or concentration in the treatment of impotence results in increasing pain and discomfort

Vasculogenic, psychogenic, or mixed etiology: Initiate dosage titration at 2.5 mcg, increasing by 2.5 mcg to a dose of 5 mcg and then in increments of 5-10 mcg depending on the erectile response until the dose produces an erection suitable for intercourse, not lasting >1 hour; if there is absolutely no response to initial 2.5 mcg dose, the second dose may be increased to 7.5 mcg, followed by increments of 5-10 mcg

Neurogenic etiology (eg, spinal cord injury): Initiate dosage titration at 1.25 mcg, increasing to a dose of 2.5 mcg and then 5 mcg; increase further in increments 5 mcg until the dose is reached that produces an erection suitable for intercourse, not lasting >1 hour

Maintenance: Once appropriate dose has been determined, patient may self-administer injections at a frequency of no more than 3 times/week with at least 24 hours between doses

Muse® Pellet: Intraurethral:

Initial: 125-250 mcg

Maintenance: Administer as needed to achieve an erection; duration of action is about 30-60 minutes; use only two systems per 24-hour period

Dosage Forms

Injection, powder for reconstitution:

Caverject®: 20 mcg, 40 mcg [contains lactose; diluent contains benzyl alcohol]

Caverject Impulse®: 10 mcg, 20 mcg [prefilled injection system; contains lactose; diluent contains benzyl alcohol]

Edex®: 10 mcg, 20 mcg, 40 mcg [contains lactose; packaged in kits containing diluent, syringe, and alcohol swab]

Injection, solution: 500 mcg/mL (1 mL)

Prostin VR Pediatric®: 500 mcg/mL (1 mL) [contains dehydrated alcohol]

Pellet, urethral (Muse®): 125 mcg (6s), 250 mcg (6s), 500 mcg (6s), 1000 mcg (6s)

Alrex® [US/Can] *see* loteprednol *on page 507*

AL-Rr® Oral *(Discontinued)* *see* chlorpheniramine *on page 175*

Altace® [US/Can] *see* ramipril *on page 731*

Altachlore [US-OTC] *see* sodium chloride *on page 777*

Altafrin [US] *see* phenylephrine *on page 660*

Altamist [US-OTC] *see* sodium chloride *on page 777*

Altarussin DM [US-OTC] *see* guaifenesin and dextromethorphan *on page 394*

Altaryl [US-OTC] *see* diphenhydramine *on page 261*

alteplase (AL te plase)

Sound-Alike/Look-Alike Issues
alteplase may be confused with Altace®
"tPA" abbreviation should not be used when writing orders for this medication; has been misread as TNKase (tenecteplase)

Synonyms alteplase, recombinant; alteplase, tissue plasminogen activator, recombinant; tPA

U.S./Canadian Brand Names Activase® rt-PA [Can]; Activase® [US]; Cathflo™ Activase® [US/Can]

Therapeutic Category Fibrinolytic Agent

Use Management of acute myocardial infarction for the lysis of thrombi in coronary arteries; management of acute ischemic stroke

Acute myocardial infarction (AMI): Chest pain ≥20 minutes, ≤12-24 hours; S-T elevation ≥0.1 mV in at least two ECG leads

Acute pulmonary embolism (APE): Age ≤75 years: Documented massive pulmonary embolism by pulmonary angiography or echocardiography or high probability lung scan with clinical shock

Cathflo® Activase®: Restoration of central venous catheter function

Usual Dosage

I.V.:

Coronary artery thrombi: Front loading dose (weight-based):

Patients >67 kg: Total dose: 100 mg over 1.5 hours; infuse 15 mg over 1-2 minutes. Infuse 50 mg over 30 minutes. See "Note."

Patients ≤67 kg: Total dose: 1.25 mg/kg; infuse 15 mg I.V. bolus over 1-2 minutes, then infuse 0.75 mg/kg (not to exceed 50 mg) over next 30 minutes, followed by 0.5 mg/kg over next 60 minutes (not to exceed 35 mg). See "Note."

Note: Concurrently, begin heparin 60 units/kg bolus (maximum: 4000 units) followed by continuous infusion of 12 units/kg/hour (maximum: 1000 units/hour) and adjust to aPTT target of 1.5-2 times the upper limit of control. Infuse remaining 35 mg of alteplase over the next hour.

Acute pulmonary embolism: 100 mg over 2 hours.

Acute ischemic stroke: Doses should be given within the first 3 hours of the onset of symptoms; recommended total dose: 0.9 mg/kg (maximum dose should not exceed 90 mg) infused over 60 minutes.

Load with 0.09 mg/kg (10% of the 0.9 mg/kg dose) as an I.V. bolus over 1 minute, followed by 0.81 mg/kg (90% of the 0.9 mg/kg dose) as a continuous infusion over 60 minutes. Heparin should not be started for 24 hours or more after starting alteplase for stroke.

Intracatheter: Central venous catheter clearance: Cathflo® Activase® 1 mg/mL:

Patients <30 kg: 110% of the internal lumen volume of the catheter, not to exceed 2 mg/2 mL; retain in catheter for 0.5-2 hours; may instill a second dose if catheter remains occluded

Patients ≥30 kg: 2 mg (2 mL); retain in catheter for 0.5-2 hours; may instill a second dose if catheter remains occluded

Dosage Forms

Injection, powder for reconstitution, recombinant:

Activase®: 50 mg [29 million int. units; contains polysorbate 80; packaged with diluent]; 100 mg [58 million int. units; contains polysorbate 80; packaged with diluent and transfer device]

Cathflo® Activase®: 2 mg [contains polysorbate 80]

alteplase, recombinant *see* alteplase *on this page*

alteplase, tissue plasminogen activator, recombinant *see* alteplase *on this page*

ALternaGel® [US-OTC] *see* aluminum hydroxide *on page 36*

Alti-Alprazolam [Can] *see* alprazolam *on page 32*

Alti-Amiodarone [Can] *see* amiodarone *on page 43*

Alti-Amoxi-Clav [Can] *see* amoxicillin and clavulanate potassium *on page 49*

Alti-Azathioprine [Can] *see* azathioprine *on page 86*

Alti-Captopril [Can] *see* captopril *on page 143*

Alti-Clindamycin [Can] *see* clindamycin *on page 198*

Alti-Clobazam [Can] *see* clobazam *(Canada only) on page 200*

Alti-Clonazepam [Can] *see* clonazepam *on page 203*

Alti-Desipramine [Can] *see* desipramine *on page 236*

Alti-Diltiazem CD [Can] *see* diltiazem *on page 257*

Alti-Divalproex [Can] *see* valproic acid and derivatives *on page 864*

Alti-Domperidone [Can] *see* domperidone *(Canada only) on page 273*

Alti-Doxazosin [Can] *see* doxazosin *on page 275*

Alti-Flunisolide [Can] *see* flunisolide *on page 352*

Alti-Fluoxetine [Can] *see* fluoxetine *on page 357*

Alti-Flurbiprofen [Can] *see* flurbiprofen *on page 360*

Alti-Fluvoxamine [Can] *see* fluvoxamine *on page 364*

Alti-Ipratropium [Can] *see* ipratropium *on page 460*

Alti-Metformin [Can] *see* metformin *on page 535*

Alti-Minocycline [Can] *see* minocycline *on page 558*

Alti-Moclobemide [Can] *see* moclobemide *(Canada only) on page 562*

Alti-MPA [Can] *see* medroxyprogesterone *on page 524*

Alti-Nadolol [Can] *see* nadolol *on page 573*

Alti-Nortriptyline [Can] *see* nortriptyline *on page 600*

Alti-Ranitidine [Can] *see* ranitidine *on page 732*

Alti-Salbutamol [Can] *see* albuterol *on page 23*

Alti-Sotalol [Can] *see* sotalol *on page 787*

Alti-Sulfasalazine [Can] *see* sulfasalazine *on page 799*

Alti-Terazosin [Can] *see* terazosin *on page 810*

Alti-Ticlopidine [Can] *see* ticlopidine *on page 827*

Alti-Timolol [Can] *see* timolol *on page 828*

Alti-Trazodone [Can] *see* trazodone *on page 843*

Alti-Verapamil [Can] *see* verapamil *on page 870*

Alti-Zopiclone [Can] *see* zopiclone *(Canada only) on page 890*

Altocor™ *(Discontinued)* *see* lovastatin *on page 508*

Altoprev® [US] *see* lovastatin *on page 508*

altretamine (al TRET a meen)

Synonyms hexamethylmelamine; HEXM; HMM; HXM; NSC-13875

U.S./Canadian Brand Names Hexalen® [US/Can]

Therapeutic Category Antineoplastic Agent

Use Palliative treatment of persistent or recurrent ovarian cancer

Usual Dosage Refer to individual protocols. Oral: Adults: Ovarian cancer: 260 mg/m^2/day in 4 divided doses for 14 or 21 days of a 28-day cycle

Dosage Forms

Gelcap:

Hexalen®: 50 mg

Alu-Cap® *(Discontinued)* *see* aluminum hydroxide *on next page*

Aludrox® *(Discontinued)* *see* aluminum hydroxide and magnesium hydroxide *on next page*

aluminum chloride hexahydrate (a LOO mi num KLOR ide heks a HYE drate)

Sound-Alike/Look-Alike Issues

Drysol™ may be confused with Drisdol®

U.S./Canadian Brand Names Certain Dri® [US-OTC]; Drysol™ [US]; Xerac AC™ [US]

Therapeutic Category Topical Skin Product

Use Astringent in the management of hyperhidrosis

Usual Dosage Topical: Adults: Apply once daily at bedtime; once excessive sweating has stopped, may decrease to once or twice weekly, or as needed. Wash treated area in the morning.

Dosage Forms

Solution, topical:

Certain Dri®: 12% (36 mL)

Drysol™: 20% (35 mL, 37.5 mL, 60 mL) [contains ethyl alcohol 93%]

Xerac AC™: 6.25% (35 mL, 60 mL) [contains ethyl alcohol 95%]

aluminum hydroxide (a LOO mi num hye DROKS ide)

U.S./Canadian Brand Names ALternaGel® [US-OTC]; Amphojel® [Can]; Basaljel® [Can]; Dermagran® [US-OTC]

Therapeutic Category Antacid

Use Treatment of hyperacidity; hyperphosphatemia; temporary protection of minor cuts, scrapes, and burns

Usual Dosage

Oral:

Hyperphosphatemia:

Children: 50-150 mg/kg/24 hours in divided doses every 4-6 hours, titrate dosage to maintain serum phosphorus within normal range

Adults: Initial: 300-600 mg 3 times/day with meals

Antacid: Adults: 600-1200 mg between meals and at bedtime

Topical: Apply to affected area as needed; reapply at least every 12 hours

Dosage Forms

Ointment:

Dermagran®: 0.275% (120 g)

Suspension, oral: 320 mg/5 mL (473 mL)

ALternaGel®: 600 mg/5 mL (360 mL)

aluminum hydroxide and magnesium carbonate

(a LOO mi num hye DROKS ide & mag NEE zhum KAR bun nate)

Synonyms magnesium carbonate and aluminum hydroxide

U.S./Canadian Brand Names Gaviscon® Extra Strength [US-OTC]; Gaviscon® Liquid [US-OTC]

Therapeutic Category Antacid

Use Temporary relief of symptoms associated with gastric acidity

Usual Dosage Oral: Adults:

Liquid:

Gaviscon® Regular Strength: 15-30 mL 4 times/day after meals and at bedtime

Gaviscon® Extra Strength Relief: 15-30 mL 4 times/day after meals

Tablet (Gaviscon® Extra Strength Relief): Chew 2-4 tablets 4 times/day

Dosage Forms

Liquid:

Gaviscon®: Aluminum hydroxide 31.7 mg and magnesium carbonate 119.3 mg per 5 mL (355 mL) [contains sodium 0.57 mEq/5 mL]

Gaviscon® Extra Strength: Aluminum hydroxide 84.6 mg and magnesium carbonate 79.1 mg per 5 mL (355 mL) [contains sodium 0.9 mEq/5 mL]

Tablet, chewable (Gaviscon® Extra Strength): Aluminum hydroxide 160 mg and magnesium carbonate 105 mg [contains sodium 1.3 mEq/tablet]

aluminum hydroxide and magnesium hydroxide

(a LOO mi num hye DROKS ide & mag NEE zhum hye DROK side)

Sound-Alike/Look-Alike Issues

Maalox® may be confused with Maox®, Monodox®

Synonyms magnesium hydroxide and aluminum hydroxide

U.S./Canadian Brand Names Alamag [US-OTC]; Diovol® Ex [Can]; Diovol® [Can]; Gelusil® Extra Strength [Can]; Mylanta™ [Can]; Rulox [US-OTC]

Therapeutic Category Antacid

Use Antacid, hyperphosphatemia in renal failure

Usual Dosage Oral: 5-10 mL 4-6 times/day, between meals and at bedtime; may be used every hour for severe symptoms

Dosage Forms [DSC] = Discontinued product

Suspension: Aluminum hydroxide 225 mg and magnesium hydroxide 200 mg per 5 mL (360 mL)

Alamag, Rulox: Aluminum hydroxide 225 mg and magnesium hydroxide 200 mg per 5 mL (360 mL)

Tablet, chewable:

Alamag: Aluminum hydroxide 300 mg and magnesium hydroxide 150 mg

Rulox No. 1: Aluminum hydroxide 200 mg and magnesium hydroxide 200 mg [DSC]

aluminum hydroxide and magnesium trisilicate

(a LOO mi num hye DROKS ide & mag NEE zhum trye SIL i kate)

Synonyms magnesium trisilicate and aluminum hydroxide

U.S./Canadian Brand Names Alenic Alka Tablet [US-OTC]; Gaviscon® Tablet [US-OTC]; Genaton Tablet [US-OTC]

Therapeutic Category Antacid
Use Temporary relief of hyperacidity
Usual Dosage Oral: Adults: Chew 2-4 tablets 4 times/day or as directed by healthcare provider
Dosage Forms
Tablet, chewable: Aluminum hydroxide 80 mg and magnesium trisilicate 20 mg
Alenic Alka: Aluminum hydroxide 80 mg and magnesium trisilicate 20 mg [butterscotch flavor]
Gaviscon®: Aluminum hydroxide 80 mg and magnesium trisilicate 20 mg [contains sodium 0.8 mEq/tablet; butterscotch flavor]
Genaton: Aluminum hydroxide 80 mg and magnesium trisilicate 20 mg

aluminum hydroxide, magnesium hydroxide, and simethicone

(a LOO mi num hye DROKS ide, mag NEE zhum hye DROKS ide, & sye METH i kone)
Sound-Alike/Look-Alike Issues
Maalox® may be confused with Maox®, Monodox®
Mylanta® may be confused with Mynatal®
Synonyms magnesium hydroxide, aluminum hydroxide, and simethicone; simethicone, aluminum hydroxide, and magnesium hydroxide
U.S./Canadian Brand Names Alamag Plus [US-OTC]; Aldroxicon I [US-OTC]; Aldroxicon II [US-OTC]; Almacone Double Strength® [US-OTC]; Almacone® [US-OTC]; Diovol Plus® [Can]; Gelusil® [US-OTC/Can]; Maalox® Max [US-OTC]; Maalox® [US-OTC]; Mi-Acid™ Maximum Strength [US-OTC]; Mi-Acid™ [US-OTC]; Mintox Extra Strength [US-OTC]; Mintox Plus [US-OTC]; Mylanta® Double Strength [Can]; Mylanta® Extra Strength [Can]; Mylanta® Liquid [US-OTC]; Mylanta® Maximum Strength Liquid [US-OTC]; Mylanta® Regular Strength [Can]
Therapeutic Category Antacid; Antiflatulent
Use Temporary relief of hyperacidity associated with gas; may also be used for indications associated with other antacids
Usual Dosage Oral: Adults: 10-20 mL or 2-4 tablets 4-6 times/day between meals and at bedtime; may be used every hour for severe symptoms
Dosage Forms
Liquid: Aluminum hydroxide 200 mg, magnesium hydroxide 200 mg, and simethicone 20 mg per 5 mL (360 mL); aluminum hydroxide 400 mg, magnesium hydroxide 400 mg, and simethicone 40 mg per 5 mL (360 mL)
Aldroxicon I: Aluminum hydroxide 200 mg, magnesium hydroxide 200 mg, and simethicone 20 mg per 5 mL (30 mL)
Aldroxicon II: Aluminum hydroxide 400 mg, magnesium hydroxide 400 mg, and simethicone 40 mg per 5 mL (30 mL)
Almacone®: Aluminum hydroxide 200 mg, magnesium hydroxide 200 mg, and simethicone 20 mg per 5 mL (360 mL)
Almacone Double Strength®: Aluminum hydroxide 400 mg, magnesium hydroxide 400 mg, and simethicone 40 mg per 5 mL (360 mL)
Maalox®: Aluminum hydroxide 200 mg, magnesium hydroxide 200 mg, and simethicone 20 mg per 5 mL (360 mL, 770 mL) [lemon and mint flavors]
Maalox® Max: Aluminum hydroxide 400 mg, magnesium hydroxide 400 mg, and simethicone 40 mg per 5 mL (360 mL, 770 mL) [cherry, vanilla creme, and wild berry flavors]
Mi-Acid: Aluminum hydroxide 200 mg, magnesium hydroxide 200 mg, and simethicone 20 mg per 5 mL (360 mL)
Mi-Acid Maximum Strength: Aluminum hydroxide 400 mg, magnesium hydroxide 400 mg, and simethicone 40 mg per 5 mL (360 mL)
Mintox Extra Strength: Aluminum hydroxide 500 mg, magnesium hydroxide 450 mg, and simethicone 40 mg per 5 mL (360 mL) [lemon creme flavor]
Mylanta®: Aluminum hydroxide 200 mg, magnesium hydroxide 200 mg, and simethicone 20 mg per 5 mL (180 mL, 360 mL, 720 mL) [original, cherry, and mint flavors]
Mylanta® Maximum Strength: Aluminum hydroxide 400 mg, magnesium hydroxide 400 mg, and simethicone 40 mg per 5 mL (180 mL, 360 mL, 720 mL) [original, cherry, orange creme, and mint flavors]
Suspension (Alamag Plus): Aluminum hydroxide 225 mg, magnesium hydroxide 200 mg, and simethicone 25 mg per 5 mL (360 mL)
Tablet, chewable: Aluminum hydroxide 200 mg, magnesium hydroxide 200 mg, and simethicone 25 mg
Alamag Plus: Aluminum hydroxide 200 mg, magnesium hydroxide 200 mg, and simethicone 25 mg [cherry flavor]
Almacone®: Aluminum hydroxide 200 mg, magnesium hydroxide 200 mg, and simethicone 20 mg [peppermint flavor]
Gelusil®: Aluminum hydroxide 200 mg, magnesium hydroxide 200 mg, and simethicone 25 mg [peppermint flavor]
Mintox Plus: Aluminum hydroxide 200 mg, magnesium hydroxide 200 mg, and simethicone 25 mg

aluminum sucrose sulfate, basic *see* sucralfate *on page 793*

aluminum sulfate and calcium acetate (a LOO mi num SUL fate & KAL see um AS e tate)

Synonyms calcium acetate and aluminum sulfate

U.S./Canadian Brand Names Domeboro® [US-OTC]; Gordon Boro-Packs [US-OTC]; Pedi-Boro® [US-OTC]

Therapeutic Category Topical Skin Product

Use Astringent wet dressing for relief of inflammatory conditions of the skin; reduce weeping that may occur in dermatitis

Usual Dosage Topical: Soak affected area in the solution 2-4 times/day for 15-30 minutes or apply wet dressing soaked in the solution for more extended periods; rewet dressing with solution 2-4 times/day every 15-30 minutes

Dosage Forms

Powder, for topical solution:

Domeboro®: Aluminum sulfate 1191 mg and calcium acetate 938 mg per packet (12s, 100s)

Gordon Boro-Packs: Aluminum sulfate 49% and calcium acetate 51% per packet (100s)

Pedi-Boro®: Aluminum sulfate 49% and calcium acetate 51% per packet (12s, 100s)

Alupent® [US] *see* metaproterenol *on page 535*

Alupent® Inhalation Solution *(Discontinued)* *see* metaproterenol *on page 535*

Alu-Tab® *(Discontinued)* *see* aluminum hydroxide *on page 36*

amantadine (a MAN ta deen)

Sound-Alike/Look-Alike Issues

amantadine may be confused with ranitidine, rimantadine

Symmetrel® may be confused with Synthroid®

Synonyms adamantanamine hydrochloride; amantadine hydrochloride

U.S./Canadian Brand Names Endantadine® [Can]; PMS-Amantadine [Can]; Symmetrel® [US/Can]

Therapeutic Category Anti-Parkinson Agent; Antiviral Agent

Use Prophylaxis and treatment of influenza A viral infection (per manufacturer labeling; also refer to current CDC guidelines for recommendations during current flu season); treatment of parkinsonism; treatment of drug-induced extrapyramidal symptoms

Usual Dosage Oral:

Children:

Influenza A treatment:

1-9 years: 5 mg/kg/day in 2 divided doses (manufacturers range: 4.4-8.8 mg/kg/day); maximum dose: 150 mg/day

≥10 years and <40 kg: 5 mg/kg/day; maximum dose: 150 mg/day

≥10 years and ≥40 kg: 100 mg twice daily

Note: Initiate within 24-48 hours after onset of symptoms; discontinue as soon as possible based on clinical response (generally within 3-5 days or within 24-48 hours after symptoms disappear)

Influenza A prophylaxis: Refer to "Influenza A treatment" dosing

Note: Continue treatment throughout the peak influenza activity in the community or throughout the entire influenza season in patients who cannot be vaccinated. Development of immunity following vaccination takes ~2 weeks; amantadine therapy should be considered for high-risk patients from the time of vaccination until immunity has developed. For children <9 years receiving influenza vaccine for the first time, amantadine prophylaxis should continue for 6 weeks (4 weeks after the first dose and 2 weeks after the second dose)

Adults:

Drug-induced extrapyramidal symptoms: 100 mg twice daily; may increase to 300-400 mg/day, if needed

Influenza A viral infection: 100 mg twice daily; initiate within 24-48 hours after onset of symptoms; discontinue as soon as possible based on clinical response (generally within 3-5 days or within 24-48 hours after symptoms disappear)

Influenza A prophylaxis: 100 mg twice daily

Note: Continue treatment throughout the peak influenza activity in the community or throughout the entire influenza season in patients who cannot be vaccinated. Development of immunity following vaccination takes ~2 weeks; amantadine therapy should be considered for high-risk patients from the time of vaccination until immunity has developed

Dosage Forms
Capsule, as hydrochloride: 100 mg
Syrup, as hydrochloride: 50 mg/5 mL (480 mL)
Tablet, as hydrochloride: 100 mg
Symmetrel®: 100 mg

amantadine hydrochloride *see* amantadine *on previous page*

Amaphen® *(Discontinued)*

Amaryl® [US/Can] *see* glimepiride *on page 384*

Amatine® [Can] *see* midodrine *on page 556*

ambenonium (am be NOE nee um)

Synonyms ambenonium chloride
U.S./Canadian Brand Names Mytelase® [US/Can]
Therapeutic Category Cholinergic Agent
Use Treatment of myasthenia gravis
Usual Dosage Oral: Adults: 5-25 mg 3-4 times/day
Dosage Forms
Caplet, as chloride [scored]:
Mytelase®: 10 mg

ambenonium chloride *see* ambenonium *on this page*

Ambi 10® *(Discontinued)* *see* benzoyl peroxide *on page 102*

Ambien® [US] *see* zolpidem *on page 890*

Ambien CR™ [US] *see* zolpidem *on page 890*

Ambifed-G [US] *see* guaifenesin and pseudoephedrine *on page 398*

Ambifed-G DM [US] *see* guaifenesin, pseudoephedrine, and dextromethorphan *on page 401*

Ambi® Skin Tone *(Discontinued)* *see* hydroquinone *on page 430*

AmBisome® [US/Can] *see* amphotericin B liposomal *on page 52*

amcinonide (am SIN oh nide)

U.S./Canadian Brand Names Amcort® [Can]; Cyclocort® [US/Can]; ratio-Amcinonide [Can]; Taro-Amcinonide [Can]
Therapeutic Category Corticosteroid, Topical
Use Relief of the inflammatory and pruritic manifestations of corticosteroid-responsive dermatoses (high potency corticosteroid)
Usual Dosage Topical: Adults: Apply in a thin film 2-3 times/day. Therapy should be discontinued when control is achieved; if no improvement is seen, reassessment of diagnosis may be necessary.
Dosage Forms
Cream: 0.1% (15 g, 30 g, 60 g) [contains benzyl alcohol]
Lotion: 0.1% (60 mL)
Cyclocort®: 0.1% (20 mL, 60 mL) [contains benzyl alcohol]
Ointment: 0.1% (30 g, 60 g) [contains benzyl alcohol]
Cyclocort®: 0.1% (15 g, 30 g, 60 g) [contains benzyl alcohol]

Amcort® [Can] *see* amcinonide *on this page*

Amcort® Injection *(Discontinued)*

Amerge® [US/Can] *see* naratriptan *on page 579*

Americaine® [US-OTC] *see* benzocaine *on page 99*

Americaine® Anesthetic Lubricant *(Discontinued)* *see* benzocaine *on page 99*

Americaine® Hemorrhoidal [US-OTC] *see* benzocaine *on page 99*

A-methapred *see* methylprednisolone *on page 547*

amethocaine hydrochloride *see* tetracaine *on page 815*

amethopterin *see* methotrexate *on page 540*

Ametop™ [Can] *see* tetracaine *on page 815*

Amevive® [US/Can] *see* alefacept *on page 26*

amfepramone *see* diethylpropion *on page 253*

AMG 073 *see* cinacalcet *on page 189*

Amibid DM [US] *see* guaifenesin and dextromethorphan *on page 394*

Amibid LA *(Discontinued)* *see* guaifenesin *on page 392*

Amicar® [US] *see* aminocaproic acid *on page 42*

Amidal [US] *see* guaifenesin and phenylephrine *on page 396*

Amidate® [US/Can] *see* etomidate *on page 330*

Amidrine [US] *see* acetaminophen, isometheptene, and dichloralphenazone *on page 13*

amifostine (am i FOS teen)

Sound-Alike/Look-Alike Issues

Ethyol® may be confused with ethanol

Synonyms ethiofos; gammaphos; WR-2721; YM-08310

U.S./Canadian Brand Names Ethyol® [US/Can]

Therapeutic Category Antidote

Use Reduce the incidence of moderate to severe xerostomia in patients undergoing postoperative radiation treatment for head and neck cancer, where the radiation port includes a substantial portion of the parotid glands; reduce the cumulative renal toxicity associated with repeated administration of cisplatin in patients with advanced ovarian cancer

Usual Dosage Note: Antiemetic medication, including dexamethasone 20 mg I.V. and a serotonin 5-HT_3 receptor antagonist, is recommended prior to and in conjunction with amifostine.

Adults:

Cisplatin-induced renal toxicity, reduction: I.V.: 740-910 mg/m^2 once daily 30 minutes prior to cytotoxic therapy

Note: Doses >740 mg/m^2 are associated with a higher incidence of hypotension and may require interruption of therapy or dose modification for subsequent cycles. For 910 mg/m^2 doses, the manufacturer suggests the following blood pressure-based adjustment schedule:

The infusion of amifostine should be interrupted if the systolic blood pressure decreases significantly from baseline, as defined below:

Decrease of 20 mm Hg if baseline systolic blood pressure <100

Decrease of 25 mm Hg if baseline systolic blood pressure 100-119

Decrease of 30 mm Hg if baseline systolic blood pressure 120-139

Decrease of 40 mm Hg if baseline systolic blood pressure 140-179

Decrease of 50 mm Hg if baseline systolic blood pressure ≥180

If the blood pressure returns to normal within 5 minutes (assisted by fluid administration and postural management) and the patient is asymptomatic, the infusion may be restarted so that the full dose of amifostine may be administered. If the full dose of amifostine cannot be administered, the dose of amifostine for subsequent cycles should be 740 mg/m^2.

Xerostomia from head and neck cancer, reduction: I.V.: 200 mg/m^2/day during radiation therapy

Dosage Forms

Injection, powder for reconstitution:

Ethyol®: 500 mg

Amigesic® [US/Can] *see* salsalate *on page 761*

amikacin (am i KAY sin)

Sound-Alike/Look-Alike Issues

amikacin may be confused with Amicar®, anakinra

Amikin® may be confused with Amicar®

Synonyms amikacin sulfate

U.S./Canadian Brand Names Amikacin Sulfate Injection, USP [Can]; Amikin® [US/Can]

Therapeutic Category Aminoglycoside (Antibiotic)

Use Treatment of serious infections due to organisms resistant to gentamicin and tobramycin, including *Pseudomonas*, *Proteus*, *Serratia*, and other gram-negative bacilli (bone infections, respiratory tract infections, endocarditis, and septicemia); documented infection of mycobacterial organisms susceptible to amikacin

Usual Dosage Note: Individualization is critical because of the low therapeutic index

Use of ideal body weight (IBW) for determining the mg/kg/dose appears to be more accurate than dosing on the basis of total body weight (TBW)

In morbid obesity, dosage requirement may best be estimated using a dosing weight of IBW + 0.4 (TBW - IBW)

Initial and periodic peak and trough plasma drug levels should be determined, particularly in critically-ill patients with serious infections or in disease states known to significantly alter aminoglycoside pharmacokinetics (eg, cystic fibrosis, burns, or major surgery)

Usual dosage range:

Infants and Children: I.M., I.V.: 5-7.5 mg/kg/dose every 8 hours

Adults: I.M., I.V.: 5-7.5 mg/kg/dose every 8 hours

Note: Some clinicians suggest a daily dose of 15-20 mg/kg for all patients with normal renal function. This dose is at least as efficacious with similar, if not less, toxicity than conventional dosing.

Indication-specific dosing:

Adults: I.V.:

Hospital-acquired pneumonia (HAP): 20 mg/kg/day with antipseudomonal beta-lactam or carbapenem (American Thoracic Society/ATS guidelines)

Meningitis *(Pseudomonas aeruginosa):* 5 mg/kg every 8 hours (administered with another bactericidal drug)

Mycobacterium fortuitum, M. chelonae, or M. abscessus: 10-15 mg/kg twice daily for at least 2 weeks with high dose cefoxitin

Dosage Forms [DSC] = Discontinued product

Injection, solution, as sulfate: 50 mg/mL (2 mL, 4 mL); 62.5 mg/mL (8 mL) [DSC]; 250 mg/mL (2 mL, 4 mL)

Amikin®: 50 mg/mL (2 mL); 250 mg/mL (2 mL, 4 mL) [contains metabisulfite]

amikacin sulfate *see* amikacin *on previous page*

Amikacin Sulfate Injection, USP [Can] *see* amikacin *on previous page*

Amikin® [US/Can] *see* amikacin *on previous page*

amiloride (a MIL oh ride)

Sound-Alike/Look-Alike Issues

amiloride may be confused with amiodarone, amlodipine, amrinone

Synonyms amiloride hydrochloride

U.S./Canadian Brand Names Apo-Amiloride® [Can]

Therapeutic Category Diuretic, Potassium Sparing

Use Counteracts potassium loss induced by other diuretics in the treatment of hypertension or edematous conditions including CHF, hepatic cirrhosis, and hypoaldosteronism; usually used in conjunction with more potent diuretics such as thiazides or loop diuretics

Usual Dosage Oral:

Children: Although safety and efficacy in children have not been established by the FDA, a dosage of 0.625 mg/kg/day has been used in children weighing 6-20 kg.

Adults: 5-10 mg/day (up to 20 mg)

Hypertension (JNC 7): 5-10 mg/day in 1-2 divided doses

Dosage Forms Tablet, as hydrochloride: 5 mg

amiloride and hydrochlorothiazide (a MIL oh ride & hye droe klor oh THYE a zide)

Synonyms hydrochlorothiazide and amiloride

U.S./Canadian Brand Names Apo-Amilzide® [Can]; Gen-Amilazide [Can]; Moduret [Can]; Novamilor [Can]; Nu-Amilzide [Can]

Therapeutic Category Diuretic, Combination

Use Potassium-sparing diuretic; antihypertensive

Usual Dosage Adults: Oral: Start with 1 tablet/day, then may be increased to 2 tablets/day if needed; usually given in a single dose

Dosage Forms Tablet: 5/50: Amiloride hydrochloride 5 mg and hydrochlorothiazide 50 mg

amiloride hydrochloride *see* amiloride *on this page*

Aminate Fe-90 [US] *see* vitamins (multiple/prenatal) *on page 879*

2-amino-6-mercaptopurine *see* thioguanine *on page 822*

2-amino-6-methoxypurine arabinoside *see* nelarabine *on page 582*

2-amino-6-trifluoromethoxy-benzothiazole *see* riluzole *on page 746*

aminobenzylpenicillin *see* ampicillin *on page 53*

aminocaproic acid (a mee noe ka PROE ik AS id)

Sound-Alike/Look-Alike Issues

Amicar® may be confused with amikacin, Amikin®, Omacor®

Synonyms epsilon aminocaproic acid

U.S./Canadian Brand Names Amicar® [US]

Therapeutic Category Hemostatic Agent

Use Treatment of excessive bleeding from fibrinolysis

Usual Dosage Acute bleeding syndrome: Adults: Oral, I.V.: 4-5 g during the first hour, followed by 1 g/hour for 8 hours or until bleeding controlled (maximum daily dose: 30 g)

Dosage Forms

Injection, solution: 250 mg/mL (20 mL)

Amicar®: 250 mg/mL (20 mL) [contains benzyl alcohol]

Solution, oral: 1.25 g/5 mL (240 mL, 480 mL)

Syrup:

Amicar®: 1.25 g/5 mL (480 mL) [raspberry flavor]

Tablet [scored]: 500 mg, 1000 mg

Amicar®: 500 mg, 1000 mg

Amino-Cerv™ [US] *see* urea *on page 861*

aminoglutethimide (a mee noe gloo TETH i mide)

Sound-Alike/Look-Alike Issues

Cytadren® may be confused with cytarabine

Synonyms AG; AGT; BA-16038; elipten

U.S./Canadian Brand Names Cytadren® [US]

Therapeutic Category Antineoplastic Agent

Use Suppression of adrenal function in selected patients with Cushing syndrome

Usual Dosage Oral: Adults: Adrenal suppression: 250 mg every 6 hours may be increased at 1- to 2-week intervals to a total of 2 g/day

Dosage Forms Tablet [scored]: 250 mg

aminolevulinic acid (a MEE noh lev yoo lin ik AS id)

Synonyms aminolevulinic acid hydrochloride

U.S./Canadian Brand Names Levulan® Kerastick® [US]; Levulan® [Can]

Therapeutic Category Photosensitizing Agent, Topical; Porphyrin Agent, Topical

Use Treatment of minimally to moderately thick actinic keratoses (grade 1 or 2) of the face or scalp; to be used in conjunction with blue light illumination

Usual Dosage Adults: Topical: Apply to actinic keratoses (**not** perilesional skin) followed 14-18 hours later by blue light illumination. Application/treatment may be repeated at a treatment site after 8 weeks.

Dosage Forms

Powder for topical solution:

Levulan® Kerastick®: 20% (6s) [2-component system containing aminolevulinic acid hydrochloride 354 mg (powder) and diluent containing ethanol 48% (1.5 mL) packaged together in an applicator tube]

aminolevulinic acid hydrochloride *see* aminolevulinic acid *on this page*

aminophylline (am in OFF i lin)

Sound-Alike/Look-Alike Issues

aminophylline may be confused with amitriptyline, ampicillin

Synonyms theophylline ethylenediamine

U.S./Canadian Brand Names Phyllocontin® [Can]; Phyllocontin®-350 [Can]

Therapeutic Category Theophylline Derivative

Use Bronchodilator in reversible airway obstruction due to asthma or COPD; increase diaphragmatic contractility

Usual Dosage

Treatment of acute bronchospasm: I.V.:

Loading dose (in patients not currently receiving aminophylline or theophylline): 6 mg/kg (based on aminophylline) administered I.V. over 20-30 minutes; administration rate should not exceed 25 mg/minute (aminophylline)

Approximate I.V. maintenance dosages are based upon **continuous infusions**; bolus dosing (often used in children <6 months of age) may be determined by multiplying the hourly infusion rate by 24 hours and dividing by the desired number of doses/day

6 weeks to 6 months: 0.5 mg/kg/hour
6 months to 1 year: 0.6-0.7 mg/kg/hour
1-9 years: 1 mg/kg/hour
9-16 years and smokers: 0.8 mg/kg/hour
Adults, nonsmoking: 0.5 mg/kg/hour
Older patients and patients with cor pulmonale: 0.3 mg/kg/hour
Patients with congestive heart failure: 0.1-0.2 mg/kg/hour

Dosage should be adjusted according to serum level measurements during the first 12- to 24-hour period.

Bronchodilator: Oral: Children ≥45 kg and Adults: Initial: 380 mg/day (equivalent to theophylline 300 mg/day) in divided doses every 6-8 hours; may increase dose after 3 days; maximum dose: 928 mg/day (equivalent to theophylline 800 mg/day)

Dosage Forms

Injection, solution, as dihydrate: 25 mg/mL (10 mL, 20 mL)
Tablet, as dihydrate: 100 mg, 200 mg

aminosalicylate sodium *see* aminosalicylic acid *on this page*

aminosalicylic acid (a mee noe sal i SIL ik AS id)

Synonyms aminosalicylate sodium; 4-aminosalicylic acid; para-aminosalicylate sodium; PAS; sodium PAS

U.S./Canadian Brand Names Paser® [US]

Therapeutic Category Nonsteroidal Antiinflammatory Drug (NSAID)

Use Adjunctive treatment of tuberculosis used in combination with other antitubercular agents

Usual Dosage Tuberculosis: Oral:

Children: 200-300 mg/kg/day in 3-4 equally divided doses
Adults: 150 mg/kg/day in 2-3 equally divided doses

Dosage Forms

Granules, delayed release:
Paser®: 4 g/packet (30s)

4-aminosalicylic acid *see* aminosalicylic acid *on this page*

5-aminosalicylic acid *see* mesalamine *on page 533*

Aminoxin® [US-OTC] *see* pyridoxine *on page 721*

amiodarone (a MEE oh da rone)

Sound-Alike/Look-Alike Issues

amiodarone may be confused with amiloride, amrinone
Cordarone® may be confused with Cardura®, Cordran®

Synonyms amiodarone hydrochloride

U.S./Canadian Brand Names Alti-Amiodarone [Can]; Amiodarone Hydrochloride for Injection® [Can]; Apo-Amiodarone® [Can]; Cordarone® [US/Can]; Gen-Amiodarone [Can]; Novo-Amiodarone [Can]; Pacerone® [US]; Rhoxal-amiodarone [Can]; Sandoz-Amiodarone [Can]

Therapeutic Category Antiarrhythmic Agent, Class III

Use Management of life-threatening recurrent ventricular fibrillation (VF) or hemodynamically-unstable ventricular tachycardia (VT) refractory to other antiarrhythmic agents or in patients intolerant of other agents used for these conditions

Usual Dosage Note: Lower loading and maintenance doses are preferable in women and all patients with low body weight.

Oral: Adults: Ventricular arrhythmias: 800-1600 mg/day in 1-2 doses for 1-3 weeks, then when adequate arrhythmia control is achieved, decrease to 600-800 mg/day in 1-2 doses for 1 month; maintenance: 400 mg/day. Lower doses are recommended for supraventricular arrhythmias.

I.V.:

Children:

Pulseless VF or VT (PALS dosing): 5 mg/kg rapid I.V. bolus or I.O.; repeat up to a maximum dose of 15 mg/kg (300 mg)

Perfusing tachycardias (PALS dosing): Loading dose: 5 mg/kg I.V. over 20-60 minutes or I.O.; may repeat up to maximum dose of 15 mg/kg/day

Adults:

Breakthrough VF or VT: 150 mg supplemental doses in 100 mL D_5W over 10 minutes

Pulseless VF or VT: I.V. push: Initial: 300 mg in 20-30 mL NS or D_5W; if VF or VT recurs, supplemental dose of 150 mg followed by infusion of 1 mg/minute for 6 hours, then 0.5 mg/minute (maximum daily dose: 2.1 g)

(Continued)

amiodarone *(Continued)*

Note: When switching from I.V. to oral therapy, use the following as a guide:

<1-week I.V. infusion: 800-1600 mg/day

1- to 3-week I.V. infusion: 600-800 mg/day

>3-week I.V. infusion: 400 mg/day

Recommendations for conversion to intravenous amiodarone after oral administration: During long-term amiodarone therapy (ie, ≥4 months), the mean plasma-elimination half-life of the active metabolite of amiodarone is 61 days. Replacement therapy may not be necessary in such patients if oral therapy is discontinued for a period <2 weeks, since any changes in serum amiodarone concentrations during this period may **not** be clinically significant.

Dosage Forms [DSC] = Discontinued product

Injection, solution, as hydrochloride: 50 mg/mL (3 mL, 9 mL, 18 mL) [contains benzyl alcohol and polysorbate (Tween®) 80] [DSC]

Cordarone®: 50 mg/mL (3 mL) [contains benzyl alcohol and polysorbate (Tween®) 80]

Tablet, as hydrochloride [scored]: 200 mg, 400 mg

Cordarone®: 200 mg

Pacerone®: 100 mg [not scored], 200 mg, 300 mg [DSC], 400 mg

amiodarone hydrochloride *see* amiodarone *on previous page*

Amiodarone Hydrochloride for Injection® [Can] *see* amiodarone *on previous page*

Ami-Tex LA [US] *see* guaifenesin and phenylephrine *on page 396*

Ami-Tex PSE [US] *see* guaifenesin and pseudoephedrine *on page 398*

Amitiza™ [US] *see* lubiprostone *on page 509*

Amitone® ***(Discontinued)*** *see* calcium carbonate *on page 135*

amitriptyline (a mee TRIP ti leen)

Sound-Alike/Look-Alike Issues

amitriptyline may be confused with aminophylline, imipramine, nortriptyline

Elavil® may be confused with Aldoril®, Eldepryl®, enalapril, Equanil®, Mellaril®, Oruvail®, Plavix®

Synonyms amitriptyline hydrochloride

U.S./Canadian Brand Names Apo-Amitriptyline® [Can]; Levate® [Can]; Novo-Triptyn [Can]; PMS-Amitriptyline [Can]

Therapeutic Category Antidepressant, Tricyclic (Tertiary Amine)

Use Relief of symptoms of depression

Usual Dosage Oral:

Adolescents: Depressive disorders: Initial: 25-50 mg/day; may administer in divided doses; increase gradually to 100 mg/day in divided doses

Adults: Depression: 50-150 mg/day single dose at bedtime or in divided doses; dose may be gradually increased up to 300 mg/day

Dosage Forms

Tablet, as hydrochloride: 10 mg, 25 mg, 50 mg, 75 mg, 100 mg, 150 mg

amitriptyline and chlordiazepoxide (a mee TRIP ti leen & klor dye az e POKS ide)

Synonyms chlordiazepoxide and amitriptyline hydrochloride

U.S./Canadian Brand Names Limbitrol® DS [US]; Limbitrol® [US/Can]

Therapeutic Category Antidepressant, Tricyclic (Tertiary Amine)

Controlled Substance C-IV

Use Treatment of moderate to severe anxiety and/or agitation and depression

Usual Dosage Initial: 3-4 tablets in divided doses; this may be increased to 6 tablets/day as required; some patients respond to smaller doses and can be maintained on 2 tablets

Dosage Forms

Tablet: 12.5/5: Amitriptyline hydrochloride 12.5 mg and chlordiazepoxide 5 mg; 25/10: Amitriptyline hydrochloride 25 mg and chlordiazepoxide 10 mg

Limbitrol®: 12.5/5: Amitriptyline hydrochloride 12.5 mg and chlordiazepoxide 5 mg

Limbitrol® DS: 25/10: Amitriptyline hydrochloride 25 mg and chlordiazepoxide 10 mg

amitriptyline and perphenazine (a mee TRIP ti leen & per FEN a zeen)

Synonyms perphenazine and amitriptyline hydrochloride

U.S./Canadian Brand Names Etrafon® [Can]

Therapeutic Category Antidepressant/Phenothiazine

Use Treatment of patients with moderate to severe anxiety and depression

Usual Dosage Oral: 1 tablet 2-4 times/day

Dosage Forms Tablet:

2-10: Amitriptyline hydrochloride 10 mg and perphenazine 2 mg
2-25: Amitriptyline hydrochloride 25 mg and perphenazine 2 mg
4-10: Amitriptyline hydrochloride 10 mg and perphenazine 4 mg
4-25: Amitriptyline hydrochloride 25 mg and perphenazine 4 mg
4-50: Amitriptyline hydrochloride 50 mg and perphenazine 4 mg

amitriptyline hydrochloride *see* amitriptyline *on previous page*

AMJ 9701 *see* palifermin *on page 632*

AmLactin® [US-OTC] *see* lactic acid and ammonium hydroxide *on page 477*

amlexanox (am LEKS an oks)

U.S./Canadian Brand Names Aphthasol® [US]

Therapeutic Category Antiinflammatory Agent, Locally Applied

Use Treatment of aphthous ulcers (ie, canker sores)

Usual Dosage Topical: Administer (0.5 cm - 1/4") directly on ulcers 4 times/day following oral hygiene, after meals, and at bedtime

Dosage Forms Paste: 5% (5 g) [contains benzyl alcohol]

amlodipine (am LOE di peen)

Sound-Alike/Look-Alike Issues

amlodipine may be confused with amiloride
Norvasc® may be confused with Navane®, Norvir®, Vascor®

Synonyms amlodipine besylate

U.S./Canadian Brand Names Norvasc® [US/Can]

Therapeutic Category Calcium Channel Blocker

Use Treatment of hypertension; treatment of symptomatic chronic stable angina, vasospastic (Prinzmetal) angina (confirmed or suspected); prevention of hospitalization due to angina with documented CAD (limited to patients without heart failure or ejection fraction <40%)

Usual Dosage Oral:

Children 6-17 years: Hypertension: 2.5-5 mg once daily

Adults:

Hypertension: Initial dose: 5 mg once daily; maximum dose: 10 mg once daily. In general, titrate in 2.5 mg increments over 7-14 days. Usual dosage range (JNC 7): 2.5-10 mg once daily.

Angina: Usual dose: 5-10 mg

Dosage Forms

Tablet:

Norvasc®: 2.5 mg, 5 mg, 10 mg

amlodipine and atorvastatin (am LOW di peen & a TORE va sta tin)

Synonyms atorvastatin calcium and amlodipine besylate

U.S./Canadian Brand Names Caduet® [US/Can]

Therapeutic Category Antilipemic Agent, HMG-CoA Reductase Inhibitor; Calcium Channel Blocker

Use For use when treatment with both amlodipine and atorvastatin is appropriate:

Amlodipine: Treatment of hypertension; treatment of symptomatic chronic stable angina, vasospastic (Prinzmetal) angina (confirmed or suspected); prevention of hospitalization due to angina with documented CAD (limited to patients without heart failure or ejection fraction <40%)

Atorvastatin: Treatment of dyslipidemias or primary prevention of cardiovascular disease (atherosclerotic) as detailed here:

Primary prevention of cardiovascular disease (high-risk for CVD): To reduce the risk of MI or stroke in patients without evidence of heart disease who have multiple CVD risk factors or type 2 diabetes. Treatment reduces the risk for angina or revascularization procedures in patients with multiple risk factors.

Treatment of dyslipidemias: To reduce elevations in total cholesterol, LDL-C, apolipoprotein B, and triglycerides in patients with elevations of one or more components, and/or to increase HDL-C as present

(Continued)

amlodipine and atorvastatin *(Continued)*

in heterozygous hypercholesterolemia (Fredrickson type IIa hyperlipidemias); treatment of primary dysbetalipoproteinemia (Fredrickson type III), elevated serum TG levels (Fredrickson type IV), and homozygous familial hypercholesterolemia

Treatment of heterozygous familial hypercholesterolemia (HeFH) in adolescent patients (10-17 years of age, females >1 year postmenarche) having LDL-C ≥190 mg/dL or LDL-C ≥160 mg/dL with positive family history of premature cardiovascular disease (CVD) or with two or more CVD risk factors.

Usual Dosage Oral:

Amlodipine:

Children >10 years: Hypertension: 2.5-5 mg once daily. **Note:** Use in ages >10 years because of atorvastatin content.

Adults:

Hypertension: Initial dose: 5 mg once daily; maximum dose: 10 mg once daily; in general, titrate in 2.5 mg increments over 7-14 days. Usual dosage range (JNC 7): 2.5-10 mg once daily

Angina: Usual dose: 5-10 mg; lower dose suggested in elderly or hepatic impairment; most patients require 10 mg for adequate effect

Atorvastatin:

Children 10-17 years (females >1 year postmenarche): HeFH: 10 mg once daily (maximum: 20 mg/day)

Adults:

Hyperlipidemias: Initial: 10-20 mg once daily; patients requiring >45% reduction in LDL-C may be started at 40 mg once daily; range: 10-80 mg once daily

Primary prevention of CVD: 10 mg once daily

Dosage Forms Tablet:

2.5/10: Amlodipine 2.5 mg and atorvastatin 10 mg
2.5/20: Amlodipine 2.5 mg and atorvastatin 20 mg
2.5/40: Amlodipine 2.5 mg and atorvastatin 40 mg
5/10: Amlodipine 5 mg and atorvastatin 10 mg
5/20: Amlodipine 5 mg and atorvastatin 20 mg
5/40: Amlodipine 5 mg and atorvastatin 40 mg
5/80: Amlodipine 5 mg and atorvastatin 80 mg
10/10: Amlodipine 10 mg and atorvastatin 10 mg
10/20: Amlodipine 10 mg and atorvastatin 20 mg
10/40: Amlodipine 10 mg and atorvastatin 40 mg
10/80: Amlodipine 10 mg and atorvastatin 80 mg

amlodipine and benazepril (am LOE di peen & ben AY ze pril)

Synonyms benazepril hydrochloride and amlodipine besylate

U.S./Canadian Brand Names Lotrel® [US]

Therapeutic Category Antihypertensive Agent, Combination

Use Treatment of hypertension

Usual Dosage Oral: Adults: 2.5-10 mg (amlodipine) and 10-40 mg (benazepril) once daily; maximum: Amlodipine: 10 mg/day; benazepril: 40 mg/day

Dosage Forms Capsule:

Lotrel® 2.5/10: Amlodipine 2.5 mg and benazepril hydrochloride 10 mg
Lotrel® 5/10: Amlodipine 5 mg and benazepril hydrochloride 10 mg
Lotrel® 5/20: Amlodipine 5 mg and benazepril hydrochloride 20 mg
Lotrel® 5/40: Amlodipine 5 mg and benazepril hydrochloride 40 mg
Lotrel® 10/20: Amlodipine 10 mg and benazepril hydrochloride 20 mg
Lotrel® 10/40: Amlodipine 10 mg and benazepril hydrochloride 40 mg

amlodipine besylate *see* amlodipine *on previous page*

Ammens® Medicated Deodorant [US-OTC] *see* zinc oxide *on page 887*

ammonapse *see* sodium phenylbutyrate *on page 781*

ammonia spirit (aromatic) (a MOE nee ah SPEAR it, air oh MAT ik)

Synonyms smelling salts

Therapeutic Category Respiratory Stimulant

Use Respiratory and circulatory stimulant; treatment of fainting

Usual Dosage Used as "smelling salts" to treat or prevent fainting

Dosage Forms Solution for inhalation [ampul]: 1.7% to 2.1% (0.33 mL)

ammonium chloride (a MOE nee um KLOR ide)

Therapeutic Category Electrolyte Supplement, Oral

Use Treatment of hypochloremic states or metabolic alkalosis

Usual Dosage Metabolic alkalosis: The following equations represent different methods of correction utilizing either the serum HCO_3^-, the serum chloride, or the base excess

Dosing of mEq NH_4Cl via the chloride-deficit method (hypochloremia):

Dose of mEq NH_4Cl = [0.2 L/kg x body weight (kg)] x [103 - observed serum chloride]; administer 50% of dose over 12 hours, then re-evaluate

Note: 0.2 L/kg is the estimated chloride volume of distribution and 103 is the average normal serum chloride concentration (mEq/L)

Dosing of mEq NH_4Cl via the bicarbonate-excess method (refractory hypochloremic metabolic alkalosis):

Dose of NH_4Cl = [0.5 L/kg x body weight (kg)] x (observed serum HCO_3^- - 24); administer 50% of dose over 12 hours, then re-evaluate

Note: 0.5 L/kg is the estimated bicarbonate volume of distribution and 24 is the average normal serum bicarbonate concentration (mEq/L)

These equations will yield different requirements of ammonium chloride

Dosage Forms Injection, solution: Ammonium 5 mEq/mL and chloride 5 mEq/mL (20 mL) [equivalent to ammonium chloride 267.5 mg/mL]

ammonium lactate *see* lactic acid and ammonium hydroxide *on page 477*

Ammonul® [US] *see* sodium phenylacetate and sodium benzoate *on page 780*

Amnesteem™ [US] *see* isotretinoin *on page 466*

amobarbital (am oh BAR bi tal)

Synonyms amobarbital sodium; amylobarbitone

U.S./Canadian Brand Names Amytal® [US]

Therapeutic Category Barbiturate

Controlled Substance C-II

Use Hypnotic in short-term treatment of insomnia; reduce anxiety and provide sedation preoperatively

Usual Dosage

Children:

Sedative: I.M., I.V.: 6-12 years: Manufacturer's dosing range: 65- 500 mg

Hypnotic: I.M.: 2-3 mg/kg (maximum: 500 mg)

Adults:

Hypnotic: I.M., I.V.: 65-200 mg at bedtime (maximum I.M. dose: 500 mg)

Sedative: I.M., I.V.: 30-50 mg 2-3 times/day

Dosage Forms Injection, powder for reconstitution, as sodium: 500 mg

amobarbital sodium *see* amobarbital *on this page*

AMO Vitrax® *(Discontinued)* *see* hyaluronate and derivatives *on page 416*

amoxapine (a MOKS a peen)

Sound-Alike/Look-Alike Issues

amoxapine may be confused with amoxicillin, Amoxil®

Asendin may be confused with aspirin

Therapeutic Category Antidepressant, Tricyclic (Secondary Amine)

Use Treatment of depression, psychotic depression, depression accompanied by anxiety or agitation

Usual Dosage Oral:

Adolescents: Initial: 25-50 mg/day; increase gradually to 100 mg/day; may administer as divided doses or as a single dose at bedtime

Adults: Initial: 25 mg 2-3 times/day, if tolerated, dosage may be increased to 100 mg 2-3 times/day; may be given in a single bedtime dose when dosage <300 mg/day

Maximum daily dose:

Inpatient: 600 mg

Outpatient: 400 mg

Dosage Forms Tablet: 25 mg, 50 mg, 100 mg, 150 mg

amoxicillin (a moks i SIL in)

Sound-Alike/Look-Alike Issues

amoxicillin may be confused with amoxapine, Amoxil®, Atarax®

(Continued)

amoxicillin *(Continued)*

Amoxil® may be confused with amoxapine, amoxicillin
Trimox® may be confused with Diamox®, Tylox®

Synonyms amoxicillin trihydrate; amoxycillin; *p*-hydroxyampicillin

U.S./Canadian Brand Names Amoxil® [US]; Apo-Amoxi® [Can]; Gen-Amoxicillin [Can]; Lin-Amox [Can]; Novamoxin® [Can]; Nu-Amoxi [Can]; PHL-Amoxicillin [Can]; PMS-Amoxicillin [Can]

Therapeutic Category Penicillin

Use Treatment of otitis media, sinusitis, and infections caused by susceptible organisms involving the respiratory tract, skin, and urinary tract; prophylaxis of bacterial endocarditis in patients undergoing surgical or dental procedures; as part of a multidrug regimen for *H. pylori* eradication

Usual Dosage

Usual dosage range:

Children ≤3 months: Oral: 20-30 mg/kg/day divided every 12 hours
Children >3 months and <40 kg: Oral: 20-50 mg/kg/day in divided doses every 8-12 hours
Adults: Oral: 250-500 mg every 8 hours or 500-875 mg twice daily

Indication-specific dosing:

Children >3 months and <40 kg: Oral:

Acute otitis media: 80-90 mg/kg/day divided every 12 hours

Anthrax exposure (CDC guidelines): Note: Postexposure prophylaxis only with documented susceptible organisms: 80 mg/kg/day in divided doses every 8 hours (maximum: 500 mg/dose)

Ear, nose, throat, genitourinary tract, or skin/skin structure infections:

Mild to moderate: 25 mg/kg/day in divided doses every 12 hours **or** 20 mg/kg/day in divided doses every 8 hours

Severe: 45 mg/kg/day in divided doses every 12 hours **or** 40 mg/kg/day in divided doses every 8 hours

Endocarditis (subacute bacterial) prophylaxis: 50 mg/kg 1 hour before procedure

Lower respiratory tract infections: 45 mg/kg/day in divided doses every 12 hours **or** 40 mg/kg/day in divided doses every 8 hours

Lyme disease: 25-50 mg/kg/day divided every 8 hours (maximum: 500 mg)

Pneumonia:

4 months to 5 years: 100 mg/kg/day divided every 8 hours
5-15 years: 100 mg/kg/day divided every 8 hours with clarithromycin, azithromycin, or doxycycline

Adults: Oral:

Anthrax exposure (CDC guidelines): Note: Postexposure prophylaxis in pregnant or nursing women only with documented susceptible organisms: 500 mg every 8 hours

Ear, nose, throat, genitourinary tract, or skin/skin structure infections:

Mild to moderate: 500 mg every 12 hours **or** 250 mg every 8 hours

Severe: 875 mg every 12 hours **or** 500 mg every 8 hours

Endocarditis prophylaxis: 2 g 1 hour before procedure

***Helicobacter pylori* eradication:** 1000 mg twice daily; requires combination therapy with at least one other antibiotic and an acid-suppressing agent (proton pump inhibitor or H_2 blocker)

Lower respiratory tract infections: 875 mg every 12 hours **or** 500 mg every 8 hours

Lyme disease: 500 mg every 6-8 hours (depending on size of patient) for 21-30 days

Dosage Forms [DSC] = Discontinued product

Capsule, as trihydrate: 250 mg, 500 mg
Amoxil®: 500 mg
Trimox®: 250 mg, 500 mg [DSC]

Powder for oral suspension, as trihydrate: 125 mg/5 mL (80 mL, 100 mL, 150 mL); 200 mg/5 mL (50 mL, 75 mL, 100 mL); 250 mg/5 mL (80 mL, 100 mL, 150 mL); 400 mg/5 mL (50 mL, 75 mL, 100 mL)
Amoxil®: 200 mg/5 mL (5 mL, 50 mL, 75 mL, 100 mL) [contains sodium benzoate; bubble gum flavor]; 250 mg/5 mL (100 mL, 150 mL) [contains sodium benzoate; bubble gum flavor]; 400 mg/5 mL (5 mL, 50 mL, 75 mL, 100 mL) [contains sodium benzoate; bubble gum flavor]
Trimox®: 125 mg/5 mL (80 mL, 100 mL, 150 mL); 250 mg/5 mL (80 mL, 100 mL, 150 mL) [contains sodium benzoate; raspberry-strawberry flavor] [DSC]

Powder for oral suspension, as trihydrate [drops]:
Amoxil®: 50 mg/mL (30 mL) [contains sodium benzoate; bubble gum flavor]

Tablet, as trihydrate: 500 mg, 875 mg
Amoxil®: 500 mg, 875 mg

Tablet, chewable, as trihydrate: 125 mg, 200 mg, 250 mg, 400 mg
Amoxil®: 200 mg [contains phenylalanine 1.82 mg/tablet; cherry banana peppermint flavor]; 400 mg [contains phenylalanine 3.64 mg/tablet; cherry banana peppermint flavor]

Tablet, for oral suspension, as trihydrate:
DisperMox™: 200 mg [contains phenylalanine 5.6 mg; strawberry flavor]; 400 mg [contains phenylalanine 5.6 mg; strawberry flavor]; 600 mg [contains phenylalanine 11.23 mg; strawberry flavor] [DSC]

amoxicillin and clavulanate potassium

(a moks i SIL in & klav yoo LAN ate poe TASS ee um)

Sound-Alike/Look-Alike Issues

Augmentin® may be confused with Azulfidine®

Synonyms amoxicillin and clavulanic acid; clavulanic acid and amoxicillin

U.S./Canadian Brand Names Alti-Amoxi-Clav [Can]; Apo-Amoxi-Clav® [Can]; Augmentin ES-600® [US]; Augmentin XR™ [US]; Augmentin® [US/Can]; Clavulin® [Can]; Novo-Clavamoxin [Can]; ratio-Aclavulanate [Can]

Therapeutic Category Penicillin

Use Treatment of otitis media, sinusitis, and infections caused by susceptible organisms involving the lower respiratory tract, skin and skin structure, and urinary tract; spectrum same as amoxicillin with additional coverage of beta-lactamase producing *B. catarrhalis, H. influenzae, N. gonorrhoeae*, and *S. aureus* (not MRSA). The expanded coverage of this combination makes it a useful alternative when amoxicillin resistance is present and patients cannot tolerate alternative treatments.

Usual Dosage Note: Dose is based on the amoxicillin component

Usual dosage range:

Infants <3 months: Oral: 30 mg/kg/day divided every 12 hours using the 125 mg/5 mL suspension

Children ≥3 months and <40 kg: Oral: 20-90 mg/kg/day divided every 8-12 hours

Children >40 kg and Adults: Oral: 250-500 mg every 8 hours or 875 mg every 12 hours

Indication-specific dosing:

Children ≥3 months and <40 kg: Oral:

Lower respiratory tract infections, severe infections, sinusitis: 45 mg/kg/day divided every 12 hours **or** 40 mg/kg/day divided every 8 hours

Mild-to-moderate infections: 25 mg/kg/day divided every 12 hours or 20 mg/kg/day divided every 8 hours

Otitis media (Augmentin® ES-600): 90 mg/kg/day divided every 12 hours for 10 days in children with severe illness and when coverage for β-lactamase-positive *H. influenzae* and *M. catarrhalis* is needed.

Children ≥16 years and Adults: Oral:

Acute bacterial sinusitis: Extended release tablet: Two 1000 mg tablets every 12 hours for 10 days

Bite wounds (animal/human): 875 mg every 12 hours **or** 500 mg every 8 hours

Chronic obstructive pulmonary disease: 875 mg every 12 hours **or** 500 mg every 8 hours

Diabetic foot: Extended release tablet: Two 1000 mg tablets every 12 hours for 7-14 days

Diverticulitis, perirectal abscess: Extended release tablet: Two 1000 mg tablets every 12 hours for 7-10 days

Erysipelas: 875 mg every 12 hours **or** 500 mg every 8 hours

Febrile neutropenia: 875 mg every 12 hours

Pneumonia:

Aspiration: 875 mg every 12 hours

Community-acquired: Extended release tablet: Two 1000 mg tablets every 12 hours for 7-10 days

Pyelonephritis (acute, uncomplicated): 875 mg every 12 hours **or** 500 mg every 8 hours

Skin abscess: 875 mg every 12 hours

Dosage Forms

Powder for oral suspension: 200: Amoxicillin 200 mg and clavulanate potassium 28.5 mg per 5 mL (50 mL, 75 mL, 100 mL) [contains phenylalanine]; 400: Amoxicillin 400 mg and clavulanate potassium 57 mg per 5 mL (50 mL, 75 mL, 100 mL) [contains phenylalanine]; 600: Amoxicillin 600 mg and clavulanic potassium 42.9 mg per 5 mL (75 mL, 125 mL, 200 mL) [contains phenylalanine]

Amoclan:

200: Amoxicillin 200 mg and clavulanate potassium 28.5 mg per 5 mL (50 mL, 75 mL, 100 mL) [contains phenylalanine 7 mg/5 mL and potassium 0.14 mEq/5 mL; fruit flavor]

400: Amoxicillin 400 mg and clavulanate potassium 57 mg per 5 mL (50 mL, 75 mL, 100 mL) [contains phenylalanine 7 mg/5 mL and potassium 0.29 mEq/5 mL; fruit flavor]

Augmentin®:

125: Amoxicillin 125 mg and clavulanate potassium 31.25 mg per 5 mL (75 mL, 100 mL, 150 mL) [contains potassium 0.16 mEq/5 mL; banana flavor]

200: Amoxicillin 200 mg and clavulanate potassium 28.5 mg per 5 mL (50 mL, 75 mL, 100 mL) [contains phenylalanine 7 mg/5 mL and potassium 0.14 mEq/5 mL; orange flavor]

250: Amoxicillin 250 mg and clavulanate potassium 62.5 mg per 5 mL (75 mL, 100 mL, 150 mL) [contains potassium 0.32 mEq/5 mL; orange flavor]

400: Amoxicillin 400 mg and clavulanate potassium 57 mg per 5 mL (50 mL, 75 mL, 100 mL) [contains phenylalanine 7 mg/5 mL and potassium 0.29 mEq/5 mL; orange flavor]

Augmentin ES-600®: Amoxicillin 600 mg and clavulanic potassium 42.9 mg per 5 mL (75 mL, 125 mL, 200 mL) [contains phenylalanine 7 mg/5 mL and potassium 0.23 mEq/5 mL; strawberry cream flavor]

(Continued)

amoxicillin and clavulanate potassium *(Continued)*

Tablet: 250: Amoxicillin 250 mg and clavulanate potassium 125 mg; 500: Amoxicillin 500 mg and clavulanate potassium 125 mg; 875: Amoxicillin 875 mg and clavulanate potassium 125 mg

Augmentin®:

250: Amoxicillin 250 mg and clavulanate potassium 125 mg [contains potassium 0.63 mEq/tablet]

500: Amoxicillin 500 mg and clavulanate potassium 125 mg [contains potassium 0.63 mEq/tablet]

875: Amoxicillin 875 mg and clavulanate potassium 125 mg [contains potassium 0.63 mEq/tablet]

Tablet, chewable: 200: Amoxicillin 200 mg and clavulanate potassium 28.5 mg [contains phenylalanine]; 400: Amoxicillin 400 mg and clavulanate potassium 57 mg [contains phenylalanine]

Augmentin®:

125: Amoxicillin 125 mg and clavulanate potassium 31.25 mg [contains potassium 0.16 mEq/tablet; lemon-lime flavor]

200: Amoxicillin 200 mg and clavulanate potassium 28.5 mg [contains phenylalanine 2.1 mg/tablet and potassium 0.14 mEq/tablet; cherry-banana flavor]

250: Amoxicillin 250 mg and clavulanate potassium 62.5 mg [contains potassium 0.32 mEq/tablet; lemon-lime flavor]

400: Amoxicillin 400 mg and clavulanate potassium 57 mg [contains phenylalanine 4.2 mg/tablet and potassium 0.29 mEq/tablet; cherry-banana flavor]

Tablet, extended release:

Augmentin XR®: Amoxicillin 1000 mg and clavulanic acid 62.5 mg [contains potassium 29.3 mg (1.27 mEq) and sodium 12.6 mg (0.32 mEq) per tablet; packaged in either a 7-day or 10-day package]

amoxicillin and clavulanic acid *see* amoxicillin and clavulanate potassium *on previous page*

amoxicillin, lansoprazole, and clarithromycin *see* lansoprazole, amoxicillin, and clarithromycin *on page 482*

amoxicillin trihydrate *see* amoxicillin *on page 47*

Amoxil® [US] *see* amoxicillin *on page 47*

amoxycillin *see* amoxicillin *on page 47*

Amphadase™ [US] *see* hyaluronidase *on page 417*

amphetamine and dextroamphetamine *see* dextroamphetamine and amphetamine *on page 244*

Amphocin® [US] *see* amphotericin B (conventional) *on next page*

Amphojel® [Can] *see* aluminum hydroxide *on page 36*

Amphojel® ***(Discontinued)*** *see* aluminum hydroxide *on page 36*

Amphotec® [US/Can] *see* amphotericin B cholesteryl sulfate complex *on this page*

amphotericin B cholesteryl sulfate complex

(am foe TER i sin bee kole LES te ril SUL fate KOM plecks)

Synonyms ABCD; amphotericin B colloidal dispersion

U.S./Canadian Brand Names Amphotec® [US/Can]

Therapeutic Category Antifungal Agent

Use Treatment of invasive aspergillosis in patients who have failed amphotericin B deoxycholate treatment, or who have renal impairment or experience unacceptable toxicity which precludes treatment with amphotericin B deoxycholate in effective doses.

Usual Dosage Children and Adults: I.V.:

Premedication: For patients who experience chills, fever, hypotension, nausea, or other nonanaphylactic infusion-related immediate reactions, premedicate with the following drugs, 30-60 minutes prior to drug administration: a nonsteroidal (eg, ibuprofen, choline magnesium trisalicylate) with or without diphenhydramine; **or** acetaminophen with diphenhydramine; **or** hydrocortisone 50-100 mg. If the patient experiences rigors during the infusion, meperidine may be administered.

Range: 3-4 mg/kg/day (infusion of 1 mg/kg/hour); maximum: 7.5 mg/kg/day

Dosage Forms Injection, powder for reconstitution: 50 mg, 100 mg

amphotericin B colloidal dispersion *see* amphotericin B cholesteryl sulfate complex *on this page*

amphotericin B (conventional) (am foe TER i sin bee con VEN sha nal)

Synonyms amphotericin B desoxycholate

U.S./Canadian Brand Names Amphocin® [US]; Fungizone® [Can]

Therapeutic Category Antifungal Agent

Use Treatment of severe systemic and central nervous system infections caused by susceptible fungi such as *Candida* species, *Histoplasma capsulatum*, *Cryptococcus neoformans*, *Aspergillus* species, *Blastomyces dermatitidis*, *Torulopsis glabrata*, and *Coccidioides immitis*; fungal peritonitis; irrigant for bladder fungal infections; used in fungal infection in patients with bone marrow transplantation, amebic meningoencephalitis, ocular aspergillosis (intraocular injection), candidal cystitis (bladder irrigation), chemoprophylaxis (low-dose I.V.), immunocompromised patients at risk of aspergillosis (intranasal/nebulized), refractory meningitis (intrathecal), coccidioidal arthritis (intra-articular/I.M.).

Low-dose amphotericin B has been administered after bone marrow transplantation to reduce the risk of invasive fungal disease.

Usual Dosage

Premedication: For patients who experience infusion-related immediate reactions, premedicate with the following drugs 30-60 minutes prior to drug administration: NSAID (with or without diphenhydramine) **or** acetaminophen with diphenhydramine **or** hydrocortisone 50-100 mg. If the patient experiences rigors during the infusion, meperidine may be administered.

Usual dosage ranges:

Infants and Children:

Test dose: I.V.: 0.1 mg/kg/dose to a maximum of 1 mg; infuse over 30-60 minutes. Many clinicians believe a test dose is unnecessary.

Maintenance dose: 0.25-1 mg/kg/day given once daily; infuse over 2-6 hours. Once therapy has been established, amphotericin B can be administered on an every-other-day basis at 1-1.5 mg/kg/dose; cumulative dose: 1.5-2 g over 6-10 weeks.

Duration of therapy: Varies with nature of infection, usual duration is 4-12 weeks or cumulative dose of 1-4 g

Adults:

Test dose: 1 mg infused over 20-30 minutes. Many clinicians believe a test dose is unnecessary.

Maintenance dose: Usual: 0.05-1.5 mg/kg/day; 1-1.5 mg/kg over 4-6 hours every other day may be given once therapy is established; aspergillosis, rhinocerebral mucormycosis, often require 1-1.5 mg/kg/day; do not exceed 1.5 mg/kg/day

Indication-specific dosing:

Children: Meningitis, coccidioidal or cryptococcal: I.T.: 25-100 mcg every 48-72 hours; increase to 500 mcg as tolerated

Adults:

Aspergillosis, disseminated: I.V.: 0.6-0.7 mg/kg/day for 3-6 months

Bone marrow transplantation (prophylaxis): I.V.: Low-dose amphotericin B 0.1-0.25 mg/kg/day has been administered after bone marrow transplantation to reduce the risk of invasive fungal disease.

Candidemia (neutropenic or non-neutropenic): I.V.: 0.6-1 mg/kg/day until 14 days after last positive blood culture and resolution of signs and symptoms

Candidiasis, chronic, disseminated: I.V.: 0.6-0.7 mg/kg/day for 3-6 months and resolution of radiologic lesions

Cystitis: Candidal: Bladder irrigation: Irrigate with 50 mcg/mL solution instilled periodically or continuously for 5-10 days or until cultures are clear

Dematiaceous fungi: I.V.: 0.7 mg/kg/day in combination with an azole

Endocarditis: I.V.: 0.6-1 mg/kg/day (with or without flucytosine) for 1 week, then 0.8 mg/kg/day every other day for 6-8 weeks postoperatively

Endophthalmitis, fungal: I.V.: 0.7-1 mg/kg/day (with or without flucytosine) for at least 4 weeks

Esophagitis: I.V.: 0.3-0.7 mg/kg/day for 14-21 after clinical improvement

Histoplasmosis: Chronic, severe pulmonary or disseminated: I.V.: 0.5-1 mg/kg/day for 7 days, then 0.8 mg/kg every other day (or 3 times/week) until total dose of 10-15 mg/kg; may continue itraconazole as suppressive therapy (lifelong for immunocompromised patients)

Meningitis:

Candidal: I.V.: 0.7-1 mg/kg/day (with or without flucytosine) for at least 4 weeks

Cryptococcal or *Coccidioides*: I.T.: Initial: 25-300 mcg every 48-72 hours; increase to 500 mcg to 1 mg as tolerated; maximum total dose: 15 mg has been suggested

Histoplasma: I.V.: 0.5-1 mg/kg/day for 7 days, then 0.8 mg/kg every other day (or 3 times/week) for 3 months total duration; follow with fluconazole suppressive therapy for up to 12 months

Meningoencephalitis, cryptococcal: I.V.:

HIV positive: 0.7-1 mg/kg/day (plus flucytosine 100 mg/kg/day) for 2 weeks, then change to oral fluconazole for at least 10 weeks; alternatively, amphotericin and flucytosine may be continued uninterrupted for 6-10 weeks

(Continued)

amphotericin B (conventional) *(Continued)*

HIV negative: 0.5-0.7 mg/kg/day (plus flucytosine) for 2 weeks
Osteomyelitis: Candidal: I.V.: 0.5-1 mg/kg/day for 6-10 weeks
Penicillium marneffei: I.V.: 0.6 mg/kg/day for 2 weeks
Pneumonia: Cryptococcal (mild to moderate): I.V.:
HIV positive: 0.5-1 mg/kg/day
HIV negative: 0.5-0.7 mg/kg/day (plus flucytosine) for 2 weeks
Sporotrichosis: Pulmonary, meningeal, osteoarticular, or disseminated: I.V.: Total dose of 1-2 g, then change to oral itraconazole or fluconazole for suppressive therapy

Dosage Forms Injection, powder for reconstitution, as desoxycholate: 50 mg

amphotericin B desoxycholate *see* amphotericin B (conventional) *on previous page*

amphotericin B lipid complex (am foe TER i sin bee LIP id KOM pleks)

Synonyms ABLC

U.S./Canadian Brand Names Abelcet® [US/Can]

Therapeutic Category Antifungal Agent

Use Treatment of aspergillosis or any type of progressive fungal infection in patients who are refractory to or intolerant of conventional amphotericin B therapy

Usual Dosage Children and Adults: I.V.:

Premedication: For patients who experience infusion-related immediate reactions, premedicate with the following drugs, 30-60 minutes prior to drug administration: a nonsteroidal antiinflammatory agent ± diphenhydramine; or acetaminophen with diphenhydramine; **or** hydrocortisone 50-100 mg. If the patient experiences rigors during the infusion, meperidine may be administered.

Range: 2.5-5 mg/kg/day as a single infusion

Dosage Forms Injection, suspension [preservative free]: 5 mg/mL (20 mL)

amphotericin B liposomal (am foe TER i sin bee lye po SO mal)

Synonyms L-AmB

U.S./Canadian Brand Names AmBisome® [US/Can]

Therapeutic Category Antifungal Agent, Systemic

Use Empirical therapy for presumed fungal infection in febrile, neutropenic patients; treatment of patients with *Aspergillus* species, *Candida* species, and/or *Cryptococcus* species infections refractory to amphotericin B desoxycholate, or in patients where renal impairment or unacceptable toxicity precludes the use of amphotericin B desoxycholate; treatment of cryptococcal meningitis in HIV-infected patients; treatment of visceral leishmaniasis

Usual Dosage

Usual dosage range:

Children: I.V.: 3-5 mg/kg/day

Adults: I.V.: 2-6 mg/kg/day; **Note:** Higher doses (15 mg/kg/day) have been used clinically.

Note: Premedication: For patients who experience nonanaphylactic infusion-related immediate reactions, premedicate with the following drugs 30-60 minutes prior to drug administration: A nonsteroidal antiinflammatory agent ± diphenhydramine; **or** acetaminophen with diphenhydramine; **or** hydrocortisone 50-100 mg. If the patient experiences rigors during the infusion, meperidine may be administered.

Indication-specific dosing:

Children: I.V.:

Candidal infection:

Endocarditis: 3-6 mg/kg/day with flucytosine 25-37.5 mg/kg 4 times daily
Meningitis: 5 mg/kg/day with flucytosine 100 mg/kg/day

Cryptococcal meningitis (HIV-positive): 6 mg/kg/day

Note: IDSA guidelines (April, 2000) report doses of 3-6 mg/kg/day, noting that 4 mg/kg/day was effective in a small, open-label trial. The manufacturer's labeled dose of 6 mg/kg/day was approved in June, 2000.

Empiric therapy: 3 mg/kg/day

Systemic fungal infections *(Aspergillus, Candida, Cryptococcus)*: 3-5 mg/kg/day

Visceral leishmaniasis:

Immunocompetent: 3 mg/kg/day on days 1-5, and 3 mg/kg/day on days 14 and 21; a repeat course may be given in patients who do not achieve parasitic clearance

Note: Alternate regimen of 10 mg/kg/day for 2 days has been reportedly effective.

Immunocompromised: 4 mg/kg/day on days 1-5, and 4 mg/kg/day on days 10, 17, 24, 31, and 38

Adults: I.V.:

Candidal infection:

Endocarditis: 3-6 mg/kg/day with flucytosine 25-37.5 mg/kg 4 times daily

Meningitis: 5 mg/kg/day with flucytosine 100 mg/kg/day

Cryptococcal meningitis (HIV-positive): 6 mg/kg/day

Note: IDSA guidelines (April, 2000) report doses of 3-6 mg/kg/day, noting that 4 mg/kg/day was effective in a small, open-label trial. The manufacturer's labeled dose of 6 mg/kg/day was approved in June, 2000.

Empiric therapy: 3 mg/kg/day

Fungal sinusitis: 5-7.5 mg/kg/day

Note: Use azole antifungal if causative organism is *Pseudallescheria boydii* (*Scedosporium* sp).

Systemic fungal infections *(Aspergillus, Candida, Cryptococcus)*: 3-5 mg/kg/day

Visceral leishmaniasis:

Immunocompetent: 3 mg/kg/day on days 1-5, and 3 mg/kg/day on days 14 and 21; a repeat course may be given in patients who do not achieve parasitic clearance

Note: Alternate regimen of 2 mg/kg/day for 5 days has been reportedly effective.

Immunocompromised: 4 mg/kg/day on days 1-5, and 4 mg/kg/day on days 10, 17, 24, 31, and 38

Dosage Forms

Injection, powder for reconstitution:

AmBisome®: 50 mg [contains soy and sucrose]

ampicillin (am pi SIL in)

Sound-Alike/Look-Alike Issues

ampicillin may be confused with aminophylline

Synonyms aminobenzylpenicillin; ampicillin sodium; ampicillin trihydrate

U.S./Canadian Brand Names Apo-Ampi® [Can]; Novo-Ampicillin [Can]; Nu-Ampi [Can]

Therapeutic Category Penicillin

Use Treatment of susceptible bacterial infections (nonbeta-lactamase-producing organisms); susceptible bacterial infections caused by streptococci, pneumococci, nonpenicillinase-producing staphylococci, *Listeria*, meningococci; some strains of *H. influenzae*, *Salmonella*, *Shigella*, *E. coli*, *Enterobacter*, and *Klebsiella*

Usual Dosage

Usual dosage range:

Infants and Children:

Oral: 50-100 mg/kg/day in doses divided every 6 hours (maximum: 2-4 g/day)

I.M., I.V.: 100-400 mg/kg/day in divided doses every 6 hours (maximum: 12 g/day)

Adults: Oral, I.M., I.V.: 250-500 mg every 6 hours

Indication-specific dosing:

Infants and Children:

Endocarditis prophylaxis:

Dental, oral, respiratory tract, or esophageal procedures: I.M., I.V.: 50 mg/kg within 30 minutes prior to procedure in patients unable to take oral amoxicillin

Genitourinary and gastrointestinal tract (except esophageal) procedures: I.M., I.V.:

High-risk patients: 50 mg/kg (maximum: 2 g) within 30 minutes prior to procedure, followed by ampicillin 25 mg/kg (or amoxicillin 25 mg/kg orally) 6 hours later; must be used in combination with gentamicin.

Moderate-risk patients: 50 mg/kg within 30 minutes prior to procedure

Mild-to-moderate infections:

Oral: 50-100 mg/kg/day in doses divided every 6 hours (maximum: 2-4 g/day)

I.M., I.V.: 100-150 mg/kg/day in divided doses every 6 hours (maximum: 2-4 g/day)

Severe infections, meningitis: I.M., I.V.: 200-400 mg/kg/day in divided doses every 6 hours (maximum: 6-12 g/day)

Adults:

Actinomycosis: I.V.: 50 mg/kg/day for 4-6 weeks then oral amoxicillin

Cholangitis (acute): I.V.: 2 g every 4 hours with gentamicin

Diverticulitis: I.M., I.V.: 2 g every 6 hours with metronidazole

Endocarditis:

Infective: I.V.: 12 g/day via continuous infusion or divided every 4 hours

Prophylaxis: Dental, oral, respiratory tract, or esophageal procedures: I.M., I.V.: 2 g within 30 minutes prior to procedure in patients unable to take oral amoxicillin

Genitourinary and gastrointestinal tract (except esophageal) procedures:

High-risk patients: I.M., I.V.: 2 g within 30 minutes prior to procedure, followed by ampicillin 1 g (or amoxicillin 1g orally) 6 hours later; must be used in combination with gentamicin.

Moderate-risk patients: I.M., I.V.: 2 g within 30 minutes prior to procedure

(Continued)

ampicillin *(Continued)*

Group B strep prophylaxis (intrapartum): I.V.: 2 g initial dose, then 1 g every 4 hours until delivery
***Listeria* infections:** I.V.: 200 mg/kg/day divided every 6 hours
Sepsis/meningitis: I.M., I.V.: 150-250 mg/kg/day divided every 3-4 hours (range: 6-12 g/day)
Urinary tract infections (enterococcus suspected): I.V.: 1-2 g every 6 hours with gentamicin

Dosage Forms
Capsule: 250 mg, 500 mg
Injection, powder for reconstitution, as sodium: 125 mg, 250 mg, 500 mg, 1 g, 2 g, 10 g
Powder for oral suspension: 125 mg/5 mL (100 mL, 200 mL); 250 mg/5 mL (100 mL, 200 mL)

ampicillin and sulbactam (am pi SIL in & SUL bak tam)

Synonyms sulbactam and ampicillin
U.S./Canadian Brand Names Unasyn® [US/Can]
Therapeutic Category Penicillin
Use Treatment of susceptible bacterial infections involved with skin and skin structure, intraabdominal infections, gynecological infections; spectrum is that of ampicillin plus organisms producing beta-lactamases such as *S. aureus*, *H. influenzae*, *E. coli*, *Klebsiella*, *Acinetobacter*, *Enterobacter*, and anaerobes
Usual Dosage Note: Unasyn® (ampicillin/sulbactam) is a combination product. Dosage recommendations for Unasyn® are based on the ampicillin component.

Usual dosage range:
Children ≥1 year: I.V.: 100-400 mg ampicillin/kg/day divided every 6 hours (maximum: 8 g ampicillin/day, 12 g Unasyn®). **Note:** The American Academy of Pediatrics recommends a dose of up to 300 mg/kg/day for severe infection in infants >1 month of age.
Adults: I.M., I.V.: 1-2 g ampicillin (1.5-3 g Unasyn®) every 6 hours (maximum: 8 g ampicillin/day, 12 g Unasyn®)

Indication-specific dosing:
Children:
Epiglottitis: I.V.: 100-200 mg ampicillin/kg/day divided in 4 doses
Mild-to-moderate infections: I.M., I.V.: 100-200 mg ampicillin/kg/day (150-300 mg Unasyn®) divided every 6 hours (maximum: 8 g ampicillin/day, 12 g Unasyn®)
Peritonsillar and retropharyngeal abscess: I.V.: 50 mg ampicillin/kg/dose every 6 hours
Severe infections: I.M., I.V.: 200-400 mg ampicillin/kg/day divided every 6 hours (maximum: 8 g ampicillin/day, 12 g Unasyn®)
Adults: Doses expressed as ampicillin/sulbactam combination:
Amnionitis, cholangitis, diverticulitis, endometritis, endophthalmitis, epididymitis/orchitis, liver abscess, osteomyelitis (diabetic foot), peritonitis: I.V.: 3 g every 6 hours
Endocarditis: I.V.: 3 g every 6 hours with gentamicin or vancomycin for 4-6 weeks
Orbital cellulitis: I.V.: 1.5 g every 6 hours
Parapharyngeal space infections: I.V.: 3 g every 6 hours
***Pasteurella multocida* (human, canine/feline bites):** I.V.: 1.5-3 g every 6 hours
Pelvic inflammatory disease: I.V.: 3 g every 6 hours with doxycycline
Peritonitis (CAPD): Intraperitoneal:
Anuric, intermittent: 3 g every 12 hours
Anuric, continuous: Loading dose: 1.5 g; maintenance dose: 150 mg
Pneumonia:
Aspiration, community-acquired: I.V.: 1.5-3 g every 6 hours
Hospital-acquired: I.V.: 3 g every 6 hours
Urinary tract infections, pyelonephritis: I.V.: 3 g every 6 hours for 14 days

Dosage Forms
Injection, powder for reconstitution: Injection, powder for reconstitution: 1.5 g: Ampicillin 1 g and sulbactam 0.5 g [contains sodium 115 mg (5 mEq)/1.5 g)]; 3 g: Ampicillin 2 g and sulbactam 1 g [contains sodium 115 mg (5 mEq)/1.5 g)]; 15 g: Ampicillin 10 g and sulbactam 5 g [bulk package; contains sodium 115 mg (5 mEq)/1.5 g)]
Unasyn®:
1.5 g: Ampicillin 1 g and sulbactam 0.5 g [contains sodium 115 mg (5 mEq)/1.5 g)]
3 g: Ampicillin 2 g and sulbactam 1 g [contains sodium 115 mg (5 mEq)/1.5 g)]
15 g: Ampicillin 10 g and sulbactam 5 g [bulk package; contains sodium 115 mg (5 mEq)/1.5 g)]

ampicillin sodium *see* ampicillin *on previous page*
ampicillin trihydrate *see* ampicillin *on previous page*

amprenavir (am PREN a veer)

U.S./Canadian Brand Names Agenerase® [US/Can]

Therapeutic Category Protease Inhibitor

Use Treatment of HIV infections in combination with at least two other antiretroviral agents; oral solution should only be used when capsules or other protease inhibitors are not therapeutic options

Usual Dosage Oral: **Note:** Capsule and oral solution are **not** interchangeable on a mg-per-mg basis.

Capsule:

Children 4-12 years **or** 13-16 years (<50 kg): 20 mg/kg twice daily or 15 mg/kg 3 times daily; maximum: 2400 mg/day

Children >13 years (≥50 kg) and Adults: 1200 mg twice daily

Note: Dosage adjustments for amprenavir when administered in combination therapy:

Efavirenz: Adjustments necessary for both agents:

Amprenavir 1200 mg 3 times/day (single protease inhibitor) **or**

Amprenavir 1200 mg twice daily plus ritonavir 200 mg twice daily

Ritonavir: Adjustments necessary for both agents:

Amprenavir 1200 mg plus ritonavir 200 mg once daily **or**

Amprenavir 600 mg plus ritonavir 100 mg twice daily

Note: Oral solution of ritonavir and amprenavir should not be coadministered.

Solution:

Children 4-12 years **or** 13-16 years (<50 kg): 22.5 mg/kg twice daily or 17 mg/kg 3 times daily; maximum: 2800 mg/day

Children >13 years (≥50 kg) and Adults: 1400 mg twice daily

Dosage Forms

Capsule:

Agenerase®: 50 mg [contains vitamin E 36.3 int. units (as TPGS)]

Solution, oral:

Agenerase®: 15 mg/mL (240 mL) [contains propylene glycol 550 mg/mL and vitamin E 46 int. units/mL; grape-bubble gum-peppermint flavor]

AMPT *see* metyrosine *on page 552*

amrinone lactate *see* inamrinone *on page 445*

Amvisc® *(Discontinued)* *see* hyaluronate and derivatives *on page 416*

Amvisc® Plus *(Discontinued)* *see* hyaluronate and derivatives *on page 416*

amyl nitrite (AM il NYE trite)

Synonyms isoamyl nitrite

Therapeutic Category Vasodilator

Use Coronary vasodilator in angina pectoris; adjunct in treatment of cyanide poisoning; produce changes in the intensity of heart murmurs

Usual Dosage Nasal inhalation:

Cyanide poisoning: Children and Adults: Inhale the vapor from a 0.3 mL crushed ampul every minute for 15-30 seconds until I.V. sodium nitrite infusion is available

Angina: Adults: 1-6 inhalations from 1 crushed ampul; may repeat in 3-5 minutes

Dosage Forms Vapor for inhalation [crushable covered glass capsules]: Amyl nitrite USP (0.3 mL)

amyl nitrite, sodium thiosulfate, and sodium nitrite *see* sodium nitrite, sodium thiosulfate, and amyl nitrite *on page 780*

amylobarbitone *see* amobarbital *on page 47*

Amytal® [US] *see* amobarbital *on page 47*

AN100226 *see* natalizumab *on page 580*

Anabolin® *(Discontinued)* *see* nandrolone *on page 577*

Anacin® PM Aspirin Free *(Discontinued)* *see* acetaminophen and diphenhydramine *on page 7*

Anadrol® [US] *see* oxymetholone *on page 629*

Anafranil® [US/Can] *see* clomipramine *on page 202*

anagrelide (an AG gre lide)

Synonyms 1370-999-397; anagrelide hydrochloride; BL4162A; 6,7-dichloro-1,5-dihydroimidazo [2,1b] quinazolin-2(3H)-one monohydrochloride

(Continued)

anagrelide *(Continued)*

U.S./Canadian Brand Names Agrylin® [US/Can]; Gen-Anagrelide [Can]; PMS-Anagrelide [Can]; Rhoxal-anagrelide [Can]; Sandoz-Anagrelide [Can]

Therapeutic Category Platelet Reducing Agent

Use Treatment of essential thrombocythemia (ET) and thrombocythemia associated with chronic myelogenous leukemia (CML), polycythemia vera, and other myeloproliferative disorders

Usual Dosage Note: Maintain for ≥1 week, then adjust to the lowest effective dose to reduce and maintain platelet count <600,000/µL ideally to the normal range; the dose must not be increased by >0.5 mg/day in any 1 week; maximum dose: 10 mg/day or 2.5 mg/dose

Oral:

Children: Initial: 0.5 mg/day (range: 0.5 mg 1-4 times/day)

Adults: 0.5 mg 4 times/day or 1 mg twice daily

Dosage Forms Capsule: 0.5 mg, 1 mg

anagrelide hydrochloride *see* anagrelide *on previous page*

anakinra (an a KIN ra)

Sound-Alike/Look-Alike Issues

anakinra may be confused with amikacin

Synonyms IL-1Ra; interleukin-1 receptor antagonist

U.S./Canadian Brand Names Kineret® [US/Can]

Therapeutic Category Antirheumatic, Disease Modifying

Use Reduction of signs and symptoms of moderately- to severely-active rheumatoid arthritis in adult patients who have failed one or more disease-modifying antirheumatic drugs (DMARDs); may be used alone or in combination with DMARDs (other than tumor necrosis factor-blocking agents)

Usual Dosage Adults: SubQ: Rheumatoid arthritis: 100 mg once daily (administer at approximately the same time each day)

Dosage Forms Injection, solution [preservative free]: 100 mg/0.67 mL (1 mL) [prefilled syringe]

Ana-Kit® [US] *see* epinephrine and chlorpheniramine *on page 297*

Analpram-HC® [US] *see* pramoxine and hydrocortisone *on page 691*

AnaMantle® HC [US] *see* lidocaine and hydrocortisone *on page 496*

Anamine® Syrup *(Discontinued)* *see* chlorpheniramine and pseudoephedrine *on page 177*

Anandron® [Can] *see* nilutamide *on page 593*

Anaplex® DM [US] *see* brompheniramine, pseudoephedrine, and dextromethorphan *on page 120*

Anaplex® DMX [US] *see* brompheniramine, pseudoephedrine, and dextromethorphan *on page 120*

Anaplex® Liquid *(Discontinued)* *see* chlorpheniramine and pseudoephedrine *on page 177*

Anaprox® [US/Can] *see* naproxen *on page 578*

Anaprox® DS [US/Can] *see* naproxen *on page 578*

Anaspaz® [US] *see* hyoscyamine *on page 434*

anastrozole (an AS troe zole)

Synonyms ICI-D1033; ZD1033

U.S./Canadian Brand Names Arimidex® [US/Can]

Therapeutic Category Antineoplastic Agent

Use Treatment of locally-advanced or metastatic breast cancer (ER-positive or hormone receptor unknown) in postmenopausal women; treatment of advanced breast cancer in postmenopausal women with disease progression following tamoxifen therapy; adjuvant treatment of early ER-positive breast cancer in postmenopausal women

Usual Dosage Breast cancer: Adults: Oral (refer to individual protocols): 1 mg once daily

Dosage Forms Tablet: 1 mg

Anatrast® [US] *see* radiological/contrast media (ionic) *on page 728*

Anbesol® [US-OTC] *see* benzocaine *on page 99*

Anbesol® Baby [US-OTC/Can] *see* benzocaine *on page 99*

Anbesol® Cold Sore Therapy [US-OTC] *see* benzocaine *on page 99*

Anbesol® Jr. [US-OTC] *see* benzocaine *on page 99*

Anbesol® Maximum Strength [US-OTC] *see* benzocaine *on page 99*

Ancef® [US] *see* cefazolin *on page 156*

Ancobon® [US/Can] *see* flucytosine *on page 350*

Andehist DM NR [US] *see* brompheniramine, pseudoephedrine, and dextromethorphan *on page 120*

Andehist DM NR Drops *(Discontinued)* *see* carbinoxamine, pseudoephedrine, and dextromethorphan *on page 150*

Andehist NR Drops *(Discontinued)* *see* carbinoxamine and pseudoephedrine *on page 149*

Andehist NR Syrup [US] *see* brompheniramine and pseudoephedrine *on page 118*

Andriol® [Can] *see* testosterone *on page 812*

Androcur® [Can] *see* cyproterone *(Canada only) on page 223*

Androcur® Depot [Can] *see* cyproterone *(Canada only) on page 223*

Androderm® [US/Can] *see* testosterone *on page 812*

AndroGel® [US/Can] *see* testosterone *on page 812*

Android® [US] *see* methyltestosterone *on page 548*

Andro-L.A.® Injection *(Discontinued)* *see* testosterone *on page 812*

Androlone®-D *(Discontinued)* *see* nandrolone *on page 577*

Androlone® *(Discontinued)* *see* nandrolone *on page 577*

Andropository [Can] *see* testosterone *on page 812*

Andropository® Injection *(Discontinued)* *see* testosterone *on page 812*

Anectine® *(Discontinued)* *see* succinylcholine *on page 793*

Anestacon® [US] *see* lidocaine *on page 493*

aneurine hydrochloride *see* thiamine *on page 821*

Anexate® [Can] *see* flumazenil *on page 351*

Anexsia® [US] *see* hydrocodone and acetaminophen *on page 420*

Anextuss [US] *see* guaifenesin, dextromethorphan, and phenylephrine *on page 400*

Angeliq® [US/Can] *see* drospirenone and estradiol *on page 282*

Angio Conray® [US] *see* radiological/contrast media (ionic) *on page 728*

Angiomax® [US/Can] *see* bivalirudin *on page 113*

Angiovist® [US] *see* radiological/contrast media (ionic) *on page 728*

Angiscein® [US] *see* fluorescein sodium *on page 354*

anidulafungin (ay nid yoo la FUN jin)

Synonyms LY303366

U.S./Canadian Brand Names Eraxis™ [US]

Therapeutic Category Antifungal Agent, Parenteral; Echinocandin

Use Treatment of candidemia and other forms of *Candida* infections (including those of intraabdominal, peritoneal, and esophageal locus)

Usual Dosage I.V.: Adults:

Candidemia, intraabdominal or peritoneal candidiasis: 200 mg loading dose on day 1, followed by 100 mg daily for at least 14 days after last positive culture

Esophageal candidiasis: 100 mg loading dose on day 1, followed by 50 mg daily for at least 14 days and for at least 7 days after symptom resolution

Dosage Forms

Injection, powder for reconstitution [preservative free]:

Eraxis™: 50 mg [contains polysorbate 80; packaged with 20% (w/w) dehydrated alcohol (15 mL) as diluent]

Anodynos-DHC® *(Discontinued)* *see* hydrocodone and acetaminophen *on page 420*

Anolor 300 [US] *see* butalbital, acetaminophen, and caffeine *on page 129*

Anoquan® *(Discontinued)*

Ansaid® [Can] *see* flurbiprofen *on page 360*

Ansaid® *(Discontinued)* *see* flurbiprofen *on page 360*

ansamycin *see* rifabutin *on page 744*

Antabuse® [US] *see* disulfiram *on page 268*

Antagon® [US/Can] *see* ganirelix *on page 375*

Antara™ [US] *see* fenofibrate *on page 338*

Antazoline-V® Ophthalmic *(Discontinued)*

Anthra-Derm® *(Discontinued)* *see* anthralin *on this page*

Anthraforte® [Can] *see* anthralin *on this page*

anthralin (AN thra lin)

Synonyms dithranol

U.S./Canadian Brand Names Anthraforte® [Can]; Anthranol® [Can]; Anthrascalp® [Can]; Dritho-Scalp® [US]; Micanol® [Can]; Psoriatec™ [US]

Therapeutic Category Keratolytic Agent

Use Treatment of psoriasis (quiescent or chronic psoriasis)

Usual Dosage Adults: Topical: Generally, apply once a day or as directed. The irritant potential of anthralin is directly related to the strength being used and each patient's individual tolerance. Always commence treatment using a short, daily contact time (5-10 minutes) for at least 1 week using the lowest strength possible. Contact time may be gradually increased (to 20-30 minutes) as tolerated.

Skin application: Apply sparingly only to psoriatic lesions and rub gently and carefully into the skin until absorbed. Avoid applying an excessive quantity which may cause unnecessary soiling and staining of the clothing or bed linen.

Scalp application: Comb hair to remove scalar debris, wet hair and, after suitably parting, rub cream well into the lesions, taking care to prevent the cream from spreading onto the forehead,

Remove by washing or showering; optimal period of contact will vary according to the strength used and the patient's response to treatment. Continue treatment until the skin is entirely clear (ie, when there is nothing to feel with the fingers and the texture is normal).

Dosage Forms

Cream:

Dritho-Scalp®: 0.5% (50 g)

Psoriatec™: 1% (50 g)

Anthranol® [Can] *see* anthralin *on this page*

Anthrascalp® [Can] *see* anthralin *on this page*

anthrax vaccine, adsorbed (AN thraks vak SEEN ad SORBED)

Synonyms AVA

U.S./Canadian Brand Names BioThrax™ [US]

Therapeutic Category Vaccine

Use Immunization against *Bacillus anthracis.* Recommended for individuals who may come in contact with animal products which come from anthrax endemic areas and may be contaminated with *Bacillus anthracis* spores; recommended for high-risk persons such as veterinarians and other handling potentially infected animals. Routine immunization for the general population is not recommended.

The Department of Defense is implementing an anthrax vaccination program against the biological warfare agent anthrax, which will be administered to all active duty and reserve personnel.

Usual Dosage SubQ: Children ≥18 years and Adults:

Primary immunization: Three injections of 0.5 mL each given 2 weeks apart, followed by three additional injections given at 6-, 12-, and 18 months; it is not necessary to restart the series if a dose is not given on time; resume as soon as practical

Subsequent booster injections: 0.5 mL at 1-year intervals are recommended for immunity to be maintained

Dosage Forms Injection, suspension: 5 mL [vial stopper contains dry natural rubber]

anti-4 alpha integrin *see* natalizumab *on page 580*

131 I anti-B1 antibody *see* tositumomab and iodine I 131 tositumomab *on page 837*

131 I-anti-B1 monoclonal antibody *see* tositumomab and iodine I 131 tositumomab *on page 837*

Antiben® *(Discontinued)* *see* antipyrine and benzocaine *on page 62*

anti-CD11a *see* efalizumab *on page 288*

anti-CD20 monoclonal antibody *see* rituximab *on page 749*

anti-CD20-murine monoclonal antibody I-131 *see* tositumomab and iodine I 131 tositumomab *on page 837*

antidigoxin fab fragments, ovine *see* digoxin immune Fab *on page 255*

antidiuretic hormone *see* vasopressin *on page 868*

antihemophilic factor (human) (an tee hee moe FIL ik FAK tor HYU man)

Synonyms AHF (human); factor VIII (human)

U.S./Canadian Brand Names Alphanate® [US]; Hemofil M [US/Can]; Koāte®-DVI [US]; Monarc-M™ [US]; Monoclate-P® [US]

Therapeutic Category Blood Product Derivative

Use Prevention and treatment of hemorrhagic episodes in patients with hemophilia A (classic hemophilia); perioperative management of hemophilia A; can be of significant therapeutic value in patients with acquired factor VIII inhibitors not exceeding 10 Bethesda units/mL

Orphan status: Alphanate®: Management of von Willebrand disease

Usual Dosage Children and Adults: I.V.: Individualize dosage based on coagulation studies performed prior to treatment and at regular intervals during treatment. In general, administration of factor VIII 1 int. unit/kg will increase circulating factor VIII levels by ~2 int. units/dL. (General guidelines presented; consult individual product labeling for specific dosing recommendations.)

Dosage based on desired factor VIII increase (%):

To calculate dosage needed based on desired factor VIII increase (%):

Body weight (kg) x 0.5 int. units/kg x desired factor VIII increase (%) = int. units factor VIII required

For example:

50 kg x 0.5 int. units/kg x 30 (% increase) = 750 int. units factor VIII

Dosage based on expected factor VIII increase (%):

It is also possible to calculate the **expected** % factor VIII increase:

(# int. units administered x 2%/int. units/kg) divided by body weight (kg) = expected % factor VIII increase

For example:

(1400 int. units x 2%/int. units/kg) divided by 70 kg = 40%

General guidelines:

Minor hemorrhage: 10-20 int. units/kg as a single dose to achieve FVIII plasma level ~20% to 40% of normal. Mild superficial or early hemorrhages may respond to a single dose; may repeat dose every 12-24 hours for 1-3 days until bleeding is resolved or healing achieved.

Moderate hemorrhage/minor surgery: 15-25 int. units/kg to achieve FVIII plasma level 30% to 50% of normal. If needed, may continue with a maintenance dose of 10-15 int. units/kg every 8-12 hours.

Major to life-threatening hemorrhage: Initial dose 40-50 int. units/kg, followed by a maintenance dose of 20-25 int. units/kg every 8-12 hours until threat is resolved, to achieve FVIII plasma level 80% to 100% of normal.

Major surgery: 50 int. units/kg given preoperatively to raise factor VIII level to 100% before surgery begins. May repeat as necessary after 6-12 hours initially and for a total of 10-14 days until healing is complete. Intensity of therapy may depend on type of surgery and postoperative regimen.

Bleeding prophylaxis: May be administered on a regular basis for bleeding prophylaxis. Doses of 24-40 int. units/kg 3 times/week have been reported in patients with severe hemophilia to prevent joint bleeding.

If bleeding is not controlled with adequate dose, test for presence of inhibitor. It may not be possible or practical to control bleeding if inhibitor titers are >10 Bethesda units/mL.

Dosage Forms

Injection, powder for reconstitution:

Alphanate®: Vial labeled with international units [contains sodium ≤10 mEq/vial and albumin]

Hemofil M: Vial labeled with international units [contains albumin; derived from mouse proteins; packaging may contain natural rubber latex]

Koate®-DVI: ~250 int. units, ~500 int. units, ~1000 int. units [contains albumin]

Monarc-M™: Vial labeled with international units [contains albumin; derived from mouse proteins; packaging may contain natural rubber latex]

Monoclate-P®: ~250 int. units, ~500 int. units, ~1000 int. units, ~1500 int. units [contains albumin; derived from mouse proteins]

antihemophilic factor (recombinant) (an tee hee moe FIL ik FAK tor ree KOM be nant)

Synonyms AHF (recombinant); factor VIII (recombinant); rAHF

U.S./Canadian Brand Names Advate [US]; Helixate® FS [US/Can]; Kogenate® FS [US/Can]; Kogenate® [Can]; Recombinate [US/Can]; ReFacto® [US/Can]

(Continued)

antihemophilic factor (recombinant) *(Continued)*

Therapeutic Category Blood Product Derivative

Use Prevention and treatment of hemorrhagic episodes in patients with hemophilia A (classic hemophilia); perioperative management of hemophilia A; can be of significant therapeutic value in patients with acquired factor VIII inhibitors ≤10 Bethesda units/mL

Usual Dosage Children and Adults: I.V.: Individualize dosage based on coagulation studies performed prior to treatment and at regular intervals during treatment. In general, administration of factor VIII 1 int. unit/kg will increase circulating factor VIII levels by ~2 int. units/dL. (General guidelines presented; consult individual product labeling for specific dosing recommendations.)

Dosage based on desired factor VIII increase (%):

To calculate dosage needed based on desired factor VIII increase (%):

[Body weight (kg) x desired factor VIII increase (%)] divided by 2%/int. units/kg = int. units factor VIII required

For example:

50 kg x 30 (% increase) divided by 2%/int. units/kg = 750 int. units factor VIII

Dosage based on expected factor VIII increase (%):

It is also possible to calculate the **expected** % factor VIII increase:

(# int. units administered x 2%/int. units/kg) divided by body weight (kg) = expected % factor VIII increase

For example:

(1400 int. units x 2%/int. units/kg) divided by 70 kg = 40%

General guidelines:

Minor hemorrhage: 10-20 int. units/kg as a single dose to achieve FVIII plasma level ~20% to 40% of normal. Mild superficial or early hemorrhages may respond to a single dose; may repeat dose every 12-24 hours for 1-3 days until bleeding is resolved or healing achieved.

Moderate hemorrhage/minor surgery: 15-30 int. units/kg to achieve FVIII plasma level 30% to 60% of normal. May repeat 1 dose at 12-24 hours if needed. Some products suggest continuing for ≥3 days until pain and disability are resolved

Major to life-threatening hemorrhage: Initial dose 40-50 int. units/kg followed by a maintenance dose of 20-25 int. units/kg every 8-12 hours until threat is resolved, to achieve FVIII plasma level 80% to 100% of normal.

Major surgery: 50 int. units/kg given preoperatively to raise factor VIII level to 100% before surgery begins. May repeat as necessary after 6-12 hours initially and for a total of 10-14 days until healing is complete. Intensity of therapy may depend on type of surgery and postoperative regimen.

Bleeding prophylaxis: May be administered on a regular basis for bleeding prophylaxis. Doses of 24-40 int. units/kg 3 times/week have been reported in patients with severe hemophilia to prevent joint bleeding.

If bleeding is not controlled with adequate dose, test for presence of inhibitor. It may not be possible or practical to control bleeding if inhibitor titers >10 Bethesda units/mL.

Dosage Forms

Injection, powder for reconstitution, recombinant [preservative free]:

Advate: 250 int. units, 500 int. units, 1000 int. units, 1500 int. units, 2000 int. units [plasma/albumin free; contains sodium 108 mEq/L, mannitol; derived from hamster or mouse proteins]

Helixate® FS, Kogenate® FS: 250 int. units, 500 int. units, 1000 int. units [albumin free; contains sucrose 28 mg/vial, sodium 27-36 mEq/L; derived from hamster or mouse protein]

Recombinate: 250 int. units, 500 units, 1000 int. units [contains human albumin, sodium 180 mEq/L; derived from bovine, hamster or mouse proteins; packaging contains natural rubber latex]

ReFacto®: 250 int. units, 500 units, 1000 int. units, 2000 int. units [contains sucrose; derived from hamster or mouse proteins]

antihemophilic factor/von Willebrand factor complex (human)

(an tee hee moe FIL ik FAK tor von WILL le brand FAK tor KOM plex HYU man)

Synonyms FVIII/vWF

U.S./Canadian Brand Names Humate-P® [US]

Therapeutic Category Antihemophilic Agent; Blood Product Derivative

Use Prevention and treatment of hemorrhagic episodes in patients with hemophilia A (classical hemophilia); treatment of spontaneous bleeding in patients with severe von Willebrand disease (vWD) and in mild or moderate vWD where use of desmopressin is known or suspected to be inadequate

Usual Dosage Children and Adults: I.V.:

Hemophilia A: Individualize dosage based on coagulation studies performed prior to treatment and at regular intervals during treatment; in general, administration of factor VIII 1 int. unit/kg will increase circulating factor VIII levels by ~2 int. units/dL.

Minor hemorrhage: Loading dose: FVIII:C 15 int. units/kg to achieve FVIII:C plasma level ~30% of normal. If second infusion is needed, half the loading dose may be given once or twice daily for 1-2 days.

Moderate hemorrhage: Loading dose: FVIII:C 25 int. units/kg to achieve FVIII:C plasma level ~50% of normal; Maintenance: FVIII:C 15 int. units/kg every 8-12 hours for 1-2 days in order to maintain FVIII:C plasma levels at 30% of normal. Repeat the same dose once or twice daily for up to 7 days or until adequate wound healing.

Life-threatening hemorrhage: Loading dose: FVIII:C 40-50 int. units/kg; Maintenance: FVIII:C 20-25 int. units/kg every 8 hours to maintain FVIII:C plasma levels at 80% to 100% of normal for 7 days. Continue same dose once or twice daily for another 7 days in order to maintain FVIII:C levels at 30% to 50% of normal.

von Willebrand disease (vWD): Individualize dosage based on coagulation studies performed prior to treatment and at regular intervals during treatment; in general, administration of factor VIII 1 int. unit/kg would be expected to raise circulating vWF:RCo approximately 3.5-4 int. units/dL

Type 1, mild (if desmopressin is not appropriate): Major hemorrhage:

Loading dose: vWF:RCo 40-60 int. units/kg

Maintenance dose: vWF:RCo 40-50 int. units/kg every 8-12 hours for 3 days, keeping VWF:RCo nadir >50%; follow with 40-50 int. units/kg daily for up to 7 days

Type 1, moderate or severe:

Minor hemorrhage: vWF:RCo 40-50 int. units/kg for 1-2 doses

Major hemorrhage:

Loading dose: vWF:RCo 50-75 int. units/kg

Maintenance dose: vWF:RCo 40-60 int. units/kg every 8-12 hours for 3 days to keep the VWF:RCo nadir >50%, then 40-60 int. units/kg daily for a total of up to 7 days

Types 2 and 3:

Minor hemorrhage: vWF:RCo 40-50 int. units/kg for 1-2 doses

Major hemorrhage:

Loading dose: vWF:RCo 60-80 int. units/kg

Maintenance dose: vWF:RCo 40-60 int. units/kg every 8-12 hours for 3 days, keeping the VWF:RCo nadir >50%; follow with 40-60 int. units/kg daily for a total of up to 7 days

Dosage Forms

Injection, powder for reconstitution:

Humate-P®: FVIII 250 int. units and vWF:RCo 600 int. units [human derived; contains albumin; packaged with diluent]; FVIII 500 int. units and vWF:RCo 1200 int. units [human derived; contains albumin; packed with diluent]; FVIII 1000 int. units and vWF:RCo 2400 int. units [human derived; contains albumin; packaged with diluent]

Antihist-1® ***(Discontinued)*** *see* clemastine *on page 197*

anti-inhibitor coagulant complex (an tee-in HI bi tor coe AG yoo lant KOM pleks)

Synonyms AICC; coagulant complex inhibitor

U.S./Canadian Brand Names Feiba VH Immuno [Can]; Feiba VH [US]

Therapeutic Category Hemophilic Agent

Use Hemophilia A & B patients with factor VIII inhibitors who are to undergo surgery or those who are bleeding

Usual Dosage I.V.: Children and Adults:

Autoplex® T: Dosage range: 25-100 factor VIII correctional units per kg depending on the severity of hemorrhage; may repeat in ~6 hours if needed. Adjust dose based on patient response.

Feiba VH: General dosing guidelines: 50-100 units/kg (maximum 200 units/kg)

Joint hemorrhage: 50 units/kg every 12 hours; may increase to 100 units/kg; continue until signs of clinical improvement occur

Mucous membrane bleeding: 50 units/kg every 6 hours; may increase to 100 units/kg (maximum: 2 administrations/day or 200 units/kg/day

Soft tissue hemorrhage: 100 units/kg every 12 hours (maximum: 200 units/kg/day)

Other severe hemorrhage: 100 units/kg every 12 hours; may be used every 6 hours if needed; continue until clinical improvement

Dosage Forms [DSC] = Discontinued product

Injection, powder for reconstitution:

Autoplex® T: Each bottle is labeled with correctional units of factor VIII [contains heparin 2 units/mL and sodium 162-192 mEg/L; packaging contains natural rubber latex] [DSC]

Feiba VH: Each bottle is labeled with Immuno units of factor VIII [heparin free; contains sodium 8 mg/mL; packaging contains natural rubber latex]

Antilirium® ***(Discontinued)*** *see* physostigmine *on page 666*

Antiminth® ***(Discontinued)*** *see* pyrantel pamoate *on page 719*

Antiphlogistine Rub A-535 No Odour [Can] *see* trolamine *on page 855*

antipyrine and benzocaine (an tee PYE reen & BEN zoe kane)

Sound-Alike/Look-Alike Issues

Auralgan® may be confused with Ophthalgan®

Synonyms benzocaine and antipyrine

U.S./Canadian Brand Names A/B Otic [US]; Allergen® [US]; Auralgan® [Can]; Aurodex [US]

Therapeutic Category Otic Agent, Analgesic; Otic Agent, Ceruminolytic

Use Temporary relief of pain and reduction of swelling associated with acute congestive and serous otitis media, swimmer's ear, otitis externa; facilitates ear wax removal

Usual Dosage Children and Adults: Otic: Fill ear canal; moisten cotton pledget, place in external ear, repeat every 1-2 hours until pain and congestion are relieved; for ear wax removal instill drops 3-4 times/day for 2-3 days

Dosage Forms

Solution, otic [drops]: Antipyrine 5.4% and benzocaine 1.4% (10 mL)

A/B Otic, Allergen®, Aurodex: Antipyrine 5.4% and benzocaine 1.4% (15 mL)

Antispas® Injection *(Discontinued)* *see* dicyclomine *on page 251*

antithrombin III (an tee THROM bin three)

Synonyms AT-III; heparin cofactor I

U.S./Canadian Brand Names Thrombate III® [US/Can]

Therapeutic Category Blood Product Derivative

Use Treatment of hereditary antithrombin III deficiency in connection with surgical procedures, obstetrical procedures, or thromboembolism

Usual Dosage Adults:

Initial dose: Dosing is individualized based on pretherapy AT-III levels. The initial dose should raise antithrombin III levels (AT-III) to 120% and may be calculated based on the following formula:

[desired AT-III level % - baseline AT-III level %] x body weight (kg) divided by 1.4%/int. units/kg

For example, if a 70 kg adult patient had a baseline AT-III level of 57%, the initial dose would be [(120% - 57%) x 70] divided by 1.4 = 3150 int. units

Maintenance dose: Subsequent dosing should be targeted to keep levels between 80% to 120% which may be achieved by administering 60% of the initial dose every 24 hours. Adjustments may be made by adjusting dose or interval. Maintain level within normal range for 2-8 days depending on type of procedure.

Dosage Forms Injection, powder for reconstitution [preservative free]: 500 int. units, 1000 int. units [contains heparin, sodium chloride 110-210 mEq/L; packaged with diluent]

antithymocyte globulin (equine) (an te THY moe site GLOB yu lin, E kwine)

Sound-Alike/Look-Alike Issues

Atgam® may be confused with Ativan®

Synonyms antithymocyte immunoglobulin; ATG; horse antihuman thymocyte gamma globulin; lymphocyte immune globulin

U.S./Canadian Brand Names Atgam® [US/Can]

Therapeutic Category Immunosuppressant Agent

Use Prevention and treatment of acute renal allograft rejection; treatment of moderate to severe aplastic anemia in patients not considered suitable candidates for bone marrow transplantation

Usual Dosage An intradermal skin test is recommended prior to administration of the initial dose of ATG; use 0.1 mL of a 1:1000 dilution of ATG in normal saline. A positive skin reaction consists of a wheal ≥10 mm in diameter. If a positive skin test occurs, the first infusion should be administered in a controlled environment with intensive life support immediately available. A systemic reaction precludes further administration of the drug. The absence of a reaction does **not** preclude the possibility of an immediate sensitivity reaction.

Premedication with diphenhydramine, hydrocortisone, and acetaminophen is recommended prior to first dose.

Children: I.V.:

Aplastic anemia protocol: 10-20 mg/kg/day for 8-14 days; then administer every other day for 7 more doses; addition doses may be given every other day for 21 total doses in 28 days

Renal allograft: 5-25 mg/kg/day

Adults: I.V.:

Aplastic anemia protocol: 10-20 mg/kg/day for 8-14 days, then administer every other day for 7 more doses, for a total of 21 doses in 28 days

Renal allograft:

Rejection prophylaxis: 15 mg/kg/day for 14 days followed by 14 days of alternative day therapy at the same dose; the first dose should be administered within 24 hours before or after transplantation

Rejection treatment: 10-15 mg/kg/day for 14 days, then administer every other day for 10-14 days up to 21 doses in 28 days

Dosage Forms Injection, solution: 50 mg/mL (5 mL)

antithymocyte globulin (rabbit) (an te THY moe site GLOB yu lin (RAB bit)

U.S./Canadian Brand Names Thymoglobulin® [US]

Therapeutic Category Immunosuppressant Agent

Use Treatment of renal transplant acute rejection in conjunction with concomitant immunosuppression

Usual Dosage I.V.: 1.5 mg/kg/day for 7-14 days

Dosage Forms Injection, powder for reconstitution: 25 mg [packaged with diluent]

antithymocyte immunoglobulin *see* antithymocyte globulin (equine) *on previous page*

antitumor necrosis factor apha (human) *see* adalimumab *on page 19*

Anti-Tuss® Expectorant *(Discontinued)* *see* guaifenesin *on page 392*

anti-VEGF monoclonal antibody *see* bevacizumab *on page 109*

antivenin *(Crotalidae)* polyvalent (an tee VEN in (kroe TAL ih die) pol i VAY lent)

Synonyms crotalidae antivenin; crotaline antivenin, polyvalent; North and South American antisnake-bite serum; pit viper antivenin; snake (pit vipers) antivenin

U.S./Canadian Brand Names Antivenin Polyvalent [Equine] [US]; CroFab™ [Ovine] [US]

Therapeutic Category Antivenin

Use Neutralization of venoms of North and South American crotalids: Rattlesnake, copperhead, cottonmouth, tropical moccasins, fer-de-lance, bushmaster

Usual Dosage Children and Adults: Crotalid envenomation:

Antivenin polyvalent (equine): I.M., I.V.: Initial sensitivity test: 0.02-0.03 mL of a 1:10 dilution of normal horse serum or antivenin given intracutaneously; also give a control test using normal saline in the opposite extremity. A positive reaction occurs within 5-30 minutes. A negative reaction does not rule out the possibility of an immediate or delayed reaction with treatment.

Minimal envenomation: 20-40 mL (2-4 vials)

Moderate envenomation: 50-90 mL (5-9 vials)

Severe envenomation: 100-150 mL (10-15 vials) or more

Note: The entire initial dose of antivenin should be administered as soon as possible to be most effective (within 4 hours after the bite). I.V. is the preferred route of administration. When administered I.V., infuse the initial 5-10 mL dilution over 3-5 minutes while carefully observing the patient for signs and symptoms of sensitivity reactions. If no reaction occurs, continue infusion at a safe I.V. fluid delivery rate. Additional doses of antivenin are based on clinical response to the initial dose. If swelling continues to progress, symptoms increase in severity, hypotension occurs, or decrease in hematocrit appears, an additional 10-50 mL (1-5 vials) should be administered.

Antivenin polyvalent (ovine): I.V.: Minimal or moderate envenomation:

Initial dose: 4-6 vials, dependent upon patient response. Treatment should begin within 6 hours of snakebite; monitor for 1 hour following infusion. Repeat with an additional 4-6 vials if control is not achieved with initial dose. Continue to treat with 4- to 6-vial doses until complete arrest of local manifestations, coagulation tests, and systemic signs are normal. Administer I.V. over 60 minutes at a rate of 25-50 mL/hour for the first 10 minutes. If no allergic reaction is observed, increase rate to 250 mL/hour. Monitor closely

Maintenance dose: Once control is achieved, administer 2 vials every 6 hours for up to 18 hours; optimal dosing past 18 hours has not been established; however, treatment may be continued if deemed necessary based on the patients condition

Dosage Forms Injection, powder for reconstitution:

Antivenin (Crotalidae) polyvalent [equine]: Derived from *Crotalus adamanteus*, *C. atrox*, *C. durissus terrificus*, and *Bothrops atrox* snake venoms [equine origin; contains phenol and thimerosal; packaged with diluent and normal horse serum for sensitivity testing]

CroFab™ [ovine]: Derived from *Crotalus adamanteus*, *C. atrox*, *C. scutulatus*, and *Agkistrodon piscivorus* snake venoms [ovine origin; contains thimerosal; manufactured with papain]

antivenin *(Latrodectus mactans)* (an tee VEN in lak tro DUK tus MAK tans)

Synonyms black widow spider species antivenin (*Latrodectus mactans*)

Therapeutic Category Antivenin

Use Treatment of patients with symptoms of black widow spider bites

Usual Dosage

Skin test: Intradermal: Children and Adults: 0.02 mL of a 1:10 dilution in NS (also use a control solution of NS); evaluate in 10 minutes. Positive reaction is urticarial wheal surrounded by zone of erythema

Conjunctival test: Ophthalmic:

Children: Instill 1 drop of a 1:100 dilution into the conjunctival sac

Adults: Instill 1 drop of a 1:10 dilution into the conjunctival sac

Note: Itching of the eye and/or reddening of conjunctiva indicates a positive reaction, usually occurring within 10 minutes.

Desensitization: Children and Adults: **Note:** In separate vials or syringes, prepare 1:10 and 1:100 dilutions of antivenin in NS.

SubQ: Inject 0.1, 0.2, and 0.5 mL of the 1:100 dilution at 15- to 30- minute intervals. Proceed with the next dose only if no reaction has occurred following the previous. Repeat procedure using the 1:10 dilution and then undiluted antivenin.

If a reaction occurs, apply tourniquet proximal to the injection site and administer epinephrine 1:1000. Wait at least 30 minutes, then administer another antivenin injection at the last dose which did not evoke a reaction.

If no reaction has occurred following 0.5 mL of undiluted antivenin, continue the dose at 15 minute intervals until entire dose has been administered.

Treatment of symptoms due to black widow spider bite: Administer only following the skin test or conjunctival test:

Children <12 years: I.V.: 2.5 mL

Children >12 years and Adults: I.M., I.V.: 2.5 mL

Dosage Forms Injection, powder for reconstitution: 6000 antivenin units [equine origin; contains thimerosal; packaged with diluent and normal horse serum for sensitivity testing]

antivenin *(Micrurus fulvius)* (an tee VEN in mye KRU rus FUL vee us)

Synonyms North American coral snake antivenin

Therapeutic Category Antivenin

Use Neutralization of venoms of Eastern coral snake and Texas coral snake, but does **not** neutralize venom of Arizona or Sonoran coral snake

Usual Dosage I.V.: Children and Adults: 3-5 vials by slow injection (dependent on severity of signs/symptoms; some patients may need more than 10 vials)

Dosage Forms Injection, powder for reconstitution: Derived from *Micrurus fulvius* venom [equine origin; contains phenol and thimerosal; packaged with diluent] [DSC]

Antivenin Polyvalent [Equine] [US] *see* antivenin *(Crotalidae)* polyvalent *on previous page*

Antivert® [US] *see* meclizine *on page 522*

Antizol® [US] *see* fomepizole *on page 366*

Antrizine® *(Discontinued)* *see* meclizine *on page 522*

Anturane® *(Discontinued)* *see* sulfinpyrazone *on page 799*

Anucort-HC® [US] *see* hydrocortisone (rectal) *on page 426*

Anu-Med [US-OTC] *see* phenylephrine *on page 660*

Anusol-HC® [US] *see* hydrocortisone (rectal) *on page 426*

Anusol® HC-1 [US-OTC] *see* hydrocortisone (rectal) *on page 426*

Anusol® Ointment [US-OTC] *see* pramoxine *on page 691*

Anuzinc [Can] *see* zinc sulfate *on page 888*

Anxanil® Oral *(Discontinued)* *see* hydroxyzine *on page 433*

Anzemet® [US/Can] *see* dolasetron *on page 271*

Apacet® *(Discontinued)* *see* acetaminophen *on page 5*

APAP *see* acetaminophen *on page 5*

APAP and tramadol *see* acetaminophen and tramadol *on page 10*

Apaphen® *(Discontinued)* *see* acetaminophen and phenyltoloxamine *on page 8*

Apatate® [US-OTC] *see* vitamin B complex combinations *on page 876*

ApexiCon™ [US] *see* diflorasone *on page 253*
ApexiCon™ E [US] *see* diflorasone *on page 253*
Aphedrid™ [US-OTC] *see* triprolidine and pseudoephedrine *on page 853*
Aphrodyne® [US] *see* yohimbine *on page 883*
Aphthasol® [US] *see* amlexanox *on page 45*
Apidra® [US] *see* insulin glulisine *on page 450*
A.P.L.® ***(Discontinued)*** *see* chorionic gonadotropin (human) *on page 186*
Aplisol® [US] *see* tuberculin tests *on page 857*
Aplitest® ***(Discontinued)*** *see* tuberculin tests *on page 857*
aplonidine *see* apraclonidine *on page 71*
Apo-Acebutolol® [Can] *see* acebutolol *on page 4*
Apo-Acetaminophen® [Can] *see* acetaminophen *on page 5*
Apo-Acetazolamide® [Can] *see* acetazolamide *on page 14*
Apo-Acyclovir® [Can] *see* acyclovir *on page 18*
Apo-Alendronate® [Can] *see* alendronate *on page 27*
Apo-Allopurinol® [Can] *see* allopurinol *on page 30*
Apo-Alpraz® [Can] *see* alprazolam *on page 32*
Apo-Amiloride® [Can] *see* amiloride *on page 41*
Apo-Amilzide® [Can] *see* amiloride and hydrochlorothiazide *on page 41*
Apo-Amiodarone® [Can] *see* amiodarone *on page 43*
Apo-Amitriptyline® [Can] *see* amitriptyline *on page 44*
Apo-Amoxi® [Can] *see* amoxicillin *on page 47*
Apo-Amoxi-Clav® [Can] *see* amoxicillin and clavulanate potassium *on page 49*
Apo-Ampi® [Can] *see* ampicillin *on page 53*
Apo-Atenol® [Can] *see* atenolol *on page 80*
Apo-Azathioprine® [Can] *see* azathioprine *on page 86*
Apo-Azithromycin® [Can] *see* azithromycin *on page 88*
Apo-Baclofen® [Can] *see* baclofen *on page 91*
Apo-Beclomethasone® [Can] *see* beclomethasone *on page 95*
Apo-Benazepril® [Can] *see* benazepril *on page 97*
Apo-Benztropine® [Can] *see* benztropine *on page 104*
Apo-Benzydamine® [Can] *see* benzydamine *(Canada only) on page 104*
Apo-Bisacodyl® [Can] *see* bisacodyl *on page 111*
Apo-Bisoprolol® [Can] *see* bisoprolol *on page 113*
Apo-Bromazepam® [Can] *see* bromazepam *(Canada only) on page 117*
Apo-Bromocriptine® [Can] *see* bromocriptine *on page 117*
Apo-Buspirone® [Can] *see* buspirone *on page 127*
Apo-Butorphanol® [Can] *see* butorphanol *on page 130*
Apo-Cal® [Can] *see* calcium carbonate *on page 135*
Apo-Calcitonin® [Can] *see* calcitonin *on page 133*
Apo-Capto® [Can] *see* captopril *on page 143*
Apo-Carbamazepine® [Can] *see* carbamazepine *on page 144*
Apo-Carvedilol® [Can] *see* carvedilol *on page 154*
Apo-Cefaclor® [Can] *see* cefaclor *on page 155*
Apo-Cefadroxil® [Can] *see* cefadroxil *on page 156*
Apo-Cefuroxime® [Can] *see* cefuroxime *on page 163*
Apo-Cephalex® [Can] *see* cephalexin *on page 166*
Apo-Cetirizine® [Can] *see* cetirizine *on page 167*

Apo-Levobunolol® [Can] *see* levobunolol *on page 488*
Apo-Levocarb® [Can] *see* levodopa and carbidopa *on page 489*
Apo-Levocarb® CR [Can] *see* levodopa and carbidopa *on page 489*
Apo-Lisinopril® [Can] *see* lisinopril *on page 500*
Apo-Lithium® Carbonate [Can] *see* lithium *on page 501*
Apo-Lithium® Carbonate SR [Can] *see* lithium *on page 501*
Apo-Loperamide® [Can] *see* loperamide *on page 503*
Apo-Loratadine® [Can] *see* loratadine *on page 505*
Apo-Lorazepam® [Can] *see* lorazepam *on page 506*
Apo-Lovastatin® [Can] *see* lovastatin *on page 508*
Apo-Loxapine® [Can] *see* loxapine *on page 509*
Apo-Medroxy® [Can] *see* medroxyprogesterone *on page 524*
Apo-Mefenamic® [Can] *see* mefenamic acid *on page 525*
Apo-Mefloquine® [Can] *see* mefloquine *on page 525*
Apo-Megestrol® [Can] *see* megestrol *on page 525*
Apo-Meloxicam® [Can] *see* meloxicam *on page 526*
Apo-Metformin® [Can] *see* metformin *on page 535*
Apo-Methazide® [Can] *see* methyldopa and hydrochlorothiazide *on page 545*
Apo-Methazolamide® [Can] *see* methazolamide *on page 538*
Apo-Methoprazine® [Can] *see* methotrimeprazine *(Canada only) on page 542*
Apo-Methotrexate® [Can] *see* methotrexate *on page 540*
Apo-Methyldopa® [Can] *see* methyldopa *on page 544*
Apo-Methylphenidate® [Can] *see* methylphenidate *on page 546*
Apo-Methylphenidate® SR [Can] *see* methylphenidate *on page 546*
Apo-Metoclop® [Can] *see* metoclopramide *on page 549*
Apo-Metoprolol® [Can] *see* metoprolol *on page 550*
Apo-Metronidazole® [Can] *see* metronidazole *on page 551*
Apo-Midazolam® [Can] *see* midazolam *on page 555*
Apo-Midodrine® [Can] *see* midodrine *on page 556*
Apo-Minocycline® [Can] *see* minocycline *on page 558*
Apo-Misoprostol® [Can] *see* misoprostol *on page 560*
Apo-Moclobemide® [Can] *see* moclobemide *(Canada only) on page 562*

apomorphine (a poe MOR feen)

Synonyms apomorphine hydrochloride; apomorphine hydrochloride hemihydrate
U.S./Canadian Brand Names Apokyn™ [US]
Therapeutic Category Anti-Parkinson Agent (Dopamine Agonist)
Use Treatment of hypomobility, "off" episodes with Parkinson disease
Usual Dosage SubQ: Adults: Begin antiemetic therapy 3 days prior to initiation and continue for 2 months before reassessing need.

Parkinson disease, "off" episode: Initial test dose 2 mg, **medical supervision required; see "Note"**. Subsequent dosing is based on both tolerance and response to initial test dose.

If patient tolerates test dose and responds: Starting dose: 2 mg as needed; may increase dose in 1 mg increments every few days; maximum dose: 6 mg

If patient tolerates but does not respond to 2 mg test dose: Second test dose: 4 mg

If patient tolerates and responds to 4 mg test dose: Starting dose: 3 mg, as needed for "off" episodes; may increase dose in 1 mg increments every few days; maximum dose 6 mg

If patient does not tolerate 4 mg test dose: Third test dose: 3 mg

If patient tolerates 3 mg test dose: Starting dose: 2 mg as needed for "off" episodes; may increase dose in 1 mg increments to a maximum of 3 mg

If therapy is interrupted for >1 week, restart at 2 mg and gradually titrate dose.

Note: Medical supervision is required for all test doses with standing and supine blood pressure monitoring predose and 20-, 40-, and 60 minutes postdose. If subsequent test doses are required, wait >2 hours before another test dose is given; next test dose should be timed with another "off" episode. If a single dose is ineffective for a particular "off" episode, then a second dose should not be given. The average dosing frequency was 3 times/day in the development program with limited experience in dosing >5 times/day and with total daily doses >20 mg. Apomorphine is intended to treat the "off" episodes associated with levodopa therapy of Parkinson disease and has not been studied in levodopa-naive Parkinson patients.

Dosage Forms

Injection, solution, as hydrochloride:

Apokyn®: 10 mg/mL (2 mL) [ampul; contains sodium metabisulfite]; (3 mL) [multidose cartridge; contains sodium metabisulfite and benzyl alcohol]

apomorphine hydrochloride *see* apomorphine *on previous page*

apomorphine hydrochloride hemihydrate *see* apomorphine *on previous page*

Apo-Nabumetone® [Can] *see* nabumetone *on page 572*

Apo-Nadol® [Can] *see* nadolol *on page 573*

Apo-Napro-Na® [Can] *see* naproxen *on page 578*

Apo-Napro-Na DS® [Can] *see* naproxen *on page 578*

Apo-Naproxen® [Can] *see* naproxen *on page 578*

Apo-Naproxen EC® [Can] *see* naproxen *on page 578*

Apo-Naproxen SR® [Can] *see* naproxen *on page 578*

Apo-Nifed® [Can] *see* nifedipine *on page 592*

Apo-Nifed PA® [Can] *see* nifedipine *on page 592*

Apo-Nitrofurantoin® [Can] *see* nitrofurantoin *on page 594*

Apo-Nizatidine® [Can] *see* nizatidine *on page 597*

Apo-Norflox® [Can] *see* norfloxacin *on page 599*

Apo-Nortriptyline® [Can] *see* nortriptyline *on page 600*

Apo-Oflox® [Can] *see* ofloxacin *on page 611*

Apo-Ofloxacin® [Can] *see* ofloxacin *on page 611*

Apo-Omeprazole® [Can] *see* omeprazole *on page 615*

Apo-Orciprenaline® [Can] *see* metaproterenol *on page 535*

Apo-Oxaprozin® [Can] *see* oxaprozin *on page 623*

Apo-Oxazepam® [Can] *see* oxazepam *on page 623*

Apo-Oxybutynin® [Can] *see* oxybutynin *on page 625*

Apo-Paclitaxel® [Can] *see* paclitaxel *on page 631*

Apo-Paroxetine® [Can] *see* paroxetine *on page 639*

Apo-Pentoxifylline SR® [Can] *see* pentoxifylline *on page 653*

Apo-Pen VK® [Can] *see* penicillin V potassium *on page 649*

Apo-Perphenazine® [Can] *see* perphenazine *on page 655*

Apo-Pimozide® [Can] *see* pimozide *on page 668*

Apo-Pindol® [Can] *see* pindolol *on page 669*

Apo-Piroxicam® [Can] *see* piroxicam *on page 671*

Apo-Pravastatin® [Can] *see* pravastatin *on page 692*

Apo-Prazo® [Can] *see* prazosin *on page 693*

Apo-Prednisone® [Can] *see* prednisone *on page 695*

Apo-Primidone® [Can] *see* primidone *on page 699*

Apo-Procainamide® [Can] *see* procainamide *on page 700*

Apo-Prochlorperazine® [Can] *see* prochlorperazine *on page 701*

Apo-Propafenone® [Can] *see* propafenone *on page 706*

Apo-Propranolol® [Can] *see* propranolol *on page 709*

Apo-Quinidine® [Can] *see* quinidine *on page 725*

Apo-Quinine® [Can] *see* quinine *on page 726*
Apo-Ranitidine® [Can] *see* ranitidine *on page 732*
Apo-Risperidone® [Can] *see* risperidone *on page 748*
Apo-Salvent® [Can] *see* albuterol *on page 23*
Apo-Salvent® CFC Free [Can] *see* albuterol *on page 23*
Apo-Salvent® Respirator Solution [Can] *see* albuterol *on page 23*
Apo-Salvent® Sterules [Can] *see* albuterol *on page 23*
Apo-Selegiline® [Can] *see* selegiline *on page 766*
Apo-Sertraline® [Can] *see* sertraline *on page 769*
Apo-Simvastatin® [Can] *see* simvastatin *on page 773*
Apo-Sotalol® [Can] *see* sotalol *on page 787*
Apo-Sulfatrim® [Can] *see* sulfamethoxazole and trimethoprim *on page 797*
Apo-Sulfatrim® DS [Can] *see* sulfamethoxazole and trimethoprim *on page 797*
Apo-Sulfatrim® Pediatric [Can] *see* sulfamethoxazole and trimethoprim *on page 797*
Apo-Sulfinpyrazone® [Can] *see* sulfinpyrazone *on page 799*
Apo-Sulin® [Can] *see* sulindac *on page 800*
Apo-Sumatriptan® [Can] *see* sumatriptan *on page 801*
Apo-Tamox® [Can] *see* tamoxifen *on page 804*
Apo-Temazepam® [Can] *see* temazepam *on page 808*
Apo-Terazosin® [Can] *see* terazosin *on page 810*
Apo-Tetra® [Can] *see* tetracycline *on page 816*
Apo-Theo LA® [Can] *see* theophylline *on page 818*
Apo-Tiaprofenic® [Can] *see* tiaprofenic acid *(Canada only) on page 826*
Apo-Ticlopidine® [Can] *see* ticlopidine *on page 827*
Apo-Timol® [Can] *see* timolol *on page 828*
Apo-Timop® [Can] *see* timolol *on page 828*
Apo-Tizanidine® [Can] *see* tizanidine *on page 831*
Apo-Tolbutamide® [Can] *see* tolbutamide *on page 834*
Apo-Trazodone® [Can] *see* trazodone *on page 843*
Apo-Trazodone D® [Can] *see* trazodone *on page 843*
Apo-Triazide® [Can] *see* hydrochlorothiazide and triamterene *on page 420*
Apo-Triazo® [Can] *see* triazolam *on page 848*
Apo-Trifluoperazine® [Can] *see* trifluoperazine *on page 849*
Apo-Trihex® [Can] *see* trihexyphenidyl *on page 850*
Apo-Trimebutine® [Can] *see* trimebutine *(Canada only) on page 850*
Apo-Trimethoprim® [Can] *see* trimethoprim *on page 851*
Apo-Trimip® [Can] *see* trimipramine *on page 852*
Apo-Valproic® [Can] *see* valproic acid and derivatives *on page 864*
Apo-Verap® [Can] *see* verapamil *on page 870*
Apo-Verap® SR [Can] *see* verapamil *on page 870*
Apo-Warfarin® [Can] *see* warfarin *on page 881*
Apo-Zidovudine® [Can] *see* zidovudine *on page 886*
Apo-Zopiclone® [Can] *see* zopiclone *(Canada only) on page 890*
APPG *see* penicillin G procaine *on page 649*
Apra Children's [US-OTC] *see* acetaminophen *on page 5*

apraclonidine (a pra KLOE ni deen)

Sound-Alike/Look-Alike Issues
Iopidine® may be confused with indapamide, iodine, Lodine®

Synonyms aplonidine; apraclonidine hydrochloride; p-aminoclonidine

U.S./Canadian Brand Names Iopidine® [US/Can]

Therapeutic Category Alpha$_2$-Adrenergic Agonist Agent, Ophthalmic

Use Prevention and treatment of postsurgical intraocular pressure (IOP) elevation; short-term, adjunctive therapy in patients who require additional reduction of IOP

Usual Dosage Adults: Ophthalmic:
0.5%: Instill 1-2 drops in the affected eye(s) 3 times/day
1%: Instill 1 drop in operative eye 1 hour prior to anterior segment laser surgery, second drop in eye immediately upon completion of procedure

Dosage Forms
Solution, ophthalmic:
Iopidine®: 0.5% (5 mL, 10 mL); 1% (0.1 mL) [contains benzalkonium chloride]

apraclonidine hydrochloride *see* apraclonidine *on this page*

aprepitant (ap RE pi tant)

Synonyms L 754030; MK 869

U.S./Canadian Brand Names Emend® [US]

Therapeutic Category Antiemetic

Use Prevention of acute and delayed nausea and vomiting associated with moderately- and highly-emetogenic chemotherapy in combination with a corticosteroid and 5-HT$_3$ receptor antagonist; prevention of postoperative nausea and vomiting (PONV)

Usual Dosage Oral: Adults:
Prevention of chemotherapy induced nausea/vomiting: 125 mg on day 1, followed by 80 mg on days 2 and 3 in combination with a corticosteroid and 5-HT$_3$ receptor antagonist
In clinical trials, the following regimens were used:
For highly-emetogenic chemotherapy:
Aprepitant: Oral: 125 mg on day 1, followed by 80 mg on days 2 and 3
Dexamethasone: Oral: 12 mg on day 1, followed 8 mg on days 2, 3, and 4
Ondansetron: I.V.: 32 mg on day 1
For moderately-emetogenic chemotherapy:
Aprepitant: Oral: 125 mg on day 1, followed by 80 mg on days 2 and 3
Dexamethasone: Oral: 12 mg on day 1 only
Ondansetron: Oral: Two 8 mg doses on day 1 only
Prevention of PONV: 40 mg within 3 hours prior to induction

Dosage Forms
Capsule:
Emend®: 40 mg, 80 mg, 125 mg
Combination package: Capsule 80 mg (2s), capsule 125 mg (1s)

Apresoline® [Can] *see* hydralazine *on page 418*

Apresoline® *(Discontinued)* *see* hydralazine *on page 418*

Apri® [US] *see* ethinyl estradiol and desogestrel *on page 317*

Aprodine® [US-OTC] *see* triprolidine and pseudoephedrine *on page 853*

aprotinin (a proe TYE nin)

U.S./Canadian Brand Names Trasylol® [US/Can]

Therapeutic Category Hemostatic Agent

Use Reduction of blood loss in patients undergoing cardiopulmonary bypass in coronary artery bypass graft surgery

Usual Dosage Adults:
Test dose: **All** patients should receive a 1 mL (1.4 mg) I.V. test dose at least 10 minutes prior to the loading dose to assess the potential for allergic reactions. **Note:** To avoid physical incompatibility with heparin when adding to pump-prime solution, each agent should be added during recirculation to assure adequate dilution.
Regimen A (standard dose):
2 million KIU (280 mg; 200 mL) loading dose I.V. over 20-30 minutes
2 million KIU (280 mg; 200 mL) into pump prime volume
500,000 KIU/hour (70 mg/hour; 50 mL/hour) I.V. during operation
(Continued)

aprotinin *(Continued)*

Regimen B (low dose):

1 million KIU (140 mg; 100 mL) loading dose I.V. over 20-30 minutes

1 million KIU (140 mg; 100 mL) into pump prime volume

250,000 KIU/hour (35 mg/hour; 25 mL/hour) I.V. during operation

Dosage Forms Injection, solution: 1.4 mg/mL [10,000 KIU/mL] (100 mL, 200 mL) [bovine derived]

Aptivus® [US/Can] *see* tipranavir *on page 830*

Aquacare® [US-OTC] *see* urea *on page 861*

Aquachloral® Supprettes® [US] *see* chloral hydrate *on page 171*

Aquacort® [Can] *see* hydrocortisone (topical) *on page 428*

AquaLase™ [US] *see* balanced salt solution *on page 92*

AquaMEPHYTON® [Can] *see* phytonadione *on page 667*

AquaMEPHYTON® *(Discontinued)* *see* phytonadione *on page 667*

Aquanil™ HC [US-OTC] *see* hydrocortisone (topical) *on page 428*

Aquaphilic® With Carbamide [US-OTC] *see* urea *on page 861*

Aquaphyllin® *(Discontinued)* *see* theophylline *on page 818*

AquaSite® [US-OTC] *see* artificial tears *on page 75*

Aquasol A® [US] *see* vitamin A *on page 874*

Aquasol E® [US-OTC] *see* vitamin E *on page 876*

Aquatab® C *(Discontinued)* *see* guaifenesin, pseudoephedrine, and dextromethorphan *on page 401*

Aquatab® D *(Discontinued)* *see* guaifenesin and pseudoephedrine *on page 398*

Aquatab® DM *(Discontinued)* *see* guaifenesin and dextromethorphan *on page 394*

AquaTar® *(Discontinued)* *see* coal tar *on page 207*

Aquatensen® [Can] *see* methyclothiazide *on page 543*

Aquavit-E® [US-OTC] *see* vitamin E *on page 876*

aqueous procaine penicillin G *see* penicillin G procaine *on page 649*

ara-C *see* cytarabine *on page 224*

arabinosylcytosine *see* cytarabine *on page 224*

Aralast [US] *see* $alpha_1$-proteinase inhibitor *on page 31*

Aralen® [US] *see* chloroquine *on page 175*

Aranelle™ [US] *see* ethinyl estradiol and norethindrone *on page 323*

Aranesp® [US/Can] *see* darbepoetin alfa *on page 230*

Arava® [US/Can] *see* leflunomide *on page 484*

Arduan® *(Discontinued)*

Aredia® [US/Can] *see* pamidronate *on page 633*

argatroban (ar GA troh ban)

Sound-Alike/Look-Alike Issues

argatroban may be confused with Aggrastat®

Therapeutic Category Anticoagulant, Thrombin Inhibitor

Use Prophylaxis or treatment of thrombosis in adults with heparin-induced thrombocytopenia; adjunct to percutaneous coronary intervention (PCI) in patients who have or are at risk of thrombosis associated with heparin-induced thrombocytopenia

Usual Dosage I.V.: Adults:

Heparin-induced thrombocytopenia:

Initial dose: 2 mcg/kg/minute

Maintenance dose: Measure aPTT after 2 hours, adjust dose until the steady-state aPTT is 1.5-3.0 times the initial baseline value, not exceeding 100 seconds; dosage should not exceed 10 mcg/kg/minute

Conversion to oral anticoagulant: Because there may be a combined effect on the INR when argatroban is combined with warfarin, loading doses of warfarin should not be used. Warfarin therapy should be started at the expected daily dose.

Patients receiving ≤2 mcg/kg/minute of argatroban: Argatroban therapy can be stopped when the combined INR on warfarin and argatroban is >4; repeat INR measurement in 4-6 hours; if INR is below therapeutic level, argatroban therapy may be restarted. Repeat procedure daily until desired INR on warfarin alone is obtained.

Patients receiving >2 mcg/kg/minute of argatroban: Reduce dose of argatroban to 2 mcg/kg/minute; measure INR for argatroban and warfarin 4-6 hours after dose reduction; argatroban therapy can be stopped when the combined INR on warfarin and argatroban is >4. Repeat INR measurement in 4-6 hours; if INR is below therapeutic level, argatroban therapy may be restarted. Repeat procedure daily until desired INR on warfarin alone is obtained.

Note: Critically-ill patients with normal hepatic function became excessively anticoagulated with FDA-approved or lower starting doses of argatroban. Doses between 0.15-1.3 mcg/kg/minute were required to maintain aPTTs in the target range. Another report of a cardiac patient with anasarca secondary to acute renal failure had a reduction in argatroban clearance similar to patients with hepatic dysfunction. Reduced clearance may have been attributed to reduced perfusion to the liver. Consider reducing starting dose to 0.5-1 mcg/kg/minute in critically-ill patients who may have impaired hepatic perfusion (eg, patients requiring vasopressors, having decreased cardiac output, having fluid overload). In a retrospective review of critical care patients, patients with three organ system failure required 0.5 mcg/kg/minute. The mean argatroban dose of ICU patients was 0.9 mcg/kg/minute.

Percutaneous coronary intervention (PCI):

Initial: Begin infusion of 25 mcg/kg/minute and administer bolus dose of 350 mcg/kg (over 3-5 minutes). ACT should be checked 5-10 minutes after bolus infusion; proceed with procedure if ACT >300 seconds. Following initial bolus:

ACT <300 seconds: Give an additional 150 mcg/kg bolus, and increase infusion rate to 30 mcg/kg/minute (recheck ACT in 5-10 minutes)

ACT >450 seconds: Decrease infusion rate to 15 mcg/kg/minute (recheck ACT in 5-10 minutes)

Once a therapeutic ACT (300-450 seconds) is achieved, infusion should be continued at this dose for the duration of the procedure.

If dissection, impending abrupt closure, thrombus formation during PCI, or inability to achieve ACT >300 sec: An additional bolus of 150 mcg/kg, followed by an increase in infusion rate to 40 mcg/kg/minute may be administered.

Note: Post-PCI anticoagulation, if required, may be achieved by continuing infusion at a reduced dose of 2-10 mcg/kg/minute, with close monitoring of aPTT.

Dosage Forms Injection, solution: 100 mg/mL (2.5 mL) [contains dehydrated alcohol 1000 mg/mL]

arginine (AR ji neen)

Synonyms arginine hydrochloride

U.S./Canadian Brand Names R-Gene® [US]

Therapeutic Category Diagnostic Agent

Use Pituitary function test (growth hormone)

Usual Dosage I.V.: Pituitary function test:

Children: 500 mg/kg/dose administered over 30 minutes

Adults: 30 g (300 mL) administered over 30 minutes

Dosage Forms Injection, solution, as hydrochloride: 10% [100 mg/mL = 950 mOsm/L] (300 mL) [contains chloride 0.475 mEq/mL]

arginine hydrochloride *see* arginine *on this page*

8-arginine vasopressin *see* vasopressin *on page 868*

Aricept® [US/Can] *see* donepezil *on page 273*

Aricept® ODT [US] *see* donepezil *on page 273*

Aricept® RDT [Can] *see* donepezil *on page 273*

Arimidex® [US/Can] *see* anastrozole *on page 56*

aripiprazole (ay ri PIP ray zole)

Sound-Alike/Look-Alike Issues

aripiprazole may be confused with rabeprazole

Synonyms BMS 337039; OPC-14597

U.S./Canadian Brand Names Abilify® [US]

Therapeutic Category Antipsychotic Agent, Quinolone

Use Treatment of schizophrenia; stabilization and maintenance therapy of bipolar disorder (with acute manic or mixed episodes)

(Continued)

aripiprazole *(Continued)*

Usual Dosage Oral: **Note:** Oral solution may be substituted for the oral tablet on a mg-per-mg basis, up to 25 mg. Patients receiving 30 mg tablets should be given 25 mg oral solution.
Adults:
Schizophrenia: 10-15 mg once daily; may be increased to a maximum of 30 mg once daily (efficacy at dosages above 10-15 mg has not been shown to be increased). Dosage titration should not be more frequent than every 2 weeks.
Bipolar disorder (acute manic or mixed episodes):
Stabilization: 30 mg once daily; may require a decrease to 15 mg based on tolerability (15% of patients had dose decreased); safety of doses >30 mg/day has not been evaluated
Maintenance: Continue stabilization dose for up to 6 weeks; efficacy of continued treatment >6 weeks has not been established

Dosage Forms
Solution, oral:
Abilify®: 1 mg/mL (150 mL) [contains sucrose 400 mg/mL and fructose 200 mg/mL; orange cream flavor]
Tablet:
Abilify®: 2 mg, 5 mg, 10 mg, 15 mg, 20 mg, 30 mg
Tablet, orally disintegrating:
Abilify® Discmelt™: 10 mg [contains phenylalanine 1.12 mg; creme de vanilla flavor]; 15 mg [contains phenylalanine 1.68 mg; creme de vanilla flavor]; 20 mg [contains phenylalanine 2.25 mg; creme de vanilla flavor]; 30 mg [contains phenylalanine 3.37 mg; creme de vanilla flavor]

Aristocort® [US/Can] *see* triamcinolone (systemic) *on page 846*
Aristocort® A [US] *see* triamcinolone (topical) *on page 846*
Aristospan® [US/Can] *see* triamcinolone (systemic) *on page 846*
Arixtra® [US/Can] *see* fondaparinux *on page 367*
A.R.M® [US-OTC] *see* chlorpheniramine and pseudoephedrine *on page 177*
Arm-a-Med® Isoproterenol *(Discontinued)* *see* isoproterenol *on page 464*
Arm-a-Med® Metaproterenol *(Discontinued)*
Armour® Thyroid [US] *see* thyroid *on page 824*
Aromasin® [US/Can] *see* exemestane *on page 331*
Arranon® [US] *see* nelarabine *on page 582*
Arrestin® *(Discontinued)* *see* trimethobenzamide *on page 851*

arsenic trioxide (AR se nik tri OKS id)

Synonyms As_2O_3; NSC-706363
U.S./Canadian Brand Names Trisenox® [US]
Therapeutic Category Antineoplastic Agent, Miscellaneous
Use Induction of remission and consolidation in patients with relapsed or refractory acute promyelocytic leukemia (APL) which is specifically characterized by t(15;17) translocation or PML/RAR-alpha gene expression.
Orphan drug: Treatment of myelodysplastic syndrome; multiple myeloma; chronic myeloid leukemia (CML); acute myelocytic leukemia (AML)
Usual Dosage I.V.: Children >5 years and Adults:
Induction: 0.15 mg/kg/day; administer daily until bone marrow remission; maximum induction: 60 doses
Consolidation: 0.15 mg/kg/day starting 3-6 weeks after completion of induction therapy; maximum consolidation: 25 doses over 5 weeks
Dosage Forms
Injection, solution [preservative free]:
Trisenox®: 1 mg/mL (10 mL)

Artane® *(Discontinued)* *see* trihexyphenidyl *on page 850*
Artha-G® *(Discontinued)* *see* salsalate *on page 761*
ArthriCare® for Women Extra Moisturizing [US-OTC] *see* capsaicin *on page 142*
ArthriCare® for Women Multi-Action [US-OTC] *see* capsaicin *on page 142*
ArthriCare® for Women Silky Dry [US-OTC] *see* capsaicin *on page 142*
ArthriCare® for Women Ultra Strength *(Discontinued)* *see* capsaicin *on page 142*
Arthropan® *(Discontinued)*

Arthrotec® [US/Can] *see* diclofenac and misoprostol *on page 251*

articaine and epinephrine (AR ti kane & ep i NEF rin)

Synonyms epinephrine and articaine hydrochloride

U.S./Canadian Brand Names Astracaine® Forte [Can]; Astracaine® [Can]; Septanest® N [Can]; Septanest® SP [Can]; Septocaine® [US]; Ultracaine® D-S Forte [Can]; Ultracaine® D-S [Can]; Zorcaine™ [US]

Therapeutic Category Local Anesthetic

Usual Dosage Summary of recommended volumes and concentrations for various types of anesthetic procedures; dosages (administered by submucosal injection and/or nerve block) apply to normal healthy adults:

Infiltration: Injection volume of 4% solution: 0.5-2.5 mL; total dose: 20-100 mg

Nerve block: Injection volume of 4% solution: 0.5-3.4 mL; total dose: 20-136 mg

Oral surgery: Injection volume of 4% solution: 1-5.1 mL; total dose: 40-204 mg

Note: These dosages are guides only; other dosages may be used; however, do not exceed maximum recommended dose

Dosage Forms [CAN] = Canadian brand name

Injection, solution:

Septocaine®: Articaine hydrochloride 4% and epinephrine bitartrate 1:100,000 (1.7 mL) [contains sodium metabisulfite]; articaine hydrochloride 4% and epinephrine bitartrate 1:200,000 (1.7 mL) [contains sodium metabisulfite]

Ultracaine DS® [CAN]: Articaine hydrochloride 4% and epinephrine 1:200,000 (1.7 mL) [contains sodium metabisulfite; not available in the U.S.]

Ultracaine DS Forte® [CAN]: Articaine hydrochloride 4% and epinephrine 1:100,000 (1.7 mL) [contains sodium metabisulfite; not available in the U.S.]

Zorcaine™: Articaine hydrochloride 4% and epinephrine bitartrate 1:100,000 (1.7 mL) [contains sodium metabisulfite]

artificial tears (ar ti FISH il tears)

Sound-Alike/Look-Alike Issues

Isopto® Tears may be confused with Isoptin®

Murocel® may be confused with Murocoll-2®

Synonyms hydroxyethylcellulose; polyvinyl alcohol

U.S./Canadian Brand Names Akwa Tears® [US-OTC]; AquaSite® [US-OTC]; Bion® Tears [US-OTC]; HypoTears PF [US-OTC]; HypoTears [US-OTC]; Isopto® Tears [US-OTC]; Liquifilm® Tears [US-OTC]; Moisture® Eyes PM [US-OTC]; Moisture® Eyes [US-OTC]; Murine® Tears [US-OTC]; Murocel® [US-OTC]; Nature's Tears® [US-OTC]; Nu-Tears® II [US-OTC]; Nu-Tears® [US-OTC]; OcuCoat® PF [US-OTC]; OcuCoat® [US-OTC]; Puralube® Tears [US-OTC]; Refresh Plus® [US-OTC]; Refresh Tears® [US-OTC]; Refresh® [US-OTC]; Teardrops® [Can]; Teargen® II [US-OTC]; Teargen® [US-OTC]; Tearisol® [US-OTC]; Tears Again® [US-OTC]; Tears Naturale® Free [US-OTC]; Tears Naturale® II [US-OTC]; Tears Naturale® [US-OTC]; Tears Plus® [US-OTC]; Tears Renewed® [US-OTC]; Ultra Tears® [US-OTC]; Viva-Drops® [US-OTC]

Therapeutic Category Ophthalmic Agent, Miscellaneous

Use Ophthalmic lubricant; for relief of dry eyes and eye irritation

Usual Dosage Children and Adults: Ophthalmic: Use as needed to relieve symptoms, 1-2 drops into eye(s) 3-4 times/day

Dosage Forms Solution, ophthalmic: 15 mL and 30 mL dropper bottles

As_2O_3 *see* arsenic trioxide *on previous page*

ASA *see* aspirin *on page 77*

5-ASA *see* mesalamine *on page 533*

Asacol® [US/Can] *see* mesalamine *on page 533*

Asacol® 800 [Can] *see* mesalamine *on page 533*

A.S.A.® *(Discontinued)* *see* aspirin *on page 77*

Asaphen [Can] *see* aspirin *on page 77*

Asaphen E.C. [Can] *see* aspirin *on page 77*

ascorbic acid (a SKOR bik AS id)

Synonyms vitamin C

U.S./Canadian Brand Names C-500-GR™ [US-OTC]; C-Gram [US-OTC]; Cecon® [US-OTC]; Cevi-Bid® [US-OTC]; Dull-C® [US-OTC]; Proflavanol C™ [Can]; Revitalose C-1000® [Can]; Vita-C® [US-OTC]

Therapeutic Category Vitamin, Water Soluble

Use Prevention and treatment of scurvy; acidify the urine

Usual Dosage Oral, I.M., I.V., SubQ:

Recommended daily allowance (RDA):
- <6 months: 30 mg
- 6 months to 1 year: 35 mg
- 1-3 years: 15 mg; upper limit of intake should not exceed 400 mg/day
- 4-8 years: 25 mg; upper limit of intake should not exceed 650 mg/day
- 9-13 years: 45 mg; upper limit of intake should not exceed 1200 mg/day
- 14-18 years: Upper limit of intake should not exceed 1800 mg/day
  - Male: 75 mg
  - Female: 65 mg
- Adults: Upper limit of intake should not exceed 2000 mg/day
  - Male: 90 mg
  - Female: 75 mg
- Pregnant female:
  - ≤18 years: 80 mg; upper limit of intake should not exceed 1800 mg/day
  - 19-50 years: 85 mg; upper limit of intake should not exceed 2000 mg/day
- Lactating female:
  - ≤18 years: 15 mg; upper limit of intake should not exceed 1800 mg/day
  - 19-50 years: 20 mg; upper limit of intake should not exceed 2000 mg/day
- Adult smoker: Add an additional 35 mg/day

Children:
- Scurvy: 100-300 mg/day in divided doses for at least 2 weeks
- Urinary acidification: 500 mg every 6-8 hours
- Dietary supplement: 35-100 mg/day

Adults:
- Scurvy: 100-250 mg 1-2 times/day for at least 2 weeks
- Urinary acidification: 4-12 g/day in 3-4 divided doses
- Prevention and treatment of colds: 1-3 g/day
- Dietary supplement: 50-200 mg/day

Dosage Forms
- Capsule: 500 mg, 1000 mg
  - C-500-GR™: 500 mg
- Capsule, timed release: 500 mg
- Crystal (Vita-C®): 4 g/teaspoonful (100 g)
- Injection, solution: 250 mg/mL (2 mL, 30 mL); 500 mg/mL (50 mL)
  - Cenolate®: 500 mg/mL (1 mL, 2 mL) [contains sodium hydrosulfite]
- Powder, solution (Dull-C®): 4 g/teaspoonful (100 g, 500 g)
- Solution, oral (Cecon®): 90 mg/mL (50 mL)
- Tablet: 100 mg, 250 mg, 500 mg, 1000 mg
  - C-Gram: 1000 mg
- Tablet, chewable: 100 mg, 250 mg, 500 mg [some products may contain aspartame]
- Tablet, timed release: 500 mg, 1000 mg, 1500 mg
  - Cevi-Bid®: 500 mg

ascorbic acid and ferrous sulfate *see* ferrous sulfate and ascorbic acid *on page 343*

Ascorbicap® ***(Discontinued)*** *see* ascorbic acid *on this page*

Ascriptin® [US-OTC] *see* aspirin *on next page*

Ascriptin® Extra Strength [US-OTC] *see* aspirin *on next page*

Asendin® ***(Discontinued)*** *see* amoxapine *on page 47*

Asmalix® ***(Discontinued)*** *see* theophylline *on page 818*

Asmanex® Twisthaler® [US] *see* mometasone furoate *on page 563*

asparaginase (a SPEAR a ji nase)

Sound-Alike/Look-Alike Issues

asparaginase may be confused with pegaspargase

Synonyms *E. coli* asparaginase; *Erwinia* asparaginase; L-asparaginase; NSC-106977 (*Erwinia*); NSC-109229 (*E. coli*)

U.S./Canadian Brand Names Elspar® [US/Can]; Erwinase® [Can]; Kidrolase® [Can]

Therapeutic Category Antineoplastic Agent

Use Treatment of acute lymphocytic leukemia, lymphoma

Usual Dosage Refer to individual protocols.

Children:

I.V.:

Infusion for induction: 1000 units/kg/day for 10 days

Consolidation: 6000-10,000 units/m²/day for 14 days

I.M.: 6000 units/m² on days 4, 7, 10, 13, 16, 19, 22, 25, 28

Adults:

I.V. infusion single agent for induction:

200 units/kg/day for 28 days **or**

5000-10,000 units/m²/day for 7 days every 3 weeks **or**

10,000-40,000 units every 2-3 weeks

I.M. as single agent: 6000-12,000 units/m²; reconstitution to 10,000 units/mL may be necessary

Some institutions recommended the following precautions for asparaginase administration: Have parenteral epinephrine, diphenhydramine, and hydrocortisone available at the bedside. Have a freely running I.V. in place. Have a physician readily accessible. Monitor the patient closely for 30-60 minutes. Avoid administering the drug at night.

Some practitioners recommend a desensitization regimen for patients who react to a test dose, or are being retreated following a break in therapy. Doses are doubled and given every 10 minutes until the total daily dose for that day has been administered.

Dosage Forms Injection, powder for reconstitution: 10,000 units

aspart insulin *see* insulin aspart *on page 449*

A-Spas® *(Discontinued)* *see* hyoscyamine *on page 434*

Aspercin [US-OTC] *see* aspirin *on this page*

Aspercin Extra [US-OTC] *see* aspirin *on this page*

Aspercreme® [US-OTC] *see* trolamine *on page 855*

Aspergum® [US-OTC] *see* aspirin *on this page*

aspirin (AS pir in)

Sound-Alike/Look-Alike Issues

aspirin may be confused with Afrin®, Asendin®

Ascriptin® may be confused with Aricept®

Ecotrin® may be confused with Akineton®, Edecrin®, Epogen®

Halfprin® may be confused with Halfan®, Haltran®

ZORprin® may be confused with Zyloprim®

Synonyms acetylsalicylic acid; ASA

U.S./Canadian Brand Names Asaphen E.C. [Can]; Asaphen [Can]; Ascriptin® Extra Strength [US-OTC]; Ascriptin® [US-OTC]; Aspercin Extra [US-OTC]; Aspercin [US-OTC]; Aspergum® [US-OTC]; Bayer® Aspirin Extra Strength [US-OTC]; Bayer® Aspirin Regimen Adult Low Strength [US-OTC]; Bayer® Aspirin Regimen Children's [US-OTC]; Bayer® Aspirin Regimen Regular Strength [US-OTC]; Bayer® Aspirin [US-OTC]; Bayer® Extra Strength Arthritis Pain Regimen [US-OTC]; Bayer® Plus Extra Strength [US-OTC]; Bayer® Women's Aspirin Plus Calcium [US-OTC]; Bufferin® Extra Strength [US-OTC]; Bufferin® [US-OTC]; Buffinol Extra [US-OTC]; Buffinol [US-OTC]; Easprin® [US]; Ecotrin® Low Strength [US-OTC]; Ecotrin® Maximum Strength [US-OTC]; Ecotrin® [US-OTC]; Entrophen® [Can]; Halfprin® [US-OTC]; Novasen [Can]; St. Joseph® Adult Aspirin [US-OTC]; Sureprin 81™ [US-OTC]; ZORprin® [US]

Therapeutic Category Analgesic, Nonnarcotic; Antiplatelet Agent; Antipyretic; Nonsteroidal Antiinflammatory Drug (NSAID)

Use Treatment of mild-to-moderate pain, inflammation, and fever; may be used as prophylaxis of myocardial infarction; prophylaxis of stroke and/or transient ischemic episodes; management of rheumatoid arthritis, rheumatic fever, osteoarthritis, and gout (high dose); adjunctive therapy in revascularization procedures (coronary artery bypass graft [CABG], percutaneous transluminal coronary angioplasty [PTCA], carotid endarterectomy), stent implantation

Usual Dosage

Children:

Analgesic and antipyretic: Oral, rectal: 10-15 mg/kg/dose every 4-6 hours, up to a total of 4 g/day

(Continued)

aspirin *(Continued)*

Antiinflammatory: Oral: Initial: 60-90 mg/kg/day in divided doses; usual maintenance: 80-100 mg/kg/day divided every 6-8 hours; monitor serum concentrations

Antiplatelet effects: Adequate pediatric studies have not been performed; pediatric dosage is derived from adult studies and clinical experience and is not well established; suggested doses have ranged from 3-5 mg/kg/day to 5-10 mg/kg/day given as a single daily dose. Doses are rounded to a convenient amount (eg, 1/2 of 80 mg tablet).

Mechanical prosthetic heart valves: 6-20 mg/kg/day given as a single daily dose (used in combination with an oral anticoagulant in children who have systemic embolism despite adequate oral anticoagulation therapy (INR 2.5-3.5) and used in combination with low-dose anticoagulation (INR 2-3) and dipyridamole when full-dose oral anticoagulation is contraindicated)

Blalock-Taussig shunts: 3-5 mg/kg/day given as a single daily dose

Kawasaki disease: Oral: 80-100 mg/kg/day divided every 6 hours; monitor serum concentrations; after fever resolves: 3-5 mg/kg/day once daily; in patients without coronary artery abnormalities, give lower dose for at least 6-8 weeks or until ESR and platelet count are normal; in patients with coronary artery abnormalities, low-dose aspirin should be continued indefinitely

Antirheumatic: Oral: 60-100 mg/kg/day in divided doses every 4 hours

Adults:

Analgesic and antipyretic: Oral, rectal: 325-650 mg every 4-6 hours up to 4 g/day

Antiinflammatory: Oral: Initial: 2.4-3.6 g/day in divided doses; usual maintenance: 3.6-5.4 g/day; monitor serum concentrations

Myocardial infarction prophylaxis: 75-325 mg/day; use of a lower aspirin dosage has been recommended in patients receiving ACE inhibitors

Acute myocardial infarction: 160-325 mg/day (have patient chew tablet if not taking aspirin before presentation)

CABG: 75-325 mg/day starting 6 hours following procedure; if bleeding prevents administration at 6 hours after CABG, initiate as soon as possible

PTCA: Initial: 80-325 mg/day starting 2 hours before procedure; longer pretreatment durations (up to 24 hours) should be considered if lower dosages (80-100 mg) are used

Stent implantation: Oral: 325 mg 2 hours prior to implantation and 160-325 mg daily thereafter

Carotid endarterectomy: 81-325 mg/day preoperatively and daily thereafter

Acute stroke: 160-325 mg/day, initiated within 48 hours (in patients who are not candidates for thrombolytics and are not receiving systemic anticoagulation)

Stroke prevention/TIA: 30-325 mg/day (dosages up to 1300 mg/day in 2-4 divided doses have been used in clinical trials)

Dosage Forms

Caplet:

Bayer® Aspirin: 325 mg

Bayer® Aspirin Extra Strength: 500 mg

Bayer® Extra Strength Arthritis Pain Regimen: 500 mg [enteric coated]

Bayer® Women's Aspirin Plus Calcium: 81 mg [contains elemental calcium 300 mg]

Caplet, buffered (Ascriptin® Extra Strength): 500 mg [contains aluminum hydroxide, calcium carbonate, and magnesium hydroxide]

Gelcap (Bayer® Aspirin Extra Strength): 500 mg

Gum (Aspergum®): 227 mg [cherry or orange flavor]

Suppository, rectal: 300 mg, 600 mg

Tablet: 325 mg

Aspercin: 325 mg

Aspercin Extra: 500 mg

Bayer® Aspirin: 325 mg [film coated]

Tablet, buffered: 325 mg

Ascriptin®: 325 mg [contains aluminum hydroxide, calcium carbonate, and magnesium hydroxide]

Bayer® Plus Extra Strength: 500 mg [contains calcium carbonate]

Bufferin®: 325 mg [contains citric acid]

Bufferin® Extra Strength: 500 mg [contains citric acid]

Buffinol: 325 mg [contains magnesium oxide]

Buffinol Extra: 500 mg [contains magnesium oxide]

Tablet, chewable: 81 mg

Bayer® Aspirin Regimen Children's Chewable: 81 mg [cherry, mint or orange flavor]

St. Joseph® Adult Aspirin: 81 mg [orange flavor]

Tablet, controlled release (ZORprin®): 800 mg

Tablet, enteric coated: 81 mg, 325 mg, 500 mg, 650 mg

Bayer® Aspirin Regimen Adult Low Strength, Ecotrin® Low Strength, St. Joseph Adult Aspirin: 81 mg

Bayer® Aspirin Regimen Regular Strength, Ecotrin®: 325 mg
Easprin®: 975 mg
Ecotrin® Maximum Strength: 500 mg
Halfprin®: 81 mg, 162 mg
Sureprin 81™: 81 mg

aspirin, acetaminophen, and caffeine *see* acetaminophen, aspirin, and caffeine *on page 10*

aspirin and carisoprodol *see* carisoprodol and aspirin *on page 152*

aspirin and dipyridamole (AS pir in & dye peer ID a mole)

Sound-Alike/Look-Alike Issues
Aggrenox® may be confused with Aggrastat®

Synonyms aspirin and extended-release dipyridamole; dipyridamole and aspirin

U.S./Canadian Brand Names Aggrenox® [US/Can]

Therapeutic Category Antiplatelet Agent

Use Reduction in the risk of stroke in patients who have had transient ischemia of the brain or completed ischemic stroke due to thrombosis

Usual Dosage Adults: Oral: 1 capsule (dipyridamole 200 mg, aspirin 25 mg) twice daily.

Dosage Forms
Capsule, variable release:
Aggrenox®: Aspirin 25 mg (immediate release) and dipyridamole 200 mg (extended release)

aspirin and extended-release dipyridamole *see* aspirin and dipyridamole *on this page*

aspirin and hydrocodone *see* hydrocodone and aspirin *on page 422*

aspirin and meprobamate (AS pir in & me proe BA mate)

Synonyms meprobamate and aspirin

U.S./Canadian Brand Names 292 MEP® [Can]; Equagesic® [US]

Therapeutic Category Skeletal Muscle Relaxant

Controlled Substance C-IV

Use Adjunct to treatment of skeletal muscular disease in patients exhibiting tension and/or anxiety

Usual Dosage Oral: 1 tablet 3-4 times/day

Dosage Forms Tablet: Aspirin 325 mg and meprobamate 200 mg

aspirin and oxycodone *see* oxycodone and aspirin *on page 628*

aspirin, caffeine, and acetaminophen *see* acetaminophen, aspirin, and caffeine *on page 10*

aspirin, caffeine, and butalbital *see* butalbital, aspirin, and caffeine *on page 129*

aspirin, caffeine, and propoxyphene *see* propoxyphene, aspirin, and caffeine *on page 708*

aspirin, caffeine, codeine, and butalbital *see* butalbital, aspirin, caffeine, and codeine *on page 129*

aspirin, carisoprodol, and codeine *see* carisoprodol, aspirin, and codeine *on page 152*

Aspirin Free Anacin® *(Discontinued)* *see* acetaminophen *on page 5*

Aspirin Free Anacin® Maximum Strength [US-OTC] *see* acetaminophen *on page 5*

aspirin, orphenadrine, and caffeine *see* orphenadrine, aspirin, and caffeine *on page 620*

Astelin® [US/Can] *see* azelastine *on page 87*

AsthmaHaler® Mist *(Discontinued)* *see* epinephrine *on page 295*

AsthmaNefrin® *(Discontinued)* *see* epinephrine *on page 295*

Astracaine® [Can] *see* articaine and epinephrine *on page 75*

Astracaine® Forte [Can] *see* articaine and epinephrine *on page 75*

Astramorph/PF™ [US] *see* morphine sulfate *on page 565*

AT-III *see* antithrombin III *on page 62*

Atacand® [US/Can] *see* candesartan *on page 141*

Atacand HCT™ [US] *see* candesartan and hydrochlorothiazide *on page 141*

Atacand® Plus [Can] *see* candesartan and hydrochlorothiazide *on page 141*

Atapryl® *(Discontinued)*

Atarax® [Can] *see* hydroxyzine *on page 433*

Atarax® *(Discontinued)* *see* hydroxyzine *on page 433*

Atasol® [Can] *see* acetaminophen *on page 5*

atazanavir (at a za NA veer)

Synonyms atazanavir sulfate; BMS-232632

U.S./Canadian Brand Names Reyataz® [US/Can]

Therapeutic Category Antiretroviral Agent, Protease Inhibitor

Use Treatment of HIV-1 infections in combination with at least two other antiretroviral agents

Note: In patients with prior virologic failure, coadministration with ritonavir is recommended.

Usual Dosage Oral: Adolescents ≥16 years and Adults:

Antiretroviral-naive patients: 400 mg once daily; administer with food

Antiretroviral-experienced patients: 300 mg once daily **plus** ritonavir 100 mg once daily; administer with food

Coadministration with efavirenz:

Antiretroviral-naive patients: It is recommended that atazanavir 300 mg plus ritonavir 100 mg be given with efavirenz 600 mg (all as a single daily dose); administer with food

Antiretroviral-experienced patients: Recommendations have not been established.

Coadministration with didanosine buffered formulations: Administer atazanavir 2 hours before or 1 hour after didanosine buffered formulations

Coadministration with tenofovir: The manufacturer recommends that atazanavir 300 mg plus ritonavir 100 mg be given with tenofovir 300 mg (all as a single daily dose); administer with food

Dosage Forms

Capsule, as sulfate:

Reyataz®: 100 mg, 150 mg, 200 mg

atazanavir sulfate *see* atazanavir *on this page*

atenolol (a TEN oh lole)

Sound-Alike/Look-Alike Issues

atenolol may be confused with albuterol, Altenol®, timolol, Tylenol®

Tenormin® may be confused with Imuran®, Norpramin®, thiamine, Trovan®

U.S./Canadian Brand Names Apo-Atenol® [Can]; Gen-Atenolol [Can]; Novo-Atenol [Can]; Nu-Atenol [Can]; PMS-Atenolol [Can]; Rhoxal-atenolol [Can]; Riva-Atenolol [Can]; Sandoz-Atenolol [Can]; Tenolin [Can]; Tenormin® [US/Can]

Therapeutic Category Beta-Adrenergic Blocker

Use Treatment of hypertension, alone or in combination with other agents; management of angina pectoris, postmyocardial infarction patients

Usual Dosage

Oral:

Children: 0.8-1 mg/kg/dose given daily; range of 0.8-1.5 mg/kg/day; maximum dose: 2 mg/kg/day

Adults:

Hypertension: 25-50 mg once daily, may increase to 100 mg/day. Doses >100 mg are unlikely to produce any further benefit.

Angina pectoris: 50 mg once daily, may increase to 100 mg/day. Some patients may require 200 mg/day.

Postmyocardial infarction: Follow I.V. dose with 100 mg/day or 50 mg twice daily for 6-9 days postmyocardial infarction.

I.V.:

Hypertension: Dosages of 1.25-5 mg every 6-12 hours have been used in short-term management of patients unable to take oral enteral beta-blockers

Postmyocardial infarction: Early treatment: 5 mg slow I.V. over 5 minutes; may repeat in 10 minutes. If both doses are tolerated, may start oral atenolol 50 mg every 12 hours or 100 mg/day for 6-9 days postmyocardial infarction.

Dosage Forms

Injection, solution: 0.5 mg/mL (10 mL)

Tablet: 25 mg, 50 mg, 100 mg

atenolol and chlorthalidone (a TEN oh lole & klor THAL i done)

Synonyms chlorthalidone and atenolol

U.S./Canadian Brand Names Tenoretic® [US/Can]

Therapeutic Category Antihypertensive Agent, Combination

Use Treatment of hypertension with a cardioselective beta-blocker and a diuretic

Usual Dosage Adults: Oral: Initial (based on atenolol component): 50 mg once daily, then individualize dose until optimal dose is achieved

Dosage Forms Tablet:

50: Atenolol 50 mg and chlorthalidone 25 mg

100: Atenolol 100 mg and chlorthalidone 25 mg

ATG *see* antithymocyte globulin (equine) *on page 62*

Atgam® [US/Can] *see* antithymocyte globulin (equine) *on page 62*

Ativan® [US/Can] *see* lorazepam *on page 506*

Atolone® Oral *(Discontinued)*

atomoxetine (AT oh mox e teen)

Synonyms atomoxetine hydrochloride; LY139603; methylphenoxy-benzene propanamine; tomoxetine

U.S./Canadian Brand Names Strattera® [US/Can]

Therapeutic Category Norepinephrine Reuptake Inhibitor, Selective

Use Treatment of attention deficit/hyperactivity disorder (ADHD)

Usual Dosage Oral: **Note:** Atomoxetine may be discontinued without the need for tapering dose.

Children and Adolescents ≤70 kg: ADHD: Initial: 0.5 mg/kg/day, increase after minimum of 3 days to ~1.2 mg/kg/day; may administer as either a single daily dose or 2 evenly divided doses in morning and late afternoon/early evening. Maximum daily dose: 1.4 mg/kg or 100 mg, whichever is less.

Dosage adjustment in patients receiving strong CYP2D6 inhibitors (eg, paroxetine, fluoxetine, quinidine), do not exceed 1.2 mg/kg/day; dose adjustments should occur only after 4 weeks.

Children and Adolescents >70 kg and Adults: ADHD: Initial: 40 mg/day, increased after minimum of 3 days to ~80 mg/day; may administer as either a single daily dose or two evenly divided doses in morning and late afternoon/early evening. May increase to 100 mg in 2-4 additional weeks to achieve optimal response.

Dosage adjustment in patients receiving strong CYP2D6 inhibitors (eg, paroxetine, fluoxetine, quinidine), do not exceed 80 mg/day; dose adjustments should occur only after 4 weeks.

Dosage Forms

Capsule:

Strattera®: 10 mg, 18 mg, 25 mg, 40 mg, 60 mg, 80 mg, 100 mg

atomoxetine hydrochloride *see* atomoxetine *on this page*

atorvastatin (a TORE va sta tin)

Sound-Alike/Look-Alike Issues

Lipitor® may be confused with Levatol®

U.S./Canadian Brand Names Lipitor® [US/Can]

Therapeutic Category HMG-CoA Reductase Inhibitor

Use Treatment of dyslipidemias or primary prevention of cardiovascular disease (atherosclerotic) as detailed below:

Primary prevention of cardiovascular disease (high-risk for CVD): To reduce the risk of MI or stroke in patients without evidence of heart disease who have multiple CVD risk factors or type 2 diabetes. Treatment reduces the risk for angina or revascularization procedures in patients with multiple risk factors.

Treatment of dyslipidemias: To reduce elevations in total cholesterol, LDL-C, apolipoprotein B, and triglycerides in patients with elevations of one or more components, and/or to increase HDL-C as present in Fredrickson type IIa, IIb, III, and IV hyperlipidemias; treatment of primary dysbetalipoproteinemia, homozygous familial hypercholesterolemia

Treatment of heterozygous familial hypercholesterolemia (HeFH) in adolescent patients (10-17 years of age, females >1 year postmenarche) having LDL-C ≥190 mg/dL or LDL-C ≥160 mg/dL with positive family history of premature cardiovascular disease (CVD) or with two or more CVD risk factors.

Usual Dosage Oral: **Note:** Doses should be individualized according to the baseline LDL-cholesterol levels, the recommended goal of therapy, and patient response; adjustments should be made at intervals of 2-4 weeks

Children 10-17 years (females >1 year postmenarche): HeFH: 10 mg once daily (maximum: 20 mg/day)

Adults:

Hyperlipidemias: Initial: 10-20 mg once daily; patients requiring >45% reduction in LDL-C may be started at 40 mg once daily; range: 10-80 mg once daily

Primary prevention of CVD: 10 mg once daily

Dosage Forms Tablet: 10 mg, 20 mg, 40 mg, 80 mg

atorvastatin calcium and amlodipine besylate *see* amlodipine and atorvastatin *on page 45*

atovaquone (a TOE va kwone)

U.S./Canadian Brand Names Mepron® [US/Can]

Therapeutic Category Antiprotozoal

Use Acute oral treatment of mild-to-moderate *Pneumocystis carinii* pneumonia (PCP) in patients who are intolerant to co-trimoxazole; prophylaxis of PCP in patients intolerant to co-trimoxazole; treatment/suppression of *Toxoplasma gondii* encephalitis; primary prophylaxis of HIV-infected persons at high risk for developing *Toxoplasma gondii* encephalitis

Usual Dosage Oral: Adolescents 13-16 years and Adults:

Prevention of PCP: 1500 mg once daily with food

Treatment of mild-to-moderate PCP: 750 mg twice daily with food for 21 days

Dosage Forms Suspension, oral: 750 mg/5 mL (5 mL, 210 mL) [contains benzyl alcohol; citrus flavor]

atovaquone and proguanil (a TOE va kwone & pro GWA nil)

Synonyms proguanil and atovaquone

U.S./Canadian Brand Names Malarone® Pediatric [Can]; Malarone® [US/Can]

Therapeutic Category Antimalarial Agent

Use Prevention or treatment of acute, uncomplicated *P. falciparum* malaria

Usual Dosage Oral:

Children (dosage based on body weight):

Prevention of malaria: Start 1-2 days prior to entering a malaria-endemic area, continue throughout the stay and for 7 days after returning. Take as a single dose, once daily.

11-20 kg: Atovaquone/proguanil 62.5 mg/25 mg
21-30 kg: Atovaquone/proguanil 125 mg/50 mg
31-40 kg: Atovaquone/proguanil 187.5 mg/75 mg
>40 kg: Atovaquone/proguanil 250 mg/100 mg

Treatment of acute malaria: Take as a single dose, once daily for 3 consecutive days.

5-8 kg: Atovaquone/proguanil 125 mg/50 mg
9-10 kg: Atovaquone/proguanil 187.5 mg/75 mg
11-20 kg: Atovaquone/proguanil 250 mg/100 mg
21-30 kg: Atovaquone/proguanil 500 mg/200 mg
31-40 kg: Atovaquone/proguanil 750 mg/300 mg
>40 kg: Atovaquone/proguanil 1 g/400 mg

Adults:

Prevention of malaria: Atovaquone/proguanil 250 mg/100 mg once daily; start 1-2 days prior to entering a malaria-endemic area, continue throughout the stay and for 7 days after returning

Treatment of acute malaria: Atovaquone/proguanil 1 g/400 mg as a single dose, once daily for 3 consecutive days

Dosage Forms

Tablet: Atovaquone 250 mg and proguanil hydrochloride 100 mg

Tablet, pediatric: Atovaquone 62.5 mg and proguanil hydrochloride 25 mg

Atozine® Oral *(Discontinued)* *see* hydroxyzine *on page 433*

ATRA *see* tretinoin (oral) *on page 844*

atracurium (a tra KYOO ree um)

Synonyms atracurium besylate

U.S./Canadian Brand Names Tracrium® [US]

Therapeutic Category Skeletal Muscle Relaxant

Use Adjunct to general anesthesia to facilitate endotracheal intubation and to relax skeletal muscles during surgery; to facilitate mechanical ventilation in ICU patients; does not relieve pain or produce sedation

Usual Dosage I.V. (not to be used I.M.): Dose to effect; doses must be individualized due to interpatient variability; use ideal body weight for obese patients

Children 1 month to 2 years: Initial: 0.3-0.4 mg/kg followed by maintenance doses as needed to maintain neuromuscular blockade

Children >2 years to Adults: 0.4-0.5 mg/kg, then 0.08-0.1 mg/kg 20-45 minutes after initial dose to maintain neuromuscular block, followed by repeat doses of 0.08-0.1 mg/kg at 15- to 25-minute intervals

Initial dose after succinylcholine for intubation (balanced anesthesia): Adults: 0.2-0.4 mg/kg

Pretreatment/priming: 10% of intubating dose given 3-5 minutes before initial dose

Continuous infusion:

Surgery: Initial: 9-10 mcg/kg/minute at initial signs of recovery from bolus dose; block usually maintained by a rate of 5-9 mcg/kg/minute under balanced anesthesia

ICU: Block usually maintained by rate of 11-13 mcg/kg/minute (rates for pediatric patients may be higher)

Dosage Forms

Injection, as besylate: 10 mg/mL (10 mL) [contains benzyl alcohol]

Injection, as besylate [preservative free]: 10 mg/mL (5 mL)

atracurium besylate *see* atracurium *on previous page*

Atropair® *(Discontinued)* *see* atropine *on this page*

AtroPen® [US] *see* atropine *on this page*

atropine (A troe peen)

Synonyms atropine sulfate

U.S./Canadian Brand Names AtroPen® [US]; Atropine-Care® [US]; Dioptic's Atropine Solution [Can]; Isopto® Atropine [US/Can]; Sal-Tropine™ [US]

Therapeutic Category Anticholinergic Agent

Use

Injection: Preoperative medication to inhibit salivation and secretions; treatment of symptomatic sinus bradycardia; AV block (nodal level); ventricular asystole; antidote for organophosphate pesticide poisoning

Ophthalmic: Produce mydriasis and cycloplegia for examination of the retina and optic disc and accurate measurement of refractive errors; uveitis

Oral: Inhibit salivation and secretions

Usual Dosage

Neonates, Infants, and Children: Doses <0.1 mg have been associated with paradoxical bradycardia.

Inhibit salivation and secretions (preanesthesia): Oral, I.M., I.V., SubQ:

<5 kg: 0.02 mg/kg/dose 30-60 minutes preop then every 4-6 hours as needed. Use of a minimum dosage of 0.1 mg in neonates <5 kg will result in dosages >0.02 mg/kg. There is no documented minimum dosage in this age group.

>5 kg: 0.01-0.02 mg/kg/dose to a maximum 0.4 mg/dose 30-60 minutes preop; minimum dose: 0.1 mg

Alternate dosing:

3-7 kg (7-16 lb): 0.1 mg

8-11 kg (17-24 lb): 0.15 mg

11-18 kg (24-40 lb): 0.2 mg

18-29 kg (40-65 lb): 0.3 mg

>30 kg (>65 lb): 0.4 mg

Bradycardia: I.V., intratracheal: 0.02 mg/kg, minimum dose 0.1 mg, maximum single dose: 0.5 mg in children and 1 mg in adolescents; may repeat in 5-minute intervals to a maximum total dose of 1 mg in children or 2 mg in adolescents. (**Note:** For intratracheal administration, the dosage must be diluted with normal saline to a total volume of 1-5 mL). When treating bradycardia in neonates, reserve use for those patients unresponsive to improved oxygenation and epinephrine.

Children: Organophosphate or carbamate poisoning:

I.V.: 0.03-0.05 mg/kg every 10-20 minutes until atropine effect, then every 1-4 hours for at least 24 hours

I.M. (AtroPen®): Mild symptoms: Administer dose listed below as soon as exposure is known or suspected. If severe symptoms develop after first dose, 2 additional doses should be repeated in 10 minutes; do not administer more than 3 doses. Severe symptoms: Immediately administer 3 doses as follows:

<6.8 kg (15 lb): Use of **AtroPen® formulation not recommended;** administer atropine 0.05 mg/kg

6.8-18 kg (15-40 lb): 0.5 mg/dose

18-41 kg (40-90 lb): 1 mg/dose

>41 kg (>90 lb): 2 mg/dose

Adults (doses <0.5 mg have been associated with paradoxical bradycardia):

Asystole or pulseless electrical activity:

I.V.: 1 mg; repeat in 3-5 minutes if asystole persists; total dose of 0.04 mg/kg.

Intratracheal: Administer 2-2.5 times the recommended I.V. dose; dilute in 10 mL NS or distilled water. **Note:** Absorption is greater with distilled water, but causes more adverse effects on PaO_2.

Inhibit salivation and secretions (preanesthesia):

I.M., I.V., SubQ: 0.4-0.6 mg 30-60 minutes preop and repeat every 4-6 hours as needed

Oral: 0.4 mg; may repeat in 4 hours if necessary; 0.4 mg initial dose may be exceeded in certain cases and may repeat in 4 hours if necessary

Bradycardia: I.V.: 0.5-1 mg every 5 minutes, not to exceed a total of 3 mg or 0.04 mg/kg; may give intratracheally in 10 mL NS (intratracheal dose should be 2-2.5 times the I.V. dose)

Neuromuscular blockade reversal: I.V.: 25-30 mcg/kg 30-60 seconds before neostigmine or 7-10 mcg/kg 30-60 seconds before edrophonium

(Continued)

atropine *(Continued)*

Organophosphate or carbamate poisoning:

I.V.: 2 mg, followed by 2 mg every 5-60 minutes until adequate atropinization has occurred; initial doses of up to 6 mg may be used in life-threatening cases

I.M. (AtroPen®): Mild symptoms: Administer 2 mg as soon as exposure is known or suspected. If severe symptoms develop after first dose, 2 additional doses should be repeated in 10 minutes; do not administer more than 3 doses. Severe symptoms: Immediately administer three 2 mg doses.

Mydriasis, cycloplegia (preprocedure): Ophthalmic (1% solution): Instill 1-2 drops 1 hour before procedure.

Uveitis: Ophthalmic:

1% solution: Instill 1-2 drops 4 times/day

Ointment: Apply a small amount in the conjunctival sac up to 3 times/day; compress the lacrimal sac by digital pressure for 1-3 minutes after instillation

Dosage Forms

Injection, solution, as sulfate: 0.05 mg/mL (5 mL); 0.1 mg/mL (5 mL, 10 mL); 0.4 mg/0.5 mL (0.5 mL); 0.4 mg/mL (0.5 mL, 1 mL, 20 mL); 1 mg/mL (1 mL)

AtroPen® [prefilled autoinjector]: 0.5 mg/0.7 mL (0.7 mL); 1 mg/0.7 mL (0.7 mL); 2 mg/0.7 mL (0.7 mL)

Ointment, ophthalmic, as sulfate: 1% (3.5 g)

Solution, ophthalmic, as sulfate: 1% (2 mL, 5 mL, 15 mL)

Atropine-Care®: 1% (2 mL) [contains benzalkonium chloride]

Isopto® Atropine: 1% (5 mL, 15 mL) [contains benzalkonium chloride]

Tablet, as sulfate (Sal-Tropine™): 0.4 mg

atropine and difenoxin *see* difenoxin and atropine *on page 253*

atropine and diphenoxylate *see* diphenoxylate and atropine *on page 264*

Atropine-Care® [US] *see* atropine *on previous page*

atropine, hyoscyamine, scopolamine, and phenobarbital *see* hyoscyamine, atropine, scopolamine, and phenobarbital *on page 435*

atropine soluble tablet ***(Discontinued)***

atropine sulfate *see* atropine *on previous page*

Atropisol® ***(Discontinued)*** *see* atropine *on previous page*

Atrosept® [US] *see* methenamine, phenyl salicylate, atropine, hyoscyamine, benzoic acid, and methylene blue *on page 539*

Atrovent® [US/Can] *see* ipratropium *on page 460*

Atrovent® HFA [US/Can] *see* ipratropium *on page 460*

A/T/S® [US] *see* erythromycin *on page 303*

attapulgite (at a PULL gite)

Sound-Alike/Look-Alike Issues

Kaopectate® may be confused with Kayexalate®

U.S./Canadian Brand Names Diasorb® [US-OTC]; Kaopectate® [Can]

Therapeutic Category Antidiarrheal

Use Symptomatic treatment of diarrhea

Usual Dosage Adequate controlled clinical studies documenting the efficacy of attapulgite are lacking; its usage and dosage has been primarily empiric; the following are manufacturer's recommended dosages

Oral: Give after each bowel movement

Children:

3-6 years: 300-750 mg/dose; maximum dose: 7 doses/day or 2250 mg/day

6-12 years: 600-1500 mg/dose; maximum dose: 7 doses/day or 4500 mg/day

Children >12 years and Adults: 1200-3000 mg/dose; maximum dose: 8 doses/day or 9000 mg/day

Dosage Forms [DSC] = Discontinued product

Caplet (Kaopectate® Maximum Strength [DSC]): 750 mg

Liquid, oral concentrate: Activated attapulgite 600 mg/15 mL (120 mL, 180 mL, 240 mL); activated attapulgite 750 mg/15 mL (120 mL, 360 mL)

Children's Kaopectate® [DSC]: Activated attapulgite 300 mg/7.5 mL (180 mL) [cherry flavor]

Diasorb®: Activated attapulgite 750 mg/5 mL (120 mL) [cola flavor; sugar free]

Kaopectate® Advanced Formula [DSC]: Activated attapulgite 750 mg/15 mL (90 mL, 240 mL, 360 mL) [peppermint flavor]

Attenuvax® [US] *see* measles virus vaccine (live) *on page 521*

Atuss® HD [US] *see* pseudoephedrine, hydrocodone, and chlorpheniramine *on page 716*

Atuss® HX [US] *see* hydrocodone and guaifenesin *on page 422*

Augmentin® [US/Can] *see* amoxicillin and clavulanate potassium *on page 49*

Augmentin ES-600® [US] *see* amoxicillin and clavulanate potassium *on page 49*

Augmentin XR™ [US] *see* amoxicillin and clavulanate potassium *on page 49*

Auralgan® [Can] *see* antipyrine and benzocaine *on page 62*

auranofin (au RANE oh fin)

Sound-Alike/Look-Alike Issues

Ridaura® may be confused with Cardura®

U.S./Canadian Brand Names Ridaura® [US/Can]

Therapeutic Category Gold Compound

Use Management of active stage of classic or definite rheumatoid arthritis in patients who do not respond to or tolerate other agents; psoriatic arthritis; adjunctive or alternative therapy for pemphigus

Usual Dosage Oral:

Children: Initial: 0.1 mg/kg/day divided daily; usual maintenance: 0.15 mg/kg/day in 1-2 divided doses; maximum: 0.2 mg/kg/day in 1-2 divided doses

Adults: 6 mg/day in 1-2 divided doses; after 3 months may be increased to 9 mg/day in 3 divided doses; if still no response after 3 months at 9 mg/day, discontinue drug

Dosage Forms Capsule: 3 mg [29% gold]

Aurodex [US] *see* antipyrine and benzocaine *on page 62*

Aurolate® [US] *see* gold sodium thiomalate *on page 390*

Autoplex® T *(Discontinued)* *see* anti-inhibitor coagulant complex *on page 61*

AVA *see* anthrax vaccine, adsorbed *on page 58*

Avagard™ [US-OTC] *see* chlorhexidine gluconate *on page 173*

Avage™ [US] *see* tazarotene *on page 806*

Avalide® [US/Can] *see* irbesartan and hydrochlorothiazide *on page 461*

Avandamet™ [US/Can] *see* rosiglitazone and metformin *on page 754*

Avandia® [US/Can] *see* rosiglitazone *on page 754*

Avapro® [US/Can] *see* irbesartan *on page 461*

Avapro® HCT *see* irbesartan and hydrochlorothiazide *on page 461*

AVAR™ [US] *see* sulfur and sulfacetamide *on page 800*

AVAR™-e [US] *see* sulfur and sulfacetamide *on page 800*

AVAR™-e Green [US] *see* sulfur and sulfacetamide *on page 800*

AVAR™ Green [US] *see* sulfur and sulfacetamide *on page 800*

Avastin® [US] *see* bevacizumab *on page 109*

Avaxim® [Can] *see* hepatitis A vaccine *on page 410*

Avaxim®-Pediatric [Can] *see* hepatitis A vaccine *on page 410*

Avelox® [US/Can] *see* moxifloxacin *on page 568*

Avelox® I.V. [US/Can] *see* moxifloxacin *on page 568*

Aventyl® [Can] *see* nortriptyline *on page 600*

Aventyl® HCl *(Discontinued)* *see* nortriptyline *on page 600*

Aviane™ [US] *see* ethinyl estradiol and levonorgestrel *on page 320*

Avinza™ [US] *see* morphine sulfate *on page 565*

Avita® [US] *see* tretinoin (topical) *on page 844*

Avitene® [US] *see* collagen hemostat *on page 212*

Avitene® Flour [US] *see* collagen hemostat *on page 212*

Avitene® Ultrafoam [US] *see* collagen hemostat *on page 212*

Avitene® UltraWrap™ [US] *see* collagen hemostat *on page 212*

Avlosulfon® *(Discontinued)* *see* dapsone *on page 229*

Avodart™ [US/Can] *see* dutasteride *on page 284*

Avonex® [US/Can] *see* interferon beta-1a *on page 457*

Axert™ [US/Can] *see* almotriptan *on page 30*

Axid® [US/Can] *see* nizatidine *on page 597*

Axid® AR [US-OTC] *see* nizatidine *on page 597*

AY-25650 *see* triptorelin *on page 854*

Aygestin® [US] *see* norethindrone *on page 598*

Ayr® Baby Saline [US-OTC] *see* sodium chloride *on page 777*

Ayr® Saline [US-OTC] *see* sodium chloride *on page 777*

Ayr® Saline No-Drip [US-OTC] *see* sodium chloride *on page 777*

5-aza-2'-deoxycytidine *see* decitabine *on page 233*

5-azaC *see* decitabine *on page 233*

azacitidine (ay za SYE ti deen)

Synonyms AZA-CR; 5-azacytidine; 5-AZC; ladakamycin; NSC-102816

U.S./Canadian Brand Names Vidaza™ [US]

Therapeutic Category Antineoplastic Agent, Antimetabolite (Pyrimidine)

Use Treatment of myelodysplastic syndrome (MDS)

Usual Dosage SubQ: Adults: MDS: 75 mg/m^2/day for 7 days repeated every 4 weeks. Dose may be increased to 100 mg/m^2/day if no benefit is observed after 2 cycles and no toxicity other than nausea and vomiting have occurred. Treatment is recommended for at least 4 cycles.

Dosage Forms

Injection, powder for suspension [preservative free]:

Vidaza™: 100 mg [contains mannitol 100 mg]

AZA-CR *see* azacitidine *on this page*

Azactam® [US/Can] *see* aztreonam *on page 89*

5-azacytidine *see* azacitidine *on this page*

Azasan® [US] *see* azathioprine *on this page*

azatadine *(Canada only)* (a ZA ta deen)

Synonyms azatadine maleate

U.S./Canadian Brand Names Optimine® [Can]

Therapeutic Category Antihistamine

Use Treatment of perennial and seasonal allergic rhinitis and chronic urticaria

Usual Dosage Children >12 years and Adults: Oral: 1-2 mg twice daily

Dosage Forms Tablet, as maleate: 1 mg

azatadine maleate *see* azatadine *(Canada only) on this page*

azathioprine (ay za THYE oh preen)

Sound-Alike/Look-Alike Issues

azathioprine may be confused with azatadine, azidothymidine, Azulfidine®

Imuran® may be confused with Elmiron®, Enduron®, Imdur®, Inderal®, Tenormin®

Synonyms azathioprine sodium

U.S./Canadian Brand Names Alti-Azathioprine [Can]; Apo-Azathioprine® [Can]; Azasan® [US]; Gen-Azathioprine [Can]; Imuran® [US/Can]; Novo-Azathioprine [Can]

Therapeutic Category Immunosuppressant Agent

Use Adjunctive therapy in prevention of rejection of kidney transplants; active rheumatoid arthritis

Usual Dosage I.V. dose is equivalent to oral dose (dosing should be based on ideal body weight):

Adults:

Renal transplantation: Oral, I.V.: Initial: 3-5 mg/kg/day usually given as a single daily dose, then 1-3 mg/kg/day maintenance

Rheumatoid arthritis: Oral:

Initial: 1 mg/kg/day given once daily or divided twice daily for 6-8 weeks; increase by 0.5 mg/kg every 4 weeks until response or up to 2.5 mg/kg/day; an adequate trial should be a minimum of 12 weeks

Maintenance dose: Reduce dose by 0.5 mg/kg every 4 weeks until lowest effective dose is reached; optimum duration of therapy not specified; may be discontinued abruptly

Dosage Forms

Injection, powder for reconstitution: 100 mg

Tablet [scored]: 50 mg

Azasan®: 75 mg, 100 mg

Imuran®: 50 mg

azathioprine sodium *see* azathioprine *on previous page*

5-AZC *see* azacitidine *on previous page*

Azdone® ***(Discontinued)*** *see* hydrocodone and aspirin *on page 422*

azelaic acid (a zeh LAY ik AS id)

U.S./Canadian Brand Names Azelex® [US]; Finacea™ [US]

Therapeutic Category Topical Skin Product

Use Topical treatment of inflammatory papules and pustules of mild-to-moderate rosacea; mild-to-moderate inflammatory acne vulgaris

Finacea®: Not FDA-approved for the treatment of acne

Usual Dosage Topical:

Adolescents ≥12 years and Adults: Acne vulgaris: Cream 20%: After skin is thoroughly washed and patted dry, gently but thoroughly massage a thin film of azelaic acid cream into the affected areas twice daily, in the morning and evening. The duration of use can vary and depends on the severity of the acne. In the majority of patients with inflammatory lesions, improvement of the condition occurs within 4 weeks.

Adults: Rosacea: Gel 15%: Massage gently into affected areas of the face twice daily; use beyond 12 weeks has not been studied

Dosage Forms

Cream:

Azelex®: 20% (30 g, 50 g) [contains benzoic acid and propylene glycol]

Gel:

Finacea®: 15% (30 g) [contains benzoic acid and propylene glycol]

azelastine (a ZEL as teen)

Sound-Alike/Look-Alike Issues

Optivar® may be confused with Optiray®

Synonyms azelastine hydrochloride

U.S./Canadian Brand Names Astelin® [US/Can]; Optivar® [US]

Therapeutic Category Antihistamine; Antihistamine, Ophthalmic

Use

Nasal spray: Treatment of the symptoms of seasonal allergic rhinitis such as rhinorrhea, sneezing, and nasal pruritus in children ≥5 years of age and adults; treatment of the symptoms of vasomotor rhinitis in children ≥12 years of age and adults

Ophthalmic: Treatment of itching of the eye associated with seasonal allergic conjunctivitis in children ≥3 years of age and adults

Usual Dosage

Children 5-11 years: Seasonal allergic rhinitis: Intranasal: 1 spray each nostril twice daily

Children ≥3 years and Adults: Itching eyes due to seasonal allergic conjunctivitis: Ophthalmic: Instill 1 drop into affected eye(s) twice daily

Children ≥12 years and Adults:

Seasonal allergic rhinitis: Intranasal: 1-2 sprays (137 mcg/spray) each nostril twice daily

Vasomotor rhinitis: Intranasal: 2 sprays each nostril twice daily.

Dosage Forms

Solution, intranasal, as hydrochloride [spray]:

Astelin®: 1 mg/mL(30 mL) [contains benzalkonium chloride; 137 mcg/spray; 200 metered sprays]

Solution, ophthalmic, as hydrochloride:

Optivar®: 0.05% (6 mL) [contains benzalkonium chloride]

azelastine hydrochloride *see* azelastine *on this page*

Azelex® [US] *see* azelaic acid *on this page*

azidothymidine *see* zidovudine *on page 886*

azidothymidine, abacavir, and lamivudine *see* abacavir, lamivudine, and zidovudine *on page 2*

Azilect® [US] *see* rasagiline *on page 733*

azithromycin (az ith roe MYE sin)

Sound-Alike/Look-Alike Issues

azithromycin may be confused with erythromycin

Zithromax® may be confused with Zinacef®

Synonyms azithromycin dihydrate; Zithromax® TRI-PAK™; Zithromax® Z-PAK®

U.S./Canadian Brand Names Apo-Azithromycin® [Can]; CO Azithromycin [Can]; GMD-Azithromycin [Can]; Novo-Azithromycin [Can]; PMS-Azithromycin [Can]; ratio-Azithromycin [Can]; Sandoz-Azithromycin [Can]; Zithromax® [US/Can]; Zmax™ [US]

Therapeutic Category Macrolide (Antibiotic)

Use Treatment of acute otitis media due to *H. influenzae*, *M. catarrhalis*, or *S. pneumoniae*; pharyngitis/tonsillitis due to *S. pyogenes*; treatment of mild-to-moderate upper and lower respiratory tract infections, infections of the skin and skin structure, community-acquired pneumonia, pelvic inflammatory disease (PID), sexually-transmitted diseases (urethritis/cervicitis), pharyngitis/tonsillitis (alternative to first-line therapy), and genital ulcer disease (chancroid) due to susceptible strains of *C. trachomatis, M. catarrhalis, H. influenzae, S. aureus, S. pneumoniae, Mycoplasma pneumoniae*, and *C. psittaci*; acute bacterial exacerbations of chronic obstructive pulmonary disease (COPD) due to *H. influenzae, M. catarrhalis,* or *S. pneumoniae*; acute bacterial sinusitis

Usual Dosage Note: Extended release suspension (Zmax™) is not interchangeable with immediate release formulations. Use should be limited to approved indications. All doses are expressed as immediate release azithromycin unless otherwise specified.

Usual dosage range:

Children ≥6 months: Oral: 5-12 mg/kg given once daily (maximum: 500 mg/day) **or** 30 mg/kg as a single dose (maximum: 1500 mg)

Adolescents ≥16 years and Adults:

Oral: 250-600 mg once daily **or** 1-2 g as a single dose

I.V.: 250-500 mg once daily

Indication-specific dosing:

Children: Oral:

Bacterial sinusitis: 10 mg/kg once daily for 3 days (maximum: 500 mg/day)

Community-acquired pneumonia: 10 mg/kg on day 1 (maximum: 500 mg/day) followed by 5 mg/kg/day once daily on days 2-5 (maximum: 250 mg/day)

Otitis media:

1-day regimen: 30 mg/kg as a single dose (maximum: 1500 mg)

3-day regimen: 10 mg/kg once daily for 3 days (maximum: 500 mg/day)

5-day regimen: 10 mg/kg on day 1 (maximum: 500 mg/day) followed by 5 mg/kg/day once daily on days 2-5 (maximum: 250 mg/day)

Pharyngitis, tonsillitis: Children ≥2 years: 12 mg/kg/day once daily for 5 days (maximum: 500 mg/day)

Pertussis (CDC guidelines):

Children <6 months: 10 mg/kg/day for 5 days

Children ≥6 months: 10 mg/kg on day 1 (maximum: 500 mg/day) followed by 5 mg/kg/day once daily on days 2-5 (maximum: 250 mg/day)

Adolescents ≥16 years and Adults:

Bacterial sinusitis: Oral: 500 mg/day for a total of 3 days

Extended release suspension (Zmax™): 2 g as a single dose

Chancroid due to *H. ducreyi*: Oral: 1 g as a single dose

Community-acquired pneumonia:

Oral (Zmax™): 2 g as a single dose

I.V.: 500 mg as a single dose for at least 2 days, follow I.V. therapy by the oral route with a single daily dose of 500 mg to complete a 7- to 10-day course of therapy.

Mild-to-moderate respiratory tract, skin, and soft tissue infections: Oral: 500 mg in a single loading dose on day 1 followed by 250 mg/day as a single dose on days 2-5

Alternative regimen: Bacterial exacerbation of COPD: 500 mg/day for a total of 3 days

Pelvic inflammatory disease (PID): I.V.: 500 mg as a single dose for 1-2 days, follow I.V. therapy by the oral route with a single daily dose of 250 mg to complete a 7-day course of therapy

Pertussis (CDC guidelines): Oral: 500 mg on day 1 followed by 250 mg/day on days 2-5 (maximum: 500 mg/day)

Urethritis/cervicitis: Oral:

Due to C. trachomatis: 1 g as a single dose

Due to N. gonorrhoeae: 2 g as a single dose

Dosage Forms Note: Strength expressed as base

Injection, powder for reconstitution, as dihydrate: 500 mg

Zithromax®: 500 mg [contains sodium 114 mg (4.96 mEq) per vial]

Injection, powder for reconstitution, as monohydrate: 500 mg

Microspheres for oral suspension, extended release, as dihydrate:
Zmax™: 2 g [single-dose bottle; contains sodium 148 mg per bottle; cherry and banana flavor]
Injection, powder for reconstitution, as monohydrate: 500 mg
Powder for oral suspension, as monohydrate: 100 mg/5 mL (15 mL); 200 mg/5 mL (15 mL, 22.5 mL, 30 mL)
Powder for oral suspension, immediate release, as dihydrate:
Zithromax®: 100 mg/5 mL (15 mL) [contains sodium 3.7 mg/ 5 mL; cherry creme de vanilla and banana flavor]; 200 mg/5 mL (15 mL, 22.5 mL, 30 mL) [contains sodium 7.4 mg/5 mL; cherry creme de vanilla and banana flavor]; 1 g [single-dose packet; contains sodium 37 mg per packet; cherry creme de vanilla and banana flavor]
Tablet, as dihydrate:
Zithromax®: 250 mg [contains sodium 0.9 mg per tablet]; 500 mg [contains sodium 1.8 mg per tablet]; 600 mg [contains sodium 2.1 mg per tablet]
Zithromax® TRI-PAK™ [unit-dose pack]: 500 mg (3s) [contains sodium 1.8 mg per tablet]
Zithromax® Z-PAK® [unit-dose pack]: 250 mg (6s) [contains sodium 0.9 mg per tablet]
Tablet, as monohydrate: 250 mg, 500 mg, 600 mg

azithromycin dihydrate *see* azithromycin *on previous page*

Azmacort® [US] *see* triamcinolone (inhalation, oral) *on page 845*

AZO-Gesic® [US-OTC] *see* phenazopyridine *on page 656*

Azopt® [US/Can] *see* brinzolamide *on page 117*

AZO-Standard® [US-OTC] *see* phenazopyridine *on page 656*

AZT™ [Can] *see* zidovudine *on page 886*

AZT, abacavir, and lamivudine *see* abacavir, lamivudine, and zidovudine *on page 2*

azthreonam *see* aztreonam *on this page*

aztreonam (AZ tree oh nam)

Sound-Alike/Look-Alike Issues
aztreonam may be confused with azidothymidine

Synonyms azthreonam

U.S./Canadian Brand Names Azactam® [US/Can]

Therapeutic Category Antibiotic, Miscellaneous

Use Treatment of patients with urinary tract infections, lower respiratory tract infections, septicemia, skin/skin structure infections, intraabdominal infections, and gynecological infections caused by susceptible gram-negative bacilli

Usual Dosage
Children >1 month: I.M., I.V.:
Mild-to-moderate infections: I.M., I.V.: 30 mg/kg every 8 hours
Moderate-to-severe infections: I.M., I.V.: 30 mg/kg every 6-8 hours; maximum: 120 mg/kg/day (8 g/day)
Cystic fibrosis: I.V.: 50 mg/kg/dose every 6-8 hours (ie, up to 200 mg/kg/day); maximum: 8 g/day
Adults:
Urinary tract infection: I.M., I.V.: 500 mg to 1 g every 8-12 hours
Moderately-severe systemic infections: 1 g I.V. or I.M. or 2 g I.V. every 8-12 hours
Severe systemic or life-threatening infections (especially caused by *Pseudomonas aeruginosa*): I.V.: 2 g every 6-8 hours; maximum: 8 g/day
Meningitis (gram-negative): I.V.: 2 g every 6-8 hours

Dosage Forms
Infusion [premixed]: 1 g (50 mL); 2 g (50 mL)
Injection, powder for reconstitution: 500 mg, 1 g, 2 g

Azulfidine® [US] *see* sulfasalazine *on page 799*

Azulfidine® EN-tabs® [US] *see* sulfasalazine *on page 799*

B1 *see* tositumomab and iodine I 131 tositumomab *on page 837*

B1 antibody *see* tositumomab and iodine I 131 tositumomab *on page 837*

B-D™ Glucose [US-OTC] *see* glucose (instant) *on page 386*

B2036-PEG *see* pegvisomant *on page 645*

B 9273 *see* alefacept *on page 26*

BA-16038 *see* aminoglutethimide *on page 42*

Babee® Cof Syrup [US-OTC] *see* dextromethorphan *on page 245*

BabyBIG® [US] *see* botulism immune globulin (intravenous-human) *on page 116*

BAC *see* benzalkonium chloride *on page 99*

Bacid® [US-OTC/Can] *see* Lactobacillus *on page 477*

Baciguent® [US-OTC/Can] *see* bacitracin *on this page*

BaciiM® [US] *see* bacitracin *on this page*

Baciject® [Can] *see* bacitracin *on this page*

bacillus calmette-Guérin (BCG) live *see* BCG vaccine *on page 94*

bacitracin (bas i TRAY sin)

Sound-Alike/Look-Alike Issues

bacitracin may be confused with Bactrim®, Bactroban®

U.S./Canadian Brand Names Baciguent® [US-OTC/Can]; BaciiM® [US]; Baciject® [Can]

Therapeutic Category Antibiotic, Miscellaneous; Antibiotic, Ophthalmic; Antibiotic, Topical

Use Treatment of susceptible bacterial infections mainly; has activity against gram-positive bacilli; due to toxicity risks, systemic and irrigant uses of bacitracin should be limited to situations where less toxic alternatives would not be effective

Usual Dosage Do not administer I.V.:

Infants: I.M.:

≤2.5 kg: 900 units/kg/day in 2-3 divided doses

>2.5 kg: 1000 units/kg/day in 2-3 divided doses

Children: I.M.: 800-1200 units/kg/day divided every 8 hours

Adults: Oral: Antibiotic-associated colitis: 25,000 units 4 times/day for 7-10 days

Children and Adults:

Topical: Apply 1-5 times/day

Ophthalmic, ointment: Instill ¹/₄" to ¹/₂" ribbon every 3-4 hours into conjunctival sac for acute infections, or 2-3 times/day for mild-to-moderate infections for 7-10 days

Irrigation, solution: 50-100 units/mL in normal saline, lactated Ringer's, or sterile water for irrigation; soak sponges in solution for topical compresses 1-5 times/day or as needed during surgical procedures

Dosage Forms [DSC] = Discontinued product

Injection, powder for reconstitution (BaciiM®): 50,000 units

Ointment, ophthalmic (AK-Tracin® [DSC]): 500 units/g (3.5 g)

Ointment, topical: 500 units/g (0.9 g, 15 g, 30 g, 120 g, 454 g)

Baciguent®: 500 units/g (15 g, 30 g)

bacitracin and polymyxin B (bas i TRAY sin & pol i MIKS in bee)

Sound-Alike/Look-Alike Issues

Betadine® may be confused with Betagan®, betaine

Synonyms polymyxin B and bacitracin

U.S./Canadian Brand Names AK-Poly-Bac® [US]; LID-Pack® [Can]; Optimyxin® [Can]; Polysporin® Ophthalmic [US]; Polysporin® Topical [US-OTC]

Therapeutic Category Antibiotic, Ophthalmic; Antibiotic, Topical

Use Treatment of superficial infections caused by susceptible organisms

Usual Dosage Children and Adults:

Ophthalmic ointment: Instill ¹/₂" ribbon in the affected eye(s) every 3-4 hours for acute infections or 2-3 times/day for mild-to-moderate infections for 7-10 days

Topical ointment/powder: Apply to affected area 1-4 times/day; may cover with sterile bandage if needed

Dosage Forms [DSC] = Discontinued product

Ointment, ophthalmic: Bacitracin 500 units and polymyxin B 10,000 units per g (3.5 g)

AK-Poly-Bac™: Bacitracin 500 units and polymyxin B 10,000 units per g (3.5 g)

Ointment, topical: Bacitracin 500 units and polymyxin B 10,000 units per g in white petrolatum (15 g, 30 g)

Betadine® First Aid Antibiotics + Moisturizer: Bacitracin 500 units and polymyxin B 10,000 units per g (14 g) [DSC]

Polysporin®: Bacitracin 500 units and polymyxin B 10,000 units per g (0.9 g, 15 g, 30 g)

Powder, topical:

Polysporin®: Bacitracin 500 units and polymyxin B 10,000 units per g (10 g)

bacitracin, neomycin, and polymyxin B

(bas i TRAY sin, nee oh MYE sin, & pol i MIKS in bee)

Synonyms neomycin, bacitracin, and polymyxin B; polymyxin B, bacitracin, and neomycin; triple antibiotic

U.S./Canadian Brand Names Neosporin® Neo To Go® [US-OTC]; Neosporin® Ophthalmic Ointment [Can]; Neosporin® Topical [US-OTC]

Therapeutic Category Antibiotic, Ophthalmic; Antibiotic, Topical

Use Helps prevent infection in minor cuts, scrapes, and burns; short-term treatment of superficial external ocular infections caused by susceptible organisms

Usual Dosage Children and Adults:

Ophthalmic: Ointment: Instill $^1/_2$" into the conjunctival sac every 3-4 hours for 7-10 days for acute infections

Topical: Apply 1-3 times/day to infected area; may cover with sterile bandage as needed

Dosage Forms [DSC] = Discontinued product

Ointment, ophthalmic (Neosporin® [DSC]): Bacitracin 400 units, neomycin 3.5 mg, and polymyxin B 10,000 units per g (3.5 g)

Ointment, topical: Bacitracin 400 units, neomycin 3.5 mg, and polymyxin B 5000 units per g (0.9 g, 15 g, 30 g, 454 g)

Neosporin®: Bacitracin 400 units, neomycin 3.5 mg, and polymyxin B 5000 units per g (15 g, 30 g)

Neosporin® Neo To Go®: Bacitracin 400 units, neomycin 3.5 mg, and polymyxin B 5000 units per g (0.9 g)

bacitracin, neomycin, polymyxin B, and hydrocortisone

(bas i TRAY sin, nee oh MYE sin, pol i MIKS in bee, & hye droe KOR ti sone)

Synonyms hydrocortisone, bacitracin, neomycin, and polymyxin B; neomycin, bacitracin, polymyxin B, and hydrocortisone; polymyxin B, bacitracin, neomycin, and hydrocortisone

U.S./Canadian Brand Names Cortisporin® Ointment [US]; Cortisporin® Topical Ointment [Can]

Therapeutic Category Antibiotic/Corticosteroid, Ophthalmic; Antibiotic/Corticosteroid, Topical

Use Prevention and treatment of susceptible inflammatory conditions where bacterial infection (or risk of infection) is present

Usual Dosage Children and Adults:

Ophthalmic: Ointment: Instill $^1/_2$" ribbon to inside of lower lid every 3-4 hours until improvement occurs

Topical: Apply sparingly 2-4 times/day. Therapy should be discontinued when control is achieved; if no improvement is seen, reassessment of diagnosis may be necessary.

Dosage Forms

Ointment, ophthalmic: Bacitracin 400 units, neomycin 3.5 mg, polymyxin B 10,000 units, and hydrocortisone 10 mg per g (3.5 g)

Ointment, topical:

Cortisporin®: Bacitracin 400 units, neomycin 3.5 mg, polymyxin B 5000 units, and hydrocortisone 10 mg per g (15 g)

bacitracin, neomycin, polymyxin B, and pramoxine

(bas i TRAY sin, nee oh MYE sin, pol i MIKS in bee, & pra MOKS een)

Synonyms neomycin, bacitracin, polymyxin B, and pramoxine; polymyxin B, neomycin, bacitracin, and pramoxine; pramoxine, neomycin, bacitracin, and polymyxin B

U.S./Canadian Brand Names Neosporin® + Pain Ointment [US-OTC]; Spectrocin Plus™ [US-OTC]

Therapeutic Category Antibiotic, Topical

Use Prevention and treatment of susceptible superficial topical infections and provide temporary relief of pain or discomfort

Usual Dosage Children ≥2 years and Adults: Apply 1-3 times/day to infected areas; cover with sterile bandage if needed

Dosage Forms

Ointment, topical: Bacitracin 500 units, neomycin base 3.5 mg, polymyxin B sulfate 10,000 units, and pramoxine hydrochloride 10 mg (15 g, 30 g)

Neosporin® + Pain Ointment: Bacitracin 500 units, neomycin base 3.5 mg, polymyxin B sulfate 10,000 units, and pramoxine hydrochloride 10 mg (15 g, 30 g)

Spectrocin Plus™: Bacitracin 500 units, neomycin base 3.5 mg, polymyxin B sulfate 10,000 units, and pramoxine hydrochloride 10 mg (30 g)

baclofen (BAK loe fen)

Sound-Alike/Look-Alike Issues

baclofen may be confused with Bactroban®

Lioresal® may be confused with lisinopril, Loniten®, Lotensin®

U.S./Canadian Brand Names Apo-Baclofen® [Can]; Gen-Baclofen [Can]; Lioresal® [US/Can]; Liotec [Can]; Nu-Baclo [Can]; PMS-Baclofen [Can]

(Continued)

baclofen *(Continued)*

Therapeutic Category Skeletal Muscle Relaxant

Use Treatment of reversible spasticity associated with multiple sclerosis or spinal cord lesions

Orphan drug: Intrathecal: Treatment of intractable spasticity caused by spinal cord injury, multiple sclerosis, and other spinal disease (spinal ischemia or tumor, transverse myelitis, cervical spondylosis, degenerative myelopathy)

Usual Dosage

Oral (avoid abrupt withdrawal of drug):

Children:

2-7 years: Initial: 10-15 mg/24 hours divided every 8 hours; titrate dose every 3 days in increments of 5-15 mg/day to a maximum of 40 mg/day

≥8 years: Maximum: 60 mg/day in 3 divided doses

Adults: 5 mg 3 times/day, may increase 5 mg/dose every 3 days to a maximum of 80 mg/day

Hiccups: Adults: Usual effective dose: 10-20 mg 2-3 times/day

Intrathecal: Children and Adults:

Test dose: 50-100 mcg, doses >50 mcg should be given in 25 mcg increments, separated by 24 hours. A screening dose of 25 mcg may be considered in very small patients. Patients not responding to screening dose of 100 mcg should not be considered for chronic infusion/implanted pump.

Maintenance: After positive response to test dose, a maintenance intrathecal infusion can be administered via an implanted intrathecal pump. Initial dose via pump: Infusion at a 24-hour rate dosed at twice the test dose. Avoid abrupt discontinuation.

Dosage Forms

Injection, solution, intrathecal [preservative free]:

Lioresal®: 50 mcg/mL (1 mL); 500 mcg/mL (20 mL); 2000 mcg/mL (5 mL, 20 mL)

Tablet: 10 mg, 20 mg

BactoShield® CHG [US-OTC] *see* chlorhexidine gluconate *on page 173*

BactoShield® ***(Discontinued)*** *see* chlorhexidine gluconate *on page 173*

Bactrim™ [US] *see* sulfamethoxazole and trimethoprim *on page 797*

Bactrim™ DS [US] *see* sulfamethoxazole and trimethoprim *on page 797*

Bactrim™ I.V. Infusion ***(Discontinued)*** *see* sulfamethoxazole and trimethoprim *on page 797*

Bactroban® [US/Can] *see* mupirocin *on page 569*

Bactroban® Nasal [US] *see* mupirocin *on page 569*

baking soda *see* sodium bicarbonate *on page 776*

BAL *see* dimercaprol *on page 259*

Balacet 325™ [US] *see* propoxyphene and acetaminophen *on page 708*

balanced salt solution (BAL anced salt soe LOO shun)

U.S./Canadian Brand Names AquaLase™ [US]; BSS Plus® [US/Can]; BSS® [US/Can]; Eye-Stream® [Can]

Therapeutic Category Ophthalmic Agent, Miscellaneous

Use

Irrigation solution for ophthalmic surgery:

AquaLase™, BSS®: Intraocular or extraocular irrigating solution

BSS® Plus: Intraocular irrigating solution

Irrigation solution for eyes, ears, nose, or throat

Usual Dosage Adults: Ophthalmic irrigation: Based on standard for each surgical procedure

Dosage Forms

Solution, irrigation [preservative free]: Sodium chloride 0.64%, potassium chloride 0.075%, calcium chloride 0.048%, magnesium chloride 0.03%, sodium acetate 0.39%, sodium citrate 0.17% (500 mL)

Solution, ophthalmic [irrigation; preservative free]: Sodium chloride 0.64%, potassium chloride 0.075%, calcium chloride 0.048%, magnesium chloride 0.03%, sodium acetate 0.39%, sodium citrate 0.17% (18 mL, 500 mL)

AquaLase™: Sodium chloride 0.64%, potassium chloride 0.075%, calcium chloride 0.048%, magnesium chloride 0.03%, sodium acetate 0.39%, sodium citrate 0.17% (90 mL)

BSS®: Sodium chloride 0.64%, potassium chloride 0.075%, calcium chloride 0.048%, magnesium chloride 0.03%, sodium acetate 0.39%, sodium citrate 0.17% (15 mL, 30 mL, 250 mL, 500 mL)

BSS Plus®: Sodium chloride 0.71%, potassium chloride 0.038%, calcium chloride 0.015%, magnesium chloride 0.02%, sodium phosphate 0.042%, sodium bicarbonate 0.21%, dextrose 0.092%, glutathione 0.018% (250 mL, 500 mL)

Baldex® *(Discontinued)*

BAL in Oil® [US] *see* dimercaprol *on page 259*

Balmex® [US-OTC] *see* zinc oxide *on page 887*

Balminil Decongestant [Can] *see* pseudoephedrine *on page 712*

Balminil DM D [Can] *see* pseudoephedrine and dextromethorphan *on page 714*

Balminil DM + Decongestant + Expectorant [Can] *see* guaifenesin, pseudoephedrine, and dextromethorphan *on page 401*

Balminil DM E [Can] *see* guaifenesin and dextromethorphan *on page 394*

Balminil Expectorant [Can] *see* guaifenesin *on page 392*

Balnetar® [US-OTC/Can] *see* coal tar *on page 207*

balsalazide (bal SAL a zide)

Sound-Alike/Look-Alike Issues
Colazal® may be confused with Clozaril®

Synonyms balsalazide disodium

U.S./Canadian Brand Names Colazal® [US]

Therapeutic Category 5-Aminosalicylic Acid Derivative; Antiinflammatory Agent

Use Treatment of mild-to-moderate active ulcerative colitis

Usual Dosage Oral: Adults: 2.25 g (three 750 mg capsules) 3 times/day for 8-12 weeks

Dosage Forms
Capsule, as disodium:
Colazal®: 750 mg

balsalazide disodium *see* balsalazide *on this page*

balsam peru, trypsin, and castor oil *see* trypsin, balsam peru, and castor oil *on page 856*

Bancap HC® [US] *see* hydrocodone and acetaminophen *on page 420*

Band-Aid® Hurt-Free™ Antiseptic Wash [US-OTC] *see* lidocaine *on page 493*

Banophen® [US-OTC] *see* diphenhydramine *on page 261*

Banophen® Anti-Itch [US-OTC] *see* diphenhydramine *on page 261*

Banophen® Decongestant Capsule *(Discontinued)* *see* diphenhydramine and pseudoephedrine *on page 263*

Baraclude™ [US] *see* entecavir *on page 294*

Barbidonna® *(Discontinued)* *see* hyoscyamine, atropine, scopolamine, and phenobarbital *on page 435*

Barbita® *(Discontinued)* *see* phenobarbital *on page 658*

Barc™ Liquid *(Discontinued)*

Baricon® [US] *see* radiological/contrast media (ionic) *on page 728*

Baridium® [US-OTC] *see* phenazopyridine *on page 656*

barium sulfate *see* radiological/contrast media (ionic) *on page 728*

Barobag® [US] *see* radiological/contrast media (ionic) *on page 728*

Baro-CAT® [US] *see* radiological/contrast media (ionic) *on page 728*

Baroflave® [US] *see* radiological/contrast media (ionic) *on page 728*

Barosperse® [US] *see* radiological/contrast media (ionic) *on page 728*

Bar-Test® [US] *see* radiological/contrast media (ionic) *on page 728*

Basaljel® [Can] *see* aluminum hydroxide *on page 36*

base ointment *see* zinc oxide *on page 887*

basiliximab (ba si LIK si mab)

U.S./Canadian Brand Names Simulect® [US/Can]

Therapeutic Category Immunosuppressant Agent

Use Prophylaxis of acute organ rejection in renal transplantation

Usual Dosage **Note:** Patients previously administered basiliximab should only be reexposed to a subsequent course of therapy with extreme caution.

(Continued)

basiliximab *(Continued)*

I.V.:

Children <35 kg: Renal transplantation: 10 mg within 2 hours prior to transplant surgery, followed by a second 10 mg dose 4 days after transplantation; the second dose should be withheld if complications occur (including severe hypersensitivity reactions or graft loss)

Children ≥35 kg and Adults: Renal transplantation: 20 mg within 2 hours prior to transplant surgery, followed by a second 20 mg dose 4 days after transplantation; the second dose should be withheld if complications occur (including severe hypersensitivity reactions or graft loss)

Dosage Forms

Injection, powder for reconstitution [preservative free]:

Simulect®: 10 mg, 20 mg

Bausch & Lomb® Computer Eye Drops [US-OTC] *see* glycerin *on page 388*

BAY 43-9006 *see* sorafenib *on page 787*

Bayer® Aspirin [US-OTC] *see* aspirin *on page 77*

Bayer® Aspirin Extra Strength [US-OTC] *see* aspirin *on page 77*

Bayer® Aspirin Regimen Adult Low Strength [US-OTC] *see* aspirin *on page 77*

Bayer® Aspirin Regimen Children's [US-OTC] *see* aspirin *on page 77*

Bayer® Aspirin Regimen Regular Strength [US-OTC] *see* aspirin *on page 77*

Bayer® Extra Strength Arthritis Pain Regimen [US-OTC] *see* aspirin *on page 77*

Bayer® Plus Extra Strength [US-OTC] *see* aspirin *on page 77*

Bayer® Women's Aspirin Plus Calcium [US-OTC] *see* aspirin *on page 77*

BayGam® [Can] *see* immune globulin (intramuscular) *on page 443*

BayGam® *(Discontinued)* *see* immune globulin (intramuscular) *on page 443*

BayHep B® [Can] *see* hepatitis B immune globulin *on page 411*

BayHepB® *(Discontinued)* *see* hepatitis B immune globulin *on page 411*

BayRab® [Can] *see* rabies immune globulin (human) *on page 727*

BayRab® *(Discontinued)* *see* rabies immune globulin (human) *on page 727*

BayRho-D® Full-Dose [Can] *see* Rh_o(D) immune globulin *on page 740*

BayRho-D® Full Dose *(Discontinued)* *see* Rh_o(D) immune globulin *on page 740*

BayRho-D® Mini Dose *(Discontinued)* *see* Rh_o(D) immune globulin *on page 740*

BayTet™ [Can] *see* tetanus immune globulin (human) *on page 814*

BayTet™ *(Discontinued)* *see* tetanus immune globulin (human) *on page 814*

Baza® Antifungal [US-OTC] *see* miconazole *on page 553*

Baza® Clear [US-OTC] *see* vitamin A and vitamin D *on page 876*

B-Caro-T™ [US] *see* beta-carotene *on page 106*

BCG, live *see* BCG vaccine *on this page*

BCG vaccine (bee see jee vak SEEN)

Synonyms bacillus calmette-Guérin (BCG) live; BCG, live; BCG vaccine U.S.P. *(percutaneous use product)*

U.S./Canadian Brand Names ImmuCyst® [Can]; Oncotice™ [Can]; Pacis™ [Can]; TheraCys® [US]; TICE® BCG [US]

Therapeutic Category Biological Response Modulator

Use Immunization against tuberculosis and immunotherapy for cancer; treatment and prophylaxis of carcinoma *in situ* of the bladder; prophylaxis of primary or recurrent superficial papillary tumors following transurethral resection

Usual Dosage

Immunization against tuberculosis: Percutaneous: **Note:** Initial lesion usually appears after 10-14 days consisting of small, red papule at injection site and reaches maximum diameter of 3 mm in 4-6 weeks.

Children <1 month: 0.2-0.3 mL (half-strength dilution). Administer tuberculin test (5 TU) after 2-3 months; repeat vaccination after 1 year of age for negative tuberculin test if indications persist.

Children >1 month and Adults: 0.2-0.3 mL (full strength dilution); conduct postvaccinal tuberculin test (5 TU of PPD) in 2-3 months; if test is negative, repeat vaccination.

Immunotherapy for bladder cancer: Intravesicular Adults:

TheraCys®: One dose instilled into bladder (for 2 hours) once weekly for 6 weeks followed by one treatment at 3, 6, 12, 18, and 24 months after initial treatment

TICE® BCG: One dose instilled into the bladder (for 2 hours) once weekly for 6 weeks followed by once monthly for 6-12 months

Dosage Forms

Injection, powder for reconstitution, intravesical:

TheraCys®: 81 mg [with diluent]

TICE® BCG: 50 mg

Injection, powder for reconstitution, percutaneous:

BCG Vaccine U.S.P.: 50 mg

BCG vaccine U.S.P. *(percutaneous use product)* *see* BCG vaccine *on previous page*

BCI-Fluoxetine [Can] *see* fluoxetine *on page 357*

BCI-Gabapentin [Can] *see* gabapentin *on page 373*

BCI-Metformin [Can] *see* metformin *on page 535*

BCI-Ranitidine [Can] *see* ranitidine *on page 732*

BCI-Simvastatin [Can] *see* simvastatin *on page 773*

BCNU *see* carmustine *on page 153*

B complex combinations *see* vitamin B complex combinations *on page 876*

Bebulin® VH [US] *see* factor IX complex (human) *on page 334*

becaplermin (be KAP ler min)

Sound-Alike/Look-Alike Issues

Regranex® may be confused with Granulex®, Repronex®

Synonyms recombinant human platelet-derived growth factor B; rPDGF-BB

U.S./Canadian Brand Names Regranex® [US/Can]

Therapeutic Category Topical Skin Product

Use Debridement adjunct for the treatment of diabetic ulcers that occur on the lower limbs and feet

Usual Dosage Topical: Adults:

Diabetic ulcers: Apply appropriate amount of gel once daily with a cotton swab or similar tool, as a coating over the ulcer

The amount of becaplermin to be applied will vary depending on the size of the ulcer area. To calculate the length of gel applied to the ulcer, measure the greatest length of the ulcer by the greatest width of the ulcer in inches. Tube size will determine the formula used in the calculation. For a 15 or 7.5 g tube, multiply length x width x 0.6. For a 2 g tube, multiply length x width x 1.3.

Note: If the ulcer does not decrease in size by ~30% after 10 weeks of treatment or complete healing has not occurred in 20 weeks, continued treatment with becaplermin gel should be reassessed.

Dosage Forms Gel, topical: 0.01% (15 g)

beclomethasone (be kloe METH a sone)

Sound-Alike/Look-Alike Issues

Vanceril® may be confused with Vancenase®

Synonyms beclomethasone dipropionate

U.S./Canadian Brand Names Apo-Beclomethasone® [Can]; Beconase® AQ [US]; Gen-Beclo [Can]; Nu-Beclomethasone [Can]; Propaderm® [Can]; QVAR® [US/Can]; Rivanase AQ [Can]; Vanceril® AEM [Can]

Therapeutic Category Adrenal Corticosteroid

Use

Oral inhalation: Maintenance and prophylactic treatment of asthma; includes those who require corticosteroids and those who may benefit from a dose reduction/elimination of systemically-administered corticosteroids. Not for relief of acute bronchospasm.

Nasal aerosol: Symptomatic treatment of seasonal or perennial rhinitis; prevent recurrence of nasal polyps following surgery.

Usual Dosage Nasal inhalation and oral inhalation dosage forms are not to be used interchangeably

Inhalation, nasal: Rhinitis, nasal polyps (Beconase® AQ): Children ≥6 years and Adults: 1-2 inhalations each nostril twice daily; total dose 168-336 mcg/day

Inhalation, oral: Asthma (doses should be titrated to the lowest effective dose once asthma is controlled) (QVAR®):

Children 5-11 years: Initial: 40 mcg twice daily; maximum dose: 80 mcg twice daily

(Continued)

beclomethasone *(Continued)*

Children ≥12 years and Adults:

Patients previously on bronchodilators only: Initial dose 40-80 mcg twice daily; maximum dose: 320 mcg twice day

Patients previously on inhaled corticosteroids: Initial dose 40-160 mcg twice daily; maximum dose: 320 mcg twice daily

NIH Asthma Guidelines (NAEPP, 2002; NIH, 1997): HFA formulation (eg, QVAR®): Administer in divided doses:

Children ≤12 years:
"Low" dose: 80-160 mcg/day
"Medium" dose: 160-320 mcg/day
"High" dose: >320 mcg/day

Children >12 years and Adults:
"Low" dose: 80-240 mcg/day
"Medium" dose: 240-480 mcg/day
"High" dose: >480 mcg/day

Dosage Forms

Aerosol for oral inhalation, as dipropionate:

QVAR®: 40 mcg/inhalation [100 metered actuations] (7.3 g); 80 mcg/inhalation [100 metered actuations] (7.3 g)

Suspension, intranasal, as dipropionate [aqueous spray]:

Beconase® AQ: 42 mcg/inhalation [180 metered sprays (25 g)

beclomethasone dipropionate *see* beclomethasone *on previous page*

Beclovent® *(Discontinued)* *see* beclomethasone *on previous page*

Beconase® AQ [US] *see* beclomethasone *on previous page*

Beconase® *(Discontinued)* *see* beclomethasone *on previous page*

Becotin® Pulvules® *(Discontinued)*

Beepen-VK® *(Discontinued)* *see* penicillin V potassium *on page 649*

behenyl alcohol *see* docosanol *on page 270*

Belix® Oral *(Discontinued)* *see* diphenhydramine *on page 261*

belladonna alkaloids with phenobarbital *see* hyoscyamine, atropine, scopolamine, and phenobarbital *on page 435*

belladonna and opium (bel a DON a & OH pee um)

Synonyms opium and belladonna

U.S./Canadian Brand Names B&O Supprettes® [US]

Therapeutic Category Analgesic, Narcotic

Controlled Substance C-II

Use Relief of moderate-to-severe pain associated with ureteral spasms not responsive to nonopioid analgesics and to space intervals between injections of opiates

Usual Dosage Rectal: Children >12 years and Adults: 1 suppository 1-2 times/day, up to 4 doses/day

Dosage Forms

Suppository: Belladonna extract 16.2 mg and opium 30 mg; belladonna extract 16.2 mg and opium 60 mg

B&O Supprettes® #15 A: Belladonna extract 16.2 mg and opium 30 mg

B&O Supprettes® #16 A: Belladonna extract 16.2 mg and opium 60 mg

belladonna, phenobarbital, and ergotamine

(bel a DON a, fee noe BAR bi tal, & er GOT a meen)

Synonyms ergotamine tartrate, belladonna, and phenobarbital; phenobarbital, belladonna, and ergotamine tartrate

U.S./Canadian Brand Names Bel-Tabs [US]; Bellamine S [US]; Bellergal® Spacetabs® [Can]

Therapeutic Category Ergot Derivative

Use Management and treatment of menopausal disorders, GI disorders, and recurrent throbbing headache

Usual Dosage Oral: 1 tablet each morning and evening

Dosage Forms Tablet: Belladonna alkaloids 0.2 mg, phenobarbital 40 mg, and ergotamine tartrate 0.6 mg

Bellamine S [US] *see* belladonna, phenobarbital, and ergotamine *on this page*

Bellatal® *(Discontinued)* *see* hyoscyamine, atropine, scopolamine, and phenobarbital *on page 435*

Bellergal-S® ***(Discontinued)***

Bellergal® Spacetabs® [Can] *see* belladonna, phenobarbital, and ergotamine *on previous page*

Bel-Tabs [US] *see* belladonna, phenobarbital, and ergotamine *on previous page*

Benadryl® [Can] *see* diphenhydramine *on page 261*

Benadryl® Allergy [US-OTC] *see* diphenhydramine *on page 261*

Benadryl® Allergy and Sinus Fastmelt™ [US-OTC] *see* diphenhydramine and pseudoephedrine *on page 263*

Benadryl® Allergy/Sinus [US-OTC] *see* diphenhydramine and pseudoephedrine *on page 263*

Benadryl® Children's Allergy [US-OTC] *see* diphenhydramine *on page 261*

Benadryl® Children's Allergy and Cold Fastmelt™ [US-OTC] *see* diphenhydramine and pseudoephedrine *on page 263*

Benadryl® Children's Allergy and Sinus [US-OTC] *see* diphenhydramine and pseudoephedrine *on page 263*

Benadryl® Children's Allergy Fastmelt® [US-OTC] *see* diphenhydramine *on page 261*

Benadryl® Dye-Free Allergy [US-OTC] *see* diphenhydramine *on page 261*

Benadryl® Injection [US] *see* diphenhydramine *on page 261*

Benadryl® Itch Stopping [US-OTC] *see* diphenhydramine *on page 261*

Benadryl® Itch Stopping Extra Strength [US-OTC] *see* diphenhydramine *on page 261*

Ben-Allergin-50® Injection ***(Discontinued)*** *see* diphenhydramine *on page 261*

Ben-Aqua® ***(Discontinued)*** *see* benzoyl peroxide *on page 102*

benazepril (ben AY ze pril)

Sound-Alike/Look-Alike Issues

benazepril may be confused with Benadryl®

Lotensin® may be confused with Lioresal®, Loniten®, lovastatin

Synonyms benazepril hydrochloride

U.S./Canadian Brand Names Apo-Benazepril® [Can]; Lotensin® [US/Can]

Therapeutic Category Angiotensin-Converting Enzyme (ACE) Inhibitor

Use Treatment of hypertension, either alone or in combination with other antihypertensive agents

Usual Dosage Oral: Hypertension:

Children ≥6 years: Initial: 0.2 mg/kg/day as monotherapy; dosing range: 0.1-0.6 mg/kg/day (maximum dose: 40 mg/day)

Adults: Initial: 10 mg/day in patients not receiving a diuretic; 20-40 mg/day as a single dose or 2 divided doses; the need for twice-daily dosing should be assessed by monitoring peak (2-6 hours after dosing) and trough responses.

Note: Patients taking diuretics should have them discontinued 2-3 days prior to starting benazepril. If they cannot be discontinued, then initial dose should be 5 mg; restart after blood pressure is stabilized if needed.

Dosage Forms

Tablet, as hydrochloride: 5 mg, 10 mg, 20 mg, 40 mg

Lotensin®: 5 mg, 10 mg, 20 mg, 40 mg

benazepril and hydrochlorothiazide (ben AY ze pril & hye droe klor oh THYE a zide)

Synonyms hydrochlorothiazide and benazepril

U.S./Canadian Brand Names Lotensin® HCT [US]

Therapeutic Category Antihypertensive Agent, Combination

Use Treatment of hypertension

Usual Dosage Oral: Dose is individualized (range: benazepril: 5-20 mg; hydrochlorothiazide: 6.25-25 mg/day)

Dosage Forms

Tablet: 5/6.25: Benazepril hydrochloride 5 mg and hydrochlorothiazide 6.25 mg; 10/12.5: Benazepril hydrochloride 10 mg and hydrochlorothiazide 12.5 mg; 20/12.5: Benazepril hydrochloride 20 mg and hydrochlorothiazide 12.5 mg; 20/25: Benazepril hydrochloride 20 mg and hydrochlorothiazide 25 mg

Lotensin® HCT 5/6.25: Benazepril hydrochloride 5 mg and hydrochlorothiazide 6.25 mg

Lotensin® HCT 10/12.5: Benazepril hydrochloride 10 mg and hydrochlorothiazide 12.5 mg

Lotensin® HCT 20/12.5: Benazepril hydrochloride 20 mg and hydrochlorothiazide 12.5 mg

Lotensin® HCT 20/25: Benazepril hydrochloride 20 mg and hydrochlorothiazide 25 mg

benazepril hydrochloride *see* benazepril *on previous page*

benazepril hydrochloride and amlodipine besylate *see* amlodipine and benazepril *on page 46*

BeneFix® [US/Can] *see* factor IX *on page 333*

Beneflur® [Can] *see* fludarabine *on page 350*

Benemid® *(Discontinued)* *see* probenecid *on page 699*

Benicar® [US] *see* olmesartan *on page 614*

Benicar HCT® [US] *see* olmesartan and hydrochlorothiazide *on page 614*

Benoquin® [US] *see* monobenzone *on page 564*

Benoxyl® [Can] *see* benzoyl peroxide *on page 102*

benserazide and levodopa *(Canada only)* (ben SER a zide & lee voe DOE pa)

Synonyms levodopa and benserazide

U.S./Canadian Brand Names Prolopa® [Can]

Therapeutic Category Anti-Parkinson Agent

Use Treatment of Parkinson disease (except drug-induced parkinsonism)

Usual Dosage Oral: Adults: **Note:** Dosage expressed as levodopa/benserazide:

Initial: 100/25 mg 1-2 times/day, increase every 3-4 days until therapeutic effect; optimal dosage: 400/100 mg to 800/200 mg/day divided into 4-6 doses

Note: 200/50 mg used only when maintenance therapy is reached and not to exceed levodopa 1000-1200 mg/benserazide 250-300 mg per day

Patients previously on levodopa: Allow 12 hours or more to lapse between last dose of levodopa; start at 15% of previous levodopa dosage

Note: Dosages should be introduced gradually, individualized, and continued for 3-6 weeks before assessing benefit. Decrease dosage in patients with dystonia.

Dosage Forms [CAN] = Canadian brand name

Capsule:

Prolopa® [CAN]:

50-12.5: Levodopa 50 mg and benserazide 12.5 mg [not available in the U.S.]

100-25: Levodopa 100 mg and benserazide 25 mg [not available in the U.S.]

200-50: Levodopa 200 mg and benserazide 50 mg [not available in the U.S.]

bentoquatam (BEN toe kwa tam)

Synonyms quaternium-18 bentonite

U.S./Canadian Brand Names IvyBlock® [US-OTC]

Therapeutic Category Protectant, Topical

Use Skin protectant for the prevention of allergic contact dermatitis to poison oak, ivy, and sumac

Usual Dosage Children >6 years and Adults: Topical: Apply to skin 15 minutes prior to potential exposure to poison ivy, poison oak, or poison sumac, and reapply every 4 hours

Dosage Forms Lotion: 5% (120 mL) [contains benzyl alcohol]

Bentyl® [US] *see* dicyclomine *on page 251*

Bentyl® Injection *(Discontinued)* *see* dicyclomine *on page 251*

Bentylol® [Can] *see* dicyclomine *on page 251*

Benuryl™ [Can] *see* probenecid *on page 699*

Benylin® 3.3 mg-D-E [Can] *see* guaifenesin, pseudoephedrine, and codeine *on page 401*

Benylin® D for Infants [Can] *see* pseudoephedrine *on page 712*

Benylin® Adult *(Discontinued)* *see* dextromethorphan *on page 245*

Benylin® Cough Syrup *(Discontinued)* *see* diphenhydramine *on page 261*

Benylin® DM-D [Can] *see* pseudoephedrine and dextromethorphan *on page 714*

Benylin® DM-D-E [Can] *see* guaifenesin, pseudoephedrine, and dextromethorphan *on page 401*

Benylin® DM *(Discontinued)* *see* dextromethorphan *on page 245*

Benylin® DM-E [Can] *see* guaifenesin and dextromethorphan *on page 394*

Benylin® E Extra Strength [Can] *see* guaifenesin *on page 392*

Benylin® Expectorant *(Discontinued)* *see* guaifenesin and dextromethorphan *on page 394*

Benylin® Pediatric *(Discontinued)* *see* dextromethorphan *on page 245*

Benza® [US-OTC] *see* benzalkonium chloride *on this page*

Benzac® [US] *see* benzoyl peroxide *on page 102*

Benzac® AC [US/Can] *see* benzoyl peroxide *on page 102*

Benzac® AC Gel *(Discontinued)* *see* benzoyl peroxide *on page 102*

Benzac® AC Wash [US] *see* benzoyl peroxide *on page 102*

BenzaClin® [US/Can] *see* clindamycin and benzoyl peroxide *on page 199*

Benzac® W [US] *see* benzoyl peroxide *on page 102*

Benzac® W Gel [Can] *see* benzoyl peroxide *on page 102*

Benzac® W Gel *(Discontinued)* *see* benzoyl peroxide *on page 102*

Benzac® W Wash [US/Can] *see* benzoyl peroxide *on page 102*

Benzagel® [US] *see* benzoyl peroxide *on page 102*

Benzagel® Wash *(Discontinued)* *see* benzoyl peroxide *on page 102*

benzalkonium chloride (benz al KOE nee um KLOR ide)

Sound-Alike/Look-Alike Issues

Benza® may be confused with Benzac®

Synonyms BAC

U.S./Canadian Brand Names 3M™ Cavilon™ Skin Cleanser [US-OTC]; Benza® [US-OTC]; HandClens® [US-OTC]; Zephiran® [US-OTC]

Therapeutic Category Antibacterial, Topical

Use Surface antiseptic and germicidal preservative

Usual Dosage Thoroughly rinse anionic detergents and soaps from the skin or other areas prior to use of solutions because they reduce the antibacterial activity of BAC. To protect metal instruments stored in BAC solution, add crushed Anti-Rust Tablets, 4 tablets/quart, to antiseptic solution, change solution at least once weekly. Not to be used for storage of aluminum or zinc instruments, instruments with lenses fastened by cement, lacquered catheters, or some synthetic rubber goods.

Dosage Forms [DSC] = Discontinued product

Solution, topical:

Benza®: 1:750 (60 mL, 240 mL, 480 mL, 3840 mL)

HandClens®: 0.13% (120 mL, 480 mL, 800 mL)

Ony-Clear [DSC]: 1% (30 mL)

Zephiran®: 1:750 (240 mL, 3840 mL) [aqueous]

Solution, topical spray (3M™ Cavilon™ Skin Cleanser): 0.11% (240 mL)

benzalkonium chloride, benzocaine, butyl aminobenzoate, and tetracaine hydrochloride *see* benzocaine, butyl aminobenzoate, tetracaine, and benzalkonium chloride *on page 101*

Benzamycin® [US] *see* erythromycin and benzoyl peroxide *on page 305*

Benzamycin® Pak [US] *see* erythromycin and benzoyl peroxide *on page 305*

Benzashave® [US] *see* benzoyl peroxide *on page 102*

benzathine benzylpenicillin *see* penicillin G benzathine *on page 646*

benzathine penicillin G *see* penicillin G benzathine *on page 646*

Benzedrex® [US-OTC] *see* propylhexedrine *on page 710*

benzene hexachloride *see* lindane *on page 497*

benzhexol hydrochloride *see* trihexyphenidyl *on page 850*

Benziq™ [US] *see* benzoyl peroxide *on page 102*

Benziq™ LS [US] *see* benzoyl peroxide *on page 102*

benzmethyzin *see* procarbazine *on page 701*

benzocaine (BEN zoe kane)

Sound-Alike/Look-Alike Issues

Orabase®-B may be confused with Orinase®

Synonyms ethyl aminobenzoate

U.S./Canadian Brand Names Americaine® Hemorrhoidal [US-OTC]; Americaine® [US-OTC]; Anbesol® Baby [US-OTC/Can]; Anbesol® Cold Sore Therapy [US-OTC]; Anbesol® Jr. [US-OTC]; Anbesol® Maximum

(Continued)

benzocaine *(Continued)*

Strength [US-OTC]; Anbesol® [US-OTC]; Benzodent® [US-OTC]; Cepacol® Sore Throat [US-OTC]; Chiggerex® [US-OTC]; Chiggertox® [US-OTC]; Cylex® [US-OTC]; Dent's Extra Strength Toothache [US-OTC]; Dent's Maxi-Strength Toothache [US-OTC]; Dentapaine [US-OTC]; Dermoplast® Antibacterial [US-OTC]; Dermoplast® Pain Relieving [US-OTC]; Detane® [US-OTC]; Foille® [US-OTC]; HDA® Toothache [US-OTC]; Hurricaine® [US-OTC]; Ivy-Rid® [US-OTC]; Kanka® Soft Brush™ [US-OTC]; Lanacane® Maximum Strength [US-OTC]; Lanacane® [US-OTC]; Mycinettes® [US-OTC]; Orabase® with Benzocaine [US-OTC]; Orajel PM® [US-OTC]; Orajel® Baby Teething Daytime and Nighttime [US-OTC]; Orajel® Baby Teething Nighttime [US-OTC]; Orajel® Baby Teething [US-OTC]; Orajel® Denture Plus [US-OTC]; Orajel® Maximum Strength [US-OTC]; Orajel® Medicated Toothache [US-OTC]; Orajel® Mouth Sore [US-OTC]; Orajel® Multi-Action Cold Sore [US-OTC]; Orajel® Ultra Mouth Sore [US-OTC]; Oticaine [US]; Otocaine™ [US]; Outgro® [US-OTC]; Red Cross™ Canker Sore [US-OTC]; Rid-A-Pain Dental Drops [US-OTC]; Skeeter Stik [US-OTC]; Sting-Kill [US-OTC]; Tanac® [US-OTC]; Thorets [US-OTC]; Trocaine® [US-OTC]; Zilactin Baby® [Can]; Zilactin Toothache and Gum Pain® [US-OTC]; Zilactin®-B [US-OTC/Can]

Therapeutic Category Local Anesthetic

Use Temporary relief of pain associated with pruritic dermatosis, pruritus, minor burns, acute congestive and serous otitis media, swimmer's ear, otitis externa, bee stings, insect bites; mouth and gum irritations (toothache, minor sore throat pain, canker sores, dentures, orthodontia, teething, mucositis, stomatitis); sunburn; hemorrhoids; anesthetic lubricant for passage of catheters and endoscopic tubes

Usual Dosage Note: These are general dosing guidelines; Refer to specific product labeling for dosing instructions.

Children ≥4 months: Topical (oral): Teething pain: 7.5% to 10%: Apply to affected gum area up to 4 times daily

Children ≥2 years and Adults:

Topical:

Bee stings, insect bites, minor burns, sunburn: 5% to 20%: Apply to affected area 3-4 times a day as needed. In cases of bee stings, remove stinger before treatment.

Lubricant for passage of catheters and instruments: 20%: Apply evenly to exterior of instrument prior to use.

Topical (oral): Mouth and gum irritation: 10% to 20%: Apply thin layer to affected area up to 4 times daily

Children ≥5 years and Adults: Oral: Sore throat: Allow one lozenge (10-15 mg) to dissolve slowly in mouth; may repeat every 2 hours as needed

Children ≥12 years and Adults: Rectal: Hemorrhoids: 5% to 20%: Apply externally to affected area up to 6 times daily

Adults: Otic: 20%: Instill 4-5 drops into external auditory canal; may repeat in 1-2 hours if needed

Dosage Forms

Aerosol, oral spray (Hurricaine®): 20% (60 mL) [dye free; cherry flavor]

Aerosol, topical spray:

Americaine®: 20% (60 mL)

Dermoplast® Antibacterial: 20% (83 mL) [contains aloe vera, benzethonium chloride, menthol]

Dermoplast® Pain Relieving: 20% (60 mL, 83 mL) [contains menthol]

Foille®: 5% (92 g) [contains chloroxylenol 0.63% and corn oil]

Ivy-Rid®: 2% (83 mL)

Lanacane® Maximum Strength: 20% (120 mL) [contains alcohol]

Solarcaine®: 20% (120 mL) [contains triclosan 0.13%, alcohol 35%]

Combination package (Orajel® Baby Daytime and Nighttime):

Gel, oral [Daytime Regular Formula]: 7.5% (5.3 g)

Gel, oral [Nighttime Formula]: 10% (5.3 g)

Cream, oral:

Benzodent®: 20% (7.5 g, 30 g)

Orajel PM®: 20% (5.3 g, 7 g)

Cream, topical:

Lanacane®: 6% (30 g, 60 g)

Lanacane® Maximum Strength: 20% (30 g)

Gel, oral:

Anbesol®: 10% (7.5 g) [contains benzyl alcohol; cool mint flavor]

Anbesol® Baby: 7.5% (7.5 g) [contains benzoic acid; grape flavor]

Anbesol® Jr.: 10% (7 g) [contains benzyl alcohol; bubble gum flavor]

Anbesol® Maximum Strength: 20% (7.5 g, 10 g) [contains benzyl alcohol]

Dentapaine: 20% (11 g) [contains clove oil]

HDA® Toothache: 6.5% (15 mL) [contains benzyl alcohol]

Hurricaine®: 20% (5 g) [dye free; wild cherry flavor]; (30 g) [dye free; mint, pina colada, watermelon, and wild cherry flavors]

Kanka® Soft Brush™: 20% (2 mL) [packaged in applicator with brush tip]
Orabase® with Benzocaine®: 20% (7 g) [contains ethyl alcohol 48%; mild mint flavor]
Orajel®: 10% (5.3 g, 7 g, 9.4 g)
Orajel® Baby Teething: 7.5% (9.4 g, 11.9 g) [cherry flavor]
Orajel® Baby Teething Nighttime: 10% (5.3 g)
Orajel® Denture Plus: 15% (9 g) [contains menthol 2%, ethyl alcohol 66.7%]
Orajel® Maximum Strength: 20% (5.3 g, 7 g, 9.4 g, 11.9 g)
Orajel® Mouth Sore: 20% (5.3 g, 9.4 g, 11.9 g) [contains benzalkonium chloride 0.02%, zinc chloride 0.1%]
Orajel® Multi-Action Cold Sore: 20% (9.4 g) [contains allantoin 0.5%, camphor 3%, dimethicone 2%]
Orajel® Ultra Mouth Sore: 15% (9.4 g) [contains ethyl alcohol 66.7%, menthol 2%]
Zilactin®-B: 10% (7.5 g)

Gel, topical (Detane®): 7.5% (15 g)

Liquid, oral:
Anbesol®: 10% (9 mL) [cool mint flavor]
Anbesol® Maximum Strength: 20% (9 mL) [contains benzyl alcohol]
Hurricaine®: 20% (30 mL) [pina colada and wild cherry flavors]
Orajel® Baby Teething: 7.5% (13 mL) [very berry flavor]
Orajel® Maximum Strength: 20% (13 mL) [contains ethyl alcohol 44%, tartrazine]

Liquid, oral drop:
Dent's Maxi-Strength Toothache: 20% (3.7 mL) [contains alcohol 74%]
Rid-A-Pain Dental Drops: 6.3% (30 mL) [contains alcohol 70%]

Liquid, topical:
Chiggertox®: 2% (30 mL)
Outgro®: 20% (9 mL)
Skeeter Stik: 5% (14 mL) [contains menthol]
Tanac®: 10% (13 mL) [contains benzalkonium chloride]

Lozenge: 6 mg (18s) [contains menthol]; 15 mg (10s)
Cepacol® Sore Throat: 10 mg (18s) [contains cetylpyridinium, menthol; cherry, citrus, honey lemon, and menthol flavors]
Cepacol® Sore Throat: 10 mg (16s) [sugar free; contains cetylpyridinium, menthol; cherry and menthol flavors]
Cylex®: 15 mg [sugar free; contains cetylpyridinium chloride 5 mg; cherry flavor]
Mycinettes®: 15 mg (12s) [sugar free; contains sodium 9 mg; cherry or regular flavor]
Thorets: 18 mg (500s) [sugar free]
Trocaine®: 10 mg (40s, 400s)

Ointment, oral:
Anbesol® Cold Sore Therapy: 20% (7.1 g) [contains benzyl alcohol, allantoin, aloe, camphor, menthol, vitamin E]
Red Cross™ Canker Sore: 20% (7.5 g) [contains coconut oil]

Ointment, rectal (Americaine® Hemorrhoidal): 20% (30 g)

Ointment, topical:
Chiggerex®: 2% (50 g) [contains aloe vera]
Foille®: 5% (3.5 g, 14 g, 28 g) [contains chloroxylenol 0.1%, benzyl alcohol; corn oil base]

Pads, topical (Sting-Kill): 20% (8s) [contains menthol and tartrazine]

Paste, oral (Orabase® with Benzocaine): 20% (6 g)

Solution, otic drops (Oticaine, Otocaine™): 20% (15 mL)

Swabs, oral:
Hurricaine®: 20% (6s, 100s) [dye free; wild cherry flavor]
Orajel® Baby Teething: 7.5% (12s) [berry flavor]
Orajel® Medicated Mouth Sore, Orajel® Medicated Toothache: 20% (8s, 12s) [contains tartrazine]
Zilactin® Toothache and Gum Pain: 20% (8s) [grape flavor]

Swabs, topical (Sting-Kill): 20% (5s) [contains menthol and tartrazine]

Wax, oral (Dent's Extra Strength Toothache Gum): 20% (1 g)

benzocaine and antipyrine *see* antipyrine and benzocaine *on page 62*

benzocaine, butyl aminobenzoate, tetracaine, and benzalkonium chloride

(BEN zoe kane, BYOO til a meen oh BENZ oh ate, TET ra kane, & benz al KOE nee um KLOR ide)

Synonyms benzalkonium chloride, benzocaine, butyl aminobenzoate, and tetracaine hydrochloride; butyl aminobenzoate, tetracaine hydrochloride, benzocaine, and benzalkonium chloride; tetracaine hydrochloride, benzocaine, butyl aminobenzoate, and benzalkonium chloride

(Continued)

benzocaine, butyl aminobenzoate, tetracaine, and benzalkonium chloride *(Continued)*

U.S./Canadian Brand Names Cetacaine® [US]

Therapeutic Category Local Anesthetic

Use Topical anesthetic to control pain or gagging, pain in surgical or endocscopic procedures; anesthetic for accessible mucous membranes except for the eyes.

Usual Dosage Apply to affected area for approximately 1 second

Dosage Forms

Aerosol, topical: Benzocaine 14%, butyl aminobenzoate 2%, tetracaine hydrochloride 2%, and benzalkonium chloride 0.5% (56 g) [also packaged in a kit with various sized cannulas]

Gel, topical: Benzocaine 14%, butyl aminobenzoate 2%, tetracaine hydrochloride 2%, and benzalkonium chloride 0.5% (29 g)

Liquid, topical: Benzocaine 14%, butyl aminobenzoate 2%, tetracaine hydrochloride 2%, and benzalkonium chloride 0.5% (56 mL)

Benzocol® *(Discontinued)* *see* benzocaine *on page 99*

Benzodent® [US-OTC] *see* benzocaine *on page 99*

benzoin (BEN zoin)

Synonyms gum benjamin

Therapeutic Category Pharmaceutical Aid; Protectant, Topical

Use Protective application for irritations of the skin; sometimes used in boiling water as steam inhalants for its expectorant and soothing action

Usual Dosage Apply 1-2 times/day

Dosage Forms [DSC] = Discontinued product

Tincture, USP: (15 mL, 60 mL, 120 mL, 480 mL, 4000 mL)

TinBen®: 120 mL [DSC]

Tincture, USP [spray]: 120 mL

benzonatate (ben ZOE na tate)

U.S./Canadian Brand Names Tessalon® [US/Can]

Therapeutic Category Antitussive

Use Symptomatic relief of nonproductive cough

Usual Dosage Children >10 years and Adults: Oral: 100 mg 3 times/day or every 4 hours up to 600 mg/day

Dosage Forms

Capsule: 100 mg

Tessalon®: 100 mg, 200 mg

benzoyl peroxide (BEN zoe il peer OKS ide)

Sound-Alike/Look-Alike Issues

Benoxyl® may be confused with Brevoxyl®, Peroxyl®

Benzac® may be confused with Benza®

Benzac® W may be confused with Benzac® W Wash

Brevoxyl® may be confused with Benoxyl®

Fostex® may be confused with pHisoHex®

U.S./Canadian Brand Names Acetoxyl® [Can]; Benoxyl® [Can]; Benzac® AC Wash [US]; Benzac® AC [US/Can]; Benzac® W Gel [Can]; Benzac® W Wash [US/Can]; Benzac® W [US]; Benzac® [US]; Benzagel® [US]; Benzashave® [US]; Benziq™ LS [US] ; Benziq™ [US]; Brevoxyl® Cleansing [US]; Brevoxyl® Wash [US]; Brevoxyl® [US]; Clearplex [US-OTC]; Clinac™ BPO [US]; Del Aqua® [US]; Desquam-E™ [US]; Desquam-X® [US/Can]; Exact® Acne Medication [US-OTC]; Fostex® 10% BPO [US-OTC]; Loroxide® [US-OTC]; Neutrogena® Acne Mask [US-OTC]; Neutrogena® On The Spot® Acne Treatment [US-OTC]; Oxy 10® Balance Spot Treatment [US-OTC]; Oxy 10® Balanced Medicated Face Wash [US-OTC]; Oxyderm™ [Can]; Palmer's® Skin Success Acne [US-OTC]; PanOxyl® Aqua Gel [US]; PanOxyl® Bar [US-OTC]; PanOxyl® [US/Can]; PanOxyl®-AQ [US]; Seba-Gel™ [US]; Solugel® [Can]; Triaz® Cleanser [US]; Triaz® [US]; Zapzyt® [US-OTC]; Zoderm® [US]

Therapeutic Category Acne Products

Use Adjunctive treatment of mild-to-moderate acne vulgaris and acne rosacea

Usual Dosage Children and Adults:

Cleansers: Wash once or twice daily; control amount of drying or peeling by modifying dose frequency or concentration

Topical: Apply sparingly once daily; gradually increase to 2-3 times/day if needed. If excessive dryness or peeling occurs, reduce dose frequency or concentration; if excessive stinging or burning occurs, remove with mild soap and water; resume use the next day.

Dosage Forms [DSC] = Discontinued product

Cream, topical:

BenzaShave®: 5% (120 g); 10% (120 g) [contains sodium coconut sulfate and coconut acid]
Exact® Acne Medication: 5% (18 g)
Neutrogena® Acne Mask: 5% (60 g)
Neutrogena® On The Spot® Acne Treatment: 2.5% (22.5 g)
Zoderm®: 4.5% (125 mL) [contains urea 10%]; 6.5% (125 mL) [contains urea 10%]; 8.5% (125 mL) [contains urea 10%]

Emulsion, topical [cleanser]:

Zoderm®: 4.5% (400 mL) [contains urea 10%]; 6.5% (400 mL) [contains urea 10%]; 8.5% (400 mL) [contains urea 10%]

Gel, topical: 2.5% (60 g); 5% (45 g, 60 g, 90 g); 10% (45 g, 60 g, 90 g)

Benzac® AC [water based]: 5% (60 g); 10% (60 g)
Benzac® W [water based]: 2.5% (60 g); 5% (60 g); 10% (60 g) [DSC]
Benzagel®: 5% (45 g); 10% (45 g)
Benzagel® Wash [water based]: 10% (60 g) [DSC]
Benziq™: 5.25% (50 g)
Benziq™ LS: 2.75% (50 g)
Brevoxyl®: 4% (43 g, 90 g); 8% (43 g, 90 g)
Clearplex: 5% (45 g); 10% (45 g)
Clinac™ BPO: 7% (45 g)
Desquam-E™ [water based]: 2.5% (42.5 g); 5% (42.5 g) [emollient gel]
Desquam-X®: 5% (42.5 g, 90 g); 10% (42.5 g, 90 g)
Fostex® 10% BPO: 10% (45 g)
Oxy 10® Balance Spot Treatment: 5% (30 g); 10% (30 g)
PanOxyl® [alcohol based]: 5% (57 g, 113 g); 10% (57 g, 113 g)
PanOxyl® AQ [water based]: 2.5% (57 g, 113 g); 5% (57 g, 113 g); 10% (57 g, 113 g)
PanOxyl® Aqua Gel [water based]: 10% (42.5 g)
Seba-Gel™: 5% (90 g); 10% (90 g)
Triaz®: 3% (42.5 g) [DSC]; 6% (42.5 g) [DSC]
Triaz® Cleanser: 3% (170 g, 340 g); 6% (170 g, 340 g); 10% (170 g, 340 g)
Zapzyt®: 10% (30 g)
Zoderm®: 4.5% (125 mL) [contains urea 10%]; 6.5% (125 mL) [contains urea 10%]; 8.5% (125 mL) [contains urea 10%]

Liquid, topical: 2.5% (240 mL); 5% (120 mL, 150 mL, 240 mL); 10% (150 mL, 240 mL)

Benzac® AC Wash [water based]: 5% (240 mL); 10% (240 mL)
Benzac® W Wash [water based]: 5% (240 mL)
Benziq™ [wash]: 5.25% (175 g)
Del-Aqua®: 5% (45 mL); 10% (45 mL)
Desquam-X®: 5% (150 mL)
Oxy-10® Balance Medicated Face Wash: 10% (240 mL)

Lotion, topical: 5% (30 mL); 10% (30 mL)

Brevoxyl® Cleansing: 4% (297 g); 8% (297 g) [in a lathering vehicle]
Brevoxyl® Wash: 4% (170 g); 8% (170 g) [in a lathering vehicle]
Fostex® 10% BPO: 10% (150 mL)
Loroxide®: 5.5% (26 mL)
Palmer's® Skin Success Acne: 10% (30 mL) [contains vitamin E and aloe]

Pad, topical:

Triaz®: 3% (30s, 60s); 6% (30s, 60s); 9% (30s)
Zoderm®: 4.5% (30s); 6.5% (30s); 8.5% (30s)

Soap, topical [bar]:

Fostex® 10% BPO: 10% (113 g)
PanOxyl® Bar: 5% (113 g); 10% (113 g)

benzoyl peroxide and clindamycin *see* clindamycin and benzoyl peroxide *on page 199*

benzoyl peroxide and erythromycin *see* erythromycin and benzoyl peroxide *on page 305*

benzoyl peroxide and hydrocortisone (BEN zoe il peer OKS ide & hye droe KOR ti sone)

Synonyms hydrocortisone and benzoyl peroxide
U.S./Canadian Brand Names Vanoxide-HC® [US/Can]
Therapeutic Category Acne Products
Use Treatment of acne vulgaris and oily skin
Usual Dosage Adolescents and Adults: Topical: Shake well; apply thin film 1-3 times/day, gently massage into skin
Dosage Forms Lotion: Benzoyl peroxide 5% and hydrocortisone acetate 0.5% (25 mL)

benzphetamine (benz FET a meen)

Synonyms benzphetamine hydrochloride
U.S./Canadian Brand Names Didrex® [US/Can]
Therapeutic Category Anorexiant
Controlled Substance C-III
Use Short-term adjunct in exogenous obesity
Usual Dosage Children ≥12 years and Adults: Oral: Dose should be individualized based on patient response: Initial: 25-50 mg once daily; titrate to 25-50 mg 1-3 times/day; once-daily dosing should be administered midmorning or midafternoon; maximum dose: 50 mg 3 times/day
Dosage Forms Tablet, as hydrochloride: 50 mg

benzphetamine hydrochloride *see* benzphetamine *on this page*

benztropine (BENZ troe peen)

Sound-Alike/Look-Alike Issues
benztropine may be confused with bromocriptine
Synonyms benztropine mesylate
U.S./Canadian Brand Names Apo-Benztropine® [Can]; Cogentin® [US]
Therapeutic Category Anti-Parkinson Agent; Anticholinergic Agent
Use Adjunctive treatment of Parkinson disease; treatment of drug-induced extrapyramidal symptoms (except tardive dyskinesia)
Usual Dosage Use in children ≤3 years of age should be reserved for life-threatening emergencies
Drug-induced extrapyramidal symptom: Oral, I.M., I.V.:
Children >3 years: 0.02-0.05 mg/kg/dose 1-2 times/day
Adults: 1-4 mg/dose 1-2 times/day
Acute dystonia: Adults: I.M., I.V.: 1-2 mg
Parkinsonism: Adults: Oral: 0.5-6 mg/day in 1-2 divided doses; if one dose is greater, administer at bedtime; titrate dose in 0.5 mg increments at 5- to 6-day intervals
Dosage Forms
Injection, solution, as mesylate (Cogentin®): 1 mg/mL (2 mL)
Tablet, as mesylate: 0.5 mg, 1 mg, 2 mg

benztropine mesylate *see* benztropine *on this page*

benzydamine *(Canada only)* (ben ZID a meen)

Synonyms benzydamine hydrochloride
U.S./Canadian Brand Names Apo-Benzydamine® [Can]; Dom-Benzydamine [Can]; Novo-Benzydamine [Can]; PMS-Benzydamine [Can]; ratio-Benzydamine [Can]; Sun-Benz® [Can]; Tantum® [Can]
Therapeutic Category Analgesic, Topical
Use Symptomatic treatment of pain associated with acute pharyngitis; treatment of pain associated with radiation-induced oropharyngeal mucositis
Usual Dosage Oral rinse: Adults:
Acute pharyngitis: Gargle with 15 mL of undiluted solution every 1½-3 hours until symptoms resolve. Patient should expel solution from mouth following use; solution should not be swallowed.
Mucositis: 15 mL of undiluted solution as a gargle or rinse 3-4 times/day; contact should be maintained for at least 30 seconds, followed by expulsion from the mouth. Clinical studies maintained contact for ~2 minutes, up to 8 times/day. Patient should not swallow the liquid. Begin treatment 1day prior to initiation of radiation therapy and continue daily during treatment. Continue oral rinse treatments after the completion of radiation therapy until desired result/healing is achieved.
Dosage Forms [CAN] = Canadian brand name
Oral rinse: 0.15% (100 mL, 250 mL) [not available in the U.S.]

benzydamine hydrochloride *see* benzydamine *(Canada only) on this page*

benzylpenicillin benzathine *see* penicillin G benzathine *on page 646*

benzylpenicillin potassium *see* penicillin G (parenteral/aqueous) *on page 648*

benzylpenicillin sodium *see* penicillin G (parenteral/aqueous) *on page 648*

benzylpenicilloyl-polylysine (BEN zil pen i SIL oyl pol i LIE seen)

Synonyms penicilloyl-polylysine; PPL

Therapeutic Category Diagnostic Agent

Use Adjunct in assessing the risk of administering penicillin (penicillin or benzylpenicillin) in adults with a history of clinical penicillin hypersensitivity

Usual Dosage PPL is administered by a scratch technique or by intradermal injection. For initial testing, PPL should always be applied via the scratch technique. **Do not administer intradermally to patients who have positive reactions to a scratch test.** PPL test alone does not identify those patients who react to a minor antigenic determinant and does not appear to predict reliably the occurrence of late reactions.

Scratch test: Use scratch technique with a 20-gauge needle to make 3-5 mm nonbleeding scratch on epidermis, apply a small drop of solution to scratch, rub in gently with applicator or toothpick. A positive reaction consists of a pale wheal surrounding the scratch site which develops within 10 minutes and ranges from 5-15 mm or more in diameter.

Intradermal test: Use intradermal test with a tuberculin syringe with a 26- to 30-gauge short bevel needle; a dose of 0.01-0.02 mL is injected intradermally. A control of 0.9% sodium chloride should be injected at least 1.5" from the PPL test site. Most skin responses to the intradermal test will develop within 5-15 minutes.

Interpretation:

(-) Negative: No reaction

(±) Ambiguous: Wheal only slightly larger than original bleb with or without erythematous flare and larger than control site

(+) Positive: Itching and marked increase in size of original bleb

Control site should be reactionless

Dosage Forms [DSC] = Discontinued product

Injection, solution: 6 x 10^{-5} M (0.25 mL) [DSC]

beractant (ber AKT ant)

Sound-Alike/Look-Alike Issues

Survanta® may be confused with Sufenta®

Synonyms bovine lung surfactant; natural lung surfactant

U.S./Canadian Brand Names Survanta® [US/Can]

Therapeutic Category Lung Surfactant

Use Prevention and treatment of respiratory distress syndrome (RDS) in premature infants

Prophylactic therapy: Body weight <1250 g in infants at risk for developing, or with evidence of, surfactant deficiency (administer within 15 minutes of birth)

Rescue therapy: Treatment of infants with RDS confirmed by x-ray and requiring mechanical ventilation (administer as soon as possible - within 8 hours of age)

Usual Dosage

Prophylactic treatment: Administer 100 mg phospholipids (4 mL/kg) intratracheal as soon as possible; as many as 4 doses may be administered during the first 48 hours of life, no more frequently than 6 hours apart. The need for additional doses is determined by evidence of continuing respiratory distress; if the infant is still intubated and requiring at least 30% inspired oxygen to maintain a PaO_2 ≤80 torr.

Rescue treatment: Administer 100 mg phospholipids (4 mL/kg) as soon as the diagnosis of RDS is made; may repeat if needed, no more frequently than every 6 hours to a maximum of 4 doses

Dosage Forms Suspension for inhalation: 25 mg/mL (4 mL, 8 mL)

Berocca® ***(Discontinued)***

Berocca® Plus ***(Discontinued)***

Berotec® [Can] *see* fenoterol *(Canada only) on page 339*

Berubigen® ***(Discontinued)*** *see* cyanocobalamin *on page 219*

Betacaine® [Can] *see* lidocaine *on page 493*

beta-carotene (BAY ta KARE oh teen)

U.S./Canadian Brand Names A-Caro-25® [US]; B-Caro-T™ [US]; Lumitene™ [US]

Therapeutic Category Vitamin, Fat Soluble

Usual Dosage Oral:

Children <14 years: 30-150 mg/day

Adults: 30-300 mg/day

Dosage Forms

Capsule: 10,000 int. units (6 mg); 25,000 int. units (15 mg)

A-Caro-25®, B-Caro-T™: 25,000 int. units (15 mg)

Lumitene™: 50,000 int. units (30 mg)

Tablet: 10,000 int. units

Betachron® *(Discontinued)* *see* propranolol *on page 709*

Betaderm [Can] *see* betamethasone (topical) *on next page*

Betadine® [US-OTC/Can] *see* povidone-iodine *on page 689*

Betadine® First Aid Antibiotics + Moisturizer *(Discontinued)* *see* bacitracin and polymyxin B *on page 90*

Betadine® Ophthalmic [US] *see* povidone-iodine *on page 689*

Betagan® [US/Can] *see* levobunolol *on page 488*

Beta-HC® [US] *see* hydrocortisone (topical) *on page 428*

betahistine *(Canada only)* (bay ta HISS teen)

Synonyms betahistine dihydrochloride

U.S./Canadian Brand Names Serc® [Can]

Therapeutic Category Antihistamine

Use Treatment of Ménière disease (to decrease episodes of vertigo)

Usual Dosage Oral: Adults: 8-16 mg 3 times/day; administration with meals is recommended

Dosage Forms [CAN] = Canadian brand name

Tablet:

Serc® [CAN]: 16 mg, 24 mg [not available in the U.S.]

betahistine dihydrochloride *see* betahistine *(Canada only)* *on this page*

betaine (BAY ta een)

Sound-Alike/Look-Alike Issues

betaine may be confused with Betadine®

Synonyms betaine anhydrous

U.S./Canadian Brand Names Cystadane® [US/Can]

Therapeutic Category Homocystinuria Agent

Use Treatment of homocystinuria (eg, deficiencies or defects in cystathionine beta-synthase [CBS], 5,10-methylene tetrahydrofolate reductase [MTHFR], and cobalamin cofactor metabolism [CBL])

Usual Dosage

Children <3 years: Dosage may be started at 100 mg/kg/day and then increased weekly by 100 mg/kg increments.

Children ≥3 years and Adults: Oral: 6 g/day administered in divided doses of 3 g twice daily. Dosages of up to 20 g/day have been necessary to control homocysteine levels in some patients.

Note: Dosage in all patients can be gradually increased until plasma homocysteine is undetectable or present only in small amounts.

Dosage Forms

Powder for oral solution:

Cystadane®: 1 g/scoop (180 g) [1 scoop = 1.7 mL]

betaine anhydrous *see* betaine *on this page*

Betaject™ [Can] *see* betamethasone (systemic) *on next page*

Betalin® S *(Discontinued)* *see* thiamine *on page 821*

Betaloc® [Can] *see* metoprolol *on page 550*

Betaloc® Durules® [Can] *see* metoprolol *on page 550*

BetaMed [US-OTC] *see* pyrithione zinc *on page 723*

betamethasone and clotrimazole (bay ta METH a sone & kloe TRIM a zole)

Sound-Alike/Look-Alike Issues
Lotrisone® may be confused with Lotrimin®

Synonyms clotrimazole and betamethasone

U.S./Canadian Brand Names Lotriderm® [Can]; Lotrisone® [US]

Therapeutic Category Antifungal/Corticosteroid

Use Topical treatment of various dermal fungal infections (including tinea pedis, cruris, and corpora in patients ≥17 years of age)

Usual Dosage Children ≥17 years and Adults:
Allergic or inflammatory diseases: Topical: Apply to affected area twice daily, morning and evening
Tinea corporis, tinea cruris: Topical: Massage into affected area twice daily, morning and evening; do not use for longer than 2 weeks; re-evaluate after 1 week if no clinical improvement; do not exceed 45 g cream/week or 45 mL lotion/week
Tinea pedis: Topical: Massage into affected area twice daily, morning and evening; do not use for longer than 4 weeks; re-evaluate after 2 weeks if no clinical improvement; do not exceed 45 g cream/week or 45 mL lotion/week

Dosage Forms
Cream: Betamethasone dipropionate 0.05% and clotrimazole 1% (15 g, 45 g) [contains benzyl alcohol]
Lotion: Betamethasone dipropionate 0.05% and clotrimazole 1% (30 mL) [contains benzyl alcohol]

betamethasone dipropionate *see* betamethasone (topical) *on this page*

betamethasone dipropionate and calcipotriene hydrate *see* calcipotriene and betamethasone *on page 133*

betamethasone dipropionate, augmented *see* betamethasone (topical) *on this page*

betamethasone sodium phosphate *see* betamethasone (systemic) *on this page*

betamethasone (systemic) (bay ta METH a sone sis TEM ik)

Sound-Alike/Look-Alike Issues
Luxiq® may be confused with Lasix®

Synonyms betamethasone sodium phosphate

U.S./Canadian Brand Names Betaject™ [Can]; Celestone® Soluspan® [US/Can]; Celestone® [US]

Therapeutic Category Adrenal Corticosteroid

Use Antiinflammatory; immunosuppressant agent; corticosteroid replacement

Usual Dosage Base dosage on severity of disease and patient response
Children: Use lowest dose listed as initial dose for adrenocortical insufficiency (physiologic replacement)
I.M.: 0.0175-0.125 mg base/kg/day divided every 6-12 hours **or** 0.5-7.5 mg base/m²/day divided every 6-12 hours
Oral: 0.0175-0.25 mg/kg/day divided every 6-8 hours **or** 0.5-7.5 mg/m²/day divided every 6-8 hours
Adolescents and Adults:
Oral: 2.4-4.8 mg/day in 2-4 doses; range: 0.6-7.2 mg/day
I.M.: Betamethasone sodium phosphate and betamethasone acetate: 0.6-9 mg/day (generally, 1/3 to 1/2 of oral dose) divided every 12-24 hours
Adults:
Intrabursal, intra-articular, intradermal: 0.25-2 mL
Intralesional: Rheumatoid arthritis/osteoarthritis:
Very large joints: 1-2 mL
Large joints: 1 mL
Medium joints: 0.5-1 mL
Small joints: 0.25-0.5 mL

Dosage Forms Note: Potency expressed as betamethasone base.
Injection, suspension (Celestone® Soluspan®): Betamethasone sodium phosphate 3 mg/mL and betamethasone acetate 3 mg/mL [6 mg/mL] (5 mL)
Syrup, as base (Celestone®): 0.6 mg/5 mL (118 mL)

betamethasone (topical) (bay ta METH a sone TOP i kal)

Sound-Alike/Look-Alike Issues
Luxiq® may be confused with Lasix®

Synonyms betamethasone dipropionate; betamethasone dipropionate, augmented; betamethasone valerate; flubenisolone

U.S./Canadian Brand Names Beta-Val® [US]; Betaderm [Can]; Betnesol® [Can]; Betnovate® [Can]; Diprolene® AF [US]; Diprolene® Glycol [Can]; Diprolene® [US]; Diprosone® [Can]; Ectosone [Can]; Luxiq®
(Continued)

betamethasone (topical) *(Continued)*

[US]; Maxivate® [US]; Prevex® B [Can]; Taro-Sone® [Can]; Topilene® [Can]; Topisone® [Can]; Valisone® Scalp Lotion [Can]

Therapeutic Category Corticosteroid, Topical

Use Inflammatory dermatoses such as seborrheic or atopic dermatitis, neurodermatitis, anogenital pruritus, psoriasis, inflammatory phase of xerosis

Usual Dosage Topical:

≤12 years: Use is not recommended.

≥13 years: Use minimal amount for shortest period of time to avoid HPA axis suppression

Gel, augmented formulation: Apply once or twice daily; rub in gently. **Note:** Do not exceed 2 weeks of treatment or 50 g/week.

Lotion: Apply a few drops twice daily

Augmented formulation: Apply a few drops once or twice daily; rub in gently. **Note:** Do not exceed 2 weeks of treatment or 50 mL/week.

Cream/ointment: Apply one or twice daily.

Augmented formulation: Apply once or twice daily. **Note:** Do not exceed 2 weeks of treatment or 45 g/week.

Adults:

Foam: Apply to the scalp twice daily, once in the morning and once at night

Gel, augmented formulation: Apply once or twice daily; rub in gently. **Note:** Do not exceed 2 weeks of treatment or 50 g/week.

Lotion: Apply a few drops twice daily

Augmented formulation: Apply a few drops once or twice daily; runb in gently. **Note:** Do not exceed 2 weeks of treatment or 50 mL/week.

Cream/ointment: Apply once or twice daily

Augmented formulation: Apply once or twice daily. **Note:** Do not exceed 2 weeks of treatment or 45 g/week.

Dosage Forms [DSC] = Discontinued product

Note: Potency expressed as betamethasone base.

Cream, topical, as dipropionate: 0.05% (15 g, 45 g)

Maxivate®: 0.05% (45 g)

Cream, topical, as dipropionate augmented (Diprolene® AF): 0.05% (15 g, 50 g)

Cream, topical, as valerate (Beta-Val®): 0.1% (15 g, 45 g)

Foam, topical, as valerate (Luxiq®): 0.12% (50 g, 100 g, 150 g) [contains alcohol 60.4%]

Gel, topical, as dipropionate augmented (Diprolene® [DSC]): 0.05% (15 g, 50 g)

Lotion, topical, as dipropionate (Maxivate®): 0.05% (60 mL)

Lotion, topical, as dipropionate augmented (Diprolene®): 0.05% (30 mL, 60 mL)

Lotion, topical, as valerate (Beta-Val®): 0.1% (60 mL)

Ointment, topical, as dipropionate: 0.05% (15 g, 45 g)

Maxivate®: 0.05% (45 g)

Ointment, topical, as dipropionate augmented (Diprolene®): 0.05% (15 g, 50 g)

Ointment, topical, as valerate: 0.1% (15 g, 45 g)

betamethasone valerate *see* betamethasone (topical) *on previous page*

Betapace® [US] *see* sotalol *on page 787*

Betapace AF® [US/Can] *see* sotalol *on page 787*

Betasept® [US-OTC] *see* chlorhexidine gluconate *on page 173*

Betaseron® [US/Can] *see* interferon beta-1b *on page 457*

Betatar® Gel [US-OTC] *see* coal tar *on page 207*

Beta-Val® [US] *see* betamethasone (topical) *on previous page*

Betaxin® [Can] *see* thiamine *on page 821*

betaxolol (be TAKS oh lol)

Sound-Alike/Look-Alike Issues

betaxolol may be confused with bethanechol, labetalol

Synonyms betaxolol hydrochloride

U.S./Canadian Brand Names Betoptic® S [US/Can]; Kerlone® [US]; Sandoz-Betaxolol [Can]

Therapeutic Category Beta-Adrenergic Blocker

Use Treatment of chronic open-angle glaucoma and ocular hypertension; management of hypertension

Usual Dosage Adults:

Ophthalmic: Instill 1-2 drops twice daily.

Oral: 5-10 mg/day; may increase dose to 20 mg/day after 7-14 days if desired response is not achieved.

Dosage Forms

Solution, ophthalmic, as hydrochloride: 0.5% (5 mL, 10 mL, 15 mL) [contains benzalkonium chloride]

Suspension, ophthalmic, as hydrochloride (Betoptic® S): 0.25% (2.5 mL, 5 mL, 10 mL, 15 mL) [contains benzalkonium chloride]

Tablet, as hydrochloride (Kerlone®): 10 mg, 20 mg

betaxolol hydrochloride *see* betaxolol *on previous page*

bethanechol (be THAN e kole)

Sound-Alike/Look-Alike Issues

bethanechol may be confused with betaxolol

Synonyms bethanechol chloride

U.S./Canadian Brand Names Duvoid® [Can]; Myotonachol® [Can]; PMS-Bethanechol [Can]; Urecholine® [US]

Therapeutic Category Cholinergic Agent

Use Nonobstructive urinary retention and retention due to neurogenic bladder

Usual Dosage Adults: Urinary retention, neurogenic bladder, and/or bladder atony:

Oral: Initial: 10-50 mg 2-4 times/day (some patients may require dosages of 50-100 mg 4 times/day). To determine effective dose, may initiate at a dose of 5-10 mg, with additional doses of 5-10 mg hourly until an effective cumulative dose is reached. Cholinergic effects at higher oral dosages may be cumulative.

SubQ: Initial: 2.575 mg, may repeat in 15-30 minutes (maximum cumulative initial dose: 10.3 mg); subsequent doses may be given 3-4 times daily as needed (some patients may require more frequent dosing at 2.5- to 3-hour intervals). Chronic neurogenic atony may require doses of 7.5-10 every 4 hours.

Dosage Forms Tablet, as chloride: 5 mg, 10 mg, 25 mg, 50 mg

bethanechol chloride *see* bethanechol *on this page*

Betimol® [US] *see* timolol *on page 828*

Betnesol® [Can] *see* betamethasone (topical) *on page 107*

Betnovate® [Can] *see* betamethasone (topical) *on page 107*

Betoptic® S [US/Can] *see* betaxolol *on previous page*

bevacizumab (be vuh SIZ uh mab)

Sound-Alike/Look-Alike Issues

bevacizumab may be confused with cetuximab

Synonyms anti-VEGF monoclonal antibody; NSC-704865; rhuMAb-VEGF

U.S./Canadian Brand Names Avastin® [US]

Therapeutic Category Antineoplastic Agent, Monoclonal Antibody; Vaccine, Recombinant

Use Treatment of metastatic colorectal cancer; treatment of nonsquamous, nonsmall cell lung cancer

Usual Dosage I.V.: Adults: Colorectal cancer: 5 or 10 mg/kg every 2 weeks (5 mg/kg in combination with fluorouracil based or irinotecan/fluorouracil/ leucovorin treatment; 10 mg/kg when given in combination with FOLFOX4 regimen)

Dosage Forms

Injection, solution [preservative free]:

Avastin®: 25 mg/mL (4 mL, 16 mL)

bexarotene (beks AIR oh teen)

U.S./Canadian Brand Names Targretin® [US/Can]

Therapeutic Category Retinoic Acid Derivative; Vitamin A Derivative; Vitamin, Fat Soluble

Use

Oral: Treatment of cutaneous manifestations of cutaneous T-cell lymphoma in patients who are refractory to at least one prior systemic therapy

Topical: Treatment of cutaneous lesions in patients with refractory cutaneous T-cell lymphoma (stage 1A and 1B) or who have not tolerated other therapies

Usual Dosage Adults:

Oral: 300-400 mg/m²/day taken as a single daily dose.

Topical: Apply once every other day for first week, then increase on a weekly basis to once daily, 2 times/day, 3 times/day, and finally 4 times/day, according to tolerance

(Continued)

bexarotene *(Continued)*

Dosage Forms
Capsule: 75 mg
Gel: 1% (60 g)

Bextra® *(Discontinued)*

Bexxar® [US] *see* tositumomab and iodine I 131 tositumomab *on page 837*

bezafibrate *(Canada only)* (be za FYE brate)

U.S./Canadian Brand Names Bezalip® [Can]; PMS-Bezafibrate [Can]

Therapeutic Category Antihyperlipidemic Agent, Miscellaneous

Use Adjunct to diet and other therapeutic measures for treatment of type IIa and IIb mixed hyperlipidemia, to regulate lipid and apoprotein levels (reduce serum TG, LDL-cholesterol, and apolipoprotein B, increase HDL-cholesterol and apolipoprotein A); treatment of adult patients with high to very high triglyceride levels (Fredrickson classification type IV and V hyperlipidemias) who are at high risk of sequelae and complications from their dyslipidemia

Usual Dosage Oral: Adults:
Immediate release: 200 mg 2-3 times/day; may reduce to 200 mg twice daily in patients with good response
Sustained release: 400 mg once daily

Dosage Forms [CAN] = Canadian brand name
Tablet, immediate release: 200 mg [not available in the U.S.]
PMA-Bezafibrate [CAN]: 200 mg [not available in the U.S.]
Tablet, sustained release:
Bezalip® [CAN]: 400 mg [not available in the U.S.]

Bezalip® [Can] *see* bezafibrate *(Canada only) on this page*

BG 9273 *see* alefacept *on page 26*

BI-007 *see* paclitaxel (protein bound) *on page 631*

Biavax® II *(Discontinued)*

Biaxin® [US/Can] *see* clarithromycin *on page 195*

Biaxin® XL [US/Can] *see* clarithromycin *on page 195*

bicalutamide (bye ka LOO ta mide)

Synonyms CDX; ICI-176334; NC-722665

U.S./Canadian Brand Names Casodex® [US/Can]; CO Bicalutamide [Can]; Novo-Bicalutamide [Can]; PMS-Bicalutamide [Can]; ratio-Bicalutamide [Can]; Sandoz-Bicalutamide [Can]

Therapeutic Category Androgen

Use In combination therapy with LHRH agonist analogues in treatment of metastatic prostate cancer

Usual Dosage Adults: Oral: Metastatic prostate cancer: 50 mg once daily (in combination with an LHRH analogue)

Dosage Forms Tablet: 50 mg

Bicillin® L-A [US] *see* penicillin G benzathine *on page 646*

Bicillin® C-R [US] *see* penicillin G benzathine and penicillin G procaine *on page 647*

Bicillin® C-R 900/300 [US] *see* penicillin G benzathine and penicillin G procaine *on page 647*

BiCNu® [US/Can] *see* carmustine *on page 153*

BiDil® [US] *see* isosorbide dinitrate and hydralazine *on page 465*

BIG-IV *see* botulism immune globulin (intravenous-human) *on page 116*

Bilopaque® *(Discontinued)* *see* radiological/contrast media (ionic) *on page 728*

Biltricide® [US/Can] *see* praziquantel *on page 693*

bimatoprost (bi MAT oh prost)

U.S./Canadian Brand Names Lumigan® [US/Can]

Therapeutic Category Ophthalmic Agent, Miscellaneous

Use Reduction of intraocular pressure (IOP) in patients with open-angle glaucoma or ocular hypertension

Usual Dosage Ophthalmic: Adults: Open-angle glaucoma or ocular hypertension: Instill 1 drop into affected eye(s) once daily in the evening; do not exceed once-daily dosing (may decrease IOP-lowering effect). If used with other topical ophthalmic agents, separate administration by at least 5 minutes.

Dosage Forms

Solution, ophthalmic:

Lumigan®: 0.03% (2.5 mL, 5 mL, 7.5 mL) [contains benzalkonium chloride]

Biobase™ [Can] *see* alcohol (ethyl) *on page 25*

Biobase-G™ [Can] *see* alcohol (ethyl) *on page 25*

Biocef® [US] *see* cephalexin *on page 166*

Bioclate® ***(Discontinued)*** *see* antihemophilic factor (recombinant) *on page 59*

Biodine® ***(Discontinued)*** *see* povidone-iodine *on page 689*

Biofed [US-OTC] *see* pseudoephedrine *on page 712*

Biolon™ [US] *see* hyaluronate and derivatives *on page 416*

Bion® Tears [US-OTC] *see* artificial tears *on page 75*

Biopatch® ***(Discontinued)*** *see* chlorhexidine gluconate *on page 173*

BioQuin® Durules™ [Can] *see* quinidine *on page 725*

Bio-Statin® [US] *see* nystatin *on page 609*

BioThrax™ [US] *see* anthrax vaccine, adsorbed *on page 58*

Biozyme-C® ***(Discontinued)*** *see* collagenase *on page 212*

biperiden (bye PER i den)

Sound-Alike/Look-Alike Issues

Akineton® may be confused with Ecotrin®

Synonyms biperiden hydrochloride; biperiden lactate

U.S./Canadian Brand Names Akineton® [US/Can]

Therapeutic Category Anti-Parkinson Agent; Anticholinergic Agent

Use Adjunct in the therapy of all forms of parkinsonism; control of extrapyramidal symptoms secondary to antipsychotics

Usual Dosage Oral: Adults:

Parkinsonism: 2 mg 3-4 times/day

Extrapyramidal: 2 mg 1-3 times/day

Dosage Forms Tablet, as hydrochloride: 2 mg

biperiden hydrochloride *see* biperiden *on this page*

biperiden lactate *see* biperiden *on this page*

Biphentin® [Can] *see* methylphenidate *on page 546*

Bisac-Evac™ [US-OTC] *see* bisacodyl *on this page*

bisacodyl (bis a KOE dil)

Sound-Alike/Look-Alike Issues

Doxidan® may be confused with doxepin

Modane® may be confused with Matulane®, Moban®

U.S./Canadian Brand Names Alophen® [US-OTC]; Apo-Bisacodyl® [Can]; Bisac-Evac™ [US-OTC]; Bisacodyl Uniserts® [US-OTC]; Carter's Little Pills® [Can]; Correctol® Tablets [US-OTC]; Doxidan® *(reformulation)* [US-OTC]; Dulcolax® [US-OTC/Can]; Femilax™ [US-OTC]; Fleet® Bisacodyl Enema [US-OTC]; Fleet® Stimulant Laxative [US-OTC]; Gentlax® [Can]; Modane Tablets® [US-OTC]; Veracolate [US-OTC]

Therapeutic Category Laxative

Use Treatment of constipation; colonic evacuation prior to procedures or examination

Usual Dosage

Children:

Oral: >6 years: 5-10 mg (0.3 mg/kg) at bedtime or before breakfast

Rectal suppository:

<2 years: 5 mg as a single dose

>2 years: 10 mg

Adults:

Oral: 5-15 mg as single dose (up to 30 mg when complete evacuation of bowel is required)

Rectal suppository: 10 mg as single dose

(Continued)

bisacodyl *(Continued)*

Dosage Forms [DSC] = Discontinued product
Enema (Fleet® Bisacodyl Enema): 10 mg/30 mL (37 mL)
Suppository, rectal (Bisac-Evac™, Bisacodyl Uniserts®, Dulcolax®): 10 mg
Tablet, enteric coated (Alophen®, Bisac-Evac™, Correctol®, Dulcolax®, Femilax™, Fleet® Stimulant Laxative, Gentlax® [DSC], Modane®, Veracolate): 5 mg
Tablet, delayed release (Doxidan®): 5 mg

Bisacodyl Uniserts® [US-OTC] *see* bisacodyl *on previous page*

bis-chloronitrosourea *see* carmustine *on page 153*

bismuth subgallate (BIZ muth sub GAL ate)

Therapeutic Category Gastrointestinal Agent, Miscellaneous
Use Symptomatic treatment of mild, nonspecific diarrhea
Usual Dosage Oral: 1-2 tablets 3 times/day with meals
Dosage Forms Tablet, chewable: 200 mg

bismuth subsalicylate (BIZ muth sub sa LIS i late)

Synonyms pink bismuth
U.S./Canadian Brand Names Children's Kaopectate® (reformulation) [US-OTC]; Colo-Fresh™ [US-OTC]; Diotame® [US-OTC]; Kaopectate® Extra Strength [US-OTC]; Kaopectate® [US-OTC]; Pepto-Bismol® Maximum Strength [US-OTC]; Pepto-Bismol® [US-OTC]
Therapeutic Category Gastrointestinal Agent, Miscellaneous
Use Symptomatic treatment of mild, nonspecific diarrhea including traveler's diarrhea; chronic infantile diarrhea
Usual Dosage Oral:
Nonspecific diarrhea:
Children: Up to 8 doses/24 hours:
3-6 years: 1/3 tablet or 5 mL every 30 minutes to 1 hour as needed
6-9 years: 2/3 tablet or 10 mL every 30 minutes to 1 hour as needed
9-12 years: 1 tablet or 15 mL every 30 minutes to 1 hour as needed
Adults: 2 tablets or 30 mL every 30 minutes to 1 hour as needed up to 8 doses/24 hours
Prevention of traveler's diarrhea: 2.1 g/day or 2 tablets 4 times/day before meals and at bedtime
Dosage Forms
Liquid: 262 mg/15 mL (240 mL, 360 mL, 480 mL); 525 mg/15 mL (240 mL, 360 mL)
Children's Kaopectate®: 87 mg/5 mL (180 mL) [cherry flavor]
Diotame®: 262 mg/15 mL (30 mL)
Kaopectate®: 262 mg/15 mL (240 mL) [regular and peppermint flavor]
Kaopectate® Extra Strength: 525 mg/15 mL (240 mL) [peppermint flavor]
Pepto-Bismol®: 262 mg/15 mL (120 mL, 240 mL, 360 mL, 480 mL) [wintergreen flavor]
Pepto-Bismol® Maximum Strength: 525 mg/15 mL (120 mL, 240 mL, 360 mL) [wintergreen flavor]
Tablet, chewable (Diotame®, Pepto-Bismol®): 262 mg

bismuth subsalicylate, metronidazole, and tetracycline

(BIZ muth sub sa LIS i late, me troe NI da zole, & tet ra SYE kleen)
Synonyms bismuth subsalicylate, tetracycline, and metronidazole; metronidazole, bismuth subsalicylate, and tetracycline; tetracycline, metronidazole, and bismuth subsalicylate
U.S./Canadian Brand Names Helidac® [US]
Therapeutic Category Antidiarrheal
Use In combination with an H_2 antagonist, as part of a multidrug regimen for *H. pylori* eradication to reduce the risk of duodenal ulcer recurrence
Usual Dosage Adults: Chew 2 bismuth subsalicylate 262.4 mg tablets, swallow 1 metronidazole 250 mg tablet, and swallow 1 tetracycline 500 mg capsule 4 times/day at meals and bedtime, plus an H_2 antagonist (at the appropriate dose) for 14 days; follow with 8 oz of water; the H_2 antagonist should be continued for a total of 28 days
Dosage Forms Combination package [each package contains 14 blister cards (2-week supply); each card contains the following]:
Capsule: Tetracycline hydrochloride: 500 mg (4)
Tablet: Bismuth subsalicylate [chewable]: 262.4 mg (8)
Tablet: Metronidazole: 250 mg (4)

bismuth subsalicylate, tetracycline, and metronidazole *see* bismuth subsalicylate, metronidazole, and tetracycline *on previous page*

bisoprolol (bis OH proe lol)

Sound-Alike/Look-Alike Issues
Zebeta® may be confused with DiaBeta®
Synonyms bisoprolol fumarate
U.S./Canadian Brand Names Apo-Bisoprolol® [Can]; Monocor® [Can]; Novo-Bisoprolol [Can]; Sandoz-Bisoprolol [Can]; Zebeta® [US/Can]
Therapeutic Category Beta-Adrenergic Blocker
Use Treatment of hypertension, alone or in combination with other agents
Usual Dosage Oral: Adults: 2.5-5 mg once daily, may be increased to 10 mg, and then up to 20 mg once daily, if necessary
Hypertension (JNC 7): 2.5-10 mg once daily
Dosage Forms Tablet, as fumarate: 5 mg, 10 mg

bisoprolol and hydrochlorothiazide (bis OH proe lol & hye droe klor oh THYE a zide)

Sound-Alike/Look-Alike Issues
Ziac® may be confused with Tiazac®, Zerit®
Synonyms hydrochlorothiazide and bisoprolol
U.S./Canadian Brand Names Ziac® [US/Can]
Therapeutic Category Antihypertensive Agent, Combination
Use Treatment of hypertension
Usual Dosage Oral: Adults: Dose is individualized, given once daily
Dosage Forms Tablet:
2.5/6.25: Bisoprolol fumarate 2.5 mg and hydrochlorothiazide 6.25 mg
5/6.25: Bisoprolol fumarate 5 mg and hydrochlorothiazide 6.25 mg
10/6.25: Bisoprolol fumarate 10 mg and hydrochlorothiazide 6.25 mg

bisoprolol fumarate *see* bisoprolol *on this page*

bistropamide *see* tropicamide *on page 856*

bivalirudin (bye VAL i roo din)

Synonyms hirulog
U.S./Canadian Brand Names Angiomax® [US/Can]
Therapeutic Category Anticoagulant (Other)
Use Anticoagulant used in conjunction with aspirin for patients with unstable angina undergoing percutaneous transluminal coronary angioplasty (PTCA) or percutaneous coronary intervention (PCI) with provisional glycoprotein IIb/IIIa inhibitor; anticoagulant used in patients undergoing PCI with (or at risk of) heparin-induced thrombocytopenia (HIT) / thrombosis syndrome (HITTS)
Usual Dosage I.V.: Adults: Anticoagulant in patients undergoing PTCA/PCI or PCI with HITS/HITTS (treatment should be started just prior to procedure): Initial: Bolus: 0.75 mg/kg, followed by continuous infusion: 1.75 mg/kg/hour for the duration of procedure and up to 4 hours post-procedure if needed; determine ACT 5 minutes after bolus dose; may administer additional bolus of 0.3 mg/kg if necessary.
A glycoprotein IIb/IIIa inhibitor may be administered concomitantly during the procedure.
If needed, infusion may be continued beyond initial 4 hours at 0.2 mg/kg/hour for up to 20 hours.
Dosage Forms Injection, powder for reconstitution: 250 mg

BL4162A *see* anagrelide *on page 55*

Black Draught Tablets [US-OTC] *see* senna *on page 767*

black widow spider species antivenin (*Latrodectus mactans*) *see* antivenin *(Latrodectus mactans)* *on page 64*

BlemErase® Lotion *(Discontinued)* *see* benzoyl peroxide *on page 102*

Blenoxane® [US/Can] *see* bleomycin *on this page*

bleo *see* bleomycin *on this page*

bleomycin (blee oh MYE sin)

Sound-Alike/Look-Alike Issues
bleomycin may be confused with Cleocin®
(Continued)

bleomycin *(Continued)*

Synonyms bleo; bleomycin sulfate; BLM; NSC-125066

U.S./Canadian Brand Names Blenoxane® [US/Can]; Bleomycin Injection, USP [Can]

Therapeutic Category Antineoplastic Agent

Use Treatment of squamous cell carcinomas, melanomas, sarcomas, testicular carcinoma, Hodgkin lymphoma, and non-Hodgkin lymphoma

Orphan drug: Sclerosing agent for malignant pleural effusion

Usual Dosage Maximum cumulative lifetime dose: 400 units; refer to individual protocols; 1 unit = 1 mg

May be administered I.M., I.V., SubQ, or intracavitary

Children and Adults:

Test dose for lymphoma patients: I.M., I.V., SubQ: Because of the possibility of an anaphylactoid reaction, ≤2 units of bleomycin for the first 2 doses; monitor vital signs every 15 minutes; wait a minimum of 1 hour before administering remainder of dose; if no acute reaction occurs, then the regular dosage schedule may be followed. **Note:** Test doses may produce false-negative results.

Single-agent therapy:

I.M./I.V./SubQ: Squamous cell carcinoma, lymphoma, testicular carcinoma: 0.25-0.5 units/kg (10-20 units/m^2) 1-2 times/week

CIV: 15 units/m^2 over 24 hours daily for 4 days

Pleural sclerosing: Intrapleural: 60 units as a single instillation (some recommend limiting the dose in the elderly to 40 units/m^2; usual maximum: 60 units). Dose may be repeated at intervals of several days if fluid continues to accumulate (mix in 50-100 mL of NS); may add lidocaine 100-200 mg to reduce local discomfort.

Dosage Forms Injection, powder for reconstitution, as sulfate: 15 units, 30 units

Bleomycin Injection, USP [Can] *see* bleomycin *on previous page*

bleomycin sulfate *see* bleomycin *on previous page*

Bleph®-10 [US] *see* sulfacetamide *on page 795*

Blephamide® [US/Can] *see* sulfacetamide and prednisolone *on page 796*

Blis-To-Sol® [US-OTC] *see* tolnaftate *on page 834*

BLM *see* bleomycin *on previous page*

Blocadren® [US] *see* timolol *on page 828*

BMS-232632 *see* atazanavir *on page 80*

BMS 337039 *see* aripiprazole *on page 73*

BMS-354825 *see* dasatinib *on page 231*

Bonamine™ [Can] *see* meclizine *on page 522*

Bondronat® [Can] *see* ibandronate *on page 436*

Bonefos® [Can] *see* clodronate *(Canada only) on page 201*

Bonine® [US-OTC/Can] *see* meclizine *on page 522*

Boniva® [US] *see* ibandronate *on page 436*

Bontril® [Can] *see* phendimetrazine *on page 657*

Bontril® PDM [US] *see* phendimetrazine *on page 657*

Bontril® Slow-Release [US] *see* phendimetrazine *on page 657*

Boostrix® [US] *see* diphtheria, tetanus toxoids, and acellular pertussis vaccine *on page 265*

bortezomib (bore TEZ oh mib)

Synonyms LDP-341; MLN341; NSC-681239; PS-341

U.S./Canadian Brand Names Velcade® [US/Can]

Therapeutic Category Proteasome Inhibitor

Use Treatment of multiple myeloma in patients who have had at least one prior therapy

Usual Dosage I.V.: Adults: Multiple myeloma: 1.3 mg/m^2 twice weekly for 2 weeks on days 1, 4, 8, 11of a 21-day treatment regimen. Consecutive doses should be separated by at least 72 hours. Therapy extending beyond 8 cycles may be given once weekly for 4 weeks (days 1, 8, 15, and 22), followed by a 13-day rest (days 22 through 35).

Dosage Forms

Injection, powder for reconstitution [preservative free]:

Velcade®: 3.5 mg [contains mannitol 35 mg]

bosentan (boe SEN tan)

U.S./Canadian Brand Names Tracleer® [US/Can]

Therapeutic Category Endothelin Antagonist

Use Treatment of pulmonary artery hypertension (PAH) (WHO Group I) in patients with World Health Organization (WHO) Class III or IV symptoms to improve exercise capacity and decrease the rate of clinical deterioration

Usual Dosage Oral: Adolescents >12 years and ≥40 kg and Adults: Initial: 62.5 mg twice daily for 4 weeks; increase to maintenance dose of 125 mg twice daily; adults <40 kg should be maintained at 62.5 mg twice daily. Doses >125 mg twice daily do not appear to confer additional clinical benefit but may increase risk of liver toxicity.

Note: When discontinuing treatment, consider a reduction in dosage to 62.5 mg twice daily for 3-7 days (to avoid clinical deterioration).

Dosage Forms

Tablet:

Tracleer®: 62.5 mg, 125 mg

B&O Supprettes® [US] *see* belladonna and opium *on page 96*

Botox® [US/Can] *see* botulinum toxin type A *on this page*

Botox® Cosmetic [US/Can] *see* botulinum toxin type A *on this page*

botulinum toxin type A (BOT yoo lin num TOKS in type aye)

Synonyms BTX-A

U.S./Canadian Brand Names Botox® Cosmetic [US/Can]; Botox® [US/Can]

Therapeutic Category Ophthalmic Agent, Toxin

Use Treatment of strabismus and blepharospasm associated with dystonia (including benign essential blepharospasm or VII nerve disorders in patients ≥12 years of age); cervical dystonia (spasmodic torticollis) in patients ≥16 years of age; temporary improvement in the appearance of lines/wrinkles of the face (moderate to severe glabellar lines associated with corrugator and/or procerus muscle activity) in adult patients ≤65 years of age; treatment of severe primary axillary hyperhidrosis in adults not adequately controlled with topical treatments

Orphan drug: Treatment of dynamic muscle contracture in pediatric cerebral palsy patients

Usual Dosage

Cervical dystonia: Children ≥16 years and Adults: I.M.: For dosing guidance, the mean dose is 236 units (25th to 75th percentile range 198-300 units) divided among the affected muscles in patients previously treated with botulinum toxin. Initial dose in previously untreated patients should be lower. Sequential dosing should be based on the patient's head and neck position, localization of pain, muscle hypertrophy, patient response, and previous adverse reactions. The total dose injected into the sternocleidomastoid muscles should be ≤100 units to decrease the occurrence of dysphagia.

Blepharospasm: Children ≥12 years and Adults: I.M.: Initial dose: 1.25-2.5 units injected into the medial and lateral pretarsal orbicularis oculi of the upper and lower lid; dose may be increased up to twice the previous dose if the response from the initial dose lasted ≤2 months; maximum dose per site: 5 units; cumulative dose in a 30-day period: ≤200 units. Tolerance may occur if treatments are given more often than every 3 months, but the effect is not usually permanent.

Strabismus: Children ≥12 years and Adults: I.M.:

Initial dose:

- Vertical muscles and for horizontal strabismus <20 prism diopters: 1.25-2.5 units in any one muscle
- Horizontal strabismus of 20-50 prism diopters: 2.5-5 units in any one muscle
- Persistent VI nerve palsy >1 month: 1.5-2.5 units in the medial rectus muscle

Re-examine patients 7-14 days after each injection to assess the effect of that dose. Subsequent doses for patients experiencing incomplete paralysis of the target may be increased up to twice the previous administered dose. The maximum recommended dose as a single injection for any one muscle is 25 units. Do not administer subsequent injections until the effects of the previous dose are gone.

Primary axillary hyperhidrosis: Adults ≥18 years: Intradermal: 50 units/axilla. Injection area should be defined by standard staining techniques. Injections should be evenly distributed into multiple sites (10-15), administered in 0.1-0.2 mL aliquots, ~1-2 cm apart.

Reduction of glabellar lines: Adults ≤65 years: I.M.: An effective dose is determined by gross observation of the patient's ability to activate the superficial muscles injected. The location, size and use of muscles may vary markedly among individuals. Inject 0.1 mL dose into each of five sites, two in each corrugator muscle and one in the procerus muscle (total dose 0.5 mL).

Dosage Forms Injection, powder for reconstitution [preservative free]: *Clostridium botulinum* toxin type A 100 units [contains human albumin]

botulinum toxin type B (BOT yoo lin num TOKS in type bee)

U.S./Canadian Brand Names Myobloc® [US]

Therapeutic Category Neuromuscular Blocker Agent, Toxin

Use Treatment of cervical dystonia (spasmodic torticollis)

Usual Dosage Adults: Cervical dystonia: I.M.: Initial: 2500-5000 units divided among the affected muscles in patients **previously treated** with botulinum toxin; initial dose in **previously untreated** patients should be lower. Subsequent dosing should be optimized according to patient's response.

Dosage Forms Injection, solution [single-dose vial]: 5000 units/mL (0.5 mL, 1 mL, 2 mL) [contains albumin 0.05%]

botulism immune globulin (intravenous-human)

(BOT yoo lism i MYUN GLOB you lin, in tra VEE nus, YU man)

Synonyms BIG-IV

U.S./Canadian Brand Names BabyBIG® [US]

Therapeutic Category Immune Globulin

Use Treatment of infant botulism caused by toxin type A or B

Usual Dosage I.V.: Children <1 year: Infant botulism: 1 mL/kg (50 mg/kg) as a single dose; infuse at 0.5 mL/kg/hour (25 mg/kg/hour) for the first 15 minutes; if well tolerated, may increase to 1 mL/kg/hour (50 mg/kg/hour)

Dosage Forms Injection, powder for reconstitution [preservative free]: ~100 mg [contains albumin 1% and sucrose 5%; packaged with SWFI]

Boudreaux's® Butt Paste [US-OTC] *see* zinc oxide *on page 887*

bovine lung surfactant *see* beractant *on page 105*

Breathe Right® Saline [US-OTC] *see* sodium chloride *on page 777*

Breezee® Mist Antifungal *(Discontinued)* *see* miconazole *on page 553*

Breonesin® *(Discontinued)* *see* guaifenesin *on page 392*

Brethaire® *(Discontinued)* *see* terbutaline *on page 811*

Brethine® [US] *see* terbutaline *on page 811*

Brevibloc® [US/Can] *see* esmolol *on page 306*

Brevicon® [US] *see* ethinyl estradiol and norethindrone *on page 323*

Brevicon® 0.5/35 [Can] *see* ethinyl estradiol and norethindrone *on page 323*

Brevicon® 1/35 [Can] *see* ethinyl estradiol and norethindrone *on page 323*

Brevital® [Can] *see* methohexital *on page 540*

Brevital® Sodium [US] *see* methohexital *on page 540*

Brevoxyl® [US] *see* benzoyl peroxide *on page 102*

Brevoxyl® Cleansing [US] *see* benzoyl peroxide *on page 102*

Brevoxyl® Wash [US] *see* benzoyl peroxide *on page 102*

Bricanyl® [Can] *see* terbutaline *on page 811*

Bricanyl® *(Discontinued)* *see* terbutaline *on page 811*

brimonidine (bri MOE ni deen)

Sound-Alike/Look-Alike Issues

brimonidine may be confused with bromocriptine

Synonyms brimonidine tartrate

U.S./Canadian Brand Names Alphagan® P [US]; Alphagan® [Can]; PMS-Brimonidine Tartrate [Can]; ratio-Brimonidine [Can]

Therapeutic Category Alpha$_2$-Adrenergic Agonist Agent, Ophthalmic

Use Lowering of intraocular pressure (IOP) in patients with open-angle glaucoma or ocular hypertension

Usual Dosage Ophthalmic: Children ≥2 years of age and Adults: Glaucoma: Instill 1 drop in affected eye(s) 3 times/day (approximately every 8 hours)

Dosage Forms

Solution, ophthalmic, as tartrate: 0.2% (5 mL, 10 mL, 15 mL) [may contain benzalkonium chloride]

Alphagan® P: 0.1% (5 mL, 10 mL, 15 mL) [contains Purite® as preservative]; 0.15% (5 mL, 10 mL, 15 mL) [contains Purite® as preservative]

brimonidine tartrate *see* brimonidine *on this page*

brinzolamide (brin ZOH la mide)

U.S./Canadian Brand Names Azopt® [US/Can]

Therapeutic Category Carbonic Anhydrase Inhibitor

Use Lowers intraocular pressure in patients with ocular hypertension or open-angle glaucoma

Usual Dosage Ophthalmic: Adults: Instill 1 drop in affected eye(s) 3 times/day

Dosage Forms Suspension, ophthalmic: 1% (5 mL, 10 mL, 15 mL) [contains benzalkonium chloride]

Brioschi® [US-OTC] *see* sodium bicarbonate *on page 776*

British anti-lewisite *see* dimercaprol *on page 259*

BRL 43694 *see* granisetron *on page 391*

Brofed® [US] *see* brompheniramine and pseudoephedrine *on next page*

Bromaline® [US-OTC] *see* brompheniramine and pseudoephedrine *on next page*

Bromaline® DM [US-OTC] *see* brompheniramine, pseudoephedrine, and dextromethorphan *on page 120*

Bromarest® *(Discontinued)* *see* brompheniramine *on next page*

Bromatane DX [US] *see* brompheniramine, pseudoephedrine, and dextromethorphan *on page 120*

Bromaxefed DM RF [US] *see* brompheniramine, pseudoephedrine, and dextromethorphan *on page 120*

Bromaxefed RF [US] *see* brompheniramine and pseudoephedrine *on next page*

bromazepam *(Canada only)* (broe MA ze pam)

U.S./Canadian Brand Names Apo-Bromazepam® [Can]; Gen-Bromazepam [Can]; Lectopam® [Can]; Novo-Bromazepam [Can]; Nu-Bromazepam [Can]

Therapeutic Category Benzodiazepine; Sedative

Use Short-term, symptomatic treatment of anxiety

Usual Dosage Oral: Adults: Initial: 6-18 mg/day in equally divided doses; initial course of treatment should not last longer than 1 week; optimal dosage range: 6-30 mg/day

Dosage Forms [CAN] = Canadian brand name

Tablet: 1.5 mg, 3 mg, 6 mg [not available in the U.S.]

Brombay® *(Discontinued)* *see* brompheniramine *on next page*

Brometane DX [US] *see* brompheniramine, pseudoephedrine, and dextromethorphan *on page 120*

Bromfed® *(Discontinued)* *see* brompheniramine and pseudoephedrine *on next page*

Bromfed-PD® *(Discontinued)* *see* brompheniramine and pseudoephedrine *on next page*

bromfenac (BROME fen ak)

Synonyms bromfenac sodium

U.S./Canadian Brand Names Xibrom™ [US]

Therapeutic Category Analgesic, Nonnarcotic; Nonsteroidal Antiinflammatory Drug (NSAID), Oral

Use Treatment of postoperative inflammation and reduction in ocular pain following cataract removal

Usual Dosage Ophthalmic: Adults: Instill 1 drop into affected eye(s) twice daily beginning 24 hours after surgery and continuing for 2 weeks postoperatively

Dosage Forms Solution, ophthalmic: 0.09% (5 mL) [contains benzoic acid and sodium sulfite]

bromfenac sodium *see* bromfenac *on this page*

Bromfenex® [US] *see* brompheniramine and pseudoephedrine *on next page*

Bromfenex® PD [US] *see* brompheniramine and pseudoephedrine *on next page*

Bromhist-DM [US] *see* brompheniramine, pseudoephedrine, and dextromethorphan *on page 120*

Bromhist-NR [US] *see* brompheniramine and pseudoephedrine *on next page*

Bromhist PDX [US] *see* brompheniramine, pseudoephedrine, and dextromethorphan *on page 120*

Bromhist Pediatric [US] *see* brompheniramine and pseudoephedrine *on next page*

bromocriptine (broe moe KRIP teen)

Sound-Alike/Look-Alike Issues

bromocriptine may be confused with benztropine, brimonidine

(Continued)

bromocriptine *(Continued)*

Parlodel® may be confused with pindolol, Provera®

Synonyms bromocriptine mesylate

U.S./Canadian Brand Names Apo-Bromocriptine® [Can]; Parlodel® [US/Can]; PMS-Bromocriptine [Can]

Therapeutic Category Anti-Parkinson Agent; Ergot Alkaloid and Derivative

Use Treatment of hyperprolactinemia associated with amenorrhea with or without galactorrhea, infertility, or hypogonadism; treatment of prolactin-secreting adenomas; treatment of acromegaly; treatment of Parkinson disease

Usual Dosage Oral:

Children: Hyperprolactinemia:

11-15 years (based on limited information): Initial: 1.25-2.5 mg daily; dosage may be increased as tolerated to achieve a therapeutic response (range: 2.5-10 mg daily).

≥16 years: Refer to adult dosing

Adults:

Parkinsonism: 1.25 mg twice daily, increased by 2.5 mg/day in 2- to 4-week intervals (usual dose range is 30-90 mg/day in 3 divided doses), though elderly patients can usually be managed on lower doses

Acromegaly: Initial: 1.25-2.5 mg daily increasing by 1.25-2.5 mg daily as necessary every 3-7 days; usual dose: 20-30 mg/day (maximum: 100 mg/day)

Hyperprolactinemia: Initial: 1.25-2.5 mg/day; may be increased by 2.5 mg/day as tolerated every 2-7 days until optimal response (range: 2.5-15 mg/day)

Dosage Forms

Capsule, as mesylate: 5 mg

Parlodel®: 5 mg

Tablet, as mesylate: 2.5 mg

Parlodel®: 2.5 mg

bromocriptine mesylate *see* bromocriptine *on previous page*

Bromophed DX [US] *see* brompheniramine, pseudoephedrine, and dextromethorphan *on page 120*

Bromphen® *(Discontinued)* *see* brompheniramine *on this page*

Bromphenex DM [US] *see* brompheniramine, pseudoephedrine, and dextromethorphan *on page 120*

brompheniramine (brome fen IR a meen)

Synonyms parabromdylamine

U.S./Canadian Brand Names Colhist® Solution [US-OTC]; Dimetane® Extentabs® [US-OTC]; Dimetapp® Allergy Children's [US-OTC]; Dimetapp® Allergy [US-OTC]; Lodrane® 12 Hour [US-OTC]; ND-Stat® Solution [US-OTC]; Polytapp® Allergy Dye-Free Medication [US-OTC]

Therapeutic Category Antihistamine

Use Perennial and seasonal allergic rhinitis and other allergic symptoms including urticaria

Usual Dosage

Oral:

Children:

<6 years: 0.125 mg/kg/dose administered every 6 hours; maximum: 6-8 mg/day

6-12 years: 2-4 mg every 6-8 hours; maximum: 12-16 mg/day

Adults: 4 mg every 4-6 hours or 8 mg of sustained release form every 8-12 hours or 12 mg of sustained release every 12 hours; maximum: 24 mg/day

I.M., I.V., SubQ:

Children <12 years: 0.5 mg/kg/24 hours divided every 6-8 hours

Adults: 5-50 mg every 4-12 hours, maximum: 40 mg/24 hours

Dosage Forms

Capsule, as maleate: 4 mg

Elixir, as maleate: 2 mg/5 mL with 3% alcohol (120 mL)

Liquid, as maleate: 2 mg/5 mL (60 mL, 120 mL, 240 mL)

Solution, as maleate: 2 mg/5 mL (10 mL)

Tablet, as maleate: 4 mg

Tablet, sustained release, as maleate: 6 mg, 12 mg

brompheniramine and pseudoephedrine (brome fen IR a meen & soo doe e FED rin)

Sound-Alike/Look-Alike Issues

Bromfed® may be confused with Bromphen®

Synonyms brompheniramine maleate and pseudoephedrine hydrochloride; brompheniramine maleate and pseudoephedrine sulfate; pseudoephedrine and brompheniramine

U.S./Canadian Brand Names Andehist NR Syrup [US]; Brofed® [US]; Bromaline® [US-OTC]; Bromaxefed RF [US]; Bromfenex® PD [US]; Bromfenex® [US]; Bromhist Pediatric [US]; Bromhist-NR [US]; Children's Dimetapp® Elixir Cold & Allergy [US-OTC]; Histex™ SR [US]; Lodrane® 12D [US]; Lodrane® LD [US]; Lodrane® [US]; Touro™ Allergy [US]

Therapeutic Category Antihistamine/Decongestant Combination

Use Temporary relief of symptoms of seasonal and perennial allergic rhinitis, and vasomotor rhinitis, including nasal obstruction

Usual Dosage Oral:

Capsule, long acting:

Based on 60 mg pseudoephedrine:

Children 6-12 years: 1 capsule every 12 hours

Children ≥12 years and Adults: 1-2 capsules every 12 hours

Based on 120 mg pseudoephedrine: Children ≥12 years and Adults: 1 capsule every 12 hours

Liquid:

Based on brompheniramine 1 mg/pseudoephedrine 15 mg per 1 mL: Children:

1-3 months: 0.25 mL 4 times/day

3-6 months: 0.5 mL 4 times/day

6-12 months: 0.75 mL 4 times/day

12-24 months: 1 mL 4 times/day

Based on brompheniramine 1 mg/pseudoephedrine 15 mg per 5 mL: Children:

6-11 months (6-8 kg): 2.5 mL every 6-8 hours (maximum: 4 doses/24 hours)

12-23 months (8-10 kg): 3.75 mL every 6-8 hours (maximum: 4 doses/24 hours)

2-6 years: 5 mL every 6-8 hours (maximum: 4 doses/24 hours)

6-12 years: 10 mL every 6-8 hours (maximum: 4 doses/24 hours)

>12 years and Adults: 20 mg every 4 hours (maximum: 4 doses/24 hours)

Based on brompheniramine 4 mg/pseudoephedrine 30 mg:

Children 2-6 years: 2.5 mL 3 times/day

Children >6 years and Adults: 5 mL 3 times/day

Brompheniramine 4 mg/pseudoephedrine 45 mg per 5 mL:

Children 2-6 years: 2.5 mL 4 times/day

Children >6 years and Adults: 5 mL 4 times/day

Tablet, extended release: Based on pseudoephedrine 45 mg:

Children 6-12 years: 1 tablet every 12 hours

Children ≥12 years and Adults: 1-2 tablets every 12 hours

Dosage Forms [DSC] = Discontinued product

Capsule, extended release: Brompheniramine maleate 6 mg and pseudoephedrine hydrochloride 60 mg; brompheniramine maleate 12 mg and pseudoephedrine hydrochloride 120 mg

Bromfenex®: Brompheniramine maleate 12 mg and pseudoephedrine hydrochloride 120 mg

Bromfenex® PD, Lodrane® LD: Brompheniramine maleate 6 mg and pseudoephedrine hydrochloride 60 mg

Histex™ SR: Brompheniramine maleate 10 mg and pseudoephedrine hydrochloride 120 mg

Capsule, sustained release (Touro™ Allergy): Brompheniramine maleate 5.75 mg and pseudoephedrine hydrochloride 60 mg

Elixir: Brompheniramine maleate 1 mg and pseudoephedrine hydrochloride 15 mg per 5 mL (120 mL, 480 mL)

Children's Dimetapp® Elixir Cold & Allergy: Brompheniramine maleate 1 mg and pseudoephedrine hydrochloride 15 mg per 5 mL (240 mL) [alcohol free; contains sodium benzoate; grape flavor]

Liquid (Lodrane®): Brompheniramine maleate 4 mg and pseudoephedrine hydrochloride 60 mg per 5 mL (480 mL) [alcohol free, dye free, sugar free; cherry flavor]

Liquid, oral drops:

Bromhist NR: Brompheniramine maleate 1 mg and pseudoephedrine hydrochloride 12.5 mg per 1 mL (30 mL) [cherry flavor]

Bromhist Pediatric: Brompheniramine maleate 1 mg and pseudoephedrine hydrochloride 15 mg per 1 mL (30 mL) [cherry flavor]

Solution (Bromaline®): Brompheniramine maleate 1 mg and pseudoephedrine hydrochloride 15 mg per 5 mL (120 mL, 480 mL) [alcohol free; contains sodium benzoate; grape flavor]

Syrup: Brompheniramine maleate 4 mg and pseudoephedrine sulfate 45 mg per 5 mL (120 mL, 480 mL)

Andehist NR: Brompheniramine maleate 4 mg and pseudoephedrine sulfate 45 mg per 5 mL (473 mL) [raspberry flavor]

Brofed®: Brompheniramine maleate 4 mg and pseudoephedrine hydrochloride 30 mg per 5 mL (480 mL) [mint flavor]

(Continued)

brompheniramine and pseudoephedrine *(Continued)*

Bromaxefed RF: Brompheniramine maleate 4 mg and pseudoephedrine hydrochloride 45 mg per 5 mL (120 mL, 480 mL) [alcohol free; cherry flavor]

Rondec®: Brompheniramine maleate 4 mg and pseudoephedrine hydrochloride 45 mg per 5 mL (120 mL, 480 mL) [cherry flavor] [DSC]

Tablet, extended release (Lodrane® 12D): Brompheniramine maleate 6 mg and pseudoephedrine hydrochloride 45 mg

brompheniramine maleate and pseudoephedrine hydrochloride *see* brompheniramine and pseudoephedrine *on page 118*

brompheniramine maleate and pseudoephedrine sulfate *see* brompheniramine and pseudoephedrine *on page 118*

brompheniramine, pseudoephedrine, and dextromethorphan

(brome fen IR a meen, soo doe e FED rin, & deks troe meth OR fan)

Synonyms dextromethorphan hydrobromide, brompheniramine maleate, and pseudoephedrine hydrochloride; pseudoephedrine tannate, dextromethorphan tannate, and brompheniramine tannate

U.S./Canadian Brand Names AccuHist® PDX Drops [US]; AllanHist PDX [US]; Anaplex® DM [US]; Anaplex® DMX [US]; Andehist DM NR [US]; Bromaline® DM [US-OTC]; Bromatane DX [US]; Bromaxefed DM RF [US]; Brometane DX [US]; Bromhist PDX [US]; Bromhist-DM [US]; Bromophed DX [US]; Bromphenex DM [US]; Brotapp-DM [US]; Carbofed DM [US]; Cardec DM [US]; Dimaphen DM [US-OTC]; Dimetapp® DM Children's Cold and Cough [US-OTC]; EndaCof-DM [US]; EndaCof-PD [US]; Histacol DM Pediatric [US]; Myphetane DX [US]; PediaHist DM [US]; Q-Tapp DM [OTC]

Therapeutic Category Antihistamine; Cough Preparation; Decongestant

Use Relief of cough and upper respiratory symptoms (including nasal congestion) associated with allergy or the common cold

Usual Dosage

Children:

- 1-3 months (AccuHist® PDX, EndaCof-PD): 0.25 mL 4 times/day
- 3-6 months (AccuHist® PDX, EndaCof-PD): 0.5 mL 4 times/day
- 6-12 months (AccuHist® PDX, EndaCof-PD): 0.75 mL 4 times/day
- 12-24 months (AccuHist® PDX, EndaCof-PD): 1 mL 4 times/day
- 2-6 years:
  - Anaplex® DM, EndaCof-DM: 1.25 mL every 4-6 hours (maximum: 4 doses/24 hours)
  - Anaplex® DMX: 1.25 mL every 12 hours (maximum: 2.5 mL/24 hours)
  - Rondec®-DM: 2.5 mL 4 times/day
- 6-12 years:
  - Anaplex® DM, EndaCof-DM: 2.5 mL every 4-6 hours (maximum: 4 doses/24 hours)
  - Anaplex® DMX: 2.5 mL every 12 hours (maximum: 5 mL/24 hours)
  - Bromaline® DM, Dimaphen DM, Dimetapp® DM Children's Cough and Cold: 10 mL every 4-6 hours (maximum: 4 doses/24 hours)
  - Rondec®-DM: Refer to Adults dosing

Children ≥12 years and Adults:

- Anaplex® DM: 5 mL every 4-6 hours (maximum: 4 doses/24 hours)
- Anaplex® DMX: 5 mL every 12 hours (maximum: 10 mL/24 hours)
- Bromaline® DM, Dimaphen DM, Dimetapp® DM Children's Cough and Cold: 20 mL every 4-6 hours (maximum: 4 doses/24 hours)
- Rondec®-DM: 5 mL 4 times/day

Dosage Forms [DSC] = Discontinued product

Elixir:

Bromaline® DM: Brompheniramine maleate 1 mg, pseudoephedrine hydrochloride 15 mg, and dextromethorphan hydrobromide 5 mg per 5 mL (120 mL, 480 mL) [alcohol free; contains sodium benzoate; grape flavor]

Dimetapp® DM Children's Cold and Cough: Brompheniramine maleate 1 mg, pseudoephedrine hydrochloride 15 mg, and dextromethorphan hydrobromide 5 mg per 5 mL (120 mL, 240 mL, 360 mL) [alcohol free; contains sodium benzoate; grape flavor]

Dimaphen DM: Brompheniramine maleate 1 mg, pseudoephedrine hydrochloride 15 mg, and dextromethorphan hydrobromide 5 mg per 5 mL (120 mL)

Q-Tapp DM: Brompheniramine maleate 1 mg, pseudoephedrine hydrochloride 15 mg, and dextromethorphan hydrobromide 5 mg per 5 mL (120 mL) [grape flavor]

Liquid:

Brotapp-DM: Brompheniramine maleate 1 mg, pseudoephedrine hydrochloride 15 mg, and dextromethorphan hydrobromide 5 mg per 5 mL (120 mL, 240 mL) [grape flavor]

Bromophed DX: Brompheniramine maleate 2 mg, pseudoephedrine hydrochloride 30 mg, and dextromethorphan hydrobromide 10 mg per 5 mL (480 mL) [butterscotch flavor]

Solution, oral drops: Brompheniramine maleate 1 mg, pseudoephedrine hydrochloride 15 mg, and dextromethorphan hydrobromide 4 mg per 1 mL (30 mL); brompheniramine maleate 1 mg, pseudoephedrine hydrochloride 12.5 mg, and dextromethorphan hydrobromide 3 mg per 1 mL (30 mL)

AccuHist® PDX, AllanHist PDX: Brompheniramine maleate 1 mg, pseudoephedrine hydrochloride 12.5 mg, and dextromethorphan hydrobromide 3 mg per 1 mL (30 mL) [alcohol free, sugar free; contains sodium benzoate; grape flavor]

Bromhist DM, PediaHist DM: Brompheniramine maleate 1 mg, pseudoephedrine hydrochloride 15 mg, and dextromethorphan hydrobromide 4 mg per 1 mL (30 mL) [grape flavor]

Bromhist PDX, EndaCof-PD: Brompheniramine maleate 1 mg, pseudoephedrine hydrochloride 12.5 mg, and dextromethorphan hydrobromide 3 mg per 1 mL (30 mL) [grape flavor]

Histacol DM Pediatric: Brompheniramine maleate 1 mg, pseudoephedrine hydrochloride 15 mg, and dextromethorphan hydrobromide 4 mg per 1 mL (30 mL)

Suspension (Anaplex® DMX): Brompheniramine tannate 8 mg, pseudoephedrine tannate 90 mg, and dextromethorphan tannate 60 mg per 5 mL (480 mL) [alcohol free, sugar free; grape flavor]

Syrup: Brompheniramine maleate 4 mg, pseudoephedrine hydrochloride 60 mg, and dextromethorphan hydrobromide 30 mg per 5 mL (480 mL)

Anaplex® DM: Brompheniramine maleate 4 mg, pseudoephedrine hydrochloride 60 mg, and dextromethorphan hydrobromide 30 mg per 5 mL (480 mL) [alcohol free, dye free, sugar free; fruit flavor]

Andehist DM NR: Brompheniramine maleate 4 mg, pseudoephedrine hydrochloride 45 mg, and dextromethorphan hydrobromide 15 mg per 5 mL (480 mL) [grape flavor]

Bromatane DX, Brometane DX: Brompheniramine maleate 2 mg, pseudoephedrine hydrochloride 30 mg, and dextromethorphan hydrobromide 10 mg per 5 mL (480 mL)

Bromaxefed DM RF: Brompheniramine maleate 4 mg, pseudoephedrine hydrochloride 45 mg, and dextromethorphan hydrobromide 15 mg per 5 mL (120 mL, 240 mL, 480 mL) [alcohol free; grape flavor]

Bromphenex DM: Brompheniramine maleate 4 mg, pseudoephedrine hydrochloride 60 mg, and dextromethorphan hydrobromide 30 mg per 5 mL (480 mL)

Carbofed DM: Brompheniramine maleate 4 mg, pseudoephedrine hydrochloride 45 mg, and dextromethorphan hydrobromide 15 mg per 5 mL (480 mL) [alcohol free, sugar free; grape flavor]

Cardec DM: Brompheniramine maleate 4 mg, pseudoephedrine hydrochloride 45 mg, and dextromethorphan hydrobromide 15 mg per 5 mL (120 mL, 480 mL) [grape flavor]

EndaCof-DM: Brompheniramine maleate 4 mg, pseudoephedrine hydrochloride 60 mg, and dextromethorphan hydrobromide 30 mg per 5 mL (480 mL) [alcohol free, dye free, sugar free; fruit flavor]

Myphetane DX: Brompheniramine maleate 2 mg, pseudoephedrine hydrochloride 30 mg, and dextromethorphan hydrobromide 10 mg per 5 mL (480 mL) [contains alcohol <1%; butterscotch flavor]

Rondec®-DM: Brompheniramine maleate 4 mg, pseudoephedrine hydrochloride 45 mg, and dextromethorphan hydrobromide 15 mg per 5 mL (120 mL, 480 mL) [contains sodium benzoate; grape flavor] [DSC]

Sildec-DM: Brompheniramine maleate 4 mg, pseudoephedrine hydrochloride 45 mg, and dextromethorphan hydrobromide 15 mg per 5 mL (480 mL) [grape flavor]

Brompheril® *(Discontinued)* *see* dexbrompheniramine and pseudoephedrine *on page 241*

Bronchial® *(Discontinued)* *see* theophylline and guaifenesin *on page 820*

Bronchial Mist® *(Discontinued)* *see* epinephrine *on page 295*

Broncho Saline® [US-OTC] *see* sodium chloride *on page 777*

Bronitin® Mist *(Discontinued)* *see* epinephrine *on page 295*

Brontex® [US] *see* guaifenesin and codeine *on page 393*

Brotane® *(Discontinued)* *see* brompheniramine *on page 118*

Brotapp-DM [US] *see* brompheniramine, pseudoephedrine, and dextromethorphan *on previous page*

BSS® [US/Can] *see* balanced salt solution *on page 92*

BSS Plus® [US/Can] *see* balanced salt solution *on page 92*

BTX-A *see* botulinum toxin type A *on page 115*

B-type natriuretic peptide (human) *see* nesiritide *on page 587*

Bubbli-Pred™ [US] *see* prednisolone (systemic) *on page 695*

Budeprion™ SR [US] *see* bupropion *on page 126*

budesonide (byoo DES oh nide)

U.S./Canadian Brand Names Entocort® EC [US]; Entocort® [Can]; Gen-Budesonide AQ [Can]; Pulmicort Respules® [US]; Pulmicort Turbuhaler® [US]; Pulmicort® [Can]; Rhinocort® Aqua® [US]; Rhinocort® Turbuhaler® [Can]

Therapeutic Category Adrenal Corticosteroid

Use

Intranasal: Children ≥6 years of age and Adults: Management of symptoms of seasonal or perennial rhinitis

Nebulization: Children 12 months to 8 years: Maintenance and prophylactic treatment of asthma

Oral capsule: Treatment of active Crohn disease (mild to moderate) involving the ileum and/or ascending colon; maintenance of remission (for up to 3 months) of Crohn disease (mild to moderate) involving the ileum and/or ascending colon

Oral inhalation: Maintenance and prophylactic treatment of asthma; includes patients who require corticosteroids and those who may benefit from systemic dose reduction/elimination

Usual Dosage

Nasal inhalation: (Rhinocort® Aqua®): Children ≥6 years and Adults: 64 mcg/day as a single 32 mcg spray in each nostril. Some patients who do not achieve adequate control may benefit from increased dosage. A reduced dosage may be effective after initial control is achieved.

Maximum dose: Children <12 years: 128 mcg/day; Adults: 256 mcg/day

Nebulization: Children 12 months to 8 years: Pulmicort Respules®: Titrate to lowest effective dose once patient is stable; start at 0.25 mg/day or use as follows:

Previous therapy of bronchodilators alone: 0.5 mg/day administered as a single dose or divided twice daily (maximum daily dose: 0.5 mg)

Previous therapy of inhaled corticosteroids: 0.5 mg/day administered as a single dose or divided twice daily (maximum daily dose: 1 mg)

Previous therapy of oral corticosteroids: 1 mg/day administered as a single dose or divided twice daily (maximum daily dose: 1 mg)

Oral inhalation:

Children ≥6 years:

Previous therapy of bronchodilators alone: 200 mcg twice initially which may be increased up to 400 mcg twice daily

Previous therapy of inhaled corticosteroids: 200 mcg twice initially which may be increased up to 400 mcg twice daily

Previous therapy of oral corticosteroids: The highest recommended dose in children is 400 mcg twice daily

Adults:

Previous therapy of bronchodilators alone: 200-400 mcg twice initially which may be increased up to 400 mcg twice daily

Previous therapy of inhaled corticosteroids: 200-400 mcg twice initially which may be increased up to 800 mcg twice daily

Previous therapy of oral corticosteroids: 400-800 mcg twice daily which may be increased up to 800 mcg twice daily

NIH Guidelines (NIH, 1997) (give in divided doses twice daily):

Children:

"Low" dose: 100-200 mcg/day

"Medium" dose: 200-400 mcg/day (1-2 inhalations/day)

"High" dose: >400 mcg/day (>2 inhalation/day)

Adults:

"Low" dose: 200-400 mcg/day (1-2 inhalations/day)

"Medium" dose: 400-600 mcg/day (2-3 inhalations/day)

"High" dose: >600 mcg/day (>3 inhalation/day)

Oral: Adults: Crohn disease (active): 9 mg once daily in the morning for up to 8 weeks; recurring episodes may be treated with a repeat 8-week course of treatment

Note: Patients receiving CYP3A4 inhibitors should be monitored closely for signs and symptoms of hypercorticism; dosage reduction may be required. If switching from oral prednisolone, prednisolone dosage should be tapered while budesonide (Entocort™ EC) treatment is initiated.

Maintenance of remission: Following treatment of active disease (control of symptoms with CDAI <150), treatment may be continued at a dosage of 6 mg once daily for up to 3 months. If symptom control is maintained for 3 months, tapering of the dosage to complete cessation is recommended. Continued dosing beyond 3 months has not been demonstrated to result in substantial benefit.

Dosage Forms [CAN] = Canadian brand name

Capsule, enteric coated (Entocort® EC): 3 mg

Powder for oral inhalation:

Pulmicort Turbuhaler®: 200 mcg/inhalation (104 g) [delivers ~160 mcg/inhalation; 200 metered actuations]

Pulmicort Turbuhaler® [CAN]: 100 mcg/inhalation [delivers 200 metered actuations]; 200 mcg/inhalation [delivers 200 metered actuations]; 400 mcg/inhalation [delivers 200 metered actuations] [not available in the U.S.]

Suspension, intranasal [spray]:

Rhinocort® Aqua®: 32 mcg/inhalation (8.6 g) [120 metered actuations]

Suspension for nebulization:

Pulmicort Respules®: 0.25 mg/2 mL (30s), 0.5 mg/2 mL (30s)

budesonide and eformoterol *see* budesonide and formoterol *(Canada only)* *on this page*

budesonide and formoterol *(Canada only)* (byoo DES oh nide & for MOH te rol)

Synonyms budesonide and eformoterol; eformoterol and budesonide; formoterol fumarate dehydrate and budesonide

U.S./Canadian Brand Names Symbicort® [Can]

Therapeutic Category Beta$_2$-Adrenergic Agonist Agent; Corticosteroid, Inhalant (Oral)

Use Treatment of asthma in patients ≥12 years of age where combination therapy is indicated

Usual Dosage Oral inhalation: Children ≥12 years and Adults:

Symbicort® 80/4.5, Symbicort® 160/4.5: 2 inhalations twice daily. Patients currently receiving a low-to-medium dose inhaled corticosteroid may be started on the lower strength combination; those receiving a medium-to-high dose inhaled corticosteroid may be started on the higher strength combination. Consider the higher dose combination for patients not adequately controlled on the lower combination following 1-2 weeks of therapy. Do not use more than 2 inhalations twice daily of either strength.

Symbicort® Turbuhaler®: 1-2 inhalations once or twice daily

Maximum long-term maintenance dose: 4 inhalations/day; in periods of worsening asthma, this may be temporarily increased to 4 inhalations twice daily

Manufacturer's recommendation: Initial: Symbicort® 200 once or twice daily to establish symptom control. Following the establishment of response/symptom control: Titrate to the lowest dosage possible to maintain control (may substitute Symbicort® 100).

Dosage Forms [CAN] = Canadian brand name

Powder for oral inhalation:

Symbicort® 80/4.5: Budesonide 80 mcg and formoterol fumarate dehydrate 4. 5mcg per actuation (10.2 g) [120 metered inhalations]

Symbicort® 160/4.5: Budesonide 160 mcg and formoterol fumarate dehydrate 4. 5mcg per actuation (10.2 g) [120 metered inhalations]

Symbicort® 100 Turbuhaler® [CAN]: Budesonide 100 mcg and formoterol dehydrate 6 mcg per inhalation (available in 60 or 120 metered doses) [delivers ~80 mcg budesonide and 4.5 mcg formoterol per inhalation; contains lactose] [not available in the U.S.]

Symbicort® 200 Turbuhaler® [CAN]: Budesonide 200 mcg and formoterol dehydrate 6 mcg per inhalation (available in 60 or 120 metered doses) [delivers ~160 mcg budesonide and 4.5 mcg formoterol per inhalation; contains lactose] [not available in the U.S.]

Bufferin® [US-OTC] *see* aspirin *on page 77*

Bufferin® Extra Strength [US-OTC] *see* aspirin *on page 77*

Buffinol [US-OTC] *see* aspirin *on page 77*

Buffinol Extra [US-OTC] *see* aspirin *on page 77*

bumetanide (byoo MET a nide)

Sound-Alike/Look-Alike Issues

bumetanide may be confused with Buminate®

Bumex® may be confused with Brevibloc®, Buprenex®, Permax®

U.S./Canadian Brand Names Bumex® [US/Can]; Burinex® [Can]

Therapeutic Category Diuretic, Loop

Use Management of edema secondary to congestive heart failure or hepatic or renal disease including nephrotic syndrome; may be used alone or in combination with antihypertensives in the treatment of hypertension; can be used in furosemide-allergic patients

Usual Dosage

Oral, I.M., I.V.:

Neonates: 0.01-0.05 mg/kg/dose every 24-48 hours

Infants and Children: 0.015-0.1 mg/kg/dose every 6-24 hours (maximum dose: 10 mg/day)

(Continued)

bumetanide *(Continued)*

Adults:
Edema:
Oral: 0.5-2 mg/dose (maximum dose: 10 mg/day) 1-2 times/day
I.M., I.V.: 0.5-1 mg/dose; may repeat in 2-3 hours for up to 2 doses if needed (maximum dose: 10 mg/day)
Continuous I.V. infusion: Initial: 1 mg I.V. load then 0.5-2 mg/hour (ACC/AHA 2005 practice guidelines for chronic heart failure)
Hypertension: Oral: 0.5 mg daily (maximum dose: 5 mg/day); usual dosage range (JNC 7): 0.5-2 mg/day in 2 divided doses

Dosage Forms
Injection, solution: 0.25 mg/mL (2 mL, 4 mL, 10 mL) [contains benzyl alcohol]
Tablet (Bumex®): 0.5 mg, 1 mg, 2 mg

Bumex® [US/Can] *see* bumetanide *on previous page*

Bumex® Injection *(Discontinued)* *see* bumetanide *on previous page*

Buminate® [US] *see* albumin *on page 22*

Buphenyl® [US] *see* sodium phenylbutyrate *on page 781*

bupivacaine (byoo PIV a kane)

Sound-Alike/Look-Alike Issues
bupivacaine may be confused with mepivacaine, ropivacaine
Marcaine® may be confused with Narcan®

Synonyms bupivacaine hydrochloride

U.S./Canadian Brand Names Marcaine® Spinal [US]; Marcaine® [US/Can]; Sensorcaine® [US/Can]; Sensorcaine®-MPF [US]

Therapeutic Category Local Anesthetic

Use Local anesthetic (injectable) for peripheral nerve block, infiltration, sympathetic block, caudal or epidural block, retrobulbar block

Usual Dosage Dose varies with procedure, depth of anesthesia, vascularity of tissues, duration of anesthesia and condition of patient; do not use solutions containing preservatives for caudal or epidural block.
Children >12 years and Adults:
Local anesthesia: Infiltration: 0.25% infiltrated locally; maximum: 175 mg
Caudal block (preservative free): 15-30 mL of 0.25% or 0.5%
Epidural block (other than caudal block - preservative free): Administer in 3-5 mL increments, allowing sufficient time to detect toxic manifestations of inadvertent I.V. or I.T. administration: 10-20 mL of 0.25% or 0.5%
Surgical procedures requiring a high degree of muscle relaxation and prolonged effects **only**: 10-20 mL of 0.75% (**Note:** Not to be used in obstetrical cases)
Peripheral nerve block: 5 mL of 0.25 or 0.5%; maximum: 400 mg/day
Sympathetic nerve block: 20-50 mL of 0.25%
Retrobulbar anesthesia: 2-4 mL of 0.75%
Adults: Spinal anesthesia: Preservative free solution of 0.75% bupivacaine in 8.25% dextrose:
Lower extremity and perineal procedures: 1 mL
Lower abdominal procedures: 1.6 mL
Normal vaginal delivery: 0.8 mL (higher doses may be required in some patients)
Cesarean section: 1-1.4 mL

Dosage Forms
Injection, solution, as hydrochloride [preservative free]: 0.25% [2.5 mg/mL] (10 mL, 20 mL, 30 mL, 50 mL); 0.5% [5 mg/mL] (10 mL, 20 mL, 30 mL); 0.75% [7.5 mg/mL] (10 mL, 20 mL, 30 mL)
Marcaine®: 0.25% [2.5 mg/mL] (10 mL, 30 mL); 0.5% [5 mg/mL] (10 mL, 30 mL); 0.75% [7.5 mg/mL] (10 mL, 30 mL)
Marcaine® Spinal: 0.75% [7.5 mg/mL] (2 mL) [in dextrose 8.25%]
Sensorcaine®-MPF: 0.25% [2.5 mg/mL] (10 mL, 30 mL); 0.5% [5 mg/mL] (10 mL, 30 mL); 0.75% [7.5 mg/mL] (10 mL, 30 mL)
Injection, solution, as hydrochloride (Marcaine®, Sensorcaine®): 0.25% [2.5 mg/mL] (50 mL); 0.5% [5 mg/mL] (50 mL) [contains methylparaben]

bupivacaine and epinephrine (byoo PIV a kane & ep i NEF rin)

Synonyms epinephrine bitartrate and bupivacaine hydrochloride

U.S./Canadian Brand Names Marcaine® with Epinephrine [US]; Sensorcaine® with Epinephrine [US/Can]; Sensorcaine®-MPF with Epinephrine [US]

Therapeutic Category Local Anesthetic

Use Local anesthetic (injectable) for peripheral nerve block, infiltration, sympathetic block, caudal or epidural block, retrobulbar block

Usual Dosage Dose varies with procedure, depth of anesthesia, vascularity of tissues, duration of anesthesia, and condition of patient. Do not use solutions containing preservatives for caudal or epidural block.

Children >12 years and Adults:

Caudal block (preservative free): 15-30 mL of 0.25% or 0.5%

Epidural block (other than caudal block, preservative free): 10-20 mL of 0.25% or 0.5%. Administer in 3-5 mL increments, allowing sufficient time to detect toxic manifestations of inadvertent I.V. or I.T. administration.

Surgical procedures requiring a high degree of muscle relaxation and prolonged effects only: 10-20 mL of 0.75% (**Note:** Not to be used in obstetrical cases)

Local anesthesia: Infiltration: 0.25% infiltrated locally (maximum: 175 mg of bupivacaine)

Peripheral nerve block: 5 mL of 0.25 or 0.5% (maximum: 400 mg/day of bupivacaine)

Retrobulbar anesthesia: 2-4 mL of 0.75%

Sympathetic nerve block: 20-50 mL of 0.25%

Infiltration and nerve block in maxillary and mandibular area: 9 mg (1.8 mL) of bupivacaine as a 0.5% solution with epinephrine 1:200,000 per injection site. A second dose may be administered if necessary to produce adequate anesthesia after allowing up to 10 minutes for onset. Up to a maximum of 90 mg of bupivacaine hydrochloride per dental appointment. The effective anesthetic dose varies with procedure, intensity of anesthesia needed, duration of anesthesia required, and physical condition of the patient; always use the lowest effective dose along with careful aspiration.

Dosage Forms

Injection, solution [preservative free]: Bupivacaine hydrochloride 0.25% and epinephrine bitartrate 1:200,000 (10 mL, 30 mL); bupivacaine hydrochloride 0.5% and epinephrine bitartrate 1:200,000 (10 mL, 30 mL)

Marcaine® with Epinephrine Preservative Free: Bupivacaine hydrochloride 0.25% and epinephrine bitartrate 1:200,000 (10 mL, 30 mL) [contains sodium metabisulfite]; bupivacaine hydrochloride 0.5% and epinephrine bitartrate 1:200,000 (1.8 mL, 3 mL, 10 mL, 30 mL) [contains sodium metabisulfite]; bupivacaine hydrochloride 0.75% and epinephrine bitartrate 1:200,000 (30 mL) [contains sodium metabisulfite]

Sensorcaine® MPF with Epinephrine: Bupivacaine hydrochloride 0.25% and epinephrine bitartrate 1:200,000 (10 mL, 30 mL) [contains sodium metabisulfite]; bupivacaine hydrochloride 0.5% and epinephrine bitartrate 1:200,000 (10 mL, 30 mL) [contains sodium metabisulfite]

Injection, solution: Bupivacaine hydrochloride 0.25% and epinephrine bitartrate 1:200,000 (50 mL); bupivacaine hydrochloride 0.5% and epinephrine bitartrate 1:200,000 (1.8 mL, 50 mL)

Marcaine® with Epinephrine, Sensorcaine® with Epinephrine: Bupivacaine hydrochloride 0.25% and epinephrine bitartrate 1:200,000 (50 mL) [contains methylparaben]; bupivacaine hydrochloride 0.5% and epinephrine bitartrate 1:200,000 (50 mL) [contains methylparaben]

bupivacaine and lidocaine *see* lidocaine and bupivacaine *on page 495*

bupivacaine hydrochloride *see* bupivacaine *on previous page*

Buprenex® [US/Can] *see* buprenorphine *on this page*

buprenorphine (byoo pre NOR feen)

Sound-Alike/Look-Alike Issues

Buprenex® may be confused with Brevibloc®, Bumex®

Synonyms buprenorphine hydrochloride

U.S./Canadian Brand Names Buprenex® [US/Can]; Subutex® [US/Can]

Therapeutic Category Analgesic, Narcotic

Controlled Substance Injection: C-V; Tablet: C-III

Use

Injection: Management of moderate to severe pain

Tablet: Treatment of opioid dependence

Usual Dosage Long-term use is not recommended

Note: These are guidelines and do not represent the maximum doses that may be required in all patients. Doses should be titrated to pain relief/prevention. In high-risk patients (eg, elderly, debilitated, presence of respiratory disease) and/or concurrent CNS depressant use, reduce dose by one-half. Buprenorphine has an analgesic ceiling.

Acute pain (moderate to severe):

Children 2-12 years: I.M., slow I.V.: 2-6 mcg/kg every 4-6 hours

(Continued)

buprenorphine *(Continued)*

Children ≥13 years and Adults:

I.M.: Initial: Opiate-naive: 0.3 mg every 6-8 hours as needed; initial dose (up to 0.3 mg) may be repeated once in 30-60 minutes after the initial dose if needed; usual dosage range: 0.15-0.6 mg every 4-8 hours as needed

Slow I.V.: Initial: Opiate-naive: 0.3 mg every 6-8 hours as needed; initial dose (up to 0.3 mg) may be repeated once in 30-60 minutes after the initial dose if needed

Sublingual: Children ≥16 years and Adults: Opioid dependence:

Induction: Range: 12-16 mg/day (doses during an induction study used 8 mg on day 1, followed by 16 mg on day 2; induction continued over 3-4 days). Treatment should begin at least 4 hours after last use of heroin or short-acting opioid, preferably when first signs of withdrawal appear. Titrating dose to clinical effectiveness should be done as rapidly as possible to prevent undue withdrawal symptoms and patient drop-out during the induction period.

Maintenance: Target dose: 16 mg/day; range: 4-24 mg/day; patients should be switched to the buprenorphine/naloxone combination product for maintenance and unsupervised therapy

Dosage Forms

Injection, solution (Buprenex®): 0.3 mg/mL (1 mL)

Tablet, sublingual (Subutex®): 2 mg, 8 mg

Additional dosage strength available in Canada: 0.4 mg

buprenorphine and naloxone (byoo pre NOR feen & nal OKS one)

Synonyms buprenorphine hydrochloride and naloxone hydrochloride dihydrate; naloxone and buprenorphine; naloxone hydrochloride dihydrate and buprenorphine hydrochloride

U.S./Canadian Brand Names Suboxone® [US]

Therapeutic Category Analgesic, Narcotic

Controlled Substance C-III

Use Treatment of opioid dependence

Usual Dosage Sublingual: Children ≥16 years and Adults: Opioid dependence: **Note:** This combination product is not recommended for use during the induction period; initial treatment should begin using buprenorphine oral tablets. Patients should be switched to the combination product for maintenance and unsupervised therapy.

Maintenance: Target dose (based on buprenorphine content): 16 mg/day; range: 4-24 mg/day

Dosage Forms Tablet, sublingual: Buprenorphine 2 mg and naloxone 0.5 mg; buprenorphine 8 mg and naloxone 2 mg [lemon-lime flavor]

buprenorphine hydrochloride *see* buprenorphine *on previous page*

buprenorphine hydrochloride and naloxone hydrochloride dihydrate *see* buprenorphine and naloxone *on this page*

Buproban™ [US] *see* bupropion *on this page*

bupropion (byoo PROE pee on)

Sound-Alike/Look-Alike Issues

buPROPion may be confused with busPIRone

Wellbutrin SR® may be confused with Wellbutrin XL™

Wellbutrin XL™ may be confused with Wellbutrin SR®

Zyban® may be confused with Zagam®

Tall-Man bu**PROP**ion

U.S./Canadian Brand Names Budeprion™ SR [US]; Buproban™ [US]; Novo-Bupropion SR [Can]; Wellbutrin SR® [US]; Wellbutrin XL™ [US/Can]; Wellbutrin® [US/Can]; Zyban® [US/Can]

Therapeutic Category Antidepressant, Aminoketone

Use Treatment of major depressive disorder, including seasonal affective disorder (SAD); adjunct in smoking cessation

Usual Dosage Oral: Adults:

Depression:

Immediate release: 100 mg 3 times/day; begin at 100 mg twice daily; may increase to a maximum dose of 450 mg/day

Sustained release: Initial: 150 mg/day in the morning; may increase to 150 mg twice daily by day 4 if tolerated; target dose: 300 mg/day given as 150 mg twice daily; maximum dose: 400 mg/day given as 200 mg twice daily

Extended release: Initial: 150 mg/day in the morning; may increase as early as day 4 of dosing to 300 mg/day; maximum dose: 450 mg/day

SAD (Wellbutrin XL™): Initial: 150 mg/day in the morning; if tolerated, may increase after 1 week to 300 mg/day

Note: Prophylactic treatment should be reserved for those patients with frequent depressive episodes and/or significant impairment. Initiate treatment in the Autumn prior to symptom onset, and discontinue in early Spring with dose tapering to 150 mg/day for 2 weeks

Smoking cessation (Zyban®): Initiate with 150 mg once daily for 3 days; increase to 150 mg twice daily; treatment should continue for 7-12 weeks

Dosage Forms

Tablet, as hydrochloride (Wellbutrin®): 75 mg, 100 mg

Tablet, extended release, as hydrochloride:

Budeprion™ SR: 100 mg [contains tartrazine; equivalent to Wellbutrin® SR], 150 mg [equivalent to Wellbutrin® SR]

Buproban™: 150 mg [equivalent to Zyban®]

Wellbutrin XL™: 150 mg, 300 mg

Tablet, sustained release, as hydrochloride: 100 mg, 150 mg [equivalent to Wellbutrin® SR], 150 mg [equivalent to Zyban®]

Wellbutrin® SR: 100 mg, 150 mg, 200 mg

Zyban®: 150 mg

Burinex® [Can] *see* bumetanide *on page 123*

Burnamycin [US-OTC] *see* lidocaine *on page 493*

Burn Jel [US-OTC] *see* lidocaine *on page 493*

Burn-O-Jel [US-OTC] *see* lidocaine *on page 493*

Buscopan® [Can] *see* scopolamine derivatives *on page 764*

buserelin acetate *(Canada only)* (BYOO se rel in AS e tate)

Therapeutic Category Luteinizing Hormone-Releasing Hormone Analog

Use For the palliative treatment of patients with hormone-dependent advanced carcinoma of the prostate gland (Stage D). Buserelin is also indicated for the treatment of endometriosis in patients who do not require surgery as primary therapy. The duration of treatment is usually 6 months and should not exceed 9 months. Experience with buserelin for the management of endometriosis has been limited to women 18 years of age and older.

Usual Dosage Buserelin should be administered at approximately equal time intervals to ensure that the desired therapeutic effect is maintained.

Prostatic Cancer: Initial Treatment: For the first 7 days of treatment give buserelin 500 mcg (0.5 mL) every 8 hours by SubQ injection. For patient comfort, vary the injection site.

Maintenance Treatment: Depending upon patient preference, or physician recommendation, maintenance treatment may be by daily SubQ injection or by intranasal administration 3 times daily. During maintenance dosing by the SubQ route, the buserelin dose is 200 mcg (0.2 mL) daily. For patient comfort, vary the site of injection.

During maintenance dosing by the intranasal administration route, the buserelin dose is 400 mcg (200 mcg into each nostril) 3 times daily using the metered-dose pump (nebulizer) provided. Each pump action delivers 100 mcg buserelin acetate or 0.1mL solution.

Endometriosis: The dose of buserelin in patients with endometriosis is 400 mcg (200 mcg into each nostril) 3 times daily using the metered-dose pump (nebulizer) provided. Each pump action delivers 100 mcg or 0.1 mL solution. The treatment duration is usually 6 months and should not exceed 9 months.

Dosage Forms Injection, depot: 6.6 mg [2 month]; 9.9 mg [3 month]

BuSpar® [US/Can] *see* buspirone *on this page*

Buspirex [Can] *see* buspirone *on this page*

buspirone (byoo SPYE rone)

Sound-Alike/Look-Alike Issues

busPIRone may be confused with buPROPion

Synonyms buspirone hydrochloride

Tall-Man bus**PIR**one

U.S./Canadian Brand Names Apo-Buspirone® [Can]; BuSpar® [US/Can]; Buspirex [Can]; Gen-Buspirone [Can]; Lin-Buspirone [Can]; Novo-Buspirone [Can]; Nu-Buspirone [Can]; PMS-Buspirone [Can]

Therapeutic Category Antianxiety Agent

Use Management of generalized anxiety disorder (GAD)

(Continued)

buspirone *(Continued)*

Usual Dosage Oral: Generalized anxiety disorder:

Children and Adolescents: Initial: 5 mg daily; increase in increments of 5 mg/day at weekly intervals as needed, to a maximum dose of 60 mg/day divided into 2-3 doses

Adults: 15 mg/day (7.5 mg twice daily); may increase in increments of 5 mg/day every 2-4 days to a maximum of 60 mg/day; target dose for most people is 30 mg/day (15 mg twice daily)

Dosage Forms

Tablet, as hydrochloride: 5 mg, 7.5 mg, 10 mg, 15 mg, 30 mg

BuSpar®: 5 mg, 10 mg, 15 mg, 30 mg

buspirone hydrochloride *see* buspirone *on previous page*

busulfan (byoo SUL fan)

Sound-Alike/Look-Alike Issues

busulfan may be confused with Butalan®

Myleran® may be confused with melphalan, Mylicon®

U.S./Canadian Brand Names Busulfex® [US/Can]; Myleran® [US/Can]

Therapeutic Category Antineoplastic Agent

Use

Oral: Chronic myelogenous leukemia; conditioning regimens for bone marrow transplantation

I.V.: Combination therapy with cyclophosphamide as a conditioning regimen prior to allogeneic hematopoietic progenitor cell transplantation for chronic myelogenous leukemia

Usual Dosage

Children:

For remission induction of CML: Oral: 0.06-0.12 mg/kg/day **or** 1.8-4.6 mg/m^2/day; titrate dosage to maintain leukocyte count above 40,000/mm^3; reduce dosage by 50% if the leukocyte count reaches 30,000-40,000/mm^3; discontinue drug if counts fall to ≤20,000/mm^3

BMT marrow-ablative conditioning regimen:

Oral: 1 mg/kg/dose (ideal body weight) every 6 hours for 16 doses

I.V.:

≤12 kg: 1.1 mg/kg/dose (ideal body weight) every 6 hours for 16 doses

>12 kg: 0.8 mg/kg/dose (ideal body weight) every 6 hours for 16 doses

Adjust dose to desired AUC [1125 μmol(min)] using the following formula:

Adjusted dose (mg) = Actual dose (mg) x [target AUC μmol(min) / actual AUC μmol(min)]

Adults:

For remission induction of CML: Oral: 4-8 mg/day (may be as high as 12 mg/day); Maintenance doses: 1-4 mg/day to 2 mg/week to maintain WBC 10,000-20,000 cells/mm^3

BMT marrow-ablative conditioning regimen:

Oral: 1 mg/kg/dose (ideal body weight) every 6 hours for 16 doses

I.V.: 0.8 mg/kg (ideal body weight or actual body weight, whichever is lower) every 6 hours for 4 days (a total of 16 doses)

Dosage Forms

Injection, solution (Busulfex®): 6 mg/mL (10 mL)

Tablet (Myleran®): 2 mg

Busulfex® [US/Can] *see* busulfan *on this page*

butabarbital (byoo ta BAR bi tal)

Sound-Alike/Look-Alike Issues

butabarbital may be confused with butalbital

U.S./Canadian Brand Names Butisol Sodium® [US]

Therapeutic Category Barbiturate

Controlled Substance C-III

Use Sedative; hypnotic

Usual Dosage Oral:

Children: Preoperative sedation: 2-6 mg/kg/dose (maximum: 100 mg)

Adults:

Sedative: 15-30 mg 3-4 times/day

Hypnotic: 50-100 mg

Preop: 50-100 mg 1-1½ hours before surgery

Dosage Forms

Elixir, as sodium: 30 mg/5 mL (480 mL) [contains alcohol 7% and tartrazine]

Tablet, as sodium: 30 mg, 50 mg [contains tartrazine]

Butalan® *(Discontinued)*

butalbital, acetaminophen, and caffeine (byoo TAL bi tal, a seet a MIN oh fen, & KAF een)

Sound-Alike/Look-Alike Issues

Fioricet® may be confused with Fiorinal®, Lorcet®

Repan® may be confused with Riopan®

Synonyms acetaminophen, butalbital, and caffeine

U.S./Canadian Brand Names Anolor 300 [US]; Dolgic® LQ [US]; Dolgic® Plus [US]; Esgic-Plus™ [US]; Esgic® [US]; Fioricet® [US]; Medigesic® [US]; Repan® [US]; Zebutal™ [US]

Therapeutic Category Barbiturate/Analgesic

Use Relief of the symptomatic complex of tension or muscle contraction headache

Usual Dosage Adults: Oral: 1-2 tablets or capsules (or 15-30 mL elixir) every 4 hours; not to exceed 6 tablets or capsules (or 180 mL elixir) daily

Dosage Forms

Capsule:

Anolor 300, Esgic®, Medigesic®: Butalbital 50 mg, acetaminophen 325 mg, and caffeine 40 mg

Dolgic® Plus: Butalbital 50 mg, acetaminophen 750 mg, and caffeine 40 mg

Esgic-Plus™, Zebutal™: Butalbital 50 mg, acetaminophen 500 mg, and caffeine 40 mg

Elixir:

Dolgic® LQ: Butalbital 50 mg, acetaminophen 325 mg, and caffeine 40 mg per 15 mL (480 mL) [contains alcohol 7%; fruit flavor]

Tablet: Butalbital 50 mg, acetaminophen 325 mg, and caffeine 40 mg; butalbital 50 mg, acetaminophen 500 mg, and caffeine 40 mg

Esgic®, Fioricet®, Repan®: Butalbital 50 mg, acetaminophen 325 mg, and caffeine 40 mg

butalbital, aspirin, and caffeine (byoo TAL bi tal, AS pir in, & KAF een)

Sound-Alike/Look-Alike Issues

Fiorinal® may be confused with Fioricet®, Florical®, Florinef®

Synonyms aspirin, caffeine, and butalbital; butalbital compound

U.S./Canadian Brand Names Fiorinal® [US/Can]

Therapeutic Category Barbiturate/Analgesic

Controlled Substance C-III

Use Relief of the symptomatic complex of tension or muscle contraction headache

Usual Dosage Oral: Adults: 1-2 tablets or capsules every 4 hours; not to exceed 6/day

Dosage Forms Capsule: Butalbital 50 mg, caffeine 40 mg, and aspirin 325 mg

butalbital, aspirin, caffeine, and codeine

(byoo TAL bi tal, AS pir in, KAF een, & KOE deen)

Sound-Alike/Look-Alike Issues

Fiorinal® may be confused with Fioricet®, Florical®, Florinef®

Phrenilin® may be confused with Phenergan®, Trinalin®

Synonyms aspirin, caffeine, codeine, and butalbital; butalbital compound and codeine; codeine and butalbital compound; codeine, butalbital, aspirin, and caffeine

U.S./Canadian Brand Names Fiorinal® With Codeine [US]; Fiorinal®-C 1/2 [Can]; Fiorinal®-C 1/4 [Can]; Phrenilin® With Caffeine and Codeine [US]; Tecnal C 1/2 [Can]; Tecnal C 1/4 [Can]

Therapeutic Category Analgesic, Narcotic; Barbiturate

Controlled Substance C-III

Use Mild-to-moderate pain when sedation is needed

Usual Dosage Adults: Oral: 1-2 capsules every 4 hours as needed for pain; up to 6/day

Dosage Forms

Capsule: Butalbital 50 mg, caffeine 40 mg, aspirin 325 mg, and codeine phosphate 30 mg

Fioricet® with Codeine: Butalbital 50 mg, caffeine 40 mg, acetaminophen 325 mg, and codeine phosphate 30 mg [may contain benzyl alcohol]

Phrenilin® with Caffeine and Codeine: Butalbital 50 mg, caffeine 40 mg, acetaminophen 325 mg, and codeine phosphate 30 mg [contains benzyl alcohol and lactose]

butalbital compound *see* butalbital, aspirin, and caffeine *on this page*

butalbital compound and codeine *see* butalbital, aspirin, caffeine, and codeine *on this page*

butenafine (byoo TEN a feen)

Sound-Alike/Look-Alike Issues

lotrimin may be confused with Lotrisone®, Otrivin®

Synonyms butenafine hydrochloride

U.S./Canadian Brand Names Lotrimin® Ultra™ [US-OTC]; Mentax® [US]

Therapeutic Category Antifungal Agent

Use Topical treatment of tinea pedis (athlete's foot), tinea cruris (jock itch), tinea corporis (ringworm), and tinea versicolor

Usual Dosage Children >12 years and Adults: Topical:

Tinea corporis, tinea cruris, or tinea versicolor: Apply once daily for 2 weeks to affected area and surrounding skin

Tinea pedis: Apply once daily for 4 weeks or twice daily for 7 days to affected area and surrounding skin (7-day regimen may have lower efficacy)

Dosage Forms Cream, as hydrochloride:

Lotrimin® Ultra™: 1% (12 g, 24 g) [contains benzyl alcohol and sodium benzoate]

Mentax®: 1% (15 g, 30 g) [contains benzyl alcohol and sodium benzoate]

butenafine hydrochloride *see* butenafine *on this page*

Buticaps® *(Discontinued)*

Butisol Sodium® [US] *see* butabarbital *on page 128*

butoconazole (byoo toe KOE na zole)

Sound-Alike/Look-Alike Issues

Mycelex® may be confused with Myoflex®

Synonyms butoconazole nitrate

U.S./Canadian Brand Names Femstat® One [Can]; Gynazole-1® [US/Can]; Mycelex®-3 [US-OTC]

Therapeutic Category Antifungal Agent

Use Local treatment of vulvovaginal candidiasis

Usual Dosage Adults: Female:

Femstat®-3 [OTC]: Insert 1 applicatorful (~5 g) intravaginally at bedtime for 3 consecutive days

Gynazole-1®: Insert 1 applicatorful (~5 g) intravaginally as a single dose; treatment may need to be extended for up to 6 days in pregnant women (use in pregnancy during 2nd or 3rd trimester only)

Dosage Forms Cream, vaginal, as nitrate:

Mycelex®-3: 2% (5 g) [prefilled applicator], (20 g) [with disposable applicator]

Gynazole-1®: 2% (5 g) [prefilled applicator]

butoconazole nitrate *see* butoconazole *on this page*

butorphanol (byoo TOR fa nole)

Sound-Alike/Look-Alike Issues

Stadol® may be confused with Haldol®, sotalol

Synonyms butorphanol tartrate

U.S./Canadian Brand Names Apo-Butorphanol® [Can]; PMS-Butorphanol [Can]; Stadol® [US]

Therapeutic Category Analgesic, Narcotic

Controlled Substance C-IV

Use

Parenteral: Management of moderate-to-severe pain; preoperative medication; supplement to balanced anesthesia; management of pain during labor

Nasal spray: Management of moderate-to-severe pain, including migraine headache pain

Usual Dosage Note: These are guidelines and do not represent the maximum doses that may be required in all patients. Doses should be titrated to pain relief/prevention. Butorphanol has an analgesic ceiling. Adults:

Parenteral:

Acute pain (moderate to severe):

I.M.: Initial: 2 mg, may repeat every 3-4 hours as needed; usual range: 1-4 mg every 3-4 hours as needed

I.V.: Initial: 1 mg, may repeat every 3-4 hours as needed; usual range: 0.5-2 mg every 3-4 hours as needed

Preoperative medication: I.M.: 2 mg 60-90 minutes before surgery

Supplement to balanced anesthesia: I.V.: 2 mg shortly before induction and/or an incremental dose of 0.5-1 mg (up to 0.06 mg/kg), depending on previously administered sedative, analgesic, and hypnotic medications

Pain during labor (fetus >37 weeks gestation and no signs of fetal distress):
I.M., I.V.: 1-2 mg; may repeat in 4 hours
Note: Alternative analgesia should be used for pain associated with delivery or if delivery is anticipated within 4 hours

Nasal spray:
Moderate to severe pain (including migraine headache pain): Initial: 1 spray (~1 mg per spray) in 1 nostril; if adequate pain relief is not achieved within 60-90 minutes, an additional 1 spray in 1 nostril may be given; may repeat initial dose sequence in 3-4 hours after the last dose as needed
Alternatively, an initial dose of 2 mg (1 spray in each nostril) may be used in patients who will be able to remain recumbent (in the event drowsiness or dizziness occurs); additional 2 mg doses should not be given for 3-4 hours
Note: In some clinical trials, an initial dose of 2 mg (as 2 doses 1 hour apart or 2 mg initially - 1 spray in each nostril) has been used, followed by 1 mg in 1 hour; side effects were greater at these dosages

Dosage Forms
Injection, solution, as tartrate [preservative free] (Stadol®): 1 mg/mL (1 mL); 2 mg/mL (1 mL, 2 mL)
Injection, solution, as tartrate [with preservative] (Stadol®): 2 mg/mL (10 mL)
Solution, intranasal, as tartrate [spray]: 10 mg/mL (2.5 mL) [14-15 doses]

butorphanol tartrate *see* butorphanol *on previous page*

butyl aminobenzoate, tetracaine hydrochloride, benzocaine, and benzalkonium chloride *see* benzocaine, butyl aminobenzoate, tetracaine, and benzalkonium chloride *on page 101*

B vitamin combinations *see* vitamin B complex combinations *on page 876*

BW-430C *see* lamotrigine *on page 480*

BW524W91 *see* emtricitabine *on page 290*

Byclomine® Injection *(Discontinued)* *see* dicyclomine *on page 251*

Bydramine® Cough Syrup *(Discontinued)* *see* diphenhydramine *on page 261*

Byetta™ [US] *see* exenatide *on page 332*

C1H *see* alemtuzumab *on page 26*

C2B8 *see* rituximab *on page 749*

C2B8 monoclonal antibody *see* rituximab *on page 749*

C7E3 *see* abciximab *on page 3*

C8-CCK *see* sincalide *on page 774*

311C90 *see* zolmitriptan *on page 889*

C225 *see* cetuximab *on page 168*

C-500-GR™ [US-OTC] *see* ascorbic acid *on page 76*

cabergoline (ca BER goe leen)

U.S./Canadian Brand Names Dostinex® [US/Can]

Therapeutic Category Ergot-like Derivative

Use Treatment of hyperprolactinemic disorders, either idiopathic or due to pituitary adenomas

Usual Dosage Oral: Initial dose: 0.25 mg twice weekly; the dose may be increased by 0.25 mg twice weekly up to a maximum of 1 mg twice weekly according to the patient's serum prolactin level. Dosage increases should not occur more rapidly than every 4 weeks. Once a normal serum prolactin level is maintained for 6 months, the dose may be discontinued and prolactin levels monitored to determine if cabergoline is still required. The durability of efficacy beyond 24 months of therapy has not been established.

Dosage Forms
Tablet: 0.5 mg
Dostinex®: 0.5 mg

Ca-DTPA *see* diethylene triamine penta-acetic acid *on page 252*

Caduet® [US/Can] *see* amlodipine and atorvastatin *on page 45*

CaEDTA *see* edetate calcium disodium *on page 286*

Caelyx® [Can] *see* doxorubicin (liposomal) *on page 278*

Cafatine-PB® *(Discontinued)* *see* ergotamine *on page 302*

Cafcit® [US] *see* caffeine *on next page*

Cafetrate® *(Discontinued)* *see* ergotamine *on page 302*

Caffedrine® [US-OTC] *see* caffeine *on this page*

caffeine (KAF een)

Synonyms caffeine and sodium benzoate; caffeine citrate; sodium benzoate and caffeine

U.S./Canadian Brand Names Cafcit® [US]; Caffedrine® [US-OTC]; Enerjets [US-OTC]; Lucidex [US-OTC]; No Doz® Maximum Strength [US-OTC]; Vivarin® [US-OTC]

Therapeutic Category Stimulant

Use

Caffeine citrate: Treatment of idiopathic apnea of prematurity

Caffeine and sodium benzoate: Treatment of acute respiratory depression (not a preferred agent)

Caffeine [OTC labeling]: Restore mental alertness or wakefulness when experiencing fatigue

Usual Dosage

Note: Caffeine citrate should not be interchanged with the caffeine sodium benzoate formulation.

Caffeine citrate: Neonates: Apnea of prematurity: Oral, I.V.:

Loading dose: 10-20 mg/kg as caffeine citrate (5-10 mg/kg as caffeine base). If theophylline has been administered to the patient within the previous 3 days, a full or modified loading dose (50% to 75% of a loading dose) may be given.

Maintenance dose: 5 mg/kg/day as caffeine citrate (2.5 mg/kg/day as caffeine base) once daily starting 24 hours after the loading dose. Maintenance dose is adjusted based on patient's response and serum caffeine concentrations.

Caffeine and sodium benzoate:

Children: Stimulant: I.M., I.V., SubQ: 8 mg/kg every 4 hours as needed

Children ≥12 years and Adults: OTC labeling (stimulant): Oral: 100-200 mg every 3-4 hours as needed

Adults: Respiratory depression: I.M., I.V.: 250 mg as a single dose; may repeat as needed. Maximum single dose should be limited to 500 mg; maximum amount in any 24-hour period should generally be limited to 2500 mg.

Dosage Forms

Caplet (Caffedrine®, Vivarin®): 200 mg [OTC]

Injection, solution, as citrate [preservative free] (Cafcit®): 20 mg/mL (3 mL) [equivalent to 10 mg/mL caffeine base]

Injection, solution [with sodium benzoate]: Caffeine 125 mg/mL and sodium benzoate 125 mg/mL (2 mL); caffeine 121 mg/mL and sodium benzoate 129 mg/mL (2 mL)

Lozenge (Enerjets): 75 mg [OTC; Hazelnut coffee or mochamint flavor]

Solution, oral, as citrate (Cafcit®): 20 mg/mL (3 mL) [equivalent to 10 mg/mL caffeine base]

Tablet:

Lucidex: 100 mg [OTC]

NoDoz® Maximum Strength, Vivarin®: 200 mg [OTC]

caffeine, acetaminophen, and aspirin *see* acetaminophen, aspirin, and caffeine *on page 10*

caffeine and sodium benzoate *see* caffeine *on this page*

caffeine, aspirin, and acetaminophen *see* acetaminophen, aspirin, and caffeine *on page 10*

caffeine citrate *see* caffeine *on this page*

caffeine, dihydrocodeine, and acetaminophen *see* acetaminophen, caffeine, and dihydrocodeine *on page 10*

caffeine, hydrocodone, chlorpheniramine, phenylephrine, and acetaminophen *see* hydrocodone, chlorpheniramine, phenylephrine, acetaminophen, and caffeine *on page 424*

caffeine, orphenadrine, and aspirin *see* orphenadrine, aspirin, and caffeine *on page 620*

caffeine, propoxyphene, and aspirin *see* propoxyphene, aspirin, and caffeine *on page 708*

Caladryl® Clear [US-OTC] *see* pramoxine *on page 691*

CalaMycin® Cool and Clear [US-OTC] *see* pramoxine *on page 691*

Calan® [US/Can] *see* verapamil *on page 870*

Calan® SR [US] *see* verapamil *on page 870*

Calcarb 600 [US-OTC] *see* calcium carbonate *on page 135*

Calcibind® [US/Can] *see* cellulose sodium phosphate *on page 165*

Calci-Chew® [US-OTC] *see* calcium carbonate *on page 135*

Calciday-667® *(Discontinued)* *see* calcium carbonate *on page 135*

Calciferol™ [US] *see* ergocalciferol *on page 301*

Calciferol™ Injection *(Discontinued)* *see* ergocalciferol *on page 301*

Calcijex® [US/Can] *see* calcitriol *on next page*

Calcimar® [Can] *see* calcitonin *on this page*

Calcimar® *(Discontinued)* *see* calcitonin *on this page*

Calci-Mix® [US-OTC] *see* calcium carbonate *on page 135*

calcipotriene (kal si POE try een)

U.S./Canadian Brand Names Dovonex® [US]

Therapeutic Category Antipsoriatic Agent

Use Treatment of plaque psoriasis

Usual Dosage Topical: Adults: Apply in a thin film to the affected skin twice daily and rub in gently and completely

Dosage Forms

Cream: 0.005% (60 g, 120 g)

Ointment: 0.005% (60 g, 120 g)

Solution, topical: 0.005% (60 mL)

calcipotriene and betamethasone (kal si POE try een & bay ta METH a sone)

Synonyms betamethasone dipropionate and calcipotriene hydrate; calcipotriol and betamethasone dipropionate

U.S./Canadian Brand Names Dovobet® [Can]; Taclonex® [US]

Therapeutic Category Corticosteroid, Topical; Vitamin D Analog

Use Treatment of psoriasis vulgaris

Usual Dosage Topical: Adults: Psoriasis vulgaris: Apply to affected area once daily for up to 4 weeks (maximum recommended dose: 100 g/week). Application to >30% of body surface area is not recommended.

Dosage Forms [CAN] = Canadian brand name

Cream, topical:

Dovobet® [CAN]: Calcipotriol 50 mcg and betamethasone 0.5 mg per gram (3 g, 30 g, 60 g, 100 g, 120 g) [not available in the U.S.]

Ointment, topical:

Taclonex®: Calcipotriene 0.005% and betamethasone 0.064% (60 g)

calcipotriol and betamethasone dipropionate *see* calcipotriene and betamethasone *on this page*

Calcite-500 [Can] *see* calcium carbonate *on page 135*

calcitonin (kal si TOE nin)

Sound-Alike/Look-Alike Issues

calcitonin may be confused with calcitriol

Miacalcin® may be confused with Micatin®

Synonyms calcitonin (salmon)

U.S./Canadian Brand Names Apo-Calcitonin® [Can]; Calcimar® [Can]; Caltine® [Can]; Fortical® [US]; Miacalcin® NS [Can]; Miacalcin® [US]

Therapeutic Category Polypeptide Hormone

Use Calcitonin (salmon): Treatment of Paget disease of bone (osteitis deformans); adjunctive therapy for hypercalcemia; postmenopausal osteoporosis

Usual Dosage Adults:

Paget's disease (Miacalcin®): Initial: I.M., SubQ: 100 units/day; maintenance: 50 units/day or 50-100 units every 1-3 days

Hypercalcemia (Miacalcin®): Initial: I.M., SubQ: 4 units/kg every 12 hours; may increase up to 8 units/kg every 12 hours to a maximum of every 6 hours

Postmenopausal osteoporosis:

I.M., SubQ: Miacalcin®: 100 units/every other day

Intranasal: Fortical®, Miacalcin®: 200 units (1 spray)/day

Dosage Forms

Injection, solution, calcitonin-salmon: (Miacalcin®): 200 int. units/mL (2 mL)

Solution, nasal spray, calcitonin-salmon:

Fortical®: 200 int. units/0.09 mL (3.7 mL) [rDNA origin; contains benzyl alcohol; delivers 30 doses, 200 units/actuation]

(Continued)

calcitonin *(Continued)*

Miacalcin®: 200 int. units/0.09 mL (3.7 mL) [contains benzalkonium chloride; delivers 30 doses, 200 units/actuation]

calcitonin (salmon) *see* calcitonin *on previous page*

Cal-Citrate® 250 [US-OTC] *see* calcium citrate *on page 137*

calcitriol (kal si TRYE ole)

Sound-Alike/Look-Alike Issues

calcitriol may be confused with calcifediol, Calciferol®, calcitonin

Synonyms 1,25 dihydroxycholecalciferol

U.S./Canadian Brand Names Calcijex® [US/Can]; Rocaltrol® [US/Can]

Therapeutic Category Vitamin D Analog

Use Management of hypocalcemia in patients on chronic renal dialysis; management of secondary hyperparathyroidism in moderate-to-severe chronic renal failure; management of hypocalcemia in hypoparathyroidism and pseudohypoparathyroidism

Usual Dosage Individualize dosage to maintain calcium levels of 9-10 mg/dL

Renal failure:

Children:

Oral: 0.25-2 mcg/day have been used (with hemodialysis); 0.014-0.041 mcg/kg/day (not receiving hemodialysis); increases should be made at 4- to 8-week intervals

I.V.: 0.01-0.05 mcg/kg 3 times/week if undergoing hemodialysis

Adults:

Oral: 0.25 mcg/day or every other day (may require 0.5-1 mcg/day); increases should be made at 4- to 8-week intervals

I.V.: 0.5 mcg/day 3 times/week (may require from 0.5-3 mcg/day given 3 times/week) if undergoing hemodialysis

Hypoparathyroidism/pseudohypoparathyroidism: Oral (evaluate dosage at 2- to 4-week intervals):

Children:

<1 year: 0.04-0.08 mcg/kg once daily

1-5 years: 0.25-0.75 mcg once daily

Children ≥6 years and Adults: 0.5-2 mcg once daily

Vitamin D-dependent rickets: Children and Adults: Oral: 1 mcg once daily

Vitamin D-resistant rickets (familial hypophosphatemia): Children and Adults: Oral: Initial: 0.015-0.02 mcg/kg once daily; maintenance: 0.03-0.06 mcg/kg once daily; maximum dose: 2 mcg once daily

Hypocalcemia in premature infants: Oral: 1 mcg once daily for 5 days

Hypocalcemic tetany in premature infants: I.V.: 0.05 mcg/kg once daily for 5-12 days

Dosage Forms

Capsule (Rocaltrol®): 0.25 mcg, 0.5 mcg [each strength contains coconut oil]

Injection, solution: 1 mcg/mL (1 mL); 2 mcg/mL (2 mL)

Calcijex®: 1 mcg/mL (1 mL)

Solution, oral (Rocaltrol®): 1 mcg/mL (15 mL) [contains palm seed oil]

calcium acetate (KAL see um AS e tate)

Sound-Alike/Look-Alike Issues

PhosLo® may be confused with Phos-Flur®, ProSom™

U.S./Canadian Brand Names PhosLo® [US]

Therapeutic Category Electrolyte Supplement, Oral

Use

Oral: Control of hyperphosphatemia in end-stage renal failure; does not promote aluminum absorption

I.V.: Calcium supplementation in parenteral nutrition therapy

Usual Dosage

Dietary Reference Intake:

0-6 months: 210 mg/day

7-12 months: 270 mg/day

1-3 years: 500 mg/day

4-8 years: 800 mg/day

Adults, Male/Female:

9-18 years: 1300 mg/day

19-50 years: 1000 mg/day

≥51 years: 1200 mg/day

Female: Pregnancy/Lactating: Same as for Adults, Male/Female

Oral: Adults, on dialysis: Initial: 1334 mg with each meal, can be increased gradually to bring the serum phosphate value <6 mg/dL as long as hypercalcemia does not develop (usual dose: 2001-2868 mg calcium acetate with each meal); do not give additional calcium supplements

I.V.: Dose is dependent on the requirements of the individual patient; in central venous total parental nutrition (TPN), calcium is administered at a concentration of 5 mEq (10 mL)/L of TPN solution; the additive maintenance dose in neonatal TPN is 0.5 mEq calcium/kg/day (1 mL/kg/day)

Neonates: 70-200 mg/kg/day
Infants and Children: 70-150 mg/kg/day
Adolescents: 18-35 mg/kg/day

Dosage Forms [DSC] = Discontinued product. **Note:** Elemental calcium listed in brackets:

Gelcap (PhosLo®): 667 mg [169 mg]
Injection, solution: 0.5 mEq/mL (10 mL, 50 mL, 100 mL)
Tablet (PhosLo®): 667 mg [169 mg] [DSC]

calcium acetate and aluminum sulfate *see* aluminum sulfate and calcium acetate *on page 38*

calcium acetylhomotaurinate *see* acamprosate *on page 3*

calcium and risedronate *see* risedronate and calcium *on page 747*

calcium carbonate (KAL see um KAR bun ate)

Sound-Alike/Look-Alike Issues

Florical® may be confused with Fiorinal®
Mylanta® may be confused with Mynatal®
Nephro-Calci® may be confused with Nephrocaps®
Os-Cal® may be confused with Asacol®

U.S./Canadian Brand Names Alcalak [US-OTC]; Alka-Mints® [US-OTC]; Apo-Cal® [Can]; Cal-Gest [US-OTC]; Cal-Mint [US-OTC]; Calcarb 600 [US-OTC]; Calci-Chew® [US-OTC]; Calci-Mix® [US-OTC]; Calcite-500 [Can]; Caltrate® 600 [US-OTC]; Caltrate® Select [Can]; Caltrate® [Can]; Children's Pepto [US-OTC]; Chooz® [US-OTC]; Florical® [US-OTC]; Maalox® Quick Dissolve [US-OTC] ; Mylanta® Children's [US-OTC]; Nephro-Calci® [US-OTC]; Nutralox® [US-OTC]; Os-Cal® 500 [US-OTC]; Os-Cal® [Can]; Oysco 500 [US-OTC]; Oyst-Cal 500 [US-OTC]; Rolaids® Softchews [US-OTC]; Titralac™ Extra Strength [US-OTC]; Titralac™ [US-OTC]; Tums® E-X [US-OTC]; Tums® Extra Strength Sugar Free [US-OTC]; Tums® Smoothies™ [US-OTC]; Tums® Ultra [US-OTC]; Tums® [US-OTC]

Therapeutic Category Antacid; Electrolyte Supplement, Oral

Use As an antacid; treatment and prevention of calcium deficiency or hyperphosphatemia (eg, osteoporosis, osteomalacia, mild/moderate renal insufficiency, hypoparathyroidism, postmenopausal osteoporosis, rickets); has been used to bind phosphate

Usual Dosage Oral (dosage is in terms of elemental calcium):

Dietary Reference Intake:

0-6 months: 210 mg/day
7-12 months: 270 mg/day
1-3 years: 500 mg/day
4-8 years: 800 mg/day
Adults, Male/Female:
9-18 years: 1300 mg/day
19-50 years: 1000 mg/day
≥51 years: 1200 mg/day
Female: Pregnancy/Lactating: Same as for Adults, Male/Female

Hypocalcemia (dose depends on clinical condition and serum calcium level): Dose expressed in mg of **elemental calcium**

Neonates: 50-150 mg/kg/day in 4-6 divided doses; not to exceed 1 g/day
Children: 45-65 mg/kg/day in 4 divided doses
Adults: 1-2 g or more/day in 3-4 divided doses

Antacid:

Children 2-5 years (24-47 lb): Elemental calcium 161 mg as needed; maximum 483 mg per 24 hours
Children 6-11 years (48-95 lb): Elemental calcium 322 mg as needed; maximum: 966 mg per 24 hours
Adults: Dosage based on acid-neutralizing capacity of specific product; generally, 1-2 tablets or 5-10 mL every 2 hours; maximum: 7000 mg calcium carbonate per 24 hours; specific product labeling should be consulted

Dietary supplementation: Adults: 500 mg to 2 g divided 2-4 times/day

Osteoporosis: Adults >51 years: 1200 mg/day

Dosage Forms

[DSC] = Discontinued product
(Continued)

calcium carbonate *(Continued)*

Capsule:
Calci-Mix®: 1250 mg [equivalent to elemental calcium 500 mg]
Florical®: 364 mg [equivalent to elemental calcium 145.6 mg; contains sodium fluoride 3.75 mg]
Gum, chewing: 250 mg (30s)
Chooz®: 500 mg [equivalent to elemental calcium 200 mg; mint flavor]
Powder: 4000 mg/teaspoonful (480 g) [equivalent to 1600 mg elemental calcium/teaspoonful]
Suspension, oral: 1250 mg/5 mL (5 mL, 500 mL) [equivalent to elemental calcium 500 mg/5 mL; mint flavor]
Tablet: 1250 mg [equivalent to elemental calcium 500 mg]; 1500 mg [equivalent to elemental calcium 600 mg]
Calcarb 600, Caltrate® 600, Nephro-Calci®: 1500 mg [equivalent to elemental calcium 600 mg]
Florical®: 364 mg [equivalent to elemental calcium 145.6 mg; contains sodium fluoride 8.3 mg]
Os-Cal® 500: 1250 mg [equivalent to elemental calcium 500 mg; contains tartrazine]
Oysco 500, Oyst-Cal 500: 1250 mg [equivalent to elemental calcium 500 mg]
Tablet, chewable: 500 mg [equivalent to elemental calcium 200 mg]; 650 mg [equivalent to elemental calcium 260 mg]; 750 mg [equivalent to elemental calcium 300 mg]
Alcalak: 420 mg [equivalent to elemental calcium 168 mg; mint flavor]
Alka-Mints®: 850 mg [equivalent to elemental calcium 340 mg; spearmint flavor]
Cal-Gest: 500 mg [equivalent to elemental calcium 200 mg; assorted flavors]
Calci-Chew®: 1250 mg [equivalent to elemental calcium 500 mg; cherry, lemon, and orange flavors]
Cal-Mint: 650 mg [equivalent to elemental calcium 260 mg; mint flavor]
Children's Pepto: 400 mg [equivalent to elemental calcium 161 mg; bubble gum or watermelon flavors]
Maalox® Quick Dissolve: 600 mg [equivalent to elemental calcium 222 mg; contains phenylalanine 0.5 mg/tablet; lemon flavor]
Mylanta® Children's: 400 mg [equivalent to elemental calcium 160 mg; bubble gum flavor]
Nutralox®: 420 mg [equivalent to elemental calcium 168 mg; sugar free; mint flavor]
Os-Cal® 500: 1250 mg [equivalent to elemental calcium 500 mg; Bavarian cream flavor] [DSC]
Titralac™: 420 mg [equivalent to elemental calcium 168 mg; sugar free; contains sodium 1.1 mg/tablet; spearmint flavor]
Titralac™ Extra Strength: 750 mg [equivalent to elemental calcium 300 mg; sugar free; contains sodium 1.1 mg/tablet; spearmint flavor] [DSC]
Tums®: 500 mg [equivalent to elemental calcium 200 mg; contains tartrazine; assorted fruit and peppermint flavors]
Tums® E-X: 750 mg [equivalent to elemental calcium 300 mg; contains tartrazine; assorted fruit, cool relief mint, fresh blend, tropical assorted fruit, wintergreen, and assorted berry flavors]
Tums® Extra Strength Sugar Free: 750 mg [equivalent to elemental calcium 300 mg; sugar free; contains phenylalanine <1 mg/tablet; orange cream flavor]
Tums® Smoothies™: 750 mg [equivalent to elemental calcium 300 mg; contains tartrazine; assorted fruit, assorted tropical fruit, peppermint flavors]
Tums® Ultra®: 1000 mg [equivalent to elemental calcium 400 mg; contains tartrazine; assorted berry, assorted fruit, assorted tropical fruit, peppermint, and spearmint flavors]
Tablet, softchew (Rolaids®): 1177 mg [equivalent to elemental calcium 471 mg; contains coconut oil and soy lecithin; vanilla creme and wild cherry flavors]

calcium carbonate and etidronate disodium *see* etidronate and calcium *on page 329*

calcium carbonate and magnesium hydroxide

(KAL see um KAR bun ate & mag NEE zhum hye DROKS ide)

Sound-Alike/Look-Alike Issues
Mylanta® may be confused with Mynatal®

Synonyms magnesium hydroxide and calcium carbonate

U.S./Canadian Brand Names Mi-Acid™ Double Strength [US-OTC]; Mylanta® Gelcaps® [US-OTC]; Mylanta® Supreme [US-OTC]; Mylanta® Ultra [US-OTC]; Rolaids® Extra Strength [US-OTC]; Rolaids® [US-OTC]

Therapeutic Category Antacid

Use Hyperacidity

Usual Dosage Adults: Oral: 2-4 tablets between meals, at bedtime, or as directed by healthcare provider

Dosage Forms
Gelcap (Mylanta® Gelcaps®): Calcium carbonate 550 mg and magnesium hydroxide 125 mg
Liquid (Mylanta® Supreme): Calcium carbonate 400 mg and magnesium hydroxide 135 mg per 5 mL (360 mL, 720 mL) [cherry flavor]

Tablet, chewable:

Mi-Acid™ Double Strength: Calcium carbonate 700 mg and magnesium hydroxide 300 mg

Mylanta® Ultra: Calcium carbonate 700 mg and magnesium hydroxide 300 mg [cherry créme and cool mint flavors]

Rolaids®: Calcium carbonate 550 mg and magnesium hydroxide 110 mg [sodium free; contains elemental calcium 220 mg and elemental magnesium 45 mg; original (peppermint), cherry, and spearmint flavors]

Rolaids® Extra Strength: Calcium carbonate 675 mg and magnesium hydroxide 135 mg [sodium free; contains elemental calcium 271 mg and elemental magnesium 56 mg, fruit flavor contains tartrazine; cool strawberry, fresh mint, fruit, and tropical fruit punch flavors]

calcium carbonate and simethicone (KAL see um KAR bun ate & sye METH i kone)

Synonyms simethicone and calcium carbonate

U.S./Canadian Brand Names Gas Ban™ [US-OTC]; Titralac® Plus [US-OTC]

Therapeutic Category Antacid; Antiflatulent

Use Relief of acid indigestion, heartburn

Usual Dosage Oral (OTC labeling): Adults: Two tablets every 2-3 hours as needed (maximum: 19 tablets/ 24 hours)

Dosage Forms Tablet, chewable:

Gas Ban™: Calcium carbonate 300 mg and simethicone 40 mg

Titralac® Plus: Calcium carbonate 420 mg and simethicone 21 mg [equivalent to elemental calcium 168 mg; sugar free; spearmint flavor]

calcium carbonate, magnesium hydroxide, and famotidine *see* famotidine, calcium carbonate, and magnesium hydroxide *on page 336*

calcium chloride (KAL see um KLOR ide)

Therapeutic Category Electrolyte Supplement, Oral

Use Cardiac resuscitation when epinephrine fails to improve myocardial contractions, cardiac disturbances of hyperkalemia, hypocalcemia; emergent treatment of hypocalcemic tetany; treatment of hypermagnesemia

Usual Dosage **Note:** Calcium chloride has 3 times more elemental calcium than calcium gluconate. Calcium chloride is 27% elemental calcium; calcium gluconate is 9% elemental calcium. One gram of calcium chloride is equal to 270 mg of elemental calcium; one gram of calcium gluconate is equal to 90 mg of elemental calcium. Dosages are expressed in terms of the calcium chloride salt based on a solution concentration of 100 mg/mL (10%) containing 1.4 mEq (27.3 mg)/mL elemental calcium.

Cardiac arrest in the presence of hyperkalemia or hypocalcemia, magnesium toxicity: I.V.:

Infants and Children: 20 mg/kg; may repeat in 10 minutes if necessary

Adolescents and Adults: 2-4 mg/kg, repeated every 10 minutes if necessary

Hypocalcemia: I.V.:

Children (manufacturer's recommendation): 2.7-5 mg/kg/dose every 4-6 hours

Alternative pediatric dosing: Infants and Children: 10-20 mg/kg/dose, repeat every 4-6 hours if needed

Adults: 500 mg to 1 g/dose repeated every 4-6 hours if needed

Hypocalcemic tetany: I.V.:

Neonates: Divided doses totaling approximately 170 mg/kg/24 hours

Infants and Children: 10 mg/kg over 5-10 minutes; may repeat after 6-8 hours or follow with an infusion with a maximum dose of 200 mg/kg/day; alternatively, higher doses of 35-50 mg/kg/dose repeated every 6-8 hours have been used

Adults: 1 g over 10-30 minutes; may repeat after 6 hours

Hypocalcemia secondary to citrated blood transfusion: I.V.: **Note:** Routine administration of calcium, in the absence of signs/symptoms of hypocalcemia, is generally not recommended. A number of recommendations have been published seeking to address potential hypocalcemia during massive transfusion of citrated blood; however, many practitioners recommend replacement only as guided by clinical evidence of hypocalcemia and/or serial monitoring of ionized calcium.

Neonates, Infants, and Children: Give 32 mg (0.45 mEq elemental calcium) for each 100 mL citrated blood infused

Adults: 200-500 mg per 500 mL of citrated blood (infused into another vein)

Dosage Forms Injection, solution [preservative free]: 10% [100 mg/mL] (10 mL) [equivalent to elemental calcium 27.2 mg/mL, calcium 1.36 mEq/mL]

calcium citrate (KAL see um SIT rate)

Sound-Alike/Look-Alike Issues

Citracal® may be confused with Citrucel®

(Continued)

calcium citrate *(Continued)*

U.S./Canadian Brand Names Cal-Citrate® 250 [US-OTC]; Citracal® [US-OTC]; Osteocit® [Can]

Therapeutic Category Electrolyte Supplement, Oral

Use Antacid; treatment and prevention of calcium deficiency or hyperphosphatemia (eg, osteoporosis, osteomalacia, mild/moderate renal insufficiency, hypoparathyroidism, postmenopausal osteoporosis, rickets)

Usual Dosage Oral: Dosage is in terms of elemental calcium

Dietary Reference Intake:

0-6 months: 210 mg/day
7-12 months: 270 mg/day
1-3 years: 500 mg/day
4-8 years: 800 mg/day
Adults, Male/Female:
9-18 years: 1300 mg/day
19-50 years: 1000 mg/day
≥51 years: 1200 mg/day
Female: Pregnancy/Lactating: Same as for Adults, Male/Female

Dietary supplement: Usual dose: 500 mg to 2 g 2-4 times/day

Dosage Forms

Granules: 760 mg/teaspoonful (480 g)
Tablet: Elemental calcium 200 mg, 250 mg
Cal-Citrate®: Elemental calcium 250 mg
Citracal®: 950 mg [equivalent to elemental calcium 200 mg]

calcium disodium edetate *see* edetate calcium disodium *on page 286*

Calcium Disodium Versenate® [US] *see* edetate calcium disodium *on page 286*

calcium EDTA *see* edetate calcium disodium *on page 286*

calcium glubionate (KAL see um gloo BYE oh nate)

Sound-Alike/Look-Alike Issues

calcium glubionate may be confused with calcium gluconate

Therapeutic Category Electrolyte Supplement, Oral

Use Dietary supplement

Usual Dosage Dosage is in terms of **elemental** calcium

Dietary Reference Intake:

0-6 months: 210 mg/day
7-12 months: 270 mg/day
1-3 years: 500 mg/day
4-8 years: 800 mg/day
Adults, Male/Female:
9-18 years: 1300 mg/day
19-50 years: 1000 mg/day
≥51 years: 1200 mg/day
Female: Pregnancy/Lactating: Same as for Adults, Male/Female

Dietary supplement: Oral:
Infants <12 months: 1 teaspoonful 5 times a day; may mix with juice or formula
Children <4 years: 2 teaspoonsful 3 times a day
Children ≥4 years and Adults: 1 tablespoonful 3 times a day
Pregnant or lactating women: 1 tablespoonful 4 times a day

Dosage Forms

Syrup:
Calcionate: 1.8 g/5 mL (480 mL) [equivalent to elemental calcium 115 mg/5 mL; contains benzoic acid; caramel and orange flavor]

calcium gluconate (KAL see um GLOO koe nate)

Sound-Alike/Look-Alike Issues

calcium gluconate may be confused with calcium glubionate

Therapeutic Category Electrolyte Supplement, Oral

Use Treatment and prevention of hypocalcemia; treatment of tetany, cardiac disturbances of hyperkalemia, cardiac resuscitation when epinephrine fails to improve myocardial contractions, hypocalcemia; calcium supplementation

Usual Dosage

Adequate Intake (as elemental calcium):

0-6 months: 210 mg/day
7-12 months: 270 mg/day
1-3 years: 500 mg/day
4-8 years: 800 mg/day
9-18 years: 1300 mg/day
Adults, Male/Female:
19-50 years: 1000 mg/day
≥51 years: 1200 mg/day
Female: Pregnancy/Lactating: Same as for Adults, Male/Female

Dosage note: Calcium chloride has 3 times more elemental calcium than calcium gluconate. Calcium chloride is 27% elemental calcium; calcium gluconate is 9% elemental calcium. One gram of calcium chloride is equal to 270 mg of elemental calcium; 1 gram of calcium gluconate is equal to 90 mg of elemental calcium. The following dosages are expressed in terms of the calcium gluconate salt based on a solution concentration of 100 mg/mL (10%) containing 0.465 mEq (9.3 mg)/mL elemental calcium:

Hypocalcemia: I.V.:
Neonates: 200-800 mg/kg/day as a continuous infusion or in 4 divided doses (maximum: 1 g/dose)
Infants and Children: 200-500 mg/kg/day as a continuous infusion or in 4 divided doses (maximum: 2-3 g/dose)
Adults: 2-15 g/24 hours as a continuous infusion or in divided doses

Hypocalcemia: Oral:
Children: 200-500 mg/kg/day divided every 6 hours
Adults: 500 mg to 2 g 2-4 times/day

Hypocalcemia secondary to citrated blood infusion: I.V.: **Note:** Routine administration of calcium, in the absence of signs/symptoms of hypocalcemia, is generally not recommended. A number of recommendations have been published seeking to address potential hypocalcemia during massive transfusion of citrated blood; however, many practitioners recommend replacement only as guided by clinical evidence of hypocalcemia and/or serial monitoring of ionized calcium.
Neonates, Infants, and Children: Give 98 mg (0.45 mEq **elemental** calcium) for each 100 mL citrated blood infused
Adults: 500 mg to 1 g per 500 mL of citrated blood (infused into another vein). Single doses up to 2 g have also been recommended.

Hypocalcemic tetany: I.V.:
Neonates, Infants, and Children: 100-200 mg/kg/dose over 5-10 minutes; may repeat every 6-8 hours **or** follow with an infusion of 500 mg/kg/day
Adults: 1-3 g may be administered until therapeutic response occurs

Magnesium intoxication, cardiac arrest in the presence of hyperkalemia or hypocalcemia: I.V.:
Infants and Children: 60-100 mg/kg/dose (maximum: 3 g/dose)
Adults: 500-800 mg/dose (maximum: 3 g/dose)

Maintenance electrolyte requirements for total parenteral nutrition: I.V.: Daily requirements: Adults: 1.7-3.4 g/1000 kcal/24 hours

Dosage Forms

Injection, solution [preservative free]: 10% [100 mg/mL] (10 mL, 50 mL, 100 mL, 200 mL) [equivalent to elemental calcium 9 mg/mL; calcium 0.46 mEq/mL]
Powder: 347 mg/tablespoonful (480 g)
Tablet: 500 mg [equivalent to elemental calcium 45 mg]; 650 mg [equivalent to elemental calcium 58.5 mg]; 975 mg [equivalent to elemental calcium 87.75 mg]

calcium lactate (KAL see um LAK tate)

Therapeutic Category Electrolyte Supplement, Oral

Use Adjunct in prevention of postmenopausal osteoporosis; treatment and prevention of calcium depletion

Usual Dosage Oral (in terms of calcium lactate):

Dietary Reference Intake (in terms of elemental calcium):

0-6 months: 210 mg/day
7-12 months: 270 mg/day
1-3 years: 500 mg/day
4-8 years: 800 mg/day
9-18 years: 1300 mg/day
Adults, Male/Female:
19-50 years: 1000 mg/day
≥51 years: 1200 mg/day
Female: Pregnancy/Lactating: Same as Adults, Male/Female

Dosage Forms Tablet: 650 mg [equivalent to elemental calcium 84.5 mg]

calcium leucovorin *see* leucovorin *on page 485*

calcium pantothenate *see* pantothenic acid *on page 637*

calcium phosphate (tribasic) (KAL see um FOS fate tri BAY sik)

Synonyms tricalcium phosphate

U.S./Canadian Brand Names Posture® [US-OTC]

Therapeutic Category Electrolyte Supplement, Oral

Use Dietary supplement

Usual Dosage Oral:

Adequate Intake (as elemental calcium):

0-6 months: 210 mg/day

7-12 months: 270 mg/day

1-3 years: 500 mg/day

4-8 years: 800 mg/day

9-18 years: 1300 mg/day

Adults, Male/Female:

19-50 years: 1000 mg/day

≥51 years: 1200 mg/day

Female: Pregnancy/Lactating: Same as for Adults, Male/Female

Dietary supplement: Adults: 2 tablets daily

Dosage Forms Tablet: 1565.2 mg [equivalent to elemental calcium 600 mg; sugar free]

Caldecort® [US-OTC] *see* hydrocortisone (topical) *on page 428*

calfactant (kaf AKT ant)

U.S./Canadian Brand Names Infasurf® [US]

Therapeutic Category Lung Surfactant

Use Prevention of respiratory distress syndrome (RDS) in premature infants at high risk for RDS and for the treatment ("rescue") of premature infants who develop RDS

Prophylaxis: Therapy at birth with calfactant is indicated for premature infants <29 weeks of gestational age at significant risk for RDS. Should be administered as soon as possible, preferably within 30 minutes after birth.

Treatment: For infants ≤72 hours of age with RDS (confirmed by clinical and radiologic findings) and requiring endotracheal intubation.

Usual Dosage Intratracheal administration **only**: Each dose is 3 mL/kg body weight at birth; should be administered every 12 hours for a total of up to 3 doses

Dosage Forms Suspension, intratracheal [preservative free]: 35 mg/mL (6 mL)

Cal-Gest [US-OTC] *see* calcium carbonate *on page 135*

Callergy Clear [US-OTC] *see* pramoxine *on page 691*

Calm-X® Oral *(Discontinued)* *see* dimenhydrinate *on page 258*

Cal-Mint [US-OTC] *see* calcium carbonate *on page 135*

Calmylin with Codeine [Can] *see* guaifenesin, pseudoephedrine, and codeine *on page 401*

Cal-Nate™ [US] *see* vitamins (multiple/prenatal) *on page 879*

Calphron® *(Discontinued)* *see* calcium acetate *on page 134*

Cal-Plus® *(Discontinued)* *see* calcium carbonate *on page 135*

Caltine® [Can] *see* calcitonin *on page 133*

Caltrate® [Can] *see* calcium carbonate *on page 135*

Caltrate® 600 [US-OTC] *see* calcium carbonate *on page 135*

Caltrate® Jr. *(Discontinued)* *see* calcium carbonate *on page 135*

Caltrate® Select [Can] *see* calcium carbonate *on page 135*

Camila™ [US] *see* norethindrone *on page 598*

Campath® [US] *see* alemtuzumab *on page 26*

campath-1H *see* alemtuzumab *on page 26*

Campho-Phenique® [US-OTC] *see* camphor and phenol *on this page*

camphor and phenol (KAM for & FEE nole)

Synonyms phenol and camphor

U.S./Canadian Brand Names Campho-Phenique® [US-OTC]

Therapeutic Category Topical Skin Product

Use Relief of pain and itching associated with minor burns, sunburn, minor cuts, insect bites, minor skin irritation; temporary relief of pain from cold sores

Usual Dosage Topical: Adults: Relief of pain/itching: Apply 1-3 times/day

Dosage Forms

Gel, topical: Camphor 10.8% and phenol 4.7% (7 g, 15 g)

Liquid, topical: Camphor 10.8% and phenol 4.7% (45 mL)

Campho-Phenique®: Camphor 10.8% and phenol 4.7% (22.5 mL, 45 mL)

Campral® [US] *see* acamprosate *on page 3*

Camptosar® [US/Can] *see* irinotecan *on page 461*

camptothecin-11 *see* irinotecan *on page 461*

Canasa™ [US] *see* mesalamine *on page 533*

Cancidas® [US/Can] *see* caspofungin *on page 154*

candesartan (kan de SAR tan)

Synonyms candesartan cilexetil

U.S./Canadian Brand Names Atacand® [US/Can]

Therapeutic Category Angiotensin II Receptor Antagonist

Use Alone or in combination with other antihypertensive agents in treating essential hypertension; treatment of heart failure (NYHA class II-IV)

Usual Dosage Adults: Oral:

Hypertension: Usual dose is 4-32 mg once daily; dosage must be individualized. Blood pressure response is dose-related over the range of 2-32 mg. The usual recommended starting dose of 16 mg once daily when it is used as monotherapy in patients who are not volume depleted. It can be administered once or twice daily with total daily doses ranging from 8-32 mg. Larger doses do not appear to have a greater effect and there is relatively little experience with such doses.

Congestive heart failure: Initial: 4 mg once daily; double the dose at 2-week intervals, as tolerated; target dose: 32 mg

Note: In selected cases, concurrent therapy with an ACE inhibitor may provide additional benefit.

Dosage Forms

Tablet, as cilexetil:

Atacand®: 4 mg, 8 mg, 16 mg, 32 mg

candesartan and hydrochlorothiazide (kan de SAR tan & hye droe klor oh THYE a zide)

Synonyms candesartan cilexetil and hydrochlorothiazide

U.S./Canadian Brand Names Atacand HCT™ [US]; Atacand® Plus [Can]

Therapeutic Category Antihypertensive Agent, Combination

Use Treatment of hypertension; combination product should not be used for initial therapy

Usual Dosage Oral: Adults: Replacement therapy: Combination product can be substituted for individual agents; maximum therapeutic effect would be expected within 4 weeks

Usual dosage range:

Candesartan: 16-32 mg/day, given once daily or twice daily in divided doses

Hydrochlorothiazide: 12.5-25 mg once daily

Dosage Forms

Tablet:

Atacand HCT™:

16-12.5: Candesartan cilexetil 16 mg and hydrochlorothiazide 12.5 mg

32-12.5: Candesartan cilexetil 32 mg and hydrochlorothiazide 12.5 mg

candesartan cilexetil *see* candesartan *on this page*

candesartan cilexetil and hydrochlorothiazide *see* candesartan and hydrochlorothiazide *on this page*

Candida albicans (Monilia) (KAN dee da AL bi kans mo NIL ya)

Synonyms *Monilia* skin test

U.S./Canadian Brand Names Candin® [US]

Therapeutic Category Diagnostic Agent

Use Screen for detection of nonresponsiveness to antigens in immunocompromised individuals

Usual Dosage Intradermal: 0.1 mL, examine reaction site in 24-48 hours; induration of ≥5 mm in diameter is a positive reaction

Dosage Forms Injection, solution: 0.1 mL/dose (1 mL)

Candin® [US] *see Candida albicans (Monilia) on this page*

Candistatin® [Can] *see* nystatin *on page 609*

Canesten® Topical [Can] *see* clotrimazole *on page 205*

Canesten® Vaginal [Can] *see* clotrimazole *on page 205*

Cankaid® [US-OTC] *see* carbamide peroxide *on page 145*

cannabidiol and tetrahydrocannabinol *see* tetrahydrocannabinol and cannabidiol *(Canada only) on page 816*

Cantil® [Can] *see* mepenzolate *on page 529*

Cantil® *(Discontinued)* *see* mepenzolate *on page 529*

Capastat® Sulfate [US] *see* capreomycin *on this page*

capecitabine (ka pe SITE a been)

Sound-Alike/Look-Alike Issues

Xeloda® may be confused with Xenical®

Synonyms NSC-712807

U.S./Canadian Brand Names Xeloda® [US/Can]

Therapeutic Category Antineoplastic Agent, Antimetabolite

Use Treatment of metastatic colorectal cancer; adjuvant therapy of Dukes C colon cancer; treatment of metastatic breast cancer

Usual Dosage Oral: Adults: 1250 mg/m^2 twice daily (morning and evening) for 2 weeks, every 21-28 days

Adjuvant therapy of Dukes C colon cancer: Recommended for a total of 24 weeks (8 cycles of 2 weeks of drug administration and 1 week rest period.

Dosage Forms Tablet: 150 mg, 500 mg

Capex™ [US/Can] *see* fluocinolone *on page 352*

Capital® and Codeine [US] *see* acetaminophen and codeine *on page 6*

Capoten® [US/Can] *see* captopril *on next page*

Capozide® [US/Can] *see* captopril and hydrochlorothiazide *on next page*

capreomycin (kap ree oh MYE sin)

Sound-Alike/Look-Alike Issues

Capastat® may be confused with Cepastat®

Synonyms capreomycin sulfate

U.S./Canadian Brand Names Capastat® Sulfate [US]

Therapeutic Category Antibiotic, Miscellaneous

Use Treatment of tuberculosis in conjunction with at least one other antituberculosis agent

Usual Dosage I.M., I.V.:

Infants and Children: 15-30 mg/kg/day, up to 1 g/day maximum

Adults: 1 g/day (not to exceed 20 mg/kg/day) for 60-120 days, followed by 1 g 2-3 times/week

Dosage Forms Injection, powder for reconstitution, as sulfate: 1 g

capreomycin sulfate *see* capreomycin *on this page*

Capsagel® [US-OTC] *see* capsaicin *on this page*

capsaicin (kap SAY sin)

Sound-Alike/Look-Alike Issues

Zostrix® may be confused with Zestril®, Zovirax®

U.S./Canadian Brand Names ArthriCare® for Women Extra Moisturizing [US-OTC]; ArthriCare® for Women Multi-Action [US-OTC]; ArthriCare® for Women Silky Dry [US-OTC]; Capsagel® [US-OTC]; Capzasin-HP® [US-OTC]; Capzasin-P® [US-OTC]; Zostrix® [US-OTC/Can]; Zostrix®-HP [US-OTC/Can]

Therapeutic Category Analgesic, Topical

Use Topical treatment of pain associated with postherpetic neuralgia, rheumatoid arthritis, osteoarthritis, diabetic neuropathy; postsurgical pain

Usual Dosage Children ≥2 years and Adults: Topical: Apply to affected area at least 3-4 times/day; application frequency less than 3-4 times/day prevents the total depletion, inhibition of synthesis, and transport of substance P resulting in decreased clinical efficacy and increased local discomfort

Dosage Forms [DSC] = Discontinued product

Cream, topical: 0.025% (60 g); 0.075% (60 g)

ArthriCare® for Women Multi-Action: 0.025% (42 g) [contains menthol]

ArthriCare® for Women Silky Dry: 0.025% (42 g)

ArthriCare® for Women Ultra Strength: 0.075% (42 g) [contains benzalkonium chloride and menthol] [DSC]

Capzasin-P®: 0.025% (45 g)

Capzasin-HP®: 0.075% (45 g)

Zostrix®: 0.025% (60 g)

Zostrix®-HP: 0.075% (60 g)

Gel, topical (Capsagel®): 0.025% (60 g); 0.05% (60 g); 0.075% (30 g)

Lotion, topical (ArthriCare® for Women Extra Moisturizing): 0.025% (120 mL, 240 mL)

captopril (KAP toe pril)

Sound-Alike/Look-Alike Issues

captopril may be confused with Capitrol®, carvedilol

Synonyms ACE

U.S./Canadian Brand Names Alti-Captopril [Can]; Apo-Capto® [Can]; Capoten® [US/Can]; Gen-Captopril [Can]; Novo-Captopril [Can]; Nu-Capto [Can]; PMS-Captopril [Can]

Therapeutic Category Angiotensin-Converting Enzyme (ACE) Inhibitor

Use Management of hypertension; treatment of congestive heart failure, left ventricular dysfunction after myocardial infarction, diabetic nephropathy

Usual Dosage **Note:** Titrate dose according to patient's response; use lowest effective dose. Oral:

Infants: Initial: 0.15-0.3 mg/kg/dose; titrate dose upward to maximum of 6 mg/kg/day in 1-4 divided doses; usual required dose: 2.5-6 mg/kg/day

Children: Initial: 0.5 mg/kg/dose; titrate upward to maximum of 6 mg/kg/day in 2-4 divided doses

Older Children: Initial: 6.25-12.5 mg/dose every 12-24 hours; titrate upward to maximum of 6 mg/kg/day

Adolescents: Initial: 12.5-25 mg/dose given every 8-12 hours; increase by 25 mg/dose to maximum of 450 mg/day

Adults:

Acute hypertension (urgency/emergency): 12.5-25 mg, may repeat as needed (may be given sublingually, but no therapeutic advantage demonstrated)

Hypertension:

Initial dose: 12.5-25 mg 2-3 times/day; may increase by 12.5-25 mg/dose at 1- to 2-week intervals up to 50 mg 3 times/day; maximum dose: 150 mg 3 times/day; add diuretic before further dosage increases

Usual dose range (JNC 7): 25-100 mg/day in 2 divided doses

Congestive heart failure:

Initial dose: 6.25-12.5 mg 3 times/day in conjunction with cardiac glycoside and diuretic therapy; initial dose depends upon patient's fluid/electrolyte status

Target dose: 50 mg 3 times/day

LVD after MI: Initial dose: 6.25 mg followed by 12.5 mg 3 times/day; then increase to 25 mg 3 times/day during next several days and then over next several weeks to target dose of 50 mg 3 times/day

Diabetic nephropathy: 25 mg 3 times/day; other antihypertensives often given concurrently

Dosage Forms Tablet: 12.5 mg, 25 mg, 50 mg, 100 mg

captopril and hydrochlorothiazide (KAP toe pril & hye droe klor oh THYE a zide)

Synonyms hydrochlorothiazide and captopril

U.S./Canadian Brand Names Capozide® [US/Can]

Therapeutic Category Antihypertensive Agent, Combination

Use Management of hypertension and treatment of congestive heart failure

(Continued)

captopril and hydrochlorothiazide *(Continued)*

Usual Dosage Oral: Adults: Hypertension, CHF: May be substituted for previously titrated dosages of the individual components; alternatively, may initiate as follows:

Initial: Single tablet (captopril 25 mg/hydrochlorothiazide 15 mg) taken once daily; daily dose of captopril should not exceed 150 mg; daily dose of hydrochlorothiazide should not exceed 50 mg

Dosage Forms Tablet:

25/15: Captopril 25 mg and hydrochlorothiazide 15 mg
25/25: Captopril 25 mg and hydrochlorothiazide 25 mg
50/15: Captopril 50 mg and hydrochlorothiazide 15 mg
50/25: Captopril 50 mg and hydrochlorothiazide 25 mg

Capzasin-HP® [US-OTC] *see* capsaicin *on page 142*

Capzasin-P® [US-OTC] *see* capsaicin *on page 142*

Carac™ [US] *see* fluorouracil *on page 356*

Carafate® [US] *see* sucralfate *on page 793*

Carapres® [Can] *see* clonidine *on page 203*

carbachol (KAR ba kole)

Sound-Alike/Look-Alike Issues

Isopto® Carbachol may be confused with Isopto® Carpine

Synonyms carbacholine; carbamylcholine chloride

U.S./Canadian Brand Names Isopto® Carbachol [US/Can]; Miostat® [US/Can]

Therapeutic Category Cholinergic Agent

Use Lowers intraocular pressure in the treatment of glaucoma; cause miosis during surgery

Usual Dosage Adults:

Ophthalmic: Instill 1-2 drops up to 3 times/day
Intraocular: 0.5 mL instilled into anterior chamber before or after securing sutures

Dosage Forms [DSC] = Discontinued product

Solution, intraocular (Carbastat® [DSC], Miostat®): 0.01% (1.5 mL)
Solution, ophthalmic (Isopto® Carbachol): 1.5% (15 mL); 3% (30 mL) [contains benzalkonium chloride]

carbacholine *see* carbachol *on this page*

carbamazepine (kar ba MAZ e peen)

Sound-Alike/Look-Alike Issues

Carbatrol® may be confused with Cartrol®
Epitol® may be confused with Epinal®
Tegretol® may be confused with Mebaral®, Tegrin®, Toradol®, Trental®

Synonyms CBZ; SPD417

U.S./Canadian Brand Names Apo-Carbamazepine® [Can]; Carbatrol® [US]; Epitol® [US]; Equetro™ [US]; Gen-Carbamazepine CR [Can]; Mapezine® [Can]; Novo-Carbamaz [Can]; Nu-Carbamazepine [Can]; PMS-Carbamazepine [Can]; Taro-Carbamazepine Chewable [Can]; Tegretol® [US/Can]; Tegretol®-XR [US]

Therapeutic Category Anticonvulsant

Use

Carbatrol®, Tegretol®, Tegretol®-XR: Partial seizures with complex symptomatology (psychomotor, temporal lobe), generalized tonic-clonic seizures (grand mal), mixed seizure patterns, trigeminal neuralgia

Equetro™: Acute manic and mixed episodes associated with bipolar 1 disorder

Usual Dosage Dosage must be adjusted according to patient's response and serum concentrations. Administer tablets (chewable or conventional) in 2-3 divided doses daily and suspension in 4 divided doses daily. Oral:

Epilepsy:

Children:

<6 years: Initial: 10-20 mg/kg/day divided twice or 3 times daily as tablets or 4 times/day as suspension; increase dose every week until optimal response and therapeutic levels are achieved

Maintenance dose: Divide into 3-4 doses daily (tablets or suspension); maximum recommended dose: 35 mg/kg/day

6-12 years: Initial: 100 mg twice daily (tablets or extended release tablets) or 50 mg of suspension 4 times/day (200 mg/day); increase by up to 100 mg/day at weekly intervals using a twice daily regimen of extended release tablets or 3-4 times daily regimen of other formulations until optimal response and therapeutic levels are achieved

Maintenance: Usual: 400-800 mg/day; maximum recommended dose: 1000 mg/day

Note: Children <12 years who receive ≥400 mg/day of carbamazepine may be converted to extended release capsules (Carbatrol®) using the same total daily dosage divided twice daily

Children >12 years and Adults: Initial: 200 mg twice daily (tablets, extended release tablets, or extended release capsules) or 100 mg of suspension 4 times/day (400 mg daily); increase by up to 200 mg/day at weekly intervals using a twice daily regimen of extended release tablets or capsules, or a 3-4 times/day regimen of other formulations until optimal response and therapeutic levels are achieved; usual dose: 800-1200 mg/day

Maximum recommended doses:

Children 12-15 years: 1000 mg/day

Children >15 years: 1200 mg/day

Adults: 1600 mg/day; however, some patients have required up to 1.6-2.4 g/day

Trigeminal or glossopharyngeal neuralgia: Adults: Initial: 100 mg twice daily with food, gradually increasing in increments of 100 mg twice daily as needed

Maintenance: Usual: 400-800 mg daily in 2 divided doses; maximum dose: 1200 mg/day

Bipolar disorder (Equetro™): Adults: Initial: 400 mg/day in divided doses, twice daily; may adjust by 200 mg daily increments; maximum dose: 1600 mg/day

Dosage Forms

Capsule, extended release (Carbatrol®, Equetro™): 100 mg, 200 mg, 300 mg

Suspension, oral: 100 mg/5 mL (10 mL, 450 mL)

Tegretol®: 100 mg/5 mL (450 mL) [citrus vanilla flavor]

Tablet (Epitol®, Tegretol®): 200 mg

Tablet, chewable (Tegretol®): 100 mg

Tablet, extended release (Tegretol®-XR): 100 mg, 200 mg, 400 mg

carbamide *see* urea *on page 861*

carbamide peroxide (KAR ba mide per OKS ide)

Synonyms urea peroxide

U.S./Canadian Brand Names Cankaid® [US-OTC]; Debrox® [US-OTC]; Dent's Ear Wax [US-OTC]; E•R•O [US-OTC]; Gly-Oxide® [US-OTC]; Murine® Ear Wax Removal System [US-OTC]; Orajel® Perioseptic® Spot Treatment [US-OTC]

Therapeutic Category Antiinfective Agent, Oral; Otic Agent, Ceruminolytic

Use Relief of minor inflammation of gums, oral mucosal surfaces, and lips including canker sores and dental irritation; emulsify and disperse ear wax

Usual Dosage Children and Adults:

Oral: Inflammation/dental irritation: Solution (should not be used for >7 days): Oral preparation should not be used in children <2 years of age; apply several drops undiluted on affected area 4 times/day after meals and at bedtime; expectorate after 2-3 minutes **or** place 10 drops onto tongue, mix with saliva, swish for several minutes, expectorate

Otic:

Children <12 years: Tilt head sideways and individualize the dose according to patient size; 3 drops (range: 1-5 drops) twice daily for up to 4 days, tip of applicator should not enter ear canal; keep drops in ear for several minutes by keeping head tilted and placing cotton in ear

Children ≥12 years and Adults: Tilt head sideways and instill 5-10 drops twice daily up to 4 days, tip of applicator should not enter ear canal; keep drops in ear for several minutes by keeping head tilted and placing cotton in ear

Dosage Forms

Solution, oral: 10% (60 mL)

Cankaid®: 10% (22 mL) [in anhydrous glycerol]

Gly-Oxide®: 10% (15 mL, 60 mL) [contains glycerin]

Orajel® Perioseptic® Spot Treatment: 15% (13.3 mL) [contains anhydrous glycerin]

Solution, otic: 6.5% (15 mL)

Debrox®: 6.5% (15 mL, 30 mL) [contains propylene glycol]

Dent's Ear Wax: 6.5% (3.7 mL) [contains glycerin]

E•R•O: 6.5% (15 mL)

Murine® Ear Wax Removal System: 6.5% (15 mL) [contains alcohol 6.3% and glycerin]

carbamylcholine chloride *see* carbachol *on previous page*

Carbaphen 12® [US] *see* carbetapentane, phenylephrine, and chlorpheniramine *on page 147*

Carbaphen 12 Ped® [US] *see* carbetapentane, phenylephrine, and chlorpheniramine *on page 147*

Carbastat® ***(Discontinued)*** *see* carbachol *on previous page*

Carbatrol® [US] *see* carbamazepine *on page 144*

Carbaxefed DM RF *(Discontinued)* *see* carbinoxamine, pseudoephedrine, and dextromethorphan *on page 150*

Carbaxefed RF *(Discontinued)* *see* carbinoxamine and pseudoephedrine *on page 149*

carbenicillin (kar ben i SIL in)

Synonyms carbenicillin indanyl sodium; carindacillin

U.S./Canadian Brand Names Geocillin® [US]

Therapeutic Category Penicillin

Use Treatment of serious urinary tract infections and prostatitis caused by susceptible gram-negative aerobic bacilli

Usual Dosage

Usual dosage range:

Children: Oral: 30-50 mg/kg/day divided every 6 hours (maximum dose: 2-3 g/day)

Adults: Oral: 1-2 tablets every 6 hours

Indication-specific dosing:

Adults: Oral:

Prostatitis: 2 tablets every 6 hours

Urinary tract infections: 1-2 tablets every 6 hours

Dosage Forms Tablet: 382 mg [contains sodium 23 mg/tablet]

carbenicillin indanyl sodium *see* carbenicillin *on this page*

carbetapentane and chlorpheniramine (kar bay ta PEN tane & klor fen IR a meen)

Synonyms carbetapentane tannate and chlorpheniramine tannate; chlorpheniramine and carbetapentane

U.S./Canadian Brand Names Tannate 12 S [US]; Tannic-12 S [US]; Tannic-12 [US]; Tannihist-12 RF [US]; Tussi-12 S™ [US]; Tussi-12® [US]; Tussizone-12 RF™ [US]

Therapeutic Category Antihistamine/Antitussive

Use Symptomatic relief of cough associated with upper respiratory tract conditions, such as the common cold, bronchitis, bronchial asthma

Usual Dosage Oral:

Children: Based on carbetapentane 30 mg and chlorpheniramine 4 mg per 5 mL suspension:

2-6 years: 2.5-5 mL every 12 hours

>6 years: 5-10 mL every 12 hours

Adults: Based on carbetapentane 60 mg and chlorpheniramine 5 mg per tablet: 1-2 tablets every 12 hours

Dosage Forms

Suspension:

Tannate 12 S: Carbetapentane tannate 30 mg and chlorpheniramine tannate 4 mg per 5 mL (120 mL, 480 mL)

Tannic-12 S: Carbetapentane tannate 30 mg and chlorpheniramine tannate 4 mg per 5 mL (120 mL) [contains benzoic acid; strawberry flavor]

Tannihist-12 RF: Carbetapentane tannate 30 mg and chlorpheniramine tannate 4 mg per 5 mL (120 mL, 480 mL) [strawberry-black currant flavor]

Tussi-12 S™: Carbetapentane tannate 30 mg and chlorpheniramine tannate 4 mg per 5 mL (120 mL) [contains benzoic acid and tartrazine; strawberry-currant flavor]

Tussizone-12 RF™: Carbetapentane tannate 30 mg and chlorpheniramine tannate 4 mg per 5 mL (120 mL, 480 mL) [contains benzoic acid and tartrazine; strawberry-black currant flavor]

Tablet (Tannic-12, Tussi-12®, Tussizone-12 RF™): Carbetapentane tannate 60 mg and chlorpheniramine tannate 5 mg

carbetapentane and pseudoephedrine (kar bay ta PEN tane & soo doe e FED rin)

Synonyms carbetapentane tannate and pseudoephedrine tannate; pseudoephedrine and carbetapentane

U.S./Canadian Brand Names Respi-Tann™ [US]

Therapeutic Category Antitussive/Decongestant

Use Relief of cough and congestion due to the common cold, influenza, sinusitis, or bronchitis

Usual Dosage Relief of cough and congestion: Oral:

Children:

2-6 years: $^{1}/_{2}$ tablet or 2.5 mL suspension every 12 hours (maximum: 4 doses/24 hours)

6-12 years: 1 tablet or 5 mL suspension every 12 hours (maximum: 4 doses/24 hours)

Children >12 years and Adults: 2 tablets or 10 mL suspension every 12 hours (maximum: 4 doses/24 hours)

Dosage Forms
Suspension: Carbetapentane tannate 25 mg and pseudoephedrine tannate 75 mg per 5 mL (480 mL) [dye free; contains sodium benzoate; cherry flavor]
Tablet, chewable: Carbetapentane tannate 25 mg and pseudoephedrine tannate 75 mg [dye free; cherry flavor]

carbetapentane, ephedrine, phenylephrine, and chlorpheniramine *see* chlorpheniramine, ephedrine, phenylephrine, and carbetapentane *on page 178*

carbetapentane, phenylephrine, and chlorpheniramine

(kar bay ta PEN tane, fen il EF rin, & klor fen IR a meen)
Synonyms chlorpheniramine, carbetapentane, and phenylephrine; phenylephrine, chlorpheniramine, and carbetapentane
U.S./Canadian Brand Names Carbaphen 12 Ped® [US]; Carbaphen 12® [US]; XiraTuss [US]
Therapeutic Category Antihistamine/Decongestant/Antitussive; Antitussive; Sympathomimetic
Use Symptomatic relief of cough, nasal congestion, and discharge associated with the common cold, bronchial asthma, acute and chronic bronchitis, and other respiratory tract conditions
Usual Dosage Oral: Relief of cough, congestion:
Children 2-6 years:
Carbaphen 12 Ped®: 1-2 mL every 12 hours
XiraTuss suspension: 2.5-5 mL every 12 hours
Children 6-12 years:
Carbaphen 12 Ped®: 2-4 mL every 12 hours
XiraTuss suspension: 5-10 mL every 12 hours
Children >12 years and Adults:
Carbaphen 12®: 5-10 mL every 12 hours
XiraTuss tablet: 1-2 tablets every 12 hours
Dosage Forms [DSC] = Discontinued product
Suspension:
Carbaphen 12®: Carbetapentane tannate 60 mg, phenylephrine tannate 20 mg, and chlorpheniramine tannate 8 mg per 5 mL (480 mL) [contains benzoic acid, phenylalanine 1 mg/5 mL; alcohol free, sugar free; blueberry-banana flavor]
Carbaphen 12 Ped®: Carbetapentane tannate 15 mg, phenylephrine tannate 2.5 mg, and chlorpheniramine tannate 2 mg per mL (60 mL) [contains benzoic acid, phenylalanine 1.6 mg/mL; alcohol free, sugar free; blueberry-banana flavor]
XiraTuss™: Carbetapentane tannate 30 mg, phenylephrine tannate 12.5 mg, and chlorpheniramine tannate 4 mg per 5 mL (120 mL) [strawberry flavor] [DSC]
Tablet:
XiraTuss™: Carbetapentane tannate 60 mg, phenylephrine tannate 10 mg, and chlorpheniramine tannate 5 mg

carbetapentane tannate and chlorpheniramine tannate *see* carbetapentane and chlorpheniramine *on previous page*

carbetapentane tannate and pseudoephedrine tannate *see* carbetapentane and pseudoephedrine *on previous page*

carbetocin *(Canada only)* (kar BE toe sin)

U.S./Canadian Brand Names Duratocin™ [Can]
Therapeutic Category Uteronic Agent
Use For the prevention of uterine atony and postpartum hemorrhage following elective cesarean section under epidural or spinal anesthesia.
Usual Dosage A single I.V. dose of 100 mcg (1 mL) is administered by bolus injection, over 1 minute, only when delivery of the infant has been completed by cesarean section under epidural anesthetic. Carbetocin can be administered either before or after delivery of the placenta
Dosage Forms Injection: 1 mcg/mL (1 mL)

carbidopa (kar bi DOE pa)

U.S./Canadian Brand Names Lodosyn® [US]
Therapeutic Category Anti-Parkinson Agent; Dopaminergic Agent (Anti-Parkinson)
Use Given with levodopa in the treatment of parkinsonism to enable a lower dosage of levodopa to be used and a more rapid response to be obtained and to decrease side effects; for details of administration and dosage, see Levodopa; has no effect without levodopa
(Continued)

carbidopa *(Continued)*

Usual Dosage Oral: Adults: 70-100 mg/day; maximum daily dose: 200 mg

Dosage Forms Tablet: 25 mg

carbidopa and levodopa *see* levodopa and carbidopa *on page 489*

carbidopa, levodopa, and entacapone *see* levodopa, carbidopa, and entacapone *on page 489*

Carbihist *(Discontinued)* *see* carbinoxamine *on this page*

carbinoxamine (kar bi NOKS a meen)

Synonyms carbinoxamine maleate; carbinoxamine tannate

U.S./Canadian Brand Names Histex™ PD [US]; Histex™ PD-12 [US]; Palgic [US]

Therapeutic Category Antihistamine

Use Seasonal and perennial allergic rhinitis; urticaria

Usual Dosage Oral: Allergic rhinitis/urticaria:

Children:
- 1-3 months (Pediatex™): 0.4 mg (1.25 mL) every 4-6 hours
- 3-9 months:
  - Histex™ PD: 1 mg (1.25 mL) 4 times/day
  - Pediatex™: 0.9-1.3 mg (2.5-3.75 mL) every 4-6 hours
- 9-18 months:
  - Histex™ PD: 1-2 mg (1.25-2.5 mL) 4 times/day
  - Histex™ PD-12: 1.25 mL every 12 hours
  - Pediatex™: 1.3-1.75 mg (3.75-5 mL) every 4-6 hours
- 18 months to 6 years:
  - Histex™ PD, Palgic: 2 mg (2.5 mL) 4 times/day
  - Histex™ PD-12: 2.5 mL every 12 hours
  - Pediatex™: 1.75 mg (5 mL) every 4-6 hours
- 2-6 years (Pediatex™ 12): 2.5-5 mL every 12 hours
- 6-12 years:
  - Histex™ PD, Histex™ PD-12, Palgic, Pediatex™: Refer to Adults dosing
  - Pediatex™ 12: 5-10 mL every 12 hours
- ≥12 years: Refer to Adults dosing

Adults:
- Histex™ I/E: One capsule or tablet every 12 hours; maximum: 2 doses/24 hours
- Histex™ PD, Palgic: 4 mg (5 mL) 4 times/day
- Histex™ PD-12: 5 mL every 12 hours
- Pediatex™: 3.5 mg (10 mL) every 4-6 hours
- Pediatex™ 12: 10-20 mL every 12 hours

Dosage Forms [DSC] = Discontinued product

Capsule, variable release:
- Histex™ I/E: Carbinoxamine maleate 2 mg [immediate release] and carbinoxamine maleate 8 mg [extended release] [DSC]

Liquid, as maleate:
- Carbihist: 4 mg/5 mL (120 mL) [cotton candy flavor] [DSC]
- Carbinoxamine PD: 4 mg/5 mL (480 mL) [bubble gum flavor] [DSC]
- Carboxine: 1.75 mg/5 mL (480 mL) [bubble gum flavor] [DSC]
- Histex™ PD: 4 mg/5 mL (480 mL) [alcohol free, dye free, sugar free; bubble gum flavor]
- Pediatex™: 1.75 mg/5 mL (480 mL) [alcohol free, dye free, sugar free; cotton candy flavor] [DSC]

Solution, as maleate:
- Palgic: 4 mg/5 mL (480 mL) [bubble gum flavor]

Suspension, as tannate:
- Pediatex™ 12: Carbinoxamine 3.6 mg per 5 mL (480 mL) [contains sodium benzoate; candy apple flavor] [DSC]

Suspension, variable release:
- Histex™ PD-12: Carbinoxamine maleate 2 mg [immediate release] and carbinoxamine tannate 6 mg [extended release] per 5 mL (120 mL, 480 mL) [alcohol free, dye free, sugar free; contains sodium benzoate; bubble gum flavor]

Tablet, as maleate [scored]:
- Palgic: 4 mg

carbinoxamine and pseudoephedrine (kar bi NOKS a meen & soo doe e FED rin)

Synonyms pseudoephedrine and carbinoxamine

U.S./Canadian Brand Names Hydro-Tussin™-CBX [US]; Palgic®-D [US]; Palgic®-DS [US]; Rondec-TR® [US]; Rondec® Tablets [US]

Therapeutic Category Antihistamine/Decongestant Combination

Use Seasonal and perennial allergic rhinitis; vasomotor rhinitis

Usual Dosage Oral:

Children:

Drops (Andehist NR, Carbaxefed RF, Rondec®, Sildec):

1-3 months: 0.25 mL 4 times/day

3-6 months: 0.5 mL 4 times/day

6-12 months: 0.75 mL 4 times/day

12-24 months: 1 mL 4 times/day

Liquid (Pediatex™-D):

1-3 months: 1.25 mL up to 4 times/day

3-6 months: 2.5 mL up to 4 times/day

6-9 months: 3.75 mL up to 4 times/day

9-18 months: 3.75-5 mL up to 4 times/day

18 months to 6 years: 5 mL 3-4 times/day

>6 years: Refer to Adults dosing

Syrup (Hydro-Tussin™-CBX, Palgic®-DS):

1-3 months: 1.25 mL up to 4 times/day

3-6 months: 2.5 mL up to 4 times/day

6-9 months: 3.75 mL up to 4 times/day

9-18 months: 3.75-5 mL up to 4 times/day

18 months to 6 years: 5 mL 3-4 times/day

>6 years: Refer to Adults dosing

Tablet (Rondec®): ≥6 years: Refer to Adults dosing

Tablet, timed release:

6-12 years (Palgic®-D): One-half tablet every 12 hours

≥12 years (Palgic®-D, Rondec-TR®): Refer to Adults dosing

Adults:

Liquid (Pediatex™-D): 10 mL 4 times/day

Syrup (Hydro-Tussin™-CBX, Palgic®-DS): 10 mL 4 times/day

Tablet (Rondec®): 1 tablet 4 times a day

Tablet, timed release (Palgic®-D, Rondec-TR®): 1 tablet every 12 hours

Dosage Forms [DSC] = Discontinued product

Liquid:

Cordron-D NR: Carbinoxamine maleate 2 mg and pseudoephedrine hydrochloride 12.5 mg per 5 mL (480 mL) [cotton candy flavor] [DSC]

Pediatex™-D: Carbinoxamine maleate 2 mg and pseudoephedrine hydrochloride 20 mg per 5 mL (480 mL) [alcohol free, dye free, sugar free; cotton candy flavor]

Solution: Carbinoxamine maleate 2 mg and pseudoephedrine hydrochloride 25 mg per 5 mL (480 mL) [DSC]

Carboxine-PSE: Carbinoxamine maleate 2 mg and pseudoephedrine hydrochloride 20 mg per 5 mL (480 mL) [peach flavor] [DSC]

Solution, oral drops:

Andehist NR: Carbinoxamine maleate 1 mg and pseudoephedrine hydrochloride 15 mg per mL (30 mL) [alcohol and sugar free; raspberry flavor] [DSC]

Carbaxefed RF, Rondec® [DSC]: Carbinoxamine maleate 1 mg and pseudoephedrine hydrochloride 15 mg per mL (30 mL) [alcohol free; contains sodium benzoate; cherry flavor] [DSC]

Sildec: Carbinoxamine maleate 1 mg and pseudoephedrine hydrochloride 15 mg per mL (30 mL) [raspberry flavor] [DSC]

Syrup: Carbinoxamine maleate 2 mg and pseudoephedrine hydrochloride 25 mg per 5 mL (480 mL)

Hydro-Tussin™-CBX, Palgic®-DS: Carbinoxamine maleate 2 mg and pseudoephedrine hydrochloride 25 mg per 5 mL (480 mL) [alcohol, dye, and sugar free; strawberry/pineapple flavor]

Tablet (Rondec®): Carbinoxamine maleate 4 mg and pseudoephedrine hydrochloride 60 mg

Tablet, timed release:

Palgic®-D: Carbinoxamine maleate 8 mg and pseudoephedrine hydrochloride 80 mg [dye free]

Rondec-TR®: Carbinoxamine maleate 8 mg and pseudoephedrine hydrochloride 120 mg

carbinoxamine, dextromethorphan, and pseudoephedrine *see* carbinoxamine, pseudoephedrine, and dextromethorphan *on next page*

carbinoxamine maleate *see* carbinoxamine *on page 148*

Carbinoxamine PD *(Discontinued)* *see* carbinoxamine *on page 148*

carbinoxamine, pseudoephedrine, and dextromethorphan

(kar bi NOKS a meen, soo doe e FED rin, & deks troe meth OR fan)

Sound-Alike/Look-Alike Issues

Tussafed® may be confused with Tussafin®

Synonyms carbinoxamine, dextromethorphan, and pseudoephedrine; dextromethorphan, carbinoxamine, and pseudoephedrine; dextromethorphan, pseudoephedrine, and carbinoxamine; pseudoephedrine, carbinoxamine, and dextromethorphan; pseudoephedrine, dextromethorphan, and carbinoxamine

Therapeutic Category Antihistamine/Decongestant/Antitussive

Use Relief of coughs and upper respiratory symptoms, including nasal congestion, associated with allergy or the common cold

Usual Dosage Oral:

Drops (Rondec®-DM): Infants and Children:
- 1-3 months: 1/4 mL 4 times/day
- 3-6 months: 1/2 mL 4 times/day
- 6-12 months: 3/4 mL 4 times/day
- 12-24 months: 1 mL 4 times/day

Liquid (Pediatex™-DM):
- Children 18 months to 6 years: 2.5 mL 4 times/day
- Children 6-12 years: 5 mL 4 times/day
- Children ≥12 years and Adults: 10 mL 4 times/day

Syrup (Tussafed®):
- Children 18 months to 6 years: 2.5 mL 4 times/day
- Children >6 years and Adults: 5 mL 4 times/day

Dosage Forms [DSC] = Discontinued product

Liquid:
- Cordron-DM NR: Carbinoxamine maleate 3 mg, pseudoephedrine hydrochloride 12.5 mg, and dextromethorphan hydrobromide 15 mg per 5 mL (480 mL) [cotton candy flavor] [DSC]
- Decahist-DM: Carbinoxamine maleate 2 mg, pseudoephedrine hydrochloride 15 mg, and dextromethorphan hydrobromide 15 mg per 5 mL (480 mL) [peach flavor] [DSC]
- Pediatex™ DM: Carbinoxamine maleate 2 mg, pseudoephedrine hydrochloride 15 mg, and dextromethorphan hydrobromide 15 mg per 5 mL (480 mL) [alcohol free, dye free, sugar free; cotton candy flavor] [DSC]

Liquid, oral drops: Carbinoxamine maleate 1 mg, pseudoephedrine hydrochloride 15 mg, and dextromethorphan hydrobromide 4 mg per mL (30 mL) [DSC]
- Andehist DM NR: Carbinoxamine maleate 1 mg, pseudoephedrine hydrochloride 15 mg, and dextromethorphan hydrobromide 4 mg per mL (30 mL) [alcohol and sugar free; grape flavor] [DSC]
- Carbaxefed DM RF: Carbinoxamine maleate 1 mg, pseudoephedrine hydrochloride 15 mg, and dextromethorphan hydrobromide 4 mg per mL (30 mL) [alcohol free; grape flavor] [DSC]
- Rondec®-DM: Carbinoxamine maleate 1 mg, pseudoephedrine hydrochloride 15 mg, and dextromethorphan hydrobromide 4 mg per mL (30 mL) [alcohol free; contains sodium benzoate; grape flavor] [DSC]
- Sildec-DM: Carbinoxamine maleate 1 mg, pseudoephedrine hydrochloride 15 mg, and dextromethorphan hydrobromide 4 mg per mL (30 mL) [DSC]

Syrup, oral: Carbinoxamine maleate 4 mg, pseudoephedrine hydrochloride 60 mg, and dextromethorphan hydrobromide 12.5 mg per 5 mL (480 mL) [alcohol and sugar free] [DSC]
- Tussafed®: Carbinoxamine maleate 4 mg, pseudoephedrine hydrochloride 60 mg, and dextromethorphan hydrobromide 15 mg per 5 mL (480 mL) [alcohol and sugar free] [DSC]

carbinoxamine, pseudoephedrine, and hydrocodone *see* hydrocodone, carbinoxamine, and pseudoephedrine *on page 424*

carbinoxamine tannate *see* carbinoxamine *on page 148*

Carbiset® Tablet *(Discontinued)* *see* carbinoxamine and pseudoephedrine *on previous page*

Carbiset-TR® Tablet *(Discontinued)* *see* carbinoxamine and pseudoephedrine *on previous page*

Carbocaine® [US/Can] *see* mepivacaine *on page 530*

Carbocaine® 2% with Neo-Cobefrin® [US] *see* mepivacaine and levonordefrin *on page 531*

Carbodec® Syrup *(Discontinued)* *see* carbinoxamine and pseudoephedrine *on previous page*

Carbodec® Tablet *(Discontinued)* *see* carbinoxamine and pseudoephedrine *on previous page*

Carbodec® TR Tablet *(Discontinued)* *see* carbinoxamine and pseudoephedrine *on previous page*

Carbofed DM [US] *see* brompheniramine, pseudoephedrine, and dextromethorphan *on page 120*

carbolic acid *see* phenol *on page 658*

Carbolith™ [Can] *see* lithium *on page 501*

carboplatin (KAR boe pla tin)

Sound-Alike/Look-Alike Issues

carboplatin may be confused with cisplatin

Paraplatin® may be confused with Platinol®

Synonyms CBDCA; NSC-241240

U.S./Canadian Brand Names Paraplatin-AQ [Can]; Paraplatin® [US]

Therapeutic Category Antineoplastic Agent

Use Treatment of ovarian cancer

Usual Dosage Refer to individual protocols: **Note:** Doses for adults are usually determined by the AUC using the Calvert formula.

IVPB, I.V. infusion: Adults:

Ovarian cancer: 300-360 mg/m^2 every 4 weeks

In adults, dosing is commonly calculated using the Calvert formula:

Total dose (mg) = Target AUC (mg/mL * minute) x (GFR [mL/minute] + 25)

Usual target AUCs:

Previously untreated patients: 6-8 mg/mL * minute

Previously treated patients: 4-6 mg/mL * minute

Dosage Forms [DSC] = Discontinued product

Injection, powder for reconstitution: 50 mg, 150 mg, 450 mg

Paraplatin®: 50 mg, 150 mg, 450 mg [DSC]

Injection, solution: 10 mg/mL (5 mL, 15 mL, 45 mL, 60 mL)

Paraplatin®: 10 mg/mL (5 mL, 15 mL, 45 mL, 60 mL) [DSC]

carboprost *see* carboprost tromethamine *on this page*

carboprost tromethamine (KAR boe prost tro METH a meen)

Synonyms carboprost; prostaglandin F_2

U.S./Canadian Brand Names Hemabate® [US/Can]

Therapeutic Category Prostaglandin

Use Termination of pregnancy; treatment of refractory postpartum uterine bleeding

Usual Dosage I.M.: Adults:

Abortion: Initial: 250 mcg, then 250 mcg at 1.5- to 3.5-hour intervals, depending on uterine response; a 500 mcg dose may be given if uterine response is not adequate after several 250 mcg doses; do not exceed 12 mg total dose or continuous administration for >2 days

Refractory postpartum uterine bleeding: Initial: 250 mcg; if needed, may repeat at 15- to 90-minute intervals; maximum total dose: 2 mg (8 doses)

Dosage Forms

Injection, solution:

Hemabate®: Carboprost 250 mcg and tromethamine 83 mcg per mL (1 mL) [contains benzyl alcohol]

carbose D *see* carboxymethylcellulose *on this page*

Carboxine *(Discontinued)* *see* carbinoxamine *on page 148*

Carboxine-PSE *(Discontinued)* *see* carbinoxamine and pseudoephedrine *on page 149*

carboxymethylcellulose (kar boks ee meth il SEL yoo lose)

Synonyms carbose D; carboxymethylcellulose sodium

U.S./Canadian Brand Names Celluvisc™ [Can]; Refresh Liquigel™ [US-OTC]; Refresh Plus® [US-OTC/Can]; Refresh Tears® [US-OTC/Can]; Tears Again® Gel Drops™ [US-OTC]; Tears Again® Night and Day™ [US-OTC]; Theratears® [US]

Therapeutic Category Ophthalmic Agent, Miscellaneous

Use Artificial tear substitute

Usual Dosage Ophthalmic: Adults: Instill 1-2 drops into eye(s) 3-4 times/day

Dosage Forms

Gel, ophthalmic, as sodium (Tears Again® Night and Day™): 1.5% (3.5 g)

Solution ophthalmic, as sodium:

Refresh Liquigel™: 1% (15 mL) [liquid gel formulation]

Refresh Plus® preservative free: 0.5% (0.4 mL) [available in packages of 30 or 50]

(Continued)

carboxymethylcellulose *(Continued)*

Refresh Tears®: 0.5% (15 mL)
Tears Again® Gel Drops™: 0.7% (15 mL)
Theratears®: 0.25% (0.6 mL [preservative free], 15 mL)

carboxymethylcellulose sodium *see* carboxymethylcellulose *on previous page*
Cardec DM [US] *see* brompheniramine, pseudoephedrine, and dextromethorphan *on page 120*
Cardene® [US] *see* nicardipine *on page 590*
Cardene® I.V. [US] *see* nicardipine *on page 590*
Cardene® SR [US] *see* nicardipine *on page 590*
Cardio-Green® *(Discontinued)* *see* indocyanine green *on page 446*
Cardioquin® *(Discontinued)* *see* quinidine *on page 725*
Cardizem® [US/Can] *see* diltiazem *on page 257*
Cardizem® CD [US/Can] *see* diltiazem *on page 257*
Cardizem® Injection *(Discontinued)* *see* diltiazem *on page 257*
Cardizem® LA [US] *see* diltiazem *on page 257*
Cardizem® SR [Can] *see* diltiazem *on page 257*
Cardizem® SR *(Discontinued)* *see* diltiazem *on page 257*
Cardura® [US] *see* doxazosin *on page 275*
Cardura-1™ [Can] *see* doxazosin *on page 275*
Cardura-2™ [Can] *see* doxazosin *on page 275*
Cardura-4™ [Can] *see* doxazosin *on page 275*
Cardura® XL [US] *see* doxazosin *on page 275*
Carimune™ *(Discontinued)* *see* immune globulin (intravenous) *on page 444*
Carimune™ NF [US] *see* immune globulin (intravenous) *on page 444*
carindacillin *see* carbenicillin *on page 146*
carisoprodate *see* carisoprodol *on this page*

carisoprodol (kar eye soe PROE dole)

Synonyms carisoprodate; isobamate
U.S./Canadian Brand Names Soma® [US/Can]
Therapeutic Category Skeletal Muscle Relaxant
Use Relief of discomfort associated with skeletal muscle condition
Usual Dosage Oral: Adults: 350 mg 3-4 times/day; take last dose at bedtime
Dosage Forms
Tablet: 350 mg
Soma®: 350 mg

carisoprodol and aspirin (kar eye soe PROE dole & AS pir in)

Synonyms aspirin and carisoprodol
U.S./Canadian Brand Names Soma® Compound [US]
Therapeutic Category Skeletal Muscle Relaxant
Use Skeletal muscle relaxant
Usual Dosage Oral: Adults: 1-2 tablets 4 times/day
Dosage Forms Tablet: Carisoprodol 200 mg and aspirin 325 mg

carisoprodol, aspirin, and codeine (kar eye soe PROE dole, AS pir in, and KOE deen)

Synonyms aspirin, carisoprodol, and codeine; codeine, aspirin, and carisoprodol
U.S./Canadian Brand Names Soma® Compound w/Codeine [US]
Therapeutic Category Skeletal Muscle Relaxant
Controlled Substance C-III
Use Skeletal muscle relaxant
Usual Dosage Oral: Adults: 1 or 2 tablets 4 times/day
Dosage Forms Tablet: Carisoprodol 200 mg, aspirin 325 mg, and codeine phosphate 16 mg

Carmol® 10 [US-OTC] *see* urea *on page 861*

Carmol® 20 [US-OTC] *see* urea *on page 861*

Carmol® 40 [US] *see* urea *on page 861*

Carmol® Deep Cleaning [US] *see* urea *on page 861*

Carmol-HC® [US] *see* urea and hydrocortisone *on page 861*

Carmol® Scalp [US] *see* sulfacetamide *on page 795*

carmustine (kar MUS teen)

Sound-Alike/Look-Alike Issues

carmustine may be confused with lomustine

Synonyms BCNU; bis-chloronitrosourea; carmustinum; NSC-409962; WR-139021

U.S./Canadian Brand Names BiCNu® [US/Can]; Gliadel Wafer® [Can]; Gliadel® [US]

Therapeutic Category Antineoplastic Agent

Use

Injection: Treatment of brain tumors (glioblastoma, brainstem glioma, medulloblastoma, astrocytoma, ependymoma, and metastatic brain tumors), multiple myeloma, Hodgkin disease, non-Hodgkin lymphomas, melanoma, lung cancer, colon cancer

Wafer (implant): Adjunct to surgery in patients with recurrent glioblastoma multiforme; adjunct to surgery and radiation in patients with high-grade malignant glioma

Usual Dosage

I.V. (refer to individual protocols):

Children: 200-250 mg/m^2 every 4-6 weeks as a single dose

Adults: Usual dosage (per manufacturer labeling): 150-200 mg/m^2 every 6 weeks as a single dose or divided into daily injections on 2 successive days

Alternative regimens:

75-120 mg/m^2 days 1 and 2 every 6-8 weeks **or**

50-80 mg/m^2 days 1,2,3 every 6-8 weeks

Primary brain cancer:

150-200 mg/m^2 every 6-8 weeks as a single dose **or**

75-120 mg/m^2 days 1 and 2 every 6-8 weeks **or**

20-65 mg/m^2 every 4-6 weeks **or**

0.5-1 mg/kg every 4-6 weeks **or**

40-80 mg/m^2/day for 3 days every 6-8 weeks

Autologous BMT: ALL OF THE FOLLOWING DOSES ARE FATAL WITHOUT BMT

Combination therapy: Up to 300-900 mg/m^2

Single-agent therapy: Up to 1200 mg/m^2 (fatal necrosis is associated with doses >2 g/m^2)

Implantation (wafer): Adults: Recurrent glioblastoma multiforme, malignant glioma: Up to 8 wafers may be placed in the resection cavity (total dose 62.6 mg); should the size and shape not accommodate 8 wafers, the maximum number of wafers allowed should be placed

Dosage Forms

Injection, powder for reconstitution:

BiCNu®: 100 mg [packaged with 3 mL of absolute alcohol as diluent]

Wafer, implant:

Gliadel®: 7.7 mg (8s)

carmustinum *see* carmustine *on this page*

Carnation Instant Breakfast® [US-OTC] *see* nutritional formula, enteral/oral *on page 608*

Carnitor® [US/Can] *see* levocarnitine *on page 488*

Carrington Antifungal [US-OTC] *see* miconazole *on page 553*

carteolol (KAR tee oh lole)

Sound-Alike/Look-Alike Issues

carteolol may be confused with carvedilol

Cartrol® may be confused with Carbatrol®

Ocupress® may be confused with Ocufen®

Synonyms carteolol hydrochloride

U.S./Canadian Brand Names Cartrol® [US/Can]; Ocupress® Ophthalmic [Can]

Therapeutic Category Beta-Adrenergic Blocker

Use Management of hypertension; treatment of chronic open-angle glaucoma and intraocular hypertension

(Continued)

carteolol *(Continued)*

Usual Dosage Adults:

Oral: 2.5 mg as a single daily dose, with a maintenance dose normally 2.5-5 mg once daily; doses >10 mg do not increase response and may in fact decrease effect.

Ophthalmic: Instill 1 drop in affected eye(s) twice daily.

Dosage Forms [DSC] = Discontinued product

Solution, ophthalmic, as hydrochloride: 1% (5 mL, 10 mL, 15 mL) [contains benzalkonium chloride]

Ocupress® [DSC]: 1% (5 mL, 10 mL, 15 mL) [contains benzalkonium chloride]

Tablet, as hydrochloride (Cartrol®): 2.5 mg, 5 mg

carteolol hydrochloride *see* carteolol *on previous page*

Carter's Little Pills® [Can] *see* bisacodyl *on page 111*

Carter's Little Pills® *(Discontinued)* *see* bisacodyl *on page 111*

Cartia XT™ [US] *see* diltiazem *on page 257*

Cartrol® [US/Can] *see* carteolol *on previous page*

carvedilol (KAR ve dil ole)

Sound-Alike/Look-Alike Issues

carvedilol may be confused with captopril, carteolol

U.S./Canadian Brand Names Apo-Carvedilol® [Can]; Coreg® [US/Can]; Novo-Carvedilol [Can]; PMS-Carvedilol [Can]; RAN™-Carvedilol [Can]; ratio-Carvedilol [Can]

Therapeutic Category Beta-Adrenergic Blocker

Use Mild-to-severe heart failure of ischemic or cardiomyopathic origin (usually in addition to standardized therapy); left ventricular dysfunction following myocardial infarction (MI); management of hypertension

Usual Dosage Oral: Adults: Reduce dosage if heart rate drops to <55 beats/minute.

Hypertension: 6.25 mg twice daily; if tolerated, dose should be maintained for 1-2 weeks, then increased to 12.5 mg twice daily. Dosage may be increased to a maximum of 25 mg twice daily after 1-2 weeks. Maximum dose: 50 mg/day

Congestive heart failure: 3.125 mg twice daily for 2 weeks; if this dose is tolerated, may increase to 6.25 mg twice daily. Double the dose every 2 weeks to the highest dose tolerated by patient. (Prior to initiating therapy, other heart failure medications should be stabilized and fluid retention minimized.)

Maximum recommended dose:

Mild to moderate heart failure:

<85 kg: 25 mg twice daily

>85 kg: 50 mg twice daily

Severe heart failure: 25 mg twice daily

Left ventricular dysfunction following MI: Initial 3.125-6.25 mg twice daily; increase dosage incrementally (ie, from 6.25 to 12.5 mg twice daily) at intervals of 3-10 days, based on tolerance, to a target dose of 25 mg twice daily. **Note**: Should be initiated only after patient is hemodynamically stable and fluid retention has been minimized.

Dosage Forms Tablet: 3.125 mg, 6.25 mg, 12.5 mg, 25 mg

Casodex® [US/Can] *see* bicalutamide *on page 110*

caspofungin (kas poe FUN jin)

Synonyms caspofungin acetate

U.S./Canadian Brand Names Cancidas® [US/Can]

Therapeutic Category Antifungal Agent, Systemic

Use Treatment of invasive *Aspergillus* infections in patients who are refractory or intolerant of other therapy; treatment of candidemia and other *Candida* infections (intraabdominal abscesses, esophageal, peritonitis, pleural space); empirical treatment for presumed fungal infections in febrile neutropenic patient

Usual Dosage I.V.: Adults: **Note:** Duration of caspofungin treatment should be determined by patient status and clinical response. Empiric therapy should be given until neutropenia resolves. In patients with positive cultures, treatment should continue until 14 days after last positive culture. In neutropenic patients, treatment should be given at least 7 days after both signs and symptoms of infection **and** neutropenia resolve.

Empiric therapy: Initial dose: 70 mg on day 1; subsequent dosing: 50 mg/day; may increase up to 70 mg/day if tolerated, but clinical response is inadequate

Invasive *Aspergillus*, candidiasis: Initial dose: 70 mg on day 1; subsequent dosing: 50 mg/day

Esophageal candidiasis: 50 mg/day; **Note:** The majority of patients studied for this indication also had oropharyngeal involvement.

Concomitant use of an enzyme inducer:
Patients receiving rifampin: 70 mg caspofungin daily
Patients receiving carbamazepine, dexamethasone, efavirenz, nevirapine, **or** phenytoin (and possibly other enzyme inducers) may require an increased daily dose of caspofungin (70 mg/day).
Dosage Forms Injection, powder for reconstitution, as acetate: 50 mg [contains sucrose 39 mg], 70 mg [contains sucrose 54 mg]

caspofungin acetate *see* caspofungin *on previous page*

castor oil (KAS tor oyl)

Synonyms oleum ricini
U.S./Canadian Brand Names Purge® [US-OTC]
Therapeutic Category Laxative
Use Preparation for rectal or bowel examination or surgery; rarely used to relieve constipation; also applied to skin as emollient and protectant
Usual Dosage Oral: Oil:
Children 2-11 years: 5-15 mL as a single dose
Children ≥12 years and Adults: 15-60 mL as a single dose
Dosage Forms [DSC] = Discontinued product
Emulsion, oral (Emulsoil® [DSC]): 95% (60 mL)
Oil, oral: 100% (60 mL, 120 mL, 480 mL, 3840 mL)
Purge®: 95% (30 mL, 60 mL) [lemon flavor]

castor oil, trypsin, and balsam peru *see* trypsin, balsam peru, and castor oil *on page 856*
Cataflam® [US/Can] *see* diclofenac *on page 250*
Catapres® [US] *see* clonidine *on page 203*
Catapres-TTS® [US] *see* clonidine *on page 203*
Cathflo™ Activase® [US/Can] *see* alteplase *on page 34*
Caverject® [US/Can] *see* alprostadil *on page 32*
Caverject Impulse® [US] *see* alprostadil *on page 32*
CaviRinse™ [US] *see* fluoride *on page 354*
CB-1348 *see* chlorambucil *on page 171*
CBDCA *see* carboplatin *on page 151*
CBZ *see* carbamazepine *on page 144*
CC-5013 *see* lenalidomide *on page 484*
CCNU *see* lomustine *on page 502*
C-Crystals® *(Discontinued)* *see* ascorbic acid *on page 76*
2-CdA *see* cladribine *on page 195*
CDDP *see* cisplatin *on page 193*
CDX *see* bicalutamide *on page 110*
Cebid® *(Discontinued)* *see* ascorbic acid *on page 76*
Ceclor® [Can] *see* cefaclor *on this page*
Ceclor® *(Discontinued)* *see* cefaclor *on this page*
Cecon® [US-OTC] *see* ascorbic acid *on page 76*
Cedax® [US] *see* ceftibuten *on page 162*
Cedocard®-SR [Can] *see* isosorbide dinitrate *on page 465*
CEE *see* estrogens (conjugated/equine) *on page 312*
CeeNU® [US/Can] *see* lomustine *on page 502*
Ceepryn® *(Discontinued)* *see* cetylpyridinium *on page 169*

cefaclor (SEF a klor)

Sound-Alike/Look-Alike Issues
cefaclor may be confused with cephalexin
U.S./Canadian Brand Names Apo-Cefaclor® [Can]; Ceclor® [Can]; Novo-Cefaclor [Can]; Nu-Cefaclor [Can]; PMS-Cefaclor [Can]; Raniclor™ [US]
(Continued)

cefaclor *(Continued)*

Therapeutic Category Cephalosporin (Second Generation)

Use Treatment of susceptible bacterial infections including otitis media, lower respiratory tract infections, acute exacerbations of chronic bronchitis, pharyngitis and tonsillitis, urinary tract infections, skin and skin structure infections

Usual Dosage

Usual dosage range:

Children >1 month: Oral: 20-40 mg/kg/day divided every 8-12 hours (maximum dose: 1 g/day)

Adults: Oral: 250-500 mg every 8 hours

Indication-specific dosing:

Children: Oral:

Otitis media: 40 mg/kg/day divided every 12 hours

Pharyngitis: 20 mg/kg/day divided every 12 hours

Dosage Forms

Capsule: 250 mg, 500 mg

Powder for oral suspension: 125 mg/5 mL (75 mL, 150 mL); 187 mg/5 mL (50 mL, 100 mL); 250 mg/5 mL (75 mL, 150 mL); 375 mg/5 mL (50 mL, 100 mL)

Tablet, chewable (Raniclor™): 125 mg [contains phenylalanine 2.8 mg; fruity flavor], 187 mg [contains phenylalanine 4.2 mg; fruity flavor]

cefadroxil (sef a DROKS il)

Synonyms cefadroxil monohydrate

U.S./Canadian Brand Names Apo-Cefadroxil® [Can]; Duricef® [US/Can]; Novo-Cefadroxil [Can]

Therapeutic Category Cephalosporin (First Generation)

Use Treatment of susceptible bacterial infections, including those caused by group A beta-hemolytic *Streptococcus*; prophylaxis against bacterial endocarditis in patients who are allergic to penicillin and undergoing surgical or dental procedures

Usual Dosage

Usual dosage range: Oral:

Children: 30 mg/kg/day divided twice daily up to a maximum of 2 g/day

Adults: 1-2 g/day in 2 divided doses

Indication-specific dosing:

Prophylaxis against bacterial endocarditis:

Children: Oral: 50 mg/kg 1 hour prior to the procedure

Adults: Oral: 2 g 1 hour prior to the procedure

Dosage Forms [DSC] = Discontinued product

Capsule, as monohydrate: 500 mg

Duricef®: 500 mg [DSC]

Powder for oral suspension, as monohydrate: 250 mg/5 mL (50 mL, 100 mL); 500 mg/5 mL (75 mL, 100 mL)

Duricef®: 250 mg/5 mL (50 mL, 100 mL); 500 mg/5 mL (75 mL, 100 mL) [contains sodium benzoate; orange-pineapple flavor]

Tablet, as monohydrate: 1 g

Duricef®: 1 g [DSC]

cefadroxil monohydrate *see* cefadroxil *on this page*

Cefanex® ***(Discontinued)*** *see* cephalexin *on page 166*

cefazolin (sef A zoe lin)

Sound-Alike/Look-Alike Issues

cefazolin may be confused with cefprozil, cephalexin, cephalothin

Kefzol® may be confused with Cefzil®

Synonyms cefazolin sodium

U.S./Canadian Brand Names Ancef® [US]

Therapeutic Category Cephalosporin (First Generation)

Use Treatment of respiratory tract, skin and skin structure, genital, urinary tract, biliary tract, bone and joint infections, and septicemia due to susceptible gram-positive cocci (except enterococcus); some gram-negative bacilli including *E. coli*, *Proteus*, and *Klebsiella* may be susceptible; perioperative prophylaxis

Usual Dosage

Usual dosage range: I.M., I.V.:

Children >1 month: 25-100 mg/kg/day divided every 6-8 hours; maximum: 6 g/day

Adults: 250 mg to 2 g every 6-12 (usually 8) hours, depending on severity of infection; maximum dose: 12 g/day

Indication-specific dosing:

Mild-to-moderate infections: Adults: 500 mg to 1 g every 6-8 hours

Mild infection with gram-positive cocci: Adults: 250-500 mg every 8 hours

Perioperative prophylaxis: Adults: 1 g given 30 minutes prior to surgery (repeat with 500 mg to 1 g during prolonged surgery); followed by 500 mg to 1 g every 6-9 hours for 24 hours postop

Pneumococcal pneumonia: Adults: 500 mg every 12 hours

Severe infection: Adults: 1-2 g every 6 hours

UTI (uncomplicated): Adults: 1 g every 12 hours

Dosage Forms [DSC] = Discontinued product

Infusion [premixed in D_5W]: 500 mg (50 mL); 1 g (50 mL)

Injection, powder for reconstitution: 500 mg, 1 g, 10 g, 20 g

Ancef®: 1 g; 10 g [DSC]

cefazolin sodium *see* cefazolin *on previous page*

cefdinir (SEF di ner)

Synonyms CFDN

U.S./Canadian Brand Names Omnicef® [US/Can]

Therapeutic Category Cephalosporin (Third Generation)

Use Treatment of community-acquired pneumonia, acute exacerbations of chronic bronchitis, acute bacterial otitis media, acute maxillary sinusitis, pharyngitis/tonsillitis, and uncomplicated skin and skin structure infections.

Usual Dosage

Usual dosage range:

Children 6 months to 12 years: Oral: 7 mg/kg/dose twice daily or 14 mg/kg/dose once daily (maximum: 600 mg/day)

Adolescents and Adults: Oral: 300 mg twice daily or 600 mg once daily

Indication-specific dosing:

Children 6 months to 12 years: Oral:

Acute bacterial otitis media, pharyngitis/tonsillitis: 7 mg/kg/dose twice daily for 5-10 days **or** 14 mg/kg/dose once daily for 10 days (maximum: 600 mg/day)

Acute maxillary sinusitis: 7 mg/kg/dose twice daily **or** 14 mg/kg/dose once daily for 10 days (maximum: 600 mg/day)

Uncomplicated skin and skin structure infections: 7 mg/kg/dose twice daily for 10 days (maximum: 600 mg/day)

Adolescents and Adults:

Acute exacerbations of chronic bronchitis, pharyngitis/tonsillitis: 300 mg twice daily for 5-10 days **or** 600 mg once daily for 10 days

Acute maxillary sinusitis: 300 mg twice daily **or** 600 mg once daily for 10 days

Community-acquired pneumonia, uncomplicated skin and skin structure infections: 300 mg twice daily for 10 days

Dosage Forms

Capsule: 300 mg

Powder for oral suspension: 125 mg/5 mL (60 mL, 100 mL) [contains sodium benzoate and sucrose 2.86 g/5 mL; strawberry flavor]; 250 mg/5 mL (60 mL, 100 mL) [contains sodium benzoate and sucrose 2.86 g/5 mL; strawberry flavor]

cefditoren (sef de TOR en)

Synonyms cefditoren pivoxil

U.S./Canadian Brand Names Spectracef™ [US]

Therapeutic Category Antibiotic, Cephalosporin

Use Treatment of acute bacterial exacerbation of chronic bronchitis or community-acquired pneumonia (due to susceptible organisms including *Haemophilus influenzae*, *Haemophilus parainfluenzae*, *Streptococcus pneumoniae*-penicillin susceptible only, *Moraxella catarrhalis*); pharyngitis or tonsillitis (*Streptococcus pyogenes*); and uncomplicated skin and skin-structure infections (*Staphylococcus aureus* - not MRSA, *Streptococcus pyogenes*)

Usual Dosage

Usual dosage range:

Children ≥12 years and Adults: Oral: 200-400 mg twice daily

(Continued)

cefditoren *(Continued)*

Indication-specific dosing:

Children ≥12 years and Adults: Oral:

Acute bacterial exacerbation of chronic bronchitis: 400 mg twice daily for 10 days

Community-acquired pneumonia: 400 mg twice daily for 14 days

Pharyngitis, tonsillitis, uncomplicated skin and skin structure infections: 200 mg twice daily for 10 days

Dosage Forms Tablet, as pivoxil: 200 mg [equivalent to cefditoren; contains sodium caseinate]

cefditoren pivoxil *see* cefditoren *on previous page*

cefepime (SEF e pim)

Synonyms cefepime hydrochloride

U.S./Canadian Brand Names Maxipime® [US/Can]

Therapeutic Category Cephalosporin (Fourth Generation)

Use Treatment of uncomplicated and complicated urinary tract infections, including pyelonephritis caused by typical urinary tract pathogens; monotherapy for febrile neutropenia; uncomplicated skin and skin structure infections caused by *Streptococcus pyogenes*; moderate-to-severe pneumonia caused by pneumococcus, *Pseudomonas aeruginosa*, and other gram-negative organisms; complicated intraabdominal infections (in combination with metronidazole). Also active against methicillin-susceptible staphylococci, *Enterobacter* sp, and many other gram-negative bacilli.

Children 2 months to 16 years: Empiric therapy of febrile neutropenia patients, uncomplicated skin/soft tissue infections, pneumonia, and uncomplicated/complicated urinary tract infections.

Usual Dosage

Usual dosage range:

Children: I.V.: 50 mg/kg every 8-12 hours

Adults: I.V.: 1-2 g every 6-12 hours

Indication-specific dosing:

Children >2 months: I.V.:

Febrile neutropenia: 50 mg/kg every 8 hours for 7-10 days

Uncomplicated skin/soft tissue infections, pneumonia, complicated/uncomplicated UTI: 50 mg/kg twice daily

Adults:

Brain abscess *(Pseudomonas),* meningitis (postsurgical): I.V.: 2 g every 8 hours

Hospital-acquired pneumonia (HAP): I.V.: 1-2 g every 8-12 hours (American Thoracic Society/ATS guidelines)

Monotherapy for febrile neutropenic patients: I.V: 2 g every 8 hours for 7 days or until the neutropenia resolves

Otitis externa (malignant), pneumonia: I.V.: 2 g every 12 hours

Peritonitis (spontaneous): I.V.: 2 g every 12 hours with metronidazole

Septic lateral/cavernous sinus thrombosis: I.V.: 2 g every 6 hours; with metronidazole for lateral

Urinary tract infections (mild to moderate) I.M., I.V.: 500-1000 mg every 12 hours

Dosage Forms Injection, powder for reconstitution, as hydrochloride: 500 mg, 1 g, 2 g

cefepime hydrochloride *see* cefepime *on this page*

Cefizox® [US/Can] *see* ceftizoxime *on page 162*

Cefotan® *(Discontinued)*

cefotaxime (sef oh TAKS eem)

Sound-Alike/Look-Alike Issues

cefotaxime may be confused with cefoxitin, ceftizoxime, cefuroxime

Synonyms cefotaxime sodium

U.S./Canadian Brand Names Claforan® [US/Can]

Therapeutic Category Cephalosporin (Third Generation)

Use Treatment of susceptible infection in respiratory tract, skin and skin structure, bone and joint, urinary tract, gynecologic as well as septicemia, and documented or suspected meningitis. Active against most gram-negative bacilli (not *Pseudomonas*) and gram-positive cocci (not enterococcus). Active against many penicillin-resistant pneumococci.

Usual Dosage

Usual dosage range:

Infants and Children 1 month to 12 years <50 kg: I.M., I.V.: 50-200 mg/kg/day in divided doses every 4-6 hours

Children >12 years and Adults: I.M., I.V.: 1-2 g every 4-12 hours

Indication-specific dosing:

Infants and Children 1 month to 12 years:

Epiglottitis: I.M., I.V.: 150-200 mg/kg/day in 4 divided doses with clindamycin for 7-10 days

Meningitis: I.M., I.V.: 200 mg/kg/day in divided doses every 6 hours

Pneumonia: I.V.: 200 mg/kg/day divided every 8 hours

Sepsis: I.V.: 150 mg/kg/day divided every 8 hours

Typhoid fever: I.M., I.V.: 150-200 mg/kg/day in 3-4 divided doses (maximum: 12 g/day); fluoroquinolone resistant: 80 mg/kg/day in 3-4 divided doses (maximum: 12 g/day)

Children >12 years and Adults:

Arthritis (septic): I.V.: 1 g every 8 hours

Brain abscess, meningitis: I.V.: 2 g every 4-6 hours

Caesarean section: I.M., I.V.: 1 g as soon as the umbilical cord is clamped, then 1 g at 6- and 12-hour intervals

Epiglottitis: I.V.: 2 g every 4-8 hours

Gonorrhea: I.M.: 1 g as a single dose

Disseminated: I.V.: 1 g every 8 hours

Life-threatening infections: I.V.: 2 g every 4 hours

Liver abscess: I.V.: 1-2 g every 6 hours

Lyme disease:

Cardiac manifestations: I.V.: 2 g every 4 hours

CNS manifestations: I.V.: 2 g every 8 hours for 14-28 days

Moderate-to-severe infections: I.M., I.V.: 1-2 g every 8 hours

Orbital cellulitis: I.V.: 2 g every 4 hours

Peritonitis (spontaneous): I.V.: 2 g every 8 hours, unless life-threatening then 2 g every 4 hours

Septicemia: I.V.: 2 g every 6-8 hours

Skin and soft tissue:

Mixed, necrotizing: I.V.: 2 g every 6 hours, with metronidazole or clindamycin

Bite wounds (animal): I.V.: 2 g every 6 hours

Surgical prophylaxis: I.M., I.V.: 1 g 30-90 minutes before surgery

Uncomplicated infections: I.M., I.V.: 1 g every 12 hours

Dosage Forms

Infusion, as sodium [premixed iso-osmotic solution]:

Claforan®: 1 g (50 mL); 2 g (50 mL) [contains sodium 50.5 mg (2.2 mEq) per cefotaxime 1 g]

Injection, powder for reconstitution, as sodium: 500 mg, 1 g, 2 g, 10 g, 20 g

Claforan®: 500 mg, 1 g, 2 g, 10 g [contains sodium 50.5 mg (2.2 mEq) per cefotaxime 1 g]

cefotaxime sodium *see* cefotaxime *on previous page*

cefoxitin (se FOKS i tin)

Sound-Alike/Look-Alike Issues

cefoxitin may be confused with cefotaxime, cefotetan, Cytoxan®

Mefoxin® may be confused with Lanoxin®

Synonyms cefoxitin sodium

U.S./Canadian Brand Names Mefoxin® [US]

Therapeutic Category Cephalosporin (Second Generation)

Use Less active against staphylococci and streptococci than first generation cephalosporins, but active against anaerobes including *Bacteroides fragilis*; active against gram-negative enteric bacilli including *E. coli*, *Klebsiella*, and *Proteus*; used predominantly for respiratory tract, skin and skin structure, bone and joint, urinary tract and gynecologic as well as septicemia; surgical prophylaxis; intraabdominal infections and other mixed infections; indicated for bacterial *Eikenella corrodens* infections

Usual Dosage

Usual dosage range:

Infants >3 months and Children: I.M., I.V.: 80-160 mg/kg/day in divided doses every 4-6 hours (maximum dose: 12 g/day)

Adults: I.M., I.V.: 1-2 g every 6-8 hours (maximum dose: 12 g/day)

Note: I.M. injection is painful

Indication-specific dosing:

Infants >3 months and Children:

Mild-to-moderate infection: I.M., I.V.: 80-100 mg/kg/day in divided doses every 4-6 hours

Perioperative prophylaxis: I.V.: 30-40 mg/kg 30-60 minutes prior to surgery followed by 30-40 mg/kg/dose every 6 hours for no more than 24 hours after surgery depending on the procedure

Severe infection: I.M., I.V.: 100-160 mg/kg/day in divided doses every 4-6 hours

(Continued)

cefoxitin *(Continued)*

Adolescents and Adults:

Perioperative prophylaxis: I.M., I.V.: 1-2 g 30-60 minutes prior to surgery followed by 1-2 g every 6-8 hours for no more than 24 hours after surgery depending on the procedure

Adults:

Amnionitis, endomyometritis: I.M., I.V.: 2 g every 6-8 hours

Aspiration pneumonia, empyema, orbital cellulitis, parapharyngeal space, human bites: I.M., I.V.: 2 g every 8 hours

Liver abscess: I.V.: 1 g every 4 hours

Mycobacterium species, not MTB or MAI: I.V.: 12 g/day with amikacin

Pelvic inflammatory disease:

Inpatients: I.V.: 2 g every 6 hours **plus** doxycycline 100 mg I.V. or 100 mg orally every 12 hours until improved, followed by doxycycline 100 mg orally twice daily to complete 14 days

Outpatients: I.M.: 2 g **plus** probenecid 1 g orally as a single dose, followed by doxycycline 100 mg orally twice daily for 14 days

Dosage Forms

Infusion, as sodium [premixed iso-osmotic solution]: 1 g (50 mL); 2 g (50 mL) [contains sodium 53.8 mg/g (2.3 mEq/g)]

Injection, powder for reconstitution, as sodium: 1 g, 2 g, 10 g [contains sodium 53.8 mg/g (2.3 mEq/g)]

cefoxitin sodium *see* cefoxitin *on previous page*

cefpodoxime (sef pode OKS eem)

Sound-Alike/Look-Alike Issues

Vantin® may be confused with Ventolin®

Synonyms cefpodoxime proxetil

U.S./Canadian Brand Names Vantin® [US/Can]

Therapeutic Category Cephalosporin (Second Generation)

Use Treatment of susceptible acute, community-acquired pneumonia caused by *S. pneumoniae* or nonbeta-lactamase producing *H. influenzae*; acute uncomplicated gonorrhea caused by *N. gonorrhoeae*; uncomplicated skin and skin structure infections caused by *S. aureus* or *S. pyogenes*; acute otitis media caused by *S. pneumoniae, H. influenzae*, or *M. catarrhalis*; pharyngitis or tonsillitis; and uncomplicated urinary tract infections caused by *E. coli, Klebsiella*, and *Proteus*

Usual Dosage

Usual dosage range:

Children 2 months to 12 years: Oral: 10 mg/kg/day divided every 12 hours (maximum dose: 800 mg/day)

Children ≥12 years and Adults: Oral: 100-400 mg/dose every 12 hours

Indication-specific dosing:

Children 2 months to 12 years: Oral:

Acute maxillary sinusitis: 10 mg/kg/day divided every 12 hours for 10 days (maximum: 200 mg/dose)

Acute otitis media: 10 mg/kg/day divided every 12 hours (400 mg/day) for 5 days (maximum: 200 mg/dose)

Pharyngitis/tonsillitis: 10 mg/kg/day in 2 divided doses for 5-10 days (maximum: 100 mg/dose)

Children ≥12 years and Adults: Oral:

Acute community-acquired pneumonia and bacterial exacerbations of chronic bronchitis: 200 mg every 12 hours for 14 days and 10 days, respectively

Acute maxillary sinusitis: 200 mg every 12 hours for 10 days

Pharyngitis/tonsillitis: 100 mg every 12 hours for 5-10 days

Skin and skin structure: 400 mg every 12 hours for 7-14 days

Uncomplicated gonorrhea (male and female) and rectal gonococcal infections (female): 200 mg as a single dose

Uncomplicated urinary tract infection: 100 mg every 12 hours for 7 days

Dosage Forms

Granules for oral suspension: 50 mg/5 mL (50 mL, 75 mL, 100 mL); 100 mg/5 mL (50 mL, 75 mL, 100 mL) [contains sodium benzoate; lemon creme flavor]

Tablet: 100 mg, 200 mg

cefpodoxime proxetil *see* cefpodoxime *on this page*

cefprozil (sef PROE zil)

Sound-Alike/Look-Alike Issues

cefprozil may be confused with cefazolin, cefuroxime

Cefzil® may be confused with Cefol®, Ceftin®, Kefzol®

U.S./Canadian Brand Names Cefzil® [US/Can]

Therapeutic Category Cephalosporin (Second Generation)

Use Treatment of otitis media and infections involving the respiratory tract and skin and skin structure; active against methicillin-sensitive staphylococci, many streptococci, and various gram-negative bacilli including *E. coli*, some *Klebsiella*, *P. mirabilis*, *H. influenzae*, and *Moraxella*.

Usual Dosage

Usual dosage range:

Infants and Children >6 months to 12 years: Oral: 7.5-15 mg/kg/day divided every 12 hours

Children >12 years and Adults: Oral: 250-500 mg every 12 hours or 500 mg every 24 hours

Indication-specific dosing:

Infants and Children >6 months to 12 years: Oral:

Otitis media: 15 mg/kg every 12 hours for 10 days

Children 2-12 years: Oral:

Pharyngitis/tonsillitis: 7.5-15 mg/kg/day divided every 12 hours for 10 days (administer for >10 days if due to *S. pyogenes*); maximum: 1 g/day

Uncomplicated skin and skin structure infections: 20 mg/kg every 24 hours for 10 days; maximum: 1 g/day

Children >12 years and Adults: Oral:

Pharyngitis/tonsillitis: 500 mg every 24 hours for 10 days

Secondary bacterial infection of acute bronchitis or acute bacterial exacerbation of chronic bronchitis: 500 mg every 12 hours for 10 days

Uncomplicated skin and skin structure infections: 250 mg every 12 hours or 500 mg every 12-24 hours for 10 days

Dosage Forms

Powder for oral suspension, as anhydrous: 125 mg/5 mL (50 mL, 75 mL, 100 mL); 250 mg/5 mL (50 mL, 75 mL, 100 mL)

Cefzil®: 125 mg/5 mL (50 mL, 75 mL, 100 mL) [contains phenylalanine 28 mg/5 mL and sodium benzoate; bubble gum flavor]; 250 mg/5 mL (50 mL, 75 mL, 100 mL) [contains phenylalanine 28 mg/5 mL and sodium benzoate; bubble gum flavor]

Tablet, as anhydrous: 250 mg, 500 mg

Cefzil®: 250 mg, 500 mg

ceftazidime (SEF tay zi deem)

Sound-Alike/Look-Alike Issues

ceftazidime may be confused with ceftizoxime

Ceptaz® may be confused with Septra®

Tazicef® may be confused with Tazidime®

Tazidime® may be confused with Tazicef®

U.S./Canadian Brand Names Fortaz® [US/Can]; Tazicef® [US]

Therapeutic Category Cephalosporin (Third Generation)

Use Treatment of documented susceptible *Pseudomonas aeruginosa* infection and infections due to other susceptible aerobic gram-negative organisms; empiric therapy of a febrile, granulocytopenic patient

Usual Dosage

Usual dosage range:

Infants and Children 1 month to 12 years: I.V.: 30-50 mg/kg/dose every 8 hours (maximum dose: 6 g/day)

Adults: I.M., I.V.: 500 mg to 2 g every 8-12 hours

Indication-specific dosing:

Bacterial arthritis (gram-negative bacilli): I.V.: 1-2 g every 8 hours

Cystic fibrosis: I.V.: 30-50 mg/kg every 8 hours (maximum: 6 g/day)

Melioidosis: I.V.: 40 mg/kg every 8 hours for 10 days, followed by oral therapy with doxycycline or TMP/SMX

Otitis externa: I.V.: 2 g every 8 hours

Peritonitis (CAPD):

Anuric, intermittent: 1000-1500 mg/day

Anuric, continuous (per liter exchange): Loading dose: 250 mg; maintenance dose: 125 mg

Severe infections, including meningitis, complicated pneumonia, endophthalmitis, CNS infection, osteomyelitis, intraabdominal and gynecological, skin and soft tissue: I.V.: 2 g every 8 hours

Dosage Forms [DSC] = Discontinued product

Infusion, as sodium [premixed iso-osmotic solution] (Fortaz®): 1 g (50 mL); 2 g (50 mL)

Injection, powder for reconstitution:

Ceptaz® [DSC]: 10 g [L-arginine formulation]

Fortaz®: 500 mg, 1 g, 2 g, 6 g [contains sodium carbonate]

Tazicef®: 1 g, 2 g, 6 g [contains sodium carbonate]

ceftibuten (sef TYE byoo ten)

U.S./Canadian Brand Names Cedax® [US]

Therapeutic Category Cephalosporin (Third Generation)

Use Oral cephalosporin for treatment of bronchitis, otitis media, and pharyngitis/tonsillitis due to *H. influenzae* and *M. catarrhalis*, both beta-lactamase-producing and nonproducing strains, as well as *S. pneumoniae* (weak) and *S. pyogenes*

Usual Dosage Oral:

Children <12 years: 9 mg/kg/day for 10 days (maximum dose: 400 mg/day)

Children ≥12 years and Adults: 400 mg once daily for 10 days (maximum dose: 400 mg/day)

Dosage Forms

Capsule: 400 mg

Powder for oral suspension: 90 mg/5 mL (30 mL, 60 mL, 120 mL) [contains sodium benzoate; cherry flavor]

Ceftin® [US/Can] *see* cefuroxime *on next page*

Ceftin® Tablet 125 mg *(Discontinued)* *see* cefuroxime *on next page*

ceftizoxime (sef ti ZOKS eem)

Sound-Alike/Look-Alike Issues

ceftizoxime may be confused with cefotaxime, ceftazidime, cefuroxime

Synonyms ceftizoxime sodium

U.S./Canadian Brand Names Cefizox® [US/Can]

Therapeutic Category Cephalosporin (Third Generation)

Use Treatment of susceptible bacterial infections, mainly respiratory tract, skin and skin structure, bone and joint, urinary tract and gynecologic, as well as septicemia; active against many gram-negative bacilli (not *Pseudomonas*), some gram-positive cocci (not *Enterococcus*), and some anaerobes

Usual Dosage

Usual dosage range:

Children ≥6 months: I.M., I.V.: 150-200 mg/kg/day divided every 6-8 hours (maximum: 12 g/24 hours)

Adults: I.M., I.V.: 1-4 g every 8-12 hours

Indication-specific dosing:

Adults:

Gonococcal:

Disseminated infection: I.M., I.V.: 1 g every 8 hours

Uncomplicated: I.M.: 1 g as single dose

Life-threatening infections: I.V.: 2 g every 4 hours or 4 g every 8 hours

Dosage Forms

Infusion [premixed iso-osmotic solution]: 1 g (50 mL); 2 g (50 mL)

Injection, powder for reconstitution: 1 g, 2 g, 10 g

ceftizoxime sodium *see* ceftizoxime *on this page*

ceftriaxone (sef trye AKS one)

Sound-Alike/Look-Alike Issues

Rocephin® may be confused with Roferon®

Synonyms ceftriaxone sodium

U.S./Canadian Brand Names Rocephin® [US/Can]

Therapeutic Category Cephalosporin (Third Generation)

Use Treatment of lower respiratory tract infections, acute bacterial otitis media, skin and skin structure infections, bone and joint infections, intraabdominal and urinary tract infections, pelvic inflammatory disease (PID), uncomplicated gonorrhea, bacterial septicemia, and meningitis; used in surgical prophylaxis

Usual Dosage

Usual dosage range:

Infants and Children: I.M., I.V.: 50-100 mg/kg/day in 1-2 divided doses (maximum: 4 g/day)

Adults: I.M., I.V.: 1-2 g every 12-24 hours

Indication-specific dosing:

Infants and Children:

Epiglottitis: I.M., I.V.: 50-100 mg/kg once daily for 7-10 days with clindamycin

Mild-to-moderate infections: I.M., I.V.: 50-75 mg/kg/day in 1-2 divided doses every 12-24 hours (maximum: 2 g/day); continue until at least 2 days after signs and symptoms of infection have resolved

Meningitis:
Gonococcal, complicated:
<45 kg: I.V.: 50 mg/kg/day given every 12 hours (maximum: 2 g/day); usual duration of treatment is 10-14 days
>45 kg: I.V.: 1-2 g every 12 hours; usual duration of treatment is 10-14 days
Uncomplicated: I.M., I.V.: Loading dose of 100 mg/kg (maximum: 4 g), followed by 100 mg/kg/day divided every 12-24 hours (maximum: 4 g/day); usual duration of treatment is 7-14 days
Otitis media: *Acute:* I.M., I.V.: 50 mg/kg in a single dose (maximum: 1 g)
Pneumonia: I.V.: 50-75 mg/kg once daily
Serious infections: I.V.: 80-100 mg/kg/day in 1-2 divided doses (maximum: 4 g/day)
Typhoid fever: I.V.: 100 mg/kg once daily (maximum 4 g)
Adults:
Arthritis (septic): I.V.: 1-2 g once daily
Brain abscess and necrotizing fasciitis: I.V.: 2 g every 12 hours
Cavernous sinus thrombosis: I.V.: 1 g every 12 hours with vancomycin or linezolid
Endocarditis, acute native valve: I.V.: 2 g once daily for 2-4 weeks
Lyme disease: I.V.: 2 g once daily for 14-28 days
Mastoiditis (hospitalized): I.V.: 2 g once daily; >60 years old: 1 g once daily
Meningitis: I.V.: 2 g every 12 hours for 7-14 days (longer courses may be necessary for selected organisms)
Pelvic inflammatory disease: I.M.: 250 mg in a single dose
Pneumonia, community-acquired: I.V.: 2 g once daily; >65 years of age: 1 g once daily
Septic/toxic shock: I.V.: 2 g once daily; with clindamycin for toxic shock
Surgical prophylaxis: I.V.: 1 g 30 minutes to 2 hours before surgery
Syphilis: I.M., I.V.: 1 g once daily for 8-10 days
Typhoid fever: I.V.: 2-3 g once daily for 7-14 days

Dosage Forms Note: Contains sodium 83 mg (3.6 mEq) per ceftriaxone 1 g
Infusion [premixed in dextrose]: 1 g (50 mL); 2 g (50 mL)
Injection, powder for reconstitution: 250 mg, 500 mg, 1 g, 2 g, 10 g

ceftriaxone sodium *see* ceftriaxone *on previous page*

cefuroxime (se fyoor OKS eem)

Sound-Alike/Look-Alike Issues
cefuroxime may be confused with cefotaxime, cefprozil, ceftizoxime, deferoxamine
Ceftin® may be confused with Cefotan®, cefotetan, Cefzil®, Cipro®
Zinacef® may be confused with Zithromax®

Synonyms cefuroxime axetil; cefuroxime sodium

U.S./Canadian Brand Names Apo-Cefuroxime® [Can]; Ceftin® [US/Can]; ratio-Cefuroxime [Can]; Zinacef® [US/Can]

Therapeutic Category Cephalosporin (Second Generation)

Use Treatment of infections caused by staphylococci, group B streptococci, *H. influenzae* (type A and B), *E. coli*, *Enterobacter*, *Salmonella*, and *Klebsiella*; treatment of susceptible infections of the lower respiratory tract, otitis media, urinary tract, skin and soft tissue, bone and joint, sepsis and gonorrhea

Usual Dosage Note: Cefuroxime axetil film-coated tablets and oral suspension are not bioequivalent and are not substitutable on a mg/mg basis

Usual dosage range:
Neonates: I.M., I.V.: 50-100 mg/kg/day divided every 12 hours
Children <13 years:
Oral: 20-30 mg/kg/day in 2 divided doses
I.M., I.V.: 75-150 mg/kg/day divided every 8 hours (maximum dose: 6 g/day)
Children ≥13 years and Adults:
Oral: 250-500 mg twice daily
I.M., I.V.: 750 mg to 1.5 g every 6-8 hours or 100-150 mg/kg/day in divided doses every 6-8 hours (maximum: 6 g/day)

Indication-specific dosing:
Children ≥3 months to 12 years:
Acute bacterial maxillary sinusitis, acute otitis media, and impetigo:
Oral: Suspension: 30 mg/kg/day in 2 divided doses for 10 days (maximum dose: 1 g/day); tablet: 250 mg twice daily for 10 days
I.M., I.V.: 75-150 mg/kg/day divided every 8 hours (maximum dose: 6 g/day)
Epiglottitis: Oral: 150 mg/kg/day in 3 divided doses for 7-10 days
(Continued)

cefuroxime *(Continued)*

Pharyngitis/tonsillitis:

Oral: Suspension: 20 mg/kg/day (maximum: 500 mg/day) in 2 divided doses for 10 days; tablet: 125 mg every 12 hours for 10 days

I.M., I.V.: 75-150 mg/kg day divided every 8 hours (maximum: 6 g/day)

Children ≥13 years and Adults:

Bronchitis (acute and exacerbations of chronic bronchitis):

Oral: 250-500 mg every 12 hours for 10 days

I.V.: 500-750 mg every 8 hours (complete therapy with oral dosing)

Cellulitis:

Oral: 500 mg every 12 hours

Orbital: I.V.: 1.5 g every 8 hours

Gonorrhea:

Disseminated: I.M., I.V.: 750 mg every 8 hours

Uncomplicated:

Oral: 1 g as a single dose

I.M.: 1.5 g as single dose (administer in 2 different sites with probenecid)

Lyme disease (early): Oral: 500 mg twice daily for 20 days

Pharyngitis/tonsillitis and sinusitis: Oral: 250 mg twice daily for 10 days

Pneumonia (uncomplicated): I.V.: 750 mg every 8 hours

Severe or complicated infections: I.M., I.V.: 1.5 g every 8 hours (up to 1.5 g every 6 hours in life-threatening infections)

Skin/skin structure infection (uncomplicated):

Oral: 250-500 mg every 12 hours for 10 days

I.M., I.V.: 750 mg every 8 hours

Surgical prophylaxis:

I.V.: 1.5 g 30 minutes to 1 hour prior to procedure (if procedure is prolonged can give 750 mg every 8 hours I.M.)

Open heart: I.V.: 1.5 g every 12 hours to a total of 6 g

Urinary tract infection (uncomplicated):

Oral: 125-250 mg every 12 hours for 7-10 days

I.M., I.V.: 750 mg every 8 hours

Dosage Forms Note: Strength expressed as base

Infusion, as sodium [premixed]: 750 mg (50 mL); 1.5 g (50 mL)

Zinacef®: 750 mg (50 mL); 1.5 g (50 mL) [contains sodium 4.8 mEq (111 mg) per 750 mg]

Injection, powder for reconstitution, as sodium: 750 mg, 1.5 g, 7.5 g

Zinacef®: 750 mg, 1.5 g, 7.5 g [contains sodium 4.8 mEq (111 mg) per 750 mg]

Powder for oral suspension, as axetil:

Ceftin®: 125 mg/5 mL (100 mL) [contains phenylalanine 11.8 mg/5 mL; tutti-frutti flavor]; 250 mg/5 mL (50 mL, 100 mL) [contains phenylalanine 25.2 mg/5 mL; tutti-frutti flavor]

Tablet, as axetil: 250 mg, 500 mg

Ceftin®: 250 mg, 500 mg

cefuroxime axetil *see* cefuroxime *on previous page*

cefuroxime sodium *see* cefuroxime *on previous page*

Cefzil® [US/Can] *see* cefprozil *on page 160*

Celebrex® [US/Can] *see* celecoxib *on this page*

celecoxib (se le KOKS ib)

Sound-Alike/Look-Alike Issues

Celebrex® may be confused with Celexa™, cerebra, Cerebyx®

U.S./Canadian Brand Names Celebrex® [US/Can]

Therapeutic Category Nonsteroidal Antiinflammatory Drug (NSAID), COX-2 Selective

Use Relief of the signs and symptoms of osteoarthritis, ankylosing spondylitis, and rheumatoid arthritis; management of acute pain; treatment of primary dysmenorrhea; decreasing intestinal polyps in familial adenomatous polyposis (FAP). **Note:** The Notice of Compliance for the use of celecoxib in FAP has been suspended by Health Canada.

Usual Dosage Adults: Oral:

Acute pain or primary dysmenorrhea: Initial dose: 400 mg, followed by an additional 200 mg if needed on day 1; maintenance dose: 200 mg twice daily as needed

Ankylosing spondylitis: 200 mg/day as a single dose or in divided doses twice daily; if no effect after 6 weeks, may increase to 400 mg/day. If no response following 6 weeks of treatment with 400 mg/day, consider discontinuation and alternative treatment.
Familial adenomatous polyposis: 400 mg twice daily
Osteoarthritis: 200 mg/day as a single dose or in divided dose twice daily
Rheumatoid arthritis: 100-200 mg twice daily

Dosage Forms Capsule: 100 mg, 200 mg, 400 mg

Celestone® [US] *see* betamethasone (systemic) *on page 107*

Celestone® Soluspan® [US/Can] *see* betamethasone (systemic) *on page 107*

Celexa® [US/Can] *see* citalopram *on page 194*

CellCept® [US/Can] *see* mycophenolate *on page 571*

Cellugel® [US] *see* hydroxypropyl methylcellulose *on page 432*

cellulose, oxidized regenerated (SEL yoo lose, OKS i dyzed re JEN er aye ted)

Sound-Alike/Look-Alike Issues
Surgicel® may be confused with Serentil®

Synonyms absorbable cotton; oxidized regenerated cellulose

U.S./Canadian Brand Names Surgicel® Fibrillar [US]; Surgicel® NuKnit [US]; Surgicel® [US]

Therapeutic Category Hemostatic Agent

Use Hemostatic; temporary packing for the control of capillary, venous, or small arterial hemorrhage

Usual Dosage Minimal amounts of the fabric strip are laid on the bleeding site or held firmly against the tissues until hemostasis occurs; remove excess material

Dosage Forms
Fabric, fibrous (Surgicel® Fibrillar):
1" x 2" (10s)
2" x 4" (10s)
4" x 4" (10s)
Fabric, knitted (Surgicel® NuKnit):
1" x 1" (24s)
1" x $3^1/_2$" (10s)
3" x 4" (24s)
6" x 9" (10s)
Fabric, sheer weave (Surgicel®):
$^1/_2$" x 2" (24s)
2" x 3" (24s)
2" x 14" (24s)
4" x 8" (24s)

cellulose sodium phosphate (sel yoo lose SOW dee um FOS fate)

Synonyms CSP; sodium cellulose phosphate

U.S./Canadian Brand Names Calcibind® [US/Can]

Therapeutic Category Urinary Tract Product

Use Adjunct to dietary restriction to reduce renal calculi formation in absorptive hypercalciuria type I

Usual Dosage Adults: Oral: 5 g 3 times/day with meals; decrease dose to 5 g with main meal and 2.5 g with each of two other meals when urinary calcium declines to <150 mg/day

Dosage Forms Powder: 2.5 g/scoop (45 g)

Celluvisc™ [Can] *see* carboxymethylcellulose *on page 151*

Celontin® [US/Can] *see* methsuximide *on page 543*

Cena-K® *(Discontinued)* *see* potassium chloride *on page 684*

Cenestin® [US] *see* estrogens (conjugated A/synthetic) *on page 312*

Centany™ [US] *see* mupirocin *on page 569*

Centrum® [US-OTC] *see* vitamins (multiple/oral) *on page 878*

Centrum® Kids Jimmy Neutron® Complete [US-OTC] *see* vitamins (multiple/pediatric) *on page 878*

Centrum® Kids Jimmy Neutron® Extra C [US-OTC] *see* vitamins (multiple/pediatric) *on page 878*

Centrum® Kids Rugrats™ Complete [US-OTC] *see* vitamins (multiple/pediatric) *on page 878*

Centrum® Kids Rugrats™ Extra C [US-OTC] *see* vitamins (multiple/pediatric) *on page 878*

Centrum® Kids Rugrats™ Extra Calcium [US-OTC] *see* vitamins (multiple/pediatric) *on page 878*

Centrum® Performance™ [US-OTC] *see* vitamins (multiple/oral) *on page 878*

Centrum® Silver® [US-OTC] *see* vitamins (multiple/oral) *on page 878*

Cepacol® Antibacterial Mouthwash [US-OTC] *see* cetylpyridinium *on page 169*

Cepacol® Antibacterial Mouthwash Gold [US-OTC] *see* cetylpyridinium *on page 169*

Cepacol® Dual Action Maximum Strength [US-OTC] *see* dyclonine *on page 284*

Cepacol® Sore Throat [US-OTC] *see* benzocaine *on page 99*

Cepastat® [US-OTC] *see* phenol *on page 658*

Cepastat® Extra Strength [US-OTC] *see* phenol *on page 658*

cephalexin (sef a LEKS in)

Sound-Alike/Look-Alike Issues

cephalexin may be confused with cefaclor, cefazolin, cephalothin, ciprofloxacin

Synonyms cephalexin monohydrate

U.S./Canadian Brand Names Apo-Cephalex® [Can]; Biocef® [US]; Keflex® [US]; Keftab® [Can]; Novo-Lexin [Can]; Nu-Cephalex [Can]

Therapeutic Category Cephalosporin (First Generation)

Use Treatment of susceptible bacterial infections including respiratory tract infections, otitis media, skin and skin structure infections, bone infections, and genitourinary tract infections, including acute prostatitis; alternative therapy for acute bacterial endocarditis prophylaxis

Usual Dosage

Usual dosage range:

Children >1 year: Oral: 25-100 mg/kg/day every 6-8 hours (maximum: 4 g/day)

Adults: Oral: 250-1000 mg every 6 hours; maximum: 4 g/day

Indication-specific dosing:

Children >1 year: Oral:

Furunculosis: 25-50 mg/kg/day in 4 divided doses

Impetigo: 25 mg/kg/day in 4 divided doses

Otitis media: 75-100 mg/kg/day in 4 divided doses

Prophylaxis of bacterial endocarditis (dental, oral, respiratory tract, or esophageal procedures): 50 mg/kg 1 hour prior to procedure (maximum: 2 g)

Severe infections: 50-100 mg/kg/day in divided doses every 6-8 hours

Skin abscess: 50 mg/kg/day in 4 divided doses (maximum: 4 g)

Streptococcal pharyngitis, skin and skin structure infections: 25-50 mg/kg/day divided every 12 hours

Children >15 years and Adults: Oral:

Cellulitis and mastitis: 500 mg every 6 hours

Furunculosis/skin abscess: 250 mg 4 times/day

Prophylaxis of bacterial endocarditis (dental, oral, respiratory tract, or esophageal procedures): 2 g 1 hour prior to procedure

Streptococcal pharyngitis, skin and skin structure infections: 500 mg every 12 hours

Uncomplicated cystitis: 500 mg every 12 hours for 7-14 days

Dosage Forms [DSC] = Discontinued product

Capsule: 250 mg, 500 mg

Biocef®: 500 mg

Keflex®: 250 mg, 333 mg [DSC], 500 mg, 750 mg

Powder for oral suspension: 125 mg/5 mL (100 mL, 200 mL); 250 mg/5 mL (100 mL, 200 mL)

Biocef®: 125 mg/5 mL (100 mL); 250 mg/5 mL (100 mL)

Keflex®: 125 mg/5 mL (100 mL, 200 mL); 250 mg/5 mL (100 mL, 200 mL)

Tablet, for oral suspension (Panixine DisperDose™): 125 mg [contains phenylalanine 2.8 mg; peppermint flavor], 250 mg [contains phenylalanine 5.6 mg; peppermint flavor] [DSC]

cephalexin monohydrate *see* cephalexin *on this page*

cephalothin (sef A loe thin)

Sound-Alike/Look-Alike Issues

cephalothin may be confused with cefazolin, cephalexin

Synonyms cephalothin sodium
Therapeutic Category Cephalosporin (First Generation)
Use Treatment of infections when caused by susceptible strains in respiratory, genitourinary, gastrointestinal, skin and soft tissue, bone and joint infections; septicemia; treatment of susceptible gram-positive bacilli and cocci (never enterococcus); some gram-negative bacilli including *E. coli*, *Proteus*, and *Klebsiella* may be susceptible
Usual Dosage
Usual dosage range:
Neonates: I.V.:
Postnatal age <7 days:
<2000 g: 20 mg every 12 hours
>2000 g: 20 mg every 8 hours
Postnatal age >7 days:
<2000 g: 20 mg every 8 hours
>2000 g: 20 mg every 6 hours
Children: I.V.: 75-125 mg/kg/day divided every 4-6 hours (maximum dose: 10 g/day)
Adults: I.V.: 500 mg to 2 g every 4-6 hours
Dosage Forms [DSC] = Discontinued product
Infusion, as sodium [frozen]: 1 g (50 mL); 2 g (50 mL) [DSC]

cephalothin sodium *see* cephalothin *on previous page*
Cephulac® *(Discontinued)* *see* lactulose *on page 478*
Ceptaz® *(Discontinued)* *see* ceftazidime *on page 161*
Cerebyx® [US/Can] *see* fosphenytoin *on page 370*
Ceredase® [US] *see* alglucerase *on page 28*
Cerezyme® [US/Can] *see* imiglucerase *on page 441*
Cerovel™ [US] *see* urea *on page 861*
Certain Dri® [US-OTC] *see* aluminum chloride hexahydrate *on page 35*
Certuss-D® [US] *see* guaifenesin, dextromethorphan, and phenylephrine *on page 400*
Cerubidine® [US/Can] *see* daunorubicin hydrochloride *on page 232*
Cerumenex® [Can] *see* triethanolamine polypeptide oleate-condensate *on page 849*
Cerumenex® *(Discontinued)* *see* triethanolamine polypeptide oleate-condensate *on page 849*
Cervidil® [US/Can] *see* dinoprostone *on page 260*
C.E.S. *see* estrogens (conjugated/equine) *on page 312*
Cesia™ [US] *see* ethinyl estradiol and desogestrel *on page 317*
Cetacaine® [US] *see* benzocaine, butyl aminobenzoate, tetracaine, and benzalkonium chloride *on page 101*
Cetacort® [US] *see* hydrocortisone (topical) *on page 428*
Cetafen® [US-OTC] *see* acetaminophen *on page 5*
Cetafen Cold® [US-OTC] *see* acetaminophen and pseudoephedrine *on page 9*
Cetafen Extra® [US-OTC] *see* acetaminophen *on page 5*
Cetamide™ [Can] *see* sulfacetamide *on page 795*
Ceta-Plus® [US] *see* hydrocodone and acetaminophen *on page 420*
Cetapred® Ophthalmic *(Discontinued)* *see* sulfacetamide and prednisolone *on page 796*

cetirizine (se TI ra zeen)

Sound-Alike/Look-Alike Issues
Zyrtec® may be confused with Serax®, Xanax®, Zantac®, Zyprexa®
Synonyms cetirizine hydrochloride; P-071; UCB-P071
U.S./Canadian Brand Names Apo-Cetirizine® [Can]; Reactine™ [Can]; Zyrtec® [US]
Therapeutic Category Antihistamine
Use Perennial and seasonal allergic rhinitis and other allergic symptoms including urticaria; chronic idiopathic urticaria
Usual Dosage Oral:
Children:
6-12 months: Chronic urticaria, perennial allergic rhinitis: 2.5 mg once daily
(Continued)

cetirizine *(Continued)*

12 months to <2 years: Chronic urticaria, perennial allergic rhinitis: 2.5 mg once daily; may increase to 2.5 mg every 12 hours if needed

2-5 years: Chronic urticaria, perennial or seasonal allergic rhinitis: Initial: 2.5 mg once daily; may be increased to 2.5 mg every 12 hours **or** 5 mg once daily

Children ≥6 years and Adults: Chronic urticaria, perennial or seasonal allergic rhinitis: 5-10 mg once daily, depending upon symptom severity

Dosage Forms

Syrup, as hydrochloride: 5 mg/5 mL (120 mL, 480 mL) [banana-grape flavor]

Tablet, as hydrochloride: 5 mg, 10 mg

Tablet, chewable, as hydrochloride: 5 mg, 10 mg [grape flavor]

cetirizine and pseudoephedrine (se TI ra zeen & soo doe e FED rin)

Sound-Alike/Look-Alike Issues

Zyrtec® may be confused with Serax®, Xanax®, Zantac®, Zyprexa®

Synonyms cetirizine hydrochloride and pseudoephedrine hydrochloride; pseudoephedrine hydrochloride and cetirizine hydrochloride

U.S./Canadian Brand Names Reactine® Allergy and Sinus [Can]; Zyrtec-D 12 Hour™ [US]

Therapeutic Category Antihistamine/Decongestant Combination

Use Treatment of symptoms of seasonal or perennial allergic rhinitis

Usual Dosage Oral: Children ≥12 years and Adults: Seasonal/perennial allergic rhinitis: 1 tablet twice daily

Dosage Forms Tablet, extended release: Cetirizine hydrochloride 5 mg and pseudoephedrine hydrochloride 120 mg

cetirizine hydrochloride *see* cetirizine *on previous page*

cetirizine hydrochloride and pseudoephedrine hydrochloride *see* cetirizine and pseudoephedrine *on this page*

cetrorelix (set roe REL iks)

Synonyms cetrorelix acetate

U.S./Canadian Brand Names Cetrotide® [US/Can]

Therapeutic Category Antigonadotropic Agent

Use Inhibits premature luteinizing hormone (LH) surges in women undergoing controlled ovarian stimulation

Usual Dosage Adults: Female: SubQ: Used in conjunction with controlled ovarian stimulation therapy using gonadotropins (FSH, HMG):

Single-dose regimen: 3 mg given when serum estradiol levels show appropriate stimulation response, usually stimulation day 7 (range days 5-9). If hCG is not administered within 4 days, continue cetrorelix at 0.25 mg/day until hCG is administered.

Multiple-dose regimen: 0.25 mg morning or evening of stimulation day 5, or morning of stimulation day 6; continue until hCG is administered.

Dosage Forms Injection, powder for reconstitution: 0.25 mg, 3 mg [supplied with SWFI in prefilled syringe]

cetrorelix acetate *see* cetrorelix *on this page*

Cetrotide® [US/Can] *see* cetrorelix *on this page*

cetuximab (se TUK see mab)

Sound-Alike/Look-Alike Issues

cetuximab may be confused with bevacizumab

Synonyms C225; IMC-C225; NSC-714692

U.S./Canadian Brand Names Erbitux® [US/Can]

Therapeutic Category Antineoplastic Agent, Monoclonal Antibody; Epidermal Growth Factor Receptor (EGFR) Inhibitor

Use Treatment of metastatic colorectal cancer; treatment of squamous cell cancer of the head and neck

Usual Dosage I.V.: Adults:

Colorectal cancer:

Initial loading dose: 400 mg/m^2 infused over 120 minutes

Maintenance dose: 250 mg/m^2 infused over 60 minutes weekly

Head and neck cancer:

Initial loading dose: 400 mg/m^2 infused over 120 minutes

Maintenance dose: 250 mg/m^2 infused over 60 minutes weekly

Note: If given in combination with radiation therapy, administer loading dose 1 week prior to initiation of radiation course. Administer weekly maintenance dose 1 hour prior to radiation for the duration of radiation therapy (6-7 weeks).

Dosage Forms Injection, solution [preservative free]: 2 mg/mL (50 mL) [contains sodium chloride 8.48 mg/mL]

cetylpyridinium (SEE til peer i DI nee um)

Synonyms cetylpyridinium chloride; CPC

U.S./Canadian Brand Names Cepacol® Antibacterial Mouthwash Gold [US-OTC]; Cepacol® Antibacterial Mouthwash [US-OTC]; DiabetAid Gingivitis Mouth Rinse [US-OTC]

Therapeutic Category Local Anesthetic

Use Antiseptic to aid in the prevention and reduction of plaque and gingivitis, and to freshen breath

Usual Dosage Children ≥6 years and Adults: Oral (OTC labeling): Rinse or gargle to freshen mouth; may be used before or after brushing

Dosage Forms Liquid, as chloride, oral [mouthwash/gargle]:

Cepacol® Antibacterial Mouthwash Gold: 0.05% (120 mL, 360 mL, 720 mL, 960 mL) [contains alcohol 14% and tartrazine; original flavor]

Cepacol® Antibacterial Mouthwash: 0.05% (120 mL, 360 mL, 720 mL, 960 mL) [contains alcohol 14% and tartrazine; mint flavor]

DiabetAid Gingivitis Mouth Rinse: 0.1% (480 mL) [sugar free]

cetylpyridinium chloride *see* cetylpyridinium *on this page*

Cevalin® *(Discontinued)* *see* ascorbic acid *on page 76*

Cevi-Bid® [US-OTC] *see* ascorbic acid *on page 76*

cevimeline (se vi ME leen)

Sound-Alike/Look-Alike Issues

Evoxac® may be confused with Eurax®

Synonyms cevimeline hydrochloride

U.S./Canadian Brand Names Evoxac® [US/Can]

Therapeutic Category Cholinergic Agent

Use Treatment of symptoms of dry mouth in patients with Sjögren syndrome

Usual Dosage Adults: Oral: 30 mg 3 times/day

Dosage Forms Capsule, as hydrochloride: 30 mg

cevimeline hydrochloride *see* cevimeline *on this page*

CFDN *see* cefdinir *on page 157*

CG *see* chorionic gonadotropin (human) *on page 186*

CGP-42446 *see* zoledronic acid *on page 889*

CGP-57148B *see* imatinib *on page 441*

C-Gram [US-OTC] *see* ascorbic acid *on page 76*

CGS-20267 *see* letrozole *on page 485*

Chantix™ [US] *see* varenicline *on page 867*

Charcadole® [Can] *see* charcoal *on this page*

Charcadole®, Aqueous [Can] *see* charcoal *on this page*

Charcadole® TFS [Can] *see* charcoal *on this page*

Char-Caps [US-OTC] *see* charcoal *on this page*

CharcoAid® *(Discontinued)* *see* charcoal *on this page*

CharcoAid G® *(Discontinued)* *see* charcoal *on this page*

charcoal (CHAR kole)

Sound-Alike/Look-Alike Issues

Actidose® may be confused with Actos®

Synonyms activated carbon; activated charcoal; adsorbent charcoal; liquid antidote; medicinal carbon; medicinal charcoal

U.S./Canadian Brand Names Actidose-Aqua® [US-OTC]; Actidose® with Sorbitol [US-OTC]; Char-Caps [US-OTC]; Charcadole® TFS [Can]; Charcadole® [Can]; Charcadole®, Aqueous [Can]; Charcoal Plus® DS [US-OTC]; Charcocaps® [US-OTC]; EZ-Char™ [US-OTC]; Kerr Insta-Char® [US-OTC]

(Continued)

charcoal *(Continued)*

Therapeutic Category Antidote

Use Emergency treatment in poisoning by drugs and chemicals; aids the elimination of certain drugs and improves decontamination of excessive ingestions of sustained-release products or in the presence of bezoars; repetitive doses have proven useful to enhance the elimination of certain drugs (eg, theophylline, phenobarbital, and aspirin); repetitive doses for gastric dialysis in uremia to adsorb various waste products; dietary supplement (digestive aid)

Usual Dosage Oral:

Acute poisoning: **Note:** ~10 g of activated charcoal for each 1 g of toxin is considered adequate; this may require multiple doses. If sorbitol is also used, sorbitol dose should not exceed 1.5 g/kg. When using multiple doses of charcoal, sorbitol should be given with every other dose (not to exceed 2 doses/day).

Children: 1 g/kg as a single dose; if multiple doses are needed, additional doses can be given as 0.25 g/kg every hour or equivalent (ie, 0.5 g/kg every 2 hours) **or**

>1 year-12 years: 25-50 g as a single dose; smaller doses (10-25 g) may be used in children 1-5 years due to smaller gut lumen capacity

Children >12 years and Adults: 25-100 g as a single dose; if multiple doses are needed, additional doses may be given as 12.5 g/hour or equivalent (ie, 25 g every 2 hours)

Dietary supplement: Adult: 500-520 mg after meals; may repeat in 2 hours if needed (maximum 10 g/day)

Dosage Forms

Capsule:
Char-Caps, Charcocaps®: 260 mg

Liquid:
Actidose-Aqua®: 15 g (72 mL); 25 g (120 mL); 50 g (240 mL)
Kerr Insta-Char®: 25 g (120 mL) [cherry flavor]; 50 g (240 mL) [unflavored or cherry flavor]

Liquid [with sorbitol]:
Actidose® with Sorbitol: 25 g (120 mL); 50 g (240 mL)
Kerr Insta-Char®: 25 g (120 mL); 50 g (240 mL) [cherry flavor]

Pellet:
EZ-Char™: 25 g

Powder for suspension: 30 g, 240 g

Tablet:
Charcoal Plus® DS: 250 mg

Charcoal Plus® DS [US-OTC] *see* charcoal *on previous page*

Charcocaps® [US-OTC] *see* charcoal *on previous page*

Chealamide® ***(Discontinued)*** *see* edetate disodium *on page 287*

Chemet® [US/Can] *see* succimer *on page 793*

Cheracol® [US] *see* guaifenesin and codeine *on page 393*

Cheracol® [US-OTC] *see* phenol *on page 658*

Cheracol® D [US-OTC] *see* guaifenesin and dextromethorphan *on page 394*

Cheracol® Plus [US-OTC] *see* guaifenesin and dextromethorphan *on page 394*

Cheratussin AC [US] *see* guaifenesin and codeine *on page 393*

CHG *see* chlorhexidine gluconate *on page 173*

Chibroxin® ***(Discontinued)*** *see* norfloxacin *on page 599*

chicken pox vaccine *see* varicella virus vaccine *on page 867*

Chiggerex® [US-OTC] *see* benzocaine *on page 99*

Chiggertox® [US-OTC] *see* benzocaine *on page 99*

Children's Advil® Cold [Can] *see* pseudoephedrine and ibuprofen *on page 715*

Children's Dimetapp® Elixir Cold & Allergy [US-OTC] *see* brompheniramine and pseudoephedrine *on page 118*

Children's Hold® ***(Discontinued)*** *see* dextromethorphan *on page 245*

Children's Kaopectate® ***(Discontinued)*** *see* attapulgite *on page 84*

Children's Kaopectate® (reformulation) [US-OTC] *see* bismuth subsalicylate *on page 112*

Children's Motion Sickness Liquid [Can] *see* dimenhydrinate *on page 258*

Children's Pepto [US-OTC] *see* calcium carbonate *on page 135*

children's vitamins *see* vitamins (multiple/pediatric) *on page 878*

Chlo-Amine® Oral *(Discontinued)* *see* chlorpheniramine *on page 175*

Chlorafed® Liquid *(Discontinued)* *see* chlorpheniramine and pseudoephedrine *on page 177*

chloral *see* chloral hydrate *on this page*

chloral hydrate (KLOR al HYE drate)

Synonyms chloral; hydrated chloral; trichloroacetaldehyde monohydrate

U.S./Canadian Brand Names Aquachloral® Supprettes® [US]; PMS-Chloral Hydrate [Can]; Somnote™ [US]

Therapeutic Category Hypnotic, Nonbarbiturate

Controlled Substance C-IV

Use Short-term sedative and hypnotic (<2 weeks); sedative/hypnotic for diagnostic procedures; sedative prior to EEG evaluations

Usual Dosage

Children:

Sedation or anxiety: Oral, rectal: 5-15 mg/kg/dose every 8 hours (maximum: 500 mg/dose)

Prior to EEG: Oral, rectal: 20-25 mg/kg/dose, 30-60 minutes prior to EEG; may repeat in 30 minutes to maximum of 100 mg/kg or 2 g total

Hypnotic: Oral, rectal: 20-40 mg/kg/dose up to a maximum of 50 mg/kg/24 hours or 1 g/dose or 2 g/24 hours

Conscious sedation: Oral: 50-75 mg/kg/dose 30-60 minutes prior to procedure; may repeat 30 minutes after initial dose if needed, to a total maximum dose of 120 mg/kg or 1 g total

Adults: Oral, rectal:

Sedation, anxiety: 250 mg 3 times/day

Hypnotic: 500-1000 mg at bedtime or 30 minutes prior to procedure, not to exceed 2 g/24 hours

Dosage Forms

Capsule (Somnote™): 500 mg

Suppository, rectal (Aquachloral® Supprettes®): 325 mg [contains tartrazine], 650 mg

Syrup: 500 mg/5 mL (480 mL) [contains sodium benzoate]

chlorambucil (klor AM byoo sil)

Sound-Alike/Look-Alike Issues

chlorambucil may be confused with Chloromycetin®

Leukeran® may be confused with Alkeran®, leucovorin, Leukine®

Synonyms CB-1348; chlorambucilum; chloraminophene; chlorbutinum; NSC-3088; WR-139013

U.S./Canadian Brand Names Leukeran® [US/Can]

Therapeutic Category Antineoplastic Agent

Use Management of chronic lymphocytic leukemia, Hodgkin and non-Hodgkin lymphoma; breast and ovarian carcinoma; Waldenström macroglobulinemia, testicular carcinoma, thrombocythemia, choriocarcinoma

Usual Dosage Oral (refer to individual protocols):

Children:

General short courses: 0.1-0.2 mg/kg/day **or** 4.5 mg/m^2/day for 3-6 weeks for remission induction (usual: 4-10 mg/day); maintenance therapy: 0.03-0.1 mg/kg/day (usual: 2-4 mg/day)

Nephrotic syndrome: 0.1-0.2 mg/kg/day every day for 5-15 weeks with low-dose prednisone

Chronic lymphocytic leukemia (CLL):

Biweekly regimen: Initial: 0.4 mg/kg/dose every 2 weeks; increase dose by 0.1 mg/kg every 2 weeks until a response occurs and/or myelosuppression occurs

Monthly regimen: Initial: 0.4 mg/kg, increase dose by 0.2 mg/kg every 4 weeks until a response occurs and/or myelosuppression occurs

Malignant lymphomas:

Non-Hodgkin lymphoma: 0.1 mg/kg/day

Hodgkin lymphoma: 0.2 mg/kg/day

Adults: 0.1-0.2 mg/kg/day **or**

3-6 mg/m^2/day for 3-6 weeks, then adjust dose on basis of blood counts **or**

0.4 mg/kg and increased by 0.1 mg/kg biweekly or monthly **or**

14 mg/m^2/day for 5 days, repeated every 21-28 days

Dosage Forms Tablet: 2 mg

chlorambucilum *see* chlorambucil *on this page*

chloraminophene *see* chlorambucil *on this page*

chloramphenicol (klor am FEN i kole)

Sound-Alike/Look-Alike Issues
Chloromycetin® may be confused with chlorambucil, Chlor-Trimeton®

U.S./Canadian Brand Names Chloromycetin® Sodium Succinate [US]; Chloromycetin® Succinate [Can]; Chloromycetin® [Can]; Diochloram® [Can]; Pentamycetin® [Can]

Therapeutic Category Antibiotic, Miscellaneous; Antibiotic, Ophthalmic; Antibiotic, Otic

Use Treatment of serious infections due to organisms resistant to other less toxic antibiotics or when its penetrability into the site of infection is clinically superior to other antibiotics to which the organism is sensitive; useful in infections caused by *Bacteroides, H. influenzae, Neisseria meningitidis, Salmonella*, and *Rickettsia*; active against many vancomycin-resistant enterococci

Usual Dosage
Meningitis: I.V.: Infants >30 days and Children: 50-100 mg/kg/day divided every 6 hours
Other infections: I.V.:
Infants >30 days and Children: 50-75 mg/kg/day divided every 6 hours; maximum daily dose: 4 g/day
Adults: 50-100 mg/kg/day in divided doses every 6 hours; maximum daily dose: 4 g/day

Dosage Forms Injection, powder for reconstitution: 1 g [contains sodium ~52 mg/g (2.25 mEq/g)]

ChloraPrep® [US-OTC] *see* chlorhexidine gluconate *on next page*

Chloraseptic® Gargle [US-OTC] *see* phenol *on page 658*

Chloraseptic® Mouth Pain [US-OTC] *see* phenol *on page 658*

Chloraseptic® Rinse [US-OTC] *see* phenol *on page 658*

Chloraseptic® Spray [US-OTC] *see* phenol *on page 658*

Chloraseptic® Spray for Kids [US-OTC] *see* phenol *on page 658*

Chlorate® Oral *(Discontinued)* *see* chlorpheniramine *on page 175*

chlorbutinum *see* chlorambucil *on previous page*

chlordiazepoxide (klor dye az e POKS ide)

Sound-Alike/Look-Alike Issues
Librium® may be confused with Librax®

Synonyms methaminodiazepoxide hydrochloride

U.S./Canadian Brand Names Apo-Chlordiazepoxide® [Can]; Librium® [US]

Therapeutic Category Benzodiazepine

Controlled Substance C-IV

Use Management of anxiety disorder or for the short-term relief of symptoms of anxiety; withdrawal symptoms of acute alcoholism; preoperative apprehension and anxiety

Usual Dosage
Children:
<6 years: Not recommended
>6 years: Anxiety: Oral, I.M.: 0.5 mg/kg/24 hours divided every 6-8 hours
Adults:
Anxiety:
Oral: 15-100 mg divided 3-4 times/day
I.M., I.V.: Initial: 50-100 mg followed by 25-50 mg 3-4 times/day as needed
Preoperative anxiety: I.M.: 50-100 mg prior to surgery
Ethanol withdrawal symptoms: Oral, I.V.: 50-100 mg to start, dose may be repeated in 2-4 hours as necessary to a maximum of 300 mg/24 hours
Note: Up to 300 mg may be given I.M. or I.V. during a 6-hour period, but not more than this in any 24-hour period.

Dosage Forms
Capsule, as hydrochloride: 5 mg, 10 mg, 25 mg
Injection, powder for reconstitution, as hydrochloride: 100 mg [diluent contains benzyl alcohol, polysorbate 80, and propylene glycol]

chlordiazepoxide and amitriptyline hydrochloride *see* amitriptyline and chlordiazepoxide *on page 44*

chlordiazepoxide and clidinium *see* clidinium and chlordiazepoxide *on page 198*

chlorethazine *see* mechlorethamine *on page 522*

chlorethazine mustard *see* mechlorethamine *on page 522*

chlorhexidine gluconate (klor HEKS i deen GLOO koe nate)

Sound-Alike/Look-Alike Issues
Peridex® may be confused with Precedex™

Synonyms CHG

U.S./Canadian Brand Names Avagard™ [US-OTC]; BactoShield® CHG [US-OTC]; Betasept® [US-OTC]; ChloraPrep® [US-OTC]; Dyna-Hex® [US-OTC]; Hibiclens® [US-OTC]; Hibidil® 1:2000 [Can]; Hibistat® [US-OTC]; Operand® Chlorhexidine Gluconate [US-OTC]; ORO-Clense [Can]; Peridex® [US]; PerioChip® [US]; PerioGard® [US]

Therapeutic Category Antibiotic, Oral Rinse; Antibiotic, Topical

Use Skin cleanser for surgical scrub, cleanser for skin wounds, preoperative skin preparation, germicidal hand rinse, and as antibacterial dental rinse. Chlorhexidine is active against gram-positive and gram-negative organisms, facultative anaerobes, aerobes, and yeast.

Orphan drug: Peridex®: Oral mucositis with cytoreductive therapy when used for patients undergoing bone marrow transplant

Usual Dosage Adults:

Oral rinse (Peridex®, PerioGard®):

Floss and brush teeth, completely rinse toothpaste from mouth and swish 15 mL (one capful) undiluted oral rinse around in mouth for 30 seconds, then expectorate. Caution patient not to swallow the medicine and instruct not to eat for 2-3 hours after treatment. (Cap on bottle measures 15 mL.)

Treatment of gingivitis: Oral prophylaxis: Swish for 30 seconds with 15 mL chlorhexidine, then expectorate; repeat twice daily (morning and evening). Patient should have a reevaluation followed by a dental prophylaxis every 6 months.

Periodontal chip: One chip is inserted into a periodontal pocket with a probing pocket depth ≥5 mm. Up to 8 chips may be inserted in a single visit. Treatment is recommended every 3 months in pockets with a remaining depth ≥5 mm. If dislodgment occurs 7 days or more after placement, the subject is considered to have had the full course of treatment. If dislodgment occurs within 48 hours, a new chip should be inserted. The chip biodegrades completely and does not need to be removed. Patients should avoid dental floss at the site of PerioChip® insertion for 10 days after placement because flossing might dislodge the chip.

Insertion of periodontal chip: Pocket should be isolated and surrounding area dried prior to chip insertion. The chip should be grasped using forceps with the rounded edges away from the forceps. The chip should be inserted into the periodontal pocket to its maximum depth. It may be maneuvered into position using the tips of the forceps or a flat instrument.

Cleanser:

Surgical scrub: Scrub 3 minutes and rinse thoroughly, wash for an additional 3 minutes

Hand sanitizer (Avagard™): Dispense 1 pumpful in palm of one hand; dip fingertips of opposite hand into solution and work it under nails. Spread remainder evenly over hand and just above elbow, covering all surfaces. Repeat on other hand. Dispense another pumpful in each hand and reapply to each hand up to the wrist. Allow to dry before gloving.

Hand wash: Wash for 15 seconds and rinse

Hand rinse: Rub 15 seconds and rinse

Dosage Forms

Chip, for periodontal pocket insertion (PerioChip®): 2.5 mg

Liquid, topical [surgical scrub]:

Avagard™: 1% (500 mL) [contains ethyl alcohol and moisturizers]

BactoShield® CHG: 2% (120 mL, 480 mL, 750 mL, 1000 mL, 3800 mL); 4% (120 mL, 480 mL, 750 mL, 1000 mL, 3800 mL) [contains isopropyl alcohol]

Betasept®: 4% (120 mL, 240 mL, 480 mL, 960 mL, 3840 mL) [contains isopropyl alcohol]

ChloraPrep®: 2% (0.67 mL, 1.5 mL, 3 mL, 10.5 mL) [contains isopropyl alcohol 70%; prefilled applicator]

Dyna-Hex®: 2% (120 mL, 960 mL, 3840 mL); 4% (120 mL, 960 mL, 3840 mL)

Hibiclens®: 4% (15 mL, 120 mL, 240 mL, 480 mL, 960 mL, 3840 mL) [contains isopropyl alcohol]

Operand® Chlorhexidine Gluconate: 2% (120 mL); 4% (120 mL, 240 mL, 480 mL, 960 mL, 3840 mL) [contains isopropyl alcohol]

Liquid, oral rinse: 0.12% (480 mL)

Peridex®: 0.12% (480 mL) [contains alcohol 11.6%]

PerioGard®: 0.12% (480 mL) [contains alcohol 11.6%; mint flavor]

Pad [prep pad] (Hibistat®): 0.5% (50s) [contains isopropyl alcohol]

Sponge/Brush (BactoShield® CHG): 4% per sponge/brush [contains isopropyl alcohol]

chlormeprazine *see* prochlorperazine *on page 701*

Chlor-Mes-D [US] *see* chlorpheniramine, phenylephrine, and methscopolamine *on page 180*

2-chlorodeoxyadenosine *see* cladribine *on page 195*

chloroethane *see* ethyl chloride *on page 328*

Chloromag® [US] *see* magnesium chloride *on page 512*

Chloromycetin® [Can] *see* chloramphenicol *on page 172*

Chloromycetin® Sodium Succinate [US] *see* chloramphenicol *on page 172*

Chloromycetin® Succinate [Can] *see* chloramphenicol *on page 172*

chlorophyll (KLOR oh fil)

Synonyms chlorophyllin

U.S./Canadian Brand Names Nullo® [US-OTC]

Therapeutic Category Gastrointestinal Agent, Miscellaneous

Use Control fecal odors in colostomy or ileostomy

Usual Dosage

Oral: Children >12 years and Adults: 100-200 mg/day in divided doses; may increase to 300 mg/day if odor is not controlled (maximum: 300 mg/day)

Ostomy: Tablet: May also place 1-2 tablets in empty pouch each time it is reused or changed.

Dosage Forms [DSC] = Discontinued product

Caplet: Chlorophyllin copper complex 100 mg

Tablet: Chlorophyllin copper complex 33.3 mg [DSC]

chlorophyllin *see* chlorophyll *on this page*

chloroprocaine (klor oh PROE kane)

Sound-Alike/Look-Alike Issues

Nesacaine® may be confused with Neptazane®

Synonyms chloroprocaine hydrochloride

U.S./Canadian Brand Names Nesacaine® [US]; Nesacaine®-CE [Can]; Nesacaine®-MPF [US]

Therapeutic Category Local Anesthetic

Use Infiltration anesthesia and peripheral and epidural anesthesia

Usual Dosage Dosage varies with anesthetic procedure, the area to be anesthetized, the vascularity of the tissues, depth of anesthesia required, degree of muscle relaxation required, and duration of anesthesia; range.

Children >3 years (normally developed): Maximum dose (without epinephrine): 11 mg/kg; for infiltration, concentrations of 0.5% to 1% are recommended; for nerve block, concentrations of 1% to 1.5% are recommended

Adults:

- Maximum single dose (without epinephrine): 11 mg/kg; maximum dose: 800 mg
- Maximum single dose (with epinephrine): 14 mg/kg; maximum dose: 1000 mg
- Infiltration and peripheral nerve block:
  - Mandibular: 2%: 2-3 mL; total dose 40-60 mg
  - Infraorbital: 2%: 0.5-1 mL; total dose 10-20 mg
  - Brachial plexus: 2%; 30-40 mL; total dose 600-800 mg
  - Digital (without epinephrine): 1%; 3-4 mL; total dose: 30-40 mg
  - Pudendal: 2%; 10 mL each side; total dose: 400 mg
  - Paracervical: 1%; 3 mL per each of four sites
- Caudal block: Preservative-free: 2% or 3%: 15-25 mL; may repeat at 40-60 minute intervals
- Lumbar epidural block: Preservative-free: 2% or 3%: 2-2.5 mL per segment; usual total volume: 15-25 mL; may repeat with doses that are 2-6 mL less than initial dose every 40-50 minutes.

Dosage Forms

Injection, solution, as hydrochloride (Nesacaine®): 1% (30 mL); 2% (30 mL) [contains disodium EDTA and methylparaben]

Injection, solution, as hydrochloride [preservative free] (Nesacaine®-MPF): 2% (20 mL); 3% (20 mL)

chloroprocaine hydrochloride *see* chloroprocaine *on this page*

Chloroptic® Ophthalmic Solution *(Discontinued)* *see* chloramphenicol *on page 172*

Chloroptic® SOP *(Discontinued)* *see* chloramphenicol *on page 172*

chloroquine (KLOR oh kwin)

Synonyms chloroquine phosphate

U.S./Canadian Brand Names Aralen® [US]; Novo-Chloroquine [Can]

Therapeutic Category Aminoquinoline (Antimalarial)

Use Suppression or chemoprophylaxis of malaria; treatment of uncomplicated or mild-to-moderate malaria; extraintestinal amebiasis

Usual Dosage Oral:

Suppression or prophylaxis of malaria:

Children: Administer 5 mg base/kg/week on the same day each week (not to exceed 300 mg base/dose); begin 1-2 weeks prior to exposure; continue for 4-6 weeks after leaving endemic area; if suppressive therapy is not begun prior to exposure, double the initial loading dose to 10 mg base/kg and administer in 2 divided doses 6 hours apart, followed by the usual dosage regimen

Adults: 500 mg/week (300 mg base) on the same day each week; begin 1-2 weeks prior to exposure; continue for 4-6 weeks after leaving endemic area; if suppressive therapy is not begun prior to exposure, double the initial loading dose to 1 g (600 mg base) and administer in 2 divided doses 6 hours apart, followed by the usual dosage regimen

Acute attack:

Children: 10 mg/kg (base) on day 1, followed by 5 mg/kg (base) 6 hours later and 5 mg/kg (base) on days 2 and 3

Adults: 1 g (600 mg base) on day 1, followed by 500 mg (300 mg base) 6 hours later, followed by 500 mg (300 mg base) on days 2 and 3

Extraintestinal amebiasis:

Children: 10 mg/kg (base) once daily for 2-3 weeks (up to 300 mg base/day)

Adults: 1 g/day (600 mg base) for 2 days followed by 500 mg/day (300 mg base) for at least 2-3 weeks

Dosage Forms

Tablet, as phosphate: 250 mg [equivalent to 150 mg base]; 500 mg [equivalent to 300 mg base]

Aralen®: 500 mg [equivalent to 300 mg base]

chloroquine phosphate *see* chloroquine *on this page*

chlorothiazide (klor oh THYE a zide)

U.S./Canadian Brand Names Diuril® [US/Can]

Therapeutic Category Diuretic, Thiazide

Use Management of mild-to-moderate hypertension; adjunctive treatment of edema

Usual Dosage Note: The manufacturer states that I.V. and oral dosing are equivalent. Some clinicians may use lower I.V. doses, however, because of chlorothiazide's poor oral absorption. I.V. dosing in infants and children has not been well established.

Infants <6 months: Oral: 20-40 mg/kg/day in 2 divided doses (maximum dose: 375 mg/day)

Infants >6 months and Children: Oral: 10-20 mg/kg/day in 2 divided doses (maximum dose: 375 mg/day in children <2 years or 1 g/day in children 2-12 years)

Adults:

Hypertension: Oral: 500-2000 mg/day divided in 1-2 doses (manufacturer labeling); doses of 125-500 mg/day have also been recommended

Edema: Oral, I.V.: 250-1000 mg once or twice daily; intermittent treatment (eg, therapy on alternative days) may be appropriate for some patients. Maximum daily dose: 1000 mg (ACC/AHA 2005 Heart Failure Guidelines)

Dosage Forms

Injection, powder for reconstitution, as sodium: 500 mg

Suspension, oral: 250 mg/5 mL (237 mL) [contains alcohol 0.5% and benzoic acid]

Tablet: 250 mg, 500 mg

Chlorphed® *(Discontinued)* *see* brompheniramine *on page 118*

Chlorphed®-LA Nasal Solution *(Discontinued)* *see* oxymetazoline *on page 628*

Chlorphen [US-OTC] *see* chlorpheniramine *on this page*

chlorpheniramine (klor fen IR a meen)

Sound-Alike/Look-Alike Issues

Chlor-Trimeton® may be confused with Chloromycetin®

Synonyms chlorpheniramine maleate; CTM

U.S./Canadian Brand Names Aller-Chlor® [US-OTC]; Chlor-Trimeton® [US-OTC]; Chlor-Tripolon® [Can]; Chlorphen [US-OTC]; Diabetic Tussin® Allergy Relief [US-OTC]; Novo-Pheniram [Can]; QDALL® AR [US]; Teldrin® HBP [US-OTC]

(Continued)

chlorpheniramine *(Continued)*

Therapeutic Category Antihistamine

Use Perennial and seasonal allergic rhinitis and other allergic symptoms including urticaria

Usual Dosage

Children: Oral: 0.35 mg/kg/day in divided doses every 4-6 hours

2-6 years: 1 mg every 4-6 hours, not to exceed 6 mg in 24 hours

6-12 years: 2 mg every 4-6 hours, not to exceed 12 mg/day or sustained release 8 mg at bedtime

Children >12 years and Adults: Oral: 4 mg every 4-6 hours, not to exceed 24 mg/day or sustained release 8-12 mg every 8-12 hours, not to exceed 24 mg/day

Dosage Forms

Capsule, variable release:

QDALL® AR: Chlorpheniramine maleate 12 mg [immediate release and sustained release]

Syrup, as maleate:

Aller-Chlor®: 2 mg/5 mL (120 mL) [contains alcohol 5%]

Diabetic Tussin® Allergy Relief: 2 mg/5 mL (120 mL) [alcohol free, dye free, sugar free]

Tablet, as maleate: 4 mg

Aller-Chlor®, Chlor-Trimeton®, Chlorphen, Teldrin® HBP: 4 mg

Tablet, extended release, as maleate:

Chlor-Trimeton®: 12 mg

chlorpheniramine, acetaminophen, and pseudoephedrine *see* acetaminophen, chlorpheniramine, and pseudoephedrine *on page 11*

chlorpheniramine and acetaminophen (klor fen IR a meen & a seet a MIN oh fen)

Synonyms acetaminophen and chlorpheniramine

U.S./Canadian Brand Names Coricidin HBP® Cold and Flu [US-OTC]

Therapeutic Category Antihistamine/Analgesic

Use Symptomatic relief of congestion, headache, aches and pains of colds and flu

Usual Dosage Adults: Oral: 2 tablets every 4 hours

Dosage Forms Tablet: Chlorpheniramine maleate 2 mg and acetaminophen 325 mg

chlorpheniramine and carbetapentane *see* carbetapentane and chlorpheniramine *on page 146*

chlorpheniramine and phenylephrine (klor fen IR a meen & fen il EF rin)

Sound-Alike/Look-Alike Issues

Rynatan® may be confused with Rynatuss®

Synonyms chlorpheniramine maleate and phenylephrine hydrochloride; chlorpheniramine tannate and phenylephrine tannate; phenylephrine and chlorpheniramine

U.S./Canadian Brand Names AllanTan Pediatric [US]; Allerx™ [US]; Dallergy-JR® [US]; Dec-Chlorphen [US]; Ed A-Hist® [US]; R-Tanna [US]; Rescon-Jr [US]; Rondec® *[reformulation]* [US]; Rynatan® Pediatric Suspension [US]; Rynatan® [US]

Therapeutic Category Antihistamine/Decongestant Combination

Use Temporary relief of upper respiratory conditions such as nasal congestion, runny nose, and sneezing due to the common cold, hay fever, or allergic or vasomotor rhinitis

Usual Dosage Antihistamine/decongestant: Oral:

Children:

6-12 months: Rondec® Drops: 0.75 mL 4 times/day

1-2 years: Rondec® Drops: 1 mL 4 times/day

2-6 years:

Allerx™: 1.25 -2.5 mL every 12 hours

Dallergy-JR® suspension: 2.5 mL every 12 hours

Rondec® Syrup: 1.25 mL every 4-6 hours; maximum 7.5 mL/24 hours

Rynatan® Suspension: 2.5 -5 mL every 12 hours

6-12 years:

Allerx™: 2.5- 5 mL every 12 hours

Dallergy-JR®: One capsule every 12 hours; maximum 2 capsules/24 hours

Dallergy-JR® suspension: 5 mL every 12 hours

Ed A-Hist™: One-half caplet every 12 hours

Rondec® Syrup: 2.5 mL every 4-6 hours; maximum 15 mL/24 hours

Rynatan® Suspension: 5-10 mL every 12 hours

≥12 years: Refer to adult dosing.

Adults:

Allerx™: 15 mL every 12 hours

Dallergy-JR®: Two capsules every 12 hours; maximum 4 capsules/24 hours

Dallergy-JR® suspension: 10 mL every 12 hours

Ed A-Hist™: One caplet every 12 hours

R-Tanna: 1-2 tablets every 12 hours

Rondec® Syrup: 5 mL every 4-6 hours; maximum 30 mL/24 hours

Rynatan® Tablet: 1-2 tablets every 12 hours

Dosage Forms

Caplet, prolonged release:

Ed A-Hist®: Chlorpheniramine maleate 8 mg and phenylephrine hydrochloride 20 mg

Capsule, extended release:

Dallergy-JR®: Chlorpheniramine maleate 4 mg and phenylephrine hydrochloride 20 mg

Liquid:

Ed A-Hist®: Chlorpheniramine maleate 4 mg and phenylephrine hydrochloride 10 mg per 5 mL (480 mL) [sugar free; grape flavor]

Liquid, oral drops:

Dec-Chlorphen: Chlorpheniramine maleate 1 mg and phenylephrine hydrochloride 3.5 mg per mL (30 mL) [alcohol free, sugar free; grape flavor]

Rondec®: Chlorpheniramine maleate 1 mg and phenylephrine hydrochloride 3.5 mg per mL (30 mL) [alcohol free, sugar free; bubble gum flavor]

Suspension, oral: Chlorpheniramine tannate 4.5 mg and phenylephrine tannate 5 mg per 5 mL (480 mL)

AllanTan Pediatric: Chlorpheniramine tannate 4.5 mg and phenylephrine tannate 5 mg per 5 mL (473 mL)

Allerx™: Chlorpheniramine tannate 3 mg and phenylephrine tannate 7.5 per 5 mL (480 mL) [contains benzoic acid; raspberry flavor]

Dallergy-JR®: Chlorpheniramine tannate 4 mg and phenylephrine tannate 20 mg per 5 mL (480 mL) [contains sodium benzoate; peaches and cream flavor]

Rynatan® Pediatric Suspension: Chlorpheniramine tannate 4.5 mg and phenylephrine tannate 5 mg per 5 mL (480 mL) [contains benzoic acid and tartrazine; strawberry flavor]

Syrup:

Rondec®: Chlorpheniramine maleate 4 mg and phenylephrine hydrochloride 12. 5 mg per 5 mL (120 mL, 480 mL) [alcohol free, sugar free; bubble gum flavor]

Tablet:

R-Tanna, Rynatan®: Chlorpheniramine tannate 9 mg and phenylephrine tannate 25 mg

Tablet, sustained release:

Rescon-Jr: Chlorpheniramine maleate 4 mg and phenylephrine hydrochloride 20 mg

chlorpheniramine and pseudoephedrine (klor fen IR a meen & soo doe e FED rin)

Sound-Alike/Look-Alike Issues

Allerest® may be confused with Sinarest®

Chlor-Trimeton® may be confused with Chloromycetin®

Sudafed® may be confused with Sufenta®

Synonyms chlorpheniramine maleate and pseudoephedrine hydrochloride; chlorpheniramine tannate and pseudoephedrine tannate; pseudoephedrine and chlorpheniramine

U.S./Canadian Brand Names A.R.M® [US-OTC]; Allerest® Maximum Strength Allergy and Hay Fever [US-OTC]; Chlor-Trimeton® Allergy D [US-OTC]; Deconamine® SR [US]; Deconamine® [US]; Dicel™ [US]; Dynahist-ER Pediatric® [US]; Histade™ [US]; Histex™ [US]; Kronofed-A® [US]; Kronofed-A®-Jr [US]; LoHist-D [US]; QDALL® [US]; Sudafed® Sinus & Allergy [US-OTC]; Sudal® 12 [US]; Triaminic® Cold and Allergy [US-OTC/Can]

Therapeutic Category Antihistamine/Decongestant Combination

Use Relief of nasal congestion associated with the common cold, hay fever, and other allergies, sinusitis, eustachian tube blockage, and vasomotor and allergic rhinitis

Usual Dosage General dosing guidelines; consult specific product labeling. Rhinitis/decongestant: Oral:

Children:

2-6 years:

Chlorpheniramine maleate 1 mg and pseudoephedrine hydrochloride 15 mg every 4-6 hours

Chlorpheniramine tannate 4.5 mg and pseudoephedrine tannate 75 mg: 2.5-5 mL every 12 hours (maximum: 10 mL/24 hours)

6-12 years: Chlorpheniramine maleate 2 mg and pseudoephedrine hydrochloride 30 mg every 4-6 hours (immediate release products)

Children ≥12 years and Adults:

Chlorpheniramine maleate 4 mg and pseudoephedrine hydrochloride 60 mg every 4-6 hours (immediate release products)

(Continued)

chlorpheniramine and pseudoephedrine *(Continued)*

Chlorpheniramine tannate 4.5 mg and pseudoephedrine tannate 75 mg: 10-20 mL every 12 hours (maximum: 40 mL/24 hours)
Deconamine® SR, Kronofed-A®: Chlorpheniramine maleate 8 mg and pseudoephedrine hydrochloride 120 mg every 12 hours

Dosage Forms [DSC] = Discontinued product
Caplet:
A.R.M.®: Chlorpheniramine maleate 4 mg and pseudoephedrine hydrochloride 60 mg
Capsule, extended release: Chlorpheniramine maleate 8 mg and pseudoephedrine hydrochloride 120 mg
Dynahist-ER Pediatric®: Chlorpheniramine maleate 4 mg and pseudoephedrine hydrochloride 60 mg
Histade™: Chlorpheniramine maleate 12 mg and pseudoephedrine hydrochloride 120 mg
QDALL®: Chlorpheniramine maleate 12 mg and pseudoephedrine hydrochloride 100 mg
Capsule, sustained release: Chlorpheniramine maleate 8 mg and pseudoephedrine hydrochloride 120 mg
Deconamine® SR, Kronofed-A®: Chlorpheniramine maleate 8 mg and pseudoephedrine hydrochloride 120 mg
Kronofed-A®-Jr: Chlorpheniramine maleate 4 mg and pseudoephedrine hydrochloride 60 mg
Liquid:
Histex™: Chlorpheniramine maleate 2 mg and pseudoephedrine sulfate 30 mg per 5 mL (480 mL) [peach flavor]
PediaCare® Cold and Allergy: Chlorpheniramine maleate 1 mg and pseudoephedrine sulfate 15 mg per 5 mL (120 mL) [alcohol free; contains sodium benzoate; bubble gum flavor] [DSC]
Triaminic® Cold and Allergy: Chlorpheniramine maleate 1 mg and pseudoephedrine sulfate 15 mg per 5 mL (120 mL) [contains benzoic acid; orange flavor]
Suspension:
Dicel™: Chlorpheniramine tannate 5 mg and pseudoephedrine tannate 75 mg per 5 mL (480 mL) [contains sodium benzoate; strawberry banana flavor]
Suspension, sustained release:
Sudal® 12: Chlorpheniramine maleate 6 mg and pseudoephedrine hydrochloride 30 mg per 5 mL (480 mL) [DSC]
Syrup: Chlorpheniramine maleate 2 mg and pseudoephedrine hydrochloride 30 mg per 5 mL (480 mL)
Deconamine®: Chlorpheniramine maleate 2 mg and pseudoephedrine sulfate 30 mg per 5 mL (480 mL) [alcohol free, dye free; contains sodium benzoate; grape flavor]
LoHist-D: Chlorpheniramine maleate 2 mg and pseudoephedrine hydrochloride 30 mg per 5 mL (480 mL) [alcohol free, dye free; peach flavor]
Tablet: Chlorpheniramine maleate 4 mg and pseudoephedrine hydrochloride 60 mg
Allerest® Maximum Strength Allergy and Hay Fever: Chlorpheniramine maleate 2 mg and pseudoephedrine hydrochloride 30 mg
Chlor-Trimeton® Allergy D, Sudafed® Sinus & Allergy: Chlorpheniramine maleate 4 mg and pseudoephedrine hydrochloride 60 mg
Deconamine®: Chlorpheniramine maleate 4 mg and pseudoephedrine hydrochloride 60 mg [dye free]
Tablet, chewable: Chlorpheniramine maleate 2 mg and pseudoephedrine sulfate 15 mg
Sudal® 12: Chloprheniramine polisterex (maleate) 4mg and pseudoephedrine polistirex (as hydrochloride) 30 mg [contains phenylalanine 25 mg/tablet; grape flavor]

chlorpheniramine, carbetapentane, and phenylephrine *see* carbetapentane, phenylephrine, and chlorpheniramine *on page 147*

chlorpheniramine, ephedrine, phenylephrine, and carbetapentane

(klor fen IR a meen, e FED rin, fen il EF rin, & kar bay ta PEN tane)

Sound-Alike/Look-Alike Issues
Rynatuss® may be confused with Rynatan®

Synonyms carbetapentane, ephedrine, phenylephrine, and chlorpheniramine; ephedrine, chlorpheniramine, phenylephrine, and carbetapentane; phenylephrine, ephedrine, chlorpheniramine, and carbetapentane

U.S./Canadian Brand Names Rynatuss® Pediatric [US]; Rynatuss® [US]; Tetra Tannate Pediatric [US]

Therapeutic Category Antihistamine/Decongestant/Antitussive

Use Symptomatic relief of cough with a decongestant and an antihistamine

Usual Dosage Oral:
Children:
<2 years: Titrate dose individually
2-6 years: 2.5-5 mL every 12 hours
>6 years: 5-10 mL every 12 hours
Adults: 1-2 tablets every 12 hours

Dosage Forms

Suspension:

Rynatuss® Pediatric [DSC], Tetra Tannate Pediatric: Carbetapentane tannate 30 mg, ephedrine tannate 5 mg, phenylephrine tannate 5 mg, and chlorpheniramine tannate 4 mg per 5 mL (240 mL, 480 mL) [contains tartrazine and benzoic acid; strawberry flavor]

Tablet:

Rynatuss®: Carbetapentane tannate 60 mg, ephedrine tannate 10 mg, phenylephrine tannate 10 mg, and chlorpheniramine tannate 5 mg

chlorpheniramine, hydrocodone, phenylephrine, acetaminophen, and caffeine *see* hydrocodone, chlorpheniramine, phenylephrine, acetaminophen, and caffeine *on page 424*

chlorpheniramine maleate *see* chlorpheniramine *on page 175*

chlorpheniramine maleate and hydrocodone bitartrate *see* hydrocodone and chlorpheniramine *on page 422*

chlorpheniramine maleate and phenylephrine hydrochloride *see* chlorpheniramine and phenylephrine *on page 176*

chlorpheniramine maleate and pseudoephedrine hydrochloride *see* chlorpheniramine and pseudoephedrine *on page 177*

chlorpheniramine maleate, ibuprofen, and pseudoephedrine *see* ibuprofen, pseudoephedrine, and chlorpheniramine *on page 439*

chlorpheniramine maleate, pseudoephedrine hydrochloride, and dextromethorphan hydrobromide *see* chlorpheniramine, pseudoephedrine, and dextromethorphan *on page 182*

chlorpheniramine, phenylephrine, and dextromethorphan

(klor fen IR a meen, fen il EF rin, & deks troe meth OR fan)

Synonyms dextromethorphan, chlorpheniramine, and phenylephrine; phenylephrine, chlorpheniramine, and dextromethorphan

U.S./Canadian Brand Names Alka-Seltzer® Plus® Cold and Cough [US-OTC]; Coldtuss DR [US]; Corfen DM [US]; De-Chlor DM [US]; De-Chlor DR [US]; Dec-Chlorphen DM [US]; Dex PC [US]; Phenabid DM® [US]; Rondec®-DM *[reformulation]* [US]; Tri-Vent™ DPC [US]

Therapeutic Category Antihistamine/Decongestant/Antitussive

Use Temporary relief of cough and upper respiratory symptoms associated with allergies or the common cold

Usual Dosage Oral: Relief of cough and cold symptoms:

Children:

6-12 months (Rondec®-DM drops): 0.75 mL 4 times/day

1-2 years (Rondec®-DM drops): 1 mL 4 times/day

2-6 years:

Rondec®-DM syrup: 1.25 mL every 4-6 hours (maximum: 7.5 mL/24 hours)

Tri-Vent™ DPC: 2.5 mL every 6 hours (maximum: 10 mL/24 hours)

6-12 years:

Rondec®-DM syrup: 2.5 mL every 4-6 hours (maximum: 15 mL/24 hours)

Tri-Vent™ DPC: 5 mL every 6 hours (maximum: 20 mL/24 hours)

Children ≥12 years and Adults:

Alka-Seltzer Plus® Cold and Cough: 2 tablets dissolved in water every 4 hours (maximum: 8 tablets/24 hours)

Rondec®-DM syrup: 5 mL every 4-6 hours (maximum: 30 mL/24 hours)

Tri-Vent™ DPC: 10 mL every 6 hours (maximum: 40 mL/24 hours)

Dosage Forms

Liquid: Chlorpheniramine maleate 2 mg, phenylephrine hydrochloride 10 mg, and dextromethorphan hydrobromide 15 mg per 5 mL (480 mL); chlorpheniramine maleate 4 mg, phenylephrine hydrochloride 10 mg, and dextromethorphan hydrobromide 15 mg per 5 mL (480 mL)

Corfen DM: Chlorpheniramine maleate 4 mg, phenylephrine hydrochloride 10 mg, and dextromethorphan hydrobromide 15 mg per 5 mL (480 mL) [grape flavor]

De-Chlor DM: Chlorpheniramine maleate 2 mg, phenylephrine hydrochloride 10 mg, and dextromethorphan hydrobromide 15 mg per 5 mL (480 mL) [strawberry flavor]

De-Chlor DR: Chlorpheniramine maleate 2 mg, phenylephrine hydrochloride 6 mg, and dextromethorphan hydrobromide 15 mg per 5 mL (480 mL) [strawberry flavor]

Liquid, oral drops:

Dec-Chlorphen DM: Chlorpheniramine maleate 1 mg, phenylephrine hydrochloride 3.5 mg, and dextromethorphan hydrobromide 3 mg per 1 mL (30 mL) [alcohol free, sugar free; grape flavor]

(Continued)

chlorpheniramine, phenylephrine, and dextromethorphan *(Continued)*

Rondec® DM: Chlorpheniramine maleate 1 mg, phenylephrine hydrochloride 3.5 mg, and dextromethorphan hydrobromide 3 mg per 1 mL (30 mL)

Syrup: Chlorpheniramine maleate 2 mg, phenylephrine hydrochloride 10 mg, and dextromethorphan hydrobromide 15 mg per 5 mL (480 mL)

Coldtuss DR: Chlorpheniramine maleate 4 mg, phenylephrine hydrochloride 6 mg, and dextromethorphan hydrobromide 15 mg per 5 mL (480 mL) [strawberry flavor]

Dec-Chlorphen DM: Chlorpheniramine maleate 4 mg, phenylephrine hydrochloride 12.5 mg, and dextromethorphan hydrobromide 15 mg per 5 mL (480 mL) [alcohol free, sugar free; grape flavor]

Dex PC: Chlorpheniramine maleate 2 mg, phenylephrine hydrochloride 6 mg, and dextromethorphan hydrobromide 15 mg per 5 mL (480 mL) [strawberry flavor]

Rondec®-DM: Chlorpheniramine maleate 4 mg, phenylephrine hydrochloride 12.5 mg, and dextromethorphan hydrobromide 15 mg per 5 mL (120 mL, 480 mL) [alcohol free, sugar free; grape flavor]

Tri-Vent™ DPC: Chlorpheniramine maleate 2 mg, phenylephrine hydrochloride 6 mg, and dextromethorphan hydrobromide 15 mg per 5 mL (480 mL) [alcohol free; contains sodium benzoate; strawberry flavor]

Tablet, effervescent (Alka-Seltzer Plus® Cold and Cough): Chlorpheniramine maleate 2 mg, phenylephrine hydrochloride 5 mg, and dextromethorphan hydrobromide 10 mg [contains phenylalanine 11 mg/tablet and sodium 504 mg/tablet]

Tablet, timed release (Phenabid DM®): Chlorpheniramine maleate 8 mg, phenylephrine hydrochloride 20 mg, and dextromethorphan hydrobromide 30 mg [dye free, sugar free]

chlorpheniramine, phenylephrine, and hydrocodone *see* phenylephrine, hydrocodone, and chlorpheniramine *on page 663*

chlorpheniramine, phenylephrine, and methscopolamine

(klor fen IR a meen, fen il EF rin, & meth skoe POL a meen)

Synonyms methscopolamine nitrate, chlorpheniramine maleate, and phenylephrine hydrochloride; phenylephrine tannate, chlorpheniramine tannate, and methscopolamine nitrate

U.S./Canadian Brand Names aeroKid™ [US]; AH-Chew II [US]; AH-Chew® [US]; Chlor-Mes-D [US]; Dallergy® [US]; Dehistine [US]; Duradyl® [US]; Durahist™ PE [US]; Extendryl JR [US]; Extendryl SR [US]; Extendryl [US]; Hista-Vent® DA [US]; OMNIhist® II L.A. [US]; PCM Allergy [US]; PCM [US]; Ralix [US]; Rescon® MX [US]

Therapeutic Category Antihistamine/Decongestant/Anticholinergic

Use Treatment of upper respiratory symptoms such as respiratory congestion, allergic rhinitis, vasomotor rhinitis, sinusitis, and allergic skin reactions of urticaria and angioedema

Usual Dosage

Children 6-11 years: Relief of respiratory symptoms: Oral:

aeroKid™: 2.5-5 mL every 4 hours

AH-Chew® suspension: 2.5-5 mL every 12 hours

Dallergy®, Durahist™ PE, OMNIhist® II L.A., Rescon® MX: One-half caplet/tablet every 12 hours

Duradryl® syrup, Extendryl syrup: 2.5-5 mL, may repeat up to every 4 hours depending on age and body weight

Extendryl chewable tablet: One tablet every 4 hours; do not exceed 4 doses in 24 hours

Extendryl JR: One capsule every 12 hours

Children ≥12 years and Adults: Relief of respiratory symptoms: Oral: **Note:** If disturbances in urination occur in patients without renal impairment, medication should be discontinued for 1-2 days and should then be restarted at a lower dose

aeroKid™: 5-10 mL every 3-4 hours

AH-Chew® suspension: 5-10 mL every 12 hours

Dallergy®, Durahist™ PE, Extendryl SR, OMNIhist® II L.A., Rescon® MX: One capsule/tablet every 12 hours

Duradryl® syrup, Extendryl syrup: 5-10 mL every 3-4 hours (4 times/day)

Extendryl: 1-2 chewable tablets every 4 hours

Dosage Forms [DSC] = Discontinued product

Caplet, extended release:

Dallergy®: Chlorpheniramine maleate 12 mg, phenylephrine hydrochloride 20 mg, and methscopolamine nitrate 2.5 mg

Capsule, extended release:

Extendryl JR: Chlorpheniramine maleate 4 mg, phenylephrine hydrochloride 10 mg, and methscopolamine nitrate 1.25 mg

Liquid:

Chlor-Mes-D: Chlorpheniramine maleate 2 mg, phenylephrine hydrochloride 10 mg, and methscopolamine nitrate 0.625 mg per 5 mL (480 mL)

Suspension:

AH-Chew®: Chlorpheniramine tannate [equivalent to chlorpheniramine maleate 2 mg], phenylephrine tannate [equivalent to phenylephrine hydrochloride 10 mg], and methscopalamine nitrate 1.5 mg per 5 mL (120 mL) [grape flavor]

Syrup:

aeroKid™: Chlorpheniramine maleate 4 mg, phenylephrine hydrochloride 10 mg, and methscopolamine nitrate 1.25 mg per 5 mL (120 mL, 480 mL) [blue raspberry flavor]

Dallergy®: Chlorpheniramine maleate 2 mg, phenylephrine hydrochloride 10 mg, and methscopolamine nitrate 0.625 mg per 5 mL (480 mL)

Dehistine: Chlorpheniramine maleate 2 mg, phenylephrine hydrochloride 10 mg, and methscopolamine nitrate 1.25 mg per 5 mL (480 mL) [root beer flavor]

Duradryl®: Chlorpheniramine maleate 2 mg, phenylephrine hydrochloride 10 mg, and methscopolamine nitrate 1.25 mg per 5 mL (480 mL) [contains sodium benzoate; cherry flavor]

Extendryl: Chlorpheniramine maleate 2 mg, phenylephrine hydrochloride 10 mg, and methscopolamine nitrate 1.25 mg per 5 mL (480 mL) [contains sodium benzoate; root beer flavor]

Tablet [scored]:

Dallergy®: Chlorpheniramine maleate 4 mg, phenylephrine hydrochloride 10 mg, and methscopolamine nitrate 1.25 mg

Tablet, chewable:

AH-Chew®: Chlorpheniramine maleate 2 mg, phenylephrine hydrochloride 10 mg, and methscopolamine nitrate 1.25 mg [grape flavor] [DSC]

AH-Chew II: Chlorpheniramine maleate 2 mg, phenylephrine hydrochloride 15 mg, and methscopolamine nitrate 1.25 mg [grape flavor]

Extendryl: Chlorpheniramine maleate 2 mg, phenylephrine hydrochloride 10 mg, and methscopolamine nitrate 1.25 mg [root beer flavor]

PCM: Chlorpheniramine maleate 2 mg, phenylephrine hydrochloride 10 mg, and methscopolamine nitrate 1.25 mg

Tablet, extended release: Chlorpheniramine maleate 8 mg, phenylephrine hydrochloride 20 mg, and methscopolamine nitrate 2.5 mg

Drize®-R: Chlorpheniramine maleate 8 mg, phenylephrine hydrochloride 20 mg, and methscopolamine nitrate 2.5 mg [dye free; scored] [DSC]

Durahist™ PE: Chlorpheniramine maleate 8 mg, phenylephrine hydrochloride 20 mg, and methscopolamine nitrate 1.25 mg [scored]

Extendryl SR: Chlorpheniramine maleate 8 mg, phenylephrine hydrochloride 20 mg, and methscopolamine nitrate 2.5 mg

Hista-Vent® DA: Chlorpheniramine maleate 8 mg, phenylephrine hydrochloride 20 mg, and methscopolamine nitrate 2.5 mg [scored]

PCM Allergy: Chlorpheniramine maleate 12 mg, phenylephrine hydrochloride 20 mg, and methscopolamine nitrate 2.5 mg

Tablet, long acting [scored]:

OMNIhist® II L.A.: Chlorpheniramine maleate 8 mg, phenylephrine hydrochloride 25 mg, and methscopolamine nitrate 2.5 mg

Rescon® MX: Chlorpheniramine maleate 8 mg, phenylephrine hydrochloride 40 mg, and methscopolamine nitrate 2.5 mg

Tablet, sustained release:

Ralix: Chlorpheniramine maleate 8 mg, phenylephrine hydrochloride 40 mg, and methscopolamine nitrate 2 mg

chlorpheniramine, phenylephrine, and phenyltoloxamine

(klor fen IR a meen, fen il EF rin, & fen il tole LOKS a meen)

Synonyms phenylephrine, chlorpheniramine, and phenyltoloxamine; phenyltoloxamine, chlorpheniramine, and phenylephrine

U.S./Canadian Brand Names Comhist® [US]; Nalex®-A [US]

Therapeutic Category Antihistamine/Decongestant Combination

Use Symptomatic relief of rhinitis and nasal congestion due to colds or allergy

Usual Dosage Oral:

Children:

2-6 years: Nalex®-A liquid: 1.25-2.5 mL every 4-6 hours

6-12 years:

Nalex®-A liquid: 5 mL every 4-6 hours

Nalex®-A tablet: 1/2 tablet 2-3 times/day

Children >12 years and Adults:

Nalex®-A liquid: 10 mL every 4-6 hours

(Continued)

chlorpheniramine, phenylephrine, and phenyltoloxamine *(Continued)*

Nalex®-A tablet: 1 tablet 2-3 times/day

Dosage Forms

Liquid (Nalex®-A): Chlorpheniramine maleate 2.5 mg, phenylephrine hydrochloride 5 mg, and phenyltoloxamine citrate 7.5 mg per 5 mL (480 mL) [alcohol free, sugar free; cotton candy flavor]

Tablet (Comhist®): Chlorpheniramine maleate 2 mg, phenylephrine hydrochloride 10 mg, and phenyltoloxamine citrate 25 mg

Tablet, prolonged release (Nalex®-A): Chlorpheniramine maleate 4 mg, phenylephrine hydrochloride 20 mg, and phenyltoloxamine citrate 40 mg

chlorpheniramine, phenylephrine, codeine, and potassium iodide

(klor fen IR a meen, fen il EF rin, KOE deen, & poe TASS ee um EYE oh dide)

Synonyms codeine, chlorpheniramine, phenylephrine, and potassium iodide; phenylephrine, chlorpheniramine, codeine, and potassium iodide; potassium iodide, chlorpheniramine, phenylephrine, and codeine

Therapeutic Category Antihistamine/Decongestant/Antitussive

Controlled Substance C-V

Use Symptomatic relief of rhinitis, nasal congestion and cough due to colds or allergy

Usual Dosage Children 6 months to 12 years: 1.25-10 mL every 4-6 hours

Dosage Forms Syrup: Chlorpheniramine maleate 0.75 mg, phenylephrine hydrochloride 2.5 mg, codeine phosphate 5 mg, and potassium iodide 75 mg per 5 mL (480 mL) [contains alcohol 5% and sodium benzoate; raspberry flavor] [DSC]

chlorpheniramine, pseudoephedrine, and acetaminophen *see* acetaminophen, chlorpheniramine, and pseudoephedrine *on page 11*

chlorpheniramine, pseudoephedrine, and codeine

(klor fen IR a meen, soo doe e FED rin, & KOE deen)

Synonyms codeine, chlorpheniramine, and pseudoephedrine; pseudoephedrine, chlorpheniramine, and codeine

U.S./Canadian Brand Names Dihistine® DH [US]

Therapeutic Category Antihistamine/Decongestant/Antitussive

Controlled Substance C-V

Use Temporary relief of cough associated with minor throat or bronchial irritation or nasal congestion due to common cold, allergic rhinitis, or sinusitis

Usual Dosage Oral:

Children:

25-50 lb: 1.25-2.5 mL every 4-6 hours, up to 4 doses in 24-hour period

50-90 lb: 2.5-5 mL every 4-6 hours, up to 4 doses in 24-hour period

Adults: 10 mL every 4-6 hours, up to 4 doses in 24-hour period

Dosage Forms

Elixir: Chlorpheniramine maleate 2 mg, pseudoephedrine hydrochloride 30 mg, and codeine phosphate 10 mg per 5 mL (120 mL, 480 mL)

Dihistine® DH: Chlorpheniramine maleate 2 mg, pseudoephedrine hydrochloride 30 mg, and codeine phosphate 10 mg per 5 mL (120 mL, 480 mL) [contains alcohol; grape flavor]

chlorpheniramine, pseudoephedrine, and dextromethorphan

(klor fen IR a meen, soo doe e FED rin, & deks troe meth OR fan)

Synonyms chlorpheniramine maleate, pseudoephedrine hydrochloride, and dextromethorphan hydrobromide; chlorpheniramine tannate, pseudoephedrine tannate, and dextromethorphan tannate; dexchlorpheniramine tannate, pseudoephedrine tannate, and dextromethorphan tannate; dextromethorphan, chlorpheniramine, and pseudoephedrine; pseudoephedrine, chlorpheniramine, and dextromethorphan

U.S./Canadian Brand Names Dicel™ DM [US]; DuraTan™ Forte [US]; Kidkare Cough and Cold [US-OTC]; PediaCare® Multi-Symptom Cold [US-OTC]; PediaCare® NightRest Cough and Cold [US-OTC]; Rescon DM [US-OTC]; Robitussin® Pediatric Night Relief [US-OTC]; Tanafed DMX™ [US]; Triaminic® Cold and Cough [US-OTC]; Triaminic® Night Time Cough and Cold [US-OTC]; Vicks® Children's NyQuil® [US-OTC]; Vicks® Pediatric 44®m [US-OTC]

Therapeutic Category Antihistamine/Decongestant/Antitussive

Use Temporarily relieves nasal congestion, runny nose, cough, and sneezing due to the common cold, hay fever, or allergic rhinitis

Usual Dosage General dosing guidelines; consult specific product labeling. Relief of cold symptoms: Oral:

Children:

2-6 years:

Dexchlorpheniramine tannate 2.5 mg, pseudoephedrine tannate 75 mg, and dextromethorphan tannate 25 mg (Tanafed DMX™): 2.5-5 mL every 12 hours (maximum: 10 mL/24 hours)

Dexchlorpheniramine tannate 3.5 mg, pseudoephedrine tannate 45 mg, and dextromethorphan tannate 30 mg (DuraTan™ Forte): 1.25-2.5 mL every 12 hours (maximum: 5 mL/24 hours)

6-12 years:

Chlorpheniramine maleate 1 mg, pseudoephedrine 15 mg, and dextromethorphan hydrobromide 7.5 mg per 5 mL: 10 mL every 6 hours

Chlorpheniramine maleate 1 mg, pseudoephedrine 15 mg, and dextromethorphan hydrobromide 5 mg per tablet or 5 mL: 2 tablets or 10 mL every 4-6 hours (maximum: 4 doses/24 hours)

Chlorpheniramine maleate 2 mg, pseudoephedrine 30 mg, and dextromethorphan hydrobromide 10 mg per tablet or 5 mL (Rescon DM): 5 mL every 4-6 hours (maximum: 4 doses/24 hours)

Dexchlorpheniramine tannate 2.5 mg, pseudoephedrine tannate 75 mg, and dextromethorphan tannate 25 mg (Tanafed DMX™): 5-10 mL every 12 hours (maximum: 20 mL/24 hours)

Dexchlorpheniramine tannate 3.5 mg, pseudoephedrine tannate 45 mg, and dextromethorphan tannate 30 mg (DuraTan™ Forte): 2.5-5 mL every 12 hours (maximum: 10 mL/24 hours)

>12 years: Refer to adult dosing

Adults:

Chlorpheniramine maleate 1 mg, pseudoephedrine 15 mg, and dextromethorphan hydrobromide 7.5 mg per 5 mL: 20 mL every 6 hours

Chlorpheniramine maleate 2 mg, pseudoephedrine 30 mg, and dextromethorphan hydrobromide 10 mg per tablet or 5 mL (Rescon DM): 10 mL every 4-6 hours (maximum: 4 doses/24 hours)

Dexchlorpheniramine tannate 2.5 mg, pseudoephedrine tannate 75 mg, and dextromethorphan tannate 25 mg (Tanafed DMX™): 10-20 mL every 12 hours (maximum: 40 mL/24 hours)

Dexchlorpheniramine tannate 3.5 mg, pseudoephedrine tannate 45 mg, and dextromethorphan tannate 30 mg (DuraTan™ Forte): 5-15 mL every 12 hours (maximum: 30 mL/24 hours)

Dosage Forms

Liquid: Chlorpheniramine maleate 1 mg, pseudoephedrine hydrochloride 15 mg, and dextromethorphan hydrobromide 5 mg per 5 mL (120 mL, 480 mL)

Kidkare Cough and Cold: Chlorpheniramine maleate 1 mg, pseudoephedrine hydrochloride 15 mg, and dextromethorphan hydrobromide 5 mg per 5 mL (120 mL)

PediaCare® Multi-Symptom Cold: Chlorpheniramine maleate 1 mg, pseudoephedrine hydrochloride 15 mg, and dextromethorphan hydrobromide 5 mg per 5 mL (120 mL) [contains sodium benzoate; cherry flavor]

PediaCare® NightRest Cough and Cold: Chlorpheniramine maleate 1 mg, pseudoephedrine hydrochloride 15 mg, and dextromethorphan hydrobromide 7.5 mg per 5 mL (120 mL) [contains sodium benzoate; cherry flavor]

Rescon DM: Chlorpheniramine maleate 2 mg, pseudoephedrine hydrochloride 30 mg, and dextromethorphan hydrobromide 10 mg per 5 mL (120 mL, 480 mL) [dye free; cherry flavor]

Triaminic® Cold and Cough: Chlorpheniramine maleate 1 mg, pseudoephedrine hydrochloride 15 mg, and dextromethorphan hydrobromide 5 mg per 5 mL (120 mL) [contains sodium 10 mg/5 mL and benzoic acid; cherry flavor]

Triaminic® Night Time Cough and Cold: Chlorpheniramine maleate 1 mg, pseudoephedrine hydrochloride 15 mg, and dextromethorphan hydrobromide 7.5 mg per 5 mL (120 mL, 240 mL) [contains sodium 7.5 mg/5 mL and benzoic acid; grape flavor]

Vicks® Pediatric 44®m: Chlorpheniramine maleate 2 mg, pseudoephedrine hydrochloride 30 mg, and dextromethorphan hydrobromide 15 mg per 15 mL (120 mL) [contains sodium 30 mg/15 mL and sodium benzoate; cherry flavor]

Vicks® Children's NyQuil®: Chlorpheniramine maleate 2 mg, pseudoephedrine hydrochloride 30 mg, and dextromethorphan hydrobromide 15 mg per 15 mL (120 mL) [contains sodium 71 mg/15 mL; cherry flavor]

Suspension:

Dicel™ DM: Chlorpheniramine tannate 5 mg, pseudoephedrine tannate 25 mg, and dextromethorphan tannate 5 mg per 5 mL (480 mL) [contains sodium benzoate; cotton candy flavor]

DuraTan™ Forte: Dexchlorpheniramine tannate 3.5 mg, pseudoephedrine tannate 45 mg, and dextromethorphan tannate 30 mg per 5 mL (480 mL) [contains sodium benzoate; grape flavor]

Tanafed DMX™: Dexchlorpheniramine tannate 2.5 mg, pseudoephedrine tannate 75 mg, and dextromethorphan tannate 25 mg (120 mL, 480 mL) [contains sodium benzoate; cotton candy flavor]

Syrup (Robitussin® Pediatric Night Relief): Chlorpheniramine maleate 1 mg, pseudoephedrine hydrochloride 15 mg, and dextromethorphan hydrobromide 7.5 mg per 5 mL (120 mL) [contains sodium benzoate; fruit punch flavor]

(Continued)

chlorpheniramine, pseudoephedrine, and dextromethorphan *(Continued)*

Tablet, chewable (PediaCare® Multi-Symptom Cold): Chlorpheniramine maleate 1 mg, pseudoephedrine hydrochloride 15 mg, and dextromethorphan hydrobromide 5 mg [contains phenylalanine 8.4 mg/tablet; cherry flavor]

chlorpheniramine, pseudoephedrine, and hydrocodone *see* pseudoephedrine, hydrocodone, and chlorpheniramine *on page 716*

chlorpheniramine tannate and phenylephrine tannate *see* chlorpheniramine and phenylephrine *on page 176*

chlorpheniramine tannate and pseudoephedrine tannate *see* chlorpheniramine and pseudoephedrine *on page 177*

chlorpheniramine tannate, pseudoephedrine tannate, and dextromethorphan tannate *see* chlorpheniramine, pseudoephedrine, and dextromethorphan *on page 182*

Chlor-Pro® Injection *(Discontinued)* *see* chlorpheniramine *on page 175*

chlorpromazine (klor PROE ma zeen)

Sound-Alike/Look-Alike Issues

chlorproMAZINE may be confused with chlorproPAMIDE, clomiPRAMINE, prochlorperazine, promethazine

Thorazine® may be confused with thiamine, thioridazine

Synonyms chlorpromazine hydrochloride; CPZ

Tall-Man chlorpro**MAZINE**

U.S./Canadian Brand Names Largactil® [Can]; Novo-Chlorpromazine [Can]

Therapeutic Category Phenothiazine Derivative

Use Control of mania; treatment of schizophrenia; control of nausea and vomiting; relief of restlessness and apprehension before surgery; acute intermittent porphyria; adjunct in the treatment of tetanus; intractable hiccups; combativeness and/or explosive hyperexcitable behavior in children 1-12 years of age and in short-term treatment of hyperactive children

Usual Dosage

Children ≥6 months:

Schizophrenia/psychoses:

Oral: 0.5-1 mg/kg/dose every 4-6 hours; older children may require 200 mg/day or higher

I.M., I.V.: 0.5-1 mg/kg/dose every 6-8 hours

<5 years (22.7 kg): Maximum: 40 mg/day

5-12 years (22.7-45.5 kg): Maximum: 75 mg/day

Nausea and vomiting:

Oral: 0.5-1 mg/kg/dose every 4-6 hours as needed

I.M., I.V.: 0.5-1 mg/kg/dose every 6-8 hours

<5 years (22.7 kg): Maximum: 40 mg/day

5-12 years (22.7-45.5 kg): Maximum: 75 mg/day

Adults:

Schizophrenia/psychoses:

Oral: Range: 30-2000 mg/day in 1-4 divided doses, initiate at lower doses and titrate as needed; usual dose: 400-600 mg/day; some patients may require 1-2 g/day

I.M., I.V.: Initial: 25 mg, may repeat (25-50 mg) in 1-4 hours, gradually increase to a maximum of 400 mg/dose every 4-6 hours until patient is controlled; usual dose: 300-800 mg/day

Intractable hiccups: Oral, I.M.: 25-50 mg 3-4 times/day

Nausea and vomiting:

Oral: 10-25 mg every 4-6 hours

I.M., I.V.: 25-50 mg every 4-6 hours

Dosage Forms

Injection, solution, as hydrochloride: 25 mg/mL (1 mL, 2 mL)

Tablet, as hydrochloride: 10 mg, 25 mg, 50 mg, 100 mg, 200 mg

chlorpromazine hydrochloride *see* chlorpromazine *on this page*

chlorpropamide (klor PROE pa mide)

Sound-Alike/Look-Alike Issues

chlorproPAMIDE may be confused with chlorproMAZINE

Diabinese® may be confused with DiaBeta®, Dialume®

Tall-Man chlorpro**PAMIDE**

U.S./Canadian Brand Names Apo-Chlorpropamide® [Can]; Diabinese® [US]; Novo-Propamide [Can]
Therapeutic Category Antidiabetic Agent, Oral
Use Management of blood sugar in type 2 diabetes mellitus (noninsulin dependent, NIDDM)
Usual Dosage Oral: The dosage of chlorpropamide is variable and should be individualized based upon the patient's response
Initial dose: Adults: 250 mg/day in mild-to-moderate diabetes in middle-aged, stable diabetic
Subsequent dosages may be increased or decreased by 50-125 mg/day at 3- to 5-day intervals
Maintenance dose: 100-250 mg/day; severe diabetics may require 500 mg/day; avoid doses >750 mg/day
Dosage Forms Tablet: 100 mg, 250 mg

chlorthalidone (klor THAL i done)

U.S./Canadian Brand Names Apo-Chlorthalidone® [Can]; Thalitone® [US]
Therapeutic Category Diuretic, Miscellaneous
Use Management of mild-to-moderate hypertension when used alone or in combination with other agents; treatment of edema associated with congestive heart failure or nephrotic syndrome. Recent studies have found chlorthalidone effective in the treatment of isolated systolic hypertension in the elderly.
Usual Dosage Oral: Adults:
Hypertension: 25-100 mg/day or 100 mg 3 times/week; usual dosage range (JNC 7): 12.5-25 mg/day
Edema: Initial: 50-100 mg/day or 100 mg on alternate days; maximum dose: 200 mg/day
Heart failure-associated edema: 12.5-25 mg once daily; maximum daily dose: 100 mg (ACC/AHA 2005 Heart Failure Guidelines)
Dosage Forms
Tablet: 25 mg, 50 mg, 100 mg
Thalitone®: 15 mg

chlorthalidone and atenolol *see* atenolol and chlorthalidone *on page 80*

chlorthalidone and clonidine *see* clonidine and chlorthalidone *on page 204*

Chlor-Trimeton® [US-OTC] *see* chlorpheniramine *on page 175*

Chlor-Trimeton® Allergy D [US-OTC] *see* chlorpheniramine and pseudoephedrine *on page 177*

Chlor-Trimeton® Syrup *(Discontinued)* *see* chlorpheniramine *on page 175*

Chlor-Tripolon® [Can] *see* chlorpheniramine *on page 175*

Chlor-Tripolon ND® [Can] *see* loratadine and pseudoephedrine *on page 505*

chlorzoxazone (klor ZOKS a zone)

Sound-Alike/Look-Alike Issues
Parafon Forte® may be confused with Fam-Pren Forte
U.S./Canadian Brand Names Parafon Forte® [Can]; Strifon Forte® [Can]
Therapeutic Category Skeletal Muscle Relaxant
Use Symptomatic treatment of muscle spasm and pain associated with acute musculoskeletal conditions
Usual Dosage Oral:
Children: 20 mg/kg/day or 600 mg/m^2/day in 3-4 divided doses
Adults: 250-500 mg 3-4 times/day up to 750 mg 3-4 times/day
Dosage Forms
Caplet (Parafon Forte® DSC): 500 mg
Tablet: 250 mg, 500 mg

Cholebrine® [US] *see* radiological/contrast media (ionic) *on page 728*

cholecalciferol (kole e kal SI fer ole)

Synonyms D_3
U.S./Canadian Brand Names D-Vi-Sol® [Can]; Delta-D® [US]
Therapeutic Category Vitamin D Analog
Use Dietary supplement, treatment of vitamin D deficiency, or prophylaxis of deficiency
Usual Dosage Adults: Oral: 400-1000 units/day
Dosage Forms
Tablet: 1000 int. units
Delta-D®: 400 int. units

cholecalciferol and alendronate *see* alendronate and cholecalciferol *on page 27*

cholestyramine resin (koe LES teer a meen REZ in)

U.S./Canadian Brand Names Novo-Cholamine Light [Can]; Novo-Cholamine [Can]; PMS-Cholestyramine [Can]; Prevalite® [US]; Questran® Light Sugar Free [Can]; Questran® Light [US]; Questran® [US]

Therapeutic Category Bile Acid Sequestrant

Use Adjunct in the management of primary hypercholesterolemia; pruritus associated with elevated levels of bile acids; diarrhea associated with excess fecal bile acids; binding toxicologic agents; pseudomembraneous colitis

Usual Dosage Oral (dosages are expressed in terms of anhydrous resin):

Children: 240 mg/kg/day in 3 divided doses; need to titrate dose depending on indication

Adults: 4 g 1-2 times/day to a maximum of 24 g/day and 6 doses/day

Dosage Forms

Powder for oral suspension: 4 g of resin/5 g of powder (5 g packets, 210 g can) [contains phenylalanine 14 mg/5 g]; 4 g of resin/5.7 g of powder (5.7 g packets, 240 g can) [light formulation]; 4 g of resin/9 g of powder (9 g packets, 378 g can)

Prevalite®: 4 g of resin/5.5 g of powder (5.5 g packets, 231 g can) [contains phenylalanine 14.1 mg/5.5 g; orange flavor]

Questran®: 4 g of resin/9 g of powder (9 g packets, 378 g can)

Questran® Light: 4 g of resin/6.4 g of powder (5 g packets, 268 g can) [contains phenylalanine 28.1 g/6.4 g]

choline magnesium trisalicylate (KOE leen mag NEE zhum trye sa LIS i late)

Synonyms tricosal

Therapeutic Category Analgesic, Nonnarcotic; Nonsteroidal Antiinflammatory Drug (NSAID)

Use Management of osteoarthritis, rheumatoid arthritis, and other arthritis; acute painful shoulder

Usual Dosage Oral (based on total salicylate content):

Children <37 kg: 50 mg/kg/day given in 2 divided doses; 2250 mg/day for heavier children

Adults: 500 mg to 1.5 g 2-3 times/day **or** 3 g at bedtime; usual maintenance dose: 1-4.5 g/day

Dosage Forms

Liquid: 500 mg/5 mL (240 mL) [choline salicylate 293 mg and magnesium salicylate 362 mg per 5 mL; cherry cordial flavor]

Tablet: 500 mg [choline salicylate 293 mg and magnesium salicylate 362 mg]; 750 mg [choline salicylate 440 mg and magnesium salicylate 544 mg]; 1000 mg [choline salicylate 587 mg and magnesium salicylate 725 mg]

Cholografin® Meglumine [US] *see* radiological/contrast media (ionic) *on page 728*

chondroitin sulfate and sodium hyaluronate

(kon DROY tin SUL fate & SOW de um hye al yoor ON ate)

Synonyms sodium hyaluronate and chrondroitin sulfate

U.S./Canadian Brand Names Viscoat® [US]

Therapeutic Category Ophthalmic Agent, Viscoelastic

Use Surgical aid in anterior segment procedures; protects corneal endothelium and coats intraocular lens thus protecting it

Usual Dosage Carefully introduce (using a 27-gauge needle or cannula) into anterior chamber after thoroughly cleaning the chamber with a balanced salt solution

Dosage Forms Solution, ophthalmic: Sodium chondroitin 4% and sodium hyaluronate 3% (0.5 mL)

Chooz® [US-OTC] *see* calcium carbonate *on page 135*

choriogonadotropin alfa *see* chorionic gonadotropin (recombinant) *on next page*

chorionic gonadotropin (human) (kor ee ON ik goe NAD oh troe pin, HYU man)

Synonyms CG; hCG

U.S./Canadian Brand Names Humegon® [Can]; Novarel® [US]; Pregnyl® [US]; Profasi® HP [Can]

Therapeutic Category Gonadotropin

Use Induces ovulation and pregnancy in anovulatory, infertile females; treatment of hypogonadotropic hypogonadism, prepubertal cryptorchidism; spermatogenesis induction with follitropin alfa

Usual Dosage I.M.:

Children: Various regimens:

Prepubertal cryptorchidism:

4000 units 3 times/week for 3 weeks **or**

5000 units every second day for 4 injections **or**

500 units 3 times/week for 4-6 weeks **or**

15 injections of 500-1000 units given over 6 weeks

Hypogonadotropic hypogonadism: Male:
500-1000 units 3 times/week for 3 weeks, followed by the same dose twice weekly for 3 weeks **or** 4000 units 3 times/week for 6-9 months, then reduce dosage to 2000 units 3 times/week for additional 3 months

Adults:
Induction of ovulation: Female: 5000-10,000 units one day following last dose of menotropins
Spermatogenesis induction associated with hypogonadotropic hypogonadism: Male: Treatment regimens vary (range: 1000-2000 units 2-3 times a week). Administer hCG until serum testosterone levels are normal (may require 2-3 months of therapy), then may add follitropin alfa or menopausal gonadotropin if needed to induce spermatogenesis; continue hCG at the dose required to maintain testosterone levels.

Dosage Forms
Injection, powder for reconstitution: 10,000 units [packaged with diluent; diluent contains benzyl alcohol and mannitol]
Novarel®: 10,000 units [packaged with diluent; diluent contains benzyl alcohol and mannitol]
Pregnyl®: 10,000 units [packaged with diluent; diluent contains benzyl alcohol]

chorionic gonadotropin (recombinant)

(kor ee ON ik goe NAD oh troe pin ree KOM be nant)

Synonyms choriogonadotropin alfa; r-hCG
U.S./Canadian Brand Names Ovidrel® [US/Can]
Therapeutic Category Gonadotropin; Ovulation Stimulator
Use As part of an assisted reproductive technology (ART) program, induces ovulation in infertile females who have been pretreated with follicle stimulating hormones (FSH); induces ovulation and pregnancy in infertile females when the cause of infertility is functional
Usual Dosage SubQ: Adults: Female: Assisted reproductive technologies (ART) and ovulation induction: 250 mcg given 1 day following the last dose of follicle stimulating agent. Use only after adequate follicular development has been determined. Hold treatment when there is an excessive ovarian response.
Dosage Forms [DSC] = Discontinued product
Injection, powder for reconstitution: 285 mcg [packaged with 1 mL SWFI; delivers 250 mcg r-hCG following reconstitution] [DSC]
Injection, solution: 257.5 mcg/0.515 mL (0.515 mL) [prefilled syringe; delivers 250 mcg r-hCG/0.5 mL]

Choron® *(Discontinued)* *see* chorionic gonadotropin (human) *on previous page*

Chromagen® OB [US] *see* vitamins (multiple/prenatal) *on page 879*

chromium *see* trace metals *on page 839*

Chronovera® [Can] *see* verapamil *on page 870*

Chronulac® *(Discontinued)* *see* lactulose *on page 478*

CI-1008 *see* pregabalin *on page 696*

Cialis® [US/Can] *see* tadalafil *on page 804*

Cibacalcin® *(Discontinued)* *see* calcitonin *on page 133*

ciclopirox (sye kloe PEER oks)

Sound-Alike/Look-Alike Issues
Loprox® may be confused with Lonox®
Synonyms ciclopirox olamine
U.S./Canadian Brand Names Loprox® [US/Can]; Penlac® [US/Can]
Therapeutic Category Antifungal Agent
Use
Cream/suspension: Treatment of tinea pedis (athlete's foot), tinea cruris (jock itch), tinea corporis (ringworm), cutaneous candidiasis, and tinea versicolor (pityriasis)
Gel: Treatment of tinea pedis (athlete's foot), tinea corporis (ringworm); seborrheic dermatitis of the scalp
Lacquer (solution): Topical treatment of mild-to-moderate onychomycosis of the fingernails and toenails due to *Trichophyton rubrum* (not involving the lunula) and the immediately-adjacent skin
Shampoo: Treatment of seborrheic dermatitis of the scalp
Usual Dosage Topical:
Children >10 years and Adults: Tinea pedis, tinea cruris, tinea corporis, cutaneous candidiasis, and tinea versicolor: Cream/suspension: Apply twice daily, gently massage into affected areas; if no improvement after 4 weeks of treatment, re-evaluate the diagnosis.
(Continued)

ciclopirox *(Continued)*

Children ≥12 years and Adults: Onychomycosis of the fingernails and toenails: Lacquer (solution): Apply to adjacent skin and affected nails daily (as a part of a comprehensive management program for onychomycosis). Remove with alcohol every 7 days.

Children >16 years and Adults:

Tinea pedis, tinea corporis: Gel: Apply twice daily, gently massage into affected areas and surrounding skin; if no improvement after 4 weeks of treatment, re-evaluate diagnosis

Seborrheic dermatitis of the scalp:

Gel: Apply twice daily, gently massage into affected areas and surrounding skin; if no improvement after 4 weeks of treatment, re-evaluate diagnosis.

Shampoo: Apply ~5 mL (1 teaspoonful) to wet hair; lather, and leave in place ~3 minutes; rinse. May use up to 10 mL for longer hair. Repeat twice weekly for 4 weeks; allow a minimum of 3 days between applications.

Dosage Forms

Cream, as olamine: 0.77% (15 g, 30 g, 90 g)

Loprox®: 0.77% (15 g, 30 g, 90 g)

Gel:

Loprox®: 0.77% (30 g, 45 g, 100 g)

Shampoo:

Loprox®: 1% (120 mL)

Solution, topical [nail lacquer]:

Penlac®: 8% (6.6 mL)

Suspension, topical, as olamine: 0.77% (30 mL, 60 mL)

Loprox®: 0.77% (30 mL, 60 mL)

ciclopirox olamine *see* ciclopirox *on previous page*

Cidecin *see* daptomycin *on page 230*

cidofovir (si DOF o veer)

U.S./Canadian Brand Names Vistide® [US]

Therapeutic Category Antiviral Agent

Use Treatment of cytomegalovirus (CMV) retinitis in patients with acquired immunodeficiency syndrome (AIDS). **Note:** Should be administered with probenecid.

Usual Dosage Adults:

Induction: 5 mg/kg I.V. over 1 hour once weekly for 2 consecutive weeks

Maintenance: 5 mg/kg over 1 hour once every other week

Note: Administer with probenecid 2 g orally 3 hours prior to each cidofovir dose and 1 g at 2 hours and 8 hours after completion of the infusion (total: 4 g)

Hydrate with 1 L of 0.9% NS I.V. prior to cidofovir infusion; a second liter may be administered over a 1- to 3-hour period immediately following infusion, if tolerated

Dosage Forms Injection, solution [preservative free]: 75 mg/mL (5 mL)

cilazapril *(Canada only)* (sye LAY za pril)

Synonyms cilazapril monohydrate

U.S./Canadian Brand Names Inhibace® [Can]; Novo-Cilazapril [Can]

Therapeutic Category Angiotensin-Converting Enzyme (ACE) Inhibitor

Use Management of hypertension; treatment of congestive heart failure

Usual Dosage Oral:

Hypertension: 2.5-5 mg once daily (maximum dose: 10 mg/day)

Congestive heart failure: Initial: 0.5 mg once daily; if tolerated, after 5 days increase to 1 mg/day (lowest maintenance dose); may increase to maximum of 2.5 mg once daily

Dosage Forms [CAN] = Canadian brand name

Tablet:

Inhibace® [CAN], Novo-Cilazapril [CAN]: 1 mg, 2.5 mg, 5 mg [not available in the U.S.]

cilazapril monohydrate *see* cilazapril *(Canada only) on this page*

cilostazol (sil OH sta zol)

Sound-Alike/Look-Alike Issues

Pletal® may be confused with Plendil®

Synonyms OPC-13013
U.S./Canadian Brand Names Pletal® [US/Can]
Therapeutic Category Platelet Aggregation Inhibitor
Use Symptomatic management of peripheral vascular disease, primarily intermittent claudication
Usual Dosage Adults: Oral: 100 mg twice daily taken at least one-half hour before or 2 hours after breakfast and dinner; dosage should be reduced to 50 mg twice daily during concurrent therapy with inhibitors of CYP3A4 or CYP2C19
Dosage Forms Tablet: 50 mg, 100 mg

Ciloxan® [US/Can] *see* ciprofloxacin *on next page*

cimetidine (sye MET i deen)

Sound-Alike/Look-Alike Issues
cimetidine may be confused with simethicone
U.S./Canadian Brand Names Apo-Cimetidine® [Can]; Gen-Cimetidine [Can]; Novo-Cimetidine [Can]; Nu-Cimet [Can]; PMS-Cimetidine [Can]; Tagamet® HB 200 [US-OTC]; Tagamet® HB [Can]; Tagamet® [US]
Therapeutic Category Histamine H_2 Antagonist
Use Short-term treatment of active duodenal ulcers and benign gastric ulcers; long-term prophylaxis of duodenal ulcer; gastric hypersecretory states; gastroesophageal reflux; prevention of upper GI bleeding in critically-ill patients; labeled for OTC use for prevention or relief of heartburn, acid indigestion, or sour stomach
Usual Dosage
Children: Oral, I.M., I.V.: 20-40 mg/kg/day in divided doses every 6 hours
Children ≥12 years and Adults: Oral: Heartburn, acid indigestion, sour stomach (OTC labeling): 200 mg up to twice daily; may take 30 minutes prior to eating foods or beverages expected to cause heartburn or indigestion
Adults:
Short-term treatment of active ulcers:
Oral: 300 mg 4 times/day or 800 mg at bedtime or 400 mg twice daily for up to 8 weeks
Note: Higher doses of 1600 mg at bedtime for 4 weeks may be beneficial for a subpopulation of patients with larger duodenal ulcers (>1 cm defined endoscopically) who are also heavy smokers (≥1 pack/day).
I.M., I.V.: 300 mg every 6 hours or 37.5 mg/hour by continuous infusion; I.V. dosage should be adjusted to maintain an intragastric pH ≥5
Prevention of upper GI bleed in critically-ill patients: 50 mg/hour by continuous infusion; I.V. dosage should be adjusted to maintain an intragastric pH ≥5
Note: Reduce dose by 50% if Cl_{cr} <30 mL/minute; treatment >7 days has not been evaluated.
Duodenal ulcer prophylaxis: Oral: 400 mg at bedtime
Gastric hypersecretory conditions: Oral, I.M., I.V.: 300-600 mg every 6 hours; dosage not to exceed 2.4 g/day
Gastroesophageal reflux disease: Oral: 400 mg 4 times/day or 800 mg twice daily for 12 weeks
Dosage Forms [DSC] = Discontinued product
Infusion, as hydrochloride [premixed in NS]: 300 mg (50 mL)
Injection, solution, as hydrochloride: 150 mg/mL (2 mL, 8 mL) [8 mL size contains benzyl alcohol]
Liquid, oral, as hydrochloride: 300 mg/5 mL (240 mL, 480 mL) [contains alcohol 2.8%; mint-peach flavor]
Tablet: 200 mg [OTC], 300 mg, 400 mg, 800 mg
Tagamet®: 300 mg; 400 mg [DSC]
Tagamet® HB 200: 200 mg

cinacalcet (sin a KAL cet)

Synonyms AMG 073; cinacalcet hydrochloride
U.S./Canadian Brand Names Sensipar™ [US]
Therapeutic Category Calcimimetic
Use Treatment of secondary hyperparathyroidism in dialysis patients; treatment of hypercalcemia in patients with parathyroid carcinoma
Usual Dosage Oral: Adults: **Do not titrate dose more frequently than every 2-4 weeks.**
Secondary hyperparathyroidism: Initial: 30 mg once daily (maximum daily dose: 180 mg); increase dose incrementally (60 mg, 90 mg, 120 mg, 180 mg once daily) as necessary to maintain iPTH level between 150-300 pg/mL.
Parathyroid carcinoma: Initial: 30 mg twice daily (maximum daily dose: 360 mg daily as 90 mg 4 times/day); increase dose incrementally (60 mg twice daily, 90 mg twice daily, 90 mg 4 times/day) as necessary to normalize serum calcium levels.
Dosage Forms Tablet: 30 mg, 60 mg, 90 mg

cinacalcet hydrochloride *see* cinacalcet *on previous page*

Cipralex® [Can] *see* escitalopram *on page 306*

Cipro® [US/Can] *see* ciprofloxacin *on this page*

Cipro® XL [Can] *see* ciprofloxacin *on this page*

Ciprodex® [US/Can] *see* ciprofloxacin and dexamethasone *on page 192*

ciprofloxacin (sip roe FLOKS a sin)

Sound-Alike/Look-Alike Issues

ciprofloxacin may be confused with cephalexin

Ciloxan® may be confused with cinoxacin, Cytoxan®

Cipro® may be confused with Ceftin®

Synonyms ciprofloxacin hydrochloride

U.S./Canadian Brand Names Apo-Ciproflox® [Can]; Ciloxan® [US/Can]; Cipro® XL [Can]; Cipro® XR [US]; Cipro® [US/Can]; CO Ciprofloxacin [Can]; Gen-Ciprofloxacin [Can]; Novo-Ciprofloxacin [Can]; PMS-Ciprofloxacin [Can]; Proquin® XR [US]; RAN™-Ciprofloxacin [Can]; ratio-Ciprofloxacin [Can]; Rhoxal-ciprofloxacin [Can]; Sandoz-Ciprofloxacin [Can]; Taro-Ciprofloxacin [Can]

Therapeutic Category Antibiotic, Ophthalmic; Quinolone

Use

Children: Complicated urinary tract infections and pyelonephritis due to *E. coli*. **Note:** Although effective, ciprofloxacin is not the drug of first choice in children.

Children and adults: To reduce incidence or progression of disease following exposure to aerolized *Bacillus anthracis*. Ophthalmologically, for superficial ocular infections (corneal ulcers, conjunctivitis) due to susceptible strains

Adults: Treatment of the following infections when caused by susceptible bacteria: Urinary tract infections; acute uncomplicated cystitis in females; chronic bacterial prostatitis; lower respiratory tract infections (including acute exacerbations of chronic bronchitis); acute sinusitis; skin and skin structure infections; bone and joint infections; complicated intraabdominal infections (in combination with metronidazole); infectious diarrhea; typhoid fever due to *Salmonella typhi* (eradication of chronic typhoid carrier state has not been proven); uncomplicated cervical and urethra gonorrhea (due to *N. gonorrhoeae*); nosocomial pneumonia; empirical therapy for febrile neutropenic patients (in combination with piperacillin)

Usual Dosage Note: Extended release tablets and immediate release formulations are not interchangeable. Unless otherwise specified, oral dosing reflects the use of immediate release formulations.

Usual dosage ranges:

Children:

Oral: 20-30 mg/kg/day in 2 divided doses; maximum dose: 1.5 g/day

I.V.: 20-30 mg/kg/day divided every 12 hours; maximum dose: 800 mg/day

Adults:

Oral: 250-750 mg every 12 hours

I.V.: 200-400 mg every 12 hours

Indication-specific dosing:

Children:

Anthrax:

Inhalational (postexposure prophylaxis):

Oral: 15 mg/kg/dose every 12 hours for 60 days; maximum: 500 mg/dose

I.V.: 10 mg/kg/dose every 12 hours for 60 days; do **not** exceed 400 mg/dose (800 mg/day)

Cutaneous (treatment, CDC guidelines): Oral: 10-15 mg/kg every 12 hours for 60 days (maximum: 1 g/day); amoxicillin 80 mg/kg/day divided every 8 hours is an option for completion of treatment after clinical improvement. **Note:** In the presence of systemic involvement, extensive edema, lesions on head/neck, refer to I.V. dosing for treatment of inhalational/gastrointestinal/oropharyngeal anthrax.

Inhalational/gastrointestinal/oropharyngeal (treatment, CDC guidelines): I.V.: Initial: 10-15 mg/kg every 12 hours for 60 days (maximum: 500 mg/dose); switch to oral therapy when clinically appropriate; refer to adult dosing for notes on combined therapy and duration

Bacterial conjunctivitis: See adult dosing

Corneal ulcer: See adult dosing

Urinary tract infection (complicated) or pyelonephritis:

Oral: 20-30 mg/kg/day in 2 divided doses (every 12 hours) for 10-21 days; maximum: 1.5 g/day

I.V.: 6-10 mg/kg every 8 hours for 10-21 days (maximum: 400 mg/dose)

Adults:

Anthrax:

Inhalational (postexposure prophylaxis):

Oral: 500 mg every 12 hours for 60 days

I.V.: 400 mg every 12 hours for 60 days

Cutaneous (treatment, CDC guidelines): Oral: Immediate release formulation: 500 mg every 12 hours for 60 days. **Note:** In the presence of systemic involvement, extensive edema, lesions on head/neck, refer to I.V. dosing for treatment of inhalational/gastrointestinal/oropharyngeal anthrax

Inhalational/gastrointestinal/oropharyngeal (treatment, CDC guidelines): I.V.: 400 mg every 12 hours. **Note:** Initial treatment should include two or more agents predicted to be effective (per CDC recommendations). Agents suggested for use in conjunction with ciprofloxacin or doxycycline include rifampin, vancomycin, imipenem, penicillin, ampicillin, chloramphenicol, clindamycin, and clarithromycin. May switch to oral antimicrobial therapy when clinically appropriate. Continue combined therapy for 60 days.

Bacterial conjunctivitis:

Ophthalmic solution: Instill 1-2 drops in eye(s) every 2 hours while awake for 2 days and 1-2 drops every 4 hours while awake for the next 5 days

Ophthalmic ointment: Apply a $1/2$" ribbon into the conjunctival sac 3 times/day for the first 2 days, followed by a $1/2$" ribbon applied twice daily for the next 5 days

Bone/joint infections:

Oral: 500-750 mg twice daily for 4-6 weeks, depending on severity and susceptibility

I.V.: Mild to moderate: 400 mg every 12 hours for 4-6 weeks; Severe/complicated: 400 mg every 8 hours for 4-6 weeks

Chancroid (CDC guidelines): Oral: 500 mg twice daily for 3 days

Corneal ulcer: Ophthalmic solution: Instill 2 drops into affected eye every 15 minutes for the first 6 hours, then 2 drops into the affected eye every 30 minutes for the remainder of the first day. On day 2, instill 2 drops into the affected eye hourly. On days 3-14, instill 2 drops into affected eye every 4 hours. Treatment may continue after day 14 if re-epithelialization has not occurred.

Febrile neutropenia (with piperacillin): I.V.: 400 mg every 8 hours for 7-14 days

Gonococcal infections:

Urethral/cervical gonococcal infections: Oral: 250-500 mg as a single dose (CDC recommends concomitant doxycycline or azithromycin due to developing resistance; avoid use in Asian or Western Pacific travelers)

Disseminated gonococcal infection (CDC guidelines): Oral: 500 mg twice daily to complete 7 days of therapy (initial treatment with ceftriaxone 1 g I.M./I.V. daily for 24-48 hours after improvement begins)

Infectious diarrhea: Oral:

Salmonella: 500 mg twice daily for 5-7 days

Shigella: 500 mg twice daily for 3 days

Traveler's diarrhea: Mild: 750 mg for one dose; Severe: 500 mg twice daily for 3 days

Vibrio cholerae: 1 g for one dose

Intraabdominal (in combination with metronidazole):

Oral: 500 mg every 12 hours for 7-14 days

I.V.: 400 mg every 12 hours for 7-14 days

Lower respiratory tract, skin/skin structure infections:

Oral: 500-750 mg twice daily for 7-14 days depending on severity and susceptibility

I.V.: Mild to moderate: 400 mg every 12 hours for 7-14 days; Severe/complicated: 400 mg every 8 hours for 7-14 days

Nosocomial pneumonia: I.V.: 400 mg every 8 hours for 10-14 days

Prostatitis (chronic, bacterial):

Oral: 500 mg every 12 hours for 28 days

I.V.: 400 mg every 12 hours for 28 days

Sinusitis (acute):

Oral: 500 mg every 12 hours for 10 days

I.V.: 400 mg every 12 hours for 10 days

Typhoid fever: Oral: 500 mg every 12 hours for 10 days

Urinary tract infection:

Acute uncomplicated: Oral: Immediate release formulation: 250 mg every 12 hours for 3 days; Extended release formulation (Cipro® XR, Proquin® XR): 500 mg every 24 hours for 3 days

Acute uncomplicated pyelonephritis: Oral: Extended release formulation (Cipro® XR): 1000 mg every 24 hours for 7-14 days

Mild to moderate:

Oral: Immediate release formulation: 250 mg every 12 hours for 7-14 days

I.V.: 200 mg every 12 hours for 7-14 days

Severe/complicated:

Oral:

Immediate release formulation: 500 mg every 12 hours for 7-14 days

Extended release formulation (Cipro® XR): 1000 mg every 24 hours for 7-14 days

I.V.: 400 mg every 12 hours for 7-14 days

(Continued)

ciprofloxacin *(Continued)*

Dosage Forms

Infusion [premixed in D_5W]:
Cipro®: 200 mg (100 mL); 400 mg (200 mL) [latex free]
Injection, solution: 10 mg/mL (20 mL, 40 mL)
Cipro®: 10 mg/mL (20 mL, 40 mL)
Microcapsules for suspension, oral:
Cipro®: 250 mg/5 mL (100 mL); 500 mg/5 mL (100 mL) [strawberry flavor]
Ointment, ophthalmic, as hydrochloride:
Ciloxan®: 3.33 mg/g [0.3% base] (3.5 g)
Solution, ophthalmic, as hydrochloride: 3.5 mg/mL (2.5 mL, 5mL, 10 mL) [0.3% base]
Ciloxin®: 3.5 mg/mL (2.5 mL, 5mL, 10 mL) [0.3% base; contains benzalkonium chloride]
Tablet: 250 mg, 500 mg, 750 mg
Cipro®: 250 mg, 500 mg, 750 mg
Tablet, extended release:
Cipro® XR: 500 mg [equivalent to ciprofloxacin hydrochloride 287.5 mg and ciprofloxacin base 212.6 mg]; 1000 mg [equivalent to ciprofloxacin hydrochloride 574.9 mg and ciprofloxacin base 425.2 mg]
Proquin® XR: 500 mg
Tablet, extended release [dose pack]:
Proquin® XR: 500 mg (3s)

ciprofloxacin and dexamethasone (sip roe FLOKS a sin & deks a METH a sone)

Synonyms ciprofloxacin hydrochloride and dexamethasone; dexamethasone and ciprofloxacin

U.S./Canadian Brand Names Ciprodex® [US/Can]

Therapeutic Category Antibiotic/Corticosteroid, Otic

Use Treatment of acute otitis media in pediatric patients with tympanostomy tubes or acute otitis externa in children and adults

Usual Dosage Otic:

Children: Acute otitis media in patients with tympanostomy tubes or acute otitis externa: Instill 4 drops into affected ear(s) twice daily for 7 days
Adults: Acute otitis externa: Instill 4 drops into affected ear(s) twice daily for 7 days

Dosage Forms Suspension, otic: Ciprofloxacin 0.3% and dexamethasone 0.1% (7.5 mL) [contains benzalkonium chloride]

ciprofloxacin and hydrocortisone (sip roe FLOKS a sin & hye droe KOR ti sone)

Synonyms ciprofloxacin hydrochloride and hydrocortisone; hydrocortisone and ciprofloxacin

U.S./Canadian Brand Names Cipro® HC [US/Can]

Therapeutic Category Antibiotic/Corticosteroid, Otic

Use Treatment of acute otitis externa, sometimes known as "swimmer's ear"

Usual Dosage Children >1 year of age and Adults: Otic: The recommended dosage for all patients is three drops of the suspension in the affected ear twice daily for 7 days; twice-daily dosing schedule is more convenient for patients than that of existing treatments with hydrocortisone, which are typically administered three or four times a day; a twice-daily dosage schedule may be especially helpful for parents and caregivers of young children

Dosage Forms Suspension, otic: Ciprofloxacin hydrochloride 0.2% and hydrocortisone 1% (10 mL) [contains benzyl alcohol]

ciprofloxacin hydrochloride *see* ciprofloxacin *on page 190*

ciprofloxacin hydrochloride and dexamethasone *see* ciprofloxacin and dexamethasone *on this page*

ciprofloxacin hydrochloride and hydrocortisone *see* ciprofloxacin and hydrocortisone *on this page*

Cipro® HC [US/Can] *see* ciprofloxacin and hydrocortisone *on this page*

Cipro® XR [US] *see* ciprofloxacin *on page 190*

cisapride (SIS a pride)

Sound-Alike/Look-Alike Issues

Propulsid® may be confused with propranolol

U.S./Canadian Brand Names Propulsid® [US]

Therapeutic Category Gastrointestinal Agent, Prokinetic

Use Treatment of nocturnal symptoms of gastroesophageal reflux disease (GERD); has demonstrated effectiveness for gastroparesis, refractory constipation, and nonulcer dyspepsia

Usual Dosage Oral:

Children: 0.15-0.3 mg/kg/dose 3-4 times/day; maximum: 10 mg/dose

Adults: Initial: 10 mg 4 times/day at least 15 minutes before meals and at bedtime; in some patients the dosage will need to be increased to 20 mg to obtain a satisfactory result

cisatracurium (sis a tra KYOO ree um)

Sound-Alike/Look-Alike Issues

Nimbex® may be confused with Revex®

Synonyms cisatracurium besylate

U.S./Canadian Brand Names Nimbex® [US/Can]

Therapeutic Category Skeletal Muscle Relaxant

Use Adjunct to general anesthesia to facilitate endotracheal intubation and to relax skeletal muscles during surgery; to facilitate mechanical ventilation in ICU patients; does not relieve pain or produce sedation

Usual Dosage I.V. (not to be used I.M.):

Operating room administration:

Infants 1-23 months: 0.15 mg/kg over 5-10 seconds during either halothane or opioid anesthesia

Children 2-12 years: Intubating doses: 0.1-0.15 mg/kg over 5-15 seconds during either halothane or opioid anesthesia. (**Note:** When given during stable opioid/nitrous oxide/oxygen anesthesia, 0.1 mg/kg produces maximum neuromuscular block in an average of 2.8 minutes and clinically effective block for 28 minutes.)

Adults: Intubating doses: 0.15-0.2 mg/kg as component of propofol/nitrous oxide/oxygen induction-intubation technique. (**Note:** May produce generally good or excellent conditions for tracheal intubation in 1.5-2 minutes with clinically effective duration of action during propofol anesthesia of 55-61 minutes.); initial dose after succinylcholine for intubation: 0.1 mg/kg; maintenance dose: 0.03 mg/kg 40-60 minutes after initial dose, then at ~20-minute intervals based on clinical criteria

Children ≥2 years and Adults: Continuous infusion: After an initial bolus, a diluted solution can be given by continuous infusion for maintenance of neuromuscular blockade during extended surgery; adjust the rate of administration according to the patient's response as determined by peripheral nerve stimulation. An initial infusion rate of 3 mcg/kg/minute may be required to rapidly counteract the spontaneous recovery of neuromuscular function; thereafter, a rate of 1-2 mcg/kg/minute should be adequate to maintain continuous neuromuscular block in the 89% to 99% range in most pediatric and adult patients. Consider reduction of the infusion rate by 30% to 40% when administering during stable isoflurane, enflurane, sevoflurane, or desflurane anesthesia. Spontaneous recovery from neuromuscular blockade following discontinuation of infusion of cisatracurium may be expected to proceed at a rate comparable to that following single bolus administration.

Intensive care unit administration: Follow the principles for infusion in the operating room. At initial signs of recovery from bolus dose, begin the infusion at a dose of 3 mcg/kg/minute and adjust rates accordingly; dosage ranges of 0.5-10 mcg/kg/minute have been reported. If patient is allowed to recover from neuromuscular blockade, readministration of a bolus dose may be necessary to quickly re-establish neuromuscular block prior to reinstituting the infusion.

Dosage Forms

Injection, solution: 2 mg/mL (5 mL); 10 mg/mL (20 mL)

Injection, solution: 2 mg/mL (10 mL) [contains benzyl alcohol]

cisatracurium besylate *see* cisatracurium *on this page*

cisplatin (SIS pla tin)

Sound-Alike/Look-Alike Issues

cisplatin may be confused with carboplatin

Platinol®-AQ may be confused with Paraplatin®, Patanol®, Plaquenil®

Synonyms CDDP

Therapeutic Category Antineoplastic Agent

Use Treatment of head and neck, breast, testicular, and ovarian cancer; Hodgkin and non-Hodgkin lymphoma; neuroblastoma; sarcomas, bladder, gastric, lung, esophageal, cervical, and prostate cancer; myeloma, melanoma, mesothelioma, small cell lung cancer, and osteosarcoma

Usual Dosage Refer to individual protocols. **VERIFY ANY CISPLATIN DOSE EXCEEDING 100 mg/m² PER COURSE.**

Adults:

Advanced bladder cancer: 50-70 mg/m² every 3-4 weeks

(Continued)

cisplatin *(Continued)*

Malignant pleural mesothelioma in combination with pemetrexed: 75 mg/m^2 on day 1 of each 21-day cycle; see pemetrexed monograph for additional details

Metastatic ovarian cancer: 75-100 mg/m^2 every 3-4 weeks

Intraperitoneal: Cisplatin has been administered intraperitoneal with systemic sodium thiosulfate for ovarian cancer; doses up to 90-270 mg/m^2 have been administered and retained for 4 hours before draining

Testicular cancer: 10-20 mg/m^2/day for 5 days repeated every 3-4 weeks

Dosage Forms [DSC] = Discontinued product

Injection, solution: 1 mg/mL (50 mL, 100 mL, 200 mL)

Platinol®-AQ: 1 mg/mL (50 mL, 100 mL) [contains sodium 9 mg/mL] [DSC]

13-*cis*-retinoic acid *see* isotretinoin *on page 466*

citalopram (sye TAL oh pram)

Sound-Alike/Look-Alike Issues

Celexa™ may be confused with Celebrex®, Cerebra®, Cerebyx®, Zyprexa®

Synonyms citalopram hydrobromide; nitalapram

U.S./Canadian Brand Names Apo-Citalopram® [Can]; Celexa® [US/Can]; CO Citalopram [Can]; Dom-Citalopram [Can]; Gen-Citalopram [Can]; Novo-Citalopram [Can]; PHL-Citalopram [Can]; PMS-Citalopram [Can]; RAN™-Citalopram [Can]; ratio-Citalopram [Can]; Rhoxal-citalopram [Can]; Sandoz-Citalopram [Can]

Therapeutic Category Antidepressant

Use Treatment of depression

Usual Dosage Oral: Adults: Depression: Initial: 20 mg/day, generally with an increase to 40 mg/day; doses of more than 40 mg are not usually necessary. Should a dose increase be necessary, it should occur in 20 mg increments at intervals of no less than 1 week. Maximum dose: 60 mg/day

Dosage Forms

Solution, oral: 10 mg/5 mL (240 mL) [alcohol free, sugar free; peppermint flavor]

Tablet: 10 mg, 20 mg, 40 mg

citalopram hydrobromide *see* citalopram *on this page*

Citanest® Plain [US/Can] *see* prilocaine *on page 698*

Citracal® [US-OTC] *see* calcium citrate *on page 137*

Citracal® Prenatal Rx [US] *see* vitamins (multiple/prenatal) *on page 879*

citrate of magnesia *see* magnesium citrate *on page 512*

citric acid and D-gluconic acid irrigant *see* citric acid, magnesium carbonate, and glucono-delta-lactone *on this page*

citric acid and potassium citrate *see* potassium citrate and citric acid *on page 686*

citric acid bladder mixture *see* citric acid, magnesium carbonate, and glucono-delta-lactone *on this page*

citric acid, magnesium carbonate, and glucono-delta-lactone

(SI trik AS id, mag NEE see um KAR bo nate, and GLOO kon o DEL ta LAK tone)

Sound-Alike/Look-Alike Issues

Renacidin® may be confused with Remicade®

Synonyms citric acid and D-gluconic acid irrigant; citric acid bladder mixture; citric acid, magnesium hydroxycarbonate, D-gluconic acid, magnesium acid citrate, and calcium carbonate; hemiacidrin

U.S./Canadian Brand Names Renacidin® [US]

Therapeutic Category Irrigating Solution

Use Prevention of formation of calcifications of indwelling urinary tract catheters; treatment of renal and bladder calculi of the apatite or struvite type

Usual Dosage Adults:

Dissolution or prevention of calcifications: Irrigation (indwelling urethral catheters): 30-60 mL 2-3 times/day by means of a rubber syringe

Renal calculi: Irrigation: Infuse NS at 60 mL/hour and increase until pain, elevated pressure, or maximum flow rate of 120 mL/hour is reached. Begin flow of solution at maximum rate achieved with NS.

Bladder calculi: 30 mL instilled through urinary catheter; clamp for 30-60 minutes, then release and drain; repeat 4-6 times/day

Dosage Forms Solution, irrigation: Citric acid 6.602 g, magnesium carbonate 3.177 g, glucono-delta-lactone 0.198 g per 100 mL (500 mL) [contains benzoic acid]

citric acid, magnesium hydroxycarbonate, D-gluconic acid, magnesium acid citrate, and calcium carbonate *see* citric acid, magnesium carbonate, and glucono-delta-lactone *on previous page*

citric acid, sodium citrate, and potassium citrate

(SIT rik AS id, SOW dee um SIT rate, & poe TASS ee um SIT rate)

Synonyms potassium citrate, citric acid, and sodium citrate; sodium citrate, citric acid, and potassium citrate

U.S./Canadian Brand Names Cytra-3 [US]; Polycitra® [US]; Polycitra®-LC [US]

Therapeutic Category Alkalinizing Agent

Use Conditions where long-term maintenance of an alkaline urine is desirable as in control and dissolution of uric acid and cystine calculi of the urinary tract

Usual Dosage Oral:

Children: 5-15 mL diluted in water after meals and at bedtime

Adults: 15-30 mL diluted in water after meals and at bedtime

Dosage Forms Note: Equivalent to potassium 1 mEq/mL, sodium 1 mEq/mL, and bicarbonate 2 mEq/mL

Solution, oral:

Cytra-3: Citric acid 334 mg, sodium citrate 500 mg, and potassium citrate 550 mg per 5 mL (480 mL) [alcohol free, sugar free; contains sodium benzoate; raspberry flavor]

Polycitra®-LC: Citric acid 334 mg, sodium citrate 500 mg, and potassium citrate 550 mg per 5 mL (480 mL) [alcohol free, sugar free]

Syrup, oral (Polycitra®): Citric acid 334 mg, sodium citrate 500 mg, and potassium citrate 550 mg per 5 mL (480 mL) [alcohol free]

Citro-Mag® [Can] *see* magnesium citrate *on page 512*

Citrotein® [US-OTC] *see* nutritional formula, enteral/oral *on page 608*

citrovorum factor *see* leucovorin *on page 485*

Citrucel® [US-OTC] *see* methylcellulose *on page 544*

Citrucel® Fiber Shake [US-OTC] *see* methylcellulose *on page 544*

Citrucel® Fiber Smoothie [US-OTC] *see* methylcellulose *on page 544*

CL-118,532 *see* triptorelin *on page 854*

Cl-719 *see* gemfibrozil *on page 378*

CL-825 *see* pentostatin *on page 652*

CL-184116 *see* porfimer *on page 682*

cladribine (KLA dri been)

Sound-Alike/Look-Alike Issues

Leustatin® may be confused with lovastatin

Synonyms 2-CdA; 2-chlorodeoxyadenosine; NSC-105014

U.S./Canadian Brand Names Leustatin® [US/Can]

Therapeutic Category Antineoplastic Agent

Use Treatment of hairy cell leukemia

Usual Dosage Adults: I.V. (refer to individual protocols): Hairy cell leukemia: Continuous infusion: 0.09 mg/kg/day days 1-7; may be repeated every 28-35 days

Dosage Forms Injection, solution [preservative free]: 1 mg/mL (10 mL)

Claforan® [US/Can] *see* cefotaxime *on page 158*

Claravis™ [US] *see* isotretinoin *on page 466*

Clarinex® [US] *see* desloratadine *on page 237*

Claripel™ [US] *see* hydroquinone *on page 430*

clarithromycin (kla RITH roe mye sin)

Sound-Alike/Look-Alike Issues

clarithromycin may be confused with erythromycin

U.S./Canadian Brand Names Biaxin® XL [US/Can]; Biaxin® [US/Can]; ratio-Clarithromycin [Can]

Therapeutic Category Macrolide (Antibiotic)

Use

Children:

Acute otitis media (*H. influenzae*, *M. catarrhalis*, or *S. pneumoniae*)

(Continued)

clarithromycin *(Continued)*

Community-acquired pneumonia due to susceptible *Mycoplasma pneumoniae, S. pneumoniae,* or *Chlamydia pneumoniae* (TWAR)

Pharyngitis/tonsillitis, acute maxillary sinusitis, uncomplicated skin/skin structure infections, and mycobacterial infections

Prevention of disseminated mycobacterial infections due to MAC disease in patients with advanced HIV infection

Adults:

Pharyngitis/tonsillitis due to susceptible *S. pyogenes*

Acute maxillary sinusitis and acute exacerbation of chronic bronchitis due to susceptible *H. influenzae, M. catarrhalis,* or *S. pneumoniae*

Community-acquired pneumonia due to susceptible *H. influenzae, H. parainfluenzae, Mycoplasma pneumoniae, S. pneumoniae,* or *Chlamydia pneumoniae* (TWAR)

Uncomplicated skin/skin structure infections due to susceptible *S. aureus, S. pyogenes*

Disseminated mycobacterial infections due to *M. avium* or *M. intracellulare*

Prevention of disseminated mycobacterial infections due to *M. avium* complex (MAC) disease (eg, patients with advanced HIV infection)

Duodenal ulcer disease due to *H. pylori* in regimens with other drugs including amoxicillin and lansoprazole or omeprazole, ranitidine bismuth citrate, bismuth subsalicylate, tetracycline, and/or an H_2 antagonist

Usual Dosage

Usual dosage range:

Children ≥6 months: Oral: 7.5-15 mg/kg every 12 hours (maximum: 500 mg/dose)

Adults: Oral: 250-500 mg every 12 hours **or** 1000 mg (two 500 mg extended release tablets) once daily for 7-14 days

Indication-specific dosing:

Children: Oral:

Community-acquired pneumonia, sinusitis, bronchitis, skin infections: 15 mg/kg/day divided every 12 hours for 10 days

Endocarditis, prophylaxis: 15 mg/kg 1 hour before procedure (maximum: 500 mg)

Mycobacterial infection (prevention and treatment): 7.5 mg/kg (up to 500 mg) twice daily. **Note:** Safety of clarithromycin for MAC not studied in children <20 months.

Pertussis (CDC guidelines):

Children ≥1 months: 15 mg/kg/day divided every 12 hours for 7 days (maximum: 1 g/day)

Children ≥6 months: 15 mg/kg/day divided every 12 hours for 10 days

Adults: Oral:

Acute exacerbation of chronic bronchitis:

M. catarrhalis and *S. pneumoniae*: 250 mg every 12 hours for 7-14 days **or** 1000 mg (two 500 mg extended release tablets) once daily for 7 days

H. influenzae: 500 mg every 12 hours for 7-14 days or 1000 mg (two 500 mg extended release tablets) for 7 days

H. parainfluenzae: 500 mg every 12 hours for 7 days or 1000 mg (two 500 mg extended release tablets) for 7 days

Acute maxillary sinusitis: 500 mg every 12 hours **or** 1000 mg (two 500 mg extended release tablets) once daily for 14 days

Endocarditis, prophylaxis: 500 mg 1 hour prior to procedure

Mycobacterial infection (prevention and treatment): 500 mg twice daily (use with other antimycobacterial drugs, eg, ethambutol or rifampin)

Peptic ulcer disease: Eradication of *Helicobacter pylori*: Dual or triple combination regimen with bismuth subsalicylate, tetracycline, clarithromycin, and an H_2-receptor; or combination of omeprazole and clarithromycin; 500 mg every 8-12 hours for 10-14 days

Pertussis (CDC guidelines): 500 mg twice daily for 7 days

Pharyngitis, tonsillitis: 250 mg every 12 hours for 10 days

Pneumonia:

C. pneumoniae, M. pneumoniae, and *S. pneumoniae*: 250 mg every 12 hours for 7-14 days **or** 1000 mg (two 500 mg extended release tablets) once daily for 7 days

H. influenzae: 250 mg every 12 hours for 7 days **or** 1000 mg (two 500 mg extended release tablets) once daily for 7 days

Skin and skin structure infection, uncomplicated: 250 mg every 12 hours for 7-14 days

Dosage Forms

Granules for oral suspension:

Biaxin®: 125 mg/5 mL (50 mL, 100 mL); 250 mg/5 mL (50 mL, 100 mL) [fruit punch flavor]

Tablet:
Biaxin®: 250 mg, 500 mg
Tablet, extended release:
Biaxin® XL: 500 mg

clarithromycin, lansoprazole, and amoxicillin *see* lansoprazole, amoxicillin, and clarithromycin *on page 482*

Claritin® [Can] *see* loratadine *on page 505*

Claritin® 24 Hour Allergy [US-OTC] *see* loratadine *on page 505*

Claritin-D® 12-Hour [US-OTC] *see* loratadine and pseudoephedrine *on page 505*

Claritin-D® 24-Hour [US-OTC] *see* loratadine and pseudoephedrine *on page 505*

Claritin® Allergic Decongestant [Can] *see* oxymetazoline *on page 628*

Claritin® Extra [Can] *see* loratadine and pseudoephedrine *on page 505*

Claritin® Hives Relief [US-OTC] *see* loratadine *on page 505*

Claritin® Kids [Can] *see* loratadine *on page 505*

Claritin® Liberator [Can] *see* loratadine and pseudoephedrine *on page 505*

Clasteon® [Can] *see* clodronate *(Canada only) on page 201*

clavulanic acid and amoxicillin *see* amoxicillin and clavulanate potassium *on page 49*

Clavulin® [Can] *see* amoxicillin and clavulanate potassium *on page 49*

Clear Away® Disc *(Discontinued)* *see* salicylic acid *on page 758*

Clear By Design® Gel *(Discontinued)* *see* benzoyl peroxide *on page 102*

Clear Eyes® ACR [US-OTC] *see* naphazoline *on page 577*

Clear Eyes® Extra Relief [US-OTC] *see* naphazoline *on page 577*

Clearplex [US-OTC] *see* benzoyl peroxide *on page 102*

Clearsil® Maximum Strength *(Discontinued)* *see* benzoyl peroxide *on page 102*

Clear Tussin® 30 *(Discontinued)* *see* guaifenesin and dextromethorphan *on page 394*

clemastine (KLEM as teen)

Synonyms clemastine fumarate

U.S./Canadian Brand Names Dayhist® Allergy [US-OTC]; Tavist® Allergy [US-OTC]

Therapeutic Category Antihistamine

Use Perennial and seasonal allergic rhinitis and other allergic symptoms including urticaria

Usual Dosage Oral:

Infants and Children <6 years: 0.05 mg/kg/day as **clemastine base** or 0.335-0.67 mg/day clemastine fumarate (0.25-0.5 mg base/day) divided into 2 or 3 doses; maximum daily dosage: 1.34 mg (1 mg base)

Children 6-12 years: 0.67-1.34 mg clemastine fumarate (0.5-1 mg base) twice daily; do not exceed 4.02 mg/day (3 mg/day base)

Children ≥12 years and Adults:

1.34 mg clemastine fumarate (1 mg base) twice daily to 2.68 mg (2 mg base) 3 times/day; do not exceed 8.04 mg/day (6 mg base)

OTC labeling: 1.34 mg clemastine fumarate (1 mg base) twice daily; do not exceed 2 mg base/24 hours

Dosage Forms

Syrup, as fumarate [prescription formulation]: 0.67 mg/5 mL (120 mL) [0.5 mg base/5 mL; contains alcohol 5.5%; citrus flavor]

Tablet, as fumarate: 1.34 mg [1 mg base; OTC], 2.68 mg [2 mg base; prescription formulation]

Dayhist® Allergy, Tavist® Allergy: 1.34 mg [1 mg base]

clemastine fumarate *see* clemastine *on this page*

Clenia™ [US] *see* sulfur and sulfacetamide *on page 800*

Cleocin® [US] *see* clindamycin *on next page*

Cleocin HCl® [US] *see* clindamycin *on next page*

Cleocin Pediatric® [US] *see* clindamycin *on next page*

Cleocin Phosphate® [US] *see* clindamycin *on next page*

Cleocin T® [US] *see* clindamycin *on next page*

clidinium and chlordiazepoxide (kli DI nee um & klor dye az e POKS ide)

Sound-Alike/Look-Alike Issues

Librax® may be confused with Librium®

Synonyms chlordiazepoxide and clidinium

U.S./Canadian Brand Names Apo-Chlorax® [Can]; Librax® [US/Can]

Therapeutic Category Anticholinergic Agent

Use Adjunct treatment of peptic ulcer; treatment of irritable bowel syndrome

Usual Dosage Oral: 1-2 capsules 3-4 times/day, before meals or food and at bedtime

Dosage Forms Capsule: Clidinium bromide 2.5 mg and chlordiazepoxide hydrochloride 5 mg

Climara® [US/Can] *see* estradiol *on page 308*

ClimaraPro® [US] *see* estradiol and levonorgestrel *on page 310*

Clinac™ BPO [US] *see* benzoyl peroxide *on page 102*

Clindagel® [US] *see* clindamycin *on this page*

ClindaMax™ [US] *see* clindamycin *on this page*

clindamycin (klin da MYE sin)

Sound-Alike/Look-Alike Issues

Cleocin® may be confused with bleomycin, Clinoril®, Lincocin®

Synonyms clindamycin hydrochloride; clindamycin palmitate; clindamycin phosphate

U.S./Canadian Brand Names Alti-Clindamycin [Can]; Apo-Clindamycin® [Can]; Cleocin HCl® [US]; Cleocin Pediatric® [US]; Cleocin Phosphate® [US]; Cleocin T® [US]; Cleocin® [US]; Clindagel® [US]; ClindaMax™ [US]; Clindamycin Injection, USP [Can]; Clindesse™ [US]; Clindets® [US]; Clindoxyl® [Can]; Dalacin® C [Can]; Dalacin® T [Can]; Dalacin® Vaginal [Can]; Evoclin™ [US]; Novo-Clindamycin [Can]; Taro-Clindamycin [Can]

Therapeutic Category Acne Products; Antibiotic, Miscellaneous

Use Treatment against aerobic and anaerobic streptococci (except enterococci), most staphylococci, *Bacteroides* sp and *Actinomyces*; bacterial vaginosis (vaginal cream, vaginal suppository); pelvic inflammatory disease (I.V.); topically in treatment of severe acne; vaginally for *Gardnerella vaginalis*

Usual Dosage

Usual dosage ranges:

Infants and Children:

Oral: 8-20 mg/kg/day as hydrochloride; 8-25 mg/kg/day as palmitate in 3-4 divided doses (minimum dose of palmitate: 37.5 mg 3 times/day)

I.M., I.V.:

<1 month: 15-20 mg/kg/day

>1 month: 20-40 mg/kg/day in 3-4 divided doses

Adults:

Oral: 150-450 mg/dose every 6-8 hours; maximum dose: 1.8 g/day

I.M., I.V.: 1.2-1.8 g/day in 2-4 divided doses; maximum dose: 4.8 g/day

Indication-specific dosing:

Children:

Anthrax: I.V.: 7.5 mg/kg every 6 hours

Babesiosis: Oral: 20-40 mg/kg/day divided every 8 hours for 7 days plus quinine

Orofacial infections: 8-25 mg/kg in 3-4 equally divided doses

Children ≥12 years and Adults:

Acne vulgaris: Topical:

Gel, pledget, lotion, solution: Apply a thin film twice daily

Foam (Evoclin™): Apply once daily

Adults:

Amnionitis: I.V.: 450-900 mg every 8 hours

Anthrax: I.V.: 900 mg every 8 hours with ciprofloxacin or doxycycline

Babesiosis:

Oral: 600 mg 3 times/day for 7 days with quinine

I.V.: 1.2 g twice daily

Bacterial vaginosis: Intravaginal:

Suppositories: Insert one ovule (100 mg clindamycin) daily into vagina at bedtime for 3 days

Cream:

Cleocin®: One full applicator inserted intravaginally once daily before bedtime for 3 or 7 consecutive days in nonpregnant patients or for 7 consecutive days in pregnant patients

Clindesse™: One full applicator inserted intravaginally as a single dose at anytime during the day in nonpregnant patients

Bite wounds (canine): Oral: 300 mg 4 times/day with a fluoroquinolone

Gangrenous myositis: I.V.: 900 mg every 8 hours with penicillin G

Group B streptococcus (neonatal prophylaxis): I.V.: 900 mg every 8 hours until delivery

Orofacial/parapharyngeal space infections:

Oral: 150-450 mg every 6 hours for 7 days, maximum 1.8 g/day

I.V.: 600-900 mg every 8 hours

Pelvic inflammatory disease: I.V.: 900 mg every 8 hours with gentamicin 2 mg/kg, then 1.5 mg/kg every 8 hours; continue after discharge with doxycycline 100 mg twice daily to complete 14 days of total therapy

Toxic shock syndrome: I.V.: 900 mg every 8 hours with penicillin G or ceftriaxone

Dosage Forms Note: Strength is expressed as base

Capsule, as hydrochloride: 150 mg, 300 mg

Cleocin HCl®: 75 mg [contains tartrazine], 150 mg [contains tartrazine], 300 mg

Cream, vaginal, as phosphate:

Cleocin®: 2% (40 g) [contains benzyl alcohol and mineral oil; packaged with 7 disposable applicators]

Clindesse™: 2% (5 g) [contains mineral oil; prefilled single disposable applicator]

Foam, topical, as phosphate (Evoclin™): 1% (50 g, 100 g) [contains ethanol 58%]

Gel, topical, as phosphate: 1% [10 mg/g] (30 g, 60 g)

Cleocin T®: 1% [10 mg/g] (30 g, 60 g)

Clindagel®: 1% [10 mg/g] (40 mL, 75 mL)

ClindaMax™: 1% (30 g, 60 g)

Granules for oral solution, as palmitate (Cleocin Pediatric®): 75 mg/5 mL (100 mL) [cherry flavor]

Infusion, as phosphate [premixed in D_5W] (Cleocin Phosphate®): 300 mg (50 mL); 600 mg (50 mL); 900 mg (50 mL)

Injection, solution, as phosphate (Cleocin Phosphate®): 150 mg/mL (2 mL, 4 mL, 6 mL, 60 mL) [contains benzyl alcohol and disodium edetate 0.5 mg]

Lotion, as phosphate (Cleocin T®, ClindaMax™): 1% [10 mg/mL] (60 mL)

Pledgets, topical: 1% (60s) [contains alcohol]

Cleocin T®: 1% (60s) [contains isopropyl alcohol 50%]

Clindets®: 1% (69s) [contains isopropyl alcohol 52%]

Solution, topical, as phosphate (Cleocin T®): 1% [10 mg/mL] (30 mL, 60 mL) [contains isopropyl alcohol 50%]

Suppository (ovule), vaginal, as phosphate (Cleocin®): 100 mg (3s) [contains oleaginous base; single reusable applicator]

clindamycin and benzoyl peroxide (klin da MYE sin & BEN zoe il peer OKS ide)

Synonyms benzoyl peroxide and clindamycin; clindamycin phosphate and benzoyl peroxide

U.S./Canadian Brand Names BenzaClin® [US/Can]; Duac™ [US]

Therapeutic Category Topical Skin Product; Topical Skin Product, Acne

Use Topical treatment of acne vulgaris

Usual Dosage Topical: Children ≥12 years and Adults: Apply to affected areas after skin has been cleansed and dried

BenzaClin®: Acne: Apply twice daily (morning and evening)

Duac™: Inflammatory acne: Apply once daily in the evening

Dosage Forms Gel, topical:

BenzaClin®: Clindamycin phosphate 1% and benzoyl peroxide 5% (25 g, 50 g)

Duac™: Clindamycin phosphate 1% and benzoyl peroxide 5% (45 g)

clindamycin hydrochloride *see* clindamycin *on previous page*

Clindamycin Injection, USP [Can] *see* clindamycin *on previous page*

clindamycin palmitate *see* clindamycin *on previous page*

clindamycin phosphate *see* clindamycin *on previous page*

clindamycin phosphate and benzoyl peroxide *see* clindamycin and benzoyl peroxide *on this page*

Clindesse™ [US] *see* clindamycin *on previous page*

Clindets® [US] *see* clindamycin *on previous page*

Clindex® *(Discontinued)* *see* clidinium and chlordiazepoxide *on previous page*

Clindoxyl® [Can] *see* clindamycin *on previous page*

Clinoril® [US] *see* sulindac *on page 800*

clioquinol and flumethasone *(Canada only)* (klye ok KWIN ole & floo METH a sone)

Synonyms flumethasone and clioquinol; iodochlorhydroxyquin and flumethasone

U.S./Canadian Brand Names Locacorten® Vioform® [Can]

Therapeutic Category Antibiotic, Topical; Corticosteroid, Topical

Use Treatment of corticosteroid-responsive dermatoses complicated by infection with bacterial and/or fungal agents

Usual Dosage Children >2 years and Adults:

Otic solution (drops): Instill 2-3 drops into affected ear(s) 2 times/day; generally limit duration to 10 days

Topical: Apply in a thin layer to affected area 2-3 times/day; generally limit duration to 7 days

Dosage Forms [CAN] = Canadian brand name

Cream, topical (Locacorten® Vioform® [CAN]): Clioquinol 3% and flumethasone pivalate 0.02% (15 g, 50 g) [not available in the U.S.]

Solution, otic (Locacorten® Vioform® [CAN]): Clioquinol 1% and flumethasone pivalate 0.02% (10 mL) [not available in the U.S.]

Clobazam-10 [Can] *see* clobazam *(Canada only)* *on this page*

clobazam *(Canada only)* (KLOE ba zam)

U.S./Canadian Brand Names Alti-Clobazam [Can]; Apo-Clobazam® [Can]; Clobazam-10 [Can]; Dom-Clobazam [Can]; Frisium® [Can]; Novo-Clobazam [Can]; PMS-Clobazam [Can]; ratio-Clobazam [Can]

Therapeutic Category Anticonvulsant; Antidepressant

Use Adjunctive treatment of epilepsy

Usual Dosage Oral:

Children:

<2 years: Initial 0.5-1 mg/kg/day

2-16 years: Initial: 5 mg/day; may be increased (no more frequently than every 5 days) to a maximum of 40 mg/day

Adults: Initial: 5-15 mg/day; dosage may be gradually adjusted (based on tolerance and seizure control) to a maximum of 80 mg/day

Note: Daily doses of up to 30 mg may be taken as a single dose at bedtime; higher doses should be divided.

Dosage Forms [CAN] = Canadian brand name

Tablet: 10 mg

Alti-Clobazam [CAN], Apo-Clobazam® [CAN], Clobazam-10 [CAN], Dom-Clobazam [CAN], Frisium® [CAN], Novo-Clobazam [CAN], PMS-Clobazam [CAN], ration-Clobazam [CAN]: 10 mg [not available in the U.S.]

clobetasol (kloe BAY ta sol)

Synonyms clobetasol propionate

U.S./Canadian Brand Names Clobevate® [US]; Clobex® [US/Can]; Cormax® [US]; Dermovate® [Can]; Gen-Clobetasol [Can]; Novo-Clobetasol [Can]; Olux® [US]; Taro-Clobetasol [Can]; Temovate E® [US]; Temovate® [US]

Therapeutic Category Corticosteroid, Topical

Use Short-term relief of inflammation of moderate-to-severe corticosteroid-responsive dermatoses (very high potency topical corticosteroid)

Usual Dosage Topical: Discontinue when control achieved; if improvement not seen within 2 weeks, reassessment of diagnosis may be necessary.

Children ≥12 years and Adults:

Steroid-responsive dermatoses:

Cream, emollient cream, gel, ointment: Apply twice daily for up to 2 weeks (maximum dose: 50 g/week)

Foam, solution: Apply to affected scalp twice daily for up to 2 weeks (maximum dose: 50 g/week or 50 mL/week)

Mild-to-moderate plaque-type psoriasis of nonscalp areas: Foam: Apply to affected area twice daily for up to 2 weeks (maximum dose: 50 g/week); do not apply to face or intertriginous areas

Children ≥16 years and Adults: Moderate-to-severe plaque-type psoriasis: Emollient cream, lotion: Apply twice daily for up to 2 weeks, has been used for up to 4 weeks when application is <10% of body surface area; use with caution (maximum dose: 50 g/week)

Children ≥18 years and Adults:

Moderate-to-severe plaque-type psoriasis: Spray: Apply by spraying directly onto affected area twice daily; should be gently rubbed into skin. Should be used for not longer than 4 weeks; treatment beyond 2 weeks should be limited to localized lesions which have not improved sufficiently. Total dose should not exceed 50 g/week or 59 mL/week.

Scalp psoriasis: Shampoo: Apply thin film to dry scalp once daily; leave in place for 15 minutes, then add water, lather; rinse thoroughly

Steroid-responsive dermatoses: Lotion: Apply twice daily for up to 2 weeks (maximum dose: 50 g/week)

Dosage Forms [DSC] = Discontinued product

Cream, as propionate: 0.05% (15 g, 30 g, 45 g, 60 g)
Cormax®: 0.05% (30 g)
Embeline™ [DSC], Temovate®: 0.05% (15 g, 30 g, 45 g, 60 g)
Cream, as propionate [in emollient base]: 0.05% (15 g, 30 g, 60 g)
Embeline™ E: 0.05% (15 g, 30 g, 60 g) [DSC]
Temovate E®: 0.05% (15 g [DSC], 30 g, 60 g)
Foam, topical, as propionate [for scalp application] (Olux®): 0.05% (50 g, 100 g) [contains ethanol 60%]
Gel, as propionate: 0.05% (15 g, 30 g, 60 g)
Clobevate®, Embeline™ [DSC]: 0.05% (15 g, 30 g, 60 g)
Temovate®: 0.05% (15 g [DSC], 30 g, 60 g)
Lotion, as propionate (Clobex®): 0.05% (30 mL, 59 mL)
Ointment, as propionate: 0.05% (15 g, 30 g, 45 g, 60 g)
Cormax®: 0.05% (15 g, 45 g)
Embeline™: 0.05% (15 g, 30 g, 45 g, 60 g) [DSC]
Temovate®: 0.05% (15 g, 30 g, 45 g [DSC], 60 g)
Shampoo, as propionate:
Clobex®: 0.05% (120 mL) [contains alcohol]
Solution, topical, as propionate [for scalp application]: 0.05% (25 mL, 50 mL)
Cormax®, Embeline™ [DSC], Temovate®: 0.05% (25 mL, 50 mL) [contains isopropyl alcohol 40%]
Spray, topical, as propionate (Clobex®): 0.05% (60 mL) [contains alcohol]

clobetasol propionate *see* clobetasol *on previous page*

Clobevate® [US] *see* clobetasol *on previous page*

Clobex® [US/Can] *see* clobetasol *on previous page*

clocortolone (kloe KOR toe lone)

Sound-Alike/Look-Alike Issues
Cloderm® may be confused with Clocort®

Synonyms clocortolone pivalate

U.S./Canadian Brand Names Cloderm® [US/Can]

Therapeutic Category Corticosteroid, Topical

Use Inflammation of corticosteroid-responsive dermatoses (intermediate-potency topical corticosteroid)

Usual Dosage Adults: Apply sparingly and gently; rub into affected area from 1-4 times/day. Therapy should be discontinued when control is achieved; if no improvement is seen, reassessment of diagnosis may be necessary.

Dosage Forms Cream, as pivalate: 0.1% (15 g, 45 g, 90 g)

clocortolone pivalate *see* clocortolone *on this page*

Cloderm® [US/Can] *see* clocortolone *on this page*

clodronate *(Canada only)* (KLOE droh nate)

Synonyms clodronate disodium

U.S./Canadian Brand Names Bonefos® [Can]; Clasteon® [Can]; Ostac® [Can]

Therapeutic Category Bisphosphonate Derivative

Use Management of hypercalcemia of malignancy

Usual Dosage

I.V.:
Multiple infusions: 300 mg/day; should not be prolonged beyond 10 days.
Single infusion: 1500 mg as a single dose

Oral: Recommended daily maintenance dose following I.V. therapy: Range: 1600 mg (4 capsules) to 2400 mg (6 capsules) given in single or 2 divided doses; maximum recommended daily dose: 3200 mg (8 capsules). Should be taken at least 1 hour before or after food, because food may decrease the amount of clodronate absorbed by the body.

Dosage Forms [CAN] = Canadian brand name

Injection:
Bonefos® [CAN], Ostac® [CAN]: 30 mg/mL (10 mL); 60 mg/mL (5 mL) [not available in the U.S.]
Capsule:
Bonefos® [CAN], Ostac® [CAN]: 400 mg [not available in the U.S.]

clodronate disodium *see* clodronate *(Canada only) on previous page*

clofarabine (klo FARE a been)

Synonyms Clofarex; NSC606869

U.S./Canadian Brand Names Clolar™ [US]

Therapeutic Category Antineoplastic Agent, Antimetabolite (Purine Antagonist)

Use Treatment of relapsed or refractory acute lymphoblastic leukemia

Usual Dosage I.V.: Children and Adults 1-21 years: ALL: 52 mg/m^2/day days 1 through 5; repeat every 2-6 weeks

Dosage Forms Injection, solution [preservative free]: 1 mg/mL (20 mL)

Clofarex *see* clofarabine *on this page*

Clolar™ [US] *see* clofarabine *on this page*

Clomid® [US/Can] *see* clomiphene *on this page*

clomiphene (KLOE mi feen)

Sound-Alike/Look-Alike Issues

clomiPHENE may be confused with clomiPRAMINE, clonidine
Clomid® may be confused with clonidine
Serophene® may be confused with Sarafem™

Synonyms clomiphene citrate

Tall-Man clomi**PHENE**

U.S./Canadian Brand Names Clomid® [US/Can]; Milophene® [Can]; Serophene® [US/Can]

Therapeutic Category Ovulation Stimulator

Use Treatment of ovulatory failure in patients desiring pregnancy

Usual Dosage Adults: Oral:

Male (infertility): 25 mg/day for 25 days with 5 days rest, or 100 mg every Monday, Wednesday, Friday

Female (ovulatory failure): 50 mg/day for 5 days (first course); start the regimen on or about the fifth day of cycle. The dose should be increased only in those patients who do not ovulate in response to cyclic 50 mg Clomid®. A low dosage or duration of treatment course is particularly recommended if unusual sensitivity to pituitary gonadotropin is suspected, such as in patients with polycystic ovary syndrome.

If ovulation does not appear to occur after the first course of therapy, a second course of 100 mg/day (two 50 mg tablets given as a single daily dose) for 5 days should be given. This course may be started as early as 30 days after the previous one after precautions are taken to exclude the presence of pregnancy. Increasing the dosage or duration of therapy beyond 100 mg/day for 5 days is not recommended. The majority of patients who are going to ovulate will do so after the first course of therapy. If ovulation does not occur after 3 courses of therapy, further treatment is not recommended and the patient should be reevaluated. If 3 ovulatory responses occur, but pregnancy has not been achieved, further treatment is not recommended. If menses does not occur after an ovulatory response, the patient should be reevaluated. Long-term cyclic therapy is not recommended beyond a total of about 6 cycles.

Dosage Forms Tablet, as citrate: 50 mg

clomiphene citrate *see* clomiphene *on this page*

clomipramine (kloe MI pra meen)

Sound-Alike/Look-Alike Issues

clomiPRAMINE may be confused with chlorproMAZINE, clomiPHENE, desipramine, Norpramin®
Anafranil® may be confused with alfentanil, enalapril, nafarelin

Synonyms clomipramine hydrochloride

Tall-Man clomi**PRAMINE**

U.S./Canadian Brand Names Anafranil® [US/Can]; Apo-Clomipramine® [Can]; CO Clomipramine [Can]; Gen-Clomipramine [Can]

Therapeutic Category Antidepressant, Tricyclic (Tertiary Amine)

Use Treatment of obsessive-compulsive disorder (OCD)

Usual Dosage Oral: Initial:

Children:

<10 years: Safety and efficacy have not been established.

≥10 years: OCD: 25 mg/day; gradually increase, as tolerated, to a maximum of 3 mg/kg/day or 200 mg/day (whichever is smaller)

Adults: OCD: 25 mg/day and gradually increase, as tolerated, to 100 mg/day the first 2 weeks, may then be increased to a total of 250 mg/day maximum

Dosage Forms Capsule, as hydrochloride: 25 mg, 50 mg, 75 mg

clomipramine hydrochloride *see* clomipramine *on previous page*

Clonapam [Can] *see* clonazepam *on this page*

clonazepam (kloe NA ze pam)

Sound-Alike/Look-Alike Issues

clonazepam may be confused with clofazimine, clonidine, clorazepate, clozapine, lorazepam

Klonopin® may be confused with clofazimine, clonidine, clorazepate, clozapine, lorazepam

U.S./Canadian Brand Names Alti-Clonazepam [Can]; Apo-Clonazepam® [Can]; Clonapam [Can]; CO Clonazepam [Can]; Gen-Clonazepam [Can]; Klonopin® [US/Can]; Novo-Clonazepam [Can]; Nu-Clonazepam [Can]; PMS-Clonazepam [Can]; Rho®-Clonazepam [Can]; Rivotril® [Can]; Sandoz-Clonazepam [Can]

Therapeutic Category Benzodiazepine

Controlled Substance C-IV

Use Alone or as an adjunct in the treatment of petit mal variant (Lennox-Gastaut), akinetic, and myoclonic seizures; petit mal (absence) seizures unresponsive to succimides; panic disorder with or without agoraphobia

Usual Dosage Oral:

Children <10 years or 30 kg: Seizure disorders:

Initial daily dose: 0.01-0.03 mg/kg/day (maximum: 0.05 mg/kg/day) given in 2-3 divided doses; increase by no more than 0.5 mg every third day until seizures are controlled or adverse effects seen

Usual maintenance dose: 0.1-0.2 mg/kg/day divided 3 times/day, not to exceed 0.2 mg/kg/day

Adults:

Burning mouth syndrome (dental use): 0.25-3 mg/day in 2 divided doses, in morning and evening

Seizure disorders:

Initial daily dose not to exceed 1.5 mg given in 3 divided doses; may increase by 0.5-1 mg every third day until seizures are controlled or adverse effects seen (maximum: 20 mg/day)

Usual maintenance dose: 0.05-0.2 mg/kg; do not exceed 20 mg/day

Panic disorder: 0.25 mg twice daily; increase in increments of 0.125-0.25 mg twice daily every 3 days; target dose: 1 mg/day (maximum: 4 mg/day)

Discontinuation of treatment: To discontinue, treatment should be withdrawn gradually. Decrease dose by 0.125 mg twice daily every 3 days until medication is completely withdrawn.

Dosage Forms

Tablet: 0.5 mg, 1 mg, 2 mg

Tablet, orally disintegrating [wafer]: 0.125 mg, 0.25 mg, 0.5 mg, 1 mg, 2 mg

clonidine (KLON i deen)

Sound-Alike/Look-Alike Issues

clonidine may be confused with Clomid®, clomiPHENE, clonazepam, clozapine, Klonopin™, Loniten®, quinidine

Catapres® may be confused with Cataflam®, Cetapred®, Combipres®

Synonyms clonidine hydrochloride

U.S./Canadian Brand Names Apo-Clonidine® [Can]; Carapres® [Can]; Catapres-TTS® [US]; Catapres® [US]; Dixarit® [Can]; Duraclon™ [US]; Novo-Clonidine [Can]; Nu-Clonidine [Can]

Therapeutic Category Alpha-Adrenergic Agonist

Use Management of mild-to-moderate hypertension; either used alone or in combination with other antihypertensives

Orphan drug: Duraclon™: For continuous epidural administration as adjunctive therapy with intraspinal opiates for treatment of cancer pain in patients tolerant to or unresponsive to intraspinal opiates

Usual Dosage

Children:

Oral:

Hypertension: Initial: 5-10 mcg/kg/day in divided doses every 8-12 hours; increase gradually at 5- to 7-day intervals to 25 mcg/kg/day in divided doses every 6 hours; maximum: 0.9 mg/day

Clonidine tolerance test (test of growth hormone release from pituitary): 0.15 mg/m^2 or 4 mcg/kg as single dose

Epidural infusion: Pain management: Reserved for patients with severe intractable pain, unresponsive to other analgesics or epidural or spinal opiates: Initial: 0.5 mcg/kg/hour; adjust with caution, based on clinical effect

(Continued)

clonidine *(Continued)*

Adults:

Oral:

Acute hypertension (urgency): Initial 0.1-0.2 mg; may be followed by additional doses of 0.1 mg every hour, if necessary, to a maximum total dose of 0.6 mg.

Hypertension: Initial dose: 0.1 mg twice daily (maximum recommended dose: 2.4 mg/day); usual dose range (JNC 7): 0.1-0.8 mg/day in 2 divided doses

Nicotine withdrawal symptoms: 0.1 mg twice daily to maximum of 0.4 mg/day for 3-4 weeks

Transdermal: Hypertension: Apply once every 7 days; for initial therapy start with 0.1 mg and increase by 0.1 mg at 1- to 2-week intervals (dosages >0.6 mg do not improve efficacy); usual dose range (JNC 7): 0.1-0.3 mg once weekly

Note: If transitioning from oral to transdermal therapy, overlap oral regimen for 1-2 days; transdermal route takes 2-3 days to achieve therapeutic effects.

Conversion from oral to transdermal:

Day 1: Place Catapres-TTS® 1; administer 100% of oral dose.

Day 2: Administer 50% of oral dose.

Day 3: Administer 25% of oral dose.

Day 4: Patch remains, no further oral supplement necessary.

Epidural infusion: Pain management: Starting dose: 30 mcg/hour; titrate as required for relief of pain or presence of side effects; minimal experience with doses >40 mcg/hour; should be considered an adjunct to intraspinal opiate therapy

Dosage Forms

Injection, epidural solution, as hydrochloride [preservative free] (Duraclon™): 100 mcg/mL (10 mL); 500 mcg/mL (10 mL)

Patch, transdermal [once-weekly patch]:

Catapres-TTS®-1: 0.1 mg/24 hours (4s)

Catapres-TTS®-2: 0.2 mg/24 hours (4s)

Catapres-TTS®-3: 0.3 mg/24 hours (4s)

Tablet, as hydrochloride (Catapres®): 0.1 mg, 0.2 mg, 0.3 mg

clonidine and chlorthalidone (KLON i deen & klor THAL i done)

Sound-Alike/Look-Alike Issues

Combipres® may be confused with Catapres®

Synonyms chlorthalidone and clonidine

U.S./Canadian Brand Names Clorpres® [US]

Therapeutic Category Antihypertensive Agent, Combination

Use Management of mild-to-moderate hypertension

Usual Dosage Oral: 1 tablet 1-2 times/day; maximum: 0.6 mg clonidine and 30 mg chlorthalidone

Dosage Forms Tablet:

0.1: Clonidine hydrochloride 0.1 mg and chlorthalidone 15 mg

0.2: Clonidine hydrochloride 0.2 mg and chlorthalidone 15 mg

0.3: Clonidine hydrochloride 0.3 mg and chlorthalidone 15 mg

clonidine hydrochloride *see* clonidine *on previous page*

clopidogrel (kloh PID oh grel)

Sound-Alike/Look-Alike Issues

Plavix® may be confused with Elavil®, Paxil®

Synonyms clopidogrel bisulfate

U.S./Canadian Brand Names Plavix® [US/Can]

Therapeutic Category Antiplatelet Agent

Use Reduces rate of atherothrombotic events (myocardial infarction, stroke, vascular deaths) in patients with recent MI or stroke, or established peripheral arterial disease; reduces rate of atherothrombotic events in patients with unstable angina or non-ST-segment elevation acute coronary syndromes (unstable angina and non-ST-segment elevation MI) managed medically or through PCI (with or without stent) or CABG; reduces rate of death and atherothrombotic events in patients with ST-segment elevation MI (STEMI) managed medically

Usual Dosage Oral: Adults:

Recent MI, recent stroke, or established arterial disease: 75 mg once daily

Acute coronary syndrome: Initial: 300 mg loading dose, followed by 75 mg once daily (in combination with aspirin 75-325 mg once daily). **Note:** A loading dose of 600 mg has been used in some investigations; limited research exists comparing the two doses.

Dosage Forms
Tablet:
Plavix®: 75 mg

clopidogrel bisulfate *see* clopidogrel *on previous page*

Clopixol® [Can] *see* zuclopenthixol *(Canada only) on page 891*

Clopixol-Acuphase® [Can] *see* zuclopenthixol *(Canada only) on page 891*

Clopixol® Depot [Can] *see* zuclopenthixol *(Canada only) on page 891*

clorazepate (klor AZ e pate)

Sound-Alike/Look-Alike Issues
clorazepate may be confused with clofibrate, clonazepam, lorazepam

Synonyms clorazepate dipotassium

U.S./Canadian Brand Names Apo-Clorazepate® [Can]; Novo-Clopate [Can]; Tranxene® SD™ [US]; Tranxene® SD™-Half Strength [US]; Tranxene® T-Tab® [US]

Therapeutic Category Anticonvulsant; Benzodiazepine

Controlled Substance C-IV

Use Treatment of generalized anxiety disorder; management of ethanol withdrawal; adjunct anticonvulsant in management of partial seizures

Usual Dosage Oral:
Children 9-12 years: Anticonvulsant: Initial: 3.75-7.5 mg/dose twice daily; increase dose by 3.75 mg at weekly intervals, not to exceed 60 mg/day in 2-3 divided doses
Children >12 years and Adults: Anticonvulsant: Initial: Up to 7.5 mg/dose 2-3 times/day; increase dose by 7.5 mg at weekly intervals, not to exceed 90 mg/day
Adults:
Anxiety:
Regular release tablets (Tranxene® T-Tab®): 7.5-15 mg 2-4 times/day
Sustained release (Tranxene® SD): 11.25 or 22.5 mg once daily at bedtime
Ethanol withdrawal: Initial: 30 mg, then 15 mg 2-4 times/day on first day; maximum daily dose: 90 mg; gradually decrease dose over subsequent days

Dosage Forms
Tablet, as dipotassium: 3.75 mg, 7.5 mg, 15 mg
Tranxene® SD™: 22.5 mg [once daily]
Tranxene® SD™-Half Strength: 11.25 mg [once daily]
Tranxene® T-Tab®: 3.75 mg, 7.5 mg, 15 mg

clorazepate dipotassium *see* clorazepate *on this page*

Clorpactin® WCS-90 [US-OTC] *see* oxychlorosene *on page 626*

Clorpres® [US] *see* clonidine and chlorthalidone *on previous page*

Clotrimaderm [Can] *see* clotrimazole *on this page*

clotrimazole (kloe TRIM a zole)

Sound-Alike/Look-Alike Issues
clotrimazole may be confused with co-trimoxazole
Lotrimin® may be confused with Lotrisone®, Otrivin®
Mycelex® may be confused with Myoflex®

U.S./Canadian Brand Names Canesten® Topical [Can]; Canesten® Vaginal [Can]; Clotrimaderm [Can]; Cruex® Cream [US-OTC]; Gyne-Lotrimin® 3 [US-OTC]; Lotrimin® AF Athlete's Foot Cream [US-OTC]; Lotrimin® AF Athlete's Foot Solution [US-OTC]; Lotrimin® AF Jock Itch Cream [US-OTC]; Mycelex® Twin Pack [US-OTC]; Mycelex® [US]; Mycelex®-7 [US-OTC]; Trivagizole-3® [Can]

Therapeutic Category Antifungal Agent

Use Treatment of susceptible fungal infections, including oropharyngeal candidiasis, dermatophytoses, superficial mycoses, and cutaneous candidiasis, as well as vulvovaginal candidiasis; limited data suggest that clotrimazole troches may be effective for prophylaxis against oropharyngeal candidiasis in neutropenic patients

Usual Dosage
Children >3 years and Adults:
Oral:
Prophylaxis: 10 mg troche dissolved 3 times/day for the duration of chemotherapy or until steroids are reduced to maintenance levels
Treatment: 10 mg troche dissolved slowly 5 times/day for 14 consecutive days
(Continued)

clotrimazole *(Continued)*

Topical (cream, solution): Apply twice daily; if no improvement occurs after 4 weeks of therapy, reevaluate diagnosis

Children >12 years and Adults:

Vaginal:

Cream:

1%: Insert 1 applicatorful vaginal cream daily (preferably at bedtime) for 7 consecutive days

2%: Insert 1 applicatorful vaginal cream daily (preferably at bedtime) for 3 consecutive days

Tablet: Insert 100 mg/day for 7 days or 500 mg single dose

Topical (cream, solution): Apply to affected area twice daily (morning and evening) for 7 consecutive days

Dosage Forms

Combination pack (Mycelex®-7): Vaginal tablet 100 mg (7s) and vaginal cream 1% (7 g)

Cream, topical: 1% (15 g, 30 g, 45 g)

Cruex®: 1% (15 g)

Lotrimin® AF Athlete's Foot: 1% (12 g, 24 g)

Lotrimin® AF Jock Itch: 1% (12 g)

Cream, vaginal: 2% (21 g)

Mycelex®-7: 1% (45 g)

Solution, topical: 1% (10 mL, 30 mL)

Lotrimin® AF Athlete's Foot: 1% (10 mL)

Tablet, vaginal (Gyne-Lotrimin® 3): 200 mg (3s)

Troche (Mycelex®): 10 mg

clotrimazole and betamethasone *see* betamethasone and clotrimazole *on page 107*

cloxacillin (kloks a SIL in)

Synonyms cloxacillin sodium

U.S./Canadian Brand Names Apo-Cloxi® [Can]; Novo-Cloxin [Can]; Nu-Cloxi [Can]; Riva-Cloxacillin [Can]

Therapeutic Category Penicillin

Use Treatment of susceptible bacterial infections, notably penicillinase-producing staphylococci causing respiratory tract, skin and skin structure, bone and joint, urinary tract infections

Usual Dosage Oral:

Children >1 month and <20 kg: 50-100 mg/kg/day in divided doses every 6 hours; (maximum: 4 g/day)

Children >20 kg and Adults: 250-500 mg every 6 hours

Dosage Forms

Capsule, as sodium: 250 mg, 500 mg

Powder for oral suspension, as sodium: 125 mg/5 mL (100 mL, 200 mL)

cloxacillin sodium *see* cloxacillin *on this page*

Cloxapen® ***(Discontinued)*** *see* cloxacillin *on this page*

clozapine (KLOE za peen)

Sound-Alike/Look-Alike Issues

clozapine may be confused with clofazimine, clonidine, Klonopin®

Clozaril® may be confused with Clinoril®, Colazal®

U.S./Canadian Brand Names Apo-Clozapine® [Can]; Clozaril® [US/Can]; FazaClo® [US]; Gen-Clozapine [Can]

Therapeutic Category Antipsychotic Agent, Dibenzodiazepine

Use Treatment-refractory schizophrenia; to reduce risk of recurrent suicidal behavior in schizophrenia or schizoaffective disorder

Usual Dosage Oral: Adults:

Schizophrenia: Initial: 12.5 mg once or twice daily; increased, as tolerated, in increments of 25-50 mg/day to a target dose of 300-450 mg/day after 2-4 weeks, may require doses as high as 600-900 mg/day

Reduce risk of suicidal behavior: Initial: 12.5 mg once or twice daily; increased, as tolerated, in increments of 25-50 mg/day to a target dose of 300-450 mg/day after 2-4 weeks; median dose is ~300 mg/day (range: 12.5-900 mg)

Termination of therapy: If dosing is interrupted for ≥48 hours, therapy must be reinitiated at 12.5-25 mg/day; may be increased more rapidly than with initial titration, unless cardiopulmonary arrest occurred during initial titration.

In the event of planned termination of clozapine, gradual reduction in dose over a 1- to 2-week period is recommended. If conditions warrant abrupt discontinuation (leukopenia), monitor patient for psychosis and cholinergic rebound (headache, nausea, vomiting, diarrhea).

Patients discontinued on clozapine therapy due to WBC <2000/mm^3 or ANC <1000/mm^3 should not be restarted on clozapine.

Dosage Forms

Tablet: 12.5 mg, 25 mg, 100 mg

Clozaril®: 25 mg, 100 mg

Tablet, orally disintegrating (FazaClo®): 25 mg [contains phenylalanine 1.75 mg; mint flavor], 100 mg [contains phenylalanine 6.96 mg; mint flavor]

Clozaril® [US/Can] *see* clozapine *on previous page*

Clysodrast® *(Discontinued)* *see* bisacodyl *on page 111*

CMA-676 *see* gemtuzumab ozogamicin *on page 379*

CMV-IGIV *see* cytomegalovirus immune globulin (intravenous-human) *on page 225*

CoActifed® [Can] *see* triprolidine, pseudoephedrine, and codeine *(Canada only) on page 853*

coagulant complex inhibitor *see* anti-inhibitor coagulant complex *on page 61*

coagulation factor VIIa *see* factor VIIa (recombinant) *on page 333*

CO Alendronate [Can] *see* alendronate *on page 27*

coal tar (KOLE tar)

Sound-Alike/Look-Alike Issues

Pentrax® may be confused with Permax®

Tegrin® may be confused with Tegretol®

Synonyms crude coal tar; LCD; pix carbonis

U.S./Canadian Brand Names Balnetar® [US-OTC/Can]; Betatar® Gel [US-OTC]; Cutar® [US-OTC]; Denorex® Original Therapeutic Strength [US-OTC]; DHS™ Tar [US-OTC]; DHS™ Targel [US-OTC]; Doak® Tar [US-OTC]; Estar® [Can]; Exorex® [US]; Fototar® [US-OTC]; Ionil T® Plus [US-OTC]; Ionil T® [US-OTC]; MG 217® Medicated Tar [US-OTC]; MG 217® [US-OTC]; Neutrogena® T/Gel Extra Strength [US-OTC]; Neutrogena® T/Gel Stubborn Itch Control [US-OTC]; Neutrogena® T/Gel [US-OTC]; Oxipor® VHC [US-OTC]; Polytar® [US-OTC]; Reme-T™ [US-OTC]; Targel® [Can]; Tera-Gel™ [US-OTC]; Zetar® [US-OTC]

Therapeutic Category Antipsoriatic Agent; Antiseborrheic Agent, Topical

Use Topically for controlling dandruff, seborrheic dermatitis, or psoriasis

Usual Dosage Topical:

Bath: Add appropriate amount to bath water; for adults usually 60-90 mL of a 5% to 20% solution or 15-25 mL of 30% lotion; soak 5-20 minutes, then pat dry; use once daily to 3 days

Shampoo: Rub shampoo onto wet hair and scalp, rinse thoroughly; repeat; leave on 5 minutes; rinse thoroughly; apply twice weekly for the first 2 weeks then once weekly or more often if needed

Soap: Use on affected areas in place of regular soap. Work into a lather using warm water; massage into skin; rinse.

Skin: Apply to the affected area 1-4 times/day; decrease frequency to 2-3 times/week once condition has been controlled

Scalp psoriasis: Tar oil bath or coal tar solution may be painted sparingly to the lesions 3-12 hours before each shampoo

Psoriasis of the body, arms, legs: Apply at bedtime; if thick scales are present, use product with salicylic acid and apply several times during the day

Dosage Forms [DSC] = Discontinued product

Cream:

Fototar®: Coal tar 2% (85 g, 454 g)

Emulsion, topical:

Cutar®: Coal tar solution 7.5% (180 mL, 3840 mL)

Exorex®: Coal tar 1% (240 mL)

Gel, shampoo:

DHS™ Targel: Coal tar solution 2.9% (240 mL) [equivalent to coal tar 0.5%]

Gel, topical:

PsoriGel®: Coal tar solution 7.5% (120 g) [DSC]

Liquid:

Doak® Tar Distillate: Coal tar 40% (60 mL) [for compounding use only]

Lotion, topical:

MG 217®: Coal tar solution 5% (120 mL) [equivalent to coal tar 1%; contains jojoba]

Oxipor® VHC: Coal tar solution 25% (60 mL, 120 mL) [equivalent to coal tar 5%; contains alcohol 79%]

Oil, topical:

Balnetar®: Coal tar 2.5% (225 mL) [for use in bath]

Doak® Tar: Coal tar distillate 2% (240 mL) [equivalent to coal tar 0.8%; for use in bath]

(Continued)

coal tar *(Continued)*

Ointment, topical:
MG 217®: Coal tar solution 10% (107 g, 430 g) [equivalent to coal tar 2%]
Shampoo:
Betatar Gel®: Coal tar solution 5% (240 mL) [equivalent to coal tar 2.5%; green apple scent]
Denorex® Original Therapeutic Strength: Coal tar solution 12.5% (120 mL, 240 mL, 360 mL) [equivalent to coal tar 2.5%; available with or without conditioner]
DHS™ Tar: Coal tar solution 2.9% (120 mL, 240 mL, 480 mL) [equivalent to coal tar 0.5%]
Doak® Tar: Coal tar distillate 3% (240 mL) [equivalent to coal tar 1.2%]
Ionil T®: Coal tar 1% (240 mL, 480 mL, 960 mL) [DSC]
Ionil T® Plus: Coal tar 2% (240 mL)
MG 217® Medicated Tar: Coal tar solution 15% (120 mL, 240 mL) [equivalent to coal tar 3%]
Neutrogena® T/Gel: Coal tar 0.5% (132 mL, 255 mL, 480 mL)
Neutrogena® T/Gel Extra Strength: Coal tar extract 4% (132 mL) [coal tar 1%]
Neutrogena® T/Gel Stubborn Itch Control: Coal tar extract 2% (132 mL) [coal tar 0.5%]
Pentrax®: Coal tar 5% (240 mL) [DSC]
Polytar®: Coal tar 0.5% (177 mL)
Reme-T™: Coal tar 5% (236 mL)
Tera-Gel™: Solubilized coal tar 0.5% (120 mL, 240 mL)
Zetar®: Coal tar 1% (180 mL)
Soap (Polytar®): Coal tar 0.5% (113 g)

coal tar and salicylic acid (KOLE tar & sal i SIL ik AS id)

Synonyms salicylic acid and coal tar
U.S./Canadian Brand Names Sebcur/T® [Can]; Tarsum® [US-OTC]; X-Seb T® Pearl [US-OTC]; X-Seb T® Plus [US-OTC]
Therapeutic Category Antipsoriatic Agent; Antiseborrheic Agent, Topical
Use Seborrheal dermatitis, dandruff, psoriasis
Usual Dosage Psoriasis: Scalp:
Gel: Apply directly to plaques; may leave in place for up to 1 hour. Apply water and work into a lather; rinse.
Shampoo: Apply to wet hair; massage into scalp; rinse.
Dosage Forms
Gel [shampoo] (Tarsum®): Coal tar solution 10% [equivalent to coal tar 2%] and salicylic acid (120 mL, 240 mL)
Shampoo, topical:
X-Seb T® Pearl: Coal tar solution 10% [equivalent to coal tar 2%] and salicylic acid (120 mL, 240 mL)
X-Seb T® Plus: Coal tar solution 10% [equivalent to coal tar 2%] and salicylic acid (120 mL, 240 mL) [conditioning shampoo]

CO Azithromycin [Can] *see* azithromycin *on page 88*

Cobex® ***(Discontinued)*** *see* cyanocobalamin *on page 219*

CO Bicalutamide [Can] *see* bicalutamide *on page 110*

cocaine (koe KANE)

Synonyms cocaine hydrochloride
Therapeutic Category Local Anesthetic
Controlled Substance C-II
Use Topical anesthesia for mucous membranes
Usual Dosage Topical application (ear, nose, throat, bronchoscopy): Dosage depends on the area to be anesthetized, tissue vascularity, technique of anesthesia, and individual patient tolerance; the lowest dose necessary to produce adequate anesthesia should be used; concentrations of 1% to 10% are used (not to exceed 1 mg/kg). Use reduced dosages for children, elderly, or debilitated patients.
Dosage Forms
Powder, as hydrochloride: 1 g, 5 g, 25 g
Solution, topical, as hydrochloride: 4% [40 mg/mL] (4 mL, 10 mL); 10% [100 mg/mL] (4 mL, 10 mL)

cocaine hydrochloride *see* cocaine *on this page*

CO Ciprofloxacin [Can] *see* ciprofloxacin *on page 190*

CO Citalopram [Can] *see* citalopram *on page 194*

CO Clomipramine [Can] *see* clomipramine *on page 202*

CO Clonazepam [Can] *see* clonazepam *on page 203*

Codal-DM [US-OTC] *see* phenylephrine, pyrilamine, and dextromethorphan *on page 664*

Codamine® *(Discontinued)*

Codamine® Pediatric *(Discontinued)*

Codehist® DH *(Discontinued)* *see* chlorpheniramine, pseudoephedrine, and codeine *on page 182*

codeine (KOE deen)

Sound-Alike/Look-Alike Issues

codeine may be confused with Cardene®, Cophene®, Cordran®, iodine, Lodine®

Synonyms codeine phosphate; codeine sulfate; methylmorphine

U.S./Canadian Brand Names Codeine Contin® [Can]

Therapeutic Category Analgesic, Narcotic; Antitussive

Controlled Substance C-II

Use Treatment of mild-to-moderate pain; antitussive in lower doses; dextromethorphan has equivalent antitussive activity but has much lower toxicity in accidental overdose

Usual Dosage Note: These are guidelines and do not represent the maximum doses that may be required in all patients. Doses should be titrated to pain relief/prevention. Doses >1.5 mg/kg body weight are not recommended.

Analgesic:

Children: Oral, I.M., SubQ: 0.5-1 mg/kg/dose every 4-6 hours as needed; maximum: 60 mg/dose

Adults:

Oral: 30 mg every 4-6 hours as needed; patients with prior opiate exposure may require higher initial doses. Usual range: 15-120 mg every 4-6 hours as needed

Oral, controlled release formulation (Codeine Contin®, not available in U.S.): 50-300 mg every 12 hours. **Note:** A patient's codeine requirement should be established using prompt release formulations; conversion to long acting products may be considered when chronic, continuous treatment is required. Higher dosages should be reserved for use only in opioid-tolerant patients.

I.M., SubQ: 30 mg every 4-6 hours as needed; patients with prior opiate exposure may require higher initial doses. Usual range: 15-120 mg every 4-6 hours as needed; more frequent dosing may be needed

Antitussive: Oral (for nonproductive cough):

Children: 1-1.5 mg/kg/day in divided doses every 4-6 hours as needed: Alternative dose according to age:

2-6 years: 2.5-5 mg every 4-6 hours as needed; maximum: 30 mg/day

6-12 years: 5-10 mg every 4-6 hours as needed; maximum: 60 mg/day

Adults: 10-20 mg/dose every 4-6 hours as needed; maximum: 120 mg/day

Dosage Forms [CAN] = Canadian brand name

Injection, as phosphate: 15 mg/mL (2 mL); 30 mg/mL (2 mL) [contains sodium metabisulfite]

Tablet, as phosphate: 30 mg, 60 mg

Tablet, as sulfate: 15 mg, 30 mg, 60 mg

Tablet, controlled release (Codeine Contin®) [CAN]: 50 mg, 100 mg, 150 mg, 200 mg [not available in U.S.]

codeine and acetaminophen *see* acetaminophen and codeine *on page 6*

codeine and butalbital compound *see* butalbital, aspirin, caffeine, and codeine *on page 129*

codeine and guaifenesin *see* guaifenesin and codeine *on page 393*

codeine and promethazine *see* promethazine and codeine *on page 704*

codeine, aspirin, and carisoprodol *see* carisoprodol, aspirin, and codeine *on page 152*

codeine, butalbital, aspirin, and caffeine *see* butalbital, aspirin, caffeine, and codeine *on page 129*

codeine, chlorpheniramine, and pseudoephedrine *see* chlorpheniramine, pseudoephedrine, and codeine *on page 182*

codeine, chlorpheniramine, phenylephrine, and potassium iodide *see* chlorpheniramine, phenylephrine, codeine, and potassium iodide *on page 182*

Codeine Contin® [Can] *see* codeine *on this page*

codeine, doxylamine, and acetaminophen *see* acetaminophen, codeine, and doxylamine *(Canada Only)* *on page 12*

codeine, guaifenesin, and pseudoephedrine *see* guaifenesin, pseudoephedrine, and codeine *on page 401*

codeine phosphate *see* codeine *on this page*

codeine, promethazine, and phenylephrine *see* promethazine, phenylephrine, and codeine *on page 705*

codeine, pseudoephedrine, and triprolidine *see* triprolidine, pseudoephedrine, and codeine *(Canada only) on page 853*

codeine sulfate *see* codeine *on previous page*

codeine, triprolidine, and pseudoephedrine *see* triprolidine, pseudoephedrine, and codeine *(Canada only) on page 853*

Codiclear® DH [US] *see* hydrocodone and guaifenesin *on page 422*

Codimal® DM [US-OTC] *see* phenylephrine, pyrilamine, and dextromethorphan *on page 664*

Codituss DM [US-OTC] *see* phenylephrine, pyrilamine, and dextromethorphan *on page 664*

cod liver oil *see* vitamin A and vitamin D *on page 876*

CO Fluoxetine [Can] *see* fluoxetine *on page 357*

Cogentin® [US] *see* benztropine *on page 104*

Co-Gesic® [US] *see* hydrocodone and acetaminophen *on page 420*

CO Glimepiride [Can] *see* glimepiride *on page 384*

Cognex® [US] *see* tacrine *on page 803*

CO Ipra-Sal [Can] *see* ipratropium and albuterol *on page 460*

Colace® [US-OTC/Can] *see* docusate *on page 270*

Colace® Adult/Children Suppositories [US-OTC] *see* glycerin *on page 388*

Colace® Infant/Children Suppositories [US-OTC] *see* glycerin *on page 388*

Colax-C® [Can] *see* docusate *on page 270*

Colazal® [US] *see* balsalazide *on page 93*

ColBenemid® ***(Discontinued)*** *see* colchicine and probenecid *on this page*

colchicine (KOL chi seen)

Therapeutic Category Antigout Agent

Use Treatment of acute gouty arthritis attacks and prevention of recurrences of such attacks

Usual Dosage

Gouty arthritis: Adults:

Prophylaxis of acute attacks: Oral: 0.6 mg twice daily; initial and/or subsequent dosage may be decreased (ie, 0.6 mg once daily) in patients at risk of toxicity or in those who are intolerant (including weakness, loose stools, or diarrhea); range: 0.6 mg every other day to 0.6 mg 3 times/day

Acute attacks:

Oral: Initial: 0.6-1.2 mg, followed by 0.6 every 1-2 hours; some clinicians recommend a maximum of 3 doses; more aggressive approaches have recommended a maximum dose of up to 6 mg. Wait at least 3 days before initiating another course of therapy

I.V.: Initial: 1-2 mg, then 0.5 mg every 6 hours until response, not to exceed total dose of 4 mg. If pain recurs, it may be necessary to administer additional daily doses. The amount of colchicine administered intravenously in an acute treatment period (generally ~1 week) should not exceed a total dose of 4 mg. Do not administer more colchicine by any route for at least 7 days after a full course of I.V. therapy.

Note: Many experts would avoid use because of potential for serious, life-threatening complications. Should not be administered to patients with renal insufficiency, hepatobiliary obstruction, patients >70 years of age, or recent oral colchicine use. Should be reserved for hospitalized patients who are under the care of a physician experienced in the use of intravenous colchicine.

Surgery: Gouty arthritis, prophylaxis of recurrent attacks: Adults: Oral: 0.6 mg/day or every other day; patients who are to undergo surgical procedures may receive 0.6 mg 3 times/day for 3 days before and 3 days after surgery

Dosage Forms

Injection, solution: 0.5 mg/mL (2 mL)

Tablet: 0.6 mg

colchicine and probenecid (KOL chi seen & proe BEN e sid)

Synonyms probenecid and colchicine

Therapeutic Category Antigout Agent

Use Treatment of chronic gouty arthritis when complicated by frequent, recurrent acute attacks of gout

Usual Dosage Adults: Oral: 1 tablet daily for 1 week, then 1 tablet twice daily thereafter

Dosage Forms Tablet: Colchicine 0.5 mg and probenecid 0.5 g

Coldcough HC [US] *see* pseudoephedrine, hydrocodone, and chlorpheniramine *on page 716*

Coldlac-LA® *(Discontinued)*

Coldloc® *(Discontinued)*

Coldmist DM [US] *see* guaifenesin, pseudoephedrine, and dextromethorphan *on page 401*

Coldtuss DR [US] *see* chlorpheniramine, phenylephrine, and dextromethorphan *on page 179*

colesevelam (koh le SEV a lam)

U.S./Canadian Brand Names WelChol® [US/Can]

Therapeutic Category Antihyperlipidemic Agent, Miscellaneous; Bile Acid Sequestrant

Use Adjunctive therapy to diet and exercise in the management of elevated LDL in primary hypercholesterolemia (Fredrickson type IIa) when used alone or in combination with an HMG-CoA reductase inhibitor

Usual Dosage Adults: Oral:

Monotherapy: 3 tablets twice daily with meals or 6 tablets once daily with a meal; maximum dose: 7 tablets/day

Combination therapy with an HMG-CoA reductase inhibitor: 4-6 tablets daily; maximum dose: 6 tablets/day

Dosage Forms

Tablet, as hydrochloride:

WelChol®: 625 mg

Colestid® [US/Can] *see* colestipol *on this page*

colestipol (koe LES ti pole)

Synonyms colestipol hydrochloride

U.S./Canadian Brand Names Colestid® [US/Can]

Therapeutic Category Antihyperlipidemic Agent, Miscellaneous

Use Adjunct in management of primary hypercholesterolemia; regression of arteriolosclerosis; relief of pruritus associated with elevated levels of bile acids; possibly used to decrease plasma half-life of digoxin in toxicity

Usual Dosage Adults: Oral:

Granules: 5-30 g/day given once or in divided doses 2-4 times/day; initial dose: 5 g 1-2 times/day; increase by 5 g at 1- to 2-month intervals

Tablets: 2-16 g/day; initial dose: 2 g 1-2 times/day; increase by 2 g at 1- to 2-month intervals

Dosage Forms

Granules, as hydrochloride:

5 g/7.5 g packet (30s, 90s) [unflavored]

5 g/7.5 g (300 g, 500 g) [unflavored]

5 g/7.5 g packet (60s) [contains phenylalanine 18.2 mg/7.5 g; orange flavor]

5 g/7.5 g (450 g) [contains phenylalanine 18.2 mg/7.5 g; orange flavor]

Tablet, as hydrochloride: 1 g

colestipol hydrochloride *see* colestipol *on this page*

CO Levetiracetam [Can] *see* levetiracetam *on page 487*

Colhist® Solution [US-OTC] *see* brompheniramine *on page 118*

colistimethate (koe lis ti METH ate)

Synonyms colistimethate sodium

U.S./Canadian Brand Names Coly-Mycin® M [US/Can]

Therapeutic Category Antibiotic, Miscellaneous

Use Treatment of infections due to sensitive strains of certain gram-negative bacilli which are resistant to other antibacterials or in patients allergic to other antibacterials

Usual Dosage Children and Adults:

I.M., I.V.: 2.5-5 mg/kg/day in 2-4 divided doses

Inhalation: 50-75 mg in NS (3-4 mL total) via nebulizer 2-3 times/day

Dosage Forms Injection, powder for reconstitution: 150 mg

colistimethate sodium *see* colistimethate *on this page*

colistin, neomycin, hydrocortisone, and thonzonium *see* neomycin, colistin, hydrocortisone, and thonzonium *on page 583*

collagen *see* collagen hemostat *on next page*

collagen absorbable hemostat *see* collagen hemostat *on next page*

collagenase (KOL la je nase)

U.S./Canadian Brand Names Santyl® [US]

Therapeutic Category Enzyme

Use Promotes debridement of necrotic tissue in dermal ulcers and severe burns

Orphan drug: Injection: Treatment of Peyronie disease; treatment of Dupytren disease

Usual Dosage Topical: Apply once daily (or more frequently if the dressing becomes soiled)

Dosage Forms Ointment: 250 units/g (15 g, 30 g)

collagen hemostat (KOL la jen HEE moe stat)

Sound-Alike/Look-Alike Issues

Avitene® may be confused with Ativan®

Synonyms collagen; collagen absorbable hemostat; MCH; microfibrillar collagen hemostat

U.S./Canadian Brand Names Avitene® Flour [US]; Avitene® Ultrafoam [US]; Avitene® UltraWrap™ [US]; Avitene® [US]; EndoAvitene® [US]; Helistat® [US]; Helitene® [US]; Instat™ MCH [US]; Instat™ [US]; SyringeAvitene™ [US]

Therapeutic Category Hemostatic Agent

Use Adjunct to hemostasis when control of bleeding by ligature is ineffective or impractical

Usual Dosage Apply dry directly to source of bleeding; remove excess material after ~10-15 minutes

Dosage Forms

Pad (Instat™) [bovine derived]: 1 inch x 2 inch (24s); 3 inch x 4 inch (24s)

Powder:

Avitene® Flour [microfibrillar product, bovine derived]: 0.5 g, 1 g, 5 g

Helitene® [bovine derived]: 0.5 g, 1 g

Instat™ MCH [microfibrillar product, bovine derived]: 0.5 g, 1 g

SyringeAvitene™ [microfibrillar product, bovine derived, prefilled syringe]: 1 g

Sheet:

Avitene® [microfibrillar product, bovine derived, nonwoven web]: 35 mm x 35 mm (1s); 70 mm x 35 mm (6s, 12s); 70 mm x 70 mm (6s, 12s)

EndoAvitene® [microfibrillar product, bovine derived, preloaded applicator]: 5 mm diameter (6s); 10 mm diameter (6s)

Sponge:

Avitene® Ultrafoam [microfibrillar product, bovine derived]: 2 cm x 6.25 cm x 7 mm (12s); 8 cm x 6.25 cm x 1 cm (6s); 8 cm x 12.5 cm x 1 cm (6s); 8 cm x 12.5 cm x 3 mm (6s)

Avitene® UltraWrap™ [microfibrillar product, bovine derived]: 8 cm x 12.5 cm (6s)

Helistat® [bovine derived]: 0.5 inch x 1 inch x 7 mm (18s) [packaged as 3 strips of 6 sponges]; 3 inch x 4 inch x 5 inch (10s)

Colo-Fresh™ [US-OTC] *see* bismuth subsalicylate *on page 112*

CO Lovastatin [Can] *see* lovastatin *on page 508*

Coly-Mycin® M [US/Can] *see* colistimethate *on previous page*

Coly-Mycin® S [US] *see* neomycin, colistin, hydrocortisone, and thonzonium *on page 583*

Colyte® [US/Can] *see* polyethylene glycol-electrolyte solution *on page 679*

Combantrin™ [Can] *see* pyrantel pamoate *on page 719*

CombiPatch® [US] *see* estradiol and norethindrone *on page 310*

Combipres® *(Discontinued)* *see* clonidine and chlorthalidone *on page 204*

Combivent® [US/Can] *see* ipratropium and albuterol *on page 460*

Combivir® [US/Can] *see* zidovudine and lamivudine *on page 886*

CO Meloxicam [Can] *see* meloxicam *on page 526*

Comfort® Ophthalmic *(Discontinued)* *see* naphazoline *on page 577*

Comfort® Tears Solution *(Discontinued)* *see* artificial tears *on page 75*

Comhist® [US] *see* chlorpheniramine, phenylephrine, and phenyltoloxamine *on page 181*

CO Mirtazapine [Can] *see* mirtazapine *on page 559*

Commit® [US-OTC] *see* nicotine *on page 591*

Compazine® [Can] *see* prochlorperazine *on page 701*

Compazine® *(Discontinued)* *see* prochlorperazine *on page 701*

Compound 347™ [US] *see* enflurane *on page 292*

compound E *see* cortisone acetate *on page 215*

compound F *see* hydrocortisone (systemic) *on page 427*

compound S *see* zidovudine *on page 886*

compound S, abacavir, and lamivudine *see* abacavir, lamivudine, and zidovudine *on page 2*

Compound W® [US-OTC] *see* salicylic acid *on page 758*

Compound W® One Step Wart Remover [US-OTC] *see* salicylic acid *on page 758*

Compoz® Nighttime Sleep Aid [US-OTC] *see* diphenhydramine *on page 261*

Compro™ [US] *see* prochlorperazine *on page 701*

Comtan® [US/Can] *see* entacapone *on page 294*

Comtrex® Flu Therapy Day/Night [US-OTC] *see* acetaminophen, chlorpheniramine, and pseudoephedrine *on page 11*

Comtrex® Flu Therapy Nighttime [US-OTC] *see* acetaminophen, chlorpheniramine, and pseudoephedrine *on page 11*

Comtrex® Maximum Strength Sinus and Nasal Decongestant ***(Discontinued)*** *see* acetaminophen, chlorpheniramine, and pseudoephedrine *on page 11*

Comtrex® Non-Drowsy Cold and Cough Relief [US-OTC] *see* acetaminophen, dextromethorphan, and pseudoephedrine *on page 12*

Comtrex® Sore Throat Maximum Strength [US-OTC] *see* acetaminophen *on page 5*

Comvax® [US] *see Haemophilus* B conjugate and hepatitis B vaccine *on page 404*

Conceptrol® [US-OTC] *see* nonoxynol 9 *on page 597*

Concerta® [US/Can] *see* methylphenidate *on page 546*

Condyline™ [Can] *see* podofilox *on page 677*

Condylox® [US] *see* podofilox *on page 677*

Conex® ***(Discontinued)***

Congess® Jr ***(Discontinued)*** *see* guaifenesin and pseudoephedrine *on page 398*

Congess® Sr ***(Discontinued)*** *see* guaifenesin and pseudoephedrine *on page 398*

Congestac® [US-OTC] *see* guaifenesin and pseudoephedrine *on page 398*

conivaptan (koe NYE vap tan)

Synonyms conivaptan hydrochloride; YM087

U.S./Canadian Brand Names Vaprisol® [US]

Therapeutic Category Vasopressin Antagonist

Use Treatment of euvolemic hyponatremia in hospitalized patients

Usual Dosage I.V.: Adults:

Loading dose: 20 mg infused over 30 minutes, followed by continuous infusion of 20 mg over 24 hours

Maintenance: 20 mg/day as continuous infusion over 24 hours; may titrate to maximum of 40 mg/day if serum sodium not rising sufficiently; total duration of therapy not to exceed 4 days

Dosage Forms

Injection, solution:

Vaprisol®: 5 mg/mL (4 mL) [single-use ampul; contains propylene glycol and ethanol]

conivaptan hydrochloride *see* conivaptan *on this page*

conjugated estrogen and methyltestosterone *see* estrogens (esterified) and methyltestosterone *on page 314*

CO Norfloxacin [Can] *see* norfloxacin *on page 599*

Conray® [US] *see* radiological/contrast media (ionic) *on page 728*

Constulose® [US] *see* lactulose *on page 478*

Contac® Cold 12 Hour Relief Non Drowsy [Can] *see* pseudoephedrine *on page 712*

Contac® Cold 12 Hour Relief Non Drowsy ***(Discontinued)*** *see* pseudoephedrine *on page 712*

Contac® Cold and Sore Throat, Non Drowsy, Extra Strength [Can] *see* acetaminophen and pseudoephedrine *on page 9*

Contac® Cold-Chest Congestion, Non Drowsy, Regular Strength [Can] *see* guaifenesin and pseudoephedrine *on page 398*

Contac® Complete [Can] *see* acetaminophen, dextromethorphan, and pseudoephedrine *on page 12*

Contac® Cough, Cold and Flu Day & Night™ [Can] *see* acetaminophen, dextromethorphan, and pseudoephedrine *on page 12*

Contac® Cough Formula Liquid *(Discontinued)* *see* guaifenesin and dextromethorphan *on page 394*

Contac® Severe Cold and Flu/Non-Drowsy [US-OTC] *see* acetaminophen, dextromethorphan, and pseudoephedrine *on page 12*

Contact® Cold [US-OTC] *see* pseudoephedrine *on page 712*

ControlRx® [US] *see* fluoride *on page 354*

Contuss® *(Discontinued)*

Contuss® XT *(Discontinued)*

CO Paroxetine [Can] *see* paroxetine *on page 639*

Copaxone® [US/Can] *see* glatiramer acetate *on page 384*

Copegus® [US] *see* ribavirin *on page 743*

Cophene-B® *(Discontinued)* *see* brompheniramine *on page 118*

Cophene XP® *(Discontinued)* *see* hydrocodone, pseudoephedrine, and guaifenesin *on page 425*

copolymer-1 *see* glatiramer acetate *on page 384*

copper *see* trace metals *on page 839*

CO Pravastatin [Can] *see* pravastatin *on page 692*

Co-Pyronil® 2 Pulvules® *(Discontinued)* *see* chlorpheniramine and pseudoephedrine *on page 177*

CO Ranitidine [Can] *see* ranitidine *on page 732*

Cordarone® [US/Can] *see* amiodarone *on page 43*

Cordran® [US/Can] *see* flurandrenolide *on page 359*

Cordran® SP [US] *see* flurandrenolide *on page 359*

Cordron-D NR *(Discontinued)* *see* carbinoxamine and pseudoephedrine *on page 149*

Cordron-DM NR *(Discontinued)* *see* carbinoxamine, pseudoephedrine, and dextromethorphan *on page 150*

Cordron-HC [US] *see* pseudoephedrine, hydrocodone, and chlorpheniramine *on page 716*

Coreg® [US/Can] *see* carvedilol *on page 154*

Corfen DM [US] *see* chlorpheniramine, phenylephrine, and dextromethorphan *on page 179*

Corgard® [US/Can] *see* nadolol *on page 573*

Coricidin HBP® Chest Congestion and Cough [US-OTC] *see* guaifenesin and dextromethorphan *on page 394*

Coricidin HBP® Cold and Flu [US-OTC] *see* chlorpheniramine and acetaminophen *on page 176*

Corlopam® [US/Can] *see* fenoldopam *on page 339*

Cormax® [US] *see* clobetasol *on page 200*

Coronex® [Can] *see* isosorbide dinitrate *on page 465*

Correctol® Tablets [US-OTC] *see* bisacodyl *on page 111*

Cortaid® Intensive Therapy [US-OTC] *see* hydrocortisone (topical) *on page 428*

Cortaid® Maximum Strength [US-OTC] *see* hydrocortisone (topical) *on page 428*

Cortaid® Sensitive Skin [US-OTC] *see* hydrocortisone (topical) *on page 428*

Cortamed® [Can] *see* hydrocortisone (topical) *on page 428*

Cortatrigen® Otic *(Discontinued)* *see* neomycin, polymyxin B, and hydrocortisone *on page 584*

Cortef® [US/Can] *see* hydrocortisone (systemic) *on page 427*

Cortenema® [Can] *see* hydrocortisone (rectal) *on page 426*

Corticool® [US-OTC] *see* hydrocortisone (topical) *on page 428*

corticotropin (kor ti koe TROE pin)

Sound-Alike/Look-Alike Issues

corticotropin may be confused with corticorelin

Synonyms ACTH; adrenocorticotropic hormone; corticotropin, repository

U.S./Canadian Brand Names H.P. Acthar® Gel [US]

Therapeutic Category Adrenal Corticosteroid

Use Acute exacerbations of multiple sclerosis; diagnostic aid in adrenocortical insufficiency, severe muscle weakness in myasthenia gravis

Cosyntropin is preferred over corticotropin for diagnostic test of adrenocortical insufficiency (cosyntropin is less allergenic and test is shorter in duration)

Usual Dosage

Children:

Antiinflammatory/immunosuppressant: I.M.: 0.8 units/kg/day or 25 units/m^2/day divided every 12-24 hours

Infantile spasms: Various regimens have been used. Some neurologists recommend low-dose ACTH (5-40 units/day) for short periods (1-6 weeks), while others recommend larger doses of ACTH (40-160 units/day) for long periods of treatment (3-12 months). Well designed comparative dosing studies are needed.

Example of low dose regimen:

Initial: I.M.: 20 units/day for 2 weeks, if patient responds, taper and discontinue; if patient does not respond, increase dose to 30 units/day for 4 weeks then taper and discontinue

I.M. usual dose: 20-40 units/day or 5-8 units/kg/day in 1-2 divided doses; range: 5-160 units/day

Oral prednisone (2 mg/kg/day) was as effective as I.M. ACTH gel (20 units/day) in controlling infantile spasms

Adults: Acute exacerbation of multiple sclerosis: I.M.: 80-120 units/day for 2-3 weeks

Repository injection: I.M., SubQ: 40-80 units every 24-72 hours

Dosage Forms Injection, gelatin: 80 units/mL (5 mL)

corticotropin, repository *see* corticotropin *on this page*

Cortifoam® [US/Can] *see* hydrocortisone (rectal) *on page 426*

Cortimyxin® [Can] *see* neomycin, polymyxin B, and hydrocortisone *on page 584*

cortisol *see* hydrocortisone (systemic) *on page 427*

cortisone acetate (KOR ti sone AS e tate)

Sound-Alike/Look-Alike Issues

cortisone may be confused with Cortizone®

Synonyms compound E

Therapeutic Category Adrenal Corticosteroid

Use Management of adrenocortical insufficiency

Usual Dosage If possible, administer glucocorticoids before 9 AM to minimize adrenocortical suppression; dosing depends upon the condition being treated and the response of the patient; **Note:** Supplemental doses may be warranted during times of stress in the course of withdrawing therapy

Children:

Antiinflammatory or immunosuppressive: Oral: 2.5-10 mg/kg/day **or** 20-300 mg/m^2/day in divided doses every 6-8 hours

Physiologic replacement: Oral: 0.5-0.75 mg/kg/day **or** 20-25 mg/m^2/day in divided doses every 8 hours

Adults:

Antiinflammatory or immunosuppressive: Oral: 25-300 mg/day in divided doses every 12-24 hours

Physiologic replacement: Oral: 25-35 mg/day

Dosage Forms Tablet, as acetate: 25 mg

Cortisporin® Cream [US] *see* neomycin, polymyxin B, and hydrocortisone *on page 584*

Cortisporin® Ointment [US] *see* bacitracin, neomycin, polymyxin B, and hydrocortisone *on page 91*

Cortisporin® Ophthalmic [US] *see* neomycin, polymyxin B, and hydrocortisone *on page 584*

Cortisporin® Otic [US/Can] *see* neomycin, polymyxin B, and hydrocortisone *on page 584*

Cortisporin®-TC [US] *see* neomycin, colistin, hydrocortisone, and thonzonium *on page 583*

Cortisporin® Topical Cream *(Discontinued)* *see* neomycin, polymyxin B, and hydrocortisone *on page 584*

Cortisporin® Topical Ointment [Can] *see* bacitracin, neomycin, polymyxin B, and hydrocortisone *on page 91*

Cortizone®-10 Maximum Strength [US-OTC] *see* hydrocortisone (topical) *on page 428*

Cortizone®-10 Plus Maximum Strength [US-OTC] *see* hydrocortisone (topical) *on page 428*

Cortizone®-10 Quick Shot [US-OTC] *see* hydrocortisone (topical) *on page 428*

Cortone® ***(Discontinued)***

Cortrosyn® [US/Can] *see* cosyntropin *on this page*

Corvert® [US] *see* ibutilide *on page 439*

CO Simvastatin [Can] *see* simvastatin *on page 773*

Cosmegen® [US/Can] *see* dactinomycin *on page 227*

Cosopt® [US/Can] *see* dorzolamide and timolol *on page 274*

CO Sotalol [Can] *see* sotalol *on page 787*

CO Sumatriptan [Can] *see* sumatriptan *on page 801*

cosyntropin (koe sin TROE pin)

Sound-Alike/Look-Alike Issues
Cortrosyn® may be confused with Cotazym®

Synonyms synacthen; tetracosactide

U.S./Canadian Brand Names Cortrosyn® [US/Can]

Therapeutic Category Diagnostic Agent

Use Diagnostic test to differentiate primary adrenal from secondary (pituitary) adrenocortical insufficiency

Usual Dosage Adrenocortical insufficiency: I.M., I.V. (over 2 minutes): Peak plasma cortisol concentrations usually occur 45-60 minutes after cosyntropin administration

Children <2 years: 0.125 mg

Children >2 years and Adults: 0.25-0.75 mg

When greater cortisol stimulation is needed, an I.V. infusion may be used:

Children >2 years and Adults: 0.25 mg administered at 0.04 mg/hour over 6 hours

Dosage Forms Injection, powder for reconstitution: 0.25 mg

Cotazym® [Can] *see* pancrelipase *on page 634*

Cotazym® ***(Discontinued)*** *see* pancrelipase *on page 634*

Cotazym-S® ***(Discontinued)*** *see* pancrelipase *on page 634*

CO Temazepam [Can] *see* temazepam *on page 808*

co-trimoxazole *see* sulfamethoxazole and trimethoprim *on page 797*

Coughtuss [US] *see* phenylephrine, hydrocodone, and chlorpheniramine *on page 663*

Coumadin® [US/Can] *see* warfarin *on page 881*

Covan® [Can] *see* triprolidine, pseudoephedrine, and codeine *(Canada only) on page 853*

Covera® [Can] *see* verapamil *on page 870*

Covera-HS® [US/Can] *see* verapamil *on page 870*

Coversyl® [Can] *see* perindopril erbumine *on page 655*

Coversyl® Plus [Can] *see* perindopril and indapamide *(Canada only) on page 654*

co-vidarabine *see* pentostatin *on page 652*

coviracil *see* emtricitabine *on page 290*

Cozaar® [US/Can] *see* losartan *on page 506*

CO Zopiclone [Can] *see* zopiclone *(Canada only) on page 890*

CP358774 *see* erlotinib *on page 302*

CPC *see* cetylpyridinium *on page 169*

CPM *see* cyclophosphamide *on page 220*

CPT-11 *see* irinotecan *on page 461*

CPZ *see* chlorpromazine *on page 184*

Crantex ER [US] *see* guaifenesin and phenylephrine *on page 396*

Crantex LA [US] *see* guaifenesin and phenylephrine *on page 396*

Creomulsion® Cough [US-OTC] *see* dextromethorphan *on page 245*
Creomulsion® for Children [US-OTC] *see* dextromethorphan *on page 245*
Creon® [US] *see* pancrelipase *on page 634*
Creon® 5 [Can] *see* pancrelipase *on page 634*
Creon® 10 [Can] *see* pancrelipase *on page 634*
Creon® 20 [Can] *see* pancrelipase *on page 634*
Creon® 25 [Can] *see* pancrelipase *on page 634*
Creo-Terpin® [US-OTC] *see* dextromethorphan *on page 245*
Crestor® [US/Can] *see* rosuvastatin *on page 755*
Cresylate® [US] *see* m-cresyl acetate *on page 520*
Crinone® [US/Can] *see* progesterone *on page 703*
Critic-Aid Skin Care® [US-OTC] *see* zinc oxide *on page 887*
Criticare HN® [US-OTC] *see* nutritional formula, enteral/oral *on page 608*
Crixivan® [US/Can] *see* indinavir *on page 445*
CroFab™ [Ovine] [US] *see* antivenin *(Crotalidae)* polyvalent *on page 63*
Crolom® [US] *see* cromolyn sodium *on this page*
cromoglycic acid *see* cromolyn sodium *on this page*

cromolyn sodium (KROE moe lin SOW dee um)

Sound-Alike/Look-Alike Issues

Intal® may be confused with Endal®
NasalCrom® may be confused with Nasacort®, Nasalide®

Synonyms cromoglycic acid; disodium cromoglycate; DSCG

U.S./Canadian Brand Names Apo-Cromolyn® [Can]; Crolom® [US]; Gastrocrom® [US]; Intal® [US/Can]; Nalcrom® [Can]; NasalCrom® [US-OTC]; Nu-Cromolyn [Can]; Opticrom® [US/Can]

Therapeutic Category Mast Cell Stabilizer

Use

Inhalation: May be used as an adjunct in the prophylaxis of allergic disorders, including asthma; prevention of exercise-induced bronchospasm
Nasal: Prevention and treatment of seasonal and perennial allergic rhinitis
Oral: Systemic mastocytosis
Ophthalmic: Treatment of vernal keratoconjunctivitis, vernal conjunctivitis, and vernal keratitis

Usual Dosage

Oral:

Systemic mastocytosis:

Children 2-12 years: 100 mg 4 times/day; not to exceed 40 mg/kg/day; given ½ hour prior to meals and at bedtime

Children >12 years and Adults: 200 mg 4 times/day; given ½ hour prior to meals and at bedtime; if control of symptoms is not seen within 2-3 weeks, dose may be increased to a maximum 40 mg/kg/day

Inhalation:

For chronic control of asthma, taper frequency to the lowest effective dose (ie, 4 times/day to 3 times/day to twice daily): **Note:** Not effective for immediate relief of symptoms in acute asthmatic attacks; must be used at regular intervals for 2-4 weeks to be effective.

Nebulization solution: Children >2 years and Adults: Initial: 20 mg 4 times/day; usual dose: 20 mg 3-4 times/day

Metered spray:

Children 5-12 years: Initial: 2 inhalations 4 times/day; usual dose: 1-2 inhalations 3-4 times/day

Children ≥12 years and Adults: Initial: 2 inhalations 4 times/day; usual dose: 2-4 inhalations 3-4 times/day

Prevention of allergen- or exercise-induced bronchospasm: Administer 10-15 minutes prior to exercise or allergen exposure but no longer than 1 hour before:

Nebulization solution: Children >2 years and Adults: Single dose of 20 mg

Metered spray: Children >5 years and Adults: Single dose of 2 inhalations

Ophthalmic: Children >4 years and Adults: 1-2 drops in each eye 4-6 times/day

Nasal: Allergic rhinitis (treatment and prophylaxis): Children ≥2 years and Adults: 1 spray into each nostril 3-4 times/day; may be increased to 6 times/day (symptomatic relief may require 2-4 weeks)

(Continued)

cromolyn sodium *(Continued)*

Dosage Forms

Aerosol, for oral inhalation, as sodium (Intal®): 800 mcg/inhalation (8.1 g) [112 metered inhalations; 56 doses], (14.2 g) [200 metered inhalations; 100 doses]

Solution for nebulization, as sodium (Intal®): 20 mg/2 mL (60s, 120s)

Solution, intranasal, as sodium [spray] (NasalCrom®): 40 mg/mL (13 mL, 26 mL) [5.2 mg/inhalation; contains benzalkonium chloride]

Solution, ophthalmic, as sodium (Crolom®, Opticrom®): 4% (10 mL) [contains benzalkonium chloride]

Solution, oral, as sodium (Gastrocrom®): 100 mg/5 mL (96s)

Crosseal™ [US] *see* fibrin sealant kit *on page 345*

crotalidae antivenin *see* antivenin *(Crotalidae)* polyvalent *on page 63*

crotaline antivenin, polyvalent *see* antivenin *(Crotalidae)* polyvalent *on page 63*

crotamiton (kroe TAM i tonn)

Sound-Alike/Look-Alike Issues

Eurax® may be confused with Efudex®, Eulexin®, Evoxac™, Serax®, Urex®

U.S./Canadian Brand Names Eurax® [US]

Therapeutic Category Scabicides/Pediculicides

Use Treatment of scabies (*Sarcoptes scabiei*) and symptomatic treatment of pruritus

Usual Dosage Topical:

Scabicide: Children and Adults: Wash thoroughly and scrub away loose scales, then towel dry; apply a thin layer and massage drug onto skin of the entire body from the neck to the toes (with special attention to skin folds, creases, and interdigital spaces). Repeat application in 24 hours. Take a cleansing bath 48 hours after the final application. Treatment may be repeated after 7-10 days if live mites are still present.

Pruritus: Massage into affected areas until medication is completely absorbed; repeat as necessary

Dosage Forms

Cream: 10% (60 g)

Lotion: 10% (60 mL, 480 mL)

crude coal tar *see* coal tar *on page 207*

Cruex® Cream [US-OTC] *see* clotrimazole *on page 205*

Cryselle™ [US] *see* ethinyl estradiol and norgestrel *on page 327*

crystalline penicillin *see* penicillin G (parenteral/aqueous) *on page 648*

Crystamine® ***(Discontinued)*** *see* cyanocobalamin *on next page*

Crysti 1000® ***(Discontinued)*** *see* cyanocobalamin *on next page*

CsA *see* cyclosporine *on page 221*

CSP *see* cellulose sodium phosphate *on page 165*

CTLA-4Ig *see* abatacept *on page 3*

CTM *see* chlorpheniramine *on page 175*

CTX *see* cyclophosphamide *on page 220*

Cubicin® [US] *see* daptomycin *on page 230*

Culturelle® [US-OTC] *see* Lactobacillus *on page 477*

Cuprimine® [US/Can] *see* penicillamine *on page 646*

Curasore [US-OTC] *see* pramoxine *on page 691*

Curosurf® [US/Can] *see* poractant alfa *on page 682*

Cutar® [US-OTC] *see* coal tar *on page 207*

Cutivate® [US] *see* fluticasone (topical) *on page 363*

CyA *see* cyclosporine *on page 221*

cyanide antidote kit *see* sodium nitrite, sodium thiosulfate, and amyl nitrite *on page 780*

Cyanide Antidote Package [US] *see* sodium nitrite, sodium thiosulfate, and amyl nitrite *on page 780*

cyanocobalamin (sye an oh koe BAL a min)

Synonyms vitamin B_{12}

U.S./Canadian Brand Names Nascobal® [US]; Twelve Resin-K [US]

Therapeutic Category Vitamin, Water Soluble

Use Treatment of pernicious anemia; vitamin B_{12} deficiency due to malabsorption diseases, inadequaste secretion of intrinisic factor, and inadequate utilization of B_{12} (eg, during neoplastic treatment); increased B_{12} requirements due to pregnancy, thyrotoxicosis, hemorrhage, malignancy, liver or kidney disease

Usual Dosage

Recommended daily allowance (RDA):

Children: 0.9-2.4 mcg/day

Adults: 2.4 mcg/day

Pregnancy: 2.6 mcg/day

Lactation: 2.8 mcg/day

Vitamin B_{12} deficiency:

Intranasal: 500 mcg in one nostril once weekly

Oral: 250 mcg/day

I.M., deep SubQ:

Children (dosage not well established): 0.2 mcg/kg for 2 days, followed by 1000 mcg/day for 2-7 days, followed by 100 mcg/week for one month; for malabsorptive causes of B_{12} deficiency, monthly maintenance doses of 100 mcg have been recommended **or** as an alternative 100 mcg/day for 10-15 days, then once or twice weekly for several months

Adults: Initial: 30 mcg/day for 5-10 days; maintenance: 100-200 mcg/month

Pernicious anemia: I.M., deep SubQ (administer concomitantly with folic acid if needed, 1 mg/day for 1 month):

Children: 30-50 mcg/day for 2 or more weeks (to a total dose of 1000-5000 mcg), then follow with 100 mcg/month as maintenance dosage

Adults: 100 mcg/day for 6-7 days; if improvement, administer same dose on alternate days for 7 doses, then every 3-4 days for 2-3 weeks; once hematologic values have returned to normal, maintenance dosage: 100 mcg/month. **Note:** Alternative dosing of 1000 mcg/day for 5 days (followed by 500-1000 mcg/month) has been used.

Hematologic remission (without evidence of nervous system involvement):

Intranasal gel: 500 mcg in one nostril once weekly

Oral: 1000-2000 mcg/day

I.M., SubQ: 100-1000 mcg/month

Schilling test: I.M.: 1000 mcg

Dosage Forms [DSC] = Discontinued product

Gel, intranasal (Nascobal®): 500 mcg/0.1 mL (2.3 mL) [contains benzalkonium chloride; delivers 8 doses] [DSC]

Injection, solution: 1000 mcg/mL (1 mL, 10 mL, 30 mL) [may contain benzyl alcohol and/or aluminum]

Lozenge [OTC]: 100 mcg, 250 mcg, 500 mcg

Solution, intranasal spray (Nascobal®): 500 mcg/0.1 mL actuation (2.3 mL) [contains benzalkonium chloride; delivers 8 doses]

Tablet [OTC]: 50 mcg, 100 mcg, 250 mcg, 500 mcg, 1000 mcg, 5000 mcg

Twelve Resin-K: 1000 mcg [may be used as oral, sublingual, or buccal]

Tablet, extended release [OTC]: 1500 mcg

Tablet, sublingual [OTC]: 2500 mcg

cyanocobalamin, folic acid, and pyridoxine *see* folic acid, cyanocobalamin, and pyridoxine *on page 365*

Cyanoject® *(Discontinued)* *see* cyanocobalamin *on this page*

Cyclen® [Can] *see* ethinyl estradiol and norgestimate *on page 325*

Cyclessa® [US/Can] *see* ethinyl estradiol and desogestrel *on page 317*

cyclobenzaprine (sye kloe BEN za preen)

Sound-Alike/Look-Alike Issues

cyclobenzaprine may be confused with cycloSERINE, cyproheptadine

Flexeril® may be confused with Floxin®

Synonyms cyclobenzaprine hydrochloride

U.S./Canadian Brand Names Apo-Cyclobenzaprine® [Can]; Flexeril® [US]; Flexitec [Can]; Gen-Cyclobenzaprine [Can]; Novo-Cycloprine [Can]; Nu-Cyclobenzaprine [Can]

Therapeutic Category Skeletal Muscle Relaxant

Use Treatment of muscle spasm associated with acute painful musculoskeletal conditions

(Continued)

cyclobenzaprine *(Continued)*

Usual Dosage Oral: **Note:** Do not use longer than 2-3 weeks

Adults: Initial: 5 mg 3 times/day; may increase to 10 mg 3 times/day if needed

Dosage Forms

Tablet, as hydrochloride: 5 mg, 10 mg

Flexeril®: 5 mg, 10 mg

cyclobenzaprine hydrochloride *see* cyclobenzaprine *on previous page*

Cyclocort® [US/Can] *see* amcinonide *on page 39*

Cyclogyl® [US/Can] *see* cyclopentolate *on this page*

Cyclomen® [Can] *see* danazol *on page 228*

Cyclomydril® [US] *see* cyclopentolate and phenylephrine *on this page*

cyclopentolate (sye kloe PEN toe late)

Synonyms cyclopentolate hydrochloride

U.S./Canadian Brand Names Cyclogyl® [US/Can]; Cylate® [US]; Diopentolate® [Can]

Therapeutic Category Anticholinergic Agent

Use Diagnostic procedures requiring mydriasis and cycloplegia

Usual Dosage Ophthalmic:

Neonates and Infants: **Note:** Cyclopentolate and phenylephrine combination formulation is the preferred agent for use in neonates and infants due to lower cyclopentolate concentration and reduced risk for systemic reactions

Children: Instill 1 drop of 0.5%, 1%, or 2% in eye followed by 1 drop of 0.5% or 1% in 5 minutes, if necessary

Adults: Instill 1 drop of 1% followed by another drop in 5 minutes; 2% solution in heavily pigmented iris

Dosage Forms [DSC] = Discontinued product

Solution, ophthalmic, as hydrochloride: 1% (2 mL, 15 mL)

AK-Pentolate® [DSC], Cylate®: 1% (2 mL, 15 mL) [contains benzalkonium chloride]

Cyclogyl®: 0.5% (15 mL); 1% (2 mL, 5 mL, 15 mL); 2% (2 mL, 5 mL, 15 mL) [contains benzalkonium chloride]

cyclopentolate and phenylephrine (sye kloe PEN toe late & fen il EF rin)

Synonyms phenylephrine and cyclopentolate

U.S./Canadian Brand Names Cyclomydril® [US]

Therapeutic Category Anticholinergic/Adrenergic Agonist

Use Induce mydriasis greater than that produced with cyclopentolate HCl alone

Usual Dosage Ophthalmic: Neonates, Infants, Children, and Adults: Instill 1 drop into the eye every 5-10 minutes, for up to 3 doses, approximately 40-50 minutes before the examination

Dosage Forms Solution, ophthalmic: Cyclopentolate hydrochloride 0.2% and phenylephrine hydrochloride 1% (2 mL, 5 mL) [contains benzalkonium chloride]

cyclopentolate hydrochloride *see* cyclopentolate *on this page*

cyclophosphamide (sye kloe FOS fa mide)

Sound-Alike/Look-Alike Issues

cyclophosphamide may be confused with cycloSPORINE, ifosfamide

Cytoxan® may be confused with cefoxitin, Centoxin®, Ciloxan®, cytarabine, CytoGam®, Cytosar®, Cytosar-U®, Cytotec®

Synonyms CPM; CTX; CYT; NSC-26271

U.S./Canadian Brand Names Cytoxan® [US/Can]; Procytox® [Can]

Therapeutic Category Antineoplastic Agent

Use

Oncologic: Treatment of Hodgkin and non-Hodgkin lymphoma, Burkitt lymphoma, chronic lymphocytic leukemia (CLL), chronic myelocytic leukemia (CML), acute myelocytic leukemia (AML), acute lymphocytic leukemia (ALL), mycosis fungoides, multiple myeloma, neuroblastoma, retinoblastoma, rhabdomyosarcoma, Ewing sarcoma; breast, testicular, endometrial, ovarian, and lung cancers, and in conditioning regimens for bone marrow transplantation

Nononcologic: Prophylaxis of rejection for kidney, heart, liver, and bone marrow transplants, severe rheumatoid disorders, nephrotic syndrome, Wegener granulomatosis, idiopathic pulmonary hemosideroses, myasthenia gravis, multiple sclerosis, systemic lupus erythematosus, lupus nephritis, autoimmune hemolytic anemia, idiopathic thrombocytic purpura (ITP), macroglobulinemia, and antibody-induced pure red cell aplasia

Usual Dosage Refer to individual protocols

Children:

SLE: I.V.: 500-750 mg/m² every month; maximum dose: 1 g/m²

JRA/vasculitis: I.V.: 10 mg/kg every 2 weeks

Children and Adults:

Oral: 50-100 mg/m²/day as continuous therapy or 400-1000 mg/m² in divided doses over 4-5 days as intermittent therapy

I.V.:

Single doses: 400-1800 mg/m² (30-50 mg/kg) per treatment course (1-5 days) which can be repeated at 2-4 week intervals

Continuous daily doses: 60-120 mg/m² (1-2.5 mg/kg) per day

Autologous BMT: IVPB: 50 mg/kg/dose x 4 days or 60 mg/kg/dose for 2 days; total dose is usually divided over 2-4 days

Nephrotic syndrome: Oral: 2-3 mg/kg/day every day for up to 12 weeks when corticosteroids are unsuccessful

Dosage Forms

Injection, powder for reconstitution (Cytoxan®): 500 mg, 1 g, 2 g [contains mannitol 75 mg per cyclophosphamide 100 mg]

Tablet (Cytoxan®): 25 mg, 50 mg

cycloserine (sye kloe SER een)

Sound-Alike/Look-Alike Issues

cycloSERINE may be confused with cyclobenzaprine, cycloSPORINE

Tall-Man cyclo**SERINE**

U.S./Canadian Brand Names Seromycin® [US]

Therapeutic Category Antibiotic, Miscellaneous

Use Adjunctive treatment in pulmonary or extrapulmonary tuberculosis

Usual Dosage Some of the neurotoxic effects may be relieved or prevented by the concomitant administration of pyridoxine

Tuberculosis: Oral:

Children: 10-20 mg/kg/day in 2 divided doses up to 1000 mg/day for 18-24 months

Adults: Initial: 250 mg every 12 hours for 14 days, then administer 500 mg to 1 g/day in 2 divided doses for 18-24 months (maximum daily dose: 1 g)

Dosage Forms Capsule: 250 mg

cyclosporin A *see* cyclosporine *on this page*

cyclosporine (SYE kloe spor een)

Sound-Alike/Look-Alike Issues

cycloSPORINE may be confused with cyclophosphamide, Cyklokapron®, cycloSERINE

Gengraf® may be confused with Prograf®

Neoral® may be confused with Neurontin®, Nizoral®

Sandimmune® may be confused with Sandostatin®

Synonyms CsA; CyA; cyclosporin A

Tall-Man cyclo**SPORINE**

U.S./Canadian Brand Names Gengraf® [US]; Neoral® [US/Can]; Restasis® [US]; Rhoxal-cyclosporine [Can]; Sandimmune® I.V. [Can]; Sandimmune® [US]; Sandoz-Cyclosporine [Can]

Therapeutic Category Immunosuppressant Agent

Use Prophylaxis of organ rejection in kidney, liver, and heart transplants, has been used with azathioprine and/or corticosteroids; severe, active rheumatoid arthritis (RA) not responsive to methotrexate alone; severe, recalcitrant plaque psoriasis in nonimmunocompromised adults unresponsive to or unable to tolerate other systemic therapy

Ophthalmic emulsion (Restasis®): Increase tear production when suppressed tear production is presumed to be due to keratoconjunctivitis sicca-associated ocular inflammation (in patients not already using topical anti-inflammatory drugs or punctal plugs)

Usual Dosage Note: Neoral® and Sandimmune® are not bioequivalent and cannot be used interchangeably

Children: Transplant: Refer to adult dosing; children may require, and are able to tolerate, larger doses than adults.

(Continued)

cyclosporine *(Continued)*

Adults:

Newly-transplanted patients: Adjunct therapy with corticosteroids is recommended. Initial dose should be given 4-12 hours prior to transplant or may be given postoperatively; adjust initial dose to achieve desired plasma concentration

Oral: Dose is dependent upon type of transplant and formulation:

Cyclosporine (modified):

Renal: 9 ± 3 mg/kg/day, divided twice daily

Liver: 8 ± 4 mg/kg/day, divided twice daily

Heart: 7 ± 3 mg/kg/day, divided twice daily

Cyclosporine (nonmodified): Initial dose: 15 mg/kg/day as a single dose (range 14-18 mg/kg); lower doses of 10-14 mg/kg/day have been used for renal transplants. Continue initial dose daily for 1-2 weeks; taper by 5% per week to a maintenance dose of 5-10 mg/kg/day; some renal transplant patients may be dosed as low as 3 mg/kg/day

Note: When using the non-modified formulation, cyclosporine levels may increase in liver transplant patients when the T-tube is closed; dose may need decreased

I.V.: Cyclosporine (nonmodified): Manufacturer's labeling: Initial dose: 5-6 mg/kg/day as a single dose ($^1/_3$ the oral dose), infused over 2-6 hours; use should be limited to patients unable to take capsules or oral solution; patients should be switched to an oral dosage form as soon as possible

Note: Many transplant centers administer cyclosporine as "divided dose" infusions (in 2-3 doses/day) or as a continuous (24-hour) infusion; dosages range from 3-7.5 mg/kg/day. Specific institutional protocols should be consulted.

Conversion to cyclosporine (modified) from cyclosporine (nonmodified): Start with daily dose previously used and adjust to obtain preconversion cyclosporine trough concentration. Plasma concentrations should be monitored every 4-7 days and dose adjusted as necessary, until desired trough level is obtained. When transferring patients with previously poor absorption of cyclosporine (non-modified), monitor trough levels at least twice weekly (especially if initial dose exceeds 10 mg/kg/day); high plasma levels are likely to occur.

Rheumatoid arthritis: Oral: Cyclosporine (modified): Initial dose: 2.5 mg/kg/day, divided twice daily; salicylates, NSAIDs, and oral glucocorticoids may be continued; dose may be increased by 0.5-0.75 mg/kg/day if insufficient response is seen after 8 weeks of treatment; additional dosage increases may be made again at 12 weeks (maximum dose: 4 mg/kg/day). Discontinue if no benefit is seen by 16 weeks of therapy.

Note: Increase the frequency of blood pressure monitoring after each alteration in dosage of cyclosporine. Cyclosporine dosage should be decreased by 25% to 50% in patients with no history of hypertension who develop sustained hypertension during therapy and, if hypertension persists, treatment with cyclosporine should be discontinued.

Psoriasis: Oral: Cyclosporine (modified): Initial dose: 2.5 mg/kg/day, divided twice daily; dose may be increased by 0.5 mg/kg/day if insufficient response is seen after 4 weeks of treatment. Additional dosage increases may be made every 2 weeks if needed (maximum dose: 4 mg/kg/day). Discontinue if no benefit is seen by 6 weeks of therapy. Once patients are adequately controlled, the dose should be decreased to the lowest effective dose. Doses lower than 2.5 mg/kg/day may be effective. Treatment longer than 1 year is not recommended.

Note: Increase the frequency of blood pressure monitoring after each alteration in dosage of cyclosporine. Cyclosporine dosage should be decreased by 25% to 50% in patients with no history of hypertension who develop sustained hypertension during therapy and, if hypertension persists, treatment with cyclosporine should be discontinued.

Keratoconjunctivitis sicca: Ophthalmic (Restasis®): Children ≥16 years and Adults: Instill 1 drop in each eye every 12 hours

Dosage Forms

Capsule, soft gel, modified: 25 mg, 100 mg [contains castor oil, ethanol]

Gengraf®: 25 mg, 100 mg [contains ethanol, castor oil, propylene glycol]

Neoral®: 25 mg, 100 mg [contains dehydrated ethanol, corn oil, castor oil, propylene glycol]

Capsule, soft gel, non-modified (Sandimmune®): 25 mg, 100 mg [contains dehydrated ethanol, corn oil]

Emulsion, ophthalmic [preservative free, single-use vial] (Restasis®): 0.05% (0.4 mL) [contains glycerin, castor oil, polysorbate 80, carbomer 1342; 32 vials/box]

Injection, solution, non-modified (Sandimmune®): 50 mg/mL (5 mL) [contains Cremophor® EL (polyoxyethylated castor oil), ethanol]

Solution, oral, modified:

Gengraf®: 100 mg/mL (50 mL) [contains castor oil, propylene glycol]

Neoral®: 100 mg/mL (50 mL) [contains dehydrated ethanol, corn oil, castor oil, propylene glycol]

Solution, oral, non-modified (Sandimmune®): 100 mg/mL (50 mL) [contains olive oil, ethanol]

Cycofed® Pediatric *(Discontinued)* *see* guaifenesin, pseudoephedrine, and codeine *on page 401*

Cyklokapron® [US/Can] *see* tranexamic acid *on page 842*

Cylate® [US] *see* cyclopentolate *on page 220*

Cylex® [US-OTC] *see* benzocaine *on page 99*

Cymbalta® [US] *see* duloxetine *on page 283*

Cyomin® *(Discontinued)* *see* cyanocobalamin *on page 219*

cyproheptadine (si proe HEP ta deen)

Sound-Alike/Look-Alike Issues

cyproheptadine may be confused with cyclobenzaprine
Periactin® may be confused with Perative®, Percodan®, Persantine®

Synonyms cyproheptadine hydrochloride

Therapeutic Category Antihistamine

Use Perennial and seasonal allergic rhinitis and other allergic symptoms including urticaria

Usual Dosage Oral:

Children:

Allergic conditions: 0.25 mg/kg/day or 8 mg/m^2/day in 2-3 divided doses **or**

2-6 years: 2 mg every 8-12 hours (not to exceed 12 mg/day)

7-14 years: 4 mg every 8-12 hours (not to exceed 16 mg/day)

Migraine headaches: 4 mg 2-3 times/day

Children ≥12 years and Adults: Spasticity associated with spinal cord damage: 4 mg at bedtime; increase by a 4 mg dose every 3-4 days; average daily dose: 16 mg in divided doses; not to exceed 36 mg/day

Children >13 years and Adults: Appetite stimulation (anorexia nervosa): 2 mg 4 times/day; may be increased gradually over a 3-week period to 8 mg 4 times/day

Adults:

Allergic conditions: 4-20 mg/day divided every 8 hours (not to exceed 0.5 mg/kg/day)

Cluster headaches: 4 mg 4 times/day

Migraine headaches: 4-8 mg 3 times/day

Dosage Forms

Syrup, as hydrochloride: 2 mg/5 mL (473 mL) [contains alcohol 5%; mint flavor]

Tablet, as hydrochloride: 4 mg

cyproheptadine hydrochloride *see* cyproheptadine *on this page*

cyproterone acetate *see* cyproterone *(Canada only)* *on this page*

cyproterone and ethinyl estradiol *(Canada only)*

(sye PROE ter one & ETH in il es tra DYE ole)

Synonyms ethinyl estradiol and cyproterone acetate

U.S./Canadian Brand Names Diane-35 [Can]

Therapeutic Category Acne Products; Estrogen and Androgen Combination

Use Treatment of females with severe acne, unresponsive to other therapies, with associated symptoms of androgenization (including mild hirsutism or seborrhea). **Should not be used solely for contraception;** however, will provide reliable contraception if taken as recommended for approved indications.

Usual Dosage Oral: Adults: Female: Acne: One tablet daily for 21 days, followed by 7 days off; first cycle should begin on the first day of menstrual flow. Discontinue therapy 3-4 cycles after symptoms have resolved.

Dosage Forms CAN = [Canadian brand name]

Tablet: Diane-35 [CAN]: Cyproterone 2 mg and ethinyl estradiol 0.35 mg (21s) [not available in the U.S.]

cyproterone *(Canada only)* (sye PROE ter one)

Synonyms cyproterone acetate

U.S./Canadian Brand Names Androcur® Depot [Can]; Androcur® [Can]; Apo-Cyproterone® [Can]; Gen-Cyproterone [Can]

Therapeutic Category Antiandrogen; Progestin

Use Palliative treatment of advanced prostate carcinoma

Usual Dosage Adults: Males: Prostatic carcinoma (palliative treatment):

Oral: 200-300 mg/day in 2-3 divided doses; following orchiectomy, reduce dose to 100-200 mg/day; should be taken with meals

I.M. (depot): 300 mg (3 mL) once weekly; reduce dose in orchiectomized patients to 300 mg every 2 weeks

(Continued)

cyproterone *(Canada only)* *(Continued)*

Dosage Forms

Injection, solution, as acetate (Androcur® Depot): 100 mg/mL (3 mL) [contains benzyl benzoate and castor oil]

Tablet, as acetate (Androcur®): 50 mg

Cystadane® [US/Can] *see* betaine *on page 106*

Cystagon® [US] *see* cysteamine *on this page*

cysteamine (sis TEE a meen)

Synonyms cysteamine bitartrate

U.S./Canadian Brand Names Cystagon® [US]

Therapeutic Category Urinary Tract Product

Use **Orphan drug:** Treatment of nephropathic cystinosis

Usual Dosage Oral: Initiate therapy with 1/4 to 1/6 of maintenance dose; titrate slowly upward over 4-6 weeks. **Note:** Dosage may be increased if cystine levels are <1 nmol/1/2 cystine/mg protein, although intolerance and incidence of adverse events may be increased.

Children <12 years: Maintenance: 1.3 g/m²/day or 60 mg/kg/day divided into 4 doses (maximum dose: 1.95 g/m²/day or 90 mg/kg/day)

Children >12 years and Adults (>110 lb): 2 g/day in 4 divided doses; maximum dose: 1.95 g/m²/day or 90 mg/kg/day

Dosage Forms Capsule: 50 mg, 150 mg

cysteamine bitartrate *see* cysteamine *on this page*

cysteine (SIS te een)

Synonyms cysteine hydrochloride

Therapeutic Category Nutritional Supplement

Use Supplement to crystalline amino acid solutions, in particular the specialized pediatric formulas (eg, Aminosyn® PF, TrophAmine®) to meet the intravenous amino acid nutritional requirements of infants receiving parenteral nutrition (PN)

Usual Dosage Neonates and Infants: I.V.: Added as a fixed ratio to crystalline amino acid solution: 40 mg cysteine per g of amino acids; dosage will vary with the daily amino acid dosage (eg, 0.5-2.5 g/kg/day amino acids would result in 20-100 mg/kg/day cysteine); individual doses of cysteine of 0.8-1 mmol/kg/day have also been added directly to the daily PN solution; the duration of treatment relates to the need for PN; patients on chronic PN therapy have received cysteine until 6 months of age and in some cases until 2 years of age

Dosage Forms Injection, solution, as hydrochloride: 50 mg/mL (10 mL, 50 mL)

cysteine hydrochloride *see* cysteine *on this page*

Cystistat® [Can] *see* hyaluronate and derivatives *on page 416*

Cystografin® [US] *see* radiological/contrast media (ionic) *on page 728*

Cystospaz® [US/Can] *see* hyoscyamine *on page 434*

Cystospaz-M® ***(Discontinued)*** *see* hyoscyamine *on page 434*

CYT *see* cyclophosphamide *on page 220*

Cytadren® [US] *see* aminoglutethimide *on page 42*

cytarabine (sye TARE a been)

Sound-Alike/Look-Alike Issues

cytarabine may be confused with Cytadren®, Cytosar®, Cytoxan®, vidarabine

Cytosar-U® may be confused with cytarabine, Cytovene®, Cytoxan®, Neosar®

Synonyms arabinosylcytosine; ara-C; cytarabine hydrochloride; cytosine arabinosine hydrochloride; NSC-63878

U.S./Canadian Brand Names Cytosar-U® [US]; Cytosar® [Can]

Therapeutic Category Antineoplastic Agent

Use Treatment of acute myeloid leukemia (AML), acute lymphocytic leukemia (ALL), chronic myelocytic leukemia (CML; blast phase), and lymphomas; prophylaxis and treatment of meningeal leukemia

Usual Dosage Refer to individual protocols. Children and Adults:
Remission induction:
I.V.: 100-200 mg/m^2/day for 5-10 days; a second course, beginning 2-4 weeks after the initial therapy, may be required in some patients.
or 100 mg/m^2 every 12 hours for 7 days
I.T.: 5-75 mg/m^2 every 2-7 days until CNS findings normalize; or age-based dosing:
<1 year of age: 20 mg
1-2 years of age: 30 mg
2-3 years of age: 50 mg
>3 years of age: 75 mg
Remission maintenance:
I.V.: 70-200 mg/m^2/day for 2-5 days at monthly intervals
I.M., SubQ: 1-1.5 mg/kg single dose for maintenance at 1- to 4-week intervals
High-dose therapies:
Doses as high as 1-3 g/m^2 have been used for refractory or secondary leukemias or refractory non-Hodgkin lymphoma.
Doses of 1-3 g/m^2 every 12 hours for up to 12 doses have been used for leukemia
Bone marrow transplant: 1.5 g/m^2 continuous infusion over 48 hours

Dosage Forms
Injection, powder for reconstitution: 100 mg, 500 mg, 1 g, 2 g
Injection, solution: 20 mg/mL (5 mL, 25 mL, 50 mL); 100 mg/mL (20 mL)

cytarabine hydrochloride *see* cytarabine *on previous page*

cytarabine (liposomal) (sye TARE a been lip po SOE mal)

Sound-Alike/Look-Alike Issues
cytarabine may be confused with Cytadren®, Cytosar®, Cytoxan®, vidarabine
DepoCyt™ may be confused with Depoject®

U.S./Canadian Brand Names DepoCyt® [US]

Therapeutic Category Antineoplastic Agent, Antimetabolite (Purine)

Use Treatment of neoplastic (lymphomatous) meningitis

Usual Dosage **Note: Patients should be started on dexamethasone 4 mg twice daily (oral or I.V.) for 5 days, beginning on the day of liposomal cytarabine injection.**
Adults:
Induction: 50 mg intrathecally every 14 days for a total of 2 doses (weeks 1 and 3)
Consolidation: 50 mg intrathecally every 14 days for 3 doses (weeks 5, 7, and 9), followed by an additional dose at week 13
Maintenance: 50 mg intrathecally every 28 days for 4 doses (weeks 17, 21, 25, and 29)
If drug-related neurotoxicity develops, the dose should be reduced to 25 mg. If toxicity persists, treatment with liposomal cytarabine should be discontinued.

Dosage Forms
Injection, suspension [preservative free]:
Depocyt®: 10 mg/mL (5 mL)

CytoGam® [US] *see* cytomegalovirus immune globulin (intravenous-human) *on this page*

cytomegalovirus immune globulin (intravenous-human)

(sye toe meg a low VYE rus i MYUN GLOB yoo lin in tra VEE nus HYU man)

Sound-Alike/Look-Alike Issues
CytoGam® may be confused with Cytoxan®, Gamimune® N

Synonyms CMV-IGIV

U.S./Canadian Brand Names CytoGam® [US]

Therapeutic Category Immune Globulin

Use Prophylaxis of cytomegalovirus (CMV) disease associated with kidney, lung, liver, pancreas, and heart transplants; concomitant use with ganciclovir should be considered in organ transplants (other than kidney) from CMV seropositive donors to CMV seronegative recipients

Usual Dosage I.V.: Adults:
Kidney transplant:
Initial dose (within 72 hours of transplant): 150 mg/kg/dose
2-, 4-, 6-, and 8 weeks after transplant: 100 mg/kg/dose
12 and 16 weeks after transplant: 50 mg/kg/dose
Liver, lung, pancreas, or heart transplant:
Initial dose (within 72 hours of transplant): 150 mg/kg/dose
(Continued)

cytomegalovirus immune globulin (intravenous-human) *(Continued)*

2-, 4-, 6-, and 8 weeks after transplant: 150 mg/kg/dose
12 and 16 weeks after transplant: 100 mg/kg/dose

Dosage Forms Injection, solution [preservative free]: 50 mg ± 10 mg/mL (50 mL) [contains human albumin and sucrose]

Cytomel® [US/Can] *see* liothyronine *on page 498*

Cytosar® [Can] *see* cytarabine *on page 224*

Cytosar-U® [US] *see* cytarabine *on page 224*

cytosine arabinosine hydrochloride *see* cytarabine *on page 224*

Cytotec® [US] *see* misoprostol *on page 560*

Cytovene® [US/Can] *see* ganciclovir *on page 375*

Cytoxan® [US/Can] *see* cyclophosphamide *on page 220*

Cytra-3 [US] *see* citric acid, sodium citrate, and potassium citrate *on page 195*

Cytra-K [US] *see* potassium citrate and citric acid *on page 686*

Cytuss HC [US] *see* phenylephrine, hydrocodone, and chlorpheniramine *on page 663*

D2E7 *see* adalimumab *on page 19*

D_3 *see* cholecalciferol *on page 185*

D-3-mercaptovaline *see* penicillamine *on page 646*

d4T *see* stavudine *on page 790*

DAB_{389}IL-2 *see* denileukin diftitox *on page 235*

dacarbazine (da KAR ba zeen)

Sound-Alike/Look-Alike Issues
dacarbazine may be confused with Dicarbosil®, procarbazine

Synonyms DIC; dimethyl triazeno imidazole carboxamide; DTIC; imidazole carboxamide; imidazole carboxamide dimethyltriazene; WR-139007

U.S./Canadian Brand Names DTIC-Dome® [US]; DTIC® [Can]

Therapeutic Category Antineoplastic Agent

Use Treatment of malignant melanoma, Hodgkin disease, soft-tissue sarcomas, fibrosarcomas, rhabdomyosarcoma, islet cell carcinoma, medullary carcinoma of the thyroid, and neuroblastoma

Usual Dosage Refer to individual protocols. Some dosage regimens include:
Intraarterial: 50-400 mg/m^2 for 5-10 days
I.V.:
Hodgkin disease, ABVD: 375 mg/m^2 days 1 and 15 every 4 weeks **or** 100 mg/m^2/day for 5 days
Metastatic melanoma (alone or in combination with other agents): 150-250 mg/m^2 days 1-5 every 3-4 weeks
Metastatic melanoma: 850 mg/m^2 every 3 weeks
High dose: Bone marrow/blood cell transplantation: I.V.: 1-3 g/m^2; maximum dose as a single agent: 3.38 g/m^2; generally combined with other high-dose chemotherapeutic drugs

Dosage Forms
Injection, powder for reconstitution: 100 mg, 200 mg, 500 mg
DTIC-Dome®: 200 mg

Dacex-DM [US] *see* guaifenesin, dextromethorphan, and phenylephrine *on page 400*

daclizumab (dac KLYE zue mab)

U.S./Canadian Brand Names Zenapax® [US/Can]

Therapeutic Category Immunosuppressant Agent

Use Part of an immunosuppressive regimen (including cyclosporine and corticosteroids) for the prophylaxis of acute organ rejection in patients receiving renal transplant

Usual Dosage Daclizumab is used adjunctively with other immunosuppressants (eg, cyclosporine, corticosteroids, mycophenolate mofetil, and azathioprine): I.V.:
Children: Use same weight-based dose as adults
Adults: Immunoprophylaxis against acute renal allograft rejection: 1 mg/kg infused over 15 minutes within 24 hours before transplantation (day 0), then every 14 days for 4 additional doses

Dosage Forms Injection, solution [preservative free]: 5 mg/mL (5 mL)

Dacodyl® *(Discontinued)* *see* bisacodyl *on page 111*

Dacogen™ [US] *see* decitabine *on page 233*

DACT *see* dactinomycin *on this page*

dactinomycin (dak ti noe MYE sin)

Sound-Alike/Look-Alike Issues

dactinomycin may be confused with daptomycin, DAUNOrubicin

actinomycin may be confused with Achromycin

Synonyms ACT; Act-D; actinomycin; actinomycin Cl; actinomycin D; DACT; NSC-3053

U.S./Canadian Brand Names Cosmegen® [US/Can]

Therapeutic Category Antineoplastic Agent

Use Treatment of testicular tumors, melanoma, choriocarcinoma, Wilms tumor, neuroblastoma, retinoblastoma, rhabdomyosarcoma, uterine sarcomas, Ewing sarcoma, Kaposi sarcoma, sarcoma botryoides, and soft tissue sarcoma

Usual Dosage Refer to individual protocols: I.V.:

Note: Medication orders for dactinomycin are commonly written in MICROgrams (eg, 150 mcg) although many regimens list the dose in MILLIgrams (eg, mg/kg or mg/m^2). One-time doses for >1000 mcg, or multiple-day doses for >500 mcg/day are not common. The dose intensity per 2-week cycle for adults and children should not exceed 15 mcg/kg/day for 5 days or 400-600 mcg/m^2/day for 5 days. Some practitioners recommend calculation of the dosage for obese or edematous patients on the basis of body surface area in an effort to relate dosage to lean body mass.

Children >6 months: 15 mcg/kg/day **or** 400-600 mcg/m^2/day for 5 days every 3-6 weeks

Adults: 2.5 mg/m^2 in divided doses over 1 week, repeated every 2 weeks **or**

0.75-2 mg/m^2 every 1-4 weeks **or**

400-600 mcg/m^2/day for 5 days, repeated every 3-6 weeks

Dosage Forms Injection, powder for reconstitution: 0.5 mg [contains mannitol 20 mg]

DAD *see* mitoxantrone *on page 561*

Dairyaid® [Can] *see* lactase *on page 476*

Dakin's Solution [US] *see* sodium hypochlorite solution *on page 779*

Dakrina® Ophthalmic Solution *(Discontinued)* *see* artificial tears *on page 75*

Dalacin® C [Can] *see* clindamycin *on page 198*

Dalacin® T [Can] *see* clindamycin *on page 198*

Dalacin® Vaginal [Can] *see* clindamycin *on page 198*

Dallergy® [US] *see* chlorpheniramine, phenylephrine, and methscopolamine *on page 180*

Dallergy-D® Syrup *(Discontinued)* *see* chlorpheniramine and phenylephrine *on page 176*

Dallergy-JR® [US] *see* chlorpheniramine and phenylephrine *on page 176*

Dalmane® [US/Can] *see* flurazepam *on page 359*

d-Alpha-Gems™ [US-OTC] *see* vitamin E *on page 876*

***d*-alpha tocopherol** *see* vitamin E *on page 876*

dalteparin (dal TE pa rin)

U.S./Canadian Brand Names Fragmin® [US/Can]

Therapeutic Category Anticoagulant (Other)

Use Prevention of deep vein thrombosis which may lead to pulmonary embolism, in patients requiring abdominal surgery who are at risk for thromboembolism complications (eg, patients >40 years of age, obesity, patients with malignancy, history of deep vein thrombosis or pulmonary embolism, and surgical procedures requiring general anesthesia and lasting >30 minutes); prevention of DVT in patients undergoing hip-replacement surgery; patients immobile during an acute illness; acute treatment of unstable angina or non-Q-wave myocardial infarction; prevention of ischemic complications in patients on concurrent aspirin therapy

Usual Dosage Adults: SubQ:

Abdominal surgery:

Low-to-moderate DVT risk: 2500 int. units 1-2 hours prior to surgery, then once daily for 5-10 days postoperatively

High DVT risk: 5000 int. units 1-2 hours prior to surgery and then once daily for 5-10 days postoperatively

(Continued)

dalteparin *(Continued)*

Patients undergoing total hip surgery: **Note:** Three treatment options are currently available. Dose is given for 5-10 days, although up to 14 days of treatment have been tolerated in clinical trials:

Postoperative start:

Initial: 2500 int. units 4-8 hours* after surgery

Maintenance: 5000 int. units once daily; start at least 6 hours after postsurgical dose

Preoperative (starting day of surgery):

Initial: 2500 int. units within 2 hours before surgery

Adjustment: 2500 int. units 4-8 hours* after surgery

Maintenance: 5000 int. units once daily; start at least 6 hours after postsurgical dose

Preoperative (starting evening prior to surgery):

Initial: 5000 int. units 10-14 hours before surgery

Adjustment: 5000 int. units 4-8 hours* after surgery

Maintenance: 5000 int. units once daily, allowing 24 hours between doses.

***Dose may be delayed if hemostasis is not yet achieved.**

Unstable angina or non-Q-wave myocardial infarction: 120 int. units/kg body weight (maximum dose: 10,000 int. units) every 12 hours for 5-8 days with concurrent aspirin therapy. Discontinue dalteparin once patient is clinically stable.

Immobility during acute illness: 5000 int. units once daily

Dosage Forms

Injection, solution [multidose vial]: Antifactor Xa 10,000 int. units per 1 mL (9.5 mL) [contains benzyl alcohol]; antifactor Xa 25,000 units per 1 mL (3.8 mL) [contains benzyl alcohol]

Injection, solution [preservative free; prefilled syringe]: Antifactor Xa 2500 int. units per 0.2 mL (0.2 mL); antifactor Xa 5000 int. units per 0.2 mL (0.2 mL); antifactor Xa 7500 int. units per 0.3 mL (0.3 mL); antifactor Xa 10,000 int. units per 1 mL (1 mL)

Damason-P® [US] *see* hydrocodone and aspirin *on page 422*

danaparoid (da NAP a roid)

Synonyms danaparoid sodium

U.S./Canadian Brand Names Orgaran® [Can]

Therapeutic Category Anticoagulant (Other)

Use Prevention of postoperative deep vein thrombosis following elective hip replacement surgery

Usual Dosage SubQ:

Children: Safety and effectiveness have not been established.

Adults: Prevention of DVT following hip replacement: 750 anti-Xa units twice daily; beginning 1-4 hours before surgery and then not sooner than 2 hours after surgery and every 12 hours until the risk of DVT has diminished. The average duration of therapy is 7-10 days.

Dosage Forms [CAN] = Canadian brand name

Injection, solution:

Orgaran® [CAN]: 750 anti-Xa units/0.6 mL (0.6 mL) [not available in the U.S.]

danaparoid sodium *see* danaparoid *on this page*

danazol (DA na zole)

Sound-Alike/Look-Alike Issues

danazol may be confused with Dantrium®

Danocrine® may be confused with Dacriose®

U.S./Canadian Brand Names Cyclomen® [Can]; Danocrine® [Can]

Therapeutic Category Androgen

Use Treatment of endometriosis, fibrocystic breast disease, and hereditary angioedema

Usual Dosage Adults: Oral:

Female: Endometriosis: Initial: 200-400 mg/day in 2 divided doses for mild disease; individualize dosage. Usual maintenance dose: 800 mg/day in 2 divided doses to achieve amenorrhea and rapid response to painful symptoms. Continue therapy uninterrupted for 3-6 months (up to 9 months).

Female: Fibrocystic breast disease: Range: 100-400 mg/day in 2 divided doses

Male/Female: Hereditary angioedema: Initial: 200 mg 2-3 times/day; after favorable response, decrease the dosage by 50% or less at intervals of 1-3 months or longer if the frequency of attacks dictates. If an attack occurs, increase the dosage by up to 200 mg/day.

Dosage Forms [DSC] = Discontinued product

Capsule: 50 mg, 100 mg, 200 mg

Danocrine®: 50 mg, 100 mg, 200 mg [DSC]

Danocrine® [Can] *see* danazol *on previous page*

Danocrine® *(Discontinued)* *see* danazol *on previous page*

Dantrium® [US/Can] *see* dantrolene *on this page*

dantrolene (DAN troe leen)

Sound-Alike/Look-Alike Issues

Dantrium® may be confused with danazol, Daraprim®

Synonyms dantrolene sodium

U.S./Canadian Brand Names Dantrium® [US/Can]

Therapeutic Category Skeletal Muscle Relaxant

Use Treatment of spasticity associated with spinal cord injury, stroke, cerebral palsy, or multiple sclerosis; treatment of malignant hyperthermia

Usual Dosage

Spasticity: Oral:

Children: Initial: 0.5 mg/kg/dose twice daily, increase frequency to 3-4 times/day at 4- to 7-day intervals, then increase dose by 0.5 mg/kg to a maximum of 3 mg/kg/dose 2-4 times/day up to 400 mg/day

Adults: 25 mg/day to start, increase frequency to 2-4 times/day, then increase dose by 25 mg every 4-7 days to a maximum of 100 mg 2-4 times/day or 400 mg/day

Malignant hyperthermia: Children and Adults:

Preoperative prophylaxis:

Oral: 4-8 mg/kg/day in 4 divided doses, begin 1-2 days prior to surgery with last dose 3-4 hours prior to surgery

I.V.: 2.5 mg/kg ~1¼ hours prior to anesthesia and infused over 1 hour with additional doses as needed and individualized

Crisis: I.V.: 2.5 mg/kg; may repeat dose up to cumulative dose of 10 mg/kg; if physiologic and metabolic abnormalities reappear, repeat regimen

Postcrisis follow-up: Oral: 4-8 mg/kg/day in 4 divided doses for 1-3 days; I.V. dantrolene may be used when oral therapy is not practical; individualize dosage beginning with 1 mg/kg or more as the clinical situation dictates

Dosage Forms

Capsule, as sodium: 25 mg, 50 mg, 100 mg

Dantrium®: 25 mg, 50 mg, 100 mg

Injection, powder for reconstitution, as sodium:

Dantrium®: 20 mg [contains mannitol 3 g]

dantrolene sodium *see* dantrolene *on this page*

dapcin *see* daptomycin *on next page*

dapiprazole (DA pi pray zole)

Synonyms dapiprazole hydrochloride

U.S./Canadian Brand Names Rēv-Eyes™ [US]

Therapeutic Category Alpha-Adrenergic Blocking Agent

Use Reverse dilation due to drugs (adrenergic or parasympathomimetic) after eye exams

Usual Dosage Adults: Ophthalmic: Instill 2 drops followed 5 minutes later by an additional 2 drops into the conjunctiva of each eye; should not be used more frequently than once a week in the same patient

Dosage Forms Powder, ophthalmic, as hydrochloride: 25 mg [contains benzalkonium chloride; 0.5% solution when mixed with supplied diluent]

dapiprazole hydrochloride *see* dapiprazole *on this page*

dapsone (DAP sone)

Sound-Alike/Look-Alike Issues

dapsone may be confused with Diprosone®

Synonyms diaminodiphenylsulfone

U.S./Canadian Brand Names Aczone™ [US]

Therapeutic Category Sulfone

Use Treatment of leprosy and dermatitis herpetiformis (infections caused by *Mycobacterium leprae*); treatment of acne vulgaris

Usual Dosage Oral:

Leprosy:

Children: 1-2 mg/kg/24 hours, up to a maximum of 100 mg/day

(Continued)

dapsone *(Continued)*

Adults: 50-100 mg/day for 3-10 years

Dermatitis herpetiformis: Adults: Start at 50 mg/day, increase to 300 mg/day, or higher to achieve full control, reduce dosage to minimum level as soon as possible

Topical: Acne vulgaris: Children ≥12 years and Adults: Apply pea-sized amount twice daily

Dosage Forms

Gel, topical (Aczone™): 5% (30 g)

Tablet: 25 mg, 100 mg

Daptacel® [US] *see* diphtheria, tetanus toxoids, and acellular pertussis vaccine *on page 265*

daptomycin (DAP toe mye sin)

Sound-Alike/Look-Alike Issues

daptomycin may be confused with dactinomycin

Synonyms Cidecin; dapcin; LY146032

U.S./Canadian Brand Names Cubicin® [US]

Therapeutic Category Antibiotic, Cyclic Lipopeptide

Use Treatment of complicated skin and skin structure infections caused by susceptible aerobic Gram-positive organisms; bacteremia, including right-sided infective endocarditis caused by MSSA or MRSA

Usual Dosage I.V.: Adults:

Skin and soft tissue: 4 mg/kg once daily for 7-14 days

Bacteremia, right-sided endocarditis caused by MSSA or MRSA: 6 mg/kg once daily for 2-6 weeks

Dosage Forms Injection, powder for reconstitution: 500 mg

Daraprim® [US/Can] *see* pyrimethamine *on page 722*

darbepoetin alfa (dar be POE e tin AL fa)

Sound-Alike/Look-Alike Issues

darbepoetin alfa may be confused with epoetin alfa

Synonyms erythropoiesis stimulating protein

U.S./Canadian Brand Names Aranesp® [US/Can]

Therapeutic Category Colony-Stimulating Factor; Growth Factor; Recombinant Human Erythropoietin

Use Treatment of anemia associated with chronic renal failure (CRF), including patients on dialysis (ESRD) and patients not on dialysis; anemia associated with chemotherapy for nonmyeloid malignancies

Usual Dosage Adults:

Anemia associated with CRF: I.V., SubQ: Initial: 0.45 mcg/kg once weekly; titrate to response; some patients may respond to doses given once every 2 weeks

Anemia associated with chemotherapy: SubQ: Initial: 2.25 mcg/kg once weekly; with inadequate response after 6 weeks: 4.5 mcg/kg once weekly

or

500 mcg once every 3 weeks

Inadequate response: Increase dose up to 4.5 mcg/kg when hemoglobin increase <1 g/dL after 4-6 weeks

Excessive response:

Decrease dose by ~40% when hemoglobin increases >1 g/dL in any 2-week period **or** hemoglobin exceeds 11 g/dL in any 2-week period

Hold dose, then decrease dose by ~40% when hemoglobin increases despite previous dose decrease (hold until hemoglobin decreases) **or** when hemoglobin ≥13 g/dL (hold until hemoglobin ≤12 g/dL)

Dosage Forms [DSC] = Discontinued product

Injection, solution [preservative free; contains human albumin 2.5 mg/mL; single-dose vial]:

Aranesp®: 25 mcg/mL (1 mL); 40 mcg/mL (1 mL); 60 mcg/mL (1 mL); 100 mcg/mL (1 mL); 150 mcg/0.75 mL (0.75 mL); 200 mcg/mL (1 mL); 300 mcg/mL (1 mL)

Injection, solution [preservative free; contains human albumin 2.5 mg/mL; prefilled syringe]:

Aranesp®: 25 mcg/0.42 mL (0.42 mL); 40 mcg/0.4 mL (0.4 mL); 60 mcg/0.3 mL (0.3 mL); 100 mcg/0.5 mL (0.5 mL); 150 mcg/0.3 mL (0.3 mL); 200 mcg/0.4 mL (0.4 mL); 300 mcg/0.6 mL (0.6 mL); 500 mcg/mL (1 mL) [DSC]

Injection, solution [preservative free; contains polysorbate 80; prefilled syringe]:

Aranesp®: 500 mcg/mL (1 mL)

darifenacin (dar i FEN a sin)

Synonyms darifenacin hydrobromide; UK-88,525

U.S./Canadian Brand Names Enablex® [US/Can]

Therapeutic Category Anticholinergic Agent

Use Management of symptoms of bladder overactivity (urge incontinence, urgency, and frequency)

Usual Dosage

Oral: Adults: Initial: 7.5 mg once daily. If response is not adequate after a minimum of 2 weeks, dosage may be increased to 15 mg once daily.

Dosage adjustment with concomitant potent CYP3A4 inhibitors: Daily dosage should not exceed 7.5 mg/day

Dosage Forms Tablet, extended release: 7.5 mg, 15 mg

darifenacin hydrobromide *see* darifenacin *on this page*

darunavir (dar OO na veer)

Synonyms darunavir ethanolate; TMC-114

U.S./Canadian Brand Names Prezista™ [US]

Therapeutic Category Antiretroviral Agent, Protease Inhibitor

Use Treatment of HIV-1 infections in combination with ritonavir and other antiretroviral agents; limited to highly treatment-experienced or multiprotease inhibitor-resistant patients

Usual Dosage Oral: Adults: 600 mg twice daily with meals

Note: Coadministration with ritonavir (100 mg twice daily) is required.

Dosage Forms

Tablet:

Prezista™: 300 mg

darunavir ethanolate *see* darunavir *on this page*

Darvocet A500™ [US] *see* propoxyphene and acetaminophen *on page 708*

Darvocet-N® 50 [US/Can] *see* propoxyphene and acetaminophen *on page 708*

Darvocet-N® 100 [US/Can] *see* propoxyphene and acetaminophen *on page 708*

Darvon® [US] *see* propoxyphene *on page 708*

Darvon® Compound *(Discontinued)* *see* propoxyphene, aspirin, and caffeine *on page 708*

Darvon-N® [US/Can] *see* propoxyphene *on page 708*

dasatinib (da SA ti nib)

Synonyms BMS-354825; NSC-732517

U.S./Canadian Brand Names Sprycel™ [US]

Therapeutic Category Antineoplastic Agent, Tyrosine Kinase Inhibitor

Use Treatment of chronic myelogenous leukemia (CML); treatment of Philadelphia chromosome-positive (Ph+) acute lymphoblastic leukemia (ALL)

Usual Dosage Oral: Adults: CML, Ph+ ALL: 70 mg twice daily

Dosage Forms

Tablet:

Sprycel™: 20 mg, 50 mg, 70 mg

daunomycin *see* daunorubicin hydrochloride *on next page*

daunorubicin citrate (liposomal) (daw noe ROO bi sin SI trate lip po SOE mal)

Sound-Alike/Look-Alike Issues

DAUNOrubicin may be confused with dactinomycin, DOXOrubicin, epirubicin, idarubicin

liposomal formulations (DaunoXome®) may be confused with conventional formulations (Adriamycin PFS®, Adriamycin RDF®, Cerubidine®, Rubex®)

Tall-Man DAUNOrubicin citrate (liposomal)

U.S./Canadian Brand Names DaunoXome® [US]

Therapeutic Category Antineoplastic Agent

Use First-line cytotoxic therapy for advanced HIV-associated Kaposi sarcoma

Usual Dosage Refer to individual protocols. Adults: I.V.:

20-40 mg/m^2 every 2 weeks

100 mg/m^2 every 3 weeks

Dosage Forms Injection, solution [preservative free]: 2 mg/mL (25 mL) [contains sucrose 2125 mg/25 mL]

daunorubicin hydrochloride (daw noe ROO bi sin hye droe KLOR ide)

Sound-Alike/Look-Alike Issues

DAUNOrubicin may be confused with dactinomycin, DOXOrubicin, epirubicin, idarubicin

conventional formulations (Cerubidine®) may be confused with liposomal formulations (DaunoXome®, Doxil®)

Synonyms daunomycin; DNR; NSC-82151; rubidomycin hydrochloride

Tall-Man **DAUNO**rubicin hydrochloride

U.S./Canadian Brand Names Cerubidine® [US/Can]

Therapeutic Category Antineoplastic Agent

Use Treatment of acute lymphocytic (ALL) and nonlymphocytic (ANLL) leukemias

Usual Dosage I.V. (refer to individual protocols):

Children:

ALL combination therapy: Remission induction: 25-45 mg/m^2 on day 1 every week for 4 cycles **or** 30-45 mg/m^2/day for 3 days

AML combination therapy: Induction: I.V. continuous infusion: 30-60 mg/m^2/day on days 1-3 of cycle

Note: In children <2 years or <0.5 m^2, daunorubicin should be based on weight - mg/kg: 1 mg/kg per protocol with frequency dependent on regimen employed

Cumulative dose should not exceed 300 mg/m^2 in children >2 years; maximum cumulative doses for younger children are unknown.

Adults:

Range: 30-60 mg/m^2/day for 3-5 days, repeat dose in 3-4 weeks

AML: Single agent induction: 60 mg/m^2/day for 3 days; repeat every 3-4 weeks

AML: Combination therapy induction: 45 mg/m^2/day for 3 days of the first course of induction therapy; subsequent courses: Every day for 2 days

ALL combination therapy: 45 mg/m^2/day for 3 days

Cumulative dose should not exceed 550 mg/m^2

Dosage Forms

Injection, powder for reconstitution: 20 mg, 50 mg

Cerubidine®: 20 mg

Injection, solution: 5 mg/mL (4 mL, 10 mL)

DaunoXome® [US] *see* daunorubicin citrate (liposomal) *on previous page*

1-Day™ [US-OTC] *see* tioconazole *on page 830*

Dayhist® Allergy [US-OTC] *see* clemastine *on page 197*

Daypro® [US/Can] *see* oxaprozin *on page 623*

Dayto Himbin® *(Discontinued)* *see* yohimbine *on page 883*

Daytrana™ [US] *see* methylphenidate *on page 546*

DC 240® Softgel® *(Discontinued)* *see* docusate *on page 270*

dCF *see* pentostatin *on page 652*

DDAVP® [US/Can] *see* desmopressin acetate *on page 237*

ddC *see* zalcitabine *on page 884*

ddI *see* didanosine *on page 252*

1-deamino-8-D-arginine vasopressin *see* desmopressin acetate *on page 237*

Debrox® [US-OTC] *see* carbamide peroxide *on page 145*

Decadron® [US] *see* dexamethasone (systemic) *on page 239*

Decadron® Phosphate *(Discontinued)* *see* dexamethasone (systemic) *on page 239*

Deca-Durabolin® [Can] *see* nandrolone *on page 577*

Deca-Durabolin® *(Discontinued)* *see* nandrolone *on page 577*

Decahist-DM *(Discontinued)* *see* carbinoxamine, pseudoephedrine, and dextromethorphan *on page 150*

Decavac™ [US] *see* diphtheria and tetanus toxoid *on page 264*

Dec-Chlorphen [US] *see* chlorpheniramine and phenylephrine *on page 176*

Dec-Chlorphen DM [US] *see* chlorpheniramine, phenylephrine, and dextromethorphan *on page 179*

De-Chlor DM [US] *see* chlorpheniramine, phenylephrine, and dextromethorphan *on page 179*

De-Chlor DR [US] *see* chlorpheniramine, phenylephrine, and dextromethorphan *on page 179*

De-Chlor HC [US] *see* phenylephrine, hydrocodone, and chlorpheniramine *on page 663*

De-Chlor HD [US] *see* phenylephrine, hydrocodone, and chlorpheniramine *on page 663*

decitabine (de SYE ta been)

Synonyms 5-aza-2'-deoxycytidine; 5-azaC; NSC-127716

U.S./Canadian Brand Names Dacogen™ [US]

Therapeutic Category Antineoplastic Agent, Antimetabolite (Pyrimidine)

Use Treatment of myelodysplastic syndrome (MDS)

Usual Dosage Adults: MDS: I.V.: 15 mg/m^2 over 3 hours every 8 hours (45 mg/m^2/day) for 3 days (135 mg/m^2/cycle) every 6 weeks. Treatment is recommended for at least 4 cycles and may continue until the patient no longer continues to benefit.

Dosage Forms

Injection, powder for reconstitution:

Dacogen™: 50 mg

Declomycin® [US/Can] *see* demeclocycline *on next page*

Deconamine® [US] *see* chlorpheniramine and pseudoephedrine *on page 177*

Deconamine® SR [US] *see* chlorpheniramine and pseudoephedrine *on page 177*

Deconsal® II [US] *see* guaifenesin and phenylephrine *on page 396*

Deep Sea [US-OTC] *see* sodium chloride *on page 777*

Defen-LA® *(Discontinued)* *see* guaifenesin and pseudoephedrine *on page 398*

deferasirox (de FER a sir ox)

Synonyms ICL670

U.S./Canadian Brand Names Exjade® [US]

Therapeutic Category Antidote; Chelating Agent

Use Treatment of chronic iron overload due to blood transfusions

Usual Dosage Oral: Children ≥2 years and Adults:

Initial: 20 mg/kg daily (calculate dose to nearest whole tablet)

Maintenance: Adjust dose every 3-6 months based on serum ferritin levels; increase by 5-10 mg/kg/day (calculate dose to nearest whole tablet); titrate. Maximum dose: 30 mg/kg/day; hold dose for serum ferritin <500 mcg/L. **Note:** Consider dose reduction or interruption for hearing loss or visual disturbances.

Dosage Forms Tablet, for oral suspension: 125 mg, 250 mg, 500 mg

deferoxamine (de fer OKS a meen)

Sound-Alike/Look-Alike Issues

deferoxamine may be confused with cefuroxime

Desferal® may be confused with desflurane, Dexferrum®, Disophrol®

Synonyms deferoxamine mesylate

U.S./Canadian Brand Names Desferal® [US/Can]; PMS-Deferoxamine [Can]

Therapeutic Category Antidote

Use Acute iron intoxication or when clinical signs of significant iron toxicity exist; chronic iron overload secondary to multiple transfusions

Usual Dosage

Acute iron toxicity: **Note:** I.V. route is used when severe toxicity is evidenced by systemic symptoms (coma, shock, metabolic acidosis, or severe gastrointestinal bleeding) or potentially severe intoxications (serum iron level >500 mcg/dL). When severe symptoms are not present, the I.M. route may be preferred (per manufacturer); however, the use of deferoxamine in situations where the serum iron concentration is <500 mcg/dL or when severe toxicity is not evident is a subject of some clinical debate.

Children:

I.M.: 90 mg/kg/dose every 8 hours (maximum: 6 g/24 hours)

I.V.: 15 mg/kg/hour (maximum: 6 g/24 hours)

Adults: I.M., I.V.: Initial: 1000 mg, may be followed by 500 mg every 4 hours for up to 2 doses; subsequent doses of 500 mg have been administered every 4-12 hours

Maximum recommended dose: 6 g/day (per manufacturer, however, higher doses have been administered)

Chronic iron overload:

Children: SubQ: 20-40 mg/kg/day over 8-12 hours (maximum: 1000-2000 mg/day)

(Continued)

deferoxamine *(Continued)*

Adults:

I.M., I.V.: 500-1000 mg/day I.M.; in addition, 2000 mg should be given I.V. with each unit of blood transfused (administer separately from blood); maximum: 6 g/day

SubQ: 1-2 g every day over 8-24 hours

Dosage Forms Injection, powder for reconstitution, as mesylate: 500 mg, 2 g

deferoxamine mesylate *see* deferoxamine *on previous page*

Deficol® *(Discontinued)* *see* bisacodyl *on page 111*

Definity® [US/Can] *see* perflutren lipid microspheres *on page 653*

Degest® 2 Ophthalmic *(Discontinued)* *see* naphazoline *on page 577*

Dehistine [US] *see* chlorpheniramine, phenylephrine, and methscopolamine *on page 180*

Dehydral® [Can] *see* methenamine *on page 538*

dehydrobenzperidol *see* droperidol *on page 281*

Del Aqua® [US] *see* benzoyl peroxide *on page 102*

Delatest® Injection *(Discontinued)* *see* testosterone *on page 812*

Delatestryl® [US/Can] *see* testosterone *on page 812*

delavirdine (de la VIR deen)

Synonyms U-90152S

U.S./Canadian Brand Names Rescriptor® [US/Can]

Therapeutic Category Antiviral Agent

Use Treatment of HIV-1 infection in combination with at least two additional antiretroviral agents

Usual Dosage Adolescents ≥16 years and Adults: Oral: 400 mg 3 times/day

Dosage Forms Tablet, as mesylate: 100 mg, 200 mg

Delestrogen® [US] *see* estradiol *on page 308*

Delfen® [US-OTC] *see* nonoxynol 9 *on page 597*

Delsym® [US-OTC] *see* dextromethorphan *on page 245*

delta-9-tetrahydro-cannabinol *see* dronabinol *on page 281*

delta-9-tetrahydrocannabinol and cannabinol *see* tetrahydrocannabinol and cannabidiol *(Canada only) on page 816*

delta-9 THC *see* dronabinol *on page 281*

Delta-D® [US] *see* cholecalciferol *on page 185*

deltacortisone *see* prednisone *on page 695*

deltadehydrocortisone *see* prednisone *on page 695*

deltahydrocortisone *see* prednisolone (systemic) *on page 695*

Del-Vi-A® *(Discontinued)* *see* vitamin A *on page 874*

Demadex® [US] *see* torsemide *on page 837*

demeclocycline (dem e kloe SYE kleen)

Synonyms demeclocycline hydrochloride; demethylchlortetracycline

U.S./Canadian Brand Names Declomycin® [US/Can]

Therapeutic Category Tetracycline Derivative

Use Treatment of susceptible bacterial infections (acne, gonorrhea, pertussis, and urinary tract infections) caused by both gram-negative and gram-positive organisms

Usual Dosage Oral:

Children ≥8 years: 8-12 mg/kg/day divided every 6-12 hours

Adults: 150 mg 4 times/day or 300 mg twice daily

Dosage Forms Tablet, as hydrochloride: 150 mg, 300 mg

demeclocycline hydrochloride *see* demeclocycline *on this page*

Demerol® [US/Can] *see* meperidine *on page 529*

4-demethoxydaunorubicin *see* idarubicin *on page 439*

demethylchlortetracycline *see* demeclocycline *on this page*

Demser® [US/Can] *see* metyrosine *on page 552*

Demulen® [US] *see* ethinyl estradiol and ethynodiol diacetate *on page 319*

Demulen® 30 [Can] *see* ethinyl estradiol and ethynodiol diacetate *on page 319*

Denavir® [US] *see* penciclovir *on page 646*

denileukin diftitox (de ni LOO kin DIF ti toks)

Synonyms $DAB_{389}IL$-2; NSC-714744

U.S./Canadian Brand Names ONTAK® [US]

Therapeutic Category Antineoplastic Agent, Miscellaneous

Use Treatment of persistent or recurrent cutaneous T-cell lymphoma whose malignant cells express the CD25 component of the IL-2 receptor

Usual Dosage Adults: I.V.: 9 or 18 mcg/kg/day days 1 through 5 every 21 days

Dosage Forms

Injection, solution [frozen]:

ONTAK®: 150 mcg/mL (2 mL) [contains EDTA]

Denorex® Original Therapeutic Strength [US-OTC] *see* coal tar *on page 207*

Denta 5000 Plus [US] *see* fluoride *on page 354*

DentaGel [US] *see* fluoride *on page 354*

Dentapaine [US-OTC] *see* benzocaine *on page 99*

Dent's Ear Wax [US-OTC] *see* carbamide peroxide *on page 145*

Dent's Extra Strength Toothache [US-OTC] *see* benzocaine *on page 99*

Dent's Maxi-Strength Toothache [US-OTC] *see* benzocaine *on page 99*

deoxycoformycin *see* pentostatin *on page 652*

2′-deoxycoformycin *see* pentostatin *on page 652*

Depacon® [US] *see* valproic acid and derivatives *on page 864*

Depade® [US] *see* naltrexone *on page 577*

Depakene® [US/Can] *see* valproic acid and derivatives *on page 864*

Depakote® Delayed Release [US] *see* valproic acid and derivatives *on page 864*

Depakote® ER [US] *see* valproic acid and derivatives *on page 864*

Depakote® Sprinkle® [US] *see* valproic acid and derivatives *on page 864*

depAndro® Injection *(Discontinued)* *see* testosterone *on page 812*

Depen® [US/Can] *see* penicillamine *on page 646*

depGynogen® Injection *(Discontinued)* *see* estradiol *on page 308*

depMedalone® Injection *(Discontinued)* *see* methylprednisolone *on page 547*

DepoCyt® [US] *see* cytarabine (liposomal) *on page 225*

DepoDur™ [US] *see* morphine sulfate *on page 565*

Depo®-Estradiol [US/Can] *see* estradiol *on page 308*

Depoject® Injection *(Discontinued)* *see* methylprednisolone *on page 547*

Depo-Medrol® [US/Can] *see* methylprednisolone *on page 547*

Deponit® Patch *(Discontinued)* *see* nitroglycerin *on page 595*

Depo-Prevera® [Can] *see* medroxyprogesterone *on page 524*

Depo-Provera® [US/Can] *see* medroxyprogesterone *on page 524*

Depo-Provera® Contraceptive [US] *see* medroxyprogesterone *on page 524*

depo-subQ provera 104™ [US] *see* medroxyprogesterone *on page 524*

Depotest® 100 [Can] *see* testosterone *on page 812*

Depotest® Injection *(Discontinued)* *see* testosterone *on page 812*

Depo®-Testosterone [US] *see* testosterone *on page 812*

deprenyl *see* selegiline *on page 766*

dequalinium *(Canada only)* (de kwal LI ne um)

Therapeutic Category Antibacterial, Topical; Antifungal Agent, Topical

Use Treatment of mouth and throat infections

Usual Dosage Adults:

Lozenge: One lozenge sucked slowly every 2-3 hours

Oral paint: Apply freely to infected area, every 2-3 hours, or as directed by physician

Dosage Forms

Lozenge, as chloride: 0.25 mg (20s)

Oral paint, as chloride: 0.5% (25 mL)

Dermaflex® Gel *(Discontinued)* *see* lidocaine *on page 493*

DermaFungal [US-OTC] *see* miconazole *on page 553*

Dermagran® [US-OTC] *see* aluminum hydroxide *on page 36*

Dermagran® AF [US-OTC] *see* miconazole *on page 553*

Dermamycin® [US-OTC] *see* diphenhydramine *on page 261*

Dermarest Dricort® [US-OTC] *see* hydrocortisone (topical) *on page 428*

Dermarest® Insect Bite [US-OTC] *see* diphenhydramine *on page 261*

Dermarest® Plus [US-OTC] *see* diphenhydramine *on page 261*

Dermarest® Skin Correction Cream Plus [US-OTC] *see* hydroquinone *on page 430*

Derma-Smoothe/FS® [US/Can] *see* fluocinolone *on page 352*

Dermatop® [US/Can] *see* prednicarbate *on page 694*

Dermatophytin-O *(Discontinued)*

Dermazene® [US] *see* iodoquinol and hydrocortisone *on page 459*

DermaZinc™ [US-OTC] *see* pyrithione zinc *on page 723*

Dermazole [Can] *see* miconazole *on page 553*

Dermoplast® Antibacterial [US-OTC] *see* benzocaine *on page 99*

Dermoplast® Pain Relieving [US-OTC] *see* benzocaine *on page 99*

Dermovate® [Can] *see* clobetasol *on page 200*

Dermtex® HC [US-OTC] *see* hydrocortisone (topical) *on page 428*

Desferal® [US/Can] *see* deferoxamine *on page 233*

desflurane (DES flure ane)

Sound-Alike/Look-Alike Issues

desflurane may be confused with Desferal®

U.S./Canadian Brand Names Suprane® [US/Can]

Therapeutic Category General Anesthetic

Use Maintenance of general anesthesia

Usual Dosage

Children: Maintenance: Surgical levels of anesthesia range between 5.2% to 10%

Adults: The minimum alveolar concentration (MAC), the concentration at which 50% of patients do not respond to surgical incision, ranges from 6.0% (45 years of age) to 7.3% (25 years of age). The concentration at which amnesia and loss of awareness occur (MAC - awake) is 2.4%. Surgical levels of anesthesia are achieved with concentrations between 2.5% to 8.5%.

Note: Because of the higher vapor pressure of desflurane, its vaporizer is heated in order to deliver a constant concentration

Dosage Forms Liquid, for inhalation: 240 mL

desiccated thyroid *see* thyroid *on page 824*

desipramine (des IP ra meen)

Sound-Alike/Look-Alike Issues

desipramine may be confused with clomiPRAMINE, deserpidine, diphenhydrAMINE, disopyramide, imipramine, nortriptyline

Norpramin® may be confused with clomiPRAMINE, imipramine, Norpace®, nortriptyline, Tenormin®

Synonyms desipramine hydrochloride; desmethylimipramine hydrochloride

U.S./Canadian Brand Names Alti-Desipramine [Can]; Apo-Desipramine® [Can]; Norpramin® [US/Can]; Nu-Desipramine [Can]; PMS-Desipramine [Can]

Therapeutic Category Antidepressant, Tricyclic (Secondary Amine)

Use Treatment of depression

Usual Dosage Oral (dose is generally administered at bedtime):

Adolescents: Depression: Initial: 25-50 mg/day; gradually increase to 100 mg/day in single or divided doses (maximum: 150 mg/day)

Adults: Depression: Initial: 75 mg/day in divided doses; increase gradually to 150-200 mg/day in divided or single dose (maximum: 300 mg/day)

Dosage Forms Tablet, as hydrochloride: 10 mg, 25 mg, 50 mg, 75 mg, 100 mg, 150 mg

desipramine hydrochloride *see* desipramine *on previous page*

Desitin® [US-OTC] *see* zinc oxide *on page 887*

Desitin® Creamy [US-OTC] *see* zinc oxide *on page 887*

desloratadine (des lor AT a deen)

U.S./Canadian Brand Names Aerius® [Can]; Clarinex® [US]

Therapeutic Category Antihistamine, Nonsedating

Use Relief of nasal and non-nasal symptoms of seasonal allergic rhinitis (SAR) and perennial allergic rhinitis (PAR); treatment of chronic idiopathic urticaria (CIU)

Usual Dosage Oral:

Children:

6-11 months: 1 mg once daily

12 months to 5 years: 1.25 mg once daily

6-11 years: 2.5 mg once daily

Children ≥12 years and Adults: 5 mg once daily

Dosage Forms

Syrup (Clarinex®): 0.5 mg/mL (120 mL, 480 mL) [bubble gum flavor]

Tablet (Clarinex®): 5 mg

Tablet, orally disintegrating (Clarinex® RediTabs®): 2.5 mg [contains phenylalanine 1.28 mg/tablet; tutti-frutti flavor]; 5 mg [contains phenylalanine 2.55 mg/tablet; tutti-frutti flavor]

desmethylimipramine hydrochloride *see* desipramine *on previous page*

desmopressin acetate (des moe PRES in AS e tate)

Synonyms 1-deamino-8-D-arginine vasopressin

U.S./Canadian Brand Names Apo-Desmopressin® [Can]; DDAVP® [US/Can]; Minirin® [Can]; Octostim® [Can]; Stimate™ [US]

Therapeutic Category Vasopressin Analog, Synthetic

Use

Injection: Treatment of diabetes insipidus; control of bleeding in hemophilia A, and mild-to-moderate classic von Willebrand disease (type I)

Tablet, nasal solution: Treatment of diabetes insipidus; primary nocturnal enuresis

Usual Dosage

Children:

Diabetes insipidus:

Intranasal (using 100 mcg/mL nasal solution): 3 months to 12 years: Initial: 5 mcg/day (0.05 mL/day) divided 1-2 times/day; range: 5-30 mcg/day (0.05-0.3 mL/day) divided 1-2 times/day; adjust morning and evening doses separately for an adequate diurnal rhythm of water turnover; doses <10 mcg should be administered using the rhinal tube system

Oral: ≥4 years: Initial: 0.05 mg twice daily; total daily dose should be increased or decreased as needed to obtain adequate antidiuresis (range: 0.1-1.2 mg divided 2-3 times/day)

Hemophilia A and von Willebrand disease (type I):

I.V.: >3 months: 0.3 mcg/kg by slow infusion; may repeat dose if needed; begin 30 minutes before procedure

Intranasal: ≥11 months: Refer to adult dosing.

Nocturnal enuresis:

Intranasal (using 100 mcg/mL nasal solution): ≥6 years: Initial: 20 mcg (0.2 mL) at bedtime; range: 10-40 mcg; it is recommended that ½ of the dose be given in each nostril. **Note:** The nasal spray pump can only deliver doses of 10 mcg (0.1 mL) or multiples of 10 mcg (0.1 mL); if doses other than this are needed, the rhinal tube delivery system is preferred. For 10 mcg dose, administer in one nostril.

(Continued)

desmopressin acetate *(Continued)*

Oral: 0.2 mg at bedtime; dose may be titrated up to 0.6 mg to achieve desired response. Patients previously on intranasal therapy can begin oral tablets 24 hours after the last intranasal dose.

Children ≥12 years and Adults:

Diabetes insipidus:

I.V., SubQ: 2-4 mcg/day (0.5-1 mL) in 2 divided doses or $^1/_{10}$ of the maintenance intranasal dose

Intranasal (using 100 mcg/mL nasal solution): 10-40 mcg/day (0.1-0.4 mL) divided 1-3 times/day; adjust morning and evening doses separately for an adequate diurnal rhythm of water turnover. **Note:** The nasal spray pump can only deliver doses of 10 mcg (0.1 mL) or multiples of 10 mcg (0.1 mL); if doses other than this are needed, the rhinal tube delivery system is preferred.

Oral: Initial: 0.05 mg twice daily; total daily dose should be increased or decreased as needed to obtain adequate antidiuresis (range: 0.1-1.2 mg divided 2-3 times/day)

Hemophilia A and mild to moderate von Willebrand disease (type I):

I.V.: 0.3 mcg/kg by slow infusion, begin 30 minutes before procedure

Intranasal: Using high concentration spray (1.5 mg/mL): <50 kg: 150 mcg (1 spray); >50 kg: 300 mcg (1 spray each nostril); repeat use is determined by the patient's clinical condition and laboratory work; if using preoperatively, administer 2 hours before surgery

Dosage Forms

Injection, solution, as acetate (DDAVP®): 4 mcg/mL (1 mL, 10 mL)

Solution, intranasal, as acetate (DDAVP®): 100 mcg/mL (2.5 mL) [with rhinal tube]

Solution, intranasal, as acetate [spray]: 100 mcg/mL (5 mL) [delivers 10 mcg/spray]

DDAVP®: 100 mcg/mL (5 mL) [delivers 10 mcg/spray]

Stimate™: 1.5 mg/mL (2.5 mL) [delivers 150 mcg/spray]

Tablet, as acetate (DDAVP®): 0.1 mg, 0.2 mg

Desocort® [Can] *see* desonide *on this page*

Desogen® [US] *see* ethinyl estradiol and desogestrel *on page 317*

desogestrel and ethinyl estradiol *see* ethinyl estradiol and desogestrel *on page 317*

desonide (DES oh nide)

U.S./Canadian Brand Names Desocort® [Can]; DesOwen® [US]; LoKara™ [US]; PMS-Desonide [Can]; Tridesilon® [US]

Therapeutic Category Corticosteroid, Topical

Use Adjunctive therapy for inflammation in acute and chronic corticosteroid responsive dermatosis (low potency corticosteroid); mild-to-moderate atopic dermatitis

Usual Dosage Corticosteroid responsive dermatoses: Topical: Apply 2-4 times/day sparingly. Therapy should be discontinued when control is achieved; if no improvement is seen, reassessment of diagnosis may be necessary.

Dosage Forms

Aerosol, topical [foam]:

Verdeso®: 0.05% (100 g)

Cream, topical: 0.05% (15 g, 60 g)

DesOwen®: 0.05% (15 g, 60 g, 90 g)

Gel, topical [aqueous]:

Desonate™: 0.05% (15 g, 30 g, 60g)

Lotion, topical: 0.05% (60 mL, 120 mL)

DesOwen®, LoKara™: 0.05% (60 mL, 120 mL)

Ointment, topical: 0.05% (15 g, 60 g)

DesOwen®: 0.05% (15 g, 60 g)

DesOwen® [US] *see* desonide *on this page*

desoximetasone (des oks i MET a sone)

Sound-Alike/Look-Alike Issues

desoximetasone may be confused with dexamethasone

Topicort® may be confused with Topic®

U.S./Canadian Brand Names Taro-Desoximetasone [Can]; Topicort® [US/Can]; Topicort®-LP [US]

Therapeutic Category Corticosteroid, Topical

Use Relieves inflammation and pruritic symptoms of corticosteroid-responsive dermatosis (intermediate- to high-potency topical corticosteroid)

Usual Dosage Desoximetasone is a potent fluorinated topical corticosteroid. Therapy should be discontinued when control is achieved; if no improvement is seen, reassessment of diagnosis may be necessary.

Cream, gel: Children and Adults: Apply a thin film to affected area twice daily
Ointment: Children ≥10 years and Adults: Apply a thin film to affected area twice daily

Dosage Forms

Cream, topical: 0.25% (15 g, 60 g); 0.05% (15 g, 60 g)
Topicort®: 0.25% (15 g, 60 g)
Topicort®-LP: 0.05% (15 g, 60 g)
Gel, topical (Topicort®): 0.05% (15 g, 60 g) [contains alcohol 20%]
Ointment, topical (Topicort®): 0.25% (15 g, 60 g)

desoxyephedrine hydrochloride *see* methamphetamine *on page 538*

Desoxyn® [US/Can] *see* methamphetamine *on page 538*

desoxyphenobarbital *see* primidone *on page 699*

Desquam-X® [US/Can] *see* benzoyl peroxide *on page 102*

Desquam-X® Wash *(Discontinued)* *see* benzoyl peroxide *on page 102*

Desquam-E™ [US] *see* benzoyl peroxide *on page 102*

Desyrel® [US/Can] *see* trazodone *on page 843*

Detane® [US-OTC] *see* benzocaine *on page 99*

detemir insulin *see* insulin detemir *on page 450*

Detrol® [US/Can] *see* tolterodine *on page 835*

Detrol® LA [US/Can] *see* tolterodine *on page 835*

Detuss [US] *see* pseudoephedrine, hydrocodone, and chlorpheniramine *on page 716*

Detussin® Expectorant *(Discontinued)* *see* hydrocodone, pseudoephedrine, and guaifenesin *on page 425*

Dex4 Glucose [US-OTC] *see* glucose (instant) *on page 386*

Dexacidin® *(Discontinued)* *see* neomycin, polymyxin B, and dexamethasone *on page 584*

Dexacine™ *(Discontinued)* *see* neomycin, polymyxin B, and dexamethasone *on page 584*

Dexalone® [US-OTC] *see* dextromethorphan *on page 245*

dexamethasone and ciprofloxacin *see* ciprofloxacin and dexamethasone *on page 192*

dexamethasone and tobramycin *see* tobramycin and dexamethasone *on page 833*

Dexamethasone Intensol® [US] *see* dexamethasone (systemic) *on this page*

dexamethasone, neomycin, and polymyxin B *see* neomycin, polymyxin B, and dexamethasone *on page 584*

dexamethasone (ophthalmic) (deks a METH a sone op THAL mik)

Sound-Alike/Look-Alike Issues

dexamethasone may be confused with desoximetasone
Maxidex® may be confused with Maxzide®

Synonyms dexamethasone sodium phosphate

U.S./Canadian Brand Names Maxidex® [US/Can]

Therapeutic Category Adrenal Corticosteroid

Use Inflammatory or allergic conjunctivitis

Usual Dosage Adults: Ophthalmic:

Ointment: Apply thin coating into conjunctival sac 3-4 times/day; gradually taper dose to discontinue
Suspension: Instill 2 drops into conjunctival sac every hour during the day and every other hour during the night; gradually reduce dose to every 3-4 hours, then to 3-4 times/day

Dosage Forms

Ointment, ophthalmic, as sodium phosphate: 0.05% (3.5 g)
Solution, ophthalmic, as sodium phosphate: 0.1% (5 mL)
Suspension, ophthalmic (Maxidex®): 0.1% (5 mL, 15 mL)

dexamethasone sodium phosphate *see* dexamethasone (ophthalmic) *on this page*

dexamethasone sodium phosphate *see* dexamethasone (systemic) *on this page*

dexamethasone (systemic) (deks a METH a sone sis TEM ik)

Sound-Alike/Look-Alike Issues

dexamethasone may be confused with desoximetasone
Decadron® may be confused with Percodan®

(Continued)

dexamethasone (systemic) *(Continued)*

Synonyms dexamethasone sodium phosphate

U.S./Canadian Brand Names Apo-Dexamethasone® [Can]; Decadron® [US]; Dexamethasone Intensol® [US]; Dexasone® [Can]; DexPak® TaperPak® [US]; Diodex® [Can]; PMS-Dexamethasone [Can]

Therapeutic Category Adrenal Corticosteroid

Use Systemically and locally for chronic swelling; allergic, hematologic, neoplastic, and autoimmune diseases; may be used in management of cerebral edema, septic shock, as a diagnostic agent, antiemetic

Usual Dosage

Children:

Antiemetic (prior to chemotherapy): I.V. (should be given as sodium phosphate): 5-20 mg given 15-30 minutes before treatment

Antiinflammatory immunosuppressant: Oral, I.M., I.V. (injections should be given as sodium phosphate): 0.08-0.3 mg/kg/day **or** 2.5-10 mg/m^2/day in divided doses every 6-12 hours

Extubation or airway edema: Oral, I.M., I.V. (injections should be given as sodium phosphate): 0.5-2 mg/kg/day in divided doses every 6 hours beginning 24 hours prior to extubation and continuing for 4-6 doses afterwards

Cerebral edema: I.V. (should be given as sodium phosphate): Loading dose: 1-2 mg/kg/dose as a single dose; maintenance: 1-1.5 mg/kg/day (maximum: 16 mg/day) in divided doses every 4-6 hours for 5 days then taper for 5 days, then discontinue

Bacterial meningitis in infants and children >2 months: I.V. (should be given as sodium phosphate): 0.6 mg/kg/day in 4 divided doses every 6 hours for the first 4 days of antibiotic treatment; start dexamethasone at the time of the first dose of antibiotic

Physiologic replacement: Oral, I.M., I.V.: 0.03-0.15 mg/kg/day **or** 0.6-0.75 mg/m^2/day in divided doses every 6-12 hours

Adults:

Antiemetic:

Prophylaxis: Oral, I.V.: 10-20 mg 15-30 minutes before treatment on each treatment day

Continuous infusion regimen: Oral or I.V.: 10 mg every 12 hours on each treatment day

Mildly emetogenic therapy: Oral, I.M., I.V.: 4 mg every 4-6 hours

Delayed nausea/vomiting: Oral: 4-10 mg 1-2 times/day for 2-4 days **or**

8 mg every 12 hours for 2 days; then

4 mg every 12 hours for 2 days **or**

20 mg 1 hour before chemotherapy; then

10 mg 12 hours after chemotherapy; then

8 mg every 12 hours for 4 doses; then

4 mg every 12 hours for 4 doses

Antiinflammatory:

Oral, I.M., I.V. (injections should be given as sodium phosphate): 0.75-9 mg/day in divided doses every 6-12 hours

Intra-articular, intralesional, or soft tissue (as sodium phosphate): 0.4-6 mg/day

Chemotherapy: Oral, I.V.: 40 mg every day for 4 days, repeated every 4 weeks (VAD regimen)

Cerebral edema: I.V. 10 mg stat, 4 mg I.M./I.V. (should be given as sodium phosphate) every 6 hours until response is maximized, then switch to oral regimen, then taper off if appropriate; dosage may be reduced after 24 days and gradually discontinued over 5-7 days

Cushing syndrome, diagnostic: Oral: 1 mg at 11 PM, draw blood at 8 AM; greater accuracy for Cushing syndrome may be achieved by the following:

Dexamethasone 0.5 mg by mouth every 6 hours for 48 hours (with 24-hour urine collection for 17-hydroxycorticosteroid excretion)

Differentiation of Cushing syndrome due to ACTH excess from Cushing due to other causes: Oral: Dexamethasone 2 mg every 6 hours for 48 hours (with 24-hour urine collection for 17-hydroxycorticosteroid excretion)

Multiple sclerosis (acute exacerbation): 30 mg/day for 1 week, followed by 4-12 mg/day for 1 month

Physiological replacement: Oral, I.M., I.V. (should be given as sodium phosphate): 0.03-0.15 mg/kg/day **or** 0.6-0.75 mg/m^2/day in divided doses every 6-12 hours

Treatment of shock:

Addisonian crisis/shock (ie, adrenal insufficiency/responsive to steroid therapy): I.V. (given as sodium phosphate): 4-10 mg as a single dose, which may be repeated if necessary

Unresponsive shock (ie, unresponsive to steroid therapy): I.V. (given as sodium phosphate): 1-6 mg/kg as a single I.V. dose or up to 40 mg initially followed by repeat doses every 2-6 hours while shock persists

Hemodialysis: Supplemental dose is not necessary

Peritoneal dialysis: Supplemental dose is not necessary

Dosage Forms [DSC] = Discontinued product

Elixir, as base: 0.5 mg/5 mL (240 mL) [contains alcohol 5%; raspberry flavor]

Injection, solution, as sodium phosphate: 4 mg/mL (1 mL, 5 mL, 10 mL, 25 mL, 30 mL); 10 mg/mL (1 mL, 10 mL)
Decadron® Phosphate: 4 mg/mL (5 mL, 25 mL); 24 mg/mL (5 mL) [contains sodium bisulfite] [DSC]
Tablet: 0.25 mg, 0.5 mg, 0.75 mg, 1 mg, 1.5 mg, 2 mg, 4 mg, 6 mg [some 0.5 mg tablets may contain tartrazine]
Decadron®: 0.5 mg, 0.75 mg, 4 mg
DexPak® TaperPak®: 1.5 mg [51 tablets on taper dose card]

Dexasone® [Can] *see* dexamethasone (systemic) *on page 239*

dexbrompheniramine and pseudoephedrine

(deks brom fen EER a meen & soo doe e FED rin)

Synonyms pseudoephedrine and dexbrompheniramine

U.S./Canadian Brand Names Drixoral® Cold & Allergy [US-OTC]; Drixoral® [Can]

Therapeutic Category Antihistamine/Decongestant Combination

Use Relief of symptoms of upper respiratory mucosal congestion in seasonal and perennial nasal allergies, acute rhinitis, rhinosinusitis and eustachian tube blockage

Usual Dosage Children >12 years and Adults: Oral: 1 timed release tablet every 12 hours, may require 1 tablet every 8 hours

Dosage Forms Tablet, sustained action: Dexbrompheniramine maleate 6 mg and pseudoephedrine sulfate 120 mg

Dexchlor® ***(Discontinued)*** *see* dexchlorpheniramine *on this page*

dexchlorpheniramine (deks klor fen EER a meen)

Synonyms dexchlorpheniramine maleate

Therapeutic Category Antihistamine

Use Perennial and seasonal allergic rhinitis and other allergic symptoms including urticaria

Usual Dosage Oral:

Children:
2-5 years: 0.5 mg every 4-6 hours (do not use timed release)
6-11 years: 1 mg every 4-6 hours or 4 mg timed release at bedtime
Adults: 2 mg every 4-6 hours or 4-6 mg timed release at bedtime or every 8-10 hours

Dosage Forms

Syrup, as maleate: 2 mg/5 mL (480 mL, 3840 mL) [contains alcohol 6%; orange flavor]
Tablet, sustained action, as maleate: 4 mg, 6 mg

dexchlorpheniramine maleate *see* dexchlorpheniramine *on this page*

dexchlorpheniramine tannate, pseudoephedrine tannate, and dextromethorphan tannate *see* chlorpheniramine, pseudoephedrine, and dextromethorphan *on page 182*

Dexcon-DM [US] *see* guaifenesin, dextromethorphan, and phenylephrine *on page 400*

Dexcon-PE [US] *see* guaifenesin, dextromethorphan, and phenylephrine *on page 400*

Dexedrine® [US/Can] *see* dextroamphetamine *on page 243*

Dexferrum® [US] *see* iron dextran complex *on page 462*

Dexiron™ [Can] *see* iron dextran complex *on page 462*

dexmedetomidine (deks MED e toe mi deen)

Sound-Alike/Look-Alike Issues

Precedex™ may be confused with Peridex®

Synonyms dexmedetomidine hydrochloride

U.S./Canadian Brand Names Precedex™ [US/Can]

Therapeutic Category Alpha-Adrenergic Agonist - Central-Acting (Alpha$_2$-Agonists); Sedative

Use Sedation of initially intubated and mechanically ventilated patients during treatment in an intensive care setting; duration of infusion should not exceed 24 hours

Usual Dosage Individualized and titrated to desired clinical effect

Adults: I.V.: Solution must be diluted prior to administration. Initial: Loading infusion of 1 mcg/kg over 10 minutes, followed by a maintenance infusion of 0.2-0.7 mcg/kg/hour; not indicated for infusions lasting >24 hours

Dosage Forms Injection, solution [preservative free]: 100 mcg/mL (2 mL)

dexmedetomidine hydrochloride *see* dexmedetomidine *on this page*

dexmethylphenidate (dex meth il FEN i date)

Synonyms dexmethylphenidate hydrochloride

U.S./Canadian Brand Names Focalin™ XR [US]; Focalin™ [US]

Therapeutic Category Central Nervous System Stimulant, Nonamphetamine

Controlled Substance C-II

Use Treatment of attention-deficit/hyperactivity disorder (ADHD)

Usual Dosage Treatment of ADHD: Oral:

Children ≥6 years: Patients not currently taking methylphenidate:

Tablet: Initial: 2.5 mg twice daily; dosage may be adjusted in increments of 2.5-5 mg at weekly intervals (maximum dose: 20 mg/day); doses should be taken at least 4 hours apart

Capsule: Initial: 5 mg/day; dosage may be adjusted in increments of 5 mg/day at weekly intervals (maximum dose: 20 mg/day)

Adults: Patients not currently taking methylphenidate:

Tablet: Initial: 2.5 mg twice daily; dosage may be adjusted in increments of 2.5-5 mg at weekly intervals (maximum dose: 20 mg/day); doses should be taken at least 4 hours apart

Capsule: Initial: 10 mg/day; dosage may be adjusted in increments of 10 mg/day at weekly intervals (maximum dose: 20 mg/day)

Conversion to dexmethylphenidate from methylphenidate: Tablet, capsule: Initial: Half the total daily dose of racemic methylphenidate (maximum dexmethylphenidate dose: 20 mg/day)

Conversion from dexmethylphenidate immediate release to dexmethylphenidate extended release: When changing from Focalin™ tablets to Focalin™ XR capsules, patients may be switched to the same daily dose using Focalin™ XR (maximum dose: 20 mg/day)

Dose reductions and discontinuation: Reduce dose or discontinue in patients with paradoxical aggravation of symptoms. Discontinue if no improvement is seen after one month of treatment.

Dosage Forms

Capsule, extended release:

Focalin® XR: 5 mg, 10 mg, 15 mg, 20 mg [bimodal release]

Tablet, as hydrochloride

Focalin®: 2.5 mg, 5 mg, 10 mg

dexmethylphenidate hydrochloride *see* dexmethylphenidate *on this page*

DexPak® TaperPak® [US] *see* dexamethasone (systemic) *on page 239*

dexpanthenol (deks PAN the nole)

Synonyms pantothenyl alcohol

U.S./Canadian Brand Names Panthoderm® [US-OTC]

Therapeutic Category Gastrointestinal Agent, Stimulant

Use Prophylactic use to minimize paralytic ileus; treatment of postoperative distention; topical to relieve itching and to aid healing of minor dermatoses

Usual Dosage

Children and Adults: Relief of itching and aid in skin healing: Topical: Apply to affected area 1-2 times/day

Adults:

Prevention of postoperative ileus: I.M.: 250-500 mg stat, repeat in 2 hours, followed by doses every 6 hours until danger passes

Paralytic ileus: I.M.: 500 mg stat, repeat in 2 hours, followed by doses every 6 hours, if needed

Dosage Forms

Cream, topical: 2% (30 g, 60 g)

Injection, solution: 250 mg/mL (2 mL)

Dex PC [US] *see* chlorpheniramine, phenylephrine, and dextromethorphan *on page 179*

dexrazoxane (deks ray ZOKS ane)

Sound-Alike/Look-Alike Issues

Zinecard® may be confused with Gemzar®

Synonyms ICRF-187

U.S./Canadian Brand Names Zinecard® [US/Can]

Therapeutic Category Cardiovascular Agent, Other

Use Reduction of the incidence and severity of cardiomyopathy associated with doxorubicin administration in women with metastatic breast cancer who have received a cumulative doxorubicin dose of 300 mg/m^2 and who would benefit from continuing therapy with doxorubicin. It is not recommended for use with the initiation of doxorubicin therapy.

Usual Dosage Adults: I.V.: A 10:1 ratio of dexrazoxane:doxorubicin (500 mg/m^2 dexrazoxane: 50 mg/m^2 doxorubicin)

Dosage Forms Injection, powder for reconstitution: 250 mg, 500 mg [10 mg/mL when reconstituted]

dextran (DEKS tran)

Sound-Alike/Look-Alike Issues

dextran may be confused with Dexatrim®, Dexedrine®

Synonyms dextran 40; dextran 70; dextran, high molecular weight; dextran, low molecular weight

U.S./Canadian Brand Names Gentran® [US/Can]; LMD® [US]

Therapeutic Category Plasma Volume Expander

Use Blood volume expander used in treatment of shock or impending shock when blood or blood products are not available; dextran 40 is also used as a priming fluid in cardiopulmonary bypass and for prophylaxis of venous thrombosis and pulmonary embolism in surgical procedures associated with a high risk of thromboembolic complications

Usual Dosage I.V. (requires an infusion pump): Dose and infusion rate are dependent upon the patient's fluid status and must be individualized:

Volume expansion/shock:

Children (Dextran 40 or 70): Total dose should not exceed 20 mL/kg during first 24 hours

Adults:

Dextran 40: 500-1000 mL at a rate of 20-40 mL/minute (maximum: 20 mL/kg/day for first 24 hours); 10 mL/kg/day thereafter; therapy should not be continued beyond 5 days

Dextran 70: 500-1000 mL at a rate of 20-40 mL/minute (maximum: 20 mL/kg/day for first 24 hours)

Pump prime (Dextran 40): Varies with the volume of the pump oxygenator; generally, the 10% solution is added in a dose of 1-2 g/kg

Prophylaxis of venous thrombosis/pulmonary embolism (Dextran 40): Begin during surgical procedure and give 50-100 g on the day of surgery; an additional 50 g (500 mL) should be administered every 2-3 days during the period of risk (up to 2 weeks postoperatively); usual maximum infusion rate for nonemergency use: 4 mL/minute

Dosage Forms

Infusion [premixed in D_5W; high molecular weight]: 6% Dextran 70 (500 mL)

Infusion [premixed in D_5W; low molecular weight] (Gentran®, LMD®): 10% Dextran 40 (500 mL)

Infusion [premixed in $D_{10}W$; high molecular weight]: 32% Dextran 70 (500 mL)

Infusion [premixed in NS; high molecular weight] (Gentran®): 6% Dextran 70 (500 mL)

Infusion [premixed in NS; low molecular weight] (Gentran®, LMD®): 10% Dextran (500 mL)

dextran 40 *see* dextran *on this page*

dextran 70 *see* dextran *on this page*

dextran 1 (DEKS tran won)

Sound-Alike/Look-Alike Issues

dextran may be confused with Dexatrim®, Dexedrine®

U.S./Canadian Brand Names Promit® [US]

Therapeutic Category Plasma Volume Expander

Use Prophylaxis of serious anaphylactic reactions to I.V. infusion of dextran

Usual Dosage I.V. (time between dextran 1 and dextran solution should not exceed 15 minutes):

Children: 0.3 mL/kg 1-2 minutes before I.V. infusion of dextran

Adults: 20 mL 1-2 minutes before I.V. infusion of dextran

Dosage Forms Injection, solution: 150 mg/mL (20 mL)

dextran, high molecular weight *see* dextran *on this page*

dextran, low molecular weight *see* dextran *on this page*

dextroamphetamine (deks troe am FET a meen)

Sound-Alike/Look-Alike Issues

Dexedrine® may be confused with dextran, Excedrin®

Synonyms dextroamphetamine sulfate

U.S./Canadian Brand Names Dexedrine® [US/Can]; Dextrostat® [US]

Therapeutic Category Amphetamine

Controlled Substance C-II

Use Narcolepsy; attention deficit/hyperactivity disorder (ADHD)

(Continued)

dextroamphetamine *(Continued)*

Usual Dosage Oral:

Children:

Narcolepsy: 6-12 years: Initial: 5 mg/day; may increase at 5 mg increments in weekly intervals until side effects appear (maximum dose: 60 mg/day)

ADHD:

3-5 years: Initial: 2.5 mg/day given every morning; increase by 2.5 mg/day in weekly intervals until optimal response is obtained; usual range: 0.1-0.5 mg/kg/dose every morning with maximum of 40 mg/day

≥6 years: 5 mg once or twice daily; increase in increments of 5 mg/day at weekly intervals until optimal response is obtained; usual range: 0.1-0.5 mg/kg/dose every morning (5-20 mg/day) with maximum of 40 mg/day

Children >12 years and Adults: Narcolepsy: Initial: 10 mg/day, may increase at 10 mg increments in weekly intervals until side effects appear; maximum: 60 mg/day

Dosage Forms [DSC] = Discontinued product

Capsule, sustained release, as sulfate: 5 mg, 10 mg, 15 mg

Dexedrine® Spansule®: 5 mg, 10 mg, 15 mg

Tablet, as sulfate: 5 mg, 10 mg

Dexedrine®: 5 mg [contains tartrazine] [DSC]

Dextrostat®: 5 mg, 10 mg [contains tartrazine]

dextroamphetamine and amphetamine (deks troe am FET a meen & am FET a meen)

Sound-Alike/Look-Alike Issues

Adderall® may be confused with Inderal®

Synonyms amphetamine and dextroamphetamine

U.S./Canadian Brand Names Adderall XR® [US/Can]; Adderall® [US]

Therapeutic Category Amphetamine

Controlled Substance C-II

Use Attention deficit/hyperactivity disorder (ADHD); narcolepsy

Usual Dosage Oral: **Note:** Use lowest effective individualized dose; administer first dose as soon as awake

ADHD:

Children: 3-5 years (Adderall®): Initial 2.5 mg/day given every morning; increase daily dose in 2.5 mg increments at weekly intervals until optimal response is obtained (maximum dose: 40 mg/day given in 1-3 divided doses); use intervals of 4-6 hours between additional doses

Children: ≥6 years:

Adderall®: Initial: 5 mg 1-2 times/day; increase daily dose in 5 mg increments at weekly intervals until optimal response is obtained (usual maximum dose: 40 mg/day given in 1-3 divided doses); use intervals of 4-6 hours between additional doses

Adderall XR®: 5-10 mg once daily in the morning; if needed, may increase daily dose in 5-10 mg increments at weekly intervals (maximum dose: 30 mg/day)

Adolescents 13-17 years (Adderall XR®): 10 mg once daily in the morning; may be increased to 20 mg/day after 1 week if symptoms are not controlled; higher doses (up to 60 mg)/day have been evaluated; however, there is not adequate evidence that higher doses afforded additional benefit.

Adults (Adderall XR®): Initial: 20 mg once daily in the morning; higher doses (up to 60 mg once daily) have been evaluated; however, there is not adequate evidence that higher doses afforded additional benefit,

Narcolepsy (Adderall®):

Children: 6-12 years: Initial: 5 mg/day; increase daily dose in 5 mg at weekly intervals until optimal response is obtained (maximum dose: 60 mg/day given in 1-3 divided doses with intervals of 4-6 hours between doses)

Children >12 years and Adults: Initial: 10 mg/day; increase daily dose in 10 mg increments at weekly intervals until optimal response is obtained (maximum dose: 60 mg/day given in 1-3 divided doses with intervals of 4-6 hours between doses)

Dosage Forms

Capsule, extended release (Adderall XR®):

5 mg [dextroamphetamine sulfate 1.25 mg, dextroamphetamine saccharate 1.25 mg, amphetamine aspartate monohydrate 1.25 mg, amphetamine sulfate 1.25 mg (equivalent to amphetamine base 3.1 mg)]

10 mg [dextroamphetamine sulfate 2.5 mg, dextroamphetamine saccharate 2.5 mg, amphetamine aspartate monohydrate 2.5 mg, amphetamine sulfate 2.5 mg (equivalent to amphetamine base 6.3 mg)]

15 mg [dextroamphetamine sulfate 3.75 mg, dextroamphetamine saccharate 3.75 mg, amphetamine aspartate monohydrate 3.75 mg, amphetamine sulfate 3.75 mg (equivalent to amphetamine base 9.4 mg)]

20 mg [dextroamphetamine sulfate 5 mg, dextroamphetamine saccharate 5 mg, amphetamine aspartate monohydrate 5 mg, amphetamine sulfate 5 mg (equivalent to amphetamine base 12.5 mg)]
25 mg [dextroamphetamine sulfate 6.25 mg, dextroamphetamine saccharate 6.25 mg, amphetamine aspartate monohydrate 6.25 mg, amphetamine sulfate 6.25 mg (equivalent to amphetamine base 15.6 mg)]
30 mg [dextroamphetamine sulfate 7.5 mg, dextroamphetamine saccharate 7.5 mg, amphetamine aspartate monohydrate 7.5 mg, amphetamine sulfate 7.5 mg (equivalent to amphetamine base 18.8 mg)]
Tablet (Adderall®):
5 mg [dextroamphetamine sulfate 1.25 mg, dextroamphetamine saccharate 1.25 mg, amphetamine aspartate 1.25 mg, amphetamine sulfate 1.25 mg (equivalent to amphetamine base 3.13 mg)]
7.5 mg [dextroamphetamine 1.875 mg, dextroamphetamine saccharate 1.875 mg, amphetamine aspartate 1.875 mg, amphetamine sulfate 1.875 mg (equivalent to amphetamine base 4.7 mg)]
10 mg [dextroamphetamine sulfate 2.5 mg, dextroamphetamine saccharate 2.5 mg, amphetamine aspartate 2.5 mg, amphetamine sulfate 2.5 mg (equivalent to amphetamine base 6.3 mg)]
12.5 mg [dextroamphetamine sulfate 3.125 mg, dextroamphetamine saccharate 3.125 mg, amphetamine aspartate 3.125 mg, amphetamine sulfate 3.125 mg (equivalent to amphetamine base 7.8 mg)]
15 mg [dextroamphetamine sulfate 3.75 mg, dextroamphetamine saccharate 3.75 mg, amphetamine aspartate 3.75 mg, amphetamine sulfate 3.75 mg (equivalent to amphetamine base 9.4 mg)]
20 mg [dextroamphetamine sulfate 5 mg, dextroamphetamine saccharate 5 mg, amphetamine aspartate 5 mg, amphetamine sulfate 5 mg (equivalent to amphetamine base 12.6 mg)]
30 mg [dextroamphetamine sulfate 7.5 mg, dextroamphetamine saccharate 7.5 mg, amphetamine aspartate 7.5 mg, amphetamine sulfate 7.5 mg (equivalent to amphetamine base 18.8 mg)]

dextroamphetamine sulfate *see* dextroamphetamine *on page 243*

dextromethorphan (deks troe meth OR fan)

Sound-Alike/Look-Alike Issues
Benylin® may be confused with Benadryl®, Ventolin®
Delsym® may be confused with Delfen®, Desyrel®

U.S./Canadian Brand Names Babee® Cof Syrup [US-OTC]; Creo-Terpin® [US-OTC]; Creomulsion® Cough [US-OTC]; Creomulsion® for Children [US-OTC]; Delsym® [US-OTC]; Dexalone® [US-OTC]; Elix-Sure™ Cough [US-OTC]; Hold® DM [US-OTC]; PediaCare® Children's Medicated Freezer Pops Long Acting Cough [US-OTC]; PediaCare® Infants' Long-Acting Cough [US-OTC]; Robitussin® CoughGels™ [US-OTC]; Robitussin® Honey Cough [US-OTC]; Robitussin® Maximum Strength Cough [US-OTC]; Robitussin® Pediatric Cough [US-OTC]; Scot-Tussin DM® Cough Chasers [US-OTC]; Silphen DM® [US-OTC]; Simply Cough® [US-OTC]; Triaminic® Thin Strips™ Long Acting Cough [US-OTC]; Vicks® 44® Cough Relief [US-OTC]

Therapeutic Category Antitussive

Use Symptomatic relief of coughs caused by minor viral upper respiratory tract infections or inhaled irritants; most effective for a chronic nonproductive cough

Usual Dosage Oral:
Children:
<2 years: Use only as directed by a physician
2-6 years (syrup): 2.5-7.5 mg every 4-8 hours; extended release is 15 mg twice daily (maximum: 30 mg/24 hours)
6-12 years: 5-10 mg every 4 hours or 15 mg every 6-8 hours; extended release is 30 mg twice daily (maximum: 60 mg/24 hours)
Children >12 years and Adults: 10-20 mg every 4 hours or 30 mg every 6-8 hours; extended release: 60 mg twice daily; maximum: 120 mg/day

Dosage Forms [DSC] = Discontinued product
Gelcap, as hydrobromide:
Dexalone®: 30 mg
Robitussin® CoughGels™: 15 mg [contains coconut oil]
Liquid, as hydrobromide:
Creo-Terpin®: 10 mg/15 mL (120 mL) [contains alcohol 25% and tartrazine]
Simply Cough®: 5 mg/5 mL (120 mL) [contains sodium benzoate; cherry berry flavor]
Vicks® 44® Cough Relief: 10 mg/5 mL (120 mL) [contains alcohol, sodium 10 mg/5 mL, sodium benzoate]
Liquid, oral, as hydrobromide [freezer pops] (PediaCare® Children's Medicated Freezer Pops Long Acting Cough): 7.5 mg/25 mL (8s) [alcohol free; contains sodium benzoate, berry flavor also contains benzyl alcohol; glacier grape™ and polar berry blue™ flavors]
Liquid, oral drops, as hydrobromide (PediaCare® Infants' Long-Acting Cough): 7.5 mg/0.8 mL (15 mL) [alcohol free, dye free; contains sodium benzoate; grape flavor]
Lozenge, as hydrobromide:
Hold® DM: 5 mg (10s) [cherry or original flavor]
(Continued)

dextromethorphan *(Continued)*

Scot-Tussin DM® Cough Chasers: 5 mg (20s)

Strips, oral, as hydrobromide (Triaminic® Thin Strips™ Long Acting Cough): 7.5 mg [equivalent to dextromethorphan 5 mg; cherry flavor]

Suspension, extended release, as hydrobromide (Delsym®): 30 mg/5 mL (89 mL, 148 mL) [contains alcohol 0.26%, sodium 5 mg/5 mL; orange flavor]

Syrup, as hydrobromide:

Babee® Cof Syrup: 7.5 mg/5 mL (120 mL) [alcohol free, dye free; cherry flavor]

Benylin® Adult: 15 mg/5 mL (120 mL) [alcohol free, sugar free; contains sodium benzoate; raspberry flavor] [DSC]

Benylin® Pediatric: 7.5 mg/mL (120 mL) [alcohol free, sugar free; contains sodium benzoate; grape flavor] [DSC]

Creomulsion® Cough: 20 mg/15 mL (120 mL) [alcohol free; contains sodium benzoate]

Creomulsion® for Children: 5 mg/5 mL (120 mL) [alcohol free; contains sodium benzoate; cherry flavor]

ElixSure™ Cough: 7.5 mg/5 mL (120 mL) [cherry bubble gum flavor]

Robitussin® Honey Cough: 10 mg/5 mL (120 mL) [alcohol free; contains sodium benzoate]

Robitussin® Maximum Strength Cough: 15 mg/5 mL (120 mL, 240 mL) [contains alcohol, sodium benzoate]

Robitussin® Pediatric Cough: 7.5 mg/5 mL (120 mL) [alcohol free; contains sodium benzoate; fruit punch flavor]

Silphen DM®: 10 mg/5 mL (120 mL) [strawberry flavor]

dextromethorphan, acetaminophen, and pseudoephedrine *see* acetaminophen, dextromethorphan, and pseudoephedrine *on page 12*

dextromethorphan and guaifenesin *see* guaifenesin and dextromethorphan *on page 394*

dextromethorphan and promethazine *see* promethazine and dextromethorphan *on page 704*

dextromethorphan and pseudoephedrine *see* pseudoephedrine and dextromethorphan *on page 714*

dextromethorphan, carbinoxamine, and pseudoephedrine *see* carbinoxamine, pseudoephedrine, and dextromethorphan *on page 150*

dextromethorphan, chlorpheniramine, and phenylephrine *see* chlorpheniramine, phenylephrine, and dextromethorphan *on page 179*

dextromethorphan, chlorpheniramine, and pseudoephedrine *see* chlorpheniramine, pseudoephedrine, and dextromethorphan *on page 182*

dextromethorphan, guaifenesin, and pseudoephedrine *see* guaifenesin, pseudoephedrine, and dextromethorphan *on page 401*

dextromethorphan hydrobromide, brompheniramine maleate, and pseudoephedrine hydrochloride *see* brompheniramine, pseudoephedrine, and dextromethorphan *on page 120*

dextromethorphan, pseudoephedrine, and carbinoxamine *see* carbinoxamine, pseudoephedrine, and dextromethorphan *on page 150*

dextromethorphan tannate, pyrilamine tannate, and phenylephrine tannate *see* phenylephrine, pyrilamine, and dextromethorphan *on page 664*

dextropropoxyphene *see* propoxyphene *on page 708*

dextrose and tetracaine *see* tetracaine and dextrose *on page 816*

dextrose, levulose and phosphoric acid *see* fructose, dextrose, and phosphoric acid *on page 371*

Dextrostat® [US] *see* dextroamphetamine *on page 243*

Dey-Dose® Isoproterenol *(Discontinued)* *see* isoproterenol *on page 464*

Dey-Dose® Metaproterenol *(Discontinued)*

DFMO *see* eflornithine *on page 288*

DHAD *see* mitoxantrone *on page 561*

DHAQ *see* mitoxantrone *on page 561*

DHC® *(Discontinued)* *see* hydrocodone and acetaminophen *on page 420*

DHC Plus® *(Discontinued)*

DHE *see* dihydroergotamine *on page 256*

D.H.E. 45® [US] *see* dihydroergotamine *on page 256*

DHPG sodium *see* ganciclovir *on page 375*

DHS™ Sal [US-OTC] *see* salicylic acid *on page 758*

DHS™ Tar [US-OTC] *see* coal tar *on page 207*

DHS™ Targel [US-OTC] *see* coal tar *on page 207*

DHS™ Zinc [US-OTC] *see* pyrithione zinc *on page 723*

DHT™ *(Discontinued)*

DHT™ Intensol™ *(Discontinued)*

DiabetAid™ Antifungal Foot Bath [US-OTC] *see* miconazole *on page 553*

DiabetAid Gingivitis Mouth Rinse [US-OTC] *see* cetylpyridinium *on page 169*

Diabetic Tussin C® [US] *see* guaifenesin and codeine *on page 393*

Diabetic Tussin® Allergy Relief [US-OTC] *see* chlorpheniramine *on page 175*

Diabetic Tussin® DM [US-OTC] *see* guaifenesin and dextromethorphan *on page 394*

Diabetic Tussin® DM Maximum Strength [US-OTC] *see* guaifenesin and dextromethorphan *on page 394*

Diabetic Tussin® EX [US-OTC] *see* guaifenesin *on page 392*

Diabinese® [US] *see* chlorpropamide *on page 184*

Diaβeta® [US/Can] *see* glyburide *on page 387*

Dialose® Tablet *(Discontinued)* *see* docusate *on page 270*

Dialume® *(Discontinued)* *see* aluminum hydroxide *on page 36*

Diamicron® [Can] *see* gliclazide *(Canada only) on page 384*

Diamicron® MR [Can] *see* gliclazide *(Canada only) on page 384*

Diamine T.D.® *(Discontinued)* *see* brompheniramine *on page 118*

diaminocyclohexane oxalatoplatinum *see* oxaliplatin *on page 622*

diaminodiphenylsulfone *see* dapsone *on page 229*

Diamode [US-OTC] *see* loperamide *on page 503*

Diamox® [Can] *see* acetazolamide *on page 14*

Diamox® 250 mg Tablet *(Discontinued)* *see* acetazolamide *on page 14*

Diamox® Sequels® [US] *see* acetazolamide *on page 14*

Diane-35 [Can] *see* cyproterone and ethinyl estradiol *(Canada only) on page 223*

Diaparene® [US-OTC] *see* methylbenzethonium chloride *on page 544*

Diar-aid® *(Discontinued)* *see* loperamide *on page 503*

Diarr-Eze [Can] *see* loperamide *on page 503*

Diasorb® [US-OTC] *see* attapulgite *on page 84*

Diastat® [US/Can] *see* diazepam *on next page*

Diastat® AcuDial™ [US] *see* diazepam *on next page*

Diastat® Rectal Delivery System [Can] *see* diazepam *on next page*

diatrizoate meglumine *see* radiological/contrast media (ionic) *on page 728*

diatrizoate meglumine and diatrizoate sodium *see* radiological/contrast media (ionic) *on page 728*

diatrizoate meglumine and iodipamide meglumine *see* radiological/contrast media (ionic) *on page 728*

diatrizoate sodium *see* radiological/contrast media (ionic) *on page 728*

Diatx™ [US] *see* vitamin B complex combinations *on page 876*

DiatxFe™ [US] *see* vitamin B complex combinations *on page 876*

Diazemuls® [Can] *see* diazepam *on next page*

Diazemuls® Injection *(Discontinued)* *see* diazepam *on next page*

diazepam (dye AZ e pam)

Sound-Alike/Look-Alike Issues

diazepam may be confused with diazoxide, Ditropan®, lorazepam

Valium® may be confused with Valcyte™

U.S./Canadian Brand Names Apo-Diazepam® [Can]; Diastat® AcuDial™ [US]; Diastat® Rectal Delivery System [Can]; Diastat® [US/Can]; Diazemuls® [Can]; Diazepam Intensol® [US]; Novo-Dipam [Can]; Valium® [US/Can]

Therapeutic Category Benzodiazepine

Controlled Substance C-IV

Use Management of anxiety disorders, ethanol withdrawal symptoms; skeletal muscle relaxant; treatment of convulsive disorders

Rectal gel: Management of selected, refractory epilepsy patients on stable regimens of antiepileptic drugs (AEDs) requiring intermittent use of diazepam to control episodes of increased seizure activity

Usual Dosage **Oral absorption is more reliable than I.M.**

Children:

Conscious sedation for procedures: Oral: 0.2-0.3 mg/kg (maximum: 10 mg) 45-60 minutes prior to procedure

Sedation/muscle relaxant/anxiety:

Oral: 0.12-0.8 mg/kg/day in divided doses every 6-8 hours

I.M., I.V.: 0.04-0.3 mg/kg/dose every 2-4 hours to a maximum of 0.6 mg/kg within an 8-hour period if needed

Status epilepticus:

Infants 30 days to 5 years: I.V.: 0.05-0.3 mg/kg/dose given over 2-3 minutes, every 15-30 minutes to a maximum total dose of 5 mg; repeat in 2-4 hours as needed **or** 0.2-0.5 mg/dose every 2-5 minutes to a maximum total dose of 5 mg

>5 years: I.V.: 0.05-0.3 mg/kg/dose given over 2-3 minutes every 15-30 minutes to a maximum total dose of 10 mg; repeat in 2-4 hours as needed **or** 1 mg/dose given over 2-3 minutes, every 2-5 minutes to a maximum total dose of 10 mg

Rectal: 0.5 mg/kg, then 0.25 mg/kg in 10 minutes if needed (prepare dose using parenteral formulation)

Anticonvulsant (acute treatment): Rectal gel:

Children <2 years: Safety and efficacy have not been studied

Children 2-5 years: 0.5 mg/kg

Children 6-11 years: 0.3 mg/kg

Children ≥12 years: 0.2 mg/kg

Note: Dosage should be rounded upward to the next available dose, 2.5, 5, 7.5, 10, 12.5, 15, 17.5, and 20 mg/dose; dose may be repeated in 4-12 hours if needed; do not use for more than 5 episodes per month or more than one episode every 5 days

Adolescents: Conscious sedation for procedures:

Oral: 10 mg

I.V.: 5 mg, may repeat with 1/2 dose if needed

Adults:

Anticonvulsant (acute treatment): Rectal gel: 0.2 mg/kg

Note: Dosage should be rounded upward to the next available dose, 2.5, 5, 7.5, 10, 12.5, 15, 17.5, and 20 mg/dose; dose may be repeated in 4-12 hours if needed; do not use for more than 5 episodes per month or more than one episode every 5 days.

Anxiety/sedation/skeletal muscle relaxant:

Oral: 2-10 mg 2-4 times/day

I.M., I.V.: 2-10 mg, may repeat in 3-4 hours if needed

Sedation in the ICU patient: I.V.: 0.03-0.1 mg/kg every 30 minutes to 6 hours

Status epilepticus: I.V.: 5-10 mg every 10-20 minutes, up to 30 mg in an 8-hour period; may repeat in 2-4 hours if necessary

Rapid tranquilization of agitated patient (administer every 30-60 minutes): Oral: 5-10 mg; average total dose for tranquilization: 20-60 mg

Dosage Forms

Gel, rectal:

Diastat®: Pediatric rectal tip [4.4 cm]: 5 mg/mL (2.5 mg, 5 mg) [contains ethyl alcohol 10%, sodium benzoate, benzyl alcohol 1.5%; twin pack]

Diastat® AcuDial™ delivery system:

10 mg: Pediatric/adult rectal tip [4.4 cm]: 5 mg/mL (delivers set doses of 5 mg, 7.5 mg, and 10 mg) [contains ethyl alcohol 10%, sodium benzoate, benzyl alcohol 1.5%; twin pack]

20 mg: Adult rectal tip [6 cm]: 5 mg/mL (delivers set doses of 10 mg, 12.5 mg, 15 mg, 17.5 mg, and 20 mg) [contains ethyl alcohol 10%, sodium benzoate, benzyl alcohol 1.5%; twin pack]

Injection, solution: 5 mg/mL (2 mL, 10 mL) [may contain benzyl alcohol, sodium benzoate, benzoic acid]

Solution, oral: 5 mg/5 mL (5 mL, 500 mL) [wintergreen-spice flavor]
Solution, oral concentrate:
Diazepam Intensol®: 5 mg/mL (30 mL)
Tablet: 2 mg, 5 mg, 10 mg
Valium®: 2 mg, 5 mg, 10 mg

Diazepam Intensol® [US] *see* diazepam *on previous page*

diazoxide (dye az OKS ide)

Sound-Alike/Look-Alike Issues
diazoxide may be confused with diazepam, Dyazide®
Hyperstat® may be confused with Nitrostat®

U.S./Canadian Brand Names Hyperstat® [US]; Proglycem® [US/Can]

Therapeutic Category Antihypertensive Agent; Antihypoglycemic Agent

Use
Oral: Hypoglycemia related to islet cell adenoma, carcinoma, hyperplasia, or adenomatosis, nesidioblastosis, leucine sensitivity, or extrapancreatic malignancy
I.V.: Severe hypertension

Usual Dosage
Hypertension: Children and Adults: I.V.: 1-3 mg/kg up to a maximum of 150 mg in a single injection; repeat dose in 5-15 minutes until blood pressure adequately reduced; repeat administration at intervals of 4-24 hours; monitor the blood pressure closely; do not use longer than 10 days
Hyperinsulinemic hypoglycemia: Oral: **Note:** Use lower dose listed as initial dose
Newborns and Infants: 8-15 mg/kg/day in divided doses every 8-12 hours
Children and Adults: 3-8 mg/kg/day in divided doses every 8-12 hours

Dosage Forms [DSC] = Discontinued product
Capsule:
Proglycem®: 50 mg [not available in the U.S.]
Injection, solution:
Hyperstat®: 15 mg/mL (20 mL) [DSC]
Suspension, oral:
Proglycem®: 50 mg/mL (30 mL) [contains alcohol 7.25%; chocolate-mint flavor]

Dibent® Injection *(Discontinued)* *see* dicyclomine *on page 251*

Dibenzyline® [US/Can] *see* phenoxybenzamine *on page 659*

dibucaine (DYE byoo kane)

U.S./Canadian Brand Names Nupercainal® [US-OTC]

Therapeutic Category Local Anesthetic

Use Fast, temporary relief of pain and itching due to hemorrhoids, minor burns

Usual Dosage Children and Adults: Topical: Apply gently to the affected areas; no more than 30 g for adults or 7.5 g for children should be used in any 24-hour period

Dosage Forms
Ointment: 1% (30 g, 454 g)
Nupercainal®: 1% (30 g, 60 g) [contains sodium bisulfite]

DIC *see* dacarbazine *on page 226*

Dicarbosil® *(Discontinued)* *see* calcium carbonate *on page 135*

Dicel™ [US] *see* chlorpheniramine and pseudoephedrine *on page 177*

Dicel™ DM [US] *see* chlorpheniramine, pseudoephedrine, and dextromethorphan *on page 182*

Dicetel® [Can] *see* pinaverium *(Canada only)* *on page 669*

dichloralphenazone, acetaminophen, and isometheptene *see* acetaminophen, isometheptene, and dichloralphenazone *on page 13*

dichloralphenazone, isometheptene, and acetaminophen *see* acetaminophen, isometheptene, and dichloralphenazone *on page 13*

6,7-dichloro-1,5-dihydroimidazo [2,1b] quinazolin-2(3H)-one monohydrochloride *see* anagrelide *on page 55*

dichlorodifluoromethane and trichloromonofluoromethane

(dye klor oh dye flor oh METH ane & tri klor oh mon oh flor oh METH ane)

Synonyms trichloromonofluoromethane and dichlorodifluoromethane

U.S./Canadian Brand Names Fluori-Methane® [US]

Therapeutic Category Analgesic, Topical

Use Management of pain associated with injections

Usual Dosage Invert bottle over treatment area approximately 12" away from site of application; open dispenseal spring valve completely, allowing liquid to flow in a stream from the bottle. The rate of spraying is approximately 10 cm/second and should be continued until entire muscle has been covered.

Dosage Forms Aerosol, topical: Dichlorodifluoromethane 15% and trichloromonofluoromethane 85% (103 mL) [contains chlorofluorocarbons]

dichlorotetrafluoroethane and ethyl chloride *see* ethyl chloride and dichlorotetrafluoroethane *on page 329*

Dickinson's® Witch Hazel [US-OTC] *see* witch hazel *on page 881*

Diclectin® [Can] *see* doxylamine and pyridoxine *(Canada only) on page 280*

diclofenac (dye KLOE fen ak)

Sound-Alike/Look-Alike Issues

diclofenac may be confused with Diflucan®, Duphalac®

Cataflam® may be confused with Catapres®

Voltaren® may be confused with tramadol, Ultram®, Verelan®

Synonyms diclofenac potassium; diclofenac sodium

U.S./Canadian Brand Names Apo-Diclo Rapide® [Can]; Apo-Diclo SR® [Can]; Apo-Diclo® [Can]; Cataflam® [US/Can]; Novo-Difenac K [Can]; Novo-Difenac [Can]; Novo-Difenac-SR [Can]; Nu-Diclo [Can]; Nu-Diclo-SR [Can]; Pennsaid® [Can]; PMS-Diclofenac SR [Can]; PMS-Diclofenac [Can]; Riva-Diclofenac [Can]; Riva-Diclofenac-K [Can]; Solaraze® [US]; Voltaren Ophthalmic® [US]; Voltaren Ophtha® [Can]; Voltaren Rapide® [Can]; Voltaren® [US/Can]; Voltaren®-XR [US]

Therapeutic Category Analgesic, Nonnarcotic; Nonsteroidal Antiinflammatory Drug (NSAID)

Use

Immediate release: Ankylosing spondylitis; primary dysmenorrhea; acute and chronic treatment of rheumatoid arthritis, osteoarthritis

Delayed-release tablets: Acute and chronic treatment of rheumatoid arthritis, osteoarthritis, ankylosing spondylitis

Extended-release tablets: Chronic treatment of osteoarthritis, rheumatoid arthritis

Ophthalmic solution: Postoperative inflammation following cataract extraction; temporary relief of pain and photophobia in patients undergoing corneal refractive surgery

Topical gel: Actinic keratosis (AK) in conjunction with sun avoidance

Usual Dosage Adults:

Oral:

Analgesia/primary dysmenorrhea: Starting dose: 50 mg 3 times/day; maximum dose: 150 mg/day

Rheumatoid arthritis: 150-200 mg/day in 2-4 divided doses (100 mg/day of sustained release product)

Osteoarthritis: 100-150 mg/day in 2-3 divided doses (100-200 mg/day of sustained release product)

Ankylosing spondylitis: 100-125 mg/day in 4-5 divided doses

Ophthalmic:

Cataract surgery: Instill 1 drop into affected eye 4 times/day beginning 24 hours after cataract surgery and continuing for 2 weeks

Corneal refractive surgery: Instill 1-2 drops into affected eye within the hour prior to surgery, within 15 minutes following surgery, and then continue for 4 times/day, up to 3 days

Topical: Apply gel to lesion area twice daily for 60-90 days

Dosage Forms [DSC] = Discontinued product

Gel, as sodium:

Solaraze®: 30 mg/g (50 g)

Solution, ophthalmic, as sodium:

Voltaren Ophthalmic®: 0.1% (2.5 mL, 5 mL)

Tablet, as potassium: 50 mg

Cataflam®: 50 mg

Tablet, delayed release, enteric coated, as sodium: 50 mg, 75 mg

Voltaren®: 25 mg [DSC], 50 mg [DSC], 75 mg

Tablet, extended release, as sodium: 100 mg

Voltaren®-XR: 100 mg

diclofenac and misoprostol (dye KLOE fen ak & mye soe PROST ole)

Synonyms misoprostol and diclofenac

U.S./Canadian Brand Names Arthrotec® [US/Can]

Therapeutic Category Analgesic, Nonnarcotic; Prostaglandin

Use The diclofenac component is indicated for the treatment of osteoarthritis and rheumatoid arthritis; the misoprostol component is indicated for the prophylaxis of NSAID-induced gastric and duodenal ulceration

Usual Dosage Oral: Adults:

Arthrotec® 50:

Osteoarthritis: 1 tablet 2-3 times/day

Rheumatoid arthritis: 1 tablet 3-4 times/day

For both regimens, if not tolerated by patient, the dose may be reduced to 1 tablet twice daily

Arthrotec® 75:

Patients who cannot tolerate full daily Arthrotec® 50 regimens: 1 tablet twice daily

Note: The use of these tablets may not be as effective at preventing GI ulceration

Dosage Forms Tablet: Diclofenac sodium 50 mg and misoprostol 200 mcg; diclofenac sodium 75 mg and misoprostol 200 mcg

diclofenac potassium *see* diclofenac *on previous page*

diclofenac sodium *see* diclofenac *on previous page*

dicloxacillin (dye kloks a SIL in)

Synonyms dicloxacillin sodium

U.S./Canadian Brand Names Dycill® [Can]; Pathocil® [Can]

Therapeutic Category Penicillin

Use Treatment of systemic infections such as pneumonia, skin and soft tissue infections, and osteomyelitis caused by penicillinase-producing staphylococci

Usual Dosage

Usual dosage range:

Children <40 kg: Oral: 12.5-100 mg/kg/day divided every 6 hours

Children >40 kg: Oral: 125-250 mg every 6 hours

Adults: Oral: 125-1000 mg every 6 hours

Indication-specific dosing:

Children: Oral:

Furunculosis: 25-50 mg/kg/day divided every 6 hours

Osteomyelitis: 50-100 mg/kg/day in divided doses every 6 hours

Adults: Oral:

Erysipelas, furunculosis, impetigo, mastitis, otitis externa, septic bursitis, skin abscess: 500 mg every 6 hours

Prosthetic joint (long-term suppression therapy): 250 mg twice daily

***Staphylococcus aureus*, methicillin susceptible infection if no I.V. access:** 500-1000 mg every 6-8 hours

Dosage Forms Capsule: 250 mg, 500 mg

dicloxacillin sodium *see* dicloxacillin *on this page*

dicyclomine (dye SYE kloe meen)

Sound-Alike/Look-Alike Issues

dicyclomine may be confused with diphenhydrAMINE, doxycycline, dyclonine

Bentyl® may be confused with Aventyl®, Benadryl®, Bontril®, Cantil®, Proventil®, Trental®

Synonyms dicyclomine hydrochloride; dicycloverine hydrochloride

U.S./Canadian Brand Names Bentylol® [Can]; Bentyl® [US]; Formulex® [Can]; Lomine [Can]; Riva-Dicyclomine [Can]

Therapeutic Category Anticholinergic Agent

Use Treatment of functional disturbances of GI motility such as irritable bowel syndrome

Usual Dosage

Oral:

Infants >6 months: 5 mg/dose 3-4 times/day

Children: 10 mg/dose 3-4 times/day

Adults: Begin with 80 mg/day in 4 equally divided doses, then increase up to 160 mg/day

I.M. **(should not be used I.V.)**: Adults: 80 mg/day in 4 divided doses (20 mg/dose)

(Continued)

dicyclomine *(Continued)*

Dosage Forms

Capsule, as hydrochloride: 10 mg

Injection, solution, as hydrochloride: 10 mg/mL (2 mL)

Syrup, as hydrochloride: 10 mg/5 mL (480 mL)

Tablet, as hydrochloride: 20 mg

dicyclomine hydrochloride *see* dicyclomine *on previous page*

dicycloverine hydrochloride *see* dicyclomine *on previous page*

Di-Dak-Sol [US] *see* sodium hypochlorite solution *on page 779*

didanosine (dye DAN oh seen)

Sound-Alike/Look-Alike Issues

Videx® may be confused with Lidex®

Synonyms ddI; dideoxyinosine

U.S./Canadian Brand Names Videx® EC [US/Can]; Videx® [US/Can]

Therapeutic Category Antiviral Agent

Use Treatment of HIV infection; always to be used in combination with at least two other antiretroviral agents

Usual Dosage Treatment of HIV infection: Oral (administer on an empty stomach):

Children:

2 weeks to 8 months: 100 mg/m^2 twice daily is recommended by the manufacturer; 50 mg/m^2 may be considered in infants 2 weeks to 4 months

>8 months: 120 mg/m^2 twice daily; dosing range: 90-150 mg/m^2 twice daily; patients with CNS disease may require higher dose

Note: At least 2 tablets per dose should be administered for adequate buffering and absorption; tablets should be chewed or dispersed (in 1 ounce of water).

Adolescents and Adults: Dosing based on patient weight:

Note: Preferred dosing frequency is twice daily for didanosine tablets/oral solution

Chewable tablets, powder for oral solution:

<60 kg: 125 mg twice daily or 250 mg once daily

≥60 kg: 200 mg twice daily or 400 mg once daily

Note: Adults should receive 2-4 tablets per dose for adequate buffering and absorption; tablets should be chewed or dispersed (in 1 ounce of water).

Delayed release capsule (Videx® EC):

<60 kg: 250 mg once daily

≥60 kg: 400 mg once daily

Dosing adjustment with tenofovir (didanosine tablets or delayed release capsules; based on tenofovir product labeling):

<60 kg: 200 mg once daily

≥60 kg: 250 mg once daily

Dosage Forms

Capsule, delayed release: 200 mg, 250 mg, 400 mg

Videx® EC: 125 mg, 200 mg, 250 mg, 400 mg

Powder for oral solution, pediatric:

Videx®: 2 g, 4 g [makes 10 mg/mL solution after final mixing]

Tablet, buffered, chewable/dispersible:

Videx®: 25 mg, 50 mg, 100 mg, 150 mg, 200 mg [all strengths contain phenylalanine 36.5 mg/tablet; orange flavor] [DSC]

dideoxycytidine *see* zalcitabine *on page 884*

dideoxyinosine *see* didanosine *on this page*

Didrex® [US/Can] *see* benzphetamine *on page 104*

Didrocal™ [Can] *see* etidronate and calcium *on page 329*

Didronel® [US/Can] *see* etidronate disodium *on page 329*

dietary supplements *see* nutritional formula, enteral/oral *on page 608*

diethylene triamine penta-acetic acid

(dye ETH i leen TRYE a meen PEN ta a SEE tik AS id)

Synonyms Ca-DTPA; diethylenetriamine pentaacetic acid; DTPA; pentetate calcium trisodium; pentetate zinc trisodium; trisodium calcium diethylenetriaminepentaacetate (Ca-DTPA); zinc diethylenetriaminepentaacetate (Zn-DTPA); Zn-DTPA

Therapeutic Category Antidote

Use Treatment of known or suspected internal contamination with plutonium, americium, or curium

Usual Dosage Internal contamination with plutonium, americium, or curium: Ca-DTPA is the preferred initial agent; sequential administration of Ca-DTPA then Zn-DTPA is recommended. I.V.:

Children <12 years:

Initial: Ca-DTPA: 14 mg/kg/day (maximum dose: 1 g/day)

Maintenance: Zn-DTPA: 14 mg/kg/day (maximum: 1 g/day); length of therapy depends on patient response and degree of contamination. **Note:** An equivalent dose of Ca-DTPA should be used for maintenance therapy only if Zn-DTPA is not available.

Children ≥12 years and Adults:

Initial: Ca-DTPA: 1 g/day

Pregnancy: Zn-DTPA 1 g/day should be used for the initial dose in pregnant women **except** in cases of high internal contamination

Maintenance: Zn-DTPA: 1 g/day; length of therapy depends on patient response and degree of contamination. **Note:** An equivalent dose of Ca-DTPA should be used for maintenance therapy only if Zn-DTPA is not available.

Dosage Forms Injection, solution:

Ca-DTPA: 200 mg/mL (5 mL)

Zn-DTPA: 200 mg/mL (5 mL)

diethylenetriamine pentaacetic acid *see* diethylene triamine penta-acetic acid *on previous page*

diethylpropion (dye eth il PROE pee on)

Synonyms amfepramone; diethylpropion hydrochloride

U.S./Canadian Brand Names Tenuate® Dospan® [Can]; Tenuate® [Can]

Therapeutic Category Anorexiant

Controlled Substance C-IV

Use Short-term adjunct in a regimen of weight reduction based on exercise, behavioral modification, and caloric reduction in the management of exogenous obesity for patients with an initial body mass index ≥30 kg/m^2 or ≥27 kg/m^2 in the presence of other risk factors (diabetes, hypertension)

Usual Dosage Adults: Oral:

Tablet: 25 mg 3 times/day before meals or food

Tablet, controlled release: 75 mg at midmorning

Dosage Forms [DSC] = Discontinued product

Tablet, as hydrochloride: 25 mg

Tenuate®: 25 mg [DSC]

Tablet, controlled release, as hydrochloride: 75 mg

Tenuate® Dospan®: 75 mg [DSC]

diethylpropion hydrochloride *see* diethylpropion *on this page*

difenoxin and atropine (dye fen OKS in & A troe peen)

Synonyms atropine and difenoxin

U.S./Canadian Brand Names Motofen® [US]

Therapeutic Category Antidiarrheal

Controlled Substance C-IV

Use Treatment of diarrhea

Usual Dosage Adults: Oral: Initial: 2 tablets (each tablet contains difenoxin hydrochloride 1 mg and atropine sulfate 0.025 mg), then 1 tablet after each loose stool; 1 tablet every 3-4 hours, up to 8 tablets in a 24-hour period; if no improvement after 48 hours, continued administration is not indicated

Dosage Forms Tablet: Difenoxin hydrochloride 1 mg and atropine sulfate 0.025 mg

Differin® [US/Can] *see* adapalene *on page 19*

Differin® XP [Can] *see* adapalene *on page 19*

diflorasone (dye FLOR a sone)

Sound-Alike/Look-Alike Issues

Psorcon® may be confused with Proscar®, ProSom®, Psorion®

Synonyms diflorasone diacetate

U.S./Canadian Brand Names ApexiCon™ E [US]; ApexiCon™ [US]; Florone® [US/Can]; Psorcon® e™ [US]; Psorcon® [Can]

(Continued)

diflorasone *(Continued)*

Therapeutic Category Corticosteroid, Topical

Use Relieves inflammation and pruritic symptoms of corticosteroid-responsive dermatosis (high to very high potency topical corticosteroid)

Maxiflor®: High potency topical corticosteroid
Psorcon®: Very high potency topical corticosteroid

Usual Dosage Topical: Apply ointment sparingly 1-3 times/day; apply cream sparingly 2-4 times/day. Therapy should be discontinued when control is achieved; if no improvement is seen, reassessment of diagnosis may be necessary.

Dosage Forms [DSC] = Discontinued product

Cream, as diacetate: 0.05% (15 g, 30 g, 60 g)
ApexiCon™ E, Florone®: 0.05% (30 g, 60 g)
Psorcon® e™: 0.05% (15 g, 30 g, 60 g) [DSC]
Ointment, as diacetate: 0.05% (15 g, 30 g, 60 g)
ApexiCon™: 0.05% (30 g, 60 g)
Psorcon® e™: 0.05% (15 g, 30 g, 60 g) [DSC]

diflorasone diacetate *see* diflorasone *on previous page*

Diflucan® [US/Can] *see* fluconazole *on page 349*

diflunisal (dye FLOO ni sal)

Sound-Alike/Look-Alike Issues

Dolobid® may be confused with Slo-Bid®

U.S./Canadian Brand Names Apo-Diflunisal® [Can]; Novo-Diflunisal [Can]; Nu-Diflunisal [Can]

Therapeutic Category Analgesic, Nonnarcotic; Nonsteroidal Antiinflammatory Drug (NSAID)

Use Management of inflammatory disorders usually including rheumatoid arthritis and osteoarthritis; can be used as an analgesic for treatment of mild to moderate pain

Usual Dosage Adults: Oral:

Mild-to-moderate pain: Initial: 500-1000 mg followed by 250-500 mg every 8-12 hours; maximum daily dose: 1.5 g
Arthritis: 500-1000 mg/day in 2 divided doses; maximum daily dose: 1.5 g

Dosage Forms [DSC] = Discontinued product

Tablet: 500 mg
Dolobid®: 250 mg, 500 mg [DSC]

Digibind® [US/Can] *see* digoxin immune Fab *on next page*

DigiFab™ [US] *see* digoxin immune Fab *on next page*

Digitek® [US] *see* digoxin *on this page*

digoxin (di JOKS in)

Sound-Alike/Look-Alike Issues

digoxin may be confused with Desoxyn®, doxepin
Lanoxin® may be confused with Lasix®, Levoxyl®, Levsinex®, Lomotil®, Lonox®, Mefoxin®, Xanax®

U.S./Canadian Brand Names Digitek® [US]; Digoxin CSD [Can]; Lanoxicaps® [US/Can]; Lanoxin® [US/Can]; Novo-Digoxin [Can]; Pediatric Digoxin CSD [Can]

Therapeutic Category Antiarrhythmic Agent, Miscellaneous; Cardiac Glycoside

Use Treatment of congestive heart failure and to slow the ventricular rate in tachyarrhythmias such as atrial fibrillation, atrial flutter, and supraventricular tachycardia (paroxysmal atrial tachycardia); cardiogenic shock

Usual Dosage When changing from oral (tablets or liquid) or I.M. to I.V. therapy, dosage should be reduced by 20% to 25%. Refer to the following:

Preterm infant[1]:
Total digitalizing dose[2]:
Oral: 20-30 mcg/kg[1]
I.V. or I.M.: 15-25 mcg/kg[1]
Daily maintenance dose[3]:
Oral: 5-7.5 mcg/kg[1]
I.V. or I.M.: 4-6 mcg/kg[1]
Full-term infant[1]:
Total digitalizing dose[2]:
Oral: 25-35 mcg/kg[1]
I.V. or I.M.: 20-30 mcg/kg[1]

Daily maintenance dose[3]:
Oral: 6-10 mcg/kg[1]
I.V. or I.M.: 5-8 mcg/kg[1]
1 month to 2 years[1]:
Total digitalizing dose[2]:
Oral: 35-60 mcg/kg[1]
I.V. or I.M.: 30-50 mcg/kg[1]
Daily maintenance dose[3]:
Oral: 10-15 mcg/kg[1]
I.V. or I.M.: 7.5-12 mcg/kg[1]
2-5 years[1]:
Total digitalizing dose[2]:
Oral: 30-40 mcg/kg[1]
I.V. or I.M.: 25-35 mcg/kg[1]
Daily maintenance dose[3]:
Oral: 7.5-10 mcg/kg[1]
I.V. or I.M.: 6-9 mcg/kg[1]
5-10 years[1]:
Total digitalizing dose[2]:
Oral: 20-35 mcg/kg[1]
I.V. or I.M.: 15-30 mcg/kg[1]
Daily maintenance dose[3]:
Oral: 5-10 mcg/kg[1]
I.V. or I.M.: 4-8 mcg/kg[1]
>10 years[1]:
Total digitalizing dose[2]:
Oral: 10-15 mcg/kg[1]
I.V. or I.M.: 8-12 mcg/kg[1]
Daily maintenance dose[3]:
Oral: 2.5-5 mcg/kg[1]
I.V. or I.M.: 2-3 mcg/kg[1]
Adults:
Total digitalizing dose[2]:
Oral: 0.75-1.5 mg
I.V. or I.M.: 0.5-1 mg
Daily maintenance dose[3]:
Oral: 0.125-0.5 mg
I.V. or I.M.: 0.1-0.4 mg

[1]Based on lean body weight and normal renal function for age. Decrease dose in patients with decreased renal function; digitalizing dose often not recommended in infants and children.
[2]Give one-half of the total digitalizing dose (TDD) in the initial dose, then give one-quarter of the TDD in each of two subsequent doses at 8- to 12-hour intervals. Obtain EKG 6 hours after each dose to assess potential toxicity.
[3]Divided every 12 hours in infants and children <10 years of age. Give once daily to children >10 years of age and adults.

Dosage Forms
Capsule:
Lanoxicaps®: 100 mcg, 200 mcg [contains ethyl alcohol]
Injection, solution: 250 mcg/mL (1 mL, 2 mL)
Lanoxin®: 250 mcg/mL (2 mL) [contains alcohol 10% and propylene glycol 40%]
Injection, solution [pediatric]: 100 mcg/mL (1 mL)
Solution, oral: 50 mcg/mL (2.5 mL, 5 mL, 60 mL)
Tablet: 125 mcg, 250 mcg
Digitek®, Lanoxin®: 125 mcg, 250 mcg

Digoxin CSD [Can] *see* digoxin *on previous page*

digoxin immune Fab (di JOKS in i MYUN fab)

Synonyms antidigoxin fab fragments, ovine
U.S./Canadian Brand Names Digibind® [US/Can]; DigiFab™ [US]
Therapeutic Category Antidote
Use Treatment of life-threatening or potentially life-threatening digoxin intoxication, including:
• acute digoxin ingestion (ie, >10 mg in adults or >4 mg in children)
(Continued)

digoxin immune Fab *(Continued)*

- chronic ingestions leading to steady-state digoxin concentrations >6 ng/mL in adults or >4 ng/mL in children
- manifestations of digoxin toxicity due to overdose (life-threatening ventricular arrhythmias, progressive bradycardia, second- or third-degree heart block not responsive to atropine, serum potassium >5 mEq/L in adults or >6 mEq in children)

Usual Dosage Each vial of Digibind® 38 mg or DigiFab™ 40 mg will bind ~0.5 mg of digoxin or digitoxin.

Estimation of the dose is based on the body burden of digitalis. This may be calculated if the amount ingested is known or the postdistribution serum drug level is known (round dose to the nearest whole vial).

Fab dose (in vials) based on number of tablets (0.25 mg) ingested.

5 tablets ingested: 2 vials
10 tablets ingested: 4 vials
25 tablets ingested: 10 vials
50 tablets ingested: 20 vials
75 tablets ingested: 30 vials
100 tablets ingested: 40 vials
150 tablets ingested: 60 vials
200 tablets ingested: 80 vials

Fab dose based on serum drug level postdistribution:

Digoxin: No. of vials = level (ng/mL) x body weight (kg) divided by 100
Digitoxin: No. of vials = digitoxin (ng/mL) x body weight (kg) divided by 1000

If neither amount ingested nor drug level are known, dose empirically as follows:

For acute toxicity: 20 vials, administered in 2 divided doses to decrease the possibility of a febrile reaction, and to avoid fluid overload in small children.

For chronic toxicity: 6 vials; for infants and small children (≤20kg), a single vial may be sufficient

Dosage Forms Injection, powder for reconstitution:
Digibind®: 38 mg
DigiFab™: 40 mg

dihematoporphyrin ether *see* porfimer *on page 682*

Dihistine® DH [US] *see* chlorpheniramine, pseudoephedrine, and codeine *on page 182*

dihydrocodeine, aspirin, and caffeine (dye hye droe KOE deen, AS pir in, & KAF een)

Sound-Alike/Look-Alike Issues
Synalgos®-DC may be confused with Synagis®

Synonyms dihydrocodeine compound

U.S./Canadian Brand Names Synalgos®-DC [US]

Therapeutic Category Analgesic, Narcotic

Controlled Substance C-III

Use Management of mild to moderate pain that requires relaxation

Usual Dosage Adults: Oral: 1-2 capsules every 4-6 hours as needed for pain

Dosage Forms Capsule: Dihydrocodeine bitartrate 16 mg, aspirin 356.4 mg, and caffeine 30 mg

dihydrocodeine bitartrate, acetaminophen, and caffeine *see* acetaminophen, caffeine, and dihydrocodeine *on page 10*

dihydrocodeine bitartrate, phenylephrine hydrochloride, and chlorpheniramine maleate *see* phenylephrine, hydrocodone, and chlorpheniramine *on page 663*

dihydrocodeine compound *see* dihydrocodeine, aspirin, and caffeine *on this page*

dihydroergotamine (dye hye droe er GOT a meen)

Synonyms DHE; dihydroergotamine mesylate

U.S./Canadian Brand Names D.H.E. 45® [US]; Migranal® [US/Can]

Therapeutic Category Ergot Alkaloid and Derivative

Use Treatment of migraine headache with or without aura; injection also indicated for treatment of cluster headaches

Usual Dosage Adults:

I.M., SubQ: 1 mg at first sign of headache; repeat hourly to a maximum dose of 3 mg total; maximum dose: 6 mg/week

I.V.: 1 mg at first sign of headache; repeat hourly up to a maximum dose of 2 mg total; maximum dose: 6 mg/week

Intranasal: 1 spray (0.5 mg) of nasal spray should be administered into each nostril; if needed, repeat after 15 minutes, up to a total of 4 sprays. **Note:** Do not exceed 3 mg (6 sprays) in a 24-hour period and no more than 8 sprays in a week.

Dosage Forms

Injection, solution, as mesylate (D.H.E. 45®): 1 mg/mL (1 mL) [contains ethanol 94%]

Solution, intranasal spray, as mesylate (Migranal®): 4 mg/mL [0.5 mg/spray] (1 mL) [contains caffeine 10 mg/mL]

dihydroergotamine mesylate *see* dihydroergotamine *on previous page*

dihydroergotoxine *see* ergoloid mesylates *on page 301*

dihydrogenated ergot alkaloids *see* ergoloid mesylates *on page 301*

dihydrohydroxycodeinone *see* oxycodone *on page 626*

dihydromorphinone *see* hydromorphone *on page 429*

dihydroxyanthracenedione dihydrochloride *see* mitoxantrone *on page 561*

1,25 dihydroxycholecalciferol *see* calcitriol *on page 134*

dihydroxydeoxynorvinkaleukoblastine *see* vinorelbine *on page 873*

dihydroxypropyl theophylline *see* dyphylline *on page 285*

Dihyrex® Injection *(Discontinued)* *see* diphenhydramine *on page 261*

diiodohydroxyquin *see* iodoquinol *on page 459*

Dilacor® XR [US] *see* diltiazem *on this page*

Dilantin® [US/Can] *see* phenytoin *on page 665*

Dilatrate®-SR [US] *see* isosorbide dinitrate *on page 465*

Dilaudid® [US/Can] *see* hydromorphone *on page 429*

Dilaudid® Cough Syrup *(Discontinued)* *see* hydromorphone *on page 429*

Dilaudid-HP® [US/Can] *see* hydromorphone *on page 429*

Dilaudid-HP-Plus® [Can] *see* hydromorphone *on page 429*

Dilaudid® Sterile Powder [Can] *see* hydromorphone *on page 429*

Dilaudid-XP® [Can] *see* hydromorphone *on page 429*

Dilocaine® Injection *(Discontinued)* *see* lidocaine *on page 493*

Dilomine® Injection *(Discontinued)* *see* dicyclomine *on page 251*

Dilor® [Can] *see* dyphylline *on page 285*

Diltia XT® [US] *see* diltiazem *on this page*

diltiazem (dil TYE a zem)

Sound-Alike/Look-Alike Issues

diltiazem may be confused with Dilantin®

Cardizem® may be confused with Cardene®, Cardene SR®, Cardizem CD®, Cardizem SR®, cardiem

Cartia XT™ may be confused with Procardia XL®

Tiazac® may be confused with Tigan®, Ziac®

Synonyms diltiazem hydrochloride

U.S./Canadian Brand Names Alti-Diltiazem CD [Can]; Apo-Diltiaz CD® [Can]; Apo-Diltiaz SR® [Can]; Apo-Diltiaz® Injectable [Can]; Apo-Diltiaz® [Can]; Cardizem® CD [US/Can]; Cardizem® LA [US]; Cardizem® SR [Can]; Cardizem® [US/Can]; Cartia XT™ [US]; Dilacor® XR [US]; Diltia XT® [US]; Diltiazem HCl ER® [Can]; Diltiazem Hydrochloride Injection [Can]; Gen-Diltiazem CD [Can]; Gen-Diltiazem [Can]; Med-Diltiazem [Can]; Novo-Diltazem [Can]; Novo-Diltazem-CD [Can]; Novo-Diltiazem HCl ER [Can]; Nu-Diltiaz [Can]; Nu-Diltiaz-CD [Can]; ratio-Diltiazem CD [Can]; Rhoxal-diltiazem CD [Can]; Rhoxal-diltiazem SR [Can]; Rhoxal-diltiazem T [Can]; Sandoz-Diltiazem CD [Can]; Sandoz-Diltiazem T [Can]; Syn-Diltiazem® [Can]; Taztia XT™ [US]; Tiazac® XC [Can]; Tiazac® [US/Can]

Therapeutic Category Calcium Channel Blocker

Use

Oral: Essential hypertension; chronic stable angina or angina from coronary artery spasm

Injection: Atrial fibrillation or atrial flutter; paroxysmal supraventricular tachycardia (PSVT)

(Continued)

diltiazem *(Continued)*

Usual Dosage Adults:

Oral:

Angina:

Capsule, extended release (Cardizem® CD, Cartia XT™, Dilacor® XR, Diltia XT®, Tiazac®): Initial: 120-180 mg once daily (maximum dose: 480 mg/day)

Tablet, extended release (Cardizem® LA): 180 mg once daily; may increase at 7- to 14-day intervals (maximum recommended dose: 360 mg/day)

Tablet, immediate release (Cardizem®): Usual starting dose: 30 mg 4 times/day; usual range: 180-360 mg/day

Hypertension:

Capsule, extended release (Cardizem® CD, Cartia XT™, Dilacor® XR, Diltia XT®, Tiazac®): Initial: 180-240 mg once daily; dose adjustment may be made after 14 days; usual dose range (JNC 7): 180-420 mg/day; Tiazac®: usual dose range: 120-540 mg/day

Capsule, sustained release (Cardizem® SR): Initial: 60-120 mg twice daily; dose adjustment may be made after 14 days; usual range: 240-360 mg/day

Tablet, extended release (Cardizem® LA): Initial: 180-240 mg once daily; dose adjustment may be made after 14 days; usual dose range (JNC 7): 120-540 mg/day

I.V.: Atrial fibrillation, atrial flutter, PSVT:

Initial bolus dose: 0.25 mg/kg actual body weight over 2 minutes (average adult dose: 20 mg)

Repeat bolus dose (may be administered after 15 minutes if the response is inadequate.): 0.35 mg/kg actual body weight over 2 minutes (average adult dose: 25 mg)

Continuous infusion (requires an infusion pump; infusions >24 hours or infusion rates >15 mg/hour are not recommended.): Initial infusion rate of 10 mg/hour; rate may be increased in 5 mg/hour increments up to 15 mg/hour as needed; some patients may respond to an initial rate of 5 mg/hour.

If diltiazem injection is administered by continuous infusion for >24 hours, the possibility of decreased diltiazem clearance, prolonged elimination half-life, and increased diltiazem and/or diltiazem metabolite plasma concentrations should be considered.

Conversion from I.V. diltiazem to oral diltiazem: Start oral approximately 3 hours after bolus dose. **Oral dose (mg/day) is approximately equal to [rate (mg/hour) x 3 + 3] x 10.**

3 mg/hour = 120 mg/day
5 mg/hour = 180 mg/day
7 mg/hour = 240 mg/day
11 mg/hour = 360 mg/day

Dosage Forms

Capsule, extended release, as hydrochloride [once-daily dosing]: 120 mg, 180 mg, 240 mg, 300 mg, 360 mg, 420 mg

Cardizem® CD: 120 mg, 180 mg, 240 mg, 300 mg, 360 mg
Cartia XT™: 120 mg, 180 mg, 240 mg, 300 mg
Dilacor® XR, Dilt-XR, Diltia XT®: 120 mg, 180 mg, 240 mg
Taztia XT™: 120 mg, 180 mg, 240 mg, 300 mg, 360 mg
Tiazac®: 120 mg, 180 mg, 240 mg, 300 mg, 360 mg, 420 mg

Capsule, sustained release, as hydrochloride [twice-daily dosing]: 60 mg, 90 mg, 120 mg

Injection, solution, as hydrochloride: 5 mg/mL (5 mL, 10 mL, 25 mL)

Injection, powder for reconstitution, as hydrochloride:

Cardizem®: 25 mg

Tablet, as hydrochloride: 30 mg, 60 mg, 90 mg, 120 mg

Cardizem®: 30 mg, 60 mg, 90 mg, 120 mg

Tablet, extended release, as hydrochloride:

Cardizem® LA: 120 mg, 180 mg, 240 mg, 300 mg, 360 mg, 420 mg

Diltiazem HCl ER® [Can] *see* diltiazem *on previous page*

diltiazem hydrochloride *see* diltiazem *on previous page*

Diltiazem Hydrochloride Injection [Can] *see* diltiazem *on previous page*

Dimaphen DM [US-OTC] *see* brompheniramine, pseudoephedrine, and dextromethorphan *on page 120*

dimenhydrinate (dye men HYE dri nate)

Sound-Alike/Look-Alike Issues

dimenhyDRINATE may be confused with diphenhydrAMINE

Tall-Man dimenhy**DRINATE**

U.S./Canadian Brand Names Apo-Dimenhydrinate® [Can]; Children's Motion Sickness Liquid [Can]; Dinate® [Can]; Dramamine® [US-OTC]; Gravol® [Can]; Jamp® Travel Tablet [Can]; Nauseatol [Can]; Novo-Dimenate [Can]; SAB-Dimenhydrinate [Can]

Therapeutic Category Antihistamine

Use Treatment and prevention of nausea, vertigo, and vomiting associated with motion sickness

Dosage forms available in Canada (not available in the U.S.), including parenteral formulations and suppositories, are also approved for the treatment of postoperative nausea and vomiting and treatment of radiation sickness.

Usual Dosage Oral:

Children:

2-5 years: 12.5-25 mg every 6-8 hours, maximum: 75 mg/day

6-12 years: 25-50 mg every 6-8 hours, maximum: 150 mg/day

Adults: 50-100 mg every 4-6 hours, not to exceed 400 mg/day

Gravol® L/A (not available in the U.S.): 75-150 mg every 8-12 hours, up to a maximum of five 75 mg caplets or three 100 mg caplets in 24 hours

Additional formulations/uses (approved in Canada) for parenteral/suppository formulations (not available in U.S.):

I.M., I.V., rectal: Adults:

Postoperative nausea and vomiting: 50-100 mg administered 30-60 minutes prior to radiation therapy; may be repeated as needed up to a maximum of 400 mg in 24 hours

Radiation sickness: 50-100 mg administered 30-60 minutes prior to radiation therapy. May be repeated as needed up to a maximum of 400 mg in 24 hours

Dosage Forms [CAN] = Canadian brand name

Caplet (TripTone®): 50 mg [DSC]

Capsule, softgel (Gravol®) [CAN]: 50 mg [not available in the U.S.]

Capsule, long-acting (Gravol® L/A) [CAN]: 75 mg, 100 mg [not available in the U.S.]

Injection, solution:

Gravol® I.M. [CAN]: 50 mg/mL (1 mL, 5 mL) [not available in the U.S.]

Gravol® I.V. [CAN]: 10 mg/mL (5 mL) [not available in the U.S.]

Solution, oral (Gravol® [CAN], Children's Motion Sickness [CAN]): 3 mg/mL (75 mL) [not available in the U.S.]

Suppository, rectal (Gravol® [CAN], Sab-Dimenhydrinate [CAN]): 75 mg, 100 mg [not available in the U.S.]

Tablet:

Dinate® [CAN], Jamp® Travel Tablet [CAN], Nauseatol® [CAN]: 50 mg

Dramamine®: 50 mg

Gravol® Filmkote Jr [CAN]: 25 mg [not available in the U.S.]

Gravol® Filmkote [CAN]: 50 mg [not available in the U.S.]

Tablet, chewable:

Dramamine®: 50 mg [contains phenylalanine 1.5 mg/tablet and tartrazine; orange flavor]

Gravol® Chewable for Children [CAN]: 25 mg [not available in the U.S.]

Gravol® Chewable for Adults [CAN]: 50 mg [not available in the U.S.]

dimercaprol (dye mer KAP role)

Synonyms BAL; British anti-lewisite; dithioglycerol

U.S./Canadian Brand Names BAL in Oil® [US]

Therapeutic Category Chelating Agent

Use Antidote to gold, arsenic (except arsine), and mercury poisoning (except nonalkyl mercury); adjunct to edetate calcium disodium in lead poisoning; possibly effective for antimony, bismuth, chromium, copper, nickel, tungsten, or zinc

Usual Dosage Children and Adults: Deep I.M.:

Arsenic, mercury, and gold poisoning: 3 mg/kg every 4-6 hours for 2 days, then every 12 hours for 7-10 days or until recovery (initial dose may be up to 5 mg if severe poisoning)

Lead poisoning (in conjunction with calcium EDTA): For symptomatic acute encephalopathy or blood level >100 mcg/dL: 4-5 mg/kg every 4 hours for 3-5 days

Dosage Forms Injection, oil: 100 mg/mL (3 mL) [contains benzyl benzoate and peanut oil]

Dimetabs® Oral *(Discontinued)* *see* dimenhydrinate *on previous page*

Dimetane® Extentabs® [US-OTC] *see* brompheniramine *on page 118*

Dimetapp® 12-Hour Non-Drowsy Extentabs® [US-OTC] *see* pseudoephedrine *on page 712*

Dimetapp® Allergy [US-OTC] *see* brompheniramine *on page 118*

Dimetapp® Allergy Children's [US-OTC] *see* brompheniramine *on page 118*

Dimetapp® Children's ND *(Discontinued)* *see* loratadine *on page 505*

Dimetapp® Decongestant Infant [US-OTC] *see* pseudoephedrine *on page 712*

Dimetapp® DM Children's Cold and Cough [US-OTC] *see* brompheniramine, pseudoephedrine, and dextromethorphan *on page 120*

Dimetapp® Infant Decongestant Plus Cough [US-OTC] *see* pseudoephedrine and dextromethorphan *on page 714*

Dimetapp® Sinus Caplets *(Discontinued)* *see* pseudoephedrine and ibuprofen *on page 715*

β,β-dimethylcysteine *see* penicillamine *on page 646*

dimethyl sulfoxide (dye meth il sul FOKS ide)

Synonyms DMSO

U.S./Canadian Brand Names Dimethyl Sulfoxide Irrigation, USP [Can]; Kemsol® [Can]; Rimso®-50 [US/Can]

Therapeutic Category Urinary Tract Product

Use Symptomatic relief of interstitial cystitis

Usual Dosage Instill 50 mL directly into bladder and allow to remain for 15 minutes; repeat every 2 weeks until maximum symptomatic relief is obtained

Dosage Forms Solution, intravesical: 50% [500 mg/mL] (50 mL)

Dimethyl Sulfoxide Irrigation, USP [Can] *see* dimethyl sulfoxide *on this page*

dimethyl triazeno imidazole carboxamide *see* dacarbazine *on page 226*

Dinate® [Can] *see* dimenhydrinate *on page 258*

Dinate® Injection *(Discontinued)* *see* dimenhydrinate *on page 258*

dinoprostone (dye noe PROST one)

Sound-Alike/Look-Alike Issues

Prepidil® may be confused with Bepridil®

Synonyms PGE_2; prostaglandin E_2

U.S./Canadian Brand Names Cervidil® [US/Can]; Prepidil® [US/Can]; Prostin E_2® [US/Can]

Therapeutic Category Prostaglandin

Use

Gel: Promote cervical ripening prior to labor induction; usage for gel include any patient undergoing induction of labor with an unripe cervix, most commonly for preeclampsia, eclampsia, postdates, diabetes, intrauterine growth retardation, and chronic hypertension

Suppositories: Terminate pregnancy from 12th through 28th week of gestation; evacuate uterus in cases of missed abortion or intrauterine fetal death; manage benign hydatidiform mole

Vaginal insert: Initiation and/or cervical ripening in patients at or near term in whom there is a medical or obstetrical indication for the induction of labor

Usual Dosage

Abortifacient: Insert 1 suppository high in vagina, repeat at 3- to 5-hour intervals until abortion occurs up to 240 mg (maximum dose); continued administration for longer than 2 days is not advisable

Cervical ripening:

Gel:

Intracervical: 0.25-1 mg

Intravaginal: 2.5 mg

Suppositories: Intracervical: 2-3 mg

Vaginal Insert (Cervidil®): 10 mg (to be removed at the onset of active labor or after 12 hours)

Dosage Forms

Gel, endocervical (Prepidil®): 0.5 mg/3 g syringe [each package contains a 10 mm and 20 mm shielded catheter]

Insert, vaginal (Cervidil®): 10 mg [releases 0.3 mg/hour]

Suppository, vaginal (Prostin E_2®): 20 mg

Diocaine® [Can] *see* proparacaine *on page 706*

Diocarpine [Can] *see* pilocarpine *on page 668*

Diochloram® [Can] *see* chloramphenicol *on page 172*

Diocto® [US-OTC] *see* docusate *on page 270*

Diocto C® *(Discontinued)*

Diocto-K® *(Discontinued)* *see* docusate *on page 270*

Diocto-K Plus® *(Discontinued)* *see* docusate *on page 270*

dioctyl calcium sulfosuccinate *see* docusate *on page 270*

dioctyl sodium sulfosuccinate *see* docusate *on page 270*

Diodex® [Can] *see* dexamethasone (systemic) *on page 239*

Diodoquin® [Can] *see* iodoquinol *on page 459*

Diogent® [Can] *see* gentamicin *on page 381*

Diomycin® [Can] *see* erythromycin *on page 303*

Dionephrine® [Can] *see* phenylephrine *on page 660*

Dionosil Oily® [US] *see* radiological/contrast media (ionic) *on page 728*

Diopentolate® [Can] *see* cyclopentolate *on page 220*

Diopred® [Can] *see* prednisolone (systemic) *on page 695*

Dioptic's Atropine Solution [Can] *see* atropine *on page 83*

Dioptimyd® [Can] *see* sulfacetamide and prednisolone *on page 796*

Dioptrol® [Can] *see* neomycin, polymyxin B, and dexamethasone *on page 584*

Diosulf™ [Can] *see* sulfacetamide *on page 795*

Diotame® [US-OTC] *see* bismuth subsalicylate *on page 112*

Diotrope® [Can] *see* tropicamide *on page 856*

Dioval® Injection *(Discontinued)* *see* estradiol *on page 308*

Diovan® [US/Can] *see* valsartan *on page 865*

Diovan HCT® [US/Can] *see* valsartan and hydrochlorothiazide *on page 865*

Diovol® [Can] *see* aluminum hydroxide and magnesium hydroxide *on page 36*

Diovol® Ex [Can] *see* aluminum hydroxide and magnesium hydroxide *on page 36*

Diovol Plus® [Can] *see* aluminum hydroxide, magnesium hydroxide, and simethicone *on page 37*

Dipentum® [US/Can] *see* olsalazine *on page 614*

Diphen® [US-OTC] *see* diphenhydramine *on this page*

Diphenacen 50® Injection *(Discontinued)* *see* diphenhydramine *on this page*

Diphen® AF [US-OTC] *see* diphenhydramine *on this page*

Diphenatol® *(Discontinued)* *see* diphenoxylate and atropine *on page 264*

Diphenhist [US-OTC] *see* diphenhydramine *on this page*

diphenhydramine (dye fen HYE dra meen)

Sound-Alike/Look-Alike Issues

diphenhydrAMINE may be confused with desipramine, dicyclomine, dimenhyDRINATE

Benadryl® may be confused with benazepril, Bentyl®, Benylin®, Caladryl®

Synonyms diphenhydramine citrate; diphenhydramine hydrochloride; diphenhydramine tannate

Tall-Man diphenhydr**AMINE**

U.S./Canadian Brand Names Aler-Cap [US-OTC]; Aler-Dryl [US-OTC]; Aler-Tab [US-OTC]; Allerdryl® [Can]; AllerMax® [US-OTC]; Allernix [Can]; Altaryl [US-OTC]; Banophen® Anti-Itch [US-OTC]; Banophen® [US-OTC]; Benadryl® Allergy [US-OTC]; Benadryl® Children's Allergy Fastmelt® [US-OTC]; Benadryl® Children's Allergy [US-OTC]; Benadryl® Dye-Free Allergy [US-OTC]; Benadryl® Injection [US]; Benadryl® Itch Stopping Extra Strength [US-OTC]; Benadryl® Itch Stopping [US-OTC]; Benadryl® [Can]; Compoz® Nighttime Sleep Aid [US-OTC]; Dermamycin® [US-OTC]; Dermarest® Insect Bite [US-OTC]; Dermarest® Plus [US-OTC]; Diphenhist [US-OTC]; Diphen® AF [US-OTC]; Diphen® [US-OTC]; Dytan™ [US]; Genahist® [US-OTC]; Hydramine® [US-OTC]; Nytol® Extra Strength [Can]; Nytol® Quick Caps [US-OTC]; Nytol® Quick Gels [US-OTC]; Nytol® [Can]; PMS-Diphenhydramine [Can]; Q-Dryl [US-OTC]; Quenalin [US-OTC]; Siladryl® Allergy [US-OTC]; Siladryl® DAS [US-OTC]; Silphen® [US-OTC]; Simply Sleep® [US-OTC/Can]; Sleep-ettes D [US-OTC]; Sleepinal® [US-OTC]; Sominex® Maximum Strength [US-OTC]; Sominex® [US-OTC]; Triaminic® Thin Strips™ Cough and Runny Nose [US-OTC]; Twilite® [US-OTC]; Unisom® Maximum Strength SleepGels® [US-OTC]

(Continued)

diphenhydramine *(Continued)*

Therapeutic Category Antihistamine

Use Symptomatic relief of allergic symptoms caused by histamine release which include nasal allergies and allergic dermatosis; can be used for mild nighttime sedation; prevention of motion sickness and as an antitussive; has antinauseant and topical anesthetic properties; treatment of antipsychotic-induced extrapyramidal symptoms

Usual Dosage

Children:

Oral, I.M., I.V.:

Treatment of moderate to severe allergic reactions: 5 mg/kg/day or 150 mg/m^2/day in divided doses every 6-8 hours, not to exceed 300 mg/day

Minor allergic rhinitis or motion sickness:

2 to <6 years: 6.25 mg every 4-6 hours; maximum: 37.5 mg/day

6 to <12 years: 12.5-25 mg every 4-6 hours; maximum: 150 mg/day

≥12 years: 25-50 mg every 4-6 hours; maximum: 300 mg/day

Night-time sleep aid: 30 minutes before bedtime:

2 to <12 years: 1 mg/kg/dose; maximum: 50 mg/dose

≥12 years: 50 mg

Oral: Antitussive:

2 to <6 years: 6.25 mg every 4 hours; maximum 37.5 mg/day

6 to <12 years: 12.5 mg every 4 hours; maximum 75 mg/day

≥12 years: 25 mg every 4 hours; maximum 150 mg/day

I.M., I.V.: Treatment of dystonic reactions: 0.5-1 mg/kg/dose

Adults:

Oral: 25-50 mg every 6-8 hours

Minor allergic rhinitis or motion sickness: 25-50 mg every 4-6 hours; maximum: 300 mg/day

Moderate to severe allergic reactions: 25-50 mg every 4 hours, not to exceed 400 mg/day

Nighttime sleep aid: 50 mg at bedtime

I.M., I.V.: 10-50 mg in a single dose every 2-4 hours, not to exceed 400 mg/day

Dystonic reaction: 50 mg in a single dose; may repeat in 20-30 minutes if necessary

Topical: For external application, not longer than 7 days

Dosage Forms

Caplet, as hydrochloride: 25 mg, 50 mg

Aler-Dryl, AllerMax®, Compoz® Nighttime Sleep Aid, Sleep-ettes D, Sominex® Maximum Strength, Twilite®: 50 mg

Simply Sleep®, Nytol® Quick Caps: 25 mg

Capsule, as hydrochloride: 25 mg, 50 mg

Aler-Cap, Banophen®, Benadryl® Allergy, Diphen®, Diphenhist, Genahist®, Q-Dryl: 25 mg

Sleepinal®: 50 mg

Capsule, softgel, as hydrochloride: 50 mg

Benadryl® Dye-Free Allergy: 25 mg [dye-free]

Compoz® Nighttime Sleep Aid, Nytol® Quick Gels, Sleepinal®, Unisom® Maximum Strength SleepGels®: 50 mg

Captab, as hydrochloride (Diphenhist®): 25 mg

Cream, as hydrochloride: 2% (30 g) [contains zinc acetate 0.1%]

Banophen® Anti-Itch: 2% (30 g) [contains zinc acetate 0.1%]

Benadryl® Itch Stopping: 1% (30 g) [contains zinc acetate 0.1%]

Benadryl® Itch Stopping Extra Strength: 2% (30 g) [contains zinc acetate 0.1%]

Diphenhist®: 2% (30 g) [contains zinc acetate 0.1%]

Elixir, as hydrochloride:

Altaryl: 12.5 mg/5 mL (120 mL, 480 mL, 3840 mL) [cherry flavor]

Banophen®: 12.5 mg/5 mL (120 mL)

Diphen AF: 12.5 mg/5 mL (120 mL, 240 mL, 480 mL) [alcohol free; cherry flavor]

Q-Dryl: 12.5 mg/5 mL (480 mL) [alcohol free]

Gel, topical, as hydrochloride:

Benadryl® Itch Stopping Extra Strength: 2% (120 mL)

Dermarest® Plus: 2% (28 g, 42 g) [contains menthol 1%]

Injection, solution, as hydrochloride: 50 mg/mL (1 mL)

Benadryl®: 50 mg/mL (1 mL, 10 mL)

Liquid, as hydrochloride:

AllerMax®: 12.5 mg/5 mL (120 mL)

Benadryl® Allergy: 12.5 mg/5 mL (120 mL, 240 mL) [alcohol free; contains sodium benzoate; cherry flavor]

Benadryl® Dye-Free Allergy: 12.5 mg/5 mL (120 mL) [alcohol free, dye free, sugar free; contains sodium benzoate; bubble gum flavor]
Genahist®: 12.5 mg/5 mL (120 mL) [alcohol free, sugar free; contains sodium benzoate; cherry flavor]
Hydramine®: 12.5 mg/5 mL (120 mL, 480 mL) [alcohol free]
Q-Dryl: 12.5 mg/5 mL (120 mL) [alcohol free; cherry flavor]
Quenalin: 12.5 mg/5 mL (120 mL) [fruit flavor]
Siladryl® Allergy: 12.5 mg/5 mL (120 mL, 240 mL, 480 mL) [alcohol free, sugar free; black cherry flavor]
Siladryl® DAS: 12.5 mg/5 mL (120 mL) [alcohol free, dye free, sugar free; black cherry flavor]

Liquid, topical, as hydrochloride [stick] (Benadryl® Itch Stopping Extra Strength): 2% (14 mL) [contains zinc acetate 0.1% and alcohol]

Solution, oral, as hydrochloride:
Banophen®: 12.5 mg/5mL (480 mL) [sugar free]
Diphenhist: 12.5 mg/5 mL (120 mL, 480 mL) [alcohol free; contains sodium benzoate]

Solution, topical, as hydrochloride [spray]:
Benadryl® Itch Stopping Extra Strength: 2% (60 mL) [contains zinc acetate 0.1% and alcohol]
Dermamycin®, Dermarest® Insect Bite: 2% (60 mL) [contains menthol 1%]

Strips, oral, as hydrochloride (Triaminic® Thin Strips™ Cough and Runny Nose): 12.5 mg (16s) [grape flavor]

Suspension, as tannate: 25 mg/5 mL (120 mL)
Dytan™: 25 mg/5 mL (120 mL) [strawberry flavor]

Syrup, as hydrochloride (Silphen® Cough): 12.5 mg/5 mL (120 mL, 240 mL, 480 mL) [contains alcohol; 5%; strawberry flavor]

Tablet, as hydrochloride: 25 mg, 50 mg
Aler-Tab, Benadryl® Allergy, Genahist®, Sleepinal®, Sominex®: 25 mg

Tablet, chewable, as hydrochloride (Benadryl® Children's Allergy): 12.5 mg [contains phenylalanine 4.2 mg/tablet; grape flavor]

Tablet, chewable, as tannate (Dytan™): 25 mg [contains phenylalanine; strawberry flavor]

Tablet, orally disintegrating, as citrate (Benadryl® Children's Allergy Fastmelt®): 19 mg [equivalent to diphenhydramine hydrochloride 12.5 mg; contains phenylalanine 4.5 mg/tablet and soy protein isolate; cherry flavor]

diphenhydramine and acetaminophen *see* acetaminophen and diphenhydramine *on page 7*

diphenhydramine and pseudoephedrine (dye fen HYE dra meen & soo doe e FED rin)

Sound-Alike/Look-Alike Issues

Benadryl® may be confused with benazepril, Bentyl®, Benylin®, Caladryl®

Synonyms pseudoephedrine and diphenhydramine

U.S./Canadian Brand Names Benadryl® Allergy and Sinus Fastmelt™ [US-OTC]; Benadryl® Allergy/Sinus [US-OTC]; Benadryl® Children's Allergy and Cold Fastmelt™ [US-OTC]; Benadryl® Children's Allergy and Sinus [US-OTC]

Therapeutic Category Antihistamine/Decongestant Combination

Use Relief of symptoms of upper respiratory mucosal congestion in seasonal and perennial nasal allergies, acute rhinitis, rhinosinusitis, and eustachian tube blockage

Usual Dosage Based on **pseudoephedrine** component: Adults: Oral: 60 mg every 4-6 hours, maximum: 240 mg/day

Dosage Forms

Liquid (Benadryl® Children's Allergy and Sinus): Diphenhydramine hydrochloride 12.5 mg and pseudoephedrine hydrochloride 30 mg per 5 mL [contains sodium benzoate; alcohol free, sugar free; grape flavor]

Tablet (Benadryl® Allergy/Sinus): Diphenhydramine hydrochloride 25 mg and pseudoephedrine hydrochloride 60 mg

Tablet, quick dissolving (Benadryl® Children's Allergy and Cold Fastmelt™, Benadryl® Allergy and Sinus Fastmelt™): Diphenhydramine citrate 19 mg [equivalent to diphenhydramine hydrochloride 12.5 mg] and pseudoephedrine 30 mg [contains phenylalanine 4.6 mg/tablet; cherry flavor]

diphenhydramine citrate *see* diphenhydramine *on page 261*

diphenhydramine hydrochloride *see* diphenhydramine *on page 261*

diphenhydramine, hydrocodone, and phenylephrine *see* hydrocodone, phenylephrine, and diphenhydramine *on page 425*

diphenhydramine tannate *see* diphenhydramine *on page 261*

diphenoxylate and atropine (dye fen OKS i late & A troe peen)

Sound-Alike/Look-Alike Issues

Lomotil® may be confused with Lamictal®, Lamisil®, lamotrigine, Lanoxin®, Lasix®, ludiomil

Lonox® may be confused with Lanoxin®, Loprox®

Synonyms atropine and diphenoxylate

U.S./Canadian Brand Names Lomotil® [US/Can]; Lonox® [US]

Therapeutic Category Antidiarrheal

Controlled Substance C-V

Use Treatment of diarrhea

Usual Dosage Oral:

Children 2-12 years (use with caution in young children due to variable responses): Liquid: Diphenoxylate 0.3-0.4 mg/kg/day in 4 divided doses until control achieved (maximum: 10 mg/day), then reduce dose as needed; some patients may be controlled on doses as low as 25% of the initial daily dose

Adults: Diphenoxylate 5 mg 4 times/day until control achieved (maximum: 20 mg/day), then reduce dose as needed; some patients may be controlled on doses of 5 mg/day

Dosage Forms

Solution, oral: Diphenoxylate hydrochloride 2.5 mg and atropine sulfate 0.025 mg per 5 mL (5 mL, 10 mL, 60 mL)

Lomotil®: Diphenoxylate hydrochloride 2.5 mg and atropine sulfate 0.025 mg per 5 mL (60 mL) [contains alcohol 15%; cherry flavor]

Tablet: Diphenoxylate hydrochloride 2.5 mg and atropine sulfate 0.025 mg

Lomotil®, Lonox®: Diphenoxylate hydrochloride 2.5 mg and atropine sulfate 0.025 mg

Diphenylan Sodium® *(Discontinued)* *see* phenytoin *on page 665*

diphenylhydantoin *see* phenytoin *on page 665*

diphtheria and tetanus toxoid (dif THEER ee a & TET a nus TOKS oyd)

Synonyms DT; Td; tetanus and diphtheria toxoid

U.S./Canadian Brand Names Decavac™ [US]

Therapeutic Category Toxoid

Use

Diphtheria and tetanus toxoids adsorbed for pediatric use (DT): Infants and children through 6 years of age: Active immunity against diphtheria and tetanus when pertussis vaccine is contraindicated

Tetanus and diphtheria toxoids adsorbed for adult use (Td) (Decavac™): Children ≥7 years of age and Adults: Active immunity against diphtheria and tetanus; tetanus prophylaxis in wound management

Usual Dosage I.M.:

Infants and Children ≤6 years (DT): Primary immunization:

6 weeks to 1 year: Three 0.5 mL doses at least 4 weeks apart; administer a reinforcing dose 6-12 months after the third injection

1-6 years: Two 0.5 mL doses at least 4 weeks apart; reinforcing dose 6-12 months after second injection; if final dose is given after seventh birthday, use adult preparation

4-6 years (booster immunization): 0.5 mL; not necessary if the fourth dose was given after fourth birthday; routinely administer booster doses at 10-year intervals with the adult preparation

Children ≥7 years and Adults (Td):

Primary immunization: Patients previously not immunized should receive 2 primary doses of 0.5 mL each, given at an interval of 4-6 weeks; third (reinforcing) dose of 0.5 mL 6-12 months later

Booster immunization: 0.5 mL every 10 years; to be given to children 11-12 years of age if at least 5 years have elapsed since last dose of toxoid containing vaccine. Subsequent routine doses are not recommended more often than every 10 years. The ACIP prefers Tdap for use in adolescents 11-18 years; refer to diphtheria and tetanus toxoids and acellular pertussis vaccine monograph for additional information.

Tetanus prophylaxis in wound management; use of tetanus toxoid (Td) and/or tetanus immune globulin (TIG) depends upon the number of prior tetanus toxoid doses and type of wound.

Clean, minor wounds:

- Prior number of tetanus toxoid doses is unknown or <3: Td[1]
- Prior number of tetanus toxoid doses is ≥3: Td[1] only if >10 years since last dose
- If only three doses of fluid tetanus toxoid have been received, a fourth dose of toxoid, preferably an adsorbed toxoid, should be given

All other wounds:

- Prior number of tetanus toxoid doses is unknown or <3: Td[1] and TIG
- Prior number of tetanus toxoid doses is ≥3: Td[1] only if >5 years since last dose

[1]Adult tetanus and diphtheria toxoids; use pediatric preparations (DT or DTP) if the patient is <7 years old.

Adapted from Report of the Committee on Infectious Diseases, American Academy of Pediatrics, Elk Grove Village, IL: American Academy of Pediatrics, 1986.

Dosage Forms

Injection, suspension, adult:

Decavac™: Diphtheria 2 Lf units and tetanus 5 Lf units per 0.5 mL (0.5 mL) [latex free prefilled syringe; contains thimerosal]

Injection, suspension, pediatric [preservative free]: Diphtheria 6.7 Lf units and tetanus 5 Lf units per 0.5 mL (0.5 mL)

diphtheria and tetanus toxoids and acellular pertussis adsorbed, hepatitis B (recombinant) and inactivated poliovirus vaccine combined *see* diphtheria, tetanus toxoids, acellular pertussis, hepatitis B (recombinant), and poliovirus (inactivated) vaccine *on this page*

diphtheria antitoxin (dif THEER ee a an tee TOKS in)

Therapeutic Category Antitoxin

Use Treatment of diphtheria (neutralizes unbound toxin, available from CDC)

Usual Dosage I.M. or slow I.V. infusion: Dosage varies; range: 20,000-120,000 units

Dosage Forms Injection: ≥500 units/mL (40 mL) [20,000 units/vial]

diphtheria CRM_{197} protein *see* pneumococcal conjugate vaccine (7-valent) *on page 675*

diphtheria CRM_{197} protein conjugate *see Haemophilus* B conjugate vaccine *on page 405*

diphtheria, tetanus toxoids, acellular pertussis, hepatitis B (recombinant), and poliovirus (inactivated) vaccine

(dif THEER ee a, TET a nus TOKS oyds, ay CEL yoo lar per TUS sis, hep a TYE tis bee ree KOM be nant, & POE lee oh VYE rus, in ak ti VAY ted vak SEEN)

Synonyms diphtheria and tetanus toxoids and acellular pertussis adsorbed, hepatitis B (recombinant) and inactivated poliovirus vaccine combined

U.S./Canadian Brand Names Pediarix™ [US]

Therapeutic Category Vaccine

Use Combination vaccine for the active immunization against diphtheria, tetanus, pertussis, hepatitis B virus (all known subtypes), and poliomyelitis (caused by poliovirus types 1, 2, and 3)

Usual Dosage I.M.: Children:

Immunization: 0.5 mL; repeat in 6-8 week intervals (preferably 8-week intervals) for a total of 3 doses. Vaccination usually begins at 2 months, but may be started as early as 6 weeks of age.

Use in children previously vaccinated with one or more component, and who are also scheduled to receive all vaccine components:

Hepatitis B vaccine: Infants born of HB_sAg-negative mothers who received 1 dose of hepatitis B vaccine at birth may be given Pediarix™ (safety data limited); use in infants who received more than 1 dose of hepatitis B vaccine has not been studied. Infants who received 1 or more doses of hepatitis B vaccine (recombinant) may be given Pediarix™ to complete the hepatitis B series (safety and efficacy not established).

Diphtheria and tetanus toxoids, and acellular pertussis vaccine (DTaP): Infants previously vaccinated with 1 or 2 doses of Infanrix® may use Pediarix™ to complete the first 3 doses of the series (safety and efficacy not established); use of Pediarix™ to complete DTaP vaccination started with products other than Infanrix® is not recommended.

Inactivated polio vaccine (IPV): Infants previously vaccinated with 1 or 2 doses of IPV may use Pediarix™ to complete the first 3 doses of the series (safety and efficacy not established).

Dosage Forms Injection, suspension [single-dose]: Diphtheria toxoid 25 Lf, tetanus toxoid 10 Lf, inactivated PT 25 mcg, FHA 25 mcg, pertactin 8 mcg, HB_sAg 10 mcg, poliovirus type 1 40 DU, poliovirus type 2 8 DU, and poliovirus type 3 32 DU per 0.5 mL [contains neomycin sulfate ≤0.05 ng/0.5 mL, polymyxin B ≤0.01 ng/0.5 mL, and yeast protein ≤5%; packaged in vials or prefilled syringes; the needleless prefilled syringes contain dry natural latex rubber in the tip cap and plunger]

diphtheria, tetanus toxoids, and acellular pertussis vaccine

(dif THEER ee a, TET a nus TOKS oyds & ay CEL yoo lar per TUS sis vak SEEN)

Synonyms DTaP; dTpa; Tdap; tetanus toxoid, reduced diphtheria toxoid, and acellular pertussis, adsorbed

U.S./Canadian Brand Names Adacel™ [US/Can]; Boostrix® [US]; Daptacel® [US]; Infanrix® [US]; Tripedia® [US]

(Continued)

diphtheria, tetanus toxoids, and acellular pertussis vaccine *(Continued)*

Therapeutic Category Toxoid

Use

Daptacel®, Infanrix®, Tripedia® (DTaP): Active immunization against diphtheria, tetanus, and pertussis from age 6 weeks through seventh birthday

Adacel™, Boostrix® (Tdap): Active booster immunization against diphtheria, tetanus, and pertussis

Usual Dosage

Primary immunization:

Children 6 weeks to <7 years: (Daptacel®, Infanrix®, Tripedia®): I.M.: 0.5 mL per dose, total of 5 doses administered as follows:

Three doses, usually given at 2-, 4-, and 6 months of age; may be given as early as 6 weeks of age and repeated every 4-8 weeks; use same product for all 3 doses

Fourth dose: Given at ~15-20 months of age, but at least 6 months after third dose

Fifth dose: Given at 5-6 years of age, prior to starting school or kindergarten; if the fourth dose is given at ≥4 years of age, the fifth dose may be omitted

Booster immunization:

ACIP recommendations: Adolescents 11-18 years: I.M.: 0.5 mL

A single dose of Tdap should be given instead of Td in adolescents who have completed the recommended childhood DTP/DTaP series and have not received Td or Tdap; preferred age of vaccination with Tdap is 11-12 years. Adolescents who received Td but not Tdap and who have completed the recommended childhood DTP/DTaP series are encouraged to receive Tdap; an interval of at least 5 years between Td and Tdap is recommended, but lesser intervals may be used if the benefit outweighs the risk.

Manufacturer's labeling:

Children 10-18 years (Boostrix®): I.M.: 0.5 mL as a single dose, administered 5 years after last dose of DTwP or DTaP vaccine.

Children ≥11 years and Adults ≤64 years (Adacel™): I.M.: 0.5 mL as a single dose, administered 5 years after last dose of DTwP or DTaP vaccine.

Wound management: Adacel™ (in patients 11-64 years of age) or Boostrix® (in patients 10-18 years of age) may be used as an alternative to Td vaccine when a tetanus toxoid-containing vaccine is needed for wound management, and in whom the pertussis component is also indicated. Td vaccine is the preferred agent in children ≥7 years and adults.

The ACIP prefers Tdap for adolescents 11-18 years requiring a tetanus toxoid product and who were vaccinated against tetanus ≥5 years earlier. Adolescents who completed the primary 3 dose series containing tetanus toxoid <5 years earlier are protected against tetanus and do not need a tetanus toxoid vaccine as part of wound management.

Dosage Forms Injection, suspension:

Adacel™: Diphtheria 2 Lf units, tetanus 5 Lf units, and acellular pertussis 2.5 mcg per 0.5 mL (0.5 mL) [vial stopper is latex free]

Boostrix®: Diphtheria 2.5 Lf units, tetanus 5 Lf units, and acellular pertussis 8 mcg per 0.5 mL (0.5 mL) [available in vial and prefilled syringe; preservative free; contains polysorbate 80; syringe cap and rubber plunger contain natural latex rubber]

Daptacel®: Diphtheria 15 Lf units, tetanus 5 Lf units, and acellular pertussis 10 mcg per 0.5 mL (0.5 mL) [vial stopper contains natural latex rubber]

Infanrix®: Diphtheria 25 Lf units, tetanus 10 Lf units, and acellular pertussis 25 mcg per 0.5 mL (0.5 mL) [available in vial and prefilled syringe; contains polysorbate 80; syringe cap and rubber plunger contain natural latex rubber]

Tripedia®: Diphtheria 6.7 Lf units, tetanus 5 Lf units, and acellular pertussis 46.8 mcg per 0.5 mL (7.5 mL) [contains polysorbate 80 and trace amounts of thimerosal; vial stopper contains natural latex rubber]

Note: Tripedia® vaccine is also used to reconstitute ActHIB® to prepare TriHIBit® vaccine (diphtheria, tetanus toxoids, and acellular pertussis and *Haemophilus influenzae* b conjugate vaccine combination)

diphtheria, tetanus toxoids, and acellular pertussis vaccine and *Haemophilus influenzae* b conjugate vaccine

(dif THEER ee a, TET a nus TOKS oyds & ay CEL yoo lar per TUS sis vak SEEN & hem OF fi lus in floo EN za bee KON joo gate vak SEEN)

Synonyms *Haemophilus influenzae* b conjugate vaccine and diphtheria, tetanus toxoids, and acellular pertussis vaccine

U.S./Canadian Brand Names TriHIBit® [US]

Therapeutic Category Toxoid; Vaccine, Inactivated Bacteria

Use Active immunization of children 15-18 months of age for prevention of diphtheria, tetanus, pertussis, and invasive disease caused by *H. influenzae* type b

Usual Dosage Children >15 months of age: I.M.: 0.5 mL (as part of a general vaccination schedule; see individual vaccines). Vaccine should be used within 30 minutes of reconstitution.

Dosage Forms Injection, suspension: 5 Lf units tetanus toxoid, 6.7 Lf units diphtheria toxoid, 46.8 mcg pertussis antigens, and 10 mcg *H. influenzae* type b purified capsular polysaccharide per 0.5 mL (0.5 mL) [The combination of Tripedia® vaccine used to reconstitute ActHIB® forms TriHIBit®]

diphtheria toxoid conjugate *see* Haemophilus B conjugate vaccine *on page 405*

dipivalyl epinephrine *see* dipivefrin *on this page*

dipivefrin (dye PI ve frin)

Synonyms dipivalyl epinephrine; dipivefrin hydrochloride; DPE

U.S./Canadian Brand Names Ophtho-Dipivefrin™ [Can]; PMS-Dipivefrin [Can]; Propine® [US]

Therapeutic Category Adrenergic Agonist Agent

Use Reduces elevated intraocular pressure in chronic open-angle glaucoma; also used to treat ocular hypertension, low tension, and secondary glaucomas

Usual Dosage Adults: Ophthalmic: Instill 1 drop every 12 hours into the eyes

Dosage Forms Solution, ophthalmic, as hydrochloride: 0.1% (5 mL, 10 mL, 15 mL) [contains benzalkonium chloride]

Propine®: 0.1% (5 mL [DSC], 10 mL, 15 mL) [contains benzalkonium chloride]

dipivefrin hydrochloride *see* dipivefrin *on this page*

Diprivan® [US/Can] *see* propofol *on page 707*

Diprolene® [US] *see* betamethasone (topical) *on page 107*

Diprolene® AF [US] *see* betamethasone (topical) *on page 107*

Diprolene® Glycol [Can] *see* betamethasone (topical) *on page 107*

dipropylacetic acid *see* valproic acid and derivatives *on page 864*

Diprosone® [Can] *see* betamethasone (topical) *on page 107*

dipyridamole (dye peer ID a mole)

Sound-Alike/Look-Alike Issues

dipyridamole may be confused with disopyramide

Persantine® may be confused with Periactin®, Permitil®

U.S./Canadian Brand Names Apo-Dipyridamole FC® [Can]; Persantine® [US/Can]

Therapeutic Category Antiplatelet Agent; Vasodilator

Use

Oral: Used with warfarin to decrease thrombosis in patients after artificial heart valve replacement

I.V.: Diagnostic agent in CAD

Usual Dosage

Oral: Children ≥12 years and Adults: Adjunctive therapy for prophylaxis of thromboembolism with cardiac valve replacement: 75-100 mg 4 times/day

I.V.: Adults: Evaluation of coronary artery disease: 0.14 mg/kg/minute for 4 minutes; maximum dose: 60 mg

Dosage Forms

Injection, solution: 5 mg/mL (2 mL, 10 mL)

Tablet: 25 mg, 50 mg, 75 mg

Persantine®: 25 mg, 50 mg, 75 mg

dipyridamole and aspirin *see* aspirin and dipyridamole *on page 79*

Disalcid® *(Discontinued)* *see* salsalate *on page 761*

disalicylic acid *see* salsalate *on page 761*

Disobrom® *(Discontinued)* *see* dexbrompheniramine and pseudoephedrine *on page 241*

disodium cromoglycate *see* cromolyn sodium *on page 217*

disodium thiosulfate pentahydrate *see* sodium thiosulfate *on page 783*

***d*-isoephedrine hydrochloride** *see* pseudoephedrine *on page 712*

Disonate® *(Discontinued)* *see* docusate *on page 270*

disopyramide (dye soe PEER a mide)

Sound-Alike/Look-Alike Issues

disopyramide may be confused with desipramine, dipyridamole

Norpace® may be confused with Norpramin®

Synonyms disopyramide phosphate

U.S./Canadian Brand Names Norpace® CR [US]; Norpace® [US/Can]; Rythmodan® [Can]; Rythmodan®-LA [Can]

Therapeutic Category Antiarrhythmic Agent, Class I-A

Use Suppression and prevention of unifocal and multifocal atrial and premature, ventricular premature complexes, coupled ventricular tachycardia; effective in the conversion of atrial fibrillation, atrial flutter, and paroxysmal atrial tachycardia to normal sinus rhythm and prevention of the recurrence of these arrhythmias after conversion by other methods

Usual Dosage Oral:

Children:

<1 year: 10-30 mg/kg/24 hours in 4 divided doses

1-4 years: 10-20 mg/kg/24 hours in 4 divided doses

4-12 years: 10-15 mg/kg/24 hours in 4 divided doses

12-18 years: 6-15 mg/kg/24 hours in 4 divided doses

Adults:

<50 kg: 100 mg every 6 hours or 200 mg every 12 hours (controlled release)

>50 kg: 150 mg every 6 hours or 300 mg every 12 hours (controlled release); if no response, increase to 200 mg every 6 hours. Maximum dose required for patients with severe refractory ventricular tachycardia is 400 mg every 6 hours.

Dosage Forms

Capsule (Norpace®): 100 mg, 150 mg

Capsule, controlled release (Norpace® CR): 100 mg, 150 mg

disopyramide phosphate *see* disopyramide *on this page*

Disotate® *(Discontinued)* *see* edetate disodium *on page 287*

Di-Spaz® Injection *(Discontinued)* *see* dicyclomine *on page 251*

Di-Spaz® Oral *(Discontinued)* *see* dicyclomine *on page 251*

DisperMox™ *(Discontinued)* *see* amoxicillin *on page 47*

disulfiram (dye SUL fi ram)

Sound-Alike/Look-Alike Issues

disulfiram may be confused with Diflucan®

Antabuse® may be confused with Anturane®

U.S./Canadian Brand Names Antabuse® [US]

Therapeutic Category Aldehyde Dehydrogenase Inhibitor Agent

Use Management of chronic alcoholism

Usual Dosage Adults: Oral: Do not administer until the patient has abstained from ethanol for at least 12 hours

Initial: 500 mg/day as a single dose for 1-2 weeks; maximum daily dose is 500 mg

Average maintenance dose: 250 mg/day; range: 125-500 mg; duration of therapy is to continue until the patient is fully recovered socially and a basis for permanent self control has been established; maintenance therapy may be required for months or even years

Dosage Forms Tablet: 250 mg

Dital® *(Discontinued)* *see* phendimetrazine *on page 657*

dithioglycerol *see* dimercaprol *on page 259*

dithranol *see* anthralin *on page 58*

Ditropan® [US/Can] *see* oxybutynin *on page 625*

Ditropan® XL [US/Can] *see* oxybutynin *on page 625*

Diurigen® *(Discontinued)* *see* chlorothiazide *on page 175*

Diuril® [US/Can] *see* chlorothiazide *on page 175*

divalproex sodium *see* valproic acid and derivatives *on page 864*

Dixarit® [Can] *see* clonidine *on page 203*

Dizac® Injectable Emulsion *(Discontinued)* *see* diazepam *on page 248*

Dizmiss® *(Discontinued)* *see* meclizine *on page 522*

5071-1DL(6) *see* megestrol *on page 525*

***dl*-alpha tocopherol** *see* vitamin E *on page 876*

4-DMDR *see* idarubicin *on page 439*

***D*-mannitol** *see* mannitol *on page 518*

D-Med® Injection *(Discontinued)* *see* methylprednisolone *on page 547*

DMSA *see* succimer *on page 793*

DMSO *see* dimethyl sulfoxide *on page 260*

DNA-derived humanized monoclonal antibody *see* alemtuzumab *on page 26*

DNase *see* dornase alfa *on page 274*

DNR *see* daunorubicin hydrochloride *on page 232*

Doak® Tar [US-OTC] *see* coal tar *on page 207*

Doan's® [US-OTC] *see* magnesium salicylate *on page 516*

Doan's® Extra Strength [US-OTC] *see* magnesium salicylate *on page 516*

dobutamine (doe BYOO ta meen)

Sound-Alike/Look-Alike Issues

DOBUTamine may be confused with DOPamine

Synonyms dobutamine hydrochloride

Tall-Man DOBUTamine

U.S./Canadian Brand Names Dobutamine Injection, USP [Can]; Dobutrex® [Can]

Therapeutic Category Adrenergic Agonist Agent

Use Short-term management of patients with cardiac decompensation

Usual Dosage Administration requires the use of an infusion pump; I.V. infusion:

Neonates: 2-15 mcg/kg/minute, titrate to desired response

Children and Adults: 2.5-20 mcg/kg/minute; maximum: 40 mcg/kg/minute, titrate to desired response.

Dosage Forms

Infusion, as hydrochloride [premixed in dextrose]: 1 mg/mL (250 mL, 500 mL); 2 mg/mL (250 mL); 4 mg/mL (250 mL)

Injection, solution, as hydrochloride: 12.5 mg/mL (20 mL, 40 mL, 100 mL) [contains sodium bisulfite]

dobutamine hydrochloride *see* dobutamine *on this page*

Dobutamine Injection, USP [Can] *see* dobutamine *on this page*

Dobutrex® [Can] *see* dobutamine *on this page*

docetaxel (doe se TAKS el)

Sound-Alike/Look-Alike Issues

docetaxel may be confused with paclitaxel

Taxotere® may be confused with Taxol®

Synonyms NSC-628503; RP-6976

U.S./Canadian Brand Names Taxotere® [US/Can]

Therapeutic Category Antineoplastic Agent

Use Second-line treatment of locally-advanced or metastatic breast cancer; adjuvant treatment of operable node-positive breast cancer (in combination with doxorubicin and cyclophosphamide); treatment of locally-advanced or metastatic nonsmall-cell lung cancer (NSCLC) (single agent for failure of platinum based regimen; in combination with cisplatin in treatment of patients who have not previously received chemotherapy for unresected NSCLC); treatment of hormone refractory, metastatic prostate cancer; treatment (in combination with cisplatin and fluorouracil) for chemo-naïve advanced gastric adenocarcinoma

Usual Dosage Children ≥16 years and Adults: I.V. infusion: Refer to individual protocols:

Breast cancer:

Locally-advanced or metastatic: 60-100 mg/m^2 every 3 weeks; patients initially started at 60 mg/m^2 who do not develop toxicity may tolerate higher doses

Operable, node-positive (adjuvant treatment): 75 mg/m^2 every 3 weeks for 6 courses

Nonsmall-cell lung cancer: 75 mg/m^2 every 3 weeks

Prostate cancer: 75 mg/m^2 every 3 weeks; prednisone (5 mg twice daily) is administered continuously

Gastric adenocarcinoma: 75 mg/m^2 every 3 weeks (in combination with cisplatin and fluorouracil)

(Continued)

docetaxel *(Continued)*

Dosage Forms

Injection, solution [concentrate]:

Taxotere®: 20 mg/0.5 mL (0.5 mL, 2 mL) [contains Polysorbate 80®; diluent contains ethanol 13%]

docosanol (doe KOE san ole)

Synonyms behenyl alcohol; *n*-docosanol

U.S./Canadian Brand Names Abreva® [US-OTC]

Therapeutic Category Antiviral Agent, Topical

Use Treatment of herpes simplex of the face or lips

Usual Dosage Children ≥12 years and Adults: Topical: Apply 5 times/day to affected area of face or lips. Start at first sign of cold sore or fever blister and continue until healed.

Dosage Forms Cream: 10% (2 g)

docusate (DOK yoo sate)

Sound-Alike/Look-Alike Issues

docusate may be confused with Doxinate®
Colace® may be confused with Calan®
Surfak® may be confused with Surbex®

Synonyms dioctyl calcium sulfosuccinate; dioctyl sodium sulfosuccinate; docusate calcium; docusate potassium; docusate sodium; DOSS; DSS

U.S./Canadian Brand Names Apo-Docusate-Sodium® [Can]; Colace® [US-OTC/Can]; Colax-C® [Can]; D-S-S® [US-OTC]; Diocto® [US-OTC]; Docusoft-S™ [US-OTC]; DOK™ [US-OTC]; DOS® [US-OTC]; Dulcolax® Stool Softener [US-OTC]; Enemeez® [US-OTC]; Fleet® Sof-Lax® [US-OTC]; Genasoft® [US-OTC]; Novo-Docusate Calcium [Can]; Novo-Docusate Sodium [Can]; Phillips'® Stool Softener Laxative [US-OTC]; PMS-Docusate Calcium [Can]; PMS-Docusate Sodium [Can]; Regulex® [Can]; Selax® [Can]; Silace [US-OTC]; Soflax™ [Can]; Surfak® [US-OTC]

Therapeutic Category Stool Softener

Use Stool softener in patients who should avoid straining during defecation and constipation associated with hard, dry stools; prophylaxis for straining (Valsalva) following myocardial infarction. A safe agent to be used in elderly; some evidence that doses <200 mg are ineffective; stool softeners are unnecessary if stool is well hydrated or "mushy" and soft; shown to be ineffective used long-term.

Usual Dosage Docusate salts are interchangeable; the amount of sodium or calcium per dosage unit is clinically insignificant

Infants and Children <3 years: Oral: 10-40 mg/day in 1-4 divided doses
Children: Oral:
3-6 years: 20-60 mg/day in 1-4 divided doses
6-12 years: 40-150 mg/day in 1-4 divided doses
Adolescents and Adults: Oral: 50-500 mg/day in 1-4 divided doses
Older Children and Adults: Rectal: Add 50-100 mg of docusate liquid to enema fluid (saline or water); administer as retention or flushing enema

Dosage Forms

Capsule, as calcium (Surfak®): 240 mg
Capsule, as sodium: 100 mg, 250 mg
Colace®: 50 mg [contains sodium 3 mg], 100 mg [contains sodium 5 mg]
Docusoft-S™: 100 mg [contains sodium 5 mg]
DOK™, Genasoft®: 100 mg
DOS®, D-S-S®: 100 mg, 250 mg
Dulcolax® Stool Softener: 100 mg [contains sodium 5 mg]
Phillips'® Stool Softener Laxative: 100 mg [contains sodium 5.2 mg]
Enema, rectal, as sodium (Enemeez®): 283 mg/5 mL 5 mL
Gelcap, as sodium (Fleet® Sof-Lax®): 100 mg
Liquid, as sodium: 150 mg/15 mL (480 mL)
Colace®: 150 mg/15 mL (30 mL) [contains sodium 1 mg/mL]
Diocto®: 150 mg/15 mL (480 mL) [vanilla flavor]
Silace: 150 mg/15 mL (480 mL) [lemon-vanilla flavor]
Syrup, as sodium: 60 mg/15 mL (480 mL)
Colace®, Diocto®: 60 mg/15 mL (480 mL) [alcohol free, sugar free; contains sodium 36 mg/5 mL]
Silace: 20 mg/5 mL (480 mL) [peppermint flavor]

docusate and senna (DOK yoo sate & SEN na)

Sound-Alike/Look-Alike Issues

Senokot® may be confused with Depakote®

Synonyms senna and docusate; senna-S

U.S./Canadian Brand Names Peri-Colace® *(reformulation)* [US-OTC]; Senokot-S® [US-OTC]

Therapeutic Category Laxative, Stimulant; Stool Softener

Use Short-term treatment of constipation

Usual Dosage Oral: Constipation: OTC ranges:

Children:

2-6 years: Initial: 4.3 mg sennosides plus 25 mg docusate (1/2 tablet) once daily (maximum: 1 tablet twice daily)

6-12 years: Initial: 8.6 sennosides plus 50 mg docusate (1 tablet) once daily (maximum: 2 tablets twice daily)

Children ≥12 years and Adults: Initial: 2 tablets (17.2 mg sennosides plus 100 mg docusate) once daily (maximum: 4 tablets twice daily)

Dosage Forms

Tablet: Docusate sodium 50 mg and sennosides 8.6 mg

Peri-Colace® (reformulation): Docusate sodium 50 mg and sennosides 8.6 mg

Senokot-S®: Docusate sodium 50 mg and sennosides 8.6 mg [sugar free; contains sodium 3 mg/tablet]

docusate calcium *see* docusate *on previous page*

docusate potassium *see* docusate *on previous page*

docusate sodium *see* docusate *on previous page*

Docusoft Plus™ ***(Discontinued)***

Docusoft-S™ [US-OTC] *see* docusate *on previous page*

dofetilide (doe FET il ide)

U.S./Canadian Brand Names Tikosyn™ [US/Can]

Therapeutic Category Antiarrhythmic Agent, Class III

Use Maintenance of normal sinus rhythm in patients with chronic atrial fibrillation/atrial flutter of longer than 1-week duration who have been converted to normal sinus rhythm; conversion of atrial fibrillation and atrial flutter to normal sinus rhythm

Usual Dosage Adults: Oral:

Note: QT or QT_c must be determined prior to first dose. If QT_c >440 msec (>500 msec in patients with ventricular conduction abnormalities), dofetilide is contraindicated.

Initial: 500 mcg orally twice daily. Initial dosage must be adjusted in patients with estimated Cl_{cr} <60 mL/minute. Dofetilide may be initiated at lower doses than recommended based on physician discretion.

Modification of dosage in response to initial dose: QT_c interval should be measured 2-3 hours after the initial dose. If the QT_c >15% of baseline, or if the QT_c is >500 msec (550 msec in patients with ventricular conduction abnormalities) dofetilide should be adjusted. If the starting dose is 500 mcg twice daily, then adjust to 250 mcg twice daily. If the starting dose was 250 mcg twice daily, then adjust to 125 mcg twice daily. If the starting dose was 125 mcg twice daily then adjust to 125 mcg every day.

Continued monitoring for doses 2-5: QT_c interval must be determined 2-3 hours after each subsequent dose of dofetilide for in-hospital doses 2-5. If the measured QT_c is >500 msec (550 msec in patients with ventricular conduction abnormalities) at any time, dofetilide should be discontinued.

Chronic therapy (following the 5th dose):

QT or QT_c and creatinine clearance should be evaluated every 3 months. If QT_c >500 msec (>550 msec in patients with ventricular conduction abnormalities), dofetilide should be discontinued.

Dosage Forms Capsule: 125 mcg, 250 mcg, 500 mcg

Dofus [US-OTC] *see* Lactobacillus *on page 477*

DOK™ [US-OTC] *see* docusate *on previous page*

Doktors® Nasal Solution ***(Discontinued)*** *see* phenylephrine *on page 660*

Dolacet® Forte ***(Discontinued)*** *see* hydrocodone and acetaminophen *on page 420*

dolasetron (dol A se tron)

Sound-Alike/Look-Alike Issues

dolasetron may be confused with granisetron, ondansetron, palonosetron

Anzemet® may be confused with Aldomet®

(Continued)

dolasetron *(Continued)*

Synonyms dolasetron mesylate; MDL 73,147EF

U.S./Canadian Brand Names Anzemet® [US/Can]

Therapeutic Category Selective 5-HT_3 Receptor Antagonist

Use Prevention of nausea and vomiting associated with emetogenic cancer chemotherapy; prevention of postoperative nausea and vomiting; treatment of postoperative nausea and vomiting (injectable form only)

Not recommended for treatment of existing chemotherapy-induced emesis (CIE).

Note: In Canada, the use of dolasetron is contraindicated for all uses in children <18 years of age or in the treatment of postoperative nausea and vomiting in adults. These are not labeled contraindications in the U.S.

Usual Dosage Note: In Canada, the use of dolasetron is contraindicated in children <18 years of age or in the treatment of postoperative nausea and vomiting in adults. These are not labeled contraindications in the U.S.

Nausea and vomiting prophylaxis, chemotherapy-induced (including initial and repeat courses):

Children 2-16 years:

Oral: 1.8 mg/kg within 1 hour before chemotherapy; maximum: 100 mg/dose

I.V.: 1.8 mg/kg ~30 minutes before chemotherapy; maximum: 100 mg/dose

Adults:

Oral:100 mg single dose 1 hour prior to chemotherapy

I.V.: 1.8 mg/kg or 100 mg 30 minutes prior to chemotherapy

Prevention of postoperative nausea and vomiting:

Children 2-16 years:

Oral: 1.2 mg/kg within 2 hours before surgery; maximum: 100 mg/dose

I.V.: 0.35 mg/kg (maximum: 12.5 mg) ~15 minutes before stopping anesthesia

Adults:

Oral: 100 mg within 2 hours before surgery

I.V.: 12.5 mg ~15 minutes before stopping anesthesia

Treatment of postoperative nausea and vomiting: I.V. (only):

Children: 0.35 mg/kg (maximum: 12.5 mg) as soon as needed

Adults: 12.5 mg as soon as needed

Dosage Forms

Injection, solution, as mesylate: 20 mg/mL (0.625 mL) [single-use ampul, Carpuject®, or vial]; 20 mg/mL (5 mL) [single-use vial]; 20 mg/mL (25 mL) [multidose vial]

Tablet, as mesylate: 50 mg, 100 mg

dolasetron mesylate *see* dolasetron *on previous page*

Dolene® *(Discontinued)* *see* propoxyphene *on page 708*

Dolgic® LQ [US] *see* butalbital, acetaminophen, and caffeine *on page 129*

Dolgic® Plus [US] *see* butalbital, acetaminophen, and caffeine *on page 129*

Dolobid® *(Discontinued)* *see* diflunisal *on page 254*

Dologesic® [US] *see* acetaminophen and phenyltoloxamine *on page 8*

Dolophine® [US/Can] *see* methadone *on page 537*

Dolorac™ *(Discontinued)* *see* capsaicin *on page 142*

Dolorex® *(Discontinued)* *see* capsaicin *on page 142*

Dolsed® [US] *see* methenamine, phenyl salicylate, atropine, hyoscyamine, benzoic acid, and methylene blue *on page 539*

Dom-Benzydamine [Can] *see* benzydamine *(Canada only) on page 104*

Dom-Citalopram [Can] *see* citalopram *on page 194*

Dom-Clobazam [Can] *see* clobazam *(Canada only) on page 200*

Dom-Domperidone [Can] *see* domperidone *(Canada only) on next page*

Domeboro® [US-OTC] *see* aluminum sulfate and calcium acetate *on page 38*

dome paste bandage *see* zinc gelatin *on page 887*

Dom-Fenofibrate Supra [Can] *see* fenofibrate *on page 338*

Dom-Mefenamic Acid [Can] *see* mefenamic acid *on page 525*

Dom-Methimazole [Can] *see* methimazole *on page 539*

domperidone *(Canada only)* (dom PE ri done)

Synonyms domperidone maleate

U.S./Canadian Brand Names Alti-Domperidone [Can]; Apo-Domperidone® [Can]; Dom-Domperidone [Can]; FTP-Domperidone Maleate [Can]; Motilium® [Can]; Novo-Domperidone [Can]; Nu-Domperidone [Can]; RAN™-Domperidone [Can]; ratio-Domperidone [Can]

Therapeutic Category Dopamine Antagonist

Use Symptomatic management of upper GI motility disorders associated with chronic and subacute gastritis and diabetic gastroparesis; prevention of GI symptoms associated with use of dopamine-agonist anti-Parkinson agents

Usual Dosage Oral: Adults:

GI motility disorders: 10 mg 3-4 times/day, 15-30 minutes before meals; severe/resistant cases: 20 mg 3-4 times/day, 15-30 minutes before meals

Nausea/vomiting associated with dopamine-agonist anti-Parkinson agents: 20 mg 3-4 times/day

Dosage Forms Tablet: 10 mg [domperidone maleate 12.72 mg]

domperidone maleate *see* domperidone *(Canada only)* *on this page*

Dom-Sumatriptan [Can] *see* sumatriptan *on page 801*

Dom-Tiaprofenic® [Can] *see* tiaprofenic acid *(Canada only)* *on page 826*

Dom-Topiramate [Can] *see* topiramate *on page 836*

donepezil (doh NEP e zil)

Sound-Alike/Look-Alike Issues

Aricept® may be confused with AcipHex®, Ascriptin®

Synonyms E2020

U.S./Canadian Brand Names Aricept® ODT [US]; Aricept® RDT [Can]; Aricept® [US/Can]

Therapeutic Category Acetylcholinesterase Inhibitor; Cholinergic Agent

Use Treatment of mild to moderate dementia of the Alzheimer type

Usual Dosage Oral: Adults: Dementia of Alzheimer type: Initial: 5 mg/day at bedtime; may increase to 10 mg/day at bedtime after 4-6 weeks

Dosage Forms

Tablet, as hydrochloride (Aricept®): 5 mg, 10 mg

Tablet, orally disintegrating, as hydrochloride (Aricept® ODT): 5 mg, 10 mg

Donnamar® ***(Discontinued)*** *see* hyoscyamine *on page 434*

Donnapine® ***(Discontinued)*** *see* hyoscyamine, atropine, scopolamine, and phenobarbital *on page 435*

Donnatal® [US] *see* hyoscyamine, atropine, scopolamine, and phenobarbital *on page 435*

Donnatal Extentabs® [US] *see* hyoscyamine, atropine, scopolamine, and phenobarbital *on page 435*

dopamine (DOE pa meen)

Sound-Alike/Look-Alike Issues

DOPamine may be confused with DOBUTamine, Dopram®

Synonyms dopamine hydrochloride

Tall-Man **DOP**amine

Therapeutic Category Adrenergic Agonist Agent

Use Adjunct in the treatment of shock (eg, MI, open heart surgery, renal failure, cardiac decompensation) which persists after adequate fluid volume replacement

Usual Dosage I.V. infusion (administration requires the use of an infusion pump):

Neonates: 1-20 mcg/kg/minute continuous infusion, titrate to desired response.

Children: 1-20 mcg/kg/minute, maximum: 50 mcg/kg/minute continuous infusion, titrate to desired response.

Adults: 1-5 mcg/kg/minute up to 20 mcg/kg/minute, titrate to desired response (maximum: 50 mcg/kg/minute). Infusion may be increased by 1-4 mcg/kg/minute at 10- to 30-minute intervals until optimal response is obtained.

If dosages >20-30 mcg/kg/minute are needed, a more direct-acting pressor may be more beneficial (ie, epinephrine, norepinephrine).

Dosage Forms

Infusion, as hydrochloride [premixed in D_5W]: 0.8 mg/mL (250 mL, 500 mL); 1.6 mg/mL (250 mL, 500 mL); 3.2 mg/mL (250 mL)

Injection, solution, as hydrochloride: 40 mg/mL (5 mL, 10 mL); 80 mg/mL (5 mL); 160 mg/mL (5 mL) [contains sodium metabisulfite]

(Continued)

dopamine hydrochloride *see* dopamine *on previous page*

Dopram® [US] *see* doxapram *on next page*

Doral® [US/Can] *see* quazepam *on page 724*

Dormarex® 2 Oral *(Discontinued)* *see* diphenhydramine *on page 261*

dornase alfa (DOOR nase AL fa)

Synonyms DNase; recombinant human deoxyribonuclease

U.S./Canadian Brand Names Pulmozyme® [US/Can]

Therapeutic Category Enzyme

Use Management of cystic fibrosis patients to reduce the frequency of respiratory infections that require parenteral antibiotics, and to improve pulmonary function

Usual Dosage Inhalation:

Children >3 months to Adults: 2.5 mg once daily through selected nebulizers; experience in children <5 years is limited

Patients unable to inhale or exhale orally throughout the entire treatment period may use Pari-Baby™ nebulizer. Some patients may benefit from twice daily administration.

Dosage Forms Solution for nebulization: 1 mg/mL (2.5 mL)

Doryx® [US] *see* doxycycline *on page 278*

dorzolamide (dor ZOLE a mide)

Synonyms dorzolamide hydrochloride

U.S./Canadian Brand Names Trusopt® [US/Can]

Therapeutic Category Carbonic Anhydrase Inhibitor

Use Lowers intraocular pressure in patients with ocular hypertension or open-angle glaucoma

Usual Dosage Children and Adults: Reduction of intraocular pressure: Instill 1 drop in the affected eye(s) 3 times/day

Dosage Forms [DSC] = Discontinued product

Solution, ophthalmic, as hydrochloride:

Trusopt®: 2% (5 mL [DSC]; 10 mL) [contains benzalkonium chloride]

dorzolamide and timolol (dor ZOLE a mide & TYE moe lole)

Synonyms timolol and dorzolamide

U.S./Canadian Brand Names Cosopt® [US/Can]; Preservative-Free Cosopt® [Can]

Therapeutic Category Beta-Adrenergic Blocker; Carbonic Anhydrase Inhibitor

Use Reduction of intraocular pressure in patients with ocular hypertension or open-angle glaucoma

Usual Dosage Ophthalmic: Children ≥2 years and Adults: Instill 1 drop in affected eye(s) twice daily

Dosage Forms [DSC] = Discontinued product

Solution, ophthalmic:

Cosopt®: Dorzolamide hydrochloride 2% (as base) and timolol maleate 0.5% (as base) (5 mL [DSC]; 10 mL) [contains benzalkonium chloride]

dorzolamide hydrochloride *see* dorzolamide *on this page*

DOS® [US-OTC] *see* docusate *on page 270*

DOSS *see* docusate *on page 270*

Dostinex® [US/Can] *see* cabergoline *on page 131*

Dovobet® [Can] *see* calcipotriene and betamethasone *on page 133*

Dovonex® [US] *see* calcipotriene *on page 133*

doxacurium (doks a KYOO ri um)

Sound-Alike/Look-Alike Issues

doxacurium may be confused with doxapram, DOXOrubicin

Synonyms doxacurium chloride
U.S./Canadian Brand Names Nuromax® [US]
Therapeutic Category Skeletal Muscle Relaxant
Use Adjunct to general anesthesia to facilitate endotracheal intubation and to relax skeletal muscles during surgery; to facilitate mechanical ventilation in ICU patients; does not relieve pain or produce sedation; the characteristics of this agent make it especially useful in procedures requiring careful maintenance of hemodynamic stability for prolonged periods
Usual Dosage Administer I.V.; dose to effect; doses will vary due to interpatient variability; use ideal body weight for obese patients

Surgery:

Children >2 years: Initial: 0.03-0.05 mg/kg followed by maintenance doses of 0.005-0.01 mg/kg after 30-45 minutes

Adults: 0.05-0.08 mg/kg with thiopental/narcotic or 0.025 mg/kg after initial dose of succinylcholine for intubation; initial maintenance dose of 0.005-0.01 mg/kg after 100-160 minutes followed by repeat doses every 30-45 minutes

Pretreatment/priming: 10% of intubating dose given 3-5 minutes before initial dose

ICU: 0.05 mg/kg bolus followed by 0.025 mg/kg every 2-3 hours or 0.25-0.75 mcg/kg/minute once initial recovery from bolus dose observed

Dosage Forms Injection, solution, as chloride: 1 mg/mL (5 mL) [contains benzyl alcohol]

doxacurium chloride *see* doxacurium *on previous page*

doxapram (DOKS a pram)

Sound-Alike/Look-Alike Issues

doxapram may be confused with doxacurium, doxazosin, doxepin, Doxinate®, DOXOrubicin

Dopram® may be confused with DOPamine

Synonyms doxapram hydrochloride
U.S./Canadian Brand Names Dopram® [US]
Therapeutic Category Respiratory Stimulant
Use Respiratory and CNS stimulant for respiratory depression secondary to anesthesia, drug-induced CNS depression; acute hypercapnia secondary to COPD
Usual Dosage

Respiratory depression following anesthesia:

Intermittent injection: Initial: 0.5-1 mg/kg; may repeat at 5-minute intervals (only in patients who demonstrate initial response); maximum total dose: 2 mg/kg

I.V. infusion: Initial: 5 mg/minute until adequate response or adverse effects seen; decrease to 1-3 mg/minute; maximum total dose: 4 mg/kg

Drug-induced CNS depression:

Intermittent injection: Initial: Priming dose of 1-2 mg/kg, repeat after 5 minutes; may repeat at 1-2 hour intervals (until sustained consciousness); maximum: 3 g/day. May repeat in 24 hours if necessary.

I.V. infusion: Initial: Priming dose of 1-2 mg/kg, repeat after 5 minutes. If no response, wait 1-2 hours and repeat. If some stimulation is noted, initiate infusion at 1-3 mg/minute (depending on size of patient/depth of CNS depression); suspend infusion if patient begins to awaken. Infusion should not be continued for >2 hours. May reinstitute infusion as described above, including bolus, after rest interval of 30 minutes to 2 hours; maximum: 3 g/day

Acute hypercapnia secondary to COPD: I.V. infusion: Initial: Initiate infusion at 1-2 mg/minute (depending on size of patient/depth of CNS depression); may increase to maximum rate of 3 mg/minute; infusion should not be continued for >2 hours. Monitor arterial blood gases prior to initiation of infusion and at 30-minute intervals during the infusion (to identify possible development of acidosis/CO_2 retention). Additional infusions are not recommended (per manufacturer).

Dosage Forms Injection, solution, as hydrochloride: 20 mg/mL (20 mL) [contains benzyl alcohol]

doxapram hydrochloride *see* doxapram *on this page*

doxazosin (doks AY zoe sin)

Sound-Alike/Look-Alike Issues

doxazosin may be confused with doxapram, doxepin, DOXOrubicin

Cardura® may be confused with Cardene®, Cordarone®, Cordran®, Coumadin®, K-Dur®, Ridaura®

Synonyms doxazosin mesylate
U.S./Canadian Brand Names Alti-Doxazosin [Can]; Apo-Doxazosin® [Can]; Cardura-1™ [Can]; Cardura-2™ [Can]; Cardura-4™ [Can]; Cardura® XL [US]; Cardura® [US]; Gen-Doxazosin [Can]; Novo-Doxazosin [Can]

(Continued)

doxazosin *(Continued)*

Therapeutic Category Alpha-Adrenergic Blocking Agent

Use Treatment of hypertension alone or in conjunction with diuretics, ACE inhibitors, beta blockers, or calcium antagonists; treatment of urinary outflow obstruction and/or obstructive and irritative symptoms associated with benign prostatic hyperplasia (BPH), particularly useful in patients with troublesome symptoms who are unable or unwilling to undergo invasive procedures, but who require rapid symptomatic relief; can be used in combination with finasteride

Usual Dosage Oral: Adults:

Immediate release: 1 mg once daily in morning or evening; may be increased to 2 mg once daily. Thereafter titrate upwards, if needed, over several weeks, balancing therapeutic benefit with doxazosin-induced postural hypotension.

Hypertension: Maximum dose: 16 mg/day

BPH: Goal: 4-8 mg/day; maximum dose: 8 mg/day

Extended release: BPH: 4 mg once daily with breakfast; titrate based on response and tolerability every 3-4 weeks to maximum recommended dose of 8 mg/day

Reinitiation of therapy: If therapy is discontinued for several days, restart at 4 mg dose and titrate as before.

Conversion to extended release from immediate release: Initiate with 4 mg once daily; omit final evening dose of immediate release prior to starting morning dosing with extended release product.

Dosage Forms

Tablet: 1 mg, 2 mg, 4 mg, 8 mg

Cardura®: 1 mg, 2 mg, 4 mg, 8 mg

Tablet, extended release:

Cardura® XL: 4 mg, 8 mg

doxazosin mesylate *see* doxazosin *on previous page*

doxepin (DOKS e pin)

Sound-Alike/Look-Alike Issues

doxepin may be confused with digoxin, doxapram, doxazosin, Doxidan®, doxycycline

Sinequan® may be confused with saquinavir, Serentil®, Seroquel®, Singulair®

Zonalon® may be confused with Zone-A Forte®

Synonyms doxepin hydrochloride

U.S./Canadian Brand Names Apo-Doxepin® [Can]; Novo-Doxepin [Can]; Prudoxin™ [US]; Sinequan® [Can]; Zonalon® [US/Can]

Therapeutic Category Antidepressant, Tricyclic (Tertiary Amine); Topical Skin Product

Use

Oral: Depression

Topical: Short-term (<8 days) management of moderate pruritus in adults with atopic dermatitis or lichen simplex chronicus

Usual Dosage

Oral: Topical: Burning mouth syndrome (dental use): Cream: Apply 3-4 times daily

Oral (entire daily dose may be given at bedtime):

Depression or anxiety:

Adolescents: Initial: 25-50 mg/day in single or divided doses; gradually increase to 100 mg/day

Adults: Initial: 25-150 mg/day at bedtime or in 2-3 divided doses; may gradually increase up to 300 mg/day; single dose should not exceed 150 mg; select patients may respond to 25-50 mg/day

Chronic urticaria, angioedema, nocturnal pruritus: Adults: 10-30 mg/day

Topical: Pruritus: Adults: Apply a thin film 4 times/day with at least 3- to 4-hour interval between applications; not recommended for use >8 days. **Note:** Low-dose (25-50 mg) oral administration has also been used to treat pruritus, but systemic effects are increased.

Dosage Forms [DSC] = Discontinued product

Capsule, as hydrochloride: 10 mg, 25 mg, 50 mg, 75 mg, 100 mg, 150 mg

Sinequan®: 10 mg, 25 mg, 50 mg, 75 mg, 100 mg, 150 mg [DSC]

Cream, as hydrochloride:

Prudoxin™: 5% (45 g) [contains benzyl alcohol]

Zonalon®: 5% (30 g, 45 g) [contains benzyl alcohol]

Solution, oral concentrate, as hydrochloride (Sinequan®): 10 mg/mL (120 mL)

Sinequan®: 10 mg/mL (120 mL) [DSC]

doxepin hydrochloride *see* doxepin *on this page*

doxercalciferol (doks er kal si fe FEER ole)

Synonyms 1α-hydroxyergocalciferol

U.S./Canadian Brand Names Hectorol® [US/Can]

Therapeutic Category Vitamin D Analog

Use Treatment of secondary hyperparathyroidism in patients with chronic kidney disease

Usual Dosage

Oral:

Dialysis patients: Dose should be titrated to lower iPTH to 150-300 pg/mL; dose is adjusted at 8-week intervals (maximum dose: 20 mcg 3 times/week)

Initial dose: iPTH >400 pg/mL: 10 mcg 3 times/week at dialysis

Dose titration:

iPTH level decreased by 50% and >300 pg/mL: Dose can be increased to 12.5 mcg 3 times/week for 8 more weeks; this titration process can continue at 8-week intervals; each increase should be by 2.5 mcg/dose

iPTH level 150-300 pg/mL: Maintain current dose

iPTH level <100 pg/mL: Suspend doxercalciferol for 1 week; resume at a reduced dose; decrease each dose (not weekly dose) by at least 2.5 mcg

Predialysis patients: Dose should be titrated to lower iPTH to 35-70 pg/mL with stage 3 disease or to 70-110 pg/mL with stage 4 disease: Dose may be adjusted at 2-week intervals (maximum dose: 3.5 mcg/day)

Initial dose: 1 mcg/day

Dose titration:

iPTH level >70 pg/mL with stage 3 disease or >110 pg/mL with stage 4 disease: Increase dose by 0.5 mcg every 2 weeks as necessary

iPTH level 35-70 pg/mL with stage 3 disease or 70-110 pg/mL with stage 4 disease: Maintain current dose

iPTH level is <35 pg/mL with stage 3 disease or <70 pg/mL with stage 4 disease: Suspend doxercalciferol for 1 week, then resume at a reduced dose (at least 0.5 mcg lower)

I.V.:

Dialysis patients: Dose should be titrated to lower iPTH to 150-300 pg/mL; dose is adjusted at 8-week intervals (maximum dose: 18 mcg/week)

Initial dose: iPTH level >400 pg/mL: 4 mcg 3 times/week after dialysis, administered as a bolus dose

Dose titration:

iPTH level decreased by <50% and >300 pg/mL: Dose can be increased by 1-2 mcg at 8-week intervals, as necessary

iPTH level decreased by >50% and >300 pg/mL: Maintain current dose

iPTH level 150-300 pg/mL: Maintain the current dose

iPTH level <100 pg/mL: Suspend doxercalciferol for 1 week; resume at a reduced dose (at least 1 mcg lower)

Dosage Forms

Capsule, softgel:

Hectorol®: 0.5 mcg, 2.5 mcg [contains coconut oil]

Injection, solution:

Hectorol®: 2 mcg/mL (2 mL) [contains disodium edetate]

Doxidan® *(reformulation)* [US-OTC] *see* bisacodyl *on page 111*

Doxil® [US] *see* doxorubicin (liposomal) *on next page*

doxorubicin (doks oh ROO bi sin)

Sound-Alike/Look-Alike Issues

DOXOrubicin may be confused with dactinomycin, DAUNOrubicin, doxacurium, doxapram, doxazosin, epirubicin, idarubicin

Adriamycin PFS® may be confused with achromycin, Aredia®, Idamycin®

Rubex® may be confused with Robaxin®

ADR is an error-prone abbreviation

conventional formulations (Adriamycin PFS®, Adriamycin RDF®, Rubex®) may be confused with liposomal formulations (DaunoXome®, Doxil®)

Synonyms adria; doxorubicin hydrochloride; hydroxydaunomycin hydrochloride; hydroxyldaunorubicin hydrochloride; NSC-123127

Tall-Man **DOXO**rubicin

U.S./Canadian Brand Names Adriamycin PFS® [US]; Adriamycin RDF® [US]; Adriamycin® [Can]; Rubex® [US]

(Continued)

doxorubicin *(Continued)*

Therapeutic Category Antineoplastic Agent

Use Treatment of leukemias, lymphomas, multiple myeloma, osseous and nonosseous sarcomas, mesotheliomas, germ cell tumors of the ovary or testis, and carcinomas of the head and neck, thyroid, lung, breast, stomach, pancreas, liver, ovary, bladder, prostate, uterus, neuroblastoma and Wilms tumor.

Usual Dosage Refer to individual protocols. I.V.:

Children:

35-75 mg/m^2 as a single dose, repeat every 21 days **or**

20-30 mg/m^2 once weekly **or**

60-90 mg/m^2 given as a continuous infusion over 96 hours every 3-4 weeks

Adults: Usual or typical dose: 60-75 mg/m^2 as a single dose, repeat every 21 days **or** other dosage regimens like 20-30 mg/m^2/day for 2-3 days, repeat in 4 weeks **or** 20 mg/m^2 once weekly

Dosage Forms

Injection, powder for reconstitution, as hydrochloride: 10 mg, 20 mg, 50 mg [contains lactose]

Adriamycin RDF®: 10 mg, 20 mg, 50 mg, 150 mg [contains lactose; rapid dissolution formula]

Rubex®: 50 mg, 100 mg [contains lactose]

Injection, solution, as hydrochloride [preservative free]: 2 mg/mL (5 mL, 10 mL, 25 mL, 100 mL)

Adriamycin PFS® [preservative free]: 2 mg/mL (5 mL, 10 mL, 25 mL, 37.5 mL, 100 mL)

doxorubicin hydrochloride *see* doxorubicin *on previous page*

doxorubicin hydrochloride (liposomal) *see* doxorubicin (liposomal) *on this page*

doxorubicin (liposomal) (doks oh ROO bi sin lip pah SOW mal)

Sound-Alike/Look-Alike Issues

DOXOrubicin may be confused with dactinomycin, DAUNOrubicin, doxacurium, doxapram, doxazosin, epirubicin, idarubicin

Doxil® may be confused with Doxy®, Paxil®

liposomal formulations (Doxil®) may be confused with conventional formulations (Adriamycin PFS®, Adriamycin RDF®, Cerubidine®, Rubex®).

Synonyms doxorubicin hydrochloride (liposomal)

Tall-Man DOXOrubicin (liposomal)

U.S./Canadian Brand Names Caelyx® [Can]; Doxil® [US]

Therapeutic Category Antineoplastic Agent

Use Treatment of AIDS-related Kaposi sarcoma, breast cancer, ovarian cancer, solid tumors

Usual Dosage Refer to individual protocols. **Liposomal formulations of doxorubicin should NOT be substituted for doxorubicin hydrochloride on a mg-per-mg basis.**

AIDS-KS patients: I.V.: 20 mg/m^2/dose once every 3 weeks

Ovarian cancer: I.V.: 50 mg/m^2/dose every 4 weeks

Dosage Forms Injection, solution, as hydrochloride: 2 mg/mL (10 mL, 25 mL)

Doxy-100® [US] *see* doxycycline *on this page*

Doxycin [Can] *see* doxycycline *on this page*

doxycycline (doks i SYE kleen)

Sound-Alike/Look-Alike Issues

doxycycline may be confused with dicyclomine, doxepin, doxylamine

Doxy-100® may be confused with Doxil®

Monodox® may be confused with Maalox®

Synonyms doxycycline calcium; doxycycline hyclate; doxycycline monohydrate

U.S./Canadian Brand Names Adoxa™ [US]; Apo-Doxy Tabs® [Can]; Apo-Doxy® [Can]; Doryx® [US]; Doxy-100® [US]; Doxycin [Can]; Doxytec [Can]; Monodox® [US]; Novo-Doxylin [Can]; Nu-Doxycycline [Can]; Periostat® [US/Can]; Vibra-Tabs® [US/Can]; Vibramycin® [US]

Therapeutic Category Tetracycline Derivative

Use Principally in the treatment of infections caused by susceptible *Rickettsia*, *Chlamydia*, and *Mycoplasma*; alternative to mefloquine for malaria prophylaxis; treatment for syphilis, uncomplicated *Neisseria gonorrhoeae, Listeria, Actinomyces israelii,* and *Clostridium* infections in penicillin-allergic patients; used for community-acquired pneumonia and other common infections due to susceptible organisms; anthrax due to *Bacillus anthracis,* including inhalational anthrax (postexposure); treatment of infections caused by uncommon susceptible gram-negative and gram-positive organisms including *Borrelia recurrentis, Ureaplasma urealyticum, Haemophilus ducreyi, Yersinia pestis, Francisella tularensis, Vibrio cholerae, Campylobacter fetus, Brucella* spp, *Bartonella bacilliformis,* and *Calymmatobacterium granulomatis*; treatment of inflammatory lesions associated with rosacea

Usual Dosage

Usual dosage range:

Children ≥8 years (<45 kg): Oral, I.V.: 2-5 mg/kg/day in 1-2 divided doses, not to exceed 200 mg/day

Children >8 years (>45 kg) and Adults: Oral, I.V.: 100-200 mg/day in 1-2 divided doses

Indication-specific dosing:

Children:

Anthrax: Doxycycline should be used in children if antibiotic susceptibility testing, exhaustion of drug supplies, or allergic reaction preclude use of penicillin or ciprofloxacin. For treatment, the consensus recommendation does not include a loading dose for doxycycline.

Inhalational (postexposure prophylaxis) (*MMWR*, 2001, 50:889-893): Oral, I.V. (use oral route when possible):

≤8 years: 2.2 mg/kg every 12 hours for 60 days

>8 years and ≤45 kg: 2.2 mg/kg every 12 hours for 60 days

>8 years and >45 kg: 100 mg every 12 hours for 60 days

Cutaneous (treatment): Oral: See dosing for "Inhalational (postexposure prophylaxis)"

Note: In the presence of systemic involvement, extensive edema, and/or lesions on head/neck, doxycycline should initially be administered I.V.

Inhalational/gastrointestinal/oropharyngeal (treatment): I.V.: Refer to dosing for inhalational anthrax (postexposure prophylaxis); switch to oral therapy when clinically appropriate

Note: Initial treatment should include two or more agents predicted to be effective (per CDC recommendations). Agents suggested for use in conjunction with doxycycline or ciprofloxacin include rifampin, vancomycin, imipenem, penicillin, ampicillin, chloramphenicol, clindamycin, and clarithromycin. May switch to oral antimicrobial therapy when clinically appropriate. Continue combined therapy for 60 days

Adults:

Anthrax:

Inhalational (postexposure prophylaxis): Oral, I.V. (use oral route when possible): 100 mg every 12 hours for 60 days (*MMWR*, 2001, 50:889-93); **Note:** Preliminary recommendation, FDA review and update is anticipated.

Cutaneous (treatment): Oral: 100 mg every 12 hours for 60 days. **Note:** In the presence of systemic involvement, extensive edema, lesions on head/neck, refer to I.V. dosing for treatment of inhalational/gastrointestinal/oropharyngeal anthrax

Inhalational/gastrointestinal/oropharyngeal (treatment): I.V.: Initial: 100 mg every 12 hours; switch to oral therapy when clinically appropriate; some recommend initial loading dose of 200 mg, followed by 100 mg every 8-12 hours (*JAMA*, 1997, 278:399-411). **Note:** Initial treatment should include two or more agents predicted to be effective (per CDC recommendations). Agents suggested for use in conjunction with doxycycline or ciprofloxacin include rifampin, vancomycin, imipenem, penicillin, ampicillin, chloramphenicol, clindamycin, and clarithromycin. May switch to oral antimicrobial therapy when clinically appropriate. Continue combined therapy for 60 days

Brucellosis: Oral: 100 mg twice daily for 6 weeks with rifampin or streptomycin

Chlamydial infections, uncomplicated: Oral: 100 mg twice daily for ≥7 days

Community-acquired pneumonia, bronchitis: Oral, I.V.: 100 mg twice daily

Endometritis, salpingitis, parametritis, or peritonitis: I.V.: 100 mg twice daily with cefoxitin 2 g every 6 hours for 4 days and for ≥48 hours after patient improves; then continue with oral therapy 100 mg twice daily to complete a 10- to 14-day course of therapy

Gonococcal infection, acute (PID) in combination with another antibiotic: I.V.: 100 mg every 12 hours until improved, followed by 100 mg orally twice daily to complete 14 days

Lyme disease, Q fever, or Tularemia: Oral: 100 mg twice daily for 14-21 days

Periodontitis: Oral (Periostat®): 20 mg twice daily as an adjunct following scaling and root planing; may be administered for up to 9 months. Safety beyond 12 months of treatment and efficacy beyond 9 months of treatment have not been established.

Rickettsial disease or erlichiosis: Oral, I.V.: 100 mg twice daily for 7-14 days

Rosacea: (Oracea™): Oral: 40 mg once daily in the morning

Syphilis:

Early syphilis: Oral, I.V.: 200 mg/day in divided doses for 14 days

Late syphilis: Oral, I.V.: 200 mg/day in divided doses for 28 days

***Yersinia pestis* (plague):** Oral: 100 mg twice daily for 10 days

Vibrio cholerae: Oral: 300 mg as a single dose

Dosage Forms [DSC] = Discontinued product

Capsule, as hyclate: 50 mg, 100 mg

Vibramycin®: 100 mg

Capsule, as monohydrate (Monodox®): 50 mg, 100 mg

Capsule, coated pellets, as hyclate (Doryx®): 75 mg, 100 mg [DSC]

Capsule, variable release (Oracea™): 40 mg [30 mg (immediate-release) and 10 mg (delayed-release)]

(Continued)

doxycycline *(Continued)*

Injection, powder for reconstitution, as hyclate (Doxy-100®): 100 mg
Powder for oral suspension, as monohydrate (Vibramycin®): 25 mg/5 mL (60 mL) [raspberry flavor]
Syrup, as calcium (Vibramycin®): 50 mg/5 mL (480 mL) [contains sodium metabisulfite; raspberry-apple flavor]
Tablet, as hyclate: 100 mg
Periostat®: 20 mg
Vibra-Tabs®: 100 mg
Tablet, as monohydrate:
Adoxa™: 50 mg, 75 mg, 100 mg
Adoxa® Pak™ 1/75 [unit-dose pack]: 75 mg (31s)
Adoxa® Pak™ 1/100 [unit-dose pack]: 100 mg (31s)
Adoxa® Pak™ 1/150 [unit-dose pack]: 150 mg (30s)
Adoxa® Pak™ 2/100 [unit-dose pack]: 100 mg (60s)
Tablet, delayed-release coated pellets, as hyclate (Doryx®): 75 mg [contains sodium 4.5 mg (0.196 mEq)], 100 mg [contains sodium 6 mg (0.261 mEq)]

doxycycline calcium *see* doxycycline *on page 278*

doxycycline hyclate *see* doxycycline *on page 278*

doxycycline monohydrate *see* doxycycline *on page 278*

doxylamine (dox IL a meen)

Sound-Alike/Look-Alike Issues
doxylamine may be confused with doxycycline

Synonyms doxylamine succinate

U.S./Canadian Brand Names Good Sense Sleep Aid [US-OTC]; Unisom® SleepTabs® [US-OTC]; Unisom®-2 [Can]

Therapeutic Category Antihistamine

Use Sleep aid; antihistamine for hypersensitivity reactions and antiemetic

Usual Dosage Oral: Adults: One tablet 30 minutes before bedtime; once daily or as instructed by healthcare professional

Dosage Forms Tablet, as succinate: 25 mg

doxylamine and pyridoxine *(Canada only)* (dox IL a meen & peer i DOX een)

Sound-Alike/Look-Alike Issues
doxylamine may be confused with doxycycline

Synonyms doxylamine succinate and pyridoxine hydrochloride; pyridoxine and doxylamine

U.S./Canadian Brand Names Diclectin® [Can]

Therapeutic Category Antihistamine; Vitamin

Use Treatment of pregnancy-associated nausea and vomiting

Usual Dosage Oral: Adults: Two delayed release tablets (a total of doxylamine 20 mg and pyridoxine 20 mg) at bedtime; in severe cases or in cases with nausea/vomiting during the day, dosage may be increased by 1 tablet in the morning and/or afternoon

Dosage Forms [CAN] = Canadian brand name
Tablet, delayed release:
Diclectin® [CAN]: Doxylamine 10 mg and pyridoxine 10 mg [not available in the U.S.]

doxylamine succinate *see* doxylamine *on this page*

doxylamine succinate and pyridoxine hydrochloride *see* doxylamine and pyridoxine *(Canada only) on this page*

doxylamine succinate, codeine phosphate, and acetaminophen *see* acetaminophen, codeine, and doxylamine *(Canada Only) on page 12*

Doxytec [Can] *see* doxycycline *on page 278*

DPA *see* valproic acid and derivatives *on page 864*

D-Pan® ***(Discontinued)*** *see* dexpanthenol *on page 242*

DPE *see* dipivefrin *on page 267*

D-penicillamine *see* penicillamine *on page 646*

DPH *see* phenytoin *on page 665*

DPM™ [US-OTC] *see* urea *on page 861*

Dramamine® [US-OTC] *see* dimenhydrinate *on page 258*

Dramamine® Less Drowsy Formula [US-OTC] *see* meclizine *on page 522*

Dramilin® Injection *(Discontinued)* *see* dimenhydrinate *on page 258*

dried smallpox vaccine *see* smallpox vaccine *on page 776*

Drinex® *(Discontinued)* *see* acetaminophen, chlorpheniramine, and pseudoephedrine *on page 11*

Drisdol® [US/Can] *see* ergocalciferol *on page 301*

Dristan® Long Lasting Nasal [Can] *see* oxymetazoline *on page 628*

Dristan® Long Lasting Nasal Solution *(Discontinued)* *see* oxymetazoline *on page 628*

Dristan® N.D. [Can] *see* acetaminophen and pseudoephedrine *on page 9*

Dristan® N.D., Extra Strength [Can] *see* acetaminophen and pseudoephedrine *on page 9*

Dristan® Saline Spray *(Discontinued)* *see* sodium chloride *on page 777*

Dristan® Sinus [US-OTC] *see* pseudoephedrine and ibuprofen *on page 715*

Drithocreme® HP 1% *(Discontinued)* *see* anthralin *on page 58*

Dritho-Scalp® [US] *see* anthralin *on page 58*

Drituss DM [US] *see* guaifenesin and dextromethorphan *on page 394*

Drixoral® [Can] *see* dexbrompheniramine and pseudoephedrine *on page 241*

Drixoral® Cold & Allergy [US-OTC] *see* dexbrompheniramine and pseudoephedrine *on page 241*

Drixoral® Cough & Congestion Liquid Caps *(Discontinued)* *see* pseudoephedrine and dextromethorphan *on page 714*

Drixoral® Cough Liquid Caps *(Discontinued)* *see* dextromethorphan *on page 245*

Drixoral® Nasal [Can] *see* oxymetazoline *on page 628*

Drixoral® ND [Can] *see* pseudoephedrine *on page 712*

Drixoral® Non-Drowsy *(Discontinued)* *see* pseudoephedrine *on page 712*

Drize®-R *(Discontinued)* *see* chlorpheniramine, phenylephrine, and methscopolamine *on page 180*

dronabinol (droe NAB i nol)

Sound-Alike/Look-Alike Issues

dronabinol may be confused with droperidol

Synonyms delta-9-tetrahydro-cannabinol; delta-9 THC; tetrahydrocannabinol; THC

U.S./Canadian Brand Names Marinol® [US/Can]

Therapeutic Category Antiemetic

Controlled Substance C-III

Use Chemotherapy-associated nausea and vomiting refractory to other antiemetic(s); AIDS-related anorexia

Usual Dosage Refer to individual protocols. Oral:

Antiemetic: Children and Adults: 5 mg/m^2 1-3 hours before chemotherapy, then 5 mg/m^2/dose every 2-4 hours after chemotherapy for a total of 4-6 doses/day; increase doses in increments of 2.5 mg/m^2 to a maximum of 15 mg/m^2/dose.

Appetite stimulant: Adults: Initial: 2.5 mg twice daily (before lunch and dinner); titrate up to a maximum of 20 mg/day.

Dosage Forms

Capsule, gelatin:

Marinol®: 2.5 mg, 5 mg, 10 mg [contains sesame oil]

droperidol (droe PER i dole)

Sound-Alike/Look-Alike Issues

droperidol may be confused with dronabinol

Inapsine® may be confused with Nebcin®

Synonyms dehydrobenzperidol

U.S./Canadian Brand Names Inapsine® [US]

Therapeutic Category Antiemetic; Antipsychotic Agent, Butyrophenone

Use Antiemetic in surgical and diagnostic procedures; preoperative medication in patients when other treatments are ineffective or inappropriate

(Continued)

droperidol ***(Continued)***

Usual Dosage Titrate carefully to desired effect

Children 2-12 years: Nausea and vomiting: I.M., I.V.: 0.05-0.06 mg/kg (maximum initial dose: 0.1 mg/kg); additional doses may be repeated to achieve effect; administer additional doses with caution

Adults: Nausea and vomiting: I.M., I.V.: Initial: 2.5 mg; additional doses of 1.25 mg may be administered to achieve desired effect; administer additional doses with caution

Dosage Forms Injection, solution: 2.5 mg/mL (1 mL, 2 mL)

drospirenone and estradiol (droh SPYE re none & es tra DYE ole)

Synonyms E2 and DRSP; estradiol and drospirenone

U.S./Canadian Brand Names Angeliq® [US/Can]

Therapeutic Category Estrogen and Progestin Combination

Use Treatment of moderate-to-severe vasomotor symptoms associated with menopause; treatment of vulvar and vaginal atrophy associated with menopause

Usual Dosage Oral: Adults:

Moderate-to-severe vasomotor symptoms associated with menopause: One tablet daily; reevaluate patients at 3- and 6-month intervals to determine if treatment is still necessary.

Atrophic vaginitis in females with an intact uterus: One tablet daily; re-evaluate patients at 3- and 6-month intervals to determine if treatment is still necessary.

Note: The lowest dose of estrogen/progestin that will control symptoms should be used; medication should be discontinued as soon as possible.

Dosage Forms Tablet: Drospirenone 0.5 mg and estradiol 1 mg

drospirenone and ethinyl estradiol *see* ethinyl estradiol and drospirenone *on page 318*

drotrecogin alfa (dro TRE coe jin AL fa)

Synonyms activated protein C, human, recombinant; drotrecogin alfa, activated; protein C (activated), human, recombinant

U.S./Canadian Brand Names Xigris® [US/Can]

Therapeutic Category Protein C (Activated)

Use Reduction of mortality from severe sepsis (associated with organ dysfunction) in adults at high risk of death (eg, APACHE II score ≥25)

Usual Dosage I.V.: Adults: Sepsis: 24 mcg/kg/hour for a total of 96 hours; stop infusion **immediately** if clinically-important bleeding is identified

Dosage Forms Injection, powder for reconstitution [preservative free]: 5 mg [contains sucrose 31.8 mg], 20 mg [contains sucrose 124.9 mg]

drotrecogin alfa, activated *see* drotrecogin alfa *on this page*

Droxia® [US] *see* hydroxyurea *on page 432*

Dr. Scholl's® Callus Remover [US-OTC] *see* salicylic acid *on page 758*

Dr. Scholl's® Clear Away [US-OTC] *see* salicylic acid *on page 758*

Dry Eye® Therapy Solution *(Discontinued)* *see* artificial tears *on page 75*

Dryox® Gel *(Discontinued)* *see* benzoyl peroxide *on page 102*

Dryox® Wash *(Discontinued)* *see* benzoyl peroxide *on page 102*

Drysol™ [US] *see* aluminum chloride hexahydrate *on page 35*

Dryvax® [US] *see* smallpox vaccine *on page 776*

DSCG *see* cromolyn sodium *on page 217*

D-ser(bu^t)^6,Azgly^{10}-LHRH *see* goserelin *on page 391*

D-S-S® [US-OTC] *see* docusate *on page 270*

DSS *see* docusate *on page 270*

DT *see* diphtheria and tetanus toxoid *on page 264*

DTaP *see* diphtheria, tetanus toxoids, and acellular pertussis vaccine *on page 265*

DTIC® [Can] *see* dacarbazine *on page 226*

DTIC *see* dacarbazine *on page 226*

DTIC-Dome® [US] *see* dacarbazine *on page 226*

DTPA *see* diethylene triamine penta-acetic acid *on page 252*

dTpa *see* diphtheria, tetanus toxoids, and acellular pertussis vaccine *on page 265*

D-Trp(6)-LHRH *see* triptorelin *on page 854*

Duac™ [US] *see* clindamycin and benzoyl peroxide *on page 199*

Duet® [US] *see* vitamins (multiple/prenatal) *on page 879*

Duet™ DHA [US] *see* vitamins (multiple/prenatal) *on page 879*

Dulcolax® [US-OTC/Can] *see* bisacodyl *on page 111*

Dulcolax® Milk of Magnesia [US-OTC] *see* magnesium hydroxide *on page 514*

Dulcolax® Stool Softener [US-OTC] *see* docusate *on page 270*

Dull-C® [US-OTC] *see* ascorbic acid *on page 76*

duloxetine (doo LOX e teen)

Sound-Alike/Look-Alike Issues

duloxetine may be confused with fluoxetine.

Synonyms duloxetine hydrochloride; LY248686; (+)-(*S*)-*N*-methyl-γ-(1-naphthyloxy)-2-thiophenepropylamine hydrochloride

U.S./Canadian Brand Names Cymbalta® [US]

Therapeutic Category Antidepressant, Serotonin/Norepinephrine Reuptake Inhibitor

Use Treatment of major depressive disorder; management of pain associated with diabetic neuropathy

Usual Dosage Oral: Adults:

Treatment of major depressive disorder: Initial: 40-60 mg/day; dose may be divided (ie, 20 or 30 mg twice daily) or given as a single daily dose of 60 mg; maximum dose: 60 mg/day

Management of diabetic neuropathy: 60 mg once daily; lower initial doses may be considered in patients where tolerability is a concern and/or renal impairment is present

Dosage Forms Capsule: 20 mg, 30 mg, 60 mg [contains enteric coated pellets]

duloxetine hydrochloride *see* duloxetine *on this page*

Duocaine™ [US] *see* lidocaine and bupivacaine *on page 495*

DuoCet™ *(Discontinued)* *see* hydrocodone and acetaminophen *on page 420*

DuoFilm® [US-OTC/Can] *see* salicylic acid *on page 758*

Duoforte® 27 [Can] *see* salicylic acid *on page 758*

DuoNeb™ [US] *see* ipratropium and albuterol *on page 460*

DuoPlant® *(Discontinued)* *see* salicylic acid *on page 758*

Duo-Trach® Injection *(Discontinued)* *see* lidocaine *on page 493*

DuP 753 *see* losartan *on page 506*

Duphalac® *(Discontinued)* *see* lactulose *on page 478*

Durabolin® [Can] *see* nandrolone *on page 577*

Duraclon™ [US] *see* clonidine *on page 203*

Duradrin® [US] *see* acetaminophen, isometheptene, and dichloralphenazone *on page 13*

Duradyl® [US] *see* chlorpheniramine, phenylephrine, and methscopolamine *on page 180*

Duradyne DHC® *(Discontinued)* *see* hydrocodone and acetaminophen *on page 420*

Duragesic® [US/Can] *see* fentanyl *on page 340*

Dura-Gest® *(Discontinued)*

Durahist™ PE [US] *see* chlorpheniramine, phenylephrine, and methscopolamine *on page 180*

Duralith® [Can] *see* lithium *on page 501*

Duralone® Injection *(Discontinued)* *see* methylprednisolone *on page 547*

Duramist® Plus [US-OTC] *see* oxymetazoline *on page 628*

Duramorph® [US] *see* morphine sulfate *on page 565*

Duraphen™ II DM [US] *see* guaifenesin, dextromethorphan, and phenylephrine *on page 400*

Duraphen™ DM [US] *see* guaifenesin, dextromethorphan, and phenylephrine *on page 400*

Duraphen™ Forte [US] *see* guaifenesin, dextromethorphan, and phenylephrine *on page 400*

DuraTan™ Forte [US] *see* chlorpheniramine, pseudoephedrine, and dextromethorphan *on page 182*

Duratest® Injection *(Discontinued)* *see* testosterone *on page 812*

Durathate® Injection *(Discontinued)* *see* testosterone *on page 812*

Duration® [US-OTC] *see* oxymetazoline *on page 628*

Duratocin™ [Can] *see* carbetocin *(Canada only) on page 147*

Duratuss® DM [US] *see* guaifenesin and dextromethorphan *on page 394*

Dura-Vent®/DA *(Discontinued)* *see* chlorpheniramine, phenylephrine, and methscopolamine *on page 180*

Dura-Vent® *(Discontinued)*

Duricef® [US/Can] *see* cefadroxil *on page 156*

Duricef® Oral Suspension 125 mg/5 mL *(Discontinued)* *see* cefadroxil *on page 156*

Durolane® [Can] *see* hyaluronate and derivatives *on page 416*

Durrax® Oral *(Discontinued)* *see* hydroxyzine *on page 433*

dutasteride (doo TAS teer ide)

U.S./Canadian Brand Names Avodart™ [US/Can]

Therapeutic Category Antineoplastic Agent, Anthracenedione

Use Treatment of symptomatic benign prostatic hyperplasia (BPH)

Usual Dosage Oral: Adults: Male: 0.5 mg once daily

Dosage Forms Capsule, softgel: 0.5 mg

Duvoid® [Can] *see* bethanechol *on page 109*

Duvoid® *(Discontinued)* *see* bethanechol *on page 109*

D-Vi-Sol® [Can] *see* cholecalciferol *on page 185*

DW286 *see* gemifloxacin *on page 379*

Dwelle® Ophthalmic Solution *(Discontinued)* *see* artificial tears *on page 75*

Dyazide® [US] *see* hydrochlorothiazide and triamterene *on page 420*

Dycill® [Can] *see* dicloxacillin *on page 251*

Dycill® *(Discontinued)* *see* dicloxacillin *on page 251*

Dyclone® *(Discontinued)* *see* dyclonine *on this page*

dyclonine (DYE kloe neen)

Sound-Alike/Look-Alike Issues

dyclonine may be confused with dicyclomine

Synonyms dyclonine hydrochloride

U.S./Canadian Brand Names Cēpacol® Dual Action Maximum Strength [US-OTC]; Sucrets® [US-OTC]

Therapeutic Category Local Anesthetic

Use Temporary relief of pain associated with oral mucosa

Usual Dosage Oral:

Lozenge: Children ≥2 years and Adults: One lozenge every 2 hours as needed (maximum: 10 lozenges/day)

Spray:

Children ≥3-12 years: 1-3 sprays, up to 4 times a day

Children ≥12 years and Adults: 1-4 sprays, up to 4 times a day

Dosage Forms

Lozenge, as hydrochloride (Sucrets®): 1.2 mg [children's cherry flavor]; 2 mg [wild cherry and assorted flavors]; 3 mg [vapor black cherry and wintergreen flavors]

Spray, oral, as hydrochloride (Cēpacol® Dual Action Maximum Strength): 0.1% (120 mL) [contains glycerin 33%; cherry, honey lemon and cool menthol flavors]

dyclonine hydrochloride *see* dyclonine *on this page*

Dylix [US] *see* dyphylline *on next page*

Dymenate® Injection *(Discontinued)* *see* dimenhydrinate *on page 258*

Dynabac® *(Discontinued)*

Dynacin® [US] *see* minocycline *on page 558*

DynaCirc® [Can] *see* isradipine *on page 467*

DynaCirc® CR [US] *see* isradipine *on page 467*

DynaCirc® ***(Discontinued)*** *see* isradipine *on page 467*

Dyna-Hex® [US-OTC] *see* chlorhexidine gluconate *on page 173*

Dynahist-ER Pediatric® [US] *see* chlorpheniramine and pseudoephedrine *on page 177*

Dynapen® ***(Discontinued)*** *see* dicloxacillin *on page 251*

Dynatuss-EX [US] *see* guaifenesin, dextromethorphan, and phenylephrine *on page 400*

Dynex [US] *see* guaifenesin and pseudoephedrine *on page 398*

dyphylline (DYE fi lin)

Synonyms dihydroxypropyl theophylline

U.S./Canadian Brand Names Dilor® [Can]; Dylix [US]; Lufyllin® [US/Can]

Therapeutic Category Theophylline Derivative

Use Bronchodilator in reversible airway obstruction due to asthma or COPD

Usual Dosage Adults: Oral: Up to 15 mg/kg 4 times/day, individualize dosage

Dosage Forms

Elixir:

Dylix: 100 mg/15 mL (473 mL) [contains alcohol 20%]

Tablet:

Lufyllin®: 200 mg, 400 mg

Dyrenium® [US] *see* triamterene *on page 847*

Dyrexan-OD® ***(Discontinued)*** *see* phendimetrazine *on page 657*

Dytan™ [US] *see* diphenhydramine *on page 261*

E2 and DRSP *see* drospirenone and estradiol *on page 282*

7E3 *see* abciximab *on page 3*

E2020 *see* donepezil *on page 273*

Easprin® [US] *see* aspirin *on page 77*

Ebixa® [Can] *see* memantine *on page 527*

echothiophate iodide (ek oh THYE oh fate EYE oh dide)

Synonyms ecostigmine iodide

U.S./Canadian Brand Names Phospholine Iodide® [US]

Therapeutic Category Cholinesterase Inhibitor

Use Used as miotic in treatment of chronic, open-angle glaucoma; may be useful in specific cases of angle-closure glaucoma (postiridectomy or where surgery refused/contraindicated); postcataract surgery-related glaucoma; accommodative esotropia

Usual Dosage Ophthalmic:

Children: Accommodative esotropia:

Diagnosis: Instill 1 drop (0.125%) once daily into both eyes at bedtime for 2-3 weeks

Treatment: Usual dose: Instill 1 drop of 0.06% once daily or 0.125% every other day (maximum: 0.125% daily). **Note:** Use lowest concentration and frequency which gives satisfactory response; if necessary, doses >0.125% daily may be used for short periods of time.

Adults: Open-angle or secondary glaucoma:

Initial: Instill 1 drop (0.03%) twice daily into eyes with 1 dose just prior to bedtime

Maintenance: Some patients have been treated with 1 dose daily or every other day

Conversion from other ophthalmic agents: If IOP control was unsatisfactory, patients may be expected to require higher doses of echothiophate (eg, ≥0.06%); however, patients should be initially started on the 0.03% strength for a short period to better tolerance.

Dosage Forms

Powder for reconstitution, ophthalmic: 6.25 mg [0.125%]

Phospholine Iodide®: 6.25 mg [0.125%] (5 mL) [packaged with sterile diluent containing mannitol]

EC-Naprosyn® [US] *see* naproxen *on page 578*

E. coli **asparaginase** *see* asparaginase *on page 76*

econazole (e KONE a zole)

Synonyms econazole nitrate

U.S./Canadian Brand Names Ecostatin® [Can]; Spectazole® [US/Can]

Therapeutic Category Antifungal Agent

Use Topical treatment of tinea pedis (athlete's foot), tinea cruris (jock itch), tinea corporis (ringworm), tinea versicolor, and cutaneous candidiasis

Usual Dosage Children and Adults: Topical:

Tinea pedis, tinea cruris, tinea corporis, tinea versicolor: Apply sufficient amount to cover affected areas once daily

Cutaneous candidiasis: Apply sufficient quantity twice daily (morning and evening)

Duration of treatment: Candidal infections and tinea cruris, versicolor, and corporis should be treated for 2 weeks and tinea pedis for 1 month; occasionally, longer treatment periods may be required

Dosage Forms Cream, topical, as nitrate: 1% (15 g, 30 g, 85 g)

econazole nitrate *see* econazole *on this page*

Econopred® Plus [US] *see* prednisolone (ophthalmic) *on page 694*

Ecostatin® [Can] *see* econazole *on this page*

ecostigmine iodide *see* echothiophate iodide *on previous page*

Ecotrin® [US-OTC] *see* aspirin *on page 77*

Ecotrin® Low Strength [US-OTC] *see* aspirin *on page 77*

Ecotrin® Maximum Strength [US-OTC] *see* aspirin *on page 77*

Ectosone [Can] *see* betamethasone (topical) *on page 107*

Ed A-Hist® [US] *see* chlorpheniramine and phenylephrine *on page 176*

edathamil disodium *see* edetate disodium *on next page*

Edecrin® [US/Can] *see* ethacrynic acid *on page 315*

edetate calcium disodium (ED e tate KAL see um dye SOW dee um)

Sound-Alike/Look-Alike Issues

Edetate calcium disodium (CaEDTA) may be confused with edetate disodium (Na_2EDTA). CDC recommends that edetate disodium should **never** be used for chelation therapy in children. Fatal hypocalcemia may result if edetate disodium is used for chelation therapy instead of edetate calcium disodium.

Synonyms CaEDTA; calcium disodium edetate; calcium EDTA; EDTA (calcium disodium)

U.S./Canadian Brand Names Calcium Disodium Versenate® [US]

Therapeutic Category Chelating Agent

Use Treatment of symptomatic acute and chronic lead poisoning or for symptomatic patients with high blood lead levels; used as an aid in the diagnosis of lead poisoning; possibly useful in poisoning by zinc, manganese, and certain heavy radioisotopes

Usual Dosage Several regimens have been recommended:

Diagnosis of lead poisoning: Mobilization test (not recommended by AAP guidelines): I.M., I.V.:

Children: 500 mg/m^2/dose (maximum dose: 1 g) as a single dose or divided into 2 doses

Adults: 500 mg/m^2/dose

Note: Urine is collected for 24 hours after first EDTA dose and analyzed for lead content; if the ratio of mcg of lead in urine to mg calcium EDTA given is >1, then test is considered positive; for convenience, an 8-hour urine collection may be done after a single 50 mg/kg I.M. (maximum dose: 1 g) or 500 mg/m^2 I.V. dose; a positive test occurs if the ratio of lead excretion to mg calcium EDTA >0.5-0.6.

Treatment of lead poisoning: Children and Adults (each regimen is specific for route):

Symptoms of lead encephalopathy and/or blood lead level >70 mcg/dL: Treat 5 days; give in conjunction with dimercaprol; wait a minimum of 2 days with no treatment before considering a repeat course:

I.M.: 250 mg/m^2/dose every 4 hours

I.V.: 50 mg/kg/day as 24-hour continuous I.V. infusion **or** 1-1.5 g/m^2 I.V. as either an 8- to 24-hour infusion or divided into 2 doses every 12 hours

Symptomatic lead poisoning **without** encephalopathy **or** asymptomatic with blood lead level >70 mcg/dL: Treat 3-5 days; treatment with dimercaprol is recommended until the blood lead level concentration <50 mcg/dL:

I.M.: 167 mg/m^2 every 4 hours

I.V.: 1 g/m^2 as an 8- to 24-hour infusion or divided every 12 hours

Asymptomatic **children** with blood lead level 45-69 mcg/dL: I.V.: 25 mg/kg/day for 5 days as an 8- to 24-hour infusion or divided into 2 doses every 12 hours

Depending upon the blood lead level, additional courses may be necessary; repeat at least 2-4 days and preferably 2-4 weeks apart

Adults with lead nephropathy: An alternative dosing regimen reflecting the reduction in renal clearance is based upon the serum creatinine. Refer to the following:

Dose of Ca EDTA based on serum creatinine:

S_{cr} ≤2 mg/dL: 1 g/m^2/day for 5 days*

S_{cr} 2-3 mg/dL: 500 mg/m^2/day for 5 days*

S_{cr} 3-4 mg/dL: 500 mg/m^2/dose every 48 hours for 3 doses*

S_{cr} >4 mg/dL: 500 mg/m^2/week*

*Repeat these regimens monthly until lead excretion is reduced toward normal.

Dosage Forms Injection, solution: 200 mg/mL (5 mL)

edetate disodium (ED e tate dye SOW dee um)

Sound-Alike/Look-Alike Issues

Edetate disodium (Na_2EDTA) may be confused with edetate calcium disodium (CaEDTA). CDC recommends that edetate disodium should **never** be used for chelation therapy in children. Fatal hypocalcemia may result if edetate disodium is used for chelation therapy instead of edetate calcium disodium.

Synonyms edathamil disodium; EDTA (disodium); Na2EDTA; sodium edetate

U.S./Canadian Brand Names Endrate® [US]

Therapeutic Category Chelating Agent

Use Emergency treatment of hypercalcemia; control digitalis-induced cardiac dysrhythmias (ventricular arrhythmias)

Usual Dosage Hypercalcemia: I.V.:

Children: 40-70 mg/kg/day slow infusion over 3-4 hours or more to a maximum of 3 g/24 hours; administer for 5 days and allow 5 days between courses of therapy

Adults: 50 mg/kg/day over 3 or more hours to a maximum of 3 g/24 hours; a suggested regimen of 5 days followed by 2 days without drug and repeated courses up to 15 total doses

Digitalis-induced arrhythmias: Children and Adults: 15 mg/kg/hour (maximum dose: 60 mg/kg/day) as continuous infusion

Dosage Forms Injection, solution: 150 mg/mL (20 mL)

Edex® [US] *see* alprostadil *on page 32*

edrophonium (ed roe FOE nee um)

Synonyms edrophonium chloride

U.S./Canadian Brand Names Enlon® [US/Can]; Reversol® [US]

Therapeutic Category Cholinergic Agent

Use Diagnosis of myasthenia gravis; differentiation of cholinergic crises from myasthenia crises; reversal of nondepolarizing neuromuscular blockers; adjunct treatment of respiratory depression caused by curare overdose

Usual Dosage Usually administered I.V., however, if not possible, I.M. or SubQ may be used:

Infants:

I.M.: 0.5-1 mg

I.V.: Initial: 0.1 mg, followed by 0.4 mg if no response; total dose = 0.5 mg

Children:

Diagnosis: Initial: 0.04 mg/kg over 1 minute followed by 0.16 mg/kg if no response, to a maximum total dose of 5 mg for children <34 kg, or 10 mg for children >34 kg **or**

Alternative dosing (manufacturer's recommendation):

≤34 kg: 1 mg; if no response after 45 seconds, repeat dosage in 1 mg increments every 30-45 seconds, up to a total of 5 mg

>34 kg: 2 mg; if no response after 45 seconds, repeat dosage in 1 mg increments every 30-45 seconds, up to a total of 10 mg

I.M.:

<34 kg: 1 mg

>34 kg: 5 mg

Titration of oral anticholinesterase therapy: 0.04 mg/kg once given 1 hour after oral intake of the drug being used in treatment; if strength improves, an increase in neostigmine or pyridostigmine dose is indicated

Adults:

Diagnosis:

I.V.: 2 mg test dose administered over 15-30 seconds; 8 mg given 45 seconds later if no response is seen; test dose may be repeated after 30 minutes

(Continued)

edrophonium *(Continued)*

I.M.: Initial: 10 mg; if no cholinergic reaction occurs, administer 2 mg 30 minutes later to rule out false-negative reaction

Titration of oral anticholinesterase therapy: 1-2 mg given 1 hour after oral dose of anticholinesterase; if strength improves, an increase in neostigmine or pyridostigmine dose is indicated

Reversal of nondepolarizing neuromuscular blocking agents (neostigmine with atropine usually preferred): I.V.: 10 mg over 30-45 seconds; may repeat every 5-10 minutes up to 40 mg

Termination of paroxysmal atrial tachycardia: I.V. rapid injection: 5-10 mg

Differentiation of cholinergic from myasthenic crisis: I.V.: 1 mg; may repeat after 1 minute. **Note:** Intubation and controlled ventilation may be required if patient has cholinergic crisis

Dosage Forms Injection, solution, as chloride:

Enlon®: 10 mg/mL (15 mL) [contains sodium sulfite]

Reversol®: 10 mg/mL (10 mL) [contains sodium sulfite]

edrophonium chloride *see* edrophonium *on previous page*

ED-SPAZ® *(Discontinued)* *see* hyoscyamine *on page 434*

EDTA (calcium disodium) *see* edetate calcium disodium *on page 286*

EDTA (disodium) *see* edetate disodium *on previous page*

E.E.S.® [US/Can] *see* erythromycin *on page 303*

efalizumab (e fa li ZOO mab)

Synonyms anti-CD11a; hu1124

U.S./Canadian Brand Names Raptiva® [US]

Therapeutic Category Immunosuppressant Agent; Monoclonal Antibody

Use Treatment of chronic moderate-to-severe plaque psoriasis in patients who are candidates for systemic therapy or phototherapy

Usual Dosage SubQ: Adults: Psoriasis: Initial: 0.7 mg/kg, followed by weekly dose of 1 mg/kg (maximum: 200 mg/dose)

Dosage Forms Injection, powder for reconstitution: 150 mg [contains sucrose 123.2 mg/vial; delivers 125 mg/1.25 mL; packaged with prefilled syringe containing sterile water for injection]

efavirenz (e FAV e renz)

U.S./Canadian Brand Names Sustiva® [US/Can]

Therapeutic Category Nonnucleoside Reverse Transcriptase Inhibitor (NNRTI)

Use Treatment of HIV-1 infections in combination with at least two other antiretroviral agents

Usual Dosage Oral: Dosing at bedtime is recommended to limit central nervous system effects; should not be used as single-agent therapy

Children ≥3 years: Dosage is based on body weight
- 10 kg to <15 kg: 200 mg once daily
- 15 kg to <20 kg: 250 mg once daily
- 20 kg to <25 kg: 300 mg once daily
- 25 kg to <32.5 kg: 350 mg once daily
- 32.5 kg to <40 kg: 400 mg once daily
- ≥40 kg: 600 mg once daily

Adults: 600 mg once daily

Dosage Forms

Capsule: 50 mg, 100 mg, 200 mg

Tablet: 600 mg

Effer-K™ [US] *see* potassium bicarbonate and potassium citrate *on page 683*

Effer-Syllium® *(Discontinued)* *see* psyllium *on page 717*

Effexor® [US] *see* venlafaxine *on page 869*

Effexor® XR [US/Can] *see* venlafaxine *on page 869*

Eflone® *(Discontinued)* *see* fluorometholone *on page 356*

eflornithine (ee FLOR ni theen)

Sound-Alike/Look-Alike Issues

Vaniqa™ may be confused with Viagra®

Synonyms DFMO; eflornithine hydrochloride
U.S./Canadian Brand Names Vaniqa™ [US/Can]
Therapeutic Category Antiprotozoal; Topical Skin Product
Use Cream: Females ≥12 years: Reduce unwanted hair from face and adjacent areas under the chin
Orphan status: Injection: Treatment of meningoencephalitic stage of *Trypanosoma brucei gambiense* infection (sleeping sickness)
Usual Dosage
Children ≥12 years and Adults: Females: Topical: Apply thin layer of cream to affected areas of face and adjacent chin twice daily, at least 8 hours apart
Adults: I.V. infusion: 100 mg/kg/dose given every 6 hours (over at least 45 minutes) for 14 days
Dosage Forms
Cream, topical, as hydrochloride: 13.9% (30 g)
Injection, solution, as hydrochloride: 200 mg/mL (100 mL) [orphan drug status]

eflornithine hydrochloride *see* eflornithine *on previous page*
Efodine® *(Discontinued)* *see* povidone-iodine *on page 689*
eformoterol and budesonide *see* budesonide and formoterol *(Canada only) on page 123*
Efudex® [US/Can] *see* fluorouracil *on page 356*
E-Gems® [US-OTC] *see* vitamin E *on page 876*
E-Gems Elite® [US-OTC] *see* vitamin E *on page 876*
E-Gems Plus® [US-OTC] *see* vitamin E *on page 876*
EHDP *see* etidronate disodium *on page 329*
Elavil® *(Discontinued)* *see* amitriptyline *on page 44*
Eldepryl® [US] *see* selegiline *on page 766*
Eldopaque® [US-OTC/Can] *see* hydroquinone *on page 430*
Eldopaque Forte® [US] *see* hydroquinone *on page 430*
Eldoquin® [US-OTC/Can] *see* hydroquinone *on page 430*
Eldoquin Forte® [US] *see* hydroquinone *on page 430*
electrolyte lavage solution *see* polyethylene glycol-electrolyte solution *on page 679*
Elestat™ [US] *see* epinastine *on page 295*

eletriptan (el e TRIP tan)

Synonyms eletriptan hydrobromide
U.S./Canadian Brand Names Relpax® [US/Can]
Therapeutic Category Serotonin 5-$HT_{1B, 1D}$ Receptor Agonist
Use Acute treatment of migraine, with or without aura
Usual Dosage Oral: Adults: Acute migraine: 20-40 mg; if the headache improves but returns, dose may be repeated after 2 hours have elapsed since first dose; maximum 80 mg/day.
Note: If the first dose is ineffective, diagnosis needs to be reevaluated. Safety of treating >3 headaches/month has not been established.
Dosage Forms Tablet, as hydrobromide: 20 mg, 40 mg [as base]

eletriptan hydrobromide *see* eletriptan *on this page*
Elidel® [US/Can] *see* pimecrolimus *on page 668*
Eligard® [US/Can] *see* leuprolide *on page 486*
Elimite® [US] *see* permethrin *on page 655*
elipten *see* aminoglutethimide *on page 42*
Elitek™ [US] *see* rasburicase *on page 734*
Elixomin® *(Discontinued)* *see* theophylline *on page 818*
Elixophyllin® [US] *see* theophylline *on page 818*
Elixophyllin-GG® [US] *see* theophylline and guaifenesin *on page 820*
ElixSure™ Congestion [US-OTC] *see* pseudoephedrine *on page 712*
ElixSure™ Cough [US-OTC] *see* dextromethorphan *on page 245*
ElixSure™ Fever/Pain *(Discontinued)* *see* acetaminophen *on page 5*

ElixSure™ IB [US-OTC] *see* ibuprofen *on page 437*
Ellence® [US/Can] *see* epirubicin *on page 297*
Elmiron® [US/Can] *see* pentosan polysulfate sodium *on page 652*
Elocom® [Can] *see* mometasone furoate *on page 563*
Elocon® [US] *see* mometasone furoate *on page 563*
Eloxatin® [US] *see* oxaliplatin *on page 622*
Elspar® [US/Can] *see* asparaginase *on page 76*
Eltor® [Can] *see* pseudoephedrine *on page 712*
Eltroxin® [Can] *see* levothyroxine *on page 491*
Emadine® [US] *see* emedastine *on this page*
Embeline™ *(Discontinued)* *see* clobetasol *on page 200*
Embeline™ E *(Discontinued)* *see* clobetasol *on page 200*
Emcyt® [US/Can] *see* estramustine *on page 311*
Emecheck® *(Discontinued)*

emedastine (em e DAS teen)

Synonyms emedastine difumarate
U.S./Canadian Brand Names Emadine® [US]
Therapeutic Category Antihistamine, H_1 Blocker, Ophthalmic
Use Treatment of allergic conjunctivitis
Usual Dosage Ophthalmic: Children ≥3 years and Adults: Instill 1 drop in affected eye up to 4 times/day
Dosage Forms Solution, ophthalmic, as difumarate: 0.05% (5 mL) [contains benzalkonium chloride]

emedastine difumarate *see* emedastine *on this page*
Emend® [US] *see* aprepitant *on page 71*
Emetrol® [US-OTC] *see* fructose, dextrose, and phosphoric acid *on page 371*
Emitrip® *(Discontinued)* *see* amitriptyline *on page 44*
Emko® *(Discontinued)* *see* nonoxynol 9 *on page 597*
EMLA® [US/Can] *see* lidocaine and prilocaine *on page 496*
Emsam® [US] *see* selegiline *on page 766*

emtricitabine (em trye SYE ta been)

Synonyms BW524W91; coviracil; FTC
U.S./Canadian Brand Names Emtriva® [US/Can]
Therapeutic Category Antiretroviral Agent, Reverse Transcriptase Inhibitor (Nucleoside)
Use Treatment of HIV infection in combination with at least two other antiretroviral agents
Usual Dosage Oral:
Children: 3 months to 17 years:
Capsule: Children >33 kg: 200 mg once daily
Solution: 6 mg/kg once daily; maximum: 240 mg/day
Adults:
Capsule: 200 mg once daily
Solution: 240 mg once daily
Dosage Forms
Capsule: 200 mg
Solution: 10 mg/mL (170 mL) [cotton candy flavor]

emtricitabine and tenofovir (em trye SYE ta been & te NOE fo veer)

Synonyms tenofovir and emtricitabine
U.S./Canadian Brand Names Truvada® [US/Can]
Therapeutic Category Antiretroviral Agent, Reverse Transcriptase Inhibitor (Nucleoside); Antiretroviral Agent, Reverse Transcriptase Inhibitor (Nucleotide)
Use Treatment of HIV infection in combination with other antiretroviral agents
Usual Dosage Adults: Oral: One tablet (emtricitabine 200 mg and tenofovir 300 mg) once daily
Dosage Forms Tablet: Emtricitabine 200 mg and tenofovir disoproxil fumarate 300 mg

Emtriva® **[US/Can]** *see* emtricitabine *on previous page*

Emulsoil® ***(Discontinued)*** *see* castor oil *on page 155*

E-Mycin® ***(Discontinued)***

E-Mycin-E® ***(Discontinued)***

ENA 713 *see* rivastigmine *on page 750*

Enablex® **[US/Can]** *see* darifenacin *on page 231*

enalapril (e NAL a pril)

Sound-Alike/Look-Alike Issues

enalapril may be confused with Anafranil®, Elavil®, Eldepryl®, nafarelin, ramipril

Synonyms enalaprilat; enalapril maleate

U.S./Canadian Brand Names Vasotec® [US/Can]

Therapeutic Category Angiotensin-Converting Enzyme (ACE) Inhibitor

Use Management of mild to severe hypertension; treatment of congestive heart failure, left ventricular dysfunction after myocardial infarction

Usual Dosage Use lower listed initial dose in patients with hyponatremia, hypovolemia, severe congestive heart failure, decreased renal function, or in those receiving diuretics.

Oral: **Enalapril**: Children 1 month to 16 years: Hypertension: Initial: 0.08 mg/kg (up to 5 mg) once daily; adjust dosage based on patient response; doses >0.58 mg/kg (40 mg) have not been evaluated in pediatric patients

Adults:

Oral: **Enalapril:**

Hypertension: 2.5-5 mg/day then increase as required, usually at 1- to 2-week intervals; usual dose range (JNC 7): 2.5-40 mg/day in 1-2 divided doses. **Note:** Initiate with 2.5 mg if patient is taking a diuretic which cannot be discontinued. May add a diuretic if blood pressure cannot be controlled with enalapril alone.

Heart failure: Initial: 2.5 mg once or twice daily (usual range: 5-40 mg/day in 2 divided doses). Titrate slowly at 1- to 2-week intervals. Target dose: 10-20 mg twice daily (ACC/AHA 2005 Heart Failure Guidelines)

Asymptomatic left ventricular dysfunction: 2.5 mg twice daily, titrated as tolerated to 20 mg/day

I.V.: **Enalaprilat:**

Hypertension: 1.25 mg/dose, given over 5 minutes every 6 hours; doses as high as 5 mg/dose every 6 hours have been tolerated for up to 36 hours. **Note:** If patients are concomitantly receiving diuretic therapy, begin with 0.625 mg I.V. over 5 minutes; if the effect is not adequate after 1 hour, repeat the dose and administer 1.25 mg at 6-hour intervals thereafter; if adequate, administer 0.625 mg I.V. every 6 hours.

Heart failure: Avoid I.V. administration in patients with unstable heart failure or those suffering acute myocardial infarction.

Conversion from I.V. to oral therapy if not concurrently on diuretics: 5 mg once daily; subsequent titration as needed; if concurrently receiving diuretics and responding to 0.625 mg I.V. every 6 hours, initiate with 2.5 mg/day.

Dosage Forms

Injection, solution, as enalaprilat: 1.25 mg/mL (1 mL, 2 mL) [contains benzyl alcohol]

Tablet, as maleate (Vasotec®): 2.5 mg, 5 mg, 10 mg, 20 mg

enalapril and felodipine (e NAL a pril & fe LOE di peen)

Synonyms felodipine and enalapril

U.S./Canadian Brand Names Lexxel® [US/Can]

Therapeutic Category Antihypertensive Agent, Combination

Use Treatment of hypertension, however, not indicated for initial treatment of hypertension; replacement therapy in patients receiving separate dosage forms (for patient convenience); when monotherapy with one component fails to achieve desired antihypertensive effect, or when dose-limiting adverse effects limit upward titration of monotherapy

Usual Dosage Oral: Adults: Enalapril 5-20 mg and felodipine 2.5-10 mg once daily

Dosage Forms Tablet, extended release:

Enalapril maleate 5 mg and felodipine 2.5 mg

Enalapril maleate 5 mg and felodipine 5 mg

enalapril and hydrochlorothiazide (e NAL a pril & hye droe klor oh THYE a zide)

Synonyms hydrochlorothiazide and enalapril

U.S./Canadian Brand Names Vaseretic® [US/Can]

Therapeutic Category Antihypertensive Agent, Combination

Use Treatment of hypertension

Usual Dosage Oral: Adults: Enalapril 5-10 mg and hydrochlorothiazide 12.5-25 mg once daily (maximum: 20 mg/day [enalapril]; 50 mg/day [hydrochlorothiazide])

Dosage Forms Tablet:

5-12.5: Enalapril maleate 5 mg and hydrochlorothiazide 12.5 mg

10-25: Enalapril maleate 10 mg and hydrochlorothiazide 25 mg

enalaprilat *see* enalapril *on previous page*

enalapril maleate *see* enalapril *on previous page*

Enbrel® [US/Can] *see* etanercept *on page 315*

Encare® [US-OTC] *see* nonoxynol 9 *on page 597*

EndaCof-DM [US] *see* brompheniramine, pseudoephedrine, and dextromethorphan *on page 120*

EndaCof-PD [US] *see* brompheniramine, pseudoephedrine, and dextromethorphan *on page 120*

Endagen™-HD *(Discontinued)* *see* phenylephrine, hydrocodone, and chlorpheniramine *on page 663*

Endal® [US] *see* guaifenesin and phenylephrine *on page 396*

Endal® HD [US] *see* hydrocodone, phenylephrine, and diphenhydramine *on page 425*

Endal® HD Plus [US] *see* phenylephrine, hydrocodone, and chlorpheniramine *on page 663*

Endantadine® [Can] *see* amantadine *on page 38*

EndoAvitene® [US] *see* collagen hemostat *on page 212*

Endocet® [US/Can] *see* oxycodone and acetaminophen *on page 627*

Endocodone® *(Discontinued)* *see* oxycodone *on page 626*

Endodan® [US/Can] *see* oxycodone and aspirin *on page 628*

Endo®-Levodopa/Carbidopa [Can] *see* levodopa and carbidopa *on page 489*

Endolor® *(Discontinued)*

Endrate® [US] *see* edetate disodium *on page 287*

Enduron® [Can] *see* methyclothiazide *on page 543*

Enduron® *(Discontinued)* *see* methyclothiazide *on page 543*

Enduronyl® Forte *(Discontinued)*

Enecat® [US] *see* radiological/contrast media (ionic) *on page 728*

Enemeez® [US-OTC] *see* docusate *on page 270*

Ener-B® *(Discontinued)* *see* cyanocobalamin *on page 219*

Enerjets [US-OTC] *see* caffeine *on page 132*

enflurane (EN floo rane)

Sound-Alike/Look-Alike Issues

enflurane may be confused with isoflurane

U.S./Canadian Brand Names Compound 347™ [US]; Ethrane® [US]

Therapeutic Category General Anesthetic

Use Maintenance of general anesthesia

Usual Dosage Minimum alveolar concentration (MAC), the concentration at which 50% of patients do not respond to surgical incision, is 1.6% for enflurane. The concentration at which amnesia and loss of awareness occur (MAC - awake) is 0.4%. Surgical levels of anesthesia are achieved with concentrations between 0.5% to 3%.

Dosage Forms Liquid, for inhalation: >99.9% (250 mL)

enfuvirtide (en FYOO vir tide)

Synonyms T-20

U.S./Canadian Brand Names Fuzeon® [US/Can]

Therapeutic Category Antiretroviral Agent, Fusion Protein Inhibitor

Use Treatment of HIV-1 infection in combination with other antiretroviral agents in treatment-experienced patients with evidence of HIV-1 replication despite ongoing antiretroviral therapy

Usual Dosage SubQ:

Children ≥6 years: 2 mg/kg twice daily (maximum dose: 90 mg twice daily)

Adults: 90 mg twice daily

Dosage Forms Injection, powder for reconstitution [preservative free]:

Fuzeon®: 108 mg [90 mg/mL following reconstitution; available in convenience kit of 60 vials, SWFI, syringes, alcohol wipes, patient instructions]

Engerix-B® [US/Can] *see* hepatitis B vaccine *on page 411*

Engerix-B® and Havrix® *see* hepatitis A inactivated and hepatitis B (recombinant) vaccine *on page 410*

enhanced-potency inactivated poliovirus vaccine *see* poliovirus vaccine (inactivated) *on page 677*

Enisyl® ***(Discontinued)*** *see* l-lysine *on page 501*

Enlon® [US/Can] *see* edrophonium *on page 287*

Enomine® ***(Discontinued)***

Enovil® ***(Discontinued)*** *see* amitriptyline *on page 44*

enoxaparin (ee noks a PA rin)

Sound-Alike/Look-Alike Issues

Lovenox® may be confused with Lotronex®, Protonix®

Synonyms enoxaparin sodium

U.S./Canadian Brand Names Enoxaparin Injection [Can]; Lovenox® HP [Can]; Lovenox® [US/Can]

Therapeutic Category Anticoagulant (Other)

Use

DVT treatment (acute): Inpatient treatment (patients with and without pulmonary embolism) and outpatient treatment (patients without pulmonary embolism)

DVT prophylaxis: Following hip or knee replacement surgery, abdominal surgery, or in medical patients with severely-restricted mobility during acute illness in patients at risk of thromboembolic complications

Note: High-risk patients include those with one or more of the following risk factors: >40 years of age, obesity, general anesthesia lasting >30 minutes, malignancy, history of deep vein thrombosis or pulmonary embolism

Unstable angina and non-Q-wave myocardial infarction (to prevent ischemic complications)

Usual Dosage Adults:

DVT prophylaxis:

Hip replacement surgery:

Twice-daily dosing: 30 mg twice daily, with initial dose within 12-24 hours after surgery, and every 12 hours until risk of DVT has diminished or the patient is adequately anticoagulated on warfarin.

Once-daily dosing: 40 mg once daily, with initial dose within 9-15 hours before surgery, and daily until risk of DVT has diminished or the patient is adequately anticoagulated on warfarin.

Knee replacement surgery: 30 mg twice daily, with initial dose within 12-24 hours after surgery, and every 12 hours until risk of DVT has diminished (usually 7-10 days).

Abdominal surgery: 40 mg once daily, with initial dose given 2 hours prior to surgery; continue until risk of DVT has diminished (usual 7-10 days).

Medical patients with severely-restricted mobility during acute illness: 40 mg once daily; continue until risk of DVT has diminished

DVT treatment (acute): **Note:** Start warfarin within 72 hours and continue enoxaparin until INR is between 2.0 and 3.0 (usually 7 days).

Inpatient treatment (with or without pulmonary embolism): 1 mg/kg/dose every 12 hours or 1.5 mg/kg once daily.

Outpatient treatment (without pulmonary embolism): 1 mg/kg/dose every 12 hours.

Unstable angina or non-Q-wave MI: 1 mg/kg twice daily in conjunction with oral aspirin therapy (100-325 mg once daily); continue until clinical stabilization (a minimum of at least 2 days)

Dosage Forms

Injection, solution, as sodium [graduated prefilled syringe; preservative free]: 60 mg/0.6 mL (0.6 mL); 80 mg/0.8 mL (0.8 mL); 100 mg/mL (1 mL); 120 mg/0.8 mL (0.8 mL); 150 mg/mL (1 mL)

(Continued)

enoxaparin *(Continued)*

Injection, solution, as sodium [multidose vial]: 100 mg/mL (3 mL) [contains benzyl alcohol]

Injection, solution, as sodium [prefilled syringe; preservative free]: 30 mg/0.3 mL (0.3 mL); 40 mg/0.4 mL (0.4 mL)

Enoxaparin Injection [Can] *see* enoxaparin *on previous page*

enoxaparin sodium *see* enoxaparin *on previous page*

Enpresse™ [US] *see* ethinyl estradiol and levonorgestrel *on page 320*

Ensure® [US-OTC] *see* nutritional formula, enteral/oral *on page 608*

Ensure Plus® [US-OTC] *see* nutritional formula, enteral/oral *on page 608*

entacapone (en TA ka pone)

U.S./Canadian Brand Names Comtan® [US/Can]

Therapeutic Category Anti-Parkinson Agent; Reverse COMT Inhibitor

Use Adjunct to levodopa/carbidopa therapy in patients with idiopathic Parkinson disease who experience "wearing-off" symptoms at the end of a dosing interval

Usual Dosage Oral: Adults: 200 mg with each dose of levodopa/carbidopa, up to a maximum of 8 times/day (maximum daily dose: 1600 mg/day). To optimize therapy, the dosage of levodopa may need reduced or the dosing interval may need extended. Patients taking levodopa ≥800 mg/day or who had moderate-to-severe dyskinesias prior to therapy required an average decrease of 25% in the daily levodopa dose.

Dosage Forms Tablet: 200 mg

entacapone, carbidopa, and levodopa *see* levodopa, carbidopa, and entacapone *on page 489*

entecavir (en TE ka veer)

U.S./Canadian Brand Names Baraclude™ [US]

Therapeutic Category Antiretroviral Agent, Reverse Transcriptase Inhibitor (Nucleoside)

Use Treatment of chronic hepatitis B infection in adults with evidence of active viral replication and either evidence of persistent transaminase elevations or histologically-active disease

Usual Dosage Oral: Adolescents ≥16 years and Adults:

Nucleoside treatment naive: 0.5 mg daily

Lamivudine-resistant viremia (or known lamivudine-resistant mutations): 1 mg daily

Dosage Forms

Oral solution: 0.05 mg/mL (210 mL) [orange flavor]

Tablet: 0.5 mg, 1 mg

Entertainer's Secret® [US-OTC] *see* saliva substitute *on page 760*

Entex® [US] *see* guaifenesin and phenylephrine *on page 396*

Entex® ER [US] *see* guaifenesin and phenylephrine *on page 396*

Entex® LA [US] *see* guaifenesin and phenylephrine *on page 396*

Entex® PSE [US] *see* guaifenesin and pseudoephedrine *on page 398*

Entocort® [Can] *see* budesonide *on page 122*

Entocort® EC [US] *see* budesonide *on page 122*

Entrobar® [US] *see* radiological/contrast media (ionic) *on page 728*

Entrophen® [Can] *see* aspirin *on page 77*

Entsol® [US-OTC] *see* sodium chloride *on page 777*

Entuss-D® Liquid *(Discontinued)* *see* hydrocodone and pseudoephedrine *on page 424*

Enulose® [US] *see* lactulose *on page 478*

Enzone® [US] *see* pramoxine and hydrocortisone *on page 691*

ephedrine (e FED rin)

Sound-Alike/Look-Alike Issues

ephedrine may be confused with Epifrin®, epinephrine

Synonyms ephedrine sulfate

U.S./Canadian Brand Names Pretz-D® [US-OTC]

Therapeutic Category Adrenergic Agonist Agent

Use Treatment of bronchial asthma, nasal congestion, acute bronchospasm, idiopathic orthostatic hypotension, hypotension induced by spinal anesthesia

Usual Dosage

Children:

Oral, SubQ: 3 mg/kg/day or 25-100 mg/m^2/day in 4-6 divided doses every 4-6 hours

I.M., slow I.V. push: 0.2-0.3 mg/kg/dose every 4-6 hours

Adults:

Oral: 25-50 mg every 3-4 hours as needed

I.M., SubQ: 25-50 mg, parenteral adult dose should not exceed 150 mg in 24 hours

I.M.: Hypotension induced by anesthesia: 25 mg

I.V.: 5-25 mg/dose slow I.V. push repeated after 5-10 minutes as needed, then every 3-4 hours not to exceed 150 mg/24 hours

Nasal spray:

Children 6-12 years: 1-2 sprays into each nostril, not more frequently than every 4 hours

Children ≥12 years and Adults: 2-3 sprays into each nostril, not more frequently than every 4 hours

Dosage Forms

Capsule, as sulfate: 25 mg

Injection, solution, as sulfate: 50 mg/mL (1 mL, 10 mL)

Solution, intranasal spray, as sulfate (Pretz-D®): 0.25% (50 mL)

ephedrine, chlorpheniramine, phenylephrine, and carbetapentane *see* chlorpheniramine, ephedrine, phenylephrine, and carbetapentane *on page 178*

ephedrine sulfate *see* ephedrine *on previous page*

Epi-C® [US] *see* radiological/contrast media (ionic) *on page 728*

EpiClenz™ [US-OTC] *see* alcohol (ethyl) *on page 25*

epidermal thymocyte activating factor *see* aldesleukin *on page 26*

Epifoam® [US] *see* pramoxine and hydrocortisone *on page 691*

Epifrin® *(Discontinued)* *see* epinephrine *on this page*

epinastine (ep i NAS teen)

Synonyms epinastine hydrochloride

U.S./Canadian Brand Names Elestat™ [US]

Therapeutic Category Antihistamine, H_1 Blocker, Ophthalmic

Use Treatment of allergic conjunctivitis

Usual Dosage Ophthalmic: Allergic conjunctivitis: Children ≥3 years and Adults: Instill 1 drop into each eye twice daily; continue throughout period of exposure, even in the absence of symptoms

Dosage Forms Solution, ophthalmic, as hydrochloride: 0.05% (5 mL) [contains benzalkonium chloride]

epinastine hydrochloride *see* epinastine *on this page*

epinephrine (ep i NEF rin)

Sound-Alike/Look-Alike Issues

epinephrine may be confused with ephedrine

Epifrin® may be confused with ephedrine, EpiPen®

EpiPen® may be confused with Epifrin®

Synonyms adrenaline; epinephrine bitartrate; epinephrine hydrochloride; racepinephrine

U.S./Canadian Brand Names Adrenalin® [US/Can]; EpiPen® Jr [US/Can]; EpiPen® [US/Can]; Primatene® Mist [US-OTC]; Raphon [US-OTC]; S2® [US-OTC]; Twinject™ [US]

Therapeutic Category Adrenergic Agonist Agent

Use Treatment of bronchospasms, bronchial asthma, nasal congestion, viral croup, anaphylactic reactions, cardiac arrest; added to local anesthetics to decrease systemic absorption of local anesthetics and increase duration of action; decrease superficial hemorrhage

Usual Dosage

Neonates: Cardiac arrest: I.V.: 0.01-0.03 mg/kg (0.1-0.3 mL/kg of **1:10,000** solution) every 3-5 minutes as needed. Although I.V. route is preferred, may consider administration of doses up to 0.1 mg/kg through the endotracheal tube until I.V. access established; dilute intratracheal doses to 1-2 mL with normal saline.

(Continued)

epinephrine *(Continued)*

Infants and Children:

Asystole/pulseless arrest, bradycardia, VT/VF (after failed defibrillations):

I.V., I.O.: 0.01 mg/kg (0.1 mL/kg of **1:10,000** solution) every 3-5 minutes as needed (maximum: 1 mg)

Intratracheal: 0.1 mg/kg (0.1 mL/kg of **1:1000** solution) every 3-5 minutes (maximum: 10 mg)

Continuous I.V. infusion: 0.1-1 mcg/kg/minute; doses <0.3 mcg/kg/minute generally produce β-adrenergic effects and higher doses generally produce α-adrenergic vasoconstriction; titrate dosage to desired effect

Bronchodilator: SubQ: 0.01 mg/kg (0.01 mL/kg of **1:1000**) (single doses not to exceed 0.5 mg) every 20 minutes for 3 doses

Nebulization: 1-3 inhalations up to every 3 hours using solution prepared with 10 drops of 1:100

Children <4 years: S2® (racepinephrine, OTC labeling): Croup: 0.05 mL/kg (max 0.5 mL/dose); dilute in NS 3 mL. Administer over ~15 minutes; do not administer more frequently than every 2 hours.

Inhalation: Children ≥4 years: Primatene® Mist: Refer to Adults dosing.

Decongestant: Children ≥6 years: Refer to Adults dosing

Hypersensitivity reaction:

SubQ, I.V.: 0.01 mg/kg every 20 minutes; larger doses or continuous infusion may be needed for some anaphylactic reactions

SubQ, I.M.:

15-30 kg: Twinject™: 0.15 mg (for self-administration following severe allergic reactions to insect stings, food, etc)

>30 kg: Refer to Adults dosing

I.M.:

<30 kg: Epipen® Jr: 0.15 mg (for self-administration following severe allergic reactions to insect stings, food, etc)

≥30 kg: Refer to Adults dosing

Adults:

Asystole/pulseless arrest, bradycardia, VT/VF:

I.V., I.O.: 1 mg every 3-5 minutes; if this approach fails, higher doses of epinephrine (up to 0.2 mg/kg) may be indicated for treatment of specific problems (eg, beta-blocker or calcium channel blocker overdose)

Intratracheal: Administer 2-2.5 mg for VF or pulseless VT if I.V./I.O. access is delayed or cannot be established; dilute in 5-10 mL NS or distilled water. **Note:** Absorption is greater with distilled water, but causes more adverse effects on PaO_2.

Bradycardia (symptomatic) or hypotension (not responsive to atropine or pacing): I.V. infusion: 2-10 mcg/minute; titrate to desired effect

Bronchodilator:

SubQ: 0.3-0.5 mg **(1:1000)** every 20 minutes for 3 doses

Nebulization: 1-3 inhalations up to every 3 hours using solution prepared with 10 drops of the **1:100** product

S2® (racepinephrine, OTC labeling): 0.5 mL (~10 drops). Dose may be repeated not more frequently than very 3-4 hours if needed. Solution should be diluted if using jet nebulizer.

Inhalation: Primatene® Mist (OTC labeling): One inhalation, wait at least 1 minute; if relieved, may use once more. Do not use again for at least 3 hours.

Decongestant: Intranasal: Apply 1:1000 locally as drops or spray or with sterile swab

Hypersensitivity reaction:

I.M., SubQ: 0.3-0.5 mg (1:1000) every 15-20 minutes if condition requires (I.M route is preferred)

>30 kg: Twinject™: 0.3 mg (for self-administration following severe allergic reactions to insect stings, food, etc)

I.M.: ≥30 kg: Epipen®: 0.3 mg (for self-administration following severe allergic reactions to insect stings, food, etc)

I.V.: 0.1 mg (1:10,000) over 5 minutes. May infuse at 1-4 mcg/minute to prevent the need to repeat injections frequently.

Dosage Forms

Aerosol for oral inhalation:

Primatene® Mist: 0.22 mg/inhalation (15 mL, 22.5 mL) [contains CFCs]

Injection, solution [prefilled auto injector]:

EpiPen®: 0.3 mg/0.3 mL [1:1000] (2 mL) [contains sodium metabisulfite; available as single unit or in double-unit pack with training unit]

EpiPen® Jr: 0.15 mg/0.3 mL [1:2000] (2 mL) [contains sodium metabisulfite; available as single unit or in double-unit pack with training unit]

Twinject™: 0.15 mg/0.15 mL [1:1000] (1.1 mL) [contains sodium bisulfite; two 0.15 mg doses per injector]; 0.3 mg/0.3 mL [1:1000] (1.1 mL) [contains sodium bisulfite; two 0.3 mg doses per injector]

Injection, solution, as hydrochloride: 0.1 mg/mL [1:10,000] (10 mL); 1 mg/mL [1:1000] (1 mL) [products may contain sodium metabisulfite]

Adrenalin®: 1 mg/mL [1:1000] (1 mL, 30 mL) [contains sodium bisulfite]

Solution for oral inhalation, as hydrochloride:

Adrenalin®: 1% [10 mg/mL, 1:100] (7.5 mL) [contains sodium bisulfite]

Solution for oral inhalation [racepinephrine]:

S2®: 2.25% (0.5 mL, 15 mL) [as d-epinephrine 1.125% and l-epinephrine 1.125%; contains metabisulfites]

Solution, topical [racepinephrine]:

Raphon: 2.25% (15 mL) [as d-epinephrine 1.125% and l-epinephrine 1.125%; contains metabisulfites]

epinephrine and articaine hydrochloride *see* articaine and epinephrine *on page 75*

epinephrine and chlorpheniramine (ep i NEF rin & klor fen IR a meen)

Synonyms insect sting kit

U.S./Canadian Brand Names Ana-Kit® [US]

Therapeutic Category Antidote

Use Anaphylaxis emergency treatment of insect bites or stings by the sensitive patient that may occur within minutes of insect sting or exposure to an allergic substance

Usual Dosage Children and Adults: I.M. or SubQ:

Epinephrine:

<2 years: 0.05-0.1 mL

2-6 years: 0.15 mL

6-12 years: 0.2 mL

>12 years : 0.3 mL

Chlorpheniramine:

<6 years: 1 tablet

6-12 years: 2 tablets

>12 years: 4 tablets

Dosage Forms Kit: Epinephrine hydrochloride 1:1000 [prefilled syringe, delivers two 0.3 mL doses; contains sodium bisulfite] (1 mL), chlorpheniramine maleate chewable tablet 2 mg (4), sterile alcohol pads [isopropyl alcohol 70%] (2), tourniquet (1)

epinephrine and lidocaine *see* lidocaine and epinephrine *on page 495*

epinephrine bitartrate *see* epinephrine *on page 295*

epinephrine bitartrate and bupivacaine hydrochloride *see* bupivacaine and epinephrine *on page 124*

epinephrine hydrochloride *see* epinephrine *on page 295*

EpiPen® [US/Can] *see* epinephrine *on page 295*

EpiPen® Jr [US/Can] *see* epinephrine *on page 295*

epipodophyllotoxin *see* etoposide *on page 330*

EpiQuin™ Micro [US] *see* hydroquinone *on page 430*

epirubicin (ep i ROO bi sin)

Sound-Alike/Look-Alike Issues

epirubicin may be confused with DAUNOrubicin, DOXOrubicin, idarubicin

Ellence® may be confused with Elase®

Synonyms pidorubicin; pidorubicin hydrochloride

U.S./Canadian Brand Names Ellence® [US/Can]; Pharmorubicin® [Can]

Therapeutic Category Antineoplastic Agent, Anthracycline; Antineoplastic Agent, Antibiotic

Use Adjuvant therapy for primary breast cancer

Usual Dosage Adults: I.V.: 100-120 mg/m^2 once every 3-4 weeks **or** 50-60 mg/m^2 days 1 and 8 every 3-4 weeks

Breast cancer:

CEF-120: 60 mg/m^2 on days 1 and 8 every 28 days for 6 cycles

FEC-100: 100 mg/m^2 on day 1 every 21 days for 6 cycles

Note: Patients receiving 120 mg/m^2/cycle as part of combination therapy should also receive prophylactic therapy with sulfamethoxazole/trimethoprim or a fluoroquinolone.

Dosage modifications:

Delay day 1 dose until platelets are ≥100,000/mm^3, ANC ≥1500/mm^3, and nonhematologic toxicities have recovered to ≤grade 1

(Continued)

epirubicin *(Continued)*

Reduce day 1 dose in subsequent cycles to 75% of previous day 1 dose if patient experiences nadir platelet counts <50,000/mm^3, ANC <250/mm^3, neutropenic fever, or grade 3/4 nonhematologic toxicity during the previous cycle

For divided doses (day 1 and day 8), reduce day 8 dose to 75% of day 1 dose if platelet counts are 75,000-100,000/mm^3 and ANC is 1000-1499/mm^3; omit day 8 dose if platelets are <75,000/mm^3, ANC <1000/mm^3, or grade 3/4 nonhematologic toxicity

Dosage adjustment in bone marrow dysfunction: Heavily-treated patients, patients with preexisting bone marrow depression or neoplastic bone marrow infiltration: Lower starting doses (75-90 mg/mm^2) should be considered.

Dosage Forms Injection, solution [preservative free]: 2 mg/mL (25 mL, 100 mL)

Epitol® [US] *see* carbamazepine *on page 144*

Epival® I.V. [Can] *see* valproic acid and derivatives *on page 864*

Epivir® [US] *see* lamivudine *on page 479*

Epivir-HBV® [US] *see* lamivudine *on page 479*

eplerenone (e PLER en one)

Sound-Alike/Look-Alike Issues

Inspra™ may be confused with Spiriva®

U.S./Canadian Brand Names Inspra™ [US]

Therapeutic Category Antihypertensive Agent; Selective Aldosterone Blocker

Use Treatment of hypertension (may be used alone or in combination with other antihypertensive agents); treatment of CHF following acute MI

Usual Dosage Oral: Adults:

Hypertension: Initial: 50 mg once daily; may increase to 50 mg twice daily if response is not adequate; may take up to 4 weeks for full therapeutic response. Doses >100 mg/day are associated with increased risk of hyperkalemia and no greater therapeutic effect.

Concurrent use with moderate CYP3A4 inhibitors: Initial: 25 mg once daily

Congestive heart failure (post-MI): Initial: 25 mg once daily; dosage goal: titrate to 50 mg once daily within 4 weeks, as tolerated

Dosage adjustment per serum potassium concentrations for CHF:

<5.0 mEq/L:

Increase dose from 25 mg every other day to 25 mg daily **or**

Increase dose from 25 mg daily to 50 mg daily

5.0-5.4 mEq/L: No adjustment needed

5.5-5.9 mEq/L:

Decrease dose from 50 mg daily to 25 mg daily **or**

Decrease dose from 25 mg daily to 25 mg every other day **or**

Decrease does from 25 mg every other day to withhold medication

≥6.0 mEq/L: Withhold medication until potassium <5.5 mEq/L, then restart at 25 mg every other day

Dosage Forms Tablet: 25 mg, 50 mg

EPO *see* epoetin alfa *on this page*

epoetin alfa (e POE e tin AL fa)

Sound-Alike/Look-Alike Issues

epoetin alfa may be confused with darbepoetin alfa

Synonyms EPO; erythropoietin; NSC-724223; *r*HuEPO-α

U.S./Canadian Brand Names Epogen® [US]; Eprex® [Can]; Procrit® [US]

Therapeutic Category Colony-Stimulating Factor

Use Treatment of anemia related to HIV therapy, chronic renal failure, antineoplastic therapy (for nonmyeloid malignancies); reduction of allogeneic blood transfusion for elective, noncardiac, nonvascular surgery

Usual Dosage

Chronic renal failure patients: I.V., SubQ:

Children: Initial dose: 50 units/kg 3 times/week

Adults: Initial dose: 50-100 units/kg 3 times/week

Dose adjustment: Children and Adults: Reduce dose by 25% when hemoglobin approaches 12 g/dL **or** hemoglobin increases 1 g/dL in any 2-week period. Increase dose by 25% if hemoglobin does not increase by 2 g/dL after 8 weeks of therapy (with adequate iron stores, may increase dose by 25% if hemoglobin increase <1 g/dL over 4 weeks) and hemoglobin is below suggested target range.

Suggested target hemoglobin range: 10-12 g/dL. Do not increase dose more frequently than at 4-week intervals.

Maintenance dose: Individualize to target range; limit additional dosage increases to every 4 weeks (or longer)

Dialysis patients: Median dose:

Children: 167 units/kg/week (hemodialysis) **or** 76 units/kg/week (peritoneal dialysis)

Adults: 75 units/kg 3 times/week

Nondialysis patients:

Children: Dosing range: 50-250 units/kg 1-3 times/week

Adults: Median dose: 75-150 units/kg/week

Zidovudine-treated, HIV-infected patients (patients with erythropoietin levels >500 mU/mL are **unlikely** to respond): I.V., SubQ:

Children: Initial dose: Reported dosing range: 50-400 units/kg 2-3 times/week

Adults: 100 units/kg 3 times/week for 8 weeks. **Dose adjustment:** Increase dose by 50-100 units/kg 3 times/week if response is not satisfactory in terms of reducing transfusion requirements or increasing hemoglobin after 8 weeks of therapy. Evaluate response every 4-8 weeks thereafter and adjust the dose accordingly by 50-100 units/kg increments 3 times/week. If patient has not responded satisfactorily to a 300 unit/kg dose 3 times/week, a response to higher doses is unlikely. Stop dose if hemoglobin exceeds 13 g/dL and resume treatment at a 25% dose reduction when hemoglobin drops to 12 g/dL.

Cancer patient on chemotherapy: Treatment of patients with erythropoietin levels >200 mU/mL is **not recommended**

Children: I.V.: 600 units/kg once weekly (maximum: 40,000 units)

Adults: SubQ: Initial dose: 150 units/kg 3 times/week or 40,000 units once weekly; commonly used doses range from 10,000 units 3 times/week to 40,000-60,000 units once weekly.

Dose adjustment: Children and Adults: If response is not satisfactory after a sufficient period of evaluation (8 weeks of 3 times/week and 4 weeks of once-weekly therapy), the dose may be increased every 4 weeks (or longer) up to 300 units/kg 3 times/week, **or** when dosed weekly, increased all at once to 60,000 units weekly (adults) or 900 units/kg/week; maximum 60,000 units (pediatrics). If patient does not respond, a response to higher doses is unlikely. Stop dose if hemoglobin exceeds 13 g/dL and resume treatment at a 25% dose reduction when hemoglobin drops to 12 g/dL; reduce dose by 25% if hemoglobin increases by 1 g/dL in any 2-week period, or if hemoglobin approaches 12 g/dL.

Surgery patients: Prior to initiating treatment, obtain a hemoglobin to establish that is >10 mg/dL or ≤13 mg/dL: Adults: SubQ: Initial dose: 300 units/kg/day for 10 days before surgery, on the day of surgery, and for 4 days after surgery

Alternative dose: 600 units/kg in once weekly doses (21, 14, and 7 days before surgery) plus a fourth dose on the day of surgery

Dosage Forms

Injection, solution [preservative free]: 2000 units/mL (1 mL); 3000 units/mL (1 mL); 4000 units/mL (1 mL); 10,000 units/mL (1 mL); 40,000 units/mL (1 mL) [contains human albumin]

Injection, solution [with preservative]: 10,000 units/mL (2 mL); 20,000 units/mL (1 mL) [contains human albumin and benzyl alcohol]

Epogen® [US] *see* epoetin alfa *on previous page*

epoprostenol (e poe PROST en ole)

Synonyms epoprostenol sodium; PGI_2; PGX; prostacyclin

U.S./Canadian Brand Names Flolan® [US/Can]

Therapeutic Category Platelet Inhibitor

Use Treatment of idiopathic pulmonary arterial hypertension [IPAH]; pulmonary hypertension associated with the scleroderma spectrum of disease [SSD] in NYHA Class III and Class IV patients who do not respond adequately to conventional therapy

Usual Dosage Adults: I.V.: Initial: 1-2 ng/kg/minute, increase dose in increments of 1-2 ng/kg/minute every 15 minutes or longer until dose-limiting side effects are noted or tolerance limit to epoprostenol is observed

Dosage Forms Injection, powder for reconstitution, as sodium: 0.5 mg, 1.5 mg [provided with 50 mL sterile diluent]

epoprostenol sodium *see* epoprostenol *on this page*

Eprex® [Can] *see* epoetin alfa *on previous page*

eprosartan (ep roe SAR tan)

U.S./Canadian Brand Names Teveten® [US/Can]

Therapeutic Category Angiotensin II Receptor Antagonist

Use Treatment of hypertension; may be used alone or in combination with other antihypertensives

(Continued)

eprosartan *(Continued)*

Usual Dosage Adults: Oral: Dosage must be individualized; can administer once or twice daily with total daily doses of 400-800 mg. Usual starting dose is 600 mg once daily as monotherapy in patients who are euvolemic. Limited clinical experience with doses >800 mg.

Dosage Forms Tablet: 400 mg, 600 mg

eprosartan and hydrochlorothiazide (ep roe SAR tan & hye droe klor oh THYE a zide)

Synonyms eprosartan mesylate and hydrochlorothiazide; hydrochlorothiazide and eprosartan

U.S./Canadian Brand Names Teveten® HCT [US/Can]; Teveten® Plus [Can]

Therapeutic Category Angiotensin II Antagonist Combination; Antihypertensive Agent, Combination; Diuretic, Thiazide

Use Treatment of hypertension (not indicated for initial treatment)

Usual Dosage Oral: Adults: Dose is individualized (combination substituted for individual components)

Usual recommended dose: Eprosartan 600 mg/hydrochlorothiazide 12.5 mg once daily (maximum dose: Eprosartan 600 mg/hydrochlorothiazide 25 mg once daily)

Dosage Forms Tablet:

600 mg/12.5 mg: Eprosartan 600 mg and hydrochlorothiazide 12.5 mg

600 mg/25 mg: Eprosartan 600 mg and hydrochlorothiazide 25 mg

eprosartan mesylate and hydrochlorothiazide *see* eprosartan and hydrochlorothiazide *on this page*

epsilon aminocaproic acid *see* aminocaproic acid *on page 42*

epsom salts *see* magnesium sulfate *on page 516*

EPT *see* teniposide *on page 810*

eptacog alfa (activated) *see* factor VIIa (recombinant) *on page 333*

eptifibatide (ep TIF i ba tide)

Synonyms intrifiban

U.S./Canadian Brand Names Integrilin® [US/Can]

Therapeutic Category Antiplatelet Agent

Use Treatment of patients with acute coronary syndrome (unstable angina/non-Q wave myocardial infarction [UA/NQMI]), including patients who are to be managed medically and those undergoing percutaneous coronary intervention (PCI including angioplasty, intracoronary stenting)

Usual Dosage I.V.: Adults:

Acute coronary syndrome: Bolus of 180 mcg/kg (maximum: 22.6 mg) over 1-2 minutes, begun as soon as possible following diagnosis, followed by a continuous infusion of 2 mcg/kg/minute (maximum: 15 mg/hour) until hospital discharge or initiation of CABG surgery, up to 72 hours. Concurrent aspirin and heparin therapy (target aPTT 50-70 seconds) are recommended.

Percutaneous coronary intervention (PCI) with or without stenting: Bolus of 180 mcg/kg (maximum: 22.6 mg) administered immediately before the initiation of PCI, followed by a continuous infusion of 2 mcg/kg/minute (maximum: 15 mg/hour). A second 180 mcg/kg bolus (maximum: 22.6 mg) should be administered 10 minutes after the first bolus. Infusion should be continued until hospital discharge or for up to 18-24 hours, whichever comes first. Concurrent aspirin (160-325 mg 1-24 hours before PCI and daily thereafter) and heparin therapy (ACT 200-300 seconds during PCI) are recommended. Heparin infusion after PCI is discouraged. In patients who undergo coronary artery bypass graft surgery, discontinue infusion prior to surgery.

Dosage Forms Injection, solution: 0.75 mg/mL (100 mL); 2 mg/mL (10 mL, 100 mL)

Epzicom™ [US] *see* abacavir and lamivudine *on page 2*

Equagesic® [US] *see* aspirin and meprobamate *on page 79*

Equalactin® [US-OTC] *see* polycarbophil *on page 678*

Equalizer Gas Relief [US-OTC] *see* simethicone *on page 772*

Equanil® ***(Discontinued)*** *see* meprobamate *on page 531*

Equetro™ [US] *see* carbamazepine *on page 144*

Equilet® ***(Discontinued)*** *see* calcium carbonate *on page 135*

Eraxis™ [US] *see* anidulafungin *on page 57*

Erbitux® [US/Can] *see* cetuximab *on page 168*

ergocalciferol (er goe kal SIF e role)

Sound-Alike/Look-Alike Issues

Calciferol™ may be confused with calcitriol

Drisdol® may be confused with Drysol™

Synonyms activated ergosterol; viosterol; vitamin D_2

U.S./Canadian Brand Names Calciferol™ [US]; Drisdol® [US/Can]; Ostoforte® [Can]

Therapeutic Category Vitamin D Analog

Use Treatment of refractory rickets, hypophosphatemia, hypoparathyroidism; dietary supplement

Usual Dosage Oral dosing is preferred; I.M. therapy required with GI, liver, or biliary disease associated with malabsorption

Dietary supplementation (each 1 mcg = 40 int. units):

Infants and Children: 5 mcg/day (200 int. units/day)

Adults:

18-50 years: 5 mcg/day (200 int. units/day)

51-70 years: 10 mcg/day (400 int. units/day)

Renal failure:

Children: 100-1000 mcg/day (4000-40,000 int. units)

Adults: 500 mcg/day (20,000 int. units)

Hypoparathyroidism:

Children: 1.25-5 mg/day (50,000-200,000 int. units) and calcium supplements

Adults: 625 mcg to 5 mg/day (25,000-200,000 int. units) and calcium supplements

Vitamin D-dependent rickets:

Children: 75-125 mcg/day (3000-5000 int. units); maximum: 1500 mcg/day

Adults: 250 mcg to 1.5 mg/day (10,000-60,000 int. units)

Nutritional rickets and osteomalacia:

Children and Adults (with normal absorption): 25-125 mcg/day (1000-5000 int. units)

Children with malabsorption: 250-625 mcg/day (10,000-25,000 int. units)

Adults with malabsorption: 250-7500 mcg (10,000-300,000 int. units)

Vitamin D-resistant rickets:

Children: Initial: 1000-2000 mcg/day (40,000-80,000 int. units) with phosphate supplements; daily dosage is increased at 3- to 4-month intervals in 250-500 mcg (10,000-20,000 int. units) increments

Adults: 250-1500 mcg/day (10,000-60,000 int. units) with phosphate supplements

Familial hypophosphatemia: 10,000-80,000 int. units daily plus 1-2 g/day elemental phosphorus

Osteoporosis prophylaxis: Adults:

51-70 years: 400 int. units/day

>70 years: 600 int. units/day

Maximum daily dose: 2000 int. units/day

Dosage Forms [DSC] = Discontinued product

Capsule (Drisdol®): 50,000 int. units [1.25 mg; contains tartrazine and soybean oil]

Injection, solution (Calciferol™): 500,000 int. units/mL [12.5 mg/mL] (1 mL) [contains sesame oil] [DSC]

Liquid, drops (Calciferol™, Drisdol®): 8000 int. units/mL [200 mcg/mL] (60 mL) [OTC]

ergoloid mesylates (ER goe loid MES i lates)

Synonyms dihydroergotoxine; dihydrogenated ergot alkaloids

U.S./Canadian Brand Names Hydergine® [Can]

Therapeutic Category Ergot Alkaloid and Derivative

Use Treatment of cerebrovascular insufficiency in primary progressive dementia, Alzheimer dementia, and senile onset

Usual Dosage Adults: Oral: 1 mg 3 times/day up to 4.5-12 mg/day; up to 6 months of therapy may be necessary

Dosage Forms

Tablet: 1 mg

Tablet, sublingual: 1 mg

Ergomar® [US] *see* ergotamine *on next page*

ergometrine maleate *see* ergonovine *on next page*

ergonovine (er goe NOE veen)

Synonyms ergometrine maleate; ergonovine maleate

U.S./Canadian Brand Names Ergotrate® [US]

Therapeutic Category Ergot Alkaloid and Derivative

Use Prevention and treatment of postpartum and postabortion hemorrhage caused by uterine atony or subinvolution

Usual Dosage Adults:

I.M., I.V. (I.V. should be reserved for emergency use only): 0.2 mg, may repeat dose in 2-4 hours if needed

Oral, SL:

Immediate post-partum: 0.2 mg (usually given I.M. or I.V)

Late post-partum: 0.2-0.4 mg every 6-12 hours until danger of uterine atony has passed (usually ~48 hours)

Dosage Forms

Injection, as maleate:

Ergotrate®: 0.2 mg/mL (1 mL)

Tablet, as maleate:

Ergotrate®: 0.2 mg

ergonovine maleate *see* ergonovine *on this page*

ergotamine (er GOT a meen)

Synonyms ergotamine tartrate

U.S./Canadian Brand Names Ergomar® [US]

Therapeutic Category Ergot Alkaloid and Derivative

Use Abort or prevent vascular headaches, such as migraine, migraine variants, or so-called "histaminic cephalalgia"

Usual Dosage Sublingual: One tablet under tongue at first sign, then 1 tablet every 30 minutes if needed; maximum dose: 3 tablets/24 hours, 5 tablets/week

Dosage Forms Tablet, sublingual: Ergotamine tartrate 2 mg

ergotamine tartrate *see* ergotamine *on this page*

Ergotamine Tartrate and Caffeine Cafatine® *(Discontinued)* *see* ergotamine *on this page*

ergotamine tartrate, belladonna, and phenobarbital *see* belladonna, phenobarbital, and ergotamine *on page 96*

Ergotrate® [US] *see* ergonovine *on this page*

erlotinib (er LOE tye nib)

Sound-Alike/Look-Alike Issues

erlotinib may be confused with gefitinib

Synonyms CP358774; erlotinib hydrochloride; NSC-718781; OSI-774; R 14-15

U.S./Canadian Brand Names Tarceva® [US/Can]

Therapeutic Category Antineoplastic, Tyrosine Kinase Inhibitor

Use Salvage therapy of advanced or metastatic nonsmall cell lung cancer

Usual Dosage Oral: Adults: **Note:** Treatment should continue until disease progression or unacceptable toxicity occurs.

NSCLC: 150 mg/day

Pancreatic cancer: 100 mg/day in combination with gemcitabine

Note: Dose reductions are more likely to be needed when erlotinib is administered concomitantly with strong CYP3A4 inhibitors. Dose reduction (if required) should be done in increments of 50 mg. Likewise, the CYP3A4 inducers may require increased doses; doses of >150 mg/day should be considered with rifampin.

Dosage Forms

Tablet:

Tarceva®: 25 mg, 100 mg, 150 mg

erlotinib hydrochloride *see* erlotinib *on this page*

Errin™ [US] *see* norethindrone *on page 598*

Ertaczo™ [US] *see* sertaconazole *on page 769*

ertapenem (er ta PEN em)

Sound-Alike/Look-Alike Issues
Invanz® may be confused with Avinza™

Synonyms ertapenem sodium; L-749,345; MK0826

U.S./Canadian Brand Names Invanz® [US/Can]

Therapeutic Category Antibiotic, Carbapenem

Use Treatment of the following moderate-severe infections: Complicated intraabdominal infections, complicated skin and skin structure infections (including diabetic foot infections without osteomyelitis), complicated UTI (including pyelonephritis), acute pelvic infections, and community-acquired pneumonia. Antibacterial coverage includes aerobic gram-positive organisms, aerobic gram-negative organisms, anaerobic organisms.

Note: Methicillin-resistant *Staphylococcus*, *Enterococcus* spp, penicillin-resistant strains of *Streptococcus pneumoniae*, beta-lactamase-positive strains of *Haemophilus influenzae* are **resistant** to ertapenem, as are most *Pseudomonas aeruginosa*.

Usual Dosage

Usual dosage ranges:
Children 3 months to 12 years: I.M., I.V.: 15 mg/kg twice daily (maximum: 1 g/day)
Children ≥13 years and Adults: I.M., I.V.: 1 g/day

Indication-specific dosing:
Children 3 months to 12 years: I.M., I.V.:
Community-acquired pneumonia, urinary tract infections/pyelonephritis: 15 mg/kg twice daily (maximum: 1 g/day); duration of total antibiotic treatment: 10-14 days (**Note:** Duration includes possible switch to appropriate oral therapy after at least 3 days of parenteral treatment, once clinical improvement demonstrated.)
Intraabdominal infection: 15 mg/kg twice daily (maximum: 1 g/day) for 5-14 days
Pelvic infections (acute): 15 mg/kg twice daily (maximum: 1 g/day) for 3-10 days
Skin and skin structure infections: 15 mg/kg twice daily (maximum: 1 g/day) for 7-14 days
Children ≥13 years and Adults: I.M., I.V.:
Community-acquired pneumonia, urinary tract infections/pyelonephritis: 1 g/day; duration of total antibiotic treatment: 10-14 days (**Note:** Duration includes possible switch to appropriate oral therapy after at least 3 days of parenteral treatment, once clinical improvement demonstrated.)
Intraabdominal infection: 1 g/day for 5-14 days
Pelvic infections (acute): 1 g/day for 3-10 days
Skin and skin structure infections (including diabetic foot infections): 1 g/day for 7-14 days
Adults: I.V.:
Prophylaxis of surgical site following colorectal surgery: 1 g given 1 hour preoperatively

Dosage Forms Injection, powder for reconstitution: 1 g [contains sodium 137 mg/g (~6 mEq/g)]

ertapenem sodium *see* ertapenem *on this page*

Erwinase® [Can] *see* asparaginase *on page 76*

***Erwinia* asparaginase** *see* asparaginase *on page 76*

Erybid™ [Can] *see* erythromycin *on this page*

Eryc® [US/Can] *see* erythromycin *on this page*

Eryderm® [US] *see* erythromycin *on this page*

Erygel® [US] *see* erythromycin *on this page*

EryPed® [US] *see* erythromycin *on this page*

Ery-Tab® [US] *see* erythromycin *on this page*

Erythrocin® [US] *see* erythromycin *on this page*

erythromycin (er ith roe MYE sin)

Sound-Alike/Look-Alike Issues
erythromycin may be confused with azithromycin, clarithromycin, Ethmozine®
Akne-Mycin® may be confused with AK-Mycin®
E.E.S.® may be confused with DES®
Eryc® may be confused with Emcyt®, Ery-Tab®
Ery-Tab® may be confused with Eryc®
Erythrocin® may be confused with Ethmozine®

Synonyms erythromycin base; erythromycin estolate; erythromycin ethylsuccinate; erythromycin gluceptate; erythromycin lactobionate; erythromycin stearate
(Continued)

erythromycin *(Continued)*

U.S./Canadian Brand Names A/T/S® [US]; Akne-Mycin® [US]; Apo-Erythro Base® [Can]; Apo-Erythro E-C® [Can]; Apo-Erythro-ES® [Can]; Apo-Erythro-S® [Can]; Diomycin® [Can]; E.E.S.® [US/Can]; Ery-Tab® [US]; Erybid™ [Can]; Eryc® [US/Can]; Eryderm® [US]; Erygel® [US]; EryPed® [US]; Erythrocin® [US]; Novo-Rythro Estolate [Can]; Novo-Rythro Ethylsuccinate [Can]; Nu-Erythromycin-S [Can]; PCE® [US/Can]; PMS-Erythromycin [Can]; Romycin® [US]; Sans Acne® [Can]; Theramycin Z® [US]

Therapeutic Category Acne Products; Antibiotic, Ophthalmic; Antibiotic, Topical; Macrolide (Antibiotic)

Use

Systemic: Treatment of susceptible bacterial infections including *S. pyogenes*, some *S. pneumoniae,* some *S. aureus, M. pneumoniae, Legionella pneumophila*, diphtheria, pertussis, *Chlamydia*, erythrasma, *N. gonorrhoeae, E. histolytica*, syphilis and nongonococcal urethritis, and *Campylobacter* gastroenteritis; used in conjunction with neomycin for decontaminating the bowel

Ophthalmic: Treatment of superficial eye infections involving the conjunctiva or cornea; neonatal ophthalmia

Topical: Treatment of acne vulgaris

Usual Dosage

Usual dosage range:

Neonates: Ophthalmic: Prophylaxis of neonatal gonococcal or chlamydial conjunctivitis: 0.5-1 cm ribbon of ointment should be instilled into each conjunctival sac

Infants and Children:

Oral (**Note:** Due to differences in absorption, 400 mg erythromycin ethylsuccinate produces the same serum levels as 250 mg erythromycin base, sterate or estolate):

Base: 30-50 mg/kg/day in 2-4 divided doses; do not exceed 2 g/day

Estolate: 30-50 mg/kg/day in 2-4 divided doses; do not exceed 2 g/day

Ethylsuccinate: 30-50 mg/kg/day in 2-4 divided doses; do not exceed 3.2 g/day

Stearate: 30-50 mg/kg/day in 2-4 divided doses; do not exceed 2 g/day

I.V.: Lactobionate: 15-50 mg/kg/day divided every 6 hours, not to exceed 4 g/day

Children and Adults:

Ophthalmic: Instill ½" (1.25 cm) 2-6 times/day depending on the severity of the infection

Topical: Apply over the affected area twice daily after the skin has been thoroughly washed and patted dry

Adults:

Oral:

Base: 250-500 mg every 6-12 hours

Ethylsuccinate: 400-800 mg every 6-12 hours

I.V.: Lactobionate: 15-20 mg/kg/day divided every 6 hours or 500 mg to 1 g every 6 hours, or given as a continuous infusion over 24 hours (maximum: 4 g/24 hours)

Indication-specific dosing:

Children: Oral:

Pharyngitis: 40 mg/kg/day in 2 doses; maximum: 1600 mg/day; short-course therapy for 5 days may be considered

Pertussis (CDC guidelines): Oral: 40-50 mg/kg/day in 4 divided doses for 14 days; maximum 2 g/day (not preferred agent for infants <1 month)

Preop bowel preparation: 20 mg/kg erythromycin base at 1, 2, and 11 PM on the day before surgery combined with mechanical cleansing of the large intestine and oral neomycin

Adults:

Cervicitis: Oral: 500 mg 4 times/day for 7 days

Community-acquired pneumonia, bronchitis: Oral, I.V.: 500-1000 mg 4 times/day for 10-14 days. If *Legionella* is suspected/confirmed, 750-1000 mg 4 times/day for 21 days or more may be recommended. **Note:** Other macrolides and/or fluoroquinolones may be preferred and better tolerated.

Lymphogranuloma venereum: Oral: 500 mg 4 times/day for 21 days

Nongonococcal urethritis (recurrent): Oral: CDC Guidelines for the Treatment of Sexually Transmitted Diseases recommendation: Metronidazole (2 g as a single dose) plus 7 days of erythromycin base (500 mg 4 times/day) or erythromycin ethylsuccinate (800 mg 4 times/day)

Pertussis (CDC guidelines): 500 mg every 6 hours for 14 days

Dosage Forms [DSC] = Discontinued product; [CAN] = Canadian brand name; **Note:** Strength expressed as base

Capsule, delayed release, enteric-coated pellets, as base: 250 mg

Eryc®: 250 mg

Gel, topical: 2% (30 g, 60 g)

A/T/S®: 2% (30 g) [contains alcohol 92%]

Erygel®: 2% (30 g, 60 g) [contains alcohol 92%]

Granules for oral suspension, as ethylsuccinate:
E.E.S.®: 200 mg/5 mL (100 mL, 200 mL) [contains sodium 25.9 mg (1.1 mEq)/5 mL; cherry flavor]
Injection, powder for reconstitution, as lactobionate:
Erythrocin®: 500 mg, 1 g
Ointment, ophthalmic: 0.5% [5 mg/g] (1 g, 3.5 g)
Romycin®: 0.5% [5 mg/g] (3.5 g)
Ointment, topical:
Akne-Mycin®: 2% (25 g)
Powder for oral suspension, as ethylsuccinate:
EryPed®: 200 mg/5 mL (100 mL, 200 mL) [contains sodium 117.5 mg (5.1 mEq)/5 mL; fruit flavor]; 400 mg/5 mL (100 mL, 200 mL) [contains sodium 117.5 mg (5.1 mEq)/5 mL; banana flavor]
Powder for oral suspension, as ethylsuccinate [drops]:
EryPed®: 100 mg/2.5 mL (50 mL) [contains sodium 58.8 mg (2.6 mEq)/dropperful; fruit flavor]
Solution, topical: 2% (60 mL)
A/T/S®: 2% (60 mL) [contains alcohol 66%]
Eryderm®, T-Stat® [DSC], Theramycin Z®: 2% (60 mL) [contain alcohol]
Sans Acne® [CAN]: 2% (60 mL) [contains ethyl alcohol 44%; not available in U.S.]
Staticin®: 1.5% (60 mL) [DSC]
Suspension, oral, as ethylsuccinate: 200 mg/5 mL (480 mL); 400 mg/5 mL (480 mL)
E.E.S.®: 200 mg/5 mL (100 mL, 480 mL) [fruit flavor]; 400 mg/5 mL (100 mL, 480 mL) [orange flavor]
Swab (T-Stat® [DSC]): 2% (60s)
Tablet, as base: 250 mg, 500 mg
Tablet, as base [polymer-coated particles]:
PCE®: 333 mg, 500 mg
Tablet, as ethylsuccinate: 400 mg
E.E.S.®: 400 mg
Tablet, as stearate: 250 mg, 500 mg
Erythrocin®: 250 mg, 500 mg
Tablet, chewable, as ethylsuccinate:
EryPed®: 200 mg [fruit flavor] [DSC]
Tablet, delayed release, enteric coated, as base:
Ery-Tab®: 250 mg, 333 mg, 500 mg

erythromycin and benzoyl peroxide (er ith roe MYE sin & BEN zoe il per OKS ide)

Synonyms benzoyl peroxide and erythromycin

U.S./Canadian Brand Names Benzamycin® Pak [US]; Benzamycin® [US]

Therapeutic Category Acne Products

Use Topical control of acne vulgaris

Usual Dosage Apply twice daily, morning and evening

Dosage Forms Gel, topical:
Benzamycin®: Erythromycin 30 mg and benzoyl peroxide 50 mg per g (47 g)
Benzamycin® Pak: Erythromycin 30 mg and benzoyl peroxide 50 mg per 0.8 g packet (60s) [supplied with diluent containing alcohol]

erythromycin and sulfisoxazole (er ith roe MYE sin & sul fi SOKS a zole)

Sound-Alike/Look-Alike Issues
Pediazole® may be confused with Pediapred®

Synonyms sulfisoxazole and erythromycin

U.S./Canadian Brand Names Pediazole® [US/Can]

Therapeutic Category Macrolide (Antibiotic); Sulfonamide

Use Treatment of susceptible bacterial infections of the upper and lower respiratory tract, otitis media in children caused by susceptible strains of *Haemophilus influenzae*, and many other infections in patients allergic to penicillin

Usual Dosage Oral (dosage recommendation is based on the product's erythromycin content):
Children ≥2 months: 50 mg/kg/day erythromycin and 150 mg/kg/day sulfisoxazole in divided doses every 6 hours; not to exceed 2 g erythromycin/day or 6 g sulfisoxazole/day for 10 days
Adults >45 kg: 400 mg erythromycin and 1200 mg sulfisoxazole every 6 hours

Dosage Forms [DSC] = Discontinued product
Powder for oral suspension: Erythromycin ethylsuccinate 200 mg and sulfisoxazole acetyl 600 mg per 5 mL (100 mL, 200 mL)
Pediazole®: Erythromycin ethylsuccinate 200 mg and sulfisoxazole acetyl 600 mg per 5 mL (100 mL, 150 mL, 200 mL) [strawberry-banana flavor] [DSC]

erythromycin base *see* erythromycin *on page 303*

erythromycin estolate *see* erythromycin *on page 303*

erythromycin ethylsuccinate *see* erythromycin *on page 303*

erythromycin gluceptate *see* erythromycin *on page 303*

erythromycin lactobionate *see* erythromycin *on page 303*

erythromycin stearate *see* erythromycin *on page 303*

erythropoiesis stimulating protein *see* darbepoetin alfa *on page 230*

erythropoietin *see* epoetin alfa *on page 298*

escitalopram (es sye TAL oh pram)

Synonyms escitalopram oxalate; Lu-26-054; S-citalopram

U.S./Canadian Brand Names Cipralex® [Can]; Lexapro® [US]

Therapeutic Category Antidepressant, Selective Serotonin Reuptake Inhibitor

Use Treatment of major depressive disorder; generalized anxiety disorders (GAD)

Usual Dosage Oral: Adults: Depression, GAD: Initial: 10 mg/day; dose may be increased to 20 mg/day after at least 1 week

Dosage Forms

Solution, oral: 1 mg/mL (240 mL) [peppermint flavor]

Tablet: 5 mg, 10 mg, 20 mg

Note: Cipralex® [CAN] is available only in 10 mg and 20 mg strengths.

escitalopram oxalate *see* escitalopram *on this page*

Esclim® [US] *see* estradiol *on page 308*

Eserine® [Can] *see* physostigmine *on page 666*

eserine salicylate *see* physostigmine *on page 666*

Esgic® [US] *see* butalbital, acetaminophen, and caffeine *on page 129*

Esgic-Plus™ [US] *see* butalbital, acetaminophen, and caffeine *on page 129*

Esidrix Tablets *(Discontinued)* *see* hydrochlorothiazide *on page 419*

Eskalith CR® *(Discontinued)* *see* lithium *on page 501*

Eskalith® *(Discontinued)* *see* lithium *on page 501*

esmolol (ES moe lol)

Sound-Alike/Look-Alike Issues

esmolol may be confused with Osmitrol®

Brevibloc® may be confused with bretylium, Brevital®, Bumex®, Buprenex®

Synonyms esmolol hydrochloride

U.S./Canadian Brand Names Brevibloc® [US/Can]

Therapeutic Category Antiarrhythmic Agent, Class II; Beta-Adrenergic Blocker

Use Treatment of supraventricular tachycardia (SVT) and atrial fibrillation/flutter (control ventricular rate); treatment of tachycardia and/or hypertension (especially intraoperative or postoperative); treatment of noncompensatory sinus tachycardia

Usual Dosage **I.V. infusion requires an infusion pump** (must be adjusted to individual response and tolerance):

Adults:

Intraoperative tachycardia and/or hypertension (immediate control): Initial bolus: 80 mg (~1 mg/kg) over 30 seconds, followed by a 150 mcg/kg/minute infusion, if necessary. Adjust infusion rate as needed to maintain desired heart rate and/or blood pressure, up to 300 mcg/kg/minute.

For control of postoperative hypertension, as many as one-third of patients may require higher doses (250-300 mcg/kg/minute) to control blood pressure; the safety of doses >300 mcg/kg/minute has not been studied.

Supraventricular tachycardia or gradual control of postoperative tachycardia/hypertension: Loading dose: 500 mcg/kg over 1 minute; follow with a 50 mcg/kg/minute infusion for 4 minutes; response to this initial infusion rate may be a rough indication of the responsiveness of the ventricular rate.

Infusion may be continued at 50 mcg/kg/minute or, if the response is inadequate, titrated upward in 50 mcg/kg/minute increments (increased no more frequently than every 4 minutes) to a maximum of 200 mcg/kg/minute.

To achieve more rapid response, following the initial loading dose and 50 mcg/kg/minute infusion, rebolus with a second 500 mcg/kg loading dose over 1 minute, and increase the maintenance infusion to

100 mcg/kg/minute for 4 minutes. If necessary, a third (and final) 500 mcg/kg loading dose may be administered, prior to increasing to an infusion rate of 150 mcg/minute. After 4 minutes of the 150 mcg/kg/minute infusion, the infusion rate may be increased to a maximum rate of 200 mcg/kg/minute (without a bolus dose).

Usual dosage range (SVT): 50-200 mcg/kg/minute with average dose of 100 mcg/kg/minute.

Guidelines for transfer to oral therapy (beta blocker, calcium channel blocker):

Infusion should be reduced by 50% 30 minutes following the first dose of the alternative agent

Manufacturer suggests following the second dose of the alternative drug, patient's response should be monitored and if control is adequate for the first hours, esmolol may be discontinued.

Dosage Forms

Infusion [premixed in sodium chloride; preservative free]:

Brevibloc®: 2000 mg (100 mL) [20 mg/mL; double strength]; 2500 mg (250 mL) [10 mg/mL]

Injection, solution, as hydrochloride: 10 mg/mL (10 mL) [premixed in sodium chloride]

Brevibloc®: 10 mg/mL (10 mL) [alcohol free; premixed in sodium chloride]; 20 mg/mL (5 mL, 100 mL) [alcohol free; double strength; premixed in sodium chloride]; 250 mg/mL (10 mL) [contains alcohol 25%, propylene glycol 25%; concentrate]

esmolol hydrochloride *see* esmolol *on previous page*

E-Solve-2® Topical *(Discontinued)*

esomeprazole (es oh ME pray zol)

Synonyms esomeprazole magnesium

U.S./Canadian Brand Names Nexium® [US/Can]

Therapeutic Category Proton Pump Inhibitor

Use

Oral: Short-term (4-8 weeks) treatment of erosive esophagitis; maintaining symptom resolution and healing of erosive esophagitis; treatment of symptomatic gastroesophageal reflux disease (GERD); as part of a multidrug regimen for *Helicobacter pylori* eradication in patients with duodenal ulcer disease (active or history of within the past 5 years); prevention of gastric ulcers in patients at risk (age ≥60 years and/or history of gastric ulcer) associated with continuous NSAID therapy

I.V.: Short-term (≤10 days) treatment of gastroesophageal reflux disease (GERD) when oral therapy is not possible or appropriate

Usual Dosage Note: Delayed-release capsules should be swallowed whole and taken at least 1 hour before eating

Adolescents 12-17 years: Oral: GERD: 20-40 mg once daily for up to 8 weeks

Adults:

Oral:

Erosive esophagitis (healing): Initial: 20-40 mg once daily for 4-8 weeks; if incomplete healing, may continue for an additional 4-8 weeks; maintenance: 20 mg once daily

Symptomatic GERD: 20 mg once daily for 4 weeks; may continue an additional 4 weeks if symptoms persist

Helicobacter pylori eradication: 40 mg once daily for 10 days; requires combination therapy

Prevention of NSAID-induced gastric ulcers: 20-40 mg once daily for up to 6 months

I.V.: GERD: 20 mg or 40 mg once daily for ≤10 days; change to oral therapy as soon as appropriate

Dosage Forms Note: Strength expressed as base

Capsule, delayed release, as magnesium:

Nexium®: 20 mg, 40 mg

Injection, powder for reconstitution, as sodium:

Nexium®: 20 mg, 40 mg [contains edetate sodium]

esomeprazole magnesium *see* esomeprazole *on this page*

Esoterica® Regular [US-OTC] *see* hydroquinone *on page 430*

Especol® [US-OTC] *see* fructose, dextrose, and phosphoric acid *on page 371*

Estalis® [Can] *see* estradiol and norethindrone *on page 310*

Estalis-Sequi® [Can] *see* estradiol and norethindrone *on page 310*

Estar® [Can] *see* coal tar *on page 207*

estazolam (es TA zoe lam)

Sound-Alike/Look-Alike Issues

ProSom® may be confused with PhosLo®, Proscar®, Pro-Sof® Plus, Prozac®, Psorcon®

(Continued)

estazolam *(Continued)*

U.S./Canadian Brand Names ProSom® [US]

Therapeutic Category Benzodiazepine

Controlled Substance C-IV

Use Short-term management of insomnia

Usual Dosage Adults: Oral: 1 mg at bedtime, some patients may require 2 mg; start at doses of 0.5 mg in debilitated patients

Dosage Forms Tablet: 1 mg, 2 mg

Ester-E™ [US-OTC] *see* vitamin E *on page 876*

esterified estrogen and methyltestosterone *see* estrogens (esterified) and methyltestosterone *on page 314*

esterified estrogens *see* estrogens (esterified) *on page 313*

Estivin® II Ophthalmic *(Discontinued)* *see* naphazoline *on page 577*

Estra-L® Injection *(Discontinued)* *see* estradiol *on this page*

Estrace® [US/Can] *see* estradiol *on this page*

Estraderm® [US/Can] *see* estradiol *on this page*

estradiol (es tra DYE ole)

Sound-Alike/Look-Alike Issues

Alora® may be confused with Aldara™

Estraderm® may be confused with Testoderm®

Synonyms estradiol acetate; estradiol cypionate; estradiol hemihydrate; estradiol transdermal; estradiol valerate

U.S./Canadian Brand Names Alora® [US]; Climara® [US/Can]; Delestrogen® [US]; Depo®-Estradiol [US/Can]; Esclim® [US]; Estrace® [US/Can]; Estraderm® [US/Can]; Estradot® [Can]; Estrasorb™ [US]; Estring® [US/Can]; EstroGel® [US/Can]; Femring™ [US]; Femtrace® [US]; Gynodiol® [US]; Menostar™ [US/Can]; Oesclim® [Can]; Sandoz-Estradiol Derm 100 [Can]; Sandoz-Estradiol Derm 50 [Can]; Sandoz-Estradiol Derm 75 [Can]; Vagifem® [US/Can]; Vivelle-Dot® [US]; Vivelle® [US]

Therapeutic Category Estrogen Derivative

Use Treatment of moderate-to-severe vasomotor symptoms associated with menopause; treatment of vulvar and vaginal atrophy; hypoestrogenism (due to hypogonadism, castration, or primary ovarian failure); prostatic cancer (palliation), breast cancer (palliation), osteoporosis (prophylaxis); abnormal uterine bleeding due to hormonal imbalance; postmenopausal urogenital symptoms of the lower urinary tract (urinary urgency, dysuria)

Usual Dosage All dosage needs to be adjusted based upon the patient's response

Oral:

Prostate cancer (androgen-dependent, inoperable, progressing): 10 mg 3 times/day for at least 3 months

Breast cancer (inoperable, progressing in appropriately selected patients): 10 mg 3 times/day for at least 3 months

Osteoporosis prophylaxis in postmenopausal females: 0.5 mg/day in a cyclic regimen (3 weeks on and 1 week off)

Female hypoestrogenism (due to hypogonadism, castration, or primary ovarian failure): 1-2 mg/day; titrate as necessary to control symptoms using minimal effective dose for maintenance therapy

Moderate to severe vasomotor symptoms associated with menopause: 1-2 mg/day, adjusted as necessary to limit symptoms; administration should be cyclic (3 weeks on, 1 week off). Patients should be re-evaluated at 3- to 6-month intervals to determine if treatment is still necessary.

I.M.

Prostate cancer: Valerate: ≥30 mg or more every 1-2 weeks

Moderate to severe vasomotor symptoms associated with menopause:

Cypionate: 1-5 mg every 3-4 weeks

Valerate: 10-20 mg every 4 weeks

Female hypoestrogenism (due to hypogonadism):

Cypionate: 1.5-2 mg monthly

Valerate: 10-20 mg every 4 weeks

Topical:

Emulsion: Moderate-to-severe vasomotor symptoms associated with menopause: 3.84 g applied once daily in the morning

Gel: Moderate-to-severe vasomotor symptoms associated with menopause, vulvar and vaginal atrophy: 1.25 g/day applied at the same time each day

Transdermal: Indicated dose may be used continuously in patients without an intact uterus. May be given continuously or cyclically (3 weeks on, 1 week off) in patients with an intact uterus **(exception - Menostar™, see specific dosing instructions).** When changing patients from oral to transdermal therapy, start transdermal patch 1 week after discontinuing oral hormone (may begin sooner if symptoms reappear within 1 week):

Once-weekly patch:

Moderate to severe vasomotor symptoms associated with menopause (Climara®): Apply 0.025 mg/day patch once weekly. Adjust dose as necessary to control symptoms. Patients should be reevaluated at 3- to 6-month intervals to determine if treatment is still necessary.

Osteoporosis prophylaxis in postmenopausal women:

Climara®: Apply patch once weekly; minimum effective dose 0.025 mg/day; adjust response to therapy by biochemical markers and bone mineral density

Menostar™: Apply patch once weekly. In women with a uterus, also administer a progestin for 14 days every 6-12 months

Twice-weekly patch:

Moderate to severe vasomotor symptoms associated with menopause, vulvar/vaginal atrophy, female hypogonadism: Titrate to lowest dose possible to control symptoms, adjusting initial dose after the first month of therapy; re-evaluate therapy at 3- to 6-month intervals to taper or discontinue medication:

Alora®, Esclim®, Estraderm®, Vivelle-Dot®: Apply 0.05 mg patch twice weekly

Vivelle®: Apply 0.0375 mg patch twice weekly

Prevention of osteoporosis in postmenopausal women:

Alora®, Vivelle®, Vivelle-Dot®: Apply 0.025 mg patch twice weekly, increase dose as necessary

Estraderm®: Apply 0.05 mg patch twice weekly

Vaginal cream: Vulvar and vaginal atrophy: Insert 2-4 g/day intravaginally for 2 weeks, then gradually reduce to 1/2 the initial dose for 2 weeks, followed by a maintenance dose of 1 g 1-3 times/week

Vaginal ring:

Postmenopausal vaginal atrophy, urogenital symptoms: Estring®: 2 mg intravaginally; following insertion, ring should remain in place for 90 days

Moderate to severe vasomotor symptoms associated with menopause; vulvar/vaginal atrophy: Femring™: 0.05 mg intravaginally; following insertion, ring should remain in place for 3 months; dose may be increased to 0.1 mg if needed

Vaginal tablets: Atrophic vaginitis: Vagifem®: Initial: Insert 1 tablet once daily for 2 weeks; maintenance: Insert 1 tablet twice weekly; attempts to discontinue or taper medication should be made at 3- to 6-month intervals

Dosage Forms

Cream, vaginal:

Estrace®: 0.1 mg/g (12 g) [refill]; 0.1 mg/g (42.5 g) [packaged with applicator]

Emulsion, topical, as hemihydrate:

Estrasorb™: 2.5 mg/g (56s) [each pouch contains 4.35 mg estradiol hemihydrate; contents of two pouches delivers estradiol 0.05 mg/day]

Gel, topical:

EstroGel®: 0.06% (93 g) [pump; delivers estradiol 0.75 mg/1.25 g; 64 doses]

Injection, oil, as cypionate:

Depo®-Estradiol: 5 mg/mL (5 mL) [contains chlorobutanol; in cottonseed oil]

Injection, oil, as valerate:

Delestrogen®:

10 mg/mL (5 mL) [contains chlorobutanol; in sesame oil]

20 mg/mL (5 mL) [contains benzyl alcohol; in castor oil]

40 mg/mL (5 mL) [contains benzyl alcohol; in castor oil]

Ring, vaginal, as base:

Estring®: 2 mg [total estradiol 2 mg; releases 7.5 mcg/day over 90 days] (1s)

Ring, vaginal, as acetate:

Femring™: 0.05 mg [total estradiol 12.4 mg; releases 0.05 mg/day over 3 months] (1s); 0.1 mg [total estradiol 24.8 mg; releases 0.1 mg/day over 3 months] (1s)

Tablet, oral, as acetate:

Femtrace®: 0.45 mg, 0.9 mg, 1.8 mg

Tablet, oral, micronized: 0.5 mg, 1 mg, 2 mg

Estrace®: 0.5 mg, 1 mg, 2 mg [2 mg tablets contain tartrazine]

Gynodiol®: 0.5 mg, 1 mg, 1.5 mg, 2 mg

Tablet, vaginal, as base:

Vagifem®: 25 mcg [contains lactose]

Transdermal system: 0.025 mg/24 hours [once-weekly patch] (4s); 0.0375 mg/24 hours (4s) [once-weekly patch]; 0.05 mg/24 hours (4s) [once-weekly patch]; 0.06 mg/24 hours (4s) [once-weekly patch] ; 0.075 mg/24 hours [once-weekly patch]; 0.1 mg/24 hours (4s) [once-weekly patch]

(Continued)

estradiol *(Continued)*

Alora® [twice-weekly patch]:
0.025 mg/24 hours [9 cm^2, total estradiol 0.77 mg] (8s)
0.05 mg/24 hours [18 cm^2, total estradiol 1.5 mg] (8s, 24s)
0.075 mg/24 hours [27 cm^2, total estradiol 2.3 mg] (8s)
0.1 mg/24 hours [36 cm^2, total estradiol 3.1 mg] (8s)

Climara® [once-weekly patch]:
0.025 mg/24 hours [6.5 cm^2, total estradiol 2.04 mg] (4s)
0.0375 mg/24 hours [9.375 cm^2, total estradiol 2.85 mg] (4s)
0.05 mg/24 hours [12.5 cm^2, total estradiol 3.8 mg] (4s)
0.06 mg/24 hours [15 cm^2, total estradiol 4.55 mg] (4s)
0.075 mg/24 hours [18.75 cm^2, total estradiol 5.7 mg] (4s)
0.1 mg/24 hours [25 cm^2, total estradiol 7.6 mg] (4s)

Esclim® [twice-weekly patch]:
0.025 mg/day [11 cm^2, total estradiol 5 mg] (8s)
0.0375 mg/day [16.5 cm^2, total estradiol 7.5 mg] (8s)
0.05 mg/day [22 cm^2, total estradiol 10 mg] (8s)
0.075 mg/day [33 cm^2, total estradiol 15 mg] (8s)
0.1 mg/day [44 cm^2, total estradiol 20 mg] (8s)

Estraderm® [twice-weekly patch]:
0.05 mg/24 hours [10 cm^2, total estradiol 4 mg] (8s)
0.1 mg/24 hours [20 cm^2, total estradiol 8 mg] (8s)

Menostar™ [once-weekly patch]: 0.014 mg/24 hours [3.25 cm^2, total estradiol 1 mg] (4s)

Vivelle® [twice-weekly patch]:
0.05 mg/24 hours [14.5 cm^2, total estradiol 4.33 mg] (8s)
0.1 mg/24 hours [29 cm^2, total estradiol 8.66 mg] (8s)

Vivelle-Dot® [twice-weekly patch]:
0.025 mg/day [2.5 cm^2, total estradiol 0.39 mg] (8s)
0.0375 mg/day [3.75 cm^2, total estradiol 0.585 mg] (8s)
0.05 mg/day [5 cm^2, total estradiol 0.78 mg] (8s)
0.075 mg/day [7.5 cm^2, total estradiol 1.17 mg] (8s)
0.1 mg/day [10 cm^2, total estradiol 1.56 mg] (8s)

estradiol acetate *see* estradiol *on page 308*

estradiol and drospirenone *see* drospirenone and estradiol *on page 282*

estradiol and levonorgestrel (es tra DYE ole & LEE voe nor jes trel)

Synonyms levonorgestrel and estradiol

U.S./Canadian Brand Names ClimaraPro® [US]

Therapeutic Category Estrogen and Progestin Combination

Use Women with an intact uterus: Treatment of moderate-to-severe vasomotor symptoms associated with menopause; prevention of postmenopausal osteoporosis

Usual Dosage Topical: Adult females with an intact uterus: Treatment of moderate-to-severe vasomotor symptoms associated with menopause or prevention of postmenopausal osteoporosis:
Estradiol 0.045 mg/levonorgestrel 0.015 mg: Apply one patch weekly

Dosage Forms Transdermal system: Estradiol 0.045 mg/24 hours and levonorgestrel 0.015 mg/24 hours (4s) [once-weekly patch; 22 cm^2; contains estradiol 4.4 mg and levonorgestrel 1.39 mg]

estradiol and NGM *see* estradiol and norgestimate *on next page*

estradiol and norethindrone (es tra DYE ole & nor eth IN drone)

Synonyms norethindrone and estradiol

U.S./Canadian Brand Names Activella® [US]; CombiPatch® [US]; Estalis-Sequi® [Can]; Estalis® [Can]

Therapeutic Category Estrogen and Progestin Combination

Use Women with an intact uterus:
Tablet: Treatment of moderate-to-severe vasomotor symptoms associated with menopause; treatment of vulvar and vaginal atrophy; prophylaxis for postmenopausal osteoporosis
Transdermal patch: Treatment of moderate-to-severe vasomotor symptoms associated with menopause; treatment of vulvar and vaginal atrophy; treatment of hypoestrogenism due to hypogonadism, castration, or primary ovarian failure

Usual Dosage Adults:
Oral (Activella®): 1 tablet daily

Transdermal patch (CombiPatch®):

Continuous combined regimen: Apply one patch twice weekly

Continuous sequential regimen: Apply estradiol-only patch for first 14 days of cycle, followed by one CombiPatch® applied twice weekly for the remaining 14 days of a 28-day cycle

Transdermal patch, combination pack (product-specific dosing for Canadian formulation):

Estalis®: Continuous combined regimen: Apply a new patch twice weekly during a 28-day cycle

Estalis-Sequi®: Continuous sequential regimen: Apply estradiol-only patch (Vivelle®) for first 14 days, followed by one Estalis® patch applied twice weekly during the last 14 days of a 28-day cycle

Note: In women previously receiving oral estrogens, initiate upon reappearance of menopausal symptoms following discontinuation of oral therapy.

Dosage Forms [CAN] = Canadian brand name

Combination pack (Estalis-Sequi® [CAN; not available in U.S.]):

140/50:

Transdermal system (Vivelle®): Estradiol 50 mcg per day (4s) [14.5 sq cm; total estradiol 4.33 mg]

Transdermal system (Estalis®): Norethindrone acetate 140 mcg and estradiol 50 mcg per day (4s) [9 sq cm; total norethindrone acetate 2.7 mg, total estradiol 0.62 mg; not available in U.S.]

250/50:

Transdermal system (Vivelle®): Estradiol 50 mcg per day (4s) [14.5 sq cm; total estradiol 4.33 mg]

Transdermal system (Estalis®): Norethindrone acetate 250 mcg and estradiol 50 mcg per day (4s) [16 sq cm; total norethindrone acetate 4.8 mg, total estradiol 0.51 mg; not available in U.S.]

Tablet (Activella®): Estradiol 1 mg and norethindrone acetate 0.5 mg (28s)

Transdermal system:

CombiPatch®:

0.05/0.14: Estradiol 0.05 mg and norethindrone acetate 0.14 mg per day (8s) [9 sq cm]

0.05/0.25: Estradiol 0.05 mg and norethindrone acetate 0.25 mg per day (8s) [16 sq cm]

Estalis® [CAN]:

140/50: Norethindrone acetate 140 mcg and estradiol 50 mcg per day (8s) [9 sq cm; total norethindrone acetate 2.7 mg, total estradiol 0.62 mg; not available in U.S.]

250/50 Norethindrone acetate 250 mcg and estradiol 50 mcg per day (8s) [16 sq cm; total norethindrone acetate 4.8 mg, total estradiol 0.51 mg; not available in U.S.]

estradiol and norgestimate (es tra DYE ole & nor JES ti mate)

Synonyms estradiol and NGM; norgestimate and estradiol; ortho prefest

U.S./Canadian Brand Names Prefest™ [US]

Therapeutic Category Estrogen and Progestin Combination

Use Women with an intact uterus: Treatment of moderate to severe vasomotor symptoms associated with menopause; treatment of atrophic vaginitis; prevention of osteoporosis

Usual Dosage Oral: Adults: Females with an intact uterus:

Treatment of menopausal symptoms, atrophic vaginitis, prevention of osteoporosis: Treatment is cyclical and consists of the following: One tablet of estradiol 1 mg (pink tablet) once daily for 3 days, followed by 1 tablet of estradiol 1 mg and norgestimate 0.09 mg (white tablet) once daily for 3 days; repeat sequence continuously. **Note:** This dose may not be the lowest effective combination for these indications. In case of a missed tablet, restart therapy with next available tablet in sequence (taking only 1 tablet each day).

Dosage Forms Tablet: Estradiol 1 mg [15 pink tablets] and estradiol 1 mg and norgestimate 0.09 mg [15 white tablets] (supplied in blister card of 30)

estradiol cypionate *see* estradiol *on page 308*

estradiol hemihydrate *see* estradiol *on page 308*

estradiol transdermal *see* estradiol *on page 308*

estradiol valerate *see* estradiol *on page 308*

Estradot® [Can] *see* estradiol *on page 308*

estramustine (es tra MUS teen)

Sound-Alike/Look-Alike Issues

Emcyt® may be confused with Eryc®

Synonyms estramustine phosphate sodium; NSC-89199

U.S./Canadian Brand Names Emcyt® [US/Can]

Therapeutic Category Antineoplastic Agent

Use Palliative treatment of prostatic carcinoma (progressive or metastatic)

Usual Dosage Refer to individual protocols.

Oral: 10-16 mg/kg/day (14 mg/kg/day is most common) or 140 mg 4 times/day (some patients have been maintained for >3 years on therapy)

Dosage Forms Capsule, as phosphate sodium: 140 mg

estramustine phosphate sodium *see* estramustine *on previous page*

Estrasorb™ [US] *see* estradiol *on page 308*

Estratab® [Can] *see* estrogens (esterified) *on next page*

Estratab® *(Discontinued)* *see* estrogens (esterified) *on next page*

Estratest® [US/Can] *see* estrogens (esterified) and methyltestosterone *on page 314*

Estratest® H.S. [US] *see* estrogens (esterified) and methyltestosterone *on page 314*

Estring® [US/Can] *see* estradiol *on page 308*

Estro-Cyp® Injection *(Discontinued)* *see* estradiol *on page 308*

EstroGel® [US/Can] *see* estradiol *on page 308*

estrogenic substances, conjugated *see* estrogens (conjugated/equine) *on this page*

estrogens (conjugated A/synthetic) (ES troe jenz, KON joo gate ed, aye, sin THET ik)

Sound-Alike/Look-Alike Issues

Cenestin® may be confused with Senexon®

U.S./Canadian Brand Names Cenestin® [US]

Therapeutic Category Estrogen Derivative

Use Treatment of moderate-to-severe vasomotor symptoms of menopause; treatment of vulvar and vaginal atrophy

Usual Dosage The lowest dose that will control symptoms should be used; medication should be discontinued as soon as possible. Oral: Adults:

Moderate-to-severe vasomotor symptoms: 0.45 mg/day; may be titrated up to 1.25 mg/day. Attempts to discontinue medication should be made at 3- to 6-month intervals.

Vulvar and vaginal atrophy: 0.3 mg/day

Dosage Forms Tablet: 0.3 mg, 0.45 mg, 0.625 mg, 0.9 mg, 1.25 mg

estrogens (conjugated/equine) (ES troe jenz KON joo gate ed, EE kwine)

Sound-Alike/Look-Alike Issues

Premarin® may be confused with Primaxin®, Provera®, Remeron®

Synonyms CEE; C.E.S.; estrogenic substances, conjugated

U.S./Canadian Brand Names Premarin® [US/Can]

Therapeutic Category Estrogen Derivative

Use Treatment of moderate-to-severe vasomotor symptoms associated with menopause; treatment of vulvar and vaginal atrophy; hypoestrogenism (due to hypogonadism, castration, or primary ovarian failure); prostatic cancer (palliation); breast cancer (palliation); osteoporosis (prophylaxis, postmenopausal women at significant risk only); abnormal uterine bleeding

Usual Dosage Adults:

Male: Androgen-dependent prostate cancer palliation: Oral: 1.25-2.5 mg 3 times/day

Female:

Prevention of postmenopausal osteoporosis: Oral: Initial: 0.3 mg/day cyclically* or daily, depending on medical assessment of patient. Dose may be adjusted based on bone mineral density and clinical response. The lowest effective dose should be used.

Moderate to severe vasomotor symptoms associated with menopause: Oral: Initial: 0.3 mg/day, cyclically* or daily, depending on medical assessment of patient. The lowest dose that will control symptoms should be used. Medication should be discontinued as soon as possible.

Vulvar and vaginal atrophy:

Oral: Initial: 0.3 mg/day; the lowest dose that will control symptoms should be used. May be given cyclically* or daily, depending on medical assessment of patient. Medication should be discontinued as soon as possible.

Vaginal cream: Intravaginal: ½ to 2 g/day given cyclically*

Abnormal uterine bleeding:

Acute/heavy bleeding:

I.M., I.V.: 25 mg, may repeat in 6-12 hours if needed

Note: Treatment should be followed by a low-dose oral contraceptive; medroxyprogesterone acetate along with or following estrogen therapy can also be given

Female hypogonadism: Oral: 0.3-0.625 mg/day given cyclically*; dose may be titrated in 6- to 12-month intervals; progestin treatment should be added to maintain bone mineral density once skeletal maturity is achieved.

Female castration, primary ovarian failure: Oral: 1.25 mg/day given cyclically*; adjust according to severity of symptoms and patient response. For maintenance, adjust to the lowest effective dose.

***Cyclic administration:** Either 3 weeks on, 1 week off **or** 25 days on, 5 days off

Male and Female: Breast cancer palliation, metastatic disease in selected patients: Oral: 10 mg 3 times/day for at least 3 months

Dosage Forms

Cream, vaginal: 0.625 mg/g (42.5 g)

Injection, powder for reconstitution: 25 mg [contains lactose 200 mg; diluent contains benzyl alcohol]

Tablet: 0.3 mg, 0.45 mg, 0.625 mg, 0.9 mg, 1.25 mg

estrogens (conjugated/equine) and medroxyprogesterone

(ES troe jenz KON joo gate ed/EE kwine & me DROKS ee proe JES te rone)

Sound-Alike/Look-Alike Issues

Premphase® may be confused with Prempro™

Prempro™ may be confused with Premphase®

Synonyms medroxyprogesterone and estrogens (conjugated); MPA and estrogens (conjugated)

U.S./Canadian Brand Names Premphase® [US/Can]; Premplus® [Can]; Prempro™ [US/Can]

Therapeutic Category Estrogen and Progestin Combination

Use Women with an intact uterus: Treatment of moderate-to-severe vasomotor symptoms associated with menopause; treatment of atrophic vaginitis; osteoporosis (prophylaxis)

Usual Dosage Oral: Adults:

Treatment of moderate-to-severe vasomotor symptoms associated with menopause or treatment of atrophic vaginitis in females with an intact uterus. (The lowest dose that will control symptoms should be used; medication should be discontinued as soon as possible):

Premphase®: One maroon conjugated estrogen 0.625 mg tablet daily on days 1 through 14 and one light blue conjugated estrogen 0.625 mg/MPA 5 mg tablet daily on days 15 through 28; re-evaluate patients at 3- and 6-month intervals to determine if treatment is still necessary; monitor patients for signs of endometrial cancer; rule out malignancy if unexplained vaginal bleeding occurs

Prempro™: One conjugated estrogen 0.3 mg/MPA 1.5 mg tablet daily; re-evaluate at 3-and 6-month intervals to determine if therapy is still needed; dose may be increased to a maximum of one conjugated estrogen 0.625 mg/MPA 5 mg tablet daily in patients with bleeding or spotting, once malignancy has been ruled out

Osteoporosis prophylaxis in females with an intact uterus:

Premphase®: One maroon conjugated estrogen 0.625 tablet daily on days 1 through 14 and one light blue conjugated estrogen 0.625 mg/MPA 5 mg tablet daily on days 15 through 28; monitor patients for signs of endometrial cancer; rule out malignancy if unexplained vaginal bleeding occurs

Prempro™: One conjugated estrogen 0.3 mg/MPA 1.5 mg tablet daily; dose may be increased to one conjugated estrogen 0.625 mg/MPA 5 mg tablet daily; in patients with bleeding or spotting, once malignancy has been ruled out

Dosage Forms Tablet:

Premphase® [therapy pack contains 2 separate tablet formulations]: Conjugated estrogens 0.625 mg [14 maroon tablets] and conjugated estrogen 0.625 mg/medroxyprogesterone acetate 5 mg [14 light blue tablets] (28s)

Prempro™:

0.3/1.5: Conjugated estrogens 0.3 mg and medroxyprogesterone acetate 1.5 mg (28s)

0.45/1.5: Conjugated estrogens 0.45 mg and medroxyprogesterone acetate 1.5 mg (28s)

0.625/2.5: Conjugated estrogens 0.625 mg and medroxyprogesterone acetate 2.5 mg (28s)

0.625/5: Conjugated estrogens 0.625 mg and medroxyprogesterone acetate 5 mg (28s)

estrogens (esterified) (ES troe jenz, es TER i fied)

Sound-Alike/Look-Alike Issues

Estratab® may be confused with Estratest®, Estratest® H.S.

Synonyms esterified estrogens

U.S./Canadian Brand Names Estratab® [Can]; Menest® [US/Can]

Therapeutic Category Estrogen Derivative

Use Treatment of moderate to severe vasomotor symptoms associated with menopause; treatment of vulvar and vaginal atrophy; hypoestrogenism (due to hypogonadism, castration, or primary ovarian failure); prostatic cancer (palliation); breast cancer (palliation); osteoporosis (prophylaxis, in women at significant risk only)

(Continued)

estrogens (esterified) *(Continued)*

Usual Dosage Oral: Adults:

Prostate cancer (palliation): 1.25-2.5 mg 3 times/day

Female hypogonadism: 2.5-7.5 mg of estrogen daily for 20 days followed by a 10-day rest period. Administer cyclically (3 weeks on and 1 week off). If bleeding does not occur by the end of the 10-day period, repeat the same dosing schedule; the number of courses is dependent upon the responsiveness of the endometrium. If bleeding occurs before the end of the 10-day period, begin an estrogen-progestin cyclic regimen of 2.5-7.5 mg esterified estrogens daily for 20 days. During the last 5 days of estrogen therapy, give an oral progestin. If bleeding occurs before regimen is concluded, discontinue therapy and resume on the fifth day of bleeding.

Moderate to severe vasomotor symptoms associated with menopause: 1.25 mg/day administered cyclically (3 weeks on and 1 week off). If patient has not menstruated within the last 2 months or more, cyclic administration is started arbitrary. If the patient is menstruating, cyclical administration is started on day 5 of the bleeding. For short-term use only and should be discontinued as soon as possible. Re-evaluate at 3- to 6-month intervals for tapering or discontinuation of therapy.

Atopic vaginitis and kraurosis vulvae: 0.3 to ≥1.25 mg/day, depending on the tissue response of the individual patient. Administer cyclically. For short-term use only and should be discontinued as soon as possible. Re-evaluate at 3- to 6-month intervals for tapering or discontinuation of therapy.

Breast cancer (palliation): 10 mg 3 times/day for at least 3 months

Osteoporosis in postmenopausal women: Initial: 0.3 mg/day and increase to a maximum daily dose of 1.25 mg/day; initiate therapy as soon as possible after menopause; cyclically or daily, depending on medical assessment of patient. Monitor patients with an intact uterus for signs of endometrial cancer; rule out malignancy if unexplained vaginal bleeding occurs

Female castration and primary ovarian failure: 1.25 mg/day, cyclically. Adjust dosage upward or downward, according to the severity of symptoms and patient response. For maintenance, adjust dosage to lowest level that will provide effective control.

Dosage Forms Tablet: 0.3 mg, 0.625 mg, 1.25 mg, 2.5 mg

estrogens (esterified) and methyltestosterone

(ES troe jenz es TER i fied & meth il tes TOS te rone)

Sound-Alike/Look-Alike Issues

Estratest® may be confused with Eskalith®, Estratab®, Estratest® H.S.

Estratest® H.S. may be confused with Eskalith®, Estratab®, Estratest®

Synonyms conjugated estrogen and methyltestosterone; esterified estrogen and methyltestosterone

U.S./Canadian Brand Names Estratest® H.S. [US]; Estratest® [US/Can]; Syntest D.S. [US]; Syntest H.S. [US]

Therapeutic Category Estrogen and Androgen Combination

Use Vasomotor symptoms of menopause

Usual Dosage Adults: Female: Oral: Lowest dose that will control symptoms should be chosen, normally given 3 weeks on and 1 week off

Dosage Forms Tablet:

Estratest®: Esterified estrogen 1.25 mg and methyltestosterone 2.5 mg [contains sodium benzoate]

Estratest® H.S.: Esterified estrogen 0.625 mg and methyltestosterone 1.25 mg [contains sodium benzoate]

Syntest D.S.: Esterified estrogen 1.25 mg and methyltestosterone 2.5 mg

Syntest H.S.: Esterified estrogen 0.625 mg and methyltestosterone 1.25 mg

estropipate (ES troe pih pate)

Synonyms piperazine estrone sulfate

U.S./Canadian Brand Names Ogen® [US/Can]; Ortho-Est® [US]

Therapeutic Category Estrogen Derivative

Use Treatment of moderate to severe vasomotor symptoms associated with menopause; treatment of vulvar and vaginal atrophy; hypoestrogenism (due to hypogonadism, castration, or primary ovarian failure); osteoporosis (prophylaxis, in women at significant risk only)

Usual Dosage Adults: Oral:

Moderate to severe vasomotor symptoms associated with menopause: Usual dosage range: 0.75-6 mg estropipate daily; use the lowest dose and regimen that will control symptoms, and discontinue as soon as possible. Attempt to discontinue or taper medication at 3- to 6-month intervals. If a patient with vasomotor symptoms has not menstruated within the last ≥2 months, start the cyclic administration arbitrarily. If the patient has menstruated, start cyclic administration on day 5 of bleeding.

Female hypogonadism: 1.5-9 mg estropipate daily for the first 3 weeks, followed by a rest period of 8-10 days; use the lowest dose and regimen that will control symptoms. Repeat if bleeding does not occur by the end of the rest period. The duration of therapy necessary to product the withdrawal bleeding will vary according to the responsiveness of the endometrium. If satisfactory withdrawal bleeding does not occur, give an oral progestin in addition to estrogen during the third week of the cycle.

Female castration or primary ovarian failure: 1.5-9 mg estropipate daily for the first 3 weeks of a theoretical cycle, followed by a rest period of 8-10 days; use the lowest dose and regimen that will control symptoms

Osteoporosis prophylaxis: 0.75 mg estropipate daily for 25 days of a 31-day cycle

Atrophic vaginitis or kraurosis vulvae: 0.75-6 mg estropipate daily; administer cyclically. Use the lowest dose and regimen that will control symptoms; discontinue as soon as possible.

Dosage Forms

Tablet: 0.625 mg [estropipate 0.75 mg]; 1.25 mg [estropipate 1.5 mg]; 2.5 mg [estropipate 3 mg]

Ogen®: 0.625 mg [estropipate 0.75 mg]; 1.25 mg [estropipate 1.5 mg]; 2.5 mg [estropipate 3 mg]

Ortho-Est®: 0.625 mg [estropipate 0.75 mg]; 1.25 mg [estropipate 1.5 mg]

Estrostep® 21 *(Discontinued)* *see* ethinyl estradiol and norethindrone *on page 323*

Estrostep® Fe [US] *see* ethinyl estradiol and norethindrone *on page 323*

eszopiclone (es zoe PIK lone)

Sound-Alike/Look-Alike Issues

Lunesta™ may be confused with Neulasta®

U.S./Canadian Brand Names Lunesta™ [US]

Therapeutic Category Hypnotic, Nonbenzodiazepine

Controlled Substance C-IV

Use Treatment of insomnia

Usual Dosage Oral: Adults: Insomnia: Initial: 2 mg before bedtime (maximum dose: 3 mg)

Concurrent use with strong CYP3A4 inhibitor: 1 mg before bedtime; if needed, dose may be increased to 2 mg

Dosage Forms Tablet: 1 mg, 2 mg, 3 mg

ETAF *see* aldesleukin *on page 26*

etanercept (et a NER sept)

U.S./Canadian Brand Names Enbrel® [US/Can]

Therapeutic Category Antirheumatic, Disease Modifying

Use Treatment of moderately- to severely-active rheumatoid arthritis, moderately- to severely-active polyarticular juvenile arthritis (in patients with inadequate response to at least one disease-modifying antirheumatic drug), psoriatic arthritis, active ankylosing spondylitis (AS); moderate-to-severe chronic plaque psoriasis

Usual Dosage SubQ:

Children 4-17 years: Juvenile rheumatoid arthritis:

Once-weekly dosing: 0.8 mg/kg (maximum: 50 mg/dose) once weekly

Twice-weekly dosing: 0.4 mg/kg (maximum: 25 mg/dose) twice weekly (individual doses should be separated by 72-96 hours)

Adults:

Rheumatoid arthritis, psoriatic arthritis, ankylosing spondylitis:

Once-weekly dosing: 50 mg once weekly

Twice weekly dosing: 25 mg given twice weekly (individual doses should be separated by 72-96 hours)

Note: If the physician determines that it is appropriate, patients may self-inject after proper training in injection technique.

Plaque psoriasis:

Initial: 50 mg twice weekly, 3-4 days apart (starting doses of 25 or 50 mg once weekly have also been used successfully); maintain initial dose for 3 months

Maintenance dose: 50 mg weekly

Dosage Forms

Injection, powder for reconstitution:

Enbrel®: 25 mg [diluent contains benzyl alcohol]

Injection, solution:

Enbrel®: 50 mg/mL (0.98 mL) [packaging may contain dry natural rubber (latex)]

ethacrynate sodium *see* ethacrynic acid *on this page*

ethacrynic acid (eth a KRIN ik AS id)

Sound-Alike/Look-Alike Issues

Edecrin® may be confused with Eulexin®, Ecotrin®

(Continued)

ethacrynic acid *(Continued)*

Synonyms ethacrynate sodium

U.S./Canadian Brand Names Edecrin® [US/Can]

Therapeutic Category Diuretic, Loop

Use Management of edema associated with congestive heart failure; hepatic cirrhosis or renal disease; short-term management of ascites due to malignancy, idiopathic edema, and lymphedema

Usual Dosage I.V. formulation should be diluted in D_5W or NS (1 mg/mL) and infused over several minutes.

Children: Oral: 1 mg/kg/dose once daily; increase at intervals of 2-3 days as needed, to a maximum of 3 mg/kg/day.

Adults:

Oral: 50-200 mg/day in 1-2 divided doses; may increase in increments of 25-50 mg at intervals of several days; doses up to 200 mg twice daily may be required with severe, refractory edema.

I.V.: 0.5-1 mg/kg/dose (maximum: 100 mg/dose); repeat doses not routinely recommended; however, if indicated, repeat doses every 8-12 hours.

Dosage Forms

Injection, powder for reconstitution, as ethacrynate sodium: 50 mg

Tablet: 25 mg

ethambutol (e THAM byoo tole)

Sound-Alike/Look-Alike Issues

Myambutol® may be confused with Nembutal®

Synonyms ethambutol hydrochloride

U.S./Canadian Brand Names Etibi® [Can]; Myambutol® [US]

Therapeutic Category Antimycobacterial Agent

Use Treatment of tuberculosis and other mycobacterial diseases in conjunction with other antituberculosis agents

Usual Dosage Oral:

Treatment of tuberculosis: **Note:** Used as part of a multidrug regimen. Treatment regimens consist of an initial 2 month phase, followed by a continuation phase of 4 or 7 additional months; frequency of dosing may differ depending on phase of therapy.

Children:

Daily therapy: 15-20 mg/kg/day (maximum: 1 g/day)

Twice weekly directly observed therapy (DOT): 50 mg/kg (maximum: 4 g/dose)

Adults (suggested doses by lean body weight):

Daily therapy: 15-25 mg/kg

40-55 kg: 800 mg

56-75 kg: 1200 mg

76-90 kg: 1600 mg (maximum dose regardless of weight)

Twice weekly directly observed therapy (DOT): 50 mg/kg

40-55 kg: 2000 mg

56-75 kg: 2800 mg

76-90 kg: 4000 mg (maximum dose regardless of weight)

Three times/week DOT: 25-30 mg/kg (maximum: 2.5 g)

40-55 kg: 1200 mg

56-75 kg: 2000 mg

76-90 kg: 2400 mg (maximum dose regardless of weight)

Disseminated *Mycobacterium avium* complex (MAC) in patients with advanced HIV infection: 15 mg/kg ethambutol in combination with azithromycin 600 mg daily

Dosage Forms Tablet, as hydrochloride: 100 mg, 400 mg

ethambutol hydrochloride *see* ethambutol *on this page*

Ethamolin® [US] *see* ethanolamine oleate *on this page*

ethanoic acid *see* acetic acid *on page 14*

ethanol *see* alcohol (ethyl) *on page 25*

ethanolamine oleate (ETH a nol a meen OH lee ate)

Sound-Alike/Look-Alike Issues

Ethamolin® may be confused with ethanol

Synonyms monoethanolamine
U.S./Canadian Brand Names Ethamolin® [US]
Therapeutic Category Sclerosing Agent
Use **Orphan drug:** Sclerosing agent used for bleeding esophageal varices
Usual Dosage Adults: 1.5-5 mL per varix, up to 20 mL total or 0.4 mL/kg for a 50 kg patient; doses should be decreased in patients with severe hepatic dysfunction and should receive less than recommended maximum dose
Dosage Forms Injection, solution: 5% [50 mg/mL] (2 mL) [contains benzyl alcohol]

EtheDent™ [US] *see* fluoride *on page 354*

Ethezyme™ [US] *see* papain and urea *on page 637*

Ethezyme™ 830 [US] *see* papain and urea *on page 637*

ethinyl estradiol and cyproterone acetate *see* cyproterone and ethinyl estradiol *(Canada only) on page 223*

ethinyl estradiol and desogestrel (ETH in il es tra DYE ole & des oh JES trel)

Sound-Alike/Look-Alike Issues
Ortho-Cept® may be confused with Ortho-Cyclen®
Synonyms desogestrel and ethinyl estradiol
U.S./Canadian Brand Names Apri® [US]; Cesia™ [US]; Cyclessa® [US/Can]; Desogen® [US]; Kariva™ [US]; Linessa® [Can]; Marvelon® [Can]; Mircette® [US]; Ortho-Cept® [US/Can]; Reclipsen™ [US]; Solia™ [US]; Velivet™ [US]
Therapeutic Category Contraceptive, Oral
Use Prevention of pregnancy
Usual Dosage Oral: Adults: Female: Contraception:
Schedule 1 (Sunday starter): Dose begins on first Sunday after onset of menstruation; if the menstrual period starts on Sunday, take first tablet that very same day. **With a Sunday start, an additional method of contraception should be used until after the first 7 days of consecutive administration.**
For 21-tablet package: Dosage is 1 tablet daily for 21 consecutive days, followed by 7 days off of the medication; a new course begins on the 8th day after the last tablet is taken.
For 28-tablet package: Dosage is 1 tablet daily without interruption.
Schedule 2 (Day 1 starter): Dose starts on first day of menstrual cycle taking 1 tablet daily.
For 21-tablet package: Dosage is 1 tablet daily for 21 consecutive days, followed by 7 days off of the medication; a new course begins on the 8th day after the last tablet is taken.
For 28-tablet package: Dosage is 1 tablet daily without interruption.
If all doses have been taken on schedule and one menstrual period is missed, continue dosing cycle. If two consecutive menstrual periods are missed, pregnancy test is required before new dosing cycle is started.
Missed doses **monophasic formulations** (refer to package insert for complete information):
One dose missed: Take as soon as remembered or take 2 tablets next day
Two consecutive doses missed in the first 2 weeks: Take 2 tablets as soon as remembered or 2 tablets next 2 days. **An additional method of contraception should be used for 7 days after missed dose.**
Two consecutive doses missed in week 3 or three consecutive doses missed at any time:
Schedule 1 (Sunday starter): Continue to take 1 tablet daily until Sunday, then discard the rest of the pack, and a new pack is started that same day.
Schedule 2 (Day 1 starter): Current pack should be discarded, and a new pack started that same day. **An additional method of contraception should be used for 7 days after missed dose.**
Missed doses **biphasic/triphasic formulations** (refer to package insert for complete information):
One dose missed: Take as soon as remembered or take 2 tablets next day.
Two consecutive doses missed in week 1 or week 2 of the pack: Take 2 tablets as soon as remembered and 2 tablets the next day. Resume taking 1 tablet daily until the pack is empty. **An additional method of contraception should be used for 7 days after a missed dose.**
Two consecutive doses missed in week 3 of the pack; **an additional method of contraception must be used for 7 days after a missed dose**:
Schedule 1 (Sunday starter): Take 1 tablet every day until Sunday. Discard the remaining pack and start a new pack of pills on the same day.
Schedule 2 (Day 1 starter): Discard the remaining pack and start a new pack the same day.
Three or more consecutive doses missed; **an additional method of contraception must be used for 7 days after a missed dose**:
Schedule 1 (Sunday starter): Take 1 tablet every day until Sunday; on Sunday, discard the pack and start a new pack.
Schedule 2 (Day 1 starter): Discard the remaining pack and begin new pack of tablets starting on the same day.
(Continued)

ethinyl estradiol and desogestrel *(Continued)*

Dosage Forms

Tablet, low-dose formulations:

Kariva™:

Day 1-21: Ethinyl estradiol 0.02 mg and desogestrel 0.15 mg [21 white tablets]

Day 22-23: 2 inactive light green tablets

Day 24-28: Ethinyl estradiol 0.01 mg [5 light blue tablets] (28s)

Mircette®:

Day 1-21: Ethinyl estradiol 0.02 mg and desogestrel 0.15 mg [21 white tablets]

Day 22-23: 2 inactive green tablets

Day 24-28: Ethinyl estradiol 0.01 mg [5 yellow tablets] (28s)

Tablet, monophasic formulations:

Apri® 28: Ethinyl estradiol 0.03 mg and desogestrel 0.15 mg [21 rose tablets and 7 white inactive tablets] (28s)

Desogen®, Reclipsen™, Solia™: Ethinyl estradiol 0.03 mg and desogestrel 0.15 mg [21 white tablets and 7 green inactive tablets] (28s)

Ortho-Cept® 28: Ethinyl estradiol 0.03 mg and desogestrel 0.15 mg [21 orange tablets and 7 green inactive tablets] (28s)

Tablet, triphasic formulations:

Cesia™, Cyclessa®:

Day 1-7:Ethinyl estradiol 0.025 mg and desogestrel 0.1 mg [7 light yellow tablets]

Day 8-14: Ethinyl estradiol 0.025 mg and desogestrel 0.125 mg [7 orange tablets]

Day 14-21: Ethinyl estradiol 0.025 mg and desogestrel 0.15 mg [7 red tablets]

Day 21-28: 7 green inactive tablets (28s)

Velivet™:

Day 1-7: Ethinyl estradiol 0.025 mg and desogestrel 0.1 mg [7 beige tablets]

Day 8-14: Ethinyl estradiol 0.025 mg and desogestrel 0.125 mg [7 orange tablets]

Day 14-21: Ethinyl estradiol 0.025 mg and desogestrel 0.15 mg [7 pink tablets]

Day 21-28: 7 white inactive tablets (28s)

ethinyl estradiol and drospirenone (ETH in il es tra DYE ole & droh SPYE re none)

Synonyms drospirenone and ethinyl estradiol

U.S./Canadian Brand Names Yasmin® [US/Can]; Yaz [US]

Therapeutic Category Contraceptive

Use Prevention of pregnancy

Usual Dosage Oral: Adults: Female: Contraception: Dosage is 1 tablet daily for 28 consecutive days. Dose should be taken at the same time each day, either after the evening meal or at bedtime. Dosing may be started on the first day of menstrual period (Day 1 starter) or on the first Sunday after the onset of the menstrual period (Sunday starter).

Day 1 starter: Dose starts on first day of menstrual cycle taking 1 tablet daily.

Sunday starter: Dose begins on first Sunday after onset of menstruation; if the menstrual period starts on Sunday, take first tablet that very same day. **With a Sunday start, an additional method of contraception should be used until after the first 7 days of consecutive administration.**

If all doses have been taken on schedule and one menstrual period is missed, continue dosing cycle. If two consecutive menstrual periods are missed, pregnancy test is required before new dosing cycle is started.

If doses have been missed during the first 3 weeks and the menstrual period is missed, pregnancy should be ruled out prior to continuing treatment.

Missed doses (monophasic formulations) (refer to package insert for complete information):

One dose missed: Take as soon as remembered or take 2 tablets next day

Two consecutive doses missed in the first 2 weeks: Take 2 tablets as soon as remembered or 2 tablets next 2 days. **An additional method of contraception should be used for 7 days after missed dose.**

Two consecutive doses missed in week 3 or three consecutive doses missed at any time: **An additional method of contraception must be used for 7 days after a missed dose.**

Day 1 starter: Current pack should be discarded, and a new pack should be started that same day.

Sunday starter: Continue dose of 1 tablet daily until Sunday, then discard the rest of the pack, and a new pack should be started that same day.

Any number of doses missed in week 4: Continue taking one pill each day until pack is empty; no back-up method of contraception is needed

Dosage Forms

Tablet:

Yasmin®: Ethinyl estradiol 0.03 mg and drospirenone 3 mg [21 yellow active tablets and 7 white inactive tablets] (28s)

Yaz: Ethinyl estradiol 0.02 mg and drospirenone 3 mg [24 light pink tablets and 4 white inactive tablets] (28s)

ethinyl estradiol and ethynodiol diacetate

(ETH in il es tra DYE ole & e thye noe DYE ole dye AS e tate)

Sound-Alike/Look-Alike Issues

Demulen® may be confused with Dalmane®, Demerol®

Synonyms ethynodiol diacetate and ethinyl estradiol

U.S./Canadian Brand Names Demulen® 30 [Can]; Demulen® [US]; Kelnor™ [US]; Zovia™ [US]

Therapeutic Category Contraceptive, Oral

Use Prevention of pregnancy

Usual Dosage Oral: Adults: Female: Contraception:

Schedule 1 (Sunday starter): Dose begins on first Sunday after onset of menstruation; if the menstrual period starts on Sunday, take first tablet that very same day. **With a Sunday start, an additional method of contraception should be used until after the first 7 days of consecutive administration.**

For 21-tablet package: 1 tablet/day for 21 consecutive days, followed by 7 days off of the medication; a new course begins on the 8th day after the last tablet is taken.

For 28-tablet package: 1 tablet/day without interruption.

Schedule 2 (Day 1 starter): Dose starts on first day of menstrual cycle taking 1 tablet daily.

For 21-tablet package: 1 tablet/day for 21 consecutive days, followed by 7 days off of the medication; a new course begins on the 8th day after the last tablet is taken.

For 28-tablet package: 1 tablet/day without interruption.

If all doses have been taken on schedule and one menstrual period is missed, continue dosing cycle. If two consecutive menstrual periods are missed, pregnancy test is required before new dosing cycle is started.

Missed doses **monophasic formulations** (refer to package insert for complete information):

One dose missed: Take as soon as remembered or take 2 tablets next day

Two consecutive doses missed in the first 2 weeks: Take 2 tablets as soon as remembered or 2 tablets next 2 days. **An additional method of contraception should be used for 7 days after missed dose.**

Two consecutive doses missed in week 3 or three consecutive doses missed at any time: **An additional method of contraception should be used for 7 days after missed dose:**

Schedule 1 (Sunday starter): Continue dose of 1 tablet daily until Sunday, then discard the rest of the pack, and a new pack should be started that same day.

Schedule 2 (Day 1 starter): Current package should be discarded, and a new pack should be started that same day.

Dosage Forms [DSC] = Discontinued products

Tablet, monophasic formulations:

Demulen® 1/35-28: Ethinyl estradiol 0.035 mg and ethynodiol diacetate 1 mg [21 white tablets and 7 blue inactive tablets] (28s) [DSC]

Kelnor™ 1/35: Ethinyl estradiol 0.035 mg and ethynodiol diacetate 1 mg [21 light yellow tablets and 7 white inactive tablets] (28s)

Zovia™ 1/35-28: Ethinyl estradiol 0.035 mg and ethynodiol diacetate 1 mg [21 light pink tablets and 7 white inactive tablets] (28s)

Zovia™ 1/50-28: Ethinyl estradiol 0.05 mg and ethynodiol diacetate 1 mg [21 pink tablets and 7 white inactive tablets] (28s)

ethinyl estradiol and etonogestrel (ETH in il es tra DYE ole & et oh noe JES trel)

Synonyms etonogestrel and ethinyl estradiol

U.S./Canadian Brand Names NuvaRing® [US/Can]

Therapeutic Category Contraceptive; Estrogen and Progestin Combination

Use Prevention of pregnancy

Usual Dosage Vaginal: Adults: Female: Contraception: One ring, inserted vaginally and left in place for 3 consecutive weeks, then removed for 1 week. A new ring is inserted 7 days after the last was removed (even if bleeding is not complete) and should be inserted at approximately the same time of day the ring was removed the previous week.

Initial treatment should begin as follows (pregnancy should always be ruled out first):

No hormonal contraceptive use in the past month: Using the first day of menstruation as "Day 1," insert the ring on or prior to "Day 5," even if bleeding is not complete. **An additional form of contraception should be used for the following 7 days.***

Switching from combination oral contraceptive: Ring can be inserted on any day within 7 days after the last **active** tablet in the cycle was taken and no later than the first day a new cycle of tablets would begin. Additional forms of contraception are not needed.

Switching from progestin-only contraceptive: **An additional form of contraception should be used for the following 7 days with any of the following.***

(Continued)

ethinyl estradiol and etonogestrel *(Continued)*

If previously using a progestin-only mini-pill, insert the ring on any day of the month; do not skip days between the last pill and insertion of the ring.

If previously using an implant, insert the ring on the same day of implant removal.

If previously using a progestin-containing IUD, insert the ring on day of IUD removal.

If previously using a progestin injection, insert the ring on the day the next injection would be given.

Following complete 1st trimester abortion: Insert ring within the first five days of abortion. If not inserted within five days, follow instructions for "No hormonal contraceptive use within the past month" and instruct patient to use a nonhormonal contraceptive in the interim.

Following delivery or 2nd trimester abortion: Insert ring 4 weeks postpartum (in women who are not breast-feeding) or following 2nd trimester abortion. **An additional form of contraception should be used for the following 7 days.***

If the ring is accidentally removed from the vagina at anytime during the 3-week period of use, it may be rinsed with cool or lukewarm water (not hot) and reinserted as soon as possible. If the ring is not reinserted within three hours, contraceptive effectiveness will be decreased. **An additional form of contraception should be used until the ring has been in place for 7 consecutive days.***

If the ring has been removed for longer than 1 week, pregnancy must be ruled out prior to restarting therapy. **An additional form of contraception should be used for the following 7 days.***

If the ring has been left in place for >3 weeks, a new ring should be inserted following a 1-week (ring-free) interval. Pregnancy must be ruled out prior to insertion and **an additional form of contraception should be used for the following 7 days.***

Disconnected ring: In the event the ring disconnects at the weld joint, discard and replace with a new ring.

***Note:** Diaphragms may interfere with proper ring placement, and therefore, are not recommended for use as an additional form of contraception.

Dosage Forms Ring, vaginal: Ethinyl estradiol 0.015 mg/day and etonogestrel 0.12 mg/day (1s) [3-week duration]

ethinyl estradiol and levonorgestrel (ETH in il es tra DYE ole & LEE voe nor jes trel)

Sound-Alike/Look-Alike Issues

Alesse® may be confused with Aleve®

Nordette® may be confused with Nicorette®

PREVEN® may be confused with Prevnar®

Tri-Levlen® may be confused with Trilafon®

Triphasil® may be confused with Tri-Norinyl®

Synonyms levonorgestrel and ethinyl estradiol

U.S./Canadian Brand Names Alesse® [US/Can]; Aviane™ [US]; Enpresse™ [US]; Lessina™ [US]; Levlen® [US]; Levlite™ [US]; Levora® [US]; Lutera™ [US]; Min-Ovral® [Can]; Nordette® [US]; Portia™ [US]; PREVEN® [US]; Seasonale® [US]; Seasonique™ [US]; Tri-Levlen® [US]; Triphasil® [US/Can]; Triquilar® [Can]; Trivora® [US]

Therapeutic Category Contraceptive, Oral

Use Prevention of pregnancy; postcoital contraception

Usual Dosage Oral: Adults: Female:

Contraception, 28-day cycle:

Schedule 1 (Sunday starter): Dose begins on first Sunday after onset of menstruation; if the menstrual period starts on Sunday, take first tablet that very same day. With a Sunday start, an additional method of contraception should be used until after the first 7 days of consecutive administration:

For 21-tablet package: 1 tablet/day for 21 consecutive days, followed by 7 days off of the medication; a new course begins on the 8th day after the last tablet is taken

For 28-tablet package: 1 tablet/day without interruption

Schedule 2 (Day 1 starter): Dose starts on first day of menstrual cycle taking 1 tablet/day:

For 21-tablet package: 1 tablet/day for 21 consecutive days, followed by 7 days off of the medication; a new course begins on the 8th day after the last tablet is taken

For 28-tablet package: 1 tablet/day without interruption

If all doses have been taken on schedule and one menstrual period is missed, continue dosing cycle. If two consecutive menstrual periods are missed, pregnancy test is required before new dosing cycle is started.

Missed doses **monophasic formulations** (refer to package insert for complete information):

One dose missed: Take as soon as remembered or take 2 tablets next day

Two consecutive doses missed in the first 2 weeks: Take 2 tablets as soon as remembered or 2 tablets next 2 days. An additional method of contraception should be used for 7 days after missed dose.

Two consecutive doses missed in week 3 or three consecutive doses missed at any time: An additional method of contraception must be used for 7 days after a missed dose:

Schedule 1 (Sunday starter): Continue dose of 1 tablet daily until Sunday, then discard the rest of the pack, and a new pack should be started that same day.

Schedule 2 (Day 1 starter): Current pack should be discarded, and a new pack should be started that same day.

Missed doses **biphasic/triphasic formulations** (refer to package insert for complete information):

One dose missed: Take as soon as remembered or take 2 tablets next day.

Two consecutive doses missed in week 1 or week 2 of the pack: Take 2 tablets as soon as remembered and 2 tablets the next day. Resume taking 1 tablet daily until the pack is empty. An additional method of contraception should be used for 7 days after a missed dose.

Two consecutive doses missed in week 3 of the pack: An additional method of contraception must be used for 7 days after a missed dose.

Schedule 1 (Sunday starter): Take 1 tablet every day until Sunday. Discard the remaining pack and start a new pack of pills on the same day.

Schedule 2 (Day 1 starter): Discard the remaining pack and start a new pack the same day.

Three or more consecutive doses missed: An additional method of contraception must be used for 7 days after a missed dose.

Schedule 1 (Sunday starter): Take 1 tablet every day until Sunday; on Sunday, discard the pack and start a new pack.

Schedule 2 (Day 1 starter): Discard the remaining pack and begin new pack of tablets starting on the same day.

Contraception, 91-day cycle (extended cycle regimen): Dose begins on first Sunday after onset of menstruation; if the menstrual period starts on Sunday, take first tablet that very same day. An additional method of contraception should be used until after the first 7 days of consecutive administration:

Seasonale®: One active tablet/day for 84 consecutive days, followed by 1 inactive tablet/day for 7 days; if all doses have been taken on schedule and one menstrual period is missed, pregnancy should be ruled out prior to continuing therapy.

Sesonique™: One active tablet/day for 84 consecutive days, followed by 1 low dose estrogen tablet/day for 7 days; if all doses have been taken on schedule and one menstrual period is missed, pregnancy should be ruled out prior to continuing therapy.

Missed doses:

One dose missed: Take as soon as remembered or take 2 tablets the next day

Two consecutive doses missed: Take 2 tablets as soon as remembered or 2 tablets the next 2 days. An additional nonhormonal method of contraception should be used for 7 consecutive days after the missed dose.

Three or more consecutive doses missed: Do not take the missed doses; continue taking 1 tablet/day until pack is complete. Bleeding may occur during the following week. An additional nonhormonal method of contraception should be used for 7 consecutive days after the missed dose.

Any number of pills during week 13: Throw away the missed pills and keep taking scheduled pills until the pack is finished. A back-up method of contraception is not needed

Emergency contraception (PREVEN®): Initial: 2 tablets as soon as possible (but within 72 hours of unprotected intercourse), followed by a second dose of 2 tablets 12 hours later. Repeat dose or use antiemetic if vomiting occurs within 1 hour of dose.

Dosage Forms

Tablet, low-dose formulations:

Alesse® 28: Ethinyl estradiol 0.02 mg and levonorgestrel 0.1 mg [21 pink tablets and 7 light green inactive tablets] (28s)

Aviane™ 28: Ethinyl estradiol 0.02 mg and levonorgestrel 0.1 mg [21 orange tablets and 7 light green inactive tablets] (28s)

Lessina™ 28, Levlite™ 28: Ethinyl estradiol 0.02 mg and levonorgestrel 0.1 mg [21 pink tablets and 7 white inactive tablets] (28s)

Lutera™, Sronyx™: Ethinyl estradiol 0.02 mg and levonorgestrel 0.1 mg [21 white tablets and 7 peach inactive tablets] (28s)

Tablet, monophasic formulations:

Levlen® 28: Ethinyl estradiol 0.03 mg and levonorgestrel 0.15 mg [21 light orange tablets and 7 pink inactive tablets] (28s)

Levora® 28: Ethinyl estradiol 0.03 mg and levonorgestrel 0.15 mg [21 white tablets and 7 peach inactive tablets] (28s)

Nordette® 28: Ethinyl estradiol 0.03 mg and levonorgestrel 0.15 mg [21 light orange tablets and 7 pink inactive tablets] (28s)

Portia™ 28: Ethinyl estradiol 0.03 mg and levonorgestrel 0.15 mg [21 pink tablets and 7 white inactive tablets] (28s)

(Continued)

ethinyl estradiol and levonorgestrel *(Continued)*

Tablet, monophasic formulations [extended cycle regimen]:

Quasense™: Ethinyl estradiol 0.03 mg and levonorgestrel 0.15 mg [84 white tablets and 7 peach inactive tablets] (91s)

Seasonale®: Ethinyl estradiol 0.03 mg and levonorgestrel 0.15 mg [84 pink tablets and 7 white inactive tablets] (91s)

Seasonique™: Ethinyl estradiol 0.03 mg and levonorgestrel 0.15 mg [84 light blue-green tablets] and ethinyl estradiol 0.01 mg [7 yellow tablets] (91s)

Tablet, triphasic formulations:

Enpresse™:

Day 1-6: Ethinyl estradiol 0.03 mg and levonorgestrel 0.05 mg [6 pink tablets]
Day 7-11: Ethinyl estradiol 0.04 mg and levonorgestrel 0.075 mg [5 white tablets]
Day 12-21: Ethinyl estradiol 0.03 mg and levonorgestrel 0.125 mg [10 orange tablets]
Day 22-28: 7 light green inactive tablets (28s)

Tri-Levlen® 28, Triphasil® 28:

Day 1-6: Ethinyl estradiol 0.03 mg and levonorgestrel 0.05 mg [6 brown tablets]
Day 7-11: Ethinyl estradiol 0.04 mg and levonorgestrel 0.075 mg [5 white tablets]
Day 12-21: Ethinyl estradiol 0.03 mg and levonorgestrel 0.125 mg [10 light yellow tablets]
Day 22-28: 7 light green inactive tablets (28s)

Trivora® 28:

Day 1-6: Ethinyl estradiol 0.03 mg and levonorgestrel 0.05 mg [6 blue tablets]
Day 7-11: Ethinyl estradiol 0.04 mg and levonorgestrel 0.075 mg [5 white tablets]
Day 12-21: Ethinyl estradiol 0.03 mg and levonorgestrel 0.125 mg [10 pink tablets]
Day 22-28: 7 peach inactive tablets (28s)

ethinyl estradiol and NGM *see* ethinyl estradiol and norgestimate *on page 325*

ethinyl estradiol and norelgestromin (ETH in il es tra DYE ole & nor el JES troe min)

Synonyms norelgestromin and ethinyl estradiol

U.S./Canadian Brand Names Evra® [Can]; Ortho Evra® [US]

Therapeutic Category Contraceptive; Estrogen and Progestin Combination

Use Prevention of pregnancy

Usual Dosage Topical: Adults: Female:

Contraception: Apply one patch each week for 3 weeks (21 total days); followed by one week that is patch-free. Each patch should be applied on the same day each week ("patch change day") and only one patch should be worn at a time. No more than 7 days should pass during the patch-free interval.

Schedule 1 (Sunday starter): Dose begins on first Sunday after onset of menstruation; if the menstrual period starts on Sunday, apply one patch that very same day. **With a Sunday start, an additional method of contraception (nonhormonal) should be used until after the first 7 days of consecutive administration.** Each patch change will then occur on Sunday.

Schedule 2 (Day 1 starter): Dose starts on first day of menstrual cycle, applying one patch during the first 24 hours of menstrual cycle. No back-up method of contraception is needed as long as the patch is applied on the first day of cycle. Each patch change will then occur on that same day of the week.

Additional dosing considerations:

No bleeding during patch-free week/missed menstrual period: If patch has been applied as directed, continue treatment on usual "patch change day". If used correctly, no bleeding during patch-free week does not necessarily indicate pregnancy. However, if no withdrawal bleeding occurs for 2 consecutive cycles, pregnancy should be ruled out. If patch has not been applied as directed, and one menstrual period is missed, pregnancy should be ruled out prior to continuing treatment.

If a patch becomes partially or completely detached for <24 hours: Try to reapply to same place, or replace with a new patch immediately. Do not reapply if patch is no longer sticky, if it is sticking to itself or another surface, or if it has material sticking to it.

If a patch becomes partially or completely detached for >24 hours (or time period is unknown): Apply a new patch and use this day of the week as the new "patch change day" from this point on. **An additional method of contraception (nonhormonal) should be used until after the first 7 days of consecutive administration.**

Switching from oral contraceptives: Apply first patch on the first day of withdrawal bleeding. If there is no bleeding within 5 days of taking the last active tablet, pregnancy must first be ruled out. If patch is applied later than the first day of bleeding, **an additional method of contraception (nonhormonal) should be used until after the first 7 days of consecutive administration**

Use after childbirth: Therapy should not be started <4 weeks after childbirth. Pregnancy should be ruled out prior to treatment if menstrual periods have not restarted. **An additional method of contraception (nonhormonal) should be used until after the first 7 days of consecutive administration.**

Use after abortion or miscarriage: Therapy may be started immediately if abortion/miscarriage occur within the first trimester. If therapy is not started within 5 days, follow instructions for first time use. If abortion/miscarriage occur during the second trimester, therapy should not be started for at least 4 weeks. Follow directions for use after childbirth.

Dosage Forms [CAN] = Canadian brand name

Note: The formulation available in Canada differs from the U.S. product in both composition and the manufacturing process (although delivery rates appear similar).

Patch, transdermal:

Ortho Evra®: Ethinyl estradiol 0.75 mg and norelgestromin 6 mg [releases ethinyl estradiol 20 mcg and norelgestromin 150 mcg per day] (1s, 3s)

Evra® [CAN]: Ethinyl estradiol 0.6 mg and norelgestromin 6 mg [releases ethinyl estradiol 20 mcg and norelgestromin 150 mcg per day] (1s, 3s) [Not available in U.S.]

ethinyl estradiol and norethindrone (ETH in il es tra DYE ole & nor eth IN drone)

Sound-Alike/Look-Alike Issues

femhrt® may be confused with Femara®
Modicon® may be confused with Mylicon®
Norinyl® may be confused with Nardil®
Tri-Norinyl® may be confused with Triphasil®

Synonyms norethindrone acetate and ethinyl estradiol

U.S./Canadian Brand Names Aranelle™ [US]; Brevicon® 0.5/35 [Can]; Brevicon® 1/35 [Can]; Brevicon® [US]; Estrostep® Fe [US]; femhrt® [US/Can]; Junel™ Fe [US]; Junel™ [US]; Leena™ [US]; Loestrin® 24 Fe [US]; Loestrin® Fe [US]; Loestrin® [US]; Loestrin™ 1.5/30 [Can]; Microgestin™ Fe [US]; Microgestin™ [US]; Minestrin™ 1/20 [Can]; Modicon® [US]; Necon® 0.5/35 [US]; Necon® 1/35 [US]; Necon® 10/11 [US]; Necon® 7/7/7 [US]; Norinyl® 1+35 [US]; Nortrel™ 7/7/7 [US]; Nortrel™ [US]; Ortho-Novum® [US]; Ortho® 0.5/35 [Can]; Ortho® 1/35 [Can]; Ortho® 7/7/7 [Can]; Ovcon® [US]; Select™ 1/35 [Can]; Synphasic® [Can]; Tri-Norinyl® [US]

Therapeutic Category Contraceptive, Oral

Use Prevention of pregnancy; treatment of acne; moderate to severe vasomotor symptoms associated with menopause; prevention of osteoporosis (in women at significant risk only)

Usual Dosage Oral:

Adolescents ≥15 years and Adults: Female: Acne: Estrostep®: Refer to dosing for contraception

Adults: Female:

Moderate-to-severe vasomotor symptoms associated with menopause: Initial: femhrt® 0.5/2.5: 1 tablet daily; patient should be reevaluated at 3- to 6-month intervals to determine if treatment is still necessary; patient should be maintained at the lowest effective dose

Prevention of osteoporosis: Initial: femhrt® 0.5/2.5: 1 tablet daily; patient should be maintained on the lowest effective dose

Contraception:

Schedule 1 (Sunday starter): Dose begins on first Sunday after onset of menstruation; if the menstrual period starts on Sunday, take first tablet that very same day. With a Sunday start, an additional method of contraception should be used until after the first 7 days of consecutive administration.

For 21-tablet package: Dosage is 1 tablet daily for 21 consecutive days, followed by 7 days off of the medication; a new course begins on the 8th day after the last tablet is taken.

For 28-tablet package: Dosage is 1 tablet daily without interruption.

Schedule 2 (Day 1 starter): Dose starts on first day of menstrual cycle taking 1 tablet daily.

For 21-tablet package: Dosage is 1 tablet daily for 21 consecutive days, followed by 7 days off of the medication; a new course begins on the 8th day after the last tablet is taken.

For 28-tablet package: Dosage is 1 tablet daily without interruption.

If all doses have been taken on schedule and one menstrual period is missed, continue dosing cycle. If two consecutive menstrual periods are missed, pregnancy test is required before new dosing cycle is started.

Missed doses **monophasic formulations** (refer to package insert for complete information):

One dose missed: Take as soon as remembered or take 2 tablets next day Two consecutive doses missed in the first 2 weeks: Take 2 tablets as soon as remembered or 2 tablets next 2 days. An additional method of contraception should be used for 7 days after missed dose.

Two consecutive doses missed in week 3 or three consecutive doses missed at any time: An additional method of contraception must be used for 7 days after a missed dose.

Schedule 1 (Sunday starter): Continue dose of 1 tablet daily until Sunday, then discard the rest of the pack, and a new pack should be started that same day.

(Continued)

ethinyl estradiol and norethindrone *(Continued)*

Schedule 2 (Day 1 starter): Current pack should be discarded, and a new pack should be started that same day.

Missed doses **biphasic/triphasic formulations** (refer to package insert for complete information):

One dose missed: Take as soon as remembered or take 2 tablets next day.

Two consecutive doses missed in week 1 or week 2 of the pack: Take 2 tablets as soon as remembered and 2 tablets the next day. Resume taking 1 tablet daily until the pack is empty. An additional method of contraception should be used for 7 days after a missed dose.

Two consecutive doses missed in week 3 of the pack: An additional method of contraception must be used for 7 days after a missed dose.

Schedule 1 (Sunday Starter): Take 1 tablet every day until Sunday. Discard the remaining pack and start a new pack of pills on the same day.

Schedule 2 (Day 1 starter): Discard the remaining pack and start a new pack the same day.

Three or more consecutive doses missed: An additional method of contraception must be used for 7 days after a missed dose.

Schedule 1 (Sunday Starter): Take 1 tablet every day until Sunday; on Sunday, discard the pack and start a new pack.

Schedule 2 (Day 1 Starter): Discard the remaining pack and begin new pack of tablets starting on the same day.

Dosage Forms

Tablet (femhrt®):

1/5: Ethinyl estradiol 5 mcg and norethindrone acetate 1 mg [white tablets]

0.5/2.5: Ethinyl estradiol 2.5 mcg and norethindrone acetate 0.5 mg [white tablets]

Tablet, monophasic formulations:

Brevicon®: Ethinyl estradiol 0.035 mg and norethindrone 0.5 mg [21 blue tablets and 7 orange inactive tablets] (28s)

Junel™ 21 1/20: Ethinyl estradiol 0.02 mg and norethindrone acetate 1 mg [yellow tablets] (21s)

Junel™ 21 1.5/30: Ethinyl estradiol 0.03 mg and norethindrone acetate 1.5 mg [pink tablets] (21s)

Junel™ Fe 1/20: Ethinyl estradiol 0.02 mg and norethindrone acetate 1 mg [21 yellow tablets] and ferrous fumarate 75 mg [7 brown tablets] (28s)

Junel™ Fe 1.5/30: Ethinyl estradiol 0.03 mg and norethindrone acetate 1.5 mg [21 pink tablets] and ferrous fumarate 75 mg [7 brown tablets] (28s)

Loestrin® 21 1/20, Microgestin™ 1/20: Ethinyl estradiol 0.02 mg and norethindrone acetate 1 mg [white tablets] (21s)

Loestrin® 21 1.5/30, Microgestin™ 1.5/30: Ethinyl estradiol 0.03 mg and norethindrone acetate 1.5 mg [green tablets] (21s)

Loestrin® 24 Fe: 1/20: Ethinyl estradiol 0.02 mg and norethindrone acetate 1 mg [24 white tablets] and ferrous fumarate 75 mg [4 brown tablets] (28s)

Loestrin® Fe 1/20, Microgestin™ Fe 1/20: Ethinyl estradiol 0.02 mg and norethindrone acetate 1 mg [21 white tablets] and ferrous fumarate 75 mg [7 brown tablets] (28s)

Loestrin® Fe 1.5/30, Microgestin™ Fe 1.5/30: Ethinyl estradiol 0.03 mg and norethindrone acetate 1.5 mg [21 green tablets] and ferrous fumarate 75 mg [7 brown tablets] (28s)

Modicon® 28: Ethinyl estradiol 0.035 mg and norethindrone 0.5 mg [21 white tablets and 7 green inactive tablets] (28s)

Necon® 0.5/35-28: Ethinyl estradiol 0.035 mg and norethindrone 0.5 mg [21 light yellow tablets and 7 white inactive tablets] (28s)

Necon® 1/35-28: Ethinyl estradiol 0.035 mg and norethindrone 1 mg [21 dark yellow tablets and 7 white inactive tablets] (28s)

Norinyl® 1+35: Ethinyl estradiol 0.035 mg and norethindrone 1 mg [21 yellow-green tablets and 7 orange inactive tablets] (28s)

Nortrel™ 0.5/35 mg:

Ethinyl estradiol 0.035 mg and norethindrone 0.5 mg [light yellow tablets] (21s)

Ethinyl estradiol 0.035 mg and norethindrone 0.5 mg [21 light yellow tablets and 7 white inactive tablets] (28s)

Nortrel™ 1/35 mg:

Ethinyl estradiol 0.035 mg and norethindrone 1 mg [yellow tablets] (21s)

Ethinyl estradiol 0.035 mg and norethindrone 1 mg [21 yellow tablets and 7 white inactive tablets] (28s)

Ortho-Novum® 1/35 28: Ethinyl estradiol 0.035 mg and norethindrone 1 mg [21 peach tablets and 7 green inactive tablets] (28s)

Ovcon® 35 21-day: Ethinyl estradiol 0.035 mg and norethindrone 0.4 mg [peach tablets] (21s)

Ovcon® 35 28-day: Ethinyl estradiol 0.035 mg and norethindrone 0.4 mg [21 peach tablets and 7 green inactive tablets] (28s)

Ovcon® 50: Ethinyl estradiol 0.05 mg and norethindrone 1 mg [21 yellow tablets and 7 green inactive tablets] (28s)

Tablet, biphasic formulations:

Necon® 10/11-28:

Day 1-10: Ethinyl estradiol 0.035 mg and norethindrone 0.5 mg [10 light yellow tablets]
Day 11-21: Ethinyl estradiol 0.035 mg and norethindrone 1 mg [11 dark yellow tablets]
Day 22-28: 7 white inactive tablets (28s)

Ortho-Novum® 10/11-28:

Day 1-10: Ethinyl estradiol 0.035 mg and norethindrone 0.5 mg [10 white tablets]
Day 11-21: Ethinyl estradiol 0.035 mg and norethindrone 1 mg [11 peach tablets]
Day 22-28: 7 green inactive tablets (28s)

Tablet, triphasic formulations:

Aranelle™:

Day 1-7: Ethinyl estradiol 0.035 mg and norethindrone 0.5 mg [7 light yellow tablets]
Day 8-16: Ethinyl estradiol 0.035 mg and norethindrone 1 mg [9 white tablets]
Day 17-21: Ethinyl estradiol 0.035 mg and norethindrone 0.5 mg [5 light yellow tablets]
Day 22-28: 7 peach inactive tablets (28s)

Estrostep® Fe:

Day 1-5: Ethinyl estradiol 0.02 mg and norethindrone acetate 1 mg [5 white triangular tablets]
Day 6-12: Ethinyl estradiol 0.03 mg and norethindrone acetate 1 mg [7 white square tablets]
Day 13-21: Ethinyl estradiol 0.035 mg and norethindrone acetate 1 mg [9 white round tablets]
Day 22-28: Ferrous fumarate 75 mg [7 brown tablets] (28s)

Leena™:

Day 1-7: Ethinyl estradiol 0.035 mg and norethindrone 0.5 mg [7 light blue tablets]
Day 8-16: Ethinyl estradiol 0.035 mg and norethindrone 1 mg [9 light yellow-green tablets]
Day 17-21: Ethinyl estradiol 0.035 mg and norethindrone 0.5 mg [5 light blue tablets]
Day 22-28: 7 orange inactive tablets (28s)

Necon® 7/7/7, Ortho-Novum® 7/7/7 28:

Day 1-7: Ethinyl estradiol 0.035 mg and norethindrone 0.5 mg [7 white tablets]
Day 8-14: Ethinyl estradiol 0.035 mg and norethindrone 0.75 mg [7 light peach tablets]
Day 15-21: Ethinyl estradiol 0.035 mg and norethindrone 1 mg [7 peach tablets]
Day 22-28: 7 green inactive tablets (28s)

Nortrel™ 7/7/7 28:

Day 1-7: Ethinyl estradiol 0.035 mg and norethindrone 0.5 mg [7 light yellow tablets]
Day 8-14: Ethinyl estradiol 0.035 mg and norethindrone 0.75 mg [7 blue tablets]
Day 15-21: Ethinyl estradiol 0.035 mg and norethindrone 1 mg [7 peach tablets]
Day 22-28: 7 white inactive tablets (28s)

Ortho-Novum® 7/7/7 28:

Day 1-7: Ethinyl estradiol 0.035 mg and norethindrone 0.5 mg [7 white tablets]
Day 8-14: Ethinyl estradiol 0.035 mg and norethindrone 0.75 mg [7 light peach tablets]
Day 15-21: Ethinyl estradiol 0.035 mg and norethindrone 1 mg [7 peach tablets]
Day 22-28: 7 green inactive tablets (28s)

Tri-Norinyl® 28:

Day 1-7: Ethinyl estradiol 0.035 mg and norethindrone 0.5 mg [7 blue tablets]
Day 8-16: Ethinyl estradiol 0.035 mg and norethindrone 1 mg [9 yellow-green tablets]
Day 17-21: Ethinyl estradiol 0.035 mg and norethindrone 0.5 mg [5 blue tablets]
Day 22-28: 7 orange inactive tablets (28s)

ethinyl estradiol and norgestimate (ETH in il es tra DYE ole & nor JES ti mate)

Sound-Alike/Look-Alike Issues

Ortho-Cyclen® may be confused with Ortho-Cept®

Synonyms ethinyl estradiol and NGM; norgestimate and ethinyl estradiol

U.S./Canadian Brand Names Cyclen® [Can]; MonoNessa™ [US]; Ortho Tri-Cyclen® Lo [US]; Ortho Tri-Cyclen® [US]; Ortho-Cyclen® [US]; Previfem™ [US]; Sprintec™ [US]; Tri-Cyclen® Lo [Can]; Tri-Cyclen® [Can]; Tri-Previfem™ [US]; Tri-Sprintec™ [US]; TriNessa™ [US]

Therapeutic Category Contraceptive, Oral

Use Prevention of pregnancy; treatment of acne

Usual Dosage Oral:

Children ≥15 years and Adults: Female: Acne (Ortho Tri-Cyclen®): Refer to dosing for contraception
(Continued)

ethinyl estradiol and norgestimate *(Continued)*

Adults: Female:

Contraception:

Schedule 1 (Sunday starter): Dose begins on first Sunday after onset of menstruation; if the menstrual period starts on Sunday, take first tablet that very same day. **With a Sunday start, an additional method of contraception should be used until after the first 7 days of consecutive administration.**

For 21-tablet package: Dosage is 1 tablet daily for 21 consecutive days, followed by 7 days off of the medication; a new course begins on the 8th day after the last tablet is taken.

For 28-tablet package: Dosage is 1 tablet daily without interruption.

Schedule 2 (Day 1 starter): Dose starts on first day of menstrual cycle taking 1 tablet daily.

For 21-tablet package: Dosage is 1 tablet daily for 21 consecutive days, followed by 7 days off of the medication; a new course begins on the 8th day after the last tablet is taken.

For 28-tablet package: Dosage is 1 tablet daily without interruption.

If all doses have been taken on schedule and one menstrual period is missed, continue dosing cycle. If two consecutive menstrual periods are missed, pregnancy test is required before new dosing cycle is started.

Missed doses **monophasic formulations** (refer to package insert for complete information):

One dose missed: Take as soon as remembered or take 2 tablets next day

Two consecutive doses missed in the first 2 weeks: Take 2 tablets as soon as remembered or 2 tablets next 2 days. **An additional method of contraception should be used for 7 days after missed dose.**

Two consecutive doses missed in week 3 or three consecutive doses missed at any time: **An additional method of contraception must be used for 7 days after a missed dose:**

Schedule 1 (Sunday starter): Continue dose of 1 tablet daily until Sunday, then discard the rest of the pack, and a new pack should be started that same day.

Schedule 2 (Day 1 starter): Current pack should be discarded, and a new pack should be started that same day.

Missed doses **biphasic/triphasic formulations** (refer to package insert for complete information):

One dose missed: Take as soon as remembered or take 2 tablets next day.

Two consecutive doses missed in week 1 or week 2 of the pack: Take 2 tablets as soon as remembered and 2 tablets the next day. Resume taking 1 tablet daily until the pack is empty. **An additional method of contraception must be used for 7 days after a missed dose.**

Two consecutive doses missed in week 3 of the pack. **An additional method of contraception must be used for 7 days after a missed dose.**

Schedule 1 (Sunday starter): Take 1 tablet every day until Sunday. Discard the remaining pack and start a new pack of pills on the same day.

Schedule 2 (Day 1 starter): Discard the remaining pack and start a new pack the same day.

Three or more consecutive doses missed. **An additional method of contraception must be used for 7 days after a missed dose.**

Schedule 1 (Sunday starter): Take 1 tablet every day until Sunday; on Sunday, discard the pack and start a new pack.

Schedule 2 (Day 1 starter): Discard the remaining pack and begin new pack of tablets starting on the same day.

Dosage Forms

Tablet, monophasic formulations:

MonoNessa™, Ortho-Cyclen®: Ethinyl estradiol 0.035 mg and norgestimate 0.25 mg [21 blue tablets and 7 green inactive tablets] (28s)

Previfem™: Ethinyl estradiol 0.035 mg and norgestimate 0.25 mg [21 blue tablets and 7 teal inactive tablets] (28s)

Sprintec™: Ethinyl estradiol 0.035 mg and norgestimate 0.25 mg [21 blue tablets and 7 white inactive tablets] (28s)

Tablet, triphasic formulations:

Ortho Tri-Cyclen®, TriNessa™:

Day 1-7: Ethinyl estradiol 0.035 mg and norgestimate 0.18 mg [7 white tablets]

Day 8-14: Ethinyl estradiol 0.035 mg and norgestimate 0.215 mg [7 light blue tablets]

Day 15-21: Ethinyl estradiol 0.035 mg and norgestimate 0.25 mg [7 blue tablets]

Day 22-28: 7 green inactive tablets (28s)

Tri-Previfem™:

Day 1-7: Ethinyl estradiol 0.035 mg and norgestimate 0.18 mg [7 white tablets]

Day 8-14: Ethinyl estradiol 0.035 mg and norgestimate 0.215 mg [7 light blue tablets]

Day 15-21: Ethinyl estradiol 0.035 mg and norgestimate 0.25 mg [7 blue tablets]

Day 22-28: 7 teal inactive tablets (28s)

Tri-Sprintec™:

Day 1-7: Ethinyl estradiol 0.035 mg and norgestimate 0.18 mg [7 gray tablets]

Day 8-14: Ethinyl estradiol 0.035 mg and norgestimate 0.215 mg [7 light blue tablets]
Day 15-21: Ethinyl estradiol 0.035 mg and norgestimate 0.25 mg [7 blue tablets]
Day 22-28: 7 white inactive tablets (28s)

Ortho Tri-Cyclen® Lo:
Day 1-7: Ethinyl estradiol 0.025 mg and norgestimate 0.18 mg [7 white tablets]
Day 8-14: Ethinyl estradiol 0.025 mg and norgestimate 0.215 mg [7 light blue tablets]
Day 15-21: Ethinyl estradiol 0.025 mg and norgestimate 0.25 mg [7 dark blue tablets]
Day 22-28: 7 green inactive tablets (28s)

ethinyl estradiol and norgestrel (ETH in il es tra DYE ole & nor JES trel)

Synonyms morning after pill; norgestrel and ethinyl estradiol

U.S./Canadian Brand Names Cryselle™ [US]; Lo/Ovral® [US]; Low-Ogestrel® [US]; Ogestrel® [US]; Ovral® [Can]

Therapeutic Category Contraceptive, Oral

Use Prevention of pregnancy; postcoital contraceptive or "morning after" pill

Usual Dosage Oral: Adults: Female:

Contraception:

Schedule 1 (Sunday starter): Dose begins on first Sunday after onset of menstruation; if the menstrual period starts on Sunday, take first tablet that very same day. **With a Sunday start, an additional method of contraception should be used until after the first 7 days of consecutive administration.**

For 21-tablet package: Dosage is 1 tablet daily for 21 consecutive days, followed by 7 days off of the medication; a new course begins on the 8th day after the last tablet is taken.

For 28-tablet package: Dosage is 1 tablet daily without interruption.

Schedule 2 (Day 1 starter): Dose starts on first day of menstrual cycle taking 1 tablet daily.

For 21-tablet package: Dosage is 1 tablet daily for 21 consecutive days, followed by 7 days off of the medication; a new course begins on the 8th day after the last tablet is taken.

For 28-tablet package: Dosage is 1 tablet daily without interruption.

If all doses have been taken on schedule and one menstrual period is missed, continue dosing cycle. If two consecutive menstrual periods are missed, pregnancy test is required before new dosing cycle is started.

Missed doses **monophasic formulations** (refer to package insert for complete information):

One dose missed: Take as soon as remembered or take 2 tablets next day

Two consecutive doses missed in the first 2 weeks: Take 2 tablets as soon as remembered or 2 tablets next 2 days. **An additional method of contraception should be used for 7 days after missed dose.**

Two consecutive doses missed in week 3 or three consecutive doses missed at any time:

Schedule 1 (Sunday starter): Continue to take 1 tablet daily until Sunday, then discard the rest of the pack, and a new pack is started that same day.

Schedule 2 (Day 1 starter): Current pack should be discarded, and a new pack started that same day. **An additional method of contraception should be used for 7 days after missed dose.**

Postcoital contraception:

Ethinyl estradiol 0.03 mg and norgestrel 0.3 mg formulation: 4 tablets within 72 hours of unprotected intercourse and 4 tablets 12 hours after first dose

Ethinyl estradiol 0.05 mg and norgestrel 0.5 mg formulation: 2 tablets within 72 hours of unprotected intercourse and 2 tablets 12 hours after first dose

Dosage Forms

Tablet, monophasic formulations:

Cryselle™: Ethinyl estradiol 0.03 mg and norgestrel 0.3 mg [21 white tablets and 7 light green inactive tablets] (28s)

Low-Ogestrel® 28: Ethinyl estradiol 0.03 mg and norgestrel 0.3 mg [21 white tablets and 7 peach inactive tablets] (28s)

Lo/Ovral® 28: Ethinyl estradiol 0.03 mg and norgestrel 0.3 mg [21 white tablets and 7 pink inactive tablets] (28s)

Ogestrel® 28: Ethinyl estradiol 0.05 mg and norgestrel 0.5 mg [21 white tablets and 7 peach inactive tablets] (28s)

ethiodized oil *see* radiological/contrast media (ionic) *on page 728*

Ethiodol® [US] *see* radiological/contrast media (ionic) *on page 728*

ethiofos *see* amifostine *on page 40*

ethionamide (e thye on AM ide)

U.S./Canadian Brand Names Trecator® [US/Can]

Therapeutic Category Antimycobacterial Agent

Use Treatment of tuberculosis and other mycobacterial diseases, in conjunction with other antituberculosis agents, when first-line agents have failed or resistance has been demonstrated

Usual Dosage Oral:

Children: 15-20 mg/kg/day in 2-3 divided doses, not to exceed 1 g/day

Adults: 15-20 mg/kg/day; initiate dose at 250 mg/day for 1-2 days, then increase to 250 mg twice daily for 1-2 days, with gradual increases to highest tolerated dose; average adult dose: 750 mg/day (maximum: 1 g/day in 3-4 divided doses)

Dosage Forms Tablet: 250 mg

Ethmozine® [US/Can] *see* moricizine *on page 565*

ethosuximide (eth oh SUKS i mide)

Sound-Alike/Look-Alike Issues

ethosuximide may be confused with methsuximide

Zarontin® may be confused with Xalatan®, Zantac®, Zaroxolyn®

U.S./Canadian Brand Names Zarontin® [US/Can]

Therapeutic Category Anticonvulsant

Use Management of absence (petit mal) seizures

Usual Dosage Oral:

Children 3-6 years: Initial: 250 mg/day (or 15 mg/kg/day) in 2 divided doses; increase every 4-7 days; usual maintenance dose: 15-40 mg/kg/day in 2 divided doses

Children >6 years and Adults: Initial: 250 mg twice daily; increase by 250 mg as needed every 4-7 days, up to 1.5 g/day in 2 divided doses; usual maintenance dose: 20-40 mg/kg/day in 2 divided doses

Dosage Forms

Capsule: 250 mg

Syrup: 250 mg/5 mL (473 mL) [contains sodium benzoate; raspberry flavor]

ethotoin (ETH oh toyn)

Synonyms ethylphenylhydantoin

U.S./Canadian Brand Names Peganone® [US/Can]

Therapeutic Category Hydantoin

Use Generalized tonic-clonic or complex-partial seizures

Usual Dosage Oral:

Children: 30-60 mg/kg/day or 250 mg twice daily, may be increased up to 2-3 g/day

Adults: 250 mg 4 times/day after meals, may be increased up to 3 g/day in divided doses 4 times/day

Dosage Forms Tablet: 250 mg

ETH-Oxydose™ [Can] *see* oxycodone *on page 626*

ethoxynaphthamido penicillin sodium *see* nafcillin *on page 574*

Ethrane® [US] *see* enflurane *on page 292*

ethyl alcohol *see* alcohol (ethyl) *on page 25*

ethyl aminobenzoate *see* benzocaine *on page 99*

ethyl chloride (ETH il KLOR ide)

Synonyms chloroethane

U.S./Canadian Brand Names Gebauer's Ethyl Chloride® [US]

Therapeutic Category Local Anesthetic

Use Local anesthetic in minor operative procedures and to relieve pain caused by insect stings and burns, and irritation caused by myofascial and visceral pain syndromes

Usual Dosage Dosage varies with use

Dosage Forms Aerosol: 100% (103 mL) [available as a fine-point or medium spray]

ethyl chloride and dichlorotetrafluoroethane

(ETH il KLOR ide & dye klor oh te tra floo or oh ETH ane)

Synonyms dichlorotetrafluoroethane and ethyl chloride

U.S./Canadian Brand Names Fluro-Ethyl® [US]

Therapeutic Category Local Anesthetic

Use Topical refrigerant anesthetic to control pain associated with minor surgical procedures, dermabrasion, injections, contusions, and minor strains

Usual Dosage Press gently on side of spray valve allowing the liquid to emerge as a fine mist approximately 2" to 4" from site of application

Dosage Forms Aerosol: Ethyl chloride 25% and dichlorotetrafluoroethane 75% (148 mL)

ethyl esters of omega-3 fatty acids *see* omega-3-acid ethyl esters *on page 615*

ethylphenylhydantoin *see* ethotoin *on previous page*

ethynodiol diacetate and ethinyl estradiol *see* ethinyl estradiol and ethynodiol diacetate *on page 319*

Ethyol® [US/Can] *see* amifostine *on page 40*

Etibi® [Can] *see* ethambutol *on page 316*

etidronate and calcium *(Canada only)* (e ti DROE nate & KAL see um)

Synonyms calcium carbonate and etidronate disodium

U.S./Canadian Brand Names Didrocal™ [Can]

Therapeutic Category Bisphosphonate Derivative; Calcium Salt

Use Treatment and prevention of postmenopausal osteoporosis; prevention of corticosteroid-induced osteoporosis

Usual Dosage Note: 90-day treatment regimen involves sequential administration of two products within the packaging; not to be taken concurrently. The first blister card contains white tablets containing etidronate disodium, while the remaining four blister cards contains blue, capsule-shaped tablets containing calcium carbonate.

Oral: Adults: Etidronate disodium 400 mg once daily for 14 days, followed by calcium carbonate 1250 mg (500 mg elemental calcium) once daily for 76 days

Dosage Forms [CAN] = Canadian brand name

Combination package [each package contains five blister cards (90-day supply)]:

Didrocal™ [CAN; not available in the U.S.]:

Tablet, etidronate disodium 400 mg (14s) [first card (white tablets)]

Tablet, calcium carbonate: 1250 mg (76s) [equivalent to elemental calcium 500 mg; remaining cards (blue tablets)]

etidronate disodium (e ti DROE nate dye SOW dee um)

Sound-Alike/Look-Alike Issues

etidronate may be confused with etidocaine, etomidate, etretinate

Synonyms EHDP; sodium etidronate

U.S./Canadian Brand Names Didronel® [US/Can]; Gen-Etidronate [Can]

Therapeutic Category Bisphosphonate Derivative

Use Symptomatic treatment of Paget disease and heterotopic ossification due to spinal cord injury or after total hip replacement, hypercalcemia associated with malignancy

Usual Dosage Oral: Adults:

Paget's disease:

Initial: 5-10 mg/kg/day (not to exceed 6 months) or 11-20 mg/kg/day (not to exceed 3 months). Doses >20 mg/kg/day are **not** recommended.

Retreatment: Initiate only after etidronate-free period ≥90 days. Monitor patients every 3-6 months. Retreatment regimens are the same as for initial treatment.

Heterotopic ossification:

Caused by spinal cord injury: 20 mg/kg/day for 2 weeks, then 10 mg/kg/day for 10 weeks; total treatment period: 12 weeks

Complicating total hip replacement: 20 mg/kg/day for 1 month preoperatively then 20 mg/kg/day for 3 months postoperatively; total treatment period is 4 months

Dosage Forms Tablet: 200 mg, 400 mg

etodolac (ee toe DOE lak)

Sound-Alike/Look-Alike Issues

Lodine® may be confused with codeine, iodine, Iopidine®, Lopid®

(Continued)

etodolac *(Continued)*

Synonyms etodolic acid

U.S./Canadian Brand Names Apo-Etodolac® [Can]; Lodine® [Can]; Utradol™ [Can]

Therapeutic Category Analgesic, Nonnarcotic; Nonsteroidal Antiinflammatory Drug (NSAID)

Use Acute and long-term use in the management of signs and symptoms of osteoarthritis; rheumatoid arthritis and juvenile rheumatoid arthritis; management of acute pain

Usual Dosage Note: For chronic conditions, response is usually observed within 2 weeks.

Children 6-16 years: Oral: Juvenile rheumatoid arthritis (Lodine® XL):

20-30 kg: 400 mg once daily
31-45 kg: 600 mg once daily
46-60 kg: 800 mg once daily
>60 kg: 1000 mg once daily

Adults: Oral:

Acute pain: 200-400 mg every 6-8 hours, as needed, not to exceed total daily doses of 1000 mg
Rheumatoid arthritis, osteoarthritis: 400 mg 2 times/day **or** 300 mg 2-3 times/day **or** 500 mg 2 times/day (doses >1000 mg/day have not been evaluated)
Lodine® XL: 400-1000 mg once daily

Dosage Forms [DSC] = Discontinued product

Capsule: 200 mg, 300 mg
Lodine®: 200 mg, 300 mg [DSC]
Tablet: 400 mg, 500 mg
Tablet, extended release (Lodine® XL): 400 mg, 500 mg [DSC]

etodolic acid *see* etodolac *on previous page*

EtOH *see* alcohol (ethyl) *on page 25*

etomidate (e TOM i date)

Sound-Alike/Look-Alike Issues

etomidate may be confused with etidronate

U.S./Canadian Brand Names Amidate® [US/Can]

Therapeutic Category General Anesthetic

Use Induction and maintenance of general anesthesia

Usual Dosage Children >10 years and Adults: I.V.: Initial: 0.2-0.6 mg/kg over 30-60 seconds for induction of anesthesia; maintenance: 5-20 mcg/kg/minute

Dosage Forms Injection, solution: 2 mg/mL (10 mL, 20 mL) [contains propylene glycol 35% v/v]

etonogestrel and ethinyl estradiol *see* ethinyl estradiol and etonogestrel *on page 319*

Etopophos® [US] *see* etoposide phosphate *on next page*

etoposide (e toe POE side)

Sound-Alike/Look-Alike Issues

etoposide may be confused with teniposide
VePesid® may be confused with Versed

Synonyms epipodophyllotoxin; VP-16; VP-16-213

U.S./Canadian Brand Names Toposar® [US]; VePesid® [US/Can]

Therapeutic Category Antineoplastic Agent

Use Treatment of lymphomas, ANLL, lung, testicular, bladder, and prostate carcinoma, hepatoma, rhabdomyosarcoma, uterine carcinoma, neuroblastoma, mycosis fungoides, Kaposi sarcoma, histiocytosis, gestational trophoblastic disease, Ewing sarcoma, Wilms tumor, and brain tumors

Usual Dosage Refer to individual protocols:

Adults:

Small cell lung cancer (in combination with other approved chemotherapeutic drugs):

Oral: Due to poor bioavailability, oral doses should be twice the I.V. dose, rounded to the nearest 50 mg given once daily
I.V.: 35 mg/m²/day for 4 days or 50 mg/m²/day for 5 days every 3-4 weeks
IVPB: 60-100 mg/m²/day for 3 days (with cisplatin)
CIV: 500 mg/m² over 24 hours every 3 weeks

Testicular cancer (in combination with other approved chemotherapeutic drugs):

IVPB: 50-100 mg/m²/day for 5 days repeated every 3-4 weeks
I.V.: 100 mg/m² every other day for 3 doses repeated every 3-4 weeks

Dosage Forms
Capsule, softgel:
VePesid®: 50 mg
Injection, solution: 20 mg/mL (5 mL, 25 mL, 50 mL)
Toposar®: 20 mg/mL (5 mL, 25 mL, 50 mL) [contains alcohol 33% and polysorbate 80]

etoposide phosphate (e toe POE side FOS fate)

Sound-Alike/Look-Alike Issues
etoposide may be confused with teniposide

U.S./Canadian Brand Names Etopophos® [US]

Therapeutic Category Antineoplastic Agent

Use Treatment of refractory testicular tumors; treatment of small cell lung cancer

Usual Dosage Refer to individual protocols. Adults: **Note:** Etoposide phosphate is a prodrug of etoposide, doses should be expressed as the desired **ETOPOSIDE** dose; **not** as the etoposide phosphate dose. (eg, etoposide phosphate equivalent to ____ mg etoposide).

Small cell lung cancer (in combination with other approved chemotherapeutic drugs): I.V.: Etoposide 35 mg/m^2/day for 4 days to 50 mg/m^2/day for 5 days. Courses are repeated at 3- to 4-week intervals after adequate recovery from any toxicity.

Testicular cancer (in combination with other approved chemotherapeutic agents): I.V.: Etoposide 50-100 mg/m^2/day on days 1-5 to 100 mg/m^2/day on days 1, 3, and 5. Courses are repeated at 3- to 4-week intervals after adequate recovery from any toxicity.

Dosage Forms Injection, powder for reconstitution, as base: 100 mg

Etrafon® [Can] *see* amitriptyline and perphenazine *on page 45*

ETS-2% Topical *(Discontinued)*

Eudal®-SR [US] *see* guaifenesin and pseudoephedrine *on page 398*

Euflex® [Can] *see* flutamide *on page 360*

Euflexxa™ [US] *see* hyaluronate and derivatives *on page 416*

Euglucon® [Can] *see* glyburide *on page 387*

Eulexin® [US/Can] *see* flutamide *on page 360*

Eurax® [US] *see* crotamiton *on page 218*

Evac-Q-Mag® *(Discontinued)* *see* magnesium citrate *on page 512*

Evac-U-Gen [US-OTC] *see* senna *on page 767*

Evalose® *(Discontinued)* *see* lactulose *on page 478*

Everone® 200 [Can] *see* testosterone *on page 812*

Everone® Injection *(Discontinued)* *see* testosterone *on page 812*

Evista® [US/Can] *see* raloxifene *on page 730*

Evoclin™ [US] *see* clindamycin *on page 198*

Evoxac® [US/Can] *see* cevimeline *on page 169*

Evra® [Can] *see* ethinyl estradiol and norelgestromin *on page 322*

Exact® Acne Medication [US-OTC] *see* benzoyl peroxide *on page 102*

Excedrin® Extra Strength [US-OTC] *see* acetaminophen, aspirin, and caffeine *on page 10*

Excedrin® IB *(Discontinued)* *see* ibuprofen *on page 437*

Excedrin® Migraine [US-OTC] *see* acetaminophen, aspirin, and caffeine *on page 10*

Excedrin® P.M. [US-OTC] *see* acetaminophen and diphenhydramine *on page 7*

Exelderm® [US/Can] *see* sulconazole *on page 795*

Exelon® [US/Can] *see* rivastigmine *on page 750*

exemestane (ex e MES tane)

U.S./Canadian Brand Names Aromasin® [US/Can]

Therapeutic Category Antineoplastic Agent, Miscellaneous

Use Treatment of advanced breast cancer in postmenopausal women whose disease has progressed following tamoxifen therapy; adjuvant treatment of postmenopausal estrogen receptor-positive early breast cancer following 2-3 years of tamoxifen (for a total of 5 years of adjuvant therapy)

Usual Dosage Adults: Oral: 25 mg once daily

Dosage Forms Tablet: 25 mg

exenatide (ex EN a tide)

Synonyms AC002993; exendin-4; LY2148568

U.S./Canadian Brand Names Byetta™ [US]

Therapeutic Category Antidiabetic Agent, Incretin Mimetic

Use Management (adjunctive) of type 2 diabetes mellitus (noninsulin dependent, NIDDM)

Usual Dosage SubQ: Adults: Initial: 5 mcg twice daily within 60 minutes prior to a meal (morning and evening); after 1 month, may be increased to 10 mcg twice daily (based on response)

Dosage Forms Injection, solution [prefilled pen]: 250 mcg/mL (1.2 mL [provides 5 mcg/dose]; 2.4 mL [provides 10 mcg/dose])

exendin-4 *see* exenatide *on this page*

Exidine® Scrub *(Discontinued)* *see* chlorhexidine gluconate *on page 173*

Exjade® [US] *see* deferasirox *on page 233*

ex-lax® [US-OTC] *see* senna *on page 767*

ex-lax® Maximum Strength [US-OTC] *see* senna *on page 767*

Exorex® [US] *see* coal tar *on page 207*

Exsel® *(Discontinued)* *see* selenium sulfide *on page 767*

Extendryl [US] *see* chlorpheniramine, phenylephrine, and methscopolamine *on page 180*

Extendryl JR [US] *see* chlorpheniramine, phenylephrine, and methscopolamine *on page 180*

Extendryl SR [US] *see* chlorpheniramine, phenylephrine, and methscopolamine *on page 180*

Extra Action Cough Syrup *(Discontinued)* *see* guaifenesin and dextromethorphan *on page 394*

Exubera® [US] *see* insulin inhalation *on page 451*

EYE001 *see* pegaptanib *on page 642*

Eye-Lube-A® Solution *(Discontinued)* *see* artificial tears *on page 75*

Eye-Sed® Ophthalmic *(Discontinued)* *see* zinc sulfate *on page 888*

Eye-Sine™ [US-OTC] *see* tetrahydrozoline *on page 817*

Eyestil [Can] *see* hyaluronate and derivatives *on page 416*

Eye-Stream® [Can] *see* balanced salt solution *on page 92*

EZ-Char™ [US-OTC] *see* charcoal *on page 169*

ezetimibe (ez ET i mibe)

Sound-Alike/Look-Alike Issues

Zetia™ may be confused with Zestril®

U.S./Canadian Brand Names Ezetrol® [Can]; Zetia™ [US]

Therapeutic Category Antilipemic Agent, 2-Azetidinone

Use Use in combination with dietary therapy for the treatment of primary hypercholesterolemia (as monotherapy or in combination with HMG-CoA reductase inhibitors); homozygous sitosterolemia; homozygous familial hypercholesterolemia (in combination with atorvastatin or simvastatin); mixed hyperlipidemia (in combination with fenofibrate)

Usual Dosage Oral:

Hyperlipidemias: Children ≥10 years and Adults: 10 mg/day

Sitosterolemia: Adults: 10 mg/day

Dosage Forms Tablet: 10 mg [capsule shaped]

ezetimibe and simvastatin (ez ET i mibe & SIM va stat in)

U.S./Canadian Brand Names Vytorin™ [US]

Therapeutic Category Antilipemic Agent, 2-Azetidinone

Use Used in combination with dietary modification for the treatment of primary hypercholesterolemia and homozygous familial hypercholesterolemia

Usual Dosage Oral: Adults:

Homozygous familial hypercholesterolemia: Ezetimibe 10 mg and simvastatin 40 mg once daily or ezetimibe 10 mg and simvastatin 80 mg once daily in the evening

Hyperlipidemias: Initial: Ezetimibe 10 mg and simvastatin 20 mg once daily in the evening

Patients who require >55% reduction in LDL-C: Initial: Ezetimibe 10 mg and simvastatin 40 mg once daily

Dosage Forms Tablet:

10/10: Ezetimibe 10 mg and simvastatin 10 mg
10/20: Ezetimibe 10 mg and simvastatin 20 mg
10/40: Ezetimibe 10 mg and simvastatin 40 mg
10/80: Ezetimibe 10 mg and simvastatin 80 mg

Ezetrol® [Can] *see* ezetimibe *on previous page*

Ezide® ***(Discontinued)*** *see* hydrochlorothiazide *on page 419*

E•R•O [US-OTC] *see* carbamide peroxide *on page 145*

F_3T *see* trifluridine *on page 849*

Fabrazyme® [US/Can] *see* agalsidase beta *on page 21*

Factive® [US] *see* gemifloxacin *on page 379*

factor VIII (human) *see* antihemophilic factor (human) *on page 59*

factor VIII (recombinant) *see* antihemophilic factor (recombinant) *on page 59*

factor VIIa (recombinant) (FAK ter SEV en aye ree KOM be nant)

Sound-Alike/Look-Alike Issues

NovoSeven® may be confused with Novacet®

Synonyms coagulation factor VIIa; eptacog alfa (activated); rFVIIa

U.S./Canadian Brand Names Niastase® [Can]; NovoSeven® [US]

Therapeutic Category Antihemophilic Agent; Blood Product Derivative

Use Treatment of bleeding episodes and prevention of bleeding in surgical interventions in patients with hemophilia A or B with inhibitors to factor VIII or factor IX and in patients with congenital factor VII deficiency

Usual Dosage Children and Adults: I.V. administration only: Hemophilia A or B with inhibitors:

Bleeding episodes: 90 mcg/kg every 2 hours until hemostasis is achieved or until the treatment is judged ineffective. The dose and interval may be adjusted based upon the severity of bleeding and the degree of hemostasis achieved. For patients experiencing severe bleeds, dosing should be continued at 3- to 6-hour intervals after hemostasis has been achieved and the duration of dosing should be minimized.

Surgical interventions: 90 mcg/kg immediately before surgery, repeat at 2-hour intervals for the duration of surgery. Continue every 2 hours for 48 hours, then every 2-6 hours until healed for minor surgery; continue every 2 hours for 5 days, then every 4 hours until healed for major surgery.

Congenital factor VII deficiency: Bleeding episodes and surgical interventions: 15-30 mcg/kg every 4-6 hours until hemostasis. Doses as low as 10 mcg/kg have been effective.

Dosage Forms Injection, powder for reconstitution [preservative free]: 1.2 mg, 2.4 mg, 4.8 mg [latex free; contains sodium 0.44 mEq/mg rFVIIa, polysorbate 80]

factor IX (FAK ter nyne)

U.S./Canadian Brand Names AlphaNine® SD [US]; BeneFix® [US/Can]; Immunine® VH [Can]; Mononine® [US/Can]

Therapeutic Category Antihemophilic Agent

Use Control bleeding in patients with factor IX deficiency (hemophilia B or Christmas disease)

Usual Dosage Dosage is expressed in units of factor IX activity and must be individualized. I.V. only:

Formula for units required to raise blood level %:

AlphaNine® SD, Mononine®: Children and Adults:

Number of Factor IX Units Required = body weight (in kg) x desired Factor IX level increase (% normal) x 1 unit/kg

For example, for a 100% level a patient who has an actual level of 20%: Number of Factor IX Units needed = 70 kg x 80% x 1 Unit/kg = 5600 Units

BeneFix®:

Children <15 years:

Number of Factor IX Units Required = body weight (in kg) x desired Factor IX level increase (% normal) x 1.4 units/kg

Adults:

Number of Factor IX Units Required = body weight (in kg) x desired Factor IX level increase (% normal) x 1.2 units/kg

(Continued)

factor IX *(Continued)*

Guidelines: As a general rule, the level of factor IX required for treatment of different conditions is listed below:

Minor spontaneous hemorrhage, prophylaxis:
- Desired levels of factor IX for hemostasis: 15% to 25%
- Initial loading dose to achieve desired level: 20-30 units/kg
- Frequency of dosing: Every 12-24 hours if necessary
- Duration of treatment: 1-2 days

Moderate hemorrhage:
- Desired levels of factor IX for hemostasis: 25% to 50%
- Initial loading dose to achieve desired level: 25-50 units/kg
- Frequency of dosing: Every 12-24 hours
- Duration of treatment: 2-7 days

Major hemorrhage:
- Desired levels of factor IX for hemostasis: >50%
- Initial loading dose to achieve desired level: 30-50 units/kg
- Frequency of dosing: Every 12-24 hours, depending on half-life and measured factor IX levels (after 3-5 days, maintain at least 20% activity)
- Duration of treatment: 7-10 days, depending upon nature of insult

Surgery:
- Desired levels of factor IX for hemostasis: 50% to 100%
- Initial loading dose to achieve desired level: 50-100 units/kg
- Frequency of dosing: Every 12-24 hours, depending on half-life and measured factor IX levels
- Duration of treatment: 7-10 days, depending upon nature of insult

Dosage Forms Injection, powder for reconstitution (**Note:** Exact potency labeled on each vial):

AlphaNine® SD [human derived; solvent detergent treated; virus filtered; contains nondetectable levels of factors II, VII, X; supplied with diluent]

BeneFix® [recombinant formulation; supplied with diluent]

Mononine® [human derived; monoclonal antibody purified; contains nondetectable levels of factors II, VII, X; supplied with diluent]

factor IX complex (human) (FAK ter nyne KOM pleks HYU man)

Synonyms prothrombin complex concentrate

U.S./Canadian Brand Names Bebulin® VH [US]; Profilnine® SD [US]; Proplex® T [US]

Therapeutic Category Antihemophilic Agent

Use

Control bleeding in patients with factor IX deficiency (hemophilia B or Christmas disease) **Note:** Factor IX concentrate containing **only** factor IX is also available and preferable for this indication.

Prevention/control of bleeding in hemophilia A patients with inhibitors to factor VIII

Prevention/control of bleeding in patients with factor VII deficiency

Emergency correction of the coagulopathy of warfarin excess in critical situations.

Usual Dosage Children and Adults: Dosage is expressed in units of factor IX activity and must be individualized. I.V. only:

Formula for units required to raise blood level %:

Total blood volume (mL blood/kg) = 70 mL/kg (adults), 80 mL/kg (children)

Plasma volume = total blood volume (mL) x [1 - Hct (in decimals)]

For example, for a 70 kg adult with a Hct = 40%: Plasma volume = [70 kg x 70 mL/kg] x [1 - 0.4] = 2940 mL

To calculate number of units needed to increase level to desired range (highly individualized and dependent on patient's condition): Number of units = desired level increase [desired level - actual level] x plasma volume (in mL)

For example, for a 100% level in the above patient who has an actual level of 20%: Number of units needed = [1 (for a 100% level) - 0.2] x 2940 mL = 2352 units

As a general rule, the level of factor IX required for treatment of different conditions is listed below:

Minor Spontaneous Hemorrhage, Prophylaxis:
- Desired levels of factor IX for hemostasis: 15% to 25%
- Initial loading dose to achieve desired level: <20-30 units/kg
- Frequency of dosing: Once; repeated in 24 hours if necessary
- Duration of treatment: Once; repeated if necessary

Major Trauma or Surgery:
- Desired levels of factor IX for hemostasis: 25% to 50%
- Initial loading dose to achieve desired level: <75 units/kg

Frequency of dosing: Every 18-30 hours, depending on half-life and measured factor IX levels
Duration of treatment: Up to 10 days, depending upon nature of insult

Factor VIII inhibitor patients: 75 units/kg/dose; may be given every 6-12 hours
Anticoagulant overdosage: I.V.: 15 units/kg

Dosage Forms Injection, powder for reconstitution (**Note:** Exact potency labeled on each vial):
Bebulin® VH [single-dose vial; vapor heated; supplied with sterile water for injection]
Profilnine® SD [single-dose vial; solvent detergent treated]
Proplex® T [single-dose vial; heat treated; supplied with sterile water for injection]

Factrel® [US] *see* gonadorelin *on page 390*

famciclovir (fam SYE kloe veer)

U.S./Canadian Brand Names Famvir® [US/Can]
Therapeutic Category Antiviral Agent
Use Treatment of acute herpes zoster (shingles); treatment and suppression of recurrent episodes of genital herpes in immunocompetent patients; treatment of herpes labialis (cold sores) in immunocompetent patients; treatment of recurrent mucocutaneous/genital herpes simplex in HIV-infected patients
Usual Dosage Adults: Oral:
Acute herpes zoster: 500 mg every 8 hours for 7 days (**Note:** Initiate therapy within 72 hours of rash onset.)
Recurrent genital herpes simplex in immunocompetent patients:
Initial: 1000 mg twice daily for 1 day (**Note:** initiate therapy within 6 hours of symptoms/lesions.)
Suppressive therapy: 250 mg twice daily for up to 1 year
Recurrent herpes labialis (cold sores): 1500 mg as a single dose; initiate therapy at first sign or symptom such as tingling, burning, or itching (initiated within 1 hour in clinical studies)
Recurrent mucocutaneous/genital herpes simplex in HIV patients: 500 mg twice daily for 7 days
Dosage Forms Tablet: 125 mg, 250 mg, 500 mg [contains lactose]

famotidine (fa MOE ti deen)

U.S./Canadian Brand Names Apo-Famotidine® Injectable [Can]; Apo-Famotidine® [Can]; Famotidine Omega [Can]; Gen-Famotidine [Can]; Novo-Famotidine [Can]; Nu-Famotidine [Can]; Pepcid® AC [US-OTC/Can]; Pepcid® I.V. [Can]; Pepcid® [US/Can]; Riva-Famotidine [Can]; Ulcidine [Can]
Therapeutic Category Histamine H_2 Antagonist
Use Therapy and treatment of duodenal ulcer, gastric ulcer, control gastric pH in critically-ill patients, symptomatic relief in gastritis, gastroesophageal reflux, active benign ulcer, and pathological hypersecretory conditions
OTC labeling: Relief of heartburn, acid indigestion, and sour stomach
Usual Dosage
Children: Treatment duration and dose should be individualized
Peptic ulcer: 1-16 years:
Oral: 0.5 mg/kg/day at bedtime or divided twice daily (maximum dose: 40 mg/day); doses of up to 1 mg/kg/day have been used in clinical studies
I.V.: 0.25 mg/kg every 12 hours (maximum dose: 40 mg/day); doses of up to 0.5 mg/kg have been used in clinical studies
GERD: Oral:
<3 months: 0.5 mg/kg once daily
3-12 months: 0.5 mg/kg twice daily
1-16 years: 1 mg/kg/day divided twice daily (maximum dose: 40 mg twice daily); doses of up to 2 mg/kg/day have been used in clinical studies

Children ≥12 years and Adults: Heartburn, indigestion, sour stomach: OTC labeling: Oral: 10-20 mg every 12 hours; dose may be taken 15-60 minutes before eating foods known to cause heartburn

Adults:
Duodenal ulcer: Oral: Acute therapy: 40 mg/day at bedtime for 4-8 weeks; maintenance therapy: 20 mg/day at bedtime
Gastric ulcer: Oral: Acute therapy: 40 mg/day at bedtime
Hypersecretory conditions: Oral: Initial: 20 mg every 6 hours, may increase in increments up to 160 mg every 6 hours
GERD: Oral: 20 mg twice daily for 6 weeks
Esophagitis and accompanying symptoms due to GERD: Oral: 20 mg or 40 mg twice daily for up to 12 weeks
Patients unable to take oral medication: I.V.: 20 mg every 12 hours
(Continued)

famotidine *(Continued)*

Dosage Forms [DSC] = Discontinued product

Gelcap:

Pepcid® AC: 10 mg

Infusion [premixed in NS]: 20 mg (50 mL)

Pepcid®: 20 mg (50 mL)

Injection, solution: 10 mg/mL (4 mL, 20 mL)

Pepcid®: 10 mg/mL (20 mL) [contains benzyl alcohol]

Injection, solution [preservative free]: 10 mg/mL (2 mL)

Pepcid®: 10 mg/mL (2 mL)

Powder for oral suspension:

Pepcid®: 40 mg/5 mL (50 mL) [contains sodium benzoate; cherry-banana-mint flavor]

Tablet: 10 mg [OTC], 20 mg, 40 mg

Pepcid®: 20 mg, 40 mg

Pepcid® AC: 10 mg, 20 mg

Tablet, chewable:

Pepcid® AC: 10 mg [contains phenylalanine 1.4 mg/tablet; mint flavor]

famotidine, calcium carbonate, and magnesium hydroxide

(fa MOE ti deen, KAL see um KAR bun ate, & mag NEE zhum hye DROKS ide)

Synonyms calcium carbonate, magnesium hydroxide, and famotidine; magnesium hydroxide, famotidine, and calcium carbonate

U.S./Canadian Brand Names Pepcid® Complete [US-OTC/Can]

Therapeutic Category Antacid; Histamine H_2 Antagonist

Use Relief of heartburn due to acid indigestion

Usual Dosage Children ≥12 years and Adults: Relief of heartburn due to acid indigestion: Oral: Pepcid® Complete: 1 tablet as needed; no more than 2 tablets in 24 hours; do **not** swallow whole, chew tablet completely before swallowing; do not use for longer than 14 days

Dosage Forms Tablet, chewable: Famotidine 10 mg, calcium carbonate 800 mg, and magnesium hydroxide 165 mg [berry blend and mint flavors]

Famotidine Omega [Can] *see* famotidine *on previous page*

Famvir® [US/Can] *see* famciclovir *on previous page*

Fansidar® [US] *see* sulfadoxine and pyrimethamine *on page 797*

Fareston® [US/Can] *see* toremifene *on page 837*

Faslodex® [US] *see* fulvestrant *on page 372*

Fasturtec® [Can] *see* rasburicase *on page 734*

fat emulsion (fat e MUL shun)

Synonyms intravenous fat emulsion

U.S./Canadian Brand Names Intralipid® [US/Can]; Liposyn® II [Can]; Liposyn® III [US]

Therapeutic Category Intravenous Nutritional Therapy

Use Source of calories and essential fatty acids for patients requiring parenteral nutrition of extended duration

Usual Dosage Fat emulsion should not exceed 60% of the total daily calories

Premature Infants: Initial dose: 0.25-0.5 g/kg/day, increase by 0.25-0.5 g/kg/day to a maximum of 3 g/kg/day depending on needs/nutritional goals; limit to 1 g/kg/day if on phototherapy; maximum rate of infusion: 0.15 g/kg/hour (0.75 mL/kg/hour of 20% solution)

Infants and Children: Initial dose: 0.5-1 g/kg/day, increase by 0.5 g/kg/day to a maximum of 3 g/kg/day depending on needs/nutritional goals; maximum rate of infusion: 0.25 g/kg/hour (1.25 mL/kg/hour of 20% solution)

Adolescents and Adults: Initial dose: 1 g/kg/day, increase by 0.5-1 g/kg/day to a maximum of 2.5 g/kg/day of 10% and 3 g/kg/day of 20% depending on needs/nutritional goals; maximum rate of infusion: 0.25 g/kg/hour (1.25 mL/kg/hour of 20% solution); do not exceed 50 mL/hour (20%) or 100 mL/hour (10%)

Prevention of essential fatty acid deficiency (8% to 10% of total caloric intake): 0.5-1 g/kg/24 hours

Children: 5-10 mL/kg/day at 0.1 mL/minute then up to 100 mL/hour

Adults: 500 mL (10%) twice weekly at rate of 1 mL/minute for 30 minutes, then increase to 42 mL/hour (500 mL over 12 hours)

Note: At the onset of therapy, the patient should be observed for any immediate allergic reactions such as dyspnea, cyanosis, and fever; slower initial rates of infusion may be used for the first 10-15 minutes of the infusion (eg, 0.1 mL/minute of 10% or 0.05 mL/minute of 20% solution)

Dosage Forms Injection, emulsion [soybean oil]:

Intralipid®: 10% [100 mg/mL] (100 mL, 250 mL, 500 mL); 20% [200 mg/mL] (50 mL, 100 mL, 250 mL, 500 mL, 1000 mL); 30% [300 mg/mL] (500 mL)

Liposyn® III: 10% [100 mg/mL] (200 mL, 500 mL); 20% [200 mg/mL] (200 mL, 500 mL); 30% [300 mg/mL] (500 mL)

FazaClo® [US] *see* clozapine *on page 206*

5-FC *see* flucytosine *on page 350*

FC1157a *see* toremifene *on page 837*

Fedahist® Expectorant *(Discontinued)* *see* guaifenesin and pseudoephedrine *on page 398*

Fedahist® Expectorant Pediatric *(Discontinued)* *see* guaifenesin and pseudoephedrine *on page 398*

Fedahist® Tablet *(Discontinued)* *see* chlorpheniramine and pseudoephedrine *on page 177*

Feen-A-Mint® *(Discontinued)* *see* bisacodyl *on page 111*

Feiba VH [US] *see* anti-inhibitor coagulant complex *on page 61*

Feiba VH Immuno [Can] *see* anti-inhibitor coagulant complex *on page 61*

felbamate (FEL ba mate)

U.S./Canadian Brand Names Felbatol® [US]

Therapeutic Category Anticonvulsant

Use Not as a first-line antiepileptic treatment; only in those patients who respond inadequately to alternative treatments and whose epilepsy is so severe that a substantial risk of aplastic anemia and/or liver failure is deemed acceptable in light of the benefits conferred by its use. Patient must be fully advised of risk and provide signed written informed consent. Felbamate can be used as either monotherapy or adjunctive therapy in the treatment of partial seizures (with and without generalization) and in adults with epilepsy.

Orphan drug: Adjunctive therapy in the treatment of partial and generalized seizures associated with Lennox-Gastaut syndrome in children

Usual Dosage Anticonvulsant:

Monotherapy: Children >14 years and Adults:

Initial: 1200 mg/day in divided doses 3 or 4 times/day; titrate previously untreated patients under close clinical supervision, increasing the dosage in 600 mg increments every 2 weeks to 2400 mg/day based on clinical response and thereafter to 3600 mg/day as clinically indicated

Conversion to monotherapy: Initiate at 1200 mg/day in divided doses 3 or 4 times/day, reduce the dosage of the concomitant anticonvulsant(s) by 20% to 33% at the initiation of felbamate therapy; at week 2, increase the felbamate dosage to 2400 mg/day while reducing the dosage of the other anticonvulsant(s) up to an additional 33% of their original dosage; at week 3, increase the felbamate dosage up to 3600 mg/day and continue to reduce the dosage of the other anticonvulsant(s) as clinically indicated

Adjunctive therapy: Children with Lennox-Gastaut and ages 2-14 years:

Week 1:

Felbamate: 15 mg/kg/day divided 3-4 times/day

Concomitant anticonvulsant(s): Reduce original dosage by 20% to 30%

Week 2:

Felbamate: 30 mg/kg/day divided 3-4 times/day

Concomitant anticonvulsant(s): Reduce original dosage up to an additional 33%

Week 3:

Felbamate: 45 mg/kg/day divided 3-4 times/day

Concomitant anticonvulsant(s): Reduce dosage as clinically indicated

Adjunctive therapy: Children >14 years and Adults:

Week 1:

Felbamate: 1200 mg/day initial dose

Concomitant anticonvulsant(s): Reduce original dosage by 20% to 33%

Week 2:

Felbamate: 2400 mg/day (therapeutic range)

Concomitant anticonvulsant(s): Reduce original dosage by up to an additional 33%

Week 3:

Felbamate: 3600 mg/day (therapeutic range)

Concomitant anticonvulsant(s): Reduce original dosage as clinically indicated

Dosage Forms [DSC] = Discontinued product

Suspension, oral:

Felbatol®: 600 mg/5 mL (240 mL, 960 mL)

Tablet:

Felbatol®: 400 mg; 600 mg [DSC]

Felbatol® [US] *see* felbamate *on previous page*

Feldene® [US] *see* piroxicam *on page 671*

felodipine (fe LOE di peen)

Sound-Alike/Look-Alike Issues
Plendil® may be confused with Isordil®, pindolol, Pletal®, Prilosec®, Prinivil®

U.S./Canadian Brand Names Plendil® [US/Can]; Renedil® [Can]

Therapeutic Category Calcium Channel Blocker

Use Treatment of hypertension

Usual Dosage Adults: Oral: 2.5-10 mg once daily; usual initial dose: 5 mg; increase by 5 mg at 2-week intervals, as needed, to a maximum of 20 mg/day

Usual dose range (JNC 7) for hypertension: 2.5-20 mg once daily

Dosage Forms Tablet, extended release: 2.5 mg, 5 mg, 10 mg

felodipine and enalapril *see* enalapril and felodipine *on page 291*

Femara® [US/Can] *see* letrozole *on page 485*

Femcet® ***(Discontinued)***

Femguard® ***(Discontinued)*** *see* sulfabenzamide, sulfacetamide, and sulfathiazole *on page 795*

femhrt® [US/Can] *see* ethinyl estradiol and norethindrone *on page 323*

Femilax™ [US-OTC] *see* bisacodyl *on page 111*

Femiron® [US-OTC] *see* ferrous fumarate *on page 342*

Fem-Prin® [US-OTC] *see* acetaminophen, aspirin, and caffeine *on page 10*

Femring™ [US] *see* estradiol *on page 308*

Femstat® One [Can] *see* butoconazole *on page 130*

FemTabs® [US] *see* vitamins (multiple/oral) *on page 878*

Femtrace® [US] *see* estradiol *on page 308*

fenofibrate (fen oh FYE brate)

Synonyms procetofene; proctofene

U.S./Canadian Brand Names Antara™ [US]; Apo-Feno-Micro® [Can]; Apo-Fenofibrate® [Can]; Dom-Fenofibrate Supra [Can]; Gen-Fenofibrate Micro [Can]; Lipidil EZ® [Can]; Lipidil Micro® [Can]; Lipidil Supra® [Can]; Lipofen™ [US]; Lofibra™ [US]; Novo-Fenofibrate [Can]; Nu-Fenofibrate [Can]; PHL-Fenofibrate Supra [Can]; PMS-Fenofibrate Micro [Can]; PMS-Fenofibrate Supra [Can]; ratio-Fenofibrate MC [Can]; TriCor® [US/Can]; Triglide™ [US]

Therapeutic Category Antihyperlipidemic Agent, Miscellaneous

Use Adjunct to dietary therapy for the treatment of adults with elevations of serum triglyceride levels (types IV and V hyperlipidemia); adjunct to dietary therapy for the reduction of low density lipoprotein cholesterol (LDL-C), total cholesterol (total-C), triglycerides, and apolipoprotein B (apo B) in adult patients with primary hypercholesterolemia or mixed dyslipidemia (Fredrickson types IIa and IIb)

Usual Dosage Oral:

Adults:

Hypertriglyceridemia: Initial:

Antara™: 43-130 mg/day

Lipofen™: 50-150 mg/day; maximum dose: 150 mg/day

Lofibra™: 67 mg/day with meals, up to 200 mg/day

TriCor®: 48 mg/day, up to 145 mg/day

Triglide™: 50-160 mg/day

Hypercholesterolemia or mixed hyperlipidemia:

Antara™: 130 mg/day

Lipofen™: 150 mg/day

Lofibra™: 200 mg/day with meals

TriCor®: 145 mg/day

Triglide™: 160 mg/day

Dosage Forms
Capsule:
Lipofen™: 50 mg, 100 mg, 150 mg
Capsule [micronized]: 67 mg, 134 mg, 200 mg
Antara™: 43 mg, 87 mg, 130 mg
Lofibra™: 67 mg, 134 mg, 200 mg
Tablet: 54 mg, 160 mg
TriCor®: 48 mg, 145 mg
Triglide™: 50 mg, 160 mg

fenoldopam (fe NOL doe pam)

Synonyms fenoldopam mesylate
U.S./Canadian Brand Names Corlopam® [US/Can]
Therapeutic Category Antihypertensive Agent
Use Treatment of severe hypertension (up to 48 hours in adults), including in patients with renal compromise; short-term (up to 4 hours) blood pressure reduction in pediatric patients
Usual Dosage I.V.: Hypertension, severe:
Children: Initial: 0.2 mcg/kg/minute; may be increased to dosages of 0.3-0.5 mcg/kg/minute every 20-30 minutes (maximum dose: 0.8 mcg/kg/minute); limited to short-term (4 hours) use
Adults: Initial: 0.1-0.3 mcg/kg/minute (lower initial doses may be associated with less reflex tachycardia); may be increased in increments of 0.05-0.1 mcg/kg/minute every 15 minutes until target blood pressure is reached; the maximal infusion rate reported in clinical studies was 1.6 mcg/kg/minute
Dosage Forms Injection, solution: 10 mg/mL (1 mL, 2 mL) [contains sodium metabisulfite and propylene glycol]

fenoldopam mesylate *see* fenoldopam *on this page*

fenoprofen (fen oh PROE fen)

Sound-Alike/Look-Alike Issues
fenoprofen may be confused with flurbiprofen
Nalfon® may be confused with Naldecon®
Synonyms fenoprofen calcium
U.S./Canadian Brand Names Nalfon® [US]
Therapeutic Category Analgesic, Nonnarcotic; Nonsteroidal Antiinflammatory Drug (NSAID)
Use Symptomatic treatment of acute and chronic rheumatoid arthritis and osteoarthritis; relief of mild to moderate pain
Usual Dosage Adults: Oral:
Rheumatoid arthritis: 300-600 mg 3-4 times/day up to 3.2 g/day
Mild to moderate pain: 200 mg every 4-6 hours as needed
Dosage Forms
Capsule, as calcium (Nalfon®): 200 mg, 300 mg
Tablet, as calcium: 600 mg

fenoprofen calcium *see* fenoprofen *on this page*

fenoterol *(Canada only)* (fen oh TER ole)

Synonyms fenoterol hydrobromide
U.S./Canadian Brand Names Berotec® [Can]
Therapeutic Category $Beta_2$-Adrenergic Agonist Agent
Use Treatment and prevention of symptoms of reversible obstructive pulmonary disease (including asthma and acute bronchospasm), chronic bronchitis, emphysema
Usual Dosage Inhalation: Children ≥12 years and Adults:
MDI:
Acute treatment: 1 puff initially; may repeat in 5 minutes; if relief is not evident, additional doses and/or other therapy may be necessary
Intermittent/long-term treatment: 1-2 puffs 3-4 times/day (maximum of 8 puffs/24 hours)
Solution: 0.5-1 mg (up to maximum of 2.5 mg)
Dosage Forms
Aerosol for inhalation, as hydrobromide: MDI: 100 mcg/dose [200 doses]
Solution for inhalation, as hydrobromide: 0.625 mg/mL (2 mL); 0.25 mg/mL (2 mL)

fenoterol hydrobromide *see* fenoterol *(Canada only) on this page*

fentanyl (FEN ta nil)

Sound-Alike/Look-Alike Issues
fentanyl may be confused with alfentanil, sufentanil

Synonyms fentanyl citrate; fentanyl hydrocholoride

U.S./Canadian Brand Names Actiq® [US/Can]; Duragesic® [US/Can]; Fentanyl Citrate Injection, USP [Can]; Ionsys™ [US]; Sublimaze® [US]

Therapeutic Category Analgesic, Narcotic; General Anesthetic

Controlled Substance C-II

Use

Injection: Sedation, relief of pain, preoperative medication, adjunct to general or regional anesthesia

Iontophoretic transdermal system (Ionsys™): Short-term in-hospital management of acute postoperative pain

Transdermal patch (eg, Duragesic®): Management of moderate-to-severe chronic pain

Transmucosal lozenge (eg, Actiq®), buccal tablet (Fentora™): Management of breakthrough cancer pain

Usual Dosage Note: These are guidelines and do not represent the maximum doses that may be required in all patients. Doses should be titrated to pain relief/prevention. Monitor vital signs routinely. Single I.M. doses have a duration of 1-2 hours, single I.V. doses last 0.5-1 hour.

Sedation for minor procedures/analgesia:

Children 1-12 years:

Sedation for minor procedures/analgesia: I.M., I.V.: 1-2 mcg/kg/dose; may repeat at 30- to 60-minute intervals. **Note:** Children 18-36 months of age may require 2-3 mcg/kg/dose

Continuous sedation/analgesia: Initial I.V. bolus: 1-2 mcg/kg; then 1-3 mcg/kg/hour to a maximum dose of 5 mcg/kg/hour

Children >12 years and Adults: I.V.: 25-50 mcg; may repeat every 3-5 minutes to desired effect or adverse event; maximum dose of 500 mcg/4 hours; higher doses are used for major procedures

Surgery: Adults:

Premedication: I.M., slow I.V.: 25-100 mcg/dose 30-60 minutes prior to surgery

Adjunct to regional anesthesia: Slow I.V.: 25-100 mcg/dose over 1-2 minutes. **Note:** An I.V. should be in place with regional anesthesia so the I.M. route is rarely used but still maintained as an option in the package labeling.

Adjunct to general anesthesia: Slow I.V.:

Low dose: 0.5-2 mcg/kg/dose depending on the indication. For example, 0.5 mcg/kg will provide analgesia or reduce the amount of propofol needed for laryngeal mask airway insertion with minimal respiratory depression. However, to blunt the hemodynamic response to intubation 2 mcg/kg is often necessary.

Moderate dose: Initial: 2-15 mcg/kg/dose; maintenance (bolus or infusion): 1-2 mcg/kg/hour. Discontinuing fentanyl infusion 30-60 minutes prior to the end of surgery will usually allow adequate ventilation upon emergence from anesthesia. For "fast-tracking" and early extubation following major surgery, total fentanyl doses are limited to 10-15 mcg/kg.

High dose: **Note:** High-dose (20-50 mcg/kg/dose) fentanyl is rarely used, but is still maintained in the package labeling.

Acute pain management: Adults:

Severe: I.M, I.V.: 50-100 mcg/dose every 1-2 hours as needed; patients with prior opiate exposure may tolerate higher initial doses

Patient-controlled analgesia (PCA): I.V.: Usual concentration: 10 mcg/mL

Demand dose: Usual: 10 mcg; range: 10-50 mcg

Lockout interval: 5-8 minutes

Mechanically-ventilated patients (based on 70 kg patient): Slow I.V.: 0.35-1.5 mcg/kg every 30-60 minutes as needed; infusion: 0.7-10 mcg/kg/hour

Iontophoretic transdermal system: 40 mcg per activation on-demand (maximum: 6 doses/hour). **Note:** Patient's pain should be controlled prior to initiating system. Instruct patient how to operate system. Only the patient should initiate system. Each system operates for 24 hours or until 80 doses have been administered, whichever comes first.

Breakthrough cancer pain:

Adults: Transmucosal: Actiq® dosing should be individually titrated to provide adequate analgesia with minimal side effects. For patients who are tolerant to and currently receiving opioid therapy for persistent cancer pain. Initial starting dose: 200 mcg; the second dose may be started 15 minutes after completion of the first dose. Consumption should be limited to 4 units/day or less. Patients needing more than 4 units/day should have the dose of their long-term opioid re-evaluated.

Chronic pain management: Children ≥2 years and Adults (opioid-tolerant patients): Transdermal:

Initial: To convert patients from oral or parenteral opioids to transdermal formulation, a 24-hour analgesic requirement should be calculated (based on prior opiate use). Using the tables, the appropriate initial dose can be determined. The initial fentanyl dosage may be approximated from the 24-hour morphine dosage and titrated to minimize adverse effects and provide analgesia. Change patch every 72 hours.

Titration: Short-acting agents may be required until analgesic efficacy is established and/or as supplements for "breakthrough" pain. The amount of supplemental doses should be closely monitored. Appropriate dosage increases may be based on daily supplemental dosage using the ratio of 45 mg/24 hours of oral morphine to a 12.5 mcg/hour increase in fentanyl dosage.

Frequency of adjustment: The dosage should not be titrated more frequently than every 3 days after the initial dose or every 6 days thereafter. Patients should wear a consistent fentanyl dosage through two applications (6 days) before dosage increase based on supplemental opiate dosages can be estimated.

Frequency of application: The majority of patients may be controlled on every 72-hour administration; however, a small number of patients require every 48-hour administration.

Dosage Forms

Buccal tablet, effervescent [oral transmucosal]:

Fentora™: 100 mcg, 200 mcg, 400 mcg, 600 mcg, 800 mcg

Infusion [premixed in NS]: 0.05 mg (10 mL); 1 mg (100 mL); 1.25 mg (250 mL); 2 mg (100 mL); 2.5 mg (250 mL)

Injection, solution [preservative free]: 0.05 mg/mL (2 mL, 5 mL, 10 mL, 20 mL, 30 mL, 50 mL)

Sublimaze®: 0.05 mg/mL (2 mL, 5 mL, 10 mL, 20 mL)

Lozenge [oral transmucosal]:

Actiq®: 200 mcg, 400 mcg, 600 mcg, 800 mcg, 1200 mcg, 1600 mcg [mounted on a plastic radiopaque handle; contains sugar 2 g/unit; raspberry flavor]

Transdermal patch: 25 mcg/hour [6.25 cm^2] (5s); 50 mcg/hour [12.5 cm^2] (5s); 75 mcg/hour [18.75 cm^2]; 100 mcg/hour [25 cm^2] (5s)

Duragesic®: 12 [delivers 12.5 mcg/hour; 5 cm^2; contains alcohol 0.1 mL/10 cm^2] (5s); 25 [delivers 25 mcg/hour; 10 cm^2; contains alcohol 0.1 mL/10 cm^2] (5s); 50 [delivers 50 mcg/hour; 20 cm^2; contains alcohol 0.1 mL/10 cm^2] (5s); 75 [delivers 75 mcg/hour; 30 cm^2; contains alcohol 0.1 mL/10 cm^2]; 100 [delivers 100 mcg/hour; 40 cm^2; contains alcohol 0.1 mL/10 cm^2] (5s)

Transdermal iontophoretic system:

Ionsys™: Fentanyl 40 mcg/dose [80 doses/patch; contains 3-volt lithium battery]

fentanyl citrate *see* fentanyl *on previous page*

Fentanyl Citrate Injection, USP [Can] *see* fentanyl *on previous page*

fentanyl hydrocholoride *see* fentanyl *on previous page*

Fentanyl Oralet® ***(Discontinued)*** *see* fentanyl *on previous page*

Feosol® [US-OTC] *see* ferrous sulfate *on page 343*

Feosol® Elixir ***(Discontinued)*** *see* ferrous sulfate *on page 343*

Feostat® ***(Discontinued)*** *see* ferrous fumarate *on next page*

Ferancee® ***(Discontinued)*** *see* ferrous sulfate and ascorbic acid *on page 343*

Feratab® [US-OTC] *see* ferrous sulfate *on page 343*

Fer-Gen-Sol [US-OTC] *see* ferrous sulfate *on page 343*

Fergon® [US-OTC] *see* ferrous gluconate *on page 343*

Feridex I.V.® [US] *see* ferumoxides *on page 344*

Fer-In-Sol® [US-OTC/Can] *see* ferrous sulfate *on page 343*

Fer-In-Sol® Syrup ***(Discontinued)*** *see* ferrous sulfate *on page 343*

Fer-Iron® [US-OTC] *see* ferrous sulfate *on page 343*

Fermalac [Can] *see* Lactobacillus *on page 477*

Ferodan™ [Can] *see* ferrous sulfate *on page 343*

Fero-Grad 500® [US-OTC] *see* ferrous sulfate and ascorbic acid *on page 343*

Fero-Gradumet® ***(Discontinued)*** *see* ferrous sulfate *on page 343*

Ferospace® ***(Discontinued)*** *see* ferrous sulfate *on page 343*

Ferralet® ***(Discontinued)*** *see* ferrous gluconate *on page 343*

Ferralyn® Lanacaps® ***(Discontinued)*** *see* ferrous sulfate *on page 343*

Ferra-TD® ***(Discontinued)*** *see* ferrous sulfate *on page 343*

Ferretts [US-OTC] *see* ferrous fumarate *on next page*

Ferrex 150 [US-OTC] *see* polysaccharide-iron complex *on page 681*

ferric (III) hexacyanoferrate (II) *see* ferric hexacyanoferrate *on this page*

ferric gluconate (FER ik GLOO koe nate)

Sound-Alike/Look-Alike Issues

Ferrlecit® may be confused with Ferralet®

Synonyms sodium ferric gluconate

U.S./Canadian Brand Names Ferrlecit® [US/Can]

Therapeutic Category Iron Salt

Use Repletion of total body iron content in patients with iron-deficiency anemia who are undergoing hemodialysis in conjunction with erythropoietin therapy

Usual Dosage I.V.: Repletion of iron in hemodialysis patients:

Children ≥6 years: 1.5 mg/kg (maximum: 125 mg/dose) diluted in NS 25 mL, administered over 60 minutes at 8 sequential dialysis sessions

Adults: **Note:** A test dose of 2 mL diluted in NS 50 mL administered over 60 minutes was previously recommended (not in current manufacturer labeling).

125 mg elemental iron per 10 mL (either by I.V. infusion or slow I.V. injection). Most patients will require a cumulative dose of 1 g elemental iron over approximately 8 sequential dialysis treatments to achieve a favorable response.

Dosage Forms Injection, solution: Elemental iron 12.5 mg/mL (5 mL) [contains benzyl alcohol and sucrose 20%]

ferric hexacyanoferrate (FER ik hex a SYE an oh fer ate)

Synonyms ferric (III) hexacyanoferrate (II); insoluble prussian blue; prussian blue

U.S./Canadian Brand Names Radiogardase™ [US]

Therapeutic Category Antidote

Use Treatment of known or suspected internal contamination with radioactive cesium and/or radioactive or nonradioactive thallium

Usual Dosage Oral: Internal contamination with radioactive cesium and/or radioactive or nonradioactive thallium:

Children 2-12 years: 1 g 3 times/day; treatment should begin as soon as possible following exposure, but is also effective if therapy is delayed

Children >12 years and Adults: 3 g 3 times/day; treatment should begin as soon as possible following exposure, but is also effective if therapy is delayed

Note: Cesium exposure: Once internal radioactivity is substantially decreased, dosage may be reduced to 1-2 g 3 times/day to improve gastrointestinal tolerance

Dosage Forms Capsule: 0.5 g

Ferrlecit® [US/Can] *see* ferric gluconate *on this page*

Ferro-Sequels® [US-OTC] *see* ferrous fumarate *on this page*

ferrous fumarate (FER us FYOO ma rate)

Sound-Alike/Look-Alike Issues

Feostat® may be confused with Feosol®

Synonyms iron fumarate

U.S./Canadian Brand Names Femiron® [US-OTC]; Ferretts [US-OTC]; Ferro-Sequels® [US-OTC]; Hemocyte® [US-OTC]; Ircon® [US-OTC]; Nephro-Fer® [US-OTC]; Palafer® [Can]

Therapeutic Category Electrolyte Supplement, Oral

Use Prevention and treatment of iron-deficiency anemias

Usual Dosage Oral **(dose expressed in terms of elemental iron):**

Children:

Severe iron-deficiency anemia: 4-6 mg Fe/kg/day in 3 divided doses

Mild to moderate iron deficiency anemia: 3 mg Fe/kg/day in 1-2 divided doses

Prophylaxis: 1-2 mg Fe/kg/day

Adults:

Iron deficiency: 60-100 mg twice daily up to 60 mg 2 times/day

Prophylaxis: 60-100 mg/day

To avoid GI upset, start with a single daily dose and increase by 1 tablet/day each week or as tolerated until desired daily dose is achieved

Dosage Forms [DSC] = Discontinued product

Tablet: 324 mg [elemental iron 106 mg]

Femiron®: 63 mg [elemental iron 20 mg]

Ferretts: 325 mg [elemental iron 106 mg]

Hemocyte®: 324 mg [elemental iron 106 mg]
Ircon®: 200 mg [elemental iron 66 mg]
Nephro-Fer®: 350 mg [elemental iron 115 mg; contains tartrazine]
Tablet, chewable (Feostat®): 100 mg [elemental iron 33 mg; chocolate flavor] [DSC]
Tablet, timed release (Ferro-Sequels®): 150 mg [elemental iron 50 mg; contains docusate sodium and sodium benzoate]

ferrous gluconate (FER us GLOO koe nate)

Synonyms iron gluconate
U.S./Canadian Brand Names Apo-Ferrous Gluconate® [Can]; Fergon® [US-OTC]; Novo-Ferrogluc [Can]
Therapeutic Category Electrolyte Supplement, Oral
Use Prevention and treatment of iron-deficiency anemias
Usual Dosage Oral **(dose expressed in terms of elemental iron):**
Children:
Severe iron-deficiency anemia: 4-6 mg Fe/kg/day in 3 divided doses
Mild to moderate iron deficiency anemia: 3 mg Fe/kg/day in 1-2 divided doses
Prophylaxis: 1-2 mg Fe/kg/day
Adults:
Iron deficiency: 60 mg twice daily up to 60 mg 4 times/day
Prophylaxis: 60 mg/day
Dosage Forms
Tablet: 246 mg [elemental iron 28 mg]; 300 mg [elemental iron 34 mg]; 325 mg [elemental iron 36 mg]
Fergon®: 240 mg [elemental iron 27 mg]

ferrous sulfate (FER us SUL fate)

Sound-Alike/Look-Alike Issues
Feosol® may be confused with Feostat®, Fer-In-Sol®
Fer-In-Sol® may be confused with Feosol®
Slow FE® may be confused with Slow-K®
Synonyms $FeSO_4$; iron sulfate
U.S./Canadian Brand Names Apo-Ferrous Sulfate® [Can]; Feosol® [US-OTC]; Fer-Gen-Sol [US-OTC]; Fer-In-Sol® [US-OTC/Can]; Fer-Iron® [US-OTC]; Feratab® [US-OTC]; Ferodan™ [Can]; Slow FE® [US-OTC]
Therapeutic Category Electrolyte Supplement, Oral
Use Prevention and treatment of iron-deficiency anemias
Usual Dosage Oral:
Children **(dose expressed in terms of elemental iron)**:
Severe iron-deficiency anemia: 4-6 mg Fe/kg/day in 3 divided doses
Mild to moderate iron deficiency anemia: 3 mg Fe/kg/day in 1-2 divided doses
Prophylaxis: 1-2 mg Fe/kg/day up to a maximum of 15 mg/day
Adults **(dose expressed in terms of ferrous sulfate)**:
Iron deficiency: 300 mg twice daily up to 300 mg 4 times/day or 250 mg (extended release) 1-2 times/day
Prophylaxis: 300 mg/day
Dosage Forms
Elixir: 220 mg/5 mL (480 mL) [elemental iron 44 mg/5 mL; contains alcohol]
Liquid, oral drops: 75 mg/0.6 mL (50 mL) [elemental iron 15 mg/0.6 mL]
Fer-Gen-Sol: 75 mg/0.6 mL (50 mL) [elemental iron 15 mg/0.6 mL]
Fer-In-Sol®: 75 mg/0.6 mL (50 mL) [elemental iron 15 mg/0.6 mL; contains alcohol 0.2% and sodium bisulfite]
Fer-Iron®: 75 mg/0.6 mL (50 mL) [elemental iron 15 mg/0.6 mL]
Tablet: 324 mg [elemental iron 65 mg]; 325 mg [elemental iron 65 mg]
Feratab®: 300 mg [elemental iron 60 mg]
Tablet, exsiccated (Feosol®): 200 mg [elemental iron 65 mg]
Tablet, exsiccated, timed release (Slow FE®): 160 mg [elemental iron 50 mg]

ferrous sulfate and ascorbic acid (FER us SUL fate & a SKOR bik AS id)

Synonyms ascorbic acid and ferrous sulfate; iron sulfate and vitamin C
U.S./Canadian Brand Names Fero-Grad 500® [US-OTC]
Therapeutic Category Vitamin
Use Treatment of iron deficiency in nonpregnant adults; treatment and prevention of iron deficiency in pregnant adults
Usual Dosage Adults: Oral: 1 tablet daily
(Continued)

ferrous sulfate and ascorbic acid *(Continued)*

Dosage Forms [DSC] = Discontinued product

Capsule, extended release (Vitelle™ Irospan®): Ferrous sulfate [elemental iron 65 mg] and ascorbic acid 150 mg [DSC]

Tablet, controlled release (Fero-Grad 500®): Ferrous sulfate 525 mg [elemental iron 105 mg] and ascorbic acid 500 mg

Tablet, extended release (Vitelle™ Irospan®): Ferrous sulfate [elemental iron 65 mg] and ascorbic acid 150 mg [DSC]

ferumoxides (fer yoo MOX ides)

Sound-Alike/Look-Alike Issues

Feridex I.V.® may be confused with Fertinex®

U.S./Canadian Brand Names Feridex I.V.® [US]

Therapeutic Category Radiopaque Agents

Use For I.V. administration as an adjunct to MRI (in adult patients) to enhance the T2 weighted images used in the detection and evaluation of lesions of the liver

Usual Dosage Adults: 0.56 mg of iron (0.05 mL Feridex I.V.®)/kg body weight diluted in 100 mL of 5% dextrose and infused over 30 minutes; a 5-micron filter is recommended; do not administer undiluted

Dosage Forms Injection, solution: Iron 11.2 mg/mL (5 mL) [contains mannitol 61.3 mg/mL]

$FeSO_4$ *see* ferrous sulfate *on previous page*

Fe-Tinic™ 150 *(Discontinued)* *see* polysaccharide-iron complex *on page 681*

FeverAll® [US-OTC] *see* acetaminophen *on page 5*

fexofenadine (feks oh FEN a deen)

Sound-Alike/Look-Alike Issues

Allegra® may be confused with Viagra®

Synonyms fexofenadine hydrochloride

U.S./Canadian Brand Names Allegra® [US/Can]

Therapeutic Category Antihistamine

Use Relief of symptoms associated with seasonal allergic rhinitis; treatment of chronic idiopathic urticaria

Usual Dosage Oral: Chronic idiopathic urticaria, seasonal allergic rhinitis:

Children 6-11 years: 30 mg twice daily

Children ≥12 years and Adults: 60 mg twice daily **or** 180 mg once daily

Dosage Forms Tablet, as hydrochloride: 30 mg, 60 mg, 180 mg

fexofenadine and pseudoephedrine (feks oh FEN a deen & soo doe e FED rin)

Sound-Alike/Look-Alike Issues

Allegra-D® may be confused with Viagra®

Synonyms pseudoephedrine and fexofenadine

U.S./Canadian Brand Names Allegra-D® 12 Hour [US]; Allegra-D® 24 Hour [US]; Allegra-D® [Can]

Therapeutic Category Antihistamine/Decongestant Combination

Use Relief of symptoms associated with seasonal allergic rhinitis in adults and children ≥12 years of age

Usual Dosage Oral: Children ≥12 years and Adults:

Allegra-D® 12 Hour: One tablet twice daily

Allegra-D® 24 Hour: One tablet once daily

Dosage Forms Tablet, extended release:

Allegra-D® 12 Hour: Fexofenadine hydrochloride 60 mg [immediate release] and pseudoephedrine hydrochloride 120 mg [extended release]

Allegra-D® 24 Hour: Fexofenadine hydrochloride 180 mg [immediate release] and pseudoephedrine hydrochloride 240 mg [extended release]

fexofenadine hydrochloride *see* fexofenadine *on this page*

Fiberall® [US] *see* psyllium *on page 717*

FiberCon® [US-OTC] *see* polycarbophil *on page 678*

Fiber-Lax® [US-OTC] *see* polycarbophil *on page 678*

fibrin sealant kit (FI brin SEEL ent kit)

Synonyms FS

U.S./Canadian Brand Names Crosseal™ [US]; Tisseel® VH [US/Can]

Therapeutic Category Hemostatic Agent

Use

Crosseal™: Adjunct to hemostasis in liver surgery

Tisseel® VH: Adjunct to hemostasis in cardiopulmonary bypass surgery and splenic injury (due to blunt or penetrating trauma to the abdomen) when the control of bleeding by conventional surgical techniques is ineffective or impractical; adjunctive sealant for closure of colostomies; hemostatic agent in heparinized patients undergoing cardiopulmonary bypass

Usual Dosage Adjunct to hemostasis: Apply topically; actual dose is based on size of surface to be covered:

Crosseal™: Children and Adults: To cover a layer of 1 mm thickness:

Maximum area to be sealed: 20 cm^2

Required size of Crosseal™ kit: 1 mL

Maximum area to be sealed: 40 cm^2

Required size of Crosseal™ kit: 2 mL

Maximum area to be sealed: 100 cm^2

Required size of Crosseal™ kit: 5 mL

Note: If hemostatic effect is not complete, apply a second layer.

Tisseel® VH: Adults:

Maximum area to be sealed: 4 cm^2

Required size of Tisseel® VH kit: 0.5 mL

Maximum area to be sealed: 8 cm^2

Required size of Tisseel® VH kit: 1 mL

Maximum area to be sealed: 16 cm^2

Required size of Tisseel® VH kit: 2 mL

Maximum area to be sealed: 40 cm^2

Required size of Tisseel® VH kit: 5 mL

Apply in thin layers to avoid excess formation of granulation tissue and slow absorption of the sealant. Following application, hold the sealed parts in the desired position for 3-5 minutes. To prevent sealant from adhering to gloves or surgical instruments, wet them with saline prior to contact.

Dosage Forms Topical: Kit [each kit contains]:

Crosseal™: Fibrinogen 40-60 mg/mL [human; also contains tranexamic acid]; thrombin 800-1200 int. units/mL [human; also contains human albumin and mannitol]; spray application device (1 mL, 2 mL, 5 mL)

Tisseel® VH: Fibrinogen 75-115 mg/mL [sealer protein concentrate, human]; aprotinin 3000 KIU/mL [fibrinolysis inhibitor solution, bovine]; thrombin 500 int. units/mL [human]; calcium chloride solution 40 micromoles/mL (0.5 mL, 1 mL, 2 mL, 5 mL)

Fibro-XL [US-OTC] *see* psyllium *on page 717*

Fibro-Lax [US-OTC] *see* psyllium *on page 717*

filgrastim (fil GRA stim)

Sound-Alike/Look-Alike Issues

Neupogen® may be confused with Epogen®, Neumega®, Nutramigen®

Synonyms G-CSF; granulocyte colony stimulating factor

U.S./Canadian Brand Names Neupogen® [US/Can]

Therapeutic Category Colony-Stimulating Factor

Use Stimulation of granulocyte production in chemotherapy-induced neutropenia (nonmyeloid malignancies, acute myeloid leukemia, and bone marrow transplantation); severe chronic neutropenia (SCN); patients undergoing peripheral blood progenitor cell (PBPC) collection

Usual Dosage Refer to individual protocols.

Dosing, even in morbidly obese patients, should be based on actual body weight. Rounding doses to the nearest vial size often enhances patient convenience and reduces costs without compromising clinical response.

SubQ, I.V.:

Myelosuppressive therapy: 5 mcg/kg/day; doses may be increased by 5 mcg/kg according to the duration and severity of the neutropenia; continue for up to 14 days or until the ANC reaches 10,000/mm^3

Bone marrow transplantation: 10 mcg/kg/day; doses may be increased by 5 mcg/kg according to the duration and severity of neutropenia; recommended steps based on neutrophil response:

When ANC >1000/mm^3 for 3 consecutive days: Reduce filgrastim dose to 5 mcg/kg/day

If ANC remains >1000/mm^3 for 3 more consecutive days: Discontinue filgrastim

(Continued)

filgrastim *(Continued)*

If ANC decreases to <1000/mm^3: Resume at 5 mcg/kg/day

If ANC decreases <1000/mm^3 during the 5 mcg/kg/day dose, increase filgrastim to 10 mcg/kg/day and follow the above steps

SubQ:

Peripheral blood progenitor cell (PBPC) collection: 10 mcg/kg/day **or** 5-8 mcg/kg twice daily in donors. Begin at least 4 days before the first leukopheresis and continue until the last leukopheresis; the optimal timing and duration of growth factor stimulation has not been determined.

Severe chronic neutropenia:

Congenital: 6 mcg/kg twice daily

Idiopathic/cyclic: 5 mcg/kg/day

Dosage Forms

Injection, solution [preservative free]: 300 mcg/mL (1 mL, 1.6 mL) [vial; contains sodium 0.035 mg/mL and sorbitol]

Injection, solution [preservative free]: 600 mcg/mL (0.5 mL, 0.8 mL) [prefilled Singleject® syringe; contains sodium 0.035 mg/mL and sorbitol]

Finacea™ [US] *see* azelaic acid *on page 87*

finasteride (fi NAS teer ide)

Sound-Alike/Look-Alike Issues

Proscar® may be confused with ProSom®, Prozac®, Psorcon®

U.S./Canadian Brand Names Propecia® [US/Can]; Proscar® [US/Can]

Therapeutic Category Antiandrogen

Use

Propecia®: Treatment of male pattern hair loss in **men only**. Safety and efficacy were demonstrated in men between 18-41 years of age.

Proscar®: Treatment of symptomatic benign prostatic hyperplasia (BPH); can be used in combination with an alpha blocker, doxazosin

Usual Dosage Oral: Adults: Male:

Benign prostatic hyperplasia (Proscar®): 5 mg/day as a single dose; clinical responses occur within 12 weeks to 6 months of initiation of therapy; long-term administration is recommended for maximal response

Male pattern baldness (Propecia®): 1 mg daily

Dosage Forms

Tablet: 5 mg

Propecia®: 1 mg

Proscar®: 5 mg

Fiorgen PF® ***(Discontinued)***

Fioricet® [US] *see* butalbital, acetaminophen, and caffeine *on page 129*

Fiorinal® [US/Can] *see* butalbital, aspirin, and caffeine *on page 129*

Fiorinal®-C 1/2 [Can] *see* butalbital, aspirin, caffeine, and codeine *on page 129*

Fiorinal®-C 1/4 [Can] *see* butalbital, aspirin, caffeine, and codeine *on page 129*

Fiorinal® With Codeine [US] *see* butalbital, aspirin, caffeine, and codeine *on page 129*

First® Testosterone [US] *see* testosterone *on page 812*

First® Testosterone MC [US] *see* testosterone *on page 812*

fisalamine *see* mesalamine *on page 533*

fish oil *see* omega-3-acid ethyl esters *on page 615*

FK506 *see* tacrolimus *on page 803*

Flagyl® [US/Can] *see* metronidazole *on page 551*

Flagyl ER® [US] *see* metronidazole *on page 551*

Flagyl® I.V. RTU™ [US] *see* metronidazole *on page 551*

Flamazine® [Can] *see* silver sulfadiazine *on page 772*

Flarex® [US/Can] *see* fluorometholone *on page 356*

Flavorcee® ***(Discontinued)*** *see* ascorbic acid *on page 76*

flavoxate (fla VOKS ate)

Sound-Alike/Look-Alike Issues

flavoxate may be confused with fluvoxamine

Urispas® may be confused with Urised®

Synonyms flavoxate hydrochloride

U.S./Canadian Brand Names Apo-Flavoxate® [Can]; Urispas® [US/Can]

Therapeutic Category Antispasmodic Agent, Urinary

Use Antispasmodic to provide symptomatic relief of dysuria, nocturia, suprapubic pain, urgency, and incontinence due to detrusor instability and hyperreflexia in elderly with cystitis, urethritis, urethrocystitis, urethrotrigonitis, and prostatitis

Usual Dosage Children >12 years and Adults: Oral: 100-200 mg 3-4 times/day; reduce the dose when symptoms improve

Dosage Forms Tablet, as hydrochloride: 100 mg

flavoxate hydrochloride *see* flavoxate *on this page*

flecainide (fle KAY nide)

Sound-Alike/Look-Alike Issues

flecainide may be confused with fluconazole

Tambocor™ may be confused with tamoxifen

Synonyms flecainide acetate

U.S./Canadian Brand Names Apo-Flecainide® [Can]; Tambocor™ [US/Can]

Therapeutic Category Antiarrhythmic Agent, Class I-C

Use Prevention and suppression of documented life-threatening ventricular arrhythmias (eg, sustained ventricular tachycardia); controlling symptomatic, disabling supraventricular tachycardias in patients without structural heart disease in whom other agents fail

Usual Dosage Oral:

Children:

Initial: 3 mg/kg/day or 50-100 mg/m^2/day in 3 divided doses

Usual: 3-6 mg/kg/day or 100-150 mg/m^2/day in 3 divided doses; up to 11 mg/kg/day or 200 mg/m^2/day for uncontrolled patients with subtherapeutic levels

Adults:

Life-threatening ventricular arrhythmias:

Initial: 100 mg every 12 hours

Increase by 50-100 mg/day (given in 2 doses/day) every 4 days; maximum: 400 mg/day.

Use of higher initial doses and more rapid dosage adjustments have resulted in an increased incidence of proarrhythmic events and congestive heart failure, particularly during the first few days. Do not use a loading dose. Use very cautiously in patients with history of congestive heart failure or myocardial infarction.

Prevention of paroxysmal supraventricular arrhythmias in patients with disabling symptoms but no structural heart disease:

Initial: 50 mg every 12 hours

Increase by 50 mg twice daily at 4-day intervals; maximum: 300 mg/day.

Dosage Forms Tablet, as acetate: 50 mg, 100 mg, 150 mg

flecainide acetate *see* flecainide *on this page*

Fleet® Accu-Prep® [US-OTC] *see* sodium phosphates *on page 781*

Fleet® Babylax® [US-OTC] *see* glycerin *on page 388*

Fleet® Bisacodyl Enema [US-OTC] *see* bisacodyl *on page 111*

Fleet Enema® [Can] *see* sodium phosphates *on page 781*

Fleet® Flavored Castor Oil *(Discontinued)* *see* castor oil *on page 155*

Fleet® Glycerin Suppositories [US-OTC] *see* glycerin *on page 388*

Fleet® Glycerin Suppositories Maximum Strength [US-OTC] *see* glycerin *on page 388*

Fleet® Laxative *(Discontinued)* *see* bisacodyl *on page 111*

Fleet® Liquid Glycerin Suppositories [US-OTC] *see* glycerin *on page 388*

Fleet® Phospho-Soda® [US-OTC] *see* sodium phosphates *on page 781*

Fleet® Phospho-Soda® Oral Laxative [Can] *see* sodium phosphates *on page 781*

Fleet® Sof-Lax® [US-OTC] *see* docusate *on page 270*

Fleet® Stimulant Laxative [US-OTC] *see* bisacodyl *on page 111*

Fletcher's® Castoria® [US-OTC] *see* senna *on page 767*

Flexaphen® *(Discontinued)* *see* chlorzoxazone *on page 185*

Flexbumin [US] *see* albumin *on page 22*

Flexeril® [US] *see* cyclobenzaprine *on page 219*

Flexitec [Can] *see* cyclobenzaprine *on page 219*

Flex-Power [US-OTC] *see* trolamine *on page 855*

Flextra 650 [US] *see* acetaminophen and phenyltoloxamine *on page 8*

Flextra-DS [US] *see* acetaminophen and phenyltoloxamine *on page 8*

Flintstones® Complete [US-OTC] *see* vitamins (multiple/pediatric) *on page 878*

Flintstones® Plus Calcium [US-OTC] *see* vitamins (multiple/pediatric) *on page 878*

Flintstones® Plus Extra C [US-OTC] *see* vitamins (multiple/pediatric) *on page 878*

Flintstones® Plus Iron [US-OTC] *see* vitamins (multiple/pediatric) *on page 878*

Flo-Coat® [US] *see* radiological/contrast media (ionic) *on page 728*

floctafenine *(Canada only)* (flok ta FEN een)

U.S./Canadian Brand Names Idarac® [Can]

Therapeutic Category Nonsteroidal Antiinflammatory Drug (NSAID), Oral

Use Short-term use in acute pain of mild and moderate severity

Usual Dosage Adults: Oral: 200-400 mg every 6-8 hours as required; maximum recommended daily dose: 1200 mg

Dosage Forms Tablet: 200 mg, 400 mg

Flolan® [US/Can] *see* epoprostenol *on page 299*

Flomax® [US/Can] *see* tamsulosin *on page 805*

Flomax® CR [Can] *see* tamsulosin *on page 805*

Flonase® [US/Can] *see* fluticasone (nasal) *on page 362*

Flora-Q™ [US-OTC] *see* Lactobacillus *on page 477*

Florazole® ER [Can] *see* metronidazole *on page 551*

Florical® [US-OTC] *see* calcium carbonate *on page 135*

Florinef® [US/Can] *see* fludrocortisone *on page 350*

Florone® [US/Can] *see* diflorasone *on page 253*

Florone E® *(Discontinued)* *see* diflorasone *on page 253*

Flovent® Diskus® [Can] *see* fluticasone (oral inhalation) *on page 362*

Flovent® HFA [US/Can] *see* fluticasone (oral inhalation) *on page 362*

Floxin® [US/Can] *see* ofloxacin *on page 611*

floxuridine (floks YOOR i deen)

Sound-Alike/Look-Alike Issues

floxuridine may be confused with Fludara®, fludarabine

FUDR® may be confused with Fludara®

Synonyms fluorodeoxyuridine; 5-FUDR; NSC-27640

U.S./Canadian Brand Names FUDR® [US/Can]

Therapeutic Category Antineoplastic Agent

Use Management of hepatic metastases of colorectal and gastric cancers

Usual Dosage Refer to individual protocols.

Intra-arterial:

0.1-0.6 mg/kg/day

4-20 mg/day

Dosage Forms Injection, powder for reconstitution: 500 mg

Fluanxol® [Can] *see* flupenthixol *(Canada only)* *on page 358*

Fluarix™ [US] *see* influenza virus vaccine *on page 448*

flubenisolone *see* betamethasone (topical) *on page 107*

Flucaine® [US] *see* proparacaine and fluorescein *on page 706*

fluconazole (floo KOE na zole)

Sound-Alike/Look-Alike Issues

fluconazole may be confused with flecainide

Diflucan® may be confused with diclofenac, Diprivan®, disulfiram

U.S./Canadian Brand Names Apo-Fluconazole® [Can]; Diflucan® [US/Can]; Fluconazole Injection [Can]; Fluconazole Omega [Can]; Gen-Fluconazole [Can]; GMD-Fluconazole [Can]; Novo-Fluconazole [Can]; Riva-Fluconazole [Can]

Therapeutic Category Antifungal Agent

Use Treatment of candidiasis (vaginal, oropharyngeal, esophageal, urinary tract infections, peritonitis, pneumonia, and systemic infections); cryptococcal meningitis; antifungal prophylaxis in allogeneic bone marrow transplant recipients

Usual Dosage The daily dose of fluconazole is the same for oral and I.V. administration

Usual dosage ranges:

Neonates: First 2 weeks of life, especially premature neonates: Same dose as older children every 72 hours

Children: Loading dose: 6-12 mg/kg; maintenance: 3-12 mg/kg/day; duration and dosage depends on severity of infection

Adults: 200-400 mg/day; duration and dosage depends on severity of infection

Indication-specific dosing:

Children:

Candidiasis:

Oropharyngeal: Loading dose: 6 mg/kg; maintenance: 3 mg/kg/day for 2 weeks

Esophageal: Loading dose: 6 mg/kg; maintenance: 3-12 mg/kg/day for 21 days and at least 2 weeks following resolution of symptoms

Systemic infection: 6 mg/kg every 12 hours for 28 days

Meningitis, cryptococcal: Loading dose: 12 mg/kg; maintenance: 6-12 mg/kg/day for 10-12 weeks following negative CSF culture; relapse suppression: 6 mg/kg/day

Adults:

Candidiasis:

Candidemia, primary therapy, non-neutropenic: 400-800 mg/day for 14 days after last positive blood culture and resolution of signs/symptoms

Alternate therapy: 800 mg/day with amphotericin B for 4-7 days followed by 800 mg/day for 14 days after last positive blood culture and resolution of signs/symptoms

Candidemia, secondary, neutropenic: 6-12 mg/kg/day for 14 days after last positive blood culture and resolution of signs/symptoms

Chronic, disseminated: 6 mg/kg/day for 3-6 months

Oropharyngeal (long-term suppression): 200 mg/day; chronic therapy is recommended in immunocompromised patients with history of oropharyngeal candidiasis (OPC)

Osteomyelitis: 6 mg/kg/day for 6-12 months

Esophageal: 200 mg on day 1, then 100-200 mg/day for 2-3 weeks after clinical improvement

Prophylaxis in bone marrow transplant: 400 mg/day; begin 3 days before onset of neutropenia and continue for 7 days after neutrophils >1000 cells/mm^3

Urinary: 200 mg/day for 1-2 weeks

Vaginal: 150 mg as a single dose

Coccidiomycosis: 400 mg/day; doses of 800-1000 mg/day have been used for meningeal disease; usual duration of therapy ranges from 3-6 months for primary uncomplicated infections and up to 1 year for pulmonary (chronic and diffuse) infection

Endocarditis, prosthetic valve, early: 6-12 mg/kg/day for 6 weeks after valve replacement

Endophthalmitis: 6-12 mg/kg/day or 400-800 mg/day for 6-12 weeks after surgical intervention. **Note:** *C. krusei* and *C. galbrata* infection acquired exogenously should be treated with voriconazole.

Meningitis, cryptococcal: 400-800 mg/day for 10-12 weeks or with flucytosine 100-150 mg/day for 6 weeks; maintenance: 200-400 mg/day

Pneumonia, cryptococcal (mild-to-moderate): 200-400 mg/day for 6-12 months (life-long in HIV-positive patients)

Dosage Forms

Infusion [premixed in sodium chloride or dextrose]: 200 mg (100 mL); 400 mg (200 mL)

Diflucan® [premixed in sodium chloride or dextrose]: 200 mg (100 mL); 400 mg (200 mL)

Powder for oral suspension: 10 mg/mL (35 mL); 40 mg/mL (35 mL)

Diflucan®: 10 mg/mL (35 mL); 40 mg/mL (35 mL) [contains sodium benzoate; orange flavor]

Tablet: 50 mg, 100 mg, 150 mg, 200 mg

Diflucan®: 50 mg, 100 mg, 150 mg, 200 mg

Fluconazole Injection [Can] *see* fluconazole *on previous page*

Fluconazole Omega [Can] *see* fluconazole *on previous page*

flucytosine (floo SYE toe seen)

Sound-Alike/Look-Alike Issues

flucytosine may be confused with fluorouracil

Ancobon® may be confused with Oncovin®

Synonyms 5-FC; 5-fluorocytosine; 5-flurocytosine

U.S./Canadian Brand Names Ancobon® [US/Can]

Therapeutic Category Antifungal Agent

Use Adjunctive treatment of systemic fungal infections (eg, septicemia, endocarditis, UTI, meningitis, or pulmonary) caused by susceptible strains of *Candida* or *Cryptococcus*

Usual Dosage

Usual dosage ranges: Adults: Oral: 50-150 mg/kg/day in divided doses every 6 hours

Indication-specific dosing:

Adults:

Endocarditis: Oral: 25-37.5 mg/kg 4 times/day (with amphotericin B) for at least 6 weeks after valve replacement

Meningoencephalitis, cryptococcal: Induction: Oral: 100 mg/kg/day (with amphotericin B) divided every 6 hours for 2 weeks; if clinical improvement, may discontinue both amphotericin and flucytosine and follow with an extended course of fluconazole; alternatively, may continue flucytosine for 6-10 weeks (with amphotericin B) without conversion to fluconazole treatment

Pneumonia, cryptococcal: HIV positive: Oral: 100-150 mg/kg/day for 10 weeks (with fluconazole 400 mg/day)

Dosage Forms Capsule: 250 mg, 500 mg

Fludara® [US/Can] *see* fludarabine *on this page*

fludarabine (floo DARE a been)

Sound-Alike/Look-Alike Issues

fludarabine may be confused with floxuridine, Flumadine®

Fludara® may be confused with FUDR®

Synonyms fludarabine phosphate

U.S./Canadian Brand Names Beneflur® [Can]; Fludara® [US/Can]

Therapeutic Category Antineoplastic Agent

Use

I.V.: Treatment of chronic lymphocytic leukemia (CLL) (including refractory CLL); non-Hodgkin's lymphoma in adults

Oral (formulation not available in U.S.): Approved in Canada for treatment of CLL

Usual Dosage

I.V.: Adults:

Chronic lymphocytic leukemia: 25 mg/m^2/day for 5 days every 28 days

Non-hodgkin's lymphoma: Loading dose: 20 mg/m^2 followed by 30 mg/m^2/day for 48 hours

Oral: Adults: **Note:** Formulation available in Canada; not available in U.S.:

CLL: 40 mg/m^2 once daily for 5 days every 28 days

Dosage Forms [CAN] = Canadian brand name

Injection, powder for reconstitution, as phosphate: 50 mg

Tablet, as phosphate [CAN]: 10 mg [not available in U.S.]

fludarabine phosphate *see* fludarabine *on this page*

fludrocortisone (floo droe KOR ti sone)

Sound-Alike/Look-Alike Issues

Florinef® may be confused with Fiorinal®

Synonyms 9α-fluorohydrocortisone acetate; fludrocortisone acetate; fluohydrisone acetate; fluohydrocortisone acetate

U.S./Canadian Brand Names Florinef® [US/Can]

Therapeutic Category Adrenal Corticosteroid (Mineralocorticoid)

Use Partial replacement therapy for primary and secondary adrenocortical insufficiency in Addison's disease; treatment of salt-losing adrenogenital syndrome

Usual Dosage Oral:

Infants and Children: 0.05-0.1 mg/day

Adults: 0.1-0.2 mg/day with ranges of 0.1 mg 3 times/week to 0.2 mg/day

Addison's disease: Initial: 0.1 mg/day; if transient hypertension develops, reduce the dose to 0.05 mg/day. Preferred administration with cortisone (10-37.5 mg/day) or hydrocortisone (10-30 mg/day).

Salt-losing adrenogenital syndrome: 0.1-0.2 mg/day

Dosage Forms Tablet, as acetate: 0.1 mg

fludrocortisone acetate *see* fludrocortisone *on previous page*

Flumadine® [US/Can] *see* rimantadine *on page 746*

flumazenil (FLOO may ze nil)

U.S./Canadian Brand Names Anexate® [Can]; Flumazenil Injection [Can]; Flumazenil Injection, USP [Can]; Romazicon® [US/Can]

Therapeutic Category Antidote

Use Benzodiazepine antagonist; reverses sedative effects of benzodiazepines used in conscious sedation and general anesthesia; treatment of benzodiazepine overdose

Usual Dosage I.V.:

Children: Reversal of conscious sedation and general anesthesia:

Initial: 0.01 mg/kg over 15 seconds (maximum: 0.2 mg)

Repeat doses (maximum: 4 doses): 0.005-0.01 mg/kg (maximum: 0.2 mg) repeated at 1-minute intervals

Maximum total cumulative dose: 1 mg or 0.05 mg/kg (whichever is lower)

Adults:

Reversal of conscious sedation and general anesthesia:

Initial: 0.2 mg over 15 seconds

Repeat doses: If desired level of consciousness is not obtained, 0.2 mg may be repeated at 1-minute intervals.

Maximum total cumulative dose: 1 mg (usual dose: 0.6-1 mg). In the event of resedation: Repeat doses may be given at 20-minute intervals with maximum of 1 mg/dose and 3 mg/hour

Suspected benzodiazepine overdose:

Initial: 0.2 mg over 30 seconds; if the desired level of consciousness is not obtained, 0.3 mg can be given over 30 seconds

Repeat doses: 0.5 mg over 30 seconds repeated at 1-minute intervals

Maximum total cumulative dose: 3 mg (usual dose: 1-3 mg). Patients with a partial response at 3 mg may require additional titration up to a total dose of 5 mg. If a patient has not responded 5 minutes after cumulative dose of 5 mg, the major cause of sedation is not likely due to benzodiazepines. In the event of resedation: May repeat doses at 20-minute intervals with maximum of 1 mg/dose and 3 mg/hour.

Resedation: Repeated doses may be given at 20-minute intervals as needed; repeat treatment doses of 1 mg (at a rate of 0.5 mg/minute) should be given at any time and no more than 3 mg should be given in any hour. After intoxication with high doses of benzodiazepines, the duration of a single dose of flumazenil is not expected to exceed 1 hour; if desired, the period of wakefulness may be prolonged with repeated low intravenous doses of flumazenil, or by an infusion of 0.1-0.4 mg/hour. Most patients with benzodiazepine overdose will respond to a cumulative dose of 1-3 mg and doses >3 mg do not reliably produce additional effects. Rarely, patients with a partial response at 3 mg may require additional titration up to a total dose of 5 mg. **If a patient has not responded 5 minutes after receiving a cumulative dose of 5 mg, the major cause of sedation is not likely to be due to benzodiazepines.**

Dosage Forms Injection, solution: 0.1 mg/mL (5 mL, 10 mL) [contains edetate sodium]

Flumazenil Injection [Can] *see* flumazenil *on this page*

Flumazenil Injection, USP [Can] *see* flumazenil *on this page*

flumethasone and clioquinol *see* clioquinol and flumethasone *(Canada only) on page 200*

fluMist® [US] *see* influenza virus vaccine *on page 448*

flunarizine *(Canada only)* (floo NAR i zeen)

U.S./Canadian Brand Names Sibelium® [Can]

Therapeutic Category Calcium-Entry Blocker (Selective)

Use Prophylaxis of migraine with and without aura; the safety of flunarizine in long-term use (ie, >4 months) has not been systematically evaluated in controlled clinical trials. Flunarizine is not indicated in the treatment of acute migraine attacks.

Usual Dosage The usual adult dosage is 10 mg/day administered in the evening. Patients who experience side effects may be maintained on 5 mg at bedtime.

Duration of therapy: Clinical experience indicates that the onset of effect of flunarizine is gradual and maximum benefits may not be seen before the patient has completed several weeks of continuous

(Continued)

flunarizine *(Canada only) (Continued)*

treatment. Therapy, therefore, should not be discontinued for lack of response before an adequate time period has elapsed (ie, 6-8 weeks).

Dosage Forms Capsule, as hydrochloride: 5 mg

flunisolide (floo NISS oh lide)

Sound-Alike/Look-Alike Issues

flunisolide may be confused with Flumadine®, fluocinonide

Nasarel® may be confused with Nizoral®

U.S./Canadian Brand Names AeroBid® [US]; AeroBid®-M [US]; Aerospan™ [US]; Alti-Flunisolide [Can]; Apo-Flunisolide® [Can]; Nasalide® [Can]; Nasarel® [US]; PMS-Flunisolide [Can]; Rhinalar® [Can]

Therapeutic Category Adrenal Corticosteroid

Use Steroid-dependent asthma; nasal solution is used for seasonal or perennial rhinitis

Usual Dosage Note: AeroBid® and Aerospan™ are not interchangeable; dosing changes when switching from one to another.

Oral Inhalation: Asthma:

AeroBid®:

Children 6-15 years: 2 inhalations twice daily (morning and evening); up to 4 inhalations/day

Children ≥16 years and Adults: 2 inhalations twice daily (morning and evening); up to 8 inhalations/day maximum

Aerospan™:

Children 6-11 years: 1 inhalation twice daily; up to 4 inhalations/day

Children ≥12 years and Adults: 2 inhalations twice daily; up to 8 inhalations/day

Intranasal: Rhinitis:

Children 6-14 years: 1 spray each nostril 3 times daily **or** 2 sprays in each nostril twice daily; not to exceed 4 sprays/day in each nostril (200 mcg/day)

Children ≥15 years and Adults: 2 sprays each nostril twice daily (morning and evening); may increase to 2 sprays 3 times daily; maximum dose: 8 sprays/day in each nostril (400 mcg/day)

Dosage Forms

Aerosol for oral inhalation:

AeroBid®: 250 mcg/actuation (7 g) [100 metered inhalations; contains CFCs]

AeroBid®-M: 250 mcg/actuation (7 g) [100 metered inhalations; contains CFCs; menthol flavor]

Aerospan™: 80 mcg/actuation (5.1 g) [60 metered inhalations; CFC free]; 80 mcg/actuation (8.9 g) [120 metered inhalations; CFC free]

Solution, intranasal [spray]: 29 mcg/actuation (25 mL) [200 sprays]

Nasarel®: 29 mcg/actuation (25 mL) [200 sprays; contains benzalkonium chloride]

fluocinolone (floo oh SIN oh lone)

Sound-Alike/Look-Alike Issues

fluocinolone may be confused with fluocinonide

Synonyms fluocinolone acetonide

U.S./Canadian Brand Names Capex™ [US/Can]; Derma-Smoothe/FS® [US/Can]; Retisert™ [US]; Synalar® [US/Can]

Therapeutic Category Corticosteroid, Topical

Use Relief of susceptible inflammatory dermatosis [low, medium, high potency topical corticosteroid]; psoriasis of the scalp; atopic dermatitis in children ≥2 years of age

Ocular implant (Retisert™): Treatment of chronic, noninfectious uveitis affecting the posterior segment of the eye.

Usual Dosage

Children ≥2 years: Topical: Atopic dermatitis (Derma-Smoothe/FS®): Moisten skin; apply to affected area twice daily; do not use for longer than 4 weeks

Children and Adults: Topical: Corticosteroid-responsive dermatoses: Cream, ointment, solution: Apply a thin layer to affected area 2-4 times/day; may use occlusive dressings to manage psoriasis or recalcitrant conditions

Adults:

Topical:

Atopic dermatitis (Derma-Smoothe/FS®): Apply thin film to affected area 3 times/day

Inflammatory and pruritic manifestations (dental use): Apply to oral lesion 4 times/day , after meals and at bedtime

Scalp psoriasis (Derma-Smoothe/FS®): Massage thoroughly into wet or dampened hair/scalp; cover with shower cap. Leave on overnight (or for at least 4 hours). Remove by washing hair with shampoo and rinsing thoroughly.

Seborrheic dermatitis of the scalp (Capex™): Apply no more than 1 ounce to scalp once daily; work into lather and allow to remain on scalp for ~5 minutes. Remove from hair and scalp by rinsing thoroughly with water.

Ocular implant: Chronic uveitis: One silicone-encased tablet (0.59 mg) surgically implanted into the posterior segment of the eye is designed to release 0.6 mcg/day, decreasing over 30 days to a steady-state release rate of 0.3-0.4 mcg/day for 30 months. Recurrence of uveitis denotes depletion of tablet, requiring reimplantation.

Dosage Forms

Cream, as acetonide: 0.01% (15 g, 60 g); 0.025% (15 g, 60 g)
Synalar®: 0.025% (15 g, 60 g)
Oil, as acetonide:
Derma-Smoothe/FS® [eczema oil]: 0.01% (120 mL) [contains peanut oil]
Derma-Smoothe/FS® [scalp oil]: 0.01% (120 mL) [contains peanut oil; packaged with shower caps]
Ointment, as acetonide (Synalar®): 0.025% (15 g, 60 g)
Shampoo, as acetonide (Capex™): 0.01% (120 mL)
Solution, as acetonide: 0.01% (60 mL)
Synalar®: 0.01% (20 mL, 60 mL)
Tablet, ocular implant, as acetonide (Retisert™): 0.59 mg [enclosed in silicone elastomer]

fluocinolone acetonide *see* fluocinolone *on previous page*

fluocinolone, hydroquinone, and tretinoin

(floo oh SIN oh lone, HYE droe kwin one, & TRET i noyn)

Synonyms hydroquinone, fluocinolone acetonide, and tretinoin; tretinoin, fluocinolone acetonide, and hydroquinone

U.S./Canadian Brand Names Tri-Luma™ [US]

Therapeutic Category Corticosteroid, Topical; Depigmenting Agent; Retinoic Acid Derivative

Use Short-term treatment of moderate to severe melasma of the face

Usual Dosage Topical: Adults: Melasma: Apply a thin film once daily to hyperpigmented areas of melasma (including 1/2 inch of normal-appearing surrounding skin). Apply 30 minutes prior to bedtime; not indicated for use beyond 8 weeks. Do not use occlusive dressings.

Dosage Forms Cream, topical: Hydroquinone 4%, tretinoin 0.05%, fluocinolone acetonide 0.01% (30 g) [contains sodium metabisulfite]

fluocinonide (floo oh SIN oh nide)

Sound-Alike/Look-Alike Issues

fluocinonide may be confused with flunisolide, fluocinolone
Lidex® may be confused with Lasix®, Videx®, Wydase®

U.S./Canadian Brand Names Lidemol® [Can]; Lidex-E® [US]; Lidex® [US/Can]; Lyderm® [Can]; Tiamol® [Can]; Topsyn® [Can]; Vanos™ [US]

Therapeutic Category Corticosteroid, Topical

Use Antiinflammatory, antipruritic; treatment of plaque-type psoriasis (up to 10% of body surface area) [high-potency topical corticosteroid]

Usual Dosage

Children and Adults: Pruritus and inflammation: Topical (0.5% cream): Apply thin layer to affected area 2-4 times/day depending on the severity of the condition. Therapy should be discontinued when control is achieved; if no improvement is seen, reassessment of diagnosis may be necessary.

Children ≥12 years and Adults: Plaque-type psoriasis (Vanos™): Topical (0.1% cream): Apply a thin layer once or twice daily to affected areas (limited to <10% of body surface area). **Note:** Not recommended for use >2 consecutive weeks or >60 g/week total exposure. Discontinue when control is achieved.

Dosage Forms

Cream, anhydrous, emollient (Lidex®): 0.05% (15 g, 30 g, 60 g)
Cream, aqueous, emollient (Lidex-E®): 0.05% (15 g, 30 g, 60 g)
Cream (Vanos™): 0.1% (30 g, 60 g)
Gel (Lidex®): 0.05% (15 g, 30 g, 60 g)
Ointment (Lidex®): 0.05% (15 g, 30 g, 60 g)
Solution (Lidex®): 0.05% (60 mL) [contains alcohol 35%]

fluohydrisone acetate *see* fludrocortisone *on page 350*

fluohydrocortisone acetate *see* fludrocortisone *on page 350*

Fluonid® Topical *(Discontinued)* *see* fluocinolone *on previous page*

Fluor-I-Strip® [US] *see* fluorescein sodium *on next page*

Fluor-I-Strip-AT® [US] *see* fluorescein sodium *on this page*

Fluoracaine® [US] *see* proparacaine and fluorescein *on page 706*

Fluor-A-Day [US-OTC/Can] *see* fluoride *on this page*

FluorCare® Neutral *(Discontinued)* *see* fluoride *on this page*

fluorescein and proparacaine *see* proparacaine and fluorescein *on page 706*

fluorescein sodium (FLURE e seen SOW dee um)

Synonyms soluble fluorescein

U.S./Canadian Brand Names AK-Fluor [US]; Angiscein® [US]; Fluor-I-Strip-AT® [US]; Fluor-I-Strip® [US]; Fluorescite® [US/Can]; Fluorets® [US]; Ful-Glo® [US]

Therapeutic Category Diagnostic Agent

Use Demonstrates defects of corneal epithelium; diagnostic aid in ophthalmic angiography

Usual Dosage

Ophthalmic:

Solution: Instill 1-2 drops of 2% solution and allow a few seconds for staining; wash out excess with sterile water or irrigating solution

Strips: Moisten strip with sterile water. Place moistened strip at the fornix into the lower cul-de-sac close to the punctum. For best results, patient should close lid tightly over strip until desired amount of staining is obtained. Patient should blink several times after application.

Removal of foreign bodies, sutures or tonometry (Fluress®): Instill 1 or 2 drops (single instillations) into each eye before operating

Deep ophthalmic anesthesia (Fluress®): Instill 2 drops into each eye every 90 seconds up to 3 doses

Injection: Prior to use, perform intradermal skin test; have epinephrine 1:1000, an antihistamine, and oxygen available

Children: 3.5 mg/lb (7.5 mg/kg) injected rapidly into antecubital vein

Adults: 500-750 mg injected rapidly into antecubital vein

Dosage Forms

Injection, solution:

AK-Fluor, Fluorescite®: 10% (5 mL); 25% (2 mL)

Angiscein®: 10% (5 mL)

Strip, ophthalmic:

Fluorets®, Fluor-I-Strip-AT®: 1 mg

Fluor-I-Strip®: 9 mg

Ful-Glo®: 0.6 mg

Fluorescite® [US/Can] *see* fluorescein sodium *on this page*

Fluorets® [US] *see* fluorescein sodium *on this page*

fluoride (FLOR ide)

Sound-Alike/Look-Alike Issues

Luride® may be confused with Lortab®

Phos-Flur® may be confused with PhosLo®

Thera-Flur-N® may be confused with Thera-Flu®

Synonyms acidulated phosphate fluoride; sodium fluoride; stannous fluoride

U.S./Canadian Brand Names ACT® Plus [US-OTC]; ACT® x2™ [US-OTC]; ACT® [US-OTC]; CaviRinse™ [US]; ControlRx® [US]; Denta 5000 Plus [US]; DentaGel [US]; EtheDent™ [US]; Fluor-A-Day [US-OTC/Can]; Fluorigard® [US-OTC]; Fluorinse® [US]; Fluotic® [Can]; Flura-Drops® [US]; Gel-Kam® Rinse [US]; Gel-Kam® [US-OTC]; Just for Kids™ [US-OTC]; Lozi-Flur™ [US]; Luride® Lozi-Tab® [US]; Luride® [US]; NeutraCare® [US]; NeutraGard® Advanced [US] ; NeutraGard® Plus [US]; NeutraGard® [US-OTC]; Omnii Gel™ [US-OTC]; PerioMed™ [US]; Pharmaflur® 1.1 [US]; Pharmaflur® [US]; Phos-Flur® Rinse [US-OTC]; Phos-Flur® [US]; PreviDent® 5000 Plus™ [US]; PreviDent® [US]; StanGard® Perio [US]; StanGard® [US]; Stop® [US]; Thera-Flur-N® [US]

Therapeutic Category Mineral, Oral

Use Prevention of dental caries

Usual Dosage Oral:

The recommended daily dose of oral fluoride supplement (mg), based on fluoride ion content (ppm) in drinking water (2.2 mg of sodium fluoride is equivalent to 1 mg of fluoride ion): Adapted from Recommeded Dosage Schedule of The American Dental Association, The American Academy of Pediatric Dentistry, and The American Academy of Pediatrics:

Less than 0.3 ppm:

Birth to 6 months: 0 mg

6 months to 3 years: 0.25 mg
3-6 years: 0.5 mg
6-16 years: 1 mg
0.3-0.6 ppm:
Birth to 3 years: 0 mg
3-6 years: 0.25 mg
6-16 years: 0.5 mg

Cream: Children ≥6 years and Adults: Brush teeth with cream once daily regardless of fluoride content of drinking water

Dental rinse or gel:

Children 6-12 years: 5-10 mL rinse or apply to teeth and spit daily after brushing

Adults: 10 mL rinse or apply to teeth and spit daily after brushing

PreviDent® rinse: Children >6 years and Adults: Once weekly, rinse 10 mL vigorously around and between teeth for 1 minute, then spit; this should be done preferably at bedtime, after thoroughly brushing teeth; for maximum benefit, do not eat, drink, or rinse mouth for at least 30 minutes after treatment; do not swallow

Fluorinse®: Children >6 years and Adults: Once weekly, vigorously swish 5-10 mL in mouth for 1 minute, then spit

Lozenge (Lozi-Flur™): Adults: One lozenge daily regardless of fluoride content of drinking water

Dosage Forms [DSC] = Discontinued product

Cream, oral, as sodium [toothpaste]: 1.1% (51 g) [fluoride 2.5 mg/dose]
Denta 5000 Plus: 1.1% (51g) [fluoride 2.5 mg/dose; spearmint flavor]
EtheDent™: 1.1% (51g) [fluoride 2.5 mg/dose]

Gel-drops, as sodium fluoride (Thera-Flur-N®): 1.1% (24 mL) [fluoride 0.5%; neutral pH; no artificial color or flavor]

Gel, topical, as acidulated phosphate fluoride (Phos-Flur®): 1.1% (60 g) [fluoride 0.5%; cherry and mint flavors]

Gel, topical, as sodium fluoride: 1.1% (56 g) [fluoride 2 mg/dose]
DentaGel, EtheDent™: 1.1% (56 g) [fluoride 2 mg/dose; fresh mint flavor]
NeutraCare®: 1.1% (60 g) [neutral pH; grape and mint flavors]
NeutraGard® Advanced: 1.1% (60 g) [cinnamon and mint flavors]
PreviDent®: 1.1% (60 g) [fluoride 2 mg/dose; berry, cherry, and mint flavors]

Gel, topical, as stannous fluoride:
Gel-Kam®: 0.4% (129 g) [bubble gum, cinnamon, fruit/berry, and mint flavors]
Just for Kids™: 0.4% (122 g) [bubble gum, fruit punch, and grapey grape flavors]
Omnii Gel™: 0.4% (122 g) [cinnamon, grape, natural, mint, and raspberry flavors]
StanGard®: 0.4% (122 g) [bubble gum, cherry, mint, and raspberry flavors]
Stop®: 0.4% (120 g) [bubble gum, cinnamon, grape, and mint flavors]

Lozenge, as sodium (Lozi-Flur™): 2.21 mg [fluoride 1 mg; cherry flavor]

Paste, oral, as sodium [toothpaste] (ControlRx®): 1.1% (56 g) [vanilla mint flavor]

Solution, oral drops, as sodium: 1.1 mg/mL (50 mL) [fluoride 0.5 mg/mL]
Flura-Drops®: 0.55 mg/drop (24 mL) [fluoride 0.25 mg/drop; dye free, sugar free]
Luride®: 1.1 mg/mL (50 mL) [fluoride 0.5 mg/mL; sugar free]
Pediaflor®: 1.1 mg/mL (50 mL) [fluoride 0.5 mg/mL; contains alcohol <0.5%; sugar free; cherry flavor] [DSC]

Solution, oral rinse, as sodium:
ACT®: 0.05% (530 mL) [fluoride 0.02%; bubble gum, cinnamon (contains tartrazine), and mint flavors]
ACT® Plus: 0.05% (530 mL) [fluoride 0.02%; alcohol free; icy cool mint flavor]
ACT® x2™: 0.5% (530 mL) [fluoride 0.02%; contains alcohol 11%; icy cool mint and spearmint flavors]
CaviRinse™: 0.2% (240 mL) [mint flavor]
Fluorigard®: 0.05% (480 mL) [alcohol free, sugar free; contains sodium benzoate and tartrazine; mint flavor]
Fluorinse®: 0.2% (480 mL) [alcohol free; cinnamon and mint flavors]
NeutraGard®: 0.05% (480 mL) [neutral pH; mint and tropical blast flavors]
NeutraGard® Plus: 0.2% (480 mL) [neutral pH; mint and tropical blast flavors]
Phos-Flur®: 0.44% (500 mL) [bubble gum, cherry, grape, and mint flavors]
PreviDent®: 0.2% (250 mL) [contains alcohol; mint flavor]

Solution, oral rinse concentrate, as stannous fluoride:
Gel-Kam®: 0.63% (300 mL) [fluoride 0.1%/dose; cinnamon and mint flavors]
PerioMed™: 0.63% (284 mL) [fluoride 7 mg/30 mL; alcohol free; cinnamon, mint and tropical fruit flavors]
StanGard® Perio: 0.63% (284 mL) [mint flavor]

Tablet, chewable, as sodium: 0.5 mg [fluoride 0.25 mg]; 1.1 mg [fluoride 0.5 mg]; 2.2 mg [fluoride 1 mg]

(Continued)

fluoride *(Continued)*

EtheDent™:

0.55 mg [fluoride 0.25 mg; sugar free; contains aspartame; vanilla flavor]

1.1 mg [fluoride 0.5 mg; sugar free; contains aspartame; grape flavor]

2.2 mg [fluoride 1 mg; sugar free; contains aspartame; cherry flavor]

Fluor-A-Day:

0.56 mg [fluoride 0.25 mg; raspberry flavor]

1.1 mg [fluoride 0.5 mg; raspberry flavor]

2.21 mg [fluoride 1 mg; raspberry flavor]

Luride® Lozi-Tab®:

0.55 mg [fluoride 0.25 mg; sugar free; vanilla flavor]

1.1 mg [fluoride 0.5 mg; sugar free; grape flavor]

2.2 mg [fluoride 1 mg; sugar free; cherry flavor]

Pharmaflur®: 2.2 mg [fluoride 1 mg; dye free, sugar free; cherry flavor]

Pharmaflur® 1.1: 1.1 mg [fluoride 0.5 mg; dye free, sugar free; grape flavor]

Fluorigard® [US-OTC] *see* fluoride *on page 354*

Fluori-Methane® [US] *see* dichlorodifluoromethane and trichloromonofluoromethane *on page 250*

Fluorinse® [US] *see* fluoride *on page 354*

Fluoritab® *(Discontinued)* *see* fluoride *on page 354*

5-fluorocytosine *see* flucytosine *on page 350*

fluorodeoxyuridine *see* floxuridine *on page 348*

9α-fluorohydrocortisone acetate *see* fludrocortisone *on page 350*

fluorometholone (flure oh METH oh lone)

Sound-Alike/Look-Alike Issues

Fluor-Op® may be confused with Fluoron® which is a brand name for fluorine in Canada

U.S./Canadian Brand Names Flarex® [US/Can]; FML® Forte [US/Can]; FML® [US/Can]; PMS-Fluorometholone [Can]

Therapeutic Category Adrenal Corticosteroid

Use Treatment of steroid-responsive inflammatory conditions of the eye

Usual Dosage Children >2 years and Adults: Ophthalmic: Re-evaluate therapy if improvement is not seen within 2 days; use care not to discontinue prematurely; in chronic conditions, gradually decrease dosing frequency prior to discontinuing treatment

Ointment: Apply small amount (~1/2 inch ribbon) to conjunctival sac every 4 hours in severe cases; 1-3 times/day in mild to moderate cases

Solution: Instill 1-2 drops into conjunctival sac every hour during day, every 2 hours at night until favorable response is obtained, then use 1 drop every 4 hours; for mild to moderate inflammation, instill 1-2 drops into conjunctival sac 2-4 times/day

Dosage Forms [DSC] = Discontinued product

Ointment, ophthalmic, as base (FML®): 0.1% (3.5 g)

Suspension, ophthalmic, as base: 0.1% (5 mL, 10 mL, 15 mL)

Fluor-Op®: 0.1% (5 mL, 10 mL, 15 mL) [contains benzalkonium chloride and polyvinyl alcohol] [DSC]

FML®: 0.1% (5 mL, 10 mL, 15 mL) [contains benzalkonium chloride]

FML® Forte: 0.25% (2 mL, 5 mL, 10 mL, 15 mL) [contains benzalkonium chloride]

Suspension, ophthalmic, as acetate:

Eflone®: 0.1% (5 mL, 10 mL) [DSC]

Flarex®: 0.1% (5 mL, 10 mL) [contains benzalkonium chloride]

fluorometholone and sulfacetamide *see* sulfacetamide sodium and fluorometholone *on page 796*

Fluor-Op® *(Discontinued)* *see* fluorometholone *on this page*

Fluoroplex® [US] *see* fluorouracil *on this page*

fluorouracil (flure oh YOOR a sil)

Sound-Alike/Look-Alike Issues

fluorouracil may be confused with flucytosine

Efudex® may be confused with Efidac (Efidac 24®), Eurax®

Synonyms 5-fluorouracil; FU; 5-FU

U.S./Canadian Brand Names Adrucil® [US]; Carac™ [US]; Efudex® [US/Can]; Fluoroplex® [US]

Therapeutic Category Antineoplastic Agent

Use Treatment of carcinomas of the breast, colon, head and neck, pancreas, rectum, or stomach; topically for the management of actinic or solar keratoses and superficial basal cell carcinomas

Usual Dosage Adults:

Refer to individual protocols:

I.V. bolus: 500-600 mg/m^2 every 3-4 weeks **or** 425 mg/m^2 on days 1-5 every 4 weeks

Continuous I.V. infusion: 1000 mg/m^2/day for 4-5 days every 3-4 weeks **or**
2300-2600 mg/m^2 on day 1 every week **or**
300-400 mg/m^2/day **or**
225 mg/m^2/day for 5-8 weeks (with radiation therapy)

Actinic keratoses: Topical:

Carac™: Apply thin film to lesions once daily for up to 4 weeks, as tolerated

Efudex®: Apply to lesions twice daily for 2-4 weeks; complete healing may not be evident for 1-2 months following treatment

Fluoroplex®: Apply to lesions twice daily for 2-6 weeks

Superficial basal cell carcinoma: Topical: Efudex® 5%: Apply to affected lesions twice daily for 3-6 weeks; treatment may be continued for up to 10-12 weeks

Dosage Forms

Cream, topical:

Carac™: 0.5% (30 g)

Efudex®: 5% (25 g, 40 g)

Fluoroplex®: 1% (30 g) [contains benzyl alcohol]

Injection, solution: 50 mg/mL (10 mL, 20 mL, 50 mL, 100 mL)

Adrucil®: 50 mg/mL (10 mL, 50 mL, 100 mL)

Solution, topical (Efudex®): 2% (10 mL); 5% (10 mL)

5-fluorouracil *see* fluorouracil *on previous page*

Fluothane® ***(Discontinued)*** *see* halothane *on page 407*

Fluotic® [Can] *see* fluoride *on page 354*

fluoxetine (floo OKS e teen)

Sound-Alike/Look-Alike Issues

fluoxetine may be confused with duloxetine, fluvastatin, fluvoxamine

Prozac® may be confused with Prilosec®, Proscar®, ProSom®, ProStep®

Sarafem™ may be confused with Serophene®

Synonyms fluoxetine hydrochloride

U.S./Canadian Brand Names Alti-Fluoxetine [Can]; Apo-Fluoxetine® [Can]; BCI-Fluoxetine [Can]; CO Fluoxetine [Can]; FXT [Can]; Gen-Fluoxetine [Can]; Novo-Fluoxetine [Can]; Nu-Fluoxetine [Can]; PMS-Fluoxetine [Can]; Prozac® Weekly™ [US]; Prozac® [US/Can]; Rhoxal-fluoxetine [Can]; Sandoz-Fluoxetine [Can]; Sarafem® [US]

Therapeutic Category Antidepressant, Selective Serotonin Reuptake Inhibitor

Use Treatment of major depressive disorder (MDD); treatment of binge-eating and vomiting in patients with moderate-to-severe bulimia nervosa; obsessive-compulsive disorder (OCD); premenstrual dysphoric disorder (PMDD); panic disorder with or without agoraphobia

Usual Dosage Oral: **Note:** Upon discontinuation of fluoxetine therapy, gradually taper dose. If intolerable symptoms occur following a dose reduction, consider resuming the previously prescribed dose and/or decrease dose at a more gradual rate.

Children:

Depression: 8-18 years: 10-20 mg/day; lower-weight children can be started at 10 mg/day, may increase to 20 mg/day after 1 week if needed

OCD: 7-18 years: Initial: 10 mg/day; in adolescents and higher-weight children, dose may be increased to 20 mg/day after 2 weeks. Range: 10-60 mg/day

Adults: 20 mg/day in the morning; may increase after several weeks by 20 mg/day increments; maximum: 80 mg/day; doses >20 mg may be given once daily or divided twice daily. **Note:** Lower doses of 5-10 mg/day have been used for initial treatment.

Usual dosage range:

Bulimia nervosa: 60-80 mg/day

Depression: 20-40 mg/day; patients maintained on Prozac® 20 mg/day may be changed to Prozac® Weekly™ 90 mg/week, starting dose 7 days after the last 20 mg/day dose

OCD: 40-80 mg/day

(Continued)

fluoxetine *(Continued)*

Panic disorder: Initial: 10 mg/day; after 1 week, increase to 20 mg/day; may increase after several weeks; doses >60 mg/day have not been evaluated

PMDD (Sarafem™): 20 mg/day continuously, **or** 20 mg/day starting 14 days prior to menstruation and through first full day of menses (repeat with each cycle)

Dosage Forms [DSC] = Discontinued product

Capsule, as hydrochloride: 10 mg, 20 mg, 40 mg

Prozac®: 10 mg, 20 mg, 40 mg

Sarafem®: 10 mg, 20 mg

Capsule, delayed release, as hydrochloride (Prozac® Weekly™): 90 mg

Solution, oral, as hydrochloride (Prozac®): 20 mg/5 mL (120 mL) [contains alcohol 0.23% and benzoic acid; mint flavor]

Tablet, as hydrochloride: 10 mg, 20 mg

Prozac® [scored]: 10 mg [DSC]

fluoxetine and olanzapine *see* olanzapine and fluoxetine *on page 613*

fluoxetine hydrochloride *see* fluoxetine *on previous page*

fluoxymesterone (floo oks i MES te rone)

Sound-Alike/Look-Alike Issues

Halotestin® may be confused with Haldol®, haloperidol, halothane, Halotussin®

Therapeutic Category Androgen

Controlled Substance C-III

Use Replacement of endogenous testicular hormone; in females, palliative treatment of breast cancer

Usual Dosage Adults: Oral:

Male:

Hypogonadism: 5-20 mg/day

Delayed puberty: 2.5-20 mg/day for 4-6 months

Female: Inoperable breast carcinoma: 10-40 mg/day in divided doses for 1-3 months

Dosage Forms [DSC] = Discontinued product

Tablet: 10 mg

Halotestin®: 2 mg, 5 mg, 10 mg [contains tartrazine; 10 mg tablet DSC]

flupenthixol *(Canada only)* (floo pen THIKS ol)

Synonyms flupenthixol decanoate; flupenthixol dihydrochloride

U.S./Canadian Brand Names Fluanxol® [Can]

Therapeutic Category Antipsychotic Agent; Thioxanthene Derivative

Use Maintenance therapy of chronic schizophrenic patients whose main manifestations do **not** include excitement, agitation, or hyperactivity

Usual Dosage

I.M. (depot): Flupenthixol is administered by deep I.M. injection, preferably in the gluteus maximus, **NOT for I.V. use**; maintenance dosages are given at 2- to 3-week intervals

Patients not previously treated with long-acting depot neuroleptics should be given an initial test dose of 5-20 mg. An initial dose of 20 mg is usually well tolerated; however, a 5 mg test dose is recommended in elderly, frail, and cachectic patients, and in patients whose individual or family history suggests a predisposition to extrapyramidal reactions. In the subsequent 5-10 days, the therapeutic response and the appearance of extrapyramidal symptoms should be carefully monitored. Oral neuroleptic drugs may be continued, but dosage should be reduced during this overlapping period and eventually discontinued.

Oral: Initial: 1 mg 3 times/day; dose must be individualized. May be increased by 1 mg every 2-3 days based on tolerance and control of symptoms. Usual maintenance dosage: 3-6 mg/day in divided doses (doses ≥12 mg/day used in some patients).

Dosage Forms

Injection, solution, as decanoate [depot]: 20 mg/mL (10 mL); 100 mg/mL (2 mL)

Tablet, as dihydrochloride: 0.5 mg, 3 mg

flupenthixol decanoate *see* flupenthixol *(Canada only)* *on this page*

flupenthixol dihydrochloride *see* flupenthixol *(Canada only)* *on this page*

fluphenazine (floo FEN a zeen)

Sound-Alike/Look-Alike Issues

Prolixin® may be confused with Proloprim®

Synonyms fluphenazine decanoate

U.S./Canadian Brand Names Apo-Fluphenazine Decanoate® [Can]; Apo-Fluphenazine® [Can]; Modecate® Concentrate [Can]; Modecate® [Can]; PMS-Fluphenazine Decanoate [Can]; Prolixin Decanoate® [US]

Therapeutic Category Phenothiazine Derivative

Use Management of manifestations of psychotic disorders and schizophrenia; depot formulation may offer improved outcome in individuals with psychosis who are nonadherent with oral antipsychotics

Usual Dosage Adults: Psychoses:

Oral: 0.5-10 mg/day in divided doses at 6- to 8-hour intervals; some patients may require up to 40 mg/day

I.M.: 2.5-10 mg/day in divided doses at 6- to 8-hour intervals (parenteral dose is $^1/_3$ to $^1/_2$ the oral dose for the hydrochloride salts)

I.M. (decanoate): 12.5 mg every 2 weeks

Conversion from hydrochloride to decanoate I.M. 0.5 mL (12.5 mg) decanoate every 3 weeks is approximately equivalent to 10 mg hydrochloride/day

Dosage Forms [DSC] = Discontinued product

Elixir, as hydrochloride (Prolixin®): 2.5 mg/5 mL (60 mL) [contains alcohol 14% and sodium benzoate] [DSC]

Injection, oil, as decanoate: 25 mg/mL (5 mL) [may contain benzyl alcohol, sesame oil]

Prolixin Decanoate®: 25 mg/mL (5 mL) [contains benzyl alcohol, sesame oil]

Injection, solution, as hydrochloride (Prolixin® [DSC]): 2.5 mg/mL (10 mL)

Solution, oral concentrate, as hydrochloride (Prolixin®): 5 mg/mL (120 mL) [contains alcohol 14%] [DSC]

Tablet, as hydrochloride: 1 mg, 2.5 mg, 5 mg, 10 mg

Prolixin®: 1 mg, 2.5 mg, 5 mg [contains tartrazine], 10 mg [DSC]

fluphenazine decanoate *see* fluphenazine *on previous page*

Flura® *(Discontinued)* *see* fluoride *on page 354*

Flura-Drops® [US] *see* fluoride *on page 354*

flurandrenolide (flure an DREN oh lide)

Sound-Alike/Look-Alike Issues

Cordran® may be confused with Cardura®, codeine, Cordarone®

Synonyms flurandrenolone

U.S./Canadian Brand Names Cordran® SP [US]; Cordran® [US/Can]

Therapeutic Category Corticosteroid, Topical

Use Inflammation of corticosteroid-responsive dermatoses [medium potency topical corticosteroid]

Usual Dosage Topical: Therapy should be discontinued when control is achieved; if no improvement is seen, reassessment of diagnosis may be necessary.

Children:

Ointment, cream: Apply sparingly 1-2 times/day

Tape: Apply once daily

Adults: Cream, lotion, ointment: Apply sparingly 2-3 times/day

Dosage Forms

Cream, emulsified, as base (Cordran® SP): 0.025% (30 g, 60 g); 0.05% (15 g, 30 g, 60 g)

Lotion (Cordran®): 0.05% (15 mL, 60 mL)

Ointment (Cordran®): 0.025% (30 g, 60 g); 0.05% (15 g, 30 g, 60 g)

Tape, topical [roll] (Cordran®): 4 mcg/cm^2 (7.5 cm x 60 cm, 7.5 cm x 200 cm)

flurandrenolone *see* flurandrenolide *on this page*

Flurate® Ophthalmic Solution *(Discontinued)* *see* fluorescein sodium *on page 354*

flurazepam (flure AZ e pam)

Sound-Alike/Look-Alike Issues

flurazepam may be confused with temazepam

Dalmane® may be confused with Demulen®, Dialume®

Synonyms flurazepam hydrochloride

U.S./Canadian Brand Names Apo-Flurazepam® [Can]; Dalmane® [US/Can]; Som Pam [Can]

Therapeutic Category Benzodiazepine

Controlled Substance C-IV

Use Short-term treatment of insomnia

Usual Dosage Oral:

Children: Insomnia:

≤15 years: Dose not established

(Continued)

flurazepam *(Continued)*

>15 years: 15 mg at bedtime
Adults: Insomnia: 15-30 mg at bedtime

Dosage Forms Capsule, as hydrochloride: 15 mg, 30 mg

flurazepam hydrochloride *see* flurazepam *on previous page*

flurbiprofen (flure BI proe fen)

Sound-Alike/Look-Alike Issues

flurbiprofen may be confused with fenoprofen
Ansaid® may be confused with Asacol®, Axid®
Ocufen® may be confused with Ocuflox®, Ocupress®

Synonyms flurbiprofen sodium

U.S./Canadian Brand Names Alti-Flurbiprofen [Can]; Ansaid® [Can]; Apo-Flurbiprofen® [Can]; Froben-SR® [Can]; Froben® [Can]; Novo-Flurprofen [Can]; Nu-Flurprofen [Can]; Ocufen® [US/Can]

Therapeutic Category Analgesic, Nonnarcotic; Nonsteroidal Antiinflammatory Drug (NSAID)

Use

Oral: Treatment of rheumatoid arthritis and osteoarthritis
Ophthalmic: Inhibition of intraoperative miosis

Usual Dosage

Oral:
Rheumatoid arthritis and osteoarthritis: 200-300 mg/day in 2-, 3-, or 4 divided doses; do not administer more than 100 mg for any single dose; maximum: 300 mg/day
Dental: Management of postoperative pain: 100 mg every 12 hours
Ophthalmic: Instill 1 drop every 30 minutes, beginning 2 hours prior to surgery (total of 4 drops in each affected eye)

Dosage Forms [DSC] = Discontinued product

Solution, ophthalmic, as sodium (Ocufen®): 0.03% (2.5 mL) [contains thimerosal]
Tablet: 50 mg, 100 mg
Ansaid®: 50 mg, 100 mg [DSC]

flurbiprofen sodium *see* flurbiprofen *on this page*

5-flurocytosine *see* flucytosine *on page 350*

Fluro-Ethyl® [US] *see* ethyl chloride and dichlorotetrafluoroethane *on page 329*

Flurosyn® Topical *(Discontinued)* *see* fluocinolone *on page 352*

FluShield® *(Discontinued)* *see* influenza virus vaccine *on page 448*

flutamide (FLOO ta mide)

Sound-Alike/Look-Alike Issues

flutamide may be confused with Flumadine®, thalidomide
Eulexin® may be confused with Edecrin®, Eurax®

Synonyms niftolid; NSC-147834; 4′-nitro-3′-trifluoromethylisobutyrantide; SCH 13521

U.S./Canadian Brand Names Apo-Flutamide® [Can]; Euflex® [Can]; Eulexin® [US/Can]; Novo-Flutamide [Can]

Therapeutic Category Antiandrogen

Use Treatment of metastatic prostatic carcinoma in combination therapy with LHRH agonist analogues

Usual Dosage Oral: Adults: Prostatic carcinoma: 250 mg 3 times/day

Dosage Forms Capsule: 125 mg

fluticasone and salmeterol (floo TIK a sone & sal ME te role)

Sound-Alike/Look-Alike Issues

Advair may be confused with Advicor®

Synonyms fluticasone propionate and salmeterol xinafoate; salmeterol and fluticasone

U.S./Canadian Brand Names Advair Diskus® [US/Can]

Therapeutic Category Beta$_2$-Adrenergic Agonist Agent; Corticosteroid, Inhalant

Use Maintenance treatment of asthma; maintenance treatment of COPD associated with chronic bronchitis

Usual Dosage Oral inhalation: **Note:** Do not use to transfer patients from systemic corticosteroid therapy.

COPD: Adults: Advair Diskus®: Fluticasone 250 mcg/salmeterol 50 mcg twice daily, 12 hours apart. **Note:** This is the maximum dose.

Asthma:

Children 4-11 years: Advair Diskus®: Fluticasone 100 mcg/salmeterol 50 mcg twice daily, 12 hours apart. **Note:** This is the maximum dose.

Children ≥12 and Adults:

Advair Diskus®: One inhalation twice daily, morning and evening, 12 hours apart

Maximum dose: Fluticasone 500 mcg/salmeterol 50 mcg per inhalation

Advair® HFA: Two inhalations twice daily, morning and evening, 12 hours apart

Maximum dose: Fluticasone 230 mcg/salmeterol 21 mcg per inhalation

Note: Initial dose prescribed should be based upon previous dose of inhaled-steroid asthma therapy. Dose should be increased after 2 weeks if adequate response is not achieved. Patients should be titrated to lowest effective dose once stable. Each suggestion below specifies the product strength to use; remember to **use 1 inhalation for Diskus® and 2 inhalations for HFA.**

Patients not currently on inhaled corticosteroids:

Advair Diskus®: Fluticasone 100 mcg/salmeterol 50 mcg **or** fluticasone 250 mcg/salmeterol 50 mcg

Advair® HFA: Fluticasone 45 mcg/salmeterol 21 mcg **or** fluticasone 115 mcg/salmeterol 21 mcg

Patients currently using inhaled beclomethasone dipropionate:

≤160 mcg/day: Advair Diskus®: Fluticasone 100 mcg/salmeterol 50 mcg **or** Advair® HFA: Fluticasone 45 mcg/salmeterol 21 mcg

320 mcg/day: Advair Diskus®: Fluticasone 250 mcg/salmeterol 50 mcg **or** Advair® HFA: Fluticasone 115 mcg/salmeterol 21 mcg

640 mcg/day: Advair Diskus®: Fluticasone 500 mcg/salmeterol 50 mcg **or** Advair® HFA: Fluticasone 230 mcg/salmeterol 21 mcg

Patients currently using inhaled budesonide:

≤400 mcg/day: Advair Diskus®: Fluticasone 100 mcg/salmeterol 50 mcg **or** Advair® HFA: Fluticasone 45 mcg/salmeterol 21 mcg

800-1200 mcg/day: Advair Diskus®: Fluticasone 250 mcg/salmeterol 50 mcg **or** Advair® HFA: Fluticasone 115 mcg/salmeterol 21mcg

1600 mcg/day: Advair Diskus®: Fluticasone 500 mcg/salmeterol 50 mcg **or** Advair® HFA: Fluticasone 230 mcg/salmeterol 21 mcg

Patients currently using inhaled flunisolide CFC aerosol:

1000 mcg/day: Advair Diskus®: Fluticasone 100 mcg/salmeterol 50 mcg **or** Advair® HFA: Fluticasone 45 mcg/salmeterol 21 mcg

1250-2000 mcg/day: Advair Diskus®: Fluticasone 250 mcg/salmeterol 50 mcg **or** Advair® HFA: Fluticasone 115 mcg/salmeterol 21 mcg

Patients currently using inhaled fluticasone HFA aerosol:

≤176 mcg/day: Advair Diskus®: Fluticasone 100 mcg/salmeterol 50 mcg **or** Advair® HFA: Fluticasone 45 mcg/salmeterol 21 mcg

440 mcg/day: Advair Diskus®: Fluticasone 250 mcg/salmeterol 50 mcg **or** Advair® HFA: Fluticasone 115 mcg/salmeterol 21 mcg

660-880 mcg/day: Advair Diskus®: Fluticasone 500 mcg/salmeterol 50 mcg **or** Advair® HFA: Fluticasone 230 mcg/salmeterol 21 mcg

Patients currently using inhaled fluticasone propionate powder:

≤200 mcg/day: Advair Diskus®: Fluticasone 100 mcg/salmeterol 50 mcg **or** Advair® HFA: Fluticasone 45 mcg/salmeterol 21 mcg

500 mcg/day: Advair Diskus®: Fluticasone 250 mcg/salmeterol 50 mcg **or** Advair® HFA: Fluticasone 115 mcg/salmeterol 21 mcg

1000 mcg/day: Advair Diskus®: Fluticasone 500 mcg/salmeterol 50 mcg **or** Advair® HFA: Fluticasone 230 mcg/salmeterol 21 mcg

Patients currently using inhaled mometasone furoate powder:

220 mcg/day: Advair Diskus®: Fluticasone 100 mcg/salmeterol 50 mcg **or** Advair® HFA: Fluticasone 45 mcg/salmeterol 21 mcg

440 mcg/day: Advair Diskus®: Fluticasone 250 mcg/salmeterol 50 mcg **or** Advair® HFA: Fluticasone 115 mcg/salmeterol 21 mcg

880 mcg/day: Advair Diskus®: Fluticasone 500 mcg/salmeterol 50 mcg **or** Advair® HFA: Fluticasone 230 mcg/salmeterol 21 mcg

Patients currently using inhaled triamcinolone acetonide:

≤1000 mcg/day: Advair Diskus®: Fluticasone 100 mcg/salmeterol 50 mcg **or** Advair® HFA: Fluticasone 45 mcg/salmeterol 21 mcg

1100-1600 mcg/day: Advair Diskus®: Fluticasone 250 mcg/salmeterol 50 mcg **or** Advair® HFA: Fluticasone 115 mcg/salmeterol 21 mcg

(Continued)

fluticasone and salmeterol *(Continued)*

Dosage Forms

Aerosol, for oral inhalation:

Advair® HFA:

45/21: Fluticasone propionate 45 mcg and salmeterol xinafoate 30.45 mcg (12 g) [120 metered inhalations]

115/21: Fluticasone propionate 115 mcg and salmeterol xinafoate 30.45 mcg (12 g) [120 metered inhalations]

230/21: Fluticasone propionate 230 mcg and salmeterol xinafoate 30.45 mcg (12 g) [120 metered inhalations]

Powder, for oral inhalation:

Advair Diskus®:

100/50: Fluticasone propionate 100 mcg and salmeterol xinafoate 50 mcg (28s, 60s) [contains lactose; chlorfluorocarbon free]

250/50: Fluticasone propionate 250 mcg and salmeterol xinafoate 50 mcg (28s, 60s) [contains lactose; chlorfluorocarbon free]

500/50: Fluticasone propionate 500 mcg and salmeterol xinafoate 50 mcg (28s, 60s) [contains lactose; chlorfluorocarbon free]

fluticasone (nasal) (floo TIK a sone NAY sal)

U.S./Canadian Brand Names Flonase® [US/Can]

Therapeutic Category Adrenal Corticosteroid

Use Intranasal: Management of seasonal and perennial allergic rhinitis and nonallergic rhinitis in patients ≥4 years of age

Usual Dosage Rhinitis: Intranasal:

Children ≥4 years and Adolescents: Initial: 1 spray (50 mcg/spray) per nostril once daily; patients not adequately responding or patients with more severe symptoms may use 2 sprays (100 mcg) per nostril. Depending on response, dosage may be reduced to 100 mcg daily. Total daily dosage should not exceed 2 sprays in each nostril (200 mcg)/day. Dosing should be at regular intervals.

Adults: Initial: 2 sprays (50 mcg/spray) per nostril once daily; may also be divided into 100 mcg twice a day. After the first few days, dosage may be reduced to 1 spray per nostril once daily for maintenance therapy. Dosing should be at regular intervals.

Dosage Forms Spray, intranasal: 50 mcg/actuation (16 g = 120 actuations)

fluticasone (oral inhalation) (floo TIK a sone or al in ha LAY shun)

U.S./Canadian Brand Names Flovent® Diskus® [Can]; Flovent® HFA [US/Can]

Therapeutic Category Adrenal Corticosteroid

Use Inhalation: Maintenance treatment of asthma as prophylactic therapy. It is also indicated for patients requiring oral corticosteroid therapy for asthma to assist in total discontinuation or reduction of total oral dose. NOT indicated for the relief of acute bronchospasm.

Usual Dosage Inhalation, oral: Asthma:

Flovent®, Flovent® HFA: Children ≥12 years: Refer to Adults dosing.

Flovent® Diskus® [Can]:

Children 4-16 years: Usual starting dose: 50-100 mcg twice daily; may increase to 200 mcg twice daily in patients not adequately controlled; titrate to the lowest effective dose once asthma stability is achieved

Children ≥16 years: Refer to Adults dosing.

Adults: **Note:** Titrate to the lowest effective dose once asthma stability is achieved

Flovent®, Flovent® HFA: Manufacturers labeling: Dosing based on previous therapy

Bronchodilator alone: Recommended starting dose: 88 mcg twice daily; highest recommended dose: 440 mcg twice daily

Inhaled corticosteroids: Recommended starting dose: 88-220 mcg twice daily; highest recommended dose: 440 mcg twice daily; a higher starting dose may be considered in patients previously requiring higher doses of inhaled corticosteroids

Oral corticosteroids: Recommended starting dose:

Flovent®: 880 mcg twice daily

Flovent® HFA: 440 mcg twice daily

Highest recommended dose: 880 mcg twice daily; starting dose is patient dependent. In patients on chronic oral corticosteroids therapy, reduce prednisone dose no faster than 2.5-5 mg/day on a weekly basis; begin taper after 1 week of fluticasone therapy

NIH Asthma Guidelines (administer in divided doses twice daily).

"Low" dose: 88-264 mcg/day

"Medium" dose: 264-660 mcg/day

"High" dose: >660 mcg/day

Flovent® Diskus® [CAN]:
Mild asthma: 100-250 mcg twice daily
Moderate asthma: 250-500 mcg twice da
Severe asthma: 500 mcg twice daily; may increase to 1000 mcg twice daily in very severe patients requiring high doses of corticosteroids

Dosage Forms [DSC] = Discontinued product; [CAN] = Canadian brand name

Aerosol for oral inhalation, as propionate [contains CFCs] (Flovent®):
44 mcg/inhalation (7.9 g) [60 metered doses], (13 g) [120 metered doses] [DSC]
110 mcg/inhalation (7.9 g) [60 metered doses], (13 g) [120 metered doses] [DSC]
220 mcg/inhalation (7.9 g) [60 metered doses], (13 g) [120 metered doses] [DSC]

Aerosol for oral inhalation, as propionate [CFC free] (Flovent® HFA):
44 mcg/inhalation (10.6 g) [120 metered doses]
110 mcg/inhalation (12 g) [120 metered doses]
220 mcg/inhalation (12 g) [120 metered doses]

Powder for oral inhalation, as propionate [prefilled blister pack] (Flovent® Diskus®) [CAN; not available in the United States]:
50 mcg (28s, 60s) [contains lactose]
100 mcg (28s, 60s) [contains lactose]
250 mcg (28s, 60s) [contains lactose]
500 mcg (28s, 60s) [contains lactose]

fluticasone propionate and salmeterol xinafoate *see* fluticasone and salmeterol *on page 360*

fluticasone (topical) (floo TIK a sone TOP i kal)

Sound-Alike/Look-Alike Issues
Cutivate® may be confused with Ultravate®

U.S./Canadian Brand Names Cutivate® [US]

Therapeutic Category Adrenal Corticosteroid; Corticosteroid, Topical

Use Relief of inflammation and pruritus associated with corticosteroid-responsive dermatoses; atopic dermatitis

Usual Dosage Topical:

Corticosteroid-responsive dermatoses:
Children ≥3 months: Cream: Apply sparingly to affected area twice daily. If no improvement is seen within 2 weeks, reassessment of diagnosis may be necessary
Adults: Cream, lotion, ointment: Apply sparingly to affected area twice daily. If no improvement is seen within 2 weeks, reassessment of diagnosis may be necessary.

Atopic dermatitis:
Children ≥3 months: Cream: Apply sparingly to affected area twice daily. If no improvement is seen within 2 weeks, reassessment of diagnosis may be necessary.
Children ≥1 year: Lotion: Apply sparingly to affected area twice daily
Adults: Cream, lotion: Apply sparingly to affected area once or twice daily. If no improvement is seen within 2 weeks, reassessment of diagnosis may be necessary

Dosage Forms
Cream, as propionate (Cutivate®): 0.05% (15 g, 30 g, 60 g)
Lotion, as propionate (Cutivate®): 0.05% (60 mL)
Ointment, as propionate (Cutivate®): 0.005% (15 g, 30 g, 60 g)

fluvastatin (FLOO va sta tin)

Sound-Alike/Look-Alike Issues
fluvastatin may be confused with fluoxetine

U.S./Canadian Brand Names Lescol® XL [US]; Lescol® [US/Can]

Therapeutic Category HMG-CoA Reductase Inhibitor

Use To be used as a component of multiple risk factor intervention in patients at risk for atherosclerosis vascular disease due to hypercholesterolemia

Adjunct to dietary therapy to reduce elevated total cholesterol (total-C), LDL-C, triglyceride, and apolipoprotein B (apo-B) levels and to increase HDL-C in primary hypercholesterolemia and mixed dyslipidemia (Fredrickson types IIa and IIb); to slow the progression of coronary atherosclerosis in patients with coronary heart disease; reduce risk of coronary revascularization procedures in patients with coronary heart disease

Usual Dosage
Adolescents 10-16 years: Oral: Heterozygous familial hypercholesterolemia: Initial: 20 mg once daily; may increase every 6 weeks based on tolerability and response to a maximum recommended dose of 80 mg/day,
(Continued)

fluvastatin *(Continued)*

given in 2 divided doses (immediate release capsule) or as a single daily dose (extended release tablet)

Note: Indicated only for adjunctive therapy when diet alone cannot reduce LDL-C below 190 mg/dL, or 160 mg/dL (with cardiovascular risk factors). Female patients must be 1 year postmenarche.

Adults: Oral:

Patients requiring ≥25% decrease in LDL-C: 40 mg capsule once daily in the evening, 80 mg extended release tablet once daily (anytime), or 40 mg capsule twice daily

Patients requiring <25% decrease in LDL-C: Initial: 20 mg capsule once daily in the evening; may increase based on tolerability and response to a maximum recommended dose of 80 mg/day, given in 2 divided doses (immediate release capsule) or as a single daily dose (extended release tablet)

Dosage Forms

Capsule (Lescol®): 20 mg, 40 mg

Tablet, extended release (Lescol® XL): 80 mg

Fluviral S/F® [Can] *see* influenza virus vaccine *on page 448*

Fluvirin® [US] *see* influenza virus vaccine *on page 448*

fluvoxamine (floo VOKS a meen)

Sound-Alike/Look-Alike Issues

fluvoxamine may be confused with flavoxate, fluoxetine

Luvox® may be confused with Lasix®, Levoxyl®

U.S./Canadian Brand Names Alti-Fluvoxamine [Can]; Apo-Fluvoxamine® [Can]; Luvox® [Can]; Novo-Fluvoxamine [Can]; Nu-Fluvoxamine [Can]; PMS-Fluvoxamine [Can]; Rhoxal-fluvoxamine [Can]; Sandoz-Fluvoxamine [Can]

Therapeutic Category Antidepressant, Selective Serotonin Reuptake Inhibitor

Use Treatment of obsessive-compulsive disorder (OCD) in children ≥8 years of age and adults

Usual Dosage Oral: **Note:** When total daily dose exceeds 50 mg, the dose should be given in 2 divided doses:

Children 8-17 years: Initial: 25 mg at bedtime; adjust in 25 mg increments at 4- to 7-day intervals, as tolerated, to maximum therapeutic benefit: Range: 50-200 mg/day

Maximum: Children 8-11 years: 200 mg/day, adolescents: 300 mg/day; lower doses may be effective in female versus male patients

Adults: Initial: 50 mg at bedtime; adjust in 50 mg increments at 4- to 7-day intervals; usual dose range: 100-300 mg/day; divide total daily dose into 2 doses; administer larger portion at bedtime

Dosage Forms Tablet: 25 mg, 50 mg, 100 mg

Fluzone® [US] *see* influenza virus vaccine *on page 448*

FML® [US/Can] *see* fluorometholone *on page 356*

FML® Forte [US/Can] *see* fluorometholone *on page 356*

FML-S® [US] *see* sulfacetamide sodium and fluorometholone *on page 796*

Focalin™ [US] *see* dexmethylphenidate *on page 242*

Focalin™ XR [US] *see* dexmethylphenidate *on page 242*

Foille® [US-OTC] *see* benzocaine *on page 99*

folacin *see* folic acid *on this page*

folacin, vitamin B_{12}, and vitamin B_6 *see* folic acid, cyanocobalamin, and pyridoxine *on next page*

folate *see* folic acid *on this page*

Folbee [US] *see* folic acid, cyanocobalamin, and pyridoxine *on next page*

Folex® PFS™ *(Discontinued)* *see* methotrexate *on page 540*

Folgard® [US-OTC] *see* folic acid, cyanocobalamin, and pyridoxine *on next page*

Folgard RX 2.2® *(Discontinued)* *see* folic acid, cyanocobalamin, and pyridoxine *on next page*

folic acid (FOE lik AS id)

Sound-Alike/Look-Alike Issues

folic acid may be confused with folinic acid

Synonyms folacin; folate; pteroylglutamic acid

U.S./Canadian Brand Names Apo-Folic® [Can]

Therapeutic Category Vitamin, Water Soluble

Use Treatment of megaloblastic and macrocytic anemias due to folate deficiency; dietary supplement to prevent neural tube defects

Usual Dosage

Oral, I.M., I.V., SubQ: Anemia:

Infants: 0.1 mg/day

Children <4 years: Up to 0.3 mg/day

Children >4 years and Adults: 0.4 mg/day

Pregnant and lactating women: 0.8 mg/day

Oral:

RDA: Expressed as dietary folate equivalents:

Children:

1-3 years: 150 mcg/day

4-8 years: 200 mcg/day

9-13 years: 300 mcg/day

Children ≥14 years and Adults: 400 mcg/day

Prevention of neural tube defects:

Females of childbearing potential: 400 mcg/day

Females at high risk or with family history of neural tube defects: 4 mg/day

Dosage Forms

Injection, solution, as sodium folate: 5 mg/mL (10 mL) [contains benzyl alcohol]

Tablet: 0.4 mg, 0.8 mg, 1 mg

folic acid, cyanocobalamin, and pyridoxine

(FOE lik AS id, sye an oh koe BAL a min, & peer i DOKS een)

Synonyms cyanocobalamin, folic acid, and pyridoxine; folacin, vitamin B_{12}, and vitamin B_6; pyridoxine, folic acid, and cyanocobalamin

U.S./Canadian Brand Names AllanFol RX [US]; Folbee [US]; Folgard® [US-OTC]; Foltx® [US]; Tricardio B [US]

Therapeutic Category Vitamin

Use Nutritional supplement in end-stage renal failure, dialysis, hyperhomocysteinemia, homocystinuria, malabsorption syndromes, dietary deficiencies

Usual Dosage Oral: Adults: 1 tablet daily

Dosage Forms [DSC] = Discontinued product

Tablet: Folic acid 0.8 mg, cyanocobalamin 1000 mcg, and pyridoxine hydrochloride 50 mg

AllanFol RX: Folic acid 2.2 mg, cyanocobalamin 1000 mcg, and pyridoxine hydrochloride 25 mg

Folbee: Folic acid 2.5 mg, cyanocobalamin 1000 mcg, and pyridoxine hydrochloride 25 mg [dye free, lactose free, and sugar free]

Folgard®: Folic acid 0.8 mg, cyanocobalamin 115 mcg, and pyridoxine hydrochloride 10 mg

Folgard RX 2.2®: Folic acid 2.2 mg, cyanocobalamin 500 mcg, and pyridoxine hydrochloride 25 mg [DSC]

Foltx®: Folic acid 2.5 mg, cyanocobalamin 2000 mcg, and pyridoxine hydrochloride 25 mg

Tricardio B: Folic acid 0.4 mg, cyanocobalamin 250 mcg, and pyridoxine hydrochloride 25 mg

folinic acid *see* leucovorin *on page 485*

follitropin alfa (foe li TRO pin AL fa)

U.S./Canadian Brand Names Gonal-f® [US/Can]

Therapeutic Category Ovulation Stimulator

Use Induction of ovulation in the anovulatory infertile patient in whom the cause of infertility is functional and not caused by primary ovarian failure

Usual Dosage Adults (women): SubQ.: Initial: 75 units/day for the first cycle; an incremental dose adjustment of up to 37.5 units may be considered after 14 days; treatment duration should not exceed 35 days unless an E2 rise indicates follicular development

Dosage Forms Injection: 37.5 FSH units, 75 FSH units, 150 FSH units

follitropin beta (foe li TRO pin BAY ta)

Therapeutic Category Ovulation Stimulator

Use The development of multiple follicles in infertility patients treated in Assisted Reproductive Technology (ART) program and for the induction of ovulation

(Continued)

follitropin beta *(Continued)*

Usual Dosage Adults (female): I.M./SubQ:

Ovulation: In general, a sequential treatment scheme is recommended. This usually starts with daily administration of 75 int. units (International Units) FSH activity. The starting dose is maintained for at least seven days. If there is no ovarian response, the daily dose is then gradually increased until follicle growth and/or plasma estradiol levels indicate an adequate pharmacodynamic response. A daily increase in estradiol levels of 40% to 100% is considered to be optimal. The daily dose is then maintained until preovulatory conditions are reached. Preovulatory conditions are reached when there ultrasonographic evidence of a dominant follicle of at least 18 mm in diameter and/or when plasma estradiol levels of 300-900 picograms/mL (1000-3000 pmol/L) are attained; usually, 7-14 days of treatment are sufficient to reach this state. The administration is then discontinued and ovulation can be induced by administering human chorionic gonadotropin (hCG). If the number of responding follicles is too high or estradiol levels increase too rapidly (ie, more than a daily doubling of estradiol for 2-3 consecutive days), the daily dose should be decreased. Since follicles of >14 mm may lead to pregnancies, multiple preovulatory follicles exceeding 14 mm carry the risk of multiple gestations. In that case, hCG should be withheld and pregnancy should be avoided in order to prevent multiple gestations.

ART: Various stimulation protocols are applied; starting dose of 150-225 units is recommended for at least the first four days; thereafter, the dose may be adjusted individually, based upon ovarian response. In clinical studies, it was shown that maintenance dosages ranging from 75-375 units for 6-12 days are sufficient, although longer treatment may be necessary. May be given either alone, or in combination with a GnRH agonist to prevent premature luteinization; in the latter case, a higher total treatment dose of Follistim® may be required. Ovarian response is monitored by ultrasonography and measurement of plasma estradiol levels; when ultrasonographic evaluation indicates the presence of at least three follicles of 16-20 mm, and there is evidence of a good estradiol (plasma levels of about 300-400 picogram/mL (1000-1300 pmol/L) for each follicle with a diameter >18 mm), the final phase of maturation of the follicles is induced by administration of hCG. Oocyte retrieval is performed 34-35 hours later.

Dosage Forms Injection: 75 FSH units

Foltx® [US] *see* folic acid, cyanocobalamin, and pyridoxine *on previous page*

Folvite® *(Discontinued)* *see* folic acid *on page 364*

fomepizole (foe ME pi zole)

Synonyms 4-methylpyrazole; 4-MP

U.S./Canadian Brand Names Antizol® [US]

Therapeutic Category Antidote

Use **Orphan drug:** Treatment of methanol or ethylene glycol poisoning alone or in combination with hemodialysis

Usual Dosage Adults: Ethylene glycol and methanol toxicity: I.V.: A loading dose of 15 mg/kg should be administered, followed by doses of 10 mg/kg every 12 hours for 4 doses, then 15 mg/kg every 12 hours thereafter until ethylene glycol levels have been reduced <20 mg/dL and patient is asymptomatic with normal pH

Dosage Forms Injection, solution [preservative free]: 1 g/mL (1.5 mL)

fomivirsen *(Canada only)* (foe MI vir sen)

Synonyms fomivirsen sodium

U.S./Canadian Brand Names Vitravene™ [Can]

Therapeutic Category Antiviral Agent, Ophthalmic

Use Local treatment of cytomegalovirus (CMV) retinitis in patients with acquired immunodeficiency syndrome who are intolerant or insufficiently responsive to other treatments for CMV retinitis or when other treatments for CMV retinitis are contraindicated

Usual Dosage Adults: Intravitreal injection: Induction: 330 mcg (0.05 mL) every other week for 2 doses, followed by maintenance dose of 330 mcg (0.05 mL) every 4 weeks

If progression occurs during maintenance, a repeat of the induction regimen may be attempted to establish resumed control. Unacceptable inflammation during therapy may be managed by temporary interruption, provided response has been established. Topical corticosteroids have been used to reduce inflammation.

Dosage Forms [DSC] = Discontinued product

Injection, solution, intravitreal, as sodium: 6.6 mg/mL (0.25 mL) [DSC]

fomivirsen sodium *see* fomivirsen *(Canada only)* *on this page*

fondaparinux (fon da PARE i nuks)

Synonyms fondaparinux sodium

U.S./Canadian Brand Names Arixtra® [US/Can]

Therapeutic Category Factor Xa Inhibitor

Use Prophylaxis of deep vein thrombosis (DVT) in patients undergoing surgery for hip replacement, knee replacement, hip fracture (including extended prophylaxis following hip fracture surgery), or abdominal surgery (in patients at risk for thromboembolic complications); treatment of acute pulmonary embolism (PE); treatment of acute DVT without PE

Usual Dosage SubQ:

DVT prophylaxis: Adults ≥50 kg: 2.5 mg once daily. **Note:** Initiate dose after hemostasis has been established, 6-8 hours postoperatively.

Usual duration: 5-9 days (up to 10 days following abdominal surgery or up to 11 days following hip replacement or knee replacement)

Extended prophylaxis is recommended following hip fracture surgery (has been tolerated for up to 32 days).

Acute DVT/PE treatment: SubQ: Adults: **Note:** Concomitant treatment with warfarin sodium should be initiated as soon as possible, usually within 72 hours:

<50 kg: 5 mg once daily

50-100 kg: 7.5 mg once daily

>100 kg: 10 mg once daily

Usual duration: 5-9 days (has been administered up to 26 days)

Dosage Forms Injection, solution, as sodium [preservative free]: 2.5 mg/0.5 mL (0.5 mL); 5 mg/0.4 mL (0.4 mL); 7.5 mg/0.6 mL (0.6 mL); 10 mg/0.8 mL (0.8 mL) [prefilled syringe]

fondaparinux sodium *see* fondaparinux *on this page*

Foradil® [Can] *see* formoterol *on this page*

Foradil® Aerolizer™ [US] *see* formoterol *on this page*

Forane® [US] *see* isoflurane *on page 463*

formoterol (for MOH te rol)

Sound-Alike/Look-Alike Issues

Foradil® may be confused with Toradol®

Synonyms formoterol fumarate

U.S./Canadian Brand Names Foradil® Aerolizer™ [US]; Foradil® [Can]; Oxeze® Turbuhaler® [Can]

Therapeutic Category $Beta_2$-Adrenergic Agonist Agent

Use Maintenance treatment of asthma and prevention of bronchospasm in patients ≥5 years of age with reversible obstructive airway disease, including patients with symptoms of nocturnal asthma, who require regular treatment with inhaled, short-acting $beta_2$-agonists; maintenance treatment of bronchoconstriction in patients with COPD; prevention of exercise-induced bronchospasm in patients ≥5 years of age

Note: Oxeze® is also approved in Canada for acute relief of symptoms ("on demand" treatment) in patients ≥6 years of age.

Usual Dosage

Asthma maintenance treatment: Children ≥5 years and Adults: Inhalation: 12 mcg capsule every 12 hours

Oxeze® (CAN): **Note:** Not labeled for use in the U.S.: Children ≥6 years and Adults: Inhalation: 6 mcg or 12 mcg every 12 hours. Maximum dose: Children: 24 mcg/day; Adults: 48 mcg/day

Prevention of exercise-induced bronchospasm: Children ≥5 years and Adults: Inhalation: 12 mcg capsule at least 15 minutes before exercise on an "as needed" basis; additional doses should not be used for another 12 hours. **Note:** If already using for asthma maintenance then should not use additional doses for exercise-induced bronchospasm.

Oxeze® (CAN): **Note:** Not labeled for use in the U.S.: Children ≥6 years and Adults: Inhalation: 6 mcg or 12 mcg at least 15 minutes before exercise.

COPD maintenance treatment: Adults: Inhalation: 12 mcg capsule every 12 hours

Additional indication for Oxeze® (approved in Canada): Acute ("on demand") relief of bronchoconstriction: Children ≥12 years and Adults: 6 mcg or 12 mcg as a single dose (maximum dose: 72 mcg in any 24-hour period). The prolonged use of high dosages (48 mcg/day for ≥3 consecutive days) may be a sign of suboptimal control, and should prompt the re-evaluation of therapy.

Dosage Forms [CAN] = Canadian brand name

Powder for oral inhalation, as fumarate:

Foradil® Aerolizer™ [capsule]: 12 mcg (12s, 60s) [contains lactose 25 mg]

(Continued)

formoterol *(Continued)*

Oxeze® Turbuhaler® [CAN]: 6 mcg/inhalation [delivers 60 metered doses; contains lactose 600 mcg/dose]; 12 mcg/inhalation [delivers 60 metered doses; contains lactose 600 mcg/dose] [not available in the U.S.]

formoterol fumarate *see* formoterol *on previous page*

formoterol fumarate dehydrate and budesonide *see* budesonide and formoterol *(Canada only) on page 123*

Formula EM [US-OTC] *see* fructose, dextrose, and phosphoric acid *on page 371*

Formula Q® ***(Discontinued)*** *see* quinine *on page 726*

Formulation R™ [US-OTC] *see* phenylephrine *on page 660*

Formulex® [Can] *see* dicyclomine *on page 251*

5-formyl tetrahydrofolate *see* leucovorin *on page 485*

Fortamet™ [US] *see* metformin *on page 535*

Fortaz® [US/Can] *see* ceftazidime *on page 161*

Forteo™ [US/Can] *see* teriparatide *on page 812*

Fortical® [US] *see* calcitonin *on page 133*

Fortovase® [Can] *see* saquinavir *on page 763*

Fortovase® ***(Discontinued)*** *see* saquinavir *on page 763*

Fosamax® [US/Can] *see* alendronate *on page 27*

Fosamax Plus D™ [US] *see* alendronate and cholecalciferol *on page 27*

fosamprenavir (FOS am pren a veer)

Sound-Alike/Look-Alike Issues

Lexiva™ may be confused with Levitra®

Synonyms fosamprenavir calcium; GW433908G

U.S./Canadian Brand Names Lexiva® [US]; Telzir® [Can]

Therapeutic Category Antiretroviral Agent, Protease Inhibitor

Use Treatment of HIV infections in combination with at least two other antiretroviral agents

Usual Dosage Oral: Adults: HIV infection:

Antiretroviral therapy-naive patients:

Unboosted regimen: 1400 mg twice daily (without ritonavir)

Ritonavir-boosted regimens:

Once-daily regimen: Fosamprenavir 1400 mg plus ritonavir 200 mg once daily

Twice-daily regimen: Fosamprenavir 700 mg plus ritonavir 100 mg twice daily

Protease inhibitor-experienced patients: Fosamprenavir 700 mg plus ritonavir 100 mg twice daily. **Note:** Once-daily administration is not recommended in protease inhibitor-experienced patients.

Combination therapy with efavirenz (ritonavir-boosted regimen):

Once-daily regimen: Fosamprenavir 1400 mg daily plus ritonavir 300 mg once daily

Twice-daily regimen: No dosage adjustment recommended for twice-daily regimen

Combination therapy with nevirapine (ritonavir-boosted regimen): Fosamprenavir 700 mg plus ritonavir 100 mg twice daily

Dosage Forms [CAN] = Canadian brand name

Tablet, as calcium:

Lexiva®: 700 mg

Suspension, oral, as calcium:

Telzir® [CAN]: 50 mg/mL (225 mL) [not available in the U.S.]

fosamprenavir calcium *see* fosamprenavir *on this page*

Fosavance [Can] *see* alendronate and cholecalciferol *on page 27*

foscarnet (fos KAR net)

Synonyms PFA; phosphonoformate; phosphonoformic acid

U.S./Canadian Brand Names Foscavir® [US/Can]

Therapeutic Category Antiviral Agent

Use

Treatment of mucotaneous herpes virus infections suspected to be caused by acyclovir-resistant (HSV, VZV) or ganciclovir-resistant (CMV) strains; this occurs almost exclusively in immunocompromised persons (eg, with advanced AIDS) who have received prolonged treatment for a herpes virus infection

Treatment of CMV retinitis in persons with AIDS

Usual Dosage

CMV retinitis: I.V.:

Induction treatment: 60 mg/kg/dose every 8 hours **or** 100 mg/kg every 12 hours for 14-21 days

Maintenance therapy: 90-120 mg/kg/day as a single infusion

Herpes simplex infections (acyclovir-resistant): Induction: I.V.: 40 mg/kg/dose every 8-12 hours for 14-21 days

Dosage Forms

Injection, solution: 24 mg/mL (250 mL, 500 mL)

Foscavir®: 24 mg/mL (500 mL)

Foscavir® [US/Can] *see* foscarnet *on this page*

fosfomycin (fos foe MYE sin)

Sound-Alike/Look-Alike Issues

Monurol™ may be confused with Monopril®

Synonyms fosfomycin tromethamine

U.S./Canadian Brand Names Monurol™ [US/Can]

Therapeutic Category Antibiotic, Miscellaneous

Use Single oral dose in the treatment of uncomplicated urinary tract infections in women due to susceptible strains of *E. coli* and *Enterococcus*; may have an advantage over other agents since it maintains high concentration in the urine for up to 48 hours

Usual Dosage Adults: Oral: Female: Uncomplicated UTI: Single dose of 3 g in 4 oz of water

Dosage Forms Powder, as tromethamine: 3 g

fosfomycin tromethamine *see* fosfomycin *on this page*

fosinopril (foe SIN oh pril)

Sound-Alike/Look-Alike Issues

fosinopril may be confused with lisinopril

Monopril® may be confused with Accupril®, minoxidil, moexipril, Monoket®, Monurol™, ramipril

Synonyms fosinopril sodium

U.S./Canadian Brand Names Apo-Fosinopril® [Can]; Monopril® [US/Can]; Novo-Fosinopril [Can]; ratio-Fosinopril [Can]; Riva-Rosinopril [Can]

Therapeutic Category Angiotensin-Converting Enzyme (ACE) Inhibitor

Use Treatment of hypertension, either alone or in combination with other antihypertensive agents; treatment of congestive heart failure, left ventricular dysfunction after myocardial infarction

Usual Dosage Oral:

Children >50 kg: Hypertension: Initial: 5-10 mg once daily

Adults:

Hypertension: Initial: 10 mg/day; most patients are maintained on 20-40 mg/day. May need to divide the dose into two if trough effect is inadequate; discontinue the diuretic, if possible 2-3 days before initiation of therapy; resume diuretic therapy carefully, if needed.

Heart failure: Initial: 10 mg/day (5 mg if renal dysfunction present) and increase, as needed, to a maximum of 40 mg once daily over several weeks; usual dose: 20-40 mg/day. If hypotension, orthostasis, or azotemia occur during titration, consider decreasing concomitant diuretic dose, if any.

Dosage Forms

Tablet, as sodium: 10 mg, 20 mg, 40 mg

Monopril®: 10 mg, 20 mg, 40 mg

fosinopril and hydrochlorothiazide (foe SIN oh pril & hye droe klor oh THYE a zide)

Sound-Alike/Look-Alike Issues

Monopril® may be confused with Accupril®, minoxidil, moexipril, Monoket®, Monurol™, ramipril

(Continued)

fosinopril and hydrochlorothiazide *(Continued)*

Synonyms hydrochlorothiazide and fosinopril

U.S./Canadian Brand Names Monopril-HCT® [US/Can]

Therapeutic Category Angiotensin-Converting Enzyme (ACE) Inhibitor

Use Treatment of hypertension; not indicated for first-line treatment

Usual Dosage **Note:** A patient whose blood pressure is not adequately controlled with fosinopril or hydrochlorothiazide monotherapy may be switched to combination therapy; **not** for initial treatment.

Adults: Oral: Hypertension: Fosinopril 10-80 mg per day, hydrochlorothiazide 12.5-50 mg per day

Dosage Forms

Tablet: 10/12.5: Fosinopril sodium 10 mg and hydrochlorothiazide 12.5 mg; 20/12.5: Fosinopril sodium 20 mg and hydrochlorothiazide 12.5 mg

Monopril-HCT® 10/12.5: Fosinopril sodium 10 mg and hydrochlorothiazide 12.5 mg

Monopril-HCT® 20/12.5: Fosinopril sodium 20 mg and hydrochlorothiazide 12.5 mg

fosinopril sodium *see* fosinopril *on previous page*

fosphenytoin (FOS fen i toyn)

Sound-Alike/Look-Alike Issues

Cerebyx® may be confused with Celebrex®, Celexa™, Cerezyme®

Synonyms fosphenytoin sodium

U.S./Canadian Brand Names Cerebyx® [US/Can]

Therapeutic Category Hydantoin

Use Used for the control of generalized convulsive status epilepticus and prevention and treatment of seizures occurring during neurosurgery; indicated for short-term parenteral administration when other means of phenytoin administration are unavailable, inappropriate or deemed less advantageous (the safety and effectiveness of fosphenytoin in this use has not been systematically evaluated for more than 5 days)

Usual Dosage **The dose, concentration in solutions, and infusion rates for fosphenytoin are expressed as phenytoin sodium equivalents (PE); fosphenytoin should always be prescribed and dispensed in phenytoin sodium equivalents (PE)**

Adults:

Status epilepticus: I.V.: Loading dose: 15-20 mg PE/kg I.V. administered at 100-150 mg PE/minute

Nonemergent loading and maintenance dosing: I.V. or I.M.:

Loading dose: 10-20 mg PE/kg I.V. or I.M. (maximum I.V. rate: 150 mg PE/minute)

Initial daily maintenance dose: 4-6 mg PE/kg/day I.V. or I.M.

I.M. or I.V. substitution for oral phenytoin therapy: May be substituted for oral phenytoin sodium at the same total daily dose; however, Dilantin® capsules are ~90% bioavailable by the oral route; phenytoin, supplied as fosphenytoin, is 100% bioavailable by both the I.M. and I.V. routes; for this reason, plasma phenytoin concentrations may increase when I.M. or I.V. fosphenytoin is substituted for oral phenytoin sodium therapy; in clinical trials I.M. fosphenytoin was administered as a single daily dose utilizing either 1 or 2 injection sites; some patients may require more frequent dosing

Dosage Forms Injection, solution, as sodium: 75 mg/mL [equivalent to phenytoin sodium 50 mg/mL] (2 mL, 10 mL)

fosphenytoin sodium *see* fosphenytoin *on this page*

Fosrenol™ [US] *see* lanthanum *on page 483*

Fostex® 10% BPO [US-OTC] *see* benzoyl peroxide *on page 102*

Fototar® [US-OTC] *see* coal tar *on page 207*

Fragmin® [US/Can] *see* dalteparin *on page 227*

framycetin *(Canada only)* (fra mye CEE tin)

U.S./Canadian Brand Names Sofra-Tulle® [Can]

Therapeutic Category Antibiotic, Topical

Use Treatment of infected or potentially infected burns, wounds, ulcers, and graft sites

Usual Dosage A single layer to be applied directly to the wound and covered with an appropriate dressing. If exudative, dressings should be changed at least daily. In case of leg ulcers, cut dressing accurately to size of ulcer to decrease the risk of sensitization and to avoid contact with surrounding healthy skin.

Dosage Forms Dressing, gauze: 1% (10 cm x 10 cm, 10 cm x 30 cm)

Fraxiparine™ [Can] *see* nadroparin *(Canada only) on page 573*

Fraxiparine™ Forte [Can] *see* nadroparin *(Canada only) on page 573*

Freezone® [US-OTC] *see* salicylic acid *on page 758*

Frisium® [Can] *see* clobazam *(Canada only) on page 200*

Froben® [Can] *see* flurbiprofen *on page 360*

Froben-SR® [Can] *see* flurbiprofen *on page 360*

Frova® [US] *see* frovatriptan *on this page*

frovatriptan (froe va TRIP tan)

Synonyms frovatriptan succinate

U.S./Canadian Brand Names Frova® [US]

Therapeutic Category Antimigraine Agent; Serotonin 5-$HT_{1B, 1D}$ Receptor Agonist

Use Acute treatment of migraine with or without aura in adults

Usual Dosage Oral: Adults: Migraine: 2.5 mg; if headache recurs, a second dose may be given if first dose provided some relief and at least 2 hours have elapsed since the first dose (maximum daily dose: 7.5 mg)

Dosage Forms Tablet, as base: 2.5 mg

frovatriptan succinate *see* frovatriptan *on this page*

fructose, dextrose, and phosphoric acid (FRUK tose, DEKS trose, & foss FOR ik AS id)

Sound-Alike/Look-Alike Issues

Emetrol® may be confused with emetine

Synonyms dextrose, levulose and phosphoric acid; levulose, dextrose and phosphoric acid; phosphorated carbohydrate solution; phosphoric acid, levulose and dextrose

U.S./Canadian Brand Names Emetrol® [US-OTC]; Especol® [US-OTC]; Formula EM [US-OTC]; Kalmz [US-OTC]; Nausea Relief [US-OTC]

Therapeutic Category Antiemetic

Use Relief of nausea associated with upset stomach that occurs with intestinal or stomach flu, and food indiscretions

Usual Dosage Oral: Nausea:

Children 2-12 years: 5-10 mL; repeat dose every 15 minutes until distress subsides; do not take for more than 1 hour (5 doses)

Children ≥12 years and Adults: 15-30 mL; repeat dose every 15 minutes until distress subsides; do not take for more than 1 hour (5 doses)

Dosage Forms

Liquid, oral: Fructose 1.87 g, dextrose 1.87 g, and phosphoric acid 21.5 mg per 5 mL (120 mL)

Emetrol®: Fructose 1.87 g, dextrose 1.87 g, and phosphoric acid 21.5 mg per 5 mL (120 mL, 240 mL) [cherry and lemon mint flavors]

Especol®: Fructose 1.87 g, dextrose 1.87 g, and phosphoric acid 21.5 mg per 5 mL (120 mL) [cherry and lemon-lime flavors]

Formula EM, Nausea Relief: Fructose 1.87 g, dextrose 1.87 g, and phosphoric acid 21.5 mg per 5 mL (120 mL)

Kalmz, Nausetrol®: Fructose 1.87 g, dextrose 1.87 g, and phosphoric acid 21.5 mg per 5 mL (120 mL) [cherry flavor]

frusemide *see* furosemide *on next page*

FS *see* fibrin sealant kit *on page 345*

FS Shampoo® Topical *(Discontinued)* *see* fluocinolone *on page 352*

FTC *see* emtricitabine *on page 290*

FTP-Domperidone Maleate [Can] *see* domperidone *(Canada only) on page 273*

FU *see* fluorouracil *on page 356*

5-FU *see* fluorouracil *on page 356*

Fucidin® [Can] *see* fusidic acid *(Canada only) on page 373*

Fucithalmic® [Can] *see* fusidic acid *(Canada only) on page 373*

FUDR® [US/Can] *see* floxuridine *on page 348*

5-FUDR *see* floxuridine *on page 348*

Ful-Glo® [US] *see* fluorescein sodium *on page 354*

fulvestrant (fool VES trant)

Synonyms ICI-182,780; zeneca 182,780; ZM-182,780

U.S./Canadian Brand Names Faslodex® [US]

Therapeutic Category Antineoplastic Agent, Estrogen Receptor Antagonist

Use Treatment of hormone receptor positive metastatic breast cancer in postmenopausal women with disease progression following antiestrogen therapy.

Usual Dosage I.M.: Adults (postmenopausal women): 250 mg at 1-month intervals

Dosage Forms Injection, solution: 50 mg/mL (2.5 mL, 5 mL) [prefilled syringe; contains alcohol, benzyl alcohol, benzyl stearate, castor oil]

Fumasorb® *(Discontinued)* *see* ferrous fumarate *on page 342*

Fumerin® *(Discontinued)* *see* ferrous fumarate *on page 342*

Funduscein® Injection *(Discontinued)* *see* fluorescein sodium *on page 354*

Fungi-Guard [US-OTC] *see* tolnaftate *on page 834*

Fungi-Nail® [US-OTC] *see* undecylenic acid and derivatives *on page 860*

Fungizone® [Can] *see* amphotericin B (conventional) *on page 51*

Fung-O® [US-OTC] *see* salicylic acid *on page 758*

Fungoid® Tincture [US-OTC] *see* miconazole *on page 553*

Furacin® Topical *(Discontinued)* *see* nitrofurazone *on page 595*

Furadantin® [US] *see* nitrofurantoin *on page 594*

Furalan® *(Discontinued)* *see* nitrofurantoin *on page 594*

Furan® *(Discontinued)* *see* nitrofurantoin *on page 594*

Furanite® *(Discontinued)* *see* nitrofurantoin *on page 594*

furazosin *see* prazosin *on page 693*

furosemide (fyoor OH se mide)

Sound-Alike/Look-Alike Issues

furosemide may be confused with torsemide

Lasix® may be confused with Esidrix®, Lanoxin®, Lidex®, Lomotil®, Luvox®, Luxiq®

Synonyms frusemide

U.S./Canadian Brand Names Apo-Furosemide® [Can]; Furosemide Injection, USP [Can]; Furosemide Special [Can]; Lasix® Special [Can]; Lasix® [US/Can]; Novo-Semide [Can]

Therapeutic Category Diuretic, Loop

Use Management of edema associated with congestive heart failure and hepatic or renal disease; alone or in combination with antihypertensives in treatment of hypertension

Usual Dosage

Infants and Children:

Oral: 1-2 mg/kg/dose increased in increments of 1 mg/kg/dose with each succeeding dose until a satisfactory effect is achieved to a maximum of 6 mg/kg/dose no more frequently than 6 hours.

I.M., I.V.: 1 mg/kg/dose, increasing by each succeeding dose at 1 mg/kg/dose at intervals of 6-12 hours until a satisfactory response up to 6 mg/kg/dose.

Adults:

Oral: 20-80 mg/dose initially increased in increments of 20-40 mg/dose at intervals of 6-8 hours; usual maintenance dose interval is twice daily or every day; may be titrated up to 600 mg/day with severe edematous states.

Hypertension (JNC 7): 20-80 mg/day in 2 divided doses

I.M., I.V.: 20-40 mg/dose, may be repeated in 1-2 hours as needed and increased by 20 mg/dose until the desired effect has been obtained. Usual dosing interval: 6-12 hours; for acute pulmonary edema, the usual dose is 40 mg I.V. over 1-2 minutes. If not adequate, may increase dose to 80 mg. **Note:** ACC/AHA 2005 guidelines for chronic congestive heart failure recommend a maximum single dose of 160-200 mg.

Continuous I.V. infusion: Initial I.V. bolus dose 20-40 mg, followed by continuous I.V. infusion doses of 10-40 mg/hour. If urine output is <1 mL/kg/hour, double as necessary to a maximum of 80-160 mg/hour. The risk associated with higher infusion rates (80-160 mg/hour) must be weighed against alternative strategies. **Note:** ACC/AHA 2005 guidelines for chronic congestive heart failure recommend 40 mg I.V. load, then 10-40 mg/hour infusion.

Refractory heart failure: Oral, I.V.: Doses up to 8 g/day have been used.

Dosage Forms

Injection, solution: 10 mg/mL (2 mL, 4 mL, 8 mL, 10 mL)

Solution, oral: 10 mg/mL (60 mL, 120 mL) [orange flavor]; 40 mg/5 mL (5 mL, 500 mL) [pineapple-peach flavor]
Tablet (Lasix®): 20 mg, 40 mg, 80 mg

Furosemide Injection, USP [Can] *see* furosemide *on previous page*

Furosemide Special [Can] *see* furosemide *on previous page*

fusidic acid *(Canada only)* (fyoo SI dik AS id)

Synonyms sodium fusidate

U.S./Canadian Brand Names Fucidin® [Can]; Fucithalmic® [Can]

Therapeutic Category Antifungal Agent, Systemic

Use

Systemic: Treatment of skin and soft tissue infections, or osteomyelitis, caused by susceptible organisms, including *Staphylococcus aureus* (penicillinase-producing or nonpenicillinase strains); may be used in the treatment of pneumonia, septicemia, endocarditis, burns, and cystic fibrosis caused by susceptible organisms when other antibiotics have failed

Topical: Treatment of primary and secondary skin infections caused by susceptible organisms

Ophthalmic: Treatment of superficial infections of the eye and conjunctiva caused by susceptible organisms

Usual Dosage

I.V.:

Children ≤12 years: 20 mg/kg/day in 3 divided doses

Children >12 years and Adults: 500 mg sodium fusidate 3 times/day

Ophthalmic: Children ≥2 years and Adults: Instill 1 drop in each eye every 12 hours for 7 days

Topical: Children and Adults: Apply to affected area 3-4 times/day until favorable results are achieved. If a gauze dressing is used, frequency of application may be reduced to 1-2 times/day.

Oral: Adults: 500 mg sodium fusidate 3 times/day. (**Note:** Oral dosage may be increased to 1000 mg 3 times/day in fulminating infections.)

Dosage Forms [CAN] = Canadian brand name

Cream, as fusidic acid:
Fucidin®: 2% (15 g, 30 g)

Injection, powder for reconstitution, as sodium fusidate:
Fucidin®: 500 mg [packaged with 10 mL diluent/buffer solution]

Ointment, topical, as sodium fusidate:
Fucidin®: 2% (15 g, 30 g) [contains lanolin]

Suspension, ophthalmic, as fusidic acid:
Fucithalmic®: 10 mg/g [1%] (0.2 g) [unit-dose, without preservative]; (3 g, 5 g) [multidose, contains benzalkonium chloride]

Tablet, as sodium fusidate:
Fucidin®: 250 mg

Fuzeon® [US/Can] *see* enfuvirtide *on page 293*

FVIII/vWF *see* antihemophilic factor/von Willebrand factor complex (human) *on page 60*

FXT [Can] *see* fluoxetine *on page 357*

GAA *see* alglucosidase alfa *on page 28*

gabapentin (GA ba pen tin)

Sound-Alike/Look-Alike Issues

Neurontin® may be confused with Neoral®, Noroxin®

U.S./Canadian Brand Names Apo-Gabapentin® [Can]; BCI-Gabapentin [Can]; Gen-Gabapentin [Can]; Neurontin® [US/Can]; Novo-Gabapentin [Can]; Nu-Gabapentin [Can]; PMS-Gabapentin [Can]

Therapeutic Category Anticonvulsant

Use Adjunct for treatment of partial seizures with and without secondary generalized seizures in patients >12 years of age with epilepsy; adjunct for treatment of partial seizures in pediatric patients 3-12 years of age; management of postherpetic neuralgia (PHN) in adults

Usual Dosage Oral:

Children: Anticonvulsant:

3-12 years: Initial: 10-15 mg/kg/day in 3 divided doses; titrate to effective dose over ~3 days; dosages of up to 50 mg/kg/day have been tolerated in clinical studies

3-4 years: Effective dose: 40 mg/kg/day in 3 divided doses

≥5-12 years: Effective dose: 25-35 mg/kg/day in 3 divided doses

See "Note" in Adults dosing.

(Continued)

gabapentin *(Continued)*

Children >12 years and Adults:

Anticonvulsant: Initial: 300 mg 3 times/day; if necessary the dose may be increased up to 1800 mg/day. Doses of up to 2400 mg/day have been tolerated in long-term clinical studies; up to 3600 mg/day has been tolerated in short-term studies.

Note: If gabapentin is discontinued or if another anticonvulsant is added to therapy, it should be done slowly over a minimum of 1 week

Adults: Postherpetic neuralgia or neuropathic pain: Day 1: 300 mg, Day 2: 300 mg twice daily, Day 3: 300 mg 3 times/day; dose may be titrated as needed for pain relief (range: 1800-3600 mg/day, daily doses >1800 mg do not generally show greater benefit)

Dosage Forms

Capsule (Neurontin®): 100 mg, 300 mg, 400 mg

Solution, oral (Neurontin®): 250 mg/5 mL (480 mL) [cool strawberry anise flavor]

Tablet: 100 mg, 300 mg, 400 mg

Neurontin®: 600 mg, 800 mg

Gabitril® [US/Can] *see* tiagabine *on page 825*

gadopentetate dimeglumine *see* radiological/contrast media (ionic) *on page 728*

gadoteridol *see* radiological/contrast media (nonionic) *on page 730*

galantamine (ga LAN ta meen)

Sound-Alike/Look-Alike Issues

Razadyne™ may be confused with Rozerem™

Reminyl® may be confused with Amaryl®

Synonyms galantamine hydrobromide

U.S./Canadian Brand Names Razadyne™ ER [US]; Razadyne™ [US]; Reminyl® ER [Can]; Reminyl® [Can]

Therapeutic Category Acetylcholinesterase Inhibitor (Central)

Use Treatment of mild-to-moderate dementia of Alzheimer disease

Usual Dosage Oral: Adults:

Note: Oral solution and tablet should be taken with breakfast and dinner; capsule should be taken with breakfast. If therapy is interrupted for ≥3 days, restart at the lowest dose and increase to current dose.

Immediate release tablet or solution: Mild-to-moderate dementia of Alzheimer: Initial: 4 mg twice a day for 4 weeks; if tolerated, increase to 8 mg twice daily for ≥4 weeks; if tolerated, increase to 12 mg twice daily

Range: 16-24 mg/day in 2 divided doses

Extended-release capsule: Initial: 8 mg once daily for 4 weeks; if tolerated, increase to 16 mg once daily for ≥4 weeks; if tolerated, increase to 24 mg once daily

Range: 16-24 mg once daily

Conversion to galantamine from other cholinesterase inhibitors: Patients experiencing poor tolerability with donepezil or rivastigmine should wait until side effects subside or allow a 7-day washout period prior to beginning galantamine. Patients not experiencing side effects with donepezil or rivastigmine may begin galantamine therapy the day immediately following discontinuation of previous therapy.

Dosage Forms

Capsule, extended release, as hydrobromide (Razadyne™ ER): 8 mg, 16 mg, 24 mg [contains gelatin]

Solution, oral, as hydrobromide (Razadyne™): 4 mg/mL (100 mL) [with calibrated pipette]

Tablet, as hydrobromide (Razadyne™): 4 mg, 8 mg, 12 mg

galantamine hydrobromide *see* galantamine *on this page*

galsulfase (gal SUL fase)

Synonyms recombinant N-acetylgalactosamine 4-sulfatase; rhASB

U.S./Canadian Brand Names Naglazyme™ [US]

Therapeutic Category Enzyme

Use Replacement therapy in mucopolysaccharidosis VI (MPS VI; Maroteaux-Lamy Syndrome) for improvement of walking and stair-climbing capacity

Usual Dosage MPS VI: Children >5 years: I.V.: 1 mg/kg once weekly

Dosage Forms Injection, solution [preservative free]: 5 mg/5 mL (5 mL)

Gamimune® N Injection *(Discontinued)* *see* immune globulin (intravenous) *on page 444*

gamma benzene hexachloride *see* lindane *on page 497*

Gamma E-Gems® [US-OTC] *see* vitamin E *on page 876*

Gamma-E Plus [US-OTC] *see* vitamin E *on page 876*

Gammagard® Liquid [US/Can] *see* immune globulin (intravenous) *on page 444*

Gammagard® S/D [US/Can] *see* immune globulin (intravenous) *on page 444*

gamma globulin *see* immune globulin (intramuscular) *on page 443*

gamma hydroxybutyric acid *see* sodium oxybate *on page 780*

gammaphos *see* amifostine *on page 40*

Gammar®-P I.V. [US] *see* immune globulin (intravenous) *on page 444*

Gamulin® Rh *(Discontinued)*

Gamunex® [US/Can] *see* immune globulin (intravenous) *on page 444*

ganciclovir (gan SYE kloe veer)

Sound-Alike/Look-Alike Issues

Cytovene® may be confused with Cytosar®, Cytosar-U®

Synonyms DHPG sodium; GCV sodium; nordeoxyguanosine

U.S./Canadian Brand Names Cytovene® [US/Can]; Vitrasert® [US/Can]

Therapeutic Category Antiviral Agent

Use

Parenteral: Treatment of CMV retinitis in immunocompromised individuals, including patients with acquired immunodeficiency syndrome; prophylaxis of CMV infection in transplant patients

Oral: Alternative to the I.V. formulation for maintenance treatment of CMV retinitis in immunocompromised patients, including patients with AIDS, in whom retinitis is stable following appropriate induction therapy and for whom the risk of more rapid progression is balanced by the benefit associated with avoiding daily I.V. infusions.

Implant: Treatment of CMV retinitis

Usual Dosage

CMV retinitis: Slow I.V. infusion (dosing is based on total body weight):

Children >3 months and Adults:

Induction therapy: 5 mg/kg/dose every 12 hours for 14-21 days followed by maintenance therapy

Maintenance therapy: 5 mg/kg/day as a single daily dose for 7 days/week or 6 mg/kg/day for 5 days/week

CMV retinitis: Oral: 1000 mg 3 times/day with food **or** 500 mg 6 times/day with food

Prevention of CMV disease in patients with advanced HIV infection and normal renal function: Oral: 1000 mg 3 times/day with food

Prevention of CMV disease in transplant patients: Same initial and maintenance dose as CMV retinitis except duration of initial course is 7-14 days, duration of maintenance therapy is dependent on clinical condition and degree of immunosuppression

Intravitreal implant: One implant for 5- to 8-month period; following depletion of ganciclovir, as evidenced by progression of retinitis, implant may be removed and replaced

Dosage Forms [DSC] = Discontinued product

Capsule: 250 mg, 500 mg

Cytovene®: 250 mg, 500 mg [DSC]

Implant, intravitreal (Vitrasert®): 4.5 mg [released gradually over 5-8 months]

Injection, powder for reconstitution, as sodium (Cytovene®): 500 mg

Ganidin NR [US] *see* guaifenesin *on page 392*

ganirelix (ga ni REL ix)

Synonyms ganirelix acetate

U.S./Canadian Brand Names Antagon® [US/Can]; Orgalutran® [Can]

Therapeutic Category Antigonadotropic Agent

Use Inhibits premature luteinizing hormone (LH) surges in women undergoing controlled ovarian hyperstimulation in fertility clinics.

Usual Dosage Adult: SubQ: 250 mcg/day during the mid-to-late phase after initiating follicle-stimulating hormone on day 2 or 3 of cycle. Treatment should be continued daily until the day of chorionic gonadotropin administration.

Dosage Forms Injection, solution, as acetate: 250 mcg/0.5 mL [prefilled glass syringe with 27-gauge x 1/2 inch needle]

ganirelix acetate *see* ganirelix *on this page*

Gani-Tuss DM NR [US] *see* guaifenesin and dextromethorphan *on page 394*

Gani-Tuss® NR [US] *see* guaifenesin and codeine *on page 393*

GannaSTAN™ S/D [US] *see* immune globulin (intramuscular) *on page 443*
Gantrisin® [US] *see* sulfisoxazole *on page 799*
GAR-936 *see* tigecycline *on page 828*
Garamycin® [Can] *see* gentamicin *on page 381*
Garamycin® *(Discontinued)* *see* gentamicin *on page 381*
Gardasil® [US] *see* papillomavirus (Types 6, 11, 16, 18) recombinant vaccine *on page 638*
Gas-X® [US-OTC] *see* simethicone *on page 772*
Gas-X® Extra Strength [US-OTC] *see* simethicone *on page 772*
Gas-X® Maximum Strength [US-OTC] *see* simethicone *on page 772*
GasAid [US-OTC] *see* simethicone *on page 772*
Gas Ban™ [US-OTC] *see* calcium carbonate and simethicone *on page 137*
Gas-Ban DS® *(Discontinued)* *see* aluminum hydroxide, magnesium hydroxide, and simethicone *on page 37*
Gastrocrom® [US] *see* cromolyn sodium *on page 217*
Gastrografin® [US] *see* radiological/contrast media (ionic) *on page 728*
Gastrosed™ *(Discontinued)* *see* hyoscyamine *on page 434*

gatifloxacin (gat i FLOKS a sin)

U.S./Canadian Brand Names Tequin® [Can]; Zymar™ [US/Can]

Therapeutic Category Antibiotic, Quinolone

Use

Oral, I.V.: Treatment of the following infections when caused by susceptible bacteria: Acute bacterial exacerbation of chronic bronchitis; acute sinusitis; community-acquired pneumonia including pneumonia caused by multidrug-resistant *S. pneumoniae* (MDRSP); uncomplicated skin and skin structure infection; uncomplicated urinary tract infections (cystitis); complicated urinary tract infections; pyelonephritis; uncomplicated urethral and cervical gonorrhea; acute, uncomplicated rectal infections in women caused by gonorrhea

Ophthalmic: Bacterial conjunctivitis

Usual Dosage

Usual dosage range:

Adults: Oral, I.V.: 400 mg once daily

Indication-specific dosing:

Children ≥1 year and Adults:

Bacterial conjunctivitis: Ophthalmic:

Days 1 and 2: Instill 1 drop into affected eye(s) every 2 hours while awake (maximum: 8 times/day)

Days 3-7: Instill 1 drop into affected eye(s) up to 4 times/day while awake

Adults: Oral, I.V.:

Acute bacterial exacerbation of chronic bronchitis: 400 mg every 24 hours for 5 days

Acute sinusitis: 400 mg every 24 hours for 10 days

Community-acquired pneumonia (including atypical organisms): 400 mg every 24 hours for 7-14 days

Pyelonephritis (acute): 400 mg every 24 hours for 7-10 days

Skin/skin structure infections (uncomplicated): 400 mg every 24 hours for 7-10 days

Urinary tract infections:

Complicated: 400 mg every 24 hours for 7-10 days

Uncomplicated, cystitis: 400 mg single dose or 200 mg every 24 hours for 3 days

Urethral gonorrhea in men (uncomplicated), cervical or rectal gonorrhea in women and pharyngitis (gonococcal): 400 mg single dose

Dosage Forms [DSC] = Discontinued product

Injection, infusion [premixed in D_5W]:

Tequin®: 200 mg (100 mL), 400 mg (200 mL) [DSC]

Injection, solution [preservative free]:

Tequin®: 10 mg/mL (40 mL) [DSC]

Solution, ophthalmic:

Zymar™: 0.3% (2.5 mL, 5 mL) [contains benzalkonium chloride]

Tablet:

Tequin®: 200 mg, 400 mg [DSC]

Tequin® Teq-paq™ [unit-dose pack]: 400 mg (5s) [DSC]

Gaviscon® Extra Strength [US-OTC] *see* aluminum hydroxide and magnesium carbonate *on page 36*

Gaviscon® Liquid [US-OTC] *see* aluminum hydroxide and magnesium carbonate *on page 36*

Gaviscon® Tablet [US-OTC] *see* aluminum hydroxide and magnesium trisilicate *on page 36*

G-CSF *see* filgrastim *on page 345*

G-CSF (PEG conjugate) *see* pegfilgrastim *on page 643*

GCV sodium *see* ganciclovir *on page 375*

Gebauer's Ethyl Chloride® [US] *see* ethyl chloride *on page 328*

Gee Gee® *(Discontinued)* *see* guaifenesin *on page 392*

gefitinib (ge FI tye nib)

Sound-Alike/Look-Alike Issues
gefitinib may be confused with erlotinib

Synonyms NSC-715055; ZD1839

U.S./Canadian Brand Names IRESSA® [US]

Therapeutic Category Antineoplastic, Tyrosine Kinase Inhibitor

Use

U.S. Labeling: Monotherapy for continued treatment of locally advanced or metastatic nonsmall cell lung cancer after failure of platinum-based and docetaxel therapies. Treatment is limited to patients who are benefiting or have benefited from treatment with gefitinib.

Note: Due to the lack of improved survival data from clinical trials of gefitinib, and in response to positive survival data with another EGFR inhibitor, physicians are advised to use other treatment options in advanced nonsmall cell lung cancer patients following one or two prior chemotherapy regimens when they are refractory/intolerant to their most recent regimen.

Canada labeling: Approved indication is limited to NSCLC patients with epidermal growth factor receptor (EGFR) expression status positive or unknown.

Usual Dosage Note: In response to the lack of improved survival data from the ISEL trial, AstraZeneca has temporarily suspended promotion of this drug.

Oral: Adults: 250 mg/day; consider 500 mg/day in patients receiving effective CYP3A4 inducers (eg, rifampin, phenytoin)

Dosage Forms Tablet: 250 mg

gelatin (absorbable) (JEL a tin, ab SORB a ble)

Synonyms absorbable gelatin sponge

U.S./Canadian Brand Names Gelfilm® [US]; Gelfoam® [US]

Therapeutic Category Hemostatic Agent

Use Adjunct to provide hemostasis in surgery; open prostatic surgery

Usual Dosage Hemostasis: Apply packs or sponges dry or saturated with sodium chloride. When applied dry, hold in place with moderate pressure. When applied wet, squeeze to remove air bubbles. The powder is applied as a paste prepared by adding approximately 4 mL of sterile saline solution to the powder.

Dosage Forms

Film, ophthalmic (Gelfilm®): 25 mm x 50 mm (6s)
Film, topical (Gelfilm®): 100 mm x 125 mm (1s)
Powder, topical (Gelfoam®): 1 g
Sponge, dental (Gelfoam®): Size 4 (12s)
Sponge, topical (Gelfoam®):
Size 50 (4s)
Size 100 (6s)
Size 200 (6s)
Size 2 cm (1s)
Size 6 cm (6s)
Size 12-7 mm (12s)

gelatin, pectin, and methylcellulose (JEL a tin, PEK tin, & meth il SEL yoo lose)

Synonyms methylcellulose, gelatin, and pectin; pectin, gelatin, and methylcellulose

Therapeutic Category Protectant, Topical

Use Temporary relief from minor oral irritations

Usual Dosage Press small dabs into place until the involved area is coated with a thin film; do not try to spread onto area; may be used as often as needed

Gelclair® [US] *see* maltodextrin *on page 518*

Gelfilm® [US] *see* gelatin (absorbable) *on previous page*

Gelfoam® [US] *see* gelatin (absorbable) *on previous page*

Gel-Kam® [US-OTC] *see* fluoride *on page 354*

Gel-Kam® Rinse [US] *see* fluoride *on page 354*

GelRite [US-OTC] *see* alcohol (ethyl) *on page 25*

Gel-Stat™ [US-OTC] *see* alcohol (ethyl) *on page 25*

Gel-Tin® *(Discontinued)* *see* fluoride *on page 354*

Gelucast® [US] *see* zinc gelatin *on page 887*

Gelusil® [US-OTC/Can] *see* aluminum hydroxide, magnesium hydroxide, and simethicone *on page 37*

Gelusil® Extra Strength [Can] *see* aluminum hydroxide and magnesium hydroxide *on page 36*

gemcitabine (jem SITE a been)

Sound-Alike/Look-Alike Issues

Gemzar® may be confused with Zinecard®

Synonyms gemcitabine hydrochloride

U.S./Canadian Brand Names Gemzar® [US/Can]

Therapeutic Category Antineoplastic Agent

Use

Adenocarcinoma of the pancreas: First-line therapy in locally-advanced (nonresectable stage II or stage III) or metastatic (stage IV) adenocarcinoma of the pancreas

Breast cancer: First-line therapy in metastatic breast cancer

Nonsmall-cell lung cancer: First-line therapy in locally-advanced (stage IIIA or IIIB) or metastatic (stage IV) nonsmall-cell lung cancer (NSLC)

Ovarian cancer: Treatment of relapsed ovarian cancer

Usual Dosage Refer to individual protocols. **Note**: Prolongation of the infusion time >60 minutes and administration more frequently than once weekly have been shown to increase toxicity. I.V.:

Pancreatic cancer: Initial: 1000 mg/m^2 over 30 minutes once weekly for up to 7 weeks followed by 1 week rest; subsequent cycles once weekly for 3 consecutive weeks out of every 4 weeks.

Dose adjustment: Patients who complete an entire cycle of therapy may have the dose in subsequent cycles increased by 25% as long as the absolute granulocyte count (AGC) nadir is >1500 x 10^6/L, platelet nadir is >100,000 x 10^6/L, and nonhematologic toxicity is less than WHO Grade 1. If the increased dose is tolerated (with the same parameters) the dose in subsequent cycles may again be increased by 20%.

Nonsmall-cell lung cancer (combination therapy with cisplatin):

28-day cycle: 1000 mg/m^2 over 30 minutes on days 1, 8, 15; repeat cycle every 28 days

or

21-day cycle: 1250 mg/m^2 over 30 minutes on days 1, 8; repeat cycle every 21 days

Breast cancer (combination therapy with paclitaxel): 1250 mg/m^2 over 30 minutes on days 1 and 8 of each 21-day cycle

Ovarian cancer (combination therapy with carboplatin): 1000 mg/m^2 over 30 minutes on days 1 and 8 of each 21-day cycle

Dosage Forms

Injection, powder for reconstitution:

Gemzar®: 200 mg, 1 g

gemcitabine hydrochloride *see* gemcitabine *on this page*

gemfibrozil (jem FI broe zil)

Sound-Alike/Look-Alike Issues

Lopid® may be confused with Levbid®, Lodine®, Lorabid®, Slo-bid™

Synonyms CI-719

U.S./Canadian Brand Names Apo-Gemfibrozil® [Can]; Gen-Gemfibrozil [Can]; GMD-Gemfibrozil [Can]; Lopid® [US/Can]; Novo-Gemfibrozil [Can]; Nu-Gemfibrozil [Can]; PMS-Gemfibrozil [Can]

Therapeutic Category Antihyperlipidemic Agent, Miscellaneous

Use Treatment of hypertriglyceridemia in types IV and V hyperlipidemia for patients who are at greater risk for pancreatitis and who have not responded to dietary intervention

Usual Dosage Adults: Oral: 1200 mg/day in 2 divided doses, 30 minutes before breakfast and dinner

Dosage Forms Tablet: 600 mg

gemifloxacin (je mi FLOKS a sin)

Synonyms DW286; gemifloxacin mesylate; LA 20304a; SB-265805

U.S./Canadian Brand Names Factive® [US]

Therapeutic Category Antibiotic, Quinolone

Use Treatment of acute exacerbation of chronic bronchitis; treatment of community-acquired pneumonia, including pneumonia caused by multidrug-resistant strains of *S. pneumoniae* (MDRSP)

Usual Dosage

Usual dosage range:

Adults: Oral: 320 mg once daily

Indication-specific dosing:

Adults: Oral:

Acute exacerbations of chronic bronchitis: 320 mg once daily for 5 days

Community-acquired pneumonia (mild to moderate): 320 mg once daily for 7 days

Dosage Forms Tablet, as mesylate: 320 mg

gemifloxacin mesylate *see* gemifloxacin *on this page*

gemtuzumab ozogamicin (gem TOO zoo mab oh zog a MY sin)

Synonyms CMA-676; NSC-720568

U.S./Canadian Brand Names Mylotarg® [US/Can]

Therapeutic Category Antineoplastic Agent, Natural Source (Plant) Derivative

Use Treatment of relapsed CD33 positive acute myeloid leukemia (AML) in patients ≥60 years of age who are not candidates for cytotoxic chemotherapy

Usual Dosage I.V.:

Adults: **Note:** Patients should receive diphenhydramine 50 mg orally and acetaminophen 650-1000 mg orally 1 hour prior to administration of each dose. Acetaminophen dosage should be repeated as needed every 4 hours for 2 additional doses. Pretreatment with methylprednisolone may ameliorate infusion-related symptoms.

AML: ≥60 years: 9 mg/m^2 infused over 2 hours. A full treatment course is a total of 2 doses administered with 14 days between doses. Full hematologic recovery is not necessary for administration of the second dose. There has been only limited experience with repeat courses of gemtuzumab ozogamicin.

Dosage Forms

Injection, powder for reconstitution:

Mylotarg®: 5 mg

Gemzar® [US/Can] *see* gemcitabine *on previous page*

Genabid® *(Discontinued)*

Genac® [US-OTC] *see* triprolidine and pseudoephedrine *on page 853*

Gen-Acebutolol [Can] *see* acebutolol *on page 4*

Genaced™ [US-OTC] *see* acetaminophen, aspirin, and caffeine *on page 10*

Gen-Acyclovir [Can] *see* acyclovir *on page 18*

Genahist® [US-OTC] *see* diphenhydramine *on page 261*

Gen-Alendronate [Can] *see* alendronate *on page 27*

Gen-Alprazolam [Can] *see* alprazolam *on page 32*

Gen-Amilazide [Can] *see* amiloride and hydrochlorothiazide *on page 41*

Genamin® Expectorant *(Discontinued)*

Gen-Amiodarone [Can] *see* amiodarone *on page 43*

Gen-Amoxicillin [Can] *see* amoxicillin *on page 47*

Gen-Anagrelide [Can] *see* anagrelide *on page 55*

Genapap™ [US-OTC] *see* acetaminophen *on page 5*

Genapap™ Children [US-OTC] *see* acetaminophen *on page 5*

Genapap™ Extra Strength [US-OTC] *see* acetaminophen *on page 5*

Genapap™ Infant [US-OTC] *see* acetaminophen *on page 5*

Genapap® Sinus Maximum Strength [US-OTC] *see* acetaminophen and pseudoephedrine *on page 9*

Genaphed® [US-OTC] *see* pseudoephedrine *on page 712*

Genasal [US-OTC] *see* oxymetazoline *on page 628*
Genasoft® [US-OTC] *see* docusate *on page 270*
Genasyme® [US-OTC] *see* simethicone *on page 772*
Gen-Atenolol [Can] *see* atenolol *on page 80*
Genaton Tablet [US-OTC] *see* aluminum hydroxide and magnesium trisilicate *on page 36*
Genatuss® *(Discontinued)* *see* guaifenesin *on page 392*
Genatuss DM® [US-OTC] *see* guaifenesin and dextromethorphan *on page 394*
Gen-Azathioprine [Can] *see* azathioprine *on page 86*
Gen-Baclofen [Can] *see* baclofen *on page 91*
Gen-Beclo [Can] *see* beclomethasone *on page 95*
Gen-Bromazepam [Can] *see* bromazepam *(Canada only) on page 117*
Gen-Budesonide AQ [Can] *see* budesonide *on page 122*
Gen-Buspirone [Can] *see* buspirone *on page 127*
Gencalc® 600 *(Discontinued)* *see* calcium carbonate *on page 135*
Gen-Captopril [Can] *see* captopril *on page 143*
Gen-Carbamazepine CR [Can] *see* carbamazepine *on page 144*
Gen-Cimetidine [Can] *see* cimetidine *on page 189*
Gen-Ciprofloxacin [Can] *see* ciprofloxacin *on page 190*
Gen-Citalopram [Can] *see* citalopram *on page 194*
Gen-Clobetasol [Can] *see* clobetasol *on page 200*
Gen-Clomipramine [Can] *see* clomipramine *on page 202*
Gen-Clonazepam [Can] *see* clonazepam *on page 203*
Gen-Clozapine [Can] *see* clozapine *on page 206*
Gen-Combo Sterinebs [Can] *see* ipratropium and albuterol *on page 460*
Gen-Cyclobenzaprine [Can] *see* cyclobenzaprine *on page 219*
Gen-Cyproterone [Can] *see* cyproterone *(Canada only) on page 223*
Gen-Diltiazem [Can] *see* diltiazem *on page 257*
Gen-Diltiazem CD [Can] *see* diltiazem *on page 257*
Gen-Divalproex [Can] *see* valproic acid and derivatives *on page 864*
Gen-Doxazosin [Can] *see* doxazosin *on page 275*
Genebs [US-OTC] *see* acetaminophen *on page 5*
Genebs Extra Strength [US-OTC] *see* acetaminophen *on page 5*
Generlac [US] *see* lactulose *on page 478*
Genesec™ [US-OTC] *see* acetaminophen and phenyltoloxamine *on page 8*
Gen-Etidronate [Can] *see* etidronate disodium *on page 329*
Geneye® [US-OTC] *see* tetrahydrozoline *on page 817*
Gen-Famotidine [Can] *see* famotidine *on page 335*
Gen-Fenofibrate Micro [Can] *see* fenofibrate *on page 338*
Genfiber® [US-OTC] *see* psyllium *on page 717*
Gen-Fluconazole [Can] *see* fluconazole *on page 349*
Gen-Fluoxetine [Can] *see* fluoxetine *on page 357*
Gen-Gabapentin [Can] *see* gabapentin *on page 373*
Gen-Gemfibrozil [Can] *see* gemfibrozil *on page 378*
Gen-Glybe [Can] *see* glyburide *on page 387*
Gengraf® [US] *see* cyclosporine *on page 221*
Gen-Hydroxychloroquine [Can] *see* hydroxychloroquine *on page 431*
Gen-Hydroxyurea [Can] *see* hydroxyurea *on page 432*
Gen-Indapamide [Can] *see* indapamide *on page 445*

Gen-Ipratropium [Can] *see* ipratropium *on page 460*

Gen-K® *(Discontinued)* *see* potassium chloride *on page 684*

Gen-Lamotrigine [Can] *see* lamotrigine *on page 480*

Gen-Levothyroxine [Can] *see* levothyroxine *on page 491*

Gen-Lovastatin [Can] *see* lovastatin *on page 508*

Gen-Medroxy [Can] *see* medroxyprogesterone *on page 524*

Gen-Meloxicam [Can] *see* meloxicam *on page 526*

Gen-Metformin [Can] *see* metformin *on page 535*

Gen-Minocycline [Can] *see* minocycline *on page 558*

Gen-Mirtazapine [Can] *see* mirtazapine *on page 559*

Gen-Nabumetone [Can] *see* nabumetone *on page 572*

Gen-Naproxen EC [Can] *see* naproxen *on page 578*

Gen-Nitro [Can] *see* nitroglycerin *on page 595*

Gen-Nizatidine [Can] *see* nizatidine *on page 597*

Gen-Nortriptyline [Can] *see* nortriptyline *on page 600*

Genoptic® *(Discontinued)* *see* gentamicin *on this page*

Genora® 0.5/35 *(Discontinued)* *see* ethinyl estradiol and norethindrone *on page 323*

Genora® 1/35 *(Discontinued)* *see* ethinyl estradiol and norethindrone *on page 323*

Genora® 1/50 *(Discontinued)* *see* mestranol and norethindrone *on page 534*

Genotropin® [US] *see* somatropin *on page 785*

Genotropin Miniquick® [US] *see* somatropin *on page 785*

Gen-Oxybutynin [Can] *see* oxybutynin *on page 625*

Gen-Paroxetine [Can] *see* paroxetine *on page 639*

Gen-Pindolol [Can] *see* pindolol *on page 669*

Gen-Piroxicam [Can] *see* piroxicam *on page 671*

Genpril® [US-OTC] *see* ibuprofen *on page 437*

Gen-Ranidine [Can] *see* ranitidine *on page 732*

Gen-Salbutamol [Can] *see* albuterol *on page 23*

Gen-Selegiline [Can] *see* selegiline *on page 766*

Gen-Sertraline [Can] *see* sertraline *on page 769*

Gen-Simvastatin [Can] *see* simvastatin *on page 773*

Gen-Sotalol [Can] *see* sotalol *on page 787*

Gen-Sumatriptan [Can] *see* sumatriptan *on page 801*

Gentacidin® *(Discontinued)* *see* gentamicin *on this page*

Gentak® [US] *see* gentamicin *on this page*

gentamicin (jen ta MYE sin)

Sound-Alike/Look-Alike Issues

gentamicin may be confused with kanamycin

Garamycin® may be confused with kanamycin, Terramycin®

Synonyms gentamicin sulfate

U.S./Canadian Brand Names Alcomicin® [Can]; Diogent® [Can]; Garamycin® [Can]; Gentak® [US]; Gentamicin Injection, USP [Can]; SAB-Gentamicin [Can]

Therapeutic Category Aminoglycoside (Antibiotic); Antibiotic, Ophthalmic; Antibiotic, Topical

Use Treatment of susceptible bacterial infections, normally gram-negative organisms including *Pseudomonas*, *Proteus*, *Serratia*, and gram-positive *Staphylococcus*; treatment of bone infections, respiratory tract infections, skin and soft tissue infections, as well as abdominal and urinary tract infections, endocarditis, and septicemia; used topically to treat superficial infections of the skin or ophthalmic infections caused by susceptible bacteria; prevention of bacterial endocarditis prior to dental or surgical procedures (Continued)

gentamicin *(Continued)*

Usual Dosage Note: Dosage Individualization is **critical** because of the low therapeutic index.

Use of ideal body weight (IBW) for determining the mg/kg/dose appears to be more accurate than dosing on the basis of total body weight (TBW). In morbid obesity, dosage requirement may best be estimated using a dosing weight of IBW + 0.4 (TBW - IBW).

Initial and periodic plasma drug levels (eg, peak and trough with conventional dosing) should be determined, particularly in critically-ill patients with serious infections or in disease states known to significantly alter aminoglycoside pharmacokinetics (eg, cystic fibrosis, burns, or major surgery).

Usual dosage ranges:

Infants and Children <5 years: I.M., I.V.: 2.5 mg/kg/dose every 8 hours*

Children ≥5 years: I.M., I.V.: 2-2.5 mg/kg/dose every 8 hours*

***Note:** Higher individual doses and/or more frequent intervals (eg, every 6 hours) may be required in selected clinical situations (cystic fibrosis) or serum levels document the need

Children and Adults:

Intrathecal: 4-8 mg/day

Ophthalmic:

Ointment: Instill 1/2" (1.25 cm) 2-3 times/day to every 3-4 hours

Solution: Instill 1-2 drops every 2-4 hours, up to 2 drops every hour for severe infections

Topical: Apply 3-4 times/day to affected area

Adults: I.M., I.V.:

Conventional: 1-2.5 mg/kg/dose every 8-12 hours; to ensure adequate peak concentrations early in therapy, higher initial dosage may be considered in selected patients when extracellular water is increased (edema, septic shock, postsurgical, or trauma)

Once daily: 4-7 mg/kg/dose once daily; some clinicians recommend this approach for all patients with normal renal function; this dose is at least as efficacious with similar, if not less, toxicity than conventional dosing

Indication-specific dosing:

Neonates: I.V.:

Meningitis:

0-7 days of age: <2000 g: 2.5 mg/kg every 18-24 hours; >2000 g: 2.5 mg/kg every 12 hours

8-28 days of age: <2000 g: 2.5 mg/kg every 8-12 hours; >2000 g: 2.5 mg/kg every 8 hours

Children and Adults: I.M., I.V.:

Brucellosis: 240 mg (I.M.) daily or 5 mg/kg (I.V.) daily for 7 days; either regimen recommended in combination with doxycycline

Cholangitis: 4-6 mg/kg once daily with ampicillin

Diverticulitis (complicated): 1.5-2 mg/kg every 8 hours (with ampicillin and metronidazole)

Endocarditis prophylaxis: Dental, oral, upper respiratory procedures, GI/GU procedures: 1.5 mg/kg with ampicillin (50 mg/kg) 30 minutes prior to procedure

Endocarditis or synergy (for Gram-positive infections): 1 mg/kg every 8 hours (with ampicillin)

Meningitis:

(Enterococcus sp or *Pseudomonas aeruginosa)*: Loading dose 2 mg/kg, then 1.7 mg/kg/dose every 8 hours (administered with another bacteriocidal drug)

Listeria: 5-7 mg/kg/day (with penicillin) for 1 week

Pelvic inflammatory disease: Loading dose: 2 mg/kg, then 1.5 mg/kg every 8 hours

Alternate therapy: 4.5 mg/kg once daily

Plague (*Yersinia pestis*): Treatment: 5 mg/kg/day, followed by postexposure prophylaxis with doxycycline

Pneumonia, hospital- or ventilator-associated: 7 mg/kg/day (with antipseudomonal beta-lactam or carbapenem)

Tularemia: 5 mg/kg/day divided every 8 hours for 1-2 weeks

Urinary tract infection: 1.5 mg/kg/dose every 8 hours

Dosage Forms [DSC] = Discontinued product

Cream, topical, as sulfate: 0.1% (15 g, 30 g)

Infusion, as sulfate [premixed in NS]: 40 mg (50 mL); 60 mg (50 mL, 100 mL); 70 mg (50 mL); 80 mg (50 mL, 100 mL); 90 mg (100 mL); 100 mg (50 mL, 100 mL); 120 mg (100 mL)

Injection, solution, as sulfate [ADD-Vantage® vial]: 10 mg/mL (6 mL, 8 mL, 10 mL)

Injection, solution, as sulfate: 40 mg/mL (2 mL, 20 mL) [may contain sodium metabisulfite]

Injection, solution, pediatric, as sulfate: 10 mg/mL (2 mL) [may contain sodium metabisulfite]

Injection, solution, pediatric, as sulfate [preservative free]: 10 mg/mL (2 mL)

Ointment, ophthalmic, as sulfate (Gentak®): 0.3% [3 mg/g] (3.5 g)

Ointment, topical, as sulfate: 0.1% (15 g, 30 g)

Solution, ophthalmic, as sulfate: 0.3% (5 mL, 15 mL) [contains benzalkonium chloride]

Genoptic®: 0.3% (1 mL) [contains benzalkonium chloride] [DSC]

Gentak®: 0.3% (5 mL; 15 mL [DSC]) [contains benzalkonium chloride]

glatiramer acetate (gla TIR a mer AS e tate)

Sound-Alike/Look-Alike Issues

Copaxone® may be confused with Compazine®

Synonyms copolymer-1

U.S./Canadian Brand Names Copaxone® [US/Can]

Therapeutic Category Biological, Miscellaneous

Use Treatment of relapsing-remitting type multiple sclerosis; studies indicate that it reduces the frequency of attacks and the severity of disability; appears to be most effective for patients with minimal disability

Usual Dosage Adults: SubQ: 20 mg daily

Dosage Forms Injection, solution [preservative free]: 20 mg/mL (1 mL) [prefilled syringe; contains mannitol; packaged with alcohol pads]

Glaucon® ***(Discontinued)*** *see* epinephrine *on page 295*

Gleevec® [US/Can] *see* imatinib *on page 441*

Gliadel® [US] *see* carmustine *on page 153*

Gliadel Wafer® [Can] *see* carmustine *on page 153*

glibenclamide *see* glyburide *on page 387*

gliclazide *(Canada only)* (GLYE kla zide)

U.S./Canadian Brand Names Apo-Gliclazide® [Can]; Diamicron® MR [Can]; Diamicron® [Can]; Novo-Gliclazide [Can]; Rhoxal-gliclazide [Can]; Sandoz-Gliclazide [Can]

Therapeutic Category Antidiabetic Agent; Hypoglycemic Agent, Oral; Sulfonylurea Agent

Use Management of type 2 diabetes mellitus (noninsulin-dependent, NIDDM)

Usual Dosage Oral: Adults:

Immediate release tablet: Initial: 80-160 mg/day; typical dose range 80-320 mg/day; dosage of ≥160 mg should be divided into 2 equal parts for twice-daily administration; maximum dose: 320 mg/day; should be taken with meals

Sustained release tablet: 30-120 mg once daily

Note: There is no fixed dosage regimen for the management of diabetes mellitus with gliclazide or any other hypoglycemic agent. Dose must be individualized based on frequent determinations of blood glucose during dose titration and throughout maintenance.

Dosage Forms [CAN] = Canadian brand name

Tablet: 80 mg [not available in the U.S.]

Diamicron® [CAN]: 80 mg [not available in the U.S.]

Tablet, sustained release:

Diamicron® MR [CAN]: 30 mg [not available in the U.S.]

glimepiride (GLYE me pye ride)

Sound-Alike/Look-Alike Issues

glimepiride may be confused with glipiZIDE

Amaryl® may be confused with Altace®, Amerge®, Reminyl®

U.S./Canadian Brand Names Amaryl® [US/Can]; CO Glimepiride [Can]; Novo-Glimepiride [Can]; ratio-Glimepiride [Can]; Rhoxal-glimepiride [Can]; Sandoz-Glimepiride [Can]

Therapeutic Category Antidiabetic Agent, Oral

Use Management of type 2 diabetes mellitus (noninsulin-dependent, NIDDM) as an adjunct to diet and exercise to lower blood glucose; may be used in combination with metformin or insulin in patients whose hyperglycemia cannot be controlled by diet and exercise in conjunction with a single oral hypoglycemic agent

Usual Dosage

Oral: Adults: Initial: 1-2 mg once daily, administered with breakfast or the first main meal; usual maintenance dose: 1-4 mg once daily; after a dose of 2 mg once daily, increase in increments of 2 mg at 1- to 2-week intervals based upon the patient's blood glucose response to a maximum of 8 mg once daily. If inadequate response to maximal dose, combination therapy with metformin may be considered.

Combination with insulin therapy (fasting glucose level for instituting combination therapy is in the range of >150 mg/dL in plasma or serum depending on the patient): initial recommended dose: 8 mg once daily with the first main meal

After starting with low-dose insulin, upward adjustments of insulin can be done approximately weekly as guided by frequent measurements of fasting blood glucose. Once stable, combination-therapy patients should monitor their capillary blood glucose on an ongoing basis, preferably daily.

Conversion from therapy with long half-life agents: Observe patient carefully for 1-2 weeks when converting from a longer half-life agent (eg, chlorpropamide) to glimepiride due to overlapping hypoglycemic effects.

Dosage Forms Tablet: 1 mg, 2 mg, 4 mg

glipizide (GLIP i zide)

Sound-Alike/Look-Alike Issues

glipiZIDE may be confused with glimepiride, glyBURIDE

Glucotrol® may be confused with Glucophage®, Glucotrol® XL, glyBURIDE

Glucotrol® XL may be confused with Glucotrol®

Synonyms glydiazinamide

Tall-Man glipi**ZIDE**

U.S./Canadian Brand Names Glucotrol® XL [US]; Glucotrol® [US]

Therapeutic Category Antidiabetic Agent, Oral

Use Management of type 2 diabetes mellitus (noninsulin-dependent, NIDDM)

Usual Dosage Oral (allow several days between dose titrations): Adults: Initial: 5 mg/day; adjust dosage at 2.5-5 mg daily increments as determined by blood glucose response at intervals of several days.

Immediate release tablet: Maximum recommended once-daily dose: 15 mg; maximum recommended total daily dose: 40 mg

Extended release tablet (Glucotrol® XL): Maximum recommended dose: 20 mg

When transferring from insulin to glipizide:

Current insulin requirement ≤20 units: Discontinue insulin and initiate glipizide at usual dose

Current insulin requirement >20 units: Decrease insulin by 50% and initiate glipizide at usual dose; gradually decrease insulin dose based on patient response. Several days should elapse between dosage changes.

Dosage Forms

Tablet (Glucotrol®): 5 mg, 10 mg

Tablet, extended release: 5 mg, 10 mg

Glucotrol® XL: 2.5 mg, 5 mg, 10 mg

glipizide and metformin (GLIP i zide & met FOR min)

Synonyms glipizide and metformin hydrochloride; metformin and glipizide

U.S./Canadian Brand Names Metaglip™ [US]

Therapeutic Category Antidiabetic Agent (Biguanide); Antidiabetic Agent (Sulfonylurea)

Use Initial therapy for management of type 2 diabetes mellitus (noninsulin-dependent, NIDDM) when hyperglycemia cannot be managed with diet and exercise alone. Second-line therapy for management of type 2 diabetes (NIDDM) when hyperglycemia cannot be managed with a sulfonylurea or metformin along with diet and exercise.

Usual Dosage Oral: Adults:

Type 2 diabetes, first-line therapy: Initial: Glipizide 2.5 mg/metformin 250 mg once daily with a meal. Dose adjustment: Increase dose by 1 tablet/day every 2 weeks, up to a maximum of glipizide 10 mg/metformin 1000 mg daily

Patients with fasting plasma glucose (FPG) 280-320 mg/dL: Consider glipizide 2.5 mg/metformin 500 mg twice daily. Dose adjustment: Increase dose by 1 tablet/day every 2 weeks, up to a maximum of glipizide 10 mg/metformin 2000 mg daily in divided doses

Type 2 diabetes, second-line therapy: Glipizide 2.5 mg/metformin 500 mg **or** glipizide 5 mg/metformin 500 mg twice daily with morning and evening meals; starting dose should not exceed current daily dose of glipizide (or sulfonylurea equivalent) or metformin. Dose adjustment: Titrate dose in increments of no more than glipizide 5 mg/metformin 500 mg, up to a maximum dose of glipizide 20 mg/metformin 2000 mg daily.

Dosage Forms

Tablet: 2.5/250: Glipizide 2.5 mg and metformin hydrochloride 250 mg; 2.5/500: Glipizide 2.5 mg and metformin hydrochloride 500 mg; 5/500: Glipizide 5 mg and metformin hydrochloride 500 mg

Metaglip™ 2.5/250: Glipizide 2.5 mg and metformin hydrochloride 250 mg

Metaglip™ 2.5/500: Glipizide 2.5 mg and metformin hydrochloride 500 mg

Metaglip™ 5/500: Glipizide 5 mg and metformin hydrochloride 500 mg

glipizide and metformin hydrochloride *see* glipizide and metformin *on this page*

glivec *see* imatinib *on page 441*

GlucaGen® [US] *see* glucagon *on next page*

GlucaGen® Diagnostic Kit [US] *see* glucagon *on next page*

GlucaGen® HypoKit™ [US] *see* glucagon *on this page*

glucagon (GLOO ka gon)

Sound-Alike/Look-Alike Issues
glucagon may be confused with Glaucon®

Synonyms glucagon hydrochloride

U.S./Canadian Brand Names GlucaGen® Diagnostic Kit [US]; GlucaGen® HypoKit™ [US]; GlucaGen® [US]; Glucagon Emergency Kit [US]

Therapeutic Category Antihypoglycemic Agent

Use Management of hypoglycemia; diagnostic aid in radiologic examinations to temporarily inhibit GI tract movement

Usual Dosage
Hypoglycemia or insulin shock therapy: I.M., I.V., SubQ:
Children <20 kg: 0.5 mg or 20-30 mcg/kg/dose; repeated in 20 minutes as needed
Children ≥20 kg and Adults: 1 mg; may repeat in 20 minutes as needed
Note: If patient fails to respond to glucagon, I.V. dextrose must be given.
Diagnostic aid: Adults: I.M., I.V.: 0.25-2 mg 10 minutes prior to procedure

Dosage Forms Injection, powder for reconstitution, as hydrochloride:
GlucaGen®: 1 mg [equivalent to 1 unit; contains lactose 107 mg]
GlucaGen® Diagnostic Kit: 1 mg [equivalent to 1 unit; contains lactose 107 mg; packaged with sterile water]
GlucaGen® HypoKit™: 1 mg [equivalent to 1 unit; contains lactose 107 mg; packaged with prefilled syringe containing sterile water]
Glucagon®: 1 mg [equivalent to 1 unit; contains lactose 49 mg]
Glucagon Diagnostic Kit, Glucagon Emergency Kit: 1 mg [equivalent to 1 unit; contains lactose 49 mg; packaged with diluent syringe containing glycerin 12 mg/mL and water for injection]

Glucagon Diagnostic Kit *(Discontinued)* *see* glucagon *on this page*

Glucagon Emergency Kit [US] *see* glucagon *on this page*

glucagon hydrochloride *see* glucagon *on this page*

glucocerebrosidase *see* alglucerase *on page 28*

GlucoNorm® [Can] *see* repaglinide *on page 737*

Glucophage® [US/Can] *see* metformin *on page 535*

Glucophage® XR [US] *see* metformin *on page 535*

glucose (instant) (GLOO kose IN stant)

Sound-Alike/Look-Alike Issues
Glutose™ may be confused with Glutofac®

U.S./Canadian Brand Names B-D™ Glucose [US-OTC]; Dex4 Glucose [US-OTC]; Glutol™ [US-OTC]; Glutose™ [US-OTC]; Insta-Glucose® [US-OTC]

Therapeutic Category Antihypoglycemic Agent

Use Management of hypoglycemia

Usual Dosage Adults: Oral: 10-20 g

Dosage Forms
Gel, oral:
Glutose™: 40% (15 g, 45 g)
Insta-Glucose®: 40% (30 g)
Solution, oral (Glutol™): 55% [100 g dextrose/180 mL] (180 mL)
Tablet, chewable:
B-D™ Glucose: 5 g
Dex4 Glucose: 4 g

glucose polymers (GLOO kose POL i merz)

U.S./Canadian Brand Names Moducal® [US-OTC]; Polycose® [US-OTC]

Therapeutic Category Nutritional Supplement

Use Supplies calories for those persons not able to meet the caloric requirement with usual food intake

Usual Dosage Adults: Oral: Add to foods or beverages or mix in water

Dosage Forms
Liquid (Polycose®): 43% (126 mL)
Powder:
Moducal®: 368 g
Polycose®: 350 g

Glucotrol® [US] *see* glipizide *on page 385*

Glucotrol® XL [US] *see* glipizide *on page 385*

Glucovance® [US] *see* glyburide and metformin *on next page*

Glu-K® [US-OTC] *see* potassium gluconate *on page 686*

glulisine insulin *see* insulin glulisine *on page 450*

Glumetza™ [US/Can] *see* metformin *on page 535*

glutamic acid (gloo TAM ik AS id)

Synonyms glutamic acid hydrochloride

Therapeutic Category Gastrointestinal Agent, Miscellaneous

Use Treatment of hypochlorhydria and achlorhydria

Usual Dosage Adults: Oral:

Tablet/powder: 500-1000 mg/day before meals or food

Capsule: 1-3 capsules 3 times/day before meals

Dosage Forms

Capsule, as hydrochloride: 340 mg

Tablet: 500 mg

glutamic acid hydrochloride *see* glutamic acid *on this page*

Glutofac®-MX [US] *see* vitamins (multiple/oral) *on page 878*

Glutofac®-ZX [US] *see* vitamins (multiple/oral) *on page 878*

Glutol™ [US-OTC] *see* glucose (instant) *on previous page*

Glutose™ [US-OTC] *see* glucose (instant) *on previous page*

Glyate® ***(Discontinued)*** *see* guaifenesin *on page 392*

glybenclamide *see* glyburide *on this page*

glybenzcyclamide *see* glyburide *on this page*

glyburide (GLYE byoor ide)

Sound-Alike/Look-Alike Issues

glyBURIDE may be confused with glipiZIDE, Glucotrol®

Diaβeta® may be confused with Diabinese®, Zebeta®

Micronase® may be confused with microK®, miconazole, Micronor®

Synonyms glibenclamide; glybenclamide; glybenzcyclamide

Tall-Man gly**BURIDE**

U.S./Canadian Brand Names Albert® Glyburide [Can]; Apo-Glyburide® [Can]; Diaβeta® [US/Can]; Euglucon® [Can]; Gen-Glybe [Can]; Glynase® PresTab® [US]; Micronase® [US]; Novo-Glyburide [Can]; Nu-Glyburide [Can]; PMS-Glyburide [Can]; ratio-Glyburide [Can]; Sandoz-Glyburide [Can]

Therapeutic Category Antidiabetic Agent, Oral

Use Management of type 2 diabetes mellitus (noninsulin-dependent, NIDDM)

Usual Dosage Oral:

Adults:

Initial: 2.5-5 mg/day, administered with breakfast or the first main meal of the day. In patients who are more sensitive to hypoglycemic drugs, start at 1.25 mg/day.

Increase in increments of no more than 2.5 mg/day at weekly intervals based on the patient's blood glucose response

Maintenance: 1.25-20 mg/day given as single or divided doses; maximum: 20 mg/day

Micronized tablets (Glynase® PresTab®): Adults:

Initial: 1.5-3 mg/day, administered with breakfast or the first main meal of the day in patients who are more sensitive to hypoglycemic drugs, start at 0.75 mg/day. Increase in increments of no more than 1.5 mg/day in weekly intervals based on the patient's blood glucose response.

Maintenance: 0.75-12 mg/day given as a single dose or in divided doses. Some patients (especially those receiving >6 mg/day) may have a more satisfactory response with twice-daily dosing.

Dosage Forms [DSC] = Discontinued product

Tablet (Diaβeta®, Micronase®): 1.25 mg, 2.5 mg, 5 mg

Tablet, micronized: 1.5 mg, 3 mg, 6 mg

Glynase® PresTab®: 1.5 mg [DSC], 3 mg, 6 mg

glyburide and metformin (GLYE byoor ide & met FOR min)

Synonyms glyburide and metformin hydrochloride; metformin and glyburide

U.S./Canadian Brand Names Glucovance® [US]

Therapeutic Category Antidiabetic Agent (Sulfonylurea); Antidiabetic Agent, Oral

Use Initial therapy for management of type 2 diabetes mellitus (noninsulin-dependent, NIDDM). Second-line therapy for management of type 2 diabetes (NIDDM) when hyperglycemia cannot be managed with a sulfonylurea or metformin; combination therapy with a thiazolidinedione may be required to achieve additional control.

Usual Dosage Note: Dose must be individualized. Dosages expressed as glyburide/metformin components.

Adults: Oral:

Initial therapy (no prior treatment with sulfonylurea or metformin): 1.25 mg/250 mg once daily with a meal; patients with Hb A_{1c} >9% or fasting plasma glucose (FPG) >200 mg/dL may start with 1.25 mg/250 mg twice daily

Dosage may be increased in increments of 1.25 mg/250 mg, at intervals of not less than 2 weeks; maximum daily dose: 10 mg/2000 mg (limited experience with higher doses)

Previously treated with a sulfonylurea or metformin alone: Initial: 2.5 mg/500 mg or 5 mg/500 mg twice daily; increase in increments no greater than 5 mg/500 mg; maximum daily dose: 20 mg/2000 mg

When switching patients previously on a sulfonylurea and metformin together, do not exceed the daily dose of glyburide (or glyburide equivalent) or metformin.

Note: May combine with a thiazolidinedione in patients with an inadequate response to glyburide/metformin therapy (risk of hypoglycemia may be increased).

Dosage Forms Tablet:

1.25 mg/250 mg: Glyburide 1.25 mg and metformin hydrochloride 250 mg

2.5 mg/500 mg: Glyburide 2.5 mg and metformin hydrochloride 500 mg

5 mg/500 mg: Glyburide 5 mg and metformin hydrochloride 500 mg

glyburide and metformin hydrochloride *see* glyburide and metformin *on this page*

glycerin (GLIS er in)

Synonyms glycerol

U.S./Canadian Brand Names Bausch & Lomb® Computer Eye Drops [US-OTC]; Colace® Adult/Children Suppositories [US-OTC]; Colace® Infant/Children Suppositories [US-OTC]; Fleet® Babylax® [US-OTC]; Fleet® Glycerin Suppositories Maximum Strength [US-OTC]; Fleet® Glycerin Suppositories [US-OTC]; Fleet® Liquid Glycerin Suppositories [US-OTC]; Sani-Supp® [US-OTC]

Therapeutic Category Laxative; Ophthalmic Agent, Miscellaneous

Use Constipation; reduction of intraocular pressure; reduction of corneal edema; glycerin has been administered orally to reduce intracranial pressure

Usual Dosage

Constipation: Rectal:

Children <6 years: 1 infant suppository 1-2 times/day as needed or 2-5 mL as an enema

Children >6 years and Adults: 1 adult suppository 1-2 times/day as needed or 5-15 mL as an enema

Children and Adults:

Reduction of intraocular pressure: Oral: 1-1.8 g/kg 1-1½ hours preoperatively; additional doses may be administered at 5-hour intervals

Reduction of intracranial pressure: Oral: 1.5 g/kg/day divided every 4 hours; 1 g/kg/dose every 6 hours has also been used

Reduction of corneal edema: Ophthalmic solution: Instill 1-2 drops in eye(s) prior to examination OR for lubricant effect, instill 1-2 drops in eye(s) every 3-4 hours

Dosage Forms [DSC] = Discontinued product

Solution, ophthalmic, sterile (Bausch & Lomb® Computer Eye Drops): 1% (15 mL) [contains benzalkonium chloride]

Solution, oral (Osmoglyn®): 50% (220 mL) [lime flavor] [DSC]

Solution, rectal:

Fleet® Babylax®: 2.3 g/2.3 mL (4 mL) [6 units per box]

Fleet® Liquid Glycerin Suppositories: 5.6 g/5.5 mL (7.5 mL) [4 units per box]

Suppository, rectal: 82.5% (12s, 25s) [pediatric size]; 82.5% (12s, 24s, 25s, 50s, 100s) [adult size]

Colace® Adult/Children: 2.1 g (12s, 24s, 48s, 100s)

Colace® Infant/Children: 1.2 g (12s, 24s)

Fleet® Glycerin Suppositories: 1 g (12s) [pediatric size]; 2g (12s, 24s, 50s) [adult size]

Fleet® Glycerin Suppositories Maximum Strength: 3g (18s) [adult size]

Sani-Supp®: 82.5% (10s, 25s) [pediatric size]; 82.5% (10s, 25s, 50s) [adult size]

glycerol *see* glycerin *on previous page*

glycerol guaiacolate *see* guaifenesin *on page 392*

Glycerol-T® *(Discontinued)* *see* theophylline and guaifenesin *on page 820*

glycerol triacetate *see* triacetin *on page 845*

glyceryl trinitrate *see* nitroglycerin *on page 595*

Glycofed® *(Discontinued)* *see* guaifenesin and pseudoephedrine *on page 398*

GlycoLax™ [US] *see* polyethylene glycol 3350 *on page 678*

Glycon [Can] *see* metformin *on page 535*

glycopyrrolate (glye koe PYE roe late)

Synonyms glycopyrronium bromide

U.S./Canadian Brand Names Robinul® Forte [US]; Robinul® [US]

Therapeutic Category Anticholinergic Agent

Use Inhibit salivation and excessive secretions of the respiratory tract preoperatively; reversal of neuromuscular blockade; control of upper airway secretions; adjunct in treatment of peptic ulcer

Usual Dosage

Children:

Reduction of secretions (preanesthetic):

Oral: 40-100 mcg/kg/dose 3-4 times/day

I.M., I.V.: 4-10 mcg/kg/dose every 3-4 hours; maximum: 0.2 mg/dose or 0.8 mg/24 hours

Intraoperative: I.V.: 4 mcg/kg not to exceed 0.1 mg; repeat at 2- to 3-minute intervals as needed

Preoperative: I.M.:

<2 years: 4-9 mcg/kg 30-60 minutes before procedure

>2 years: 4 mcg/kg 30-60 minutes before procedure

Children and Adults: Reverse neuromuscular blockade: I.V.: 0.2 mg for each 1 mg of neostigmine or 5 mg of pyridostigmine administered or 5-15 mcg/kg glycopyrrolate with 25-70 mcg/kg of neostigmine or 0.1-0.3 mg/kg of pyridostigmine (agents usually administered simultaneously, but glycopyrrolate may be administered first if bradycardia is present)

Adults:

Reduction of secretions:

Intraoperative: I.V.: 0.1 mg repeated as needed at 2- to 3-minute intervals

Preoperative: I.M.: 4 mcg/kg 30-60 minutes before procedure

Peptic ulcer:

Oral: 1-2 mg 2-3 times/day

I.M., I.V.: 0.1-0.2 mg 3-4 times/day

Dosage Forms [DSC] = Discontinued product

Injection, solution: 0.2 mg/mL (1 mL, 2 mL, 5 mL, 20 mL)

Robinul®: 0.2 mg/mL (1 mL, 2 mL, 5 mL; 20 mL [DSC]) [contains benzoyl alcohol]

Tablet: 1 mg, 2 mg

Robinul®: 1 mg

Robinul® Forte: 2 mg

glycopyrronium bromide *see* glycopyrrolate *on this page*

Glycotuss® *(Discontinued)* *see* guaifenesin *on page 392*

Glycotuss-dM® *(Discontinued)* *see* guaifenesin and dextromethorphan *on page 394*

glydiazinamide *see* glipizide *on page 385*

Glynase® PresTab® [US] *see* glyburide *on page 387*

Gly-Oxide® [US-OTC] *see* carbamide peroxide *on page 145*

Glyquin® [US] *see* hydroquinone *on page 430*

Glyquin-XM™ [US/Can] *see* hydroquinone *on page 430*

Glyset® [US/Can] *see* miglitol *on page 557*

GM-CSF *see* sargramostim *on page 763*

GMD-Azithromycin [Can] *see* azithromycin *on page 88*

GMD-Fluconazole [Can] *see* fluconazole *on page 349*

GMD-Gemfibrozil [Can] *see* gemfibrozil *on page 378*

GMD-Sertraline [Can] *see* sertraline *on page 769*

G-myticin® *(Discontinued)* *see* gentamicin *on page 381*

GnRH *see* gonadorelin *on this page*

Gold Bond® Antifungal [US-OTC] *see* tolnaftate *on page 834*

gold sodium thiomalate (gold SOW dee um thye oh MAL ate)

U.S./Canadian Brand Names Aurolate® [US]; Myochrysine® [Can]

Therapeutic Category Gold Compound

Use Treatment of progressive rheumatoid arthritis

Usual Dosage I.M.:

Children: Initial: Test dose of 10 mg is recommended, followed by 1 mg/kg/week for 20 weeks; maintenance: 1 mg/kg/dose at 2- to 4-week intervals thereafter for as long as therapy is clinically beneficial and toxicity does not develop. Administration for 2-4 months is usually required before clinical improvement is observed.

Adults: 10 mg first week; 25 mg second week; then 25-50 mg/week until 1 g cumulative dose has been given; if improvement occurs without adverse reactions, administer 25-50 mg every 2-3 weeks for 2-20 weeks, then every 3-4 weeks indefinitely

Dosage Forms Injection, solution: 50 mg/mL (1 mL, 10 mL) [contains benzyl alcohol]

GoLYTELY® [US] *see* polyethylene glycol-electrolyte solution *on page 679*

gonadorelin (goe nad oh RELL in)

Sound-Alike/Look-Alike Issues

gonadorelin may be confused with gonadotropin, guanadrel

Factrel® may be confused with Sectral®

Gonadotropin may be confused with gonadorelin

Synonyms GnRH; gonadorelin acetate; gonadorelin hydrochloride; gonadotropin releasing hormone; LHRH; LRH; luteinizing hormone releasing hormone

U.S./Canadian Brand Names Factrel® [US]; Lutrepulse™ [Can]

Therapeutic Category Diagnostic Agent; Gonadotropin

Use Evaluation of functional capacity and response of gonadotrophic hormones; evaluate abnormal gonadotropin regulation as in precocious puberty and delayed puberty.

Orphan drug: Lutrepulse®: Induction of ovulation in females with hypothalamic amenorrhea

Usual Dosage

Diagnostic test: Children >12 years and Female Adults: I.V., SubQ hydrochloride salt: 100 mcg administered in women during early phase of menstrual cycle (day 1-7)

Primary hypothalamic amenorrhea: Female Adults: Acetate: I.V.: 5 mcg every 90 minutes via Lutrepulse® pump kit at treatment intervals of 21 days (pump will pulsate every 90 minutes for 7 days)

Dosage Forms Injection, powder for reconstitution, as hydrochloride: 100 mcg [diluent contains benzyl alcohol]

gonadorelin acetate *see* gonadorelin *on this page*

gonadorelin hydrochloride *see* gonadorelin *on this page*

gonadotropin releasing hormone *see* gonadorelin *on this page*

Gonak™ [US-OTC] *see* hydroxypropyl methylcellulose *on page 432*

Gonal-f® [US/Can] *see* follitropin alfa *on page 365*

gonioscopic ophthalmic solution *see* hydroxypropyl methylcellulose *on page 432*

Goniosoft™ [US] *see* hydroxypropyl methylcellulose *on page 432*

Goniosol® *(Discontinued)* *see* hydroxypropyl methylcellulose *on page 432*

Good Sense Sleep Aid [US-OTC] *see* doxylamine *on page 280*

Goody's® Extra Strength Headache Powder [US-OTC] *see* acetaminophen, aspirin, and caffeine *on page 10*

Goody's® Extra Strength Pain Relief [US-OTC] *see* acetaminophen, aspirin, and caffeine *on page 10*

Goody's PM® [US-OTC] *see* acetaminophen and diphenhydramine *on page 7*

Gordofilm® [US-OTC] *see* salicylic acid *on page 758*

Gordon Boro-Packs [US-OTC] *see* aluminum sulfate and calcium acetate *on page 38*

Gormel® [US-OTC] *see* urea *on page 861*

goserelin (GOE se rel in)

Synonyms D-ser(bu^t)^6,Azgly^{10}-LHRH; goserelin acetate; ICI-118630; NSC-606864

U.S./Canadian Brand Names Zoladex® LA [Can]; Zoladex® [US/Can]

Therapeutic Category Gonadotropin-Releasing Hormone Analog

Use Palliative treatment of advanced breast cancer and carcinoma of the prostate; treatment of endometriosis, including pain relief and reduction of endometriotic lesions; endometrial thinning agent as part of treatment for dysfunctional uterine bleeding

Usual Dosage SubQ: Adults:

Prostate cancer:

Monthly implant: 3.6 mg injected into upper abdomen every 28 days

3-month implant: 10.8 mg injected into the upper abdominal wall every 12 weeks

Breast cancer, endometriosis, endometrial thinning: Monthly implant: 3.6 mg injected into upper abdomen every 28 days

Note: For breast cancer, treatment may continue indefinitely; for endometriosis, it is recommended that duration of treatment not exceed 6 months. Only 1-2 doses are recommended for endometrial thinning.

Dosage Forms

Injection, solution, 1-month implant [disposable syringe; single-dose]: 3.6 mg [with 16-gauge hypodermic needle]

Injection, solution, 3-month implant [disposable syringe; single-dose]: 10.8 mg [with 14-gauge hypodermic needle]

goserelin acetate *see* goserelin *on this page*

GP 47680 *see* oxcarbazepine *on page 624*

G-Phed [US] *see* guaifenesin and pseudoephedrine *on page 398*

GR38032R *see* ondansetron *on page 616*

gramicidin, neomycin, and polymyxin B *see* neomycin, polymyxin B, and gramicidin *on page 584*

granisetron (gra NI se tron)

Sound-Alike/Look-Alike Issues

granisetron may be confused with dolasetron, ondansetron, palonosetron

Synonyms BRL 43694

U.S./Canadian Brand Names Kytril® [US/Can]

Therapeutic Category Selective 5-HT_3 Receptor Antagonist

Use Prophylaxis of nausea and vomiting associated with emetogenic chemotherapy and radiation therapy, (including total body irradiation and fractionated abdominal radiation); prophylaxis and treatment of postoperative nausea and vomiting (PONV)

Generally **not** recommended for treatment of existing chemotherapy-induced emesis (CIE) or for prophylaxis of nausea from agents with a low emetogenic potential.

Usual Dosage

Oral: Adults:

Prophylaxis of chemotherapy-related emesis: 2 mg once daily up to 1 hour before chemotherapy or 1 mg twice daily; the first 1 mg dose should be given up to 1 hour before chemotherapy.

Prophylaxis of radiation therapy-associated emesis: 2 mg once daily given 1 hour before radiation therapy.

I.V.:

Children ≥2 years and Adults: Prophylaxis of chemotherapy-related emesis:

Within U.S.: 10 mcg/kg/dose (maximum: 1 mg/dose) given 30 minutes prior to chemotherapy; for some drugs (eg, carboplatin, cyclophosphamide) with a later onset of emetic action, 10 mcg/kg every 12 hours may be necessary.

Outside U.S.: 40 mcg/kg/dose (or 3 mg/dose); maximum: 9 mg/24 hours

Breakthrough: Granisetron has not been shown to be effective in teminating nausea or vomiting once it occurs and should not be used for this purpose.

Adults: PONV:

Prevention: 1 mg given undiluted over 30 seconds; administer before induction of anesthesia or immediately before reversal of anesthesia

Treatment: 1 mg given undiluted over 30 seconds

Dosage Forms

Injection, solution: 1 mg/mL (1 mL, 4 mL) [contains benzyl alcohol]

Injection, solution [preservative free]: 0.1 mg/mL (1 mL)

Solution, oral: 2 mg/10 mL (30 mL) [contains sodium benzoate; orange flavor]

Tablet: 1 mg

Granulex® [US] *see* trypsin, balsam peru, and castor oil *on page 856*

granulocyte colony stimulating factor *see* filgrastim *on page 345*

granulocyte colony stimulating factor (PEG conjugate) *see* pegfilgrastim *on page 643*

granulocyte-macrophage colony stimulating factor *see* sargramostim *on page 763*

Gravol® [Can] *see* dimenhydrinate *on page 258*

Grifulvin® V [US] *see* griseofulvin *on this page*

Grifulvin® V Tablet 250 mg and 500 mg *(Discontinued)* *see* griseofulvin *on this page*

Grisactin® Ultra *(Discontinued)* *see* griseofulvin *on this page*

griseofulvin (gri see oh FUL vin)

Sound-Alike/Look-Alike Issues
Fulvicin® may be confused with Furacin®

Synonyms griseofulvin microsize; griseofulvin ultramicrosize

U.S./Canadian Brand Names Grifulvin® V [US]; Gris-PEG® [US]

Therapeutic Category Antifungal Agent

Use Treatment of susceptible tinea infections of the skin, hair, and nails

Usual Dosage Oral:

Children >2 years:
- Microsize: 10-20 mg/kg/day in single or 2 divided doses.
- Ultramicrosize: >2 years: 5-10 mg/kg/day in single or 2 divided doses.

Adults:
- Microsize: 500-1000 mg/day in single or divided doses
- Ultramicrosize: 330-375 mg/day in single or divided doses; doses up to 750 mg/day have been used for infections more difficult to eradicate such as tinea unguium

Duration of therapy depends on the site of infection:
- Tinea corporis: 2-4 weeks
- Tinea capitis: 4-6 weeks or longer (up to 8-12 weeks)
- Tinea pedis: 4-8 weeks
- Tinea unguium: 3-6 months or longer

Dosage Forms
Suspension, oral, microsize (Grifulvin® V): 125 mg/5 mL (120 mL) [contains alcohol 0.2%]
Tablet, microsize (Grifulvin® V): 500 mg
Tablet, ultramicrosize: 125 mg, 250 mg, 330 mg
Gris-PEG®: 125 mg, 250 mg

griseofulvin microsize *see* griseofulvin *on this page*

griseofulvin ultramicrosize *see* griseofulvin *on this page*

Gris-PEG® [US] *see* griseofulvin *on this page*

Guaicon DM [US-OTC] *see* guaifenesin and dextromethorphan *on page 394*

Guaifed® [US] *see* guaifenesin and phenylephrine *on page 396*

Guaifed-PD® [US] *see* guaifenesin and phenylephrine *on page 396*

Guaifen-C [US] *see* guaifenesin and codeine *on next page*

Guaifen™ DM [US] *see* guaifenesin, dextromethorphan, and phenylephrine *on page 400*

guaifenesin (gwye FEN e sin)

Sound-Alike/Look-Alike Issues
guaifenesin may be confused with guanfacine
Mucinex® may be confused with Mucomyst®
Naldecon® may be confused with Nalfon®

Synonyms GG; glycerol guaiacolate

U.S./Canadian Brand Names Allfen Jr [US]; Balminil Expectorant [Can]; Benylin® E Extra Strength [Can]; Diabetic Tussin® EX [US-OTC]; Ganidin NR [US]; Guiatuss™ [US-OTC]; Humibid® Maximum Strength [US]; Iophen NR [US]; Koffex Expectorant [Can]; Mucinex® [US-OTC]; Organ-1 NR [US]; Organidin® NR [US]; Phanasin [US-OTC]; Phanasin® Diabetic Choice [US-OTC]; Q-Tussin [US-OTC]; Robitussin®

[US-OTC/Can]; Scot-Tussin® Expectorant [US-OTC]; Siltussin DAS [US-OTC]; Siltussin SA [US-OTC]; Tussin [US-OTC]; Vicks® Casero™ [US-OTC]; XPECT™ [US-OTC]

Therapeutic Category Expectorant

Use Help loosen phlegm and thin bronchial secretions to make coughs more productive

Usual Dosage Oral:

Children:

6 months to 2 years: 25-50 mg every 4 hours, not to exceed 300 mg/day

2-5 years: 50-100 mg every 4 hours, not to exceed 600 mg/day

6-11 years: 100-200 mg every 4 hours, not to exceed 1.2 g/day

Children >12 years and Adults: 200-400 mg every 4 hours to a maximum of 2.4 g/day

Extended release tablet: 600-1200 mg every 12 hours, not to exceed 2.4 g/day

Dosage Forms [DSC] = Discontinued product

Liquid: 100 mg/5 mL (120 mL, 480 mL)

Diabetic Tussin EX®: 100 mg/5 mL (120 mL) [alcohol free, sugar free, dye free; contains phenylalanine 8.4 mg/5 mL]

Ganidin NR: 100 mg/5 mL (480 mL) [raspberry flavor]

Iophen NR: 100 mg/5 mL (480 mL)

Organidin® NR: 100 mg/5 mL (480 mL) [contains sodium benzoate; raspberry flavor]

Q-Tussin: 100 mg/5 mL (120 mL, 240 mL, 480 mL, 3840 mL) [alcohol free; cherry flavor]

Siltussin DAS: 100 mg/5 mL (120 mL) [alcohol free, dye free, sugar free; strawberry flavor]

Syrup: 100 mg/5 mL (120 mL, 480 mL)

Guiatuss™: 100 mg/5 mL (120 mL, 480 mL) [alcohol free; fruit-mint flavor]

Phanasin®: 100 mg/5 mL (120 mL, 240 mL) [alcohol free, sugar free; mint flavor]

Phanasin® Diabetic Choice: 100 mg/5 mL (120 mL) [alcohol free, sugar free; mint flavor]

Robitussin®: 100 mg/5 mL (5 mL, 10 mL, 15 mL, 30 mL, 120 mL, 240 mL, 480 mL) [alcohol free; contains sodium benzoate]

Scot-Tussin® Expectorant: 100 mg/5 mL (120 mL) [alcohol free, dye free, sugar free; contains benzoic acid; grape flavor]

Siltussin SA: 100 mg/5 mL (120 mL, 240 mL, 480 mL) [alcohol free, sugar free; strawberry flavor]

Tussin: 100 mg/5 mL (120 mL, 240 mL)

Vicks® Casero™: 100 mg/6.25 mL (120 mL, 480 mL) [contains phenylalanine 5.5 mg/12.5 mL, sodium 32 mg/12.5 mL, and sodium benzoate; honey menthol flavor]

Syrup, oral drops (Phanasin®): 50 mg/mL (50 mL) [alcohol free, sugar free; fruit flavor]

Tablet: 200 mg

Allfen Jr: 400 mg [dye free]

Humibid® *e*: 400 mg [DSC]

Organ-1 NR, Organidin® NR: 200 mg

XPECT™: 400 mg

Tablet, extended release:

Humibid® Maximum Strength: 1200 mg

Mucinex®: 600 mg

Guaifenesin AC [US] *see* guaifenesin and codeine *on this page*

guaifenesin and codeine (gwye FEN e sin & KOE deen)

Sound-Alike/Look-Alike Issues

Halotussin® may be confused with Halotestin®

Synonyms codeine and guaifenesin

U.S./Canadian Brand Names Brontex® [US]; Cheracol® [US]; Cheratussin AC [US]; Diabetic Tussin C® [US]; Gani-Tuss® NR [US]; Guaifen-C [US]; Guaifenesin AC [US]; Guaituss AC® [US]; Iophen-C NR [US]; Kolephrin® #1 [US]; Mytussin® AC [US]; Robafen® AC [US]; Romilar® AC [US]; Tussi-Organidin® NR [US]; Tussi-Organidin® S-NR [US]

Therapeutic Category Antitussive/Expectorant

Controlled Substance C-V

Use Temporary control of cough due to minor throat and bronchial irritation

Usual Dosage Oral: **Note:** Also refer to specific product labeling:

Children:

2-6 years (Diabetic Tussin C® liquid, Tussi-Organidin® NR): Codeine 1 mg/kg/day in 4 divided doses

6-12 years (Diabetic Tussin C®, Kolephrin® #1, Romilar® AC, Tussi-Organidin® NR liquid): 5 mL every 4 hours; maximum 30 mL/24 hours

Children ≥12 years and Adults:

Brontex® tablets: 1 tablet every 4 hours; maximum 6 tablets/24 hours

(Continued)

guaifenesin and codeine *(Continued)*

Diabetic Tussin C®, Kolephrin® #1, Romilar® AC, Tussi-Organidin® NR liquid: 10 mL every 4 hours; maximum 60 mL/24 hours

Dosage Forms

Liquid:

Brontex®: Guaifenesin 75 mg and codeine phosphate 2.5 mg per 5 mL (480 mL) [alcohol free; strawberry mint flavor]

Diabetic Tussin C®: Guaifenesin 200 mg and codeine phosphate 10 mg per 5 mL (480 mL) [contains phenylalanine 0.03 mcg/5 mL; cherry vanilla flavor]

Gani-Tuss® NR: Guaifenesin 100 mg and codeine phosphate 10 mg per 5 mL (480 mL) [raspberry flavor]

Guaifen-C: Guaifenesin 75 mg and codeine phosphate 2.5 mg per 5 mL (480 mL) [cherry flavor]

Guaifenesin AC: Guaifenesin 100 mg and codeine phosphate 10 mg per 5 mL (120 mL, 480 mL) [alcohol free, sugar free; raspberry flavor]

Iophen-C NR: Guaifenesin 100 mg and codeine phosphate 10 mg per 5 mL (480 mL) [raspberry flavor]

Kolephrin® #1: Guaifenesin 100 mg and codeine phosphate 10 mg per 5 mL (120 mL) [contains sodium 1.1 mg/5 mL and sodium benzoate]

Tussi-Organidin® NR: Guaifenesin 100 mg and codeine phosphate 10 mg per 5 mL (480 mL) [contains sodium benzoate; raspberry flavor]

Tussi-Organidin® S-NR: Guaifenesin 100 mg and codeine phosphate 10 mg per 5 mL (120 mL) [contains sodium benzoate; raspberry flavor]

Syrup:

Cheracol®: Guaifenesin 100 mg and codeine phosphate 10 mg per 5 mL (120 mL) [contains alcohol 4.75% and benzoic acid]

Cheratussin AC: Guaifenesin 100 mg and codeine phosphate 10 mg per 5 mL (120 mL, 240 mL, 480 mL)

Guaituss AC: Guaifenesin 100 mg and codeine phosphate 10 mg per 5 mL (120 mL, 480 mL) [contains alcohol; sugar free; fruit-mint flavor]

Mytussin® AC: Guaifenesin 100 mg and codeine phosphate 10 mg per 5 mL (120 mL, 480 mL) [contains alcohol; sugar free; fruit flavor]

Robafen® AC: Guaifenesin 100 mg and codeine phosphate 10 mg per 5 mL (120 mL, 480 mL)

Romilar® AC: Guaifenesin 100 mg and codeine phosphate 10 mg per 5 mL (480 mL) [contains benzoic acid and phenylalanine; alcohol free, sugar free, dye free; grape flavor]

Tablet: Guaifenesin 300 mg and codeine phosphate 10 mg

Brontex®: Guaifenesin 300 mg and codeine phosphate 10 mg

guaifenesin and dextromethorphan (gwye FEN e sin & deks troe meth OR fan)

Sound-Alike/Look-Alike Issues

Benylin® may be confused with Benadryl®, Ventolin®

Synonyms dextromethorphan and guaifenesin

U.S./Canadian Brand Names Allfen-DM [US]; Altarussin DM [US-OTC]; Amibid DM [US]; Balminil DM E [Can]; Benylin® DM-E [Can]; Cheracol® D [US-OTC]; Cheracol® Plus [US-OTC]; Coricidin HBP® Chest Congestion and Cough [US-OTC]; Diabetic Tussin® DM Maximum Strength [US-OTC]; Diabetic Tussin® DM [US-OTC]; Drituss DM [US]; Duratuss® DM [US]; Gani-Tuss DM NR [US]; Genatuss DM® [US-OTC]; Guaicon DM [US-OTC]; Guaifenex® DM [US]; Guia-D [US]; Guiacon DMS [US-OTC]; Guiatuss-DM® [US-OTC]; Hydro-Tussin™ DM [US]; Iophen DM NR [US]; Koffex DM-Expectorant [Can]; Kolephrin® GG/DM [US-OTC]; Mintab DM [US]; Mucinex® DM [US-OTC]; Phanatuss® DM [US-OTC]; Q-Bid DM [US]; Q-Tussin DM [US-OTC]; Respa-DM® [US]; Robafen DM [US-OTC]; Robitussin® Cough and Congestion [US-OTC]; Robitussin® DM Infant [US-OTC]; Robitussin® DM [US-OTC/Can]; Robitussin® Sugar Free Cough [US-OTC]; Safe Tussin® [US-OTC]; Scot-Tussin® Senior [US-OTC]; Silexin® [US-OTC]; Siltussin DM DAS [US-OTC]; Siltussin DM [US-OTC]; Su-Tuss DM [US]; Touro® DM [US]; Vicks® 44E [US-OTC]; Vicks® Pediatric Formula 44E [US-OTC]; Z-Cof LA™ [US]

Therapeutic Category Antitussive/Expectorant

Use Temporary control of cough due to minor throat and bronchial irritation

Usual Dosage Oral:

Children 2-6 years:

General dosing guidelines: Guaifenesin 50-100 mg and dextromethorphan 2.5-5 mg every 4 hours (maximum dose: Guaifenesin 600 mg and dextromethorphan 30 mg per day)

Product-specific labeling:

Benylin®: 5 mL every 4 hours (maximum: 6 doses/24 hours)

Guaifenex® DM, Touro® DM: 1/2 tablet every 12 hours (maximum: 1 tablet/24 hour)

Robitussin® DM, Robitussin® DM Infant, Robitussin® Sugar Free Cough: 2.5 mL every 4 hours (maximum: 6 doses/24 hours)

Vicks® Pediatric Formula 44E: 7.5 mL every 4 hours (maximum: 6 doses/24 hours)

Children: 6-12 years:
General dosing guidelines: Guaifenesin 100-200 mg and dextromethorphan 5-10 mg every 4 hours (maximum dose: Guaifenesin 1200 mg and dextromethorphan 60 mg per day)
Product-specific labeling:
Benylin®: 10 mL every 4 hours (maximum: 6 doses/24 hours)
Guaifenex® DM, Touro® DM: 1 tablet every 12 hours (maximum: 2 tablets/24 hours)
Humibid® CS: 1/2 tablet every 4 hours (maximum: 6 doses/24 hours)
Robitussin® DM, Robitussin® Sugar Free Cough: 5 mL every 4 hours (maximum: 6 doses/24 hours)
Vicks® 44E: 7.5 mL every 4 hours (maximum: 6 doses/24 hours)
Vicks® Pediatric Formula 44E: 15 mL every 4 hours (maximum: 6 doses/24 hours)
Z-Cof LA™: 1/2 tablet very 12 hours
Children ≥12 years and Adults:
General dosing guidelines: Guaifenesin 200-400 mg and dextromethorphan 10-20 mg every 4 hours (maximum dose: Guaifenesin 2400 mg and dextromethorphan 120 mg per day)
Product-specific labeling:
Benylin®: 20 mL every 4 hours (maximum: 6 doses/24 hours)
Guaifenex® DM, Mucinex® DM, Touro® DM: 1-2 tablets every 12 hours (maximum: 4 tablets/24 hours)
Humibid® CD: 1 tablet every 4 hours (maximum: 6 tablets/24 hours)
Robitussin® DM, Robitussin® Sugar Free Cough: 10 mL every 4 hours (maximum: 6 doses/24 hours)
Vicks® 44E: 15 mL every 4 hours (maximum: 6 doses/24 hours)
Vicks® Pediatric Formula 44E: 30 mL every 4 hours (maximum: 6 doses/24 hours)
Z-Cof LA™: 1 tablet every 12 hours

Dosage Forms [DSC] = Discontinued product

Caplet, sustained release (Mindal DM [DSC]): Guaifenesin 500 mg and dextromethorphan hydrobromide 30 mg
Capsule, softgel (Coricidin HBP® Chest Congestion and Cough): Guaifenesin 200 mg and dextromethorphan hydrobromide 10 mg
Elixir:
Duratuss DM®: Guaifenesin 225 mg and dextromethorphan hydrobromide 25 mg per 5 mL (480 mL) [contains sodium benzoate; grape flavor]
Drituss DM: Guaifenesin 200 mg and dextromethorphan hydrobromide 20 mg per 5 mL (480 mL) [grape flavor]
Su-Tuss DM: Guaifenesin 200 mg and dextromethorphan hydrobromide 20 mg per 5 mL (480 mL) [fruit flavor]
Liquid: Guaifenesin 100 mg and dextromethorphan hydrobromide 10 mg per 5 mL (480 mL)
Diabetic Tussin® DM: Guaifenesin 100 mg and dextromethorphan hydrobromide 10 mg per 5 mL (120 mL) [alcohol free, sugar free, dye free; contains phenylalanine 8.4 mg/5 mL]
Diabetic Tussin® DM Maximum Strength: Guaifenesin 200 mg and dextromethorphan hydrobromide 10 mg per 5 mL (120 mL) [alcohol free, sugar free, dye free; contains phenylalanine 8.4 mg/5 mL]
Gani-Tuss® DM NR: Guaifenesin 100 mg and dextromethorphan hydrobromide 10 mg per 5 mL (480 mL) [raspberry flavor]
Hydro-Tussin™ DM: Guaifenesin 200 mg and dextromethorphan hydrobromide 20 mg per 5 mL (480 mL) [alcohol free, sugar free; contains sodium benzoate]
Iophen DM NR: Guaifenesin 100 mg and dextromethorphan hydrobromide 10 mg per 5 mL (480 mL) [raspberry flavor]
Kolephrin® GG/DM: Guaifenesin 150 mg and dextromethorphan hydrobromide 10 mg per 5 mL (120 mL) [alcohol free; cherry flavor]
Q-Tussin DM: Guaifenesin 100 mg and dextromethorphan hydrobromide 10 mg per 5 mL (120 mL, 240 mL, 480 mL, 3840 mL) [cherry flavor]
Safe Tussin®: Guaifenesin 100 mg and dextromethorphan hydrobromide 15 mg per 5 mL (120 mL) [alcohol free, sodium free, sugar free, dye free; mint flavor]
Scot-Tussin® Senior: Guaifenesin 200 mg and dextromethorphan hydrobromide 15 mg per 5 mL (120 mL) [alcohol free, sodium free, sugar free]
Vicks® 44E: Guaifenesin 200 mg and dextromethorphan hydrobromide 20 mg per 15 mL (120 mL, 235 mL) [contains sodium 31 mg/15 mL, alcohol, sodium benzoate]
Vicks® Pediatric Formula 44E: Guaifenesin 100 mg and dextromethorphan hydrobromide 10 mg per 15 mL (120 mL) [alcohol free; contains sodium 30 mg/15 mL, sodium benzoate; cherry flavor]
Liquid, oral drops (Robitussin® DM Infant): Guaifenesin 100 mg and dextromethorphan hydrobromide 5 mg per 2.5 mL (30 mL) [alcohol free; contains sodium benzoate; fruit punch flavor]
Syrup: Guaifenesin 100 mg and dextromethorphan hydrobromide 10 mg per 5 mL (120 mL, 480 mL)
Altarussin DM: Guaifenesin 100 mg and dextromethorphan hydrobromide 10 mg per 5 mL (120 mL, 240 mL, 480 mL, 3840 mL)
Benylin® Expectorant: Guaifenesin 100 mg and dextromethorphan hydrobromide 5 mg per 5 mL (120 mL) [alcohol free, sugar free; contains sodium benzoate; raspberry flavor] [DSC]
(Continued)

guaifenesin and dextromethorphan *(Continued)*

Cheracol® D: Guaifenesin 100 mg and dextromethorphan hydrobromide 10 mg per 5 mL (120 mL, 180 mL) [contains alcohol 4.75%, benzoic acid]

Cheracol® Plus: Guaifenesin 100 mg and dextromethorphan hydrobromide 10 mg per 5 mL (120 mL) [contains alcohol 4.75%, benzoic acid]

Genatuss DM®: Guaifenesin 100 mg and dextromethorphan hydrobromide 10 mg per 5 mL (120 mL)

Guiatuss® DM: Guaifenesin 100 mg and dextromethorphan hydrobromide 10 mg per 5 mL (120 mL, 480 mL, 3840 mL) [alcohol free; contains sodium benzoate]

Guaicon DM®: Guaifenesin 100 mg and dextromethorphan hydrobromide 10 mg per 5 mL (10 mL) [alcohol free]

Guaicon DMS®: Guaifenesin 100 mg and dextromethorphan hydrobromide 10 mg per 5 mL (10 mL) [alcohol free, sugar free]

Mintab DM: Guaifenesin 200 mg and dextromethorphan hydrobromide 10 mg per 5 mL (480 mL) [alcohol free, dye free; cherry vanilla flavor]

Phanatuss® DM: Guaifenesin 100 mg and dextromethorphan hydrobromide 10 mg per 5 mL (120 mL) [alcohol free, sugar free]

Robafen® DM: Guaifenesin 100 mg and dextromethorphan hydrobromide 10 mg per 5 mL (120 mL, 240 mL, 480 mL) [cherry flavor]

Robitussin® Cough and Congestion: Guaifenesin 100 mg and dextromethorphan hydrobromide 10 mg per 5 mL (120 mL) [alcohol free; contains sodium benzoate]

Robitussin®-DM: Guaifenesin 100 mg and dextromethorphan hydrobromide 10 mg per 5 mL (5 mL, 120 mL, 340 mL, 360 mL) [alcohol free; contains sodium benzoate]

Robitussin® Sugar Free Cough: Guaifenesin 100 mg and dextromethorphan hydrobromide 10 mg per 5 mL (120 mL) [alcohol free, sugar free; contains sodium benzoate]

Silexin: Guaifenesin 100 mg and dextromethorphan hydrobromide 10 mg per 5 mL (45 mL) [alcohol free, sugar free)]

Siltussin DM: Guaifenesin 100 mg and dextromethorphan hydrobromide 10 mg per 5 mL (120 mL, 240 mL, 480 mL) [strawberry flavor]

Siltussin DM DAS: Guaifenesin 100 mg and dextromethorphan hydrobromide 10 mg per 5 mL (120 mL) [alcohol free, dye free, sugar free; strawberry flavor]

Tablet:

Humibid® CS: Guaifenesin 400 mg and dextromethorphan hydrobromide 20 mg [DSC]

Silexin: Guaifenesin 100 mg and dextromethorphan hydrobromide 10 mg

Tablet, extended release: Guaifenesin 500 mg and dextromethorphan hydrobromide 30 mg

Amibid DM, Guaifenex® DM, Mucinex® DM, Q-Bid DM, Respa-DM®: Guaifenesin 600 mg and dextromethorphan hydrobromide 30 mg

Mucophen® DM: Guaifenesin 1000 mg and dextromethorphan hydrobromide 60 mg

Touro® DM: Guaifenesin 575 mg and dextromethorphan hydrobromide 30 mg

Tablet, long-acting: Guaifenesin 500 mg and dextromethorphan hydrobromide 30 mg; guaifenesin 1000 mg and dextromethorphan hydrobromide 50 mg; guaifenesin 1000 mg and dextromethorphan hydrobromide 60 mg

Z-Cof LA [scored]: Guaifenesin 650 mg and dextromethorphan hydrobromide 30 mg

Tablet, sustained release: Guaifenesin 800 mg and dextromethorphan hydrobromide 30 mg; guaifenesin 1000 mg and dextromethorphan hydrobromide 60 mg; guaifenesin 1200 mg and dextromethorphan hydrobromide 60 mg

Allfen-DM: Guaifenesin 1000 mg and dextromethorphan hydrobromide 55 mg

Tussi-Bid®: Guaifenesin 1200 mg and dextromethorphan hydrobromide 60 mg

Tablet, timed release [scored] (Guia-D): Guaifenesin 1000 mg and dextromethorphan hydrobromide 60 mg [dye free]

guaifenesin and hydrocodone *see* hydrocodone and guaifenesin *on page 422*

guaifenesin and phenylephrine (gwye FEN e sin & fen il EF rin)

Sound-Alike/Look-Alike Issues

Endal® may be confused with Depen®, Intal®

Entex® may be confused with Tenex®

Entex® LA brand name represents a different product in the U.S. than it does in Canada. In the U.S., Entex® LA contains guaifenesin and phenylephrine, while in Canada the product bearing this brand name contains guaifenesin and pseudoephedrine.

Synonyms guaifenesin and phenylephrine tannate; phenylephrine hydrochloride and guaifenesin

U.S./Canadian Brand Names Aldex™ [US]; Ami-Tex LA [US]; Amidal [US]; Crantex ER [US]; Crantex LA [US]; Deconsal® II [US]; Endal® [US]; Entex® ER [US]; Entex® LA [US]; Entex® [US]; Guaifed-PD® [US];

Guaifed® [US]; Liquibid-D [US]; Liquibid-PD [US]; PhenaVent™ D [US]; PhenaVent™ Ped [US]; PhenaVent™ [US]; Prolex™-D [US]; Rescon GG [US]; Sil-Tex [US]; Sina-12X [US]; SINUvent® PE [US]

Therapeutic Category Cold Preparation

Use Temporary relief of nasal congestion, sinusitis, rhinitis and hay fever; temporary relief of cough associated with upper respiratory tract conditions, especially when associated with dry, nonproductive cough

Usual Dosage Oral:

Children 2-6 years:

Entex®, Rescon GG, Sil-Tex: 2.5 mL every 4-6 hours; maximum 10 mL/24 hours

Sina-12X suspension: 2.5-5 mL every 12 hours

Children 6-12 years:

Aldex™, Crantex LA, Liquibid-D, PhenaVent™ D, Sina-12X tablet: One-half tablet every 12 hours (maximum: 1 tablet/24 hours)

Deconsal® II: One capsule daily

Entex®, Rescon GG: 5 mL every 4-6 hours (maximum: 20 mL/24 hours)

Guaifed-PD®, PhenaVent™ Ped: One capsule every 12 hours

Liquibid-PD, SINUvent® PE: One tablet every 12 hours (maximum: 2 tablets/24 hours)

Prolex™-D: One-half to 1 tablet every 12 hours

Sina-12X suspension: Refer to Adults dosing.

Children ≥12 years:

Aldex™, Crantex LA, Deconsal® II, Entex®, Entex® LA, Guaifed®, Guaifed-PD®, Liquibid-D, Liquibid-PD, PhenaVent™, PhenaVent™ D, PhenaVent™ Ped, Prolex™-D, Rescon GG, Sil-Tex, Sina-12X, SINUvent® PE: Refer to Adults dosing

Crantex ER, Entex® ER: One capsule every 12 hours

Adults:

Aldex™, Crantex LA, XPECT-PE™, Liquibid-D, PhenaVent™ D: One tablet every 12 hours

Crantex ER, Entex® ER, Guaifed-PD®, PhenaVent™ Ped: 1-2 capsules every 12 hours

Deconsal® II: 1-2 capsules every 12 hours (maximum: 3 capsules/24 hours)

Endal®, Prolex™-D: 1-2 tablets every 12 hours

Entex®, Sil-Tex: 5-10 mL every 4-6 hours (maximum: 40 mL/24 hours)

Entex® LA, Guaifed®, PhenaVent™: One capsule every 12 hours (maximum: 2 capsules/24 hours)

Liquibid-PD, Sina-12X tablet: 1-2 tablets every 12 hours (maximum: 4 tablets/24 hours)

Rescon GG: 10 mL every 4-6 hours (maximum: 40 mL/24 hours)

Sina-12X suspension: 5-10 mL every 12 hours

SINUvent® PE: Two tablets every 12 hours

Dosage Forms [DSC] = Discontinued product

Capsule, variable release:

Crantex ER, Entex® ER: Guaifenesin 300 mg [immediate release] and phenylephrine hydrochloride 10 mg [extended release]

Deconsal® II: Guaifenesin 375 mg [immediate release] and phenylephrine hydrochloride 20 mg [extended release] [contains tartrazine]

Entex® LA: Guaifenesin 400 mg [immediate release] and phenylephrine hydrochloride 30 mg [extended release]

Guaifed®, PhenaVent™: Guaifenesin 400 mg [immediate release] and phenylephrine hydrochloride 15 mg [extended release]

Guaifed-PD®, PhenaVent™ Ped: Guaifenesin 200 mg [immediate release] and phenylephrine hydrochloride 7.5 mg [extended release]

Liquid: Guaifenesin 100 mg and phenylephrine hydrochloride 7.5 mg per 5 mL (480 mL)

Entex®, Sil-Tex: Guaifenesin 100 mg and phenylephrine hydrochloride 7.5 mg per 5 mL (480 mL) [alcohol free, dye-free, sugar free; punch flavor]

Rescon GG: Guaifenesin 100 mg and phenylephrine hydrochloride 5 mg per 5 mL (120 mL, 480 mL) [cherry orange-pineapple flavor]

Suspension:

Sina-12X: Guaifenesin 100 mg and phenylephrine tannate 5 mg per 5 mL (120 mL) [contains benzoic acid; grape flavor]

Tablet:

Amidal: Guaifenesin 300 mg and phenylephrine hydrochloride 20 mg

Sina-12X: Guaifenesin 200 mg and phenylephrine tannate 25 mg

Tablet, extended release: Guaifenesin 600 mg and phenylephrine hydrochloride 20 mg; guaifenesin 600 mg and phenylephrine hydrochloride 40 mg; guaifenesin 1200 mg and phenylephrine hydrochloride 40 mg

Aldex™: Guaifenesin 650 mg and phenylephrine hydrochloride 25 mg

Ami-Tex LA: Guaifenesin 600 mg and phenylephrine hydrochloride 30 mg

Liquibid-D: Guaifenesin 600 mg and phenylephrine hydrochloride 40 mg [DSC]

(Continued)

guaifenesin and phenylephrine *(Continued)*

Liquibid-PD: Guaifenesin 275 mg and phenylephrine hydrochloride 25 mg
PhenaVent™ D: Guaifenesin 1200 mg and phenylephrine hydrochloride 40 mg
SINUvent® PE: Guaifenesin 600 mg and phenylephrine hydrochloride 15 mg
Tablet, sustained release: Guaifenesin 600 mg and phenylephrine hydrochloride 30 mg
Crantex LA: Guaifenesin 600 mg and phenylephrine hydrochloride 30 mg [dye-free]
Prolex™-D: Guaifenesin 600 mg and phenylephrine hydrochloride 20 mg [dye-free]
XPECT-PE™: Guaifenesin 1200 mg and phenylephrine hydrochloride 25 mg
Tablet, timed release (Endal®): Guaifenesin 300 mg and phenylephrine hydrochloride 20 mg

guaifenesin and phenylephrine tannate *see* guaifenesin and phenylephrine *on page 396*

guaifenesin and pseudoephedrine (gwye FEN e sin & soo doe e FED rin)

Sound-Alike/Look-Alike Issues
Entex® may be confused with Tenex®
Entex® LA brand name represents a different product in the U.S. than it does in Canada. In the U.S., Entex® LA contains guaifenesin and phenylephrine, while in Canada the product bearing this brand name contains guaifenesin and pseudoephedrine.
Profen II® may be confused with Profen II DM®, Profen Forte®, Profen Forte™ DM
Profen Forte® may be confused with Profen II®, Profen II DM®, Profen Forte™ DM

Synonyms pseudoephedrine and guaifenesin

U.S./Canadian Brand Names Ambifed-G [US]; Ami-Tex PSE [US]; Congestac® [US-OTC]; Contac® Cold-Chest Congestion, Non Drowsy, Regular Strength [Can]; Dynex [US]; Entex® PSE [US]; Eudal®-SR [US]; G-Phed [US]; Guaifenex® GP [US]; Guaifenex® PSE [US]; Guaimax-D® [US]; Levall G [US]; Maxifed-G® [US]; Maxifed® [US]; Mucinex®-D [US-OTC]; Nasatab® LA [US]; Novahistex® Expectorant with Decongestant [Can]; PanMist®-JR [US]; PanMist®-LA [US]; PanMist®-S [US]; Profen Forte® [US]; Profen II® [US]; Pseudo GG TR [US]; Pseudovent™ 400 [US]; Pseudovent™ [US]; Pseudovent™-Ped [US]; Refenesen Plus [US-OTC]; Respaire®-120 SR [US]; Respaire®-60 SR [US]; Robitussin-PE® [US-OTC]; Robitussin® Severe Congestion [US-OTC]; Sudafed® Non-Drying Sinus [US-OTC]; Touro LA® [US]; Zephrex LA® [US]; Zephrex® [US]

Therapeutic Category Expectorant/Decongestant

Use Temporary relief of nasal congestion and to help loosen phlegm and thin bronchial secretions in the treatment of cough

Usual Dosage Oral:

Children 2-6 years:
Guaifenex® PSE 60: One-half tablet every 12 hours (maximum: 1 tablet/12 hours)
Maxifed-G®: One-third to $1/2$ tablet every 12 hours (maximum: 1 tablet/12 hours)
PanMist®-S: 2.5 mL 4 times/day (maximum: Pseudoephedrine 4 mg/kg/day)
Robitussin® PE: 2.5 mL every 4-6 hours (maximum: 4 doses/24 hours)

Children 6-12 years:
Ambifed-G, Dynex, Eudal®-SR, Guaimax-D®, Guaifenex® PSE 80, Guaifenex® PSE 120, Maxifed®, Nasatab® LA, PanMist®-LA, Profen II®, Profen Forte®, Zephrex® LA: One-half caplet or tablet every 12 hours (maximum: 1 tablet/24 hours)
Congestac®: One-half caplet every 4-6 hours (maximum: 2 caplets/24 hours)
Guaifenex® PSE 60, PanMist®-JR, Pseudovent™-Ped, Respaire®-60 SR: One tablet or capsule every 12 hours (maximum: 2 tablets or capsules every 24 hours)
Levall G: One capsule every 24 hours
Maxifed-G®: One-half to 1 tablet every 12 hours (maximum: 2 tablets/24 hours)
PanMist®-S: 5 mL 4 times/day (maximum: Pseudoephedrine 4 mg/kg/day)
Robitussin® PE: 5 mL every 4-6 hours (maximum: 4 doses/24 hours)
Robitussin® Severe Congestion: One capsule every 4 hours (maximum: 4 doses/24 hours)
Zephrex®: One-half tablet every 6 hours

Children >12 years and Adults:
Ambifed-G, Aquatab® D, Dynex, Entex® PSE, Eudal®- SR, G-Phed, Guaifenex® GP, Guaifenex® PSE 120, Guaimax-D®, Levall G, Mucinex®-D 1200/120, Nasatab® LA, PanMist®-LA, Profen Forte®, Pseudovent™, Respaire®-120 SR, Touro LA, Zephrex® LA: One tablet or capsule every 12 hours (maximum: 2 tablets or capsules in 24 hours)
Congestac®: One caplet every 4-6 hours (maximum: 4 caplets in 24 hours)
Guaifenex® PSE 60, Maxifed-G®, Mucinex®-D 600/60, PanMist®-JR, Pseudovent™-Ped, Respaire®-60 SR: 1-2 tablets or capsules every 12 hours (maximum: 4 tablets or capsules/24 hours)
Guaifenex® PSE 80, PanMist®-LA: One tablet every twelve hours (maximum: 3 tablets/24 hours)
Guaifenex™ RX: 1-2 of the AM tablets every morning and 1-2 of the PM tablets 12 hours following morning dose

Maxifed®, Profen II®: One to $1^1/_2$ tablets every 12 hours (maximum: 3 tablets/24 hours)
PanMist®-S: Up to 10 mL 4 times/day
Robitussin® PE: 10 mL every 4-6 hours (maximum: 4 doses/24 hours)
Robitussin® Severe Congestion, Sudafed® Non-Drying Sinus: Two capsules every 4 hours (maximum: 4 doses/24 hours)
Zephrex®: One tablet every 6 hours

Dosage Forms [DSC] = Discontinued product

Caplet (Congestac®, Refenesen Plus): Guaifenesin 400 mg and pseudoephedrine hydrochloride 60 mg
Caplet, long-acting (Touro LA®): Guaifenesin 500 mg and pseudoephedrine hydrochloride 120 mg
Caplet, prolonged release (Ambifed-G): Guaifenesin 1000 mg and pseudoephedrine hydrochloride 60 mg
Capsule, extended release:
Respaire®-60 SR: Guaifenesin 200 mg and pseudoephedrine hydrochloride 60 mg
Respaire®-120 SR: Guaifenesin 250 mg and pseudoephedrine hydrochloride 120 mg
Capsule, liquicap (Sudafed® Non-Drying Sinus): Guaifenesin 200 mg and pseudoephedrine hydrochloride 30 mg
Capsule, softgel (Robitussin® Severe Congestion): Guaifenesin 200 mg and pseudoephedrine hydrochloride 30 mg
Capsule, variable release:
Entex® PSE: Guaifenesin 400 mg [immediate release] and pseudoephedrine hydrochloride 120 mg [extended release]
G-Phed: Guaifenesin 250 mg [immediate release] and pseudoephedrine hydrochloride 120 mg [prolonged release]
Levall G: Guaifenesin 400 mg [immediate release] and pseudoephedrine hydrochloride 90 mg [extended release]
Pseudovent™: Guaifenesin 250 mg [immediate release] and pseudoephedrine hydrochloride 120 mg [prolonged release]
Pseudovent™-Ped: Guaifenesin 300 mg [immediate release] and pseudoephedrine hydrochloride 60 mg [prolonged release]
Pseudovent™ 400: Guaifenesin 400 mg [immediate release] and pseudoephedrine hydrochloride 120 mg [extended release]
Syrup: Guaifenesin 200 mg and pseudoephedrine hydrochloride 40 mg per 5 mL (480 mL)
PanMist®-S: Guaifenesin 200 mg and pseudoephedrine hydrochloride 40 mg per 5 mL (480 mL) [alcohol free; grape flavor]
Robitussin-PE®: Guaifenesin 100 mg and pseudoephedrine hydrochloride 30 mg per 5 mL (120 mL, 240 mL) [alcohol free; contains sodium benzoate]
Tablet (Zephrex®): Guaifenesin 400 mg and pseudoephedrine hydrochloride 60 mg
Tablet, extended release: Guaifenesin 550 mg and pseudoephedrine hydrochloride 60 mg; guaifenesin 595 mg and pseudoephedrine hydrochloride 48 mg; guaifenesin 600 mg and pseudoephedrine hydrochloride 60 mg; guaifenesin 600 mg and pseudoephedrine hydrochloride 120 mg; guaifenesin 795 mg and pseudoephedrine hydrochloride 85 mg; guaifenesin 800 mg and pseudoephedrine hydrochloride 45 mg; guaifenesin 800 mg and pseudoephedrine hydrochloride 60 mg; guaifenesin 800 mg and pseudoephedrine hydrochloride 90 mg; guaifenesin 1200 mg and pseudoephedrine hydrochloride 50 mg; guaifenesin 1200 mg and pseudoephedrine hydrochloride 60 mg; guaifenesin 1200 mg and pseudoephedrine hydrochloride 75 mg; guaifenesin 1200 mg and pseudoephedrine hydrochloride 90 mg; guaifenesin 1200 mg and pseudoephedrine hydrochloride 120 mg
Ami-Tex PSE, Guaimax-D®, Zephrex LA®: Guaifenesin 600 mg and pseudoephedrine hydrochloride 120 mg
Guaifenex® GP: Guaifenesin 1200 mg and pseudoephedrine hydrochloride 120 mg [dye free]
Guaifenex® PSE 60: Guaifenesin 600 mg and pseudoephedrine hydrochloride 60 mg
Guaifenex® PSE 80: Guaifenesin 800 mg and pseudoephedrine hydrochloride 80 mg
Maxifed®: Guaifenesin 700 mg and pseudoephedrine hydrochloride 80 mg
Maxifed-G®: Guaifenesin 550 mg and pseudoephedrine hydrochloride 60 mg
Mucinex®-D 600/60: Guaifenesin 600 mg and pseudoephedrine hydrochloride 60 mg
Mucinex®-D 1200/120: Guaifenesin 1200 mg and pseudoephedrine hydrochloride 120 mg
PanMist®-JR, Pseudo GG TR: Guaifenesin 595 mg and pseudoephedrine hydrochloride 48 mg
PanMist®-LA: Guaifenesin 795 mg and pseudoephedrine hydrochloride 85 mg
Profen II®: Guaifenesin 800 mg and pseudoephedrine hydrochloride 45 mg
Profen Forte®: Guaifenesin 800 mg and pseudoephedrine hydrochloride 90 mg
Tablet, long acting:
Dynex: Guaifenesin 1200 mg and pseudoephedrine hydrochloride 90 mg
Guaifenex® PSE 120: Guaifenesin 600 mg and pseudoephedrine hydrochloride 120 mg [dye free]
Tablet, sustained release (Nasatab® LA): Guaifenesin 500 mg and pseudoephedrine hydrochloride 120 mg

guaifenesin and theophylline *see* theophylline and guaifenesin *on page 820*

guaifenesin, dextromethorphan, and phenylephrine

(gwye FEN e sin, deks troe meth OR fan, & fen il EF rin)

Synonyms guaifenesin, dextromethorphan hydrobromide, and phenylephrine hydrochloride; phenylephrine hydrochloride, guaifenesin, and dextromethorphan hydrobromide

U.S./Canadian Brand Names Anextuss [US]; Certuss-D® [US]; Dacex-DM [US]; Dexcon-DM [US]; Dexcon-PE [US]; Duraphen™ DM [US]; Duraphen™ Forte [US]; Duraphen™ II DM [US]; Dynatuss-EX [US]; Giltuss Pediatric® [US]; Giltuss TR® [US]; Giltuss® [US]; Guaifen™ DM [US]; Maxiphen DM [US]; SINUtuss® DM [US]; TriTuss® ER [US]; TriTuss® [US]

Therapeutic Category Antitussive; Decongestant

Use Symptomatic relief of dry nonproductive coughs and upper respiratory symptoms associated with hay fever, colds, or the flu

Usual Dosage Also refer to specific product labeling.

Oral:

Children 6-12 years (Certuss-D, Duraphen™ DM, Duraphen™ Forte, Duraphen™ II DM, Maxiphen DM): One-half tablet every 12 hours, not to exceed 1 tablet/24 hours

Children ≥12 years and Adults:

Certuss-D, Duraphen™ DM, Duraphen™ Forte, Maxiphen DM: One tablet every 12 hours, not to exceed 2 tablets/24 hours

Duraphen™ II DM: 1-1½ tablets twice daily, not to exceed 3 tablets/24 hours

Dosage Forms

Caplet:

Dexcon-PE: Guaifenesin 550 mg, dextromethorphan hydrobromide 25 mg, and phenylephrine hydrochloride 20 mg

Caplet, extended release:

TriTuss®-ER: Guaifenesin 600 mg, dextromethorphan hydrobromide 30 mg, and phenylephrine hydrochloride 10 mg

Liquid:

Giltuss®: Guaifenesin 300 mg, dextromethorphan hydrobromide 15 mg, and phenylephrine hydrochloride 10 mg per 5 mL (237 mL) [alcohol free, sugar free; contains phenylalanine 3.75 mg per 5 mL; natural grape flavor]

Giltuss Pediatric®: Guaifenesin 50 mg, dextromethorphan hydrobromide 5 mg, and phenylephrine hydrochloride 2.5 mg per mL (60 mL) [alcohol free, dye free, sugar free; grape flavor]

Liquid, oral drops: Guaifenesin 50 mg, dextromethorphan hydrobromide 5 mg, and phenylephrine 2.5 mg per mL (30 mL) [alcohol free; cherry flavor]

Syrup: Guaifenesin 200 mg, dextromethorphan hydrobromide 30 mg, and phenylephrine hydrochloride 10 mg (473 mL) [cherry flavor]

Dacex-DM: Guaifenesin 175 mg, dextromethorphan hydrobromide 25 mg, and phenylephrine hydrochloride 12.5 mg per 5 mL (480 mL) [strawberry flavor]

Dexcon-DM: Guaifenesin 100 mg, dextromethorphan hydrobromide 20 mg, and phenylephrine hydrochloride 10 mg per 5 mL (480 mL) [strawberry flavor]

Dynatuss-Ex: Guaifenesin 200 mg, dextromethorphan hydrobromide 30 mg, and phenylephrine hydrochloride 10 mg (473 mL) [alcohol free; cherry vanilla flavor]

TriTuss®: Guaifenesin 175 mg, dextromethorphan hydrobromide 25 mg, and phenylephrine hydrochloride 12.5 mg per 5 mL (480 mL) [alcohol free, sugar free]

Tablet [scored]:

SINUtuss™ DM: Guaifenesin 600 mg, dextromethorphan hydrobromide 30 mg, and phenylephrine hydrochloride 15 mg

Tablet, extended release [scored]:

Duraphen™ II DM: Guaifenesin 800 mg, dextromethorphan hydrobromide 20 mg, and phenylephrine hydrochloride 20 mg [dye free]

Duraphen™ Forte: Guaifenesin 1200 mg, dextromethorphan hydrobromide 30 mg, and phenylephrine hydrochloride 30 mg [dye free, sugar free]

Tablet, prolonged release [scored]:

Maxiphen DM: Guaifenesin 1000 mg, dextromethorphan hydrobromide 60 mg, and phenylephrine hydrochloride 40 mg [dye free]

Tablet, sustained release: Guaifenesin 600 mg, dextromethorphan hydrobromide 60 mg, and phenylephrine hydrochloride 40 mg

Anextuss: Guaifenesin 600 mg, dextromethorphan hydrobromide 60 mg, and phenylephrine hydrochloride 40 mg

Certuss-D® [scored]: Guaifenesin 600 mg, dextromethorphan hydrobromide 60 mg, and phenylephrine hydrochloride 40 mg

Duraphen™ DM [scored]: Guaifenesin 1200 mg, dextromethorphan hydrobromide 20 mg, and phenylephrine hydrochloride 40 mg [dye free]

Guaifen™ DM [scored]: Guaifenesin 1200 mg, dextromethorphan hydrobromide 20 mg, and phenylephrine hydrochloride 40 mg [dye free]

Tablet, timed release [scored]:

Giltuss TR®: Guaifenesin 600 mg, dextromethorphan hydrobromide 30 mg, and phenylephrine hydrochloride 20 mg [dye free, sugar free]

guaifenesin, dextromethorphan hydrobromide, and phenylephrine hydrochloride *see* guaifenesin, dextromethorphan, and phenylephrine *on previous page*

guaifenesin, hydrocodone, and pseudoephedrine *see* hydrocodone, pseudoephedrine, and guaifenesin *on page 425*

guaifenesin, pseudoephedrine, and codeine

(gwye FEN e sin, soo doe e FED rin, & KOE deen)

Sound-Alike/Look-Alike Issues

Halotussin® may be confused with Halotestin®

Synonyms codeine, guaifenesin, and pseudoephedrine; pseudoephedrine, guaifenesin, and codeine

U.S./Canadian Brand Names Benylin® 3.3 mg-D-E [Can]; Calmylin with Codeine [Can]; Guiatuss™ DAC® [US]; Mytussin® DAC [US]

Therapeutic Category Antitussive/Decongestant/Expectorant

Controlled Substance C-III; C-V

Use Temporarily relieves nasal congestion and controls cough associated with upper respiratory infections and related conditions (common cold, sinusitis, bronchitis, influenza)

Usual Dosage Oral:

Children 6-12 years: 5 mL every 4 hours, not to exceed 40 mL/24 hours

Children >12 years and Adults: 10 mL every 4 hours, not to exceed 40 mL/24 hours

Dosage Forms [DSC] = Discontinued product

Syrup:

Guiatuss DAC: Guaifenesin 100 mg, pseudoephedrine hydrochloride 30 mg, and codeine phosphate 10 mg per 5 mL (480 mL)

Mytussin® DAC: Guaifenesin 100 mg, pseudoephedrine hydrochloride 30 mg, and codeine phosphate 10 mg per 5 mL (120 mL, 480 mL) [sugar free; contains alcohol 1.7%; strawberry-raspberry flavor]

Nucofed® Expectorant: Guaifenesin 200 mg, pseudoephedrine hydrochloride 60 mg, and codeine phosphate 20 mg per 5 mL (480 mL) [contains alcohol 12.5%; cherry flavor] [DSC]

Nucofed® Pediatric Expectorant: Guaifenesin 100 mg, pseudoephedrine hydrochloride 30 mg, and codeine phosphate 10 mg per 5 mL (480 mL) [contains alcohol 6%; strawberry flavor] [DSC]

guaifenesin, pseudoephedrine, and dextromethorphan

(gwye FEN e sin, soo doe e FED rin, & deks troe meth OR fan)

Sound-Alike/Look-Alike Issues

Profen II DM® may be confused with Profen II®, Profen Forte®, Profen Forte™ DM

Profen Forte™ DM may be confused with Profen II®, Profen II DM®, Profen Forte®

Synonyms dextromethorphan, guaifenesin, and pseudoephedrine; pseudoephedrine, dextromethorphan, and guaifenesin

U.S./Canadian Brand Names Ambifed-G DM [US]; Balminil DM + Decongestant + Expectorant [Can]; Benylin® DM-D-E [Can]; Coldmist DM [US]; Koffex DM + Decongestant + Expectorant [Can]; Maxifed DM [US]; Maxifed DMX [US]; Medent-DM [US]; Novahistex® DM Decongestant Expectorant [Can]; Novahistine® DM Decongestant Expectorant [Can]; Profen Forte™ DM [US]; Profen II DM® [US]; Pseudo Max DMX [US]; Pseudovent™ DM [US]; Relacon-DM NR [US]; Robitussin® Cough and Cold CF [US-OTC]; Robitussin® Cough and Cold Infant [US-OTC]; Robitussin® Cough and Cold® [US-OTC/Can]; Ru-Tuss DM [US]; Touro® CC [US]; Touro® CC-LD [US]; Tri-Vent™ DM [US]; Tusnel Pediatric® [US]; Z-Cof™ DM [US]

Therapeutic Category Cold Preparation

Use Temporarily relieves nasal congestion and controls cough due to minor throat and bronchial irritation; helps loosen phlegm and thin bronchial secretions to make coughs more productive

Usual Dosage Note: Also refer to specific product labeling.

Children 2-6 years:

Maxifed DM: $1/3$ to $1/2$ tablet every 12 hours, not to exceed 1 tablet/24 hours

Tri-Vent™ DM: 2.5 mL up to 3-4 times/day, not to exceed pseudoephedrine 4 mg/kg/day

Profen II DM (syrup): 1.25-2.5 mL every 4 hours, not to exceed 15 mL/24 hours

Robitussin® Pediatric Cough and Cold Infant: 2.5 mL every 4-6 hours, not to exceed 4 doses/24 hours

Touro® CC: $1/2$ tablet every 12 hour, not to exceed 1 tablet/24 hours

Z-Cof™ DM: 2.5 mL 2-3 times/day, not to exceed 7.5 mL/24 hours

(Continued)

guaifenesin, pseudoephedrine, and dextromethorphan *(Continued)*

Children 6-12 years:

Ambifed-G DM, Profen Forte™ DM, Profen II DM®: 1/2 tablet every 12 hours not to exceed 1 tablet/24 hours

Maxifed DM: 1/2 to 1 tablet every 12 hours, not to exceed 2 tablets/24 hours

Tri-Vent™ DM: 5 mL up to 3-4 times/day, not to exceed pseudoephedrine 4 mg/kg/day

Touro® CC, Pseudovent™ DM: 1 tablet every 12 hours, not to exceed 2 tablets/24 hours

Profen II DM (syrup): 2.5-5 mL every 4 hours, not to exceed 30 mL/24 hours

Z-Cof™ DM: 5 mL 2-3 times/day, not to exceed 15 mL/24 hours

Children ≥12 years and Adults:

Ambifed-G DM, Aquatab® C, Profen Forte™ DM: 1 tablet every 12 hours not to exceed 2 tablets/24 hours

Maxifed DM, Touro® CC, Pseudovent™ DM: 1-2 tablets every 12 hours, not to exceed 4 tablets/24 hours

Tri-Vent™ DM: Up to 10 mL 3-4 times/day, not to exceed pseudoephedrine 240 mg/24 hours

Profen II DM (tablet): 1 to 1 1/2 tablets every 12 hours, not to exceed 3 tablets/24 hours

Profen II DM (syrup): 5-10 mL every 4 hours, not to exceed 60 mL/24 hours

Z-Cof™ DM: 10 mL 2-3 times/day, not to exceed 30 mL/24 hours

Dosage Forms

Caplet, prolonged release:

Ambifed-G DM: Guaifenesin 1000 mg, pseudoephedrine hydrochloride 60 mg, and dextromethorphan hydrobromide 30 mg

Caplet, sustained release [scored]:

Touro® CC: Guaifenesin 575 mg, pseudoephedrine hydrochloride 60 mg, and dextromethorphan hydrobromide 30 mg [dye free]

Touro® CC-LD: Guaifenesin 575 mg, pseudoephedrine hydrochloride 25 mg, and dextromethorphan hydrobromide 30 mg

Capsule, softgel:

Robitussin® Cough and Cold: Guaifenesin 200 mg, pseudoephedrine hydrochloride 30 mg, and dextromethorphan hydrobromide 10 mg

Liquid: Guaifenesin 100 mg, pseudoephedrine hydrochloride 30 mg, and dextromethorphan hydrobromide 10 mg per 5 mL (120 mL)

Profen II DM®: Guaifenesin 200 mg, pseudoephedrine hydrochloride 15 mg, and dextromethorphan hydrobromide 10 mg per 5 mL (480 mL) [alcohol free, dye free, sugar free; cherry flavor]

Relacon-DM NR: Guaifenesin 200 mg, pseudoephedrine hydrochloride 32 mg, and dextromethorphan hydrobromide 15 mg (480 mL) [alcohol free, sugar free; grape flavor]

Tusnel Pediatric®: Guaifenesin 50 mg, pseudoephedrine hydrochloride 15 mg, and dextromethorphan hydrobromide 5 mg per 5 mL (120 mL) [alcohol free]

Z-Cof™ DM: Guaifenesin 200 mg, pseudoephedrine hydrochloride 40 mg, and dextromethorphan hydrobromide 15 mg per 5 mL (480 mL) [alcohol free, sugar free; contains sodium benzoate; grape flavor]

Liquid, oral drops:

Robitussin® Cough and Cold Infant CF: Guaifenesin 100 mg, pseudoephedrine hydrochloride 15 mg, and dextromethorphan hydrobromide 5 mg per 2.5 mL (30 mL) [alcohol free; contains sodium benzoate]

Syrup: Guaifenesin 100 mg, pseudoephedrine hydrochloride 45 mg, and dextromethorphan hydrobromide 15 mg per 5 mL (480 mL)

Robitussin® Cough and Cold CF: Guaifenesin 100 mg, pseudoephedrine hydrochloride 30 mg, and dextromethorphan hydrobromide 10 mg per 5 mL (120 mL, 240 mL, 360 mL) [alcohol free; contains sodium benzoate]

Ru-Tuss DM: Guaifenesin 100 mg, pseudoephedrine hydrochloride 45 mg, and dextromethorphan hydrobromide 15 mg per 5 mL (480 mL) [alcohol free, dye free; strawberry flavor]

Tri-Vent™ DM: Guaifenesin 100 mg, pseudoephedrine hydrochloride 40 mg, and dextromethorphan hydrobromide 15 mg per 5 mL (480 mL) [alcohol free, dye free, sugar free; strawberry flavor]

Tablet, extended release: Guaifenesin 100 mg, pseudoephedrine hydrochloride 30 mg, and dextromethorphan hydrobromide 10 mg; guaifenesin 800 mg, pseudoephedrine hydrochloride 60 mg, and dextromethorphan hydrobromide 30 mg; guaifenesin 1200 mg, pseudoephedrine hydrochloride 60 mg, and dextromethorphan hydrobromide 60 mg; guaifenesin 1200 mg, pseudoephedrine hydrochloride 120 mg, and dextromethorphan hydrobromide 60 mg; guaifenesin 800 mg, pseudoephedrine hydrochloride 90 mg, and dextromethorphan hydrobromide 60 mg; guaifenesin 550 mg, pseudoephedrine hydrochloride 60 mg, and dextromethorphan hydrobromide 30 mg; guaifenesin 595 mg, pseudoephedrine hydrochloride 48 mg, and dextromethorphan hydrobromide 32 mg; guaifenesin 600 mg, pseudoephedrine hydrochloride 60 mg, and dextromethorphan hydrobromide 30 mg

Coldmist DM, Pseudovent™ DM: Guaifenesin 595 mg, pseudoephedrine hydrochloride 48 mg, and dextromethorphan hydrobromide 32 mg

Profen Forte™ DM: Guaifenesin 800 mg, pseudoephedrine hydrochloride 90 mg, and dextromethorphan hydrobromide 60 mg

Profen II DM®: Guaifenesin 800 mg, pseudoephedrine hydrochloride 45 mg, and dextromethorphan hydrobromide 30 mg

Tablet, long acting [scored]:

Medent-DM: Guaifenesin 800 mg, pseudoephedrine hydrochloride 60 mg, and dextromethorphan hydrobromide 30 mg [dye free]

Tablet, sustained release:

Maxifed DM: Guaifenesin 580 mg, pseudoephedrine hydrochloride 60 mg, and dextromethorphan hydrobromide 30 mg [dye free, scored]

Maxifed DM: Guaifenesin 780 mg, pseudoephedrine hydrochloride 80 mg, and dextromethorphan hydrobromide 40 mg [dye free, scored]

Pseudo Max DMX: Guaifenesin 700 mg, pseudoephedrine hydrochloride 80 mg, and dextromethorphan hydrobromide 40 mg

Guaifenex® *(Discontinued)*

Guaifenex® DM [US] *see* guaifenesin and dextromethorphan *on page 394*

Guaifenex® GP [US] *see* guaifenesin and pseudoephedrine *on page 398*

Guaifenex® PPA 75 *(Discontinued)*

Guaifenex® PSE [US] *see* guaifenesin and pseudoephedrine *on page 398*

Guaifenex™-Rx *(Discontinued)* *see* guaifenesin and pseudoephedrine *on page 398*

Guaifenex™-Rx DM *(Discontinued)* *see* guaifenesin, pseudoephedrine, and dextromethorphan *on page 401*

Guaimax-D® [US] *see* guaifenesin and pseudoephedrine *on page 398*

Guaipax® *(Discontinued)*

Guaitab® *(Discontinued)* *see* guaifenesin and pseudoephedrine *on page 398*

Guaituss AC® [US] *see* guaifenesin and codeine *on page 393*

Guaituss CF® *(Discontinued)*

Guaivent® *(Discontinued)* *see* guaifenesin and pseudoephedrine *on page 398*

guanabenz (GWAHN a benz)

Sound-Alike/Look-Alike Issues

guanabenz may be confused with guanadrel, guanfacine

Synonyms guanabenz acetate

U.S./Canadian Brand Names Wytensin® [Can]

Therapeutic Category Alpha-Adrenergic Agonist

Use Management of hypertension

Usual Dosage Adults: Oral: Initial: 4 mg twice daily; increase in increments of 4-8 mg/day every 1-2 weeks to a maximum of 32 mg twice daily.

Dosage Forms Tablet: 4 mg, 8 mg

guanabenz acetate *see* guanabenz *on this page*

guanfacine (GWAHN fa seen)

Sound-Alike/Look-Alike Issues

guanfacine may be confused with guaifenesin, guanabenz, guanidine

Tenex® may be confused with Entex®, Ten-K®, Xanax®

Synonyms guanfacine hydrochloride

U.S./Canadian Brand Names Tenex® [US/Can]

Therapeutic Category Alpha-Adrenergic Agonist

Use Management of hypertension

Usual Dosage Oral: Adults: Hypertension: 1 mg usually at bedtime, may increase if needed at 3- to 4-week intervals; usual dose range (JNC 7): 0.5-2 mg once daily

Dosage Forms Tablet: 1 mg, 2 mg

guanfacine hydrochloride *see* guanfacine *on this page*

guanidine (GWAHN i deen)

Sound-Alike/Look-Alike Issues

guanidine may be confused with guanfacine, guanethidine

(Continued)

guanidine *(Continued)*

Synonyms guanidine hydrochloride

Therapeutic Category Cholinergic Agent

Use Reduction of the symptoms of muscle weakness associated with the myasthenic syndrome of Eaton-Lambert, not for myasthenia gravis

Usual Dosage Adults: Oral: Eaton-Lambert syndrome: Initial: 10-15 mg/kg/day in 3-4 divided doses, gradually increase to 35 mg/kg/day or up to development of side effects

Dosage Forms Tablet, as hydrochloride: 125 mg

guanidine hydrochloride *see* guanidine *on previous page*

Guia-D [US] *see* guaifenesin and dextromethorphan *on page 394*

Guiacon DMS [US-OTC] *see* guaifenesin and dextromethorphan *on page 394*

GuiaCough® *(Discontinued)* *see* guaifenesin and dextromethorphan *on page 394*

GuiaCough® Expectorant *(Discontinued)* *see* guaifenesin *on page 392*

Guiatex® *(Discontinued)*

Guiatuss™ [US-OTC] *see* guaifenesin *on page 392*

Guiatuss™ DAC® [US] *see* guaifenesin, pseudoephedrine, and codeine *on page 401*

Guiatuss-DM® [US-OTC] *see* guaifenesin and dextromethorphan *on page 394*

gum benjamin *see* benzoin *on page 102*

GW506U78 *see* nelarabine *on page 582*

GW-1000-02 *see* tetrahydrocannabinol and cannabidiol *(Canada only) on page 816*

GW433908G *see* fosamprenavir *on page 368*

G-well® *(Discontinued)* *see* lindane *on page 497*

Gynazole-1® [US/Can] *see* butoconazole *on page 130*

Gyne-Lotrimin® 3 [US-OTC] *see* clotrimazole *on page 205*

Gyne-Sulf® *(Discontinued)* *see* sulfabenzamide, sulfacetamide, and sulfathiazole *on page 795*

Gynodiol® [US] *see* estradiol *on page 308*

Gynogen L.A.® Injection *(Discontinued)* *see* estradiol *on page 308*

Gynol II® [US-OTC] *see* nonoxynol 9 *on page 597*

Gynovite® Plus [US-OTC] *see* vitamins (multiple/oral) *on page 878*

H-C Tussive [US] *see* phenylephrine, hydrocodone, and chlorpheniramine *on page 663*

Habitrol® [Can] *see* nicotine *on page 591*

Haemophilus B conjugate and hepatitis B vaccine

(he MOF i lus bee KON joo gate & hep a TYE tis bee vak SEEN)

Sound-Alike/Look-Alike Issues

Comvax® may be confused with Recombivax [Recombivax HB®]

Synonyms *Haemophilus* b (meningococcal protein conjugate) conjugate vaccine; hepatitis b vaccine (recombinant); Hib

U.S./Canadian Brand Names Comvax® [US]

Therapeutic Category Vaccine, Inactivated Virus

Use

Immunization against invasive disease caused by *H. influenzae* type b and against infection caused by all known subtypes of hepatitis B virus in infants 6 weeks to 15 months of age born of hepatitis B surface antigen (HB_sAg) negative mothers

Infants born of HB_sAg-positive mothers or mothers of unknown HB_sAg status should receive hepatitis B immune globulin and hepatitis B vaccine (recombinant) at birth and should complete the hepatitis B vaccination series given according to a particular schedule

Usual Dosage Infants: I.M.: 0.5 mL at 2, 4, and 12-15 months of age (total of 3 doses)

If the recommended schedule cannot be followed, the interval between the first two doses should be at least 6 weeks and the interval between the second and third dose should be as close as possible to 8-11 months. Minimum age for first dose is 6 weeks.

Modified Schedule: Children who receive one dose of hepatitis B vaccine at or shortly after birth may receive Comvax® on a schedule of 2, 4, and 12-15 months of age

Dosage Forms Injection, suspension [preservative free]: *Haemophilus* b PRP 7.5 mcg and HB_sAg 5 mcg per 0.5 mL (0.5 mL) [vial stopper contains latex]

Haemophilus B conjugate vaccine (he MOF fi lus bee KON joo gate vak SEEN)

Synonyms diphtheria CRM_{197} protein conjugate; diphtheria toxoid conjugate; *Haemophilus* b oligosaccharide conjugate vaccine; *Haemophilus* b polysaccharide vaccine; HbCV; HbOC; Hib polysaccharide conjugate; PRP-OMP; PRP-T

U.S./Canadian Brand Names ActHIB® [US/Can]; HibTITER® [US]; PedvaxHIB® [US/Can]

Therapeutic Category Vaccine, Inactivated Bacteria

Use Routine immunization of children 2 months to 5 years of age against invasive disease caused by *H. influenzae*

Unimmunized children ≥5 years of age with a chronic illness known to be associated with increased risk of *Haemophilus influenzae* type b disease, specifically, persons with anatomic or functional asplenia or sickle cell anemia or those who have undergone splenectomy, should receive *Haemophilus influenzae* type b (Hib) vaccine.

Haemophilus b conjugate vaccines are not indicated for prevention of bronchitis or other infections due to *H. influenzae* in adults; adults with specific dysfunction or certain complement deficiencies who are at especially high risk of *H. influenzae* type b infection (HIV-infected adults); patients with Hodgkin's disease (vaccinated at least 2 weeks before the initiation of chemotherapy or 3 months after the end of chemotherapy)

Usual Dosage Children: I.M.: 0.5 mL as a single dose should be administered; do not inject I.V.

Dosage Forms

Injection, powder for reconstitution (ActHIB®) [preservative free]: *Haemophilus* b capsular polysaccharide 10 mcg and tetanus toxoid 24 mcg per dose [may be reconstituted with provided diluent (forms solution; vial stopper contains latex) or TriHIBit® (forms suspension)]

Injection, solution [preservative free] (HibTITER®): *Haemophilus* b saccharide 10 mcg and diphtheria CRM 197 protein 25 mcg per 0.5 mL (0.5 mL) [vial stopper contains latex]

Injection, suspension (PedvaxHIB®): *Haemophilus* b capsular polysaccharide 7.5 mcg and *Neisseria meningitidis* OMPC 125 mcg per 0.5 mL (0.5 mL) [contains aluminum 225 mcg/0.5 mL]

***Haemophilus* b (meningococcal protein conjugate) conjugate vaccine** *see* *Haemophilus* B conjugate and hepatitis B vaccine *on previous page*

***Haemophilus* b oligosaccharide conjugate vaccine** *see* *Haemophilus* B conjugate vaccine *on this page*

***Haemophilus* b polysaccharide vaccine** *see* *Haemophilus* B conjugate vaccine *on this page*

***Haemophilus influenzae* b conjugate vaccine and diphtheria, tetanus toxoids, and acellular pertussis vaccine** *see* diphtheria, tetanus toxoids, and acellular pertussis vaccine and *Haemophilus influenzae* b conjugate vaccine *on page 266*

halcinonide (hal SIN oh nide)

Sound-Alike/Look-Alike Issues

halcinonide may be confused with Halcion®

Halog® may be confused with Haldol®, Mycolog®

U.S./Canadian Brand Names Halog® [US/Can]

Therapeutic Category Corticosteroid, Topical

Use Inflammation of corticosteroid-responsive dermatoses [high potency topical corticosteroid]

Usual Dosage Children and Adults: Topical: Steroid-responsive dermatoses: Apply sparingly 1-3 times/day, occlusive dressing may be used for severe or resistant dermatoses; a thin film is effective; do not overuse. Therapy should be discontinued when control is achieved; if no improvement is seen, reassessment of diagnosis may be necessary.

Dosage Forms [DSC] = Discontinued product

Cream (Halog®): 0.1% (15 g, 30 g, 60 g, 240 g) [DSC]

Ointment (Halog®): 0.1% (15 g, 30 g, 60 g, 240 g) [DSC]

Solution, topical (Halog®): 0.1% (20 mL, 60 mL)

Halcion® [US/Can] *see* triazolam *on page 848*

Haldol® [US] *see* haloperidol *on next page*

Haldol® Decanoate [US] *see* haloperidol *on next page*

Haley's M-O *see* magnesium hydroxide and mineral oil *on page 514*

HalfLytely® and Bisacodyl [US] *see* polyethylene glycol-electrolyte solution and bisacodyl *on page 680*

Halfprin® [US-OTC] *see* aspirin *on page 77*

halobetasol (hal oh BAY ta sol)

Sound-Alike/Look-Alike Issues

Ultravate® may be confused with Cutivate®

Synonyms halobetasol propionate

U.S./Canadian Brand Names Ultravate® [US/Can]

Therapeutic Category Corticosteroid, Topical

Use Relief of inflammatory and pruritic manifestations of corticosteroid-response dermatoses [super high potency topical corticosteroid]

Usual Dosage Children ≥12 years and Adults: Topical:

Inflammatory and pruritic manifestations (dental use): Cream: Apply sparingly to lesion twice daily. Treatment should not exceed 2 consecutive weeks and total dosage should not exceed 50 g/week. Therapy should be discontinued when control is achieved; if no improvement is seen, reassessment of diagnosis may be necessary.

Steroid-responsive dermatoses: Apply sparingly to skin twice daily, rub in gently and completely; treatment should not exceed 2 consecutive weeks and total dosage should not exceed 50 g/week. Therapy should be discontinued when control is achieved; if no improvement is seen, reassessment of diagnosis may be necessary.

Dosage Forms

Cream, as propionate: 0.05% (15 g, 50 g)

Ointment, as propionate: 0.05% (15 g, 50 g)

halobetasol propionate *see* halobetasol *on this page*

Halog® [US/Can] *see* halcinonide *on previous page*

Halog®-E *(Discontinued)* *see* halcinonide *on previous page*

haloperidol (ha loe PER i dole)

Sound-Alike/Look-Alike Issues

haloperidol may be confused Halotestin®

Haldol® may be confused with Halcion®, Halenol®, Halog®, Halotestin®, Stadol®

Synonyms haloperidol decanoate; haloperidol lactate

U.S./Canadian Brand Names Apo-Haloperidol LA® [Can]; Apo-Haloperidol® [Can]; Haldol® Decanoate [US]; Haldol® [US]; Haloperidol Injection, USP [Can]; Haloperidol-LA Omega [Can]; Haloperidol-LA [Can]; Novo-Peridol [Can]; Peridol [Can]; PMS-Haloperidol LA [Can]

Therapeutic Category Antipsychotic Agent, Butyrophenone

Use Management of schizophrenia; control of tics and vocal utterances of Tourette disorder in children and adults; severe behavioral problems in children

Usual Dosage

Children: 3-12 years (15-40 kg): Oral:

Initial: 0.05 mg/kg/day or 0.25-0.5 mg/day given in 2-3 divided doses; increase by 0.25-0.5 mg every 5-7 days; maximum: 0.15 mg/kg/day

Usual maintenance:

Agitation or hyperkinesia: 0.01-0.03 mg/kg/day once daily

Nonpsychotic disorders: 0.05-0.075 mg/kg/day in 2-3 divided doses

Psychotic disorders: 0.05-0.15 mg/kg/day in 2-3 divided doses

Children 6-12 years: Sedation/psychotic disorders: I.M. (as lactate): 1-3 mg/dose every 4-8 hours to a maximum of 0.15 mg/kg/day; change over to oral therapy as soon as able

Adults: Psychosis:

Oral: 0.5-5 mg 2-3 times/day; usual maximum: 30 mg/day

I.M. (as lactate): 2-5 mg every 4-8 hours as needed

I.M. (as decanoate): Initial: 10-20 times the daily oral dose administered at 4-week intervals

Maintenance dose: 10-15 times initial oral dose; used to stabilize psychiatric symptoms

Dosage Forms [DSC] = Discontinued product

Note: Strength expressed as base.

Injection, oil, as decanoate: 50 mg/mL (1 mL, 5 mL); 100 mg/mL (1 mL, 5 mL)

Haldol® Decanoate: 50 mg/mL (1 mL; 5 mL [DSC]); 100 mg/mL (1 mL; 5 mL [DSC]) [contains benzyl alcohol, sesame oil]

Injection, solution, as lactate: 5 mg/mL (1 mL, 10 mL)

Haldol®: 5 mg/mL (1 mL)

Solution, oral concentrate, as lactate: 2 mg/mL (15 mL, 120 mL)
Tablet: 0.5 mg, 1 mg, 2 mg, 5 mg, 10 mg, 20 mg

haloperidol decanoate *see* haloperidol *on previous page*

Haloperidol Injection, USP [Can] *see* haloperidol *on previous page*

Haloperidol-LA [Can] *see* haloperidol *on previous page*

haloperidol lactate *see* haloperidol *on previous page*

Haloperidol-LA Omega [Can] *see* haloperidol *on previous page*

Halotestin® *(Discontinued)* *see* fluoxymesterone *on page 358*

halothane (HA loe thane)

Sound-Alike/Look-Alike Issues
halothane may be confused with Halotestin®

Therapeutic Category General Anesthetic

Use Induction and maintenance of general anesthesia

Usual Dosage Minimum alveolar concentration (MAC), the concentration at which 50% of patients do not respond to surgical incision, is 0.74% for halothane. The concentration at which amnesia and loss of awareness occur (MAC - awake) is 0.41%. Surgical levels of anesthesia are maintained with concentrations between 0.5% to 2%; inspired concentrations of up to 3% required for induction of anesthesia.

Dosage Forms [DSC] = Discontinued product
Liquid: 125 mL [DSC], 250 mL

Halotussin® *(Discontinued)* *see* guaifenesin *on page 392*

Halotussin® DM *(Discontinued)* *see* guaifenesin and dextromethorphan *on page 394*

Halotussin® PE *(Discontinued)* *see* guaifenesin and pseudoephedrine *on page 398*

Haltran® *(Discontinued)* *see* ibuprofen *on page 437*

hamamelis water *see* witch hazel *on page 881*

HandClens® [US-OTC] *see* benzalkonium chloride *on page 99*

Havrix® [US/Can] *see* hepatitis A vaccine *on page 410*

Havrix® and Engerix-B® *see* hepatitis A inactivated and hepatitis B (recombinant) vaccine *on page 410*

HbCV *see Haemophilus* B conjugate vaccine *on page 405*

HBIG *see* hepatitis B immune globulin *on page 411*

hBNP *see* nesiritide *on page 587*

HbOC *see Haemophilus* B conjugate vaccine *on page 405*

hCG *see* chorionic gonadotropin (human) *on page 186*

HD 85® [US] *see* radiological/contrast media (ionic) *on page 728*

HD 200 Plus® [US] *see* radiological/contrast media (ionic) *on page 728*

HDA® Toothache [US-OTC] *see* benzocaine *on page 99*

HDCV *see* rabies virus vaccine *on page 728*

Head & Shoulders® Citrus Breeze [US-OTC] *see* pyrithione zinc *on page 723*

Head & Shoulders® Classic Clean [US-OTC] *see* pyrithione zinc *on page 723*

Head & Shoulders® Classic Clean 2-In-1 [US-OTC] *see* pyrithione zinc *on page 723*

Head & Shoulders® Dry Scalp Care [US-OTC] *see* pyrithione zinc *on page 723*

Head & Shoulders® Extra Volume [US-OTC] *see* pyrithione zinc *on page 723*

Head & Shoulders® Intensive Treatment [US-OTC] *see* selenium sulfide *on page 767*

Head & Shoulders® Leave-in Treatment [US-OTC] *see* pyrithione zinc *on page 723*

Head & Shoulders® Refresh [US-OTC] *see* pyrithione zinc *on page 723*

Head & Shoulders® Sensitive Care [US-OTC] *see* pyrithione zinc *on page 723*

Head & Shoulders® Smooth & Silky 2-In-1 [US-OTC] *see* pyrithione zinc *on page 723*

Healon® [US/Can] *see* hyaluronate and derivatives *on page 416*

Healon®5 [US] *see* hyaluronate and derivatives *on page 416*

Healon GV® [US/Can] *see* hyaluronate and derivatives *on page 416*

Hectorol® [US/Can] *see* doxercalciferol *on page 277*

Helidac® [US] *see* bismuth subsalicylate, metronidazole, and tetracycline *on page 112*

Helistat® [US] *see* collagen hemostat *on page 212*

Helitene® [US] *see* collagen hemostat *on page 212*

Helixate® FS [US/Can] *see* antihemophilic factor (recombinant) *on page 59*

Hemabate® [US/Can] *see* carboprost tromethamine *on page 151*

hematin *see* hemin *on this page*

hemiacidrin *see* citric acid, magnesium carbonate, and glucono-delta-lactone *on page 194*

hemin (HEE min)

Synonyms hematin

U.S./Canadian Brand Names Panhematin® [US]

Therapeutic Category Blood Modifiers

Use Treatment of recurrent attacks of acute intermittent porphyria (AIP)

Usual Dosage I.V.: Children ≥16 years and Adults: 1-4 mg/kg/day administered over 10-15 minutes for 3-14 days; may be repeated no earlier than every 12 hours; not to exceed 6 mg/kg in any 24-hour period

Dosage Forms

Injection, powder for reconstitution [preservative free]:

Panhematin®: 313 mg [provides 7 mg/mL when reconstituted]

Hemocyte® [US-OTC] *see* ferrous fumarate *on page 342*

Hemocyte Plus® [US] *see* vitamins (multiple/oral) *on page 878*

Hemofil M [US/Can] *see* antihemophilic factor (human) *on page 59*

Hemril®-30 [US] *see* hydrocortisone (rectal) *on page 426*

HepaGam B™ [US] *see* hepatitis B immune globulin *on page 411*

Hepalean® [Can] *see* heparin *on this page*

Hepalean® Leo [Can] *see* heparin *on this page*

Hepalean®-LOK [Can] *see* heparin *on this page*

heparin (HEP a rin)

Sound-Alike/Look-Alike Issues

heparin may be confused with Hespan®

Synonyms heparin calcium; heparin lock flush; heparin sodium

U.S./Canadian Brand Names Hep-Lock U/P [US]; Hep-Lock® [US]; Hepalean® Leo [Can]; Hepalean® [Can]; Hepalean®-LOK [Can]; HepFlush®-10 [US]

Therapeutic Category Anticoagulant (Other)

Use Prophylaxis and treatment of thromboembolic disorders

Note: Heparin lock flush solution is intended only to maintain patency of I.V. devices and is **not** to be used for anticoagulant therapy.

Usual Dosage

Children:

Intermittent I.V.: Initial: 50-100 units/kg, then 50-100 units/kg every 4 hours

I.V. infusion: Initial: 50 units/kg, then 15-25 units/kg/hour; increase dose by 2-4 units/kg/hour every 6-8 hours as required

Adults:

Prophylaxis (low-dose heparin): SubQ: 5000 units every 8-12 hours

Intermittent I.V.: Initial: 10,000 units, then 50-70 units/kg (5000-10,000 units) every 4-6 hours

I.V. infusion (weight-based dosing per institutional nomogram recommended):

Acute coronary syndromes: MI: Fibrinolytic therapy:

Full-dose alteplase, reteplase, or tenecteplase with dosing as follows: Concurrent bolus of 60 units/kg (maximum: 4000 units), then 12 units/kg/hour (maximum: 1000 units/hour) as continuous infusion. Check aPTT every 4-6 hours; adjust to target of 1.5-2 times the upper limit of control (50-70 seconds in clinical trials); usual range 10-30 units/kg/hour. Duration of heparin therapy depends on concurrent therapy and the specific patient risks for systemic or venous thromboembolism.

Streptokinase: Heparin use optional depending on concurrent therapy and specific patient risks for systemic or venous thromboembolism (anterior MI, CHF, previous embolus, atrial fibrillation, LV thrombus): If heparin is administered, start when aPTT <2 times the upper limit of control; do not use a bolus, but initiate infusion adjusted to a target aPTT of 1.5-2 times the upper limit of control (50-70 seconds in clinical trials). If heparin is not administered by infusion, 7500-12,500 units SubQ every 12 hours (when aPTT <2 times the upper limit of control) is recommended.

Percutaneous coronary intervention: Heparin bolus and infusion may be administered to an activated clotting time (ACT) of 300-350 seconds if no concurrent GPIIb/IIIa receptor antagonist is administered or 200-250 seconds if a GPIIb/IIIa receptor antagonist is administered.

Treatment of unstable angina (high-risk and some intermediate-risk patients): Initial bolus of 60-70 units/kg (maximum: 5000 units), followed by an initial infusion of 12-15 units/kg/hour (maximum: 1000 units/hour). The American College of Chest Physicians consensus conference has recommended dosage adjustments to correspond to a therapeutic range equivalent to heparin levels of 0.3-0.7 units/mL by antifactor Xa determinations.

Treatment of venous thromboembolism:

DVT/PE: I.V. push: 80 units/kg followed by continuous infusion of 18 units/kg/hour

DVT: SubQ: 17,500 units every 12 hours

Line flushing: When using daily flushes of heparin to maintain patency of single and double lumen central catheters, 10 units/mL is commonly used for younger infants (eg, <10 kg) while 100 units/mL is used for older infants, children, and adults. Capped PVC catheters and peripheral heparin locks require flushing more frequently (eg, every 6-8 hours). Volume of heparin flush is usually similar to volume of catheter (or slightly greater). Additional flushes should be given when stagnant blood is observed in catheter, after catheter is used for drug or blood administration, and after blood withdrawal from catheter.

Addition of heparin (0.5-3 unit/mL) to peripheral and central parenteral nutrition has not been shown to decrease catheter-related thrombosis. The final concentration of heparin used for TPN solutions may need to be decreased to 0.5 units/mL in small infants receiving larger amounts of volume in order to avoid approaching therapeutic amounts. Arterial lines are heparinized with a final concentration of 1 unit/mL.

Using a standard heparin solution (25,000 units/500 mL D_5W), the following infusion rates can be used to achieve the listed doses.

For a dose of:

400 units/hour: Infuse at 8 mL/hour
500 units/hour: Infuse at 10 mL/hour
600 units/hour: Infuse at 12 mL/hour
700 units/hour: Infuse at 14 mL/hour
800 units/hour: Infuse at 16 mL/hour
900 units/hour: Infuse at 18 mL/hour
1000 units/hour: Infuse at 20 mL/hour
1100 units/hour: Infuse at 22 mL/hour
1200 units/hour: Infuse at 24 mL/hour
1300 units/hour: Infuse at 26 mL/hour
1400 units/hour: Infuse at 28 mL/hour
1500 units/hour: Infuse at 30 mL/hour
1600 units/hour: Infuse at 32 mL/hour
1700 units/hour: Infuse at 34 mL/hour
1800 units/hour: Infuse at 36 mL/hour
1900 units/hour: Infuse at 38 mL/hour
2000 units/hour: Infuse at 40 mL/hour

Dosage Forms [DSC] = Discontinued product

Infusion, as sodium [premixed in NaCl 0.45%; porcine intestinal mucosa source]: 12,500 units (250 mL); 25,000 units (250 mL, 500 mL)

Infusion, as sodium [preservative free; premixed in D_5W; porcine intestinal mucosa source]: 10,000 units (100 mL) [contains sodium metabisulfite]; 12,500 units (250 mL) [contains sodium metabisulfite]; 20,000 units (500 mL) [contains sodium metabisulfite]; 25,000 units (250 mL, 500 mL) [contains sodium metabisulfite]

Infusion, as sodium [preservative free; premixed in NaCl 0.9%; porcine intestinal mucosa source]: 1000 units (500 mL); 2000 units (1000 mL)

Injection, solution, as sodium [lock flush preparation; porcine intestinal mucosa source; multidose vial]: 10 units/mL (1 mL, 10 mL, 30 mL) [contains parabens]; 100 units/mL (1 mL, 5 mL) [contains parabens]

Injection, solution, as sodium [lock flush preparation; porcine intestinal mucosa source; multidose vial]: 10 units/mL (10 mL, 30 mL); 100 units/mL (10 mL, 30 mL) [contains benzyl alcohol]

Hep-Lock®: 10 units/mL (1 mL, 2 mL, 10 mL, 30 mL); 100 units/mL (1 mL, 2 mL, 10 mL, 30 mL) [contains benzyl alcohol]

Injection, solution, as sodium [lock flush preparation; porcine intestinal mucosa source; prefilled syringe]: 10 units/mL (1 mL, 2 mL, 3 mL, 5 mL); 100 units/mL (1 mL, 2 mL, 3 mL, 5 mL) [contains benzyl alcohol]

Injection, solution, as sodium [preservative free; lock flush preparation; porcine intestinal mucosa source; prefilled syringe]: 100 units/mL (5 mL)

(Continued)

heparin *(Continued)*

Injection, solution, as sodium [preservative free; lock flush preparation; porcine intestinal mucosa source; vial]:
HepFlush®-10: 10 units/mL (10 mL)
Hep-Lock U/P: 10 units/mL (1 mL); 100 units/mL (1 mL)

Injection, solution, as sodium [porcine intestinal mucosa source; multidose vial]: 1000 units/mL (1 mL, 10 mL, 30 mL) [contains benzyl alcohol]; 1000 units/mL (1 mL, 10 mL, 30 mL) [contains methylparabens]; 5000 units/mL (1 mL, 10 mL) [contains benzyl alcohol]; 5000 units/mL (1 mL) [contains methylparabens]; 10,000 units/mL (1 mL, 4 mL) [contains benzyl alcohol]; 10,000 units/mL (1 mL, 5 mL) [contains methylparabens]; 20,000 units/mL (1 mL) [contains methylparabens]

Injection, solution, as sodium [porcine intestinal mucosa source; prefilled syringe]: 5000 units/mL (1 mL) [contains benzyl alcohol]

Injection, solution, as sodium [preservative free; porcine intestinal mucosa source; prefilled syringe]: 10,000 units/mL (0.5 mL)

Injection, solution, as sodium [preservative free; porcine intestinal mucosa source; vial]: 1000 units/mL (2 mL); 2000 units/mL (5 mL); 2500 units/mL (10 mL)

heparin calcium *see* heparin *on page 408*

heparin cofactor I *see* antithrombin III *on page 62*

heparin lock flush *see* heparin *on page 408*

heparin sodium *see* heparin *on page 408*

hepatitis A inactivated and hepatitis B (recombinant) vaccine

(hep a TYE tis aye in ak ti VAY ted & hep a TYE tis bee ree KOM be nant vak SEEN)

Synonyms Engerix-B® and Havrix®; Havrix® and Engerix-B®; hepatitis B (recombinant) and hepatitis A inactivated vaccine

U.S./Canadian Brand Names Twinrix® [US/Can]

Therapeutic Category Vaccine

Use Active immunization against disease caused by hepatitis A virus and hepatitis B virus (all known subtypes) in populations desiring protection against or at high risk of exposure to these viruses.

Populations include travelers to areas of intermediate/high endemicity for **both** HAV and HBV; those at increased risk of HBV infection due to behavioral or occupational factors; patients with chronic liver disease; laboratory workers who handle live HAV and HBV; healthcare workers, police, and other personnel who render first-aid or medical assistance; workers who come in contact with sewage; employees of day care centers and correctional facilities; patients/staff of hemodialysis units; male homosexuals; patients frequently receiving blood products; military personnel; users of injectable illicit drugs; close household contacts of patients with hepatitis A and hepatitis B infection.

Usual Dosage I.M.: Adults: Primary immunization: Three doses (1 mL each) given on a 0-, 1-, and 6-month schedule

Dosage Forms Injection, suspension: Inactivated hepatitis A virus 720 ELISA units and hepatitis B surface antigen 20 mcg per mL (1 mL) [prefilled syringe; single-dose vial]

hepatitis A vaccine (hep a TYE tis aye vak SEEN)

U.S./Canadian Brand Names Avaxim® [Can]; Avaxim®-Pediatric [Can]; Havrix® [US/Can]; VAQTA® [US/Can]

Therapeutic Category Vaccine, Inactivated Virus

Use

Active immunization against disease caused by hepatitis A virus in populations desiring protection against or at high risk of exposure

Populations at high risk of exposure to hepatitis A virus may include children and adolescents in selected states and regions, travelers to developing countries, household and sexual contacts of persons infected with hepatitis A, child day care employees, patients with chronic liver disease, illicit drug users, male homosexuals, institutional workers (eg, institutions for the mentally and physically handicapped persons, prisons), and healthcare workers who may be exposed to hepatitis A virus (eg, laboratory employees)

Usual Dosage I.M.:

Havrix®:

Children 12 months to 18 years: 720 ELISA units (0.5 mL) with a booster dose of 720 ELISA units 6-12 months following primary immunization

Adults: 1440 ELISA units (1 mL) with a booster dose of 1440 ELISA units 6-12 months following primary immunization

VAQTA®:

Children 12 months to 18 years: 25 units (0.5 mL) with 25 units (0.5 mL) booster dose of 25 units to be given 6-18 months after primary immunization (6-12 months if initial dose was with Havrix®)

Adults: 50 units (1 mL) with 50 units (1 mL) booster dose of 50 units to be given 6-18 months after primary immunization (6-12 months if initial dose was with Havrix®)

Dosage Forms

Injection, suspension, adult:

Havrix®: Viral antigen 1440 ELISA units/mL (1 mL) [contains trace amounts of neomycin; syringe plunger contains latex rubber; available in prefilled syringe or single-dose vial]

VAQTA®: HAV antigen 50 units/mL (1 mL) [vial stopper and syringe plunger contain latex rubber; available in prefilled syringe or single-dose vial]

Injection, suspension, pediatric (Havrix®): Viral antigen 720 ELISA units/0.5 mL (0.5 mL) [contains trace amounts of neomycin; syringe plunger contains latex rubber; available in prefilled syringe or single-dose vial]

Injection, suspension, pediatric/adolescent (VAQTA®): HAV antigen 25 units/0.5 mL (0.5 mL) [vial stopper and syringe plunger contain latex rubber; available in prefilled syringe or single-dose vial]

hepatitis B immune globulin (hep a TYE tis bee i MYUN GLOB yoo lin)

Synonyms HBIG

U.S./Canadian Brand Names BayHep B® [Can]; HepaGam B™ [US]; HyperHep B® [Can]; HyperHEP B™ S/D [US]; Nabi-HB® [US]

Therapeutic Category Immune Globulin

Use Passive prophylactic immunity to hepatitis B following: Acute exposure to blood containing hepatitis B surface antigen (HBsAg); perinatal exposure of infants born to HBsAg-positive mothers; sexual exposure to HBsAg-positive persons; household exposure to persons with acute HBV infection

Note: Hepatitis B immune globulin is not indicated for treatment of active hepatitis B infection and is ineffective in the treatment of chronic active hepatitis B infection.

Usual Dosage I.M.:

Newborns: Hepatitis B: 0.5 mL as soon after birth as possible (within 12 hours); may repeat at 3 months in order for a higher rate of prevention of the carrier state to be achieved; at this time an active vaccination program with the vaccine may begin

Infants <12 months: Household exposure prophylaxis: 0.5 mL (to be administered if mother or primary caregiver has acute HBV infection)

Adults: Postexposure prophylaxis: 0.06 mL/kg as soon as possible after exposure (ie, within 24 hours of needlestick, ocular, or mucosal exposure or within 14 days of sexual exposure); usual dose: 3-5 mL; repeat at 28-30 days after exposure in nonresponders or in patients who refuse vaccination

Note: HBIG may be administered at the same time (but at a different site) or up to 1 month preceding hepatitis B vaccination without impairing the active immune response

Dosage Forms Note: Potency expressed in international units as compared to the WHO standard

Injection, solution [preservative free]:

BayHepB® [DSC], HyperHEP B™ S/D: 15% to 18% (0.5 mL) [neonatal single-dose syringe]; (1 mL) [single-dose syringe or single-dose vial]; (5 mL) [single-dose vial]

Nabi-HB®: 5% (1 mL, 5 mL) [>312 int. units/mL; single-dose vial]

HepaGam B™: 5% (1 mL, 5 mL) [>312 int. units/mL; contains maltose, single-dose vial]

hepatitis B inactivated virus vaccine (plasma derived) *see* hepatitis B vaccine *on this page*

hepatitis B inactivated virus vaccine (recombinant DNA) *see* hepatitis B vaccine *on this page*

hepatitis B (recombinant) and hepatitis A inactivated vaccine *see* hepatitis A inactivated and hepatitis B (recombinant) vaccine *on previous page*

hepatitis B vaccine (hep a TYE tis bee vak SEEN)

Sound-Alike/Look-Alike Issues

Recombivax HB® may be confused with Comvax®

Synonyms hepatitis B inactivated virus vaccine (plasma derived); hepatitis B inactivated virus vaccine (recombinant DNA)

U.S./Canadian Brand Names Engerix-B® [US/Can]; Recombivax HB® [US/Can]

Therapeutic Category Vaccine, Inactivated Virus

Use Immunization against infection caused by all known subtypes of hepatitis B virus, in individuals considered at high risk of potential exposure to hepatitis B virus or HB_sAg-positive materials:

Healthcare workers[1]

Special patient groups (eg, adolescents, infants born to HB_s Ag-positive mothers, children born after 11/21/91, military personnel)

(Continued)

hepatitis B vaccine *(Continued)*

Hemodialysis patients[2] (see dosing recommendations), recipients of certain blood products[3]

Lifestyle factors: Homosexual and bisexual men, intravenous drug abusers, heterosexually-active persons with multiple sexual partners or recently acquired sexually-transmitted diseases

Environmental factors: Household and sexual contacts of HBV carriers; prison inmates; clients and staff of institutions for the mentally handicapped; residents, immigrants, and refugees from areas with endemic HBV infection; international travelers at increased risk of acquiring HBV infection

[1]The risk of hepatitis B virus (HBV) infection for healthcare workers varies both between hospitals and within hospitals. Hepatitis B vaccination is recommended for all healthcare workers with blood exposure.

[2]Hemodialysis patients often respond poorly to hepatitis B vaccination; higher vaccine doses or increased number of doses are required. A special formulation of one vaccine is now available for such persons (Recombivax HB®, 40 mcg/mL). The anti-HB_s(antibody to hepatitis B surface antigen) response of such persons should be tested after they are vaccinated, and those who have not responded should be revaccinated with 1-3 additional doses. Patients with chronic renal disease should be vaccinated as early as possible, ideally before they require hemodialysis. In addition, their anti-HB_s levels should be monitored at 6- to 12-month intervals to assess the need for revaccination.

[3]Patients with hemophilia should be immunized subcutaneously, not intramuscularly.

Usual Dosage I.M.:

Immunization regimen: Regimen consists of 3 doses (0, 1, and 6 months): First dose given on the elected date, second dose given 1 month later, third dose given 6 months after the first dose.

Initial dose:

Birth (infants born of HB_s Ag-negative mothers) to 19 years:
- Recombivax HB®: 0.5 mL (5 mcg/0.5 mL pediatric/adolescent formulation) **or**
- Engerix-B®: 0.5 mL (10 mcg/0.5 mL formulation)

20 years and older:
- Recombivax HB®: 1 mL (10 mcg/mL adult formulation) **or**
- Engerix-B®: 1 mL (20 mcg/mL formulation)

Dialysis or immunocompromised patients (revaccinate if anti-HB_s <10 mIU/mL ≥1-2 months after third dose):
- Recombivax HB®: 1 mL (40 mcg/mL dialysis formulation) **or**
- Engerix-B®: 2 mL (two 1 mL doses given at different sites using the 40 mcg/2 mL dialysis formulation)

1-month dose:

Birth (infants born of HB_sAg-negative mothers) to 19 years:
- Recombivax HB®: 0.5 mL (5 mcg/0.5 mL pediatric/adolescent formulation) **or**
- Engerix-B®: 0.5 mL (10 mcg/0.5 mL formulation)

20 years and older:
- Recombivax HB®: 1 mL (10 mcg/mL adult formulation) **or**
- Engerix-B®: 1 mL (20 mcg/mL formulation)

Dialysis or immunocompromised patients (revaccinate if anti-HB_s <10 mIU/mL ≥1-2 months after third dose):
- Recombivax HB®: 1 mL (40 mcg/mL dialysis formulation) **or**
- Engerix-B®: 2 mL (two 1 mL doses given at different sites using the 40 mcg/2 mL dialysis formulation)

6-month dose:

Birth (infants born of HB_sAg-negative mothers) to 19 years: 0.5 mL (5 mcg/0.5 mL pediatric/adolescent formulation) Recombivax HB® **or** 0.5 mL (10 mcg/0.5 mL formulation) Engerix-B®

20 years and older:
- Recombivax HB®: 1 mL (10 mcg/mL adult formulation) **or**
- Engerix-B®: 1 mL (20 mcg/mL formulation)

Dialysis or immunocompromised patients (revaccinate if anti-HB_s <10 mIU/mL ≥1-2 months after third dose):
- Recombivax HB®: 1 mL (40 mcg/mL dialysis formulation) **or**
- Engerix-B®: 2 mL (two 1 mL doses given at different sites using the 40 mcg/2 mL dialysis formulation)

Alternative dosing schedule for **Recombivax HB®:** Children 11-15 years (10 mcg/mL adult formulation): First dose of 1 mL given on the elected date, second dose given 4-6 months later

Alternative dosing schedules for **Engerix-B®:**

Children ≤10 years (10 mcg/0.5 mL formulation): High-risk children: 0.5 mL at 0, 1, 2, and 12 months; lower-risk children ages 5-10 who are candidates for an extended administration schedule may receive an alternative regimen of 0.5 mL at 0, 12, and 24 months. If booster dose is needed, revaccinate with 0.5 mL.

Adolescents 11-19 years (20 mcg/mL formulation): 1 mL at 0, 1, and 6 months. High-risk adolescents: 1 mL at 0, 1, 2, and 12 months; lower-risk adolescents 11-16 years who are candidates for an extended administration schedule may receive an alternative regimen of 0.5 mL (using the 10 mcg/0.5 mL) formulation at 0, 12, and 24 months. If booster dose is needed, revaccinate with 20 mcg.

Adults ≥20 years: High-risk adults (20 mcg/mL formulation): 1 mL at 0, 1, 2, and 12 months. If booster dose is needed, revaccinate with 1 mL.

Postexposure prophylaxis recommended dosage for infants born to HB_s Ag-positive mothers (by product /age):

Engerix-B® (pediatric formulation 10 mcg/0.5 mL):

Give 0.5 mL within 7 days; repeat 0.5 mL at 1 month and 6 months.

Alternately, the first dose may be given at birth at the same time as HBIG, but give in the opposite anterolateral thigh. This may better ensure vaccine absorption.

An alternate regimen is administration of the vaccine at birth, within 7 days of birth, and at 1, 2, and 12 months later.

Recombivax HB® (pediatric/adolescent formulation 5 mcg/0.5 mL):

Give 0.5 mL within 7 days; repeat 0.5 mL at 1 month and 6 months

Alternately, the first dose may be given at birth at the same time as HBIG, but give in the opposite anterolateral thigh. This may better ensure vaccine absorption.

Hepatitis B immune globulin: Give 0.5 mL at birth.

Dosage Forms Injection, suspension [preservative free] [recombinant DNA]:

Engerix-B®:

Adult: Hepatitis B surface antigen 20 mcg/mL (1 mL) [contains trace amounts of thimerosal; some dosage forms contain dry natural latex rubber]

Pediatric/adolescent: Hepatitis B surface antigen 10 mcg/0.5 mL (0.5 mL) [contains trace amounts of thimerosal; some dosage forms contain dry natural latex rubber]

Recombivax HB®:

Adult: Hepatitis B surface antigen 10 mcg/mL (1 mL, 3 mL)

Dialysis: Hepatitis B surface antigen 40 mcg/mL (1 mL)

Pediatric/adolescent: Hepatitis B surface antigen 5 mcg/0.5 mL (0.5 mL)

hepatitis b vaccine (recombinant) *see* *Haemophilus* B conjugate and hepatitis B vaccine *on page 404*

HepFlush®-10 [US] *see* heparin *on page 408*

Hep-Lock® [US] *see* heparin *on page 408*

Hep-Lock U/P [US] *see* heparin *on page 408*

Hepsera™ [US] *see* adefovir *on page 19*

Heptalac® *(Discontinued)* *see* lactulose *on page 478*

Heptovir® [Can] *see* lamivudine *on page 479*

Herceptin® [US/Can] *see* trastuzumab *on page 843*

HES *see* hetastarch *on this page*

Hespan® [US] *see* hetastarch *on this page*

hetastarch (HET a starch)

Sound-Alike/Look-Alike Issues

Hespan® may be confused with heparin

Synonyms HES; hydroxyethyl starch

U.S./Canadian Brand Names Hespan® [US]; Hextend® [US/Can]; Voluven® [Can]

Therapeutic Category Plasma Volume Expander

Use Blood volume expander used in treatment of hypovolemia

Hespan®: Adjunct in leukapheresis to improve harvesting and increasing the yield of granulocytes by centrifugal means

Usual Dosage I.V. infusion (requires an infusion pump):

Plasma volume expansion: Adults: 500-1000 mL (up to 1500 mL/day) or 20 mL/kg/day (up to 1500 mL/day); larger volumes (15,000 mL/24 hours) have been used safely in small numbers of patients

Leukapheresis: 250-700 mL; **Note:** Citrate anticoagulant is added before use.

Dosage Forms

Infusion [premixed in lactated electrolyte injection] (Hextend®): 6% (500 mL)

Infusion, solution [premixed in NaCl 0.9%] (Hespan®): 6% (500 mL)

Hexabrix™ [US] *see* radiological/contrast media (ionic) *on page 728*

hexachlorocyclohexane *see* lindane *on page 497*

hexachlorophene (heks a KLOR oh feen)

Sound-Alike/Look-Alike Issues

pHisoHex® may be confused with Fostex®, pHisoDerm®

U.S./Canadian Brand Names pHisoHex® [US/Can]

Therapeutic Category Antibacterial, Topical

Use Surgical scrub and as a bacteriostatic skin cleanser; control an outbreak of gram-positive infection when other procedures have been unsuccessful

Usual Dosage Children and Adults: Topical: Apply 5 mL cleanser and water to area to be cleansed; lather and rinse thoroughly under running water

Dosage Forms Liquid, topical: 3% (150 mL, 500 mL, 3840 mL)

Hexalen® [US/Can] *see* altretamine *on page 35*

hexamethylenetetramine *see* methenamine *on page 538*

hexamethylmelamine *see* altretamine *on page 35*

Hexit™ [Can] *see* lindane *on page 497*

HEXM *see* altretamine *on page 35*

Hextend® [US/Can] *see* hetastarch *on previous page*

hexylresorcinol (heks il re ZOR si nole)

U.S./Canadian Brand Names S.T. 37® [US-OTC]; Sucrets® Original [US-OTC]

Therapeutic Category Local Anesthetic

Use Minor antiseptic and local anesthetic for sore throat; topical antiseptic for minor cuts or abrasions

Usual Dosage Children ≥2 years and Adults:

Antiseptic: Topical: Solution: Apply to affected area 1-3 times/day

Sore throat: Oral:

Lozenge: May be used as needed, allow to dissolve slowly in mouth (maximum: 10 lozenges/day)

Solution: Gargle or swish in mouth up to 4 times/day

Dosage Forms

Lozenge (Sucrets® Original): 2.4 mg [mint flavor]

Solution (S.T. 37®): 0.1% (480 mL) [contains sodium bisulfite]

hGH *see* somatropin *on page 785*

Hib *see Haemophilus* B conjugate and hepatitis B vaccine *on page 404*

Hibiclens® [US-OTC] *see* chlorhexidine gluconate *on page 173*

Hibidil® 1:2000 [Can] *see* chlorhexidine gluconate *on page 173*

Hibistat® [US-OTC] *see* chlorhexidine gluconate *on page 173*

Hib polysaccharide conjugate *see Haemophilus* B conjugate vaccine *on page 405*

HibTITER® [US] *see Haemophilus* B conjugate vaccine *on page 405*

High Gamma Vitamin E Complete™ [US-OTC] *see* vitamin E *on page 876*

Hi-Kovite [US-OTC] *see* vitamins (multiple/oral) *on page 878*

Hiprex® [US/Can] *see* methenamine *on page 538*

hirulog *see* bivalirudin *on page 113*

Histacol DM Pediatric [US] *see* brompheniramine, pseudoephedrine, and dextromethorphan *on page 120*

Histade™ [US] *see* chlorpheniramine and pseudoephedrine *on page 177*

Histalet® X *(Discontinued)* *see* guaifenesin and pseudoephedrine *on page 398*

Histatab® Plus *(Discontinued)* *see* chlorpheniramine and phenylephrine *on page 176*

Hista-Vent® DA [US] *see* chlorpheniramine, phenylephrine, and methscopolamine *on page 180*

Histerone® Injection *(Discontinued)* *see* testosterone *on page 812*

Histex™ [US] *see* chlorpheniramine and pseudoephedrine *on page 177*

Histex™ I/E *(Discontinued)* *see* carbinoxamine *on page 148*

Histex™ HC [US] *see* hydrocodone, carbinoxamine, and pseudoephedrine *on page 424*

Histex™ PD [US] *see* carbinoxamine *on page 148*

Histex™ PD-12 [US] *see* carbinoxamine *on page 148*

Histex™ SR [US] *see* brompheniramine and pseudoephedrine *on page 118*

Histinex® D Liquid *(Discontinued)* *see* hydrocodone and pseudoephedrine *on page 424*

Histinex® HC [US] *see* phenylephrine, hydrocodone, and chlorpheniramine *on page 663*

Histinex® PV [US] *see* pseudoephedrine, hydrocodone, and chlorpheniramine *on page 716*

Histor-D® Syrup *(Discontinued)* *see* chlorpheniramine and phenylephrine *on page 176*

Histor-D® Timecelles® *(Discontinued)* *see* chlorpheniramine, phenylephrine, and methscopolamine *on page 180*

Histrodrix® *(Discontinued)* *see* dexbrompheniramine and pseudoephedrine *on page 241*

Histussin D® [US] *see* hydrocodone and pseudoephedrine *on page 424*

Histussin® HC [US] *see* phenylephrine, hydrocodone, and chlorpheniramine *on page 663*

Hi-Vegi-Lip [US-OTC] *see* pancreatin *on page 633*

Hivid® [US/Can] *see* zalcitabine *on page 884*

hMG *see* menotropins *on page 528*

HMM *see* altretamine *on page 35*

HMR 3647 *see* telithromycin *on page 807*

HMS Liquifilm® *(Discontinued)* *see* medrysone *on page 524*

HN_2 *see* mechlorethamine *on page 522*

Hold® DM [US-OTC] *see* dextromethorphan *on page 245*

homatropine (hoe MA troe peen)

Synonyms homatropine hydrobromide

U.S./Canadian Brand Names Isopto® Homatropine [US]

Therapeutic Category Anticholinergic Agent

Use Producing cycloplegia and mydriasis for refraction; treatment of acute inflammatory conditions of the uveal tract

Usual Dosage Ophthalmic:

Children:

Mydriasis and cycloplegia for refraction: Instill 1 drop of 2% solution immediately before the procedure; repeat at 10-minute intervals as needed

Uveitis: Instill 1 drop of 2% solution 2-3 times/day

Adults:

Mydriasis and cycloplegia for refraction: Instill 1-2 drops of 2% solution or 1 drop of 5% solution before the procedure; repeat at 5- to 10-minute intervals as needed; maximum of 3 doses for refraction

Uveitis: Instill 1-2 drops of 2% or 5% 2-3 times/day up to every 3-4 hours as needed

Dosage Forms Solution, ophthalmic, as hydrobromide: 2% (5 mL); 5% (5 mL, 15 mL) [contains benzalkonium chloride]

homatropine and hydrocodone *see* hydrocodone and homatropine *on page 423*

homatropine hydrobromide *see* homatropine *on this page*

horse antihuman thymocyte gamma globulin *see* antithymocyte globulin (equine) *on page 62*

H.P. Acthar® Gel [US] *see* corticotropin *on page 215*

Hp-PAC® [Can] *see* lansoprazole, amoxicillin, and clarithromycin *on page 482*

HPV vaccine *see* papillomavirus (Types 6, 11, 16, 18) recombinant vaccine *on page 638*

HTF919 *see* tegaserod *on page 807*

hu1124 *see* efalizumab *on page 288*

Humalog® [US/Can] *see* insulin lispro *on page 451*

Humalog® Mix 25 [Can] *see* insulin lispro protamine and insulin lispro *on page 451*

Humalog® Mix 50/50™ [US] *see* insulin lispro protamine and insulin lispro *on page 451*

Humalog® Mix 50/50 Insulin *(Discontinued)*

Humalog® Mix 75/25™ [US] *see* insulin lispro protamine and insulin lispro *on page 451*

human antitumor necrosis factor alpha *see* adalimumab *on page 19*

human diploid cell cultures rabies vaccine *see* rabies virus vaccine *on page 728*

human growth hormone *see* somatropin *on page 785*
humanized IgG1 anti-CD52 monoclonal antibody *see* alemtuzumab *on page 26*
human LFA-3/IgG(1) fusion protein *see* alefacept *on page 26*
human menopausal gonadotropin *see* menotropins *on page 528*
human thyroid stimulating hormone *see* thyrotropin alpha *on page 825*
Humate-P® [US] *see* antihemophilic factor/von Willebrand factor complex (human) *on page 60*
Humatin® [US/Can] *see* paromomycin *on page 639*
Humatrope® [US/Can] *see* somatropin *on page 785*
Humegon® [Can] *see* chorionic gonadotropin (human) *on page 186*
Humegon® *(Discontinued)* *see* menotropins *on page 528*
Humibid® CS *(Discontinued)* *see* guaifenesin and dextromethorphan *on page 394*
Humibid® DM *(Discontinued)* *see* guaifenesin and dextromethorphan *on page 394*
Humibid® *e (Discontinued)* *see* guaifenesin *on page 392*
Humibid® LA *(Discontinued)* *see* guaifenesin *on page 392*
Humibid® Maximum Strength [US] *see* guaifenesin *on page 392*
Humibid® Pediatric *(Discontinued)* *see* guaifenesin *on page 392*
Humibid® Sprinkle *(Discontinued)* *see* guaifenesin *on page 392*
Humira® [US/Can] *see* adalimumab *on page 19*
Humulin® 20/80 [Can] *see* insulin NPH and insulin regular *on page 452*
Humulin® 50/50 [US] *see* insulin NPH and insulin regular *on page 452*
Humulin® L *(Discontinued)*
Humulin® 70/30 [US/Can] *see* insulin NPH and insulin regular *on page 452*
Humulin® N [US/Can] *see* insulin NPH *on page 452*
Humulin® R [US/Can] *see* insulin regular *on page 453*
Humulin® R (Concentrated) U-500 [US] *see* insulin regular *on page 453*
Humulin® U *(Discontinued)*
Hurricaine® [US-OTC] *see* benzocaine *on page 99*
HXM *see* altretamine *on page 35*
Hyalgan® [US] *see* hyaluronate and derivatives *on this page*
hyaluronan *see* hyaluronate and derivatives *on this page*

hyaluronate and derivatives (hye al yoor ON ate & dah RIV ah tives)

Sound-Alike/Look-Alike Issues
Healon® may be confused with Halcion®
Synvisc® may be confused with Synagis®

Synonyms hyaluronan; hyaluronic acid; hylan polymers; sodium hyaluronate

U.S./Canadian Brand Names Biolon™ [US]; Cystistat® [Can]; Durolane® [Can]; Euflexxa™ [US]; Eyestil [Can]; Healon GV® [US/Can]; Healon® [US/Can]; Healon®5 [US]; Hyalgan® [US]; Hylaform® Plus [US]; Hylaform® [US]; IPM Wound Gel™ [US-OTC]; OrthoVisc® [US/Can]; Provisc® [US]; Restylane® [US]; Supartz™ [US]; Suplasyn® [Can]; Synvisc® [US]; Vitrax® [US]

Therapeutic Category Antirheumatic Miscellaneous; Ophthalmic Agent, Viscoelastic; Skin and Mucous Membrane Agent

Use
Intraarticular injection: Treatment of pain in osteoarthritis in knee in patients who have failed nonpharmacologic treatment and simple analgesics
Intradermal: Correction of moderate-to-severe facial wrinkles or folds
Ophthalmic: Surgical aid in cataract extraction, intraocular implantation, corneal transplant, glaucoma filtration, and retinal attachment surgery
Topical: Management of skin ulcers and wounds

Usual Dosage Adults:
Osteoarthritis of the knee: Intra-articular:
Eulexxa™: Inject 20 mg (2 mL) once weekly for 3 weeks

Hyalgan®: Inject 20 mg (2 mL) once weekly for 5 weeks; some patients may benefit with a total of 3 injections

Orthovisc®: Inject 30 mg (2 mL) once weekly for 3-4 weeks

Supartz™: Inject 25 mg (2.5 mL) once weekly for 5 weeks

Synvisc®: Inject 16 mg (2 mL) once weekly for 3 weeks (total of 3 injections)

Facial wrinkles: Intradermal (Hylaform®, Hylaform® Plus, Restylane®): Inject as required for cosmetic result; typical treatment regimen requires <2 mL; limit injection to ≤1.5 mL per injection site. Hylaform®, Hylaform® Plus: Maximum: 20 mL/60 kg/year

Ophthalmic (Biolon™, Healon®, Provisc®, Vitrax®): Depends upon procedure (slowly introduce a sufficient quantity into eye)

Topical (IPM Wound Gel™): Apply to clean dry ulcer or wound, and cover with nonstick dressing; repeat daily. Discontinue if wound size increase after 3-4 applications.

Dosage Forms

Hylan B: Injection, gel:

Hylaform® [500 micron particle]: 5.5 mg/mL (0.75 mL) [prefilled syringe; derived from avian source]

Hylaform® Plus [700 micron particle]: 5.5 mg/mL (0.75 mL) [prefilled syringe; derived from avian source]

Hylan polymers A and B (Hylan G-F 20): Injection, solution, intra-articular (Synvisc®): 8 mg/mL (2 mL) [prefilled syringe; contains trace amounts of *Streptococcus*]

Sodium Hyaluronate:

Gel, topical (IPM Wound Gel™): 2.5% (10 g)

Injection, gel, intradermal (Restylane®): 20 mg/mL [prefilled syringe]

Injection, solution, intra-articular:

Euflexxa™: 10 mg/mL (2 mL) [prefilled syringe; syringe contains latex]

Hyalgan®: 10 mg/mL (2 mL)

Orthovisc®: 15 mg/mL (2 mL) [prefilled syringe; derived from avian source]

Supartz™: 10 mg/mL (2.5 mL) [derived from avian source]

Synvisc®: 8 mg/mL (2 mL) [prefilled syringe; derived from avian source]

Injection, solution, intraocular:

Biolon™: 10 mg/mL (0.5 mL, 1 mL)

Healon®: 10 mg/mL (0.4 mL, 0.55 mL, 0.85 mL, 2 mL)

Healon®5: 23 mg/mL

Healon GV®: 14 mg/mL (0.55 mL, 0.85 mL)

Provisc®: 10 mg/mL (0.4 mL, 0.55 mL, 0.8 mL) [prefilled syringe; contains lactose]

Vitrax®: 30 mg/mL (0.65 mL)

hyaluronic acid *see* hyaluronate and derivatives *on previous page*

hyaluronidase (hye al yoor ON i dase)

Sound-Alike/Look-Alike Issues

Wydase® may be confused with Lidex®, Wyamine®

U.S./Canadian Brand Names Amphadase™ [US]; Hydase™ [US]; Hylenex™ [US]; Vitrase® [US]

Therapeutic Category Enzyme

Use Increase the dispersion and absorption of other drugs; increase rate of absorption of parenteral fluids given by hypodermoclysis; adjunct in subcutaneous urography for improving resorption of radiopaque agents

Usual Dosage Note: A preliminary skin test for hypersensitivity can be performed. ACTH, antihistamines, corticosteroids, estrogens, and salicylates, when used in large doses, may cause tissues to be partly resistant to hyaluronidase. May require larger doses of hyaluronidase for the same effect.

Skin test: Intradermal: 0.02 mL (3 units) of a 150 units/mL solution. Positive reaction consists of a wheal with pseudopods appearing within 5 minutes and persisting for 20-30 minutes with localized itching.

Hypodermoclysis: SubQ: 15 units is added to each 100 mL of I.V. fluid to be administered; 150 units facilitates absorption of >1000 mL of solution

Premature Infants and Neonates: Volume of a single clysis should not exceed 25 mL/kg and the rate of administration should not exceed 2 mL/minute

Children <3 years: Volume of a single clysis should not exceed 200 mL

Children ≥3 years and Adults: Rate and volume of a single clysis should not exceed those used for infusion of I.V. fluids

Urography: Children and Adults: SubQ: 75 units over each scapula followed by injection of contrast medium at the same site; patient should be in the prone position.

Dosage Forms

Injection, powder for reconstitution:

Vitrase®: 6200 units [ovine derived; contains lactose]

(Continued)

hyaluronidase *(Continued)*

Injection, solution:

Amphadase™: 150 units/mL (2 mL) [bovine derived; contains edetate disodium 1 mg, thimerosal ≤0.1 mg]

Injection, solution [preservative free]:

Hydase™: 150 units/mL (2 mL) [bovine derived; contains edetate disodium 1 mg]

Hylenex™: 150 units/mL (1 mL, 2 mL) [recombinant; contains human albumin and edetate disodium]

Vitrase®: 200 units/mL (2 mL) [ovine derived; contains lactulose]

hycamptamine *see* topotecan *on page 836*

Hycamtin® [US/Can] *see* topotecan *on page 836*

hycet™ [US] *see* hydrocodone and acetaminophen *on page 420*

HycoClear Tuss® *(Discontinued)* *see* hydrocodone and guaifenesin *on page 422*

Hycodan® [US] *see* hydrocodone and homatropine *on page 423*

Hycomine® Compound [US] *see* hydrocodone, chlorpheniramine, phenylephrine, acetaminophen, and caffeine *on page 424*

Hycomine® *(Discontinued)*

Hycomine® Pediatric *(Discontinued)*

Hycort™ [Can] *see* hydrocortisone (topical) *on page 428*

Hycotuss® [US] *see* hydrocodone and guaifenesin *on page 422*

Hydase™ [US] *see* hyaluronidase *on previous page*

Hydeltra T.B.A.® [Can] *see* prednisolone (systemic) *on page 695*

Hydergine® [Can] *see* ergoloid mesylates *on page 301*

Hydergine® *(Discontinued)* *see* ergoloid mesylates *on page 301*

Hyderm [Can] *see* hydrocortisone (topical) *on page 428*

hydralazine (hye DRAL a zeen)

Sound-Alike/Look-Alike Issues

hydrALAZINE may be confused with hydrochlorothiazide, hydrOXYzine

Synonyms hydralazine hydrochloride

Tall-Man hydr**ALAZINE**

U.S./Canadian Brand Names Apo-Hydralazine® [Can]; Apresoline® [Can]; Novo-Hylazin [Can]; Nu-Hydral [Can]

Therapeutic Category Vasodilator

Use Management of moderate to severe hypertension, congestive heart failure, hypertension secondary to preeclampsia/eclampsia; treatment of primary pulmonary hypertension

Usual Dosage

Children:

Oral: Initial: 0.75-1 mg/kg/day in 2-4 divided doses; increase over 3-4 weeks to maximum of 7.5 mg/kg/day in 2-4 divided doses; maximum daily dose: 200 mg/day

I.M., I.V.: 0.1-0.2 mg/kg/dose (not to exceed 20 mg) every 4-6 hours as needed, up to 1.7-3.5 mg/kg/day in 4-6 divided doses

Adults:

Oral:

Hypertension:

Initial dose: 10 mg 4 times/day for first 2-4 days; increase to 25 mg 4 times/day for the balance of the first week

Increase by 10-25 mg/dose gradually to 50 mg 4 times/day (maximum: 300 mg/day); usual dose range (JNC 7): 25-100 mg/day in 2 divided doses

Congestive heart failure:

Initial dose: 10-25 mg 3-4 times/day

Adjustment: Dosage must be adjusted based on individual response

Target dose: 225-300 mg/day in divided doses; use in combination with isosorbide dinitrate

I.M., I.V.:

Hypertension: Initial: 10-20 mg/dose every 4-6 hours as needed, may increase to 40 mg/dose; change to oral therapy as soon as possible.

Pre-eclampsia/eclampsia: 5 mg/dose then 5-10 mg every 20-30 minutes as needed.

Dosage Forms

Injection, solution, as hydrochloride: 20 mg/mL (1 mL)

Tablet, as hydrochloride: 10 mg, 25 mg, 50 mg, 100 mg

hydralazine and hydrochlorothiazide (hye DRAL a zeen & hye droe klor oh THYE a zide)

Synonyms hydrochlorothiazide and hydralazine

Therapeutic Category Antihypertensive Agent, Combination

Use Management of moderate to severe hypertension and treatment of congestive heart failure

Usual Dosage Adults: Oral: Hydralazine 25-100 mg/day and hydrochlorothiazide 25-50 mg/day in 2 divided doses (maximum: hydrochlorothiazide: 50 mg/day)

Dosage Forms Capsule:
- 25/25: Hydralazine hydrochloride 25 mg and hydrochlorothiazide 25 mg
- 50/50: Hydralazine hydrochloride 50 mg and hydrochlorothiazide 50 mg
- 100/50: Hydralazine hydrochloride 100 mg and hydrochlorothiazide 50 mg

hydralazine and isosorbide dinitrate *see* isosorbide dinitrate and hydralazine *on page 465*

hydralazine hydrochloride *see* hydralazine *on previous page*

Hydramine® [US-OTC] *see* diphenhydramine *on page 261*

hydrated chloral *see* chloral hydrate *on page 171*

Hydrate® *(Discontinued)* *see* dimenhydrinate *on page 258*

Hydrea® [US/Can] *see* hydroxyurea *on page 432*

Hydrisalic™ [US-OTC] *see* salicylic acid *on page 758*

Hydrocet® *(Discontinued)* *see* hydrocodone and acetaminophen *on next page*

hydrochlorothiazide (hye droe klor oh THYE a zide)

Sound-Alike/Look-Alike Issues
- hydrochlorothiazide may be confused with hydralazine, hydrocortisone, hydroflumethiazide
- Esidrix may be confused with Lasix®
- HCTZ is an error-prone abbreviation

U.S./Canadian Brand Names Apo-Hydro® [Can]; Microzide™ [US]; Novo-Hydrazide [Can]; PMS-Hydrochlorothiazide [Can]

Therapeutic Category Diuretic, Thiazide

Use Management of mild to moderate hypertension; treatment of edema in congestive heart failure and nephrotic syndrome

Usual Dosage Oral (effect of drug may be decreased when used every day):

Children (in pediatric patients, chlorothiazide may be preferred over hydrochlorothiazide as there are more dosage formulations [eg, suspension] available):
- <6 months: 2-3 mg/kg/day in 2 divided doses
- >6 months: 2 mg/kg/day in 2 divided doses

Adults:
- Edema: 25-100 mg/day in 1-2 doses; maximum: 200 mg/day
- Hypertension: 12.5-50 mg/day; minimal increase in response and more electrolyte disturbances are seen with doses >50 mg/day

Dosage Forms
- Capsule (Microzide™): 12.5 mg
- Tablet: 25 mg, 50 mg

hydrochlorothiazide and amiloride *see* amiloride and hydrochlorothiazide *on page 41*

hydrochlorothiazide and benazepril *see* benazepril and hydrochlorothiazide *on page 97*

hydrochlorothiazide and bisoprolol *see* bisoprolol and hydrochlorothiazide *on page 113*

hydrochlorothiazide and captopril *see* captopril and hydrochlorothiazide *on page 143*

hydrochlorothiazide and enalapril *see* enalapril and hydrochlorothiazide *on page 292*

hydrochlorothiazide and eprosartan *see* eprosartan and hydrochlorothiazide *on page 300*

hydrochlorothiazide and fosinopril *see* fosinopril and hydrochlorothiazide *on page 369*

hydrochlorothiazide and hydralazine *see* hydralazine and hydrochlorothiazide *on this page*

hydrochlorothiazide and irbesartan *see* irbesartan and hydrochlorothiazide *on page 461*

hydrochlorothiazide and lisinopril *see* lisinopril and hydrochlorothiazide *on page 501*

hydrochlorothiazide and losartan *see* losartan and hydrochlorothiazide *on page 507*

hydrochlorothiazide and methyldopa *see* methyldopa and hydrochlorothiazide *on page 545*

hydrochlorothiazide and metoprolol *see* metoprolol and hydrochlorothiazide *on page 550*

hydrochlorothiazide and metoprolol tartrate *see* metoprolol and hydrochlorothiazide *on page 550*

hydrochlorothiazide and moexipril *see* moexipril and hydrochlorothiazide *on page 563*

hydrochlorothiazide and olmesartan medoxomil *see* olmesartan and hydrochlorothiazide *on page 614*

hydrochlorothiazide and propranolol *see* propranolol and hydrochlorothiazide *on page 710*

hydrochlorothiazide and quinapril *see* quinapril and hydrochlorothiazide *on page 725*

hydrochlorothiazide and spironolactone

(hye droe klor oh THYE a zide & speer on oh LAK tone)

Sound-Alike/Look-Alike Issues

Aldactazide® may be confused with Aldactone®

Synonyms spironolactone and hydrochlorothiazide

U.S./Canadian Brand Names Aldactazide 25® [Can]; Aldactazide 50® [Can]; Aldactazide® [US]; Novo-Spirozine [Can]

Therapeutic Category Antihypertensive Agent, Combination

Use Management of mild- to-moderate hypertension; treatment of edema in congestive heart failure and nephrotic syndrome, and cirrhosis of the liver accompanied by edema and/or ascites

Usual Dosage Oral:

Children: 1.5-3 mg/kg/day in 2-4 divided doses (maximum: 200 mg/day)

Adults: Hydrochlorothiazide 12.5-50 mg/day and spironolactone 12.5-50 mg/day; manufacturer labeling states hydrochlorothiazide maximum 200 mg/day, however, usual dose in JNC-7 is 12.5-50 mg/day

Dosage Forms

Tablet: Hydrochlorothiazide 25 mg and spironolactone 25 mg

Aldactazide®:

25/25: Hydrochlorothiazide 25 mg and spironolactone 25 mg

50/50: Hydrochlorothiazide 50 mg and spironolactone 50 mg

hydrochlorothiazide and telmisartan *see* telmisartan and hydrochlorothiazide *on page 808*

hydrochlorothiazide and triamterene

(hye droe klor oh THYE a zide & trye AM ter een)

Sound-Alike/Look-Alike Issues

Dyazide® may be confused with diazoxide, Dynacin®

Maxzide® may be confused with Maxidex®

Synonyms triamterene and hydrochlorothiazide

U.S./Canadian Brand Names Apo-Triazide® [Can]; Dyazide® [US]; Maxzide® [US]; Maxzide®-25 [US]; Novo-Triamzide [Can]; Nu-Triazide [Can]; Penta-Triamterene HCTZ [Can]; Riva-Zide [Can]

Therapeutic Category Antihypertensive Agent, Combination

Use Management of mild to moderate hypertension; treatment of edema in congestive heart failure and nephrotic syndrome

Usual Dosage Adults: Oral:

Hydrochlorothiazide 25 mg and triamterene 37.5 mg: 1-2 tablets/capsules once daily

Hydrochlorothiazide 50 mg and triamterene 75 mg: $^1/_2$-1 tablet daily

Dosage Forms

Capsule (Dyazide®): Hydrochlorothiazide 25 mg and triamterene 37.5 mg

Tablet:

Maxzide®: Hydrochlorothiazide 50 mg and triamterene 75 mg

Maxzide®-25: Hydrochlorothiazide 25 mg and triamterene 37.5 mg

hydrochlorothiazide and valsartan *see* valsartan and hydrochlorothiazide *on page 865*

Hydrocil® Instant [US-OTC] *see* psyllium *on page 717*

hydrocodone and acetaminophen

(hye droe KOE done & a seet a MIN oh fen)

Sound-Alike/Look-Alike Issues

Lorcet® may be confused with Fioricet®

Lortab® may be confused with Cortef®, Lorabid®, Luride®

Vicodin® may be confused with Hycodan®, Hycomine®, Indocin®, Uridon®

Zydone® may be confused with Vytone®

Synonyms acetaminophen and hydrocodone

U.S./Canadian Brand Names Anexsia® [US]; Bancap HC® [US]; Ceta-Plus® [US]; Co-Gesic® [US]; hycet™ [US]; Lorcet® 10/650 [US]; Lorcet® Plus [US]; Lortab® [US]; Margesic® H [US]; Maxidone™ [US]; Norco® [US]; Stagesic® [US]; Vicodin® ES [US]; Vicodin® HP [US]; Vicodin® [US]; Zydone® [US]

Therapeutic Category Analgesic, Narcotic

Controlled Substance C-III

Use Relief of moderate to severe pain

Usual Dosage Oral (doses should be titrated to appropriate analgesic effect): Analgesic:

Children 2-13 years or <50 kg: Hydrocodone 0.135 mg/kg/dose every 4-6 hours; do not exceed 6 doses/day or the maximum recommended dose of acetaminophen

Children and Adults ≥50 kg: Average starting dose in opioid naive patients: Hydrocodone 5-10 mg 4 times/day; the dosage of acetaminophen should be limited to ≤4 g/day (and possibly less in patients with hepatic impairment or ethanol use).

Dosage ranges (based on specific product labeling): Hydrocodone 2.5-10 mg every 4-6 hours; maximum: 60 mg hydrocodone/day (maximum dose of hydrocodone may be limited by the acetaminophen content of specific product)

Dosage Forms

Capsule:

Bancap HC®, Ceta-Plus®, Margesic® H, Stagesic®: Hydrocodone bitartrate 5 mg and acetaminophen 500 mg

Elixir: Hydrocodone bitartrate 7.5 mg and acetaminophen 500 mg per 15 mL (480 mL)

Lortab®: Hydrocodone bitartrate 7.5 mg and acetaminophen 500 mg per 15 mL (480 mL) [contains alcohol 7%; tropical fruit punch flavor]

Solution, oral:

hycet™: Hydrocodone bitartrate 7.5 mg and acetaminophen 325 mg per 15 mL (480 mL) [contains alcohol 7%; tropical fruit punch flavor]

Tablet:

Hydrocodone bitartrate 2.5 mg and acetaminophen 500 mg
Hydrocodone bitartrate 5 mg and acetaminophen 325 mg
Hydrocodone bitartrate 5 mg and acetaminophen 500 mg
Hydrocodone bitartrate 7.5 mg and acetaminophen 325 mg
Hydrocodone bitartrate 7.5 mg and acetaminophen 500 mg
Hydrocodone bitartrate 7.5 mg and acetaminophen 650 mg
Hydrocodone bitartrate 7.5 mg and acetaminophen 750 mg
Hydrocodone bitartrate 10 mg and acetaminophen 325 mg
Hydrocodone bitartrate 10 mg and acetaminophen 500 mg
Hydrocodone bitartrate 10 mg and acetaminophen 650 mg
Hydrocodone bitartrate 10 mg and acetaminophen 660 mg

Anexsia®:

5/500: Hydrocodone bitartrate 5 mg and acetaminophen 500 mg [DSC]
7.5/650: Hydrocodone bitartrate 7.5 mg and acetaminophen 650 mg

Co-Gesic® 5/500: Hydrocodone bitartrate 5 mg and acetaminophen 500 mg

Lorcet® 10/650: Hydrocodone bitartrate 10 mg and acetaminophen 650 mg

Lorcet® Plus: Hydrocodone bitartrate 7.5 mg and acetaminophen 650 mg

Lortab®:

2.5/500: Hydrocodone bitartrate 2.5 mg and acetaminophen 500 mg
5/500: Hydrocodone bitartrate 5 mg and acetaminophen 500 mg
7.5/500: Hydrocodone bitartrate 7.5 mg and acetaminophen 500 mg
10/500: Hydrocodone bitartrate 10 mg and acetaminophen 500 mg

Maxidone™: Hydrocodone bitartrate 10 mg and acetaminophen 750 mg

Norco®:

Hydrocodone bitartrate 5 mg and acetaminophen 325 mg
Hydrocodone bitartrate 7.5 mg and acetaminophen 325 mg
Hydrocodone bitartrate 10 mg and acetaminophen 325 mg

Vicodin®: Hydrocodone bitartrate 5 mg and acetaminophen 500 mg

Vicodin® ES: Hydrocodone bitartrate 7.5 mg and acetaminophen 750 mg

Vicodin® HP: Hydrocodone bitartrate 10 mg and acetaminophen 660 mg

Zydone®:

Hydrocodone bitartrate 5 mg and acetaminophen 400 mg
Hydrocodone bitartrate 7.5 mg and acetaminophen 400 mg
Hydrocodone bitartrate 10 mg and acetaminophen 400 mg

hydrocodone and aspirin (hye droe KOE done & AS pir in)

Synonyms aspirin and hydrocodone

U.S./Canadian Brand Names Damason-P® [US]

Therapeutic Category Analgesic, Narcotic

Controlled Substance C-III

Use Relief of moderate to moderately severe pain

Usual Dosage Adults: Oral: 1-2 tablets every 4-6 hours as needed for pain

Dosage Forms Tablet: Hydrocodone bitartrate 5 mg and aspirin 500 mg

hydrocodone and chlorpheniramine (hye droe KOE done & klor fen IR a meen)

Synonyms chlorpheniramine maleate and hydrocodone bitartrate; hydrocodone tannate and chlorpheniramine tannate

U.S./Canadian Brand Names HyTan™ [US]; Tussionex® [US]

Therapeutic Category Antihistamine/Antitussive

Controlled Substance C-III

Use Symptomatic relief of cough and upper respiratory symptoms associated with cold and allergy

Usual Dosage Oral:

Children 6-12 years:

HyTan™: 5 mL every 12 hours; do not exceed 10 mL/24 hours

Tussionex®: 2.5 mL every 12 hours; do not exceed 5 mL/24 hours

Children >12 years and Adults:

HyTan™: 10 mL every 12 hours; do not exceed 20 mL/24 hours

Tussionex®: 5 mL every 12 hours; do not exceed 10 mL/24 hours

Dosage Forms

Suspension:

HyTan™: Hydrocodone tannate 5 mg and chlorpheniramine tannate 4 mg (120 mL) [contains phenylalanine 12.5 mg/5 mL; tropical fruit flavor]

Suspension, extended release:

Tussionex®: Hydrocodone polistirex [equivalent to hydrocodone bitartrate 10 mg] and chlorpheniramine polistirex [equivalent to chlorpheniramine maleate 8 mg] per 5 mL (480 mL)

hydrocodone and guaifenesin (hye droe KOE done & gwye FEN e sin)

Sound-Alike/Look-Alike Issues

Vicodin® may be confused with Hycodan®, Hycomine®, Indocin®, Uridon®

Synonyms guaifenesin and hydrocodone

U.S./Canadian Brand Names Atuss® HX [US]; Codiclear® DH [US]; Hycotuss® [US]; Hydro-Tussin™ [US]; Kwelcof® [US]; Maxi-Tuss HCG [US]; Pneumotussin® [US]; Vitussin [US]

Therapeutic Category Antitussive/Expectorant

Controlled Substance C-III

Use Symptomatic relief of nonproductive coughs associated with upper and lower respiratory tract congestion

Usual Dosage

Children:

6-12 years:

Atuss® Hx: One capsule every 8 hours

Codiclear® DH, Hycotuss®, Kwelcof®, Maxi-Tuss HCG: 2.5-5 mL every 4 hours, after meals and at bedtime

Hydro-Tussin™ HG: 2.5 mL after meals and at bedtime

Pneumotussin®: One tablet or 5 mL every 4-6 hours (maximum: 4 doses/24 hours)

>12 years:

Codiclear® DH, Hycotuss®, Kwelcof®, Maxi-Tuss HCG: 5-10 mL every 4 hours, after meals and at bedtime

Hydro-Tussin™ HG: 5 mL after meals and at bedtime; may increase to 10 mL/dose if needed (maximum: 30 mL/day)

Pneumotussin®: 1-2 tablets or 10 mL every 4-6 hours (maximum: 4 doses/24 hours)

Children ≥12 years and Adults (Atuss® HX): 1-2 capsules every 8 hours

Adults:

Codiclear® DH, Kwelcof®, Hycotuss®: 5-15 mL every 4 hours, after meals and at bedtime (maximum: 30 mL/24 hours)

Hydro-Tussin™ HG: 5 mL after meals and at bedtime; may increase to 15 mL/dose if needed (maximum: 30 mL/day)

Maxi-Tuss HCG: 5-10 mL every 4 hours, after meals and at bedtime

Pneumotussin®: 1-2 tablets or 10 mL every 4-6 hours (maximum: 4 doses/24 hours)

Dosage Forms

Caplet:

Ztuss™ ZT: Hydrocodone bitartrate 5 mg and guaifenesin 300 mg

Capsule, variable release:

Atuss® HX: Hydrocodone bitartrate 5 mg [immediate release] and guaifenesin 100 mg [sustained release]

Liquid: Hydrocodone bitartrate 5 mg and guaifenesin 100 mg per 5 mL (480 mL, 960 mL)

ExeCof-XP: Hydrocodone bitartrate 3 mg and guaifenesin 90 mg per 5 mL (3840 mL) [contains benzoic acid]

Kwelcof®: Hydrocodone bitartrate 5 mg and guaifenesin 100 mg per 5 mL (480 mL) [alcohol free, dye free, sugar free; contains benzoic acid; apricot-pineapple flavor]

Pancof-XP: Hydrocodone bitartrate 3 mg and guaifenesin 90 mg per 5 mL (3840 mL) [contains benzoic acid]

Phanatuss® HC: Hydrocodone bitartrate 5 mg and guaifenesin 100 mg per 5 mL (480 mL) [alcohol free, sugar free; mint flavor]

Vitussin: Hydrocodone bitartrate 5 mg and guaifenesin 100 mg per 5 mL (480 mL) [alcohol free, sugar free, dye free; cherry flavor]

Tablet:

EndaCof: Hydrocodone bitartrate 2.5 mg and guaifenesin 300 mg

Pneumotussin®: Hydrocodone bitartrate 2.5 mg and guaifenesin 300 mg [dye free]

Touro® HC: Hydrocodone bitartrate 5 mg and guaifenesin 575 mg

Tablet, sustained release:

Extendryl® HC: Hydrocodone bitartrate 10 mg and guaifenesin 1000 mg

Xpect-HC™: Hydrocodone bitartrate 5 mg and guaifenesin 600 mg

Syrup: Hydrocodone bitartrate 5 mg and guaifenesin 100 mg per 5 mL (480 mL)

Codiclear® DH: Hydrocodone bitartrate 3.5 mg and guaifenesin 100 mg per 5 mL (120 mL, 480 mL) [alcohol free, dye free, sugar free; contains benzoic acid; grape flavor]

EndaCof-XP: Hydrocodone bitartrate 2.5 mg and guaifenesin 200 mg per 5 mL (480 mL) [alcohol free, dye free, sugar free; contains phenylalanine; cherry punch flavor]

Hycotuss®: Hydrocodone bitartrate 5 mg and guaifenesin 100 mg per 5 mL (480 mL) [contains alcohol 10%; butterscotch flavor]

Hydro-Tussin™ HG: Hydrocodone bitartrate 3.5 mg and guaifenesin 100 mg per 5 mL (480 mL) [alcohol free, dye free, sugar free; grape flavor]

Maxi-Tuss HCG: Hydrocodone bitartrate 6 mg and guaifenesin 200 mg per 5 mL (480 mL) [alcohol free, sugar free; contains aspartame; butterscotch flavor]

Pneumotussin®: Hydrocodone bitartrate 2.5 mg and guaifenesin 200 mg per 5 mL (480 mL) [alcohol free, dye free, sugar free; cherry punch flavor]

Tusso-DF®: Hydrocodone bitartrate 2.5 mg and guaifenesin 100 mg per 5 mL (480 mL) [cherry flavor]

hydrocodone and homatropine (hye droe KOE done & hoe MA troe peen)

Sound-Alike/Look-Alike Issues

Hycodan® may be confused with Hycomine®, Vicodin®

Synonyms homatropine and hydrocodone

U.S./Canadian Brand Names Hycodan® [US]; Hydromet® [US]; Tussigon® [US]

Therapeutic Category Antitussive

Controlled Substance C-III

Use Symptomatic relief of cough

Usual Dosage Oral:

Children 6-12 years: 1/2 tablet or 2.5 mL every 4-6 hours as needed (maximum: 3 tablets or 15 mL/24 hours)

Children ≥12 years and Adults: 1 tablet or 5 mL every 4-6 hours as needed (maximum: 6 tablets/24 hours or 30 mL/24 hours)

Dosage Forms

Syrup:

Hycodan®, Hydromet®: Hydrocodone bitartrate 5 mg and homatropine methylbromide 1.5 mg per 5 mL (480 mL) [cherry flavor]

Tablet: Hydrocodone bitartrate 5 mg and homatropine methylbromide 1.5 mg

Hycodan®, Tussigon®: Hydrocodone bitartrate 5 mg and homatropine methylbromide 1.5 mg

hydrocodone and ibuprofen (hye droe KOE done & eye byoo PROE fen)

Synonyms ibuprofen and hydrocodone

U.S./Canadian Brand Names Reprexain™ [US]; Vicoprofen® [US/Can]

Therapeutic Category Analgesic, Narcotic

Controlled Substance C-III

Use Short-term (generally <10 days) management of moderate to severe acute pain; is not indicated for treatment of such conditions as osteoarthritis or rheumatoid arthritis

Usual Dosage Adults: Oral: 1 tablet every 4-6 hours as needed for pain; maximum: 5 tablets/day

Dosage Forms

Tablet: Hydrocodone bitartrate 5 mg and ibuprofen 200 mg; hydrocodone bitartrate 7.5 mg and ibuprofen 200 mg

Reprexain™: Hydrocodone bitartrate 5 mg and ibuprofen 200 mg

Vicoprofen®: Hydrocodone bitartrate 7.5 mg and ibuprofen 200 mg

hydrocodone and pseudoephedrine (hye droe KOE done & soo doe e FED rin)

Synonyms pseudoephedrine and hydrocodone

U.S./Canadian Brand Names Histussin D® [US]; P-V Tussin Tablet [US]

Therapeutic Category Cough and Cold Combination

Controlled Substance C-III

Use Symptomatic relief of cough due to colds, nasal congestion, and cough

Usual Dosage Oral: Adults: 5 mL 4 times/day

Dosage Forms

Syrup (Histussin D®): Hydrocodone bitartrate 5 mg and pseudoephedrine hydrochloride 60 mg per 5 mL (480 mL)

Tablet (P-V Tussin): Hydrocodone bitartrate 5 mg and pseudoephedrine hydrochloride 60 mg

hydrocodone bitartrate, carbinoxamine maleate, and pseudoephedrine hydrochloride *see* hydrocodone, carbinoxamine, and pseudoephedrine *on this page*

hydrocodone bitartrate, phenylephrine hydrochloride, and diphenhydramine hydrochloride *see* hydrocodone, phenylephrine, and diphenhydramine *on next page*

hydrocodone, carbinoxamine, and pseudoephedrine

(hye droe KOE done, kar bi NOKS a meen, & soo doe e FED rin)

Synonyms carbinoxamine, pseudoephedrine, and hydrocodone; hydrocodone bitartrate, carbinoxamine maleate, and pseudoephedrine hydrochloride; pseudoephedrine, hydrocodone, and carbinoxamine

U.S./Canadian Brand Names Histex™ HC [US]; Tri-Vent™ HC [US]

Therapeutic Category Antihistamine/Decongestant/Antitussive

Controlled Substance C-III

Use Symptomatic relief of cough, congestion, and rhinorrhea associated with the common cold, influenza, bronchitis, or sinusitis

Usual Dosage Oral: Relief of cough, congestion, and runny nose:

Children:

2-10 years: Dosing based on hydrocodone content: 0.6 mg/kg/day given in 4 divided doses. Alternately, the following dosing may be used based on age:

2-4 years: 1.25 mL every 4-6 hours; maximum dose: 7.5 mL/24 hours

4-10 years: 2.5 mL every 4-6 hours; maximum dose: 15 mL/24 hours

>10 years: Refer to Adults dosing

Adults: 5-10 mL every 4-6 hours; maximum dose: 30 mL/24 hours

Dosage Forms [DSC] = Discontinued product

Liquid: Hydrocodone bitartrate 5 mg, carbinoxamine maleate 2 mg, and pseudoephedrine hydrochloride 30 mg per 5 mL (480 mL) [DSC]

Histex™ HC, Tri-Vent™ HC: Hydrocodone bitartrate 5 mg, carbinoxamine maleate 2 mg, and pseudoephedrine hydrochloride 30 mg per 5 mL (480 mL) [alcohol free, sugar free; peach flavor]

hydrocodone, chlorpheniramine, and pseudoephedrine *see* pseudoephedrine, hydrocodone, and chlorpheniramine *on page 716*

hydrocodone, chlorpheniramine, phenylephrine, acetaminophen, and caffeine (hye droe KOE done, klor fen IR a meen, fen il EF rin, a seet a MIN oh fen, & KAF een)

Sound-Alike/Look-Alike Issues

Hycomine® may be confused with Byclomine®, Hycamtin®, Hycodan®, Vicodin®

Synonyms acetaminophen, caffeine, hydrocodone, chlorpheniramine, and phenylephrine; caffeine, hydrocodone, chlorpheniramine, phenylephrine, and acetaminophen; chlorpheniramine, hydrocodone, phenylephrine, acetaminophen, and caffeine; phenylephrine, hydrocodone, chlorpheniramine, acetaminophen, and caffeine

U.S./Canadian Brand Names Hycomine® Compound [US]

Therapeutic Category Antitussive

Controlled Substance C-III

Use Symptomatic relief of cough and symptoms of upper respiratory infection

Usual Dosage Adults: Oral: 1 tablet every 4 hours, up to 4 times/day

Dosage Forms Tablet: Hydrocodone bitartrate 5 mg, chlorpheniramine maleate 2 mg, phenylephrine hydrochloride 10 mg, acetaminophen 250 mg, and caffeine 30 mg [cherry flavor]

Hydrocodone PA® Syrup *(Discontinued)*

hydrocodone, phenylephrine, and chlorpheniramine *see* phenylephrine, hydrocodone, and chlorpheniramine *on page 663*

hydrocodone, phenylephrine, and diphenhydramine

(hye droe KOE done, fen il EF rin, & dye fen HYE dra meen)

Sound-Alike/Look-Alike Issues

Endal® may be confused with Depen®, Intal®

Synonyms diphenhydramine, hydrocodone, and phenylephrine; hydrocodone bitartrate, phenylephrine hydrochloride, and diphenhydramine hydrochloride; phenylephrine, diphenhydramine, and hydrocodone

U.S./Canadian Brand Names Endal® HD [US]; Hydro DP [US]; TussiNate™ [US]

Therapeutic Category Antihistamine/Decongestant/Antitussive; Antitussive; Decongestant

Controlled Substance C-III

Use Symptomatic relief of cough and congestion associated with the common cold, sinusitis, or acute upper respiratory tract infections

Usual Dosage Oral: Relief of cough, congestion:

Children 6-12 years: 5 mL every 4 hours (maximum: 20 mL/24 hours)

Children >12 years and Adults: 10 mL every 4 hours (maximum: 40 mL/24 hours)

Dosage Forms Syrup:

Endal® HD: Hydrocodone bitartrate 2 mg, phenylephrine hydrochloride 7.5 mg, and diphenhydramine hydrochloride 12.5 mg per 5 mL (480 mL) [alcohol free, sugar free; contains sodium benzoate; cherry flavor]

Hydro DP: Hydrocodone bitartrate 2 mg, phenylephrine hydrochloride 7.5 mg, and diphenhydramine hydrochloride 12.5 mg per 5 mL (480 mL) [cherry flavor]

TussiNate™: Hydrocodone bitartrate 3.5 mg, phenylephrine hydrochloride 5 mg, and diphenhydramine hydrochloride 12.5 mg per 5 mL (480 mL) [alcohol free; contains sodium benzoate; black raspberry flavor]

hydrocodone, pseudoephedrine, and guaifenesin

(hye droe KOE done, soo doe e FED rin & gwye FEN e sin)

Synonyms guaifenesin, hydrocodone, and pseudoephedrine; pseudoephedrine, hydrocodone, and guaifenesin

U.S./Canadian Brand Names Hydro-Tussin™ HD [US]; Hydro-Tussin™ XP [US]; Su-Tuss®-HD [US]; Ztuss™ Tablet [US]

Therapeutic Category Antitussive/Decongestant/Expectorant

Controlled Substance C-III

Use Symptomatic relief of irritating, nonproductive cough associated with upper respiratory conditions and allergies

Usual Dosage Oral: Cough/congestion:

Children:

2-6 years: Hydro-Tussin™ XP: 1.25-2.5 mL 4 times/day as needed

6-12 years:

Hydro-Tussin™ XP: 2.5-5 mL 4 times/day as needed

Tussend®, Hydro-Tussin™ HD: 5 mL every 4-6 hours as needed

Ztuss™: One-half to 1 tablet every 4-6 hours (maximum: 6 tablets/24 hours)

Children ≥12 years and Adults:

Hydro-Tussin™ XP: 5-10 mL 4 times/day as needed

Tussend®, Hydro-Tussin™ HD: 10 mL every 4-6 hours as needed

Ztuss™: 1-1½ tablets every 4-6 hours (maximum: 8 tablets/24 hours)

(Continued)

hydrocodone, pseudoephedrine, and guaifenesin *(Continued)*

Dosage Forms [DSC] = Discontinued product

Elixir (Su-Tuss®-HD): Hydrocodone bitartrate 2.5 mg, pseudoephedrine hydrochloride 30 mg, and guaifenesin 100 mg per 5 mL (480 mL) [contains alcohol; fruit punch flavor]

Liquid:

Hydro-Tussin™ HD: Hydrocodone bitartrate 2.5 mg, pseudoephedrine hydrochloride 30 mg, and guaifenesin 100 mg per 5 mL (480 mL) [alcohol free; contains sodium benzoate]

Hydro-Tussin® XP: Hydrocodone bitartrate 3 mg, pseudoephedrine hydrochloride 15 mg, and guaifenesin 100 mg per 5 mL (480 mL) [alcohol free, dye free]

Tussend® Expectorant: Hydrocodone bitartrate 2.5 mg, pseudoephedrine hydrochloride 30 mg, and guaifenesin 100 mg per 5 mL (480 mL) [contains alcohol; fruit punch flavor] [DSC]

Tablet (Ztuss™): Hydrocodone bitartrate 5 mg, pseudoephedrine hydrochloride 30 mg, and guaifenesin 300 mg [sugar free]

hydrocodone tannate and chlorpheniramine tannate *see* hydrocodone and chlorpheniramine *on page 422*

hydrocortisone acetate *see* hydrocortisone (rectal) *on this page*

hydrocortisone acetate *see* hydrocortisone (topical) *on page 428*

hydrocortisone, acetic acid, and propylene glycol diacetate *see* acetic acid, propylene glycol diacetate, and hydrocortisone *on page 15*

hydrocortisone and benzoyl peroxide *see* benzoyl peroxide and hydrocortisone *on page 104*

hydrocortisone and ciprofloxacin *see* ciprofloxacin and hydrocortisone *on page 192*

hydrocortisone and iodoquinol *see* iodoquinol and hydrocortisone *on page 459*

hydrocortisone and lidocaine *see* lidocaine and hydrocortisone *on page 496*

hydrocortisone and pramoxine *see* pramoxine and hydrocortisone *on page 691*

hydrocortisone and urea *see* urea and hydrocortisone *on page 861*

hydrocortisone, bacitracin, neomycin, and polymyxin B *see* bacitracin, neomycin, polymyxin B, and hydrocortisone *on page 91*

hydrocortisone butyrate *see* hydrocortisone (topical) *on page 428*

hydrocortisone, neomycin, and polymyxin B *see* neomycin, polymyxin B, and hydrocortisone *on page 584*

hydrocortisone, neomycin, colistin, and thonzonium *see* neomycin, colistin, hydrocortisone, and thonzonium *on page 583*

hydrocortisone probutate *see* hydrocortisone (topical) *on page 428*

hydrocortisone (rectal) (hye droe KOR ti sone REK tal)

Sound-Alike/Look-Alike Issues

hydrocortisone may be confused with hydrocodone, hydroxychloroquine, hydrochlorothiazide

Synonyms hydrocortisone acetate

U.S./Canadian Brand Names Anucort-HC® [US]; Anusol-HC® [US]; Anusol® HC-1 [US-OTC]; Cortenema® [Can]; Cortifoam® [US/Can]; Hemril®-30 [US]; Preparation H® Hydrocortisone [US-OTC]; Procto-Kit™ [US]; Procto-Pak™ [US]; Proctocort® [US]; ProctoCream® HC [US]; Proctosert [US]; Proctosol-HC® [US]; Proctozone-HC™ [US]

Therapeutic Category Adrenal Corticosteroid

Use Adjunctive treatment of ulcerative colitis

Usual Dosage Adults: Rectal: Ulcerative colitis: 10-100 mg 1-2 times/day for 2-3 weeks

Dosage Forms [DSC] = Discontinued product

Aerosol, rectal, as acetate (Cortifoam®): 10% (15 g) [90 mg/applicator]

Cream, rectal, as acetate (Nupercainal® Hydrocortisone Cream): 1% (30 g) [strength expressed as base]

Cream, rectal, as base:

Cortizone®-10: 1% (30 g) [contains aloe]

Preparation H® Hydrocortisone: 1% (27 g)

Suppository, rectal, as acetate: 25 mg (12s, 24s, 100s)

Anucort-HC®, Tucks® Anti-Itch: 25 mg (12s, 24s, 100s) [strength expressed as base; Anucort-HC® *renamed* Tucks® Anti-Itch]

Anusol-HC®, Proctosol-HC®: 25 mg (12s, 24s)

Encort™: 30 mg (12s)

Hemril®-30, Proctocort®, Proctosert: 30 mg (12s, 24s)

Suspension, rectal, as base: 100 mg/60 mL (7s)

Colocort®: 100 mg/60 mL (1s, 7s)

hydrocortisone sodium succinate *see* hydrocortisone (systemic) *on this page*

hydrocortisone (systemic) (hye droe KOR ti sone sis TEM ik)

Sound-Alike/Look-Alike Issues

hydrocortisone may be confused with hydrocodone, hydroxychloroquine, hydrochlorothiazide
Cortef® may be confused with Lortab®
Cortizone® may be confused with cortisone
HCT (occasional abbreviation for hydrocortisone) is an error-prone abbreviation (mistaken as hydrochlorothiazide)

Synonyms compound F; cortisol; hydrocortisone sodium succinate

U.S./Canadian Brand Names Cortef® [US/Can]; Solu-Cortef® [US/Can]

Therapeutic Category Adrenal Corticosteroid

Use Management of adrenocortical insufficiency

Usual Dosage Dose should be based on severity of disease and patient response

Acute adrenal insufficiency: I.M., I.V.:
Infants and young Children: Succinate: 1-2 mg/kg/dose bolus, then 25-150 mg/day in divided doses every 6-8 hours
Older Children: Succinate: 1-2 mg/kg bolus then 150-250 mg/day in divided doses every 6-8 hours
Adults: Succinate: 100 mg I.V. bolus, then 300 mg/day in divided doses every 8 hours or as a continuous infusion for 48 hours; once patient is stable change to oral, 50 mg every 8 hours for 6 doses, then taper to 30-50 mg/day in divided doses

Chronic adrenal corticoid insufficiency: Adults: Oral: 20-30 mg/day

Antiinflammatory or immunosuppressive:
Infants and Children:
Oral: 2.5-10 mg/kg/day **or** 75-300 mg/m^2/day every 6-8 hours
I.M., I.V.: Succinate: 1-5 mg/kg/day **or** 30-150 mg/m^2/day divided every 12-24 hours
Adolescents and Adults: Oral, I.M., I.V.: Succinate: 15-240 mg every 12 hours

Congenital adrenal hyperplasia: Oral: Initial: 10-20 mg/m^2/day in 3 divided doses; a variety of dosing schedules have been used. **Note:** Inconsistencies have occurred with liquid formulations; tablets may provide more reliable levels. Doses must be individualized by monitoring growth, bone age, and hormonal levels. Mineralocorticoid and sodium supplementation may be required based upon electrolyte regulation and plasma renin activity.

Physiologic replacement: Children:
Oral: 0.5-0.75 mg/kg/day **or** 20-25 mg/m^2/day every 8 hours
I.M.: Succinate: 0.25-0.35 mg/kg/day **or** 12-15 mg/m^2/day once daily

Shock: I.M., I.V.: Succinate:
Children: Initial: 50 mg/kg, then repeated in 4 hours and/or every 24 hours as needed
Adolescents and Adults: 500 mg to 2 g every 2-6 hours

Status asthmaticus: Children and Adults: I.V.: Succinate: 1-2 mg/kg/dose every 6 hours for 24 hours, then maintenance of 0.5-1 mg/kg every 6 hours

Adults:
Rheumatic diseases:
Intralesional, intra-articular, soft tissue injection: Acetate:
Large joints: 25 mg (up to 37.5 mg)
Small joints: 10-25 mg
Tendon sheaths: 5-12.5 mg
Soft tissue infiltration: 25-50 mg (up to 75 mg)
Bursae: 25-37.5 mg
Ganglia: 12.5-25 mg
Stress dosing (surgery) in patients known to be adrenally-suppressed or on chronic systemic steroids: I.V.:
Minor stress (ie, inguinal herniorrhaphy): 25 mg/day for 1 day
Moderate stress (ie, joint replacement, cholecystectomy): 50-75 mg/day (25 mg every 8-12 hours) for 1-2 days
Major stress (pancreatoduodenectomy, esophagogastrectomy, cardiac surgery): 100-150 mg/day (50 mg every 8-12 hours) for 2-3 days

Dosage Forms

Injection, powder for reconstitution, as sodium succinate (Solu-Cortef®): 100 mg, 250 mg, 500 mg, 1 g [diluent contains benzyl alcohol; strength expressed as base]
Tablet, as base: 20 mg
Cortef®: 5 mg, 10 mg, 20 mg

hydrocortisone (topical) (hye droe KOR ti sone TOP i kal)

Sound-Alike/Look-Alike Issues

hydrocortisone may be confused with hydrocodone, hydroxychloroquine, hydrochlorothiazide
Cortef® may be confused with Lortab®
Cortizone® may be confused with cortisone
HCT (occasional abbreviation for hydrocortisone) is an error-prone abbreviation (mistaken as hydrochlorothiazide)
Hytone® may be confused with Vytone®

Synonyms hydrocortisone acetate; hydrocortisone butyrate; hydrocortisone probutate; hydrocortisone valerate

U.S./Canadian Brand Names Aquacort® [Can]; Aquanil™ HC [US-OTC]; Beta-HC® [US]; Caldecort® [US-OTC]; Cetacort® [US]; Cortaid® Intensive Therapy [US-OTC]; Cortaid® Maximum Strength [US-OTC]; Cortaid® Sensitive Skin [US-OTC]; Cortamed® [Can]; Corticool® [US-OTC]; Cortizone®-10 Maximum Strength [US-OTC]; Cortizone®-10 Plus Maximum Strength [US-OTC]; Cortizone®-10 Quick Shot [US-OTC]; Dermarest Dricort® [US-OTC]; Dermtex® HC [US-OTC]; Hycort™ [Can]; Hyderm [Can]; HydroZone Plus [US-OTC]; Hytone® [US]; IvySoothe® [US-OTC]; Locoid Lipocream® [US]; Locoid® [US/Can]; Nupercainal® Hydrocortisone Cream [US-OTC]; Nutracort® [US]; Pandel® [US]; Post Peel Healing Balm [US-OTC]; Prevex® HC [Can]; Sarna® HC [Can]; Sarnol®-HC [US-OTC]; Summer's Eve® SpecialCare™ Medicated Anti-Itch Cream [US-OTC]; Texacort® [US]; Tucks® Anti-Itch [US-OTC]; Westcort® [US/Can]

Therapeutic Category Corticosteroid, Topical

Use Relief of inflammation of corticosteroid-responsive dermatoses (low and medium potency topical corticosteroid)

Usual Dosage Dermatosis: Children >2 years and Adults: Topical: Apply to affected area 2-4 times/day (Buteprate: Apply once or twice daily). Therapy should be discontinued when control is achieved; if no improvement is seen, reassessment of diagnosis may be necessary.

Dosage Forms [DSC] = Discontinued product

Cream, topical, as acetate: 0.5% (9 g, 30 g, 60 g) [available with aloe]; 1% (30 g, 454 g) [available with aloe]
Cream, topical, as base: 0.5% (30 g); 1% (1.5 g, 30 g, 114 g, 454 g); 2.5% (20 g, 30 g, 454 g)
Anusol-HC®: 2.5% (30 g) [contains benzyl alcohol]
Caldecort®: 1% (30 g) [contains aloe vera gel]
Cortaid® Intensive Therapy: 1% (60 g)
Cortaid® Maximum Strength: 1% (15 g, 30 g, 40 g, 60 g) [contains aloe vera gel and benzyl alcohol]
Cortaid® Sensitive Skin: 0.5% (15 g) [contains aloe vera gel]
Cortizone®-10 Maximum Strength: 1% (15 g, 30 g, 60 g) [contains aloe]
Cortizone®-10 Plus Maximum Strength: 1% (30 g, 60 g) [contains vitamins A, D, E and aloe]
Dermarest® Dricort®: 1% (15 g, 30 g)
HydroZone Plus, Proctocort®, Procto-Pak™: 1% (30 g)
Hytone®: 2.5% (30 g, 60 g)
IvySoothe®: 1% (30 g) [contains aloe]
Post Peel Healing Balm: 1% (23 g)
ProctoCream® HC: 2.5% (30 g) [contains benzyl alcohol]
Procto-Kit™: 1% (30 g) [packaged with applicator tips and finger cots]; 2.5% (30 g) [packaged with applicator tips and finger cots]
Proctosol-HC®, Proctozone-HC™: 2.5% (30 g)
Summer's Eve® SpecialCare™ Medicated Anti-Itch Cream: 1% (30 g)
Cream, topical, as butyrate (Locoid®, Locoid Lipocream®): 0.1% (15 g, 45 g)
Cream, topical, as probutate (Pandel®): 0.1% (15 g, 45 g, 80 g)
Cream, topical, as valerate (Westcort®): 0.2% (15 g, 45 g, 60 g)
Gel, topical, as base (Corticool®): 1% (45 g)
Lotion, topical, as base: 1% (120 mL); 2.5% (60 mL)
Aquanil™ HC: 1% (120 mL)
Beta-HC®, Cetacort®, Sarnol®-HC: 1% (60 mL)
HydroZone Plus: 1% (120 mL)
Hytone®: 2.5% (60 mL)
Nutracort®: 1% (60 mL, 120 mL); 2.5% (60 mL, 120 mL)
Ointment, topical, as acetate: 1% (30 g) [strength expressed as base; available with aloe]
Anusol® HC-1: 1% (21 g) [strength expressed as base]
Cortaid® Maximum Strength: 1% (15 g, 30 g) [strength expressed as base]
Ointment, topical, as base: 0.5% (30 g); 1% (30 g, 454 g); 2.5% (20 g, 30 g, 454 g)
Cortizone®-10 Maximum Strength: 1% (30 g, 60 g)
Hytone®: 2.5% (30 g)
Ointment, topical, as butyrate (Locoid®): 0.1% (15 g, 45 g)

Ointment, topical, as valerate (Westcort®): 0.2% (15 g, 45 g, 60 g)
Solution, otic, as base (EarSol® HC): 1% (30 mL) [contains alcohol 44%, benzyl benzoate, yerba santa]
Solution, topical, as base (Texacort®): 2.5% (30 mL) [contains alcohol]
Solution, topical, as butyrate (Locoid®): 0.1% (20 mL, 60 mL) [contains alcohol 50%]
Solution, topical spray, as base:
Cortaid® Intensive Therapy: 1% (60 mL) [contains alcohol]
Cortizone®-10 Quick Shot: 1% (44 mL) [contains benzyl alcohol]
Dermtex® HC: 1% (52 mL) [contains menthol 1%]

hydrocortisone valerate *see* hydrocortisone (topical) *on previous page*

HydroDIURIL® ***(Discontinued)*** *see* hydrochlorothiazide *on page 419*

Hydro DP [US] *see* hydrocodone, phenylephrine, and diphenhydramine *on page 425*

Hydrogesic® ***(Discontinued)*** *see* hydrocodone and acetaminophen *on page 420*

Hydromet® [US] *see* hydrocodone and homatropine *on page 423*

Hydromorph Contin® [Can] *see* hydromorphone *on this page*

Hydromorph-IR® [Can] *see* hydromorphone *on this page*

hydromorphone (hye droe MOR fone)

Sound-Alike/Look-Alike Issues

hydromorphone may be confused with morphine; significant overdoses have occurred when hydromorphone products have been inadvertently administered instead of morphine sulfate. Commercially available prefilled syringes of both products looks similar and are often stored in close proximity to each other. **Note:** Hydromorphone 1 mg oral is approximately equal to morphine 4 mg oral; hydromorphone 1 mg I.V. is approximately equal to morphine 5 mg I.V.

Dilaudid® may be confused with Demerol®, Dilantin®

Dilaudid®, Dilaudid-HP®: Extreme caution should be taken to avoid confusing the highly-concentrated (Dilaudid-HP®) injection with the less-concentrated (Dilaudid®) injectable product.

Synonyms dihydromorphinone; hydromorphone hydrochloride

U.S./Canadian Brand Names Dilaudid-HP-Plus® [Can]; Dilaudid-HP® [US/Can]; Dilaudid-XP® [Can]; Dilaudid® Sterile Powder [Can]; Dilaudid® [US/Can]; Hydromorph Contin® [Can]; Hydromorph-IR® [Can]; Hydromorphone HP [Can]; Hydromorphone HP® 10 [Can]; Hydromorphone HP® 20 [Can]; Hydromorphone HP® 50 [Can]; Hydromorphone HP® Forte [Can]; Hydromorphone Hydrochloride Injection, USP [Can]; PMS-Hydromorphone [Can]

Therapeutic Category Analgesic, Narcotic

Controlled Substance C-II

Use Management of moderate-to-severe pain

Usual Dosage

Acute pain (moderate to severe): **Note:** These are guidelines and do not represent the maximum doses that may be required in all patients. Doses should be titrated to pain relief/prevention.
Children ≥6 months and <50 kg:
Oral: 0.03-0.08 mg/kg/dose every 3-4 hours as needed
I.V.: 0.015 mg/kg/dose every 3-6 hours as needed
Children >50 kg and Adults:
Oral: Initial: Opiate-naive: 2-4 mg every 3-6 hours as needed; elderly/debilitated patients may require lower doses; patients with prior opiate exposure may require higher initial doses; usual dosage range: 2-8 mg every 3-4 hours as needed
I.V.: Initial: Opiate-naive: 0.2-0.6 mg every 2-3 hours as needed; patients with prior opiate exposure may tolerate higher initial doses
Note: More frequent dosing may be needed.
Mechanically-ventilated patients (based on 70 kg patient): 0.7-2 mg every 1-2 hours as needed; infusion (based on 70 kg patient): 0.5-1 mg/hour
Patient-controlled analgesia (PCA): (Opiate-naive: Consider lower end of dosing range)
Usual concentration: 0.2 mg/mL
Demand dose: Usual: 0.1-0.2 mg; range: 0.05-0.5 mg
Lockout interval: 5-15 minutes
4-hour limit: 4-6 mg
Epidural:
Bolus dose: 1-1.5 mg
Infusion concentration: 0.05-0.075 mg/mL
Infusion rate: 0.04-0.4 mg/hour
Demand dose: 0.15 mg

(Continued)

hydromorphone *(Continued)*

Lockout interval: 30 minutes

I.M., SubQ: **Note:** I.M. use may result in variable absorption and a lag time to peak effect.

Initial: Opiate-naive: 0.8-1 mg every 4-6 hours as needed; patients with prior opiate exposure may require higher initial doses; usual dosage range: 1-2 mg every 3-6 hours as needed

Rectal: 3 mg every 4-8 hours as needed

Chronic pain: Adults: Oral: **Note:** Patients taking opioids chronically may become tolerant and require doses higher than the usual dosage range to maintain the desired effect. Tolerance can be managed by appropriate dose titration. There is no optimal or maximal dose for hydromorphone in chronic pain. The appropriate dose is one that relieves pain throughout its dosing interval without causing unmanageable side effects.

Controlled release formulation (Hydromorph Contin®, not available in U.S.): 3-30 mg every 12 hours. **Note:** A patient's hydromorphone requirement should be established using prompt release formulations; conversion to long acting products may be considered when chronic, continuous treatment is required. Higher dosages should be reserved for use only in opioid-tolerant patients.

Dosage Forms [CAN] = Canadian brand name

Capsule, controlled release (Hydromorph Contin®) [CAN]: 3 mg, 6 mg, 12 mg, 18 mg, 24 mg, 30 mg [not available in U.S.]

Injection, powder for reconstitution, as hydrochloride (Dilaudid-HP®): 250 mg

Injection, solution, as hydrochloride: 1 mg/mL (1 mL); 2 mg/mL (1 mL, 20 mL); 4 mg/mL (1 mL); 10 mg/mL (1 mL, 5 mL, 10 mL)

Dilaudid®: 1 mg/mL (1 mL); 2 mg/mL (1 mL, 20 mL) [20 mL size contains edetate sodium; vial stopper contains latex]; 4 mg/mL (1 mL)

Dilaudid-HP®: 10 mg/mL (1 mL, 5 mL, 50 mL)

Liquid, oral, as hydrochloride (Dilaudid®): 1 mg/mL (480 mL) [may contain trace amounts of sodium bisulfite]

Suppository, rectal, as hydrochloride (Dilaudid®): 3 mg (6s)

Tablet, as hydrochloride (Dilaudid®): 2 mg, 4 mg, 8 mg (8 mg tablets may contain trace amounts of sodium bisulfite)

Hydromorphone HP [Can] *see* hydromorphone *on previous page*

Hydromorphone HP® 10 [Can] *see* hydromorphone *on previous page*

Hydromorphone HP® 20 [Can] *see* hydromorphone *on previous page*

Hydromorphone HP® 50 [Can] *see* hydromorphone *on previous page*

Hydromorphone HP® Forte [Can] *see* hydromorphone *on previous page*

hydromorphone hydrochloride *see* hydromorphone *on previous page*

Hydromorphone Hydrochloride Injection, USP [Can] *see* hydromorphone *on previous page*

Hydromox® *(Discontinued)*

Hydron CP [US] *see* phenylephrine, hydrocodone, and chlorpheniramine *on page 663*

Hydron PSC [US] *see* pseudoephedrine, hydrocodone, and chlorpheniramine *on page 716*

Hydro-Par® *(Discontinued)* *see* hydrochlorothiazide *on page 419*

Hydro-PC II [US] *see* phenylephrine, hydrocodone, and chlorpheniramine *on page 663*

Hydro PC II Plus [US] *see* phenylephrine, hydrocodone, and chlorpheniramine *on page 663*

hydroquinol *see* hydroquinone *on this page*

hydroquinone (HYE droe kwin one)

Sound-Alike/Look-Alike Issues

Eldopaque® may be confused with Eldoquin®

Eldoquin® may be confused with Eldopaque®

Eldopaque Forte® may be confused with Eldoquin Forte®

Eldoquin Forte® may be confused with Eldopaque Forte®

Synonyms hydroquinol; quinol

U.S./Canadian Brand Names Alphaquin HP [US]; Claripel™ [US]; Dermarest® Skin Correction Cream Plus [US-OTC]; Eldopaque Forte® [US]; Eldopaque® [US-OTC/Can]; Eldoquin Forte® [US]; Eldoquin® [US-OTC/Can]; EpiQuin™ Micro [US]; Esoterica® Regular [US-OTC]; Glyquin-XM™ [US/Can]; Glyquin® [US]; Lustra-AF™ [US]; Lustra® [US/Can]; Melanex® [US]; Melpaque HP® [US]; Melquin HP® [US]; Melquin-3® [US]; NeoStrata AHA [US-OTC]; NeoStrata® HQ [Can]; Nuquin HP® [US]; Palmer's® Skin Success Eventone® Fade Cream [US-OTC]; Solaquin Forte® [US]; Solaquin® [US-OTC/Can]; Ultraquin™ [Can]

Therapeutic Category Topical Skin Product

Use Gradual bleaching of hyperpigmented skin conditions

Usual Dosage Children >12 years and Adults: Topical: Apply thin layer and rub in twice daily

Dosage Forms

Cream, topical: 4% (30 g) [may contain sodium metabisulfite]
- Alphaquin HP®: 4% (30 g, 60 g)
- Eldoquin®: 2% (15 g, 30 g)
- Eldoquin Forte®: 4% (30 g) [contains sodium metabisulfite]
- EpiQuin™ Micro: 4% (30 g) [contains benzyl alcohol and sodium metabisulfite]
- Esoterica® Regular: 2% (85 g) [contains sodium bisulfite]
- Lustra®: 4% (30 g) [contains sodium metabisulfite]
- Melquin HP®: 4% (15 g, 30 g) [contains sodium metabisulfite]

Cream, topical [with sunscreen]: 4% (30 g) [may contain sodium metabisulfite]
- Claripel™: 4% (30 g, 45 g) [contains sodium metabisulfite]
- Dermarest® Skin Correcting Cream Plus: 2% (85 g) [contains aloe vera, sodium bisulfite]
- Eldopaque®: 2% (15 g, 30 g)
- Eldopaque Forte®: 4% (30 g) [contains sodium metabisulfite]
- Glyquin®: 4% (30 g)
- Glyquin-XM™: 4% (30 g)
- Lustra-AF™: 4% (30 g, 60 g) [contains sodium metabisulfite]
- Melpaque HP®: 4% (15 g, 30 g) [contains sodium metabisulfite; sunblocking cream base]
- Nuquin HP®: 4% (15 g, 30 g, 60 g) [contains sodium metabisulfite]
- Palmer's® Skin Success Eventone® Fade Cream: 2% (81 g, 132 g) [contains sodium sulfite; available in regular, oily skin, and dry skin formulas]
- Solaquin®: 2% (30 g)
- Solaquin Forte®: 4% (30 g) [contains sodium metabisulfite]

Gel, topical (NeoStrata® AHA): 2% (45 g) [contains glycolic acid 10%, sodium bisulfite, and sodium sulfite]

Gel, topical [with sunscreen]: 4% (30 g)
- Nuquin HP: 4% (15 g, 30 g) [contains sodium bisulfite]
- Solaquin Forte®: 4% (30 g) [contains sodium metabisulfite]

Solution, topical (Melanex®, Melquin-3®): 3% (30 mL) [contains alcohol]

hydroquinone, fluocinolone acetonide, and tretinoin *see* fluocinolone, hydroquinone, and tretinoin *on page 353*

Hydrotropine® *(Discontinued)* *see* hydrocodone and homatropine *on page 423*

Hydro-Tussin™ [US] *see* hydrocodone and guaifenesin *on page 422*

Hydro-Tussin™-CBX [US] *see* carbinoxamine and pseudoephedrine *on page 149*

Hydro-Tussin™ DM [US] *see* guaifenesin and dextromethorphan *on page 394*

Hydro-Tussin™ HC [US] *see* pseudoephedrine, hydrocodone, and chlorpheniramine *on page 716*

Hydro-Tussin™ HD [US] *see* hydrocodone, pseudoephedrine, and guaifenesin *on page 425*

Hydro-Tussin™ XP [US] *see* hydrocodone, pseudoephedrine, and guaifenesin *on page 425*

4-hydroxybutyrate *see* sodium oxybate *on page 780*

hydroxycarbamide *see* hydroxyurea *on next page*

hydroxychloroquine (hye droks ee KLOR oh kwin)

Sound-Alike/Look-Alike Issues

hydroxychloroquine may be confused with hydrocortisone

Plaquenil® may be confused with Platinol®

Synonyms hydroxychloroquine sulfate

U.S./Canadian Brand Names Apo-Hydroxyquine® [Can]; Gen-Hydroxychloroquine [Can]; Plaquenil® [US/Can]

Therapeutic Category Aminoquinoline (Antimalarial)

Use Suppression and treatment of acute attacks of malaria; treatment of systemic lupus erythematosus and rheumatoid arthritis

Usual Dosage Note: Hydroxychloroquine sulfate 200 mg is equivalent to 155 mg hydroxychloroquine base and 250 mg chloroquine phosphate. Oral:

Children:

Chemoprophylaxis of malaria: 5 mg/kg (base) once weekly; should not exceed the recommended adult dose; begin 2 weeks before exposure; continue for 4-6 weeks after leaving endemic area; if suppressive therapy is not begun prior to the exposure, double the initial dose and give in 2 doses, 6 hours apart

(Continued)

hydroxychloroquine *(Continued)*

Acute attack: 10 mg/kg (base) initial dose; followed by 5 mg/kg at 6, 24, and 48 hours
JRA or SLE: 3-5 mg/kg/day divided 1-2 times/day; avoid exceeding 7 mg/kg/day

Adults:

Chemoprophylaxis of malaria: 310 mg base weekly on same day each week; begin 2 weeks before exposure; continue for 4-6 weeks after leaving endemic area; if suppressive therapy is not begun prior to the exposure, double the initial dose and give in 2 doses, 6 hours apart

Acute attack: 620 mg first dose day 1; 310 mg in 6 hours day 1; 310 mg in 1 dose day 2; and 310 mg in 1 dose on day 3

Rheumatoid arthritis: 310-465 mg/day to start taken with food or milk; increase dose until optimum response level is reached; usually after 4-12 weeks dose should be reduced by ½ and a maintenance dose of 155-310 mg/day given

Lupus erythematosus: 310 mg every day or twice daily for several weeks depending on response; 155-310 mg/day for prolonged maintenance therapy

Dosage Forms Tablet, as sulfate: 200 mg [equivalent to 155 mg base]

hydroxychloroquine sulfate *see* hydroxychloroquine *on previous page*

hydroxydaunomycin hydrochloride *see* doxorubicin *on page 277*

1α-hydroxyergocalciferol *see* doxercalciferol *on page 277*

hydroxyethylcellulose *see* artificial tears *on page 75*

hydroxyethyl starch *see* hetastarch *on page 413*

hydroxyldaunorubicin hydrochloride *see* doxorubicin *on page 277*

hydroxypropyl cellulose (hye droks ee PROE pil SEL yoo lose)

U.S./Canadian Brand Names Lacrisert® [US/Can]

Therapeutic Category Ophthalmic Agent, Miscellaneous

Use Dry eyes (moderate to severe)

Usual Dosage Adults: Ophthalmic: Apply once daily into the inferior cul-de-sac beneath the base of tarsus, not in apposition to the cornea nor beneath the eyelid at the level of the tarsal plate

Dosage Forms Insert, ophthalmic [preservative free]: 5 mg

hydroxypropyl methylcellulose (hye droks ee PROE pil meth il SEL yoo lose)

Sound-Alike/Look-Alike Issues

Isopto® Tears may be confused with Isoptin®

Synonyms gonioscopic ophthalmic solution; hypromellose

U.S./Canadian Brand Names Cellugel® [US]; GenTeal® Mild [US-OTC]; GenTeal® [US-OTC/Can]; Gonak™ [US-OTC]; Goniosoft™ [US]; Isopto® Tears [US-OTC/Can]; Tearisol® [US-OTC]; Tears Again® MC [US-OTC]

Therapeutic Category Ophthalmic Agent, Miscellaneous

Use Relief of burning and minor irritation due to dry eyes; diagnostic agent in gonioscopic examination

Usual Dosage Adults: Dry eyes: Ophthalmic: Instill 1-2 drops in affected eye(s) as needed

Dosage Forms [DSC] = Discontinued product

Gel, ophthalmic (GenTeal®): 0.3% (10 mL)

Solution, ophthalmic: 0.4% (15 mL)
- GenTeal®: 0.3% (15 mL, 25 mL)
- GenTeal® Mild: 0.2% (15 mL, 25 mL)
- Gonak™: 2.5% (15 mL)
- Goniosoft™: 2.5% (15 mL)
- Goniosol®: 2.5% (15 mL) [contains benzalkonium chloride] [DSC]
- Isopto® Tears: 0.5% (15 mL) [contains benzalkonium chloride]
- Tearisol®: 0.5% (15 mL) [contains benzalkonium chloride]
- Tears Again® MC: 0.3% (15 mL)

Solution, ophthalmic [for injection] (Cellugel®): 2% (1 mL)

hydroxyurea (hye droks ee yoor EE a)

Sound-Alike/Look-Alike Issues

hydroxyurea may be confused with hydrOXYzine

Synonyms hydroxycarbamide

U.S./Canadian Brand Names Apo-Hydroxyurea® [Can]; Droxia® [US]; Gen-Hydroxyurea [Can]; Hydrea® [US/Can]; Mylocel™ [US]

Therapeutic Category Antineoplastic Agent

Use Treatment of melanoma, refractory chronic myelocytic leukemia (CML), relapsed and refractory metastatic ovarian cancer; radiosensitizing agent in the treatment of squamous cell head and neck cancer (excluding lip cancer); adjunct in the management of sickle cell patients who have had at least three painful crises in the previous 12 months (to reduce frequency of these crises and the need for blood transfusions)

Usual Dosage Oral (refer to individual protocols): All dosage should be based on ideal or actual body weight, whichever is less:

Adults: Dose should always be titrated to patient response and WBC counts; usual oral doses range from 10-30 mg/kg/day or 500-3000 mg/day; if WBC count falls to <2500 cells/mm^3, or the platelet count to <100,000/mm^3, therapy should be stopped for at least 3 days and resumed when values rise toward normal

Solid tumors:

Intermittent therapy: 80 mg/kg as a single dose every third day

Continuous therapy: 20-30 mg/kg/day given as a single dose/day

Concomitant therapy with irradiation: 80 mg/kg as a single dose every third day starting at least 7 days before initiation of irradiation

Resistant chronic myelocytic leukemia: Continuous therapy: 20-30 mg/kg as a single daily dose

Sickle cell anemia (moderate/severe disease): Initial: 15 mg/kg/day, increased by 5 mg/kg every 12 weeks if blood counts are in an acceptable range until the maximum tolerated dose of 35 mg/kg/day is achieved or the dose that does not produce toxic effects

Acceptable range:

Neutrophils ≥2500 cells/mm^3

Platelets ≥95,000/mm^3

Hemoglobin >5.3 g/dL, and

Reticulocytes ≥95,000/mm^3 if the hemoglobin concentration is <9 g/dL

Toxic range:

Neutrophils <2000 cells/mm^3

Platelets <80,000/mm^3

Hemoglobin <4.5 g/dL

Reticulocytes <80,000/mm^3 if the hemoglobin concentration is <9 g/dL

Monitor for toxicity every 2 weeks; if toxicity occurs, stop treatment until the bone marrow recovers; restart at 2.5 mg/kg/day less than the dose at which toxicity occurs; if no toxicity occurs over the next 12 weeks, then the subsequent dose should be increased by 2.5 mg/kg/day; reduced dosage of hydroxyurea alternating with erythropoietin may decrease myelotoxicity and increase levels of fetal hemoglobin in patients who have not been helped by hydroxyurea alone

Dosage Forms

Capsule: 500 mg

Droxia®: 200 mg, 300 mg, 400 mg

Hydrea®: 500 mg

Tablet (Mylocel™): 1000 mg

hydroxyzine (hye DROKS i zeen)

Sound-Alike/Look-Alike Issues

hydrOXYzine may be confused with hydrALAZINE, hydroxyurea

Atarax® may be confused with amoxicillin, Ativan®

Vistaril® may be confused with Restoril®, Versed, Zestril®

Synonyms hydroxyzine hydrochloride; hydroxyzine pamoate

Tall-Man hydro**OXY**zine

U.S./Canadian Brand Names Apo-Hydroxyzine® [Can]; Atarax® [Can]; Hydroxyzine Hydrochloride Injection, USP [Can]; Novo-Hydroxyzin [Can]; PMS-Hydroxyzine [Can]; Vistaril® [US/Can]

Therapeutic Category Antiemetic; Antihistamine

Use Treatment of anxiety; preoperative sedative; antipruritic

Usual Dosage

Children:

Preoperative sedation:

Oral: 0.6 mg/kg/dose every 6 hours

I.M.: 0.5-1.1 mg/kg/dose every 4-6 hours as needed

Manufacturer labeling: Pruritus, anxiety:

<6 years: 50 mg daily in divided doses

≥6 years: 50-100 mg daily in divided doses

Adults:

Antiemetic: I.M.: 25-100 mg/dose every 4-6 hours as needed

Anxiety: Oral: 25-100 mg 4 times/day; maximum dose: 600 mg/day

(Continued)

hydroxyzine *(Continued)*

Preoperative sedation:
Oral: 50-100 mg
I.M.: 25-100 mg
Management of pruritus: Oral: 25 mg 3-4 times/day

Dosage Forms

Capsule, as pamoate: 25 mg, 50 mg, 100 mg
Vistaril®: 25 mg, 50 mg
Injection, solution, as hydrochloride: 25 mg/mL (1 mL); 50 mg/mL (1 mL, 2 mL, 10 mL)
Suspension, oral, as pamoate:
Vistaril®: 25 mg/5 mL (120 mL, 480 mL) [lemon flavor]
Syrup, as hydrochloride: 10 mg/5 mL (120 mL, 480 mL)
Tablet, as hydrochloride: 10 mg, 25 mg, 50 mg

hydroxyzine hydrochloride *see* hydroxyzine *on previous page*

Hydroxyzine Hydrochloride Injection, USP [Can] *see* hydroxyzine *on previous page*

hydroxyzine pamoate *see* hydroxyzine *on previous page*

HydroZone Plus [US-OTC] *see* hydrocortisone (topical) *on page 428*

Hyflex-DS® [US] *see* acetaminophen and phenyltoloxamine *on page 8*

Hygroton® *(Discontinued)* *see* chlorthalidone *on page 185*

Hylaform® [US] *see* hyaluronate and derivatives *on page 416*

Hylaform® Plus [US] *see* hyaluronate and derivatives *on page 416*

hylan polymers *see* hyaluronate and derivatives *on page 416*

Hylenex™ [US] *see* hyaluronidase *on page 417*

Hylutin Injection *(Discontinued)*

hyoscine butylbromide *see* scopolamine derivatives *on page 764*

hyoscine hydrobromide *see* scopolamine derivatives *on page 764*

hyoscyamine (hye oh SYE a meen)

Sound-Alike/Look-Alike Issues

Anaspaz® may be confused with Anaprox®, Antispas®
Levbid® may be confused with Lithobid®, Lopid®, Lorabid®
Levsinex® may be confused with Lanoxin®

Synonyms hyoscyamine sulfate; *l*-hyoscyamine sulfate

U.S./Canadian Brand Names Anaspaz® [US]; Cystospaz® [US/Can]; Hyosine [US]; Levbid® [US]; Levsin/SL® [US]; Levsinex® [US]; Levsin® [US/Can]; NuLev™ [US]; Symax SL [US]; Symax SR [US]

Therapeutic Category Anticholinergic Agent

Use

Oral: Adjunctive therapy for peptic ulcers, irritable bowel, neurogenic bladder/bowel; treatment of infant colic, GI tract disorders caused by spasm; to reduce rigidity, tremors, sialorrhea, and hyperhidrosis associated with parkinsonism; as a drying agent in acute rhinitis

Injection: Preoperative antimuscarinic to reduce secretions and block cardiac vagal inhibitory reflexes; to improve radiologic visibility of the kidneys; symptomatic relief of biliary and renal colic; reduce GI motility to facilitate diagnostic procedures (ie, endoscopy, hypotonic duodenography); reduce pain and hypersecretion in pancreatitis, certain cases of partial heart block associated with vagal activity; reversal of neuromuscular blockade

Usual Dosage

Oral: Children: Gastrointestinal disorders: Dose as listed, based on age and weight (kg) using 0.125 mg/mL drops; repeat dose every 4 hours as needed:
Children <2 years:
3.4 kg: 4 drops; maximum: 24 drops/24 hours
5 kg: 5 drops; maximum: 30 drops/24 hours
7 kg: 6 drops; maximum: 36 drops/24 hours
10 kg: 8 drops; maximum: 48 drops/24 hours

Oral, S.L.:
Children 2-12 years: Gastrointestinal disorders: Dose as listed, based on age and weight (kg); repeat dose every 4 hours as needed:
10 kg: 0.031-0.033 mg; maximum: 0.75 mg/24 hours
20 kg: 0.0625 mg; maximum: 0.75 mg/24 hours

40 kg: 0.0938 mg; maximum: 0.75 mg/24 hours
50 kg: 0.125 mg; maximum: 0.75 mg/24 hours
Children >12 years and Adults: Gastrointestinal disorders: 0.125-0.25 mg every 4 hours or as needed (before meals or food); maximum: 1.5 mg/24 hours
Cystospaz®: 0.15-0.3 mg up to 4 times/day
Oral (timed release): Children >12 years and Adults: Gastrointestinal disorders: 0.375-0.75 mg every 12 hours; maximum: 1.5 mg/24 hours
I.M., I.V., SubQ: Children >12 years and Adults: Gastrointestinal disorders: 0.25-0.5 mg; may repeat as needed up to 4 times/day, at 4-hour intervals
I.V.: Children >2 year and Adults: I.V.: Preanesthesia: 5 mcg/kg given 30-60 minutes prior to induction of anesthesia or at the time preoperative narcotics or sedatives are administered
I.V.: Adults: Diagnostic procedures: 0.25-0.5 mg given 5-10 minutes prior to procedure
To reduce drug-induced bradycardia during surgery: 0.125 mg; repeat as needed
To reverse neuromuscular blockade: 0.2 mg for every 1 mg neostigmine (or the physostigmine/pyridostigmine equivalent)

Dosage Forms [DSC] = Discontinued product
Capsule, timed release, as sulfate (Cystospaz-M® [DSC], Levsinex®): 0.375 mg
Elixir, as sulfate: 0.125 mg/5 mL (480 mL)
Hyosine: 0.125 mg/5 mL (480 mL) [contains alcohol 20% and sodium benzoate; orange flavor]
Levsin®: 0.125 mg/5 mL (480 mL) [contains alcohol 20%; orange flavor]
Injection, solution, as sulfate (Levsin®): 0.5 mg/mL (1 mL)
Liquid, as sulfate (Spacol [DSC]): 0.125 mg/5 mL (120 mL) [sugar free, alcohol free, simethicone based, bubble gum flavor]
Solution, oral drops, as sulfate: 0.125 mg/mL (15 mL)
Hyosine: 0.125 mg/mL (15 mL) [contains alcohol 5% and sodium benzoate; orange flavor]
Levsin®: 0.125 mg/mL (15 mL) [contains alcohol 5%; orange flavor]
Tablet (Cystospaz®): 0.15 mg
Tablet, as sulfate (Anaspaz®, Levsin®, Spacol [DSC]): 0.125 mg
Tablet, extended release, as sulfate (Levbid®, Symax SR, Spacol T/S [DSC]): 0.375 mg
Tablet, orally disintegrating, as sulfate (NuLev™): 0.125 mg [contains phenylalanine 1.7 mg/tablet, mint flavor]
Tablet, sublingual, as sulfate: 0.125 mg
Levsin/SL®: 0.125 mg [peppermint flavor]
Symax SL: 0.125 mg

hyoscyamine, atropine, scopolamine, and phenobarbital

(hye oh SYE a meen, A troe peen, skoe POL a meen, & fee noe BAR bi tal)

Sound-Alike/Look-Alike Issues
Donnatal® may be confused with Donnagel®

Synonyms atropine, hyoscyamine, scopolamine, and phenobarbital; belladonna alkaloids with phenobarbital; phenobarbital, hyoscyamine, atropine, and scopolamine; scopolamine, hyoscyamine, atropine, and phenobarbital

U.S./Canadian Brand Names Donnatal Extentabs® [US]; Donnatal® [US]

Therapeutic Category Anticholinergic Agent

Use Adjunct in treatment of irritable bowel syndrome, acute enterocolitis, duodenal ulcer

Usual Dosage Oral:
Children: Donnatal® elixir: To be given every 4-6 hours; initial dose based on weight:
4.5 kg: 0.5 mL every 4 hours **or** 0.75 mL every 6 hours
10 kg: 1 mL every 4 hours **or** 1.5 mL every 6 hours
14 kg: 1.5 mL every 4 hours **or** 2 mL every 6 hours
23 kg: 2.5 mL every 4 hours **or** 3.8 mL every 6 hours
34 kg: 3.8 mL every 4 hours **or** 5 mL every 6 hours
≥45 kg: 5 mL every 4 hours **or** 7.5 mL every 6 hours
Adults:
Donnatal®: 1-2 tablets or 5-10 mL of elixir 3-4 times/day
Donnatal Extentabs®: 1 tablet every 12 hours; may increase to 1 tablet every 8 hours if needed

Dosage Forms
Elixir (Donnatal®): Hyoscyamine sulfate 0.1037 mg, atropine sulfate 0.0194 mg, scopolamine hydrobromide 0.0065 mg, and phenobarbital 16.2 mg per 5 mL (120 mL, 480 mL) [contains alcohol 95%; grape flavor]
Tablet (Donnatal®): Hyoscyamine sulfate 0.1037 mg, atropine sulfate 0.0194 mg, scopolamine hydrobromide 0.0065 mg, and phenobarbital 16.2 mg
(Continued)

hyoscyamine, atropine, scopolamine, and phenobarbital *(Continued)*

Tablet, extended release (Donnatal Extentabs®): Hyoscyamine sulfate 0.3111 mg, atropine sulfate 0.0582 mg, scopolamine hydrobromide 0.0195 mg, and phenobarbital 48.6 mg

hyoscyamine sulfate *see* hyoscyamine *on page 434*
Hyosine [US] *see* hyoscyamine *on page 434*
Hy-Pam® Oral *(Discontinued)* *see* hydroxyzine *on page 433*
Hypaque-Cysto® [US] *see* radiological/contrast media (ionic) *on page 728*
Hypaque® Meglumine [US] *see* radiological/contrast media (ionic) *on page 728*
Hypaque® Sodium [US] *see* radiological/contrast media (ionic) *on page 728*
Hyperab® *(Discontinued)* *see* rabies immune globulin (human) *on page 727*
hyperal *see* total parenteral nutrition *on page 838*
hyperalimentation *see* total parenteral nutrition *on page 838*
HyperHep B® [Can] *see* hepatitis B immune globulin *on page 411*
HyperHEP B™ S/D [US] *see* hepatitis B immune globulin *on page 411*
HyperRAB™ S/D [US] *see* rabies immune globulin (human) *on page 727*
HyperRHO™ S/D Full Dose [US] *see* Rh_o(D) immune globulin *on page 740*
HyperRHO™ S/D Mini Dose [US] *see* Rh_o(D) immune globulin *on page 740*
Hyperstat® [US] *see* diazoxide *on page 249*
HyperTET™ S/D [US] *see* tetanus immune globulin (human) *on page 814*
Hyphed [US] *see* pseudoephedrine, hydrocodone, and chlorpheniramine *on page 716*
Hy-Phen® *(Discontinued)* *see* hydrocodone and acetaminophen *on page 420*
HypoTears [US-OTC] *see* artificial tears *on page 75*
HypoTears PF [US-OTC] *see* artificial tears *on page 75*
HypRho®-D *(Discontinued)*
HypRho®-D Mini-Dose *(Discontinued)*
Hyprogest® 250 *(Discontinued)*
hypromellose *see* hydroxypropyl methylcellulose *on page 432*
Hytakerol® *(Discontinued)*
HyTan™ [US] *see* hydrocodone and chlorpheniramine *on page 422*
Hytinic® [US-OTC] *see* polysaccharide-iron complex *on page 681*
Hytone® [US] *see* hydrocortisone (topical) *on page 428*
Hytrin® [US/Can] *see* terazosin *on page 810*
Hyzaar® [US/Can] *see* losartan and hydrochlorothiazide *on page 507*
Hyzaar® DS [Can] *see* losartan and hydrochlorothiazide *on page 507*
Hyzine® *(Discontinued)* *see* hydroxyzine *on page 433*

ibandronate (eye BAN droh nate)

Synonyms ibandronate sodium
U.S./Canadian Brand Names Bondronat® [Can]; Boniva® [US]
Therapeutic Category Bisphosphonate Derivative
Use Treatment and prevention of osteoporosis in postmenopausal females
Usual Dosage
Oral:
Treatment of postmenopausal osteoporosis: 2.5 mg/day or 150 mg once a month
Prevention of postmenopausal osteoporosis: 2.5 mg/day; 150 mg once a month may be considered
I.V.: Treatment of postmenopausal osteoporosis: 3 mg every 3 months
Dosage Forms
Injection, solution: 1 mg/mL (3 mL) [prefilled syringe]
Tablet: 2.5 mg [once-daily formulation]; 150 mg [once-monthly formulation]

ibandronate sodium *see* ibandronate *on this page*

Iberet® [US-OTC] *see* vitamins (multiple/oral) *on page 878*

Iberet®-500 [US-OTC] *see* vitamins (multiple/oral) *on page 878*

ibidomide hydrochloride *see* labetalol *on page 475*

ibritumomab (ib ri TYOO mo mab)

Synonyms ibritumomab tiuxetan; In-111 zevalin; Y-90 zevalin

U.S./Canadian Brand Names Zevalin® [US]

Therapeutic Category Antineoplastic Agent, Monoclonal Antibody; Radiopharmaceutical

Use Treatment of relapsed or refractory low-grade, follicular, or transformed B-cell non-Hodgkin lymphoma (including rituximab-refractory follicular non-Hodgkin lymphoma) as part of a therapeutic regimen with rituximab (Zevalin™ therapeutic regimen); **not to be used as single-agent therapy**; must be radiolabeled prior to use

Usual Dosage I.V.: Adults: Ibritumomab is administered **only** as part of the Zevalin™ therapeutic regimen (a combined treatment regimen with rituximab). The regimen consists of two steps:

Step 1:

Rituximab infusion: 250 mg/m^2 at an initial rate of 50 mg/hour. If hypersensitivity or infusion-related events do not occur, increase infusion in increments of 50 mg/hour every 30 minutes, to a maximum of 400 mg/hour. Infusions should be temporarily slowed or interrupted if hypersensitivity or infusion-related events occur. The infusion may be resumed at one-half the previous rate upon improvement of symptoms.

In-111 ibritumomab infusion: Within 4 hours of the completion of rituximab infusion, inject 5 mCi (1.6 mg total antibody dose) over 10 minutes.

Biodistribution of In-111 ibritumomab should be assessed by imaging at 2-24 hours and at 48-72 hours postinjection. An optional third imaging may be performed 90-120 hours following injection. If biodistribution is not acceptable, the patient should not proceed to Step 2.

Step 2 (initiated 7-9 days following Step 1):

Rituximab infusion: 250 mg/m^2 at an initial rate of 100 mg/hour (50 mg/hour if infusion-related events occurred with the first infusion). If hypersensitivity or infusion-related events do not occur, increase infusion in increments of 100 mg/hour every 30 minutes, to a maximum of 400 mg/hour, as tolerated.

Y-90 ibritumomab infusion: Within 4 hours of the completion of rituximab infusion:

Platelet count >150,000 cells/mm^3: Inject 0.4 mCi/kg (14.8 MBq/kg actual body weight) over 10 minutes

Platelet count between 100,000-149,000 cells/mm^3: Inject 0.3 mCi/kg (11.1 MBq/kg actual body weight) over 10 minutes

Platelet count <100,000 cells/mm^3: Do **not** administer

Maximum dose: The prescribed, measured, and administered dose of Y-90 ibritumomab must not exceed 32 mCi (1184 MBq), regardless of the patient's body weight

Dosage Forms Each kit contains 4 vials for preparation of either In-111 or Y-90 conjugate (as indicated on container label)

Injection, solution: 1.6 mg/mL (2 mL) [supplied with sodium acetate solution, formulation buffer vial (includes albumin 750 mg), and an empty reaction vial]

ibritumomab tiuxetan *see* ibritumomab *on this page*

Ibu-200 [US-OTC] *see* ibuprofen *on this page*

Ibuprin® ***(Discontinued)*** *see* ibuprofen *on this page*

ibuprofen (eye byoo PROE fen)

Sound-Alike/Look-Alike Issues

Haltran® may be confused with Halfprin®

Synonyms ibuprofen lysine; *p*-isobutylhydratropic acid

U.S./Canadian Brand Names Advil® Children's [US-OTC]; Advil® Infants' [US-OTC]; Advil® Junior [US-OTC]; Advil® Migraine [US-OTC]; Advil® [US-OTC/Can]; Apo-Ibuprofen® [Can]; ElixSure™ IB [US-OTC]; Genpril® [US-OTC]; I-Prin [US-OTC]; Ibu-200 [US-OTC]; Midol® Cramp and Body Aches [US-OTC]; Motrin® Children's [US-OTC/Can]; Motrin® IB [US-OTC/Can]; Motrin® Infants' [US-OTC]; Motrin® Junior Strength [US-OTC]; Motrin® [US]; NeoProfen®; Novo-Profen [Can]; Nu-Ibuprofen [Can]; Proprinal [US-OTC]; Ultraprin [US-OTC]

Therapeutic Category Analgesic, Nonnarcotic; Antipyretic; Nonsteroidal Antiinflammatory Drug (NSAID)

Use

Oral: Inflammatory diseases and rheumatoid disorders including juvenile rheumatoid arthritis, mild-to-moderate pain, fever, dysmenorrhea

Injection: Ibuprofen lysine is for use in premature infants weighing between 500-1500 g and who are ≤32 weeks gestational age (GA) to induce closure of a clinically-significant patent ductus arteriosus (PDA) when usual treatments are ineffective

(Continued)

ibuprofen *(Continued)*

Usual Dosage

I.V.: Infants between 500-1500 g and ≤32 weeks GA: Patent ductus arteriosus: Initial dose: Ibuprofen 10 mg/kg, followed by two doses of 5 mg/kg at 24 and 48 hours. Dose should be based on birth weight.

Oral:

Children:

Antipyretic: 6 months to 12 years: Temperature <102.5°F (39°C): 5 mg/kg/dose; temperature >102.5°F: 10 mg/kg/dose given every 6-8 hours (maximum daily dose: 40 mg/kg/day)

Juvenile rheumatoid arthritis: 30-50 mg/kg/24 hours divided every 8 hours; start at lower end of dosing range and titrate upward (maximum: 2.4 g/day)

Analgesic: 4-10 mg/kg/dose every 6-8 hours

OTC labeling (analgesic, antipyretic):

Children 6 months to 11 years: See below; use of weight to select dose is preferred; doses may be repeated every 6-8 hours (maximum: 4 doses/day)

Children ≥12 years: 200 mg every 4-6 hours as needed (maximum: 1200 mg/24 hours)

Ibuprofen Dosing:

Weight 12-17 lbs (6-11 months of age): 50 mg
Weight 18-23 lbs (12-23 months of age): 75 mg
Weight 24-35 lbs (2-3 years of age): 100 mg
Weight 35-47 lbs (4-5 years of age): 150 mg
Weight 48-59 lbs (6-8 years of age): 200 mg
Weight 60-71 lbs (9-10 years of age): 250 mg
Weight 72-95 lbs (11 years of age): 300 mg

Adults:

Inflammatory disease: 400-800 mg/dose 3-4 times/day (maximum dose: 3.2 g/day)

Analgesia/pain/fever/dysmenorrhea: 200-400 mg/dose every 4-6 hours (maximum daily dose: 1.2 g, unless directed by physician)

OTC labeling (analgesic, antipyretic): 200 mg every 4-6 hours as needed (maximum: 1200 mg/24 hours)

Dosage Forms

Caplet: 200 mg [OTC]
Advil®: 200 mg [contains sodium benzoate]
Ibu-200, Motrin® IB: 200 mg
Motrin® Junior Strength: 100 mg

Capsule, liqui-gel:
Advil®: 200 mg
Advil® Migraine: 200 mg [solubilized ibuprofen; contains potassium 20 mg]

Gelcap:
Advil®: 200 mg [contains coconut oil]

Injection, solution, as lysine [preservative free]:
NeoProfen®: 17.1 mg/mL (2 mL) [equivalent to ibuprofen 10 mg/mL]

Suspension, oral: 100 mg/5 mL (5 mL, 120 mL, 480 mL)
Advil® Children's: 100 mg/5 mL (60 mL, 120 mL) [contains sodium benzoate; blue raspberry, fruit, and grape flavors]
ElixSure™ IB: 100 mg/5 mL (120 mL) [berry flavor]
Motrin® Children's: 100 mg/5 mL (60 mL, 120 mL) [contains sodium benzoate; berry, dye free berry, bubble gum, and grape flavors]

Suspension, oral drops: 40 mg/mL (15 mL)
Advil® Infants': 40 mg/mL (15 mL) [contains sodium benzoate; fruit and grape flavors]
Motrin® Infants': 40 mg/mL (15 mL, 30 mL) [contains sodium benzoate; berry and dye-free berry flavors]

Tablet: 200 mg [OTC], 400 mg, 600 mg, 800 mg
Advil®: 200 mg [contains sodium benzoate]
Advil® Junior: 100 mg [contains sodium benzoate; coated tablets]
Genpril®, I-Prin, Midol® Cramp and Body Aches, Motrin® IB, Proprinal, Ultraprin: 200 mg
Motrin®: 400 mg, 600 mg, 800 mg

Tablet, chewable:
Advil® Children's: 50 mg [contains phenylalanine 2.1 mg; grape flavors]
Advil® Junior: 100 mg [contains phenylalanine 4.2 mg; grape flavors]
Motrin® Children's: 50 mg [contains phenylalanine 1.4 mg; grape and orange flavor]
Motrin® Junior Strength: 100 mg [contains phenylalanine 2.1 mg; grape and orange flavors]

ibuprofen and hydrocodone *see* hydrocodone and ibuprofen *on page 424*

ibuprofen and pseudoephedrine *see* pseudoephedrine and ibuprofen *on page 715*

ibuprofen lysine *see* ibuprofen *on page 437*

ibuprofen, pseudoephedrine, and chlorpheniramine

(eye byoo PROE fen, soo doe e FED rin, & klor fen IR a meen)

Synonyms chlorpheniramine maleate, ibuprofen, and pseudoephedrine; ibuprofen, pseudoephedrine, and chlorpheniramine maleate; pseudoephedrine, chlorpheniramine, and ibuprofen

U.S./Canadian Brand Names Advil® Allergy Sinus [US]; Advil® Cold and Sinus Plus [Can]; Advil® Multi-Symptom Cold [US]

Therapeutic Category Antihistamine/Decongestant/Analgesic

Use Temporary relief of symptoms associated with the common cold, hay fever, or other respiratory allergies

Usual Dosage Oral: Children ≥12 years and Adults: One caplet every 4-6 hours while symptoms persist (maximum: 6 caplets/24 hours)

Dosage Forms Caplet: Ibuprofen 200 mg, pseudoephedrine hydrochloride 30 mg, and chlorpheniramine maleate 2 mg

ibuprofen, pseudoephedrine, and chlorpheniramine maleate *see* ibuprofen, pseudoephedrine, and chlorpheniramine *on this page*

ibutilide (i BYOO ti lide)

Synonyms ibutilide fumarate

U.S./Canadian Brand Names Corvert® [US]

Therapeutic Category Antiarrhythmic Agent, Class III

Use Acute termination of atrial fibrillation or flutter of recent onset; the effectiveness of ibutilide has not been determined in patients with arrhythmias >90 days in duration

Usual Dosage I.V.: Initial: Adults:

<60 kg: 0.01 mg/kg over 10 minutes

≥60 kg: 1 mg over 10 minutes

If the arrhythmia does not terminate within 10 minutes after the end of the initial infusion, a second infusion of equal strength may be infused over a 10-minute period

Dosage Forms Injection, solution, as fumarate: 0.1 mg/mL (10 mL)

ibutilide fumarate *see* ibutilide *on this page*

IC-Green® [US] *see* indocyanine green *on page 446*

ICI-182,780 *see* fulvestrant *on page 372*

ICI-204,219 *see* zafirlukast *on page 883*

ICI-46474 *see* tamoxifen *on page 804*

ICI-118630 *see* goserelin *on page 391*

ICI-176334 *see* bicalutamide *on page 110*

ICI-D1033 *see* anastrozole *on page 56*

ICI-D1694 *see* raltitrexed *(Canada only) on page 731*

ICL670 *see* deferasirox *on page 233*

ICRF-187 *see* dexrazoxane *on page 242*

Idamycin® [Can] *see* idarubicin *on this page*

Idamycin® *(Discontinued)* *see* idarubicin *on this page*

Idamycin PFS® [US] *see* idarubicin *on this page*

Idarac® [Can] *see* floctafenine *(Canada only) on page 348*

idarubicin (eye da ROO bi sin)

Sound-Alike/Look-Alike Issues

idarubicin may be confused with DOXOrubicin, DAUNOrubicin, epirubicin

Idamycin PFS® may be confused with Adriamycin

Synonyms 4-demethoxydaunorubicin; 4-DMDR; idarubicin hydrochloride; IDR; IMI 30; NSC-256439; SC 33428

U.S./Canadian Brand Names Idamycin PFS® [US]; Idamycin® [Can]

Therapeutic Category Antineoplastic Agent

Use Treatment of acute leukemias (AML, ANLL, ALL), accelerated phase or blast crisis of chronic myelogenous leukemia (CML), breast cancer

(Continued)

idarubicin *(Continued)*

Usual Dosage Refer to individual protocols. I.V.:
Children:
Leukemia: 10-12 mg/m^2/day for 3 days every 3 weeks
Solid tumors: 5 mg/m^2/day for 3 days every 3 weeks
Adults:
Leukemia induction: 12 mg/m^2/day for 3 days
Leukemia consolidation: 10-12 mg/m^2/day for 2 days

Dosage Forms Injection, solution, as hydrochloride [preservative free] (Idamycin PFS®): 1 mg/mL (5 mL, 10 mL, 20 mL)

idarubicin hydrochloride *see* idarubicin *on previous page*

IDEC-C2B8 *see* rituximab *on page 749*

IDR *see* idarubicin *on previous page*

Ifex® [US/Can] *see* ifosfamide *on this page*

IFLrA *see* interferon alfa-2a *on page 454*

ifosfamide (eye FOSS fa mide)

Sound-Alike/Look-Alike Issues
ifosfamide may be confused with cyclophosphamide

Synonyms isophosphamide; NSC-109724; Z4942

U.S./Canadian Brand Names Ifex® [US/Can]

Therapeutic Category Antineoplastic Agent

Use Treatment of lung cancer, Hodgkin and non-Hodgkin lymphoma, breast cancer, acute and chronic lymphocytic leukemias, ovarian cancer, sarcomas, pancreatic and gastric carcinomas
Orphan drug: Treatment of testicular cancer

Usual Dosage Refer to individual protocols. To prevent bladder toxicity, ifosfamide should be given with the urinary protector mesna and hydration of at least 2 L of oral or I.V. fluid per day. I.V.:
Children:
1200-1800 mg/m^2/day for 3-5 days every 21-28 days **or**
5 g/m^2 once every 21-28 days **or**
3 g/m^2/day for 2 days every 21-28 days
Adults:
50 mg/kg/day or 700-2000 mg/m^2 for 5 days every 3-4 weeks
Alternatives: 2400 mg/m^2/day for 3 days or 5000 mg/m^2 as a single dose every 3-4 weeks

Dosage Forms
Injection, powder for reconstitution: 1 g
Ifex®: 1 g, 3 g

IG *see* immune globulin (intramuscular) *on page 443*

IgG4-kappa monoclonal antibody *see* natalizumab *on page 580*

IGIM *see* immune globulin (intramuscular) *on page 443*

IL-1Ra *see* anakinra *on page 56*

IL-2 *see* aldesleukin *on page 26*

IL-11 *see* oprelvekin *on page 618*

Ilopan-Choline® Oral ***(Discontinued)*** *see* dexpanthenol *on page 242*

Ilopan® Injection ***(Discontinued)*** *see* dexpanthenol *on page 242*

iloprost (EYE loe prost)

Synonyms iloprost tromethamine; prostacyclin PGI_2

U.S./Canadian Brand Names Ventavis™ [US]

Therapeutic Category Prostaglandin

Use Treatment of idiopathic pulmonary arterial hypertension in patients with NYHA Class III or IV symptoms

Usual Dosage Inhalation: Adults: Initial: 2.5 mcg/dose; if tolerated, increase to 5 mcg/dose; administer 6-9 times daily (dosing at intervals ≥2 hours while awake); maintenance dose: 5 mcg/dose; maximum daily dose: 45 mcg

Dosage Forms Solution for oral inhalation [preservative-free]: 10 mcg/mL (1 mL, 2 mL) [ampul]

iloprost tromethamine *see* iloprost *on this page*

Ilozyme® *(Discontinued)* *see* pancrelipase *on page 634*

imatinib (eye MAT eh nib)

Synonyms CGP-57148B; glivec; imatinib mesylate; STI571

U.S./Canadian Brand Names Gleevec® [US/Can]

Therapeutic Category Antineoplastic, Tyrosine Kinase Inhibitor

Use Treatment of newly-diagnosed Philadelphia chromosome-positive (Ph+) chronic myeloid leukemia (CML) in chronic phase; treatment of patients with Ph+ CML in blast crisis, accelerated phase or chronic phase after failure of interferon therapy; treatment of pediatric patients with Ph+ CML (chronic phase) recurring following stem cell transplant or who are resistant to interferon-alpha therapy; treatment of Kit-positive (CD117) unresectable and/or (metastatic) malignant gastrointestinal stromal tumors (GIST)

Usual Dosage Oral:

Children ≥3 years: CML (chronic phase): 260 mg/m^2/day; may be increased to 340 mg/m^2/day

Adults:

CML:

Chronic phase: 400 mg once daily; may be increased to 600 mg daily

Accelerated phase or blast crisis: 600 mg once daily; may be increased to 800 mg daily (400 mg twice daily)

Gastrointestinal stromal tumors: 400-600 mg/day

Note: Dosage should be increased by at least 50% when used concurrently with a potent enzyme-inducing agent (ie, rifampin, phenytoin).

Dosage Forms

Tablet:

Gleevec®: 100 mg; 400 mg

imatinib mesylate *see* imatinib *on this page*

IMC-C225 *see* cetuximab *on page 168*

Imdur® [US/Can] *see* isosorbide mononitrate *on page 466*

IMI 30 *see* idarubicin *on page 439*

IMid-3 *see* lenalidomide *on page 484*

imidazole carboxamide *see* dacarbazine *on page 226*

imidazole carboxamide dimethyltriazene *see* dacarbazine *on page 226*

imiglucerase (i mi GLOO ser ace)

Sound-Alike/Look-Alike Issues

Cerezyme® may be confused with Cerebyx®, Ceredase®

U.S./Canadian Brand Names Cerezyme® [US/Can]

Therapeutic Category Enzyme

Use Long-term enzyme replacement therapy for patients with Type 1 Gaucher disease

Usual Dosage I.V.: Children ≥2 years and Adults: Initial: 30-60 units/kg every 2 weeks; dosing is individualized based on disease severity. Dosing range: 2.5 units/kg 3 times/week up to as much as 60 units/kg administered as frequently as once a week or as infrequently as every 4 weeks. Average dose: 60 units/kg administered every 2 weeks

Dosage Forms Injection, powder for reconstitution [preservative free]: 200 units, 400 units

imipemide *see* imipenem and cilastatin *on this page*

imipenem and cilastatin (i mi PEN em & sye la STAT in)

Sound-Alike/Look-Alike Issues

Primaxin® may be confused with Premarin®, Primacor®

Synonyms imipemide

U.S./Canadian Brand Names Primaxin® I.V. [Can]; Primaxin® [US/Can]

Therapeutic Category Carbapenem (Antibiotic)

Use Treatment of lower respiratory tract, urinary tract, intraabdominal, gynecologic, bone and joint, skin and skin structure, and polymicrobic infections as well as bacterial septicemia and endocarditis. Antibacterial activity includes resistant gram-negative bacilli (*Pseudomonas aeruginosa* and *Enterobacter* sp), gram-positive bacteria (methicillin-sensitive *Staphylococcus aureus* and *Streptococcus* sp) and anaerobes.

Usual Dosage

Usual dosage ranges: Note: Dosage based on **imipenem** content:

Neonates ≤3 months and weight ≥1500 g: Non-CNS infections: I.V.:

<1 week: 25 mg/kg every 12 hours

(Continued)

imipenem and cilastatin *(Continued)*

1-4 weeks: 25 mg/kg every 8 hours
4 weeks to 3 months: 25 mg/kg every 6 hours
Children >3 months: Non-CNS infections: I.V.: 15-25 mg/kg every 6 hours; maximum dosage: Susceptible infections: 2 g/day; moderately-susceptible organisms: 4 g/day
Adults:
I.M.: Weight ≥70 kg: 500-750 mg every 12 hours
I.V.: Weight ≥70 kg: 250-1000 mg every 6-8 hours; maximum: 4 g/day

Indication-specific dosing: Note: Doses based on imipenem content. I.M. administration is not intended for severe or life-threatening infections (eg, septicemia, endocarditis, shock), UTI, bone/joint or polymicrobic infections:
Children: I.V.: **Cystic fibrosis:** Doses up to 90 mg/kg/day have been used
Adults:
Intraabdominal infections:
I.V.: Mild infection: 250-500 mg every 6 hours; severe: 500 mg every 6 hours
I.M.: Mild-to-moderate infection: 750 mg every 12 hours
Liver abscess: I.V.: 500 mg every 6 hours for 2-3 weeks, then appropriate oral therapy for a total of 4-6 weeks
Lower respiratory tract, skins/skin structure, gynecologic infections: I.M.: Mild/moderate: 500-750 mg every 12 hours
Mild infection: Note: Rarely a suitable option in mild infections; normally reserved for moderate-severe cases:
I.M.: 500 mg every 12 hours
I.V.:
Fully-susceptible organisms: 250 mg every 6 hours
Moderately-susceptible organisms: 500 mg every 6 hours
Moderate infection:
I.M.: 750 mg every 12 hours
I.V.:
Fully-susceptible organisms: 500 mg every 6-8 hours
Moderately-susceptible organisms: 500 mg every 6 hours or 1 g every 8 hours
Neutropenic fever, otitis externa: I.V.: 500 mg every 6 hours
***Pseudomonas* infections:** I.V.: 500 mg every 6 hours; **Note:** Higher doses may be required based on organism sensitivity.
Severe infection: I.V.:
Fully-susceptible organisms: 500 mg every 6 hours
Moderately-susceptible organisms: 1 g every 6-8 hours
Maximum daily dose should not exceed 50 mg/kg or 4 g/day, whichever is lower
Urinary tract infection: I.V.:
Uncomplicated: 250 mg every 6 hours
Complicated: 500 mg every 6 hours

Dosage Forms
Injection, powder for reconstitution [I.M.]: Imipenem 500 mg and cilastatin 500 mg [contains sodium 32 mg (1.4 mEq)]
Injection, powder for reconstitution [I.V.]: Imipenem 250 mg and cilastatin 250 mg [contains sodium 18.8 mg (0.8 mEq)]; imipenem 500 mg and cilastatin 500 mg [contains sodium 37.5 mg (1.6 mEq)]

imipramine (im IP ra meen)

Sound-Alike/Look-Alike Issues
imipramine may be confused with amitriptyline, desipramine, Norpramin®

Synonyms imipramine hydrochloride; imipramine pamoate

U.S./Canadian Brand Names Apo-Imipramine® [Can]; Novo-Pramine [Can]; Tofranil-PM® [US]; Tofranil® [US/Can]

Therapeutic Category Antidepressant, Tricyclic (Tertiary Amine)

Use Treatment of depression; treatment of nocturnal enuresis in children

Usual Dosage Oral:
Children: Enuresis: ≥6 years: Initial: 25 mg at bedtime, if inadequate response still seen after 1 week of therapy, increase by 25 mg/day; dose should not exceed 2.5 mg/kg/day or 50 mg at bedtime if 6-12 years of age or 75 mg at bedtime if ≥12 years of age
Adolescents: Depression: Initial: 30-40 mg/day; increase gradually; maximum: 100 mg/day in single or divided doses
Adults: Depression: Initial: 25 mg 3-4 times/day, increase dose gradually, total dose may be given at bedtime; maximum: 300 mg/day

Dosage Forms
Capsule, as pamoate: 75 mg, 100 mg, 125 mg, 150 mg
Tofranil-PM®: 75 mg, 100 mg, 125 mg, 150 mg
Tablet, as hydrochloride: 10 mg, 25 mg, 50 mg
Tofranil®): 10 mg, 25 mg, 50 mg

imipramine hydrochloride *see* imipramine *on previous page*

imipramine pamoate *see* imipramine *on previous page*

imiquimod (i mi KWI mod)

Sound-Alike/Look-Alike Issues
Aldara™ may be confused with Alora®

U.S./Canadian Brand Names Aldara™ [US/Can]

Therapeutic Category Immune Response Modifier

Use Treatment of external genital and perianal warts/condyloma acuminata; nonhyperkeratotic, nonhypertrophic actinic keratosis on face or scalp; superficial basal cell carcinoma (sBCC) with a maximum tumor diameter of 2 cm located on the trunk, neck, or extremities (excluding hands or feet)

Usual Dosage Topical:
Children ≥12 years and Adults: Perianal warts/condyloma acuminata: Apply a thin layer 3 times/week prior to bedtime and leave on skin for 6-10 hours. Remove with mild soap and water. Examples of 3 times/week application schedules are: Monday, Wednesday, Friday; or Tuesday, Thursday, Saturday. Continue imiquimod treatment until there is total clearance of the genital/perianal warts for ≤16 weeks. A rest period of several days may be taken if required by the patient's discomfort or severity of the local skin reaction. Treatment may resume once the reaction subsides.
Adults:
Actinic keratosis: Apply twice weekly for 16 weeks to a treatment area on face or scalp; apply prior to bedtime and leave on skin for 8 hours. Remove with mild soap and water.
Common oral warts (dental use): Apply once daily prior to bedtime
Superficial basal cell carcinoma: Apply once daily prior to bedtime, 5 days/week for 6 weeks. Treatment area should include a 1 cm margin of skin around the tumor. Leave on skin for 8 hours. Remove with mild soap and water.

Dosage Forms Cream: 5% (12s) [contains benzyl alcohol; single-dose packets]

Imitrex® [US/Can] *see* sumatriptan *on page 801*

Imitrex® DF [Can] *see* sumatriptan *on page 801*

Imitrex® Nasal Spray [Can] *see* sumatriptan *on page 801*

ImmuCyst® [Can] *see* BCG vaccine *on page 94*

immune globulin (intramuscular) (i MYUN GLOB yoo lin, IN tra MUS kyoo ler)

Synonyms gamma globulin; IG; IGIM; immune serum globulin; ISG

U.S./Canadian Brand Names BayGam® [Can]; GannaSTAN™ S/D [US]

Therapeutic Category Immune Globulin

Use To provide passive immunity in susceptible individuals under the following circumstances:
Hepatitis A: Within 14 days of exposure and prior to manifestation of disease
Measles: For use within 6 days of exposure in an unvaccinated person, who has not previously had measles
Varicella: When Varicella Zoster Immune Globulin is not available
Rubella: Post exposure prophylaxis (within 72 hours) to reduce the risk of infection in exposed pregnant women who will not consider therapeutic abortion
Immunoglobulin deficiency: To help prevent serious infections

Usual Dosage I.M.: Children and Adults:
Hepatitis A:
Pre-exposure prophylaxis upon travel into endemic areas (hepatitis A vaccine preferred):
0.02 mL/kg for anticipated risk of exposure <3 months
0.06 mL/kg for anticipated risk of exposure ≥3 months
Repeat approximate dose every 5 months if exposure continues
Postexposure prophylaxis: 0.02 mL/kg given within 14 days of exposure. IG is not needed if at least 1 dose of hepatitis A vaccine was given at ≥1 month before exposure
Measles:
Prophylaxis, immunocompetent: 0.25 mL/kg/dose (maximum dose: 15 mL) given within 6 days of exposure followed by live attenuated measles vaccine in 5-6 months when indicated
Prophylaxis, immunocompromised: 0.5 mL/kg (maximum dose: 15 mL) immediately following exposure

(Continued)

immune globulin (intramuscular) *(Continued)*

Rubella: Prophylaxis during pregnancy: 0.55 mL/kg/dose within 72 hours of exposure

Varicella: Prophylaxis: 0.6-1.2 mL/kg (varicella zoster immune globulin preferred) within 72 hours of exposure

IgG deficiency: 0.66 mL/kg/dose every 3-4 weeks. A double dose may be given at onset of therapy; some patients may require more frequent injections.

Dosage Forms

Injection, solution [preservative free]:

BayGam® [DSC], GammaSTAN™ S/D: 15% to 18% (2 mL, 10 mL)

immune globulin (intravenous) (i MYUN GLOB yoo lin, IN tra VEE nus)

Sound-Alike/Look-Alike Issues

Gamimune® N may be confused with CytoGam®

Synonyms IVIG

U.S./Canadian Brand Names Carimune™ NF [US]; Gammagard® Liquid [US/Can]; Gammagard® S/D [US/Can]; Gammar®-P I.V. [US]; Gamunex® [US/Can]; Iveegam EN [US]; Iveegam Immuno® [Can]; Octagam® [US]; Panglobulin® NF [US]; Polygam® S/D [US]

Therapeutic Category Immune Globulin

Use

Treatment of primary immunodeficiency syndromes (congenital agammaglobulinemia, severe combined immunodeficiency syndromes [SCIDS], common variable immunodeficiency, X-linked immunodeficiency, Wiskott-Aldrich syndrome); idiopathic thrombocytopenic purpura (ITP); Kawasaki disease (in combination with aspirin)

Prevention of bacterial infection in B-cell chronic lymphocytic leukemia (CLL); pediatric HIV infection; bone marrow transplant (BMT)

Usual Dosage Approved doses and regimens may vary between brands; check manufacturer guidelines. **Note:** Some clinicians dose IVIG on ideal body weight or an adjusted ideal body weight in morbidly obese patients.

Children: I.V.: Pediatric HIV: 400 mg/kg every 28 days

Children and Adults: I.V.:

Primary immunodeficiency disorders: 200-400 mg/kg every 4 weeks or as per monitored serum IgG concentrations

Gammagard® Liquid, Gamunex®, Octagam®: 300-600 mg/kg every 3-4 weeks; adjusted based on dosage and interval in conjunction with monitored serum IgG concentrations.

B-cell chronic lymphocytic leukemia (CLL): 400 mg/kg/dose every 3 weeks

Idiopathic thrombocytopenic purpura (ITP):

Acute: 400 mg/kg/day for 5 days or 1000 mg/kg/day for 1-2 days

Chronic: 400 mg/kg as needed to maintain platelet count >30,000/mm^3; may increase dose to 800 mg/kg (1000 mg/kg if needed)

Kawasaki disease: Initiate therapy within 10 days of disease onset: 2 g/kg as a single dose administered over 10 hours, or 400 mg/kg/day for 4 days. **Note:** Must be used in combination with aspirin: 80-100 mg/kg/day in 4 divided doses for 14 days; when fever subsides, dose aspirin at 3-5 mg/kg once daily for ≥6-8 weeks

Bone marrow transplant: 500 mg/kg beginning on days 7 and 2 pretransplant, then 500 mg/kg/week for 90 days post-transplant

Dosage Forms

Injection, powder for reconstitution [preservative free]:

Gammar®-P I.V.: 5 g, 10 g [stabilized with human albumin and sucrose]

Iveegam EN: 5 g [stabilized with glucose]

Injection, powder for reconstitution [preservative free, nanofiltered]:

Carimune™ NF: 3 g, 6 g, 12 g [contains sucrose]

Panglobulin® NF: 6 g, 12 g [contains sucrose]

Injection, powder for reconstitution [preservative free, solvent detergent-treated]:

Gammagard® S/D: 2.5 g, 5 g, 10 g [stabilized with human albumin, glycine, glucose, and polyethylene glycol]

Polygam® S/D: 5 g, 10 g [stabilized with human albumin, glycine, glucose, and polyethylene glycol]

Injection, solution [preservative free; solvent detergent-treated]:

Gammagard® Liquid: 10% [100 mg/mL] (10 mL, 25 mL, 50 mL, 100 mL, 200 mL) [latex free, sucrose free; stabilized with glycine]

Octagam®: 5% [50 mg/mL] (20 mL, 50 mL, 100 mL, 200 mL) [sucrose free; contains sodium 30 mmol/L and maltose]

Injection, solution [preservative free] (Gamunex®): 10% (10 mL, 25 mL, 50 mL, 100 mL, 200 mL) [caprylate/chromatography purified]

immune serum globulin *see* immune globulin (intramuscular) *on page 443*

Immunine® VH [Can] *see* factor IX *on page 333*

Imodium® [Can] *see* loperamide *on page 503*

Imodium® A-D [US-OTC] *see* loperamide *on page 503*

Imogam® Rabies-HT [US] *see* rabies immune globulin (human) *on page 727*

Imogam® Rabies Pasteurized [Can] *see* rabies immune globulin (human) *on page 727*

Imovane® [Can] *see* zopiclone *(Canada only) on page 890*

Imovax® Rabies [US/Can] *see* rabies virus vaccine *on page 728*

Imuran® [US/Can] *see* azathioprine *on page 86*

In-111 zevalin *see* ibritumomab *on page 437*

inamrinone (eye NAM ri none)

Sound-Alike/Look-Alike Issues
amrinone may be confused with amiloride, amiodarone

Synonyms amrinone lactate

Therapeutic Category Adrenergic Agonist Agent

Use Infrequently used as a last resort, short-term therapy in patients with intractable heart failure

Usual Dosage Dosage is based on clinical response (**Note:** Dose should not exceed 10 mg/kg/24 hours).
Infants, Children, and Adults: 0.75 mg/kg I.V. bolus over 2-3 minutes followed by maintenance infusion of 5-10 mcg/kg/minute; I.V. bolus may need to be repeated in 30 minutes.

Dosage Forms Injection, solution, as lactate: 5 mg/mL (20 mL) [contains sodium metabisulfite]

I-Naphline® Ophthalmic *(Discontinued)* *see* naphazoline *on page 577*

Inapsine® [US] *see* droperidol *on page 281*

Increlex™ [US] *see* mecasermin *on page 522*

indapamide (in DAP a mide)

Sound-Alike/Look-Alike Issues
indapamide may be confused with Iopidine®

U.S./Canadian Brand Names Apo-Indapamide® [Can]; Gen-Indapamide [Can]; Lozide® [Can]; Lozol® [US/Can]; Novo-Indapamide [Can]; Nu-Indapamide [Can]; PMS-Indapamide [Can]

Therapeutic Category Diuretic, Miscellaneous

Use Management of mild to moderate hypertension; treatment of edema in congestive heart failure and nephrotic syndrome

Usual Dosage Adults: Oral:
Edema: 2.5-5 mg/day. **Note:** There is little therapeutic benefit to increasing the dose >5 mg/day; there is, however, an increased risk of electrolyte disturbances
Hypertension: 1.25 mg in the morning, may increase to 5 mg/day by increments of 1.25-2.5 mg; consider adding another antihypertensive and decreasing the dose if response is not adequate

Dosage Forms
Tablet: 1.25 mg, 2.5 mg
Lozol®: 1.25 mg

Inderal® [US/Can] *see* propranolol *on page 709*

Inderal® LA [US/Can] *see* propranolol *on page 709*

Inderide® [US] *see* propranolol and hydrochlorothiazide *on page 710*

indinavir (in DIN a veer)

Sound-Alike/Look-Alike Issues
indinavir may be confused with Denavir™

Synonyms indinavir sulfate

U.S./Canadian Brand Names Crixivan® [US/Can]

Therapeutic Category Antiviral Agent

Use Treatment of HIV infection; should always be used as part of a multidrug regimen (at least three antiretroviral agents)

Usual Dosage Adults: Oral:
Unboosted regimen: 800 mg every 8 hours
(Continued)

indinavir *(Continued)*

Ritonavir-boosted regimens:
Ritonavir 100-200 mg twice daily plus indinavir 800 mg twice daily **or**
Ritonavir 400 mg twice daily plus indinavir 400 mg twice daily

Dosage adjustments for indinavir when administered in combination therapy:
Delavirdine, itraconazole, or ketoconazole: Reduce indinavir dose to 600 mg every 8 hours
Efavirenz: Increase indinavir dose to 1000 mg every 8 hours
Lopinavir and ritonavir (Kaletra™): Indinavir 600 mg twice daily
Nelfinavir: Increase indinavir dose to 1200 mg twice daily
Nevirapine: Increase indinavir dose to 1000 mg every 8 hours
Rifabutin: Reduce rifabutin to $^1/_2$ the standard dose plus increase indinavir to 1000 mg every 8 hours

Dosage Forms
Capsule:
Crixivan®: 100 mg, 200 mg, 333 mg, 400 mg

indinavir sulfate *see* indinavir *on previous page*

Indocid® P.D.A. [Can] *see* indomethacin *on this page*

Indocin® [US/Can] *see* indomethacin *on this page*

Indocin® I.V. [US] *see* indomethacin *on this page*

Indocin® SR [US] *see* indomethacin *on this page*

indocyanine green (in doe SYE a neen green)

U.S./Canadian Brand Names IC-Green® [US]

Therapeutic Category Diagnostic Agent

Use Determining hepatic function, cardiac output, and liver blood flow; ophthalmic angiography

Usual Dosage
Angiography: Use 40 mg of dye in 2 mL of aqueous solvent, in some patients, half the volume (1 mL) has been found to produce angiograms of comparable resolution; immediately following the bolus dose of dye, a bolus of sodium chloride 0.9% is given; this regimen will deliver a spatially limited dye bolus of optimal concentration to the choroidal vasculature following I.V. injection
Determination of cardiac output: Dye is injected as rapidly as possible into the right atrium, right ventricle, or pulmonary artery through a cardiac catheter; the usual dose is 1.25 mg for infants, 2.5 mg for children, and 5 mg for adults; total dose should not exceed 2 mg/kg; the dye is diluted with sterile water for injection or sodium chloride 0.9% to make a final volume of 1 mL; doses are repeated periodically to obtain several dilution curves; the dye should be flushed from the catheter with sodium chloride 0.9% to prevent hemolysis

Dosage Forms
Injection, powder for reconstitution:
IC-Green™: 25 mg [contains sodium iodide ≤5%; supplied with diluent]

Indo-Lemmon [Can] *see* indomethacin *on this page*

indometacin *see* indomethacin *on this page*

indomethacin (in doe METH a sin)

Sound-Alike/Look-Alike Issues
Indocin® may be confused with Imodium®, Lincocin®, Minocin®, Vicodin®

Synonyms indometacin; indomethacin sodium trihydrate

U.S./Canadian Brand Names Apo-Indomethacin® [Can]; Indo-Lemmon [Can]; Indocid® P.D.A. [Can]; Indocin® I.V. [US]; Indocin® SR [US]; Indocin® [US/Can]; Indotec [Can]; Novo-Methacin [Can]; Nu-Indo [Can]; Rhodacine® [Can]

Therapeutic Category Analgesic, Nonnarcotic; Nonsteroidal Antiinflammatory Drug (NSAID)

Use Acute gouty arthritis, acute bursitis/tendonitis, moderate to severe osteoarthritis, rheumatoid arthritis, ankylosing spondylitis; I.V. form used as alternative to surgery for closure of patent ductus arteriosus in neonates

Usual Dosage
Patent ductus arteriosus:
Neonates: I.V.: Initial: 0.2 mg/kg, followed by 2 doses depending on postnatal age (PNA):
PNA **at time of first dose** <48 hours: 0.1 mg/kg at 12- to 24-hour intervals
PNA **at time of first dose** 2-7 days: 0.2 mg/kg at 12- to 24-hour intervals
PNA **at time of first dose** >7 days: 0.25 mg/kg at 12- to 24-hour intervals

In general, may use 12-hour dosing interval if urine output >1 mL/kg/hour after prior dose; use 24-hour dosing interval if urine output is <1 mL/kg/hour but >0.6 mL/kg/hour; doses should be withheld if patient has oliguria (urine output <0.6 mL/kg/hour) or anuria

Inflammatory/rheumatoid disorders: Oral: Use lowest effective dose.

Children >2 years: 1-2 mg/kg/day in 2-4 divided doses; maximum dose: 4 mg/kg/day; not to exceed 150-200 mg/day

Adults: 25-50 mg/dose 2-3 times/day; maximum dose: 200 mg/day; extended release capsule should be given on a 1-2 times/day schedule; maximum dose for sustained release is 150 mg/day. In patients with arthritis and persistent night pain and/or morning stiffness may give the larger portion (up to 100 mg) of the total daily dose at bedtime.

Bursitis/tendonitis: Oral: Adults: Initial dose: 75-150 mg/day in 3-4 divided doses; usual treatment is 7-14 days

Acute gouty arthritis: Oral: Adults: 50 mg 3 times daily until pain is tolerable then reduce dose; usual treatment <3-5 days

Dosage Forms

Capsule (Indocin®): 25 mg, 50 mg

Capsule, sustained release (Indocin® SR): 75 mg

Injection, powder for reconstitution, as sodium trihydrate (Indocin® I.V.): 1 mg

Suspension, oral (Indocin®): 25 mg/5 mL (237 mL) [contains alcohol 1%; pineapple-coconut-mint flavor]

indomethacin sodium trihydrate *see* indomethacin *on previous page*

Indotec [Can] *see* indomethacin *on previous page*

INF-alpha 2 *see* interferon alfa-2b *on page 454*

Infanrix® [US] *see* diphtheria, tetanus toxoids, and acellular pertussis vaccine *on page 265*

Infantaire [US-OTC] *see* acetaminophen *on page 5*

Infantaire Gas Drops [US-OTC] *see* simethicone *on page 772*

Infants' Tylenol® Cold Plus Cough Concentrated Drops [US-OTC] *see* acetaminophen, dextromethorphan, and pseudoephedrine *on page 12*

Infasurf® [US] *see* calfactant *on page 140*

INFeD® [US] *see* iron dextran complex *on page 462*

Infergen® [US] *see* interferon alfacon-1 *on page 456*

Inflamase® Mild [Can] *see* prednisolone (ophthalmic) *on page 694*

infliximab (in FLIKS e mab)

Sound-Alike/Look-Alike Issues

Remicade® may be confused with Renacidin®, Rituxan®

Synonyms infliximab, recombinant; NSC-728729

U.S./Canadian Brand Names Remicade® [US/Can]

Therapeutic Category Monoclonal Antibody

Use

Ankylosing spondylitis: Improving signs and symptoms of disease

Crohn disease: Induction and maintenance of remission in patients with moderate to severe disease who have an inadequate response to conventional therapy; to reduce the number of draining enterocutaneous and rectovaginal fistulas and to maintain fistula closure

Psoriatic arthritis: Improving signs and symptoms of active arthritis in patients with psoriatic arthritis

Rheumatoid arthritis: Inhibits the progression of structural damage and improves physical function in patients with moderate to severe disease; used with methotrexate

Ulcerative colitis (UC): To reduce signs and symptoms, achieve clinical remission and mucosal healing and eliminate corticosteroid use in moderately to severely active UC inadequately responsive to conventional therapy

Usual Dosage I.V.:

Children ≥6 years: Crohn disease: 5 mg/kg at 0, 2, and 6 weeks, followed by a maintenance dose of 5 mg/kg every 8 weeks

Adults:

Crohn disease: Induction regimen: 5 mg/kg at 0, 2, and 6 weeks, followed by 5 mg/kg every 8 weeks thereafter; dose may be increased to 10 mg/kg in patients who respond but then lose their response. If no response by week 14, consider discontinuing therapy.

Psoriatic arthritis (with or without methotrexate): 5 mg/kg at 0, 2, and 6 weeks, then every 8 weeks

(Continued)

infliximab *(Continued)*

Rheumatoid arthritis (in combination with methotrexate therapy): 3 mg/kg at 0, 2, and 6 weeks, then every 8 weeks thereafter; doses have ranged from 3-10 mg/kg intravenous infusion repeated at 4- to 8-week intervals

Ankylosing spondylitis: 5 mg/kg at 0, 2, and 6 weeks, followed by 5 mg/kg every 6 weeks thereafter

Ulcerative colitis: 5 mg/kg at 0, 2, and 6 weeks, followed by 5 mg/kg every 8 weeks thereafter

Dosage Forms

Injection, powder for reconstitution [preservative free]:

Remicade®: 100 mg [contains sucrose and polysorbate 80]

infliximab, recombinant *see* infliximab *on previous page*

influenza virus vaccine (in floo EN za VYE rus vak SEEN)

Sound-Alike/Look-Alike Issues

Influenza virus vaccine may be confused with tetanus toxoid and tuberculin products. Medication errors have occurred when tuberculin skin tests (PPD) have been inadvertently administered instead of tetanus toxoid products and influenza virus vaccine. These products are refrigerated and often stored in close proximity to each other.

Synonyms influenza virus vaccine (purified surface antigen); influenza virus vaccine (split-virus); influenza virus vaccine (trivalent, live); live attenuated influenza vaccine (LAIV); trivalent inactivated influenza vaccine (TIV)

U.S./Canadian Brand Names Fluarix™ [US]; fluMist® [US]; Fluviral S/F® [Can]; Fluvirin® [US]; Fluzone® [US]; Vaxigrip® [Can]

Therapeutic Category Vaccine, Inactivated Virus

Use Provide active immunity to influenza virus strains contained in the vaccine

Groups at Increased Risk for Influenza-Related Complications: Recommendations for vaccination:

- Persons ≥65 years of age
- Residents of nursing homes and other chronic-care facilities that house persons of any age with chronic medical conditions
- Adults and children with chronic disorders of the pulmonary or cardiovascular systems, including children with asthma
- Adults and children who have required regular medical follow-up or hospitalization during the preceding year because of chronic metabolic diseases (including diabetes mellitus), renal dysfunction, hemoglobinopathies, or immunosuppression (including immunosuppression caused by medications or HIV)
- Adults and children with conditions which may compromise respiratory function, the handling of respiratory secretions, or that can increase the risk of aspiration (eg, cognitive dysfunction, spinal; cord injuries, seizure disorders, other neuromuscular disorders)
- Children and adolescents (6 months to 18 years of age) who are receiving long-term aspirin therapy and therefore, may be at risk for developing Reye syndrome after influenza
- Women who will be pregnant during the influenza season
- Children 6-23 months of age

Vaccination is also recommended for persons 50-64 years of age, close contacts of children 0-23 months of age, healthy persons who may transmit influenza to those at risk, all healthcare workers, and persons who smoke.

Usual Dosage Optimal time to receive vaccine is October-November, prior to exposure to influenza; however, vaccination can continue into December and later as long as vaccine is available.

I.M.:

Fluzone®:

Children 6-35 months: 0.25 mL/dose (1 or 2 doses per season; see **Note**)

Children 3-8 years: 0.5 mL/dose (1 or 2 doses per season; see **Note**)

Children ≥9 years and Adults: 0.5 mL/dose (1 dose per season)

Fluvirin®:

Children 4-8 years: 0.5 mL/dose (1 or 2 doses per season; see **Note**)

Children ≥9 years and Adults: 0.5 mL/dose (1 dose per season)

Note: Previously unvaccinated children <9 years should receive 2 doses, given >1 month apart in order to achieve satisfactory antibody response.

Fluarix™: Adults: 0.5 mL/dose (1 dose per season)

Intranasal (fluMist®):

Children 5-8 years, previously **not vaccinated** with influenza vaccine: Initial season: Two 0.5 mL doses separated by 6-10 weeks

Children 5-8 years, previously **vaccinated** with influenza vaccine: 0.5 mL/dose (1 dose per season)

Children ≥9 years and Adults ≤49 years: 0.5 mL/dose (1 dose per season)

Dosage Forms

Injection, solution, purified split-virus [preservative free]:

Fluvirin®: (0.5 mL) [TIV; contains thimerosal (trace amounts); manufactured using chicken eggs, neomycin, and polymyxin]

Injection, suspension, purified split-virus:

FluLaval™: (5 mL) [TIV; latex-free; contains thimerosal; produced in chick embryo cell culture]

Fluzone®: (5 mL) [TIV; latex free; contains thimerosal; produced in chick embryo cell culture]

Injection, suspension, purified split-virus [preservative free]:

Fluarix®: (0.5 mL) [TIV; syringe cap and rubber plunger contain natural latex rubber; produced in chick embryo cell culture; may contain residual amounts of thimerosal, hydrocortisone, gentamicin, and ovalbumin]

Fluzone®: (0.25 mL) [TIV; latex free; produced in chick embryo cell culture]; (0.5 mL) [TIV; latex free; produced in chick embryo cell culture]

Solution, intranasal [preservative free; trivalent; live virus; spray]:

fluMist®: (0.5 mL) [LAIV; manufactured using eggs and gentamicin]

influenza virus vaccine (purified surface antigen) *see* influenza virus vaccine *on previous page*

influenza virus vaccine (split-virus) *see* influenza virus vaccine *on previous page*

influenza virus vaccine (trivalent, live) *see* influenza virus vaccine *on previous page*

Infufer® [Can] *see* iron dextran complex *on page 462*

Infumorph® [US] *see* morphine sulfate *on page 565*

Infuvite® Adult [US] *see* vitamins (multiple/injectable) *on page 878*

Infuvite® Pediatric [US] *see* vitamins (multiple/injectable) *on page 878*

INH *see* isoniazid *on page 464*

inhaled insulin *see* insulin inhalation *on page 451*

Inhibace® [Can] *see* cilazapril *(Canada only) on page 188*

Innohep® [US/Can] *see* tinzaparin *on page 829*

InnoPran XL™ [US] *see* propranolol *on page 709*

Inocor® ***(Discontinued)***

INOmax® [US/Can] *see* nitric oxide *on page 594*

insect sting kit *see* epinephrine and chlorpheniramine *on page 297*

insoluble prussian blue *see* ferric hexacyanoferrate *on page 342*

Inspra™ [US] *see* eplerenone *on page 298*

Insta-Glucose® [US-OTC] *see* glucose (instant) *on page 386*

Instat™ [US] *see* collagen hemostat *on page 212*

Instat™ MCH [US] *see* collagen hemostat *on page 212*

insulin aspart (IN soo lin AS part)

Sound-Alike/Look-Alike Issues

NovoLog® may be confused with Novolin®

Synonyms aspart insulin

U.S./Canadian Brand Names NovoLog® [US]; NovoRapid® [Can]

Therapeutic Category Antidiabetic Agent, Insulin

Use Treatment of type 1 diabetes mellitus (insulin-dependent, IDDM); type 2 diabetes mellitus (noninsulin-dependent, NIDDM) to control hyperglycemia

Usual Dosage Refer to insulin regular monograph *on page 453*. Insulin aspart is a rapid-acting insulin analog which is normally administered as a a premeal component of the insulin regimen. It is normally used along with a long-acting (basal) form of insulin.

Dosage Forms Injection, solution (NovoLog®): 100 units/mL (3 mL) [FlexPen® prefilled syringe or PenFill® prefilled cartridge]; (10 mL) [vial]

insulin aspart and insulin aspart protamine *see* insulin aspart protamine and insulin aspart *on next page*

insulin aspart protamine and insulin aspart

(IN soo lin AS part PROE ta meen & IN soo lin AS part)

Sound-Alike/Look-Alike Issues

NovoLog® Mix 70/30 may be confused with Novolin® 70/30

Synonyms insulin aspart and insulin aspart protamine

U.S./Canadian Brand Names NovoLog® Mix 70/30 [US]

Therapeutic Category Antidiabetic Agent, Insulin

Use Treatment of type 1 diabetes mellitus (insulin-dependent, IDDM); type 2 diabetes mellitus (noninsulin-dependent, NIDDM) to control hyperglycemia

Usual Dosage Refer to insulin regular monograph *on page 453*. Fixed ratio insulins (such as insulin aspart protamine and insulin aspart combination) are normally administered in 2 daily doses.

Dosage Forms Injection, suspension (NovoLog® Mix 70/30): Insulin aspart protamine suspension 70% [intermediate acting] and insulin aspart solution 30% [rapid acting]: 100 units/mL (3 mL) [PenFill® prefilled cartridge or FlexPen® prefilled syringe]; (10 mL) [vial]

insulin detemir (IN soo lin DE te mir)

Synonyms detemir insulin

U.S./Canadian Brand Names Levemir® [US/Can]

Therapeutic Category Antidiabetic Agent, Insulin

Use Treatment of type 1 diabetes mellitus (insulin-dependent, IDDM); type 2 diabetes mellitus (noninsulin-dependent, NIDDM) to control hyperglycemia

Usual Dosage Also refer to insulin regular *on page 453.*

Notes: Duration is dose-dependent. Dosage must be carefully titrated (adjustment of dose and timing. Adjustment of concomitant antidiabetic treatment (short-acting insulins or oral antidiabetic agents) may be required. In Canada, insulin detemir is not approved for use in children.

SubQ: Children ≥6 years and Adults: Type 1 or type 2 diabetes:

Basal insulin or basal-bolus: May be substituted on a unit-per-unit basis. Adjust dose to achieve glycemic targets.

Insulin-naive patients (type 2 diabetes only): 0.1-0.2 units/kg once daily in the evening or 10 units once or twice daily. Adjust dose to achieve glycemic targets. Note: Canadian labeling recommends 10 units once daily (twice daily dosing is not included).

Dosage Forms Injection, solution (Levemir®): 100 units/mL (3 mL) [Innolet® prefilled syringe, Penfill® prefilled cartridge, or FlexPen® prefilled syringe]; (10 mL) [vial]

insulin glargine (IN soo lin GLAR jeen)

Sound-Alike/Look-Alike Issues

Lantus® may be confused with Lente®

Synonyms glargine insulin

U.S./Canadian Brand Names Lantus® OptiSet® [Can]; Lantus® [US/Can]

Therapeutic Category Antidiabetic Agent, Insulin

Use Treatment of type 1 diabetes mellitus (insulin-dependent, IDDM); type 2 diabetes mellitus (noninsulin-dependent, NIDDM) requiring basal (long-acting) insulin to control hyperglycemia

Usual Dosage SubQ: Adults:

Type 1 diabetes: Refer to insulin regular monograph *on page 453.*

Type 2 diabetes:

Patient not already on insulin: 10 units once daily, adjusted according to patient response (range in clinical study: 2-100 units/day)

Patient already receiving insulin: In clinical studies, when changing to insulin glargine from once-daily NPH or Ultralente® insulin, the initial dose was not changed; when changing from twice-daily NPH to once-daily insulin glargine, the total daily dose was reduced by 20% and adjusted according to patient response

Dosage Forms Injection, solution (Lantus®): 100 units/mL (3 mL) [cartridge]; (10 mL) [vial]

insulin glulisine (IN soo lin gloo LIS een)

Synonyms glulisine insulin

U.S./Canadian Brand Names Apidra® [US]

Therapeutic Category Antidiabetic Agent, Insulin

Use Treatment of type 1 diabetes mellitus (insulin-dependent, IDDM); type 2 diabetes mellitus (noninsulin-dependent, NIDDM) to control hyperglycemia

Usual Dosage Refer to insulin regular monograph *on page 453.*

Dosage Forms

Injection, solution:

Apidra®: 100 units/mL (3 mL [cartridge], 10 mL [vial])

insulin inhalation (IN soo lin in ha LAY shun)

Synonyms inhaled insulin

U.S./Canadian Brand Names Exubera® [US]

Therapeutic Category Antidiabetic Agent, Insulin

Use Treatment of type 1 diabetes mellitus (insulin-dependent, IDDM); type 2 diabetes mellitus (noninsulin-dependent, NIDDM)

Usual Dosage Inhalation: Children ≥6 years and Adults:

Initial: 0.05 mg/kg (rounded down to nearest whole milligram) 3 times/daily administered within 10 minutes of a meal

Adjustment: Dosage may be increased or decreased based on serum glucose monitoring, meal size, nutrient composition, time of day, and exercise patterns.

Note: A 1 mg blister is approximately equivalent to 3 units of regular insulin, while a 3 mg blister is approximately equivalent to 8 units of regular insulin administered subcutaneously. Patients should combine 1 mg and 3 mg blisters so that the fewest blisters are required to achieve the prescribed dose. Consecutive inhalation of three 1 mg blisters results in significantly higher insulin levels as compared to inhalation of a single 3 mg blister (do not substitute). In a patient stabilized on a dosage which uses 3 mg blisters, if 3 mg blister is temporarily unavailable, inhalation of two 1 mg blisters may be substituted.

Dosage Forms

Combination package:

Exubera® Kit [packaged with inhaler, chamber and release unit]:

Powder for oral inhalation [prefilled blister pack]: 1 mg/blister (180s)

Powder for oral inhalation [prefilled blister pack]: 3 mg/blister (90s)

Exubera® Combination Pack 15 [packaged with 2 release units]:

Powder for oral inhalation [prefilled blister pack]: 1 mg/blister (180s)

Powder for oral inhalation [prefilled blister pack]: 3 mg/blister (90s)

Exubera® Combination Pack 12 [packaged with 2 release units]:

Powder for oral inhalation [prefilled blister pack]: 1 mg/blister (90s)

Powder for oral inhalation [prefilled blister pack]: 3 mg/blister (90s)

insulin lispro (IN soo lin LYE sproe)

Sound-Alike/Look-Alike Issues

Humalog® may be confused with Humulin®, Humira®

Synonyms lispro insulin

U.S./Canadian Brand Names Humalog® [US/Can]

Therapeutic Category Antidiabetic Agent, Insulin

Use Treatment of type 1 diabetes mellitus (insulin-dependent, IDDM); type 2 diabetes mellitus (noninsulin-dependent, NIDDM) to control hyperglycemia

Note: In type 1 diabetes mellitus (insulin dependent, IDDM), insulin lispro (Humalog®) should be used in combination with a long-acting insulin. However, in type 2 diabetes mellitus (noninsulin-dependent, NIDDM), insulin lispro (Humalog®) may be used without a long-acting insulin when used in combination with a sulfonylurea.

Usual Dosage Refer to insulin regular monograph *on page 453*. Insulin lispro is equipotent to insulin regular, but has a more rapid onset.

Dosage Forms Injection, solution (Humalog®): 100 units/mL (3 mL) [prefilled cartridge or prefilled disposable pen]; (10 mL) [vial]

insulin lispro and insulin lispro protamine *see* insulin lispro protamine and insulin lispro *on this page*

insulin lispro protamine and insulin lispro

(IN soo lin LYE sproe PROE ta meen & IN soo lin LYE sproe)

Sound-Alike/Look-Alike Issues

Humalog® Mix 75/25™ may be confused with Humulin® 70/30.

Synonyms insulin lispro and insulin lispro protamine

U.S./Canadian Brand Names Humalog® Mix 25 [Can]; Humalog® Mix 50/50™ [US]; Humalog® Mix 75/25™ [US]

(Continued)

insulin lispro protamine and insulin lispro *(Continued)*

Therapeutic Category Antidiabetic Agent, Insulin

Use Treatment of type 1 diabetes mellitus (insulin-dependent, IDDM); type 2 diabetes mellitus (noninsulin-dependent, NIDDM) to control hyperglycemia

Usual Dosage Refer to insulin regular monograph *on page 453*. Fixed ratio insulins (such as insulin lispro protamine and insulin lispro) are normally administered in 2 daily doses.

Dosage Forms Injection, suspension:

Humalog® Mix 50/50™: Insulin lispro protamine suspension 50% [intermediate acting] and insulin lispro solution 50% [rapid acting]: 100 units/mL (3 mL) [disposable pen]

Humalog® Mix 75/25™: Insulin lispro protamine suspension 75% [intermediate acting] and insulin lispro solution 25% [rapid acting]: 100 units/mL (3 mL) [disposable pen]; (10 mL) [vial]

insulin NPH (IN soo lin N P H)

Sound-Alike/Look-Alike Issues

Humulin® may be confused with Humalog®, Humira®

Novolin® may be confused with NovoLog®

Synonyms isophane insulin; NPH insulin

U.S./Canadian Brand Names Humulin® N [US/Can]; Novolin® ge NPH [Can]; Novolin® N [US]

Therapeutic Category Insulin, Intermediate-Acting

Use Treatment of type 1 diabetes mellitus (insulin-dependent, IDDM); type 2 diabetes mellitus (noninsulin-dependent, NIDDM) to control hyperglycemia

Usual Dosage Refer to insulin regular monograph *on page 453*. Insulin NPH is usually administered 1-2 times daily.

Dosage Forms [CAN] = Canadian brand name

Injection, suspension:

Humulin® N: 100 units/mL (3 mL) [disposable pen]; (10 mL) [vial]

Novolin® ge NPH [CAN]: 100 units/mL (3 mL) [NovolinSet® prefilled syringe or PenFill® prefilled cartridge]; 10 mL [vial]

Novolin® N: 100 units/mL (3 mL) [InnoLet® prefilled syringe or PenFill® prefilled cartridge]; (10 mL) [vial]

insulin NPH and insulin regular (IN soo lin N P H & IN soo lin REG yoo ler)

Sound-Alike/Look-Alike Issues

Humulin® 70/30 may be confused with Humalog® Mix 75/25

Novolin® 70/30 may be confused with NovoLog® Mix 70/30

Synonyms insulin regular and insulin NPH; isophane insulin and regular insulin; NPH insulin and regular insulin

U.S./Canadian Brand Names Humulin® 20/80 [Can]; Humulin® 50/50 [US]; Humulin® 70/30 [US/Can]; Novolin® 70/30 [US]; Novolin® ge 10/90 [Can]; Novolin® ge 20/80 [Can]; Novolin® ge 30/70 [Can]; Novolin® ge 40/60 [Can]; Novolin® ge 50/50 [Can]

Therapeutic Category Antidiabetic Agent, Insulin

Use Treatment of type 1 diabetes mellitus (insulin-dependent, IDDM); type 2 diabetes mellitus (noninsulin-dependent, NIDDM) to control hyperglycemia

Usual Dosage Refer to insulin regular monograph *on page 453*. Fixed ratio insulins are normally administered in 1-2 daily doses.

Dosage Forms

Injection, suspension:

Humulin® 50/50: Insulin NPH suspension 50% [intermediate acting] and insulin regular solution 50% [short acting]: 100 units/mL (10 mL) [vial]

Humulin® 70/30: Insulin NPH suspension 70% [intermediate acting] and insulin regular solution 30% [short acting]: 100 units/mL (3 mL) [disposable pen]; (10 mL) [vial]

Novolin® 70/30: Insulin NPH suspension 70% [intermediate acting] and insulin regular solution 30% [short acting]: 100 units/mL (3 mL) [InnoLet® prefilled syringe or PenFill® prefilled cartridge]; (10 mL) [vial]

Additional formulations available in Canada: Injection, suspension:

Humulin® 20/80: Insulin regular solution 20% [short acting] and insulin NPH suspension 80% [intermediate acting]: 100 units/mL (3 mL) [PenFill® prefilled cartridge]

Novolin® ge 10/90: Insulin regular solution 10% [short acting] and insulin NPH suspension 90% [intermediate acting]: 100 units/mL (3 mL) [PenFill® prefilled cartridge]

Novolin® ge 20/80: Insulin regular solution 20% [short acting] and insulin NPH suspension 80% [intermediate acting]: 100 units/mL (3 mL) [PenFill® prefilled cartridge]

Novolin® ge 30/70: Insulin regular solution 30% [short acting] and insulin NPH suspension 70% [intermediate acting]: 100 units/mL (3 mL) [prefilled syringe or PenFill® prefilled cartridge]; (10 mL) [vial]

Novolin® ge 40/60: Insulin regular solution 40% [short acting] and insulin NPH suspension 60% [intermediate acting]: 100 units/mL (3 mL) [PenFill® prefilled cartridge]

Novolin® ge 50/50: Insulin regular solution 50% [short acting] and insulin NPH suspension 50% [intermediate acting]: 100 units/mL (3 mL) [PenFill® prefilled cartridge]

insulin regular (IN soo lin REG yoo ler)

Sound-Alike/Look-Alike Issues

Humulin® may be confused with Humalog®, Humira®

Novolin® may be confused with NovoLog®

Synonyms regular insulin

U.S./Canadian Brand Names Humulin® R (Concentrated) U-500 [US]; Humulin® R [US/Can]; Novolin® ge Toronto [Can]; Novolin® R [US]

Therapeutic Category Antidiabetic Agent, Insulin; Antidote

Use Treatment of type 1 diabetes mellitus (insulin-dependent, IDDM); type 2 diabetes mellitus (noninsulin-dependent, NIDDM) unresponsive to treatment with diet and/or oral hypoglycemics, to control hyperglycemia; adjunct to parenteral nutrition; diabetic ketoacidosis (DKA)

Usual Dosage SubQ (regular insulin may also be administered I.V.): The number and size of daily doses, time of administration, and diet and exercise require continuous medical supervision. In addition, specific formulations may require distinct administration procedures.

Type 1 Diabetes Mellitus: Children and Adults: **Note:** Multiple daily doses guided by blood glucose monitoring are the standard of diabetes care. Combinations of insulin are commonly used.

Initial dose: 0.2-0.6 units/kg/day in divided doses. Conservative initial doses of 0.2-0.4 units/kg/day are often recommended to avoid the potential for hypoglycemia.

Division of daily insulin requirement: Generally, 50% to 75% of the daily insulin dose is given as an intermediate- or long-acting form of insulin (in 1-2 daily injections). The remaining portion of the 24-hour insulin requirement is divided and administered as a rapid-acting or short-acting form of insulin. These may be given with meals (before or at the time of meals depending on the form of insulin) or at the same time as injections of intermediate forms (some premixed combinations are intended for this purpose).

Adjustment of dose: Dosage must be titrated to achieve glucose control and avoid hypoglycemia. Adjust dose to maintain premeal and bedtime glucose of 80-140 mg/dL (children <5 years: 100-200 mg/dL). Since combinations of agents are frequently used, dosage adjustment must address the individual component of the insulin regimen which most directly influences the blood glucose value in question, based on the known onset and duration of the insulin component.

Usual maintenance range: 0.5-1.2 units/kg/day in divided doses. An estimate of anticipated needs may be based on body weight and/or activity factors as follows:

Adolescents: May require ≤1.5 units/kg/day during growth spurts

Nonobese: 0.4-0.6 units/kg/day

Obese: 0.8-1.2 units/kg/day

Renal failure: Due to alterations in pharmacokinetics of insulin, may require <0.2 units/kg/day

Type 2 Diabetes Mellitus:

Augmentation therapy: Initial dosage of 0.15 (insulin glargine, corresponding to ~10 units) to 0.2 units/kg/day (insulins other than glargine) have been recommended. Dosage must be carefully adjusted.

Note: Administered when residual beta-cell function is present, as a supplemental agent when oral hypoglycemics have not achieved goal glucose control. Twice daily NPH, or an evening dose of NPH, lente, or glargine insulin may be added to oral therapy with metformin or a sulfonylurea. Augmentation to control postprandial glucose may be accomplished with regular, glulisine, aspart, or lispro insulin.

Monotherapy: Initial dose: Highly variable: See Augmentation therapy dosing.

Note: An empirically-defined scheme for dosage estimation based on fasting plasma glucose and degree of obesity has been published with recommended doses ranging from 6-77 units/day. In the setting of glucose toxicity (loss of beta-cell sensitivity to glucose concentrations), insulin therapy may be used for short-term management to restore sensitivity of beta-cells; in these cases, the dose may need to be rapidly reduced/withdrawn when sensitivity is re-established.

Diabetic ketoacidosis:

Children <20 years:

I.V.: Regular insulin infused at 0.1 units/kg/hour; continue until acidosis clears, then decrease to 0.05 units/kg/hour until SubQ replacement dosing can be initiated

SubQ, I.M.: If no I.V. infusion access, regular insulin 0.1 units/kg I.M. bolus followed by 0.1 units/kg/hour SubQ or I.M.; continue until acidosis clears, then decrease to 0.05 units/kg/hour until SubQ replacement dosing can be initiated

Adults:

I.V.: Regular insulin 0.15 units/kg initially followed by an infusion of 0.1 units/kg/hour

SubQ, I.M.: Regular insulin 0.4 units/kg given half as I.V. bolus and half as SubQ or I.M., followed by 0.1 units/kg/hour SubQ or I.M.

(Continued)

insulin regular *(Continued)*

If serum glucose does not fall by 50-70 mg/dL in the first hour, double insulin dose hourly until glucose falls at an hourly rate of 50-70 mg/dL. Decrease dose to 0.05-0.1 units/kg/hour once serum glucose reaches 250 mg/dL.

Note: Newly-diagnosed patients with IDDM presenting in DKA and patients with blood sugars <800 mg/dL may be relatively "sensitive" to insulin and should receive loading and initial maintenance doses ~50% of those indicated.

Infusion should continue until reversal of acid-base derangement/ketonemia. Serum glucose is not a direct indicator of these abnormalities, and may decrease more rapidly than correction of the range of metabolic abnormalities.

Dosage Forms

Injection, solution:

Humulin® R: 100 units/mL (10 mL) [vial]

Novolin® R: 100 units/mL (3 mL) [InnoLet® prefilled syringe or PenFill® prefilled cartridge]; (10 mL) [vial]

Injection, solution [concentrate] (Humulin® R U-500): 500 units/mL (20 mL vial)

insulin regular and insulin NPH *see* insulin NPH and insulin regular *on page 452*

Intal® [US/Can] *see* cromolyn sodium *on page 217*

Integrilin® [US/Can] *see* eptifibatide *on page 300*

Intensol® Solution *(Discontinued)* *see* metoclopramide *on page 549*

α-2-interferon *see* interferon alfa-2b *on this page*

interferon alfa-2a (PEG conjugate) *see* peginterferon alfa-2a *on page 643*

interferon alfa-2b and ribavirin combination pack *see* interferon alfa-2b and ribavirin *on next page*

interferon alfa-2b (PEG conjugate) *see* peginterferon alfa-2b *on page 644*

interferon alfa-2a (in ter FEER on AL fa too aye)

Sound-Alike/Look-Alike Issues

interferon alfa-2a may be confused with interferon alfa-2b

Roferon-A® may be confused with Rocephin®

Synonyms IFLrA; rIFN-A

U.S./Canadian Brand Names Roferon-A® [US/Can]

Therapeutic Category Biological Response Modulator

Use

Patients >18 years of age: Hairy cell leukemia, AIDS-related Kaposi sarcoma, chronic hepatitis C

Children and Adults: Chronic myelogenous leukemia (CML), Philadelphia chromosome positive, within 1 year of diagnosis (limited experience in children)

Usual Dosage Refer to individual protocols

Children (limited data): Chronic myelogenous leukemia (CML): I.M.: 2.5-5 million units/m^2/day; **Note:** In juveniles, higher dosages (30 million units/m^2/day) have been associated with severe adverse events, including death

Adults:

Hairy cell leukemia: SubQ, I.M.: 3 million units/day for 16-24 weeks, then 3 million units 3 times/week for up to 6-24 months

Chronic myelogenous leukemia (CML): SubQ, I.M.: 9 million units/day, continue treatment until disease progression

AIDS-related Kaposi sarcoma: SubQ, I.M.: 36 million units/day for 10-12 weeks, then 36 million units 3 times/week; to minimize adverse reactions, can use escalating dose (3-, 9-, then 18 million units each day for 3 days, then 36 million units daily thereafter).

Hepatitis C: SubQ, I.M.: 3 million units 3 times/week for 12 months

Dosage Forms Injection, solution [single-dose prefilled syringe; SubQ use only]: 3 million units/0.5 mL (0.5 mL); 6 million units/0.5 mL (0.5 mL); 9 million units/0.5 mL (0.5 mL) [contains benzyl alcohol]

interferon alfa-2b (in ter FEER on AL fa too bee)

Sound-Alike/Look-Alike Issues

interferon alfa-2b may be confused with interferon alfa-2a

Synonyms α-2-interferon; INF-alpha 2; rLFN-α2

U.S./Canadian Brand Names Intron® A [US/Can]

Therapeutic Category Biological Response Modulator

Use

Patients ≥1 year of age: Chronic hepatitis B

Patients ≥18 years of age: Condyloma acuminata, chronic hepatitis C, hairy cell leukemia, malignant melanoma, AIDS-related Kaposi sarcoma, follicular non-Hodgkin lymphoma

Usual Dosage Refer to individual protocols

Children 1-17 years: Chronic hepatitis B: SubQ: 3 million units/m² 3 times/week for 1 week; then 6 million units/m² 3 times/week; maximum: 10 million units 3 times/week; total duration of therapy 16-24 weeks

Adults:

Hairy cell leukemia: I.M., SubQ: 2 million units/m² 3 times/week for 2-6 months

Lymphoma (follicular): SubQ: 5 million units 3 times/week for up to 18 months

Malignant melanoma: 20 million units/m² I.V. for 5 consecutive days per week for 4 weeks, then 10 million units/m² SubQ 3 times/week for 48 weeks

AIDS-related Kaposi's sarcoma: I.M., SubQ: 30 million units/m² 3 times/week

Chronic hepatitis B: I.M., SubQ: 5 million units/day or 10 million units 3 times/week for 16 weeks

Chronic hepatitis C: I.M., SubQ: 3 million units 3 times/week for 16 weeks. In patients with normalization of ALT at 16 weeks, continue treatment for 18-24 months; consider discontinuation if normalization does not occur at 16 weeks. **Note:** May be used in combination therapy with ribavirin in previously untreated patients or in patients who relapse following alpha interferon therapy; refer to interferon alfa-2b and ribavirin.

Condyloma acuminata: Intralesionally: 1 million units/lesion (maximum: 5 lesions/treatment) 3 times/week (on alternate days) for 3 weeks; may administer a second course at 12-16 weeks

Dosage Forms

Injection, powder for reconstitution: 10 million units; 18 million units; 50 million units [contains human albumin]

Injection, solution [multidose prefilled pen]:

Delivers 3 million units/0.2 mL (1.5 mL) [delivers 6 doses; 18 million units]

Delivers 5 million units/0.2 mL (1.5 mL) [delivers 6 doses; 30 million units]

Delivers 10 million units/0.2 mL (1.5 mL) [delivers 6 doses; 60 million units]

Injection, solution [multidose vial]: 6 million units/mL (3 mL); 10 million units/mL (2.5 mL)

Injection, solution [single-dose vial]: 10 million units/ mL (1 mL)

See also Interferon Alfa-2b and Ribavirin Combination Pack monograph.

interferon alfa-2b and ribavirin (in ter FEER on AL fa too bee & rye ba VYE rin)

Synonyms interferon alfa-2b and ribavirin combination pack; ribavirin and interferon alfa-2b combination pack

U.S./Canadian Brand Names Rebetron® [US]

Therapeutic Category Antiviral Agent; Biological Response Modulator

Use Combination therapy for the treatment of chronic hepatitis C in patients with compensated liver disease previously untreated with alpha interferon or who have relapsed after alpha interferon therapy

Usual Dosage

Children ≥3 years: Chronic hepatitis C: **Note:** Duration of therapy: genotype 1: 48 weeks; genotype 2 or 3: 24 weeks. Discontinue treatment in any patient if HCV-RNA is not below the limits of detection of the assay after 24 weeks of therapy. Combination therapy:

Intron® A: SubQ:

25-61 kg: 3 million int. units/m² 3 times/week

>61 kg: Refer to Adults dosing

Rebetol®: Oral: **Note:** Oral solution should be used in children 3-5 years of age, children ≤25 kg, or those unable to swallow capsules.

Capsule/solution: 15 mg/kg/day in 2 divided doses (morning and evening)

Capsule dosing recommendations:

25-36 kg: 400 mg/day (200 mg morning and evening)

37-49 kg: 600 mg/day (200 mg in the morning and two 200 mg capsules in the evening)

50-61 kg: 800 mg/day (two 200 mg capsules morning and evening)

>61 kg: Refer to Adults dosing

Adults: Chronic hepatitis C: Recommended dosage of combination therapy:

Intron® A: SubQ: 3 million int. units 3 times/week **and**

Rebetol® capsule: Oral:

≤75 kg (165 lb): 1000 mg/day (two 200 mg capsules in the morning and three 200 mg capsules in the evening)

>75 kg: 1200 mg/day (three 200 mg capsules in the morning and three 200 mg capsules in the evening)

(Continued)

interferon alfa-2b and ribavirin *(Continued)*

Treatment duration recommendations:

Following relapse after alpha interferon monotherapy: 24 weeks

Previously untreated: 24-48 weeks (individualized based on response, tolerance, and baseline characteristics)

Consider discontinuing therapy in any patient not achieving HCV-RNA below the limit of assay detection by 24 weeks.

Dosage Forms **Combination package:**

For patients ≤75 kg [contains single-dose vials]:

Injection, solution: Interferon alfa-2b (Intron® A): 3 million int. units/0.5 mL (0.5 mL) [6 vials (3 million int. units/vial), 6 syringes, and alcohol swabs]

Capsule: Ribavirin (Rebetol®): 200 mg (70s)

For patients ≤75 kg [contains multidose vials]:

Injection, solution: Interferon alfa-2b (Intron® A): 3 million int. units/0.5 mL (3.8 mL) [1 multidose vial (18 million int. units/vial), 6 syringes, and alcohol swabs]

Capsule: Ribavirin (Rebetol®): 200 mg (70s)

For patients ≤75 kg [contains multidose pen]:

Injection, solution: Interferon alfa-2b (Intron® A): 3 million int. units/0.2 mL (1.5 mL) [1 multidose pen (18 million int. units/pen), 6 needles, and alcohol swabs]

Capsule: Ribavirin (Rebetol®): 200 mg (70s)

For patients >75 kg [contains single-dose vials]:

Injection, solution: Interferon alfa-2b (Intron® A): 3 million int. units/0.5 mL (0.5 mL) [6 vials (3 million int. units/vial), 6 syringes, and alcohol swabs]

Capsule: Ribavirin (Rebetol®): 200 mg (84s)

For patients >75 kg [contains multidose vials]:

Injection, solution: Interferon alfa-2b (Intron® A): 3 million int. units/0.5 mL (3.8 mL) [1 multidose vial (18 million int. units/vial), 6 syringes, and alcohol swabs]

Capsule: Ribavirin (Rebetol®): 200 mg (84s)

For patients >75 kg [contains multidose pen]:

Injection, solution: Interferon alfa-2b (Intron® A): 3 million int. units/0.2 mL (1.5 mL) [1 multidose pen (18 million int. units/pen), 6 needles, and alcohol swabs]

Capsule: Ribavirin (Rebetol®): 200 mg (84s)

For Rebetol® dose reduction [contains single-dose vials]:

Injection, solution: Interferon alfa-2b (Intron® A): 3 million int. units/0.5 mL (0.5 mL) [6 vials (3 million int. units/vial), 6 syringes, and alcohol swabs]

Capsule: Ribavirin (Rebetol®): 200 mg (42s)

For Rebetol® dose reduction [contains multidose vials]:

Injection, solution: Interferon alfa-2b (Intron® A): 3 million int. units/0.5 mL (3.8 mL) [1 multidose vial (18 million int. units/vial), 6 syringes, and alcohol swabs]

Capsule: Ribavirin (Rebetol®): 200 mg (42s)

For Rebetol® dose reduction [contains multidose pen]:

Injection, solution: Interferon alfa-2b (Intron® A): 3 million int. units/0.2 mL (1.5 mL) [1 multidose pen (18 million int. units/pen), 6 needles, and alcohol swabs]

Capsule: Ribavirin (Rebetol®): 200 mg (42s)

interferon alfacon-1 (in ter FEER on AL fa con one)

U.S./Canadian Brand Names Infergen® [US]

Therapeutic Category Interferon

Use Treatment of chronic hepatitis C virus (HCV) infection in patients ≥18 years of age with compensated liver disease and anti-HCV serum antibodies or HCV RNA.

Usual Dosage Adults ≥18 years: SubQ:

Chronic HCV infection: 9 mcg 3 times/week for 24 weeks; allow 48 hours between doses

Patients who have previously tolerated interferon therapy but did not respond or relapsed: 15 mcg 3 times/week for 6 months

Dose reduction for toxicity: Dose should be held in patients who experience a severe adverse reaction, and treatment should be stopped or decreased if the reaction does not become tolerable.

Doses were reduced from 9 mcg to 7.5 mcg in the pivotal study.

For patients receiving 15 mcg/dose, doses were reduced in 3 mcg increments. Efficacy is decreased with doses <7.5 mcg

Dosage Forms Injection, solution [preservative free]: 30 mcg/mL (0.3 mL, 0.5 mL)

interferon alfa-n3 (in ter FEER on AL fa en three)

Sound-Alike/Look-Alike Issues

Alferon® may be confused with Alkeran®

U.S./Canadian Brand Names Alferon® N [US/Can]

Therapeutic Category Biological Response Modulator

Use Patients ≥18 years of age: Intralesional treatment of refractory or recurring genital or venereal warts (condylomata acuminata)

Usual Dosage Adults: Inject 250,000 units (0.05 mL) in each wart twice weekly for a maximum of 8 weeks; therapy should not be repeated for at least 3 months after the initial 8-week course of therapy

Dosage Forms Injection, solution: 5 million int. units (1 mL) [contains albumin]

interferon beta-1a (in ter FEER on BAY ta won aye)

Sound-Alike/Look-Alike Issues

Avonex® may be confused with Avelox®

Synonyms rIFN beta-1a

U.S./Canadian Brand Names Avonex® [US/Can]; Rebif® [US/Can]

Therapeutic Category Biological Response Modulator

Use Treatment of relapsing forms of multiple sclerosis (MS)

Usual Dosage Adults: **Note:** Analgesics and/or antipyretics may help decrease flulike symptoms on treatment days:

I.M. (Avonex®): 30 mcg once weekly

SubQ (Rebif®): Doses should be separated by at least 48 hours:

Target dose 44 mcg 3 times/week: 11

Initial: 8.8 mcg (20% of final dose) 3 times/week for 8 weeks

Titration: 22 mcg (50% of final dose) 3 times/week for 8 weeks

Final dose: 44 mcg 3 times/week

Target dose 22 mcg 3 times/week:

Initial: 4.4 mcg (20% of final dose) 3 times/week for 8 weeks

Titration: 11 mcg (50% of final dose) 3 times/week for 8 weeks

Final dose: 22 mcg 3 times/week

Dosage Forms

Combination package [preservative free] (Rebif® Titration Pack):

Injection, solution: 8.8 mcg/0.2 mL (0.2 mL) [6 prefilled syringes; contains albumin]

Injection, solution: 22 mcg/0.5 mL (0.5 mL) [6 prefilled syringes; contains albumin]

Injection, powder for reconstitution (Avonex®): 33 mcg [6.6 million units; provides 30 mcg/mL following reconstitution] [contains albumin; packaged with SWFI, alcohol wipes, and access pin and needle]

Injection, solution (Avonex®): 30 mcg/0.5 mL (0.5 mL) [albumin free; prefilled syringe; syringe cap contains latex; packaged with alcohol wipes, gauze pad, and adhesive bandages]

Injection, solution [preservative free] (Rebif®): 22 mcg/0.5 mL (0.5 mL) [prefilled syringe; contains albumin]; 44 mcg/0.5 mL (0.5 mL) [prefilled syringe; contains albumin]

interferon beta-1b (in ter FEER on BAY ta won bee)

Synonyms rIFN beta-1b

U.S./Canadian Brand Names Betaseron® [US/Can]

Therapeutic Category Biological Response Modulator

Use Treatment of relapsing forms of multiple sclerosis (MS)

Usual Dosage Adults: SubQ: 0.25 mg (8 million units) every other day

Dosage Forms Injection, powder for reconstitution [preservative free]: 0.3 mg [9.6 million units] [contains albumin; packaged with prefilled syringe containing diluent]

interferon gamma-1b (in ter FEER on GAM ah won bee)

U.S./Canadian Brand Names Actimmune® [US/Can]

Therapeutic Category Biological Response Modulator

Use Reduce frequency and severity of serious infections associated with chronic granulomatous disease; delay time to disease progression in patients with severe, malignant osteopetrosis

Usual Dosage If severe reactions occur, reduce dose by 50% or therapy should be interrupted until adverse reaction abates.

Chronic granulomatous disease: Children >1 year and Adults: SubQ:

BSA ≤0.5 m^2: 1.5 mcg/kg/dose 3 times/week

BSA >0.5 m^2: 50 mcg/m^2 (1 million int. units/m^2) 3 times/week

(Continued)

interferon gamma-1b *(Continued)*

Severe, malignant osteopetrosis: Children >1 year: SubQ:
BSA ≤0.5 m^2: 1.5 mcg/kg/dose 3 times/week
BSA >0.5 m^2: 50 mcg/m^2 (1 million int. units/m^2) 3 times/week

Note: Previously expressed as 1.5 million units/m^2; 50 mcg is equivalent to 1 million int. units/m^2.

Dosage Forms Injection, solution [preservative free]: 100 mcg [2 million int. units] (0.5 mL)
Previously, 100 mcg was expressed as 3 million units. This is equivalent to 2 million int. units.

interleukin-1 receptor antagonist *see* anakinra *on page 56*

interleukin-2 *see* aldesleukin *on page 26*

interleukin-11 *see* oprelvekin *on page 618*

Intralipid® [US/Can] *see* fat emulsion *on page 336*

intravenous fat emulsion *see* fat emulsion *on page 336*

intrifiban *see* eptifibatide *on page 300*

Intron® A [US/Can] *see* interferon alfa-2b *on page 454*

Intropin® *(Discontinued)* *see* dopamine *on page 273*

Invanz® [US/Can] *see* ertapenem *on page 303*

Inversine® [US/Can] *see* mecamylamine *on page 522*

Invirase® [US/Can] *see* saquinavir *on page 763*

iocetamic acid *see* radiological/contrast media (ionic) *on page 728*

iodamide meglumine *see* radiological/contrast media (ionic) *on page 728*

Iodex [US-OTC] *see* iodine *on this page*

Iodex-p® *(Discontinued)* *see* povidone-iodine *on page 689*

iodine (EYE oh dyne)

Sound-Alike/Look-Alike Issues
iodine may be confused with codeine, Iopidine®, Lodine®

U.S./Canadian Brand Names Iodex [US-OTC]; Iodoflex™ [US]; Iodosorb® [US]

Therapeutic Category Topical Skin Product

Use Used topically as an antiseptic in the management of minor, superficial skin wounds and has been used to disinfect the skin preoperatively

Usual Dosage
Topical:
Cleaning wet ulcers and wounds (Iodosorb®, Iodoflex™): Apply to clean wound; maximum: 50 g/application and 150 g/week. Change dressing ~3 times/week; reduce applications as exudate decreases. Do not use for >3 months; discontinue when wound is free of exudate.
Antiseptic for minor cuts, scrapes, burns: Apply small amount to affected area 1-3 times/day
Oral: RDA:
Children:
1-8 years: 90 mcg/day
9-13 years: 120 mcg/day
≥14 years: Refer to adult dosing
Adults: 150 mcg/day
Pregnancy: 220 mcg/day
Breast-feeding: 290 mcg/day

Dosage Forms
Dressing, topical [gel pad] (Iodoflex™): 0.9% (5 g, 10 g)
Gel, topical (Iodosorb®): 0.9% (40 g)
Ointment, topical (Iodex): 4.7% (30 g, 720 g)
Tincture, topical: 2% (30 mL, 480 mL); 7% (30 mL, 480 mL)

iodine *see* trace metals *on page 839*

iodine I 131 tositumomab and tositumomab *see* tositumomab and iodine I 131 tositumomab *on page 837*

iodipamide meglumine *see* radiological/contrast media (ionic) *on page 728*

iodochlorhydroxyquin and flumethasone *see* clioquinol and flumethasone *(Canada only) on page 200*

Iodoflex™ [US] *see* iodine *on previous page*

Iodopen® [US] *see* trace metals *on page 839*

iodoquinol (eye oh doe KWIN ole)

Synonyms diiodohydroxyquin

U.S./Canadian Brand Names Diodoquin® [Can]; Yodoxin® [US]

Therapeutic Category Amebicide

Use Treatment of acute and chronic intestinal amebiasis; asymptomatic cyst passers; *Blastocystis hominis* infections; ineffective for amebic hepatitis or hepatic abscess

Usual Dosage Oral:

Children: 30-40 mg/kg/day (maximum: 650 mg/dose) in 3 divided doses for 20 days; not to exceed 1.95 g/day

Adults: 650 mg 3 times/day after meals for 20 days; not to exceed 1.95 g/day

Dosage Forms Tablet: 210 mg, 650 mg

iodoquinol and hydrocortisone (eye oh doe KWIN ole & hye droe KOR ti sone)

Sound-Alike/Look-Alike Issues

Vytone® may be confused with Hytone®, Zydone®

Synonyms hydrocortisone and iodoquinol

U.S./Canadian Brand Names Dermazene® [US]; Vytone® [US]

Therapeutic Category Antifungal/Corticosteroid

Use Treatment of eczema; infectious dermatitis; chronic eczematoid otitis externa; mycotic dermatoses

Usual Dosage Apply 3-4 times/day

Dosage Forms

Cream: Iodoquinol 1% and hydrocortisone acetate 1% (30 g)

Dermazene®: Iodoquinol 1% and hydrocortisone acetate 1% (30 g, 45 g)

Vytone®: Iodoquinol 1% and hydrocortisone acetate 1% (30 g)

Iodosorb® [US] *see* iodine *on previous page*

iohexol *see* radiological/contrast media (nonionic) *on page 730*

Ionamin® [US/Can] *see* phentermine *on page 659*

Ionil® [US-OTC] *see* salicylic acid *on page 758*

Ionil® Plus [US-OTC] *see* salicylic acid *on page 758*

Ionil T® [US-OTC] *see* coal tar *on page 207*

Ionil T® Plus [US-OTC] *see* coal tar *on page 207*

Ionsys™ [US] *see* fentanyl *on page 340*

iopamidol *see* radiological/contrast media (nonionic) *on page 730*

iopanoic acid *see* radiological/contrast media (ionic) *on page 728*

Iophen-C NR [US] *see* guaifenesin and codeine *on page 393*

Iophen DM NR [US] *see* guaifenesin and dextromethorphan *on page 394*

Iophen NR [US] *see* guaifenesin *on page 392*

Iopidine® [US/Can] *see* apraclonidine *on page 71*

Iosat™ [US-OTC] *see* potassium iodide *on page 686*

iothalamate meglumine and iothalamate sodium *see* radiological/contrast media (ionic) *on page 728*

iothalamate sodium *see* radiological/contrast media (ionic) *on page 728*

ioversol *see* radiological/contrast media (nonionic) *on page 730*

ipecac syrup (IP e kak SIR up)

Synonyms syrup of ipecac

Therapeutic Category Antidote

Use Treatment of acute oral drug overdosage and in certain poisonings

Usual Dosage Oral:

Children:

6-12 months: 5-10 mL followed by 10-20 mL/kg of water; repeat dose one time if vomiting does not occur within 20 minutes

(Continued)

ipecac syrup *(Continued)*

1-12 years: 15 mL followed by 10-20 mL/kg of water; repeat dose one time if vomiting does not occur within 20 minutes

If emesis does not occur within 30 minutes after second dose, ipecac must be removed from stomach by gastric lavage

Adults: 15-30 mL followed by 200-300 mL of water; repeat dose one time if vomiting does not occur within 20 minutes

Dosage Forms Syrup: 70 mg/mL (30 mL) [contains alcohol]

I-Pentolate® *(Discontinued)* *see* cyclopentolate *on page 220*

I-Phrine® Ophthalmic Solution *(Discontinued)* *see* phenylephrine *on page 660*

I-Picamide® *(Discontinued)* *see* tropicamide *on page 856*

Iplex™ [US] *see* mecasermin *on page 522*

IPM Wound Gel™ [US-OTC] *see* hyaluronate and derivatives *on page 416*

ipodate calcium *see* radiological/contrast media (ionic) *on page 728*

ipodate sodium *see* radiological/contrast media (ionic) *on page 728*

IPOL® [US/Can] *see* poliovirus vaccine (inactivated) *on page 677*

ipratropium (i pra TROE pee um)

Sound-Alike/Look-Alike Issues

Atrovent® may be confused with Alupent®

Synonyms ipratropium bromide

U.S./Canadian Brand Names Alti-Ipratropium [Can]; Apo-Ipravent® [Can]; Atrovent® HFA [US/Can]; Atrovent® [US/Can]; Gen-Ipratropium [Can]; Novo-Ipramide [Can]; Nu-Ipratropium [Can]; PMS-Ipratropium [Can]

Therapeutic Category Anticholinergic Agent

Use Anticholinergic bronchodilator used in bronchospasm associated with COPD, bronchitis, and emphysema; symptomatic relief of rhinorrhea associated with the common cold and allergic and nonallergic rhinitis

Usual Dosage

Nebulization:

Infants and Children ≤12 years: 125-250 mcg 3 times/day

Children >12 years and Adults: 500 mcg (one unit-dose vial) 3-4 times/day with doses 6-8 hours apart

Oral inhalation: MDI:

Children 3-12 years: 1-2 inhalations 3 times/day, up to 6 inhalations/24 hours

Children >12 years and Adults: 2 inhalations 4 times/day, up to 12 inhalations/24 hours

Intranasal: Nasal spray:

Symptomatic relief of rhinorrhea associated with the common cold (safety and efficacy of use beyond 4 days in patients with the common cold have not been established):

Children 5-11 years: 0.06%: 2 sprays in each nostril 3 times/day

Children ≥5 years and Adults: 0.06%: 2 sprays in each nostril 3-4 times/day

Symptomatic relief of rhinorrhea associated with allergic/nonallergic rhinitis: Children ≥6 years and Adults: 0.03%: 2 sprays in each nostril 2-3 times/day

Dosage Forms [DSC] = Discontinued product

Aerosol for oral inhalation, as bromide (Atrovent®): 18 mcg/actuation (14 g) [contains soya lecithin and chlorofluorocarbons] [DSC]

Aerosol for oral inhalation, as bromide (Atrovent® HFA): 17 mcg/actuation (12.9 g)

Solution for nebulization, as bromide: 0.02% (2.5 mL)

Solution, intranasal, as bromide [spray] (Atrovent®): 0.03% (30 mL); 0.06% (15 mL)

ipratropium and albuterol (i pra TROE pee um & al BYOO ter ole)

Sound-Alike/Look-Alike Issues

Combivent® may be confused with Combivir®

Synonyms albuterol and ipratropium; salbutamol and ipratropium

U.S./Canadian Brand Names CO Ipra-Sal [Can]; Combivent® [US/Can]; DuoNeb™ [US]; Gen-Combo Sterinebs [Can]

Therapeutic Category Bronchodilator

Use Treatment of COPD in those patients that are currently on a regular bronchodilator who continue to have bronchospasms and require a second bronchodilator

Usual Dosage Adults:
Inhalation: 2 inhalations 4 times/day (maximum: 12 inhalations/24 hours)
Inhalation via nebulization: Initial: 3 mL every 6 hours (maximum: 3 mL every 4 hours)

Dosage Forms
Aerosol for oral inhalation (Combivent®): Ipratropium bromide 18 mcg and albuterol sulfate 103 mcg per actuation [200 doses] (14.7 g) [contains soya lecithin]
Solution for nebulization (DuoNeb™): Ipratropium bromide 0.5 mg [0.017%] and albuterol base 2.5 mg [0.083%] per 3 mL vial (30s, 60s)

ipratropium bromide *see* ipratropium *on previous page*

I-Prin [US-OTC] *see* ibuprofen *on page 437*

iproveratril hydrochloride *see* verapamil *on page 870*

IPV *see* poliovirus vaccine (inactivated) *on page 677*

Iquix® [US] *see* levofloxacin *on page 490*

irbesartan (ir be SAR tan)

Sound-Alike/Look-Alike Issues
Avapro® may be confused with Anaprox®

U.S./Canadian Brand Names Avapro® [US/Can]

Therapeutic Category Angiotensin II Receptor Antagonist

Use Treatment of hypertension alone or in combination with other antihypertensives; treatment of diabetic nephropathy in patients with type 2 diabetes mellitus (noninsulin-dependent, NIDDM) and hypertension

Usual Dosage Oral:
Hypertension:
Children: ≥6-12 years: Initial: 75 mg once daily; may be titrated to a maximum of 150 mg once daily
Children ≥13 years and Adults: 150 mg once daily; patients may be titrated to 300 mg once daily
Note: Starting dose in volume-depleted patients should be 75 mg
Nephropathy in patients with type 2 diabetes and hypertension: Adults: Target dose: 300 mg once daily

Dosage Forms Tablet: 75 mg, 150 mg, 300 mg

irbesartan and hydrochlorothiazide (ir be SAR tan & hye droe klor oh THYE a zide)

Sound-Alike/Look-Alike Issues
Avalide® may be confused with Avandia®

Synonyms Avapro® HCT; hydrochlorothiazide and irbesartan

U.S./Canadian Brand Names Avalide® [US/Can]

Therapeutic Category Antihypertensive Agent, Combination

Use Combination therapy for the management of hypertension

Usual Dosage Dose must be individualized. A patient who is not controlled with either agent alone may be switched to the combination product. Mean effect increases with the dose of each component. The lowest dosage available is irbesartan 150 mg/hydrochlorothiazide 12.5 mg. Dose increases should be made not more frequently than every 2-4 weeks.

Dosage Forms Tablet:
Irbesartan 150 mg and hydrochlorothiazide 12.5 mg
Irbesartan 300 mg and hydrochlorothiazide 12.5 mg
Irbesartan 300 mg and hydrochlorothiazide 25 mg

Ircon® [US-OTC] *see* ferrous fumarate *on page 342*

IRESSA® [US] *see* gefitinib *on page 377*

irinotecan (eye rye no TEE kan)

Synonyms camptothecin-11; CPT-11; NSC-616348

U.S./Canadian Brand Names Camptosar® [US/Can]; Irinotecan Hydrochloride Trihydrate [Can]

Therapeutic Category Antineoplastic Agent

Use Treatment of metastatic carcinoma of the colon or rectum

Usual Dosage I.V. (Refer to individual protocols): **Note:** A reduction in the starting dose by one dose level should be considered for patients ≥65 years of age, prior pelvic/abdominal radiotherapy, performance status of 2, homozygosity for UGT1A1*28 allele, or increased bilirubin (dosing for patients with a bilirubin >2 mg/dL cannot be recommended based on lack of data per manufacturer).
Single-agent therapy:
125 mg/m^2 over 90 minutes on days 1, 8, 15, and 22, followed by a 2-week rest
Adjusted dose level -1: 100 mg/m^2
(Continued)

irinotecan *(Continued)*

Adjusted dose level -2: 75 mg/m^2
Once-every-3-week regimen: 350 mg/m^2 over 90 minutes, once every 3 weeks
Adjusted dose level -1: 300 mg/m^2
Adjusted dose level -2: 250 mg/m^2

Depending on the patient's ability to tolerate therapy, doses should be adjusted in increments of 25-50 mg/m^2. Irinotecan doses may range from 50-150 mg/m^2 for the weekly regimen. Patients may be dosed as low as 200 mg/m^2 (in 50 mg/m^2 decrements) for the once-every-3-week regimen.

Combination therapy with fluorouracil and leucovorin: Six-week (42-day) cycle:
Regimen 1: 125 mg/m^2 over 90 minutes on days 1, 8, 15, and 22; to be given in combination with bolus leucovorin and fluorouracil (leucovorin administered immediately following irinotecan; fluorouracil immediately following leucovorin)
Adjusted dose level -1: 100 mg/m^2
Adjusted dose level -2: 75 mg/m^2
Regimen 2: 180 mg/m^2 over 90 minutes on days 1, 15, and 29; to be given in combination with infusional leucovorin and bolus/infusion fluorouracil (leucovorin administered immediately following irinotecan; fluorouracil immediately following leucovorin)
Adjusted dose level -1: 150 mg/m^2
Adjusted dose level -2: 120 mg/m^2

Note: For all regimens: It is recommended that new courses begin only after the granulocyte count recovers to ≥1500/mm^3, the platelet count recovers to ≥100,000/mm^3, and treatment-related diarrhea has fully resolved. Treatment should be delayed 1-2 weeks to allow for recovery from treatment-related toxicities. If the patient has not recovered after a 2-week delay, consideration should be given to discontinuing irinotecan.

Dosage Forms
Injection, solution, as hydrochloride:
Camptosar®: 20 mg/mL (2 mL, 5 mL) [contains sorbitol 45 mg/mL]

Irinotecan Hydrochloride Trihydrate [Can] *see* irinotecan *on previous page*

iron dextran complex (EYE ern DEKS tran KOM pleks)

Sound-Alike/Look-Alike Issues
Dexferrum® may be confused with Desferal®

U.S./Canadian Brand Names Dexferrum® [US]; Dexiron™ [Can]; INFeD® [US]; Infufer® [Can]

Therapeutic Category Electrolyte Supplement, Oral

Use Treatment of microcytic hypochromic anemia resulting from iron deficiency in patients in whom oral administration is infeasible or ineffective

Usual Dosage I.M. (Z-track method should be used for I.M. injection), I.V.:
A 0.5 mL test dose (0.25 mL in infants) should be given prior to starting iron dextran therapy; total dose should be divided into a daily schedule for I.M., total dose may be given as a single continuous infusion
Iron-deficiency anemia:
Children 5-15 kg: Should not normally be given in the first 4 months of life:
Dose (mL) = 0.0442 (desired hemoglobin - observed hemoglobin) x W + (0.26 x W)
Desired hemoglobin: Usually 12 g/dL
W = Total body weight in kg
Children >15 kg and Adults:
Dose (mL) = 0.0442 (desired hemoglobin - observed hemoglobin) x LBW + (0.26 x LBW)
Desired hemoglobin: Usually 14.8 g/dL
LBW = Lean body weight in kg
Iron replacement therapy for blood loss: Replacement iron (mg) = blood loss (mL) x hematocrit
Maximum daily dosage:
Manufacturer's labeling: **Note:** Replacement of larger estimated iron deficits may be achieved by serial administration of smaller incremental dosages. Daily dosages should be limited to:
Children:
5-15 kg: 50 mg iron (1 mL)
15-50 kg: 100 mg iron (2 mL)
Adults >50 kg: 100 mg iron (2 mL)

Dosage Forms Note: Strength expressed as elemental iron
Injection, solution:
Dexferrum®: 50 mg/mL (1 mL, 2 mL)
INFeD®: 50 mg/mL (2 mL)

iron fumarate *see* ferrous fumarate *on page 342*

iron gluconate *see* ferrous gluconate *on page 343*

iron-polysaccharide complex *see* polysaccharide-iron complex *on page 681*

iron sucrose (EYE ern SOO krose)

U.S./Canadian Brand Names Venofer® [US/Can]

Therapeutic Category Iron Salt

Use Treatment of iron-deficiency anemia in chronic renal failure, including nondialysis-dependent patients (with or without erythropoietin therapy) and dialysis-dependent patients receiving erythropoietin therapy

Usual Dosage Doses expressed in mg of **elemental** iron. **Note:** Test dose: Product labeling does not indicate need for a test dose in product-naive patients; test doses were administered in some clinical trials as 50 mg (2.5 mL) in 50 mL 0.9% NaCl administered over 3-10 minutes.

I.V.: Adults: Iron-deficiency anemia in chronic renal disease:

Hemodialysis-dependent patient: 100 mg (5 mL of iron sucrose injection) administered 1-3 times/week during dialysis; administer no more than 3 times/week to a cumulative total dose of 1000 mg (10 doses); may continue to administer at lowest dose necessary to maintain target hemoglobin, hematocrit, and iron storage parameters

Peritoneal dialysis-dependent patient: Slow intravenous infusion at the following schedule: Two infusions of 300 mg each over 1½hours 14 days apart followed by a single 400 mg infusion over 2½ hours 14 days later (total cumulative dose of 1000 mg in 3 divided doses)

Nondialysis-dependent patient: 200 mg slow injection (over 2-5 minutes) on 5 different occasions within a 14-day period. Total cumulative dose: 1000 mg in 14-day period. **Note:** Dosage has also been administered as two infusions of 500 mg in a maximum of 250 mL 0.9% NaCl infused over 3.5-4 hours on day 1 and day 14 (limited experience)

Dosage Forms Injection, solution [preservative free]: 20 mg of elemental iron/mL (5 mL)

iron sulfate *see* ferrous sulfate *on page 343*

iron sulfate and vitamin C *see* ferrous sulfate and ascorbic acid *on page 343*

Isagel® [US-OTC] *see* alcohol (ethyl) *on page 25*

ISD *see* isosorbide dinitrate *on page 465*

ISDN *see* isosorbide dinitrate *on page 465*

ISG *see* immune globulin (intramuscular) *on page 443*

ISMN *see* isosorbide mononitrate *on page 466*

Ismo® [US] *see* isosorbide mononitrate *on page 466*

isoamyl nitrite *see* amyl nitrite *on page 55*

isobamate *see* carisoprodol *on page 152*

Isocal® [US-OTC] *see* nutritional formula, enteral/oral *on page 608*

isocarboxazid (eye soe kar BOKS a zid)

U.S./Canadian Brand Names Marplan® [US]

Therapeutic Category Antidepressant, Monoamine Oxidase Inhibitor

Use Treatment of depression

Usual Dosage Adults: Oral: 10 mg 2-3 times/day; reduce to 10-20 mg/day in divided doses when condition improves

Dosage Forms Tablet: 10 mg

Isochron™ [US] *see* isosorbide dinitrate *on page 465*

isoflurane (eye soe FLURE ane)

Sound-Alike/Look-Alike Issues

isoflurane may be confused with enflurane, isoflurophate

U.S./Canadian Brand Names Forane® [US]; Terrell™ [US]

Therapeutic Category General Anesthetic

Use Maintenance of general anesthesia

Usual Dosage Minimum alveolar concentration (MAC), the concentration at which 50% of patients do not respond to surgical incision, is 1.2% for isoflurane. The concentration at which amnesia and loss of awareness occur (MAC - awake) is 0.4%. Surgical levels of anesthesia are achieved with concentrations between 1% to 2.5%.

Dosage Forms Liquid, for inhalation: >99.9% (100 mL, 250 mL)

isometheptene, acetaminophen, and dichloralphenazone *see* acetaminophen, isometheptene, and dichloralphenazone *on page 13*

isometheptene, dichloralphenazone, and acetaminophen *see* acetaminophen, isometheptene, and dichloralphenazone *on page 13*

IsonaRif™ [US] *see* rifampin and isoniazid *on page 745*

isoniazid (eye soe NYE a zid)

Synonyms INH; isonicotinic acid hydrazide

U.S./Canadian Brand Names Isotamine® [Can]; PMS-Isoniazid [Can]

Therapeutic Category Antitubercular Agent

Use Treatment of susceptible tuberculosis infections; treatment of latent tuberculosis infection (LTBI)

Usual Dosage Recommendations often change due to resistant strains and newly-developed information; consult *MMWR* for current CDC recommendations:

Oral (injectable is available for patients who are unable to either take or absorb oral therapy):

Infants and Children:

Treatment of latent TB infection (LTBI): 10-20 mg/kg/day in 1-2 divided doses (maximum: 300 mg/day) or 20-40 mg/kg (maximum: 900 mg/dose) twice weekly for 9 months

Treatment of active TB infection:

Daily therapy: 10-15 mg/kg/day in 1-2 divided doses (maximum: 300 mg/day)

Twice weekly directly observed therapy (DOT): 20-30 mg/kg (maximum: 900 mg)

Adults:

Treatment of latent tuberculosis infection (LTBI): 300 mg/day or 900 mg twice weekly for 6-9 months in patients who do not have HIV infection (9 months is optimal, 6 months may be considered to reduce costs of therapy) and 9 months in patients who have HIV infection. Extend to 12 months of therapy if interruptions in treatment occur.

Treatment of active TB infection (drug susceptible):

Daily therapy: 5 mg/kg/day given daily (usual dose: 300 mg/day); 10 mg/kg/day in 1-2 divided doses in patients with disseminated disease

Twice weekly directly observed therapy (DOT): 15 mg/kg (maximum: 900 mg); 3 times/week therapy: 15 mg/kg (maximum: 900 mg)

Note: Treatment may be defined by the number of doses administered (eg, "six-month" therapy involves 192 doses of INH and rifampin, and 56 doses of pyrazinamide). Six months is the shortest interval of time over which these doses may be administered, assuming no interruption of therapy.

Note: Concomitant administration of 6-50 mg/day pyridoxine is recommended in malnourished patients or those prone to neuropathy (eg, alcoholics, diabetics)

Dosage Forms [DSC] = Discontinued product

Injection, solution (Nydrazid®): 100 mg/mL (10 mL) [DSC]

Syrup: 50 mg/5 mL (473 mL) [orange flavor]

Tablet: 100 mg, 300 mg

isoniazid and rifampin *see* rifampin and isoniazid *on page 745*

isoniazid, rifampin, and pyrazinamide *see* rifampin, isoniazid, and pyrazinamide *on page 745*

isonicotinic acid hydrazide *see* isoniazid *on this page*

isonipecaine hydrochloride *see* meperidine *on page 529*

isophane insulin *see* insulin NPH *on page 452*

isophane insulin and regular insulin *see* insulin NPH and insulin regular *on page 452*

isophosphamide *see* ifosfamide *on page 440*

isoproterenol (eye soe proe TER e nole)

Sound-Alike/Look-Alike Issues

Isuprel® may be confused with Disophrol®, Ismelin®, Isordil®

Synonyms isoproterenol hydrochloride

U.S./Canadian Brand Names Isuprel® [US]

Therapeutic Category Adrenergic Agonist Agent

Use Ventricular arrhythmias due to AV nodal block; hemodynamically compromised bradyarrhythmias or atropine- and dopamine-resistant bradyarrhythmias (when transcutaneous/venous pacing is not available); temporary use in third-degree AV block until pacemaker insertion

Usual Dosage I.V.: Cardiac arrhythmias:

Children: Initial: 0.1 mcg/kg/minute (usual effective dose 0.2-2 mcg/kg/minute)

Adults: Initial: 2 mcg/minute; titrate to patient response (2-10 mcg/minute)

Dosage Forms Injection, solution, as hydrochloride: 0.02 mg/mL (10 mL); 0.2 mg/mL (1:5000) (1 mL, 5 mL) [contains sodium metabisulfite]

isoproterenol hydrochloride *see* isoproterenol *on previous page*

Isoptin® *(Discontinued)* *see* verapamil *on page 870*

Isoptin® SR [US/Can] *see* verapamil *on page 870*

Isopto® Atropine [US/Can] *see* atropine *on page 83*

Isopto® Carbachol [US/Can] *see* carbachol *on page 144*

Isopto® Carpine [US/Can] *see* pilocarpine *on page 668*

Isopto® Cetapred® *(Discontinued)*

Isopto® Eserine [Can] *see* physostigmine *on page 666*

Isopto® Eserine *(Discontinued)* *see* physostigmine *on page 666*

Isopto® Frin Ophthalmic Solution *(Discontinued)* *see* phenylephrine *on page 660*

Isopto® Homatropine [US] *see* homatropine *on page 415*

Isopto® Hyoscine [US] *see* scopolamine derivatives *on page 764*

Isopto® Plain Solution *(Discontinued)* *see* artificial tears *on page 75*

Isopto® Tears [US-OTC] *see* artificial tears *on page 75*

Isopto® Tears [US-OTC/Can] *see* hydroxypropyl methylcellulose *on page 432*

Isordil® [US] *see* isosorbide dinitrate *on this page*

isosorbide dinitrate (eye soe SOR bide dye NYE trate)

Sound-Alike/Look-Alike Issues

Isordil® may be confused with Inderal®, Isuprel®

Synonyms ISD; ISDN

U.S./Canadian Brand Names Apo-ISDN® [Can]; Cedocard®-SR [Can]; Coronex® [Can]; Dilatrate®-SR [US]; Isochron™ [US]; Isordil® [US]; Novo-Sorbide [Can]; PMS-Isosorbide [Can]

Therapeutic Category Vasodilator

Use Prevention and treatment of angina pectoris; for congestive heart failure; to relieve pain, dysphagia, and spasm in esophageal spasm with GE reflux

Usual Dosage Adults: Oral:

Angina: 5-40 mg 4 times/day or 40 mg every 8-12 hours in sustained-release dosage form

Sublingual: 2.5-5 mg every 5-10 minutes for maximum of 3 doses in 15-30 minutes; may also use prophylactically 15 minutes prior to activities which may provoke an attack

Congestive heart failure:

Initial dose: 20 mg 3-4 times per day

Target dose: 120-160 mg/day in divided doses; use in combination with hydralazine

Tolerance to nitrate effects develops with chronic exposure: Dose escalation does not overcome this effect. Tolerance can only be overcome by short periods of nitrate absence from the body. Short periods (10-12 hours) of nitrate withdrawal help minimize tolerance. General recommendations are to take the last dose of short-acting agents no later than 7 PM; administer 2-3 times/day rather than 4 times/day. Sustained release preparations could be administered at times to allow a 15- to 17-hour interval between first and last daily dose. Example: Administer sustained release at 8 AM and 2 PM for a twice daily regimen.

Dosage Forms [DSC] = Discontinued product

Capsule, sustained release (Dilatrate®-SR): 40 mg

Tablet: 5 mg, 10 mg, 20 mg, 30 mg

Isordil®: 5 mg, 10 mg [DSC], 20 mg [DSC], 30 mg [DSC], 40 mg

Tablet, extended release (Isochron™): 40 mg

Tablet, sublingual: 2.5 mg, 5 mg

Isordil®: 2.5 mg, 5 mg, 10 mg [DSC]

isosorbide dinitrate and hydralazine

(eye soe SOR bide dye NYE trate & hye DRAL a zeen)

Synonyms hydralazine and isosorbide dinitrate

U.S./Canadian Brand Names BiDil® [US]

Therapeutic Category Vasodilator

Use Treatment of heart failure, adjunct to standard therapy, in self-identified African-Americans

Usual Dosage Oral: Adults: Initial: 1 tablet 3 times/day; titrate to a maximum dose of 2 tablets 3 times/day

Dosage Forms Tablet: Isosorbide dinitrate 20 mg and hydralazine 37.5 mg

isosorbide mononitrate (eye soe SOR bide mon oh NYE trate)

Sound-Alike/Look-Alike Issues

Imdur® may be confused with Imuran®, Inderal LA®, K-Dur®

Monoket® may be confused with Monopril®

Synonyms ISMN

U.S./Canadian Brand Names Apo-ISMN [Can]; Imdur® [US/Can]; Ismo® [US]; Monoket® [US]

Therapeutic Category Vasodilator

Use Long-acting metabolite of the vasodilator isosorbide dinitrate used for the prophylactic treatment of angina pectoris

Usual Dosage Adults and Geriatrics (start with lowest recommended dose): Oral:

Regular tablet: 5-20 mg twice daily with the two doses given 7 hours apart (eg, 8 AM and 3 PM) to decrease tolerance development; then titrate to 10 mg twice daily in first 2-3 days.

Extended release tablet: Initial: 30-60 mg given in morning as a single dose; titrate upward as needed, giving at least 3 days between increases; maximum daily single dose: 240 mg

Tolerance to nitrate effects develops with chronic exposure. Dose escalation does not overcome this effect. Tolerance can only be overcome by short periods of nitrate absence from the body. Short periods (10-12 hours) of nitrate withdrawal help minimize tolerance. Recommended dosage regimens incorporate this interval. General recommendations are to take the last dose of short-acting agents no later than 7 PM; administer 2 times/day rather than 4 times/day. Administer sustained release tablet once daily in the morning.

Dosage Forms

Tablet: 10 mg, 20 mg

Ismo®: 20 mg

Monoket®: 10 mg, 20 mg

Tablet, extended release (Imdur®): 30 mg, 60 mg, 120 mg

isosulfan blue *see* radiological/contrast media (ionic) *on page 728*

Isotamine® [Can] *see* isoniazid *on page 464*

isotretinoin (eye soe TRET i noyn)

Sound-Alike/Look-Alike Issues

Accutane® may be confused with Accolate®, Accupril®

Synonyms 13-*cis*-retinoic acid

U.S./Canadian Brand Names Accutane® [US/Can]; Amnesteem™ [US]; Claravis™ [US]; Isotrex® [Can]; Sotret® [US]

Therapeutic Category Retinoic Acid Derivative

Use Treatment of severe recalcitrant nodular acne unresponsive to conventional therapy

Usual Dosage Oral: Children and Adults: Severe recalcitrant nodular acne: 0.5-2 mg/kg/day in 2 divided doses (dosages as low as 0.05 mg/kg/day have been reported to be beneficial) for 15-20 weeks or until the total cyst count decreases by 70%, whichever is sooner. A second course of therapy may be initiated after a period of ≥2 months off therapy.

Dosage Forms Capsule:

Accutane®: 10 mg, 20 mg, 40 mg [contains soybean oil and parabens]

Amnesteem™: 10 mg, 20 mg, 40 mg [contains soybean oil]

Claravis™: 10 mg, 20 mg, 40 mg

Sotret®: 10 mg, 20 mg, 30 mg, 40 mg [contains soybean oil]

Isotrex® [Can] *see* isotretinoin *on this page*

Isovue® [US] *see* radiological/contrast media (nonionic) *on page 730*

isoxsuprine (eye SOKS syoo preen)

Sound-Alike/Look-Alike Issues

Vasodilan® may be confused with Vasocidin®

Synonyms isoxsuprine hydrochloride

Therapeutic Category Vasodilator

Use Treatment of peripheral vascular diseases, such as arteriosclerosis obliterans and Raynaud disease

Usual Dosage Oral: Adults: 10-20 mg 3-4 times/day

Dosage Forms Tablet, as hydrochloride: 10 mg, 20 mg

isoxsuprine hydrochloride *see* isoxsuprine *on previous page*

isradipine (iz RA di peen)

Sound-Alike/Look-Alike Issues

DynaCirc® may be confused with Dynabac®, Dynacin®

U.S./Canadian Brand Names DynaCirc® CR [US]; DynaCirc® [Can]

Therapeutic Category Calcium Channel Blocker

Use Treatment of hypertension

Usual Dosage Oral: Adults:

Capsule: 2.5 mg twice daily; antihypertensive response occurs in 2-3 hours; maximal response in 2-4 weeks; increase dose at 2- to 4-week intervals at 2.5-5 mg increments; usual dose range (JNC 7): 2.5-10 mg/day in 2 divided doses. **Note:** Most patients show no improvement with doses >10 mg/day except adverse reaction rate increases; therefore, maximal dose in older adults should be 10 mg/day.

Controlled release tablet: 5 mg once daily; antihypertensive response occurs in 2 hours. Adjust dose in increments of 5 mg at 2-4 week intervals. Maximum dose 20 mg/day; adverse events are increased at doses >10 mg/day.

Dosage Forms

Capsule: 2.5 mg, 5 mg

DynaCirc®: 2.5 mg [DSC], 5 mg [DSC]

Tablet, controlled release:

DynaCirc® CR: 5 mg, 10 mg

Istalol™ [US] *see* timolol *on page 828*

Isuprel® [US] *see* isoproterenol *on page 464*

Itch-X® [US-OTC] *see* pramoxine *on page 691*

itraconazole (i tra KOE na zole)

Sound-Alike/Look-Alike Issues

Sporanox® may be confused with Suprax®

U.S./Canadian Brand Names Sporanox® [US/Can]

Therapeutic Category Antifungal Agent

Use Treatment of susceptible fungal infections in immunocompromised and immunocompetent patients including blastomycosis and histoplasmosis; indicated for aspergillosis, and onychomycosis of the toenail; treatment of onychomycosis of the fingernail without concomitant toenail infection via a pulse-type dosing regimen; has activity against *Aspergillus*, *Candida*, *Coccidioides*, *Cryptococcus*, *Sporothrix*, tinea unguium

Oral: Useful in superficial mycoses including dermatophytoses (eg, tinea capitis), pityriasis versicolor, sebopsoriasis, vaginal and chronic mucocutaneous candidiases; systemic mycoses including candidiasis, meningeal and disseminated cryptococcal infections, paracoccidioidomycosis, coccidioidomycoses; miscellaneous mycoses such as sporotrichosis, chromomycosis, leishmaniasis, fungal keratitis, alternariosis, zygomycosis

Oral solution: Treatment of oral and esophageal candidiasis

Intravenous solution: Indicated in the treatment of blastomycosis, histoplasmosis (nonmeningeal), and aspergillosis (in patients intolerant or refractory to amphotericin B therapy); empiric therapy of febrile neutropenic fever

Usual Dosage

Usual dosage ranges:

Children: Efficacy and safety have not been established; a small number of patients 3-16 years of age have been treated with 100 mg/day for systemic fungal infections with no serious adverse effects reported. A dose of 5 mg/kg once daily was used in a pharmacokinetic study using the oral solution in patients 6 months to 12 years; duration of study was 2 weeks.

Adults: Oral, I.V.: 100-400 mg/day; doses >200 mg/day are given in 2 divided doses; length of therapy varies from 1 day to >6 months depending on the condition and mycological response

Indication-specific dosing:

Adults:

Aspergillosis:

Oral: 200-400 mg/day

I.V.: 200 mg twice daily for 4 doses, followed by 200 mg daily

Blastomycosis/histoplasmosis:

Oral: 200 mg once daily, if no obvious improvement or there is evidence of progressive fungal disease, increase the dose in 100 mg increments to a maximum of 400 mg/day; doses >200 mg/day are given in 2 divided doses; length of therapy varies from 1 day to >6 months depending on the condition and mycological response

(Continued)

itraconazole *(Continued)*

I.V.: 200 mg twice daily for 4 doses, followed by 200 mg/day

Brain abscess: Cerebral phaeohyphomycosis (dematiaceous): Oral: 200 mg twice daily for at least 6 months with amphotericin

Candidiasis:

Oropharyngeal: Oral solution: 200 mg once daily for 1-2 weeks; in patients unresponsive or refractory to fluconazole: 100 mg twice daily (clinical response expected in 1-2 weeks)

Esophageal: Oral solution: 100-200 mg once daily for a minimum of 3 weeks; continue dosing for 2 weeks after resolution of symptoms

***Coccidioides*:** Oral: 200 mg twice daily

Infections, life-threatening:

Oral: 200 mg 3 times/day (600 mg/day) should be given for the first 3 days of therapy

I.V.: 200 mg twice daily for 4 doses, followed by 200 mg/day

Meningitis: *Coccidioides:* Oral: 400-800 mg/day

Onychomycosis: Oral: 200 mg once daily for 12 consecutive weeks

Pneumonia: *Coccidioides:* Mild to moderate: Oral, I.V.: 200 mg twice daily

Protothecal infection: 200 mg once daily for 2 months

Sporotrichosis: Oral:

Lymphocutaneous: 100-200 mg/day for 3-6 months

Osteoarticular and pulmonary: 200 mg twice daily for 1-2 years (may use amphotericin B initially for stabilization)

Dosage Forms

Capsule: 100 mg

Injection, solution: 10 mg/mL (25 mL) [packaged in a kit containing sodium chloride 0.9% (50 mL); filtered infusion set (1)]

Solution, oral: 100 mg/10 mL (150 mL) [cherry flavor]

I-Tropine® *(Discontinued)* *see* atropine *on page 83*

Iveegam EN [US] *see* immune globulin (intravenous) *on page 444*

Iveegam Immuno® [Can] *see* immune globulin (intravenous) *on page 444*

ivermectin (eye ver MEK tin)

U.S./Canadian Brand Names Stromectol® [US]

Therapeutic Category Antibiotic, Miscellaneous

Use Treatment of the following infections: Strongyloidiasis of the intestinal tract due to the nematode parasite *Strongyloides stercoralis.* Onchocerciasis due to the nematode parasite *Onchocerca volvulus.* Ivermectin is only active against the immature form of *Onchocerca volvulus*, and the intestinal forms of *Strongyloides stercoralis.*

Usual Dosage Oral: Children ≥15 kg and Adults:

Strongyloidiasis: 200 mcg/kg as a single dose; follow-up stool examinations

Onchocerciasis: 150 mcg/kg as a single dose; retreatment may be required every 3-12 months until the adult worms die

Dosage Forms Tablet [scored]: 3 mg

IVIG *see* immune globulin (intravenous) *on page 444*

IvyBlock® [US-OTC] *see* bentoquatam *on page 98*

Ivy-Rid® [US-OTC] *see* benzocaine *on page 99*

IvySoothe® [US-OTC] *see* hydrocortisone (topical) *on page 428*

Jamp® Travel Tablet [Can] *see* dimenhydrinate *on page 258*

Janimine® *(Discontinued)* *see* imipramine *on page 442*

Jantoven™ [US] *see* warfarin *on page 881*

Japanese encephalitis virus vaccine (inactivated)

(jap a NEESE en sef a LYE tis VYE rus vak SEEN, in ak ti VAY ted)

U.S./Canadian Brand Names JE-VAX® [US/Can]

Therapeutic Category Vaccine, Inactivated Virus

Use Active immunization against Japanese encephalitis for persons 1 year of age and older who plan to spend 1 month or more in endemic areas in Asia, especially persons traveling during the transmission season or visiting rural areas; consider vaccination for shorter trips to epidemic areas or extensive outdoor activities in rural endemic areas; elderly (>55 years of age) individuals should be considered for vaccination, since they have increased risk of developing symptomatic illness after infection; those planning travel to or residence in endemic areas should consult the Travel Advisory Service (Central Campus) for specific advice

Usual Dosage U.S. recommended primary immunization schedule:

Children 1-3 years: SubQ: Three 0.5 mL doses given on days 0, 7, and 30; abbreviated schedules should be used only when necessary due to time constraints

Children >3 years and Adults: SubQ: Three 1 mL doses given on days 0, 7, and 30. Give third dose on day 14 when time does not permit waiting; 2 doses a week apart produce immunity in about 80% of recipients; the longest regimen yields highest titers after 6 months.

Booster dose: Give after 2 years, or according to current recommendation

Note: Travel should not commence for at least 10 days after the last dose of vaccine, to allow adequate antibody formation and recognition of any delayed adverse reaction

Advise concurrent use of other means to reduce the risk of mosquito exposure when possible, including bed nets, insect repellents, protective clothing, avoidance of travel in endemic areas, and avoidance of outdoor activity during twilight and evening periods

Dosage Forms Injection, powder for reconstitution: 1 mL, 10 mL

Jenamicin® *(Discontinued)* *see* gentamicin *on page 381*

Jenest™-28 *(Discontinued)* *see* ethinyl estradiol and norethindrone *on page 323*

JE-VAX® [US/Can] *see* Japanese encephalitis virus vaccine (inactivated) *on previous page*

Jolivette™ [US] *see* norethindrone *on page 598*

Junel™ [US] *see* ethinyl estradiol and norethindrone *on page 323*

Junel™ Fe [US] *see* ethinyl estradiol and norethindrone *on page 323*

Just for Kids™ [US-OTC] *see* fluoride *on page 354*

Just Tears® Solution *(Discontinued)* *see* artificial tears *on page 75*

K-10® [Can] *see* potassium chloride *on page 684*

Kabikinase® *(Discontinued)* *see* streptokinase *on page 791*

Kadian® [US/Can] *see* morphine sulfate *on page 565*

Kala® [US-OTC] *see* Lactobacillus *on page 477*

Kalcinate® *(Discontinued)* *see* calcium gluconate *on page 138*

Kaletra® [US/Can] *see* lopinavir and ritonavir *on page 504*

Kalmz [US-OTC] *see* fructose, dextrose, and phosphoric acid *on page 371*

kanamycin (kan a MYE sin)

Sound-Alike/Look-Alike Issues

kanamycin may be confused with Garamycin®, gentamicin

Synonyms kanamycin sulfate

U.S./Canadian Brand Names Kantrex® [US/Can]

Therapeutic Category Aminoglycoside (Antibiotic)

Use Treatment of serious infections caused by susceptible strains of *E. coli*, *Proteus* species, *Enterobacter aerogenes*, *Klebsiella pneumoniae*, *Serratia marcescens*, and *Acinetobacter* species; second-line treatment of *Mycobacterium tuberculosis*

Usual Dosage Note: Dosing should be based on ideal body weight

Children: Infections: I.M., I.V.: 15 mg/kg/day in divided doses every 8-12 hours

Adults:

Infections: I.M., I.V.: 5-7.5 mg/kg/dose in divided doses every 8-12 hours (<15 mg/kg/day)

Intraperitoneal: After contamination in surgery: 500 mg

Irrigating solution: 0.25%; maximum 1.5 g/day (via all administration routes)

Aerosol: 250 mg 2-4 times/day

Dosage Forms Injection, solution, as sulfate: 1 g/3 mL (3 mL) [contains sodium bisulfate]

kanamycin sulfate *see* kanamycin *on this page*

Kanka® Soft Brush™ [US-OTC] *see* benzocaine *on page 99*

Kantrex® [US/Can] *see* kanamycin *on this page*

Kaochlor-Eff® *(Discontinued)*

Kaochlor® SF *(Discontinued)* *see* potassium chloride *on page 684*

Kaodene® *(Discontinued)* *see* kaolin and pectin *on this page*

Kaodene® NN *(Discontinued)* *see* kaolin and pectin *on this page*

kaolin and pectin (KAY oh lin & PEK tin)

Synonyms pectin and kaolin
Therapeutic Category Antidiarrheal
Use Treatment of uncomplicated diarrhea
Usual Dosage Oral:
Children:
<6 years: Do not use
6-12 years: 30-60 mL after each loose stool
Adults: 60-120 mL after each loose stool
Dosage Forms [DSC] = Discontinued product
Suspension, oral:
Kaodene® NN: Kaolin 650 mg and pectin 32.4 mg per 5 mL (120 mL) [contains bismuth subsalicylate 2.8 mg/5 mL] [DSC]
Kao-Spen®: Kaolin 860 mg and pectin 43 mg per 5 mL (3840 mL) [DSC]
Kapectolin®: Kaolin 15 g and pectin 33 mg per 5 mL (480 mL) [DSC]

Kaon-Cl-10® [US] *see* potassium chloride *on page 684*
Kaon-Cl® 20 [US] *see* potassium chloride *on page 684*
Kao-Paverin® [US-OTC] *see* loperamide *on page 503*
Kaopectate® [Can] *see* attapulgite *on page 84*
Kaopectate® [US-OTC] *see* bismuth subsalicylate *on page 112*
Kaopectate® II *(Discontinued)* *see* loperamide *on page 503*
Kaopectate® Advanced Formula *(Discontinued)* *see* attapulgite *on page 84*
Kaopectate® Extra Strength [US-OTC] *see* bismuth subsalicylate *on page 112*
Kaopectate® Maximum Strength Caplets *(Discontinued)* *see* attapulgite *on page 84*
Kao-Spen® *(Discontinued)* *see* kaolin and pectin *on this page*
Kapectolin® *(Discontinued)* *see* kaolin and pectin *on this page*
Karidium® *(Discontinued)* *see* fluoride *on page 354*
Karigel® *(Discontinued)* *see* fluoride *on page 354*
Karigel®-N *(Discontinued)* *see* fluoride *on page 354*
Kariva™ [US] *see* ethinyl estradiol and desogestrel *on page 317*
Kasof® *(Discontinued)* *see* docusate *on page 270*
Kaybovite-1000® *(Discontinued)* *see* cyanocobalamin *on page 219*
Kay Ciel® [US] *see* potassium chloride *on page 684*
Kayexalate® [US/Can] *see* sodium polystyrene sulfonate *on page 783*
K-Citra® [Can] *see* potassium citrate *on page 685*
KCl *see* potassium chloride *on page 684*
K-Dur® [Can] *see* potassium chloride *on page 684*
K-Dur® 10 [US] *see* potassium chloride *on page 684*
K-Dur® 20 [US] *see* potassium chloride *on page 684*
Keflex® [US] *see* cephalexin *on page 166*
Keftab® [Can] *see* cephalexin *on page 166*
Kefurox® Injection *(Discontinued)* *see* cefuroxime *on page 163*
Kefzol® *(Discontinued)* *see* cefazolin *on page 156*
K-Electrolyte® Effervescent *(Discontinued)* *see* potassium bicarbonate *on page 683*
Kelnor™ [US] *see* ethinyl estradiol and ethynodiol diacetate *on page 319*
Kemadrin® [US] *see* procyclidine *on page 702*
Kemsol® [Can] *see* dimethyl sulfoxide *on page 260*
Kenacort® Oral *(Discontinued)*

Kenaject® Injection *(Discontinued)*

Kenalog® [US/Can] *see* triamcinolone (systemic) *on page 846*

Kenalog® [US/Can] *see* triamcinolone (topical) *on page 846*

Kenalog-10® [US] *see* triamcinolone (systemic) *on page 846*

Kenalog-40® [US] *see* triamcinolone (systemic) *on page 846*

Kenalog® in Orabase [Can] *see* triamcinolone (topical) *on page 846*

Kenonel® Topical *(Discontinued)*

keoxifene hydrochloride *see* raloxifene *on page 730*

Kepivance™ [US] *see* palifermin *on page 632*

Keppra® [US/Can] *see* levetiracetam *on page 487*

Keralac™ [US] *see* urea *on page 861*

Keralac™ Nailstik [US] *see* urea *on page 861*

Keralyt® [US-OTC] *see* salicylic acid *on page 758*

Kerlone® [US] *see* betaxolol *on page 108*

Kerr Insta-Char® [US-OTC] *see* charcoal *on page 169*

Ketalar® [US/Can] *see* ketamine *on this page*

ketamine (KEET a meen)

Sound-Alike/Look-Alike Issues

Ketalar® may be confused with Kenalog®

Synonyms ketamine hydrochloride

U.S./Canadian Brand Names Ketalar® [US/Can]; Ketamine Hydrochloride Injection, USP [Can]

Therapeutic Category General Anesthetic

Controlled Substance C-III

Use Induction and maintenance of general anesthesia, especially when cardiovascular depression must be avoided (ie, hypotension, hypovolemia, cardiomyopathy, constrictive pericarditis); sedation; analgesia

Usual Dosage Used in combination with anticholinergic agents to decrease hypersalivation

Children:

- Oral: 6-10 mg/kg for 1 dose (mixed in 0.2-0.3 mL/kg of cola or other beverage) given 30 minutes before the procedure
- I.M.: 3-7 mg/kg
- I.V.: Range: 0.5-2 mg/kg, use smaller doses (0.5-1 mg/kg) for sedation for minor procedures; usual induction dosage: 1-2 mg/kg
- Continuous I.V. infusion: Sedation: 5-20 mcg/kg/minute

Adults:

- I.M.: 3-8 mg/kg
- I.V.: Range: 1-4.5 mg/kg; usual induction dosage: 1-2 mg/kg

Children and Adults: Maintenance: Supplemental doses of $^1/_3$ to $^1/_2$ of initial dose

Dosage Forms

Injection, solution: 50 mg/mL (10 mL); 100 mg/mL (5 mL)

Ketalar®: 10 mg/mL (20 mL); 50 mg/mL (10 mL); 100 mg/mL (5 mL)

ketamine hydrochloride *see* ketamine *on this page*

Ketamine Hydrochloride Injection, USP [Can] *see* ketamine *on this page*

Ketek® [US/Can] *see* telithromycin *on page 807*

ketoconazole (kee toe KOE na zole)

Sound-Alike/Look-Alike Issues

Nizoral® may be confused with Nasarel®, Neoral®, Nitrol®

U.S./Canadian Brand Names Apo-Ketoconazole® [Can]; Ketoderm® [Can]; Nizoral® A-D [US-OTC]; Nizoral® [US]; Novo-Ketoconazole [Can]

Therapeutic Category Antifungal Agent

Use

Systemic: Treatment of susceptible fungal infections, including candidiasis, oral thrush, blastomycosis, histoplasmosis, paracoccidioidomycosis, coccidioidomycosis, chromomycosis, candiduria, chronic mucocutaneous candidiasis, as well as certain recalcitrant cutaneous dermatophytoses

(Continued)

ketoconazole *(Continued)*

Topical: Treatment of tinea corporis, tinea cruris, tinea versicolor, cutaneous candidiasis, seborrheic dermatitis

Usual Dosage

Fungal infections:

Oral:

Children ≥2 years: 3.3-6.6 mg/kg/day as a single dose for 1-2 weeks for candidiasis, for at least 4 weeks in recalcitrant dermatophyte infections, and for up to 6 months for other systemic mycoses

Adults: 200-400 mg/day as a single daily dose for durations as stated above

Shampoo: Children >12 years and Adults: Apply twice weekly for 4 weeks with at least 3 days between each shampoo

Topical: Adults:

Tinea infections: Cream: Rub gently into the affected area once daily. Duration of treatment: Tinea corporis, cruris: 2 weeks; tinea pedis: 6 weeks

Seborrheic dermatitis:

Cream: Rub gently into the affected area twice daily for 4 weeks or until clinical response is noted

Gel: Rub gently into the affected area once daily for 2 weeks

Dosage Forms

Cream, topical: 2% (15 g, 30 g, 60 g)

Kuric™: 2%: (25 g, 75 g)

Gel, topical:

Xolegel™: 2% (15 g) [contains dehydrated alcohol 34%]

Shampoo, topical: 1% (120 mL)

Nizoral® A-D: 1% (120 mL, 210 mL)

Tablet: 200 mg

Nizoral®: 200 mg

Ketoderm® [Can] *see* ketoconazole *on previous page*

ketoprofen (kee toe PROE fen)

Sound-Alike/Look-Alike Issues

Oruvail® may be confused with Clinoril®, Elavil®

U.S./Canadian Brand Names Apo-Keto SR® [Can]; Apo-Keto-E® [Can]; Apo-Keto® [Can]; Novo-Keto [Can]; Novo-Keto-EC [Can]; Nu-Ketoprofen [Can]; Nu-Ketoprofen-E [Can]; Oruvail® [Can]; Rhodis SR™ [Can]; Rhodis-EC™ [Can]; Rhodis™ [Can]

Therapeutic Category Analgesic, Nonnarcotic; Nonsteroidal Antiinflammatory Drug (NSAID)

Use Acute and long-term treatment of rheumatoid arthritis and osteoarthritis; primary dysmenorrhea; mild to moderate pain

Usual Dosage Oral: Children ≥16 years and Adults:

Rheumatoid arthritis or osteoarthritis:

Capsule: 50-75 mg 3-4 times/day up to a maximum of 300 mg/day

Capsule, extended release: 200 mg once daily

Mild to moderate pain: Capsule: 25-50 mg every 6-8 hours up to a maximum of 300 mg/day

OTC labeling: 12.5 mg every 4-6 hours, up to a maximum of 6 tablets/24 hours

Dosage Forms [DSC] = Discontinued product

Capsule: 50 mg, 75 mg

Capsule, extended release: 200 mg

Tablet (Orudis® KT): 12.5 mg [contains tartrazine and sodium benzoate] [DSC]

ketorolac (KEE toe role ak)

Sound-Alike/Look-Alike Issues

Acular® may be confused with Acthar®, Ocular®

Toradol® may be confused with Foradil®, Inderal®, Tegretol®, Torecan®, tramadol

Synonyms ketorolac tromethamine

U.S./Canadian Brand Names Acular LS™ [US/Can]; Acular® PF [US]; Acular® [US/Can]; Apo-Ketorolac Injectable® [Can]; Apo-Ketorolac® [Can]; Ketorolac Tromethamine Injection, USP [Can]; Novo-Ketorolac [Can]; ratio-Ketorolac [Can]; Toradol® IM [Can]; Toradol® [US/Can]

Therapeutic Category Analgesic, Nonnarcotic; Nonsteroidal Antiinflammatory Drug (NSAID)

Use

Oral, injection: Short-term (≤5 days) management of moderately-severe acute pain requiring analgesia at the opioid level

Ophthalmic: Temporary relief of ocular itching due to seasonal allergic conjunctivitis; postoperative inflammation following cataract extraction; reduction of ocular pain and photophobia following incisional refractive surgery, reduction of ocular pain, burning and stinging following corneal refractive surgery

Usual Dosage

Children 2-16 years: **Do not exceed adult doses**

Single-dose treatment:

I.M.: 1 mg/kg (maximum: 30 mg)

I.V.: 0.5 mg/kg (maximum: 15 mg)

Children ≥16 years and Adults (pain relief usually begins within 10 minutes with parenteral forms): **Note:** The maximum combined duration of treatment (for parenteral and oral) is 5 days; do not increase dose or frequency; supplement with low-dose opioids if needed for breakthrough pain.

I.M.: 60 mg as a single dose or 30 mg every 6 hours (maximum daily dose: 120 mg)

I.V.: 30 mg as a single dose or 30 mg every 6 hours (maximum daily dose: 120 mg)

Oral: 20 mg, followed by 10 mg every 4-6 hours; do not exceed 40 mg/day; oral dosing is intended to be a continuation of I.M. or I.V. therapy only

Ophthalmic: Children ≥3 years and Adults:

Allergic conjunctivitis (relief of ocular itching) (Acular®): Instill 1 drop (0.25 mg) 4 times/day for seasonal allergic conjunctivitis

Inflammation following cataract extraction (Acular®): Instill 1 drop (0.25 mg) to affected eye(s) 4 times/day beginning 24 hours after surgery; continue for 2 weeks

Pain and photophobia following incisional refractive surgery (Acular® PF): Instill 1 drop (0.25 mg) 4 times/day to affected eye for up to 3 days

Pain following corneal refractive surgery (Acular LS™): Instill 1 drop 4 times/day as needed to affected eye for up to 4 days

Dosage Forms [DSC] = Discontinued product

Injection, solution, as tromethamine: 15 mg/mL (1 mL); 30 mg/mL (1 mL, 2 mL, 10 mL) [contains alcohol]

Solution, ophthalmic, as tromethamine:

Acular®: 0.5% (3 mL, 5 mL, 10 mL) [contains benzalkonium chloride]

Acular LS™: 0.4% (5 mL) [contains benzalkonium chloride]

Acular® P.F. [preservative free]: 0.5% (0.4 mL)

Tablet, as tromethamine: 10 mg

Toradol®: 10 mg [DSC]

ketorolac tromethamine *see* ketorolac *on previous page*

Ketorolac Tromethamine Injection, USP [Can] *see* ketorolac *on previous page*

ketotifen (kee toe TYE fen)

Synonyms ketotifen fumarate

U.S./Canadian Brand Names Apo-Ketotifen® [Can]; Novo-Ketotifen [Can]; Zaditen® [Can]; Zaditor™ [US/Can]

Therapeutic Category Antihistamine, H_1 Blocker, Ophthalmic

Use Temporary prevention of eye itching due to allergic conjunctivitis

Usual Dosage Children ≥3 years and Adults: Ophthalmic: Instill 1 drop into the affected eye(s) twice daily, every 8-12 hours

Dosage Forms

Solution, ophthalmic: 0.025% (5 mL)

Zaditor™: 0.025% (5 mL) [contains benzalkonium chloride]

ketotifen fumarate *see* ketotifen *on this page*

Key-E® [US-OTC] *see* vitamin E *on page 876*

Key-E® Kaps [US-OTC] *see* vitamin E *on page 876*

Keygesic [US-OTC] *see* magnesium salicylate *on page 516*

Key-Pred® ***(Discontinued)***

Key-Pred-SP® ***(Discontinued)***

K-G® ***(Discontinued)*** *see* potassium gluconate *on page 686*

K-Gen® Effervescent ***(Discontinued)*** *see* potassium bicarbonate *on page 683*

KI *see* potassium iodide *on page 686*

K-Ide® ***(Discontinued)***

Kidkare Cough and Cold [US-OTC] *see* chlorpheniramine, pseudoephedrine, and dextromethorphan *on page 182*
Kidkare Decongestant [US-OTC] *see* pseudoephedrine *on page 712*
Kidrolase® [Can] *see* asparaginase *on page 76*
Kinerase® *(Discontinued)* *see* hyaluronidase *on page 417*
Kineret® [US/Can] *see* anakinra *on page 56*
Kinesed® *(Discontinued)* *see* hyoscyamine, atropine, scopolamine, and phenobarbital *on page 435*
Kinevac® [US] *see* sincalide *on page 774*
Kionex™ [US] *see* sodium polystyrene sulfonate *on page 783*
Kivexa™ [Can] *see* abacavir and lamivudine *on page 2*
Klaron® [US] *see* sulfacetamide *on page 795*
Klean-Prep® [Can] *see* polyethylene glycol-electrolyte solution *on page 679*
K-Lease® *(Discontinued)* *see* potassium chloride *on page 684*
Klerist-D® Tablet *(Discontinued)* *see* chlorpheniramine and pseudoephedrine *on page 177*
Klonopin® [US/Can] *see* clonazepam *on page 203*
K-Lor® [US/Can] *see* potassium chloride *on page 684*
Klor-Con® [US] *see* potassium chloride *on page 684*
Klor-Con® 8 [US] *see* potassium chloride *on page 684*
Klor-Con® 10 [US] *see* potassium chloride *on page 684*
Klor-Con®/25 [US] *see* potassium chloride *on page 684*
Klor-Con® M [US] *see* potassium chloride *on page 684*
Klor-Con®/EF [US] *see* potassium bicarbonate and potassium citrate *on page 683*
Klorominr® Oral *(Discontinued)* *see* chlorpheniramine *on page 175*
Klorvess® *(Discontinued)* *see* potassium chloride *on page 684*
Klorvess® Effervescent *(Discontinued)*
K-Lyte® [US] *see* potassium bicarbonate and potassium citrate *on page 683*
K-Lyte/Cl® 50 *(Discontinued)* *see* potassium bicarbonate and potassium chloride *on page 683*
K-Lyte/Cl® [US] *see* potassium bicarbonate and potassium chloride *on page 683*
K-Lyte® DS [US] *see* potassium bicarbonate and potassium citrate *on page 683*
K-Lyte® Effervescent *(Discontinued)* *see* potassium bicarbonate *on page 683*
K-Norm® *(Discontinued)* *see* potassium chloride *on page 684*
Koate®-HP *(Discontinued)* *see* antihemophilic factor (human) *on page 59*
Kodet SE [US-OTC] *see* pseudoephedrine *on page 712*
Koffex DM-D [Can] *see* pseudoephedrine and dextromethorphan *on page 714*
Koffex DM + Decongestant + Expectorant [Can] *see* guaifenesin, pseudoephedrine, and dextromethorphan *on page 401*
Koffex DM-Expectorant [Can] *see* guaifenesin and dextromethorphan *on page 394*
Koffex Expectorant [Can] *see* guaifenesin *on page 392*
Kogenate® [Can] *see* antihemophilic factor (recombinant) *on page 59*
Kogenate® *(Discontinued)* *see* antihemophilic factor (recombinant) *on page 59*
Kogenate® FS [US/Can] *see* antihemophilic factor (recombinant) *on page 59*
Kolephrin® [US-OTC] *see* acetaminophen, chlorpheniramine, and pseudoephedrine *on page 11*
Kolephrin® #1 [US] *see* guaifenesin and codeine *on page 393*
Kolephrin® GG/DM [US-OTC] *see* guaifenesin and dextromethorphan *on page 394*
Konakion [Can] *see* phytonadione *on page 667*
Konakion® Injection *(Discontinued)* *see* phytonadione *on page 667*
Kondon's Nasal® *(Discontinued)* *see* ephedrine *on page 294*

labetalol (la BET a lole)

Sound-Alike/Look-Alike Issues
labetalol may be confused with betaxolol, Hexadrol®, lamotrigine
Trandate® may be confused with tramadol, Trendar®, Trental®, Tridrate®

Synonyms ibidomide hydrochloride; labetalol hydrochloride

U.S./Canadian Brand Names Apo-Labetalol® [Can]; Labetalol Hydrochloride Injection, USP [Can]; Normodyne® [Can]; Trandate® [US/Can]

Therapeutic Category Alpha-/Beta- Adrenergic Blocker

Use Treatment of mild to severe hypertension; I.V. for hypertensive emergencies

Usual Dosage Due to limited documentation of its use, labetalol should be initiated cautiously in pediatric patients with careful dosage adjustment and blood pressure monitoring.

Children:

Oral: Limited information regarding labetalol use in pediatric patients is currently available in literature. Some centers recommend initial oral doses of 4 mg/kg/day in 2 divided doses. Reported oral doses have started at 3 mg/kg/day and 20 mg/kg/day and have increased up to 40 mg/kg/day.

I.V., intermittent bolus doses of 0.3-1 mg/kg/dose have been reported.

For treatment of pediatric hypertensive emergencies, initial continuous infusions of 0.4-1 mg/kg/hour with a maximum of 3 mg/kg/hour have been used. Administration requires the use of an infusion pump.

Adults:

Oral: Initial: 100 mg twice daily, may increase as needed every 2-3 days by 100 mg until desired response is obtained; usual dose: 200-400 mg twice daily; may require up to 2.4 g/day.

Usual dose range (JNC 7): 200-800 mg/day in 2 divided doses

(Continued)

labetalol *(Continued)*

I.V.: 20 mg (0.25 mg/kg for an 80 kg patient) IVP over 2 minutes; may administer 40-80 mg at 10-minute intervals, up to 300 mg total dose.

I.V. infusion (acute loading): Initial: 2 mg/minute; titrate to response up to 300 mg total dose, if needed. Administration requires the use of an infusion pump.

I.V. infusion (500 mg/250 mL D_5W) rates:
- 1 mg/minute: 30 mL/hour
- 2 mg/minute: 60 mL/hour
- 3 mg/minute: 90 mL/hour
- 4 mg/minute: 120 mL/hour
- 5 mg/minute: 150 mL/hour
- 6 mg/minute: 180 mL/hour

Note: Although loading infusions are well described in the product labeling, the labeling is silent in specific clinical situations, such as in the patient who has an initial response to labetalol infusions but cannot be converted to an oral route for subsequent dosing. There is limited documentation of prolonged continuous infusions. In rare clinical situations, higher dosages (up to 6 mg/minute) have been used in the critical care setting (eg, aortic dissection). At the other extreme, continuous infusions at relatively low doses (2-6 mg/hour - note difference in units) have been used in some settings (following loading infusion in patients who are unable to be converted to oral regimens or in some cases as a continuation of outpatient oral regimens). These prolonged infusions should not be confused with loading infusions. Because of wide variation in the use of infusions, an awareness of institutional policies and practices is extremely important. Careful clarification of orders and specific infusion rates/units is required to avoid confusion. Due to the prolonged duration of action, careful monitoring should be extended for the duration of the infusion and for several hours after the infusion. Excessive administration may result in prolonged hypotension and/or bradycardia.

Dosage Forms

Injection, solution, as hydrochloride: 5 mg/mL (4 mL, 20 mL, 40 mL)
 Trandate®: 5 mg/mL (20 mL, 40 mL)

Tablet, as hydrochloride: 100 mg, 200 mg, 300 mg
 Trandate®: 100 mg, 200 mg [contains sodium benzoate], 300 mg

labetalol hydrochloride *see* labetalol *on previous page*

Labetalol Hydrochloride Injection, USP [Can] *see* labetalol *on previous page*

Lac-Hydrin® [US] *see* lactic acid and ammonium hydroxide *on next page*

Lac-Hydrin® Five [US-OTC] *see* lactic acid and ammonium hydroxide *on next page*

LAClotion™ [US] *see* lactic acid and ammonium hydroxide *on next page*

Lacril® Ophthalmic Solution *(Discontinued)* *see* artificial tears *on page 75*

Lacrisert® [US/Can] *see* hydroxypropyl cellulose *on page 432*

Lactaid® Extra Strength *(Discontinued)* *see* lactase *on this page*

Lactaid® Fast Act [US-OTC] *see* lactase *on this page*

Lactaid® Original [US-OTC] *see* lactase *on this page*

Lactaid® Ultra *(Discontinued)* *see* lactase *on this page*

lactase (LAK tase)

U.S./Canadian Brand Names Dairyaid® [Can]; Lactaid® Fast Act [US-OTC]; Lactaid® Original [US-OTC]; Lactrase® [US-OTC]

Therapeutic Category Nutritional Supplement

Use Help digest lactose in milk for patients with lactose intolerance

Usual Dosage Oral:

Capsule: 1-2 capsules taken with milk or meal; pretreat milk with 1-2 capsules/quart of milk

Liquid: 5-15 drops/quart of milk

Tablet: 1-3 tablets with meals

Dosage Forms

Caplet:
 Lactaid® Original: 3000 FCC lactase units [contains sodium 5 mg per 3 caplets]
 Lactaid® Extra Strength: 4500 FCC lactase units [DSC]
 Lactaid® Fast Act: 9000 FCC lactase units [contains sodium 5 mg]
 Lactaid® Ultra: 9000 FCC lactase units [DSC]

Capsule (Lactrase®): 250 mg standardized enzyme lactase

Tablet, chewable:
Lactaid® Fast Act: 9000 FCC lactase units [contains sodium 5 mg; vanilla twist flavor]
Lactaid® Ultra: 9000 FCC lactase units [vanilla twist flavor] [DSC]

lactic acid (LAK tik AS id)

Synonyms sodium-PCA and lactic acid

U.S./Canadian Brand Names LactiCare® [US-OTC]; Lactinol-E® [US]; Lactinol® [US]

Therapeutic Category Topical Skin Product

Use Lubricate and moisturize the skin counteracting dryness and itching

Usual Dosage Adults: Lubricant/moisturizer: Topical: Apply twice daily

Dosage Forms
Cream: 10% (120 g) [contains vitamin E]
Lactinol-E®: 10% (120 g, 240 g) [contains vitamin E 3500 int. units/ounce]
Lotion: 10% (360 mL)
LactiCare®: 5% (222 mL, 340 mL) [contains sodium PCA]
Lactinol®: 10% (360 mL, 480 mL)

lactic acid and ammonium hydroxide (LAK tik AS id & a MOE nee um hye DROKS ide)

Synonyms ammonium lactate

U.S./Canadian Brand Names AmLactin® [US-OTC]; Geri-Hydrolac™ [US-OTC]; Geri-Hydrolac™-12 [US-OTC]; Lac-Hydrin® Five [US-OTC]; Lac-Hydrin® [US]; LAClotion™ [US]

Therapeutic Category Topical Skin Product

Use Treatment of moderate to severe xerosis and ichthyosis vulgaris

Usual Dosage Children ≥2 years and Adults: Topical: Apply twice daily to affected area; rub in well

Dosage Forms
Cream, topical: Lactic acid 12% with ammonium hydroxide (140 g, 280 g, 385 g)
AmLactin®: Lactic acid 12% with ammonium hydroxide (140 g)
Lac-Hydrin®: Lactic acid 12% with ammonium hydroxide (280 g, 385 g)
Lotion, topical (AmLactin®, Lac-Hydrin®, LAClotion™): Lactic acid 12% with ammonium hydroxide (225 g, 400 g)
Geri-Hydrolac™, Lac-Hydrin® Five: Lactic acid 5% with ammonium hydroxide (120 mL, 240 mL)
Geri-Hydrolac™-12: Lactic acid 12% with ammonium hydroxide (120 mL, 240 mL)

LactiCare® [US-OTC] *see* lactic acid *on this page*
Lactinex™ [US-OTC] *see* Lactobacillus *on this page*
Lactinol® [US] *see* lactic acid *on this page*
Lactinol-E® [US] *see* lactic acid *on this page*

Lactobacillus (lak toe ba SIL us)

Synonyms *Lactobacillus acidophilus*; *Lactobacillus bifidus*; *Lactobacillus bulgaricus*; *Lactobacillus casei*; *Lactobacillus paracasei*; *Lactobacillus reuteri*; *Lactobacillus rhamnosus* GG

U.S./Canadian Brand Names Bacid® [US-OTC/Can]; Culturelle® [US-OTC]; Dofus [US-OTC]; Fermalac [Can]; Flora-Q™ [US-OTC]; Kala® [US-OTC]; Lactinex™ [US-OTC]; Lacto-Bifidus [US-OTC]; Lacto-Key [US-OTC]; Lacto-Pectin [US-OTC]; Lacto-TriBlend [US-OTC]; Megadophilus® [US-OTC]; MoreDophilus® [US-OTC]; Superdophilus® [US-OTC]

Therapeutic Category Gastrointestinal Agent, Miscellaneous

Use Promote normal bacterial flora of the intestinal tract

Usual Dosage
Dietary supplement: Oral: Dosing varies by manufacturer; consult product labeling
Children (Culturelle®): 1 capsule daily
Adults:
Bacid®: 2 caplets/day
Culturelle®: 1 capsule daily; may increase to twice daily
Flora-Q™: 1 capsule/day
Lacto-Key 100 or 600: 1-2 capsules/day
Lactinex™: 1 packet or 4 tablets 3-4 times/day

Dosage Forms
Capsule:
Culturelle®: *L. rhamnosus* GG 10 billion colony-forming units [contains casein and whey]
Dofus: *L. acidophilus* and *L. bifidus* 10:1 ratio [beet root powder base]
(Continued)

Lactobacillus *(Continued)*

Flora-Q™: *L. acidophilus* and *L. paracasei* ≥8 billion colony-forming units [also contains *Bifidobacterium* and *S. thermophilus*]
Lacto-Key:
100: *L. acidophilus* 1 billion colony-forming units [milk, soy, and yeast free; rice derived]
600: *L. acidophilus* 6 billion colony-forming units [milk, soy, and yeast free; rice derived]
Lacto-Bifidus:
100: *L. bifidus* 1 billion colony-forming units [milk, soy, and yeast free; rice derived]
600: *L. bifidus* 6 billion colony-forming units [milk, soy, and yeast free; rice derived]
Lacto-Pectin: *L. acidophilus* and *L. casei* ≥5 billion colony-forming units [also contains *Bifidobacterium lactis* and citrus pectin cellulose complex]
Lacto-TriBlend:
100: *L. acidophilus, L. bifidus,* and *L. bulgaricus* 1 billion colony-forming units [milk, soy and yeast free; rice derived]
600: *L. acidophilus, L. bifidus,* and *L. bulgaricus* 6 billion colony-forming units [milk, soy and yeast free; rice derived]
Megadophilus®, Superdophilus®: *L. acidophilus* 2 billion units [available in dairy based or dairy free formulations]
Capsule, softgel: *L. acidophilus* 100 active units
Caplet (Bacid®): *L. acidophilus 80%* and *L. bulgaricus* 10% [also contains *Bifidobacterium biffidum* 5% and *S. thermophilus* 5%]
Granules (Lactinex™): *L. acidophilus* and *L. bulgaricus* 100 million live cells per 1 g packet (12s) [contains whey, evaporated milk, soy peptone, lactose, and beef extract]
Powder:
Lacto-TriBlend: *L. acidophilus, L. bifidus,* and *L. bulgaricus* 10 billion colony-forming units per 1/4 teaspoon (60 g) [milk, soy, and yeast free; rice derived]
Megadophilus®, Superdophilus®: *L. acidophilus* 2 billion units per half-teaspoon (49 g, 70 g, 84 g, 126 g) [available in dairy based or dairy free (garbanzo bean) formulations]
MoreDophilus®: *L. acidophilus* 12.4 billion units per teaspoon (30 g, 120 g) [dairy free, yeast free; soy and carrot derived]
Tablet:
Kala®: *L. acidophilus* 200 million units [dairy free, yeast free; soy based]
Lactinex™: *L. acidophilus* and *L. bulgaricus* 1 million live cells [contains whey, evaporated milk, soy peptone, lactose, and beef extract; contains sodium 5.6 mg/4 tablets]
Tablet, chewable: *L. reuteri* 100 million organisms
Wafer: *L. acidophilus* 90 mg and *L. bifidus* 25 mg (100s) [provides 1 billion organisms/wafer at time of manufacture; milk free]

Lactobacillus acidophilus *see* Lactobacillus *on previous page*

Lactobacillus bifidus *see* Lactobacillus *on previous page*

Lactobacillus bulgaricus *see* Lactobacillus *on previous page*

Lactobacillus casei *see* Lactobacillus *on previous page*

Lactobacillus paracasei *see* Lactobacillus *on previous page*

Lactobacillus reuteri *see* Lactobacillus *on previous page*

***Lactobacillus rhamnosus* GG** *see* Lactobacillus *on previous page*

Lacto-Bifidus [US-OTC] *see* Lactobacillus *on previous page*

lactoflavin *see* riboflavin *on page 744*

Lacto-Key [US-OTC] *see* Lactobacillus *on previous page*

Lacto-Pectin [US-OTC] *see* Lactobacillus *on previous page*

Lacto-TriBlend [US-OTC] *see* Lactobacillus *on previous page*

Lactrase® [US-OTC] *see* lactase *on page 476*

lactulose (LAK tyoo lose)

Sound-Alike/Look-Alike Issues
lactulose may be confused with lactose

U.S./Canadian Brand Names Acilac [Can]; Apo-Lactulose® [Can]; Constulose® [US]; Enulose® [US]; Generlac [US]; Kristalose™ [US]; Laxilose [Can]; PMS-Lactulose [Can]

Therapeutic Category Ammonium Detoxicant; Laxative

Use Adjunct in the prevention and treatment of portal-systemic encephalopathy; treatment of chronic constipation

Usual Dosage Diarrhea may indicate overdosage and responds to dose reduction

Prevention of portal systemic encephalopathy (PSE): Oral:

Infants: 2.5-10 mL/day divided 3-4 times/day; adjust dosage to produce 2-3 stools/day

Older Children: Daily dose of 40-90 mL divided 3-4 times/day; if initial dose causes diarrhea, then reduce it immediately; adjust dosage to produce 2-3 stools/day

Constipation: Oral:

Children: 5 g/day (7.5 mL) after breakfast

Adults: 15-30 mL/day increased to 60 mL/day in 1-2 divided doses if necessary

Acute PSE: Adults:

Oral: 20-30 g (30-45 mL) every 1-2 hours to induce rapid laxation; adjust dosage daily to produce 2-3 soft stools; doses of 30-45 mL may be given hourly to cause rapid laxation, then reduce to recommended dose; usual daily dose: 60-100 g (90-150 mL) daily

Rectal administration: 200 g (300 mL) diluted with 700 mL of H_20 or NS; administer rectally via rectal balloon catheter and retain 30-60 minutes every 4-6 hours

Dosage Forms

Crystals for reconstitution:

Kristalose™: 10 g/packet (30s), 20 g/packet (30s)

Syrup: 10 g/15 mL (15 mL, 30 mL, 237 mL, 473 mL, 946 mL, 1890 mL)

Constulose: 10 g/15 mL (240 mL, 960 mL)

Enulose: 10 g/15 mL (480 mL)

Generlac: 10 g/15 mL (480 mL, 1920 mL)

Lactulose PSE® *(Discontinued)* *see* lactulose *on previous page*

ladakamycin *see* azacitidine *on page 86*

L-AmB *see* amphotericin B liposomal *on page 52*

Lamictal® [US/Can] *see* lamotrigine *on next page*

Lamisil® Oral [US/Can] *see* terbinafine (oral) *on page 811*

Lamisil® Topical [US/Can] *see* terbinafine (topical) *on page 811*

lamivudine (la MI vyoo deen)

Sound-Alike/Look-Alike Issues

lamivudine may be confused with lamotrigine

Epivir® may be confused with Combivir®

Synonyms 3TC

U.S./Canadian Brand Names 3TC® [Can]; Epivir-HBV® [US]; Epivir® [US]; Heptovir® [Can]

Therapeutic Category Antiviral Agent

Use

Epivir®: Treatment of HIV infection when antiretroviral therapy is warranted; should always be used as part of a multidrug regimen (at least three antiretroviral agents)

Epivir-HBV®: Treatment of chronic hepatitis B associated with evidence of hepatitis B viral replication and active liver inflammation

Usual Dosage Note: The formulation and dosage of Epivir-HBV® are not appropriate for patients infected with both HBV and HIV. Use with at least two other antiretroviral agents when treating HIV

Oral:

Children 3 months to 16 years: HIV: 4 mg/kg twice daily (maximum: 150 mg twice daily)

Children 2-17 years: Treatment of hepatitis B (Epivir-HBV®): 3 mg/kg once daily (maximum: 100 mg/day)

Adults:

HIV: 150 mg twice daily **or** 300 mg once daily

<50 kg: 4 mg/kg twice daily (maximum: 150 mg twice daily)

Treatment of hepatitis B (Epivir-HBV®): 100 mg/day

Dosage Forms

Solution, oral:

Epivir®: 10 mg/mL (240 mL) [strawberry-banana flavor]

Epivir-HBV®: 5 mg/mL (240 mL) [strawberry-banana flavor]

Tablet:

Epivir®: 150 mg, 300 mg

Epivir-HBV®: 100 mg

lamivudine, abacavir, and zidovudine *see* abacavir, lamivudine, and zidovudine *on page 2*

lamivudine and abacavir *see* abacavir and lamivudine *on page 2*
lamivudine and zidovudine *see* zidovudine and lamivudine *on page 886*

lamotrigine (la MOE tri jeen)

Sound-Alike/Look-Alike Issues
lamotrigine may be confused with labetalol, Lamisil®, lamivudine, Lomotil®, ludiomil
Lamictal® may be confused with Lamisil®, Lomotil®, ludiomil

Synonyms BW-430C; LTG

U.S./Canadian Brand Names Apo-Lamotrigine® [Can]; Gen-Lamotrigine [Can]; Lamictal® [US/Can]; Novo-Lamotrigine [Can]; PMS-Lamotrigine [Can]; ratio-Lamotrigine [Can]

Therapeutic Category Anticonvulsant

Use Adjunctive therapy in the treatment of generalized seizures of Lennox-Gastaut syndrome, primary generalized tonic-clonic seizures, and partial seizures in adults and children ≥2 years of age; conversion to monotherapy in adults with partial seizures who are receiving treatment with valproic acid or a single enzyme-inducing antiepileptic drug (specifically carbamazepine, phenytoin, phenobarbital or primidone); maintenance treatment of bipolar I disorder

Usual Dosage Note: Only whole tablets should be used for dosing, round calculated dose down to the nearest whole tablet: Oral:

Children 2-12 years: Lennox-Gastaut (adjunctive) or partial seizures (adjunctive): **Note:** Children 2-6 years will likely require maintenance doses at the higher end of recommended range:

Patients receiving AED regimens containing valproic acid:

Weeks 1 and 2: 0.15 mg/kg/day in 1-2 divided doses; round dose down to the nearest whole tablet. For patients >6.7 kg and <14 kg, dosing should be 2 mg every other day.

Weeks 3 and 4: 0.3 mg/kg/day in 1-2 divided doses; round dose down to the nearest whole tablet; may use combinations of 2 mg and 5 mg tablets. For patients >6.7 kg and <14 kg, dosing should be 2 mg/day.

Maintenance dose: Titrate dose to effect; after week 4, increase dose every 1-2 weeks by a calculated increment; calculate increment as 0.3 mg/kg/day rounded down to the nearest whole tablet; add this amount to the previously administered daily dose; usual maintenance: 1-5 mg/kg/day in 1-2 divided doses; maximum: 200 mg/day given in 1-2 divided doses

Patients receiving enzyme-inducing AED regimens without valproic acid:

Weeks 1 and 2: 0.6 mg/kg/day in 2 divided doses; round dose down to the nearest whole tablet

Weeks 3 and 4: 1.2 mg/kg/day in 2 divided doses; round dose down to the nearest whole tablet

Maintenance dose: Titrate dose to effect; after week 4, increase dose every 1-2 weeks by a calculated increment; calculate increment as 1.2 mg/kg/day rounded down to the nearest whole tablet; add this amount to the previously administered daily dose; usual maintenance: 5-15 mg/kg/day in 2 divided doses; maximum: 400 mg/day

Children >12 years: Lennox-Gastaut (adjunctive) or partial seizures (adjunctive): Refer to Adults dosing

Children ≥16 years: Conversion from single enzyme-inducing AED regimen to monotherapy: Refer to Adults dosing

Adults:

Lennox-Gastaut (adjunctive) or treatment of partial seizures (adjunctive):

Patients receiving AED regimens containing valproic acid: Initial dose: 25 mg every other day for 2 weeks, then 25 mg every day for 2 weeks. Dose may be increased by 25-50 mg every day for 1-2 weeks in order to achieve maintenance dose. Maintenance dose: 100-400 mg/day in 1-2 divided doses (usual range 100-200 mg/day).

Patients receiving enzyme-inducing AED regimens without valproic acid: Initial dose: 50 mg/day for 2 weeks, then 100 mg in 2 doses for 2 weeks; thereafter, daily dose can be increased by 100 mg every 1-2 weeks to be given in 2 divided doses. Usual maintenance dose: 300-500 mg/day in 2 divided doses; doses as high as 700 mg/day have been reported

Conversion to monotherapy (partial seizures in patients ≥16 years of age):

Adjunctive therapy with valproate: Initiate and titrate as per recommendations to a lamotrigine dose of 200 mg/day. Then taper valproate dose in decrements of not more than 500 mg/day at intervals of one week (or longer) to a valproate dosage of 500 mg/day; this dosage should be maintained for one week. The lamotrigine dosage should then be increased to 300 mg/day while valproate is decreased to 250 mg/day; this dosage should be maintained for one week. Valproate may then be discontinued, while the lamotrigine dose is increased by 100 mg/day at weekly intervals to achieve a lamotrigine maintenance dose of 500 mg/day.

Adjunctive therapy with enzyme-inducing AED: Initiate and titrate as per recommendations to a lamotrigine dose of 500 mg/day. Concomitant enzyme-inducing AED should then be withdrawn by 20% decrements each week over a 4-week period. Patients should be monitored for rash.

Adjunctive therapy with nonenzyme-inducing AED: No specific guidelines available

Bipolar disorder: 25 mg/day for 2 weeks, followed by 50 mg/day for 2 weeks, followed by 100 mg/day for 1 week; thereafter, daily dosage may be increased to 200 mg/day

Patients receiving valproic acid: Initial: 25 mg every other day for 2 weeks, followed by 25 mg/day for 2 weeks, followed by 50 mg/day for 1 week, followed by 100 mg/day (target dose) thereafter. **Note:** If valproate is discontinued, increase daily lamotrigine dose in 50 mg increments at weekly intervals until daily dosage of 200 mg is attained.

Patients receiving enzyme-inducing drugs (eg, carbamazepine): Initial: 50 mg/day for 2 weeks, followed by 100 mg/day (in divided doses) for 2 weeks, followed by 200 mg/day (in divided doses) for 1 week, followed by 300 mg/day (in divided doses) for 1 week. May increase to 400 mg/day (in divided doses) during week 7 and thereafter. **Note:** If carbamazepine (or other enzyme-inducing drug) is discontinued, decrease daily lamotrigine dose in 100 mg increments at weekly intervals until daily dosage of 200 mg is attained.

Discontinuing therapy: Children and Adults: Decrease dose by ~50% per week, over at least 2 weeks unless safety concerns require a more rapid withdrawal.

Restarting therapy after discontinuation: If lamotrigine has been withheld for >5 half-lives, consider restarting according to initial dosing recommendations.

Dosage Forms

Tablet:
- Lamictal®: 25 mg, 100 mg, 150 mg, 200 mg

Tablet, combination package [each unit-dose starter kit contains]:
- Lamictal® (blue kit; for patients taking valproic acid):
  - Tablet: Lamotrigine 25 mg (35s)
- Lamictal® (green kit; for patients taking carbamazepine, phenytoin, phenobarbital, primidone, or rifampin and **not** taking valproic acid):
  - Tablet: Lamotrigine 25 mg (84s)
  - Tablet: Lamotrigine 100 mg (14s)
- Lamictal® (orange kit; for patients **not** taking carbamazepine, phenytoin, phenobarbital, primidone, rifampin, or valproic acid):
  - Tablet: Lamotrigine 25 mg (42s)
  - Tablet: Lamotrigine 100 mg (7s)

Tablet, dispersible/chewable: 5 mg, 25 mg
- Lamictal®: 2 mg, 5 mg, 25 mg [black currant flavor]

Lanacane® [US-OTC] *see* benzocaine *on page 99*

Lanacane® Maximum Strength [US-OTC] *see* benzocaine *on page 99*

Lanaphilic® [US-OTC] *see* urea *on page 861*

lanolin, cetyl alcohol, glycerin, petrolatum, and mineral oil

(LAN oh lin, SEE til AL koe hol, GLIS er in, pe troe LAY tum, & MIN er al oyl)

Synonyms mineral oil, petrolatum, lanolin, cetyl alcohol, and glycerin

U.S./Canadian Brand Names Lubriderm® Fragrance Free [US-OTC]; Lubriderm® [US-OTC]

Therapeutic Category Topical Skin Product

Use Treatment of dry skin

Usual Dosage Topical: Apply to skin as necessary

Dosage Forms

Lotion, topical [bottle]: 180 mL, 300 mL, 480 mL

Lotion, topical [tube]: 100 mL

Lanorinal® ***(Discontinued)***

Lanoxicaps® [US/Can] *see* digoxin *on page 254*

Lanoxin® [US/Can] *see* digoxin *on page 254*

lansoprazole (lan SOE pra zole)

Sound-Alike/Look-Alike Issues

Prevacid® may be confused with Pravachol®, Prevpac®, Prilosec®, Prinivil®

U.S./Canadian Brand Names Prevacid® SoluTab™ [US]; Prevacid® [US/Can]

Therapeutic Category Gastric Acid Secretion Inhibitor

Use

Oral: Short-term treatment of active duodenal ulcers; maintenance treatment of healed duodenal ulcers; as part of a multidrug regimen for *H. pylori* eradication to reduce the risk of duodenal ulcer recurrence; short-term treatment of active benign gastric ulcer; treatment of NSAID-associated gastric ulcer; to reduce the

(Continued)

lansoprazole *(Continued)*

risk of NSAID-associated gastric ulcer in patients with a history of gastric ulcer who require an NSAID; short-term treatment of symptomatic GERD; short-term treatment for all grades of erosive esophagitis; to maintain healing of erosive esophagitis; long-term treatment of pathological hypersecretory conditions, including Zollinger-Ellison syndrome

I.V.: Short-term treatment (≤7 days) of erosive esophagitis in adults unable to take oral medications

Usual Dosage

Children 1-11 years: GERD, erosive esophagitis: Oral:

≤30 kg: 15 mg once daily

>30 kg: 30 mg once daily

Note: Doses were increased in some pediatric patients if still symptomatic after 2 or more weeks of treatment (maximum dose: 30 mg twice daily)

Children 12-17 years: Oral:

Nonerosive GERD: 15 mg once daily for up to 8 weeks

Erosive esophagitis: 30 mg once daily for up to 8 weeks

Adults:

Duodenal ulcer: Oral: Short-term treatment: 15 mg once daily for 4 weeks; maintenance therapy: 15 mg once daily

Gastric ulcer: Oral: Short-term treatment: 30 mg once daily for up to 8 weeks

NSAID-associated gastric ulcer (healing): Oral: 30 mg once daily for 8 weeks; controlled studies did not extend past 8 weeks of therapy

NSAID-associated gastric ulcer (to reduce risk): Oral: 15 mg once daily for up to 12 weeks; controlled studies did not extend past 12 weeks of therapy

Symptomatic GERD: Oral: Short-term treatment: 15 mg once daily for up to 8 weeks

Erosive esophagitis:

Oral: Short-term treatment: 30 mg once daily for up to 8 weeks; continued treatment for an additional 8 weeks may be considered for recurrence or for patients that do not heal after the first 8 weeks of therapy; maintenance therapy: 15 mg once daily

I.V.: 30 mg once daily for up to 7 days; patients should be switched to an oral formulation as soon as they can take oral medications

Hypersecretory conditions: Oral: Initial: 60 mg once daily; adjust dose based upon patient response and to reduce acid secretion to <10 mEq/hour (5 mEq/hour in patients with prior gastric surgery); doses of 90 mg twice daily have been used; administer doses >120 mg/day in divided doses

Helicobacter pylori eradication: Oral: Currently accepted recommendations (may differ from product labeling): Dose varies with regimen: 30 mg once daily or 60 mg/day in 2 divided doses; requires combination therapy with antibiotics

Dosage Forms

Capsule, delayed release (Prevacid®): 15 mg, 30 mg

Granules, for oral suspension, delayed release (Prevacid®): 15 mg/packet (30s), 30 mg/packet (30s) [strawberry flavor]

Injection, powder for reconstitution (Prevacid®): 30 mg

Tablet, orally disintegrating (Prevacid® SoluTab™): 15 mg [contains phenylalanine 2.5 mg; strawberry flavor]; 30 mg [contains phenylalanine 5.1 mg; strawberry flavor]

lansoprazole, amoxicillin, and clarithromycin

(lan SOE pra zole, a moks i SIL in, & kla RITH roe mye sin)

Sound-Alike/Look-Alike Issues

Prevpac® may be confused with Prevacid®

Synonyms amoxicillin, lansoprazole, and clarithromycin; clarithromycin, lansoprazole, and amoxicillin

U.S./Canadian Brand Names Hp-PAC® [Can]; Prevpac® [US/Can]

Therapeutic Category Antibiotic, Macrolide Combination; Antibiotic, Penicillin; Gastrointestinal Agent, Miscellaneous

Use Eradication of *H. pylori* to reduce the risk of recurrent duodenal ulcer

Usual Dosage Oral: Adults: Lansoprazole 30 mg, amoxicillin 1 g, and clarithromycin 500 mg taken together twice daily for 10 or 14 days

Dosage Forms

Combination package [each administration card contains]:

Prevpac®:

Capsule: Amoxicillin 500 mg (4 capsules/day)

Capsule, delayed release (Prevacid®): Lansoprazole 30 mg (2 capsules/day)

Tablet (Biaxin®): Clarithromycin 500 mg (2 tablets/day)

lansoprazole and naproxen (lan SOE pra zole & na PROKS en)

Sound-Alike/Look-Alike Issues
Prevacid® may be confused with Pravachol®, Prevpac®, Prilosec®, Prinivil®

Synonyms NapraPAC™; naproxen and lansoprazole

U.S./Canadian Brand Names Prevacid® NapraPAC™ [US]

Therapeutic Category Gastric Acid Secretion Inhibitor; Nonsteroidal Antiinflammatory Drug (NSAID)

Use Reduction of the risk of NSAID-associated gastric ulcers in patients with history of gastric ulcer who require an NSAID for the treatment of rheumatoid arthritis, osteoarthritis, and ankylosing spondylitis

Usual Dosage Oral: Adults: Reduce NSAID-associated gastric ulcers during treatment for arthritis: Lansoprazole 15 mg once daily in the morning; naproxen 375 mg or 500 mg twice daily

Dosage Forms [DSC] = Discontinued product
Combination package:
Prevacid® NapraPAC™ 375 [each administration card contains] [DSC]:
Capsule, delayed release (Prevacid®): Lansoprazole 15 mg (7 capsules per card)
Tablet (Naprosyn®): Naproxen 375 mg (14 tablets per card)
Prevacid® NapraPAC™ 500 [each administration card contains]:
Capsule, delayed release (Prevacid®): Lansoprazole 15 mg (7 capsules per card)
Tablet (Naprosyn®): Naproxen 500 mg (14 tablets per card)

lanthanum (LAN tha num)

Synonyms lanthanum carbonate

U.S./Canadian Brand Names Fosrenol™ [US]

Therapeutic Category Phosphate Binder

Use Reduction of serum phosphate in patients with stage 5 chronic kidney disease (kidney failure: GFR <15 mL/minute/1.73 m^2 or dialysis)

Usual Dosage Oral: Adults: Initial: 750-1500 mg/day divided and taken with meals; typical increases of 750 mg/day every 2-3 weeks are suggested as needed to bring the serum phosphate level <6 mg/dL; usual dosage range: 1500-3000 mg; doses of up to 3750 mg have been used

Dosage Forms Tablet, chewable: 250 mg, 500 mg, 750 mg, 1000 mg

lanthanum carbonate *see* lanthanum *on this page*

Lantus® [US/Can] *see* insulin glargine *on page 450*

Lantus® OptiSet® [Can] *see* insulin glargine *on page 450*

Lanvis® [Can] *see* thioguanine *on page 822*

Lapase [Can] *see* pancreatin *on page 633*

Largactil® [Can] *see* chlorpromazine *on page 184*

Lariam® [US/Can] *see* mefloquine *on page 525*

laronidase (lair OH ni days)

Synonyms recombinant α-L-iduronidase (glycosaminoglycan α-L-iduronohydrolase)

U.S./Canadian Brand Names Aldurazyme® [US/Can]

Therapeutic Category Enzyme

Use Treatment of Hurler and Hurler-Scheie forms of mucopolysaccharidosis I (MPS I); treatment of Scheie form of MPS I in patients with moderate to severe symptoms

Usual Dosage I.V.: Children ≥5 years and Adults: 0.58 mg/kg once weekly; dose should be rounded up to the nearest whole vial

Dosage Forms Injection, solution [preservative free]: 2.9 mg/5 mL (5 mL)

Lasix® [US/Can] *see* furosemide *on page 372*

Lasix® Special [Can] *see* furosemide *on page 372*

L-asparaginase *see* asparaginase *on page 76*

lassar's zinc paste *see* zinc oxide *on page 887*

latanoprost (la TA noe prost)

Sound-Alike/Look-Alike Issues
Xalatan® may be confused with Travatan®, Zarontin®

U.S./Canadian Brand Names Xalatan® [US/Can]

Therapeutic Category Prostaglandin

Use Reduction of elevated intraocular pressure in patients with open-angle glaucoma or ocular hypertension

(Continued)

latanoprost *(Continued)*

Usual Dosage Adults: Ophthalmic: 1 drop (1.5 mcg) in the affected eye(s) once daily in the evening; do not exceed the once daily dosage because it has been shown that more frequent administration may decrease the IOP lowering effect

Note: A medication delivery device (Xal-Ease™) is available for use with Xalatan®.

Dosage Forms Solution, ophthalmic: 0.005% (2.5 mL) [contains benzalkonium chloride]

Lavacol® [US-OTC] *see* alcohol (ethyl) *on page 25*

Laxilose [Can] *see* lactulose *on page 478*

***l*-bunolol hydrochloride** *see* levobunolol *on page 488*

L-carnitine *see* levocarnitine *on page 488*

LCD *see* coal tar *on page 207*

LCR *see* vincristine *on page 873*

L-deprenyl *see* selegiline *on page 766*

LDP-341 *see* bortezomib *on page 114*

Lectopam® [Can] *see* bromazepam *(Canada only)* *on page 117*

Leena™ [US] *see* ethinyl estradiol and norethindrone *on page 323*

leflunomide (le FLOO noh mide)

U.S./Canadian Brand Names Apo-Leflunomide® [Can]; Arava® [US/Can]; Novo-Leflunomide [Can]

Therapeutic Category Antiinflammatory Agent

Use Treatment of active rheumatoid arthritis; indicated to reduce signs and symptoms, and to retard structural damage and improve physical function

Orphan drug: Prevention of acute and chronic rejection in recipients of solid organ transplants

Usual Dosage Oral: Adults: Rheumatoid arthritis: Initial: 100 mg/day for 3 days, followed by 20 mg/day; dosage may be decreased to 10 mg/day in patients who have difficulty tolerating the 20 mg dose. Due to the long half-life of the active metabolite, plasma levels may require a prolonged period to decline after dosage reduction.

Dosage Forms

Tablet (Arava®): 10 mg, 20 mg

Legatrin PM® [US-OTC] *see* acetaminophen and diphenhydramine *on page 7*

lenalidomide (le na LID oh mide)

Synonyms CC-5013; IMid-3

U.S./Canadian Brand Names Revlimid® [US]

Therapeutic Category Angiogenesis Inhibitor; Immunosuppressant Agent; Tumor Necrosis Factor (TNF) Blocking Agent

Use Treatment of myelodysplastic syndrome (MDS) in patients with deletion 5q (del 5q) cytogenetic abnormality; treatment of multiple myeloma

Usual Dosage Oral: Adults:

Myelodysplastic syndrome (MDS): 10 mg once daily

Multiple myeloma: 25 mg once daily for 21 days of a 28-day treatment cycle (with dexamethasone 40 mg daily on days 1-4, 9-12, and 17-20 of the 28-day treatment cycle)

Dosage Forms

Capsule:

Revlimid®: 5 mg, 10 mg, 15 mg, 25 mg

Lente® Iletin® II *(Discontinued)*

lepirudin (leh puh ROO din)

Synonyms lepirudin (rDNA); recombinant hirudin

U.S./Canadian Brand Names Refludan® [US/Can]

Therapeutic Category Anticoagulant (Other)

Use Indicated for anticoagulation in patients with heparin-induced thrombocytopenia (HIT) and associated thromboembolic disease in order to prevent further thromboembolic complications

Usual Dosage Adults: Maximum dose: Do not exceed 0.21 mg/kg/hour unless an evaluation of coagulation abnormalities limiting response has been completed. **Dosing is weight-based, however, patients**

weighing >110 kg should not receive doses greater than the recommended dose for a patient weighing 110 kg (44 mg bolus and initial maximal infusion rate of 16.5 mg/hour).

Heparin-induced thrombocytopenia: Bolus dose: 0.4 mg/kg IVP (over 15-20 seconds), followed by continuous infusion at 0.15 mg/kg/hour; bolus and infusion must be reduced in renal insufficiency

Note: Due to potential renal insufficiency in critical care patients, some clinicians suggest that for isolated HIT (without thromboembolic complications), the initial infusion rate should be 0.1 mg/kg/hour (omit the initial bolus dose unless acute HITTS).

Concomitant use with thrombolytic therapy: Bolus dose: 0.2 mg/kg IVP (over 15-20 seconds), followed by continuous infusion at 0.1 mg/kg/hour

Dosing adjustments during infusions: Monitor first aPTT 4 hours after the start of the infusion. Subsequent determinations of aPTT should be obtained at least once daily during treatment. More frequent monitoring is recommended in renally impaired patients. Any aPTT ratio measurement out of range (1.5-2.5) should be confirmed prior to adjusting dose, unless a clinical need for immediate reaction exists. If the aPTT is below target range, increase infusion by 20%. If the aPTT is in excess of the target range, stop infusion for 2 hours and when re-started the infusion rate should be decreased by 50%. A repeat aPTT should be obtained 4 hours after any dosing change.

Use in patients scheduled for switch to oral anticoagulants: Reduce lepirudin dose gradually to reach aPTT ratio just above 1.5 before starting warfarin therapy; as soon as INR reaches 2.0, lepirudin therapy should be discontinued.

Dosage Forms Injection, powder for reconstitution: 50 mg

lepirudin (rDNA) *see* lepirudin *on previous page*

Lescol® [US/Can] *see* fluvastatin *on page 363*

Lescol® XL [US] *see* fluvastatin *on page 363*

Lessina™ [US] *see* ethinyl estradiol and levonorgestrel *on page 320*

letrozole (LET roe zole)

Sound-Alike/Look-Alike Issues

Femara® may be confused with femhrt®

Synonyms CGS-20267; NSC-719345

U.S./Canadian Brand Names Femara® [US/Can]

Therapeutic Category Antineoplastic Agent, Hormone (Antiestrogen)

Use First-line treatment of hormone receptor positive or hormone receptor unknown, locally advanced, or metastatic breast cancer in postmenopausal women; treatment of advanced breast cancer in postmenopausal women with disease progression following antiestrogen therapy; adjuvant treatment of postmenopausal hormone receptor positive early breast cancer; extended adjuvant treatment of early breast cancer in postmenopausal women who have received 5 years of adjuvant tamoxifen therapy

Usual Dosage Oral (refer to individual protocols): Adults: Breast cancer: 2.5 mg once daily

Dosage Forms Tablet: 2.5 mg

leucovorin (loo koe VOR in)

Sound-Alike/Look-Alike Issues

leucovorin may be confused with Leukeran®, Leukine®

folinic acid may be confused with folic acid

Synonyms calcium leucovorin; citrovorum factor; folinic acid; 5-formyl tetrahydrofolate; leucovorin calcium

Therapeutic Category Folic Acid Derivative

Use Antidote for folic acid antagonists (methotrexate, trimethoprim, pyrimethamine); treatment of megaloblastic anemias when folate is deficient as in infancy, sprue, pregnancy, and nutritional deficiency when oral folate therapy is not possible; in combination with fluorouracil in the treatment of colon cancer

Usual Dosage Children and Adults:

Treatment of folic acid antagonist overdosage: Oral: 2-15 mg/day for 3 days or until blood counts are normal, **or** 5 mg every 3 days; doses of 6 mg/day are needed for patients with platelet counts <100,000/mm^3

Folate-deficient megaloblastic anemia: I.M.: 1 mg/day

Megaloblastic anemia secondary to congenital deficiency of dihydrofolate reductase: I.M.: 3-6 mg/day

Rescue dose: Initial: I.V.: 10 mg/m^2, then:

Oral, I.M., I.V., SubQ: 10-15 mg/m^2 every 6 hours until methotrexate level <0.05 micromole/L; if methotrexate level remains >5 micromole/L at 48-72 hours after the end of the methotrexate infusion, increase to 20-100 mg/m^2 every 6 hours until methotrexate level <0.05 micromole/L

Dosage Forms

Injection, powder for reconstitution, as calcium: 50 mg, 100 mg, 200 mg, 350 mg, 500 mg

Injection, solution, as calcium: 10 mg/mL (50 mL)

Tablet, as calcium: 5 mg, 10 mg, 15 mg, 25 mg

leucovorin calcium *see* leucovorin *on previous page*

Leukeran® [US/Can] *see* chlorambucil *on page 171*

Leukine® [US/Can] *see* sargramostim *on page 763*

leuprolide (loo PROE lide)

Sound-Alike/Look-Alike Issues

Lupron® may be confused with Nuprin®

Synonyms abbott-43818; leuprolide acetate; leuprorelin acetate; NSC-377526; TAP-144

U.S./Canadian Brand Names Eligard® [US/Can]; Lupron Depot-Ped® [US]; Lupron Depot® [US/Can]; Lupron® [US/Can]; Viadur® [US/Can]

Therapeutic Category Antineoplastic Agent; Luteinizing Hormone-Releasing Hormone Analog

Use Palliative treatment of advanced prostate carcinoma; management of endometriosis; treatment of anemia caused by uterine leiomyomata (fibroids); central precocious puberty

Usual Dosage

Children: Precocious puberty (consider discontinuing by age 11 for females and by age 12 for males):

SubQ (Lupron®): Initial: 50 mcg/kg/day (per manufacturer, doses of 20-45 mcg/kg/day have also been reported); titrate dose upward by 10 mcg/kg/day if down-regulation is not achieved

I.M. (Lupron Depot-Ped®): 0.3 mg/kg/dose given every 28 days (minimum dose: 7.5 mg)

≤25 kg: 7.5 mg

>25-37.5 kg: 11.25 mg

>37.5 kg: 15 mg

Titrate dose upward in increments of 3.75 mg every 4 weeks if down-regulation is not achieved.

Adults:

Advanced prostatic carcinoma:

SubQ:

Eligard®: 7.5 mg monthly **or** 22.5 mg every 3 months **or** 30 mg every 4 months **or** 45 mg every 6 months

Lupron®: 1 mg/day

Viadur®: 65 mg implanted subcutaneously every 12 months

I.M.:

Lupron Depot®: 7.5 mg/dose given monthly (every 28-33 days) **or**

Lupron Depot®-3: 22.5 mg every 3 months **or**

Lupron Depot®-4: 30 mg every 4 months

Endometriosis: I.M.: Initial therapy may be with leuprolide alone or in combination with norethindrone; if retreatment for an additional 6 months is necessary, norethindrone should be used. Retreatment is not recommended for longer than one additional 6-month course.

Lupron Depot®: 3.75 mg/month for up to 6 months **or**

Lupron Depot®-3: 11.25 mg every 3 months for up to 2 doses (6 months total duration of treatment)

Uterine leiomyomata (fibroids): I.M. (in combination with iron):

Lupron Depot®: 3.75 mg/month for up to 3 months **or**

Lupron Depot®-3: 11.25 mg as a single injection

Dosage Forms

Implant (Viadur®): 65 mg [released over 12 months; packaged with administration kit]

Injection, solution, as acetate (Lupron®): 5 mg/mL (2.8 mL) [contains benzyl alcohol; packaged with syringes and alcohol swabs]

Injection, powder for reconstitution, as acetate [depot formulation; prefilled syringe]:

Eligard®:

7.5 mg [released over 1 month]

22.5 mg [released over 3 months]

30 mg [released over 4 months]

45 mg [released over 6 months]

Lupron Depot®: 3.75 mg, 7.5 mg [released over 1 month; contains polysorbate 80]

Lupron Depot®-3 Month: 11.25 mg, 22.5 mg [released over 3 months; contains polysorbate 80]

Lupron Depot®-4 Month: 30 mg [released over 4 months; contains polysorbate 80]

Lupron Depot-Ped®: 7.5 mg, 11.25 mg, 15 mg [released over 1 month; contains polysorbate 80]

leuprolide acetate *see* leuprolide *on this page*

leuprorelin acetate *see* leuprolide *on this page*

leurocristine sulfate *see* vincristine *on page 873*

Leustatin® [US/Can] *see* cladribine *on page 195*

levalbuterol (leve al BYOO ter ole)

Sound-Alike/Look-Alike Issues

Xopenex® may be confused with Xanax®

Synonyms levalbuterol hydrochloride; levalbuterol tartrate; R-albuterol

U.S./Canadian Brand Names Xopenex HFA™ [US]; Xopenex® [US/Can]

Therapeutic Category Adrenergic Agonist Agent; Beta$_2$-Adrenergic Agonist Agent; Bronchodilator

Use Treatment or prevention of bronchospasm in children and adults with reversible obstructive airway disease

Usual Dosage

Metered-dose inhalation: Aerosol: Children ≥4 years and Adults: 1-2 puffs every 4-6 hours

Nebulization:

Children 6-11 years: 0.31 mg 3 times/day (maximum dose: 0.63 mg 3 times/day)

Children >12 years and Adults: 0.63 mg 3 times/day at intervals of 6-8 hours; dosage may be increased to 1.25 mg 3 times/day with close monitoring for adverse effects. Most patients gain optimal benefit from regular use

Dosage Forms Note: Strength expressed as base.

Aerosol, oral, as tartrate:

Xopenex HFA™: 45 mcg/actuation (15 g) [200 doses; chlorofluorocarbon free]

Solution for nebulization, as hydrochloride:

Xopenex®: 0.31 mg/3 mL (24s); 0.63 mg/3 mL (24s); 1.25 mg/3 mL (24s)

Solution for nebulization, concentrate, as hydrochloride:

Xopenex®: 1.25 mg/0.5 mL (30s)

levalbuterol hydrochloride *see* levalbuterol *on this page*

levalbuterol tartrate *see* levalbuterol *on this page*

Levall G [US] *see* guaifenesin and pseudoephedrine *on page 398*

Levaquin® [US/Can] *see* levofloxacin *on page 490*

levarterenol bitartrate *see* norepinephrine *on page 598*

Levate® [Can] *see* amitriptyline *on page 44*

Levatol® [US/Can] *see* penbutolol *on page 645*

Levbid® [US] *see* hyoscyamine *on page 434*

Levemir® [US/Can] *see* insulin detemir *on page 450*

levetiracetam (lee va tye RA se tam)

Sound-Alike/Look-Alike Issues

Potential for dispensing errors between Keppra® and Kaletra™ (lopinavir/ritonavir)

U.S./Canadian Brand Names CO Levetiracetam [Can]; Keppra® [US/Can]

Therapeutic Category Anticonvulsant, Miscellaneous

Use Adjunctive therapy in the treatment of partial onset seizures; adjunctive treatment of myoclonic seizures

Usual Dosage

Oral:

Children 4-15 years: Partial onset seizures: 10 mg/kg/dose given twice daily; may increase every 2 weeks by 10 mg/kg/dose to a maximum of 30 mg/kg/dose twice daily

Children ≥12 years and Adults: Juvenile myoclonic epilepsy: Initial: 500 mg twice daily; may increase every 2 weeks by 500 mg/dose to the recommended dose of 1500 mg twice daily. Efficacy of doses <3000 mg/day has not been established.

Children ≥16 years and Adults: Partial onset seizure: Initial: 500 mg twice daily; may increase every 2 weeks by 500 mg/dose to a maximum of 1500 mg twice daily. Doses >3000 mg/day have been used in trials; however, there is no evidence of increased benefit.

I.V.: Children ≥16 years and Adults: Partial onset seizure: Initial: 500 mg twice daily; may increase every 2 weeks by 500 mg/dose to a maximum of 1500 mg twice daily. Doses >3000 mg/day have been used in trials; however, there is no evidence of increased benefit.

Note: When switching from oral to I.V. formulations, the total daily dose should be the same.

Dosage Forms

Injection, solution:

Keppra®: 100 mg/mL (5 mL)

Solution, oral:

Keppra®: 100 mg/mL (480 mL) [dye free; grape flavor]

Tablet:

Keppra®: 250 mg, 500 mg, 750 mg, 1000 mg

Levitra® [US/Can] *see* vardenafil *on page 867*

Levlen® [US] *see* ethinyl estradiol and levonorgestrel *on page 320*

Levlite™ [US] *see* ethinyl estradiol and levonorgestrel *on page 320*

levobunolol (lee voe BYOO noe lole)

Sound-Alike/Look-Alike Issues

levobunolol may be confused with levocabastine

Betagan® may be confused with Betadine®

Synonyms *l*-bunolol hydrochloride; levobunolol hydrochloride

U.S./Canadian Brand Names Apo-Levobunolol® [Can]; Betagan® [US/Can]; Novo-Levobunolol [Can]; Optho-Bunolol® [Can]; PMS-Levobunolol [Can]; Sandoz-Levobunolol [Can]

Therapeutic Category Beta-Adrenergic Blocker

Use To lower intraocular pressure in chronic open-angle glaucoma or ocular hypertension

Usual Dosage Adults: Ophthalmic: Instill 1 drop in the affected eye(s) 1-2 times/day

Dosage Forms

Solution, ophthalmic, as hydrochloride: 0.25% (5 mL, 10 mL); 0.5% (5 mL, 10 mL, 15 mL) [contains benzalkonium chloride and sodium metabisulfite]

Betagan®: 0.25% (5 mL, 10 mL); 0.5% (2 mL, 5 mL, 10 mL, 15 mL) [contains benzalkonium chloride and sodium metabisulfite]

levobunolol hydrochloride *see* levobunolol *on this page*

levocarnitine (lee voe KAR ni teen)

Sound-Alike/Look-Alike Issues

levocarnitine may be confused with levocabastine

Synonyms L-carnitine

U.S./Canadian Brand Names Carnitor® [US/Can]

Therapeutic Category Dietary Supplement

Use

Oral: Primary systemic carnitine deficiency; acute and chronic treatment of patients with an inborn error of metabolism which results in secondary carnitine deficiency

I.V.: Acute and chronic treatment of patients with an inborn error of metabolism which results in secondary carnitine deficiency; prevention and treatment of carnitine deficiency in patients with end-stage renal disease (ESRD) who are undergoing hemodialysis.

Usual Dosage

Carnitine deficiency:

Oral:

Infants/Children: Initial: 50 mg/kg/day; titrate to 50-100 mg/kg/day in divided doses with a maximum dose of 3 g/day

Adults: 990 mg (tablet) 2-3 times/day or 1-3 g/day (solution)

I.V.: Children and Adults: 50 mg/kg/day in divided doses; titrate based on patient response. Maximum reported dose: 300 mg/kg. An equivalent loading dose may be used in patients in severe metabolic crisis.

ESRD patients on hemodialysis: I.V.: Adults: 20 mg/kg dry body weight as a slow 2- to 3-minute bolus after each dialysis session

Note: Safety and efficacy of oral carnitine have not been established in ESRD. Chronic administration of high **oral** doses to patients with severely compromised renal function or ESRD patients on dialysis may result in accumulation of **potentially toxic** metabolites.

Dosage Forms

Capsule: 250 mg

Injection, solution: 200 mg/mL (5 mL, 12.5 mL)

Carnitor®: 200 mg/mL (5 mL)

Solution, oral: 100 mg/mL (118 mL)

Carnitor®: 100 mg/mL (118 mL) [cherry flavor]

Tablet: 330 mg, 500 mg

Carnitor®: 330 mg

levodopa and benserazide *see* benserazide and levodopa *(Canada only)* *on page 98*

levodopa and carbidopa (lee voe DOE pa & kar bi DOE pa)

Synonyms carbidopa and levodopa

U.S./Canadian Brand Names Apo-Levocarb® CR [Can]; Apo-Levocarb® [Can]; Endo®-Levodopa/Carbidopa [Can]; Novo-Levocarbidopa [Can]; Nu-Levocarb [Can]; Parcopa™ [US]; Sinemet® CR [US/Can]; Sinemet® [US/Can]

Therapeutic Category Anti-Parkinson Agent; Dopaminergic Agent (Anti-Parkinson)

Use Idiopathic Parkinson disease; postencephalitic parkinsonism; symptomatic parkinsonism

Usual Dosage Oral: Adults: Parkinson disease:

Immediate release tablet:

Initial: Carbidopa 25 mg/levodopa 100 mg 3 times/day

Dosage adjustment: Alternate tablet strengths may be substituted according to individual carbidopa/levodopa requirements. Increase by 1 tablet every other day as necessary, except when using the carbidopa 25 mg/levodopa 250 mg tablets where increases should be made using $^1/_2$-1 tablet every 1-2 days. Use of more than 1 dosage strength or dosing 4 times/day may be required (maximum: 8 tablets of any strength/day or 200 mg of carbidopa and 2000 mg of levodopa)

Sustained release tablet:

Initial: Carbidopa 50 mg/levodopa 200 mg 2 times/day, at intervals not <6 hours

Dosage adjustment: May adjust every 3 days; intervals should be between 4-8 hours during the waking day (maximum: 8 tablets/day)

Dosage Forms

Tablet immediate release (Sinemet®):

10/100: Carbidopa 10 mg and levodopa 100 mg

25/100: Carbidopa 25 mg and levodopa 100 mg

25/250: Carbidopa 25 mg and levodopa 250 mg

Tablet, immediate release, orally disintegrating (Parcopa™):

10/100: Carbidopa 10 mg and levodopa 100 mg [contains phenylalanine 3.4 mg/tablet; mint flavor]

25/100: Carbidopa 25 mg and levodopa 100 mg [contains phenylalanine 3.4 mg/tablet; mint flavor]

25/250: Carbidopa 25 mg and levodopa 250 mg [contains phenylalanine 8.4 mg/tablet; mint flavor]

Tablet, sustained release (Sinemet® CR):

Carbidopa 25 mg and levodopa 100 mg

Carbidopa 50 mg and levodopa 200 mg

levodopa, carbidopa, and entacapone (lee voe DOE pa, kar bi DOE pa, & en TA ka pone)

Synonyms carbidopa, levodopa, and entacapone; entacapone, carbidopa, and levodopa

U.S./Canadian Brand Names Stalevo™ [US]

Therapeutic Category Anti-Parkinson Agent, COMT Inhibitor; Dopaminergic Agent (Anti-Parkinson)

Use Treatment of idiopathic Parkinson disease

Usual Dosage Oral: Adults: Parkinson disease:

Note: All strengths of Stalevo™ contain a carbidopa/levodopa ratio of 1:4 plus entacapone 200 mg.

Dose should be individualized based on therapeutic response; doses may be adjusted by changing strength or adjusting interval. Fractionated doses are not recommended and only 1 tablet should be given at each dosing interval; maximum dose: 8 tablets/day (equivalent to entacapone 1600 mg/day)

Patients previously treated with carbidopa/levodopa immediate release tablets (ratio of 1:4):

With current entacapone therapy: May switch directly to corresponding strength of combination tablet. No data available on transferring patients from controlled release preparations or products with a 1:10 ratio of carbidopa/levodopa.

Without entacapone therapy:

If current levodopa dose is >600 mg/day: Levodopa dose reduction may be required when adding entacapone to therapy; therefore, titrate dose using individual products first (carbidopa/levodopa immediate release with a ratio of 1:4 plus entacapone 200 mg); then transfer to combination product once stabilized.

If current levodopa dose is <600 mg without dyskinesias: May transfer to corresponding dose of combination product; monitor, dose reduction of levodopa may be required.

Dosage Forms Tablet:

50: Carbidopa 12.5 mg, levodopa 50 mg, and entacapone 200 mg

100: Carbidopa 25 mg, levodopa 100 mg, and entacapone 200 mg

150: Carbidopa 37.5 mg, levodopa 150 mg, and entacapone 200 mg

Levo-Dromoran® [US] *see* levorphanol *on page 491*

levofloxacin (lee voe FLOKS a sin)

U.S./Canadian Brand Names Iquix® [US]; Levaquin® [US/Can]; Novo-Levofloxacin [Can]; Quixin™ [US]

Therapeutic Category Antibiotic, Ophthalmic; Antibiotic, Quinolone

Use

Systemic: Treatment of mild, moderate, or severe infections caused by susceptible organisms. Includes the treatment of community-acquired pneumonia, including multidrug resistant strains of *S. pneumoniae* (MDRSP); nosocomial pneumonia; chronic bronchitis (acute bacterial exacerbation); acute bacterial sinusitis; urinary tract infection (uncomplicated or complicated), including acute pyelonephritis caused by *E. coli*; prostatitis (chronic bacterial); skin or skin structure infections (uncomplicated or complicated); reduce incidence or disease progression of inhalational anthrax (postexposure)

Ophthalmic: Treatment of bacterial conjunctivitis caused by susceptible organisms (Quixin™ 0.5% ophthalmic solution); treatment of corneal ulcer caused by susceptible organisms (Iquix® 1.5% ophthalmic solution)

Usual Dosage Note: Sequential therapy (intravenous to oral) may be instituted based on prescriber's discretion.

Usual dosage range:

Children ≥1 year: Ophthalmic: 1-2 drops every 2-6 hours

Adults:

Ophthalmic: 1-2 drops every 2-6 hours

Oral, I.V.: 250-500 mg every 24 hours; severe or complicated infections: 750 mg every 24 hours

Indication-specific dosing:

Children ≥1 year and Adults: Ophthalmic:

Conjunctivitis (0.5% ophthalmic solution):

Treatment day 1 and day 2: Instill 1-2 drops into affected eye(s) every 2 hours while awake, up to 8 times/day

Treatment day 3 through day 7: Instill 1-2 drops into affected eye(s) every 4 hours while awake, up to 4 times/day

Children ≥6 years and Adults: Ophthalmic:

Corneal ulceration (1.5% ophthalmic solution): Treatment day 1 through day 3: Instill 1-2 drops into affected eye(s) every 30 minutes to 2 hours while awake and 4-6 hours after retiring.

Adults: Oral, I.V.:

Anthrax (inhalational): 500 mg every 24 hours for 60 days, beginning as soon as possible after exposure

Chronic bronchitis (acute bacterial exacerbation): 500 mg every 24 hours for at least 7 days

Pneumonia:

Community-acquired: 500 mg every 24 hours for 7-14 days or 750 mg every 24 hours for 5 days (efficacy of 5-day regimen for MDRSP not established)

Nosocomial: 750 mg every 24 hours for 7-14 days

Prostatitis (chronic bacterial): 500 mg every 24 hours for 28 days

Sinusitis (bacterial, acute): 500 mg every 24 hours for 10-14 days or 750 mg every 24 hours for 5 days

Skin and skin structure infections:

Uncomplicated: 500 mg every 24 hours for 7-10 days

Complicated: 750 mg every 24 hours for 7-14 days

Urinary tract infections:

Uncomplicated: 250 mg once daily for 3 days

Complicated, including pyelonephritis: 250 mg once daily for 10 days

Dosage Forms

Infusion [premixed in D_5W] (Levaquin®): 250 mg (50 mL); 500 mg (100 mL); 750 mg (150 mL)

Injection, solution [preservative free] (Levaquin®): 25 mg/mL (20 mL, 30 mL)

Solution, ophthalmic:

Iquix®: 1.5% (5 mL)

Quixin™: 0.5% (5 mL) [contains benzalkonium chloride]

Solution, oral (Levaquin®): 25 mg/mL (480 mL) [contains benzyl alcohol]

Tablet (Levaquin®): 250 mg, 500 mg, 750 mg

Levaquin® Leva-Pak: 750 mg (5s)

levomepromazine *see* methotrimeprazine *(Canada only) on page 542*

levonordefrin and mepivacaine hydrochloride *see* mepivacaine and levonordefrin *on page 531*

levonorgestrel (LEE voe nor jes trel)

Synonyms LNg 20

U.S./Canadian Brand Names Mirena® [US/Can]; Norplant® Implant [Can]; Plan B® [US/Can]

Therapeutic Category Contraceptive, Implant (Progestin); Contraceptive, Progestin Only

Use Prevention of pregnancy

Usual Dosage Adults: Females:

Long-term prevention of pregnancy: Intrauterine system: To be inserted into uterine cavity; should be inserted within 7 days of onset of menstruation or immediately after 1st trimester abortion; releases 20 mcg levonorgestrel/day over 5 years. May be removed and replaced with a new unit at anytime during menstrual cycle; do not leave any one system in place for >5 years

Emergency contraception: Oral tablet: One 0.75 mg tablet as soon as possible within 72 hours of unprotected sexual intercourse; a second 0.75 mg tablet should be taken 12 hours after the first dose; may be used at any time during menstrual cycle

Dosage Forms

Intrauterine device:

Mirena®: 52 mg levonorgestrel/unit [releases levonorgestrel 20 mcg/day]

Tablet:

Plan B®: 0.75 mg

levonorgestrel and estradiol *see* estradiol and levonorgestrel *on page 310*

levonorgestrel and ethinyl estradiol *see* ethinyl estradiol and levonorgestrel *on page 320*

Levophed® [US/Can] *see* norepinephrine *on page 598*

Levora® [US] *see* ethinyl estradiol and levonorgestrel *on page 320*

levorphanol (lee VOR fa nole)

Synonyms levorphanol tartrate; levorphan tartrate

U.S./Canadian Brand Names Levo-Dromoran® [US]

Therapeutic Category Analgesic, Narcotic

Controlled Substance C-II

Use Relief of moderate to severe pain; also used parenterally for preoperative sedation and an adjunct to nitrous oxide/oxygen anesthesia

Usual Dosage Adults: **Note:** These are guidelines and do not represent the maximum doses that may be required in all patients. Doses should be titrated to pain relief/prevention.

Acute pain (moderate to severe):

Oral: Initial: Opiate-naive: 2 mg every 6-8 hours as needed; patients with prior opiate exposure may require higher initial doses; usual dosage range: 2-4 mg every 6-8 hours as needed

I.M., SubQ: Initial: Opiate-naive: 1 mg every 6-8 hours as needed; patients with prior opiate exposure may require higher initial doses; usual dosage range: 1-2 mg every 6-8 hours as needed

Slow I.V.: Initial: Opiate-naive: Up to 1 mg/dose every 3-6 hours as needed; patients with prior opiate exposure may require higher initial doses

Chronic pain: Patients taking opioids chronically may become tolerant and require doses higher than the usual dosage range to maintain the desired effect. Tolerance can be managed by appropriate dose titration. **There is no optimal or maximal dose for levorphanol in chronic pain. The appropriate dose is one that relieves pain throughout its dosing interval without causing unmanageable side effects.**

Premedication: I.M., SubQ: 1-2 mg/dose 60-90 minutes prior to surgery; older or debilitated patients usually require less drug

Dosage Forms

Injection, solution, as tartrate: 2 mg/mL (1 mL, 10 mL)

Tablet, as tartrate: 2 mg

levorphanol tartrate *see* levorphanol *on this page*

levorphan tartrate *see* levorphanol *on this page*

Levo-T™ *(Discontinued)* *see* levothyroxine *on this page*

Levothroid® [US] *see* levothyroxine *on this page*

levothyroxine (lee voe thye ROKS een)

Sound-Alike/Look-Alike Issues

levothyroxine may be confused with liothyronine

Levoxyl® may be confused with Lanoxin®, Luvox®

Synthroid® may be confused with Symmetrel®

(Continued)

levothyroxine *(Continued)*

Synonyms levothyroxine sodium; *L*-thyroxine sodium; T_4

U.S./Canadian Brand Names Eltroxin® [Can]; Gen-Levothyroxine [Can]; Levothroid® [US]; Levoxyl® [US]; Synthroid® [US/Can]; Unithroid® [US]

Therapeutic Category Thyroid Product

Use Replacement or supplemental therapy in hypothyroidism; pituitary TSH suppression

Usual Dosage Doses should be adjusted based on clinical response and laboratory parameters.

Oral:

Children: Hypothyroidism:

Newborns: Initial: 10-15 mcg/kg/day. Lower doses of 25 mcg/day should be considered in newborns at risk for cardiac failure. Newborns with T_4 levels <5 mcg/dL should be started at 50 mcg/day. Adjust dose at 4- to 6-week intervals.

Infants and Children: Dose based on body weight and age as listed below. Children with severe or chronic hypothyroidism should be started at 25 mcg/day; adjust dose by 25 mcg every 2-4 weeks. In older children, hyperactivity may be decreased by starting with $^1/_4$ of the recommended dose and increasing by $^1/_4$ dose each week until the full replacement dose is reached. Refer to adult dosing once growth and puberty are complete.

0-3 months: 10-15 mcg/kg/day
3-6 months: 8-10 mcg/kg/day
6-12 months: 6-8 mcg/kg/day
1-5 years: 5-6 mcg/kg/day
6-12 years: 4-5 mcg/kg/day
>12 years: 2-3 mcg/kg/day

Adults:

Hypothyroidism: 1.7 mcg/kg/day in otherwise healthy adults <50 years old, children in whom growth and puberty are complete, and older adults who have been recently treated for hyperthyroidism or who have been hypothyroid for only a few months. Titrate dose every 6 weeks. Average starting dose ~100 mcg; usual doses are ≤200 mcg/day; doses ≥300 mcg/day are rare (consider poor compliance, malabsorption, and/or drug interactions).

Severe hypothyroidism: Initial: 12.5-25 mcg/day; adjust dose by 25 mcg/day every 2-4 weeks as appropriate; **Note:** Oral agents are not recommended for myxedema (see I.V. dosing).

Subclinical hypothyroidism (if treated): 1 mcg/kg/day

TSH suppression:

Well-differentiated thyroid cancer: Highly individualized; Doses >2 mcg/kg/day may be needed to suppress TSH to <0.1 mU/L.

Benign nodules and nontoxic multinodular goiter: Goal TSH suppression: 0.1-0.3 mU/L

I.M., I.V.: Children, Adults: Hypothyroidism: 50% of the oral dose

I.V.: Adults: Myxedema coma or stupor: 200-500 mcg, then 100-300 mcg the next day if necessary; smaller doses should be considered in patients with cardiovascular disease

Dosage Forms

Injection, powder for reconstitution, as sodium: 0.2 mg, 0.5 mg

Tablet, as sodium: 25 mcg, 50 mcg, 75 mcg, 88 mcg, 100 mcg, 112 mcg, 125 mcg, 150 mcg, 175 mcg, 200 mcg, 300 mcg

Levothroid®: 25 mcg, 50 mcg, 75 mcg, 88 mcg, 100 mcg, 112 mcg, 125 mcg, 150 mcg, 175 mcg, 200 mcg, 300 mcg

Levoxyl®, Synthroid®: 25 mcg, 50 mcg, 75 mcg, 88 mcg, 100 mcg, 112 mcg, 125 mcg, 137 mcg, 150 mcg, 175 mcg, 200 mcg, 300 mcg

Unithroid®: 25 mcg, 50 mcg, 75 mcg, 88 mcg, 100 mcg, 112 mcg, 125 mcg, 150 mcg, 175 mcg, 200 mcg, 300 mcg

levothyroxine sodium *see* levothyroxine *on previous page*

Levoxyl® [US] *see* levothyroxine *on previous page*

Levsin® [US/Can] *see* hyoscyamine *on page 434*

Levsinex® [US] *see* hyoscyamine *on page 434*

Levsin/SL® [US] *see* hyoscyamine *on page 434*

Levulan® [Can] *see* aminolevulinic acid *on page 42*

Levulan® Kerastick® [US] *see* aminolevulinic acid *on page 42*

levulose, dextrose and phosphoric acid *see* fructose, dextrose, and phosphoric acid *on page 371*

Lexapro® [US] *see* escitalopram *on page 306*

Lexiva® [US] *see* fosamprenavir *on page 368*

Lexxel® [US/Can] *see* enalapril and felodipine *on page 291*

LFA-3/IgG(1) fusion protein, human *see* alefacept *on page 26*

LHRH *see* gonadorelin *on page 390*

***l*-hyoscyamine sulfate** *see* hyoscyamine *on page 434*

Librax® [US/Can] *see* clidinium and chlordiazepoxide *on page 198*

Librium® [US] *see* chlordiazepoxide *on page 172*

Lice-Aid [US-OTC] *see* pyrethrins and piperonyl butoxide *on page 720*

Lice-Enz® Shampoo *(Discontinued)*

Licide® [US-OTC] *see* pyrethrins and piperonyl butoxide *on page 720*

LidaMantle® [US] *see* lidocaine *on this page*

Lida-Mantle® HC [US] *see* lidocaine and hydrocortisone *on page 496*

Lidemol® [Can] *see* fluocinonide *on page 353*

Lidex® [US/Can] *see* fluocinonide *on page 353*

Lidex-E® [US] *see* fluocinonide *on page 353*

lidocaine (LYE doe kane)

Synonyms lidocaine hydrochloride; lignocaine hydrochloride

U.S./Canadian Brand Names Anestacon® [US]; Band-Aid® Hurt-Free™ Antiseptic Wash [US-OTC]; Betacaine® [Can]; Burn Jel [US-OTC]; Burn-O-Jel [US-OTC]; Burnamycin [US-OTC]; L-M-X™ 4 [US-OTC]; L-M-X™ 5 [US-OTC]; LidaMantle® [US]; Lidodan™ [Can]; Lidoderm® [US/Can]; LTA® 360 [US]; Premjact® [US-OTC]; Solarcaine® Aloe Extra Burn Relief [US-OTC]; Topicaine® [US-OTC]; Xylocaine® MPF [US]; Xylocaine® Viscous [US]; Xylocaine® [US/Can]; Xylocard® [Can]; Zilactin-L® [US-OTC]; Zilactin® [Can]

Therapeutic Category Analgesic, Topical; Antiarrhythmic Agent, Class I-B; Local Anesthetic

Use Local anesthetic and acute treatment of ventricular arrhythmias from myocardial infarction, or cardiac manipulation

Rectal: Temporary relief of pain and itching due to anorectal disorders

Topical: Local anesthetic for use in laser, cosmetic, and outpatient surgeries; minor burns, cuts, and abrasions of the skin

Lidoderm® Patch: Relief of allodynia (painful hypersensitivity) and chronic pain in postherpetic neuralgia

Usual Dosage

Antiarrhythmic:

Children:

I.V., I.O.: **Note:** For use in pulseless VT or VF, give after defibrillation, CPR, and epinephrine:

Loading dose: 1 mg/kg (maximum 100 mg); follow with continuous infusion; may administer second bolus of 0.5-1 mg/kg if delay between bolus and start of infusion is >15 minutes

Continuous infusion: 20-50 mcg/kg/minute. Use 20 mcg/kg/minute in patients with shock, hepatic disease, cardiac arrest, mild CHF; moderate-to-severe CHF may require $^1/_2$ loading dose and lower infusion rates to avoid toxicity.

E.T. (loading dose only): 2-10 times the I.V. bolus dose; dilute with NS to a volume of 3-5 mL and follow with several positive-pressure ventilations

Adults:

Ventricular fibrillation or pulseless ventricular tachycardia (after defibrillation, CPR, and vasopressor administration): I.V.: Initial: 1-1.5 mg/kg. Refractory ventricular tachycardia or ventricular fibrillation, a repeat 0.5-0.75 mg/kg bolus may be given every 5-10 minutes after initial dose for a maximum of 3 doses. Total dose should not exceed 3 mg/kg. Follow with continuous infusion (1-4 mg/minute) after return of perfusion. Reappearance of arrhythmia during constant infusion: 0.5 mg/kg bolus and reassessment of infusion.

E.T. (loading dose only): 2-2.5 times the recommended I.V. dose; dilute in 10 mL NS or distilled water. **Note:** Absorption is greater with distilled water, but causes more adverse effects on PaO_2.

Hemodynamically stable VT: 0.5-0.75 mg/kg followed by synchronized cardioversion

Note: Decrease dose in patients with CHF, shock, or hepatic disease.

Anesthesia, topical:

Cream:

LidaMantle®: Skin irritation: Children and Adults: Apply to affected area 2-3 times/day as needed

L-M-X™ 4: Children ≥2 years and Adults: Apply $^1/_4$ inch thick layer to intact skin. Leave on until adequate anesthetic effect is obtained. Remove cream and cleanse area before beginning procedure.

(Continued)

lidocaine *(Continued)*

L-M-X™ 5: Relief of anorectal pain and itching: Children ≥12 years and Adults: Rectal: Apply topically to clean, dry area **or** using applicator, insert rectally, up to 6 times/day

Gel, ointment, solution: Adults: Apply to affected area ≤3 times/day as needed (maximum dose: 4.5 mg/kg, not to exceed 300 mg)

Jelly:

Children ≥10 years: Dose varies with age and weight (maximum dose: 4.5 mg/kg)

Adults (maximum dose: 30 mL [600 mg] in any 12-hour period):

Anesthesia of male urethra: 5-30 mL

Anesthesia of female urethra: 3-5 mL

Lubrication of endotracheal tube: Apply a moderate amount to external surface only

Liquid: Cold sores and fever blisters: Children ≥5 years and Adults: Apply to affected area every 6 hours as needed

Patch: Postherpetic neuralgia: Adults: Apply patch to most painful area. Up to 3 patches may be applied in a single application. Patch may remain in place for up to 12 hours in any 24-hour period.

Anesthetic, local injectable: Children and Adults: Varies with procedure, degree of anesthesia needed, vascularity of tissue, duration of anesthesia required, and physical condition of patient; maximum: 4.5 mg/kg/dose; do not repeat within 2 hours.

Dosage Forms [DSC] = Discontinued product

Cream, rectal (L-M-X™ 5): 5% (15 g) [contains benzyl alcohol; packaged with applicator]; (30 g) [contains benzyl alcohol]

Cream, topical (L-M-X™ 4): 4% (5 g) [contains benzyl alcohol; packaged with Tegaderm™ dressing]; (15 g, 30 g) [contains benzyl alcohol]

Cream, topical, as hydrochloride: 3% (30 g)

LidaMantle®: 3% (30 g, 85 g)

Gel, topical:

Burn-O-Jel: 0.5% (90 g)

Topicaine®: 4% (10 g, 30 g, 113 g) [contains alcohol 35%, benzyl alcohol, aloe vera, and jojoba]

Gel, topical, as hydrochloride:

Burn Jel: 2% (3.5 g, 120 g)

Solarcaine® Aloe Extra Burn Relief: 0.5% (113 g, 226 g) [contains aloe vera gel and tartrazine]

Infusion, as hydrochloride [premixed in D_5W]: 0.4% [4 mg/mL] (250 mL, 500 mL); 0.8% [8 mg/mL] (250 mL, 500 mL)

Injection, solution, as hydrochloride: 0.5% [5 mg/mL] (50 mL); 1% [10 mg/mL] (2 mL, 10 mL, 20 mL, 30 mL, 50 mL); 2% [20 mg/mL] (2 mL, 5 mL, 20 mL, 50 mL)

Xylocaine®: 0.5% [5 mg/mL] (50 mL); 1% [10 mg/mL] (10 mL, 20 mL, 50 mL); 2% [20 mg/mL] (1.8 mL, 10 mL, 20 mL, 50 mL)

Injection, solution, as hydrochloride [preservative free]: 0.5% [5 mg/mL] (50 mL); 1% [10 mg/mL] (2 mL, 5 mL, 30 mL); 1.5% [15 mg/mL] (20 mL); 2% [20 mg/mL] (2 mL, 5 mL, 10 mL); 4% [40 mg/mL] (5 mL)

Xylocaine®: 10% [100 mg/mL] (5 mL) [for ventricular arrhythmias]

Xylocaine® MPF: 0.5% [5 mg/mL] (50 mL); 1% [10 mg/mL] (2 mL, 5 mL, 10 mL, 30 mL); 1.5% [15 mg/mL] (10 mL, 20 mL); 2% [20 mg/mL] (2 mL, 5 mL, 10 mL); 4% [40 mg/mL] (5 mL)

Injection, solution, as hydrochloride [premixed in $D_{7.5}W$, preservative free]: 5% (2 mL)

Xylocaine® MPF: 1.5% (2 mL) [DSC]

Jelly, topical, as hydrochloride: 2% (5 mL, 30 mL)

Anestacon®: 2% (15 mL) [contains benzalkonium chloride]

Xylocaine®: 2% (5 mL, 30 mL)

Liquid, topical (Zilactin®-L): 2.5% (7.5 mL)

Lotion, topical, as hydrochloride (LidaMantle®): 3% (177 mL)

Ointment, topical: 5% (37 g, 50 g)

Solution, topical, as hydrochloride: 4% [40 mg/mL] (50 mL)

Band-Aid® Hurt-Free™ Antiseptic Wash: 2% (180 mL)

LTA® 360: 4% [40 mg/mL] (4 mL) [packaged with cannula for laryngotracheal administration]

Xylocaine®: 4% [40 mg/mL] (50 mL)

Solution, viscous, as hydrochloride: 2% [20 mg/mL] (20 mL, 100 mL)

Xylocaine® Viscous: 2% [20 mg/mL] (100 mL, 450 mL)

Spray, topical:

Burnamycin: 0.5% (60 mL) [contains aloe vera gel and menthol]

Premjact®: 9.6% (13 mL)

Solarcaine® Aloe Extra Burn Relief: 0.5% (127 g) [contains aloe vera]

Transdermal system, topical (Lidoderm®): 5% (30s)

lidocaine and bupivacaine (LYE doe kane & byoo PIV a kane)

Synonyms bupivacaine and lidocaine; lidocaine hydrochloride and bupivacaine hydrochloride

U.S./Canadian Brand Names Duocaine™ [US]

Therapeutic Category Local Anesthetic

Use Local or regional anesthesia in ophthalmologic surgery by peripheral nerve block techniques such as peribulbar, retrobulbar, and facial blocks; may be used with or without epinephrine

Usual Dosage Adults: **Note:** Use lowest effective dose to limit toxic effects. Dosing based on lidocaine 1% and bupivacaine 0.375%

Retrobulbar injection: 2-5 mL; a portion of dose is injected retrobulbarly and remainder may be used to block the facial nerve

Peribulbar block: 6-12 mL

Maximum dose: 0.18 mL/kg or 12 mL; if used with epinephrine, the dose should not exceed 0.28 mL/kg or 20 mL

Dosage Forms Injection, solution [preservative free]: Lidocaine hydrochloride 1% and bupivacaine hydrochloride 0.375% (10 mL)

lidocaine and epinephrine (LYE doe kane & ep i NEF rin)

Synonyms epinephrine and lidocaine

U.S./Canadian Brand Names LidoSite™ [US]; Xylocaine® MPF With Epinephrine [US]; Xylocaine® With Epinephrine [US/Can]

Therapeutic Category Local Anesthetic

Use Local infiltration anesthesia; AVS for nerve block; topical local analgesia for superficial dermatologic procedures

Usual Dosage Dosage varies with the anesthetic procedure, degree of anesthesia needed, vascularity of tissue, duration of anesthesia required, and physical condition of patient.

Dental anesthesia, infiltration, or conduction block:

Children <10 years: 20-30 mg (1-1.5 mL) of lidocaine hydrochloride as a 2% solution with epinephrine 1:100,000; maximum: 4-5 mg of lidocaine hydrochloride/kg of body weight or 100-150 mg as a single dose

Children >10 years and Adults: Do not exceed 6.6 mg/kg body weight or 300 mg of lidocaine hydrochloride and 3 mcg (0.003 mg) of epinephrine/kg of body weight or 0.2 mg epinephrine per dental appointment. The effective anesthetic dose varies with procedure, intensity of anesthesia needed, duration of anesthesia required, and physical condition of the patient. Always use the lowest effective dose along with careful aspiration.

For most routine dental procedures, lidocaine hydrochloride 2% with epinephrine 1:100,000 is preferred. When a more pronounced hemostasis is required, a 1:50,000 epinephrine concentration should be used.

Dermatologic procedure: Children ≥5 and Adults: Topical: Place 1 transdermal patch over area requiring analgesia; attach patch to iontophoretic controller and leave on for 10 minutes. Remove patch and perform procedure within 10-20 minutes of patch removal. Do not use another patch for 30 minutes.

Dosage Forms

Injection, solution:

0.5% / 1:200,000: Lidocaine hydrochloride 0.5% and epinephrine 1:200,000 (50 mL)

1% / 1:100,000: Lidocaine hydrochloride 1% and epinephrine 1:100,000 (20 mL, 30 mL, 50 mL)

1% / 1:200,000: Lidocaine hydrochloride 1% and epinephrine 1:200,000 (30 mL)

1.5% / 1:200,000: Lidocaine hydrochloride 1.5% and epinephrine 1:200,000 (30 mL)

2% / 1:50,000: Lidocaine hydrochloride 2% and epinephrine 1:50,000 (1.8 mL)

2% / 1:100,000: Lidocaine hydrochloride 2% and epinephrine 1:100,000 (1.8 mL, 30 mL, 50 mL)

2% / 1:200,000: Lidocaine hydrochloride 2% and epinephrine 1:200,000 (20 mL)

Xylocaine® with Epinephrine:

0.5% / 1:200,000: Lidocaine hydrochloride 0.5% and epinephrine 1:200,000 (50 mL) [contains methylparaben]

1% / 1:100,000: Lidocaine hydrochloride 1% and epinephrine 1:100,000 (10 mL, 20 mL, 50 mL) [contains methylparaben]

2% / 1:50,000: Lidocaine hydrochloride 2% and epinephrine 1:50,000 (1.8 mL) [contains sodium metabisulfite]

2% / 1:100,000: Lidocaine hydrochloride 2% and epinephrine 1:100,000 (1.8 mL) [contains sodium metabisulfite]; (10 mL, 20 mL, 50 mL) [contains methylparaben]

Xylocaine®-MPF with Epinephrine:

1% / 1:200,000: Lidocaine hydrochloride 1% and epinephrine 1:200,000 (5 mL, 10 mL, 30 mL) [contains sodium metabisulfite]

1.5% / 1:200,000: Lidocaine hydrochloride 1.5% and epinephrine 1:200,000 (5 mL, 10 mL, 30 mL) [contains sodium metabisulfite]

(Continued)

lidocaine and epinephrine *(Continued)*

2% / 1:200,000: Lidocaine hydrochloride 2% and epinephrine 1:200,000 (5 mL, 10 mL, 20 mL) [contains sodium metabisulfite]

Transdermal system (LidoSite™): Lidocaine hydrochloride 10% and epinephrine 0.1% (25s) [contains sodium metabisulfite; for use only with LidoSite™ controller]

lidocaine and hydrocortisone (LYE doe kane & hye droe KOR ti sone)

Synonyms hydrocortisone and lidocaine

U.S./Canadian Brand Names AnaMantle® HC [US]; Lida-Mantle® HC [US]

Therapeutic Category Anesthetic/Corticosteroid

Use Topical antiinflammatory and anesthetic for skin disorders; rectal for the treatment of hemorrhoids, anal fissures, pruritus ani, or similar conditions

Usual Dosage Adults:

Topical: Apply 2-3 times/day

Rectal: One applicatorful twice daily

Dosage Forms

Cream, rectal (AnaMantle® HC): Lidocaine hydrochloride 3% and hydrocortisone acetate 0.5% (7 g) [kit contains 14 single-use tubes (7 g each) and 14 applicators]

Cream, topical: Lidocaine hydrochloride 3% and hydrocortisone acetate 0.5% (30 g)

Lida-Mantle® HC: Lidocaine hydrochloride 3% and hydrocortisone acetate 0.5% (30 g, 85 g)

Lotion, topical (Lida-Mantle® HC): Lidocaine hydrochloride 3% and hydrocortisone acetate 0.5% (177 mL)

lidocaine and prilocaine (LYE doe kane & PRIL oh kane)

Synonyms prilocaine and lidocaine

U.S./Canadian Brand Names EMLA® [US/Can]; Oraquix®

Therapeutic Category Analgesic, Topical

Use Topical anesthetic for use on normal intact skin to provide local analgesia for minor procedures such as I.V. cannulation or venipuncture; has also been used for painful procedures such as lumbar puncture and skin graft harvesting; for superficial minor surgery of genital mucous membranes and as an adjunct for local infiltration anesthesia in genital mucous membranes.

Usual Dosage Although the incidence of systemic adverse effects with EMLA® is very low, caution should be exercised, particularly when applying over large areas and leaving on for >2 hours

Children (intact skin): EMLA® should **not** be used in neonates with a gestation age <37 weeks nor in infants <12 months of age who are receiving treatment with methemoglobin-inducing agents

Dosing is based on child's age and weight:

Age 0-3 months or <5 kg: Apply a maximum of 1 g over no more than 10 cm^2 of skin; leave on for no longer than 1 hour

Age 3 months to 12 months and >5 kg: Apply no more than a maximum 2 g total over no more than 20 cm^2 of skin; leave on for no longer than 4 hours

Age 1-6 years and >10 kg: Apply no more than a maximum of 10 g total over no more than 100 cm^2 of skin; leave on for no longer than 4 hours.

Age 7-12 years and >20 kg: Apply no more than a maximum 20 g total over no more than 200 cm^2 of skin; leave on for no longer than 4 hours.

Note: If a patient greater than 3 months old does not meet the minimum weight requirement, the maximum total dose should be restricted to the corresponding maximum based on patient weight.

Adults (intact skin):

EMLA® cream and EMLA® anesthetic disc: A thick layer of EMLA® cream is applied to intact skin and covered with an occlusive dressing, or alternatively, an EMLA® anesthetic disc is applied to intact skin

Minor dermal procedures (eg, I.V. cannulation or venipuncture): Apply 2.5 g of cream (1/2 of the 5 g tube) over 20-25 cm of skin surface area, or 1 anesthetic disc (1 g over 10 cm^2) for at least 1 hour. **Note:** In clinical trials, 2 sites were usually prepared in case there was a technical problem with cannulation or venipuncture at the first site.

Major dermal procedures (eg, more painful dermatological procedures involving a larger skin area such as split thickness skin graft harvesting): Apply 2 g of cream per 10 cm^2 of skin and allow to remain in contact with the skin for at least 2 hours.

Adult male genital skin (eg, pretreatment prior to local anesthetic infiltration): Apply a thick layer of cream (1 g/10 cm^2) to the skin surface for 15 minutes. Local anesthetic infiltration should be performed immediately after removal of EMLA® cream.

Note: Dermal analgesia can be expected to increase for up to 3 hours under occlusive dressing and persist for 1-2 hours after removal of the cream

Adult females: Genital mucous membranes: Minor procedures (eg, removal of condylomata acuminata, pretreatment for local anesthetic infiltration): Apply 5-10 g (thick layer) of cream for 5-10 minutes

Periodontal gel (Oraqix®): Adults: Apply on gingival margin around selected teeth using the blunt-tipped applicator included in package. Wait 30 seconds, then fill the periodontal pockets using the blunt-tipped applicator until gel becomes visible at the gingival margin. Wait another 30 seconds before starting treatment. Maximum recommended dose: One treatment session: 5 cartridges (8.5 g)

Dosage Forms

Cream, topical: Lidocaine 2.5% and prilocaine 2.5% (5 g, 30 g)

EMLA®: Lidocaine 2.5% and prilocaine 2.5% (5 g, 30 g) [each packaged with Tegaderm® dressings]

Disc, topical: Lidocaine 2.5% and prilocaine 2.5% per disc (2s, 10s) [each 1 g disc is 10 cm^2]

Gel, periodontal: Lidocaine 2.5% and prilocaine 2.5% (1.7 g) [cartridge]

lidocaine hydrochloride *see* lidocaine *on page 493*

lidocaine hydrochloride and bupivacaine hydrochloride *see* lidocaine and bupivacaine *on page 495*

Lidodan™ [Can] *see* lidocaine *on page 493*

Lidoderm® [US/Can] *see* lidocaine *on page 493*

LidoPen® I.M. Injection Auto-Injector *(Discontinued)* *see* lidocaine *on page 493*

LidoSite™ [US] *see* lidocaine and epinephrine *on page 495*

LID-Pack® [Can] *see* bacitracin and polymyxin B *on page 90*

lignocaine hydrochloride *see* lidocaine *on page 493*

Limbitrol® [US/Can] *see* amitriptyline and chlordiazepoxide *on page 44*

Limbitrol® DS [US] *see* amitriptyline and chlordiazepoxide *on page 44*

Lin-Amox [Can] *see* amoxicillin *on page 47*

Lin-Buspirone [Can] *see* buspirone *on page 127*

Lincocin® [US/Can] *see* lincomycin *on this page*

lincomycin (lin koe MYE sin)

Sound-Alike/Look-Alike Issues

Lincocin® may be confused with Cleocin®, Indocin®, Minocin®

Synonyms lincomycin hydrochloride

U.S./Canadian Brand Names Lincocin® [US/Can]

Therapeutic Category Antibiotic, Lincosamide

Use Treatment of serious susceptible bacterial infections, mainly those caused by streptococci and staphylococci resistant to other agents

Usual Dosage Note: Frequency may be increased if needed due to severity of infection

Children >1 month:

I.M.: 10 mg/kg every 12-24 hours

I.V.: 10-20 mg/kg/day in divided doses every 8-12 hours

Adults:

I.M.: 600 mg every 12-24 hours

I.V.: 600 mg to 1 g every 8-12 hours; maximum dose: 8 g/day

Subconjuctival injection: 75 mg (ocular fluid levels with sufficient MICs last for at least 5 hours)

Dosage Forms Injection, solution, as hydrochloride: 300 mg/mL (2 mL, 10 mL) [contains benzyl alcohol]

lincomycin hydrochloride *see* lincomycin *on this page*

lindane (LIN dane)

Synonyms benzene hexachloride; gamma benzene hexachloride; hexachlorocyclohexane

U.S./Canadian Brand Names Hexit™ [Can]; PMS-Lindane [Can]

Therapeutic Category Scabicides/Pediculicides

Use Treatment of *Sarcoptes scabiei* (scabies), *Pediculus capitis* (head lice), and *Phthirus pubis* (crab lice); FDA recommends reserving lindane as a second-line agent or with inadequate response to other therapies

Usual Dosage Children and Adults: Topical:

Scabies: Apply a thin layer of lotion and massage it on skin from the neck to the toes; after 8-12 hours, bathe and remove the drug

Head lice, crab lice: Apply shampoo to dry hair and massage into hair for 4 minutes; add small quantities of water to hair until lather forms, then rinse hair thoroughly and comb with a fine tooth comb to remove nits. Amount of shampoo needed is based on length and density of hair; most patients will require 30 mL (maximum: 60 mL).

(Continued)

lindane *(Continued)*

Dosage Forms

Lotion, topical: 1% (60 mL)

Shampoo, topical: 1% (60 mL) [contains alcohol 0.5%]

Linessa® [Can] *see* ethinyl estradiol and desogestrel *on page 317*

linezolid (li NE zoh lid)

Sound-Alike/Look-Alike Issues

Zyvox™ may be confused with Vioxx®, Zosyn®, Zovirax®

U.S./Canadian Brand Names Zyvoxam® [Can]; Zyvox™ [US]

Therapeutic Category Antibiotic, Oxazolidinone

Use Treatment of vancomycin-resistant *Enterococcus faecium* (VRE) infections, nosocomial pneumonia caused by *Staphylococcus aureus* including MRSA or *Streptococcus pneumoniae* (including multidrug-resistant strains [MDRSP]), complicated and uncomplicated skin and skin structure infections (including diabetic foot infections without concomitant osteomyelitis), and community-acquired pneumonia caused by susceptible gram-positive organisms

Usual Dosage

VRE infections: Oral, I.V.:

Preterm neonates (<34 weeks gestational age): 10 mg/kg every 12 hours; neonates with a suboptimal clinical response can be advanced to 10 mg/kg every 8 hours. By day 7 of life, all neonates should receive 10 mg/kg every 8 hours.

Infants (excluding preterm neonates <1 week) and Children ≤11 years: 10 mg/kg every 8 hours for 14-28 days

Children ≥12 years and Adults: 600 mg every 12 hours for 14-28 days

Nosocomial pneumonia, complicated skin and skin structure infections, community-acquired pneumonia including concurrent bacteremia: Oral, I.V.:

Infants (excluding preterm neonates <1 week) and Children ≤11 years: 10 mg/kg every 8 hours for 10-14 days

Children ≥12 years and Adults: 600 mg every 12 hours for 10-14 days

Uncomplicated skin and skin structure infections: Oral:

Infants (excluding preterm neonates <1 week) and Children <5 years: 10 mg/kg every 8 hours for 10-14 days

Children 5-11 years: 10 mg/kg every 12 hours for 10-14 days

Children ≥12-18 years: 600 mg every 12 hours for 10-14 days

Adults: 400 mg every 12 hours for 10-14 days

Dosage Forms

Infusion [premixed]: 200 mg (100 mL) [contains sodium 1.7 mEq]; 400 mg (200 mL) [contains sodium 3.3 mEq]; 600 mg (300 mL) [contains sodium 5 mEq]

Powder for oral suspension: 20 mg/mL (150 mL) [contains phenylalanine 20 mg/5 mL, sodium benzoate, and sodium 0.4 mEq/5 mL; orange flavor]

Tablet: 600 mg [contains sodium 0.1 mEq/tablet]

Lin-Sotalol [Can] *see* sotalol *on page 787*

Lioresal® [US/Can] *see* baclofen *on page 91*

Liotec [Can] *see* baclofen *on page 91*

liothyronine (lye oh THYE roe neen)

Sound-Alike/Look-Alike Issues

liothyronine may be confused with levothyroxine

T_3 sodium is an error-prone abbreviation

Synonyms liothyronine sodium; sodium *L*-triiodothyronine

U.S./Canadian Brand Names Cytomel® [US/Can]; Triostat® [US]

Therapeutic Category Thyroid Product

Use

Oral: Replacement or supplemental therapy in hypothyroidism; management of nontoxic goiter; a diagnostic aid

I.V.: Treatment of myxedema coma/precoma

Usual Dosage Doses should be adjusted based on clinical response and laboratory parameters.

Children: Congenital hypothyroidism: Oral: 5 mcg/day increase by 5 mcg every 3-4 days until the desired response is achieved. Usual maintenance dose: 20 mcg/day for infants, 50 mcg/day for children 1-3 years of age, and adult dose for children >3 years.

Adults:

Hypothyroidism: Oral: 25 mcg/day increase by increments of 12.5-25 mcg/day every 1-2 weeks to a maximum of 100 mcg/day; usual maintenance dose: 25-75 mcg/day.

Patients with cardiovascular disease: Oral: 5 mcg/day; increase by 5 mcg/day every 2 weeks

T_3 suppression test: Oral: 75-100 mcg/day for 7 days

Myxedema: Oral: Initial: 5 mcg/day; increase in increments of 5-10 mcg/day every 1-2 weeks. When 25 mcg/day is reached, dosage may be increased at intervals of 5-25 mcg/day every 1-2 weeks. Usual maintenance dose: 50-100 mcg/day.

Myxedema coma: I.V.: 25-50 mcg

Patients with known or suspected cardiovascular disease: 10-20 mcg

Note: Normally, at least 4 hours should be allowed between doses to adequately assess therapeutic response and no more than 12 hours should elapse between doses to avoid fluctuations in hormone levels. Oral therapy should be resumed as soon as the clinical situation has been stabilized and the patient is able to take oral medication. If levothyroxine rather than liothyronine sodium is used in initiating oral therapy, the physician should bear in mind that there is a delay of several days in the onset of levothyroxine activity and that I.V. therapy should be discontinued gradually.

Simple (nontoxic) goiter: Oral: Initial: 5 mcg/day; increase by 5-10 mcg every 1-2 weeks; after 25 mcg/day is reached, may increase dose by 12.5-25 mcg. Usual maintenance dose: 75 mcg/day

Dosage Forms

Injection, solution, as sodium (Triostat®): 10 mcg/mL (1 mL) [contains alcohol 6.8%]

Tablet, as sodium (Cytomel®): 5 mcg, 25 mcg, 50 mcg

liothyronine sodium *see* liothyronine *on previous page*

liotrix (LYE oh triks)

Sound-Alike/Look-Alike Issues

liotrix may be confused with Klotrix®

Thyrolar® may be confused with Theolair™, Thyrogen®, Thytropar®

Synonyms T_3/T_4 liotrix

U.S./Canadian Brand Names Thyrolar® [US/Can]

Therapeutic Category Thyroid Product

Use Replacement or supplemental therapy in hypothyroidism (uniform mixture of T_4:T_3 in 4:1 ratio by weight); little advantage to this product exists and cost is not justified

Usual Dosage Oral:

Congenital hypothyroidism:

Children (dose of T_4 or levothyroxine/day):

0-6 months: 8-10 mcg/kg or 25-50 mcg/day

6-12 months: 6-8 mcg/kg or 50-75 mcg/day

1-5 years: 5-6 mcg/kg or 75-100 mcg/day

6-12 years: 4-5 mcg/kg or 100-150 mcg/day

>12 years: 2-3 mcg/kg or >150 mcg/day

Hypothyroidism (dose of thyroid equivalent): Adults: 30 mg/day (15 mg/day if cardiovascular impairment), increasing by increments of 15 mg/day at 2- to 3-week intervals to a maximum of 180 mg/day (usual maintenance dose: 60-120 mg/day)

Dosage Forms Tablet:

1/4 [levothyroxine sodium 12.5 mcg and liothyronine sodium 3.1 mcg]

1/2 [levothyroxine sodium 25 mcg and liothyronine sodium 6.25 mcg]

1 [levothyroxine sodium 50 mcg and liothyronine sodium 12.5 mcg]

2 [levothyroxine sodium 100 mcg and liothyronine sodium 25 mcg]

3 [levothyroxine sodium 150 mcg and liothyronine sodium 37.5 mcg]

lipancreatin *see* pancrelipase *on page 634*

Lipidil EZ® [Can] *see* fenofibrate *on page 338*

Lipidil Micro® [Can] *see* fenofibrate *on page 338*

Lipidil Supra® [Can] *see* fenofibrate *on page 338*

Lipitor® [US/Can] *see* atorvastatin *on page 81*

Lipofen™ [US] *see* fenofibrate *on page 338*

Liposyn® II [Can] *see* fat emulsion *on page 336*

Liposyn® III [US] *see* fat emulsion *on page 336*

Lipram 4500 [US] *see* pancrelipase *on page 634*

Lipram-CR [US] *see* pancrelipase *on page 634*

Lipram-PN [US] *see* pancrelipase *on page 634*

Lipram-UL [US] *see* pancrelipase *on page 634*

Liquaemin® *(Discontinued)* *see* heparin *on page 408*

Liquibid-D [US] *see* guaifenesin and phenylephrine *on page 396*

Liquibid® 1200 *(Discontinued)* *see* guaifenesin *on page 392*

Liquibid® *(Discontinued)* *see* guaifenesin *on page 392*

Liquibid-PD [US] *see* guaifenesin and phenylephrine *on page 396*

Liqui-Char® *(Discontinued)* *see* charcoal *on page 169*

liquid antidote *see* charcoal *on page 169*

Liquid Barosperse® [US] *see* radiological/contrast media (ionic) *on page 728*

Liquid Pred® *(Discontinued)* *see* prednisone *on page 695*

Liquifilm® Forte Solution *(Discontinued)* *see* artificial tears *on page 75*

Liquifilm® Tears [US-OTC] *see* artificial tears *on page 75*

Liquifilm® Tears Solution *(Discontinued)* *see* artificial tears *on page 75*

Liquipake® [US] *see* radiological/contrast media (ionic) *on page 728*

lisinopril (lyse IN oh pril)

Sound-Alike/Look-Alike Issues

lisinopril may be confused with fosinopril, Lioresal®, Risperdal®

Prinivil® may be confused with Plendil®, Pravachol®, Prevacid®, Prilosec®, Proventil®

Zestril® may be confused with Desyrel®, Restoril®, Vistaril®, Zetia™, Zostrix®

U.S./Canadian Brand Names Apo-Lisinopril® [Can]; Prinivil® [US/Can]; Zestril® [US/Can]

Therapeutic Category Angiotensin-Converting Enzyme (ACE) Inhibitor

Use Treatment of hypertension, either alone or in combination with other antihypertensive agents; adjunctive therapy in treatment of CHF (afterload reduction); treatment of acute myocardial infarction within 24 hours in hemodynamically-stable patients to improve survival; treatment of left ventricular dysfunction after myocardial infarction

Usual Dosage Oral:

Hypertension:

Children ≥6 years: Initial: 0.07 mg/kg once daily (up to 5 mg); increase dose at 1- to 2-week intervals; doses >0.61 mg/kg or >40 mg have not been evaluated.

Adults: Usual dosage range(JNC 7): 10-40 mg/day

Not maintained on diuretic: Initial: 10 mg/day

Maintained on diuretic: Initial: 5 mg/day

Note: Antihypertensive effect may diminish toward the end of the dosing interval especially with doses of 10 mg/day. An increased dose may aid in extending the duration of antihypertensive effect. Doses up to 80 mg/day have been used, but do not appear to give greater effect (Zestril® Product Information, 12/04).

Patients taking diuretics should have them discontinued 2-3 days prior to initiating lisinopril if possible. Restart diuretic after blood pressure is stable if needed. If diuretic cannot be discontinued prior to therapy, begin with 5 mg with close supervision until stable blood pressure. In patients with hyponatremia (<130 mEq/L), start dose at 2.5 mg/day

Congestive heart failure: Adults: Initial: 2.5-5 mg once daily; then increase by no more than 10 mg increments at intervals no less than 2 weeks to a maximum daily dose of 40 mg. Usual maintenance: 5-40 mg/day as a single dose. Target dose: 20-40 mg once daily (ACC/AHA 2005 Heart Failure Guidelines)

Note: If patient has hyponatremia (serum sodium <130 meq/L) or renal impairment (Cl_{cr} <30 mL/minute or creatinine >3 mg/dL), then initial dose should be 2.5 mg/day

Acute myocardial infarction (within 24 hours in hemodynamically stable patients): Oral: 5 mg immediately, then 5 mg at 24 hours, 10 mg at 48 hours, and 10 mg every day thereafter for 6 weeks. Patients should continue to receive standard treatments such as thrombolytics, aspirin, and beta-blockers.

Dosage Forms [DSC] = Discontinued product

Tablet: 2.5 mg, 5 mg, 10 mg, 20 mg, 30 mg, 40 mg

Prinivil®: 5 mg, 10 mg, 20 mg, 30 mg; 40 mg [DSC]

Zestril®: 2.5 mg, 5 mg, 10 mg, 20 mg, 30 mg, 40 mg

lisinopril and hydrochlorothiazide (lyse IN oh pril & hye droe klor oh THYE a zide)

Synonyms hydrochlorothiazide and lisinopril

U.S./Canadian Brand Names Prinzide® [US/Can]; Zestoretic® [US/Can]

Therapeutic Category Antihypertensive Agent, Combination

Use Treatment of hypertension

Usual Dosage Adults: Oral: Dosage is individualized; see each component for appropriate dosing suggestions; doses >80 mg/day lisinopril or >50 mg/day hydrochlorothiazide are not recommended.

Dosage Forms Tablet:
- Lisinopril 10 mg and hydrochlorothiazide 12.5 mg
- Lisinopril 20 mg and hydrochlorothiazide 12.5 mg
- Lisinopril 20 mg and hydrochlorothiazide 25 mg

lispro insulin *see* insulin lispro *on page 451*

Listermint® With Fluoride *(Discontinued)* *see* fluoride *on page 354*

Lithane® [Can] *see* lithium *on this page*

Lithane® *(Discontinued)* *see* lithium *on this page*

lithium (LITH ee um)

Sound-Alike/Look-Alike Issues
- Eskalith® may be confused with Estratest®
- Lithobid® may be confused with Levbid®, Lithostat®

Synonyms lithium carbonate; lithium citrate

U.S./Canadian Brand Names Apo-Lithium® Carbonate SR [Can]; Apo-Lithium® Carbonate [Can]; Carbolith™ [Can]; Duralith® [Can]; Lithane® [Can]; Lithobid® [US]; PMS-Lithium Carbonate [Can]; PMS-Lithium Citrate [Can]

Therapeutic Category Antimanic Agent

Use Management of bipolar disorders; treatment of mania in individuals with bipolar disorder (maintenance treatment prevents or diminishes intensity of subsequent episodes)

Usual Dosage Oral: Monitor serum concentrations and clinical response (efficacy and toxicity) to determine proper dose

Children 6-12 years: Bipolar disorder: 15-60 mg/kg/day in 3-4 divided doses; dose not to exceed usual adult dosage

Adults: Bipolar disorder: 900-2400 mg/day in 3-4 divided doses or 900-1800 mg/day (sustained release) in 2 divided doses

Dosage Forms

[DSC] = Discontinued product

Capsule, as carbonate: 150 mg, 300 mg, 600 mg
- Eskalith®: 300 mg [contains benzyl alcohol] [DSC]

Solution, as citrate: 300 mg/5 mL (5 mL, 500 mL) [equivalent to amount of lithium in lithium carbonate]

Syrup, as citrate: 300 mg/5 mL (480 mL) [equivalent to amount of lithium in lithium carbonate]

Tablet, as carbonate: 300 mg

Tablet, controlled release, as carbonate: 450 mg
- Eskalith CR®: 450 mg [DSC]

Tablet, slow release, as carbonate: 300 mg
- Lithobid®: 300 mg

lithium carbonate *see* lithium *on this page*

lithium citrate *see* lithium *on this page*

Lithobid® [US] *see* lithium *on this page*

Lithonate® *(Discontinued)* *see* lithium *on this page*

Lithostat® [US/Can] *see* acetohydroxamic acid *on page 15*

Lithotabs® *(Discontinued)* *see* lithium *on this page*

live attenuated influenza vaccine (LAIV) *see* influenza virus vaccine *on page 448*

l-lysine (el LYE seen)

Synonyms l-lysine hydrochloride

U.S./Canadian Brand Names Lysinyl [US-OTC]

Therapeutic Category Dietary Supplement

Use Improves utilization of vegetable proteins

(Continued)

l-lysine *(Continued)*

Usual Dosage Oral: Adults: 334-1500 mg/day

Recurrent herpes simplex infection (dental use): 2000 mg every 4 hours until symptoms subside. Begin treatment during early stage of recurrence.

Dosage Forms

Capsule (Lysinyl): 500 mg

Tablet: 500 mg, 1000 mg

l-lysine hydrochloride *see* l-lysine *on previous page*

LMD® [US] *see* dextran *on page 243*

LNg 20 *see* levonorgestrel *on page 491*

Locacorten® Vioform® [Can] *see* clioquinol and flumethasone *(Canada only) on page 200*

LoCHOLEST® *(Discontinued)* *see* cholestyramine resin *on page 186*

LoCHOLEST® Light *(Discontinued)* *see* cholestyramine resin *on page 186*

Locoid® [US/Can] *see* hydrocortisone (topical) *on page 428*

Locoid Lipocream® [US] *see* hydrocortisone (topical) *on page 428*

Lodine® [Can] *see* etodolac *on page 329*

Lodine® XL *(Discontinued)* *see* etodolac *on page 329*

Lodine® *(Discontinued)* *see* etodolac *on page 329*

Lodosyn® [US] *see* carbidopa *on page 147*

lodoxamide (loe DOKS a mide)

Synonyms lodoxamide tromethamine

U.S./Canadian Brand Names Alomide® [US/Can]

Therapeutic Category Mast Cell Stabilizer

Use Treatment of vernal keratoconjunctivitis, vernal conjunctivitis, and vernal keratitis

Usual Dosage Ophthalmic: Instill 1-2 drops in eye(s) 4 times/day for up to 3 months

Dosage Forms Solution, ophthalmic: 0.1% (10 mL) [contains benzalkonium chloride]

lodoxamide tromethamine *see* lodoxamide *on this page*

Lodrane® [US] *see* brompheniramine and pseudoephedrine *on page 118*

Lodrane® 12D [US] *see* brompheniramine and pseudoephedrine *on page 118*

Lodrane® 12 Hour [US-OTC] *see* brompheniramine *on page 118*

Lodrane® LD [US] *see* brompheniramine and pseudoephedrine *on page 118*

Loestrin® [US] *see* ethinyl estradiol and norethindrone *on page 323*

Loestrin™ 1.5/30 [Can] *see* ethinyl estradiol and norethindrone *on page 323*

Loestrin® 24 Fe [US] *see* ethinyl estradiol and norethindrone *on page 323*

Loestrin® Fe [US] *see* ethinyl estradiol and norethindrone *on page 323*

Lofibra™ [US] *see* fenofibrate *on page 338*

Logen® *(Discontinued)* *see* diphenoxylate and atropine *on page 264*

LoHist-D [US] *see* chlorpheniramine and pseudoephedrine *on page 177*

L-OHP *see* oxaliplatin *on page 622*

LoKara™ [US] *see* desonide *on page 238*

Lomanate® *(Discontinued)* *see* diphenoxylate and atropine *on page 264*

Lomine [Can] *see* dicyclomine *on page 251*

Lomotil® [US/Can] *see* diphenoxylate and atropine *on page 264*

lomustine (loe MUS teen)

Sound-Alike/Look-Alike Issues

lomustine may be confused with carmustine

Synonyms CCNU

U.S./Canadian Brand Names CeeNU® [US/Can]

Therapeutic Category Antineoplastic Agent

Use Treatment of brain tumors and Hodgkin disease, non-Hodgkin lymphoma, melanoma, renal carcinoma, lung cancer, colon cancer

Usual Dosage Oral (refer to individual protocols):

Children: 75-150 mg/m^2 as a single dose every 6 weeks; subsequent doses are readjusted after initial treatment according to platelet and leukocyte counts

Adults: 100-130 mg/m^2 as a single dose every 6 weeks; readjust after initial treatment according to platelet and leukocyte counts

With compromised marrow function: Initial dose: 100 mg/m^2 as a single dose every 6 weeks

Repeat courses should only be administered after adequate recovery: WBC >4000 and platelet counts >100,000

Subsequent dosing adjustment based on nadir:

Leukocytes 2000-2900/mm^3, platelets 25,000-74,999/mm^3: Administer 70% of prior dose

Leukocytes <2000/mm^3, platelets <25,000/mm^3: Administer 50% of prior dose

Dosage Forms

Capsule: 10 mg, 40 mg, 100 mg

Capsule [dose pack]: 10 mg (2s); 40 mg (2s); 100 mg (2s)

Loniten® [US] *see* minoxidil *on page 559*

Loniten® 2.5 mg Tablet *(Discontinued)* *see* minoxidil *on page 559*

Lonox® [US] *see* diphenoxylate and atropine *on page 264*

Lo/Ovral® [US] *see* ethinyl estradiol and norgestrel *on page 327*

Loperacap [Can] *see* loperamide *on this page*

loperamide (loe PER a mide)

Sound-Alike/Look-Alike Issues

Imodium® A-D may be confused with Indocin®, Ionamin®

Synonyms loperamide hydrochloride

U.S./Canadian Brand Names Apo-Loperamide® [Can]; Diamode [US-OTC]; Diarr-Eze [Can]; Imodium® A-D [US-OTC]; Imodium® [Can]; K-Pek II [US-OTC]; Kao-Paverin® [US-OTC]; Loperacap [Can]; Novo-Loperamide [Can]; PMS-Loperamine [Can]; Rho®-Loperamine [Can]; Riva-Loperamine [Can]

Therapeutic Category Antidiarrheal

Use Treatment of chronic diarrhea associated with inflammatory bowel disease; acute nonspecific diarrhea; increased volume of ileostomy discharge

OTC labeling: Control of symptoms of diarrhea, including traveler's diarrhea

Usual Dosage Oral:

Children:

Acute diarrhea: Initial doses (in first 24 hours):

2-5 years (13-20 kg): 1 mg 3 times/day

6-8 years (20-30 kg): 2 mg twice daily

8-12 years (>30 kg): 2 mg 3 times/day

Maintenance: After initial dosing, 0.1 mg/kg doses after each loose stool, but not exceeding initial dosage

Traveler's diarrhea:

6-8 years: 2 mg after first loose stool, followed by 1 mg after each subsequent stool (maximum dose: 4 mg/day)

9-11 years: 2 mg after first loose stool, followed by 1 mg after each subsequent stool (maximum dose: 6 mg/day)

≥12 years: See adult dosing.

Adults:

Acute diarrhea: Initial: 4 mg, followed by 2 mg after each loose stool, up to 16 mg/day

Chronic diarrhea: Initial: Follow acute diarrhea; maintenance dose should be slowly titrated downward to minimum required to control symptoms (typically, 4-8 mg/day in divided doses)

Traveler's diarrhea: Initial: 4 mg after first loose stool, followed by 2 mg after each subsequent stool (maximum dose: 8 mg/day)

Dosage Forms

Caplet, as hydrochloride: 2 mg

Diamode, Imodium® A-D, Kao-Paverin®: 2 mg

Capsule, as hydrochloride: 2 mg

Liquid, oral, as hydrochloride: 1 mg/5 mL (5 mL, 10 mL, 120 mL)

(Continued)

loperamide *(Continued)*

Imodium® A-D: 1 mg/5 mL (60 mL, 120 mL) [contains alcohol, sodium benzoate, benzoic acid; cherry mint flavor]

Imodium® A-D [new formulation]: 1 mg/7.5 mL (60 mL, 120 mL, 360 mL) [contains sodium 10 mg/30 mL, sodium benzoate; creamy mint flavor]

Tablet, as hydrochloride: 2 mg

K-Pek II: 2 mg

loperamide hydrochloride *see* loperamide *on previous page*

Lopid® [US/Can] *see* gemfibrozil *on page 378*

lopinavir and ritonavir (loe PIN a veer & rit ON uh veer)

Sound-Alike/Look-Alike Issues

Potential for dispensing errors between Kaletra™ and Keppra® (levetiracetam)

Synonyms ritonavir and lopinavir

U.S./Canadian Brand Names Kaletra® [US/Can]

Therapeutic Category Antiretroviral Agent, Non-nucleoside Reverse Transcriptase Inhibitor (NNRTI)

Use Treatment of HIV infection in combination with other antiretroviral agents

Usual Dosage Oral: **Note:** Tablet and capsule [DSC] contain differing amounts of drug.

Children 6 months to 12 years: Dosage based on weight, presented based on mg of lopinavir (maximum dose: Lopinavir 400 mg/ritonavir 100 mg)

7-<15 kg: 12 mg/kg twice daily

15-40 kg: 10 mg/kg twice daily

>40 kg: Refer to adult dosing. **Note:** Once-daily dosing regimen has not been evaluated in pediatric patients.

Children >12 years and Adults:

Therapy-naive: Lopinavir 800 mg/ritonavir 200 mg once daily **or** lopinavir 400 mg/ritonavir 100 mg twice daily

Therapy-experienced: Lopinavir 400 mg/ritonavir 100 mg twice daily

Note: Once-daily dosing regimen has not been evaluated with concurrent indinavir or saquinavir and should not be used with concomitant phenytoin, carbamazepine, or phenobarbital therapy.

Dosage adjustment when taken with amprenavir, efavirenz, fosamprenavir, nelfinavir, or nevirapine:

Note: Once-daily dosing regimen should not be used when concomitantly taking amprenavir, efavirenz, nelfinavir, or nevirapine therapy.

Children 6 months to 12 years: Solution:

7-<15 kg: 13 mg/kg twice daily

15-45 kg: 11 mg/kg twice daily

>45 kg: Refer to adult dosing

Note: In the USHHS guidelines, the cutoff for adult dosing is 50 kg. (Pediatric Guidelines - March 24, 2005, are available at http://www.aidsinfo.nih.gov)

Children >12 years and Adults:

Therapy-naive: Tablet: Adjustment not needed with twice-daily dosing

Therapy-experienced:

Solution: Lopinavir 533 mg/ritonavir 133 mg twice daily

Tablet: Lopinavir 600 mg/ritonavir 150 mg twice daily

Dosage Forms [DSC] = Discontinued product

Capsule: Lopinavir 133.3 mg and ritonavir 33.3 mg [DSC]

Solution, oral: Lopinavir 80 mg and ritonavir 20 mg per mL (160 mL) [contains alcohol 42.4%]

Tablet: Lopinavir 200 mg and ritonavir 50 mg

Lopressor® [US/Can] *see* metoprolol *on page 550*

Lopressor HCT® [US] *see* metoprolol and hydrochlorothiazide *on page 550*

Loprox® [US/Can] *see* ciclopirox *on page 187*

Lorabid® [US/Can] *see* loracarbef *on this page*

loracarbef (lor a KAR bef)

Sound-Alike/Look-Alike Issues

Lorabid® may be confused with Levbid®, Lopid®, Lortab®, Slo-bid™

U.S./Canadian Brand Names Lorabid® [US/Can]

Therapeutic Category Antibiotic, Carbacephem

Use Treatment of infections caused by susceptible organisms involving the upper and lower respiratory tract, uncomplicated skin and skin structure, and urinary tract (including uncomplicated pyelonephritis)

Usual Dosage

Usual dosage range:

Children 6 months to 12 years: Oral: 7.5-15 mg/kg twice daily

Adults: Oral: 200-400 mg every 12-24 hours

Indication-specific dosing:

Children 6 months to 12 years: Oral:

Acute otitis media: 15 mg/kg twice daily for 10 days

Pharyngitis and impetigo: 7.5-15 mg/kg twice daily for 10 days

Adults: Oral:

Bronchitis: 200-400 mg every 12 hours for 7 days

Pharyngitis/tonsillitis: 200 mg every 12 hours for 10 days

Pneumonia: 400 mg every 12 hours for 14 days

Pyelonephritis (uncomplicated): 400 mg every 12 hours for 14 days

Sinusitis: 400 mg every 12 hours for 10 days

Skin and soft tissue: 200-400 mg every 12-24 hours

Urinary tract infections (uncomplicated): 200 mg once daily for 7 days

Dosage Forms

Capsule: 200 mg, 400 mg

Powder for oral suspension: 100 mg/5 mL (100 mL); 200 mg/5 mL (100 mL) [strawberry bubble gum flavor]

loratadine (lor AT a deen)

Sound-Alike/Look-Alike Issues

Dimetapp® may be confused with Dermatop®, Dimetabs®, Dimetane®

U.S./Canadian Brand Names Alavert® [US-OTC]; Apo-Loratadine® [Can]; Claritin® 24 Hour Allergy [US-OTC]; Claritin® Hives Relief [US-OTC]; Claritin® Kids [Can]; Claritin® [Can]; Tavist® ND [US-OTC]; Triaminic® Allerchews™ [US-OTC]

Therapeutic Category Antihistamine

Use Relief of nasal and nonnasal symptoms of seasonal allergic rhinitis; treatment of chronic idiopathic urticaria

Usual Dosage Oral: Seasonal allergic rhinitis, chronic idiopathic urticaria:

Children 2-5 years: 5 mg once daily

Children ≥6 years and Adults: 10 mg once daily

Dosage Forms

Syrup: 1 mg/mL (120 mL)

Claritin®: 1 mg/mL (120 mL) [contains sodium benzoate; fruit flavor]; (60 mL, 120 mL) [alcohol free, dye free, sugar free; contains sodium 6 mg/5 mL and sodium benzoate; grape flavor]

Tablet: 10 mg

Alavert®, Claritin®, Claritin® Hives Relief, Claritin® 24 Hour Allergy, Tavist® ND: 10 mg

Tablet, rapidly disintegrating: 10 mg

Alavert®: 10 mg [contains phenylalanine 8.4 mg/tablet; mint and citrus burst flavors]

Claritin® RediTabs®: 10 mg [mint flavor]

Triaminic® Allerchews™: 10 mg

loratadine and pseudoephedrine (lor AT a deen & soo doe e FED rin)

Synonyms pseudoephedrine and loratadine

U.S./Canadian Brand Names Alavert™ Allergy and Sinus [US-OTC]; Chlor-Tripolon ND® [Can]; Claritin-D® 12-Hour [US-OTC]; Claritin-D® 24-Hour [US-OTC]; Claritin® Extra [Can]; Claritin® Liberator [Can]

Therapeutic Category Antihistamine/Decongestant Combination

Use Temporary relief of symptoms of seasonal allergic rhinitis, other upper respiratory allergies, or the common cold

Usual Dosage Children ≥12 years and Adults: Oral:

Claritin-D® 12-Hour: 1 tablet every 12 hours

Alavert™ Allergy and Sinus, Claritin-D® 24-Hour: 1 tablet daily

Dosage Forms

Tablet, extended release: Loratadine 10 mg and pseudoephedrine sulfate 240 mg

Alavert™ Allergy and Sinus, Claritin-D® 12-hour: Loratadine 5 mg and pseudoephedrine sulfate 120 mg

Claritin-D® 24-hour: Loratadine 10 mg and pseudoephedrine sulfate 240 mg

lorazepam (lor A ze pam)

Sound-Alike/Look-Alike Issues

lorazepam may be confused with alprazolam, clonazepam, clorazepate, diazepam, temazepam

Ativan® may be confused with Atarax®, Atgam®, Avitene®

U.S./Canadian Brand Names Apo-Lorazepam® [Can]; Ativan® [US/Can]; Lorazepam Injection, USP [Can]; Lorazepam Intensol® [US]; Novo-Lorazepam [Can]; Nu-Loraz [Can]; PMS-Lorazepam [Can]; Riva-Lorazepam [Can]

Therapeutic Category Benzodiazepine

Controlled Substance C-IV

Use

Oral: Management of anxiety disorders or short-term relief of the symptoms of anxiety or anxiety associated with depressive symptoms

I.V.: Status epilepticus, preanesthesia for desired amnesia, antiemetic adjunct

Usual Dosage

Antiemetic:

Children 2-15 years: I.V.: 0.05 mg/kg (up to 2 mg/dose) prior to chemotherapy

Adults: Oral, I.V. (**Note:** May be administered sublingually; not a labeled route): 0.5-2 mg every 4-6 hours as needed

Anxiety and sedation:

Infants and Children: Oral, I.M., I.V.: Usual: 0.05 mg/kg/dose (range: 0.02-0.09 mg/kg) every 4-8 hours

I.V.: May use smaller doses (eg, 0.01-0.03 mg/kg) and repeat every 20 minutes, as needed to titrate to effect

Adults: Oral: 1-10 mg/day in 2-3 divided doses; usual dose: 2-6 mg/day in divided doses

Insomnia: Adults: Oral: 2-4 mg at bedtime

Preoperative: Adults:

I.M.: 0.05 mg/kg administered 2 hours before surgery (maximum: 4 mg/dose)

I.V.: 0.044 mg/kg 15-20 minutes before surgery (usual maximum: 2 mg/dose)

Preprocedural anxiety (dental use): Adults: Oral: 1-2 mg 1 hour before procedure

Operative amnesia: Adults: I.V.: Up to 0.05 mg/kg (maximum: 4 mg/dose)

Sedation (preprocedure): Infants and Children:

Oral, I.M., I.V.: Usual: 0.05 mg/kg (range: 0.02-0.09 mg/kg);

I.V.: May use smaller doses (eg, 0.01-0.03 mg/kg) and repeat every 20 minutes, as needed to titrate to effect

Status epilepticus: I.V.:

Infants and Children: 0.1 mg/kg slow I.V. over 2-5 minutes; do not exceed 4 mg/single dose; may repeat second dose of 0.05 mg/kg slow I.V. in 10-15 minutes if needed

Adolescents: 0.07 mg/kg slow I.V. over 2-5 minutes; maximum: 4 mg/dose; may repeat in 10-15 minutes

Adults: 4 mg/dose slow I.V. over 2-5 minutes; may repeat in 10-15 minutes; usual maximum dose: 8 mg

Rapid tranquilization of agitated patient (administer every 30-60 minutes):

Oral: 1-2 mg

I.M.: 0.5-1 mg

Average total dose for tranquilization: Oral, I.M.: 4-8 mg

Dosage Forms

Injection, solution (Ativan®): 2 mg/mL (1 mL, 10 mL); 4 mg/mL (1 mL, 10 mL) [contains benzyl alcohol]

Solution, oral concentrate (Lorazepam Intensol®): 2 mg/mL (30 mL) [alcohol free, dye free]

Tablet (Ativan®): 0.5 mg, 1 mg, 2 mg

Lorazepam Injection, USP [Can] *see* lorazepam *on this page*

Lorazepam Intensol® [US] *see* lorazepam *on this page*

Lorcet® 10/650 [US] *see* hydrocodone and acetaminophen *on page 420*

Lorcet®-HD *(Discontinued)* *see* hydrocodone and acetaminophen *on page 420*

Lorcet® Plus [US] *see* hydrocodone and acetaminophen *on page 420*

Loroxide® [US-OTC] *see* benzoyl peroxide *on page 102*

Lorsin® *(Discontinued)* *see* acetaminophen, chlorpheniramine, and pseudoephedrine *on page 11*

Lortab® [US] *see* hydrocodone and acetaminophen *on page 420*

Lortab® ASA *(Discontinued)* *see* hydrocodone and aspirin *on page 422*

losartan (loe SAR tan)

Sound-Alike/Look-Alike Issues

losartan may be confused with valsartan

Cozaar® may be confused with Hyzaar®, Zocor®

Synonyms DuP 753; losartan potassium; MK594
U.S./Canadian Brand Names Cozaar® [US/Can]
Therapeutic Category Angiotensin II Receptor Antagonist
Use Treatment of hypertension (HTN); treatment of diabetic nephropathy in patients with type 2 diabetes mellitus (noninsulin-dependent, NIDDM) and a history of hypertension; stroke risk reduction in patients with HTN and left ventricular hypertrophy (LVH)
Usual Dosage Oral:
Hypertension:
Children 6-16 years: 0.7 mg/kg once daily (maximum: 50 mg/day); adjust dose based on response; doses >1.4 mg/kg (maximum: 100 mg) have not been studied
Adults: Usual starting dose: 50 mg once daily; can be administered once or twice daily with total daily doses ranging from 25-100 mg
Patients receiving diuretics or with intravascular volume depletion: Usual initial dose: 25 mg
Nephropathy in patients with type 2 diabetes and hypertension: Adults: Initial: 50 mg once daily; can be increased to 100 mg once daily based on blood pressure response
Stroke reduction (HTN with LVH): Adults: 50 mg once daily (maximum daily dose: 100 mg); may be used in combination with a thiazide diuretic
Dosage Forms Tablet, as potassium: 25 mg, 50 mg, 100 mg

losartan and hydrochlorothiazide (loe SAR tan & hye droe klor oh THYE a zide)

Sound-Alike/Look-Alike Issues
Hyzaar® may be confused with Cozaar®
Synonyms hydrochlorothiazide and losartan
U.S./Canadian Brand Names Hyzaar® DS [Can]; Hyzaar® [US/Can]
Therapeutic Category Antihypertensive Agent, Combination
Use Treatment of hypertension; stroke risk reduction in patients with HTN and left ventricular hypertrophy (LVH)
Usual Dosage
Oral: Adults: Dose is individualized (combination substituted for individual components); dose may be titrated after 2-4 weeks of therapy
Hypertension/stroke reduction in hypertension (with LVH): Usual recommended starting dose of losartan: 50 mg once daily when used as monotherapy in patients who are not volume depleted
Dosage Forms
Tablet:
Hyzaar® 50-12.5: Losartan potassium 50 mg and hydrochlorothiazide 12.5 mg
Hyzaar® 100-12.5: Losartan potassium 100 mg and hydrochlorothiazide 12.5 mg
Hyzaar® 100-25: Losartan potassium 100 mg and hydrochlorothiazide 25 mg

losartan potassium *see* losartan *on previous page*

Losec® [Can] *see* omeprazole *on page 615*

Losec MUPS® [Can] *see* omeprazole *on page 615*

Losopan® *(Discontinued)* *see* magaldrate and simethicone *on page 511*

Lotemax® [US/Can] *see* loteprednol *on this page*

Lotensin® [US/Can] *see* benazepril *on page 97*

Lotensin® HCT [US] *see* benazepril and hydrochlorothiazide *on page 97*

loteprednol (loe te PRED nol)

Synonyms loteprednol etabonate
U.S./Canadian Brand Names Alrex® [US/Can]; Lotemax® [US/Can]
Therapeutic Category Corticosteroid, Ophthalmic
Use
Suspension, 0.2% (Alrex®): Temporary relief of signs and symptoms of seasonal allergic conjunctivitis
Suspension, 0.5% (Lotemax®): Inflammatory conditions (treatment of steroid-responsive inflammatory conditions of the palpebral and bulbar conjunctiva, cornea, and anterior segment of the globe such as allergic conjunctivitis, acne rosacea, superficial punctate keratitis, herpes zoster keratitis, iritis, cyclitis, selected infective conjunctivitis, when the inherent hazard of steroid use is accepted to obtain an advisable diminution in edema and inflammation) and treatment of postoperative inflammation following ocular surgery
Usual Dosage Adults: Ophthalmic:
Suspension, 0.2% (Alrex®): Instill 1 drop into affected eye(s) 4 times/day
(Continued)

loteprednol *(Continued)*

Suspension, 0.5% (Lotemax®):

Inflammatory conditions: Apply 1-2 drops into the conjunctival sac of the affected eye(s) 4 times/day. During the initial treatment within the first week, the dosing may be increased up to 1 drop every hour. Advise patients not to discontinue therapy prematurely. If signs and symptoms fail to improve after 2 days, re-evaluate the patient.

Postoperative inflammation: Apply 1-2 drops into the conjunctival sac of the operated eye(s) 4 times/day beginning 24 hours after surgery and continuing throughout the first 2 weeks of the postoperative period

Dosage Forms Suspension, ophthalmic, as etabonate:

Alrex®: 0.2% (5 mL, 10 mL) [contains benzalkonium chloride]

Lotemax®: 0.5% (2.5 mL, 5 mL, 10 mL, 15 mL) [contains benzalkonium chloride]

loteprednol etabonate *see* loteprednol *on previous page*

Lotrel® [US] *see* amlodipine and benazepril *on page 46*

Lotriderm® [Can] *see* betamethasone and clotrimazole *on page 107*

Lotrimin® AF Athlete's Foot Cream [US-OTC] *see* clotrimazole *on page 205*

Lotrimin® AF Athlete's Foot Solution [US-OTC] *see* clotrimazole *on page 205*

Lotrimin® AF Cream *(Discontinued)* *see* clotrimazole *on page 205*

Lotrimin® AF Jock Itch Cream [US-OTC] *see* clotrimazole *on page 205*

Lotrimin® AF Jock Itch Powder Spray [US-OTC] *see* miconazole *on page 553*

Lotrimin® AF Lotion *(Discontinued)* *see* clotrimazole *on page 205*

Lotrimin® AF Powder/Spray [US-OTC] *see* miconazole *on page 553*

Lotrimin® AF Solution *(Discontinued)* *see* clotrimazole *on page 205*

Lotrimin® Ultra™ [US-OTC] *see* butenafine *on page 130*

Lotrisone® [US] *see* betamethasone and clotrimazole *on page 107*

Lotronex® [US] *see* alosetron *on page 31*

lovastatin (LOE va sta tin)

Sound-Alike/Look-Alike Issues

lovastatin may be confused with Leustatin®, Livostin®, Lotensin®

Mevacor® may be confused with Mivacron®

Synonyms mevinolin; monacolin K

U.S./Canadian Brand Names Altoprev® [US]; Apo-Lovastatin® [Can]; CO Lovastatin [Can]; Gen-Lovastatin [Can]; Mevacor® [US/Can]; Novo-Lovastatin [Can]; Nu-Lovastatin [Can]; PMS-Lovastatin [Can]; RAN™-Lovastatin [Can]; ratio-Lovastatin [Can]; Riva-Lovastatin [Can]; Sandoz-Lovastatin [Can]

Therapeutic Category HMG-CoA Reductase Inhibitor

Use

Adjunct to dietary therapy to decrease elevated serum total and LDL-cholesterol concentrations in primary hypercholesterolemia

Primary prevention of coronary artery disease (patients without symptomatic disease with average to moderately elevated total and LDL-cholesterol and below average HDL-cholesterol); slow progression of coronary atherosclerosis in patients with coronary heart disease

Adjunct to dietary therapy in adolescent patients (10-17 years of age, females >1 year postmenarche) with heterozygous familial hypercholesterolemia having LDL >189 mg/dL, **or** LDL >160 mg/dL with positive family history of premature cardiovascular disease (CVD), **or** LDL >160 mg/dL with the presence of at least two other CVD risk factors

Usual Dosage Oral:

Adolescents 10-17 years: Immediate release tablet:

LDL reduction <20%: Initial: 10 mg/day with evening meal

LDL reduction ≥20%: Initial: 20 mg/day with evening meal

Usual range: 10-40 mg with evening meal, then adjust dose at 4-week intervals

Adults: Initial: 20 mg with evening meal, then adjust at 4-week intervals; maximum dose: 80 mg/day immediate release tablet **or** 60 mg/day extended release tablet

Dosage modification/limits based on concurrent therapy:

Cyclosporine and other immunosuppressant drugs: Initial dose: 10 mg/day with a maximum recommended dose of 20 mg/day

Concurrent therapy with fibrates, danazol, and/or lipid-lowering doses of niacin (>1 g/day): Maximum recommended dose: 20 mg/day. Concurrent use with fibrates should be avoided unless risk to benefit favors use.

Concurrent therapy with amiodarone or verapamil: Maximum recommended dose: 40 mg/day of regular release or 20 mg/day with extended release.

Dosage Forms

Tablet: 10 mg, 20 mg, 40 mg

Mevacor®: 20 mg, 40 mg

Tablet, extended release:

Altoprev®: 20 mg, 40 mg, 60 mg

lovastatin and niacin *see* niacin and lovastatin *on page 589*

Lovenox® [US/Can] *see* enoxaparin *on page 293*

Lovenox® HP [Can] *see* enoxaparin *on page 293*

Low-Ogestrel® [US] *see* ethinyl estradiol and norgestrel *on page 327*

Loxapac® IM [Can] *see* loxapine *on this page*

loxapine (LOKS a peen)

Sound-Alike/Look-Alike Issues

Loxitane® may be confused with Soriatane®

Synonyms loxapine succinate; oxilapine succinate

U.S./Canadian Brand Names Apo-Loxapine® [Can]; Loxapac® IM [Can]; Loxitane® [US]; Nu-Loxapine [Can]; PMS-Loxapine [Can]

Therapeutic Category Antipsychotic Agent, Dibenzoxazepine

Use Management of psychotic disorders

Usual Dosage Oral: Adults: 10 mg twice daily, increase dose until psychotic symptoms are controlled; usual dose range: 20-100 mg/day in divided doses 2-4 times/day; dosages >250 mg/day are not recommended

Dosage Forms Capsule, as succinate: 5 mg, 10 mg, 25 mg, 50 mg

loxapine succinate *see* loxapine *on this page*

Loxitane® [US] *see* loxapine *on this page*

Loxitane® I.M. *(Discontinued)* *see* loxapine *on this page*

Lozide® [Can] *see* indapamide *on page 445*

Lozi-Flur™ [US] *see* fluoride *on page 354*

Lozi-Tab® *(Discontinued)* *see* fluoride *on page 354*

Lozol® [US/Can] *see* indapamide *on page 445*

L-PAM *see* melphalan *on page 526*

LRH *see* gonadorelin *on page 390*

L-sarcolysin *see* melphalan *on page 526*

LTA® 360 [US] *see* lidocaine *on page 493*

LTG *see* lamotrigine *on page 480*

***L*-thyroxine sodium** *see* levothyroxine *on page 491*

Lu-26-054 *see* escitalopram *on page 306*

lubiprostone (loo bi PROS tone)

Synonyms RU 0211; SPI 0211

U.S./Canadian Brand Names Amitiza™ [US]

Therapeutic Category Gastrointestinal Agent, Miscellaneous

Use Treatment of chronic idiopathic constipation

Usual Dosage Oral: Adults: 24 mcg twice daily

Dosage Forms Capsule: 24 mcg

Lubriderm® [US-OTC] *see* lanolin, cetyl alcohol, glycerin, petrolatum, and mineral oil *on page 481*

Lubriderm® Fragrance Free [US-OTC] *see* lanolin, cetyl alcohol, glycerin, petrolatum, and mineral oil *on page 481*

LubriTears® Solution *(Discontinued)* *see* artificial tears *on page 75*

Lucentis™ [US] *see* ranibizumab *on page 732*
Lucidex [US-OTC] *see* caffeine *on page 132*
Ludiomil® *(Discontinued)* *see* maprotiline *on page 519*
Lufyllin® [US/Can] *see* dyphylline *on page 285*
Lumigan® [US/Can] *see* bimatoprost *on page 110*
Luminal® Sodium [US] *see* phenobarbital *on page 658*
Lumitene™ [US] *see* beta-carotene *on page 106*
Lunesta™ [US] *see* eszopiclone *on page 315*
LupiCare™ II Psoriasis [US-OTC] *see* salicylic acid *on page 758*
LupiCare™ Dandruff [US-OTC] *see* salicylic acid *on page 758*
LupiCare™ Psoriasis [US-OTC] *see* salicylic acid *on page 758*
Lupron® [US/Can] *see* leuprolide *on page 486*
Lupron Depot® [US/Can] *see* leuprolide *on page 486*
Lupron Depot-Ped® [US] *see* leuprolide *on page 486*
Luride® [US] *see* fluoride *on page 354*
Luride® Lozi-Tab® [US] *see* fluoride *on page 354*
Luride®-SF *(Discontinued)* *see* fluoride *on page 354*
Lustra® [US/Can] *see* hydroquinone *on page 430*
Lustra-AF™ [US] *see* hydroquinone *on page 430*
luteinizing hormone releasing hormone *see* gonadorelin *on page 390*
Lutera™ [US] *see* ethinyl estradiol and levonorgestrel *on page 320*
Lutrepulse™ [Can] *see* gonadorelin *on page 390*

lutropin alfa (LOO troe pin AL fa)

Synonyms recombinant human luteinizing hormone; r-hLH
U.S./Canadian Brand Names Luveris® [US]
Therapeutic Category Gonadotropin; Ovulation Stimulator
Use Stimulation of follicular development in infertile hypogonadotropic hypogonadal (HH) women with profound luteinizing hormone (LH) deficiency; to be used in combination with follitropin alfa
Usual Dosage SubQ: Adults: Female: Infertility: 75 int. units daily until adequate follicular development is noted; maximum duration of treatment: 14 days; to be used concomitantly with follitropin alfa
Dosage Forms Injection, powder for reconstitution: 75 int. units [contains sucrose; packaged with SWFI]

Luveris® [US] *see* lutropin alfa *on this page*
Luvox® [Can] *see* fluvoxamine *on page 364*
Luvox® *(Discontinued)* *see* fluvoxamine *on page 364*
Luxiq® [US] *see* betamethasone (topical) *on page 107*
LY139603 *see* atomoxetine *on page 81*
LY146032 *see* daptomycin *on page 230*
LY170053 *see* olanzapine *on page 613*
LY231514 *see* pemetrexed *on page 645*
LY248686 *see* duloxetine *on page 283*
LY303366 *see* anidulafungin *on page 57*
LY2148568 *see* exenatide *on page 332*
Lycolan® Elixir *(Discontinued)* *see* l-lysine *on page 501*
Lyderm® [Can] *see* fluocinonide *on page 353*
LYMErix™ *(Discontinued)*
Lymphazurin® [US/Can] *see* radiological/contrast media (ionic) *on page 728*
lymphocyte immune globulin *see* antithymocyte globulin (equine) *on page 62*
lymphocyte mitogenic factor *see* aldesleukin *on page 26*

Lyphocin® Injection *(Discontinued)* *see* vancomycin *on page 865*

Lyrica® [US/Can] *see* pregabalin *on page 696*

Lysinyl [US-OTC] *see* l-lysine *on page 501*

Lysodren® [US/Can] *see* mitotane *on page 560*

M-M-R® II [US/Can] *see* measles, mumps, and rubella vaccines, combined *on page 520*

Maalox® [US-OTC] *see* aluminum hydroxide, magnesium hydroxide, and simethicone *on page 37*

Maalox® Anti-Gas *(Discontinued)* *see* aluminum hydroxide, magnesium hydroxide, and simethicone *on page 37*

Maalox® Anti-Gas Extra Strength *(Discontinued)* *see* aluminum hydroxide, magnesium hydroxide, and simethicone *on page 37*

Maalox® Extra Strength *(Discontinued)* *see* aluminum hydroxide and magnesium hydroxide *on page 36*

Maalox® Max [US-OTC] *see* aluminum hydroxide, magnesium hydroxide, and simethicone *on page 37*

Maalox® Plus *(Discontinued)* *see* aluminum hydroxide, magnesium hydroxide, and simethicone *on page 37*

Maalox® Quick Dissolve [US-OTC] *see* calcium carbonate *on page 135*

Maalox® TC (Therapeutic Concentrate) *(Discontinued)* *see* aluminum hydroxide and magnesium hydroxide *on page 36*

Macrobid® [US/Can] *see* nitrofurantoin *on page 594*

Macrodantin® [US/Can] *see* nitrofurantoin *on page 594*

Macrodex® *(Discontinued)* *see* dextran *on page 243*

Macugen® [US/Can] *see* pegaptanib *on page 642*

mafenide (MA fe nide)

Synonyms mafenide acetate

U.S./Canadian Brand Names Sulfamylon® [US]

Therapeutic Category Antibacterial, Topical

Use Adjunct in the treatment of second- and third-degree burns to prevent septicemia caused by susceptible organisms such as *Pseudomonas aeruginosa*

Orphan drug: Prevention of graft loss of meshed autografts on excised burn wounds

Usual Dosage Children and Adults: Topical: Apply once or twice daily with a sterile gloved hand; apply to a thickness of approximately 16 mm; the burned area should be covered with cream at all times

Dosage Forms

Cream, topical, as acetate: 85 mg/g (60 g, 120 g, 454 g) [contains sodium metabisulfite]

Powder, for topical solution: 5% (5s) [50 g/packet]

mafenide acetate *see* mafenide *on this page*

Mag 64™ [US-OTC] *see* magnesium chloride *on next page*

magaldrate and simethicone (MAG al drate & sye METH i kone)

Sound-Alike/Look-Alike Issues

Riopan Plus® may be confused with Repan®

Synonyms simethicone and magaldrate

Therapeutic Category Antacid; Antiflatulent

Use Relief of hyperacidity associated with peptic ulcer, gastritis, peptic esophagitis and hiatal hernia which are accompanied by symptoms of gas

Usual Dosage Adults: Oral: 540-1080 mg magaldrate between meals and at bedtime

Dosage Forms [DSC] = Discontinued product

Suspension, oral: Magaldrate 540 mg and simethicone 20 mg per 5 mL (360 mL)

Riopan Plus®: Magaldrate 540 mg and simethicone 20 mg per 5 mL (360 mL) [DSC]

Riopan Plus® Double Strength: Magaldrate 1080 mg and simethicone 40 mg per 5 mL (360 mL) [DSC]

Magalox Plus® *(Discontinued)* *see* aluminum hydroxide, magnesium hydroxide, and simethicone *on page 37*

Magan® *(Discontinued)* *see* magnesium salicylate *on page 516*

Mag-Caps [US-OTC] *see* magnesium oxide *on page 515*

Mag Delay® [US-OTC] *see* magnesium chloride *on this page*

Mag G® [US-OTC] *see* magnesium gluconate *on next page*

MagGel™ [US-OTC] *see* magnesium oxide *on page 515*

Maginex™ [US-OTC] *see* magnesium L-aspartate hydrochloride *on page 515*

Maginex™ DS [US-OTC] *see* magnesium L-aspartate hydrochloride *on page 515*

Magnacal® [US-OTC] *see* nutritional formula, enteral/oral *on page 608*

Magnelium® [Can] *see* magnesium glucoheptonate *on next page*

magnesia magma *see* magnesium hydroxide *on page 514*

magnesium carbonate and aluminum hydroxide *see* aluminum hydroxide and magnesium carbonate *on page 36*

magnesium chloride (mag NEE zhum KLOR ide)

U.S./Canadian Brand Names Chloromag® [US]; Mag 64™ [US-OTC]; Mag Delay® [US-OTC]; Slow-Mag® [US-OTC]

Therapeutic Category Electrolyte Supplement, Oral

Use Correction or prevention of hypomagnesemia; dietary supplement

Usual Dosage Note: Serum magnesium is poor reflection of repletional status as the majority of magnesium is intracellular; serum levels may be transiently normal for a few hours after a dose is given, therefore, aim for consistently high normal serum levels in patients with normal renal function for most efficient repletion.

Dietary supplement: Adults: Oral (Mag 64™, Mag Delay®, Slow-Mag®): 2 tablets once daily

Parenteral nutrition supplementation: I.V. (elemental magnesium):

Children:
- <50 kg: 0.3-0.5 mEq/kg/day
- >50 kg: 10-30 mEq/day

Adults: 8-20 mEq/day

RDA (elemental magnesium):

Children:
- 1-3 years: 80 mg/day
- 4-8 years: 130 mg/day
- 9-13 years: 240 mg/day
- 14-18 years:
  - Female: 360 mg/day
  - Pregnant female: 400 mg/day
  - Male: 410 mg/day

Adults:
- 19-30 years:
  - Female: 310 mg/day
  - Pregnant female: 350 mg/day
  - Male: 400 mg/day
- ≥31 years:
  - Female: 320 mg/day
  - Pregnant female: 360 mg/day
  - Male: 420 mg/day

Dosage Forms

Injection, solution: 200 mg/mL [1.97 mEq/mL] (50 mL)
 Chloromag®: 200 mg/mL [1.97 mEq/mL] (50 mL)

Tablet [enteric coated]:
 Slow-Mag®: Elemental magnesium 64 mg [contains elemental calcium 106 mg]

Tablet, delayed release:
 Mag 64™, Mag Delay®: Magnesium chloride hexahydrate 535 mg [equivalent to elemental magnesium 64 mg; contains elemental calcium 110 mg]

magnesium citrate (mag NEE zhum SIT rate)

Synonyms citrate of magnesia

U.S./Canadian Brand Names Citro-Mag® [Can]

Therapeutic Category Laxative

Use Evacuation of bowel prior to certain surgical and diagnostic procedures or overdose situations

Usual Dosage Cathartic: Oral:
Children:
<6 years: 0.5 mL/kg up to a maximum of 200 mL repeated every 4-6 hours until stools are clear
6-12 years: 100-150 mL
Children ≥12 years and Adults: 1/2 to 1 full bottle (120-300 mL)

Dosage Forms
Solution, oral: 290 mg/5 mL (300 mL) [cherry and lemon flavors]
Tablet: 100 mg [as elemental magnesium]

magnesium gluceptate *see* magnesium glucoheptonate *on this page*

magnesium glucoheptonate (mag NEE zhum gloo koh HEP toh nate)

Synonyms magnesium gluceptate

U.S./Canadian Brand Names Magnelium® [Can]; Magnolex® [Can]; Magnorol® Sirop [Can]; ratio-Magnesium [Can]

Therapeutic Category Electrolyte Supplement, Parenteral; Magnesium Salt

Use Treatment and prevention of hypomagnesemia

Usual Dosage The recommended dietary allowance (RDA) of magnesium is 4.5 mg/kg which is a total daily allowance of 350-400 mg for adult men and 280-300 mg for adult women. During pregnancy the RDA is 300 mg and during lactation the RDA is 355 mg. Average daily intakes of dietary magnesium have declined in recent years due to processing of food. The latest estimate of the average American dietary intake was 349 mg/day. Dose represented as magnesium sulfate unless stated otherwise.

Note: Serum magnesium is poor reflection of repletional status as the majority of magnesium is intracellular; serum levels may be transiently normal for a few hours after a dose is given, therefore, aim for consistently high normal serum levels in patients with normal renal function for most efficient repletion

Hypomagnesemia: Adults: Oral: 100-600 mg (5-30 mg elemental magnesium) 1-2 times/day with food.
Maintenance electrolyte requirements:
Daily requirements: 0.2-0.5 mEq/kg/24 hours or 3-10 mEq/1000 kcal/24 hours
Maximum: 8-16 mEq/24 hours

Dosage Forms
Capsule:
Magnelium®, Magnorol®: 20 mg [contains 20 mg elemental magnesium]
Magnolex®: 300 mg [contains 15 mg elemental magnesium]
Solution, oral (ratio-Magnesium): 100 mg/mL (500 mL, 2000 mL) [contains 5 mg/mL elemental magnesium]
Syrup (Magnorol® Sirop): 90 mg/mL (400 mL) [contains 4.5 mg/mL elemental magnesium]

magnesium gluconate (mag NEE zhum GLOO koe nate)

U.S./Canadian Brand Names Almora® [US-OTC]; Mag G® [US-OTC]; Magonate® [US-OTC]; Magtrate® [US-OTC]

Therapeutic Category Electrolyte Supplement, Oral

Use Dietary supplement

Usual Dosage **RDA (elemental magnesium):**
Children:
1-3 years: 80 mg/day
4-8 years: 130 mg/day
9-13 years: 240 mg/day
14-18 years:
Female: 360 mg/day
Pregnant female: 400 mg/day
Male: 410 mg/day
Adults:
19-30 years:
Female: 310 mg/day
Pregnant female: 350 mg/day
Male: 400 mg/day
≥31 years:
Female: 320 mg/day
Pregnant female: 360 mg/day
Male: 420 mg/day
(Continued)

magnesium gluconate *(Continued)*

Dosage Forms

Solution:

Magonate®: 1000 mg/5 mL (480 mL) [magnesium 4.8 mEq/5 mL; equivalent to elemental magnesium 54 mg/5 mL; contains sodium benzoate]

Tablet: 500 mg [magnesium 2.4 mEq; equivalent to elemental magnesium 27 mg]

Almora®, Mag G®, Magonate®, Magtrate®): 500 mg [magnesium 2.4 mEq; equivalent to elemental magnesium 27 mg]

magnesium hydroxide (mag NEE zhum hye DROKS ide)

Synonyms magnesia magma; milk of magnesia; MOM

U.S./Canadian Brand Names Dulcolax® Milk of Magnesia [US-OTC]; Phillips'® Milk of Magnesia [US-OTC]

Therapeutic Category Antacid; Electrolyte Supplement, Oral; Laxative

Use Short-term treatment of occasional constipation and symptoms of hyperacidity, magnesium replacement therapy

Usual Dosage Oral:

Average daily intakes of dietary magnesium have declined in recent years due to processing of food; the latest estimate of the average American dietary intake was 349 mg/day

Laxative:

Liquid:

Children

<2 years: 0.5 mL/kg/dose

2-5 years: 5-15 mL/day (2.5-7.5 mL/day of liquid concentrate) or in divided doses

6-12 years: 15-30 mL/day (7.5-15 mL/day of liquid concentrate) or in divided doses

Children ≥12 years and Adults: 30-60 mL/day (15-30 mL/day of liquid concentrate) or in divided doses

Tablet:

Children:

2-5 years: 1-2 tablets before bedtime

6-11 years: 3-4 tablets before bedtime

Children ≥12 years and Adults: 6-8 tablets before bedtime

Antacid:

Liquid:

Children: 2.5-5 mL as needed up to 4 times/day

Adults: 5-15 mL (2.5-7.5 mL of liquid concentrate) as needed up to 4 times/day

Tablet:

Children 7-14 years: 1 tablet up to 4 times/day

Adults: 2-4 tablets up to 4 times/day

Dosage Forms

Liquid, oral: 400 mg/5 mL (360 mL, 480 mL, 960 mL, 3780 mL)

Dulcolax® Milk of Magnesia: 400 mg/5 mL (360 mL, 780 mL) [regular and mint flavors]

Phillips'® Milk of Magnesia: 400 mg/5 mL (120 mL, 360 mL, 780 mL) [original, French vanilla, cherry, and mint flavors]

Liquid, oral concentrate: 800 mg/5 mL (100 mL, 400 mL)

Phillips'® Milk of Magnesia [concentrate]: 800 mg/5 mL (240 mL) [strawberry créme flavor]

Tablet, chewable (Phillips'® Milk of Magnesia): 311 mg [mint flavor]

magnesium hydroxide, aluminum hydroxide, and simethicone *see* aluminum hydroxide, magnesium hydroxide, and simethicone *on page 37*

magnesium hydroxide and aluminum hydroxide *see* aluminum hydroxide and magnesium hydroxide *on page 36*

magnesium hydroxide and calcium carbonate *see* calcium carbonate and magnesium hydroxide *on page 136*

magnesium hydroxide and mineral oil (mag NEE zhum hye DROKS ide & MIN er al oyl)

Synonyms Haley's M-O; MOM/mineral oil emulsion

U.S./Canadian Brand Names Phillips'® M-O [US-OTC]

Therapeutic Category Laxative

Use Short-term treatment of occasional constipation

Usual Dosage

Children 6-11 years: 5-15 mL at bedtime or upon rising

Children ≥12 years and Adults: 30-60 mL at bedtime or upon rising

Dosage Forms Suspension, oral: Magnesium hydroxide 300 mg and mineral oil 1.25 mL per 5 mL (360 mL, 780 mL) [original and mint flavors]

magnesium hydroxide, famotidine, and calcium carbonate *see* famotidine, calcium carbonate, and magnesium hydroxide *on page 336*

magnesium L-aspartate hydrochloride (mag NEE zhum el as PAR tate hye droe KLOR ide)

Synonyms MAH

U.S./Canadian Brand Names Maginex™ DS [US-OTC]; Maginex™ [US-OTC]

Therapeutic Category Electrolyte Supplement, Oral

Use Dietary supplement

Usual Dosage

RDA (elemental magnesium):

Children:
- 1-3 years: 80 mg/day
- 4-8 years: 130 mg/day
- 9-13 years: 240 mg/day
- 14-18 years:
  - Female: 360 mg/day
  - Pregnant female: 400 mg/day
  - Male: 410 mg/day

Adults:
- 19-30 years:
  - Female: 310 mg/day
  - Pregnant female: 350 mg/day
  - Male: 400 mg/day
- ≥31 years:
  - Female: 320 mg/day
  - Pregnant female: 360 mg/day
  - Male: 420 mg/day

Dietary supplement: Adults: Oral: Magnesium-L-aspartate 1230 mg (magnesium 122 mg) up to 3 times/day

Dosage Forms

Granules:

Maginex™ DS: 1230 mg [magnesium 10 mEq; equivalent to magnesium 122 mg; lemon flavor]

Tablet [enteric coated]:

Maginex™: 615 mg [magnesium 5 mEq; equivalent to magnesium 61 mg]

magnesium oxide (mag NEE zhum OKS ide)

U.S./Canadian Brand Names Mag-Caps [US-OTC]; Mag-Ox® 400 [US-OTC]; MagGel™ [US-OTC]; Uro-Mag® [US-OTC]

Therapeutic Category Antacid; Electrolyte Supplement, Oral; Laxative

Use Electrolyte replacement

Usual Dosage

RDA (elemental magnesium):

Children:
- 1-3 years: 80 mg/day
- 4-8 years: 130 mg/day
- 9-13 years: 240 mg/day
- 14-18 years:
  - Female: 360 mg/day
  - Pregnant female: 400 mg/day
  - Male: 410 mg/day

Adults:
- 19-30 years:
  - Female: 310 mg/day
  - Pregnant female: 350 mg/day
  - Male: 400 mg/day
- ≥31 years:
  - Female: 320 mg/day
  - Pregnant female: 360 mg/day
  - Male: 420 mg/day

(Continued)

magnesium oxide *(Continued)*

Dietary supplement: Adults: Oral:
Mag-Ox 400®: 2 tablets daily with food
Mag-Caps, Uro-Mag®: 4-5 capsules daily with food

Dosage Forms
Caplet: 250 mg
Capsule:
Mag-Caps: Elemental magnesium 85 mg
Uro-Mag®: 140 mg [magnesium 7 mEq; equivalent to elemental magnesium 84.5 mg]
Capsule, softgel:
MagGel™: 600 mg [magnesium 28.64 mEq; equivalent to elemental magnesium 348 mg]
Tablet: 400 mg [magnesium 20 mEq; equivalent to elemental magnesium 242 mg], 500 mg
Mag-Ox® 400: 400 mg [magnesium 20 mEq; equivalent to elemental magnesium 242 mg]

magnesium salicylate (mag NEE zhum sa LIS i late)

U.S./Canadian Brand Names Doan's® Extra Strength [US-OTC]; Doan's® [US-OTC]; Keygesic [US-OTC]; Momentum® [US-OTC]

Therapeutic Category Nonsteroidal Antiinflammatory Drug (NSAID)

Use Mild-to-moderate pain, fever, various inflammatory conditions; relief of pain and inflammation of rheumatoid arthritis and osteoarthritis

Usual Dosage Oral: Children ≥12 years and Adults:
Doan's®: Two caplets every 4 hours as needed (maximum: 12 caplets/24 hours)
Doan's® Extra Strength, Momentum®: Two caplets every 6 hours (maximum: 8 caplets/24 hours)
Keygesic: One caplet every 4 hours as needed (maximum 4 caplets/24 hours)

Dosage Forms
Caplet, as anhydrous: 467 mg
Doan's®: 304 mg
Doan's® Extra Strength: 467 mg
Momentum®: 467 mg
Tablet, chelated:
Keygesic: 650 mg
Tablet, as tetrahydrate [scored]:
Novasal™: 600 mg

magnesium sulfate (mag NEE zhum SUL fate)

Sound-Alike/Look-Alike Issues
magnesium sulfate may be confused with manganese sulfate, morphine sulfate
$MgSO_4$ is an error-prone abbreviation (mistaken as morphine sulfate)

Synonyms epsom salts

Therapeutic Category Anticonvulsant; Electrolyte Supplement, Oral; Laxative

Use Treatment and prevention of hypomagnesemia; seizure prevention in severe pre-eclampsia or eclampsia, pediatric acute nephritis; torsade de pointes; treatment of cardiac arrhythmias (VT/VF) caused by hypomagnesemia; short-term treatment of constipation; soaking aid

Usual Dosage Dose represented as magnesium sulfate unless stated otherwise. **Note:** Serum magnesium is poor reflection of repletional status as the majority of magnesium is intracellular; serum levels may be transiently normal for a few hours after a dose is given, therefore, aim for consistently high normal serum levels in patients with normal renal function for most efficient repletion.

Hypomagnesemia: Note: Treatment depends on severity and clinical status:
Children: I.V., I.O.: 25-50 mg/kg/dose (0.2-0.4 mEq/kg/dose) over 10-20 minutes (faster in torsade); maximum single dose: 2000 mg (16 mEq)
Adults: I.V.:
Severe or smptomatic: 1-2 g over 5-60 minutes
Hypomagnesemia with seizures: 2 g over 10 minutes; calcium administration may also be appropriate

Eclampsia, pre-eclampsia: Adults: I.V.: 4-6 g over 15-20 minutes followed by 2 g/hour

Torsade de pointes: Adults: I.V.:
Pulseless: 1-2 g over 5-20 minutes
With pulse: 1-2 g over 5-60 minutes. **Note:** Slower administration preferable for stable patients.

Cathartic: Oral:
Children:
2-5 years: 2.5-5 g/kg/day in divided doses
6-11 years: 5-10 g/day in divided doses
Children ≥12 years and Adults: 10-30 g/day in divided doses

Parenteral nutrition supplementation (elemental magnesium): I.V.:
Children:
<50 kg: 0.3-0.5 mEq/kg/day
>50 kg: 10-30 mEq/day
Adults: 8-20 mEq/day

Soaking aid: Topical: Adults: Dissolve 2 cupfuls of powder per gallon of warm water

RDA (elemental magnesium):
Children:
1-3 years: 80 mg/day
4-8 years: 130 mg/day
9-13 years: 240 mg/day
14-18 years:
Female: 360 mg/day
Pregnant female: 400 mg/day
Male: 410 mg/day
Adults:
19-30 years:
Female: 310 mg/day
Pregnant female: 350 mg/day
Male: 400 mg/day
≥31 years:
Female: 320 mg/day
Pregnant female: 360 mg/day
Male: 420 mg/day

Dosage Forms
Infusion [premixed in D_5W]: 10 mg/mL (100 mL); 20 mg/mL (500 mL, 1000 mL)
Infusion [premixed in water for injection]: 40 mg/mL (100 mL, 500 mL, 1000 mL); 80 mg/mL (50 mL)
Injection, solution: 125 mg/mL (8 mL); 500 mg/mL (2 mL, 5 mL, 10 mL, 20 mL, 50 mL)
Powder: Magnesium sulfate USP (480 g, 1810 g, 1920 g)

magnesium trisilicate and aluminum hydroxide *see* aluminum hydroxide and magnesium trisilicate *on page 36*

Magnevist® [US/Can] *see* radiological/contrast media (ionic) *on page 728*

Magnolex® [Can] *see* magnesium glucoheptonate *on page 513*

Magnorol® Sirop [Can] *see* magnesium glucoheptonate *on page 513*

Magonate® [US-OTC] *see* magnesium gluconate *on page 513*

Magonate® Sport *(Discontinued)* *see* magnesium gluconate *on page 513*

Mag-Ox® 400 [US-OTC] *see* magnesium oxide *on page 515*

Magsal® *(Discontinued)* *see* magnesium salicylate *on previous page*

Magtrate® [US-OTC] *see* magnesium gluconate *on page 513*

MAH *see* magnesium L-aspartate hydrochloride *on page 515*

Majeptil® [Can] *see* thioproperazine *(Canada only) on page 823*

Malarone® [US/Can] *see* atovaquone and proguanil *on page 82*

Malarone® Pediatric [Can] *see* atovaquone and proguanil *on page 82*

malathion (mal a THYE on)

U.S./Canadian Brand Names Ovide® [US]

Therapeutic Category Scabicides/Pediculicides

Use Treatment of head lice and their ova

Usual Dosage Sprinkle Ovide® lotion on dry hair and rub gently until the scalp is thoroughly moistened; pay special attention to the back of the head and neck. Allow to dry naturally - use no heat and leave uncovered. After 8-12 hours, the hair should be washed with a nonmedicated shampoo; rinse and use a fine-toothed comb to remove dead lice and eggs. If required, repeat with second application in 7-9 days. Further treatment is generally not necessary. Other family members should be evaluated to determine if infested and if so, receive treatment.

Dosage Forms Lotion: 0.5% (59 mL) [contains isopropyl alcohol 78%]

Mallisol® *(Discontinued)* *see* povidone-iodine *on page 689*

maltodextrin (mal toe DEK strin)

U.S./Canadian Brand Names Gelclair® [US]; Multidex® [US-OTC]; OraRinse™ [US-OTC]

Therapeutic Category Skin and Mucous Membrane Agent

Use Topical: Treatment of infected or noninfected wounds

Usual Dosage Adults:

Oral: Management of pain due to oral lesions:

Gelclair®: Using contents of 1 reconstituted packet, rinse around mouth for ~1 minute, 3 times/day or more if needed; gargle and expectorate. May be used undiluted or with less dilution if adequate pain relief is not achieved.

OraRinse™: 1 tablespoonful, swish or gargle for ~1 minute, 4 times/day or more if needed

Topical: Wound dressing: Multidex®: After debridement and irrigation of wound, apply and cover with a nonadherent, nonocclusive dressing. May be applied to moist or dry, infected or noninfected wounds.

Dosage Forms

Gel, oral [concentrate] (Gelclair®): 15 mL/packet (21s) [contains benzalkonium chloride and sodium benzoate]

Gel, topical dressing (Multidex®): (4 mL, 7 mL, 14 mL, 85 mL)

Powder, for oral suspension (OraRinse™): (19 g) [contains phenylalanine; also contains aloe vera, fructose, and sodium benzoate; vanilla flavor]

Powder, topical dressing (Multidex®): (6 g, 12 g, 25 g, 45 g)

Mandelamine® [US/Can] *see* methenamine *on page 538*

mandrake *see* podophyllum resin *on page 677*

Manerix® [Can] *see* moclobemide *(Canada only) on page 562*

manganese *see* trace metals *on page 839*

mannitol (MAN i tole)

Sound-Alike/Look-Alike Issues

Osmitrol® may be confused with esmolol

Synonyms *D*-mannitol

U.S./Canadian Brand Names Osmitrol® [US/Can]; Resectisol® [US]

Therapeutic Category Diuretic, Osmotic

Use Reduction of increased intracranial pressure associated with cerebral edema; promotion of diuresis in the prevention and/or treatment of oliguria or anuria due to acute renal failure; reduction of increased intraocular pressure; promoting urinary excretion of toxic substances; genitourinary irrigant in transurethral prostatic resection or other transurethral surgical procedures

Usual Dosage

Children: I.V.:

Test dose (to assess adequate renal function): 200 mg/kg over 3-5 minutes to produce a urine flow of at least 1 mL/kg for 1-3 hours

Initial: 0.25-1 g/kg

Maintenance: 0.25-0.5 g/kg given every 4-6 hours

Adults:

I.V.:

Test dose (to assess adequate renal function): 12.5 g (200 mg/kg) over 3-5 minutes to produce a urine flow of at least 30-50 mL of urine per hour. If urine flow does not increase, a second test dose may be given. If test dose does not produce an acceptable urine output, then need to reassess management.

Initial: 0.5-1 g/kg

Maintenance: 0.25-0.5 g/kg every 4-6 hours; usual daily dose: 20-200 g/24 hours

Intracranial pressure: Cerebral edema: 0.25-1.5 g/kg/dose I.V. as a 15% to 20% solution over ≥30 minutes; maintain serum osmolality 310 to <320 mOsm/kg

Prevention of acute renal failure (oliguria): 50-100 g dose

Treatment of oliguria: 100 g dose

Preoperative for neurosurgery: 1.5-2 g/kg administered 1-1.5 hours prior to surgery

Reduction of intraocular pressure: 1.5-2 g/kg as a 15% to 20% solution; administer over 30 minutes

Topical: Transurethral irrigation: Use urogenital solution as required for irrigation

Dosage Forms

Injection, solution: 5% [50 mg/mL] (1000 mL); 10% [100 mg/mL] (500 mL, 1000 mL); 15% [150 mg/mL] (500 mL); 20% [200 mg/mL] (150 mL, 250 mL, 500 mL); 25% [250 mg/mL] (50 mL)

Osmitrol®: 5% [50 mg/mL] (1000 mL); 10% [100 mg/mL] (500 mL, 1000 mL); 15% [150 mg/mL] (500 mL); 20% [200 mg/mL] (250 mL, 500 mL)

Solution, urogenital (Resectisol®): 5% [50 mg/mL] (2000 mL, 4000 mL)

mantoux *see* tuberculin tests *on page 857*

Maox® *(Discontinued)* *see* magnesium oxide *on page 515*

Mapap [US-OTC] *see* acetaminophen *on page 5*

Mapap Children's [US-OTC] *see* acetaminophen *on page 5*

Mapap Extra Strength [US-OTC] *see* acetaminophen *on page 5*

Mapap Infants [US-OTC] *see* acetaminophen *on page 5*

Mapap Sinus Maximum Strength [US-OTC] *see* acetaminophen and pseudoephedrine *on page 9*

Mapezine® [Can] *see* carbamazepine *on page 144*

maprotiline (ma PROE ti leen)

Sound-Alike/Look-Alike Issues

Ludiomil® may be confused with Lamictal®, lamotrigine, Lomotil®

Synonyms maprotiline hydrochloride

U.S./Canadian Brand Names Novo-Maprotiline [Can]

Therapeutic Category Antidepressant, Tetracyclic

Use Treatment of depression and anxiety associated with depression

Usual Dosage Oral: Adults: Depression/anxiety: 75 mg/day to start, increase by 25 mg every 2 weeks up to 150-225 mg/day; given in 3 divided doses or in a single daily dose

Dosage Forms Tablet, as hydrochloride: 25 mg, 50 mg, 75 mg

maprotiline hydrochloride *see* maprotiline *on this page*

Marcaine® [US/Can] *see* bupivacaine *on page 124*

Marcaine® Spinal [US] *see* bupivacaine *on page 124*

Marcaine® with Epinephrine [US] *see* bupivacaine and epinephrine *on page 124*

Margesic® H [US] *see* hydrocodone and acetaminophen *on page 420*

Marinol® [US/Can] *see* dronabinol *on page 281*

Marmine® Injection *(Discontinued)* *see* dimenhydrinate *on page 258*

Marmine® Oral *(Discontinued)* *see* dimenhydrinate *on page 258*

Marplan® [US] *see* isocarboxazid *on page 463*

Marthritic® *(Discontinued)* *see* salsalate *on page 761*

Marvelon® [Can] *see* ethinyl estradiol and desogestrel *on page 317*

Matulane® [US/Can] *see* procarbazine *on page 701*

3M™ Avagard® *(Discontinued)* *see* chlorhexidine gluconate *on page 173*

Mavik® [US/Can] *see* trandolapril *on page 841*

Maxair™ Autohaler™ [US] *see* pirbuterol *on page 671*

Maxalt® [US/Can] *see* rizatriptan *on page 750*

Maxalt-MLT® [US] *see* rizatriptan *on page 750*

Maxalt RPD™ [Can] *see* rizatriptan *on page 750*

Maxaquin® *(Discontinued)*

Maxidex® [US/Can] *see* dexamethasone (ophthalmic) *on page 239*

Maxidone™ [US] *see* hydrocodone and acetaminophen *on page 420*

Maxifed® [US] *see* guaifenesin and pseudoephedrine *on page 398*

Maxifed DM [US] *see* guaifenesin, pseudoephedrine, and dextromethorphan *on page 401*

Maxifed DMX [US] *see* guaifenesin, pseudoephedrine, and dextromethorphan *on page 401*

Maxifed-G® [US] *see* guaifenesin and pseudoephedrine *on page 398*

Maxiflor® *(Discontinued)* *see* diflorasone *on page 253*

Maximum Strength Desenex® Antifungal Cream *(Discontinued)* *see* miconazole *on page 553*

Maximum Strength Dex-A-Diet® *(Discontinued)*

Maximum Strength Dexatrim® *(Discontinued)*

Maxiphen DM [US] *see* guaifenesin, dextromethorphan, and phenylephrine *on page 400*

Maxipime® [US/Can] *see* cefepime *on page 158*

Maxitrol® [US/Can] *see* neomycin, polymyxin B, and dexamethasone *on page 584*

Maxi-Tuss HC® [US] *see* phenylephrine, hydrocodone, and chlorpheniramine *on page 663*

Maxi-Tuss HCG [US] *see* hydrocodone and guaifenesin *on page 422*

Maxi-Tuss HCX [US] *see* phenylephrine, hydrocodone, and chlorpheniramine *on page 663*

Maxivate® [US] *see* betamethasone (topical) *on page 107*

Maxolon® ***(Discontinued)*** *see* metoclopramide *on page 549*

Maxzide® [US] *see* hydrochlorothiazide and triamterene *on page 420*

Maxzide®-25 [US] *see* hydrochlorothiazide and triamterene *on page 420*

may apple *see* podophyllum resin *on page 677*

3M™ Cavilon™ Skin Cleanser [US-OTC] *see* benzalkonium chloride *on page 99*

MCH *see* collagen hemostat *on page 212*

m-cresyl acetate (em-KREE sil AS e tate)

U.S./Canadian Brand Names Cresylate® [US]

Therapeutic Category Otic Agent, Antiinfective

Use Provides an acid medium; for external otitis infections caused by susceptible bacteria or fungus

Usual Dosage Otic: Instill 2-4 drops as required

Dosage Forms Solution, otic: 25% (15 mL) [with isopropanol 25%, chlorobutanol 1%, benzyl alcohol 1%, and castor oil 5% in propylene glycol]

MCT *see* medium chain triglycerides *on page 524*

MCT Oil® [US-OTC] *see* medium chain triglycerides *on page 524*

MCV4 *see* meningococcal polysaccharide (Groups A / C / Y and W-135) diphtheria toxoid conjugate vaccine *on page 527*

MD-Gastroview® [US] *see* radiological/contrast media (ionic) *on page 728*

MDL 73,147EF *see* dolasetron *on page 271*

measles, mumps, and rubella vaccines, combined

(MEE zels, mumpz & roo BEL a vak SEENS, kom BINED)

Synonyms MMR; mumps, measles and rubella vaccines, combined; rubella, measles and mumps vaccines, combined

U.S./Canadian Brand Names M-M-R® II [US/Can]; Priorix™ [Can]

Therapeutic Category Vaccine, Live Virus

Use Measles, mumps, and rubella prophylaxis

Usual Dosage SubQ:

Infants <12 months: If there is risk of exposure to measles, single-antigen measles vaccine should be administered at 6-11 months of age with a second dose (of MMR) at >12 months of age.

Children ≥12 months:

Primary immunization: 0.5 mL at 12-15 months

Revaccination: 0.5 mL at 4-6 years of age; revaccination is recommended prior to elementary school. If the second dose was not received, the schedule should be completed by the 11- to 12-year old visit. During a mumps outbreak, children ages 1-4 should consider a second dose of a live mumps virus vaccine. (Minimum interval between doses is 28 days.)

Adults:

Birth year ≥1957 without evidence of immunity: 1 or 2 doses (0.5 mL/dose); minimum interval between doses is 28 days

Routine vaccination of healthcare workers:

Birth year ≥1957 without evidence of immunity: 2 doses of a live mumps virus vaccine; minimum interval between doses is 28 days

Birth year <1957 without evidence of immunity: 1 dose of a live mumps virus vaccine.

Mumps outbreak:

Healthcare workers born <1957 without other evidence of immunity: Consider 2 doses of a live mumps virus vaccine; minimum interval between doses is 28 days

Low-risk adults: A second dose of a live mumps virus vaccine should be considered in adults who previously received 1 dose; minimum interval between doses is 28 days

Dosage Forms

Injection, powder for reconstitution [preservative free]:

M-M-R® II: Measles virus 1000 $TCID_{50}$, mumps virus 20,000 $TCID_{50}$, and , rubella virus 1000 $TCID_{50}$ [contains neomycin 25 mcg, gelatin, human albumin, and bovine serum; produced in chick embryo cell culture]

measles, mumps, rubella, and varicella virus vaccine

(MEE zels, mumpz, roo BEL a, & var i SEL a VYE rus vak SEEN)

Synonyms mumps, rubella, varicella, and measles vaccine; rubella, varicella, measles, and mumps vaccine; varicella, measles, mumps, and rubella vaccine

U.S./Canadian Brand Names ProQuad® [US]

Therapeutic Category Vaccine, Live Virus

Use To provide simultaneous active immunization against measles, mumps, rubella, and varicella

Usual Dosage SubQ: Children 12 months to 12 years: One dose (0.5 mL)

Allow at least 1 month between administering a dose of a measles containing vaccine (eg, M-M-R® II) and ProQuad®.

Allow at least 3 months between administering a varicella containing vaccine (eg, Varivax®) and ProQuad®.

Dosage Forms Injection, powder for reconstitution [preservative free] (ProQuad®): Measles virus ≥3.00 log_{10} TCID50, mumps virus ≥4.3 log_{10} TCID50, rubella virus ≥3.0 log_{10} TCID50, and varicella virus ≥3.99 log_{10} plaque-forming units [contains neomycin, sucrose, gelatin, human albumin, and bovine serum; produced in chick embryo cell culture]

measles virus vaccine (live) (MEE zels VYE rus vak SEEN, live)

Sound-Alike/Look-Alike Issues

Attenuvax® may be confused with Meruvax®

Synonyms more attenuated enders strain; rubeola vaccine

U.S./Canadian Brand Names Attenuvax® [US]

Therapeutic Category Vaccine, Live Virus

Use Adults born before 1957 are generally considered to be immune. All those born in or after 1957 without documentation of live vaccine on or after first birthday, physician-diagnosed measles, or laboratory evidence of immunity should be vaccinated, ideally with two doses of vaccine separated by no less than 1 month. For those previously vaccinated with one dose of measles vaccine, revaccination is recommended for students entering colleges and other institutions of higher education, for healthcare workers at the time of employment, and for international travelers who visit endemic areas.

MMR is the vaccine of choice if recipients are likely to be susceptible to rubella and/or mumps as well as to measles. Persons vaccinated between 1963 and 1967 with a killed measles vaccine, followed by live vaccine within 3 months, or with a vaccine of unknown type should be revaccinated with live measles virus vaccine.

Usual Dosage Children ≥15 months and Adults: SubQ: 0.5 mL in outer aspect of the upper arm, no routine boosters

Dosage Forms Injection, powder for reconstitution [preservative free]: 1000 $TCID_{50}$ [contains human albumin, bovine serum, and neomycin; produced in chick embryo cell culture]

Measurin® *(Discontinued)* *see* aspirin *on page 77*

Mebaral® [US/Can] *see* mephobarbital *on page 530*

mebendazole (me BEN da zole)

U.S./Canadian Brand Names Vermox® [Can]

Therapeutic Category Anthelmintic

Use Treatment of pinworms (*Enterobius vermicularis*), whipworms (*Trichuris trichiura*), roundworms (*Ascaris lumbricoides*), and hookworms (*Ancylostoma duodenale*)

Usual Dosage Children and Adults: Oral:

Pinworms: 100 mg as a single dose; may need to repeat after 2 weeks; treatment should include family members in close contact with patient

Whipworms, roundworms, hookworms: One tablet twice daily, morning and evening on 3 consecutive days; if patient is not cured within 3-4 weeks, a second course of treatment may be administered

Capillariasis: 200 mg twice daily for 20 days

Dosage Forms Tablet, chewable: 100 mg

mecamylamine (mek a MIL a meen)

Sound-Alike/Look-Alike Issues

mecamylamine may be confused with mesalamine

Synonyms mecamylamine hydrochloride

U.S./Canadian Brand Names Inversine® [US/Can]

Therapeutic Category Ganglionic Blocking Agent

Use Treatment of moderately severe to severe hypertension and in uncomplicated malignant hypertension

Usual Dosage Adults: Oral: 2.5 mg twice daily after meals for 2 days; increased by increments of 2.5 mg at intervals ≥2 days until desired blood pressure response is achieved; average daily dose: 25 mg (usually in 3 divided doses)

Note: Reduce dosage of other antihypertensives when combined with mecamylamine with exception of thiazide diuretics which may be maintained at usual dose while decreasing mecamylamine by 50%

Dosage Forms Tablet, as hydrochloride: 2.5 mg

mecamylamine hydrochloride *see* mecamylamine *on this page*

mecasermin (mek a SER min)

Synonyms mecasermin (rDNA origin); mecasermin rinfabate; recombinant human insulin-like growth factor-1; rhIGF-1; rhIGF-1/rhIGFBP-3

U.S./Canadian Brand Names Increlex™ [US]; Iplex™ [US]

Therapeutic Category Growth Hormone

Use Treatment of growth failure in children with severe primary insulin-like growth factor-1 deficiency (IGF-1 deficiency; primary IGFD), or with growth hormone (GH) gene deletions who have developed neutralizing antibodies to GH

Usual Dosage Primary IGFD: SubQ:

Increlex™: Children ≥2 years: Initial: 0.04-0.08 mg/kg twice daily; if tolerated for 7 days, may increase by 0.04 mg/kg/dose (maximum dose: 0.12 mg/kg given twice daily). Must be administered within 20 minutes of a meal or snack; omit dose if patient is unable to eat. Reduce dose if hypoglycemia occurs despite adequate food intake.

Iplex™: Children ≥3 years: Initial: 0.5 mg/kg once daily; dose may be increased to 1-2 mg/kg/day, given once daily. Withhold dose if hypoglycemia is present.

Dosage Forms

Injection, solution (Increlex™): 10 mg/mL (4 mL) [contains benzyl alcohol]

Injection, solution, as rinfabate [preservative free] (Iplex™): 36 mg/0.6 mL (0.6 mL)

mecasermin (rDNA origin) *see* mecasermin *on this page*

mecasermin rinfabate *see* mecasermin *on this page*

mechlorethamine (me klor ETH a meen)

Synonyms chlorethazine; chlorethazine mustard; HN_2; mechlorethamine hydrochloride; mustine; nitrogen mustard; NSC-762

U.S./Canadian Brand Names Mustargen® [US/Can]

Therapeutic Category Antineoplastic Agent

Use Combination therapy of Hodgkin disease and malignant lymphomas; non-Hodgkin lymphoma; may be used by intracavitary injection for treatment of metastatic tumors; pleural and other malignant effusions; topical treatment of mycosis fungoides

Usual Dosage Refer to individual protocols.

Children and Adults: I.V.: 6 mg/m^2 on days 1 and 8 of a 28-day cycle (MOPP regimen)

Adults:

I.V.: 0.4 mg/kg **or** 12-16 mg/m^2 for one dose **or** divided into 0.1 mg/kg/day for 4 days, repeated at 4- to 6-week intervals

Intracavitary: 0.2-0.4 mg/kg (10-20 mg) as a single dose; may be repeated if fluid continues to accumulate.

Intrapericardially: 0.2-0.4 mg/kg as a single dose; may be repeated if fluid continues to accumulate.

Topical: 0.01% to 0.02% solution, lotion, or ointment

Dosage Forms Injection, powder for reconstitution, as hydrochloride: 10 mg

mechlorethamine hydrochloride *see* mechlorethamine *on this page*

meclizine (MEK li zeen)

Sound-Alike/Look-Alike Issues

Antivert® may be confused with Axert™

Synonyms meclizine hydrochloride; meclozine hydrochloride

U.S./Canadian Brand Names Antivert® [US]; Bonamine™ [Can]; Bonine® [US-OTC/Can]; Dramamine® Less Drowsy Formula [US-OTC]

Therapeutic Category Antihistamine

Use Prevention and treatment of symptoms of motion sickness; management of vertigo with diseases affecting the vestibular system

Usual Dosage Children >12 years and Adults: Oral:

Motion sickness: 12.5-25 mg 1 hour before travel, repeat dose every 12-24 hours if needed; doses up to 50 mg may be needed

Vertigo: 25-100 mg/day in divided doses

Dosage Forms

Tablet, as hydrochloride: 12.5 mg, 25 mg

Antivert®: 12.5 mg, 25 mg, 50 mg

Dramamine® Less Drowsy Formula: 25 mg

Tablet, chewable, as hydrochloride (Bonine®): 25 mg

meclizine hydrochloride *see* meclizine *on previous page*

meclofenamate (me kloe fen AM ate)

Synonyms meclofenamate sodium

U.S./Canadian Brand Names Meclomen® [Can]

Therapeutic Category Analgesic, Nonnarcotic; Nonsteroidal Antiinflammatory Drug (NSAID)

Use Treatment of inflammatory disorders, arthritis, mild to moderate pain, dysmenorrhea

Usual Dosage Children >14 years and Adults: Oral:

Mild to moderate pain: 50 mg every 4-6 hours; increases to 100 mg may be required; maximum dose: 400 mg

Rheumatoid arthritis and osteoarthritis: 50 mg every 4-6 hours; increase, over weeks, to 200-400 mg/day in 3-4 divided doses; do not exceed 400 mg/day; maximal benefit for any dose may not be seen for 2-3 weeks

Dosage Forms Capsule, as sodium: 50 mg, 100 mg

meclofenamate sodium *see* meclofenamate *on this page*

Meclomen® [Can] *see* meclofenamate *on this page*

meclozine hydrochloride *see* meclizine *on previous page*

Med-Diltiazem [Can] *see* diltiazem *on page 257*

Medent-DM [US] *see* guaifenesin, pseudoephedrine, and dextromethorphan *on page 401*

medicinal carbon *see* charcoal *on page 169*

medicinal charcoal *see* charcoal *on page 169*

Medicone® [US-OTC] *see* phenylephrine *on page 660*

Medidin® Liquid *(Discontinued)* *see* hydrocodone and guaifenesin *on page 422*

Medigesic® [US] *see* butalbital, acetaminophen, and caffeine *on page 129*

Medihaler-Iso® *(Discontinued)* *see* isoproterenol *on page 464*

Medipain 5® *(Discontinued)* *see* hydrocodone and acetaminophen *on page 420*

Mediplast® [US-OTC] *see* salicylic acid *on page 758*

Medipren® *(Discontinued)* *see* ibuprofen *on page 437*

Medi-Quick® Topical Ointment *(Discontinued)* *see* bacitracin, neomycin, and polymyxin B *on page 91*

Medispaz® *(Discontinued)* *see* hyoscyamine *on page 434*

Medi-Synal [US-OTC] *see* acetaminophen and pseudoephedrine *on page 9*

Medi-Tuss® *(Discontinued)* *see* guaifenesin *on page 392*

medium chain triglycerides (mee DEE um chane trye GLIS er ides)

Synonyms MCT; triglycerides, medium chain

U.S./Canadian Brand Names MCT Oil® [US-OTC]

Therapeutic Category Nutritional Supplement

Use Dietary supplement for those who cannot digest long chain fats; malabsorption associated with disorders such as pancreatic insufficiency, bile salt deficiency, short bowel syndrome, and bacterial overgrowth of the small bowel; induce ketosis as a prevention for seizures

Usual Dosage Oral:

Infants: Nutritional supplement: Initial: 0.5 mL every other feeding, then advance to every feeding, then increase in increments of 0.25-0.5 mL/feeding at intervals of 2-3 days as tolerated

Children: Seizures: About 40 mL with each meal or 50% to 70% (800-1120 kcal) of total calories (1600 kcal) as the oil will induce ketosis necessary for seizure control

Children and Adults: Cystic fibrosis: 3 tablespoons/day in divided doses

Adults: Malabsorption syndromes: 15 mL 3-4 times/day

Dosage Forms Oil: 14 g/15 mL (960 mL) [115 calories/15 mL; derived from coconut oil]

Medralone® Injection *(Discontinued)* *see* methylprednisolone *on page 547*

Medrol® [US/Can] *see* methylprednisolone *on page 547*

medroxyprogesterone (me DROKS ee proe JES te rone)

Sound-Alike/Look-Alike Issues

medroxyPROGESTERone may be confused with hydroxyprogesterone, methylPREDNISolone, methylTESTOSTERone, progesterone

Provera® may be confused with Covera®, Parlodel®, Premarin®

Synonyms acetoxymethylprogesterone; medroxyprogesterone acetate; methylacetoxyprogesterone

Tall-Man medroxy**PROGESTER**one

U.S./Canadian Brand Names Alti-MPA [Can]; Apo-Medroxy® [Can]; Depo-Prevera® [Can]; Depo-Provera® Contraceptive [US]; Depo-Provera® [US/Can]; depo-subQ provera 104™ [US]; Gen-Medroxy [Can]; Novo-Medrone [Can]; Provera-Pak [Can]; Provera® [US/Can]

Therapeutic Category Contraceptive, Progestin Only; Progestin

Use Endometrial carcinoma or renal carcinoma; secondary amenorrhea or abnormal uterine bleeding due to hormonal imbalance; reduction of endometrial hyperplasia in nonhysterectomized postmenopausal women receiving conjugated estrogens; prevention of pregnancy; management of endometriosis-associated pain

Usual Dosage

Adolescents and Adults:

Amenorrhea: Oral: 5-10 mg/day for 5-10 days

Abnormal uterine bleeding: Oral: 5-10 mg for 5-10 days starting on day 16 or 21 of cycle

Contraception:

Depo-Provera® Contraceptive: I.M.: 150 mg every 3 months

depo-subQ provera 104™: SubQ: 104 mg every 3 months (every 12-14 weeks)

Endometriosis: depo-subQ provera 104™: SubQ: 104 mg every 3 months (every 12-14 weeks)

Adults:

Endometrial or renal carcinoma (Depo-Provera®): I.M.: 400-1000 mg/week

Accompanying cyclic estrogen therapy, postmenopausal: Oral: 5-10 mg for 12-14 consecutive days each month, starting on day 1 or day 16 of the cycle; lower doses may be used if given with estrogen continuously throughout the cycle

Dosage Forms

Injection, suspension, as acetate: 150 mg/mL (1 mL)

Depo-Provera®: 400 mg/mL (2.5 mL)

Depo-Provera® Contraceptive: 150 mg/mL (1 mL) [prefilled syringe or vial]

depo-subQ provera 104™: 104 mg/0.65 mL (0.65 mL) [prefilled syringe]

Tablet, as acetate (Provera®): 2.5 mg, 5 mg, 10 mg

medroxyprogesterone acetate *see* medroxyprogesterone *on this page*

medroxyprogesterone and estrogens (conjugated) *see* estrogens (conjugated/equine) and medroxyprogesterone *on page 313*

medrysone (ME dri sone)

Therapeutic Category Adrenal Corticosteroid

Use Treatment of allergic conjunctivitis, vernal conjunctivitis, episcleritis, ophthalmic epinephrine sensitivity reaction

Usual Dosage Children ≥3 years and Adults: Ophthalmic: Instill 1 drop in conjunctival sac 2-4 times/day up to every 4 hours; may use every 1-2 hours during first 1-2 days

Dosage Forms [DSC] = Discontinued product

Solution, ophthalmic: 1% (5 mL, 10 mL) [contains benzalkonium chloride] [DSC]

Mefenamic-250 [Can] *see* mefenamic acid *on this page*

mefenamic acid (me fe NAM ik AS id)

Sound-Alike/Look-Alike Issues

Ponstel® may be confused with Pronestyl®

U.S./Canadian Brand Names Apo-Mefenamic® [Can]; Dom-Mefenamic Acid [Can]; Mefenamic-250 [Can]; Nu-Mefenamic [Can]; PMS-Mefenamic Acid [Can]; Ponstan® [Can]; Ponstel® [US]

Therapeutic Category Analgesic, Nonnarcotic; Nonsteroidal Antiinflammatory Drug (NSAID)

Use Short-term relief of mild to moderate pain including primary dysmenorrhea

Usual Dosage Children >14 years and Adults: Oral: 500 mg to start then 250 mg every 4 hours as needed; maximum therapy: 1 week

Dosage Forms Capsule: 250 mg

mefloquine (ME floe kwin)

Synonyms mefloquine hydrochloride

U.S./Canadian Brand Names Apo-Mefloquine® [Can]; Lariam® [US/Can]

Therapeutic Category Antimalarial Agent

Use Treatment of acute malarial infections and prevention of malaria

Usual Dosage Oral (dose expressed as mg of mefloquine hydrochloride):

Children ≥6 months and >5 kg:

Malaria treatment: 20-25 mg/kg in 2 divided doses, taken 6-8 hours apart (maximum: 1250 mg) Take with food and an ample amount of water. If clinical improvement is not seen within 48-72 hours, an alternative therapy should be used for retreatment.

Malaria prophylaxis: 5 mg/kg/once weekly (maximum dose: 250 mg) starting 1 week before, arrival in endemic area, continuing weekly during travel and for 4 weeks after leaving endemic area. Take with food and an ample amount of water.

Adults:

Malaria treatment (mild to moderate infection): 5 tablets (1250 mg) as a single dose. Take with food and at least 8 oz of water. If clinical improvement is not seen within 48-72 hours, an alternative therapy should be used for retreatment.

Malaria prophylaxis: 1 tablet (250 mg) weekly starting 1 week before, arrival in endemic area, continuing weekly during travel and for 4 weeks after leaving endemic area. Take with food and at least 8 oz of water.

Dosage Forms Tablet, as hydrochloride: 250 mg [equivalent to 228 mg base]

mefloquine hydrochloride *see* mefloquine *on this page*

Mefoxin® [US] *see* cefoxitin *on page 159*

Megace® [US/Can] *see* megestrol *on this page*

Megace® ES [US] *see* megestrol *on this page*

Megace® OS [Can] *see* megestrol *on this page*

Megadophilus® [US-OTC] *see* Lactobacillus *on page 477*

megestrol (me JES trole)

Sound-Alike/Look-Alike Issues

Megace® may be confused with Reglan®

Synonyms 5071-1DL(6); megestrol acetate; NSC-10363

U.S./Canadian Brand Names Apo-Megestrol® [Can]; Megace® ES [US]; Megace® OS [Can]; Megace® [US/Can]; Nu-Megestrol [Can]

Therapeutic Category Antineoplastic Agent; Progestin

Use Palliative treatment of breast and endometrial carcinoma; treatment of anorexia, cachexia, or unexplained significant weight loss in patients with AIDS

Usual Dosage Adults: Oral:

Female (refer to individual protocols):

Breast carcinoma: 40 mg 4 times/day

Endometrial carcinoma: 40-320 mg/day in divided doses; use for 2 months to determine efficacy; maximum doses used have been up to 800 mg/day

(Continued)

megestrol *(Continued)*

Male/Female: HIV-related cachexia:

Megace®: Initial dose: 800 mg/day; daily doses of 400 and 800 mg/day were found to be clinically effective

Megace ES®: 625 mg/day

Dosage Forms

Suspension, oral, as acetate: 40 mg/mL (240 mL, 480 mL)

Megace®: 40 mg/mL (240 mL) [contains alcohol 0.06% and sodium benzoate; lemon-lime flavor]

Megace® ES: 125 mg/mL (150 mL) [contains alcohol 0.06% and sodium benzoate; lemon-lime flavor]

Tablet, as acetate: 20 mg, 40 mg

megestrol acetate *see* megestrol *on previous page*

Melanex® [US] *see* hydroquinone *on page 430*

Melfiat® [US] *see* phendimetrazine *on page 657*

Mellaril® [Can] *see* thioridazine *on page 823*

Mellaril® (all products) *(Discontinued)* *see* thioridazine *on page 823*

Mellaril-S® *(Discontinued)* *see* thioridazine *on page 823*

meloxicam (mel OKS i kam)

U.S./Canadian Brand Names Apo-Meloxicam® [Can]; CO Meloxicam [Can]; Gen-Meloxicam [Can]; Mobicox® [Can]; Mobic® [US/Can]; Novo-Meloxicam [Can]; PMS-Meloxicam [Can]

Therapeutic Category Nonsteroidal Antiinflammatory Drug (NSAID)

Use Relief of signs and symptoms of osteoarthritis, rheumatoid arthritis, and juvenile rheumatoid arthritis (JRA)

Usual Dosage Oral:

Children ≥2 years: JRA: 0.125 mg/kg/day; maximum dose: 7.5 mg/day

Adults: Osteoarthritis, rheumatoid arthritis: Initial: 7.5 mg once daily; some patients may receive additional benefit from an increased dose of 15 mg once daily; maximum dose: 15 mg/day

Dosage Forms

Suspension: 7.5 mg/5 mL (100 mL)

Mobic®: 7.5 mg/5 mL (100 mL) [contains sodium benzoate; raspberry flavor]

Tablet: 7.5 mg, 15 mg

Mobic®: 7.5 mg, 15 mg

Melpaque HP® [US] *see* hydroquinone *on page 430*

melphalan (MEL fa lan)

Sound-Alike/Look-Alike Issues

melphalan may be confused with Mephyton®, Myleran®

Alkeran® may be confused with Alferon®, Leukeran®

Synonyms L-PAM; L-sarcolysin; NSC-8806; phenylalanine mustard

U.S./Canadian Brand Names Alkeran® [US/Can]

Therapeutic Category Antineoplastic Agent

Use Palliative treatment of multiple myeloma and nonresectable epithelial ovarian carcinoma

Usual Dosage Adults: Refer to individual protocols.

Oral: Dose should always be adjusted to patient response and weekly blood counts:

Multiple myeloma (multiple regimens have been employed): **Note:** Response is gradual; may require repeated courses to realize benefit:

6 mg daily for 2-3 weeks initially, followed by up to 4 weeks rest, then a maintenance dose of 2 mg daily as hematologic recovery begins **or**

10 mg daily for 7-10 days; institute 2 mg daily maintenance dose after WBC >4000 cells/mcL and platelets >100,000 cells/mcL (~4-8 weeks); titrate maintenance dose to hematologic response **or**

0.15 mg/kg/day for 7 days, with a 2-6 week rest, followed by a maintenance dose of ≤0.05 mg/kg/day as hematologic recovery begins **or**

0.25 mg/kg/day for 4 days (or 0.2 mg/kg/day for 5 days); repeat at 4- to 6-week intervals as ANC and platelet counts return to normal

Ovarian carcinoma: 0.2 mg/kg/day for 5 days, repeat every 4-5 weeks.

I.V.: Multiple myeloma: 16 mg/m^2 administered at 2-week intervals for 4 doses, then administer at 4-week intervals after adequate hematologic recovery.

Dosage Forms

Injection, powder for reconstitution: 50 mg [diluent contains ethanol and propylene glycol]

Tablet: 2 mg

Melquin-3® [US] *see* hydroquinone *on page 430*

Melquin HP® [US] *see* hydroquinone *on page 430*

memantine (me MAN teen)

Synonyms memantine hydrochloride

U.S./Canadian Brand Names Ebixa® [Can]; Namenda™ [US]

Therapeutic Category N-Methyl-D-Aspartate Receptor Antagonist

Use Treatment of moderate-to-severe dementia of the Alzheimer type

Usual Dosage Oral: Adults:

Alzheimer's disease: Initial: 5 mg/day; increase dose by 5 mg/day to a target dose of 20 mg/day; wait at least 1 week between dosage changes. Doses >5 mg/day should be given in 2 divided doses.

Suggested titration: 5 mg/day for ≥1 week; 5 mg twice daily for ≥1 week; 15 mg/day given in 5 mg and 10 mg separated doses for ≥1 week; then 10 mg twice daily

Dosage Forms

Solution, oral: 2 mg/mL (360 mL) [alcohol free, dye free, sugar free; peppermint flavor]

Tablet, as hydrochloride: 5 mg, 10 mg

Combination package [titration pack contains two separate tablet formulations]: Memantine hydrochloride 5 mg (28s) and memantine hydrochloride 10 mg (21s)

memantine hydrochloride *see* memantine *on this page*

Menactra® [US] *see* meningococcal polysaccharide (Groups A / C / Y and W-135) diphtheria toxoid conjugate vaccine *on this page*

Menadol® ***(Discontinued)*** *see* ibuprofen *on page 437*

Menest® [US/Can] *see* estrogens (esterified) *on page 313*

Meni-D® ***(Discontinued)*** *see* meclizine *on page 522*

meningococcal polysaccharide (Groups A / C / Y and W-135) diphtheria toxoid conjugate vaccine

(me NIN joe kok al pol i SAK a ride groops aye, see, why & dubl yoo won thur tee fyve dif THEER ee a TOKS oyds KON joo gate vak SEEN)

Synonyms MCV4

U.S./Canadian Brand Names Menactra® [US]

Therapeutic Category Vaccine

Use Provide active immunization of adolescents and adults (11-55 years of age) against invasive meningococcal disease caused by *N. meningitidis* serogroups A, C, Y and W-135

The ACIP recommends routine vaccination of all adolescents at age 11-12 years. For adolescents not previously vaccinated, vaccine should be administered prior to high school entry (~15 years of age).

The ACIP also recommends routine vaccination for persons at increased risk for meningococcal disease. (MCV4 is preferred for persons aged 11-55 years; MPSV4 may be used if MCV4 is not available). Persons at increased risk include:

College freshmen living in dormitories

Microbiologists routinely exposed to isolates of *N. meningitides*

Military recruits

Persons traveling to or who reside in countries where *N. meningitides* is hyperendemic or epidemic, particularly if contact with local population will be prolonged

Persons with terminal complement component deficiencies

Persons with anatomic or functional asplenia

Use is also recommended during meningococcal outbreaks caused by vaccine preventable serogroups.

Usual Dosage I.M.: Adolescents 11-18 years and Adults ≤55 years: 0.5 mL

Note: Revaccination: May be indicated in patients previously vaccinated with MPSV4 who remain at increased risk for infection. The ACIP recommends the use of MCV4 for revaccination in patients 11-55 years, however use of MPSV4 is also acceptable. Consider revaccination after 3-5 years. The need for revaccination in patients previously vaccinated with MCV4 is currently under study.

Dosage Forms

Injection, solution:

Menactra®: 4 mcg each of polysaccharide antigen groups A, C, Y, and W-135 per 0.5 mL [conjugated to diphtheria toxoid protein 48 mcg; adjuvant and preservative free; vial stopper contains dry, natural latex rubber]

meningococcal polysaccharide vaccine (groups A / C / Y and W-135)

(me NIN joe kok al pol i SAK a ride vak SEEN groops aye, see, why & dubl yoo won thur tee fyve)

Synonyms MPSV4

U.S./Canadian Brand Names Menomune®-A/C/Y/W-135 [US]

Therapeutic Category Vaccine, Live Bacteria

Use Provide active immunity to meningococcal serogroups contained in the vaccine

The ACIP recommends routine vaccination for persons at increased risk for meningococcal disease. (Use of MPSV4 is recommended in children 2-10 years and adults > 55 years. MCV4 is preferred for persons aged 11-55 years; MPSV4 may be used if MCV4 is not available). Persons at increased risk include:

College freshmen living in dormitories

Microbiologists routinely exposed to isolates of *N. meningitides*

Military recruits

Persons traveling to or who reside in countries where *N. meningitides* is hyperendemic or epidemic, particularly if contact with local population will be prolonged

Persons with terminal complement component deficiencies

Persons with anatomic or functional asplenia

Use is also recommended during meningococcal outbreaks caused by vaccine preventable serogroups.

Usual Dosage SubQ:

Children <2 years: Not usually recommended. Two doses (0.5 mL/dose), 3 months apart, may be considered in children 3-18 months to elicit short-term protection against serogroup A disease. A single dose may be considered in children 19-23 months.

Children ≥2 years and Adults: 0.5 mL

Note: Revaccination: May be indicated in patients previously vaccinated with MPSV4 who remain at increased risk for infection. The ACIP recommends the use of MCV4 for revaccination in patients 11-55 years, however use of MPSV4 is also acceptable.

Children first vaccinated at <4 years: Revaccinate after 2-3 years.

Adults: Not determined, consider revaccination after 3-5 years.

Dosage Forms Injection, powder for reconstitution: 50 mcg each of polysaccharide antigen groups A, C, Y, and W-135 [contains lactose; packaged with 0.78 mL preservative free diluent or 6 mL diluent containing thimerosal; vial stoppers contain dry, natural latex rubber]

Menomune®-A/C/Y/W-135 [US] *see* meningococcal polysaccharide vaccine (groups A / C / Y and W-135) *on this page*

Menopur® [US] *see* menotropins *on this page*

Menostar™ [US/Can] *see* estradiol *on page 308*

menotropins (men oh TROE pins)

Sound-Alike/Look-Alike Issues

Repronex® may be confused with Regranex®

Synonyms hMG; human menopausal gonadotropin

U.S./Canadian Brand Names Menopur® [US]; Repronex® [US/Can]

Therapeutic Category Gonadotropin

Use Female:

In conjunction with hCG to induce ovulation and pregnancy in infertile females experiencing oligoanovulation or anovulation when the cause of anovulation is functional and not caused by primary ovarian failure (Repronex®)

Stimulation of multiple follicle development in ovulatory patients as part of an assisted reproductive technology (ART) (Menopur®, Repronex®)

Usual Dosage Adults:

Repronex®: I.M., SubQ:

Induction of ovulation in patients with oligoanovulation (Female): Initial: 150 int. units daily for the first 5 days of treatment. Adjustments should not be made more frequently than once every 2 days and should not exceed 75-150 int. units per adjustment. Maximum daily dose should not exceed 450 int. units and dosing beyond 12 days is not recommended. If patient's response is appropriate, hCG 5000-10,000 units should be given one day following the last dose of Repronex®. Hold dose if serum estradiol is >2000 pg/mL, if the ovaries are abnormally enlarged, or if abdominal pain occurs; the patient should also be advised to refrain from intercourse. May repeat process if follicular development is inadequate or if pregnancy does not occur.

Assisted reproductive technologies (Female): Initial (in patients who have received GnRH agonist or antagonist pituitary suppression): 225 int. units; adjustments in dose should not be made more frequently than once every 2 days and should not exceed more than 75-150 int. units per adjustment. The maximum daily doses of Repronex® given should not exceed 450 int. units and dosing beyond 12 days is not recommended. Once adequate follicular development is evident, hCG (5000-10,000 units) should be administered to induce final follicular maturation in preparation for oocyte retrieval. Withhold treatment when ovaries are abnormally enlarged on last day of therapy (to reduce chance of developing OHSS).

Menopur®: SubQ: *Assisted reproductive technologies (ART):* Initial (in patients who have received GnRH agonist for pituitary suppression): 225 int. units; adjustments in dose should not be made more frequently than once every 2 days and should not exceed more than 150 int. units per adjustment. The maximum daily dose given should not exceed 450 int. units and dosing beyond 20 days is not recommended. Once adequate follicular development is evident, hCG should be administered to induce final follicular maturation in preparation for oocyte retrieval. Withhold treatment when ovaries are abnormally enlarged on last day of therapy (to reduce chance of developing OHSS).

Dosage Forms

Injection, powder for reconstitution:

Menopur®: Follicle stimulating hormone activity 75 int. units and luteinizing hormone activity 75 int. units [packaged with diluent; contains lactose 21 mg]

Repronex®: Follicle stimulating hormone activity 75 int. units and luteinizing hormone activity 75 int. units [packaged with diluent]

Mentax® [US] *see* butenafine *on page 130*

292 MEP® [Can] *see* aspirin and meprobamate *on page 79*

mepenzolate (me PEN zoe late)

Sound-Alike/Look-Alike Issues

Cantil® may be confused with Bentyl®

Synonyms mepenzolate bromide

U.S./Canadian Brand Names Cantil® [Can]

Therapeutic Category Anticholinergic Agent

Use Adjunctive treatment of peptic ulcer disease

Usual Dosage Adults: Oral: 25-50 mg 4 times/day with meals and at bedtime

Dosage Forms [DSC] = Discontinued product

Tablet, as bromide: 25 mg [contains tartrazine] [DSC]

mepenzolate bromide *see* mepenzolate *on this page*

mepergan *see* meperidine and promethazine *on next page*

meperidine (me PER i deen)

Sound-Alike/Look-Alike Issues

meperidine may be confused with meprobamate

Demerol® may be confused with Demulen®, Desyrel®, dicumarol, Dilaudid®, Dymelor®, Pamelor®

Synonyms isonipecaine hydrochloride; meperidine hydrochloride; pethidine hydrochloride

U.S./Canadian Brand Names Demerol® [US/Can]; Meperitab® [US]

Therapeutic Category Analgesic, Narcotic

Controlled Substance C-II

Use Management of moderate to severe pain; adjunct to anesthesia and preoperative sedation

Usual Dosage Note: Doses should be titrated to necessary analgesic effect. When changing route of administration, note that oral doses are about half as effective as parenteral dose. Not recommended for chronic pain. These are guidelines and do not represent the maximum doses that may be required in all patients. In patients with normal renal function, doses of ≤600 mg/24 hours and use for ≤48 hours are recommended.

Children: Pain: Oral, I.M., I.V., SubQ: 1-1.5 mg/kg/dose every 3-4 hours as needed; 1-2 mg/kg as a single dose preoperative medication may be used; maximum 100 mg/dose (**Note:** Oral route is not recommended for acute pain.)

Adults: Pain:

Oral: Initial: Opiate-naive: 50 mg every 3-4 hours as needed; usual dosage range: 50-150 mg every 2-4 hours as needed (manufacturers recommendation; oral route is not recommended for acute pain)

I.M., SubQ: Initial: Opiate-naive: 50-75 mg every 3-4 hours as needed; patients with prior opiate exposure may require higher initial doses

Preoperatively: 50-100 mg given 30-90 minutes before the beginning of anesthesia

Slow I.V.: Initial: 5-10 mg every 5 minutes as needed

Patient-controlled analgesia (PCA): Usual concentration: 10 mg/mL

Initial dose: 10 mg

Demand dose: 1-5 mg (manufacturer recommendations); range 5-25 mg (American Pain Society, 1999).

Lockout interval: 5-10 minutes

(Continued)

meperidine *(Continued)*

Dosage Forms

Injection, solution, as hydrochloride [ampul]: 25 mg/0.5 mL (0.5 mL); 25 mg/mL (1 mL); 50 mg/mL (1 mL, 1.5 mL, 2 mL); 75 mg/mL (1 mL); 100 mg/mL (1 mL)

Injection, solution, as hydrochloride [prefilled syringe]: 25 mg/mL (1 mL); 50 mg/mL (1 mL); 75 mg/mL (1 mL); 100 mg/mL (1 mL)

Injection, solution, as hydrochloride [for PCA pump]: 10 mg/mL (30 mL, 50 mL, 60 mL)

Injection, solution, as hydrochloride [vial]: 25 mg/mL (1 mL); 50 mg/mL (1 mL, 30 mL); 75 mg/mL (1 mL); 100 mg/mL (1 mL, 20 mL) [may contain sodium metabisulfite]

Syrup, as hydrochloride:

Demerol®: 50 mg/5 mL (480 mL) [contains benzoic acid; banana flavor]

Tablet, as hydrochloride: 50 mg, 100 mg

Demerol®, Meperitab®: 50 mg, 100 mg

meperidine and promethazine (me PER i deen & proe METH a zeen)

Sound-Alike/Look-Alike Issues

mepergan may be confused with meprobamate

Synonyms mepergan; promethazine and meperidine

Therapeutic Category Analgesic, Narcotic

Controlled Substance C-II

Use Management of moderate pain

Usual Dosage Adults: Oral: One (1) capsule every 4-6 hours as needed

Dosage Forms Capsule: Meperidine hydrochloride 50 mg and promethazine hydrochloride 25 mg

meperidine hydrochloride *see* meperidine *on previous page*

Meperitab® [US] *see* meperidine *on previous page*

mephobarbital (me foe BAR bi tal)

Sound-Alike/Look-Alike Issues

mephobarbital may be confused with methocarbamol

Mebaral® may be confused with Medrol®, Mellaril®, Tegretol®

Synonyms methylphenobarbital

U.S./Canadian Brand Names Mebaral® [US/Can]

Therapeutic Category Barbiturate

Controlled Substance C-IV

Use Sedative; treatment of grand mal and petit mal epilepsy

Usual Dosage Oral:

Epilepsy:

Children: 6-12 mg/kg/day in 2-4 divided doses

Adults: 200-600 mg/day in 2-4 divided doses

Sedation:

Children:

<5 years: 16-32 mg 3-4 times/day

>5 years: 32-64 mg 3-4 times/day

Adults: 32-100 mg 3-4 times/day

Dosage Forms Tablet: 32 mg, 50 mg, 100 mg

Mephyton® [US/Can] *see* phytonadione *on page 667*

mepivacaine (me PIV a kane)

Sound-Alike/Look-Alike Issues

mepivacaine may be confused with bupivacaine

Polocaine® may be confused with prilocaine

Synonyms mepivacaine hydrochloride

U.S./Canadian Brand Names Carbocaine® [US/Can]; Polocaine® Dental [US]; Polocaine® MPF [US]; Polocaine® [US/Can]

Therapeutic Category Local Anesthetic

Use Local or regional analgesia; anesthesia by local infiltration, peripheral and central neural techniques including epidural and caudal blocks; **not** for use in spinal anesthesia

Usual Dosage

Injectable local anesthetic: Dose varies with procedure, degree of anesthesia needed, vascularity of tissue, duration of anesthesia required, and physical condition of patient. The smallest dose and concentration required to produce the desired effect should be used.

Children: Maximum dose: 5-6 mg/kg; only concentrations <2% should be used in children <3 years or <14 kg (30 lbs)

Adults: Maximum dose: 400 mg; do not exceed 1000 mg/24 hours

Cervical, brachial, intercostal, pudenal nerve block: 5-40 mL of a 1% solution (maximum: 400 mg) **or** 5-20 mL of a 2% solution (maximum: 400 mg). For pudenal block, inject 1/2 the total dose each side.

Transvaginal block (paracervical plus pudenal): Up to 30 mL (both sides) of a 1% solution (maximum: 300 mg). Inject 1/2 the total dose each side.

Paracervical block: Up to 20 mL (both sides) of a 1% solution (maximum: 200 mg). Inject 1/2 the total dose to each side. This is the maximum recommended dose per 90-minute procedure; inject slowly with 5 minutes between sides.

Caudal and epidural block (preservative free solutions only): 15-30 mL of a 1% solution (maximum: 300 mg) **or** 10-25 mL of a 1.5% solution (maximum: 375 mg) **or** 10-20 mL of a 2% solution (maximum: 400 mg)

Infiltration: Up to 40 mL of a 1% solution (maximum: 400 mg)

Therapeutic block (pain management): 1-5 mL of a 1% solution (maximum: 50 mg) **or** 1-5 mL of a 2% solution (maximum: 100 mg)

Dental anesthesia: Adults:

Single site in upper or lower jaw: 54 mg (1.8 mL) as a 3% solution

Infiltration and nerve block of entire oral cavity: 270 mg (9 mL) as a 3% solution. Manufacturer's maximum recommended dose is not more than 400 mg to normal healthy adults.

Dosage Forms

Injection, solution, as hydrochloride [contains methylparabens]:

Carbocaine®: 1% (50 mL); 2% (50 mL)

Polocaine®: 1% (50 mL); 2% (50 mL)

Injection, solution, as hydrochloride [preservative free]:

Carbocaine®: 1% (30 mL); 1.5% (30 mL); 2% (20 mL); 3% (1.8 mL) [dental cartridge]

Polocaine® Dental: 3% (1.8 mL) [dental cartridge]

Polocaine® MPF: 1% (30 mL); 1.5% (30 mL); 2% (20 mL)

mepivacaine and levonordefrin (me PIV a kane & lee voe nor DEF rin)

Synonyms levonordefrin and mepivacaine hydrochloride

U.S./Canadian Brand Names Carbocaine® 2% with Neo-Cobefrin® [US]; Polocaine® 2% and Levonordefrin 1:20,000 [Can]

Therapeutic Category Local Anesthetic

Usual Dosage

Children <10 years: Maximum pediatric dosage must be carefully calculated on the basis of patient's weight but should not exceed 6.6 mg/kg of body weight or 180 mg of mepivacaine hydrochloride as a 2% solution with levonordefrin 1:20,000

Children >10 years and Adults:

Dental infiltration and nerve block, single site: 36 mg (1.8 mL) of mepivacaine hydrochloride as a 2% solution with levonordefrin 1:20,000

Entire oral cavity: 180 mg (9 mL) of mepivacaine hydrochloride as a 2% solution with levonordefrin 1:20,000; up to a maximum of 6.6 mg/kg of body weight but not to exceed 400 mg of mepivacaine hydrochloride per appointment. The effective anesthetic dose varies with procedure, intensity of anesthesia needed, duration of anesthesia required, and physical condition of the patient. Always use the lowest effective dose along with careful aspiration.

Dosage Forms Injection, solution: Mepivacaine hydrochloride 2% and levonordefrin 1:20,000 (1.8 mL) [dental cartridges; contains sodium bisulfite]

mepivacaine hydrochloride *see* mepivacaine *on previous page*

meprobamate (me proe BA mate)

Sound-Alike/Look-Alike Issues

meprobamate may be confused with Mepergan, meperidine

U.S./Canadian Brand Names Novo-Mepro [Can]

Therapeutic Category Antianxiety Agent, Miscellaneous

Controlled Substance C-IV

Use Management of anxiety disorders

(Continued)

meprobamate *(Continued)*

Usual Dosage Oral:

Children 6-12 years: Anxiety: 100-200 mg 2-3 times/day

Adults: Anxiety: 400 mg 3-4 times/day, up to 2400 mg/day

Dosage Forms

[DSC] = Discontinued product

Tablet: 200 mg, 400 mg

Miltown®: 200 mg, 400 mg [DSC]

meprobamate and aspirin *see* aspirin and meprobamate *on page 79*

Mepron® [US/Can] *see* atovaquone *on page 82*

mequinol and tretinoin (ME kwi nole & TRET i noyn)

Synonyms tretinoin and mequinol

U.S./Canadian Brand Names Solagé™ [US/Can]

Therapeutic Category Retinoic Acid Derivative; Vitamin A Derivative; Vitamin, Topical

Use Treatment of solar lentigines; the efficacy of using Solagé™ daily for >24 weeks has not been established. The local cutaneous safety of Solagé™ in non-Caucasians has not been adequately established.

Usual Dosage Solar lentigines: Topical: Apply twice daily to solar lentigines using the applicator tip while avoiding application to the surrounding skin. Separate application by at least 8 hours or as directed by physician.

Dosage Forms Liquid, topical: Mequinol 2% and tretinoin 0.01% (30 mL) [contains alcohol 78%; dispensed in applicator bottle]

mercaptopurine (mer kap toe PYOOR een)

Sound-Alike/Look-Alike Issues

Purinethol® may be confused with propylthiouracil

Synonyms 6-mercaptopurine; 6-MP; NSC-755

U.S./Canadian Brand Names Purinethol® [US/Can]

Therapeutic Category Antineoplastic Agent

Use Treatment (maintenance and induction) of acute lymphoblastic leukemia (ALL)

Usual Dosage Oral (refer to individual protocols):

Children: ALL:

Induction: 2.5-5 mg/kg/day **or** 70-100 mg/m²/day given once daily

Maintenance: 1.5-2.5 mg/kg/day **or** 50-75 mg/m²/day given once daily

Adults:

ALL:

Induction: 2.5-5 mg/kg/day (100-200 mg)

Maintenance: 1.5-2.5 mg/kg/day **or** 80-100 mg/m²/day given once daily

Dosage adjustment with concurrent allopurinol: Reduce mercaptopurine dosage to 1/4 to 1/3 the usual dose.

Dosage adjustment in TPMT-deficiency: Not established; substantial reductions are generally required only in homozygous deficiency.

Dosage Forms Tablet [scored]: 50 mg

6-mercaptopurine *see* mercaptopurine *on this page*

mercapturic acid *see* acetylcysteine *on page 15*

Meridia® [US/Can] *see* sibutramine *on page 771*

meropenem (mer oh PEN em)

U.S./Canadian Brand Names Merrem® I.V. [US]; Merrem® [Can]

Therapeutic Category Carbapenem (Antibiotic)

Use Treatment of intraabdominal infections (complicated appendicitis and peritonitis); treatment of bacterial meningitis in pediatric patients ≥3 months of age caused by *S. pneumoniae*, *H. influenzae*, and *N. meningitidis*; treatment of complicated skin and skin structure infections caused by susceptible organisms

Usual Dosage

Usual dosage ranges:

Neonates: I.V.:

Postnatal age 0-7 days: 20 mg/kg/dose every 12 hours

Postnatal age >7 days:

Weight 1200-2000 g: 20 mg/kg/dose every 12 hours

Weight >2000 g: 20 mg/kg/dose every 8 hours

Children ≥3 months: I.V.: 60 mg/kg/day divided every 8 hours (maximum dose: 6 g/day)
Adults: I.V.: 1.5-6 g/day divided every 8 hours

Indication-specific dosing:

Children >3 months (<50 kg): I.V.:

Intraabdominal infections: 20 mg/kg every 8 hours (maximum dose: 1 g every 8 hours)
Meningitis: 40 mg/kg every 8 hours (maximum dose: 2 g every 8 hours)
Skin and skin structure infections (complicated): 10 mg/kg every 8 hours (maximum dose: 500 mg every 8 hours)

Children >50 kg and Adults: I.V.:

Burkholderia pseudomallei **(melioidosis),** ***Pseudomonas:*** 1 g every 8 hours
Cholangitis, intraabdominal infections, otitis externa, septic lateral sinus thrombosis: 1 g every 8 hours
Liver abscess: 1 g every 8 hours for 2-3 weeks, then oral therapy for duration of 4-6 weeks
Meningitis: 2 g every 8 hours
Mild-to-moderate infection: 1.5-3 g/day divided every 8 hours
Skin and skin structure infections (complicated): 500 mg every 8 hours; diabetic foot: 1 g every 8 hours

Dosage Forms Injection, powder for reconstitution: 500 mg [contains sodium 45.1 mg as sodium carbonate (1.96 mEq)]; 1 g [contains sodium 90.2 mg as sodium carbonate (3.92 mEq)]

Merrem® [Can] *see* meropenem *on previous page*

Merrem® I.V. [US] *see* meropenem *on previous page*

Mersol® [US-OTC] *see* thimerosal *on page 822*

Mersyndol® With Codeine [Can] *see* acetaminophen, codeine, and doxylamine *(Canada Only)* *on page 12*

Merthiolate® [US-OTC] *see* thimerosal *on page 822*

Meruvax® II [US] *see* rubella virus vaccine (live) *on page 756*

mesalamine (me SAL a meen)

Sound-Alike/Look-Alike Issues

mesalamine may be confused with mecamylamine
Asacol® may be confused with Ansaid®, Os-Cal®

Synonyms 5-aminosalicylic acid; 5-ASA; fisalamine; mesalazine

U.S./Canadian Brand Names Asacol® 800 [Can]; Asacol® [US/Can]; Canasa™ [US]; Mesasal® [Can]; Novo-5 ASA [Can]; Pendo-5 ASA [Can]; Pentasa® [US/Can]; Quintasa® [Can]; Rowasa® [US/Can]; Salofalk® [Can]

Therapeutic Category 5-Aminosalicylic Acid Derivative

Use

Oral: Treatment and maintenance of remission of mildly to moderately active ulcerative colitis
Rectal: Treatment of active mild to moderate distal ulcerative colitis, proctosigmoiditis, or proctitis

Usual Dosage Adults (usual course of therapy is 3-8 weeks):

Oral:

Treatment of ulcerative colitis:
Capsule: 1 g 4 times/day
Tablet: Initial: 800 mg (2 tablets) 3 times/day for 6 weeks

Maintenance of remission of ulcerative colitis:
Capsule: 1 g 4 times/day
Tablet: 1.6 g/day in divided doses

Rectal:

Retention enema: 60 mL (4 g) at bedtime, retained overnight, approximately 8 hours
Rectal suppository (Canasa™):
500 mg: Insert 1 suppository in rectum twice daily; may increase to 3 times/day if inadequate response is seen after 2 weeks
1000 mg: Insert 1 suppository in rectum daily at bedtime
Note: Suppositories should be retained for at least 1-3 hours to achieve maximum benefit.

Note: Some patients may require rectal and oral therapy concurrently.

Dosage Forms

Capsule, controlled release (Pentasa®): 250 mg, 500 mg
Suppository, rectal (Canasa™): 500 mg [DSC], 1000 mg [contains saturated vegetable fatty acid esters]
Suspension, rectal: 4 g/60 mL (7s, 28s) [contains potassium metabisulfite and sodium benzoate]
Rowasa®: 4 g/60 mL (7s, 28s) [contains potassium metabisulfite and sodium benzoate]
Tablet, delayed release [enteric coated] (Asacol®): 400 mg

mesalazine *see* mesalamine *on previous page*

Mesasal® [Can] *see* mesalamine *on previous page*

M-Eslon® [Can] *see* morphine sulfate *on page 565*

mesna (MES na)

Synonyms sodium 2-mercaptoethane sulfonate

U.S./Canadian Brand Names Mesnex® [US/Can]; Uromitexan [Can]

Therapeutic Category Antidote

Use Orphan drug: Prevention of hemorrhagic cystitis induced by ifosfamide

Usual Dosage Children and Adults (refer to individual protocols):

I.V.: Recommended dose is 60% of the ifosfamide dose given in 3 divided doses (0, 4, and 8 hours after the start of ifosfamide)

Alternative I.V. regimens include 80% of the ifosfamide dose given in 4 divided doses (0, 3, 6, and 9 hours after the start of ifosfamide) and continuous infusions

I.V./Oral: Recommended dose is 100% of the ifosfamide dose, given as 20% of the ifosfamide dose I.V. at hour 0, followed by 40% of the ifosfamide dose given orally 2 and 6 hours after start of ifosfamide

Dosage Forms

Injection, solution: 100 mg/mL (10 mL) [contains benzyl alcohol]

Tablet: 400 mg

Mesnex® [US/Can] *see* mesna *on this page*

Mestinon® [US/Can] *see* pyridostigmine *on page 720*

Mestinon® Injection *(Discontinued)* *see* pyridostigmine *on page 720*

Mestinon®-SR [Can] *see* pyridostigmine *on page 720*

Mestinon® Timespan® [US] *see* pyridostigmine *on page 720*

mestranol and norethindrone (MES tra nole & nor eth IN drone)

Sound-Alike/Look-Alike Issues

Norinyl® may be confused with Nardil®

Synonyms norethindrone and mestranol

U.S./Canadian Brand Names Necon® 1/50 [US]; Norinyl® 1+50 [US]; Ortho-Novum® 1/50 [US]

Therapeutic Category Contraceptive, Oral

Use Prevention of pregnancy

Usual Dosage Oral: Adults: Female: Contraception:

Schedule 1 (Sunday starter): Dose begins on first Sunday after onset of menstruation; if the menstrual period starts on Sunday, take first tablet that very same day. **With a Sunday start, an additional method of contraception should be used until after the first 7 days of consecutive administration.**

For 21-tablet package: Dosage is 1 tablet daily for 21 consecutive days, followed by 7 days off of the medication; a new course begins on the 8th day after the last tablet is taken.

For 28-tablet package: Dosage is 1 tablet daily without interruption.

Schedule 2 (Day 1 starter): Dose starts on first day of menstrual cycle taking 1 tablet daily.

For 21-tablet package: Dosage is 1 tablet daily for 21 consecutive days, followed by 7 days off of the medication; a new course begins on the 8th day after the last tablet is taken.

For 28-tablet package: Dosage is 1 tablet daily without interruption.

If all doses have been taken on schedule and one menstrual period is missed, continue dosing cycle. If two consecutive menstrual periods are missed, pregnancy test is required before new dosing cycle is started.

Missed doses **monophasic formulations** (refer to package insert for complete information):

One dose missed: Take as soon as remembered or take 2 tablets next day

Two consecutive doses missed in the first 2 weeks: Take 2 tablets as soon as remembered or 2 tablets next 2 days. **An additional method of contraception should be used for 7 days after missed dose.**

Two consecutive doses missed in week 3 or three consecutive doses missed at any time: **An additional method of contraception must be used for 7 days after a missed dose:**

Schedule 1 (Sunday starter): Continue dose of 1 tablet daily until Sunday, then discard the rest of the pack, and a new pack should be started that same day.

Schedule 2 (Day 1 starter): Current pack should be discarded, and a new pack should be started that same day.

Dosage Forms Tablet, monophasic formulations:

Necon® 1/50: Norethindrone 1 mg and mestranol 0.05 mg [21 light blue tablets and 7 white inactive tablets] (28s)

Norinyl® 1+50: Norethindrone 1 mg and mestranol 0.05 mg [21 white tablets and 7 orange inactive tablets] (28s)

Ortho-Novum® 1/50: Norethindrone 1 mg and mestranol 0.05 mg [21 yellow tablets and 7 green inactive tablets] (28s)

metacortandralone *see* prednisolone (systemic) *on page 695*

Metadate® CD [US] *see* methylphenidate *on page 546*

Metadate® ER [US] *see* methylphenidate *on page 546*

Metadol™ [Can] *see* methadone *on page 537*

Metaglip™ [US] *see* glipizide and metformin *on page 385*

Metamucil® [US-OTC/Can] *see* psyllium *on page 717*

Metamucil® Plus Calcium [US-OTC] *see* psyllium *on page 717*

Metamucil® Smooth Texture [US-OTC] *see* psyllium *on page 717*

metaproterenol (met a proe TER e nol)

Sound-Alike/Look-Alike Issues
metaproterenol may be confused with metipranolol, metoprolol
Alupent® may be confused with Atrovent®

Synonyms metaproterenol sulfate; orciprenaline sulfate

U.S./Canadian Brand Names Alupent® [US]; Apo-Orciprenaline® [Can]; Ratio-Orciprenaline® [Can]; Tanta-Orciprenaline® [Can]

Therapeutic Category Adrenergic Agonist Agent

Use Bronchodilator in reversible airway obstruction due to asthma or COPD; because of its delayed onset of action (1 hour) and prolonged effect (4 or more hours), this may not be the drug of choice for assessing response to a bronchodilator

Usual Dosage
Oral:
Children:
<2 years: 0.4 mg/kg/dose given 3-4 times/day; in infants, the dose can be given every 8-12 hours
2-6 years: 1-2.6 mg/kg/day divided every 6 hours
6-9 years: 10 mg/dose 3-4 times/day
Children >9 years and Adults: 20 mg 3-4 times/day
Inhalation: Children >12 years and Adults: 2-3 inhalations every 3-4 hours, up to 12 inhalations in 24 hours
Nebulizer:
Infants and Children: 0.01-0.02 mL/kg of 5% solution; minimum dose: 0.1 mL; maximum dose: 0.3 mL diluted in 2-3 mL normal saline every 4-6 hours (may be given more frequently according to need)
Adolescents and Adults: 5-20 breaths of full strength 5% metaproterenol **or** 0.2 to 0.3 mL 5% metaproterenol in 2.5-3 mL normal saline until nebulized every 4-6 hours (can be given more frequently according to need)

Dosage Forms
Aerosol for oral inhalation, as sulfate (Alupent®): 0.65 mg/inhalation (14 g) [200 doses]
Solution for nebulization, as sulfate [preservative free]: 0.4% [4 mg/mL] (2.5 mL); 0.6% [6 mg/mL] (2.5 mL)
Syrup, as sulfate: 10 mg/5 mL (480 mL) [may contain sodium benzoate]
Tablet, as sulfate: 10 mg, 20 mg

metaproterenol sulfate *see* metaproterenol *on this page*

Metasep® ***(Discontinued)***

Metastron® [US/Can] *see* strontium-89 *on page 792*

metaxalone (me TAKS a lone)

Sound-Alike/Look-Alike Issues
metaxalone may be confused with metolazone

U.S./Canadian Brand Names Skelaxin® [US/Can]

Therapeutic Category Skeletal Muscle Relaxant

Use Relief of discomfort associated with acute, painful musculoskeletal conditions

Usual Dosage Children >12 years and Adults: Oral: 800 mg 3-4 times/day

Dosage Forms [DSC] = Discontinued product
Tablet: 400 mg [DSC], 800 mg

metformin (met FOR min)

Sound-Alike/Look-Alike Issues
metformin may be confused with metronidazole
Glucophage® may be confused with Glucotrol®, Glutofac®

(Continued)

metformin *(Continued)*

Synonyms metformin hydrochloride

U.S./Canadian Brand Names Alti-Metformin [Can]; Apo-Metformin® [Can]; BCI-Metformin [Can]; Fortamet™ [US]; Gen-Metformin [Can]; Glucophage® XR [US]; Glucophage® [US/Can]; Glumetza™ [US/Can]; Glycon [Can]; Novo-Metformin [Can]; Nu-Metformin [Can]; PMS-Metformin [Can]; RAN™-Metformin [Can]; ratio-Metformin [Can]; Rho®-Metformin [Can]; Riomet™ [US]; Sandoz-Metformin FC [Can]

Therapeutic Category Antidiabetic Agent, Oral

Use Management of type 2 diabetes mellitus (noninsulin dependent, NIDDM) as monotherapy when hyperglycemia cannot be managed on diet alone. May be used concomitantly with a sulfonylurea or insulin to improve glycemic control.

Usual Dosage Note: Allow 1-2 weeks between dose titrations: Generally, clinically significant responses are not seen at doses <1500 mg daily; however, a lower recommended starting dose and gradual increased dosage is recommended to minimize gastrointestinal symptoms

Children 10-16 years: Management of type 2 diabetes mellitus: Oral (500 mg tablet or oral solution): Initial: 500 mg twice daily (given with the morning and evening meals); increases in daily dosage should be made in increments of 500 mg at weekly intervals, given in divided doses, up to a maximum of 2000 mg/day

Adults ≥17 years: Management of type 2 diabetes mellitus: Oral:

Immediate release tablet or oral solution: Initial: 500 mg twice daily (give with the morning and evening meals) **or** 850 mg once daily; increase dosage incrementally.

Incremental dosing recommendations based on dosage form:

500 mg tablet: One tablet/day at weekly intervals
850 mg tablet: One tablet/day every other week
Oral solution: 500 mg twice daily every other week

Doses of up to 2000 mg/day may be given twice daily. If a dose >2000 mg/day is required, it may be better tolerated in three divided doses. Maximum recommended dose 2550 mg/day.

Extended release tablet: Initial: 500 mg once daily (with the evening meal); dosage may be increased by 500 mg weekly; maximum dose: 2000 mg once daily. If glycemic control is not achieved at maximum dose, may divide dose to 1000 mg twice daily. If doses >2000 mg/day are needed, switch to regular release tablets and titrate to maximum dose of 2550 mg/day.

Transfer from other antidiabetic agents: No transition period is generally necessary except when transferring from chlorpropamide. When transferring from chlorpropamide, care should be exercised during the first 2 weeks because of the prolonged retention of chlorpropamide in the body, leading to overlapping drug effects and possible hypoglycemia.

Concomitant metformin and oral sulfonylurea therapy: If patients have not responded to 4 weeks of the maximum dose of metformin monotherapy, consider a gradual addition of an oral sulfonylurea, even if prior primary or secondary failure to a sulfonylurea has occurred. Continue metformin at the maximum dose.

Failed sulfonylurea therapy: Patients with prior failure on glyburide may be treated by gradual addition of metformin. Initiate with glyburide 20 mg and metformin 500 mg daily. Metformin dosage may be increased by 500 mg/day at weekly intervals, up to a maximum of 2500 mg/day (dosage of glyburide maintained at 20 mg/day).

Concomitant metformin and insulin therapy: Initial: 500 mg metformin once daily, continue current insulin dose; increase by 500 mg metformin weekly until adequate glycemic control is achieved

Maximum dose: 2500 mg metformin; 2000 mg metformin extended release

Decrease insulin dose 10% to 25% when FPG <120 mg/dL; monitor and make further adjustments as needed

Dosage Forms

Solution, oral, as hydrochloride:
Riomet™: 100 mg/mL (118 mL, 473 mL) [contains saccharin; cherry flavor]
Tablet, as hydrochloride: 500 mg, 850 mg, 1000 mg
Glucophage®: 500 mg, 850 mg, 1000 mg
Tablet, extended release, as hydrochloride: 500 mg, 750 mg
Fortamet®: 500 mg, 1000 mg
Glucophage® XR: 500 mg, 750 mg
Glumetza™: 500 mg

metformin and glipizide *see* glipizide and metformin *on page 385*

metformin and glyburide *see* glyburide and metformin *on page 388*

metformin and rosiglitazone *see* rosiglitazone and metformin *on page 754*

metformin hydrochloride *see* metformin *on previous page*

metformin hydrochloride and rosiglitazone maleate *see* rosiglitazone and metformin *on page 754*

methacholine (meth a KOLE leen)

Synonyms methacholine chloride

U.S./Canadian Brand Names Methacholine Omega [Can]; Provocholine® [US/Can]

Therapeutic Category Diagnostic Agent

Use Diagnosis of bronchial airway hyperactivity

Usual Dosage Before inhalation challenge, perform baseline pulmonary function tests; the patient must have an FEV_1 of at least 70% of the predicted value. The following is a suggested schedule for administration of methacholine challenge. Calculate cumulative units by multiplying number of breaths by concentration given. Total cumulative units is the sum of cumulative units for each concentration given. See table.

Methacholine

Vial	Serial Concentration (mg/mL)	No. of Breaths	Cumulative Units per Concentration	Total Cumulative Units
E	0.025	5	0.125	0.125
D	0.25	5	1.25	1.375
C	2.5	5	12.5	13.88
B	10	5	50	63.88
A	25	5	125	188.88

Dosage Forms Powder for oral inhalation, as chloride: 100 mg

methacholine chloride *see* methacholine *on this page*

Methacholine Omega [Can] *see* methacholine *on this page*

methadone (METH a done)

Sound-Alike/Look-Alike Issues

methadone may be confused with Mephyton®, methylphenidate

Synonyms methadone hydrochloride

U.S./Canadian Brand Names Dolophine® [US/Can]; Metadol™ [Can]; Methadone Diskets® [US]; Methadone Intensol™ [US]; Methadose® [US/Can]

Therapeutic Category Analgesic, Narcotic

Controlled Substance C-II

Use Management of severe pain; detoxification and maintenance treatment of narcotic addiction (if used for detoxification and maintenance treatment of narcotic addiction, it must be part of an FDA-approved program)

Usual Dosage Regulations regarding methadone use may vary by state and/or country. Obtain advice from appropriate regulatory agencies and/or consult with pain management/palliative care specialists. **Note:** These are guidelines and do not represent the maximum doses that may be required in all patients. Methadone accumulates with repeated doses and dosage may need reduction after 3-5 days to prevent CNS depressant effects. Some patients may benefit from every 8-12 hour dosing interval for chronic pain management. Doses should be titrated to appropriate effects.

Adults:

Pain (analgesia):

Oral: Initial: 5-10 mg; dosing interval may range from 4-12 hours during initial therapy; decrease in dose or frequency may be required (~days 2-5) due to accumulation with repeated doses

Manufacturer's labeling: 2.5-10 mg every 3-4 hours as needed

I.V.: Manufacturers labeling: Initial: 2.5-10 mg every 8-12 hours in opioid-naive patients; titrate slowly to effect; may also be administered by SubQ or I.M. injection

Conversion from oral to parenteral dose: Initial dose: Oral: parenteral: 2:1 ratio

Detoxification: Oral:

Initial: Should not exceed 30 mg; lower doses should be considered in patients with low tolerance at initiation (eg, absence of opioids ≥5 days); an additional 5-10 mg of methadone may be provided if withdrawal symptoms have not been suppressed or if symptoms reappear after 2-4 hours; total daily dose on the first day should not exceed 40 mg, unless the program physician documents in the patient's record that 40 mg did not control opiate abstinence symptoms.

Maintenance: Usual range: 80-120 mg/day (titration should occur cautiously)

Withdrawal: Dose reductions should be <10% of the maintenance dose, every 10-14 days

Detoxification (short-term): Oral:

Initial: Titrate to 40 mg/day in 2 divided doses

(Continued)

methadone *(Continued)*

Maintenance: Continue 40 mg dose for 2-3 days
Withdrawal: Decrease daily or every other day, keeping withdrawal symptoms tolerable; hospitalized patients may tolerate a 20% reduction/day; ambulatory patients may require a slower reduction

Dosage Forms
Injection, solution, as hydrochloride: 10 mg/mL (20 mL)
Solution, oral, as hydrochloride: 5 mg/5 mL (500 mL); 10 mg/5 mL (500 mL) [contains alcohol 8%; citrus flavor]
Solution, oral concentrate, as hydrochloride: 10 mg/mL (946 mL)
Methadone Intensol™: 10 mg/mL (30 mL)
Methadose®: 10 mg/mL (1000 mL) [cherry flavor]
Methadose®: 10 mg/mL (1000 mL) [dye free, sugar free, unflavored]
Tablet, as hydrochloride (Dolophine®, Methadose®): 5 mg, 10 mg
Tablet, dispersible, as hydrochloride:
Methadose®: 40 mg
Methadone Diskets®: 40 mg [orange-pineapple flavor]

Methadone Diskets® [US] *see* methadone *on previous page*

methadone hydrochloride *see* methadone *on previous page*

Methadone Intensol™ [US] *see* methadone *on previous page*

Methadose® [US/Can] *see* methadone *on previous page*

methaminodiazepoxide hydrochloride *see* chlordiazepoxide *on page 172*

methamphetamine (meth am FET a meen)

Sound-Alike/Look-Alike Issues
Desoxyn® may be confused with digoxin

Synonyms desoxyephedrine hydrochloride; methamphetamine hydrochloride

U.S./Canadian Brand Names Desoxyn® [US/Can]

Therapeutic Category Amphetamine

Controlled Substance C-II

Use Treatment of attention-deficit/hyperactivity disorder (ADHD); exogenous obesity (short-term adjunct)

Usual Dosage Oral:
Children >6 years and Adults: ADHD: 2.5-5 mg 1-2 times/day; may increase by 5 mg increments at weekly intervals until optimum response is achieved, usually 20-25 mg/day
Children >12 years and Adults: Exogenous obesity: 5 mg 30 minutes before each meal; treatment duration should not exceed a few weeks

Dosage Forms Tablet, as hydrochloride: 5 mg

methamphetamine hydrochloride *see* methamphetamine *on this page*

methazolamide (meth a ZOE la mide)

Sound-Alike/Look-Alike Issues
methazolamide may be confused with methenamine, metolazone
Neptazane® may be confused with Nesacaine®

U.S./Canadian Brand Names Apo-Methazolamide® [Can]

Therapeutic Category Carbonic Anhydrase Inhibitor

Use Adjunctive treatment of open-angle or secondary glaucoma; short-term therapy of narrow-angle glaucoma when delay of surgery is desired

Usual Dosage Adults: Oral: 50-100 mg 2-3 times/day

Dosage Forms Tablet: 25 mg, 50 mg

methenamine (meth EN a meen)

Sound-Alike/Look-Alike Issues
methenamine may be confused with methazolamide, methionine
Urex® may be confused with Eurax®, Serax®

Synonyms hexamethylenetetramine; methenamine hippurate; methenamine mandelate

U.S./Canadian Brand Names Dehydral® [Can]; Hiprex® [US/Can]; Mandelamine® [US/Can]; Urasal® [Can]; Urex® [US/Can]

Therapeutic Category Antibiotic, Miscellaneous

Use Prophylaxis or suppression of recurrent urinary tract infections; urinary tract discomfort secondary to hypermotility

Usual Dosage Oral:

Children:

>2-6 years: *Mandelate:* 50-75 mg/kg/day in 3-4 doses or 0.25 g/30 lb 4 times/day

6-12 years:

Hippurate: 0.5-1 g twice daily

Mandelate: 50-75 mg/kg/day in 3-4 doses or 0.5 g 4 times/day

Children >12 years and Adults:

Hippurate: 0.5-1 g twice daily

Mandelate: 1 g 4 times/day after meals and at bedtime

Dosage Forms

Tablet, as hippurate (Hiprex®, Urex®): 1 g [Hiprex® contains tartrazine dye]

Tablet, enteric coated, as mandelate (Mandelamine®): 500 mg, 1 g

methenamine hippurate *see* methenamine *on previous page*

methenamine mandelate *see* methenamine *on previous page*

methenamine, phenyl salicylate, atropine, hyoscyamine, benzoic acid, and methylene blue

(meth EN a meen, fen nil sa LIS i late, A troe peen, hye oh SYE a meen, ben ZOE ik AS id, & METH i leen bloo)

U.S./Canadian Brand Names Atrosept® [US]; Dolsed® [US]; UAA® [US]; Urelle® [US]; Uridon Modified® [US]; Urised® [US]; Uritin® [US]

Therapeutic Category Antibiotic, Urinary Antiinfective; Urinary Tract Product

Use Urinary tract infections

Usual Dosage Adults: Oral: Two tablets 4 times/day

Dosage Forms Tablet: Methenamine 40.8 mg, phenyl salicylate 18.1 mg, atropine sulfate 0.03 mg, hyoscyamine sulfate 0.03 mg, benzoic acid 4.5 mg, and methylene blue 5.4 mg

Methergine® [US/Can] *see* methylergonovine *on page 545*

methimazole (meth IM a zole)

Sound-Alike/Look-Alike Issues

methimazole may be confused with metolazone

Synonyms thiamazole

U.S./Canadian Brand Names Dom-Methimazole [Can]; PHL-Methimazole [Can]; Tapazole® [US/Can]

Therapeutic Category Antithyroid Agent

Use Palliative treatment of hyperthyroidism, return the hyperthyroid patient to a normal metabolic state prior to thyroidectomy, and to control thyrotoxic crisis that may accompany thyroidectomy. The use of antithyroid thioamides is as effective in elderly as they are in younger adults; however, the expense, potential adverse effects, and inconvenience (compliance, monitoring) make them undesirable. The use of radioiodine due to ease of administration and less concern for long-term side effects and reproduction problems (some older males) makes it a more appropriate therapy.

Usual Dosage Oral: Administer in 3 equally divided doses at approximately 8-hour intervals

Children: Initial: 0.4 mg/kg/day in 3 divided doses; maintenance: 0.2 mg/kg/day in 3 divided doses up to 30 mg/24 hours maximum

Alternatively: Initial: 0.5-0.7 mg/kg/day **or** 15-20 mg/m^2/day in 3 divided doses

Maintenance: $^1/_3$ to $^2/_3$ of the initial dose beginning when the patient is euthyroid

Maximum: 30 mg/24 hours

Adults: Initial: 15 mg/day for mild hyperthyroidism; 30-40 mg/day in moderately severe hyperthyroidism; 60 mg/day in severe hyperthyroidism; maintenance: 5-15 mg/day

Adjust dosage as required to achieve and maintain serum T_3, T_4, and TSH levels in the normal range. An elevated T_3 may be the sole indicator of inadequate treatment. An elevated TSH indicates excessive antithyroid treatment.

Dosage Forms

Tablet: 5 mg, 10 mg, 20 mg

Tapazole® 5 mg, 10 mg

Methitest™ [US] *see* methyltestosterone *on page 548*

methocarbamol (meth oh KAR ba mole)

Sound-Alike/Look-Alike Issues

methocarbamol may be confused with mephobarbital

Robaxin® may be confused with Rubex®

(Continued)

methocarbamol *(Continued)*

U.S./Canadian Brand Names Robaxin® [US/Can]

Therapeutic Category Skeletal Muscle Relaxant

Use Treatment of muscle spasm associated with acute painful musculoskeletal conditions; supportive therapy in tetanus

Usual Dosage

Tetanus: I.V.:

Children: Recommended **only** for use in tetanus: 15 mg/kg/dose or 500 mg/m^2/dose, may repeat every 6 hours if needed; maximum dose: 1.8 g/m^2/day for 3 days only

Adults: Initial dose: 1-3 g; may repeat dose every 6 hours until oral dosing is possible; injection should not be used for more than 3 consecutive days

Muscle spasm: Children ≥16 years and Adults:

Oral: 1.5 g 4 times/day for 2-3 days (up to 8 g/day may be given in severe conditions), then decrease to 4-4.5 g/day in 3-6 divided doses

I.M., I.V.: 1 g every 8 hours if oral not possible; injection should not be used for more than 3 consecutive days. If condition persists, may repeat course of therapy after a drug-free interval of 48 hours.

Dosage Forms

Injection, solution: 100 mg/mL (10 mL) [in polyethylene glycol; vial stopper contains latex]

Tablet: 500 mg, 750 mg

methohexital (meth oh HEKS i tal)

Sound-Alike/Look-Alike Issues

Brevital® may be confused with Brevibloc®

Synonyms methohexital sodium

U.S./Canadian Brand Names Brevital® Sodium [US]; Brevital® [Can]

Therapeutic Category Barbiturate

Controlled Substance C-IV

Use Induction and maintenance of general anesthesia for short procedures

Can be used in pediatric patients ≥1 month of age as follows: For rectal or intramuscular induction of anesthesia prior to the use of other general anesthetic agents, as an adjunct to subpotent inhalational anesthetic agents for short surgical procedures, or for short surgical, diagnostic, or therapeutic procedures associated with minimal painful stimuli

Usual Dosage Doses must be titrated to effect

Manufacturer's recommendations:

Infants <1 month: Safety and efficacy not established

Infants ≥1 month and Children:

I.M.: Induction: 6.6-10 mg/kg of a 5% solution

Rectal: Induction: Usual: 25 mg/kg of a 1% solution

Alternative pediatric dosing:

Children 3-12 years:

I.M.: Preoperative: 5-10 mg/kg/dose

I.V.: Induction: 1-2 mg/kg/dose

Rectal: Preoperative/induction: 20-35 mg/kg/dose; usual: 25 mg/kg/dose; maximum dose: 500 mg/dose; give as 10% aqueous solution

Adults: I.V.: Induction: 50-120 mg to start; 20-40 mg every 4-7 minutes

Dosage Forms Injection, powder for reconstitution, as sodium: 500 mg, 2.5 g, 5 g

methohexital sodium *see* methohexital *on this page*

methotrexate (meth oh TREKS ate)

Sound-Alike/Look-Alike Issues

methotrexate may be confused with metolazone, mitoxantrone

MTX is an error-prone abbreviation (mistaken as mitoxantrone)

Synonyms amethopterin; methotrexate sodium; NSC-740

U.S./Canadian Brand Names Apo-Methotrexate® [Can]; ratio-Methotrexate [Can]; Rheumatrex® [US]; Trexall™ [US]

Therapeutic Category Antineoplastic Agent

Use Treatment of trophoblastic neoplasms; leukemias; psoriasis; rheumatoid arthritis (RA), including polyarticular-course juvenile rheumatoid arthritis (JRA); breast, head and neck, and lung carcinomas; osteosarcoma; soft-tissue sarcomas; carcinoma of gastrointestinal tract, esophagus, testes; lymphomas

Usual Dosage Refer to individual protocols.

Note: Doses between 100-500 mg/m^2 **may require** leucovorin rescue. Doses >500 mg/m^2 **require** leucovorin rescue: Oral, I.M., I.V.: Leucovorin 10-15 mg/m^2 every 6 hours for 8 or 10 doses, starting 24 hours after the start of methotrexate infusion. Continue until the methotrexate level is ≤0.1 micromolar (10^{-7}M). Some clinicians continue leucovorin until the methotrexate level is <0.05 micromolar (5 x 10^{-8}M) or 0.01 micromolar (10^{-8}M).

If the 48-hour methotrexate level is >1 micromolar (10^{-7}M) or the 72-hour methotrexate level is >0.2 micromolar (2 x 10^{-7}M): I.V., I.M, Oral: Leucovorin 100 mg/m^2 every 6 hours until the methotrexate level is ≤0.1 micromolar (10^{-7}M). Some clinicians continue leucovorin until the methotrexate level is <0.05 micromolar (5 x 10^{-8}M) or 0.01 micromolar (10^{-8}M).

Children:
- Dermatomyositis: Oral: 15-20 mg/m^2/week as a single dose once weekly **or** 0.3-1 mg/kg/dose once weekly
- Juvenile rheumatoid arthritis: Oral, I.M.: 10 mg/m^2 once weekly, then 5-15 mg/m^2/week as a single dose **or** as 3 divided doses given 12 hours apart
- Antineoplastic dosage range:
  - Oral, I.M.: 7.5-30 mg/m^2/week **or** every 2 weeks
  - I.V.: 10-18,000 mg/m^2 bolus dosing **or** continuous infusion over 6-42 hours
  - Dosing schedule: **Note:** Doses between 100-500 mg/m^2 may require leucovorin rescue in some patients:
    - Conventional dose:
      - 15-20 mg/m^2 oral twice weekly
      - 30-50 mg/m^2 oral, I.V. weekly
      - 15 mg/day for 5 days oral, I.M. every 2-3 weeks
    - Intermediate dose:
      - 50-150 mg/m^2 I.V. push every 2-3 weeks
      - 240 mg/m^2 I.V. infusion every 4-7 days
      - 0.5-1 g/m^2 (followed with leucovorin rescue - refer to leucovorin monograph) I.V. infusion every 2-3 weeks
    - High dose: 1-25 g/m^2 I.V. infusion every 1-3 weeks
- Pediatric solid tumors (high-dose): I.V.:
  - <12 years: 12-25 g/m^2
  - ≥12 years: 8 g/m^2
- Acute lymphocytic leukemia (intermediate-dose): I.V.: Loading: 100 mg/m^2 bolus dose, followed by 900 mg/m^2/day infusion over 23-41 hours.
- Meningeal leukemia: I.T.: 10-15 mg/m^2 (maximum dose: 15 mg) **or** an age-based dosing regimen; one possible system is:
  - ≤3 months: 3 mg/dose
  - 4-11 months: 6 mg/dose
  - 1 year: 8 mg/dose
  - 2 years: 10 mg/dose
  - ≥3 years: 12 mg/dose

Adults: I.V.: Range is wide from 30-40 mg/m^2/week to 100-12,000 mg/m^2 with leucovorin rescue
- Trophoblastic neoplasms:
  - Oral, I.M.: 15-30 mg/day for 5 days; repeat in 7 days for 3-5 courses
  - I.V.: 11 mg/m^2 days 1 through 5 every 3 weeks
- Head and neck cancer: Oral, I.M., I.V.: 25-50 mg/m^2 once weekly
- Mycosis fungoides (cutaneous T-cell lymphoma): Oral, I.M.: Initial (early stages):
  - 5-50 mg once weekly **or**
  - 15-37.5 mg twice weekly
- Bladder cancer: I.V.:
  - 30 mg/m^2 day 1 and 8 every 3 weeks **or**
  - 30 mg/m^2 day 1, 15, and 22 every 4 weeks
- Breast cancer: I.V.: 30-60 mg/m^2 days 1 and 8 every 3-4 weeks
- Gastric cancer: I.V.:1500 mg/m^2 every 4 weeks
- Lymphoma, non-Hodgkin's: I.V.:
  - 30 mg/m^2 days 3 and 10 every 3 weeks **or**
  - 120 mg/m^2 day 8 and 15 every 3-4 weeks **or**
  - 200 mg/m^2 day 8 and 15 every 3 weeks **or**
  - 400 mg/m^2 every 4 weeks for 3 cycles **or**
  - 1 g/m^2 every 3 weeks **or**
  - 1.5 g/m^2 every 4 weeks
- Sarcoma: I.V.: 8-12 g/m^2 weekly for 2-4 weeks

(Continued)

methotrexate *(Continued)*

Rheumatoid arthritis: Oral: 7.5 mg once weekly **or** 2.5 mg every 12 hours for 3 doses/week, not to exceed 20 mg/week

Psoriasis:

Oral: 2.5-5 mg/dose every 12 hours for 3 doses given weekly **or**

Oral, I.M.: 10-25 mg/dose given once weekly

Dosage Forms

Injection, powder for reconstitution [preservative free]: 20 mg, 1 g

Injection, solution: 25 mg/mL (2 mL, 10 mL) [contains benzyl alcohol]

Injection, solution [preservative free]: 25 mg/mL (2 mL, 4 mL, 8 mL, 10 mL)

Tablet: 2.5 mg

Trexall™: 5 mg, 7.5 mg, 10 mg, 15 mg

Tablet, as sodium [dose pack] (Rheumatrex® Dose Pack): 2.5 mg (4 cards with 2, 3, 4, 5, or 6 tablets each)

methotrexate sodium *see* methotrexate *on page 540*

methotrimeprazine *(Canada only)* (meth oh trye MEP ra zeen)

Synonyms levomepromazine; methotrimeprazine hydrochloride

U.S./Canadian Brand Names Apo-Methoprazine® [Can]; Nozinan® [Can]

Therapeutic Category Neuroleptic Agent

Use Treatment of schizophrenia or psychosis; management of pain, including pain caused by neuralgia or cancer; adjunct to general anesthesia; management of nausea and vomiting; sedation

Usual Dosage

Children >2 years:

Oral: 0.25 mg/kg/day in 2-3 divided doses; may increase gradually based on response.

Maximum dose: 40 mg/day in children <12 years

I.M.: 0.06-0.125 mg/kg/day in 1-3 divided doses

Adults:

Oral:

Anxiety, mild-moderate pain: 6-25 mg/day in 3 divided doses

Psychoses, severe pain: 50-75 mg/day in 2-3 divided doses; titrate to effect (doses up to 1000 mg/day or greater have been used in treatment of some patients with psychoses). If higher dosages are used to initiate therapy (100-200 mg/day), patients should be restricted to bed for the first few days of therapy.

Sedative: 10-25 mg at bedtime

I.M.:

Psychoses, severe pain: 75-100 mg (administered in 3-4 deep I.M. injections)

Analgesia (postoperative): 10-25 mg every 8 hours (2.5-7.5 mg every 4-6 hours is suggested postoperatively if residual effects of anesthetic may be present)

Premedication: 10-25 mg every 8 hours (final preoperative dose may be 25-50 mg administered ~1 hour prior to surgery)

I.V.: During surgical procedures/labor: 20-50 mcg/minute (some patients may require up to 100 mcg/minute)

SubQ (continuous infusion): Palliative care: 25-200 mcg/day (via syringe driver)

Dosage Forms

Injection, solution, as hydrochloride: 25 mg/mL (1 mL)

Solution, oral: 5 mg/mL (500 mL) [contains ethanol 2%]

Solution, oral drops: 40 mg/mL (100 mL) [contains ethanol 16.5%]

Tablet, as maleate: 2 mg, 5 mg, 25 mg, 50 mg

methotrimeprazine hydrochloride *see* methotrimeprazine *(Canada only) on this page*

methoxsalen (meth OKS a len)

Synonyms methoxypsoralen; 8-methoxypsoralen

U.S./Canadian Brand Names 8-MOP® [US/Can]; Oxsoralen-Ultra® [US/Can]; Oxsoralen® [US/Can]; Ultramop™ [Can]; Uvadex® [US/Can]

Therapeutic Category Psoralen

Use

Oral: Symptomatic control of severe, recalcitrant disabling psoriasis; repigmentation of idiopathic vitiligo; palliative treatment of skin manifestations of cutaneous T-cell lymphoma (CTCL)

Topical: Repigmentation of idiopathic vitiligo

Extracorporeal: Palliative treatment of skin manifestations of CTCL

Usual Dosage Note: Refer to treatment protocols for UVA exposure guidelines.

Children >12 years and Adults: Vitiligo: Topical: Apply lotion 1-2 hours before exposure to UVA light, no more than once weekly

Adults:

Psoriasis: Oral: 10-70 mg 11/2-2 hours before exposure to UVA light; dose may be repeated 2-3 times per week, based on UVA exposure; doses must be given at least 48 hours apart; dosage is based upon patient's body weight and skin type:

<30 kg: 10 mg
30-50 kg: 20 mg
51-65 kg: 30 mg
66-80 kg: 40 mg
81-90 kg: 50 mg
91-115 kg: 60 mg
>115 kg: 70 mg

Vitiligo: (8-MOP®): Oral: 20 mg 2-4 hours before exposure to UVA light; dose may be repeated based on erythema and tenderness of skin; do not give on 2 consecutive days

CTCL: Extracorporeal (Uvadex®): 200 mcg injected into the photoactivation bag during the collection cycle using the UVAR® photopheresis system (consult user's guide). Treatment schedule: Two consecutive days every 4 weeks for a minimum of 7 treatment cycles

Dosage Forms

Capsule:

8-MOP®: 10 mg [hard-gelatin capsule]

Oxsoralen-Ultra®: 10 mg [soft-gelatin capsule]

Lotion (Oxsoralen®): 1% (30 mL) [contains alcohol 71%]

Solution, for extracorporeal administration (Uvadex®): 20 mcg/mL (10 mL) **[not for injection]**

methoxypsoralen *see* methoxsalen *on previous page*

8-methoxypsoralen *see* methoxsalen *on previous page*

methscopolamine (meth skoe POL a meen)

Synonyms methscopolamine bromide

U.S./Canadian Brand Names Pamine® Forte [US]; Pamine® [US/Can]

Therapeutic Category Anticholinergic Agent

Use Adjunctive therapy in the treatment of peptic ulcer

Usual Dosage Adults: Oral: 2.5 mg 30 minutes before meals or food and 2.5-5 mg at bedtime; may increase dose to 5 mg twice daily

Dosage Forms Tablet, as bromide:

Pamine®: 2.5 mg [lactose free]

Pamine® Forte: 5 mg [lactose free; dosepak]

methscopolamine bromide *see* methscopolamine *on this page*

methscopolamine nitrate, chlorpheniramine maleate, and phenylephrine hydrochloride *see* chlorpheniramine, phenylephrine, and methscopolamine *on page 180*

methsuximide (meth SUKS i mide)

Sound-Alike/Look-Alike Issues

methsuximide may be confused with ethosuximide

U.S./Canadian Brand Names Celontin® [US/Can]

Therapeutic Category Anticonvulsant

Use Control of absence (petit mal) seizures that are refractory to other drugs

Usual Dosage Oral: Anticonvulsant:

Children: Initial: 10-15 mg/kg/day in 3-4 divided doses; increase weekly up to maximum of 30 mg/kg/day

Adults: 300 mg/day for the first week; may increase by 300 mg/day at weekly intervals up to 1.2 g/day in 2-4 divided doses/day

Dosage Forms Capsule: 150 mg, 300 mg

methyclothiazide (meth i kloe THYE a zide)

Sound-Alike/Look-Alike Issues

Enduron® may be confused with Empirin®, Imuran®, Inderal®

(Continued)

methyclothiazide *(Continued)*

U.S./Canadian Brand Names Aquatensen® [Can]; Enduron® [Can]

Therapeutic Category Diuretic, Thiazide

Use Management of mild to moderate hypertension; treatment of edema in congestive heart failure and nephrotic syndrome

Usual Dosage Adults: Oral:

Edema: 2.5-10 mg/day

Hypertension: 2.5-5 mg/day; may add another antihypertensive if 5 mg is not adequate after a trial of 8-12 weeks of therapy

Dosage Forms Tablet: 5 mg

methylacetoxyprogesterone *see* medroxyprogesterone *on page 524*

methylbenzethonium chloride (meth il ben ze THOE nee um KLOR ide)

U.S./Canadian Brand Names Diaparene® [US-OTC]; Puri-Clens™ [US-OTC]

Therapeutic Category Topical Skin Product

Use Treatment of diaper rash and ammonia dermatitis

Usual Dosage Topical: Apply to area as needed

Dosage Forms

Cream, topical: 0.1% (30 g, 60 g, 120 g)

Ointment, topical: 0.1% (30 g, 60 g, 120 g)

Powder, topical: 0.055% (120 g, 270 g, 420 g)

methylcellulose (meth il SEL yoo lose)

Sound-Alike/Look-Alike Issues

Citrucel® may be confused with Citracal®

U.S./Canadian Brand Names Citrucel® Fiber Shake [US-OTC]; Citrucel® Fiber Smoothie [US-OTC]; Citrucel® [US-OTC]

Therapeutic Category Laxative

Use Adjunct in treatment of constipation

Usual Dosage Oral:

Children 6-12 years:

Citrucel® caplet: 1 caplet up to 6 times/day; follow each dose with 8 oz of water

Citrucel® powder: Half the adult dose in 4 oz of cold water, 1-3 times/day

Children ≥12 years and Adults:

Citrucel® caplet: 2-4 caplets 1-3 times/day; follow each dose with 8 oz of water

Citrucel® powder: 1 heaping tablespoon (19 g) in 8 oz of cold water, 1-3 times/day

FiberEase™: 2 tablespoonsful mixed in 7 oz of water, 1-3 times/day

Dosage Forms

Caplet:

Citrucel®: 500 mg

Powder: 2 g/level scoop (454 g)

Citrucel® Fiber Smoothie: 2 g/level scoop (275 g, 539 g) [contains sodium 3 mg/level scoop; lemon lime flavor]

Citrucel®:

2 g/level scoop (448 g, 840 g, 1418g, 1843 g) [contains sodium 3 mg and potassium 105 mg per scoop]

2 g/packet (20s) [orange flavor] [DSC]

Citrucel® [sugar free formulation]:

2 g/level scoop (473 g, 907g, 1190 g) [contains phenylalanine 52 mg/level scoop; orange flavor]

2 g/packet (20s) [contains phenylalanine 52 mg/packet; orange flavor] [DSC]

Citrucel® Fiber Shake: 2 g/level scoop (204 g, 413 g) [sugar free; contains sodium 20 mg/level scoop, phenylalanine 49 mg/level scoop and soy lecithin; chocolate flavor]

methylcellulose, gelatin, and pectin *see* gelatin, pectin, and methylcellulose *on page 377*

methyldopa (meth il DOE pa)

Sound-Alike/Look-Alike Issues

methyldopa may be confused with L-dopa, levodopa

Synonyms methyldopate hydrochloride

U.S./Canadian Brand Names Apo-Methyldopa® [Can]; Nu-Medopa [Can]

Therapeutic Category Alpha-Adrenergic Blocking Agent

Use Management of moderate to severe hypertension

Usual Dosage
Children:
Oral: Initial: 10 mg/kg/day in 2-4 divided doses; increase every 2 days as needed to maximum dose of 65 mg/kg/day; do not exceed 3 g/day.
I.V.: 5-10 mg/kg/dose every 6-8 hours up to a total dose of 65 mg/kg/24 hours or 3 g/24 hours
Adults:
Oral: Initial: 250 mg 2-3 times/day; increase every 2 days as needed (maximum dose: 3 g/day): usual dose range (JNC 7): 250-1000 mg/day in 2 divided doses
I.V.: 250-500 mg every 6-8 hours; maximum dose: 1 g every 6 hours

Dosage Forms
Injection, solution, as methyldopate hydrochloride: 50 mg/mL (5 mL) [contains sodium bisulfite]
Tablet: 250 mg, 500 mg

methyldopa and hydrochlorothiazide (meth il DOE pa & hye droe klor oh THYE a zide)

Sound-Alike/Look-Alike Issues
Aldoril® may be confused with Aldoclor®, Aldomet®, Elavil®

Synonyms hydrochlorothiazide and methyldopa

U.S./Canadian Brand Names Aldoril® [US]; Apo-Methazide® [Can]

Therapeutic Category Antihypertensive Agent, Combination

Use Management of moderate to severe hypertension

Usual Dosage Oral: Dosage titrated on individual components, then switch to combination product; no more than methyldopa 3 g/day and/or hydrochlorothiazide 50 mg/day; maintain initial dose for first 48 hours, then decrease or increase at intervals of not less than 2 days until an adequate response is achieved
Methyldopa 250 mg and hydrochlorothiazide 15 mg: 2-3 times/day
Methyldopa 250 mg and hydrochlorothiazide 25 mg: Twice daily

Dosage Forms
Tablet:
Methyldopa 250 mg and hydrochlorothiazide 15 mg
Methyldopa 250 mg and hydrochlorothiazide 25 mg
Aldoril® 25: Methyldopa 250 mg and hydrochlorothiazide 25 mg

methyldopate hydrochloride *see* methyldopa *on previous page*

methylene blue (METH i leen bloo)

U.S./Canadian Brand Names Urolene Blue® [US]

Therapeutic Category Antidote

Use Antidote for cyanide poisoning and drug-induced methemoglobinemia, indicator dye

Usual Dosage
Children: NADPH-methemoglobin reductase deficiency: Oral: 1-1.5 mg/kg/day (maximum: 300 mg/day) given with 5-8 mg/kg/day of ascorbic acid
Children and Adults: Methemoglobinemia: I.V.: 1-2 mg/kg or 25-50 mg/m^2 over several minutes; may be repeated in 1 hour if necessary
Adults: Genitourinary antiseptic: Oral: 65-130 mg 3 times/day with a full glass of water (maximum: 390 mg/day)

Dosage Forms
Injection, solution: 10 mg/mL (1 mL, 10 mL)
Tablet (Urolene Blue®): 65 mg

methylergometrine maleate *see* methylergonovine *on this page*

methylergonovine (meth il er goe NOE veen)

Sound-Alike/Look-Alike Issues
methylergonovine and terbutaline parenteral dosage forms look similar. Due to their contrasting indications, use care when administering these agents.

Synonyms methylergometrine maleate; methylergonovine maleate

U.S./Canadian Brand Names Methergine® [US/Can]

Therapeutic Category Ergot Alkaloid and Derivative

Use Prevention and treatment of postpartum and postabortion hemorrhage caused by uterine atony or subinvolution

Usual Dosage Adults:
Oral: 0.2 mg 3-4 times/day for 2-7 days
(Continued)

methylergonovine *(Continued)*

I.M., I.V.: 0.2 mg after delivery of anterior shoulder, after delivery of placenta, or during puerperium; may be repeated as required at intervals of 2-4 hours

Dosage Forms

Injection, solution, as maleate: 0.2 mg/mL (1 mL)

Tablet, as maleate: 0.2 mg

methylergonovine maleate *see* methylergonovine *on previous page*

Methylin® [US] *see* methylphenidate *on this page*

Methylin® ER [US] *see* methylphenidate *on this page*

methylmorphine *see* codeine *on page 209*

methylphenidate (meth il FEN i date)

Sound-Alike/Look-Alike Issues

methylphenidate may be confused with methadone

Ritalin® may be confused with Ismelin®, Rifadin®

Synonyms methylphenidate hydrochloride

U.S./Canadian Brand Names Apo-Methylphenidate® SR [Can]; Apo-Methylphenidate® [Can]; Biphentin® [Can]; Concerta® [US/Can]; Daytrana™ [US]; Metadate® CD [US]; Metadate® ER [US]; Methylin® ER [US]; Methylin® [US]; PMS-Methylphenidate [Can]; Riphenidate [Can]; Ritalin-SR® [US/Can]; Ritalin® LA [US]; Ritalin® [US/Can]

Therapeutic Category Central Nervous System Stimulant, Nonamphetamine

Controlled Substance C-II

Use Treatment of attention-deficit/hyperactivity disorder (ADHD); symptomatic management of narcolepsy

Usual Dosage

ADHD:

Oral:

Immediate release products Children ≥6 years and Adults: Initial: 5 mg/dose (~0.3 mg/kg/dose) given twice daily before breakfast and lunch; increase by 5-10 mg/day (0.2 mg/kg/day) at weekly intervals; maximum dose: 60 mg/day (2 mg/kg/day). **Note:** Discontinue periodically to re-evaluate or if no improvement occurs within 1 month.

Extended release products:

Children ≥6 years and Adults:

Metadate® ER, Methylin® ER, Ritalin® SR: May be given in place of immediate release products, once the daily dose is titrated and the titrated 8-hour dosage corresponds to sustained or extended release tablet size; maximum: 60 mg/day

Metadate® CD, Ritalin® LA: Initial: 20 mg once daily; may be adjusted in 10-20 mg increments at weekly intervals; maximum: 60 mg/day

Children 6-12 years and Adolescents 13-17 years: *Concerta®:*

Patients not currently taking methylphenidate: Initial dose: 18 mg once daily in the morning

Patients currently taking methylphenidate: **Note:** Initial dose: Dosing based on current regimen and clinical judgment; suggested dosing listed below:

- Patients taking methylphenidate 5 mg 2-3 times/day **or** 20 mg/day sustained release formulation: 18 mg once every morning
- Patients taking methylphenidate 10 mg 2-3 times/day **or** 40 mg/day sustained release formulation: 36 mg once every morning
- Patients taking methylphenidate 15 mg 2-3 times/day **or** 60 mg/day sustained release formulation: 54 mg once every morning

Dose adjustment: May increase dose in increments of 18 mg; dose may be adjusted at weekly intervals. A dosage strength of 27 mg is available for situations in which a dosage between 18-36 mg is desired. Maximum dose should not exceed 2 mg/kg/day **or** 54 mg/day in children 6-12 years or 72 mg/day in children 13-17 years.

Transdermal (Daytrana™): Children 6-12 years: Initial: 10 mg patch once daily; remove up to 9 hours after application. Titrate based on response and tolerability; may increase to next transdermal dose no more frequently than every week. **Note:** Application should occur 2 hours prior to desired effect. Drug absorption may continue for a period of time after patch removal.

Narcolepsy: Oral: Adults: 10 mg 2-3 times/day, up to 60 mg/day

Dosage Forms

Capsule, extended release, as hydrochloride:

Metadate® CD: 10 mg, 20 mg, 30 mg, 40 mg, 50 mg, 60 mg

Ritalin® LA: 10 mg, 20 mg, 30 mg, 40 mg

Solution, oral, as hydrochloride:
Methylin®: 5 mg/5 mL (500 mL) [grape flavor]; 10 mg/5 mL (500 mL) [grape flavor]
Tablet, as hydrochloride: 5 mg, 10 mg, 20 mg
Methylin®, Ritalin®: 5 mg, 10 mg, 20 mg
Tablet, chewable, as hydrochloride:
Methylin®: 2.5 mg [contains phenylalanine 0.42 mg; grape flavor]; 5 mg [contains phenylalanine 0.84 mg; grape flavor]; 10 mg [contains phenylalanine 1.68 mg; grape flavor]
Tablet, extended release, as hydrochloride: 20 mg
Concerta®: 18 mg, 27 mg, 36 mg, 54 mg [osmotic controlled release]
Metadate® ER, Methylin® ER: 10 mg, 20 mg
Tablet, sustained release, as hydrochloride:
Ritalin-SR®: 20 mg [dye free]
Transdermal system [once-daily patch]:
Daytrana™: 10 mg/9 hours (10s, 30s) [12.5 cm^2, total methylphenidate 27.5 mg]; 15 mg/9 hours (10s, 30s) [18.75 cm^2, total methylphenidate 41.3 mg]; 20 mg/9 hours (10s, 30s) [25 cm^2, total methylphenidate 55 mg]; 30 mg/9 hours (10s, 30s) [37.5 cm^2, total methylphenidate 82.5 mg]

methylphenidate hydrochloride *see* methylphenidate *on previous page*

methylphenobarbital *see* mephobarbital *on page 530*

methylphenoxy-benzene propanamine *see* atomoxetine *on page 81*

methylphenyl isoxazolyl penicillin *see* oxacillin *on page 622*

methylphytyl napthoquinone *see* phytonadione *on page 667*

methylprednisolone (meth il pred NIS oh lone)

Sound-Alike/Look-Alike Issues
methylPREDNISolone may be confused with medroxyPROGESTERone, predniSONE
Depo-Medrol® may be confused with Solu-Medrol®
Medrol® may be confused with Inderal®, Mebaral®
Solu-Medrol® may be confused with Depo-Medrol®

Synonyms 6-α-methylprednisolone; A-methapred; methylprednisolone acetate; methylprednisolone sodium succinate

Tall-Man methyl**PREDNIS**olone

U.S./Canadian Brand Names Depo-Medrol® [US/Can]; Medrol® [US/Can]; Solu-Medrol® [US/Can]

Therapeutic Category Adrenal Corticosteroid

Use Primarily as an antiinflammatory or immunosuppressant agent in the treatment of a variety of diseases including those of hematologic, allergic, inflammatory, neoplastic, and autoimmune origin. Prevention and treatment of graft-versus-host disease following allogeneic bone marrow transplantation.

Usual Dosage Dosing should be based on the lesser of ideal body weight or actual body weight

Only sodium succinate may be given I.V.; methylprednisolone sodium succinate is highly soluble and has a rapid effect by I.M. and I.V. routes. Methylprednisolone acetate has a low solubility and has a sustained I.M. effect.

Children:
Antiinflammatory or immunosuppressive: Oral, I.M., I.V. (sodium succinate): 0.5-1.7 mg/kg/day **or** 5-25 mg/m²/day in divided doses every 6-12 hours; "Pulse" therapy: 15-30 mg/kg/dose over ≥30 minutes given once daily for 3 days
Status asthmaticus: I.V. (sodium succinate): Loading dose: 2 mg/kg/dose, then 0.5-1 mg/kg/dose every 6 hours for up to 5 days
Acute spinal cord injury: I.V. (sodium succinate): 30 mg/kg over 15 minutes, followed in 45 minutes by a continuous infusion of 5.4 mg/kg/hour for 23 hours
Lupus nephritis: I.V. (sodium succinate): 30 mg/kg over ≥30 minutes every other day for 6 doses

Adults: **Only sodium succinate may be given I.V.;** methylprednisolone sodium succinate is highly soluble and has a rapid effect by I.M. and I.V. routes. Methylprednisolone acetate has a low solubility and has a sustained I.M. effect.
Acute spinal cord injury: I.V. (sodium succinate): 30 mg/kg over 15 minutes, followed in 45 minutes by a continuous infusion of 5.4 mg/kg/hour for 23 hours
Antiinflammatory or immunosuppressive:
Oral: 2-60 mg/day in 1-4 divided doses to start, followed by gradual reduction in dosage to the lowest possible level consistent with maintaining an adequate clinical response.
I.M. (sodium succinate): 10-80 mg/day once daily
I.M. (acetate): 10-80 mg every 1-2 weeks
(Continued)

methylprednisolone *(Continued)*

I.V. (sodium succinate): 10-40 mg over a period of several minutes and repeated I.V. or I.M. at intervals depending on clinical response; when high dosages are needed, give 30 mg/kg over a period ≥30 minutes and may be repeated every 4-6 hours for 48 hours.

Status asthmaticus: I.V. (sodium succinate): Loading dose: 2 mg/kg/dose, then 0.5-1 mg/kg/dose every 6 hours for up to 5 days

Lupus nephritis: High-dose "pulse" therapy: I.V. (sodium succinate): 1 g/day for 3 days

Aplastic anemia: I.V. (sodium succinate): 1 mg/kg/day or 40 mg/day (whichever dose is higher), for 4 days. After 4 days, change to oral and continue until day 10 or until symptoms of serum sickness resolve, then rapidly reduce over approximately 2 weeks.

Pneumocystis pneumonia in AIDs patients: I.V.: 40-60 mg every 6 hours for 7-10 days

Intra-articular (acetate): Administer every 1-5 weeks.
Large joints: 20-80 mg
Small joints: 4-10 mg

Intralesional (acetate): 20-60 mg every 1-5 weeks

Dosage Forms

Injection, powder for reconstitution, as sodium succinate: 125 mg [strength expressed as base]
Solu-Medrol®: 40 mg, 125 mg, 500 mg, 1 g, 2 g [packaged with diluent; diluent contains benzyl alcohol; strength expressed as base]
Solu-Medrol®: 500 mg, 1 g

Injection, suspension, as acetate (Depo-Medrol®): 20 mg/mL (5 mL); 40 mg/mL (5 mL); 80 mg/mL (5 mL) [contains benzyl alcohol; strength expressed as base]

Injection, suspension, as acetate [single-dose vial] (Depo-Medrol®): 40 mg/mL (1 mL, 10 mL); 80 mg/mL (1 mL)

Tablet: 4 mg
Medrol®: 2 mg, 4 mg, 8 mg, 16 mg, 32 mg

Tablet, dose-pack: 4 mg (21s)
Medrol® Dosepack™: 4 mg (21s)

6-α-methylprednisolone *see* methylprednisolone *on previous page*

methylprednisolone acetate *see* methylprednisolone *on previous page*

methylprednisolone sodium succinate *see* methylprednisolone *on previous page*

4-methylpyrazole *see* fomepizole *on page 366*

methyltestosterone (meth il tes TOS te rone)

Sound-Alike/Look-Alike Issues
methylTESTOSTERone may be confused with medroxyPROGESTERone
Virilon® may be confused with Verelan®

Tall-Man methyl**TESTOSTER**one

U.S./Canadian Brand Names Android® [US]; Methitest™ [US]; Testred® [US]; Virilon® [US]

Therapeutic Category Androgen

Controlled Substance C-III

Use
Male: Hypogonadism; delayed puberty; impotence and climacteric symptoms
Female: Palliative treatment of metastatic breast cancer

Usual Dosage Adults (buccal absorption produces twice the androgenic activity of oral tablets):

Male:
Hypogonadism, male climacteric and impotence: Oral: 10-40 mg/day
Androgen deficiency:
Oral: 10-50 mg/day
Buccal: 5-25 mg/day
Postpubertal cryptorchidism: Oral: 30 mg/day

Female:
Breast pain/engorgement:
Oral: 80 mg/day for 3-5 days
Buccal: 40 mg/day for 3-5 days
Breast cancer:
Oral: 50-200 mg/day
Buccal: 25-100 mg/day

Dosage Forms
Capsule (Android®, Testred®, Virilon®): 10 mg
Tablet (Methitest™): 10 mg

Meticorten® ***(Discontinued)*** *see* prednisone *on page 695*

Metimyd Ophthalmic Ointment ***(Discontinued)***

metipranolol (met i PRAN oh lol)

Sound-Alike/Look-Alike Issues

metipranolol may be confused with metaproterenol

Synonyms metipranolol hydrochloride

U.S./Canadian Brand Names OptiPranolol® [US/Can]

Therapeutic Category Beta-Adrenergic Blocker

Use Agent for lowering intraocular pressure in patients with chronic open-angle glaucoma

Usual Dosage Ophthalmic: Adults: Instill 1 drop in the affected eye(s) twice daily

Dosage Forms Solution, ophthalmic: 0.3% (5 mL, 10 mL) [contains benzalkonium chloride]

metipranolol hydrochloride *see* metipranolol *on this page*

metoclopramide (met oh KLOE pra mide)

Sound-Alike/Look-Alike Issues

metoclopramide may be confused with metolazone

Reglan® may be confused with Megace®, Regonol®, Renagel®

U.S./Canadian Brand Names Apo-Metoclop® [Can]; Metoclopramide Hydrochloride Injection [Can]; Nu-Metoclopramide [Can]; Reglan® [US]

Therapeutic Category Gastrointestinal Agent, Prokinetic

Use

Oral: Symptomatic treatment of diabetic gastric stasis; gastroesophageal reflux

I.V., I.M.: Symptomatic treatment of diabetic gastric stasis; postpyloric placement of enteral feeding tubes; prevention and/or treatment of nausea and vomiting associated with chemotherapy, or postsurgery; to stimulate gastric emptying and intestinal transit of barium during radiological examination

Usual Dosage

Children:

Postpyloric feeding tube placement: I.V.:

<6 years: 0.1 mg/kg

6-14 years: 2.5-5 mg

>14 years: Refer to Adults dosing.

Adults:

Gastroesophageal reflux: Oral: 10-15 mg/dose up to 4 times/day 30 minutes before meals or food and at bedtime; single doses of 20 mg are occasionally needed for provoking situations. Treatment >12 weeks has not been evaluated.

Diabetic gastric stasis:

Oral: 10 mg 30 minutes before each meal and at bedtime

I.M., I.V. (for severe symptoms): 10 mg over 1-2 minutes; 10 days of I.V. therapy may be necessary for best response

Chemotherapy-induced emesis:

I.V.: 1-2 mg/kg 30 minutes before chemotherapy and repeated every 2 hours for 2 doses, then every 3 hours for 3 doses (manufacturer labeling)

Alternate dosing (with or without diphenhydramine):

Moderate emetic risk chemotherapy: 0.5 mg/kg every 6 hours on days 2-4

Low and minimal risk chemotherapy: 1-2 mg/kg every 3-4 hours

Breakthrough treatment: 1-2 mg/kg every 3-4 hours

Postoperative nausea and vomiting: I.M., I.V.: 10-20 mg near end of surgery

Postpyloric feeding tube placement, radiological exam: I.V.: 10 mg

Dosage Forms

Injection, solution (Reglan®): 5 mg/mL (2 mL, 10 mL, 30 mL)

Syrup: 5 mg/5 mL (10 mL, 480 mL)

Tablet (Reglan®): 5 mg, 10 mg

Metoclopramide Hydrochloride Injection [Can] *see* metoclopramide *on this page*

metolazone (me TOLE a zone)

Sound-Alike/Look-Alike Issues

metolazone may be confused with metaxalone, methazolamide, methimazole, methotrexate, metoclopramide, metoprolol, minoxidil

Zaroxolyn® may be confused with Zarontin®

(Continued)

metolazone *(Continued)*

U.S./Canadian Brand Names Mykrox® [Can]; Zaroxolyn® [US/Can]

Therapeutic Category Diuretic, Miscellaneous

Use Management of mild to moderate hypertension; treatment of edema in congestive heart failure and nephrotic syndrome, impaired renal function

Usual Dosage Adults: Oral:

Edema: 2.5-20 mg/dose every 24 hours (ACC/AHA 2005 Heart Failure Guidelines)

Hypertension (Zaroxolyn®): 2.5-5 mg/dose every 24 hours

Hypertension (Mykrox®): 0.5 mg/day; if response is not adequate, increase dose to maximum of 1 mg/day

Dosage Forms

Tablet: 2.5 mg, 5 mg, 10 mg

Zaroxolyn®: 2.5 mg, 5 mg, 10 mg

Metopirone® [US] *see* metyrapone *on page 552*

metoprolol (me toe PROE lole)

Sound-Alike/Look-Alike Issues

metoprolol may be confused with metaproterenol, metolazone, misoprostol

Toprol-XL® may be confused with Topamax®

Synonyms metoprolol succinate; metoprolol tartrate

U.S./Canadian Brand Names Apo-Metoprolol® [Can]; Betaloc® Durules® [Can]; Betaloc® [Can]; Lopressor® [US/Can]; Metoprolol Tartrate Injection, USP [Can]; Novo-Metoprolol [Can]; Nu-Metop [Can]; PMS-Metoprolol [Can]; Sandoz-Metoprolol [Can]; Toprol-XL® [US/Can]

Therapeutic Category Beta-Adrenergic Blocker

Use Treatment of hypertension and angina pectoris; prevention of myocardial infarction, atrial fibrillation, flutter, symptomatic treatment of hypertrophic subaortic stenosis

Extended release: To reduce mortality/hospitalization in patients with congestive heart failure (stable NYHA Class II or III) in patients already receiving ACE inhibitors, diuretics, and/or digoxin

Usual Dosage Adults:

Hypertension: Oral: 100-450 mg/day in 2-3 divided doses, begin with 50 mg twice daily and increase doses at weekly intervals to desired effect; usual dosage range (JNC 7): 50-100 mg/day

Extended release: Initial: 25-100 mg/day (maximum: 400 mg/day)

Angina, SVT, MI prophylaxis: Oral: 100-450 mg/day in 2-3 divided doses, begin with 50 mg twice daily and increase doses at weekly intervals to desired effect

Extended release: Initial: 100 mg/day (maximum: 400 mg/day)

Hypertension/ventricular rate control: I.V. (in patients having nonfunctioning GI tract): Initial: 1.25-5 mg every 6-12 hours; titrate initial dose to response. Initially, low doses may be appropriate to establish response; however, up to 15 mg every 3-6 hours has been employed.

Congestive heart failure: Oral (extended release): Initial: 25 mg once daily (reduce to 12.5 mg once daily in NYHA class higher than class II); may double dosage every 2 weeks as tolerated, up to 200 mg/day

Myocardial infarction (acute): I.V.: 5 mg every 2 minutes for 3 doses in early treatment of myocardial infarction; thereafter give 50 mg orally every 6 hours 15 minutes after last I.V. dose and continue for 48 hours; then administer a maintenance dose of 100 mg twice daily.

Dosage Forms

Injection, solution, as tartrate: 1 mg/mL (5 mL)

Lopressor®: 1 mg/mL (5 mL)

Tablet, as tartrate: 25 mg, 50 mg, 100 mg

Lopressor®: 50 mg, 100 mg

Tablet, extended release, as succinate: 25 mg, 50 mg, 100 mg, 200 mg [expressed as mg equivalent to tartrate]

Toprol-XL®: 25 mg, 50 mg, 100 mg, 200 mg [expressed as mg equivalent to tartrate]

metoprolol and hydrochlorothiazide (me toe PROE lole & hye droe klor oh THYE a zide)

Synonyms hydrochlorothiazide and metoprolol; hydrochlorothiazide and metoprolol tartrate; metoprolol tartrate and hydrochlorothiazide

U.S./Canadian Brand Names Lopressor HCT® [US]

Therapeutic Category Beta Blocker, Beta$_1$ Selective; Diuretic, Thiazide

Use Treatment of hypertension

Usual Dosage Oral: Adults: Hypertension: Dosage should be determined by titration of the individual agents and the combination product substituted based upon the daily requirements.

Usual dose: Metoprolol 50-100 mg and hydrochlorothiazide 25-50 mg administered daily as single or divided doses (twice daily)

Note: Hydrochlorothiazide >50 mg/day is not recommended.

Concomitant therapy: It is recommended that if an additional antihypertensive agent is required, gradual titration should occur using 1/2 the usual starting dose of the other agent to avoid hypotension.

Dosage Forms Tablet:

50/25: Metoprolol tartrate 50 mg and hydrochlorothiazide 25 mg

100/25: Metoprolol tartrate 100 mg and hydrochlorothiazide 25 mg

100/50: Metoprolol tartrate 100 mg and hydrochlorothiazide 50 mg

metoprolol succinate *see* metoprolol *on previous page*

metoprolol tartrate *see* metoprolol *on previous page*

metoprolol tartrate and hydrochlorothiazide *see* metoprolol and hydrochlorothiazide *on previous page*

Metoprolol Tartrate Injection, USP [Can] *see* metoprolol *on previous page*

Metreton® *(Discontinued)*

metrizamide *see* radiological/contrast media (nonionic) *on page 730*

MetroCream® [US/Can] *see* metronidazole *on this page*

MetroGel® [US/Can] *see* metronidazole *on this page*

MetroGel-Vaginal® [US] *see* metronidazole *on this page*

Metro I.V.® Injection *(Discontinued)* *see* metronidazole *on this page*

MetroLotion® [US] *see* metronidazole *on this page*

metronidazole (met roe NYE da zole)

Sound-Alike/Look-Alike Issues

metronidazole may be confused with metformin.

Synonyms metronidazole hydrochloride

U.S./Canadian Brand Names Apo-Metronidazole® [Can]; Flagyl ER® [US]; Flagyl® I.V. RTU™ [US]; Flagyl® [US/Can]; Florazole® ER [Can]; MetroCream® [US/Can]; MetroGel-Vaginal® [US]; MetroGel® [US/Can]; MetroLotion® [US]; Nidagel™ [Can]; Noritate® [US/Can]; Trikacide [Can]; Vandazole™ [US]

Therapeutic Category Amebicide; Antibiotic, Miscellaneous; Antibiotic, Topical; Antiprotozoal

Use Treatment of susceptible anaerobic bacterial and protozoal infections in the following conditions: Amebiasis, symptomatic and asymptomatic trichomoniasis; skin and skin structure infections; CNS infections; intraabdominal infections (as part of combination regimen); systemic anaerobic infections; treatment of antibiotic-associated pseudomembranous colitis (AAPC), bacterial vaginosis; as part of a multidrug regimen for *H. pylori* eradication to reduce the risk of duodenal ulcer recurrence

Topical: Treatment of inflammatory lesions and erythema of rosacea

Usual Dosage

Infants and Children:

Amebiasis: Oral: 35-50 mg/kg/day in divided doses every 8 hours for 10 days

Trichomoniasis: Oral: 15-30 mg/kg/day in divided doses every 8 hours for 7 days

Anaerobic infections:

Oral: 15-35 mg/kg/day in divided doses every 8 hours

I.V.: 30 mg/kg/day in divided doses every 6 hours

Clostridium difficile (antibiotic-associated colitis): Oral: 20 mg/kg/day divided every 6 hours

Maximum dose: 2 g/day

Adults:

Anaerobic infections (diverticulitis, intraabdominal, peritonitis, cholangitis, or abscess): Oral, I.V.: 500 mg every 6-8 hours, not to exceed 4 g/day

Acne rosacea: Topical:

0.75%: Apply and rub a thin film twice daily, morning and evening, to entire affected areas after washing. Significant therapeutic results should be noticed within 3 weeks. Clinical studies have demonstrated continuing improvement through 9 weeks of therapy.

1%: Apply thin film to affected area once daily

Amebiasis: Oral: 500-750 mg every 8 hours for 5-10 days

Antibiotic-associated pseudomembranous colitis: Oral: 250-500 mg 3-4 times/day for 10-14 days

Giardiasis: 500 mg twice daily for 5-7 days

Helicobacter pylori eradication: Oral: 250-500 mg with meals and at bedtime for 14 days; requires combination therapy with at least one other antibiotic and an acid-suppressing agent (proton pump inhibitor or H_2 blocker)

Bacterial vaginosis or vaginitis due to *Gardnerella*, *Mobiluncus*:

Oral: 500 mg twice daily (regular release) or 750 mg once daily (extended release tablet) for 7 days

(Continued)

metronidazole *(Continued)*

Vaginal: 1 applicatorful (~37.5 mg metronidazole) intravaginally once or twice daily for 5 days; apply once in morning and evening if using twice daily, if daily, use at bedtime

Trichomoniasis: Oral: 250 mg every 8 hours for 7 days **or** 375 mg twice daily for 7 days **or** 2 g as a single dose

Dosage Forms

Capsule:
Flagyl®: 375 mg
Cream, topical: 0.75% (45 g)
MetroCream®: 0.75% (45 g) [contains benzyl alcohol]
Noritate®: 1% (60 g)
Gel, topical: 0.75% (45 g)
MetroGel®: 1% (60 g)
Gel, vaginal:
MetroGel-Vaginal®, Vandazole™: 0.75% (70 g)
Infusion [premixed iso-osmotic sodium chloride solution]: 500 mg (100 mL)
Flagyl® I.V. RTU™: 500 mg (100 mL) [contains sodium 14 mEq]
Lotion, topical: 0.75% (60 mL)
MetroLotion®: 0.75% (60 mL) [contains benzyl alcohol]
Tablet: 250 mg, 500 mg
Flagyl®: 250 mg, 500 mg
Tablet, extended release:
Flagyl® ER: 750 mg

metronidazole, bismuth subsalicylate, and tetracycline *see* bismuth subsalicylate, metronidazole, and tetracycline *on page 112*

metronidazole hydrochloride *see* metronidazole *on previous page*

metyrapone (me TEER a pone)

Sound-Alike/Look-Alike Issues
metyrapone may be confused with metyrosine

U.S./Canadian Brand Names Metopirone® [US]

Therapeutic Category Diagnostic Agent

Use Diagnostic test for hypothalamic-pituitary ACTH function

Usual Dosage Oral:
Children: 15 mg/kg every 4 hours for 6 doses; minimum dose: 250 mg
Adults: 750 mg every 4 hours for 6 doses

Dosage Forms Capsule: 250 mg

metyrosine (me TYE roe seen)

Sound-Alike/Look-Alike Issues
metyrosine may be confused with metyrapone

Synonyms AMPT; OGMT

U.S./Canadian Brand Names Demser® [US/Can]

Therapeutic Category Tyrosine Hydroxylase Inhibitor

Use Short-term management of pheochromocytoma before surgery, long-term management when surgery is contraindicated or when chronic malignant pheochromocytoma exists

Usual Dosage Children >12 years and Adults: Oral: Initial: 250 mg 4 times/day, increased by 250-500 mg/day up to 4 g/day; maintenance: 2-3 g/day in 4 divided doses; for preoperative preparation, administer optimum effective dosage for 5-7 days

Dosage Forms Capsule: 250 mg

Mevacor® [US/Can] *see* lovastatin *on page 508*

mevinolin *see* lovastatin *on page 508*

mexiletine (meks IL e teen)

U.S./Canadian Brand Names Novo-Mexiletine [Can]

Therapeutic Category Antiarrhythmic Agent, Class I-B

Use Management of serious ventricular arrhythmias; suppression of PVCs

Usual Dosage Adults: Oral: Initial: 200 mg every 8 hours (may load with 400 mg if necessary); adjust dose every 2-3 days; usual dose: 200-300 mg every 8 hours; maximum dose: 1.2 g/day (some patients respond to every 12-hour dosing). When switching from another antiarrhythmic, initiate a 200 mg dose 6-12 hours after stopping former agents, 3-6 hours after stopping procainamide.

Dosage Forms [DSC] = Discontinued product

Capsule, as hydrochloride: 150 mg, 200 mg, 250 mg

Mexitil®: 150 mg, 200 mg, 250 mg [DSC]

Mexitil® *(Discontinued)* *see* mexiletine *on previous page*

MG 217® [US-OTC] *see* coal tar *on page 207*

MG 217® Medicated Tar [US-OTC] *see* coal tar *on page 207*

MG217 Sal-Acid® [US-OTC] *see* salicylic acid *on page 758*

Miacalcin® [US] *see* calcitonin *on page 133*

Miacalcin® NS [Can] *see* calcitonin *on page 133*

Mi-Acid™ [US-OTC] *see* aluminum hydroxide, magnesium hydroxide, and simethicone *on page 37*

Mi-Acid™ Double Strength [US-OTC] *see* calcium carbonate and magnesium hydroxide *on page 136*

Mi-Acid™ Maximum Strength [US-OTC] *see* aluminum hydroxide, magnesium hydroxide, and simethicone *on page 37*

Micaderm® [US-OTC] *see* miconazole *on this page*

micafungin (mi ka FUN gin)

Synonyms micafungin sodium

U.S./Canadian Brand Names Mycamine™ [US]

Therapeutic Category Antifungal Agent, Parental; Drug-induced Neuritis, Treatment Agent

Use Esophageal candidiasis; *Candida* prophylaxis in patients undergoing hematopoietic stem cell transplant

Usual Dosage I.V.: Adults:

Esophageal candidiasis: 150 mg daily; median duration of therapy (from clinical trials) was 14 days

Prophylaxis of *Candida* infection in hematopoietic stem cell transplantation: 50 mg daily; median duration of therapy (from clinical trials) was 18 days

Dosage Forms Injection, powder for reconstitution, as sodium [preservative-free]: Micafungin 50 mg [contains lactose]

micafungin sodium *see* micafungin *on this page*

Micanol® [Can] *see* anthralin *on page 58*

Micardis® [US/Can] *see* telmisartan *on page 808*

Micardis® HCT [US] *see* telmisartan and hydrochlorothiazide *on page 808*

Micardis® Plus [Can] *see* telmisartan and hydrochlorothiazide *on page 808*

Micatin® [Can] *see* miconazole *on this page*

Micatin® Athlete's Foot [US-OTC] *see* miconazole *on this page*

Micatin® Jock Itch [US-OTC] *see* miconazole *on this page*

miconazole (mi KON a zole)

Sound-Alike/Look-Alike Issues

miconazole may be confused with Micronase®, Micronor®

Lotrimin® may be confused with Lotrisone®, Otrivin®

Micatin® may be confused with Miacalcin®

Synonyms miconazole nitrate

U.S./Canadian Brand Names Aloe Vesta® 2-n-1 Antifungal [US-OTC]; Baza® Antifungal [US-OTC]; Carrington Antifungal [US-OTC]; DermaFungal [US-OTC]; Dermagran® AF [US-OTC]; Dermazole [Can]; DiabetAid™ Antifungal Foot Bath [US-OTC]; Fungoid® Tincture [US-OTC]; Lotrimin® AF Jock Itch Powder Spray [US-OTC]; Lotrimin® AF Powder/Spray [US-OTC]; Micaderm® [US-OTC]; Micatin® Athlete's Foot [US-OTC]; Micatin® Jock Itch [US-OTC]; Micatin® [Can]; Micozole [Can]; Micro-Guard® [US-OTC]; Mitrazol™ [US-OTC]; Monistat-Derm® [US]; Monistat® 1 Combination Pack [US-OTC]; Monistat® 3 [US-OTC/Can]; Monistat® 7 [US-OTC]; Monistat® [Can]; Neosporin® AF [US-OTC]; Podactin Cream [US-OTC]; Secura® Antifungal [US-OTC]; Zeasorb®-AF [US-OTC]

Therapeutic Category Antifungal Agent

Use Treatment of vulvovaginal candidiasis and a variety of skin and mucous membrane fungal infections

(Continued)

miconazole *(Continued)*

Usual Dosage

Topical: Children and Adults: **Note:** Not for OTC use in children <2 years:

- Tinea corporis: Apply twice daily for 4 weeks
- Tinea pedis: Apply twice daily for 4 weeks
  - Effervescent tablet: Dissolve 1 tablet in ∼1 gallon of water; soak feet for 15-30 minutes; pat dry
- Tinea cruris: Apply twice daily for 2 weeks

Vaginal: Adults: Vulvovaginal candidiasis:

- Cream, 2%: Insert 1 applicatorful at bedtime for 7 days
- Cream, 4%: Insert 1 applicatorful at bedtime for 3 days
- Suppository, 100 mg: Insert 1 suppository at bedtime for 7 days
- Suppository, 200 mg: Insert 1 suppository at bedtime for 3 days
- Suppository, 1200 mg: Insert 1 suppository (a one-time dose); may be used at bedtime or during the day

Note: Many products are available as a combination pack, with a suppository for vaginal instillation and cream to relieve external symptoms. External cream may be used twice daily, as needed, for up to 7 days.

Dosage Forms [DSC] = Discontinued product

Combination products: Miconazole nitrate vaginal suppository 200 mg (3s) and miconazole nitrate external cream 2%

- Monistat® 1 Combination Pack: Miconazole nitrate vaginal insert 1200 mg (1) and miconazole nitrate external cream 2% (5 g) [Note: Do not confuse with 1-Day™ (formerly Monistat® 1) which contains tioconazole]
- Monistat® 3 Combination Pack:
  - Miconazole nitrate vaginal suppository 200 mg (3s) and miconazole nitrate external cream 2%
  - Miconazole nitrate vaginal cream 4% and miconazole nitrate external cream 2%
- Monistat® 7 Combination Pack:
  - Miconazole nitrate vaginal suppository 100 mg (7s) and miconazole nitrate external cream 2%
  - Miconazole nitrate vaginal cream 2% (7 prefilled applicators) and miconazole nitrate external cream 2%

Cream, topical, as nitrate: 2% (15 g, 30 g, 45 g)

- Baza® Antifungal: 2% (4 g, 57 g, 142 g) [zinc oxide based formula]
- Carrington Antifungal: 2% (150 g)
- Micaderm®, Neosporin® AF, Podactin: 2% (30 g)
- Micatin® Athlete's Foot, Micatin® Jock Itch: 2% (15 g)
- Micro-Guard®, Mitrazol™: 2% (60 g)
- Monistat-Derm®: 2% (15 g, 30 g, 85 g)
- Secura® Antifungal: 2% (60 g, 98 g)

Cream, vaginal, as nitrate [prefilled or refillable applicator]: 2% (45 g)

- Monistat® 3: 4% (15 g, 25 g)
- Monistat® 7: 2% (45 g)

Liquid, spray, topical, as nitrate:

- Micatin® Athlete's Foot: 2% (90 mL) [contains alcohol]
- Neosporin AF®: 2% (105 mL)

Lotion, powder, as nitrate (Zeasorb®-AF): 2% (56 g) [contains alcohol 36%]

Ointment, topical, as nitrate:

- Aloe Vesta® 2-n-1 Antifungal: 2% (60 g, 150 g)
- DermaFungal: 2% (113 g)
- Dermagran® AF: (113 g) [contains vitamin A and zinc]

Powder, topical, as nitrate:

- Lotrimin® AF: 2% (160 g)
- Micro-Guard®: 2% (90 g)
- Mitrazol™: 2% (30 g)
- Zeasorb®-AF: 2% (70 g)

Powder spray, topical, as nitrate:

- Lotrimin® AF, Lotrimin® AF Jock Itch: 2% (140 g)
- Micatin® Athlete's Foot, Micatin® Jock Itch: 2% (90 g) [contains alcohol]
- Neosporin® AF: 2% (85 g)

Suppository, vaginal, as nitrate: 100 mg (7s); 200 mg (3s)

- Monistat® 3: 200 mg (3s)
- Monistat® 7: 100 mg (7s)

Tablet, effervescent, topical, as nitrate (DiabetAid™ Antifungal Foot Bath): 2% (10s)

Tincture, topical, as nitrate (Fungoid®): 2% (30 mL, 473 mL) [contains isopropyl alcohol 30%]; 30 mL size also available in a treatment kit which contains nail scrub and nail brush]

miconazole nitrate *see* miconazole *on previous page*

Micozole [Can] *see* miconazole *on page 553*
MICRhoGAM® [US] *see* Rh_0(D) immune globulin *on page 740*
microfibrillar collagen hemostat *see* collagen hemostat *on page 212*
Microgestin™ [US] *see* ethinyl estradiol and norethindrone *on page 323*
Microgestin™ Fe [US] *see* ethinyl estradiol and norethindrone *on page 323*
Micro-Guard® [US-OTC] *see* miconazole *on page 553*
microK® [US] *see* potassium chloride *on page 684*
microK® 10 [US] *see* potassium chloride *on page 684*
Micro-K Extencaps® [Can] *see* potassium chloride *on page 684*
Micro-K® LS *(Discontinued)* *see* potassium chloride *on page 684*
Microlipid™ [US-OTC] *see* nutritional formula, enteral/oral *on page 608*
Micronase® [US] *see* glyburide *on page 387*
microNefrin® *(Discontinued)* *see* epinephrine *on page 295*
Micronor® [US/Can] *see* norethindrone *on page 598*
Microzide™ [US] *see* hydrochlorothiazide *on page 419*
Midamor® *(Discontinued)* *see* amiloride *on page 41*

midazolam (MID aye zoe lam)

Sound-Alike/Look-Alike Issues
Versed® may be confused with VePesid®, Vistaril®

Synonyms midazolam hydrochloride

U.S./Canadian Brand Names Apo-Midazolam® [Can]

Therapeutic Category Benzodiazepine

Controlled Substance C-IV

Use Preoperative sedation and provides conscious sedation prior to diagnostic or radiographic procedures; ICU sedation (continuous infusion); intravenous anesthesia (induction); intravenous anesthesia (maintenance)

Usual Dosage The dose of midazolam needs to be individualized based on the patient's age, underlying diseases, and concurrent medications. Decrease dose (by ~30%) if narcotics or other CNS depressants are administered concomitantly. **Personnel and equipment needed for standard respiratory resuscitation should be immediately available during midazolam administration.**

Children <6 years may require higher doses and closer monitoring than older children; calculate dose on ideal body weight

Conscious sedation for procedures or preoperative sedation:

Oral: 0.25-0.5 mg/kg as a single dose preprocedure, up to a maximum of 20 mg; administer 30-45 minutes prior to procedure. Children <6 years or less cooperative patients may require as much as 1 mg/kg as a single dose; 0.25 mg/kg may suffice for children 6-16 years of age.

I.M.: 0.1-0.15 mg/kg 30-60 minutes before surgery or procedure; range 0.05-0.15 mg/kg; doses up to 0.5 mg/kg have been used in more anxious patients; maximum total dose: 10 mg

I.V.:

Infants <6 months: Limited information is available in nonintubated infants; dosing recommendations not clear; infants <6 months are at higher risk for airway obstruction and hypoventilation; titrate dose in small increments to desired effect; monitor carefully

Infants 6 months to Children 5 years: Initial: 0.05-0.1 mg/kg; titrate dose carefully; total dose of 0.6 mg/kg may be required; usual maximum total dose: 6 mg

Children 6-12 years: Initial: 0.025-0.05 mg/kg; titrate dose carefully; total doses of 0.4 mg/kg may be required; usual maximum total dose: 10 mg

Children 12-16 years: Dose as adults; usual maximum total dose: 10 mg

Conscious sedation during mechanical ventilation: Children: Loading dose: 0.05-0.2 mg/kg, followed by initial continuous infusion: 0.06-0.12 mg/kg/hour (1-2 mcg/kg/minute); titrate to the desired effect; usual range: 0.4-6 mcg/kg/minute

Adults:

Preoperative sedation:

I.M.: 0.07-0.08 mg/kg 30-60 minutes prior to surgery/procedure; usual dose: 5 mg; **Note:** Reduce dose in patients with COPD, high-risk patients, patients ≥60 years of age, and patients receiving other narcotics or CNS depressants

I.V.: 0.02-0.04 mg/kg; repeat every 5 minutes as needed to desired effect or up to 0.1-0.2 mg/kg

(Continued)

midazolam *(Continued)*

Conscious sedation: I.V.: Initial: 0.5-2 mg slow I.V. over at least 2 minutes; slowly titrate to effect by repeating doses every 2-3 minutes if needed; usual total dose: 2.5-5 mg

Healthy Adults <60 years: Some patients respond to doses as low as 1 mg; no more than 2.5 mg should be administered over a period of 2 minutes. Additional doses of midazolam may be administered after a 2-minute waiting period and evaluation of sedation after each dose increment. A total dose >5 mg is generally not needed. If narcotics or other CNS depressants are administered concomitantly, the midazolam dose should be reduced by 30%.

Anesthesia: I.V.:

Induction:

Unpremedicated patients: 0.3-0.35 mg/kg (up to 0.6 mg/kg in resistant cases)

Premedicated patients: 0.15-0.35 mg/kg

Maintenance: 0.05-0.3 mg/kg as needed, or continuous infusion 0.25-1.5 mcg/kg/minute

Sedation in mechanically-ventilated patients: I.V. continuous infusion: 100 mg in 250 mL D_5W or NS (if patient is fluid-restricted, may concentrate up to a maximum of 0.5 mg/mL); initial dose: 0.02-0.08 mg/kg (~1 mg to 5 mg in 70 kg adult) initially and either repeated at 5-15 minute intervals until adequate sedation is achieved or continuous infusion rates of 0.04-0.2 mg/kg/hour and titrate to reach desired level of sedation

Dosage Forms

Injection, solution: 1 mg/mL (2 mL, 5 mL, 10 mL); 5 mg/mL (1 mL, 2 mL, 5 mL, 10 mL) [contains benzyl alcohol 1%]

Injection, solution [preservative free]: 1 mg/mL (2 mL, 5 mL); 5 mg/mL (1 mL, 2 mL)

Syrup: 2 mg/mL (118 mL) [contains sodium benzoate; cherry flavor]

midazolam hydrochloride *see* midazolam *on previous page*

midodrine (MI doe dreen)

Sound-Alike/Look-Alike Issues

ProAmatine® may be confused with protamine

Synonyms midodrine hydrochloride

U.S./Canadian Brand Names Amatine® [Can]; Apo-Midodrine® [Can]; Orvaten™ [US]; ProAmatine® [US]

Therapeutic Category Alpha-Adrenergic Agonist

Use Orphan drug: Treatment of symptomatic orthostatic hypotension

Usual Dosage Adults: Oral: 10 mg 3 times/day during daytime hours (every 3-4 hours) when patient is upright (maximum: 40 mg/day)

Dosage Forms Tablet, as hydrochloride: 2.5 mg, 5 mg, 10 mg

midodrine hydrochloride *see* midodrine *on this page*

Midol® Cramp and Body Aches [US-OTC] *see* ibuprofen *on page 437*

Midol® Extended Relief [US] *see* naproxen *on page 578*

Midrin® [US] *see* acetaminophen, isometheptene, and dichloralphenazone *on page 13*

Mifeprex® [US] *see* mifepristone *on this page*

mifepristone (mi FE pris tone)

Sound-Alike/Look-Alike Issues

mifepristone may be confused with misoprostol

Mifeprex® may be confused with Mirapex®

Synonyms RU-486; RU-38486

U.S./Canadian Brand Names Mifeprex® [US]

Therapeutic Category Abortifacient; Antineoplastic Agent, Hormone Antagonist; Antiprogestin

Use Medical termination of intrauterine pregnancy, through day 49 of pregnancy. Patients may need treatment with misoprostol and possibly surgery to complete therapy

Usual Dosage Adults: Oral:

Termination of pregnancy: Treatment consists of three office visits by the patient; the patient must read medication guide and sign patient agreement prior to treatment:

Day 1: 600 mg (three 200 mg tablets) taken as a single dose under physician supervision

Day 3: Patient must return to the healthcare provider 2 days following administration of mifepristone; unless abortion has occurred (confirmed using ultrasound or clinical examination): 400 mcg (two 200 mcg tablets) of misoprostol; patient may need treatment for cramps or gastrointestinal symptoms at this time

Day 14: Patient must return to the healthcare provider ~14 days after administration of mifepristone; confirm complete termination of pregnancy by ultrasound or clinical exam. Surgical termination is recommended to manage treatment failures.

Dosage Forms Tablet: 200 mg

miglitol (MIG li tol)

U.S./Canadian Brand Names Glyset® [US/Can]

Therapeutic Category Antidiabetic Agent, Oral

Use Type 2 diabetes mellitus (noninsulin-dependent, NIDDM):

Monotherapy adjunct to diet to improve glycemic control in patients with type 2 diabetes mellitus (noninsulin-dependent, NIDDM) whose hyperglycemia cannot be managed with diet alone

Combination therapy with a sulfonylurea when diet plus either miglitol or a sulfonylurea alone do not result in adequate glycemic control. The effect of miglitol to enhance glycemic control is additive to that of sulfonylureas when used in combination.

Usual Dosage Adults: Oral: 25 mg 3 times/day with the first bite of food at each meal; the dose may be increased to 50 mg 3 times/day after 4-8 weeks; maximum recommended dose: 100 mg 3 times/day

Dosage Forms Tablet: 25 mg, 50 mg, 100 mg

miglustat (MIG loo stat)

Synonyms OGT-918

U.S./Canadian Brand Names Zavesca® [US/Can]

Therapeutic Category Enzyme Inhibitor

Use Treatment of mild-to-moderate type 1 Gaucher disease when enzyme replacement therapy is not a therapeutic option

Usual Dosage Oral: Adults: Type 1 Gaucher disease: 100 mg 3 times/day; dose may be reduced to 100 mg 1-2 times/day in patients with adverse effects (ie, tremor, GI distress)

Dosage Forms Capsule: 100 mg

Migquin [US] *see* acetaminophen, isometheptene, and dichloralphenazone *on page 13*

Migranal® [US/Can] *see* dihydroergotamine *on page 256*

Migrapap® *(Discontinued)* *see* acetaminophen, isometheptene, and dichloralphenazone *on page 13*

Migratine [US] *see* acetaminophen, isometheptene, and dichloralphenazone *on page 13*

Migrazone® [US] *see* acetaminophen, isometheptene, and dichloralphenazone *on page 13*

Migrin-A [US] *see* acetaminophen, isometheptene, and dichloralphenazone *on page 13*

milk of magnesia *see* magnesium hydroxide *on page 514*

Milontin® *(Discontinued)*

Milophene® [Can] *see* clomiphene *on page 202*

Milophene® *(Discontinued)* *see* clomiphene *on page 202*

milrinone (MIL ri none)

Sound-Alike/Look-Alike Issues

Primacor® may be confused with Primaxin®

Synonyms milrinone lactate

U.S./Canadian Brand Names Milrinone Lactate Injection [Can]; Primacor® [US]

Therapeutic Category Cardiovascular Agent, Other

Use Short-term I.V. therapy of congestive heart failure; calcium antagonist intoxication

Usual Dosage Adults: I.V.: Loading dose: 50 mcg/kg administered over 10 minutes followed by a maintenance dose titrated according to the hemodynamic and clinical response

Dosage Forms [DSC] = Discontinued product

Infusion [premixed in D_5W] (Primacor®): 200 mcg/mL (100 mL, 200 mL)

Injection, solution: 1 mg/mL (10 mL, 20 mL, 50 mL)

Primacor®: 1 mg/mL (10 mL, 20 mL; 50 mL [DSC])

milrinone lactate *see* milrinone *on this page*

Milrinone Lactate Injection [Can] *see* milrinone *on this page*

Miltown® *(Discontinued)* *see* meprobamate *on page 531*

Mindal DM *(Discontinued)* *see* guaifenesin and dextromethorphan *on page 394*

mineral oil, petrolatum, lanolin, cetyl alcohol, and glycerin *see* lanolin, cetyl alcohol, glycerin, petrolatum, and mineral oil *on page 481*

Minestrin™ 1/20 [Can] *see* ethinyl estradiol and norethindrone *on page 323*

Minidyne® [US-OTC] *see* povidone-iodine *on page 689*

Mini-Gamulin® Rh *(Discontinued)*

Minipress® [US/Can] *see* prazosin *on page 693*

Minirin® [Can] *see* desmopressin acetate *on page 237*

Minitran™ [US/Can] *see* nitroglycerin *on page 595*

Minizide® [US] *see* prazosin and polythiazide *on page 693*

Minocin® [US/Can] *see* minocycline *on this page*

minocycline (mi noe SYE kleen)

Sound-Alike/Look-Alike Issues

Dynacin® may be confused with Dyazide®, Dynabac®, DynaCirc®, Dynapen®

Minocin® may be confused with Indocin®, Lincocin®, Minizide®, Mithracin®, niacin

Synonyms minocycline hydrochloride

U.S./Canadian Brand Names Alti-Minocycline [Can]; Apo-Minocycline® [Can]; Dynacin® [US]; Gen-Minocycline [Can]; Minocin® [US/Can]; myrac™ [US]; Novo-Minocycline [Can]; Rhoxal-minocycline [Can]; Sandoz-Minocycline [Can]; Solodyn™ [US]

Therapeutic Category Tetracycline Derivative

Use Treatment of susceptible bacterial infections of both gram-negative and gram-positive organisms; treatment of anthrax (inhalational, cutaneous, and gastrointestinal); acne; meningococcal (asymptomatic) carrier state; Rickettsial diseases (including Rocky Mountain spotted fever, Q fever); nongonococcal urethritis, gonorrhea; acute intestinal amebiasis

Usual Dosage

Usual dosage range:

Children >8 years: Oral: Initial: 4 mg/kg, followed by 2 mg/kg/dose every 12 hours

Adults: Oral: Initial: 200 mg, followed by 100 mg every 12 hours (maximum: 400 mg/day)

Indication-specific dosing:

Children ≥12 years: **Acne** *(inflammatory, nonnodular, moderate-to-severe)* (Solodyn™): Oral:

45-59 kg: 45 mg once daily

60-90 kg: 90 mg once daily

91-136 kg: 135 mg once daily

Note: Therapy should be continued for 12 weeks. Higher doses do not confer greater efficacy, and safety of use beyond 12 weeks has not been established.

Adults: Oral:

Acne: Capsule or immediate-release tablet: 50-100 mg daily

Inflammatory, nonnodular, moderate-to-severe (Solodyn™):

45-59 kg: 45 mg once daily

60-90 kg: 90 mg once daily

91-136 kg: 135 mg once daily

Note: Therapy should be continued for 12 weeks. Higher doses do not confer greater efficacy, and safety of use beyond 12 weeks has not been established.

Chlamydial or *Ureaplasma urealyticum* infection, uncomplicated: Urethral, endocervical, or rectal: 100 mg every 12 hours for at least 7 days

Gonococcal infection, uncomplicated (males):

Without urethritis or anorectal infection: Initial: 200 mg, followed by 100 mg every 12 hours for at least 4 days (cultures 2-3 days post-therapy)

Urethritis: 100 mg every 12 hours for 5 days

Meningococcal carrier state: 100 mg every 12 hours for 5 days

Mycobacterium marinum: 100 mg every 12 hours for 6-8 weeks

Nocardiosis, cutaneous (non-CNS): 100 mg every 12 hours

Syphilis: Initial: 200 mg, followed by 100 mg every 12 hours for 10-15 days

Dosage Forms

Capsule: 50 mg, 75 mg, 100 mg

Dynacin®: 75 mg, 100 mg

Capsule, pellet filled: 50 mg, 100 mg

Minocin®: 50 mg, 100 mg

Tablet: 50 mg, 75 mg, 100 mg

Dynacin®, myrac™: 50 mg, 75 mg, 100 mg

Tablet, extended release:

Solodyn™: 45 mg, 90 mg, 135 mg

minocycline hydrochloride *see* minocycline *on previous page*

Min-Ovral® [Can] *see* ethinyl estradiol and levonorgestrel *on page 320*

Minox [Can] *see* minoxidil *on this page*

minoxidil (mi NOKS i dil)

Sound-Alike/Look-Alike Issues

minoxidil may be confused with metolazone, Monopril®

Loniten® may be confused with clonidine, Lioresal®, Lotensin®

U.S./Canadian Brand Names Apo-Gain® [Can]; Loniten® [US]; Minox [Can]; Rogaine® Extra Strength for Men [US-OTC]; Rogaine® for Men [US-OTC]; Rogaine® for Women [US-OTC]; Rogaine® [Can]

Therapeutic Category Topical Skin Product; Vasodilator

Use Management of severe hypertension (usually in combination with a diuretic and beta-blocker); treatment (topical formulation) of alopecia androgenetica in males and females

Usual Dosage

Children <12 years: Hypertension: Oral: Initial: 0.1-0.2 mg/kg once daily; maximum: 5 mg/day; increase gradually every 3 days; usual dosage: 0.25-1 mg/kg/day in 1-2 divided doses; maximum: 50 mg/day

Children >12 years and Adults: Hypertension: Oral: Initial: 5 mg once daily, increase gradually every 3 days (maximum: 100 mg/day); usual dose range (JNC 7): 2.5-80 mg/day in 1-2 divided doses

Adults: Alopecia: Topical: Apply twice daily; 4 months of therapy may be necessary for hair growth.

Dosage Forms [DSC] = Discontinued product

Solution, topical: 2% [20 mg/metered dose] (60 mL); 5% [50 mg/metered dose] (60 mL)

Rogaine® for Men, Rogaine® for Women: 2% [20 mg/metered dose] (60 mL)

Rogaine® Extra Strength for Men: 5% [50 mg/metered dose] (60 mL)

Tablet: 2.5 mg, 10 mg

Loniten®: 2.5 mg [DSC], 10 mg

Mintab DM [US] *see* guaifenesin and dextromethorphan *on page 394*

Mintezol® [US] *see* thiabendazole *on page 821*

Mintox Extra Strength [US-OTC] *see* aluminum hydroxide, magnesium hydroxide, and simethicone *on page 37*

Mintox Plus [US-OTC] *see* aluminum hydroxide, magnesium hydroxide, and simethicone *on page 37*

Mintuss HC [US] *see* phenylephrine, hydrocodone, and chlorpheniramine *on page 663*

Mintuss HD [US] *see* phenylephrine, hydrocodone, and chlorpheniramine *on page 663*

Mintuss MS [US] *see* phenylephrine, hydrocodone, and chlorpheniramine *on page 663*

Minute-Gel® *(Discontinued)* *see* fluoride *on page 354*

Miochol-E® [US/Can] *see* acetylcholine *on page 15*

Miostat® [US/Can] *see* carbachol *on page 144*

MiraLax™ [US] *see* polyethylene glycol 3350 *on page 678*

Mirapex® [US/Can] *see* pramipexole *on page 690*

Mircette® [US] *see* ethinyl estradiol and desogestrel *on page 317*

Mirena® [US/Can] *see* levonorgestrel *on page 491*

mirtazapine (mir TAZ a peen)

Sound-Alike/Look-Alike Issues

Remeron® may be confused with Premarin®, Zemuron®

U.S./Canadian Brand Names CO Mirtazapine [Can]; Gen-Mirtazapine [Can]; Novo-Mirtazapine [Can]; PMS-Mirtazapine [Can]; ratio-Mirtazapine [Can]; Remeron SolTab® [US]; Remeron® RD [Can]; Remeron® [US/Can]; Rhoxal-mirtazapine FC [Can]; Rhoxal-mirtazapine [Can]; Riva-Mirtazapine [Can]; Sandoz-Mirtazapine FC [Can]; Sandoz-Mirtazapine [Can]

Therapeutic Category Antidepressant, Alpha-2 Antagonist

Use Treatment of depression

Usual Dosage Treatment of depression: Adults: Oral: Initial: 15 mg nightly, titrate up to 15-45 mg/day with dose increases made no more frequently than every 1-2 weeks; there is an inverse relationship between dose and sedation

(Continued)

mirtazapine *(Continued)*

Dosage Forms

Tablet (Remeron®): 15 mg, 30 mg, 45 mg

Tablet, orally disintegrating: 15 mg, 30 mg

Remeron SolTab®:

15 mg [contains phenylalanine 2.6 mg/tablet; orange flavor]

30 mg [contains phenylalanine 5.2 mg/tablet; orange flavor]

45 mg [contains phenylalanine 7.8 mg/tablet; orange flavor]

misoprostol (mye soe PROST ole)

Sound-Alike/Look-Alike Issues

misoprostol may be confused with metoprolol, mifepristone

Cytotec® may be confused with Cytoxan®, Sytobex®

U.S./Canadian Brand Names Apo-Misoprostol® [Can]; Cytotec® [US]; Novo-Misoprostol [Can]

Therapeutic Category Prostaglandin

Use Prevention of NSAID-induced gastric ulcers; medical termination of pregnancy of ≤49 days (in conjunction with mifepristone)

Usual Dosage Adults: Oral:

Prevention of NSAID-induced gastric ulcers: 200 mcg 4 times/day with food; if not tolerated, may decrease dose to 100 mcg 4 times/day with food or 200 mcg twice daily with food; last dose of the day should be taken at bedtime

Medical termination of pregnancy: Refer to mifepristone monograph.

Dosage Forms Tablet: 100 mcg, 200 mcg

misoprostol and diclofenac *see* diclofenac and misoprostol *on page 251*

Mito-Carn® ***(Discontinued)*** *see* levocarnitine *on page 488*

mitomycin (mye toe MYE sin)

Sound-Alike/Look-Alike Issues

mitomycin may be confused with mithramycin, mitotane, mitoxantrone, Mutamycin®

Mutamycin® may be confused with mitomycin

Synonyms mitomycin-C; mitomycin-X; MTC; NSC-26980

U.S./Canadian Brand Names Mutamycin® [US/Can]

Therapeutic Category Antineoplastic Agent

Use Treatment of adenocarcinoma of stomach or pancreas, bladder cancer, breast cancer, or colorectal cancer

Usual Dosage Refer to individual protocols. Adults:

Single agent therapy: I.V.: 20 mg/m^2 every 6-8 weeks

Combination therapy: I.V.: 10 mg/m^2 every 6-8 weeks

Bladder carcinoma: Intravesicular instillation (unapproved route): 20-40 mg/dose instilled into the bladder for 3 hours repeated up to 3 times/week for up to 20 procedures per course

Dosage Forms Injection, powder for reconstitution: 5 mg, 20 mg, 40 mg

mitomycin-X *see* mitomycin *on this page*

mitomycin-C *see* mitomycin *on this page*

mitotane (MYE toe tane)

Sound-Alike/Look-Alike Issues

mitotane may be confused with mitomycin

Synonyms NSC-38721; o,p′-DDD

U.S./Canadian Brand Names Lysodren® [US/Can]

Therapeutic Category Antineoplastic Agent

Use Treatment of adrenocortical carcinoma

Usual Dosage Adrenocortical carcinoma: Oral: Adults: Start at 2-6 g/day in 3-4 divided doses, then increase incrementally to 9-10 g/day in 3-4 divided doses (maximum daily dose: 18 g)

Dosage Forms

Tablet [scored]:

Lysodren®: 500 mg

mitoxantrone (mye toe ZAN trone)

Sound-Alike/Look-Alike Issues
mitoxantrone may be confused with methotrexate, mitomycin

Synonyms DAD; DHAD; DHAQ; dihydroxyanthracenedione dihydrochloride; mitoxantrone hydrochloride CL-232315; mitozantrone; NSC-301739

U.S./Canadian Brand Names Mitoxantrone Injection® [Can]; Novantrone® [US/Can]

Therapeutic Category Antineoplastic Agent

Use Treatment of acute leukemias, lymphoma, breast cancer, pediatric sarcoma, progressive or relapsing-remitting multiple sclerosis, prostate cancer

Usual Dosage Refer to individual protocols. I.V. (dilute in D_5W or NS):
Acute leukemias:
Children ≤2 years: 0.4 mg/kg/day once daily for 3-5 days
Children >2 years and Adults: 8-12 mg/m^2/day once daily for 4-5 days
Solid tumors:
Children: 18-20 mg/m^2 every 3-4 weeks **or** 5-8 mg/m^2 every week
Adults: 12-14 mg/m^2 every 3-4 weeks **or** 2-4 mg/m^2/day for 5 days every 4 weeks
Hormone-refractory prostate cancer: Adults: 12-14 mg/m^2
Multiple sclerosis: Adults: 12 mg/m^2 every 3 months (maximum lifetime cumulative dose: 140 mg/m^2

Dosage Forms
Injection, solution: 2 mg/mL (10 mL, 12.5 mL, 15 mL)
Novantrone®: 2 mg/mL (10 mL, 12.5 mL, 15 mL)

mitoxantrone hydrochloride CL-232315 *see* mitoxantrone *on this page*

Mitoxantrone Injection® [Can] *see* mitoxantrone *on this page*

mitozantrone *see* mitoxantrone *on this page*

Mitran® Oral *(Discontinued)* *see* chlordiazepoxide *on page 172*

Mitrazol™ [US-OTC] *see* miconazole *on page 553*

Mivacron® [Can] *see* mivacurium *on this page*

Mivacron® *(Discontinued)* *see* mivacurium *on this page*

mivacurium (mye va KYOO ree um)

Sound-Alike/Look-Alike Issues
Mivacron® may be confused with Mevacor®

Synonyms mivacurium chloride

U.S./Canadian Brand Names Mivacron® [Can]

Therapeutic Category Skeletal Muscle Relaxant

Use Adjunct to general anesthesia to facilitate endotracheal intubation and to relax skeletal muscles during surgery; to facilitate mechanical ventilation in ICU patients; does not relieve pain or produce sedation

Usual Dosage Continuous infusion requires an infusion pump; dose to effect; doses will vary due to interpatient variability; use ideal body weight for obese patients

Children 2-12 years (duration of action is shorter and dosage requirements are higher): 0.2 mg/kg I.V. followed by average infusion rate of 14 mcg/kg/minute (range: 5-31 mcg/kg/minute) upon evidence of spontaneous recovery from initial dose
Adults: Initial: I.V.: 0.15-0.25 mg/kg bolus followed by maintenance doses of 0.1 mg/kg at approximately 15-minute intervals; for prolonged neuromuscular block, initial infusion of 9-10 mcg/kg/minute is used upon evidence of spontaneous recovery from initial dose, usual infusion rate of 6-7 mcg/kg/minute (1-15 mcg/kg/minute) under balanced anesthesia; initial dose after succinylcholine for intubation (balanced anesthesia): Adults: 0.1 mg/kg
Pretreatment/priming: 10% of intubating dose given 3-5 minutes before initial dose

Dosage Forms
Injection, solution [preservative free]:
Mivacron®: 2 mg/mL (5 mL, 10 mL) [DSC]
Injection, solution:
Mivacron®: 2 mg/mL (20 mL, 50 mL) [with benzyl alcohol] [DSC]

mivacurium chloride *see* mivacurium *on this page*

MK-191 *see* pivampicillin *(Canada only) on page 671*

MK383 *see* tirofiban *on page 830*

MK462 *see* rizatriptan *on page 750*

MK594 *see* losartan *on page 506*
MK0826 *see* ertapenem *on page 303*
MK 869 *see* aprepitant *on page 71*
MLN341 *see* bortezomib *on page 114*
MMF *see* mycophenolate *on page 571*
MMR *see* measles, mumps, and rubella vaccines, combined *on page 520*
Moban® [US/Can] *see* molindone *on next page*
Mobic® [US/Can] *see* meloxicam *on page 526*
Mobicox® [Can] *see* meloxicam *on page 526*
Mobidin® *(Discontinued)* *see* magnesium salicylate *on page 516*
Mobisyl® [US-OTC] *see* trolamine *on page 855*

moclobemide *(Canada only)* (moe KLOE be mide)

U.S./Canadian Brand Names Alti-Moclobemide [Can]; Apo-Moclobemide® [Can]; Manerix® [Can]; Novo-Moclobemide [Can]; Nu-Moclobemide [Can]; PMS-Moclobemide [Can]

Therapeutic Category Antidepressant, Monoamine Oxidase Inhibitor

Use Symptomatic relief of depressive illness

Usual Dosage Oral: Adults: Initial: 300 mg/day in 2 divided doses; increase gradually to maximum of 600 mg/day; **Note:** Individual patient response may allow a reduction in daily dose in long-term therapy.

Dosage Forms Tablet: 150 mg, 300 mg

modafinil (moe DAF i nil)

U.S./Canadian Brand Names Alertec® [Can]; Provigil® [US/Can]

Therapeutic Category Central Nervous System Stimulant, Nonamphetamine

Controlled Substance C-IV

Use Improve wakefulness in patients with excessive daytime sleepiness associated with narcolepsy and shift work sleep disorder (SWSD); adjunctive therapy for obstructive sleep apnea/hypopnea syndrome (OSAHS)

Usual Dosage Oral: Adults:

Narcolepsy, OSAHS: Initial: 200 mg as a single daily dose in the morning

SWSD: Initial: 200 mg as a single dose taken ~1 hour prior to start of work shift

Note: Doses of 400 mg/day, given as a single dose, have been well tolerated, but there is no consistent evidence that this dose confers additional benefit

Dosage Forms Tablet: 100 mg, 200 mg

Modane® Bulk [US-OTC] *see* psyllium *on page 717*
Modane® Soft *(Discontinued)* *see* docusate *on page 270*
Modane Tablets® [US-OTC] *see* bisacodyl *on page 111*
Modecate® [Can] *see* fluphenazine *on page 358*
Modecate® Concentrate [Can] *see* fluphenazine *on page 358*
Modicon® [US] *see* ethinyl estradiol and norethindrone *on page 323*
modified Dakin's solution *see* sodium hypochlorite solution *on page 779*
Moducal® [US-OTC] *see* glucose polymers *on page 386*
Modulon® [Can] *see* trimebutine *(Canada only) on page 850*
Moduret [Can] *see* amiloride and hydrochlorothiazide *on page 41*
Moduretic® *(Discontinued)* *see* amiloride and hydrochlorothiazide *on page 41*

moexipril (mo EKS i pril)

Sound-Alike/Look-Alike Issues

moexipril may be confused with Monopril®

Synonyms moexipril hydrochloride

U.S./Canadian Brand Names Univasc® [US]

Therapeutic Category Angiotensin-Converting Enzyme (ACE) Inhibitor

Use Treatment of hypertension, alone or in combination with thiazide diuretics; treatment of left ventricular dysfunction after myocardial infarction

Usual Dosage Adults: Oral: Initial: 7.5 mg once daily (in patients **not** receiving diuretics), 1 hour prior to a meal **or** 3.75 mg once daily (when combined with thiazide diuretics); maintenance dose: 7.5-30 mg/day in 1 or 2 divided doses 1 hour before meals

Dosage Forms Tablet, as hydrochloride [scored]: 7.5 mg, 15 mg

moexipril and hydrochlorothiazide (mo EKS i pril & hye droe klor oh THYE a zide)

Synonyms hydrochlorothiazide and moexipril

U.S./Canadian Brand Names Uniretic® [US/Can]

Therapeutic Category Angiotensin-Converting Enzyme (ACE) Inhibitor; Diuretic, Thiazide

Use Combination therapy for hypertension, however, not indicated for initial treatment of hypertension; replacement therapy in patients receiving separate dosage forms (for patient convenience); when monotherapy with one component fails to achieve desired antihypertensive effect, or when dose-limiting adverse effects limit upward titration of monotherapy

Usual Dosage Adults: Oral: 7.5-30 mg of moexipril, taken either in a single or divided dose one hour before meals; hydrochlorothiazide dose should be ≤50 mg/day

Dosage Forms Tablet [scored]:

7.5/12.5: Moexipril hydrochloride 7.5 mg and hydrochlorothiazide 12.5 mg

15/12.5: Moexipril hydrochloride 15 mg and hydrochlorothiazide 12.5 mg

15/25: Moexipril hydrochloride 15 mg and hydrochlorothiazide 25 mg

moexipril hydrochloride *see* moexipril *on previous page*

Moi-Stir® [US-OTC] *see* saliva substitute *on page 760*

Moisture® Eyes [US-OTC] *see* artificial tears *on page 75*

Moisture® Eyes PM [US-OTC] *see* artificial tears *on page 75*

molindone (moe LIN done)

Sound-Alike/Look-Alike Issues

molindone may be confused with Mobidin®

Moban® may be confused with Mobidin®, Modane®

Synonyms molindone hydrochloride

U.S./Canadian Brand Names Moban® [US/Can]

Therapeutic Category Antipsychotic Agent, Dihydroindoline

Use Management of schizophrenia

Usual Dosage Oral:

Children: Schizophrenia/psychoses:

3-5 years: 1-2.5 mg/day in 4 divided doses

5-12 years: 0.5-1 mg/kg/day in 4 divided doses

Adults: Schizophrenia/psychoses: 50-75 mg/day increase at 3- to 4-day intervals up to 225 mg/day

Dosage Forms Tablet, as hydrochloride: 5 mg, 10 mg, 25 mg, 50 mg

molindone hydrochloride *see* molindone *on this page*

molybdenum *see* trace metals *on page 839*

Molypen® [US] *see* trace metals *on page 839*

MOM *see* magnesium hydroxide *on page 514*

Momentum® [US-OTC] *see* magnesium salicylate *on page 516*

mometasone furoate (moe MET a sone FYOOR oh ate)

Sound-Alike/Look-Alike Issues

Elocon® lotion may be confused with ophthalmic solutions. Manufacturer's labeling emphasizes the product is **NOT** for use in the eyes.

U.S./Canadian Brand Names Asmanex® Twisthaler® [US]; Elocom® [Can]; Elocon® [US]; Nasonex® [US/Can]; PMS-Mometasone [Can]; ratio-Mometasone [Can]; Taro-Mometasone [Can]

Therapeutic Category Corticosteroid, Intranasal; Corticosteroid, Topical

Use Relief of the inflammatory and pruritic manifestations of corticosteroid-responsive dermatoses (medium potency topical corticosteroid); treatment of nasal symptoms of seasonal and perennial allergic rhinitis; prevention of nasal symptoms associated with seasonal allergic rhinitis; treatment of nasal polyps in adults; maintenance treatment of asthma as prophylactic therapy or as a supplement in asthma patients requiring oral corticosteroids for the purpose of decreasing or eliminating the oral corticosteroid requirement

(Continued)

mometasone furoate *(Continued)*

Usual Dosage

Oral inhalation: Children ≥12 years and Adults: Previous therapy:

Bronchodilators or inhaled corticosteroids: Initial: 1 inhalation (220 mcg) daily (maximum 2 inhalations or 440 mcg/day); may be given in the evening or in divided doses twice daily

Oral corticosteroids: Initial: 440 mcg twice daily (maximum 880 mcg/day); prednisone should be reduced no faster than 2.5 mg/day on a weekly basis, beginning after at least 1 week of mometasone furoate use

Note: Maximum effects may not be evident for 1-2 weeks or longer; dose should be titrated to effect, using the lowest possible dose

Nasal spray:

Allergic rhinitis:

Children 2-11 years: 1 spray (50 mcg) in each nostril daily

Children ≥12 years and Adults: 2 sprays (100 mcg) in each nostril daily; when used for the prevention of allergic rhinitis, treatment should begin 2-4 weeks prior to pollen season

Nasal polyps: Adults: 2 sprays (100 mcg) in each nostril twice daily; 2 sprays (100 mcg) once daily may be effective in some patients

Topical: Apply sparingly, do not use occlusive dressings. Therapy should be discontinued when control is achieved; if no improvement is seen in 2 weeks, reassessment of diagnosis may be necessary.

Cream, ointment: Children ≥2 years and Adults: Apply a thin film to affected area once daily; do not use in pediatric patients for longer than 3 weeks

Lotion: Children ≥12 years and Adults: Apply a few drops to affected area once daily

Dosage Forms

Cream, topical:

Elocon®: 0.1% (15 g, 45 g)

Lotion, topical:

Elocon®: 0.1% (30 mL, 60 mL) [contains isopropyl alcohol 40%]

Ointment, topical: 0.1% (15 g, 45 g)

Elocon®: 0.1% (15 g, 45 g)

Powder for oral inhalation:

Asmanex® Twisthaler®: 220 mcg (14 units, 30 units, 60 units, 120 units) [contains lactose]

Suspension, intranasal [spray]:

Nasonex®: 50 mcg/spray (17 g) [delivers 120 sprays; contains benzalkonium chloride]

MOM/mineral oil emulsion *see* magnesium hydroxide and mineral oil *on page 514*

monacolin K *see* lovastatin *on page 508*

Monafed® *(Discontinued)* *see* guaifenesin *on page 392*

Monafed® DM *(Discontinued)* *see* guaifenesin and dextromethorphan *on page 394*

Monarc-M™ [US] *see* antihemophilic factor (human) *on page 59*

***Monilia* skin test** *see Candida albicans (Monilia) on page 142*

Monistat® [Can] *see* miconazole *on page 553*

Monistat® 1 Combination Pack [US-OTC] *see* miconazole *on page 553*

Monistat® 3 [US-OTC/Can] *see* miconazole *on page 553*

Monistat® 7 [US-OTC] *see* miconazole *on page 553*

Monistat-Derm® [US] *see* miconazole *on page 553*

Monistat i.v.™ Injection *(Discontinued)* *see* miconazole *on page 553*

Monitan® [Can] *see* acebutolol *on page 4*

monobenzone (mon oh BEN zone)

U.S./Canadian Brand Names Benoquin® [US]

Therapeutic Category Topical Skin Product

Use Final depigmentation in extensive vitiligo

Usual Dosage Children ≥12 years and Adults: Topical: Apply 2-3 times daily; once desired degree of pigmentation is obtained, may apply as needed (usually 2 times/week)

Dosage Forms Cream, topical: 20% (35 g)

Monocaps [US-OTC] *see* vitamins (multiple/oral) *on page 878*

Monoclate-P® [US] *see* antihemophilic factor (human) *on page 59*

monoclonal antibody *see* muromonab-CD3 *on page 570*

Monocor® [Can] *see* bisoprolol *on page 113*

Monodox® [US] *see* doxycycline *on page 278*

monoethanolamine *see* ethanolamine oleate *on page 316*

Monoket® [US] *see* isosorbide mononitrate *on page 466*

MonoNessa™ [US] *see* ethinyl estradiol and norgestimate *on page 325*

Mononine® [US/Can] *see* factor IX *on page 333*

Monopril® [US/Can] *see* fosinopril *on page 369*

Monopril-HCT® [US/Can] *see* fosinopril and hydrochlorothiazide *on page 369*

montelukast (mon te LOO kast)

Sound-Alike/Look-Alike Issues

Singulair® may be confused with Sinequan®

Synonyms montelukast sodium

U.S./Canadian Brand Names Singulair® [US/Can]

Therapeutic Category Leukotriene Receptor Antagonist

Use Prophylaxis and chronic treatment of asthma; relief of symptoms of seasonal allergic rhinitis and perennial allergic rhinitis

Usual Dosage Oral:

Children:

6-23 months: Perennial allergic rhinitis: 4 mg (oral granules) once daily

12-23 months: Asthma: 4 mg (oral granules) once daily, taken in the evening

2-5 years: Asthma, seasonal or perennial allergic rhinitis: 4 mg (chewable tablet or oral granules) once daily, taken in the evening

6-14 years: Asthma, seasonal or perennial allergic rhinitis: Chew one 5 mg chewable tablet/day, taken in the evening

Children ≥15 years and Adults: Asthma, seasonal or perennial allergic rhinitis: 10 mg/day, taken in the evening

Dosage Forms

Granules: 4 mg/packet

Tablet: 10 mg

Tablet, chewable: 4 mg [contains phenylalanine 0.674 mg; cherry flavor]; 5 mg [contains phenylalanine 0.842 mg; cherry flavor]

montelukast sodium *see* montelukast *on this page*

Monurol™ [US/Can] *see* fosfomycin *on page 369*

8-MOP® [US/Can] *see* methoxsalen *on page 542*

more attenuated enders strain *see* measles virus vaccine (live) *on page 521*

MoreDophilus® [US-OTC] *see* Lactobacillus *on page 477*

moricizine (mor I siz een)

Sound-Alike/Look-Alike Issues

Ethmozine® may be confused with Erythrocin®, erythromycin

Synonyms moricizine hydrochloride

U.S./Canadian Brand Names Ethmozine® [US/Can]

Therapeutic Category Antiarrhythmic Agent, Class I

Use Treatment of ventricular tachycardia and life-threatening ventricular arrhythmias

Usual Dosage Adults: Oral: 200-300 mg every 8 hours, adjust dosage at 150 mg/day at 3-day intervals.

Dosage Forms Tablet, as hydrochloride: 200 mg, 250 mg, 300 mg

moricizine hydrochloride *see* moricizine *on this page*

morning after pill *see* ethinyl estradiol and norgestrel *on page 327*

Morphine HP® [Can] *see* morphine sulfate *on this page*

Morphine LP® Epidural [Can] *see* morphine sulfate *on this page*

morphine sulfate (MOR feen SUL fate)

Sound-Alike/Look-Alike Issues

morphine may be confused with hydromorphone

morphine sulfate may be confused with magnesium sulfate

(Continued)

morphine sulfate *(Continued)*

MSO_4 is an error-prone abbreviation (mistaken as magnesium sulfate)
Avinza™ may be confused with Evista®, Invanz®
Roxanol™ may be confused with OxyFast®, Roxicet™

U.S./Canadian Brand Names Astramorph/PF™ [US]; Avinza™ [US]; DepoDur™ [US]; Duramorph® [US]; Infumorph® [US]; Kadian® [US/Can]; M-Eslon® [Can]; M.O.S.-S.R.® [Can]; M.O.S.-Sulfate® [Can]; M.O.S.® 10 [Can]; M.O.S.® 20 [Can]; M.O.S.® 30 [Can]; Morphine HP® [Can]; Morphine LP® Epidural [Can]; MS Contin® [US/Can]; MS-IR® [Can]; Oramorph SR® [US]; PMS-Morphine Sulfate SR [Can]; ratio-Morphine SR [Can]; RMS® [US]; Roxanol 100™ [US]; Roxanol™ [US]; Statex® [Can]; Zomorph® [Can]

Therapeutic Category Analgesic, Narcotic

Controlled Substance C-II

Use Relief of moderate to severe acute and chronic pain; relief of pain of myocardial infarction; relief of dyspnea of acute left ventricular failure and pulmonary edema; preanesthetic medication
DepoDur™: Epidural (lumbar) single-dose management of surgical pain
Infumorph®: Used in microinfusion devices for intraspinal administration in treatment of intractable chronic pain

Usual Dosage Note: These are guidelines and do not represent the doses that may be required in all patients. Doses should be titrated to pain relief/prevention.

Children >6 months and <50 kg: Acute pain (moderate-to-severe):
Oral (prompt release): 0.15-0.3 mg/kg every 3-4 hours as needed
I.M.: 0.1 mg/kg every 3-4 hours as needed
I.V.: 0.05-0.1 mg/kg every 3-4 hours as needed
I.V. infusion: Range: 10-30 mcg/kg/hour

Adolescents >12 years: Sedation/analgesia for procedures: I.V.: 3-4 mg and repeat in 5 minutes if necessary

Adults:

Acute pain (moderate-to-severe):
Oral: Prompt release formulations: Opiate-naive: Initial: 10 mg every 3-4 hours as needed; patients with prior opiate exposure may require higher initial doses: usual dosage range: 10-30 mg every 3-4 hours as needed
I.M., SubQ: **Note:** Repeated SubQ administration causes local tissue irritation, pain, and induration.
Initial: Opiate-naive: 5-10 mg every 3-4 hours as needed; patients with prior opiate exposure may require higher initial doses; usual dosage range: 5-20 mg every 3-4 hours as needed
Rectal: 10-20 mg every 3-4 hours
I.V.: Initial: Opiate-naive: 2.5-5 mg every 3-4 hours; patients with prior opiate exposure may require higher initial doses. **Note:** Repeated doses (up to every 5 minutes if needed) in small increments (eg, 1-4 mg) may be preferred to larger and less frequent doses.
I.V., SubQ continuous infusion: 0.8-10 mg/hour; usual range: Up to 80 mg/hour
Mechanically-ventilated patients (based on 70 kg patient): 0.7-10 mg every 1-2 hours as needed; infusion: 5-35 mg/hour
Patient-controlled analgesia (PCA): (Opiate-naive: Consider lower end of dosing range):
Usual concentration: 1 mg/mL
Demand dose: Usual: 1 mg; range: 0.5-2.5 mg
Lockout interval: 5-10 minutes

Intrathecal (I.T.): **Note:** Administer with extreme caution and in reduced dosage to geriatric or debilitated patients.
Opioid-naive: 0.2-0.25 mg/dose (may provide adequate relief for 24 hours); repeat doses are **not** recommended.

Epidural: **Note:** Administer with extreme caution and in reduced dosage to geriatric or debilitated patients. Vigilant monitoring is particularly important in these patients.
Pain management:
Single-dose (Duramorph®): Initial: 3-5 mg
Infusion:
Bolus dose: 1-6 mg
Infusion rate: 0.1-0.2 mg/hour
Maximum dose: 10 mg/24 hours

Surgical anesthesia: Epidural: Single-dose (extended-release, Depo-Dur™): Lumbar epidural only; not recommended in patients <18 years of age:
Cesarean section: 10 mg
Lower abdominal/pelvic surgery: 10-15 mg
Major orthopedic surgery of lower extremity: 15 mg
For Depo-Dur™: To minimize the pharmacokinetic interaction resulting in higher peak serum concentrations of morphine, administer the test dose of the local anesthetic at least 15 minutes prior to Depo-Dur™

administration. Use of Depo-Dur™ with epidural local anesthetics has not been studied. Other medications should not be administered into the epidural space for at least 48 hours after administration of DepoDur™.

Note: Some patients may benefit from a 20 mg dose, however, the incidence of adverse effects may be increased.

Chronic pain: Note: Patients taking opioids chronically may become tolerant and require doses higher than the usual dosage range to maintain the desired effect. Tolerance can be managed by appropriate dose titration. There is no optimal or maximal dose for morphine in chronic pain. The appropriate dose is one that relieves pain throughout its dosing interval without causing unmanageable side effects.

Oral: Controlled-, extended-, or sustained-release formulations: A patient's morphine requirement should be established using prompt-release formulations. Conversion to long-acting products may be considered when chronic, continuous treatment is required. Higher dosages should be reserved for use only in opioid-tolerant patients.

Capsules, extended-release (Avinza™): Daily dose administered once daily (for best results, administer at same time each day)

Capsules, sustained-release (Kadian®): Daily dose administered once daily or in 2 divided doses daily (every 12 hours)

Tablets, controlled-release (MS Contin®), sustained-release (Oramorph SR®), or extended-release: Daily dose divided and administered every 8 or every 12 hours

Dosage Forms [DSC] = Discontinued product

Capsule, extended-release (Avinza®): 30 mg, 60 mg, 90 mg, 120 mg

Capsule, sustained-release (Kadian®): 20 mg, 30 mg, 50 mg, 60 mg, 100 mg

Infusion [premixed in D_5W]: 1 mg/mL (100 mL, 250 mL)

Injection, extended-release liposomal suspension [lumbar epidural injection, preservative free] (DepoDur™): 10 mg/mL (1 mL, 1.5 mL, 2 mL)

Injection, solution: 2 mg/mL (1 mL); 4 mg/mL (1 mL); 5 mg/mL (1 mL); 8 mg/mL (1 mL); 10 mg/mL (1 mL, 10 mL); 15 mg/mL (1 mL, 20 mL); 25 mg/mL (4 mL, 10 mL, 20 mL, 40 mL, 50 mL, 100 mL, 250 mL); 50 mg/mL (20 mL, 40 mL) [some preparations contain sodium metabisulfite]

Injection, solution [epidural, intrathecal, or I.V. infusion; preservative free]:

Astramorph/PF™: 0.5 mg/mL (2 mL, 10 mL); 1 mg/mL (2 mL, 10 mL)

Duramorph®: 0.5 mg/mL (10 mL); 1 mg/mL (10 mL)

Injection, solution [epidural or intrathecal infusion via microinfusion device; preservative free] (Infumorph®): 10 mg/mL (20 mL); 25 mg/mL (20 mL)

Injection, solution [I.V. infusion via PCA pump]: 0.5 mg/mL (30 mL); 1 mg/mL (30 mL, 50 mL); 2 mg/mL (30 mL); 5 mg/mL (30 mL, 50 mL)

Injection, solution [preservative free]: 0.5 mg/mL (10 mL); 1 mg/mL (10 mL); 25 mg/mL (4 mL, 10 mL, 20 mL)

Solution, oral: 10 mg/5 mL (5 mL, 10 mL, 100 mL, 500 mL); 20 mg/5 mL (100 mL, 500 mL); 20 mg/mL (30 mL, 120 mL, 240 mL)

Roxanol™: 20 mg/mL (30 mL, 120 mL)

Roxanol 100™: 100 mg/5 mL (240 mL) [with calibrated spoon]

Roxanol™-T: 20 mg/mL (30 mL, 120 mL) [tinted, flavored] [DSC]

Suppository, rectal (RMS®): 5 mg (12s), 10 mg (12s), 20 mg (12s), 30 mg (12s)

Tablet: 15 mg, 30 mg

Tablet, controlled-release (MS Contin®): 15 mg, 30 mg, 60 mg, 100 mg, 200 mg

Tablet, extended-release: 15 mg, 30 mg, 60 mg, 100 mg, 200 mg

Tablet, sustained-release (Oramorph SR®): 15 mg, 30 mg, 60 mg, 100 mg

morrhuate sodium (MOR yoo ate SOW dee um)

U.S./Canadian Brand Names Scleromate® [US]

Therapeutic Category Sclerosing Agent

Use Treatment of small, uncomplicated varicose veins of the lower extremities

Usual Dosage Adults: I.V.: 50-250 mg, repeated at 5- to 7-day intervals (50-100 mg for small veins, 150-250 mg for large veins)

Dosage Forms Injection, solution: 50 mg/mL (30 mL)

M.O.S.® 10 [Can] *see* morphine sulfate *on page 565*

M.O.S.® 20 [Can] *see* morphine sulfate *on page 565*

M.O.S.® 30 [Can] *see* morphine sulfate *on page 565*

Mosco® Corn and Callus Remover [US-OTC] *see* salicylic acid *on page 758*

M.O.S.-S.R.® [Can] *see* morphine sulfate *on page 565*

M.O.S.-Sulfate® [Can] *see* morphine sulfate *on page 565*

Motilium® [Can] *see* domperidone *(Canada only) on page 273*

Motofen® [US] *see* difenoxin and atropine *on page 253*

Motrin® [US] *see* ibuprofen *on page 437*

Motrin® Children's [US-OTC/Can] *see* ibuprofen *on page 437*

Motrin® Cold and Sinus [US-OTC] *see* pseudoephedrine and ibuprofen *on page 715*

Motrin® Cold, Children's [US-OTC] *see* pseudoephedrine and ibuprofen *on page 715*

Motrin® IB [US-OTC/Can] *see* ibuprofen *on page 437*

Motrin® IB Sinus *(Discontinued)* *see* pseudoephedrine and ibuprofen *on page 715*

Motrin® Infants' [US-OTC] *see* ibuprofen *on page 437*

Motrin® Junior Strength [US-OTC] *see* ibuprofen *on page 437*

Mouthkote® [US-OTC] *see* saliva substitute *on page 760*

moxifloxacin (moxs i FLOKS a sin)

Sound-Alike/Look-Alike Issues
Avelox® may be confused with Avonex®

Synonyms moxifloxacin hydrochloride

U.S./Canadian Brand Names Avelox® I.V. [US/Can]; Avelox® [US/Can]; Vigamox™ [US/Can]

Therapeutic Category Antibiotic, Quinolone

Use Treatment of mild-to-moderate community-acquired pneumonia, including multidrug-resistant *Streptococcus pneumoniae* (MDRSP); acute bacterial exacerbation of chronic bronchitis; acute bacterial sinusitis; complicated and uncomplicated skin and skin structure infections; complicated intraabdominal infections; bacterial conjunctivitis (ophthalmic formulation)

Usual Dosage

Usual dosage range:
Children ≥1 year and Adults: Ophthalmic: Instill 1 drop into affected eye(s) 3 times/day for 7 days
Adults: Oral, I.V.: 400 mg every 24 hours

Indication-specific dosing:
Children ≥1 year and Adults: Ophthalmic:
Bacterial conjunctivitis: Instill 1 drop into affected eye(s) 3 times/day for 7 days
Adults: Oral, I.V.:
Acute bacterial sinusitis: 400 mg every 24 hours for 10 days
Chronic bronchitis, acute bacterial exacerbation: 400 mg every 24 hours for 5 days
Intraabdominal infections (complicated): 400 mg every 24 hours for 5-14 days (initiate with I.V.)
Pneumonia, community-acquired (including MDRSP): 400 mg every 24 hours for 7-14 days
Skin and skin structure infections:
Complicated: 400 mg every 24 hours for 7-21 days
Uncomplicated: 400 mg every 24 hours for 7 days

Dosage Forms
Infusion [premixed in sodium chloride 0.8%] (Avelox® I.V.): 400 mg (250 mL)
Solution, ophthalmic (Vigamox™): 0.5% (3 mL)
Tablet:
Avelox®: 400 mg
Avelox® ABC Pack [unit-dose pack]: 400 mg (5s)

moxifloxacin hydrochloride *see* moxifloxacin *on this page*

4-MP *see* fomepizole *on page 366*

6-MP *see* mercaptopurine *on page 532*

MPA and estrogens (conjugated) *see* estrogens (conjugated/equine) and medroxyprogesterone *on page 313*

M-Prednisol® Injection *(Discontinued)* *see* methylprednisolone *on page 547*

MPSV4 *see* meningococcal polysaccharide vaccine (groups A / C / Y and W-135) *on page 528*

MS Contin® [US/Can] *see* morphine sulfate *on page 565*

MS-IR® [Can] *see* morphine sulfate *on page 565*

MTA *see* pemetrexed *on page 645*

MTC *see* mitomycin *on page 560*

M.T.E.-4® [US] *see* trace metals *on page 839*

M.T.E.-5® [US] *see* trace metals *on page 839*

M.T.E.-6® [US] *see* trace metals *on page 839*

M.T.E.-7® [US] *see* trace metals *on page 839*

Mucinex® [US-OTC] *see* guaifenesin *on page 392*

Mucinex®-D [US-OTC] *see* guaifenesin and pseudoephedrine *on page 398*

Mucinex® DM [US-OTC] *see* guaifenesin and dextromethorphan *on page 394*

Mucomyst® [Can] *see* acetylcysteine *on page 15*

Mucosil™ *(Discontinued)* *see* acetylcysteine *on page 15*

Multidex® [US-OTC] *see* maltodextrin *on page 518*

multiple vitamins *see* vitamins (multiple/oral) *on page 878*

Multiret Folic 500 [US] *see* vitamins (multiple/oral) *on page 878*

multitargeted antifolate *see* pemetrexed *on page 645*

Multitest CMI® *(Discontinued)*

Multitrace™-4 [US] *see* trace metals *on page 839*

Multitrace™-4 Neonatal [US] *see* trace metals *on page 839*

Multitrace™-4 Pediatric [US] *see* trace metals *on page 839*

Multitrace™-5 [US] *see* trace metals *on page 839*

multivitamins/fluoride *see* vitamins (multiple/pediatric) *on page 878*

mumps, measles and rubella vaccines, combined *see* measles, mumps, and rubella vaccines, combined *on page 520*

mumps, rubella, varicella, and measles vaccine *see* measles, mumps, rubella, and varicella virus vaccine *on page 521*

Mumpsvax® [US] *see* mumps virus vaccine, live, attenuated *on this page*

mumps virus vaccine, live, attenuated (mumpz VYE rus vak SEEN, live, a ten YOO ate ed)

U.S./Canadian Brand Names Mumpsvax® [US]

Therapeutic Category Vaccine, Live Virus

Use Mumps prophylaxis by promoting active immunity

Note: Trivalent measles-mumps-rubella (MMR) vaccine is the preferred agent for most children and many adults; persons born prior to 1957 are generally considered immune and need not be vaccinated

Usual Dosage Children ≥12-15 months and Adults: SubQ: 0.5 mL as a single dose

Dosage Forms

Injection, powder for reconstitution [preservative free]:

Mumpsvax®: $TCID_{50}$ 20,000 [contains human albumin, bovine serum, gelatin, neomycin; packaged with diluent]

mupirocin (myoo PEER oh sin)

Sound-Alike/Look-Alike Issues

Bactroban® may be confused with bacitracin, baclofen

Synonyms mupirocin calcium; pseudomonic acid A

U.S./Canadian Brand Names Bactroban® Nasal [US]; Bactroban® [US/Can]; Centany™ [US]

Therapeutic Category Antibiotic, Topical

Use

Intranasal: Eradication of nasal colonization with MRSA in adult patients and healthcare workers

Topical: Treatment of impetigo or secondary infected traumatic skin lesions due to *S. aureus* and *S. pyogenes*

Usual Dosage

Intranasal: Children ≥12 years and Adults: Eradication of nasal MRSA: Approximately one-half of the ointment from the single-use tube should be applied into one nostril and the other half into the other nostril twice daily for 5 days

Topical:

Children ≥2 months and Adults: Impetigo: Ointment: Apply to affected area 3 times/day; re-evaluate after 3-5 days if no clinical response

Children ≥3 months and Adults: Secondary skin infections: Cream: Apply to affected area 3 times/day for 10 days; re-evaluate after 3-5 days if no clinical response

(Continued)

mupirocin *(Continued)*

Dosage Forms Note: Strength expressed as base
Cream, topical, as calcium:
Bactroban®: 2% (15 g, 30 g) [contains benzyl alcohol]
Ointment, intranasal, as calcium:
Bactroban® Nasal: 2% (1 g) [single-use tube]
Ointment, topical: 2% (0.9 g, 22 g)
Bactroban®: 2% (22 g) [contains polyethylene glycol]
Centany™: 2% (15 g, 30 g)

mupirocin calcium *see* mupirocin *on previous page*

Murine® Ear Wax Removal System [US-OTC] *see* carbamide peroxide *on page 145*

Murine® Tears [US-OTC] *see* artificial tears *on page 75*

Murine® Tears Plus [US-OTC] *see* tetrahydrozoline *on page 817*

Muro 128® [US-OTC] *see* sodium chloride *on page 777*

Murocel® [US-OTC] *see* artificial tears *on page 75*

Murocoll-2® [US] *see* phenylephrine and scopolamine *on page 662*

muromonab-CD3 (myoo roe MOE nab see dee three)

Synonyms monoclonal antibody; OKT3

U.S./Canadian Brand Names Orthoclone OKT® 3 [US/Can]

Therapeutic Category Immunosuppressant Agent

Use Treatment of acute allograft rejection in renal transplant patients; treatment of acute hepatic, kidney, and pancreas rejection episodes resistant to conventional treatment. Acute graft-versus-host disease following bone marrow transplantation resistant to conventional treatment.

Usual Dosage I.V. (refer to individual protocols):
Children <30 kg: 2.5 mg/day once daily for 7-14 days
Children >30 kg: 5 mg/day once daily for 7-14 days
OR
Children <12 years: 0.1 mg/kg/day once daily for 10-14 days
Children ≥12 years and Adults: 5 mg/day once daily for 10-14 days

Dosage Forms Injection, solution: 1 mg/mL (5 mL) [contains sodium 43 mg/5 mL]

Muroptic-5® ***(Discontinued)*** *see* sodium chloride *on page 777*

Muse® [US] *see* alprostadil *on page 32*

Muse® Pellet [Can] *see* alprostadil *on page 32*

Mustargen® [US/Can] *see* mechlorethamine *on page 522*

mustine *see* mechlorethamine *on page 522*

Mutamycin® [US/Can] *see* mitomycin *on page 560*

M.V.I.®-12 ***(Discontinued)*** *see* vitamins (multiple/injectable) *on page 878*

M.V.I. Adult™ [US] *see* vitamins (multiple/injectable) *on page 878*

M.V.I® Pediatric [US] *see* vitamins (multiple/injectable) *on page 878*

Myambutol® [US] *see* ethambutol *on page 316*

Mycamine™ [US] *see* micafungin *on page 553*

Mycelex® [US] *see* clotrimazole *on page 205*

Mycelex®-3 [US-OTC] *see* butoconazole *on page 130*

Mycelex®-7 [US-OTC] *see* clotrimazole *on page 205*

Mycelex®-G ***(Discontinued)*** *see* clotrimazole *on page 205*

Mycelex® Twin Pack [US-OTC] *see* clotrimazole *on page 205*

Mycifradin® Sulfate ***(Discontinued)*** *see* neomycin *on page 582*

Mycinaire™ [US-OTC] *see* sodium chloride *on page 777*

Mycinettes® [US-OTC] *see* benzocaine *on page 99*

Mycobutin® [US/Can] *see* rifabutin *on page 744*

Mycolog®-II ***(Discontinued)*** *see* nystatin and triamcinolone *on page 610*

Myco-Nail [US-OTC] *see* triacetin *on page 845*

Myconel® Topical *(Discontinued)* *see* nystatin and triamcinolone *on page 610*

mycophenolate (mye koe FEN oh late)

Synonyms MMF; mycophenolate mofetil; mycophenolate sodium; mycophenolic acid

U.S./Canadian Brand Names CellCept® [US/Can]; Myfortic® [US/Can]

Therapeutic Category Immunosuppressant Agent

Use Prophylaxis of organ rejection concomitantly with cyclosporine and corticosteroids in patients receiving allogenic renal (CellCept®, Myfortic®), cardiac (CellCept®), or hepatic (CellCept®) transplants

Usual Dosage

Children: Renal transplant: Oral:

CellCept® suspension: 600 mg/m^2/dose twice daily; maximum dose: 1 g twice daily

Alternatively, may use solid dosage forms according to BSA as follows:

BSA 1.25-1.5 m^2: 750 mg capsule twice daily

BSA >1.5 m^2: 1 g capsule or tablet twice daily

Myfortic®: 400 mg/m^2/dose twice daily; maximum dose: 720 mg twice daily

BSA <1.19 m^2: Use of this formulation is not recommended

BSA 1.19-1.58 m^2: 540 mg twice daily (maximum: 1080 mg/day)

BSA >1.58 m^2: 720 mg twice daily (maximum: 1440 mg/day)

Adults:

Renal transplant:

CellCept®:

Oral: 1 g twice daily. Doses >2 g/day are not recommended.

I.V.: 1 g twice daily

Myfortic®: Oral: 720 mg twice daily (1440 mg/day)

Cardiac transplantation:

Oral (CellCept®): 1.5 g twice daily

I.V. (CellCept®): 1.5 g twice daily

Hepatic transplantation:

Oral (CellCept®): 1.5 g twice daily

I.V. (CellCept®): 1 g twice daily

Dosage Forms

Capsule, as mofetil (CellCept®): 250 mg

Injection, powder for reconstitution, as mofetil hydrochloride (CellCept®): 500 mg [contains polysorbate 80]

Powder for oral suspension, as mofetil (CellCept®): 200 mg/mL (225 mL) [provides 175 mL suspension following reconstitution; contains phenylalanine 0.56 mg/mL; mixed fruit flavor]

Tablet, as mofetil (CellCept®): 500 mg [may contain ethyl alcohol]

Tablet, delayed release, as mycophenolic acid (Myfortic®): 180 mg, 360 mg [formulated as a sodium salt]

mycophenolate mofetil *see* mycophenolate *on this page*

mycophenolate sodium *see* mycophenolate *on this page*

mycophenolic acid *see* mycophenolate *on this page*

Mycostatin® [US] *see* nystatin *on page 609*

Mydfrin® [US/Can] *see* phenylephrine *on page 660*

Mydral™ [US] *see* tropicamide *on page 856*

Mydriacyl® [US/Can] *see* tropicamide *on page 856*

My First Flintstones® [US-OTC] *see* vitamins (multiple/pediatric) *on page 878*

Myfortic® [US/Can] *see* mycophenolate *on this page*

Mykrox® [Can] *see* metolazone *on page 549*

Mykrox® *(Discontinued)* *see* metolazone *on page 549*

Mylanta™ [Can] *see* aluminum hydroxide and magnesium hydroxide *on page 36*

Mylanta®-II *(Discontinued)* *see* aluminum hydroxide, magnesium hydroxide, and simethicone *on page 37*

Mylanta AR® *(Discontinued)* *see* famotidine *on page 335*

Mylanta® Children's [US-OTC] *see* calcium carbonate *on page 135*

Mylanta® Double Strength [Can] *see* aluminum hydroxide, magnesium hydroxide, and simethicone *on page 37*

Mylanta® Extra Strength [Can] *see* aluminum hydroxide, magnesium hydroxide, and simethicone *on page 37*

Mylanta® Gas [US-OTC] *see* simethicone *on page 772*

Mylanta® Gas Maximum Strength [US-OTC] *see* simethicone *on page 772*

Mylanta® Gelcaps® [US-OTC] *see* calcium carbonate and magnesium hydroxide *on page 136*

Mylanta® Liquid [US-OTC] *see* aluminum hydroxide, magnesium hydroxide, and simethicone *on page 37*

Mylanta® Maximum Strength Liquid [US-OTC] *see* aluminum hydroxide, magnesium hydroxide, and simethicone *on page 37*

Mylanta® Regular Strength [Can] *see* aluminum hydroxide, magnesium hydroxide, and simethicone *on page 37*

Mylanta® Supreme [US-OTC] *see* calcium carbonate and magnesium hydroxide *on page 136*

Mylanta® Ultra [US-OTC] *see* calcium carbonate and magnesium hydroxide *on page 136*

Myleran® [US/Can] *see* busulfan *on page 128*

Mylicon® Infants [US-OTC] *see* simethicone *on page 772*

Mylocel™ [US] *see* hydroxyurea *on page 432*

Mylotarg® [US/Can] *see* gemtuzumab ozogamicin *on page 379*

Myminic® Expectorant *(Discontinued)*

Myobloc® [US] *see* botulinum toxin type B *on page 116*

Myochrysine® [Can] *see* gold sodium thiomalate *on page 390*

Myoflex® [US-OTC/Can] *see* trolamine *on page 855*

Myotonachol® [Can] *see* bethanechol *on page 109*

Myotonachol® *(Discontinued)* *see* bethanechol *on page 109*

Myozyme® [US] *see* alglucosidase alfa *on page 28*

Myphetane DX [US] *see* brompheniramine, pseudoephedrine, and dextromethorphan *on page 120*

myrac™ [US] *see* minocycline *on page 558*

Mysoline® [US] *see* primidone *on page 699*

Mytelase® [US/Can] *see* ambenonium *on page 39*

Mytrex *(Discontinued)* *see* nystatin and triamcinolone *on page 610*

Mytussin® AC [US] *see* guaifenesin and codeine *on page 393*

Mytussin® DAC [US] *see* guaifenesin, pseudoephedrine, and codeine *on page 401*

N-9 *see* nonoxynol 9 *on page 597*

Na2EDTA *see* edetate disodium *on page 287*

Nabi-HB® [US] *see* hepatitis B immune globulin *on page 411*

NAB-paclitaxel *see* paclitaxel (protein bound) *on page 631*

nabumetone (na BYOO me tone)

U.S./Canadian Brand Names Apo-Nabumetone® [Can]; Gen-Nabumetone [Can]; Novo-Nabumetone [Can]; Relafen® [Can]; Rhoxal-nabumetone [Can]; Sandoz-Nabumetone [Can]

Therapeutic Category Analgesic, Nonnarcotic; Nonsteroidal Antiinflammatory Drug (NSAID)

Use Management of osteoarthritis and rheumatoid arthritis

Usual Dosage Adults: Oral: 1000 mg/day; an additional 500-1000 mg may be needed in some patients to obtain more symptomatic relief; may be administered once or twice daily (maximum dose: 2000 mg/day)
Note: Patients <50 kg are less likely to require doses >1000 mg/day.

Dosage Forms [DSC] = Discontinued product
Tablet: 500 mg, 750 mg
Relafen®: 500 mg, 750 mg [DSC]

NAC *see* acetylcysteine *on page 15*

***n*-acetyl-L-cysteine** *see* acetylcysteine *on page 15*

***n*-acetylcysteine** *see* acetylcysteine *on page 15*

***n*-acetyl-p-aminophenol** *see* acetaminophen *on page 5*

NaCl *see* sodium chloride *on page 777*

nadolol (NAY doe lol)

Sound-Alike/Look-Alike Issues

nadolol may be confused with Mandol®

Corgard® may be confused with Cognex®

U.S./Canadian Brand Names Alti-Nadolol [Can]; Apo-Nadol® [Can]; Corgard® [US/Can]; Novo-Nadolol [Can]

Therapeutic Category Beta-Adrenergic Blocker

Use Treatment of hypertension and angina pectoris; prophylaxis of migraine headaches

Usual Dosage Oral: Adults: Initial: 40 mg/day, increase dosage gradually by 40-80 mg increments at 3- to 7-day intervals until optimum clinical response is obtained with profound slowing of heart rate; doses up to 160-240 mg/day in angina and 240-320 mg/day in hypertension may be necessary.

Hypertension: Usual dosage range (JNC 7): 40-120 mg once daily

Dosage Forms [DSC] = Discontinued product

Tablet: 20 mg, 40 mg, 80 mg, 120 mg, 160 mg

Corgard®: 20 mg, 40 mg, 80 mg, 120 mg [DSC], 160 mg [DSC]

nadroparin calcium *see* nadroparin *(Canada only) on this page*

nadroparin *(Canada only)* (nad roe PA rin)

Synonyms nadroparin calcium

U.S./Canadian Brand Names Fraxiparine™ Forte [Can]; Fraxiparine™ [Can]

Therapeutic Category Low Molecular Weight Heparin

Use Prophylaxis of thromboembolic disorders (particularly deep venous thrombosis and pulmonary embolism) in general and orthopedic surgery; treatment of deep venous thrombosis; prevention of clotting during hemodialysis

Usual Dosage SubQ: Adults:

Prophylaxis of thromboembolic disorders in general surgery: 2850 anti-Xa int. units once daily; begin 2-4 hours before surgery and continue for 7 days

Prophylaxis of thromboembolic disorders in hip replacement: 38 anti-Xa int. units/kg 12 hours before and 12 hours after surgery, **followed by** 38 anti-Xa int. units/kg/day up to and including day 3, **then** 57 anti-Xa int. units/kg/day for up to 10 days total therapy

Treatment of thromboembolic disorders: 171 anti-Xa int. units/kg/day to a maximum of 17,100 int. units; plasma anti-Xa levels should be 1.2-1.8 anti-Xa int. units/mL 3-4 hours postinjection

Patients at increased risk of bleeding: 86 anti-Xa int. units/kg twice daily; plasma anti-Xa levels should be 0.5-1.1 anti-Xa int. units/mL 3-4 hours postinjection

Prevention of clotting during hemodialysis: Single dose of 65 anti-Xa int. units/kg into arterial line at start of each dialysis session; may give additional dose if session lasts longer than 4 hours

Patients at risk of hemorrhage: Administer 50% of dose

Dosage Forms [CAN] = Canadian brand name

Injection, solution, as calcium:

Fraxiparine™ [CAN]:

9500 anti-Xa int. units/mL (0.2 mL, 0.3 mL, 0.4 mL) [ungraduated prefilled syringe]

9500 anti-Xa int. units/mL (0.6 mL, 0.8 mL, 1 mL) [graduated prefilled syringe]

Fraxiparine™ Forte [CAN]: 19,000 anti-Xa int. units/mL (0.6 mL, 0.8 mL, 1 mL) [graduated prefilled syringe]

nafarelin (naf a REL in)

Sound-Alike/Look-Alike Issues

nafarelin may be confused with Anafranil®, enalapril

Synonyms nafarelin acetate

U.S./Canadian Brand Names Synarel® [US/Can]

Therapeutic Category Hormone, Posterior Pituitary

Use Treatment of endometriosis, including pain and reduction of lesions; treatment of central precocious puberty (CPP; gonadotropin-dependent precocious puberty) in children of both sexes

Usual Dosage Intranasal:

Endometriosis: Adults: Female: 1 spray (200 mcg) in 1 nostril each morning and the other nostril each evening starting on days 2-4 of menstrual cycle (total: 2 sprays/day). Dose may be increased to 2 sprays (400 mcg; 1 spray in each nostril) in the morning and evening if amenorrhea is not achieved (total: 8 sprays [1600 mcg]/day). Total duration of therapy should not exceed 6 months due to decreases in bone mineral density; retreatment is not recommended by the manufacturer.

(Continued)

nafarelin *(Continued)*

Central precocious puberty: Children: Male/Female: 2 sprays (400 mcg) into each nostril in the morning and 2 sprays (400 mcg) into each nostril in the evening (total: 8 sprays [1600 mcg]/day). If inadequate suppression, may increase dose to 3 sprays (600 mcg) into alternating nostrils 3 times/day (total: 9 sprays [1800 mcg]/day).

Dosage Forms

Solution, intranasal [spray]:

Synarel®: 2 mg/mL (8 mL) [200 mcg/spray: 60 metered sprays; contains benzalkonium chloride]

nafarelin acetate *see* nafarelin *on previous page*

Nafazair® Ophthalmic *(Discontinued)* *see* naphazoline *on page 577*

nafcillin (naf SIL in)

Synonyms ethoxynaphthamido penicillin sodium; nafcillin sodium; sodium nafcillin

U.S./Canadian Brand Names Nallpen® [Can]; Unipen® [Can]

Therapeutic Category Penicillin

Use Treatment of infections such as osteomyelitis, septicemia, endocarditis, and CNS infections caused by susceptible strains of staphylococci species

Usual Dosage

Usual dosage range:

Neonates: I.V.:

<2000 g, <7 days: 50 mg/kg/day divided every 12 hours
>2000 g, <7 days: 50 mg/kg/day divided every 8 hours
<2000 g, >7 days: 75 mg/kg/day divided every 8 hours
>2000 g, >7 days: 75 mg/kg/day divided every 6 hours

Children:

I.M.: 25 mg/kg twice daily
I.V.: 50-200 mg/kg/day in divided doses every 4-6 hours (maximum: 12 g/day)

Adults:

I.M.: 500 mg every 4-6 hours
I.V.: 500-2000 mg every 4-6 hours

Indication-specific dosing:

Neonates:

Arthritis, septic: I.V.:

<2000 g, <7 days: 50 mg/kg/day divided every 12 hours
<2000 g, >7 days: 75 mg/kg/day divided every 8 hours
>2000 g, <7 days: 75 mg/kg/day divided every 8 hours
>2000 g, >7 days: 222 mg/kg/day divided every 6 hours

Children:

Epiglottitis: I.V.: 150-200 mg/kg/day divided in 4 doses
Mild to moderate infections: I.M., I.V.: 50-100 mg/kg/day in divided doses every 6 hours
Severe infections: I.M., I.V.: 100-200 mg/kg/day in divided doses every 4-6 hours (maximum dose: 12 g/day)
Toxic epidermal necrolysis: I.V.: 150 mg/kg/day divided every 6 hours for 5-7 days

Adults: I.V.:

Endocarditis: MSSA:

Native valve: 2 g every 4 hours
Prosthetic valve: 1 g every 4 hours with rifampin for 6 weeks with gentamicin for 2 weeks
Tricuspid valve: 2 g every 4 hours with gentamicin for 2 weeks

Joint:

Bursitis, septic: 2 g every 4 hours
Prosthetic: 2 g every 4-6 hours with rifampin for 6 weeks

***Staphylococcus aureus*, methicillin-susceptible infections, including brain abscess, empyema, erysipelas, mastitis, myositis, osteomyelitis, pneumonia, toxic shock, urinary tract (perinephric abscess):** 2 g every 4 hours

Toxic epidermal necrolysis: 2 g every 4 hours

Dosage Forms

Infusion [premixed iso-osmotic dextrose solution]: 1 g (50 mL); 2 g (100 mL)
Injection, powder for reconstitution, as sodium: 1 g, 2 g, 10 g

nafcillin sodium *see* nafcillin *on this page*

naftifine (NAF ti feen)

Synonyms naftifine hydrochloride

U.S./Canadian Brand Names Naftin® [US]

Therapeutic Category Antifungal Agent

Use Topical treatment of tinea cruris (jock itch), tinea corporis (ringworm), and tinea pedis (athlete's foot)

Usual Dosage Adults: Topical: Apply cream once daily and gel twice daily (morning and evening) for up to 4 weeks

Dosage Forms

Cream, as hydrochloride: 1% (15 g, 30 g, 60 g) [contains benzyl alcohol]

Gel, as hydrochloride: 1% (20 g, 40 g, 60 g) [contains alcohol 52%]

naftifine hydrochloride *see* naftifine *on this page*

Naftin® [US] *see* naftifine *on this page*

Naglazyme™ [US] *see* galsulfase *on page 374*

$NaHCO_3$ *see* sodium bicarbonate *on page 776*

nalbuphine (NAL byoo feen)

Sound-Alike/Look-Alike Issues

Nubain® may be confused with Navane®, Nebcin®

Synonyms nalbuphine hydrochloride

U.S./Canadian Brand Names Nubain® [US]

Therapeutic Category Analgesic, Narcotic

Use Relief of moderate to severe pain; preoperative analgesia, postoperative and surgical anesthesia, and obstetrical analgesia during labor and delivery

Usual Dosage Adults:

Pain management: I.M., I.V., SubQ: 10 mg/70 kg every 3-6 hours; maximum single dose in nonopioid-tolerant patients: 20 mg; maximum daily dose: 160 mg

Surgical anesthesia supplement: I.V.: Induction: 0.3-3 mg/kg over 10-15 minutes; maintenance doses of 0.25-0.5 mg/kg may be given as required

Dosage Forms [DSC] = Discontinued product

Injection, solution, as hydrochloride: 10 mg/mL (10 mL); 20 mg/mL (10 mL)

Nubain®: 10 mg/mL (10 mL) [DSC]; 20 mg/mL (10 mL)

Injection, solution, as hydrochloride [preservative free]: 10 mg/mL (1 mL); 20 mg/mL (1 mL)

Nubain®: 10 mg/mL (1 mL); 20 mg/mL (1 mL)

nalbuphine hydrochloride *see* nalbuphine *on this page*

Nalcrom® [Can] *see* cromolyn sodium *on page 217*

Naldecon® DX Adult Liquid *(Discontinued)*

Naldecon-EX® Children's Syrup *(Discontinued)*

Naldecon Senior EX® *(Discontinued)* *see* guaifenesin *on page 392*

Nalex®-A [US] *see* chlorpheniramine, phenylephrine, and phenyltoloxamine *on page 181*

Nalfon® [US] *see* fenoprofen *on page 339*

Nallpen® [Can] *see* nafcillin *on previous page*

Nallpen® *(Discontinued)* *see* nafcillin *on previous page*

***N*-allylnoroxymorphine hydrochloride** *see* naloxone *on next page*

nalmefene (NAL me feen)

Sound-Alike/Look-Alike Issues

Revex® may be confused with Nimbex®, ReVia®

Synonyms nalmefene hydrochloride

U.S./Canadian Brand Names Revex® [US]

Therapeutic Category Antidote

Use Complete or partial reversal of opioid drug effects, including respiratory depression induced by natural or synthetic opioids; reversal of postoperative opioid depression; management of known or suspected opioid overdose

Usual Dosage I.M., I.V., SubQ:

Reversal of postoperative opioid depression: Blue-labeled product (100 mcg/mL): Titrate to reverse the undesired effects of opioids; initial dose for nonopioid dependent patients: 0.25 mcg/kg followed by 0.25

(Continued)

nalmefene *(Continued)*

mcg/kg incremental doses at 2- to 5-minute intervals; after a total dose >1 mcg/kg, further therapeutic response is unlikely

Note: In patients with increased cardiovascular risks, dilute 1:1 in NS or SWFI, and initiate/titrate with 0.1 mcg/kg doses.

Management of known/suspected opioid overdose: Green-labeled product (1 mg/mL): Initial dose: 0.5 mg/70 kg; may repeat with 1 mg/70 kg in 2-5 minutes; further increase beyond a total dose of 1.5 mg/70 kg will not likely result in improved response and may result in cardiovascular stress and precipitated withdrawal syndrome. (If opioid dependency is suspected, administer a challenge dose of 0.1 mg/70 kg; if no withdrawal symptoms are observed in 2 minutes, the recommended doses can be administered.)

Note: If recurrence of respiratory depression is noted, dose may again be titrated to clinical effect using incremental doses.

Note: If I.V. access is lost or not readily obtainable, a single SubQ or I.M. dose of 1 mg may be effective in 5-15 minutes.

Dosage Forms

Injection, solution:

Revex®: 100 mcg/mL (1 mL) [blue label]; 1 mg/mL (2 mL) [green label]

nalmefene hydrochloride *see* nalmefene *on previous page*

naloxone (nal OKS one)

Sound-Alike/Look-Alike Issues

naloxone may be confused with naltrexone

Narcan® may be confused with Marcaine®, Norcuron®

Synonyms *N*-allylnoroxymorphine hydrochloride; naloxone hydrochloride

U.S./Canadian Brand Names Naloxone Hydrochloride Injection® [Can]

Therapeutic Category Antidote

Use

Complete or partial reversal of opioid depression, including respiratory depression, induced by natural and synthetic opioids, including propoxyphene, methadone, and certain mixed agonist-antagonist analgesics: nalbuphine, pentazocine, and butorphanol

Diagnosis of suspected opioid tolerance or acute opioid overdose

Adjunctive agent to increase blood pressure in the management of septic shock

Usual Dosage I.M., I.V. (preferred), intratracheal, SubQ:

Postanesthesia narcotic reversal: Infants and Children: 0.01 mg/kg; may repeat every 2-3 minutes, as needed based on response

Opiate intoxication:

Children:

Birth (including premature infants) to 5 years or <20 kg: 0.1 mg/kg; repeat every 2-3 minutes if needed; may need to repeat doses every 20-60 minutes

>5 years or ≥20 kg: 2 mg/dose; if no response, repeat every 2-3 minutes; may need to repeat doses every 20-60 minutes

Children and Adults: Continuous infusion: I.V.: If continuous infusion is required, calculate dosage/hour based on effective intermittent dose used and duration of adequate response seen, titrate dose 0.04-0.16 mg/kg/hour for 2-5 days in children, adult dose typically 0.25-6.25 mg/hour (short-term infusions as high as 2.4 mg/kg/hour have been tolerated in adults during treatment for septic shock); alternatively, continuous infusion utilizes $^{2}/_{3}$ of the initial naloxone bolus on an hourly basis; add 10 times this dose to each liter of D_5W and infuse at a rate of 100 mL/hour; $^{1}/_{2}$ of the initial bolus dose should be readministered 15 minutes after initiation of the continuous infusion to prevent a drop in naloxone levels; increase infusion rate as needed to assure adequate ventilation

Narcotic overdose: Adults: I.V.: 0.4-2 mg every 2-3 minutes as needed; may need to repeat doses every 20-60 minutes, if no response is observed after 10 mg, question the diagnosis. **Note:** Use 0.1-0.2 mg increments in patients who are opioid dependent and in postoperative patients to avoid large cardiovascular changes.

Dosage Forms [DSC] = Discontinued product

Injection, solution, as hydrochloride: 0.4 mg/mL (1 mL, 10 mL)

Narcan®: 0.4 mg/mL (1 mL) [DSC]

naloxone and buprenorphine *see* buprenorphine and naloxone *on page 126*

naloxone hydrochloride *see* naloxone *on this page*

naloxone hydrochloride and pentazocine hydrochloride *see* pentazocine *on page 651*

naloxone hydrochloride dihydrate and buprenorphine hydrochloride *see* buprenorphine and naloxone *on page 126*

Naloxone Hydrochloride Injection® [Can] *see* naloxone *on previous page*

naltrexone (nal TREKS one)

Sound-Alike/Look-Alike Issues

naltrexone may be confused with naloxone

ReVia® may be confused with Revex®

Synonyms naltrexone hydrochloride

U.S./Canadian Brand Names Depade® [US]; ReVia® [US/Can]; Vivitrol™ [US]

Therapeutic Category Antidote

Use Treatment of ethanol dependence; blockade of the effects of exogenously administered opioids

Usual Dosage Adults: Do not give until patient is opioid-free for 7-10 days as determined by urinalysis

Oral: Alcohol dependence, opioid antidote: 25 mg; if no withdrawal signs within 1 hour give another 25 mg; maintenance regimen is flexible, variable and individualized (50 mg/day to 100-150 mg 3 times/week for 12 weeks); up to 800 mg/day has been tolerated in a small number of healthy adults without an adverse effect

I.M.: Alcohol dependence: 380 mg once every 4 weeks

Dosage Forms

Injection, powder for suspension [extended-release microspheres]:

Vivitrol™: 380 mg [diluent provided]

Tablet, as hydrochloride: 50 mg

Depade®: 25 mg, 50 mg, 100 mg

ReVia®: 50 mg

naltrexone hydrochloride *see* naltrexone *on this page*

Namenda™ [US] *see* memantine *on page 527*

nandrolone (NAN droe lone)

Synonyms nandrolone decanoate; nandrolone phenpropionate

U.S./Canadian Brand Names Deca-Durabolin® [Can]; Durabolin® [Can]

Therapeutic Category Androgen

Controlled Substance C-III

Use Control of metastatic breast cancer; management of anemia of renal insufficiency

Usual Dosage Deep I.M. (into gluteal muscle):

Children 2-13 years (decanoate): 25-50 mg every 3-4 weeks

Adults:

Male:

Breast cancer (phenpropionate): 50-100 mg/week

Anemia of renal insufficiency (decanoate): 100-200 mg/week

Female: 50-100 mg/week

Breast cancer (phenpropionate): 50-100 mg/week

Anemia of renal insufficiency (decanoate): 50-100 mg/week

Dosage Forms Injection, solution, as decanoate [in sesame oil]: 100 mg/mL (2 mL); 200 mg/mL (1 mL) [contains benzyl alcohol]

nandrolone decanoate *see* nandrolone *on this page*

nandrolone phenpropionate *see* nandrolone *on this page*

NAPA and NABZ *see* sodium phenylacetate and sodium benzoate *on page 780*

naphazoline (naf AZ oh leen)

Synonyms naphazoline hydrochloride

U.S./Canadian Brand Names AK-Con™ [US]; Albalon® [US]; Allersol® [US]; Clear Eyes® ACR [US-OTC]; Clear Eyes® Extra Relief [US-OTC]; Naphcon Forte® [Can]; Naphcon® [US-OTC]; Privine® [US-OTC]; Vasocon® [Can]

Therapeutic Category Adrenergic Agonist Agent

Use Topical ocular vasoconstrictor; temporary relief of nasal congestion associated with the common cold, upper respiratory allergies or sinusitis; relief of redness of the eye due to minor irritation

Usual Dosage

Nasal: Children ≥12 years and Adults: 0.05% instill 1-2 drops or sprays every 6 hours if needed; therapy should not exceed 3 days

(Continued)

naphazoline *(Continued)*

Ophthalmic: Adults:
0.1% (prescription): 1-2 drops into conjuctival sac every 3-4 hours as needed
0.012% (OTC): 1-2 drops into affected eye(s) up to 4 times a day; therapy should not exceed 3 days

Dosage Forms
Solution, intranasal drops, as hydrochloride:
Privine®: 0.05% (25 mL)
Solution, intranasal spray, as hydrochloride:
Privine®: 0.05% (20 mL)
Solution, ophthalmic, as hydrochloride:
AK-Con™, Albalon®, Allersol®: 0.1% (15 mL) [contains benzalkonium chloride]
Clear Eyes® ACR: 0.012% (15 mL, 30 mL) [contains glycerin 0.2%, zinc sulfate 0.25%, and benzalkonium chloride]
Clear Eyes® Extra Relief: 0.012% (6 mL, 15 mL, 30 mL) [contains glycerin 0.2% and benzalkonium chloride]
Naphcon®: 0.012% (15 mL) [contains benzalkonium chloride]

naphazoline and pheniramine (naf AZ oh leen & fen NIR a meen)

Sound-Alike/Look-Alike Issues
Visine® may be confused with Visken®

Synonyms pheniramine and naphazoline

U.S./Canadian Brand Names Naphcon-A® [US-OTC/Can]; Opcon-A® [US-OTC]; Visine-A™ [US-OTC]; Visine® Advanced Allergy [Can]

Therapeutic Category Antihistamine/Decongestant Combination

Use Treatment of ocular congestion, irritation, and itching

Usual Dosage Ophthalmic: Children ≥6 years and Adults: 1-2 drops up to 4 times/day

Dosage Forms
Solution, ophthalmic: Naphazoline hydrochloride 0.025% and pheniramine 0.3% (15 mL) [contains benzalkonium chloride]
Naphcon-A®: Naphazoline hydrochloride 0.025% and pheniramine 0.3% (5 mL) [contains benzalkonium chloride; 2 bottles/box], (15 mL) [contains benzalkonium chloride]
Opcon-A®, Visine-A™: Naphazoline hydrochloride 0.025% and pheniramine 0.3% (15 mL) [contains benzalkonium chloride]

naphazoline hydrochloride *see* naphazoline *on previous page*

Naphcon® [US-OTC] *see* naphazoline *on previous page*

Naphcon-A® [US-OTC/Can] *see* naphazoline and pheniramine *on this page*

Naphcon Forte® [Can] *see* naphazoline *on previous page*

Naphcon Forte® Ophthalmic *(Discontinued)* *see* naphazoline *on previous page*

NapraPAC™ *see* lansoprazole and naproxen *on page 483*

Naprelan® [US] *see* naproxen *on this page*

Naprosyn® [US/Can] *see* naproxen *on this page*

naproxen (na PROKS en)

Sound-Alike/Look-Alike Issues
naproxen may be confused with Natacyn®, Nebcin®
Aleve® may be confused with Alesse®
Anaprox® may be confused with Anaspaz®, Avapro®
Naprelan® may be confused with Naprosyn®
Naprosyn® may be confused with Naprelan®, Natacyn®, Nebcin®

Synonyms naproxen sodium

U.S./Canadian Brand Names Aleve® [US-OTC]; Anaprox® DS [US/Can]; Anaprox® [US/Can]; Apo-Napro-Na DS® [Can]; Apo-Napro-Na® [Can]; Apo-Naproxen EC® [Can]; Apo-Naproxen SR® [Can]; Apo-Naproxen® [Can]; EC-Naprosyn® [US]; Gen-Naproxen EC [Can]; Midol® Extended Relief [US]; Naprelan® [US]; Naprosyn® [US/Can]; Naxen® EC [Can]; Naxen® [Can]; Novo-Naproc EC [Can]; Novo-Naprox Sodium DS [Can]; Novo-Naprox Sodium [Can]; Novo-Naprox SR [Can]; Novo-Naprox [Can]; Nu-Naprox [Can]; Pamprin® Maximum Strength All Day Relief [US-OTC]; Riva-Naproxen [Can]

Therapeutic Category Analgesic, Nonnarcotic; Antipyretic; Nonsteroidal Antiinflammatory Drug (NSAID)

Use Management of ankylosing spondylitis, osteoarthritis, and rheumatoid disorders (including juvenile rheumatoid arthritis); acute gout; mild-to-moderate pain; tendonitis, bursitis; dysmenorrhea; fever

Usual Dosage Note: Dosage expressed as naproxen base; 200 mg naproxen base is equivalent to 220 mg naproxen sodium.

Oral:

Children >2 years: Juvenile arthritis: 10 mg/kg/day in 2 divided doses

Adults:

Gout, acute: Initial: 750 mg, followed by 250 mg every 8 hours until attack subsides. **Note:** EC-Naprosyn® is not recommended.

Pain (mild-to-moderate), dysmenorrhea, acute tendonitis, bursitis: Initial: 500 mg, then 250 mg every 6-8 hours; maximum: 1250 mg/day naproxen base

Rheumatoid arthritis, osteoarthritis, and ankylosing spondylitis: 500-1000 mg/day in 2 divided doses; may increase to 1.5 g/day of naproxen base for limited time period

OTC labeling: Pain/fever:

Children ≥12 years and Adults ≤65 years: 200 mg naproxen base every 8-12 hours; if needed, may take 400 mg naproxen base for the initial dose; maximum: 600 mg naproxen base/24 hours

Adults >65 years: 200 mg naproxen base every 12 hours

Dosage Forms

Caplet, as sodium (Aleve®, Midol® Extended Relief, Pamprin® Maximum Strength All Day Relief): 220 mg [equivalent to naproxen 200 mg and sodium 20 mg]

Gelcap, as sodium (Aleve®): 220 mg [equivalent to naproxen 200 mg and sodium 20 mg]

Suspension, oral (Naprosyn®): 125 mg/5 mL (480 mL) [contains sodium 0.3 mEq/mL; orange-pineapple flavor]

Tablet (Naprosyn®): 250 mg, 375 mg, 500 mg

Tablet, as sodium: 220 mg [equivalent to naproxen 200 mg and sodium 20 mg]; 275 mg [equivalent to naproxen 250 mg and sodium 25 mg]; 550 mg [equivalent to naproxen 500 mg and sodium 50 mg]

Aleve®: 220 mg [equivalent to naproxen 200 mg and sodium 20 mg]

Anaprox®: 275 mg [equivalent to naproxen 250 mg and sodium 25 mg]

Anaprox® DS: 550 mg [equivalent to naproxen 500 mg and sodium 50 mg]

Tablet, controlled release, as sodium: 550 mg [equivalent to naproxen 500 mg and sodium 50 mg]

Naprelan®: 421.5 mg [equivalent to naproxen 375 mg and sodium 37.5 mg]; 550 mg [equivalent to naproxen 500 mg and sodium 50 mg]

Tablet, delayed release (EC-Naprosyn®): 375 mg, 500 mg

naproxen and lansoprazole *see* lansoprazole and naproxen *on page 483*

naproxen sodium *see* naproxen *on previous page*

naratriptan (NAR a trip tan)

Sound-Alike/Look-Alike Issues

Amerge® may be confused with Altace®, Amaryl®

Synonyms naratriptan hydrochloride

U.S./Canadian Brand Names Amerge® [US/Can]

Therapeutic Category Antimigraine Agent; Serotonin Agonist

Use Treatment of acute migraine headache with or without aura

Usual Dosage Adults: Oral: 1-2.5 mg at the onset of headache; it is recommended to use the lowest possible dose to minimize adverse effects. If headache returns or does not fully resolve, the dose may be repeated after 4 hours; do not exceed 5 mg in 24 hours.

Dosage Forms Tablet: 1 mg, 2.5 mg

naratriptan hydrochloride *see* naratriptan *on this page*

Narcan® *(Discontinued)* *see* naloxone *on page 576*

Nardil® [US/Can] *see* phenelzine *on page 657*

Naropin® [US/Can] *see* ropivacaine *on page 753*

Nasacort® AQ [US/Can] *see* triamcinolone (inhalation, nasal) *on page 845*

Nasacort® HFA [US] *see* triamcinolone (inhalation, nasal) *on page 845*

Nasahist B® *(Discontinued)* *see* brompheniramine *on page 118*

NaSal™ [US-OTC] *see* sodium chloride *on page 777*

NasalCrom® [US-OTC] *see* cromolyn sodium *on page 217*

Nasalide® [Can] *see* flunisolide *on page 352*

Nasal Moist® [US-OTC] *see* sodium chloride *on page 777*

Nasarel® [US] *see* flunisolide *on page 352*

Nasatab® LA [US] *see* guaifenesin and pseudoephedrine *on page 398*

Nascobal® [US] *see* cyanocobalamin *on page 219*

Nasonex® [US/Can] *see* mometasone furoate *on page 563*

Natabec® *(Discontinued)*

Natabec® FA *(Discontinued)*

Natabec® Rx *(Discontinued)*

NataChew™ [US] *see* vitamins (multiple/prenatal) *on page 879*

Natacyn® [US/Can] *see* natamycin *on this page*

NataFort® [US] *see* vitamins (multiple/prenatal) *on page 879*

NatalCare® CFe 60 *(Discontinued)* *see* vitamins (multiple/prenatal) *on page 879*

NatalCare® GlossTabs™ [US] *see* vitamins (multiple/prenatal) *on page 879*

NatalCare® PIC [US] *see* vitamins (multiple/prenatal) *on page 879*

NatalCare® PIC Forte [US] *see* vitamins (multiple/prenatal) *on page 879*

NatalCare® Plus [US] *see* vitamins (multiple/prenatal) *on page 879*

NatalCare® Rx [US] *see* vitamins (multiple/prenatal) *on page 879*

NatalCare® Three [US] *see* vitamins (multiple/prenatal) *on page 879*

Natalins® Rx *(Discontinued)*

natalizumab (na ta LIZ u mab)

Synonyms AN100226; anti-4 alpha integrin; IgG4-kappa monoclonal antibody

U.S./Canadian Brand Names Tysabri® [US]

Therapeutic Category Monoclonal Antibody, Selective Adhesion-Molecule Inhibitor

Use Treatment of relapsing forms of multiple sclerosis

Usual Dosage I.V.: Adults: Multiple sclerosis: 300 mg infused over 1 hour every 4 weeks

Dosage Forms Injection, solution [preservative free]: 300 mg/15 mL (15 mL) [contains polysorbate-80]

natamycin (na ta MYE sin)

Sound-Alike/Look-Alike Issues

Natacyn® may be confused with Naprosyn®

Synonyms pimaricin

U.S./Canadian Brand Names Natacyn® [US/Can]

Therapeutic Category Antifungal Agent

Use Treatment of blepharitis, conjunctivitis, and keratitis caused by susceptible fungi (*Aspergillus*, *Candida*), *Cephalosporium, Curvularia, Fusarium, Penicillium, Microsporum, Epidermophyton, Blastomyces dermatitidis, Coccidioides immitis, Cryptococcus neoformans, Histoplasma capsulatum, Sporothrix schenckii,* and *Trichomonas vaginalis*

Usual Dosage Adults: Ophthalmic: Instill 1 drop in conjunctival sac every 1-2 hours, after 3-4 days reduce to one drop 6-8 times/day; usual course of therapy is 2-3 weeks.

Dosage Forms Suspension, ophthalmic: 5% (15 mL) [contains benzalkonium chloride]

NataTab™ CFe [US] *see* vitamins (multiple/prenatal) *on page 879*

NataTab™ FA [US] *see* vitamins (multiple/prenatal) *on page 879*

NataTab™ Rx [US] *see* vitamins (multiple/prenatal) *on page 879*

nateglinide (na te GLYE nide)

U.S./Canadian Brand Names Starlix® [US/Can]

Therapeutic Category Antidiabetic Agent

Use Management of type 2 diabetes mellitus (noninsulin-dependent, NIDDM) as monotherapy when hyperglycemia cannot be managed by diet and exercise alone; in combination with metformin or a thiazolidinedione to lower blood glucose in patients whose hyperglycemia cannot be controlled by exercise, diet, or a single agent alone

Usual Dosage Adults: Management of type 2 diabetes mellitus: Oral: Initial and maintenance dose: 120 mg 3 times/day, 1-30 minutes before meals; may be given alone or in combination with metformin or a thiazolidinedione; patients close to Hb A_{1c} goal may be started at 60 mg 3 times/day

Dosage Forms Tablet: 60 mg, 120 mg

Natelle® [US] *see* vitamins (multiple/prenatal) *on page 879*
Natelle®-ez [US] *see* vitamins (multiple/prenatal) *on page 879*
Natelle® Prefer [US] *see* vitamins (multiple/prenatal) *on page 879*
Natrecor® [US] *see* nesiritide *on page 587*
natriuretic peptide *see* nesiritide *on page 587*
Natulan® [Can] *see* procarbazine *on page 701*
Natural Fiber Therapy [US-OTC] *see* psyllium *on page 717*
natural lung surfactant *see* beractant *on page 105*
Nature's Tears® [US-OTC] *see* artificial tears *on page 75*
Nature-Throid® NT [US] *see* thyroid *on page 824*
Naus-A-Way® *(Discontinued)*
Nausea Relief [US-OTC] *see* fructose, dextrose, and phosphoric acid *on page 371*
Nauseatol [Can] *see* dimenhydrinate *on page 258*
Navane® [US/Can] *see* thiothixene *on page 824*
Navelbine® [US/Can] *see* vinorelbine *on page 873*
Naxen® [Can] *see* naproxen *on page 578*
Naxen® EC [Can] *see* naproxen *on page 578*
Na-Zone® [US-OTC] *see* sodium chloride *on page 777*
NC-722665 *see* bicalutamide *on page 110*
***n*-docosanol** *see* docosanol *on page 270*
ND-Stat® Solution [US-OTC] *see* brompheniramine *on page 118*
Nebcin® *(Discontinued)* *see* tobramycin *on page 831*
NebuPent® [US] *see* pentamidine *on page 650*
Necon® 0.5/35 [US] *see* ethinyl estradiol and norethindrone *on page 323*
Necon® 1/35 [US] *see* ethinyl estradiol and norethindrone *on page 323*
Necon® 1/50 [US] *see* mestranol and norethindrone *on page 534*
Necon® 7/7/7 [US] *see* ethinyl estradiol and norethindrone *on page 323*
Necon® 10/11 [US] *see* ethinyl estradiol and norethindrone *on page 323*

nedocromil (inhalation) (ne doe KROE mil in hil LA shun)

U.S./Canadian Brand Names Tilade® [US/Can]
Therapeutic Category Mast Cell Stabilizer
Use Maintenance therapy in patients with mild to moderate bronchial asthma
Usual Dosage Children >6 years and Adults: 2 inhalations 4 times/day; may reduce dosage to 2-3 times/day once desired clinical response to initial dose is observed
Dosage Forms Aerosol for inhalation, as sodium (Tilade®): 1.75 mg/activation (16.2 g)

nedocromil (ophthalmic) (ne doe KROE mil op THAL mik)

U.S./Canadian Brand Names Alocril® [US/Can]
Therapeutic Category Mast Cell Stabilizer
Use Treatment of itching associated with allergic conjunctivitis
Usual Dosage Adults: Ophthalmic: 1-2 drops in eye(s) twice daily
Dosage Forms Solution, ophthalmic, as sodium (Alocril®): 2% (5 mL) [contains benzalkonium chloride]

nefazodone (nef AY zoe done)

Sound-Alike/Look-Alike Issues
Serzone® may be confused with selegiline, Serentil®, Seroquel®, sertraline
Synonyms nefazodone hydrochloride
Therapeutic Category Antidepressant, Miscellaneous
Use Treatment of depression
Usual Dosage Oral: Adults: Depression: 200 mg/day, administered in 2 divided doses initially, with a range of 300-600 mg/day in 2 divided doses thereafter
Dosage Forms Tablet, as hydrochloride: 50 mg, 100 mg, 150 mg, 200 mg, 250 mg

nefazodone hydrochloride *see* nefazodone *on previous page*

NegGram® *(Discontinued)*

nelarabine (nel AY re been)

Synonyms 2-amino-6-methoxypurine arabinoside; GW506U78; 506U78

U.S./Canadian Brand Names Arranon® [US]

Therapeutic Category Antineoplastic Agent, Antimetabolite

Use Treatment of relapsed or refractory T-cell acute lymphoblastic leukemia (ALL) and T-cell lymphoblastic lymphoma

Usual Dosage I.V.: T-cell ALL, T-cell lymphoblastic lymphoma:

Children: 650 mg/m²/day on days 1 through 5; repeat every 21 days

Adults: 1500 mg/m²/day on days 1, 3, and 5; repeat every 21 days

Dosage Forms Injection, solution: 5 mg/mL (50 mL)

nelfinavir (nel FIN a veer)

Sound-Alike/Look-Alike Issues

nelfinavir may be confused with nevirapine

Viracept® may be confused with Viramune®

Synonyms NFV

U.S./Canadian Brand Names Viracept® [US/Can]

Therapeutic Category Antiviral Agent

Use In combination with other antiretroviral therapy in the treatment of HIV infection

Usual Dosage Oral:

Children 2-13 years: 45-55 mg/kg twice daily **or** 25-35 mg/kg 3 times/day (maximum: 2500 mg/day); all doses should be taken with a meal. If tablets are unable to be taken, use oral powder in small amount of water, milk, formula, or dietary supplements; do not use acidic food/juice or store for >6 hours.

Adults: 750 mg 3 times/day with meals or 1250 mg twice daily with meals in combination with other antiretroviral therapies

Dosage Forms

Powder, oral: 50 mg/g (144 g) [contains phenylalanine 11.2 mg/g]

Tablet: 250 mg, 625 mg

Nelova™ 0.5/35E *(Discontinued)* *see* ethinyl estradiol and norethindrone *on page 323*

Nelova™ 1/35E *(Discontinued)* *see* ethinyl estradiol and norethindrone *on page 323*

Nelova™ 1/50M *(Discontinued)* *see* mestranol and norethindrone *on page 534*

Nelova™ 10/11 *(Discontinued)* *see* ethinyl estradiol and norethindrone *on page 323*

Nembutal® [US] *see* pentobarbital *on page 652*

Neo-Calglucon® *(Discontinued)* *see* calcium glubionate *on page 138*

NeoCeuticals™ Acne Spot Treatment [US-OTC] *see* salicylic acid *on page 758*

Neo-Dexameth® Ophthalmic *(Discontinued)*

Neo-Durabolic® *(Discontinued)* *see* nandrolone *on page 577*

Neofed® *(Discontinued)* *see* pseudoephedrine *on page 712*

Neo-Fradin™ [US] *see* neomycin *on this page*

Neomixin® Topical *(Discontinued)* *see* bacitracin, neomycin, and polymyxin B *on page 91*

neomycin (nee oh MYE sin)

Sound-Alike/Look-Alike Issues

myciguent may be confused with Mycitracin®

Synonyms neomycin sulfate

U.S./Canadian Brand Names Neo-Fradin™ [US]; Neo-Rx [US]

Therapeutic Category Aminoglycoside (Antibiotic); Antibiotic, Topical

Use Orally to prepare GI tract for surgery; topically to treat minor skin infections; treatment of diarrhea caused by *E. coli*; adjunct in the treatment of hepatic encephalopathy; bladder irrigation; ocular infections

Usual Dosage

Children: Oral:

Preoperative intestinal antisepsis: 90 mg/kg/day divided every 4 hours for 2 days; or 25 mg/kg at 1 PM, 2 PM, and 11 PM on the day preceding surgery as an adjunct to mechanical cleansing of the intestine and in combination with erythromycin base

Hepatic encephalopathy: 50-100 mg/kg/day in divided doses every 6-8 hours or 2.5-7 g/m^2/day divided every 4-6 hours for 5-6 days not to exceed 12 g/day

Children and Adults: Topical: Topical solutions containing 0.1% to 1% neomycin have been used for irrigation

Adults: Oral:

Preoperative intestinal antisepsis: 1 g each hour for 4 doses then 1 g every 4 hours for 5 doses; or 1 g at 1 PM, 2 PM, and 11 PM on day preceding surgery as an adjunct to mechanical cleansing of the bowel and oral erythromycin; or 6 g/day divided every 4 hours for 2-3 days

Hepatic encephalopathy: 500-2000 mg every 6-8 hours or 4-12 g/day divided every 4-6 hours for 5-6 days

Chronic hepatic insufficiency: 4 g/day for an indefinite period

Dosage Forms

Powder, micronized, as sulfate [for prescription compounding] (Neo-Rx): (10 g, 100 g)

Solution, oral, as sulfate (Neo-Fradin™): 125 mg/5 mL (60 mL, 480 mL) [contains benzoic acid; cherry flavor]

Tablet, as sulfate: 500 mg

neomycin and polymyxin B (nee oh MYE sin & pol i MIKS in bee)

Synonyms polymyxin B and neomycin

U.S./Canadian Brand Names Neosporin® G.U. Irrigant [US]; Neosporin® Irrigating Solution [Can]

Therapeutic Category Antibiotic, Topical; Genitourinary Irrigant

Use Short-term as a continuous irrigant or rinse in the urinary bladder to prevent bacteriuria and gram-negative rod septicemia associated with the use of indwelling catheters; to help prevent infection in minor cuts, scrapes, and burns

Usual Dosage Children and Adults: Bladder irrigation: **Not for injection**; add 1 mL irrigant to 1 liter isotonic saline solution and connect container to the inflow of lumen of 3-way catheter. Continuous irrigant or rinse in the urinary bladder for up to a maximum of 10 days with administration rate adjusted to patient's urine output; usually no more than 1 L of irrigant is used per day.

Dosage Forms

Solution, irrigant: Neomycin 40 mg and polymyxin B 200,000 units per mL (1 mL)

Neosporin® G.U. Irrigant: Neomycin 40 mg and polymyxin B 200,000 units per mL (1 mL, 20 mL)

neomycin, bacitracin, and polymyxin B *see* bacitracin, neomycin, and polymyxin B *on page 91*

neomycin, bacitracin, polymyxin B, and hydrocortisone *see* bacitracin, neomycin, polymyxin B, and hydrocortisone *on page 91*

neomycin, bacitracin, polymyxin B, and pramoxine *see* bacitracin, neomycin, polymyxin B, and pramoxine *on page 91*

neomycin, colistin, hydrocortisone, and thonzonium

(nee oh MYE sin, koe LIS tin, hye droe KOR ti sone, & thon ZOE nee um)

Synonyms colistin, neomycin, hydrocortisone, and thonzonium; hydrocortisone, neomycin, colistin, and thonzonium; thonzonium, neomycin, colistin, and hydrocortisone

U.S./Canadian Brand Names Coly-Mycin® S [US]; Cortisporin®-TC [US]

Therapeutic Category Antibiotic/Corticosteroid, Otic

Use Treatment of superficial and susceptible bacterial infections of the external auditory canal; for treatment of susceptible bacterial infections of mastoidectomy and fenestration cavities

Usual Dosage Otic:

Calibrated dropper:

Children: 4 drops in affected ear 3-4 times/day

Adults: 5 drops in affected ear 3-4 times/day

Dropper bottle:

Children: 3 drops in affected ear 3-4 times/day

Adults: 4 drops in affected ear 3-4 times/day

Note: Alternatively, a cotton wick may be inserted in the ear canal and saturated with suspension every 4 hours; wick should be replaced at least every 24 hours

Dosage Forms Suspension, otic [drops]:

Coly-Mycin® S: Neomycin 0.33%, colistin 0.3%, hydrocortisone acetate 1%, and thonzonium bromide 0.05% (5 mL) [contains thimerosal; packaged with dropper]

Cortisporin®-TC: Neomycin 0.33%, colistin 0.3%, hydrocortisone acetate 1%, and thonzonium bromide 0.05% (10 mL) [contains thimerosal; packaged with dropper]

neomycin, polymyxin B, and dexamethasone

(nee oh MYE sin, pol i MIKS in bee, & deks a METH a sone)

Sound-Alike/Look-Alike Issues

AK-Trol® may be confused with AKTob®

Synonyms dexamethasone, neomycin, and polymyxin B; polymyxin B, neomycin, and dexamethasone

U.S./Canadian Brand Names Dioptrol® [Can]; Maxitrol® [US/Can]; Poly-Dex™ [US]

Therapeutic Category Antibiotic/Corticosteroid, Ophthalmic

Use Steroid-responsive inflammatory ocular conditions in which a corticosteroid is indicated and where bacterial infection or a risk of bacterial infection exists

Usual Dosage Children and Adults: Ophthalmic:

Ointment: Place a small amount (~1/2") in the affected eye 3-4 times/day or apply at bedtime as an adjunct wsith drops

Suspension: Instill 1-2 drops into affected eye(s) every 3-4 hours; in severe disease, drops may be used hourly and tapered to discontinuation

Dosage Forms [DSC] = Discontinued product

Ointment, ophthalmic (Maxitrol®, Poly-Dex™): Neomycin 3.5 mg, polymyxin B sulfate 10,000 units, and dexamethasone 0.1% per g (3.5 g)

Suspension, ophthalmic (AK-Trol® [DSC], Maxitrol®, Poly-Dex™): Neomycin 3.5 mg, polymyxin B sulfate 10,000 units, and dexamethasone 0.1% per mL (5 mL) [contains benzalkonium chloride]

neomycin, polymyxin B, and gramicidin

(nee oh MYE sin, pol i MIKS in bee, & gram i SYE din)

Synonyms gramicidin, neomycin, and polymyxin B; polymyxin B, neomycin, and gramicidin

U.S./Canadian Brand Names Neosporin® Ophthalmic Solution [US]; Neosporin® [Can]; Optimyxin Plus® [Can]

Therapeutic Category Antibiotic, Ophthalmic

Use Treatment of superficial ocular infection

Usual Dosage Children and Adults: Ophthalmic: Instill 1-2 drops 4-6 times/day or more frequently as required for severe infections

Dosage Forms Solution, ophthalmic: Neomycin 1.75 mg, polymyxin B 10,000 units, and gramicidin 0.025 mg per mL (10 mL) [contains alcohol 0.5% and thimerosal]

neomycin, polymyxin B, and hydrocortisone

(nee oh MYE sin, pol i MIKS in bee, & hye droe KOR ti sone)

Synonyms hydrocortisone, neomycin, and polymyxin B; polymyxin B, neomycin, and hydrocortisone

U.S./Canadian Brand Names Cortimyxin® [Can]; Cortisporin® Cream [US]; Cortisporin® Ophthalmic [US]; Cortisporin® Otic [US/Can]; PediOtic® [US]

Therapeutic Category Antibiotic/Corticosteroid, Ophthalmic; Antibiotic/Corticosteroid, Otic; Antibiotic/Corticosteroid, Topical

Use Steroid-responsive inflammatory condition for which a corticosteroid is indicated and where bacterial infection or a risk of bacterial infection exists

Usual Dosage Duration of use should be limited to 10 days unless otherwise directed by the physician

Otic solution is used **only** for swimmer's ear (infections of external auditory canal)

Otic:

Children: Instill 3 drops into affected ear 3-4 times/day

Adults: Instill 4 drops 3-4 times/day; otic suspension is the preferred otic preparation

Children and Adults:

Ophthalmic: Drops: Instill 1-2 drops 2-4 times/day, or more frequently as required for severe infections; in acute infections, instill 1-2 drops every 15-30 minutes gradually reducing the frequency of administration as the infection is controlled

Topical: Apply a thin layer 1-4 times/day. Therapy should be discontinued when control is achieved; if no improvement is seen, reassessment of diagnosis may be necessary.

Dosage Forms

Cream, topical (Cortisporin®): Neomycin 3.5 mg, polymyxin B 10,000 units, and hydrocortisone acetate 5 mg per g (7.5 g)

Solution, otic (Cortisporin®): Neomycin 3.5 mg, polymyxin B 10,000 units, and hydrocortisone 10 mg per mL (10 mL) [contains potassium metabisulfite]

Suspension, ophthalmic (Cortisporin®): Neomycin 3.5 mg, polymyxin B 10,000 units, and hydrocortisone 10 mg per mL (7.5 mL) [contains thimerosal]

Suspension, otic: Neomycin 3.5 mg, polymyxin B 10,000 units, and hydrocortisone 10 mg per mL (10 mL)

Cortisporin®: Neomycin 3.5 mg, polymyxin B 10,000 units, and hydrocortisone 10 mg per mL (10 mL) [contains thimerosal]

PediOtic®: Neomycin 3.5 mg, polymyxin B 10,000 units, and hydrocortisone 10 mg per mL (7.5 mL) [contains thimerosal]

neomycin, polymyxin B, and prednisolone

(nee oh MYE sin, pol i MIKS in bee, & pred NIS oh lone)

Synonyms polymyxin B, neomycin, and prednisolone; prednisolone, neomycin, and polymyxin B

U.S./Canadian Brand Names Poly-Pred® [US]

Therapeutic Category Antibiotic/Corticosteroid, Ophthalmic

Use Steroid-responsive inflammatory ocular condition in which bacterial infection or a risk of bacterial ocular infection exists

Usual Dosage Children and Adults: Ophthalmic: Instill 1-2 drops every 3-4 hours; acute infections may require every 30-minute instillation initially with frequency of administration reduced as the infection is brought under control. To treat the lids: Instill 1-2 drops every 3-4 hours, close the eye and rub the excess on the lids and lid margins.

Dosage Forms Suspension, ophthalmic: Neomycin 0.35%, polymyxin B 10,000 units per mL, and prednisolone acetate 0.5% (5 mL; 10 mL [DSC]) [contains thimerosal]

neomycin sulfate *see* neomycin *on page 582*

neonatal trace metals *see* trace metals *on page 839*

NeoProfen® *see* ibuprofen *on page 437*

Neoral® [US/Can] *see* cyclosporine *on page 221*

Neo-Rx [US] *see* neomycin *on page 582*

Neosporin® [Can] *see* neomycin, polymyxin B, and gramicidin *on previous page*

Neosporin® AF [US-OTC] *see* miconazole *on page 553*

Neosporin® G.U. Irrigant [US] *see* neomycin and polymyxin B *on page 583*

Neosporin® Irrigating Solution [Can] *see* neomycin and polymyxin B *on page 583*

Neosporin® Neo To Go® [US-OTC] *see* bacitracin, neomycin, and polymyxin B *on page 91*

Neosporin® Ophthalmic Ointment [Can] *see* bacitracin, neomycin, and polymyxin B *on page 91*

Neosporin® Ophthalmic Ointment *(Discontinued)* *see* bacitracin, neomycin, and polymyxin B *on page 91*

Neosporin® Ophthalmic Solution [US] *see* neomycin, polymyxin B, and gramicidin *on previous page*

Neosporin® + Pain Ointment [US-OTC] *see* bacitracin, neomycin, polymyxin B, and pramoxine *on page 91*

Neosporin® Topical [US-OTC] *see* bacitracin, neomycin, and polymyxin B *on page 91*

neostigmine (nee oh STIG meen)

Sound-Alike/Look-Alike Issues

Prostigmin® may be confused with physostigmine

Synonyms neostigmine bromide; neostigmine methylsulfate

U.S./Canadian Brand Names Prostigmin® [US/Can]

Therapeutic Category Cholinergic Agent

Use Diagnosis and treatment of myasthenia gravis; prevention and treatment of postoperative bladder distention and urinary retention; reversal of the effects of nondepolarizing neuromuscular-blocking agents after surgery

Usual Dosage

Myasthenia gravis: Diagnosis: I.M.:

Children: 0.04 mg/kg as a single dose

Adults: 0.02 mg/kg as a single dose

Myasthenia gravis: Treatment:

Children:

Oral: 2 mg/kg/day divided every 3-4 hours

I.M., I.V., SubQ: 0.01-0.04 mg/kg every 2-4 hours

Adults:

Oral: 15 mg/dose every 3-4 hours up to 375 mg/day maximum; interval between doses must be individualized to maximal response

I.M., I.V., SubQ: 0.5-2.5 mg every 1-3 hours up to 10 mg/24 hours maximum

(Continued)

neostigmine *(Continued)*

Reversal of nondepolarizing neuromuscular blockade after surgery in conjunction with atropine (must administer atropine several minutes prior to neostigmine): I.V.:

Infants: 0.025-0.1 mg/kg/dose

Children: 0.025-0.08 mg/kg/dose

Adults: 0.5-2.5 mg; total dose not to exceed 5 mg

Bladder atony: Adults: I.M., SubQ:

Prevention: 0.25 mg every 4-6 hours for 2-3 days

Treatment: 0.5-1 mg every 3 hours for 5 doses after bladder has emptied

Dosage Forms

Injection, solution, as methylsulfate: 0.5 mg/mL (1 mL, 10 mL); 1 mg/mL (10 mL)

Tablet, as bromide: 15 mg

neostigmine bromide *see* neostigmine *on previous page*

neostigmine methylsulfate *see* neostigmine *on previous page*

NeoStrata AHA [US-OTC] *see* hydroquinone *on page 430*

NeoStrata® HQ [Can] *see* hydroquinone *on page 430*

Neo-Synephrine® [Can] *see* phenylephrine *on page 660*

Neo-Synephrine® 12 Hour [US-OTC] *see* oxymetazoline *on page 628*

Neo-Synephrine® 12 Hour Extra Moisturizing [US-OTC] *see* oxymetazoline *on page 628*

Neo-Synephrine® Extra Strength [US-OTC] *see* phenylephrine *on page 660*

Neo-Synephrine® Mild [US-OTC] *see* phenylephrine *on page 660*

Neo-Synephrine® Ophthalmic *(Discontinued)* *see* phenylephrine *on page 660*

Neo-Synephrine® Regular Strength [US-OTC] *see* phenylephrine *on page 660*

Neo-Tabs® *(Discontinued)* *see* neomycin *on page 582*

Neotrace-4® [US] *see* trace metals *on page 839*

NeoVadrin® *(Discontinued)*

nepafenac (ne pa FEN ak)

U.S./Canadian Brand Names Nevanac™ [US]

Therapeutic Category Nonsteroidal Antiinflammatory Drug (NSAID), Ophthalmic

Use Treatment of pain and inflammation associated with cataract surgery

Usual Dosage Ophthalmic: Children ≥10 years and Adults: Instill 1 drop into affected eye(s) 3 times/day, beginning 1 day prior to surgery, the day of surgery, and through the first 2 weeks of the postoperative period

Dosage Forms Suspension, ophthalmic: 0.1% (3 mL) [contains benzalkonium chloride]

NephPlex® Rx [US] *see* vitamin B complex combinations *on page 876*

Nephro-Calci® [US-OTC] *see* calcium carbonate *on page 135*

Nephrocaps® [US] *see* vitamin B complex combinations *on page 876*

Nephro-Fer® [US-OTC] *see* ferrous fumarate *on page 342*

Nephron FA® [US] *see* vitamin B complex combinations *on page 876*

Nephro-Vite® [US] *see* vitamin B complex combinations *on page 876*

Nephro-Vite® Rx [US] *see* vitamin B complex combinations *on page 876*

Nephrox Suspension *(Discontinued)* *see* aluminum hydroxide *on page 36*

Neptazane® *(Discontinued)* *see* methazolamide *on page 538*

Nervocaine® Injection *(Discontinued)* *see* lidocaine *on page 493*

Nesacaine® [US] *see* chloroprocaine *on page 174*

Nesacaine®-CE [Can] *see* chloroprocaine *on page 174*

Nesacaine®-MPF [US] *see* chloroprocaine *on page 174*

nesiritide (ni SIR i tide)

Synonyms B-type natriuretic peptide (human); hBNP; natriuretic peptide

U.S./Canadian Brand Names Natrecor® [US]

Therapeutic Category Natriuretic Peptide, B-type, Human; Vasodilator

Use Treatment of acutely decompensated congestive heart failure (CHF) in patients with dyspnea at rest or with minimal activity

Usual Dosage Adults: I.V.: Initial: 2 mcg/kg (bolus); followed by continuous infusion at 0.01 mcg/kg/minute; **Note:** Should not be initiated at a dosage higher than initial recommended dose. At intervals of ≥3 hours, the dosage may be increased by 0.005 mcg/kg/minute (preceded by a bolus of 1 mcg/kg), up to a maximum of 0.03 mcg/kg/minute. Increases beyond the initial infusion rate should be limited to selected patients and accompanied by hemodynamic monitoring.

Patients experiencing hypotension during the infusion: Infusion should be interrupted. May attempt to restart at a lower dose (reduce initial infusion dose by 30% and omit bolus).

Dosage Forms Injection, powder for reconstitution: 1.5 mg

Nestabs® CBF [US] *see* vitamins (multiple/prenatal) *on page 879*

Nestabs® FA [US] *see* vitamins (multiple/prenatal) *on page 879*

Nestabs® RX [US] *see* vitamins (multiple/prenatal) *on page 879*

Nestrex® ***(Discontinued)*** *see* pyridoxine *on page 721*

Netromycin® ***(Discontinued)***

Neucalm-50® Injection ***(Discontinued)*** *see* hydroxyzine *on page 433*

Neulasta® [US/Can] *see* pegfilgrastim *on page 643*

Neuleptil® [Can] *see* pericyazine *(Canada only) on page 654*

Neumega® [US] *see* oprelvekin *on page 618*

Neupogen® [US/Can] *see* filgrastim *on page 345*

Neuramate® ***(Discontinued)*** *see* meprobamate *on page 531*

Neurontin® [US/Can] *see* gabapentin *on page 373*

Neut® [US] *see* sodium bicarbonate *on page 776*

NeutraCare® [US] *see* fluoride *on page 354*

NeutraGard® [US-OTC] *see* fluoride *on page 354*

NeutraGard® Advanced [US] *see* fluoride *on page 354*

NeutraGard® Plus [US] *see* fluoride *on page 354*

Neutra-Phos® [US-OTC] *see* potassium phosphate and sodium phosphate *on page 688*

Neutra-Phos®-K [US-OTC] *see* potassium phosphate *on page 687*

NeuTrexin® [US] *see* trimetrexate *on page 852*

Neutrogena® Acne Mask [US-OTC] *see* benzoyl peroxide *on page 102*

Neutrogena® Acne Wash [US-OTC] *see* salicylic acid *on page 758*

Neutrogena® Body Clear™ [US-OTC] *see* salicylic acid *on page 758*

Neutrogena® Clear Pore [US-OTC] *see* salicylic acid *on page 758*

Neutrogena® Clear Pore Shine Control [US-OTC] *see* salicylic acid *on page 758*

Neutrogena® Healthy Scalp [US-OTC] *see* salicylic acid *on page 758*

Neutrogena® Maximum Strength T/Sal® [US-OTC] *see* salicylic acid *on page 758*

Neutrogena® On The Spot® Acne Patch [US-OTC] *see* salicylic acid *on page 758*

Neutrogena® On The Spot® Acne Treatment [US-OTC] *see* benzoyl peroxide *on page 102*

Neutrogena® T/Gel [US-OTC] *see* coal tar *on page 207*

Neutrogena® T/Gel Extra Strength [US-OTC] *see* coal tar *on page 207*

Neutrogena® T/Gel Stubborn Itch Control [US-OTC] *see* coal tar *on page 207*

Nevanac™ [US] *see* nepafenac *on previous page*

nevirapine (ne VYE ra peen)

Sound-Alike/Look-Alike Issues

nevirapine may be confused with nelfinavir

(Continued)

nevirapine *(Continued)*

Viramune® may be confused with Viracept®

Synonyms NVP

U.S./Canadian Brand Names Viramune® [US/Can]

Therapeutic Category Antiviral Agent

Use In combination therapy with other antiretroviral agents for the treatment of HIV-1

Usual Dosage Oral:

Children 2 months to <8 years: Initial: 4 mg/kg/dose once daily for 14 days; increase dose to 7 mg/kg/dose every 12 hours if no rash or other adverse effects occur; maximum dose: 200 mg/dose every 12 hours

Children ≥8 years: Initial: 4 mg/kg/dose once daily for 14 days; increase dose to 4 mg/kg/dose every 12 hours if no rash or other adverse effects occur; maximum dose: 200 mg/dose every 12 hours

Note: Alternative pediatric dosing (AIDSinfo guidelines): 120-200 mg/m^2 every 12 hours; this dosing has been proposed due to the fact that dosing based on mg/kg may result in an abrupt decrease in dose at the 8th birthday, which may be inappropriate.

Adults: Initial: 200 mg once daily for 14 days; maintenance: 200 mg twice daily (in combination with an additional antiretroviral agent)

Note: If patient experiences a rash during the 14-day lead-in period, dose should not be increased until the rash has resolved. Discontinue if severe rash, or rash with constitutional symptoms, is noted. If therapy is interrupted for >7 days, restart with initial dose for 14 days. Use of prednisone to prevent nevirapine-associated rash is not recommended. Permanently discontinue if symptomatic hepatic events occur.

Prevention of maternal-fetal HIV transmission in women with no prior antiretroviral therapy (AIDS information guidelines):

Mother: 200 mg as a single dose at onset of labor. May be used in combination with zidovudine.

Infant: 2 mg/kg as a single dose at age 48-72 hours. If a maternal dose was given <1 hour prior to delivery, administer a 2 mg/kg dose as soon as possible after birth and repeat at 48-72 hours. May be used in combination with zidovudine.

Dosage Forms

Suspension, oral: 50 mg/5 mL (240 mL)

Tablet: 200 mg

Nexavar® [US] *see* sorafenib *on page 787*

Nexium® [US/Can] *see* esomeprazole *on page 307*

NFV *see* nelfinavir *on page 582*

N.G.A.® Topical *(Discontinued)* *see* nystatin and triamcinolone *on page 610*

niacin (NYE a sin)

Sound-Alike/Look-Alike Issues

niacin may be confused with Minocin®, Niaspan®, Nispan®

Niaspan® may be confused with niacin

Nicobid® may be confused with Nitro-Bid®

Synonyms nicotinic acid; vitamin B_3

U.S./Canadian Brand Names Niacor® [US]; Niaspan® [US/Can]; Slo-Niacin® [US-OTC]

Therapeutic Category Vitamin, Water Soluble

Use Adjunctive treatment of dyslipidemias (types IIa and IIb or primary hypercholesterolemia) to lower the risk of recurrent MI and/or slow progression of coronary artery disease, including combination therapy with other antidyslipidemic agents when additional triglyceride-lowering or HDL-increasing effects are desired; treatment of hypertriglyceridemia in patients at risk of pancreatitis; treatment of peripheral vascular disease and circulatory disorders; treatment of pellagra; dietary supplement

Usual Dosage Note: Formulations of niacin (regular release versus extended release) are not interchangeable.

Children: Oral:

Pellagra: 50-100 mg/dose 3 times/day

Recommended daily allowances:

0-0.5 years: 5 mg/day

0.5-1 year: 6 mg/day

1-3 years: 9 mg/day

4-6 years: 12 mg/day

7-10 years: 13 mg/day

Children and Adolescents: Recommended daily allowances:

Male:

11-14 years: 17 mg/day

15-18 years: 20 mg/day
19-24 years: 19 mg/day
Female: 11-24 years: 15 mg/day
Adults: Oral:
Recommended daily allowances:
Male: 25-50 years: 19 mg/day; >51 years: 15 mg/day
Female: 25-50 years: 15 mg/day; >51 years: 13 mg/day
Hyperlipidemia: Usual target dose: 1.5-6 g/day in 3 divided doses with or after meals using a dosage titration schedule; extended release: 375 mg to 2 g once daily at bedtime
Regular release formulation (Niacor®): Initial: 250 mg once daily (with evening meal); increase frequency and/or dose every 4-7 days to desired response or first-level therapeutic dose (1.5-2 g/day in 2-3 divided doses); after 2 months, may increase at 2- to 4-week intervals to 3 g/day in 3 divided doses
Extended release formulation (Niaspan®): 500 mg at bedtime for 4 weeks, then 1 g at bedtime for 4 weeks; adjust dose to response and tolerance; can increase to a maximum of 2 g/day, but only at 500 mg/day at 4-week intervals
With lovastatin: Maximum lovastatin dose: 40 mg/day
Pellagra: 50-100 mg 3-4 times/day, maximum: 500 mg/day
Niacin deficiency: 10-20 mg/day, maximum: 100 mg/day

Dosage Forms
Capsule, extended release: 125 mg, 250 mg, 400 mg, 500 mg
Capsule, timed release: 250 mg
Tablet: 50 mg, 100 mg, 250 mg, 500 mg
Niacor®: 500 mg
Tablet, controlled release (Slo-Niacin®): 250 mg, 500 mg, 750 mg
Tablet, extended release (Niaspan®): 500 mg, 750 mg, 1000 mg
Note: 500 mg and 750 mg tablets are not interchangeable (eg, three 500 mg tablets are not equivalent to two 750 mg tablets)
Tablet, timed release: 250 mg, 500 mg, 750 mg, 1000 mg

niacinamide (nye a SIN a mide)

Sound-Alike/Look-Alike Issues
niacinamide may be confused with niCARdipine
Synonyms nicotinamide; nicotinic acid amide; vitamin B_3
U.S./Canadian Brand Names Nicomide-T™ [US]
Therapeutic Category Vitamin, Water Soluble
Use
Oral: Prophylaxis and treatment of pellagra
Topical: Improve the appearance of acne and decrease visible inflammation and irritation caused by acne medications
Usual Dosage
Pellagra: Oral:
Children: 100-300 mg/day in divided doses
Adults: 300-500 mg/day
Acne: Topical: Adults: Apply to affected area on face twice daily
Dosage Forms
Cream (Nicomide-T™): 4% (30 g) [contains benzyl alcohol]
Gel (Nicomide-T™): 4% (30 g) [contains alcohol]
Tablet: 100 mg, 250 mg, 500 mg

niacin and lovastatin (NYE a sin & LOE va sta tin)

Sound-Alike/Look-Alike Issues
Advicor® may be confused with Advair, Altocor™
Synonyms lovastatin and niacin
U.S./Canadian Brand Names Advicor® [US/Can]
Therapeutic Category HMG-CoA Reductase Inhibitor; Vitamin, Water Soluble
Use Treatment of primary hypercholesterolemia (heterozygous familial and nonfamilial) and mixed dyslipidemia (Fredrickson types IIa and IIb) in patients previously treated with either agent alone (patients who require further lowering of triglycerides (TG) or increase in HDL-cholesterol (HDL-C) from addition of niacin or further lowering of LDL-cholesterol (LDL-C) from addition of lovastatin). Combination product; not intended for initial treatment.
Usual Dosage Dosage forms are a fixed combination of niacin and lovastatin.
(Continued)

niacin and lovastatin *(Continued)*

Oral: Adults: Lowest dose: Niacin 500 mg/lovastatin 20 mg; may increase by not more than 500 mg (niacin) at 4-week intervals (maximum dose: Niacin 2000 mg/lovastatin 40 mg daily); should be taken at bedtime with a low-fat snack

Not for use as initial therapy of dyslipidemias. May be substituted for equivalent dose of Niaspan®, however, manufacturer does not recommend direct substitution with other niacin products.

Dosage Forms

Tablet, variable release (Advicor®):

500/20: Niacin 500 mg [extended release] and lovastatin 20 mg [immediate release] [contains polysorbate 80]

750/20: Niacin 750 mg [extended release] and lovastatin 20 mg [immediate release] [contains polysorbate 80]

1000/20: Niacin 1000 mg [extended release] and lovastatin 20 mg [immediate release] [contains polysorbate 80]

1000/40: Niacin 1000 mg [extended release] and lovastatin 40 mg [immediate release] [contains polysorbate 80]

Niacor® [US] *see* niacin *on page 588*

Niaspan® [US/Can] *see* niacin *on page 588*

Niastase® [Can] *see* factor VIIa (recombinant) *on page 333*

nicardipine (nye KAR de peen)

Sound-Alike/Look-Alike Issues

niCARdipine may be confused with niacinamide, NIFEdipine, nimodipine

Cardene® may be confused with Cardizem®, Cardura®, codeine

Synonyms nicardipine hydrochloride

Tall-Man ni**CAR**dipine

U.S./Canadian Brand Names Cardene® I.V. [US]; Cardene® SR [US]; Cardene® [US]

Therapeutic Category Calcium Channel Blocker

Use Chronic stable angina (immediate-release product only); management of essential hypertension (immediate and sustained release; parenteral only for short time that oral treatment is not feasible)

Usual Dosage Adults:

Oral:

Immediate release: Initial: 20 mg 3 times/day; usual: 20-40 mg 3 times/day (allow 3 days between dose increases)

Sustained release: Initial: 30 mg twice daily, titrate up to 60 mg twice daily

Note: The total daily dose of immediate-release product may not automatically be equivalent to the daily sustained-release dose; use caution in converting.

I.V. (dilute to 0.1 mg/mL):

Acute hypertension: Initial: 5 mg/hour increased by 2.5 mg/hour every 15 minutes to a maximum of 15 mg/hour; consider reduction to 3 mg/hour after response is achieved. Monitor and titrate to lowest dose necessary to maintain stable blood pressure.

Substitution for oral therapy (approximate equivalents):

20 mg every 8 hours oral, equivalent to 0.5 mg/hour I.V. infusion

30 mg every 8 hours oral, equivalent to 1.2 mg/hour I.V. infusion

40 mg every 8 hours oral, equivalent to 2.2 mg/hour I.V. infusion

Dosage Forms

Capsule (Cardene®): 20 mg, 30 mg

Capsule, sustained release (Cardene® SR): 30 mg, 45 mg, 60 mg

Injection, solution (Cardene® IV): 2.5 mg/mL (10 mL)

nicardipine hydrochloride *see* nicardipine *on this page*

N'ice® *(Discontinued)* *see* ascorbic acid *on page 76*

Nicobid® *(Discontinued)* *see* niacin *on page 588*

Nicoderm® [Can] *see* nicotine *on next page*

NicoDerm® CQ® [US-OTC] *see* nicotine *on next page*

Nicolar® *(Discontinued)* *see* niacin *on page 588*

Nicomide-T™ [US] *see* niacinamide *on previous page*

Nicorette® [US-OTC/Can] *see* nicotine *on next page*

Nicorette® Plus [Can] *see* nicotine *on next page*

nicotinamide *see* niacinamide *on page 589*

nicotine (nik oh TEEN)

Sound-Alike/Look-Alike Issues

NicoDerm® may be confused with Nitroderm

Nicorette® may be confused with Nordette®

U.S./Canadian Brand Names Commit® [US-OTC]; Habitrol® [Can]; NicoDerm® CQ® [US-OTC]; Nicoderm® [Can]; Nicorette® Plus [Can]; Nicorette® [US-OTC/Can]; Nicotrol® Inhaler [US]; Nicotrol® NS [US]; Nicotrol® Patch [US-OTC]; Nicotrol® [Can]

Therapeutic Category Smoking Deterrent

Use Treatment to aid smoking cessation for the relief of nicotine withdrawal symptoms (including nicotine craving)

Usual Dosage

Smoking deterrent: Patients should be advised to completely stop smoking upon initiation of therapy.

Oral:

Gum: Chew 1 piece of gum when urge to smoke, up to 24 pieces/day. Patients who smoke <25 cigarettes/day should start with 2-mg strength; patients smoking ≥25 cigarettes/day should start with the 4-mg strength. Use according to the following 12-week dosing schedule:

Weeks 1-6: Chew 1 piece of gum every 1-2 hours; to increase chances of quitting, chew at least 9 pieces/day during the first 6 weeks

Weeks 7-9: Chew 1 piece of gum every 2-4 hours

Weeks 10-12: Chew 1 piece of gum every 4-8 hours

Inhaler: Usually 6 to 16 cartridges per day; best effect was achieved by frequent continuous puffing (20 minutes); recommended duration of treatment is 3 months, after which patients may be weaned from the inhaler by gradual reduction of the daily dose over 6-12 weeks

Lozenge: Patients who smoke their first cigarette within 30 minutes of waking should use the 4 mg strength; otherwise the 2 mg strength is recommended. Use according to the following 12-week dosing schedule:

Weeks 1-6: One lozenge every 1-2 hours

Weeks 7-9: One lozenge every 2-4 hours

Weeks 10-12: One lozenge every 4-8 hours

Note: Use at least 9 lozenges/day during first 6 weeks to improve chances of quitting; do not use more than one lozenge at a time (maximum: 5 lozenges every 6 hours, 20 lozenges/day)

Topical:

Transdermal patch: Apply new patch every 24 hours to nonhairy, clean, dry skin on the upper body or upper outer arm; each patch should be applied to a different site. **Note:** Adjustment may be required during initial treatment (move to higher dose if experiencing withdrawal symptoms; lower dose if side effects are experienced).

NicoDerm CQ®:

Patients smoking ≥10 cigarettes/day: Begin with **step 1** (21 mg/day) for 4-6 weeks, followed by **step 2** (14 mg/day) for 2 weeks; finish with **step 3** (7 mg/day) for 2 weeks

Patients smoking <10 cigarettes/day: Begin with **step 2** (14 mg/day) for 6 weeks, followed by **step 3** (7 mg/day) for 2 weeks

Note: Initial starting dose for patients <100 pounds, history of cardiovascular disease: 14 mg/day for 4-6 weeks, followed by 7 mg/day for 2-4 weeks

Note: Patients receiving >600 mg/day of cimetidine: Decrease to the next lower patch size

Nicotrol®: One patch daily for 6 weeks

Note: Benefits of use of nicotine transdermal patches beyond 3 months have not been demonstrated.

Nasal: Spray: 1-2 sprays/hour; do not exceed more than 5 doses (10 sprays) per hour [maximum: 40 doses/day (80 sprays); each dose (2 sprays) contains 1 mg of nicotine

Dosage Forms

Gum, chewing, as polacrilex: 2 mg (48s, 108s); 4 mg (48s, 108s)

Nicorette®:

2 mg (48s, 50s, 110s, 168s, 170s, 192s, 200s, 216s) [fruit chill flavor contains calcium 94 mg/gum and sodium 11 mg/gum; mint, fresh mint, fruit chill, orange, and original flavors]

4 mg (48s, 108s, 168s) [fruit chill flavor contains calcium 94 mg/gum and sodium 13 mg/gum; mint, fresh mint, fruit chill, orange, and original flavors]

Lozenge, as polacrilexL:

Commit®: 2 mg (48s, 72s) [contains phenylalanine 3.4 mg/lozenge, sodium 18 mg/lozenge; mint flavor]; 4 mg (48s, 72s) [contains phenylalanine 3.4 mg/lozenge, sodium 18 mg/lozenge; mint flavor]

(Continued)

nicotine *(Continued)*

Oral inhalation system:

Nicotrol® Inhaler: 10 mg cartridge [delivering 4 mg nicotine] (168s) [each unit consists of 5 mouthpieces, 28 storage trays each containing 6 cartridges, and 1 storage case]

Patch, transdermal: 7 mg/24 (30s); 14 mg/24 hours (30s); 21 mg/24 hours (30s)

NicoDerm® CQ®: 7 mg/24 hours (14s); 14 mg/24 hours (14s); 21 mg/24 hours (14s) [available in tan or clear patch]

Nicotrol®: 15 mg/16 hours (7s, 14s) [step 1]; 10 mg/16 hours (14s) [step 2]; 5 mg/16 hours (14s) [step 3]

Solution, intranasal spray (Nicotrol® NS): 10 mg/mL (10 mL) [delivers 0.5 mg/spray; 200 sprays]

nicotinic acid *see* niacin *on page 588*

nicotinic acid amide *see* niacinamide *on page 589*

Nicotrol® [Can] *see* nicotine *on previous page*

Nicotrol® Inhaler [US] *see* nicotine *on previous page*

Nicotrol® NS [US] *see* nicotine *on previous page*

Nicotrol® Patch [US-OTC] *see* nicotine *on previous page*

Nico-Vert® *(Discontinued)* *see* meclizine *on page 522*

Nidagel™ [Can] *see* metronidazole *on page 551*

Nifediac™ CC [US] *see* nifedipine *on this page*

Nifedical™ XL [US] *see* nifedipine *on this page*

nifedipine (nye FED i peen)

Sound-Alike/Look-Alike Issues

NIFEdipine may be confused with niCARdipine, nimodipine, nisoldipine

Procardia XL® may be confused with Cartia® XT

Tall-Man NIFEdipine

U.S./Canadian Brand Names Adalat® CC [US]; Adalat® XL® [Can]; Afeditab™ CR [US]; Apo-Nifed PA® [Can]; Apo-Nifed® [Can]; Nifediac™ CC [US]; Nifedical™ XL [US]; Novo-Nifedin [Can]; Nu-Nifed [Can]; Procardia XL® [US]; Procardia® [US/Can]

Therapeutic Category Calcium Channel Blocker

Use Angina and hypertension (sustained release only), pulmonary hypertension

Usual Dosage Oral:

Children: Hypertrophic cardiomyopathy: 0.6-0.9 mg/kg/24 hours in 3-4 divided doses

Adolescents and Adults: (**Note:** When switching from immediate release to sustained release formulations, total daily dose will start the same)

Initial: 30 mg once daily as sustained release formulation, or if indicated, 10 mg 3 times/day as capsules

Usual dose: 10-30 mg 3 times/day as capsules or 30-60 mg once daily as sustained release

Maximum dose: 120-180 mg/day

Increase sustained release at 7- to 14-day intervals

Dosage Forms

Capsule, softgel: 10 mg, 20 mg

Procardia®: 10 mg

Tablet, extended release: 30 mg, 60 mg, 90 mg

Adalat® CC, Procardia XL®: 30 mg, 60 mg, 90 mg

Afeditab™ CR, Nifedical™ XL: 30 mg, 60 mg

Nifediac™ CC: 30 mg, 60 mg, 90 mg [90 mg tablet contains tartrazine]

Niferex® [US-OTC] *see* polysaccharide-iron complex *on page 681*

Niferex® 150 [US-OTC] *see* polysaccharide-iron complex *on page 681*

Niferex®-PN [US] *see* vitamins (multiple/prenatal) *on page 879*

Niferex®-PN Forte [US] *see* vitamins (multiple/prenatal) *on page 879*

niftolid *see* flutamide *on page 360*

Nilandron® [US] *see* nilutamide *on next page*

Nilstat [Can] *see* nystatin *on page 609*

Nilstat® *(Discontinued)* *see* nystatin *on page 609*

nilutamide (ni LOO ta mide)

Synonyms RU-23908

U.S./Canadian Brand Names Anandron® [Can]; Nilandron® [US]

Therapeutic Category Antineoplastic Agent

Use Treatment of metastatic prostate cancer

Usual Dosage Refer to individual protocols.

Adults: Oral: 300 mg daily for 30 days starting the same day or day after surgical castration, then 150 mg/day

Dosage Forms Tablet: 150 mg

Nimbex® [US/Can] *see* cisatracurium *on page 193*

nimodipine (nye MOE di peen)

Sound-Alike/Look-Alike Issues

nimodipine may be confused with niCARdipine, NIFEdipine

U.S./Canadian Brand Names Nimotop® [US/Can]

Therapeutic Category Calcium Channel Blocker

Use Spasm following subarachnoid hemorrhage from ruptured intracranial aneurysms regardless of the patients neurological condition postictus (Hunt and Hess grades I-V)

Usual Dosage Note: Capsules and contents are for oral administration **ONLY.**

Adults: Oral: 60 mg every 4 hours for 21 days, start therapy within 96 hours after subarachnoid hemorrhage.

Dosage Forms Capsule, liquid filled: 30 mg

Nimotop® [US/Can] *see* nimodipine *on this page*

Nipent® [US/Can] *see* pentostatin *on page 652*

Niravam™ [US] *see* alprazolam *on page 32*

nisoldipine (nye SOL di peen)

Sound-Alike/Look-Alike Issues

nisoldipine may be confused with NIFEdipine

U.S./Canadian Brand Names Sular® [US]

Therapeutic Category Calcium Channel Blocker

Use Management of hypertension, alone or in combination with other antihypertensive agents

Usual Dosage Adults: Oral: Initial: 20 mg once daily, then increase by 10 mg/week (or longer intervals) to attain adequate control of blood pressure; usual dose range (JNC 7): 10-40 mg once daily; doses >60 mg once daily are not recommended.

Dosage Forms Tablet, extended release: 10 mg, 20 mg, 30 mg, 40 mg

nitalapram *see* citalopram *on page 194*

nitazoxanide (nye ta ZOX a nide)

Synonyms NTZ

U.S./Canadian Brand Names Alinia® [US]

Therapeutic Category Antiprotozoal

Use Treatment of diarrhea caused by *Cryptosporidium parvum* or *Giardia lamblia*

Usual Dosage Diarrhea caused by *Cryptosporidium parvum* or *Giardia lamblia*:

Children 1-3 years: 100 mg every 12 hours for 3 days

Children 4-11 years: 200 mg every 12 hours for 3 days

Children ≥12 years and Adults: 500 mg every 12 hours for 3 days

Dosage Forms

Powder for oral suspension: 100 mg/5 mL (60 mL) [contains sucrose 1.48 g/5 mL, sodium benzoate; strawberry flavor]

Tablet: 500 mg

Alinia® 3-Day Therapy Packs™ [unit-dose pack]: 500 mg (6s)

nitisinone (ni TIS i known)

U.S./Canadian Brand Names Orfadin® [US]

Therapeutic Category 4-Hydroxyphenylpyruvate Dioxygenase Inhibitor

Use Treatment of hereditary tyrosinemia type 1 (HT-1); to be used with dietary restriction of tyrosine and phenylalanine

(Continued)

nitisinone *(Continued)*

Usual Dosage Oral: **Note:** Must be used in conjunction with a low protein diet restricted in tyrosine and phenylalanine.

Infants: See dosing for Children and Adults; infants may require maximal dose once liver function has improved

Children and Adults: Initial: 1 mg/kg/day in divided doses, given in the morning and evening, 1 hour before meals; doses do not need to be divided evenly

Dosage Forms Capsule: 2 mg, 5 mg, 10 mg

Nitoman™ [Can] *see* tetrabenazine *(Canada only) on page 815*

nitrazepam *(Canada only)* (nye TRA ze pam)

Synonyms nitrozepamum

U.S./Canadian Brand Names Sandoz-Nitrazepam [Can]

Therapeutic Category Benzodiazepine

Use Short-term management of insomnia; treatment of infantile spasm and seizures

Usual Dosage Oral:

Insomnia:

Children:

1-6 years: 2.5 mg

≥7 years: 5 mg

Adults: 5-10 mg at night

Epilepsy: Children and Adults: 1-6 mg/day; dosage should be decreased in elderly, hypothyroid patients, and cirrhosis

Children maximum dose: 60 mg

Adult maximum dose: 20 mg

Dosage Forms

Capsule: 5 mg

Tablet: 5 mg

Nitrek® [US] *see* nitroglycerin *on next page*

nitric oxide (NYE trik OKS ide)

U.S./Canadian Brand Names INOmax® [US/Can]

Therapeutic Category Vasodilator, Pulmonary

Use Treatment of term and near-term (>34 weeks) neonates with hypoxic respiratory failure associated with pulmonary hypertension; used concurrently with ventilatory support and other agents

Usual Dosage Inhalation: Neonates (up to 14 days old): 20 ppm. Treatment should be maintained up to 14 days or until the underlying oxygen desaturation has resolved and the neonate is ready to be weaned from therapy. In the CINRGI trial, patients whose oxygenation improved had their dose reduced to 5 ppm at the end of 4 hours of treatment. Doses above 20 ppm should not be used because of the risk of methemoglobinemia and elevated NO_2.

Dosage Forms Gas, for inhalation:

100 ppm [nitric oxide 0.01% and nitrogen 99.99%] (353 L) [delivers 344 L], (1963 L) [delivers 1918 L]

800 ppm [nitric oxide 0.08% and nitrogen 99.92%] (353 L) [delivers 344 L], (1963 L) [delivers 1918 L]

4′-nitro-3′-trifluoromethylisobutyrantide *see* flutamide *on page 360*

Nitro-Bid® [US] *see* nitroglycerin *on next page*

Nitrodisc® Patch *(Discontinued)* *see* nitroglycerin *on next page*

Nitro-Dur® [US/Can] *see* nitroglycerin *on next page*

nitrofural *see* nitrofurazone *on next page*

nitrofurantoin (nye troe fyoor AN toyn)

U.S./Canadian Brand Names Apo-Nitrofurantoin® [Can]; Furadantin® [US]; Macrobid® [US/Can]; Macrodantin® [US/Can]; Novo-Furantoin [Can]

Therapeutic Category Antibiotic, Miscellaneous

Use Prevention and treatment of urinary tract infections caused by susceptible strains of *E. coli, S. aureus, Enterococcus, Klebsiella,* and *Enterobacter*

Usual Dosage Oral:

Children >1 month: 5-7 mg/kg/day in divided doses every 6 hours; maximum: 400 mg/day

UTI prophylaxis (chronic): 1-2 mg/kg/day in divided doses every 12-24 hours; maximum: 100 mg/day

Adults: 50-100 mg/dose every 6 hours
Macrocrystal/monohydrate: 100 mg twice daily
UTI prophylaxis (chronic): 50-100 mg/dose at bedtime

Dosage Forms
Capsule [macrocrystal]: 50 mg, 100 mg
Macrodantin®: 25 mg, 50 mg, 100 mg
Capsule [macrocrystal/monohydrate]: 100 mg [nitrofurantoin macrocrystal 25% and nitrofurantoin monohydrate 75%]
Macrobid®: 100 mg [nitrofurantoin macrocrystal 25% and nitrofurantoin monohydrate 75%]
Suspension, oral:
Furadantin®: 25 mg/5 mL (470 mL)

nitrofurazone (nye troe FYOOR a zone)

Synonyms nitrofural
Therapeutic Category Antibacterial, Topical
Use Antibacterial agent used in second- and third-degree burns and skin grafting
Usual Dosage Children and Adults: Topical: Apply once daily or every few days to lesion or place on gauze
Dosage Forms
Cream: 0.2% (28 g)
Ointment, soluble dressing: 0.2% (28 g, 56 g, 454 g, 480 g)
Solution, topical: 0.2% (480 mL)

nitrogen mustard *see* mechlorethamine *on page 522*

nitroglycerin (nye troe GLI ser in)

Sound-Alike/Look-Alike Issues
nitroglycerin may be confused with nitroprusside
Nitro-Bid® may be confused with Nicobid®
Nitroderm may be confused with NicoDerm®
Nitrol® may be confused with Nizoral®
Nitrostat® may be confused with Hyperstat®, Nilstat®, nystatin

Synonyms glyceryl trinitrate; nitroglycerol; NTG

U.S./Canadian Brand Names Gen-Nitro [Can]; Minitran™ [US/Can]; Nitrek® [US]; Nitro-Bid® [US]; Nitro-Dur® [US/Can]; Nitrolingual® [US]; Nitrol® [Can]; NitroQuick® [US]; Nitrostat® [US/Can]; NitroTime® [US]; Rho-Nitro [Can]; Transderm-Nitro® [Can]; Trinipatch® 0.2 [Can]; Trinipatch® 0.4 [Can]; Trinipatch® 0.6 [Can]

Therapeutic Category Vasodilator

Use Treatment of angina pectoris; I.V. for congestive heart failure (especially when associated with acute myocardial infarction); pulmonary hypertension; hypertensive emergencies occurring perioperatively (especially during cardiovascular surgery)

Usual Dosage Note: Hemodynamic and antianginal tolerance often develop within 24-48 hours of continuous nitrate administration. Nitrate-free interval (10-12 hours/day) is recommended to avoid tolerance development; gradually decrease dose in patients receiving NTG for prolonged period to avoid withdrawal reaction.

Children: Pulmonary hypertension: Continuous infusion: Start 0.25-0.5 mcg/kg/minute and titrate by 1 mcg/kg/minute at 20- to 60-minute intervals to desired effect; usual dose: 1-3 mcg/kg/minute; maximum: 5 mcg/kg/minute

Adults:
Oral: 2.5-9 mg 2-4 times/day (up to 26 mg 4 times/day)
I.V.: 5 mcg/minute, increase by 5 mcg/minute every 3-5 minutes to 20 mcg/minute; if no response at 20 mcg/minute increase by 10 mcg/minute every 3-5 minutes, up to 200 mcg/minute
Ointment: ½" upon rising and ½" 6 hours later; the dose may be doubled and even doubled again as needed
Patch, transdermal: Initial: 0.2-0.4 mg/hour, titrate to doses of 0.4-0.8 mg/hour; tolerance is minimized by using a patch-on period of 12-14 hours and patch-off period of 10-12 hours
Sublingual: 0.2-0.6 mg every 5 minutes for maximum of 3 doses in 15 minutes; may also use prophylactically 5-10 minutes prior to activities which may provoke an attack
Translingual: 1-2 sprays into mouth under tongue every 3-5 minutes for maximum of 3 doses in 15 minutes, may also be used 5-10 minutes prior to activities which may provoke an attack prophylactically

Dosage Forms
Capsule, extended release: 2.5 mg, 6.5 mg, 9 mg
Nitro-Time®: 2.5 mg, 6.5 mg, 9 mg
(Continued)

nitroglycerin *(Continued)*

Infusion [premixed in D_5W]: 25 mg (250 mL) [0.1 mg/mL]; 50 mg (250 mL) [0.2 mg/mL]; 50 mg (500 mL) [0.1 mg/mL]; 100 mg (250 mL) [0.4 mg/mL]; 200 mg (500 mL) [0.4 mg/mL]
Injection, solution: 5 mg/mL (5 mL, 10 mL) [contains alcohol and propylene glycol]
Ointment, topical:
Nitro-Bid®: 2% [20 mg/g] (1 g, 30 g, 60 g)
Solution, translingual [spray]:
Nitrolingual®: 0.4 mg/metered spray (4.9 g) [contains alcohol 20%; 60 metered sprays]; (12 g) [contains alcohol 20%; 200 metered sprays]
Tablet, sublingual:
NitroQuick®, Nitrostat®: 0.3 mg, 0.4 mg, 0.6 mg
Transdermal system [once-daily patch]: 0.1 mg/hour (30s); 0.2 mg/hour (30s); 0.4 mg/hour (30s); 0.6 mg/hour (30s)
Minitran™: 0.1 mg/hour (30s); 0.2 mg/hour (30s); 0.4 mg/hour (30s); 0.6 mg/hour (30s)
Nitrek®: 0.2 mg/hour (30s); 0.4 mg/hour (30s); 0.6 mg/hour (30s)
Nitro-Dur®: 0.1 mg/hour (30s); 0.2 mg/hour (30s); 0.3 mg/hour (30s); 0.4 mg/hour (30s); 0.6 mg/hour (30s); 0.8 mg/hour (30s)

nitroglycerol *see* nitroglycerin *on previous page*

Nitrol® [Can] *see* nitroglycerin *on previous page*

Nitrol® *(Discontinued)* *see* nitroglycerin *on previous page*

Nitrolingual® [US] *see* nitroglycerin *on previous page*

Nitrong® Oral Tablet *(Discontinued)* *see* nitroglycerin *on previous page*

Nitropress® [US] *see* nitroprusside *on this page*

nitroprusside (nye troe PRUS ide)

Sound-Alike/Look-Alike Issues
nitroprusside may be confused with nitroglycerin
Synonyms nitroprusside sodium; sodium nitroferricyanide; sodium nitroprusside
U.S./Canadian Brand Names Nitropress® [US]
Therapeutic Category Vasodilator
Use Management of hypertensive crises; congestive heart failure; used for controlled hypotension to reduce bleeding during surgery
Usual Dosage Administration requires the use of an infusion pump. Average dose: 5 mcg/kg/minute.
Children: Pulmonary hypertension: I.V.: Initial: 1 mcg/kg/minute by continuous I.V. infusion; increase in increments of 1 mcg/kg/minute at intervals of 20-60 minutes; titrating to the desired response; usual dose: 3 mcg/kg/minute, rarely need >4 mcg/kg/minute; maximum: 5 mcg/kg/minute.
Adults: I.V. Initial: 0.3-0.5 mcg/kg/minute; increase in increments of 0.5 mcg/kg/minute, titrating to the desired hemodynamic effect or the appearance of headache or nausea; usual dose: 3 mcg/kg/minute; rarely need >4 mcg/kg/minute; maximum: 10 mcg/kg/minute. When administered by prolonged infusion faster than 2 mcg/kg/minute, cyanide is generated faster than an unaided patient can handle.
Dosage Forms Injection, solution, as sodium: 25 mg/mL (2 mL)

nitroprusside sodium *see* nitroprusside *on this page*

NitroQuick® [US] *see* nitroglycerin *on previous page*

Nitrostat® [US/Can] *see* nitroglycerin *on previous page*

NitroTime® [US] *see* nitroglycerin *on previous page*

nitrous oxide (NYE trus OKS ide)

Therapeutic Category Anesthetic, Gas
Use Produces sedation and analgesia; principal adjunct to inhalation and intravenous general anesthesia
Usual Dosage Children and Adults:
Surgical: For sedation and analgesia: Concentrations of 25% to 50% nitrous oxide with oxygen. For general anesthesia, concentrations of 40% to 70% via mask or endotracheal tube. Minimal alveolar concentration (MAC), which can be considered the ED_{50} of inhalational anesthetics, is 105%; therefore delivery in a hyperbaric chamber is necessary to use as a complete anesthetic. When administered at 70%, reduces the MAC of other anesthetics by half.
Dental: For sedation and analgesia: Concentrations of 25% to 50% nitrous oxide with oxygen
Dosage Forms Supplied in blue cylinders

nitrozepamum *see* nitrazepam *(Canada only)* *on page 594*

Nix® [US-OTC/Can] *see* permethrin *on page 655*

nizatidine (ni ZA ti deen)

Sound-Alike/Look-Alike Issues

Axid® may be confused with Ansaid®

U.S./Canadian Brand Names Apo-Nizatidine® [Can]; Axid® AR [US-OTC]; Axid® [US/Can]; Gen-Nizatidine [Can]; Novo-Nizatidine [Can]; Nu-Nizatidine [Can]; PMS-Nizatidine [Can]

Therapeutic Category Histamine H_2 Antagonist

Use Treatment and maintenance of duodenal ulcer; treatment of benign gastric ulcer; treatment of gastroesophageal reflux disease (GERD); OTC tablet used for the prevention of meal-induced heartburn, acid indigestion, and sour stomach

Usual Dosage Oral:

Children ≥12 years:

GERD: Refer to Adults dosing

Meal-induced heartburn, acid indigestion and sour stomach: Refer to Adults dosing

Adults:

Duodenal ulcer:

Treatment of active ulcer: 300 mg at bedtime or 150 mg twice daily

Maintenance of healed ulcer: 150 mg/day at bedtime

Gastric ulcer: 150 mg twice daily or 300 mg at bedtime

GERD: 150 mg twice daily

Meal-induced heartburn, acid indigestion, and sour stomach: 75 mg tablet [OTC] twice daily, 30 to 60 minutes prior to consuming food or beverages

Dosage Forms

Capsule (Axid®): 150 mg, 300 mg

Solution, oral (Axid®): 15 mg/mL (120 mL, 480 mL) [bubble gum flavor]

Tablet (Axid® AR): 75 mg

Nizoral® [US] *see* ketoconazole *on page 471*

Nizoral® A-D [US-OTC] *see* ketoconazole *on page 471*

N-methylhydrazine *see* procarbazine *on page 701*

No Doz® Maximum Strength [US-OTC] *see* caffeine *on page 132*

Nolahist® ***(Discontinued)***

Nolex® LA ***(Discontinued)***

Nolvadex® [Can] *see* tamoxifen *on page 804*

Nolvadex®-D [Can] *see* tamoxifen *on page 804*

Nolvadex® ***(Discontinued)*** *see* tamoxifen *on page 804*

nonoxynol 9 (non OKS i nole nine)

Sound-Alike/Look-Alike Issues

Delfen® may be confused with Delsym®

Synonyms N-9

U.S./Canadian Brand Names Advantage-S™ [US-OTC]; Conceptrol® [US-OTC]; Delfen® [US-OTC]; Encare® [US-OTC]; Gynol II® [US-OTC]; Today® Sponge [US-OTC]; VCF™ [US-OTC]

Therapeutic Category Spermicide

Use Prevention of pregnancy

Usual Dosage Note: Prior to use, refer to specific product labeling for complete instructions.

Prevention of pregnancy: Vaginal:

Advantage-S®, Conceptrol®: Insert 1 applicatorful vaginally up to 1 hour prior to intercourse

Encare®: Unwrap and insert 1 suppository vaginally at least 10 minutes prior to intercourse; effective for 1 hour

Today® Sponge: Insert 1 sponge vaginally prior to intercourse; allow to remain in place for 6 hours after intercourse before removing; effective for use up to 24 continuous hours. Do not leave in place for >30 hours.

VCF®:

Film: Insert 1 film vaginally at least 15 minutes, but no more than 3 hours, prior to intercourse. Insert new film for each act of intercourse or if more than 3 hours have elapsed.

Foam: Insert 1 applicatorful at least 15 minutes prior to intercourse; effective for up to 1 hour

(Continued)

nonoxynol 9 *(Continued)*

Dosage Forms [DSC] = Discontinued product

Film, vaginal (VCF™): 28% (3s, 6s,12s)

Foam, vaginal:

Delfen®: 12.5% (18 g)

Emko®: 8% (40 g, 90 g) [DSC]

VCF™: 12.5% (40 g)

Gel, vaginal:

Advantage-S™: 3.5% (1.5 g) [packaged in 3s or with 6 prefilled applicators]; (30g) [packaged with reusable applicator]

Conceptrol®: 4% (2.7 g) [packaged in 6s and 10s with disposable applicators]

Gynol II®: 2% (85 g, 114 g)

Shur-Seal®: 2% (6 g) [packaged in 24s] [DSC]

Sponge, vaginal (Today®): 1 g (3s, 6s, 12s) [contains sodium metabisulfite]

Suppository, vaginal (Encare®): 100 mg (12s, 18s)

No Pain-HP® ***(Discontinued)*** *see* capsaicin *on page 142*

Nora-BE™ [US] *see* norethindrone *on this page*

noradrenaline *see* norepinephrine *on this page*

noradrenaline acid tartrate *see* norepinephrine *on this page*

Norcet® ***(Discontinued)*** *see* hydrocodone and acetaminophen *on page 420*

Norco® [US] *see* hydrocodone and acetaminophen *on page 420*

Norcuron® ***(Discontinued)*** *see* vecuronium *on page 869*

nordeoxyguanosine *see* ganciclovir *on page 375*

Nordette® [US] *see* ethinyl estradiol and levonorgestrel *on page 320*

Norditropin® [US] *see* somatropin *on page 785*

Norditropin® NordiFlex® [US] *see* somatropin *on page 785*

Nordryl® Injection ***(Discontinued)*** *see* diphenhydramine *on page 261*

Nordryl® Oral ***(Discontinued)*** *see* diphenhydramine *on page 261*

norelgestromin and ethinyl estradiol *see* ethinyl estradiol and norelgestromin *on page 322*

norepinephrine (nor ep i NEF rin)

Synonyms levarterenol bitartrate; noradrenaline; noradrenaline acid tartrate; norepinephrine bitartrate

U.S./Canadian Brand Names Levophed® [US/Can]

Therapeutic Category Adrenergic Agonist Agent

Use Treatment of shock which persists after adequate fluid volume replacement

Usual Dosage **Administration requires the use of an infusion pump!**

Note: Norepinephrine dosage is stated in terms of norepinephrine base and intravenous formulation is norepinephrine bitartrate

Norepinephrine bitartrate 2 mg = Norepinephrine base 1 mg

Continuous I.V. infusion:

Children: Initial: 0.05-0.1 mcg/kg/minute; titrate to desired effect; maximum dose: 1-2 mcg/kg/minute

Adults: Initial: 0.5-1 mcg/minute and titrate to desired response; 8-30 mcg/minute is usual range; range used in clinical trials: 0.01-3 mcg/kg/minute; ACLS dosage range: 0.5-30 mcg/minute

Dosage Forms Injection, solution, as bitartrate: 1 mg/mL (4 mL) [contains sodium metabisulfite]

norepinephrine bitartrate *see* norepinephrine *on this page*

Norethin™ 1/35E ***(Discontinued)*** *see* ethinyl estradiol and norethindrone *on page 323*

norethindrone (nor ETH in drone)

Sound-Alike/Look-Alike Issues

Micronor® may be confused with miconazole, Micronase®

Synonyms norethindrone acetate; norethisterone

U.S./Canadian Brand Names Aygestin® [US]; Camila™ [US]; Errin™ [US]; Jolivette™ [US]; Micronor® [US/Can]; Nor-QD® [US]; Nora-BE™ [US]; Norlutate® [Can]

Therapeutic Category Contraceptive, Progestin Only; Progestin

Use Treatment of amenorrhea; abnormal uterine bleeding; endometriosis, oral contraceptive; **higher rate of failure with progestin only contraceptives**

Usual Dosage Oral: Adolescents and Adults: Female:

Contraception: Progesterone only: Norethindrone 0.35 mg every day of the year starting on first day of menstruation; if one dose is missed, discontinue and use an alternative method of contraception

Amenorrhea and abnormal uterine bleeding:

Norethindrone: 5-20 mg/day for 5-10 days during the second half of the menstrual cycle

Norethindrone acetate: 2.5-10 mg/day for 5-10 days during the second half of the menstrual cycle

Endometriosis:

Norethindrone: 10 mg/day for 2 weeks; increase at increments of 5 mg/day every 2 weeks until 30 mg/day; continue for 6-9 months or until breakthrough bleeding demands temporary termination

Norethindrone acetate: 5 mg/day for 14 days; increase at increments of 2.5 mg/day every 2 weeks up to 15 mg/day; continue for 6-9 months or until breakthrough bleeding demands temporary termination

Dosage Forms

Tablet (Camila™, Errin™, Jolivette™, Micronor®, Nora-BE™, Nor-QD®): 0.35 mg

Tablet, as acetate (Aygestin®): 5 mg

norethindrone acetate *see* norethindrone *on previous page*

norethindrone acetate and ethinyl estradiol *see* ethinyl estradiol and norethindrone *on page 323*

norethindrone and estradiol *see* estradiol and norethindrone *on page 310*

norethindrone and mestranol *see* mestranol and norethindrone *on page 534*

norethisterone *see* norethindrone *on previous page*

Norflex™ [US/Can] *see* orphenadrine *on page 620*

norfloxacin (nor FLOKS a sin)

Sound-Alike/Look-Alike Issues

norfloxacin may be confused with Norflex™, Noroxin®

Noroxin® may be confused with Neurontin®, Norflex™, norfloxacin

U.S./Canadian Brand Names Apo-Norflox® [Can]; CO Norfloxacin [Can]; Norfloxacine® [Can]; Noroxin® [US/Can]; Novo-Norfloxacin [Can]; PMS-Norfloxacin [Can]; Riva-Norfloxacin [Can]

Therapeutic Category Quinolone

Use Uncomplicated and complicated urinary tract infections caused by susceptible gram-negative and gram-positive bacteria; sexually-transmitted disease (eg, uncomplicated urethral and cervical gonorrhea) caused by *N. gonorrhoeae*; prostatitis due to *E. coli*

Usual Dosage

Usual dosage range:

Adults: Oral: 400 mg every 12 hours (maximum: 800 mg/day)

Indication-specific dosing:

Adults: Oral:

Dysenteric enterocolitis (*Shigella* unlabeled use): 400 mg twice daily for 5 days or 800 mg as a single dose (mild infection)

Prostatitis: 400 mg every 12 hours for 4 weeks

Uncomplicated gonorrhea: 800 mg as a single dose (CDC recommends as an alternative regimen to ciprofloxacin or ofloxacin)

Urinary tract infections: 400 mg twice daily for 3-21 days depending on severity of infection or organism sensitivity

Dosage Forms

Tablet:

Noroxin®: 400 mg

Norfloxacine® [Can] *see* norfloxacin *on this page*

Norgesic™ [Can] *see* orphenadrine, aspirin, and caffeine *on page 620*

Norgesic™ *(Discontinued)* *see* orphenadrine, aspirin, and caffeine *on page 620*

Norgesic™ Forte [Can] *see* orphenadrine, aspirin, and caffeine *on page 620*

Norgesic™ Forte *(Discontinued)* *see* orphenadrine, aspirin, and caffeine *on page 620*

norgestimate and estradiol *see* estradiol and norgestimate *on page 311*

norgestimate and ethinyl estradiol *see* ethinyl estradiol and norgestimate *on page 325*

norgestrel and ethinyl estradiol *see* ethinyl estradiol and norgestrel *on page 327*

Norinyl® 1+35 [US] *see* ethinyl estradiol and norethindrone *on page 323*

Norinyl® 1+50 [US] *see* mestranol and norethindrone *on page 534*

Noritate® [US/Can] *see* metronidazole *on page 551*
Norlutate® [Can] *see* norethindrone *on page 598*
normal human serum albumin *see* albumin *on page 22*
normal saline *see* sodium chloride *on page 777*
normal serum albumin (human) *see* albumin *on page 22*
Normiflo® *(Discontinued)*
Normodyne® [Can] *see* labetalol *on page 475*
Noroxin® [US/Can] *see* norfloxacin *on previous page*
Norpace® [US/Can] *see* disopyramide *on page 268*
Norpace® CR [US] *see* disopyramide *on page 268*
Norplant® Implant [Can] *see* levonorgestrel *on page 491*
Norplant® Implant *(Discontinued)* *see* levonorgestrel *on page 491*
Norpramin® [US/Can] *see* desipramine *on page 236*
Nor-QD® [US] *see* norethindrone *on page 598*
Nortemp Children's [US-OTC] *see* acetaminophen *on page 5*
North American coral snake antivenin *see* antivenin *(Micrurus fulvius) on page 64*
North and South American antisnake-bite serum *see* antivenin *(Crotalidae)* polyvalent *on page 63*
Nortrel™ [US] *see* ethinyl estradiol and norethindrone *on page 323*
Nortrel™ 7/7/7 [US] *see* ethinyl estradiol and norethindrone *on page 323*

nortriptyline (nor TRIP ti leen)

Sound-Alike/Look-Alike Issues
nortriptyline may be confused with amitriptyline, desipramine, Norpramin®
Aventyl® HCl may be confused with Bentyl®
Pamelor® may be confused with Demerol®, Dymelor®

Synonyms nortriptyline hydrochloride

U.S./Canadian Brand Names Alti-Nortriptyline [Can]; Apo-Nortriptyline® [Can]; Aventyl® [Can]; Gen-Nortriptyline [Can]; Norventyl [Can]; Novo-Nortriptyline [Can]; Nu-Nortriptyline [Can]; Pamelor® [US]; PMS-Nortriptyline [Can]

Therapeutic Category Antidepressant, Tricyclic (Secondary Amine)

Use Treatment of symptoms of depression

Usual Dosage Oral:
Depression: Adults: 25 mg 3-4 times/day up to 150 mg/day
Myofascial pain, neuralgia, burning mouth syndrome (dental use): Initial: 10-25 mg at bedtime; dosage may be increased by 25 mg/day weekly, if tolerated; usual maintenance dose: 75 mg as a single bedtime dose or 2 divided doses

Dosage Forms
Capsule, as hydrochloride: 10 mg, 25 mg, 50 mg, 75 mg
Pamelor®: 10 mg, 25 mg, 50 mg, 75 mg [may contain benzyl alcohol; 50 mg may also contain sodium bisulfite]
Solution, as hydrochloride (Pamelor®): 10 mg/5 mL (473 mL) [contains alcohol 4% and benzoic acid]

nortriptyline hydrochloride *see* nortriptyline *on this page*
Norvasc® [US/Can] *see* amlodipine *on page 45*
Norventyl [Can] *see* nortriptyline *on this page*
Norvir® [US/Can] *see* ritonavir *on page 748*
Norvir® SEC [Can] *see* ritonavir *on page 748*
Novacet® *(Discontinued)* *see* sulfur and sulfacetamide *on page 800*
Novafed® A *(Discontinued)* *see* chlorpheniramine and pseudoephedrine *on page 177*
Novahistex® DM Decongestant [Can] *see* pseudoephedrine and dextromethorphan *on page 714*
Novahistex® DM Decongestant Expectorant [Can] *see* guaifenesin, pseudoephedrine, and dextromethorphan *on page 401*

Novo-Pirocam [Can] *see* piroxicam *on page 671*
Novo-Pramine [Can] *see* imipramine *on page 442*
Novo-Pranol [Can] *see* propranolol *on page 709*
Novo-Pravastatin [Can] *see* pravastatin *on page 692*
Novo-Prazin [Can] *see* prazosin *on page 693*
Novo-Prednisolone [Can] *see* prednisolone (systemic) *on page 695*
Novo-Prednisone [Can] *see* prednisone *on page 695*
Novo-Profen [Can] *see* ibuprofen *on page 437*
Novo-Propamide [Can] *see* chlorpropamide *on page 184*
Novo-Purol [Can] *see* allopurinol *on page 30*
Novo-Quinidin [Can] *see* quinidine *on page 725*
Novo-Quinine [Can] *see* quinine *on page 726*
Novo-Ranidine [Can] *see* ranitidine *on page 732*
NovoRapid® [Can] *see* insulin aspart *on page 449*
Novo-Rythro Estolate [Can] *see* erythromycin *on page 303*
Novo-Rythro Ethylsuccinate [Can] *see* erythromycin *on page 303*
Novo-Selegiline [Can] *see* selegiline *on page 766*
Novo-Semide [Can] *see* furosemide *on page 372*
Novo-Sertraline [Can] *see* sertraline *on page 769*
NovoSeven® [US] *see* factor VIIa (recombinant) *on page 333*
Novo-Simvastatin [Can] *see* simvastatin *on page 773*
Novo-Sorbide [Can] *see* isosorbide dinitrate *on page 465*
Novo-Sotalol [Can] *see* sotalol *on page 787*
Novo-Soxazole [Can] *see* sulfisoxazole *on page 799*
Novo-Spiroton [Can] *see* spironolactone *on page 789*
Novo-Spirozine [Can] *see* hydrochlorothiazide and spironolactone *on page 420*
Novo-Sucralate [Can] *see* sucralfate *on page 793*
Novo-Sumatriptan [Can] *see* sumatriptan *on page 801*
Novo-Sundac [Can] *see* sulindac *on page 800*
Novo-Tamoxifen [Can] *see* tamoxifen *on page 804*
Novo-Temazepam [Can] *see* temazepam *on page 808*
Novo-Terazosin [Can] *see* terazosin *on page 810*
Novo-Theophyl SR [Can] *see* theophylline *on page 818*
Novo-Tiaprofenic [Can] *see* tiaprofenic acid *(Canada only) on page 826*
Novo-Ticlopidine [Can] *see* ticlopidine *on page 827*
Novo-Topiramate [Can] *see* topiramate *on page 836*
Novo-Trazodone [Can] *see* trazodone *on page 843*
Novo-Triamzide [Can] *see* hydrochlorothiazide and triamterene *on page 420*
Novo-Trifluzine [Can] *see* trifluoperazine *on page 849*
Novo-Trimel [Can] *see* sulfamethoxazole and trimethoprim *on page 797*
Novo-Trimel D.S. [Can] *see* sulfamethoxazole and trimethoprim *on page 797*
Novo-Triptyn [Can] *see* amitriptyline *on page 44*
Novo-Veramil SR [Can] *see* verapamil *on page 870*
Novo-Warfarin [Can] *see* warfarin *on page 881*
Novoxapram® [Can] *see* oxazepam *on page 623*
Novo-Zopiclone [Can] *see* zopiclone *(Canada only) on page 890*
Nozinan® [Can] *see* methotrimeprazine *(Canada only) on page 542*
NP-27® ***(Discontinued)*** *see* tolnaftate *on page 834*

Nu-Clonazepam [Can] *see* clonazepam *on page 203*
Nu-Clonidine [Can] *see* clonidine *on page 203*
Nu-Cloxi [Can] *see* cloxacillin *on page 206*
Nucofed® Expectorant *(Discontinued)* *see* guaifenesin, pseudoephedrine, and codeine *on page 401*
Nucofed® Pediatric Expectorant *(Discontinued)* *see* guaifenesin, pseudoephedrine, and codeine *on page 401*
Nu-Cotrimox [Can] *see* sulfamethoxazole and trimethoprim *on page 797*
Nu-Cromolyn [Can] *see* cromolyn sodium *on page 217*
Nu-Cyclobenzaprine [Can] *see* cyclobenzaprine *on page 219*
Nu-Desipramine [Can] *see* desipramine *on page 236*
Nu-Diclo [Can] *see* diclofenac *on page 250*
Nu-Diclo-SR [Can] *see* diclofenac *on page 250*
Nu-Diflunisal [Can] *see* diflunisal *on page 254*
Nu-Diltiaz [Can] *see* diltiazem *on page 257*
Nu-Diltiaz-CD [Can] *see* diltiazem *on page 257*
Nu-Divalproex [Can] *see* valproic acid and derivatives *on page 864*
Nu-Domperidone [Can] *see* domperidone *(Canada only) on page 273*
Nu-Doxycycline [Can] *see* doxycycline *on page 278*
Nu-Erythromycin-S [Can] *see* erythromycin *on page 303*
Nu-Famotidine [Can] *see* famotidine *on page 335*
Nu-Fenofibrate [Can] *see* fenofibrate *on page 338*
Nu-Fluoxetine [Can] *see* fluoxetine *on page 357*
Nu-Flurprofen [Can] *see* flurbiprofen *on page 360*
Nu-Fluvoxamine [Can] *see* fluvoxamine *on page 364*
Nu-Gabapentin [Can] *see* gabapentin *on page 373*
Nu-Gemfibrozil [Can] *see* gemfibrozil *on page 378*
Nu-Glyburide [Can] *see* glyburide *on page 387*
Nu-Hydral [Can] *see* hydralazine *on page 418*
Nu-Ibuprofen [Can] *see* ibuprofen *on page 437*
Nu-Indapamide [Can] *see* indapamide *on page 445*
Nu-Indo [Can] *see* indomethacin *on page 446*
Nu-Ipratropium [Can] *see* ipratropium *on page 460*
Nu-Iron® 150 [US-OTC] *see* polysaccharide-iron complex *on page 681*
Nu-Ketoprofen [Can] *see* ketoprofen *on page 472*
Nu-Ketoprofen-E [Can] *see* ketoprofen *on page 472*
NuLev™ [US] *see* hyoscyamine *on page 434*
Nu-Levocarb [Can] *see* levodopa and carbidopa *on page 489*
Nullo® [US-OTC] *see* chlorophyll *on page 174*
Nu-Loraz [Can] *see* lorazepam *on page 506*
Nu-Lovastatin [Can] *see* lovastatin *on page 508*
Nu-Loxapine [Can] *see* loxapine *on page 509*
NuLYTELY® [US] *see* polyethylene glycol-electrolyte solution *on page 679*
Nu-Medopa [Can] *see* methyldopa *on page 544*
Nu-Mefenamic [Can] *see* mefenamic acid *on page 525*
Nu-Megestrol [Can] *see* megestrol *on page 525*
Nu-Metformin [Can] *see* metformin *on page 535*
Nu-Metoclopramide [Can] *see* metoclopramide *on page 549*

Nu-Metop [Can] *see* metoprolol *on page 550*
Nu-Moclobemide [Can] *see* moclobemide *(Canada only) on page 562*
Numorphan® [US] *see* oxymorphone *on page 629*
Numzident® ***(Discontinued)*** *see* benzocaine *on page 99*
Nu-Naprox [Can] *see* naproxen *on page 578*
Nu-Nifed [Can] *see* nifedipine *on page 592*
Nu-Nizatidine [Can] *see* nizatidine *on page 597*
Nu-Nortriptyline [Can] *see* nortriptyline *on page 600*
Nu-Oxybutyn [Can] *see* oxybutynin *on page 625*
Nu-Pentoxifylline SR [Can] *see* pentoxifylline *on page 653*
Nu-Pen-VK [Can] *see* penicillin V potassium *on page 649*
Nupercainal® [US-OTC] *see* dibucaine *on page 249*
Nupercainal® Hydrocortisone Cream [US-OTC] *see* hydrocortisone (topical) *on page 428*
Nu-Pindol [Can] *see* pindolol *on page 669*
Nu-Pirox [Can] *see* piroxicam *on page 671*
Nu-Prazo [Can] *see* prazosin *on page 693*
Nuprin® ***(Discontinued)*** *see* ibuprofen *on page 437*
Nu-Prochlor [Can] *see* prochlorperazine *on page 701*
Nu-Propranolol [Can] *see* propranolol *on page 709*
Nuquin HP® [US] *see* hydroquinone *on page 430*
Nu-Ranit [Can] *see* ranitidine *on page 732*
Nuromax® [US] *see* doxacurium *on page 274*
Nu-Selegiline [Can] *see* selegiline *on page 766*
Nu-Sertraline [Can] *see* sertraline *on page 769*
Nu-Sotalol [Can] *see* sotalol *on page 787*
Nu-Sucralate [Can] *see* sucralfate *on page 793*
Nu-Sulfinpyrazone [Can] *see* sulfinpyrazone *on page 799*
Nu-Sundac [Can] *see* sulindac *on page 800*
Nu-Tears® [US-OTC] *see* artificial tears *on page 75*
Nu-Tears® II [US-OTC] *see* artificial tears *on page 75*
Nu-Temazepam [Can] *see* temazepam *on page 808*
Nu-Terazosin [Can] *see* terazosin *on page 810*
Nu-Tetra [Can] *see* tetracycline *on page 816*
Nu-Tiaprofenic [Can] *see* tiaprofenic acid *(Canada only) on page 826*
Nu-Ticlopidine [Can] *see* ticlopidine *on page 827*
Nu-Timolol [Can] *see* timolol *on page 828*
Nutracort® [US] *see* hydrocortisone (topical) *on page 428*
Nutralox® [US-OTC] *see* calcium carbonate *on page 135*
Nutraplus® [US-OTC] *see* urea *on page 861*
Nu-Trazodone [Can] *see* trazodone *on page 843*
Nu-Triazide [Can] *see* hydrochlorothiazide and triamterene *on page 420*
Nu-Trimipramine [Can] *see* trimipramine *on page 852*
NutriNate® [US] *see* vitamins (multiple/prenatal) *on page 879*

nutritional formula, enteral/oral (noo TRISH un al FOR myoo la, EN ter al/OR al)

Synonyms dietary supplements

U.S./Canadian Brand Names Carnation Instant Breakfast® [US-OTC]; Citrotein® [US-OTC]; Criticare HN® [US-OTC]; Ensure Plus® [US-OTC]; Ensure® [US-OTC]; Isocal® [US-OTC]; Magnacal® [US-OTC]; Microlipid™ [US-OTC]; Osmolite® HN [US-OTC]; Pedialyte® [US-OTC]; Portagen® [US-OTC]; Pregestimil®

[US-OTC]; Propac™ [US-OTC]; Soyalac® [US-OTC]; Vital HN® [US-OTC]; Vitaneed™ [US-OTC]; Vivonex® T.E.N. [US-OTC]; Vivonex® [US-OTC]

Therapeutic Category Nutritional Supplement

Dosage Forms

Liquid: Calcium and sodium caseinate, maltodextrin, sucrose, partially hydrogenated soy oil, soy lecithin

Powder: Amino acids, predigested carbohydrates, safflower oil

Nutropin® [US] *see* somatropin *on page 785*

Nutropin AQ® [US] *see* somatropin *on page 785*

Nutropine® [Can] *see* somatropin *on page 785*

NuvaRing® [US/Can] *see* ethinyl estradiol and etonogestrel *on page 319*

Nu-Verap [Can] *see* verapamil *on page 870*

Nu-Zopiclone [Can] *see* zopiclone *(Canada only) on page 890*

NVB *see* vinorelbine *on page 873*

NVP *see* nevirapine *on page 587*

Nyaderm [Can] *see* nystatin *on this page*

Nyamyc™ [US] *see* nystatin *on this page*

Nydrazid® ***(Discontinued)*** *see* isoniazid *on page 464*

nystatin (nye STAT in)

Sound-Alike/Look-Alike Issues

nystatin may be confused with Nilstat®, Nitrostat®

Nilstat® may be confused with Nitrostat®, nystatin

U.S./Canadian Brand Names Bio-Statin® [US]; Candistatin® [Can]; Mycostatin® [US]; Nilstat [Can]; Nyaderm [Can]; Nyamyc™ [US]; Nystat-Rx® [US]; Nystop® [US]; Pedi-Dri® [US]; PMS-Nystatin [Can]

Therapeutic Category Antifungal Agent

Use Treatment of susceptible cutaneous, mucocutaneous, and oral cavity fungal infections normally caused by the *Candida* species

Usual Dosage

Oral candidiasis:

Suspension (swish and swallow orally):

Premature infants: 100,000 units 4 times/day

Infants: 200,000 units 4 times/day or 100,000 units to each side of mouth 4 times/day

Children and Adults: 400,000-600,000 units 4 times/day

Powder for compounding: Children and Adults: 1/8 teaspoon (500,000 units) to equal approximately 1/2 cup of water; give 4 times/day

Mucocutaneous infections: Children and Adults: Topical: Apply 2-3 times/day to affected areas; very moist topical lesions are treated best with powder

Intestinal infections: Adults: Oral: 500,000-1,000,000 units every 8 hours

Vaginal infections: Adults: Vaginal tablets: Insert 1 tablet/day at bedtime for 2 weeks

Dosage Forms

Capsule (Bio-Statin®): 500,000 units, 1 million units

Cream: 100,000 units/g (15 g, 30 g)

Mycostatin®: 100,000 units/g (30 g)

Ointment, topical: 100,000 units/g (15 g, 30 g)

Powder, for prescription compounding: 50 million units (10 g); 150 million units (30 g); 500 million units (100 g); 2 billion units (400 g)

Nystat-Rx®: 50 million units (10 g); 150 million units (30 g); 500 million units (100 g); 1 billion units (190 g); 2 billion units (350 g)

Powder, topical:

Mycostatin®: 100,000 units/g (15 g)

Nyamyc™: 100,000 units/g (15 g, 30 g)

Nystop®: 100,000 units/g (15 g, 30 g, 60 g)

Pedi-Dri®: 100,000 units/g (56.7 g)

Suspension, oral: 100,000 units/mL (5 mL, 60 mL, 480 mL)

Tablet: 500,000 units

Tablet, vaginal: 100,000 units (15s) [packaged with applicator]

nystatin and triamcinolone (nye STAT in & trye am SIN oh lone)

Sound-Alike/Look-Alike Issues

Mycolog®-II may be confused with Halog®

Synonyms triamcinolone and nystatin

Therapeutic Category Antifungal/Corticosteroid

Use Treatment of cutaneous candidiasis

Usual Dosage Children and Adults: Topical: Apply sparingly 2-4 times/day. Therapy should be discontinued when control is achieved; if no improvement is seen, reassessment of diagnosis may be necessary.

Dosage Forms [DSC] = Discontinued product

Cream (Mycolog®-II [DSC]): Nystatin 100,000 units and triamcinolone acetonide 0.1% (15 g, 30 g, 60 g)

Ointment: Nystatin 100,000 units and triamcinolone acetonide 0.1% (15 g, 30 g, 60 g)

Mycolog®-II: Nystatin 100,000 units and triamcinolone acetonide 0.1% (15 g, 30 g, 60 g) [DSC]

Nystat-Rx® [US] *see* nystatin *on previous page*

Nystex® *(Discontinued)* *see* nystatin *on previous page*

Nystop® [US] *see* nystatin *on previous page*

Nytol® [Can] *see* diphenhydramine *on page 261*

Nytol® Extra Strength [Can] *see* diphenhydramine *on page 261*

Nytol® Quick Caps [US-OTC] *see* diphenhydramine *on page 261*

Nytol® Quick Gels [US-OTC] *see* diphenhydramine *on page 261*

Nāsop™ [US] *see* phenylephrine *on page 660*

Nōstrilla® [US-OTC] *see* oxymetazoline *on page 628*

O-V Staticin® *(Discontinued)* *see* nystatin *on previous page*

OB-20 [US] *see* vitamins (multiple/prenatal) *on page 879*

Obegyn® [US] *see* vitamins (multiple/prenatal) *on page 879*

Obezine® *(Discontinued)* *see* phendimetrazine *on page 657*

OCBZ *see* oxcarbazepine *on page 624*

Occlusal®-HP [US-OTC/Can] *see* salicylic acid *on page 758*

Ocean® [US-OTC] *see* sodium chloride *on page 777*

Ocean® for Kids [US-OTC] *see* sodium chloride *on page 777*

OCL® *(Discontinued)* *see* polyethylene glycol-electrolyte solution *on page 679*

Octagam® [US] *see* immune globulin (intravenous) *on page 444*

Octamide® *(Discontinued)* *see* metoclopramide *on page 549*

Octicair® Otic *(Discontinued)* *see* neomycin, polymyxin B, and hydrocortisone *on page 584*

Octocaine® *(Discontinued)* *see* lidocaine and epinephrine *on page 495*

Octostim® [Can] *see* desmopressin acetate *on page 237*

octreotide (ok TREE oh tide)

Sound-Alike/Look-Alike Issues

Sandostatin® may be confused with Sandimmune®

Synonyms NSC-671663; octreotide acetate

U.S./Canadian Brand Names Octreotide Acetate Injection [Can]; Octreotide Acetate Omega [Can]; Sandostatin LAR® [US/Can]; Sandostatin® [US/Can]

Therapeutic Category Somatostatin Analog

Use Control of symptoms in patients with metastatic carcinoid and vasoactive intestinal peptide-secreting tumors (VIPomas); acromegaly

Usual Dosage Adults: SubQ, I.V.: Initial: 50 mcg 2-3 times/day and titrate dose based on patient tolerance, response, and indication

Carcinoid: Initial 2 weeks: 100-600 mcg/day in 2-4 divided doses; usual range 50-1500 mcg/day

VIPomas: Initial 2 weeks: 200-300 mcg/day in 2-4 divided doses; usual range 150-750 mcg/day

Acromegaly: Initial: SubQ: 50 mcg 3 times/day; titrate to achieve growth hormone levels <5 ng/mL or IGF-I (somatomedin C) levels <1.9 U/mL in males and <2.2 U/mL in females; usual effective dose 100 mcg 3 times/day; range 300-1500 mcg/day

Note: Should be withdrawn yearly for a 4-week interval (8 weeks for depot injection) in patients who have received irradiation. Resume if levels increase and signs/symptoms recur.

Acromegaly, carcinoid tumors, and VIPomas (depot injection): Patients must be stabilized on subcutaneous octreotide for at least 2 weeks before switching to the long-acting depot: Upon switch: 20 mg I.M. intragluteally every 4 weeks for 2-3 months, then the dose may be modified based upon response. Patients receiving depot injection for carcinoid tumor or VIPoma should continue to receive their SubQ injections for the first 2 weeks at the same dose in order to maintain therapeutic levels.

Dosage adjustment for acromegaly: After 3 months of depot injections the dosage may be continued or modified as follows:

GH ≤2.5 ng/mL, IGF-1 is normal, symptoms controlled: Maintain octreotide LAR® at 20 mg I.M. every 4 weeks

GH >2.5 ng/mL, IGF-1 is elevated, and/or symptoms uncontrolled: Increase octreotide LAR® to 30 mg I.M. every 4 weeks

GH ≤1 ng/mL, IGF-1 is normal, symptoms controlled: Reduce octreotide LAR® to 10 mg I.M. every 4 weeks

Note: Patients not adequately controlled may increase dose to 40 mg every 4 weeks. Dosages >40 mg are not recommended

Dosage adjustment for carcinoid tumors and VIPomas: After 2 months of depot injections the dosage may be continued or modified as follows:

Increase to 30 mg I.M. every 4 weeks if symptoms are inadequately controlled

Decrease to 10 mg I.M. every 4 weeks, for a trial period, if initially responsive to 20 mg dose

Dosage >30 mg is not recommended

Dosage Forms

Injection, microspheres for suspension, as acetate [depot formulation]:
Sandostatin LAR®: 10 mg, 20 mg, 30 mg [with diluent and syringe]

Injection, solution, as acetate: 0.2 mg/mL (5 mL); 1 mg/mL (5 mL)
Sandostatin®: 0.2 mg/mL (5 mL); 1 mg/mL (5 mL)

Injection, solution, as acetate [preservative free]: 0.05 mg/mL (1 mL); 0.1 mg/mL (1 mL); 0.5 mg/mL (1 mL)
Sandostatin®: 0.05 mg/mL (1 mL); 0.1 mg/mL (1 mL); 0.5 mg/mL (1 mL)

octreotide acetate *see* octreotide *on previous page*

Octreotide Acetate Injection [Can] *see* octreotide *on previous page*

Octreotide Acetate Omega [Can] *see* octreotide *on previous page*

OcuClear® *(Discontinued)* *see* oxymetazoline *on page 628*

OcuCoat® [US-OTC] *see* artificial tears *on page 75*

OcuCoat® PF [US-OTC] *see* artificial tears *on page 75*

Ocufen® [US/Can] *see* flurbiprofen *on page 360*

Ocuflox® [US/Can] *see* ofloxacin *on this page*

Ocupress® *(Discontinued)* *see* carteolol *on page 153*

Ocupress® Ophthalmic [Can] *see* carteolol *on page 153*

Ocusert Pilo-20® *(Discontinued)* *see* pilocarpine *on page 668*

Ocusert Pilo-40® *(Discontinued)* *see* pilocarpine *on page 668*

Ocu-Sul® *(Discontinued)* *see* sulfacetamide *on page 795*

Ocutricin® Topical Ointment *(Discontinued)* *see* bacitracin, neomycin, and polymyxin B *on page 91*

Ocuvite® [US-OTC] *see* vitamins (multiple/oral) *on page 878*

Ocuvite® Extra® [US-OTC] *see* vitamins (multiple/oral) *on page 878*

Ocuvite® Lutein [US-OTC] *see* vitamins (multiple/oral) *on page 878*

Oesclim® [Can] *see* estradiol *on page 308*

ofloxacin (oh FLOKS a sin)

Sound-Alike/Look-Alike Issues

Floxin® may be confused with Flexeril®
Ocuflox® may be confused with Ocufen®

U.S./Canadian Brand Names Apo-Ofloxacin® [Can]; Apo-Oflox® [Can]; Floxin® [US/Can]; Novo-Ofloxacin [Can]; Ocuflox® [US/Can]; PMS-Ofloxacin [Can]

Therapeutic Category Antibiotic, Ophthalmic; Antibiotic, Otic; Quinolone

Use Quinolone antibiotic for the treatment of acute exacerbations of chronic bronchitis, community-acquired pneumonia, skin and skin structure infections (uncomplicated), urethral and cervical gonorrhea (acute,
(Continued)

ofloxacin *(Continued)*

uncomplicated), urethritis and cervicitis (nongonococcal), mixed infections of the urethra and cervix, pelvic inflammatory disease (acute), cystitis (uncomplicated), urinary tract infections (complicated), prostatitis

Ophthalmic: Treatment of superficial ocular infections involving the conjunctiva or cornea due to strains of susceptible organisms

Otic: Otitis externa, chronic suppurative otitis media, acute otitis media

Usual Dosage

Usual dosage range:

Children ≥6 months: Otic: 5 drops daily

Children >1 year: Ophthalmic: 1-2 drops every 30 minutes to 4 hours initially, decreasing to every 4-6 hours

Children >12 years: Otic: 10 drops once or twice daily

Adults:

Ophthalmic: 1-2 drops every 30 minutes to 4 hours initially, decreasing to every 4-6 hours

Oral: 200-400 mg every 12 hours

Otic: 10 drops once or twice daily

Indication-specific dosing:

Acute otitis media with tympanostomy tubes: Children 1-12 years: Otic: Instill 5 drops (or the contents of 1 single-dose container) into affected ear(s) twice daily for 10 days

Otitis externa: Children 6 months to 13 years: Otic: Instill 5 drops (or the contents of 1 single-dose container) into affected ear(s) once daily for 7 days

Children >1 year and Adults: Ophthalmic:

Conjunctivitis: Instill 1-2 drops in affected eye(s) every 2-4 hours for the first 2 days, then use 4 times/day for an additional 5 days

Corneal ulcer: Instill 1-2 drops every 30 minutes while awake and every 4-6 hours after retiring for the first 2 days; beginning on day 3, instill 1-2 drops every hour while awake for 4-6 additional days; thereafter, 1-2 drops 4 times/day until clinical cure.

Children >12 years and Adults:

Otitis media, chronic suppurative with perforated tympanic membranes: Otic: Instill 10 drops (or the contents of 2 single-dose containers) into affected ear twice daily for 14 days

Children ≥13 years and Adults:

Otitis externa: Otic: Instill 10 drops (or the contents of 2 single-dose containers) into affected ear(s) once daily for 7 days

Adults: Oral:

Cervicitis/urethritis (nongonococcal) due to *C. trachomatis,* mixed infection of urethra and cervix due to *C. trachomatis* and *N. gonorrhoea:* 300 mg every 12 hours for 7 days

Chronic bronchitis (acute exacerbation), community-acquired pneumonia, skin and skin structure infections (uncomplicated): 400 mg every 12 hours for 10 days

Cystitis (uncomplicated), *E. coli* or *K. pneumoniae:* 200 mg every 12 hours for 3 days or up to 7 days for other organisms

Pelvic inflammatory disease (acute): 400 mg every 12 hours for 10-14 days

Prostatitis:

Acute: 400 mg for 1 dose, then 300 mg twice daily for 10 days

Chronic: 200 mg every 12 hours for 6 weeks

Urethral and cervical gonorrhea (acute, uncomplicated): 400 mg as a single dose

UTI (complicated): 200 mg every 12 hours for 10 days

Dosage Forms [DSC] = Discontinued product

Solution, ophthalmic (Ocuflox®): 0.3% (5 mL; 10 mL [DSC]) [contains benzalkonium chloride]

Solution, otic:

Floxin®: 0.3% (5 mL, 10 mL) [contains benzalkonium chloride]

Floxin® Otic Singles™: 0.3% (0.25 mL) [contains benzalkonium chloride; packaged as 2 single-dose containers per pouch, 10 pouches per carton, total net volume 5 mL]

Tablet (Floxin®): 200 mg, 300 mg, 400 mg

Ogen® [US/Can] *see* estropipate *on page 314*

Ogestrel® [US] *see* ethinyl estradiol and norgestrel *on page 327*

OGMT *see* metyrosine *on page 552*

OGT-918 *see* miglustat *on page 557*

OKT3 *see* muromonab-CD3 *on page 570*

olanzapine (oh LAN za peen)

Sound-Alike/Look-Alike Issues

olanzapine may be confused with olsalazine

Zyprexa® may be confused with Celexa™, Zyrtec®

Synonyms LY170053

U.S./Canadian Brand Names Zyprexa® Zydis® [US/Can]; Zyprexa® [US/Can]

Therapeutic Category Antipsychotic Agent

Use Treatment of the manifestations of schizophrenia; treatment of acute or mixed mania episodes associated with Bipolar I Disorder (as monotherapy or in combination with lithium or valproate); maintenance treatment of bipolar disorder; acute agitation (patients with schizophrenia or bipolar mania)

Usual Dosage

Children: Schizophrenia/bipolar disorder: Oral: Initial: 2.5 mg/day; titrate as necessary to 20 mg/day (0.12-0.29 mg/kg/day)

Adults:

Schizophrenia: Oral:

Initial: 5-10 mg once daily (increase to 10 mg once daily within 5-7 days); thereafter, adjust by 5 mg/day at 1-week intervals, up to a recommended maximum of 20 mg/day. Maintenance: 10-20 mg once daily. **Note:** Doses of 30-50 mg/day have been used; however, doses >10 mg/day have not demonstrated better efficacy, and safety and efficacy of doses >20 mg/day have not been evaluated.

Bipolar I acute mixed or manic episodes: Oral:

Monotherapy: Initial: 10-15 mg once daily; increase by 5 mg/day at intervals of not less than 24 hours. Maintenance: 5-20 mg/day; recommended maximum dose: 20 mg/day

Combination therapy (with lithium or valproate): Initial: 10 mg once daily; dosing range: 5-20 mg/day

Agitation (acute, associated with bipolar I mania or schizophrenia): I.M.: Initial dose: 5-10 mg (a lower dose of 2.5 mg may be considered when clinical factors warrant); additional doses (2.5-10 mg) may be considered; however, 2-4 hours should be allowed between doses to evaluate response (maximum total daily dose: 30 mg, per manufacturer's recommendation)

Dosage Forms

Injection, powder for reconstitution (Zyprexa® IntraMuscular): 10 mg [contains lactose 50 mg]

Tablet (Zyprexa®): 2.5 mg, 5 mg, 7.5 mg, 10 mg, 15 mg, 20 mg

Tablet, orally disintegrating (Zyprexa® Zydis®): 5 mg [contains phenylalanine 0.34 mg/tablet], 10 mg [contains phenylalanine 0.45 mg/tablet], 15 mg [contains phenylalanine 0.67 mg/tablet], 20 mg [contains phenylalanine 0.9 mg/tablet]

olanzapine and fluoxetine (oh LAN za peen & floo OKS e teen)

Synonyms fluoxetine and olanzapine; olanzapine and fluoxetine hydrochloride

U.S./Canadian Brand Names Symbyax™ [US]

Therapeutic Category Antidepressant, Selective Serotonin Reuptake Inhibitor; Antipsychotic Agent, Thienobenzodiaepine

Use Treatment of depressive episodes associated with bipolar disorder

Usual Dosage Oral: Adults: Depression associated with bipolar disorder: Initial: Olanzapine 6 mg/fluoxetine 25 mg once daily in the evening. Dosing range: Olanzapine 6-12 mg/fluoxetine 25-50 mg. Use caution adjusting dose in patients predisposed to hypotension, in females, and in nonsmokers (metabolism may be decreased). Safety of daily doses of olanzapine >18 mg/fluoxetine >75 mg have not been evaluated.

Dosage Forms Capsule:

6/25: Olanzapine 6 mg and fluoxetine 25 mg

6/50: Olanzapine 6 mg and fluoxetine 50 mg

12/25: Olanzapine 12 mg and fluoxetine 25 mg

12/50: Olanzapine 12 mg and fluoxetine 50 mg

olanzapine and fluoxetine hydrochloride *see* olanzapine and fluoxetine *on this page*

Olay® Vitamins Complete Women's [US-OTC] *see* vitamins (multiple/oral) *on page 878*

Olay® Vitamins Complete Women's 50+ [US-OTC] *see* vitamins (multiple/oral) *on page 878*

Olay® Vitamins Even Complexion [US-OTC] *see* vitamins (multiple/oral) *on page 878*

oleovitamin A *see* vitamin A *on page 874*

oleum ricini *see* castor oil *on page 155*

olmesartan (ole me SAR tan)

Synonyms olmesartan medoxomil

U.S./Canadian Brand Names Benicar® [US]

Therapeutic Category Angiotensin II Receptor Antagonist

Use Treatment of hypertension with or without concurrent use of other antihypertensive agents

Usual Dosage Oral: Adults: Initial: Usual starting dose is 20 mg once daily; if initial response is inadequate, may be increased to 40 mg once daily after 2 weeks. May administer with other antihypertensive agents if blood pressure inadequately controlled with olmesartan. Consider lower starting dose in patients with possible depletion of intravascular volume (eg, patients receiving diuretics).

Dosage Forms Tablet, as medoxomil: 5 mg, 20 mg, 40 mg

olmesartan and hydrochlorothiazide (ole me SAR tan & hye droe klor oh THYE a zide)

Synonyms hydrochlorothiazide and olmesartan medoxomil; olmesartan medoxomil and hydrochlorothiazide

U.S./Canadian Brand Names Benicar HCT® [US]

Therapeutic Category Angiotensin II Receptor Antagonist; Diuretic, Thiazide

Use Treatment of hypertension (not recommended for initial treatment)

Usual Dosage Oral: Adults: One tablet daily; dosage must be individualized (see below). May be titrated at 2- to 4-week intervals.

Replacement therapy: May be substituted for previously titrated dosages of the individual components.

Patients not controlled with single-agent therapy: Initiate by adding the lowest available dose of the alternative component (hydrochlorothiazide 12.5 mg or olmesartan 20 mg). Titrate to effect (maximum daily hydrochlorothiazide dose: 25 mg; maximum daily olmesartan dose: 40 mg).

Dosage Forms Tablet:

20/12.5: Olmesartan medoxomil 20 mg and hydrochlorothiazide 12.5 mg

40/12.5: Olmesartan medoxomil 40 mg and hydrochlorothiazide 12.5 mg

40/25: Olmesartan medoxomil 40 mg and hydrochlorothiazide 25 mg

olmesartan medoxomil *see* olmesartan *on this page*

olmesartan medoxomil and hydrochlorothiazide *see* olmesartan and hydrochlorothiazide *on this page*

olopatadine (oh la PAT a deen)

Sound-Alike/Look-Alike Issues

Patanol® may be confused with Platinol®

U.S./Canadian Brand Names Patanol® [US/Can]

Therapeutic Category Antihistamine

Use Treatment of the signs and symptoms of allergic conjunctivitis

Usual Dosage Adults: Ophthalmic: Instill 1 to 2 drops into affected eye(s) twice daily (allowing 6-8 hours between doses); results from an environmental study demonstrated that olopatadine was effective when dosed twice daily for up to 6 weeks

Dosage Forms Solution, ophthalmic: 0.1% (5 mL) [contains benzalkonium chloride]

olsalazine (ole SAL a zeen)

Sound-Alike/Look-Alike Issues

olsalazine may be confused with olanzapine

Dipentum® may be confused with Dilantin®

Synonyms olsalazine sodium

U.S./Canadian Brand Names Dipentum® [US/Can]

Therapeutic Category 5-Aminosalicylic Acid Derivative

Use Maintenance of remission of ulcerative colitis in patients intolerant to sulfasalazine

Usual Dosage Adults: Oral: 1 g/day in 2 divided doses

Dosage Forms Capsule, as sodium: 250 mg

olsalazine sodium *see* olsalazine *on this page*

Olux® [US] *see* clobetasol *on page 200*

Omacor® [US] *see* omega-3-acid ethyl esters *on next page*

omalizumab (oh mah lye ZOO mab)

Synonyms rhuMAb-E25

U.S./Canadian Brand Names Xolair® [US/Can]

Therapeutic Category Monoclonal Antibody

Use Treatment of moderate-to-severe, persistent allergic asthma not adequately controlled with inhaled corticosteroids

Usual Dosage SubQ: Children ≥12 years and Adults: Asthma: Dose is based on pretreatment IgE serum levels and body weight. Dosing should not be adjusted based on IgE levels taken during treatment or <1 year following discontinuation of therapy; doses should be adjusted during treatment for significant changes in body weight

IgE ≥30-100 int. units/mL:
- 30-90 kg: 150 mg every 4 weeks
- >90-150 kg: 300 mg every 4 weeks

IgE >100-200 int. units/mL:
- 30-90 kg: 300 mg every 4 weeks
- >90-150 kg: 225 mg every 2 weeks

IgE >200-300 int. units/mL:
- 30-60 kg: 300 mg every 4 weeks
- >60-90 kg: 225 mg every 2 weeks
- >90-150 kg: 300 mg every 2 weeks

IgE >300-400 int. units/mL:
- 30-70 kg: 225 mg every 2 weeks
- >70-90 kg: 300 mg every 2 weeks
- >90 kg: Do not administer dose

IgE >400-500 int. units/mL:
- 30-70 kg: 300 mg every 2 weeks
- >70-90 kg: 375 mg every 2 weeks
- >90 kg: Do not administer dose

IgE >500-600 int. units/mL:
- 30-60 kg: 300 mg every 2 weeks
- >60-70 kg: 375 mg every 2 weeks
- >70 kg: Do not administer dose

IgE >600-700 int. units/mL:
- 30-60 kg: 375 mg every 2 weeks
- >60 kg: Do not administer dose

Dosage Forms

Injection, powder for reconstitution [preservative free]:
- Xolair®: 150 mg [contains sucrose 145.5 g]

omega-3-acid ethyl esters (oh MEG a three AS id ETH il ES ters)

Sound-Alike/Look-Alike Issues

Omacor® may be confused with Amicar®

Synonyms ethyl esters of omega-3 fatty acids; fish oil

U.S./Canadian Brand Names Omacor® [US]

Therapeutic Category Antilipemic Agent, Miscellaneous

Use Omacor®: Treatment of hypertriglyceridemia (≥500 mg/dL)

Note: A number of OTC formulations containing omega-3 fatty acids are marketed as nutritional supplements; these do not have FDA-approved indications.

Usual Dosage Oral: Adults: Hypertriglyceridemia: 4 g/day as a single daily dose or in 2 divided doses

Dosage Forms Capsule: 1 g [contains EPA ~465 mg and DHA ~375 mg]

omeprazole (oh MEP ra zole)

Sound-Alike/Look-Alike Issues

Prilosec® may be confused with Plendil®, Prevacid®, predniSONE, prilocaine, Prinivil®, Proventil®, Prozac®

U.S./Canadian Brand Names Apo-Omeprazole® [Can]; Losec MUPS® [Can]; Losec® [Can]; Prilosec OTC™ [US-OTC]; Prilosec® [US]

Therapeutic Category Gastric Acid Secretion Inhibitor

Use Short-term (4-8 weeks) treatment of active duodenal ulcer disease or active benign gastric ulcer; treatment of heartburn and other symptoms associated with gastroesophageal reflux disease (GERD); short-term (4-8 weeks) treatment of endoscopically-diagnosed erosive esophagitis; maintenance healing of

(Continued)

omeprazole *(Continued)*

erosive esophagitis; long-term treatment of pathological hypersecretory conditions; as part of a multidrug regimen for *H. pylori* eradication to reduce the risk of duodenal ulcer recurrence

OTC labeling: Short-term treatment of frequent, uncomplicated heartburn occurring ≥2 days/week

Usual Dosage Oral:

Children ≥2 years: GERD or other acid-related disorders:
- <20 kg: 10 mg once daily
- ≥20 kg: 20 mg once daily

Adults:
- Active duodenal ulcer: 20 mg/day for 4-8 weeks
- Gastric ulcers: 40 mg/day for 4-8 weeks
- Symptomatic GERD: 20 mg/day for up to 4 weeks
- Erosive esophagitis: 20 mg/day for 4-8 weeks; maintenance of healing: 20 mg/day for up to 12 months total therapy (including treatment period of 4-8 weeks)
- *Helicobacter pylori* eradication: Dose varies with regimen: 20 mg once daily **or** 40 mg/day as single dose or in 2 divided doses; requires combination therapy with antibiotics
- Pathological hypersecretory conditions: Initial: 60 mg once daily; doses up to 120 mg 3 times/day have been administered; administer daily doses >80 mg in divided doses
- Frequent heartburn (OTC labeling): 20 mg/day for 14 days; treatment may be repeated after 4 months if needed

Dosage Forms

Capsule, delayed release: 10 mg, 20 mg
- Prilosec®: 10 mg, 20 mg, 40 mg

Tablet, delayed release:
- Prilosec OTC™: 20 mg

Omnicef® [US/Can] *see* cefdinir *on page 157*

OMNIhist® II L.A. [US] *see* chlorpheniramine, phenylephrine, and methscopolamine *on page 180*

Omnii Gel™ [US-OTC] *see* fluoride *on page 354*

Omnipaque® [US] *see* radiological/contrast media (nonionic) *on page 730*

Omnipen® *(Discontinued)* *see* ampicillin *on page 53*

Omnipen®-N *(Discontinued)* *see* ampicillin *on page 53*

Omnitrope™ [US] *see* somatropin *on page 785*

Oncaspar® [US] *see* pegaspargase *on page 642*

Oncet® *(Discontinued)* *see* hydrocodone and homatropine *on page 423*

Oncotice™ [Can] *see* BCG vaccine *on page 94*

Oncovin® *(Discontinued)* *see* vincristine *on page 873*

ondansetron (on DAN se tron)

Sound-Alike/Look-Alike Issues

ondansetron may be confused with dolasetron, granisetron, palonosetron

Zofran® may be confused with Zantac®, Zosyn®

Synonyms GR38032R; ondansetron hydrochloride

U.S./Canadian Brand Names Zofran® ODT [US/Can]; Zofran® [US/Can]

Therapeutic Category Selective 5-HT_3 Receptor Antagonist

Use Prevention of nausea and vomiting associated with moderately- to highly-emetogenic cancer chemotherapy [not recommended for treatment of **existing** chemotherapy-induced emesis (CIE)]; radiotherapy in patients receiving total body irradiation or fractions to the abdomen; prevention of postoperative nausea and vomiting (PONV); treatment of PONV if no prophylactic dose received

Usual Dosage Note: Studies in adults have shown a single daily dose of 8-12 mg I.V. or 8-24 mg orally to be as effective as mg/kg dosing, and should be considered for **all** patients whose mg/kg dose exceeds 8-12 mg I.V.; oral solution and ODT formulations are bioequivalent to corresponding doses of tablet formulation

Children:

I.V.:
- Prevention of chemotherapy-induced emesis: 6 months to 18 years: 0.15 mg/kg/dose administered 30 minutes prior to chemotherapy, 4 and 8 hours after the first dose **or** 0.45 mg/kg/day as a single dose
- Prevention of postoperative nausea and vomiting: 1 month to 12 years:
  - ≤40 kg: 0.1 mg/kg as a single dose

>40 kg: 4 mg as a single dose
Oral: Prevention of chemotherapy-induced emesis:
4-11 years: 4 mg 30 minutes before chemotherapy; repeat 4 and 8 hours after initial dose, then 4 mg every 8 hours for 1-2 days after chemotherapy completed
≥12 years: Refer to adult dosing.

Adults:
I.V.:
Prevention of chemotherapy-induced emesis:
0.15 mg/kg 3 times/day beginning 30 minutes prior to chemotherapy **or**
0.45 mg/kg once daily **or**
8-10 mg 1-2 times/day **or**
24 mg or 32 mg once daily
I.M., I.V.: Postoperative nausea and vomiting: 4 mg as a single dose approximately 30 minutes before the end of anesthesia, or as treatment if vomiting occurs after surgery
Note: Repeat doses given in response to inadequate control of nausea/vomiting from preoperative doses are generally ineffective.
Oral:
Chemotherapy-induced emesis:
Highly-emetogenic agents/single-day therapy: 24 mg given 30 minutes prior to the start of therapy
Moderately-emetogenic agents: 8 mg every 12 hours beginning 30 minutes before chemotherapy, continuously for 1-2 days after chemotherapy completed
Total body irradiation: 8 mg 1-2 hours before daily each fraction of radiotherapy
Single high-dose fraction radiotherapy to abdomen: 8 mg 1-2 hours before irradiation, then 8 mg every 8 hours after first dose for 1-2 days after completion of radiotherapy
Daily fractionated radiotherapy to abdomen: 8 mg 1-2 hours before irradiation, then 8 mg 8 hours after first dose for each day of radiotherapy
Postoperative nausea and vomiting: 16 mg given 1 hour prior to induction of anesthesia

Dosage Forms [DSC] = Discontinued product
Infusion [premixed in D_5W, preservative free]:
Zofran®: 32 mg (50 mL)
Injection, solution:
Zofran®: 2 mg/mL (2 mL, 20 mL)
Solution, oral:
Zofran®: 4 mg/5 mL (50 mL) [contains sodium benzoate; strawberry flavor]
Tablet:
Zofran®: 4 mg; 8 mg; 24 mg [DSC]
Tablet, orally disintegrating:
Zofran® ODT: 4 mg, 8 mg [each strength contains phenylalanine <0.03 mg/tablet; strawberry flavor]

ondansetron hydrochloride *see* ondansetron *on previous page*

One-A-Day® 50 Plus Formula [US-OTC] *see* vitamins (multiple/oral) *on page 878*

One-A-Day® Active Formula [US-OTC] *see* vitamins (multiple/oral) *on page 878*

One-A-Day® Carb Smart [US-OTC] *see* vitamins (multiple/oral) *on page 878*

One-A-Day® Cholesterol Plus™ [US-OTC] *see* vitamins (multiple/oral) *on page 878*

One-A-Day® Essential Formula [US-OTC] *see* vitamins (multiple/oral) *on page 878*

One-A-Day® Kids Bugs Bunny and Friends Complete [US-OTC] *see* vitamins (multiple/pediatric) *on page 878*

One-A-Day® Kids Bugs Bunny and Friends Plus Extra C [US-OTC] *see* vitamins (multiple/pediatric) *on page 878*

One-A-Day® Kids Extreme Sports [US-OTC] *see* vitamins (multiple/pediatric) *on page 878*

One-A-Day® Kids Scooby-Doo! Complete [US-OTC] *see* vitamins (multiple/pediatric) *on page 878*

One-A-Day® Kids Scooby-Doo! Fizzy Vites [US-OTC] *see* vitamins (multiple/pediatric) *on page 878*

One-A-Day® Kids Scooby-Doo! Plus Calcium [US-OTC] *see* vitamins (multiple/pediatric) *on page 878*

One-A-Day® Maximum Formula [US-OTC] *see* vitamins (multiple/oral) *on page 878*

One-A-Day® Men's Formula [US-OTC] *see* vitamins (multiple/oral) *on page 878*

One-A-Day® Today [US-OTC] *see* vitamins (multiple/oral) *on page 878*

One-A-Day® Weight Smart [US-OTC] *see* vitamins (multiple/oral) *on page 878*

One-A-Day® Women's Formula [US-OTC] *see* vitamins (multiple/oral) *on page 878*

ONTAK® [US] *see* denileukin diftitox *on page 235*

Onxol™ [US] *see* paclitaxel *on page 631*

Ony-Clear *(Discontinued)* *see* benzalkonium chloride *on page 99*

OPC-13013 *see* cilostazol *on page 188*

OPC-14597 *see* aripiprazole *on page 73*

OP-CCK *see* sincalide *on page 774*

Opcon-A® [US-OTC] *see* naphazoline and pheniramine *on page 578*

Opcon® Ophthalmic *(Discontinued)* *see* naphazoline *on page 577*

Operand® [US-OTC] *see* povidone-iodine *on page 689*

Operand® Chlorhexidine Gluconate [US-OTC] *see* chlorhexidine gluconate *on page 173*

Ophthalgan® Ophthalmic *(Discontinued)* *see* glycerin *on page 388*

Ophthetic® [US] *see* proparacaine *on page 706*

Ophthifluor® *(Discontinued)* *see* fluorescein sodium *on page 354*

Ophthochlor® Ophthalmic *(Discontinued)* *see* chloramphenicol *on page 172*

Ophtho-Dipivefrin™ [Can] *see* dipivefrin *on page 267*

Ophtho-Tate® [Can] *see* prednisolone (ophthalmic) *on page 694*

opium and belladonna *see* belladonna and opium *on page 96*

opium tincture (OH pee um TING chur)

Sound-Alike/Look-Alike Issues

opium tincture may be confused with camphorated tincture of opium (paregoric)

DTO is an error-prone abbreviation (mistaken as Diluted Tincture of Opium; dose equivalency of paregoric)

Synonyms opium tincture, deodorized

Therapeutic Category Analgesic, Narcotic

Controlled Substance C-II

Use Treatment of diarrhea or relief of pain

Usual Dosage Oral: **Note:** Opium tincture 10% contains morphine 10 mg/mL. Use caution in ordering, dispensing, and/or administering.

Children:

Diarrhea: 0.005-0.01 mL/kg/dose every 3-4 hours for a maximum of 6 doses/24 hours

Analgesia: 0.01-0.02 mL/kg/dose every 3-4 hours

Adults:

Diarrhea: 0.3-1 mL/dose every 2-6 hours to maximum of 6 mL/24 hours

Analgesia: 0.6-1.5 mL/dose every 3-4 hours

Dosage Forms Liquid: 10% (120 mL, 480 mL) [0.6 mL equivalent to morphine 6 mg; contains alcohol 19%]

opium tincture, deodorized *see* opium tincture *on this page*

oprelvekin (oh PREL ve kin)

Sound-Alike/Look-Alike Issues

oprelvekin may be confused with aldesleukin, Proleukin®

Neumega® may be confused with Neupogen®

Synonyms IL-11; interleukin-11; NSC-722848; recombinant human interleukin-11; recombinant interleukin-11; rhIL-11; rIL-11

U.S./Canadian Brand Names Neumega® [US]

Therapeutic Category Platelet Growth Factor

Use Prevention of severe thrombocytopenia and the reduction of the need for platelet transfusions following myelosuppressive chemotherapy

Usual Dosage SubQ: Administer first dose ~6-24 hours after the end of chemotherapy. Discontinue at least 48 hours before beginning the next cycle of chemotherapy.

Adults: 50 mcg/kg once daily for ~10-21 days (until postnadir platelet count ≥50,000 cells/μL)

Dosage Forms

Injection, powder for reconstitution:

Neumega®: 5 mg [packaged with diluent]

Optase™ [US] *see* trypsin, balsam peru, and castor oil *on page 856*

Optho-Bunolol® [Can] *see* levobunolol *on page 488*

Opticrom® [US/Can] *see* cromolyn sodium *on page 217*

Optigene® 3 [US-OTC] *see* tetrahydrozoline *on page 817*

Optimine® [Can] *see* azatadine *(Canada only) on page 86*

Optimine® ***(Discontinued)***

Optimoist® Solution ***(Discontinued)*** *see* saliva substitute *on page 760*

Optimyxin® [Can] *see* bacitracin and polymyxin B *on page 90*

Optimyxin Plus® [Can] *see* neomycin, polymyxin B, and gramicidin *on page 584*

OptiPranolol® [US/Can] *see* metipranolol *on page 549*

Optiray® [US] *see* radiological/contrast media (nonionic) *on page 730*

Optivar® [US] *see* azelastine *on page 87*

Optivite® P.M.T. [US-OTC] *see* vitamins (multiple/oral) *on page 878*

o,p′-DDD *see* mitotane *on page 560*

Orabase® with Benzocaine [US-OTC] *see* benzocaine *on page 99*

Oracort [Can] *see* triamcinolone (systemic) *on page 846*

Oradex-C® ***(Discontinued)*** *see* dyclonine *on page 284*

Oragrafin® Calcium [US] *see* radiological/contrast media (ionic) *on page 728*

Oragrafin® Sodium [US] *see* radiological/contrast media (ionic) *on page 728*

Orajel® Baby Teething [US-OTC] *see* benzocaine *on page 99*

Orajel® Baby Teething Daytime and Nighttime [US-OTC] *see* benzocaine *on page 99*

Orajel® Baby Teething Nighttime [US-OTC] *see* benzocaine *on page 99*

Orajel® Brace-Aid Oral Anesthetic ***(Discontinued)*** *see* benzocaine *on page 99*

Orajel® Denture Plus [US-OTC] *see* benzocaine *on page 99*

Orajel® Maximum Strength [US-OTC] *see* benzocaine *on page 99*

Orajel® Medicated Toothache [US-OTC] *see* benzocaine *on page 99*

Orajel® Mouth Sore [US-OTC] *see* benzocaine *on page 99*

Orajel® Multi-Action Cold Sore [US-OTC] *see* benzocaine *on page 99*

Orajel® Perioseptic® Spot Treatment [US-OTC] *see* carbamide peroxide *on page 145*

Orajel PM® [US-OTC] *see* benzocaine *on page 99*

Orajel® Ultra Mouth Sore [US-OTC] *see* benzocaine *on page 99*

Oramorph SR® [US] *see* morphine sulfate *on page 565*

Oranyl [US-OTC] *see* pseudoephedrine *on page 712*

Orap® [US/Can] *see* pimozide *on page 668*

Orapred® [US] *see* prednisolone (systemic) *on page 695*

Oraquix® *see* lidocaine and prilocaine *on page 496*

OraRinse™ [US-OTC] *see* maltodextrin *on page 518*

Orasone® ***(Discontinued)*** *see* prednisone *on page 695*

Orazinc® [US-OTC] *see* zinc sulfate *on page 888*

orciprenaline sulfate *see* metaproterenol *on page 535*

Orencia® [US] *see* abatacept *on page 3*

Oreton® Methyl ***(Discontinued)*** *see* methyltestosterone *on page 548*

Orfadin® [US] *see* nitisinone *on page 593*

ORG 946 *see* rocuronium *on page 751*

Orgalutran® [Can] *see* ganirelix *on page 375*

Organ-1 NR [US] *see* guaifenesin *on page 392*

Organidin® NR [US] *see* guaifenesin *on page 392*

Orgaran® [Can] *see* danaparoid *on page 228*

Orgaran® *(Discontinued)* *see* danaparoid *on page 228*

ORG NC 45 *see* vecuronium *on page 869*

Orinase Diagnostic® *(Discontinued)* *see* tolbutamide *on page 834*

Orinase® Oral *(Discontinued)* *see* tolbutamide *on page 834*

ORLAAM® *(Discontinued)*

orlistat (OR li stat)

Sound-Alike/Look-Alike Issues
Xenical® may be confused with Xeloda®

U.S./Canadian Brand Names Xenical® [US/Can]

Therapeutic Category Lipase Inhibitor

Use Management of obesity, including weight loss and weight management when used in conjunction with a reduced-calorie diet; reduce the risk of weight regain after prior weight loss; indicated for obese patients with an initial body mass index (BMI) ≥30 kg/m^2 or ≥27 kg/m^2 in the presence of other risk factors

Usual Dosage Oral: Children ≥12 years and Adults: 120 mg 3 times/day with each main meal containing fat (during or up to 1 hour after the meal); omit dose if meal is occasionally missed or contains no fat.

Dosage Forms Capsule: 120 mg

Ormazine® *(Discontinued)* *see* chlorpromazine *on page 184*

Ornex® [US-OTC] *see* acetaminophen and pseudoephedrine *on page 9*

Ornex® Maximum Strength [US-OTC] *see* acetaminophen and pseudoephedrine *on page 9*

Ornidyl® Injection *(Discontinued)* *see* eflornithine *on page 288*

ORO-Clense [Can] *see* chlorhexidine gluconate *on page 173*

Orphenace® [Can] *see* orphenadrine *on this page*

orphenadrine (or FEN a dreen)

Sound-Alike/Look-Alike Issues
Norflex™ may be confused with norfloxacin, Noroxin®

Synonyms orphenadrine citrate

U.S./Canadian Brand Names Norflex™ [US/Can]; Orphenace® [Can]; Rhoxal-orphendrine [Can]

Therapeutic Category Skeletal Muscle Relaxant

Use Treatment of muscle spasm associated with acute painful musculoskeletal conditions; supportive therapy in tetanus

Usual Dosage Adults:
Oral: 100 mg twice daily
I.M., I.V.: 60 mg every 12 hours

Dosage Forms
Injection, solution, as citrate: 30 mg/mL (2 mL)
Norflex™: 30 mg/mL (2 mL) [contains sodium bisulfite]
Tablet, extended release, as citrate: 100 mg
Norflex™: 100 mg

orphenadrine, aspirin, and caffeine (or FEN a dreen, AS pir in, & KAF een)

Sound-Alike/Look-Alike Issues
Norgesic™ Forte may be confused with Norgesic 40®

Synonyms aspirin, orphenadrine, and caffeine; caffeine, orphenadrine, and aspirin

U.S./Canadian Brand Names Norgesic™ Forte [Can]; Norgesic™ [Can]

Therapeutic Category Analgesic, Nonnarcotic; Skeletal Muscle Relaxant

Use Relief of discomfort associated with skeletal muscular conditions

Usual Dosage Oral: 1-2 tablets 3-4 times/day

Dosage Forms [DSC] = Discontinued product
Tablet: Orphenadrine citrate 25 mg, aspirin 385 mg, and caffeine 30 mg; orphenadrine citrate 50 mg, aspirin 770 mg, and caffeine 60 mg
Norgesic™, Orphengesic: Orphenadrine citrate 25 mg, aspirin 385 mg, and caffeine 30 mg [DSC]
Norgesic™ Forte, Orphengesic Forte: Orphenadrine citrate 50 mg, aspirin 770 mg, and caffeine 60 mg [DSC]

orphenadrine citrate *see* orphenadrine *on this page*

Orphengesic *(Discontinued)* *see* orphenadrine, aspirin, and caffeine *on this page*

Orphengesic Forte ***(Discontinued)*** *see* orphenadrine, aspirin, and caffeine *on previous page*

Ortho® 0.5/35 [Can] *see* ethinyl estradiol and norethindrone *on page 323*

Ortho® 1/35 [Can] *see* ethinyl estradiol and norethindrone *on page 323*

Ortho® 7/7/7 [Can] *see* ethinyl estradiol and norethindrone *on page 323*

Ortho-Cept® [US/Can] *see* ethinyl estradiol and desogestrel *on page 317*

Orthoclone OKT® 3 [US/Can] *see* muromonab-CD3 *on page 570*

Ortho-Cyclen® [US] *see* ethinyl estradiol and norgestimate *on page 325*

Ortho-Est® [US] *see* estropipate *on page 314*

Ortho Evra® [US] *see* ethinyl estradiol and norelgestromin *on page 322*

Ortho-Novum® [US] *see* ethinyl estradiol and norethindrone *on page 323*

Ortho-Novum® 1/50 [US] *see* mestranol and norethindrone *on page 534*

ortho prefest *see* estradiol and norgestimate *on page 311*

Ortho Tri-Cyclen® [US] *see* ethinyl estradiol and norgestimate *on page 325*

Ortho Tri-Cyclen® Lo [US] *see* ethinyl estradiol and norgestimate *on page 325*

OrthoVisc® [US/Can] *see* hyaluronate and derivatives *on page 416*

Or-Tyl® Injection ***(Discontinued)*** *see* dicyclomine *on page 251*

Orudis® KT ***(Discontinued)*** *see* ketoprofen *on page 472*

Oruvail® [Can] *see* ketoprofen *on page 472*

Orvaten™ [US] *see* midodrine *on page 556*

Os-Cal® [Can] *see* calcium carbonate *on page 135*

Os-Cal® 500 [US-OTC] *see* calcium carbonate *on page 135*

oseltamivir (oh sel TAM i vir)

Sound-Alike/Look-Alike Issues

Tamiflu® may be confused with Thera-Flu®

U.S./Canadian Brand Names Tamiflu® [US/Can]

Therapeutic Category Antiviral Agent, Oral

Use Treatment of uncomplicated acute illness due to influenza (A or B) infection in children ≥1 year of age and adults who have been symptomatic for no more than 2 days; prophylaxis against influenza (A or B) infection in children ≥1 year of age and adults

Usual Dosage Oral:

Treatment: Initiate treatment within 2 days of onset of symptoms; duration of treatment: 5 days:

Children: 1-12 years:

≤15 kg: 30 mg twice daily

>15 kg to ≤23 kg: 45 mg twice daily

>23 kg to ≤40 kg: 60 mg twice daily

>40 kg: 75 mg twice daily

Adolescents ≥13 years and Adults: 75 mg twice daily

Prophylaxis: Initiate treatment within 2 days of contact with an infected individual; duration of treatment: 10 days

Children: 1-12 years:

≤15 kg: 30 mg once daily

>15 kg to ≤23 kg: 45 mg once daily

>23 kg to ≤40 kg: 60 mg once daily

>40 kg: 75 mg once daily

Adolescents ≥13 years and Adults: 75 mg once daily. During community outbreaks, dosing is 75 mg once daily. May be used for up to 6 weeks; duration of protection lasts for length of dosing period

Dosage Forms

Capsule, as phosphate:

Tamiflu®: 75 mg

Powder for oral suspension:

Tamiflu®: 12 mg/mL (25 mL) [contains sodium benzoate; tutti-frutti flavor]

OSI-774 *see* erlotinib *on page 302*

Osmitrol® [US/Can] *see* mannitol *on page 518*

Osmoglyn® ***(Discontinued)*** *see* glycerin *on page 388*

Osmolite® HN [US-OTC] *see* nutritional formula, enteral/oral *on page 608*

OsmoPrep™ [US] *see* sodium phosphates *on page 781*

Ostac® [Can] *see* clodronate *(Canada only) on page 201*

Osteocalcin® *(Discontinued)* *see* calcitonin *on page 133*

Osteocit® [Can] *see* calcium citrate *on page 137*

Ostoforte® [Can] *see* ergocalciferol *on page 301*

Oticaine [US] *see* benzocaine *on page 99*

Otic-Care® Otic *(Discontinued)* *see* neomycin, polymyxin B, and hydrocortisone *on page 584*

Otobiotic Otic Solution *(Discontinued)*

Otocaine™ [US] *see* benzocaine *on page 99*

Otocort® Otic *(Discontinued)* *see* neomycin, polymyxin B, and hydrocortisone *on page 584*

Otosporin® Otic *(Discontinued)* *see* neomycin, polymyxin B, and hydrocortisone *on page 584*

Outgro® [US-OTC] *see* benzocaine *on page 99*

Ovace™ [US] *see* sulfacetamide *on page 795*

Ovcon® [US] *see* ethinyl estradiol and norethindrone *on page 323*

Ovide® [US] *see* malathion *on page 517*

Ovidrel® [US/Can] *see* chorionic gonadotropin (recombinant) *on page 187*

Ovol® [Can] *see* simethicone *on page 772*

Ovral® [Can] *see* ethinyl estradiol and norgestrel *on page 327*

Ovral® *(Discontinued)* *see* ethinyl estradiol and norgestrel *on page 327*

Ovrette® *(Discontinued)*

oxacillin (oks a SIL in)

Synonyms methylphenyl isoxazolyl penicillin; oxacillin sodium

Therapeutic Category Penicillin

Use Treatment of infections such as osteomyelitis, septicemia, endocarditis, and CNS infections caused by susceptible strains of *Staphylococcus*

Usual Dosage

Usual dosage range:

Infants and Children: I.M., I.V.: 100-200 mg/kg/day in divided doses every 6 hours (maximum: 12 g/day)

Adults: I.M., I.V.: 250-2000 mg every 4-6 hours

Indication-specific dosing:

Children:

Arthritis (septic): I.V.: 37 mg/kg every 6 hours

Epiglottitis: I.V.: 150-200 mg/kg/day divided every 6 hours

Mild-to-moderate infections: I.M., I.V.: 100-150 mg/kg/day in divided doses every 6 hours (maximum: 4 g/day)

Severe infections: I.M., I.V.: 150-200 mg/kg/day in divided doses every 6 hours (maximum: 12 g/day)

Staphylococcal scalded-skin syndrome: I.V.: 150 mg/kg/day divided every 6 hours for 5-7 days

Adults:

Endocarditis: I.V.: 2 g every 4 hours with gentamicin

Mild-to-moderate infections: I.M., I.V.: 250-500 mg every 4-6 hours

Prosthetic joint infection: I.V.: 2 g every 4 hours with rifampin

Severe infections: I.M., I.V.: 1-2 g every 4-6 hours

***Staphylococcus aureus*, methicillin-susceptible infections, including brain abscess, bursitis, erysipelas, mastitis, mastoiditis, osteomyelitis, perinephric abscess, pneumonia, pyomyositis, scalded skin syndrome, toxic shock syndrome:** I.V.: 2 g every 4 hours

Dosage Forms

Infusion [premixed iso-osmotic dextrose solution]: 1 g (50 mL); 2 g (50 mL)

Injection, powder for reconstitution, as sodium: 1 g, 2 g, 10 g

oxacillin sodium *see* oxacillin *on this page*

oxaliplatin (ox AL i pla tin)

Sound-Alike/Look-Alike Issues

oxaliplatin may be confused with Aloxi™

Synonyms diaminocyclohexane oxalatoplatinum; L-OHP; NSC-266046
U.S./Canadian Brand Names Eloxatin® [US]
Therapeutic Category Antineoplastic Agent, Alkylating Agent
Use Treatment of advanced colon cancer and advanced rectal carcinoma
Usual Dosage Refer to individual protocols.
Adults: Stage III colon cancer and colorectal cancer: I.V.: 85 mg/m^2 every 2 weeks
Dosage Forms [DSC] = Discontinued product
Injection, powder for reconstitution:
Eloxatin®: 50 mg, 100 mg [contains lactose] [DSC]
Injection, solution [preservative free]:
Eloxatin®: 5 mg/mL (10 mL, 20 mL)

Oxandrin® [US] *see* oxandrolone *on this page*

oxandrolone (oks AN droe lone)

U.S./Canadian Brand Names Oxandrin® [US]
Therapeutic Category Androgen
Controlled Substance C-III
Use Adjunctive therapy to promote weight gain after weight loss following extensive surgery, chronic infections, or severe trauma, and in some patients who, without definite pathophysiologic reasons, fail to gain or to maintain normal weight; to offset protein catabolism with prolonged corticosteroid administration; relief of bone pain associated with osteoporosis
Usual Dosage
Children: Total daily dose: ≤0.1 mg/kg **or** ≤0.045 mg/lb
Adults: 2.5-20 mg in divided doses 2-4 times/day based on individual response; a course of therapy of 2-4 weeks is usually adequate. This may be repeated intermittently as needed.
Dosage Forms Tablet: 2.5 mg, 10 mg

oxaprozin (oks a PROE zin)

Sound-Alike/Look-Alike Issues
oxaprozin may be confused with oxazepam
Daypro® may be confused with Diupres®
U.S./Canadian Brand Names Apo-Oxaprozin® [Can]; Daypro® [US/Can]
Therapeutic Category Analgesic, Nonnarcotic; Nonsteroidal Antiinflammatory Drug (NSAID)
Use Acute and long-term use in the management of signs and symptoms of osteoarthritis and rheumatoid arthritis; juvenile rheumatoid arthritis
Usual Dosage Oral (individualize dosage to lowest effective dose to minimize adverse effects):
Children 6-16 years: Juvenile rheumatoid arthritis:
22-31 kg: 600 mg once daily
32-54 kg: 900 mg once daily
≥55 kg: 1200 mg once daily
Adults:
Osteoarthritis: 600-1200 mg once daily; patients should be titrated to lowest dose possible; patients with low body weight should start with 600 mg daily
Rheumatoid arthritis: 1200 mg once daily; a one-time loading dose of up to 1800 mg/day or 26 mg/kg (whichever is lower) may be given
Maximum doses:
Patient <50 kg: Maximum: 1200 mg/day
Patient >50 kg with normal renal/hepatic function and low risk of peptic ulcer: Maximum: 1800 mg or 26 mg/kg (whichever is lower) in divided doses
Dosage Forms Tablet: 600 mg

oxazepam (oks A ze pam)

Sound-Alike/Look-Alike Issues
oxazepam may be confused with oxaprozin, quazepam
Serax® may be confused with Eurax®, Urex®, Zyrtec®
U.S./Canadian Brand Names Apo-Oxazepam® [Can]; Novoxapram® [Can]; Oxpam® [Can]; Oxpram® [Can]; PMS-Oxazepam [Can]; Riva-Oxazepam [Can]; Serax® [US]
Therapeutic Category Anticonvulsant; Benzodiazepine
Controlled Substance C-IV
Use Treatment of anxiety; management of ethanol withdrawal
(Continued)

oxazepam *(Continued)*

Usual Dosage Oral:

Children: Anxiety: 1 mg/kg/day has been administered

Adults:

Anxiety: 10-30 mg 3-4 times/day

Ethanol withdrawal: 15-30 mg 3-4 times/day

Hypnotic: 15-30 mg

Dosage Forms

Capsule: 10 mg, 15 mg, 30 mg

Tablet: 15 mg [contains tartrazine]

oxcarbazepine (ox car BAZ e peen)

Synonyms GP 47680; OCBZ

U.S./Canadian Brand Names Trileptal® [US/Can]

Therapeutic Category Anticonvulsant, Miscellaneous

Use Monotherapy or adjunctive therapy in the treatment of partial seizures in adults and children ≥4 years of age with epilepsy; adjunctive therapy in the treatment of partial seizures in children ≥2 years of age with epilepsy.

Usual Dosage Oral:

Children 2-3 years:

Adjunctive therapy: 8-10 mg/kg/day, not to exceed 600 mg/day, given in 2 divided daily doses. Maintenance dose should be achieved over 2 weeks, and is dependent upon patient weight.

<20 kg: Consider initiating dose at 16-20 mg/kg/day; maximum maintenance dose should be achieved over 2-4 weeks and should not exceed 60 mg/kg/day

Children 4-16 years:

Adjunctive therapy: 8-10 mg/kg/day, not to exceed 600 mg/day, given in 2 divided daily doses. Maintenance dose should be achieved over 2 weeks, and is dependent upon patient weight, according to the following:

20-29 kg: 900 mg/day in 2 divided doses

29.1-39 kg: 1200 mg/day in 2 divided doses

>39 kg: 1800 mg/day in 2 divided doses

Children 4-16 years:

Conversion to monotherapy: Oxcarbazepine 8-10 mg/kg/day in twice daily divided doses, while simultaneously initiating the reduction of the dose of the concomitant antiepileptic drug; the concomitant drug should be withdrawn over 3-6 weeks. Oxcarbazepine dose may be increased by a maximum of 10 mg/kg/day at weekly intervals. See below for recommended total daily dose by weight.

Initiation of monotherapy: Oxcarbazepine should be initiated at 8-10 mg/kg/day in twice daily divided doses; doses may be titrated by 5 mg/kg/day every third day. See below for recommended total daily dose by weight.

Range of maintenance doses by weight during monotherapy:

20 kg: 600-900 mg/day

25-30 kg: 900-1200 mg/day

35-40 kg: 900-1500 mg/day

45 kg: 1200-1500 mg/day

50-55 kg: 1200-1800 mg/day

60-65 kg: 1200-2100 mg/day

70 kg: 1500-2100 mg/day

Adults:

Adjunctive therapy: Initial: 300 mg twice daily; dose may be increased by as much as 600 mg/day at weekly intervals; recommended daily dose: 1200 mg/day in 2 divided doses. Although daily doses >1200 mg/day demonstrated greater efficacy, most patients were unable to tolerate 2400 mg/day (due to CNS effects).

Conversion to monotherapy: Oxcarbazepine 600 mg/day in twice daily divided doses while simultaneously initiating the reduction of the dose of the concomitant antiepileptic drug. The concomitant dosage should be withdrawn over 3-6 weeks, while the maximum dose of oxcarbazepine should be reached in about 2-4 weeks. Recommended daily dose: 2400 mg/day.

Initiation of monotherapy: Oxcarbazepine should be initiated at a dose of 600 mg/day in twice daily divided doses; doses may be titrated upward by 300 mg/day every third day to a final dose of 1200 mg/day given in 2 daily divided doses

Dosage Forms

Suspension, oral: 300 mg/5 mL (250 mL) [contains ethanol; packaged with oral syringe]

Tablet: 150 mg, 300 mg, 600 mg

Oxeze® Turbuhaler® [Can] *see* formoterol *on page 367*

oxiconazole (oks i KON a zole)

Synonyms oxiconazole nitrate

U.S./Canadian Brand Names Oxistat® [US/Can]

Therapeutic Category Antifungal Agent

Use Treatment of tinea pedis (athlete's foot), tinea cruris (jock itch), and tinea corporis (ringworm)

Usual Dosage Topical:

Children and Adults:

Tinea corporis/tinea cruris: Cream, lotion: Apply to affected areas 1-2 times daily for 2 weeks

Tinea pedis: Cream, lotion: Apply to affected areas 1-2 times daily for 1 month

Adults: Tinea versicolor: Cream: Apply to affected areas once daily for 2 weeks

Dosage Forms

Cream: 1% (15 g, 30 g, 60 g) [contains benzoic acid]

Lotion: 1% (30 mL) [contains benzoic acid]

oxiconazole nitrate *see* oxiconazole *on this page*

oxidized regenerated cellulose *see* cellulose, oxidized regenerated *on page 165*

oxilapine succinate *see* loxapine *on page 509*

Oxipor® VHC [US-OTC] *see* coal tar *on page 207*

Oxistat® [US/Can] *see* oxiconazole *on this page*

Oxpam® [Can] *see* oxazepam *on page 623*

oxpentifylline *see* pentoxifylline *on page 653*

Oxpram® [Can] *see* oxazepam *on page 623*

oxprenolol *(Canada only)* (ox PREN oh lole)

Synonyms oxprenolol hydrochloride

U.S./Canadian Brand Names Slow-Trasicor® [Can]; Trasicor® [Can]

Therapeutic Category Beta-Adrenergic Blocker

Use Treatment of mild or moderate hypertension

Usual Dosage Oral: Adults:

Initial: 20 mg 3 times/day (regular-release formulation); increase by 60 mg/day (in 3 divided doses) at 1-2 week intervals until adequate control is obtained

Maintenance: 120-320 mg/day; do not exceed 480 mg; may switch to slow-release formulation once-daily dosing at this time

Dosage Forms

Tablet (Trasicor®): 40 mg, 80 mg

Tablet, slow release (Slow-Trasicor®): 80 mg, 160 mg

oxprenolol hydrochloride *see* oxprenolol *(Canada only) on this page*

Oxsoralen® [US/Can] *see* methoxsalen *on page 542*

Oxsoralen-Ultra® [US/Can] *see* methoxsalen *on page 542*

Oxy-5® ***(Discontinued)*** *see* benzoyl peroxide *on page 102*

Oxy 10® Balanced Medicated Face Wash [US-OTC] *see* benzoyl peroxide *on page 102*

Oxy 10® Balance Spot Treatment [US-OTC] *see* benzoyl peroxide *on page 102*

Oxy Balance® [US-OTC] *see* salicylic acid *on page 758*

Oxy Balance® Deep Pore [US-OTC] *see* salicylic acid *on page 758*

oxybutynin (oks i BYOO ti nin)

Sound-Alike/Look-Alike Issues

oxybutynin may be confused with OxyContin®

Ditropan® may be confused with Detrol®, diazepam, Diprivan®, dithranol

Synonyms oxybutynin chloride

U.S./Canadian Brand Names Apo-Oxybutynin® [Can]; Ditropan® XL [US/Can]; Ditropan® [US/Can]; Gen-Oxybutynin [Can]; Novo-Oxybutynin [Can]; Nu-Oxybutyn [Can]; Oxytrol® [US/Can]; PMS-Oxybutynin [Can]; Uromax® [Can]

Therapeutic Category Antispasmodic Agent, Urinary

Use Antispasmodic for neurogenic bladder (urgency, frequency, urge incontinence) and uninhibited bladder

(Continued)

oxybutynin *(Continued)*

Usual Dosage

Oral:

Children:

>5 years: 5 mg twice daily, up to 5 mg 3 times/day maximum

>6 years: Extended release: 5 mg once daily; maximum dose: 20 mg/day

Adults: 5 mg 2-3 times/day up to 5 mg 4 times/day maximum

Extended release: Initial: 5-10 mg once daily, may increase in 5-10 mg increments; maximum: 30 mg daily

Transdermal: Adults: Apply one 3.9 mg/day patch twice weekly (every 3-4 days)

Note: Should be discontinued periodically to determine whether the patient can manage without the drug and to minimize resistance to the drug

Dosage Forms

Syrup, as chloride: 5 mg/5 mL (473 mL)

Ditropan®: 5 mg/5 mL (473 ml)

Tablet, as chloride: 5 mg

Ditropan®: 5 mg

Tablet, extended release, as chloride:

Ditropan® XL: 5 mg, 10 mg, 15 mg

Transdermal system:

Oxytrol®: 3.9 mg/day (8s) [39 cm^2; total oxybutynin 36 mg]

oxybutynin chloride *see* oxybutynin *on previous page*

oxychlorosene (oks i KLOR oh seen)

Synonyms oxychlorosene sodium

U.S./Canadian Brand Names Clorpactin® WCS-90 [US-OTC]

Therapeutic Category Antibiotic, Topical

Use Treatment of localized infections

Usual Dosage Topical (0.1% to 0.5% solutions): Apply by irrigation, instillation, spray, soaks, or wet compresses

Dosage Forms Powder for solution, as sodium: 2 g

oxychlorosene sodium *see* oxychlorosene *on this page*

Oxycocet® [Can] *see* oxycodone and acetaminophen *on next page*

Oxycodan® [Can] *see* oxycodone and aspirin *on page 628*

oxycodone (oks i KOE done)

Sound-Alike/Look-Alike Issues

oxycodone may be confused with OxyContin®

OxyContin® may be confused with oxybutynin, oxycodone

OxyFast® may be confused with Roxanol™

Synonyms dihydrohydroxycodeinone; oxycodone hydrochloride

U.S./Canadian Brand Names ETH-Oxydose™ [Can]; Oxy.IR® [Can]; OxyContin® [US/Can]; OxyFast® [US]; OxyIR® [US]; Roxicodone® [US]; Supeudol® [Can]

Therapeutic Category Analgesic, Narcotic

Controlled Substance C-II

Use Management of moderate to severe pain, normally used in combination with nonopioid analgesics

OxyContin® is indicated for around-the-clock management of moderate to severe pain when an analgesic is needed for an extended period of time. **Note:** OxyContin® is not intended for use as an "as needed" analgesic or for immediately-postoperative pain management (should be used postoperatively only if the patient has received it prior to surgery or if severe, persistent pain is anticipated).

Usual Dosage Oral:

Immediate release:

Children:

6-12 years: 1.25 mg every 6 hours as needed

>12 years: 2.5 mg every 6 hours as needed

Adults: 5 mg every 6 hours as needed

Controlled release: Adults:

Opioid naive (not currently on opioid): 10 mg every 12 hours

Currently on opioid/ASA or acetaminophen or NSAID combination:
1-5 tablets: 10-20 mg every 12 hours
6-9 tablets: 20-30 mg every 12 hours
10-12 tablets: 30-40 mg every 12 hours
May continue the nonopioid as a separate drug.

Currently on opioids: Use standard conversion chart to convert daily dose to oxycodone equivalent. Divide daily dose in 2 (for every 12-hour dosing) and round down to nearest dosage form.

Note: 80 mg or 160 mg tablets are for use **only** in opioid-tolerant patients. Special safety considerations must be addressed when converting to OxyContin® doses ≥160 mg every 12 hours. Dietary caution must be taken when patients are initially titrated to 160 mg tablets.

Dosage Forms

Capsule, immediate release, as hydrochloride: 5 mg
OxyIR®: 5 mg
Solution, oral, as hydrochloride: 5 mg/5 mL (500 mL)
Roxicodone®: 5 mg/5 mL (5 mL, 500 mL) [contains alcohol]
Solution, oral concentrate, as hydrochloride: 20 mg/mL (30 mL)
ETH-Oxydose™: 20 mg/mL (30 mL) [contains sodium benzoate; berry flavor]
OxyFast®: 20 mg/mL (30 mL) [contains sodium benzoate and dry natural rubber]
Roxicodone®: 20 mg/mL (30 mL) [contains sodium benzoate]
Tablet, as hydrochloride: 5 mg, 15 mg, 30 mg
Roxicodone®: 5 mg, 15 mg, 30 mg
Tablet, controlled release, as hydrochloride:
OxyContin®: 10 mg, 20 mg, 40 mg, 80 mg, 160 mg
Tablet, extended release, as hydrochloride: 10 mg, 20 mg, 40 mg, 80 mg

oxycodone and acetaminophen (oks i KOE done & a seet a MIN oh fen)

Sound-Alike/Look-Alike Issues

Percocet® may be confused with Percodan®
Roxicet™ may be confused with Roxanol™
Tylox® may be confused with Trimox®, Tylenol®, Wymox®, Xanax®

Synonyms acetaminophen and oxycodone

U.S./Canadian Brand Names Endocet® [US/Can]; Oxycocet® [Can]; Percocet® [US/Can]; Percocet®-Demi [Can]; PMS-Oxycodone-Acetaminophen [Can]; Roxicet™ 5/500 [US]; Roxicet™ [US]; Tylox® [US]

Therapeutic Category Analgesic, Narcotic

Controlled Substance C-II

Use Management of moderate to severe pain

Usual Dosage Oral: Doses should be given every 4-6 hours as needed and titrated to appropriate analgesic effects. **Note:** Initial dose is based on the **oxycodone** content; however, the maximum daily dose is based on the **acetaminophen** content.

Children: Maximum acetaminophen dose: Children <45 kg: 90 mg/kg/day; children >45 kg: 4 g/day
Mild to moderate pain: Initial dose, **based on oxycodone content:** 0.05-0.1 mg/kg/dose
Severe pain: Initial dose, **based on oxycodone content:** 0.3 mg/kg/dose
Adults:
Mild to moderate pain: Initial dose, **based on oxycodone content:** 5 mg
Severe pain: Initial dose, **based on oxycodone content:** 15-30 mg. Do not exceed acetaminophen 4 g/day.

Dosage Forms

Caplet:
Roxicet™ 5/500: Oxycodone hydrochloride 5 mg and acetaminophen 500 mg
Capsule: 5/500: Oxycodone hydrochloride 5 mg and acetaminophen 500 mg
Tylox®: 5/500: Oxycodone hydrochloride 5 mg and acetaminophen 500 mg [contains sodium benzoate and sodium metabisulfite]
Solution, oral:
Roxicet™: Oxycodone hydrochloride 5 mg and acetaminophen 325 mg per 5 mL (5 mL, 500 mL) [contains alcohol <0.5%]
Tablet: 5/325: Oxycodone hydrochloride 5 mg and acetaminophen 325 mg; 7.5/325: Oxycodone hydrochloride 7.5 mg and acetaminophen 325 mg; 7.5/500: Oxycodone hydrochloride 7.5 mg and acetaminophen 500 mg; 10/325: Oxycodone hydrochloride 10 mg and acetaminophen 325 mg; 10/650: Oxycodone hydrochloride 10 mg and acetaminophen 650 mg
Endocet® 5/325 [scored]: Oxycodone hydrochloride 5 mg and acetaminophen 325 mg
Endocet® 7.5/325: Oxycodone hydrochloride 7.5 mg and acetaminophen 325 mg
Endocet® 7.5/500: Oxycodone hydrochloride 7.5 mg and acetaminophen 500 mg
Endocet® 10/325: Oxycodone hydrochloride 10 mg and acetaminophen 325 mg

(Continued)

oxycodone and acetaminophen *(Continued)*

Endocet® 10/650: Oxycodone hydrochloride 10 mg and acetaminophen 650 mg
Percocet® 2.5/325: Oxycodone hydrochloride 2.5 mg and acetaminophen 325 mg
Percocet® 5/325 [scored]: Oxycodone hydrochloride 5 mg and acetaminophen 325 mg
Percocet® 7.5/325: Oxycodone hydrochloride 7.5 mg and acetaminophen 325 mg
Percocet® 7.5/500: Oxycodone hydrochloride 7.5 mg and acetaminophen 500 mg
Percocet® 10/325: Oxycodone hydrochloride 10 mg and acetaminophen 325 mg
Percocet® 10/650: Oxycodone hydrochloride 10 mg and acetaminophen 650 mg
Roxicet™ [scored]: Oxycodone hydrochloride 5 mg and acetaminophen 325 mg

oxycodone and aspirin (oks i KOE done & AS pir in)

Sound-Alike/Look-Alike Issues

Percodan® may be confused with Decadron®, Percocet®, Percogesic®, Periactin®

Synonyms aspirin and oxycodone

U.S./Canadian Brand Names Endodan® [US/Can]; Oxycodan® [Can]; Percodan® [US/Can]

Therapeutic Category Analgesic, Narcotic

Controlled Substance C-II

Use Management of moderate to severe pain

Usual Dosage Oral (based on oxycodone combined salts):

Children: Maximum oxycodone: 5 mg/dose; maximum aspirin dose should not exceed 4 g/day. Doses should be given every 6 hours as needed.

Mild-to-moderate pain: Initial dose, **based on oxycodone content:**: 0.05-0.1 mg/kg/dose

Severe pain: Initial dose, **based on oxycodone content**: 0.3 mg/kg/dose

Adults: Percodan®: 1 tablet every 6 hours as needed for pain; maximum aspirin dose should not exceed 4 g/day.

Dosage Forms

Tablet: Oxycodone hydrochloride 4.5 mg, oxycodone terephthalate 0.38 mg, and aspirin 325 mg

Endodan®, Percodan®: Oxycodone hydrochloride 4.8355 mg and aspirin 325 mg

oxycodone hydrochloride *see* oxycodone *on page 626*

OxyContin® [US/Can] *see* oxycodone *on page 626*

Oxyderm™ [Can] *see* benzoyl peroxide *on page 102*

OxyFast® [US] *see* oxycodone *on page 626*

Oxy.IR® [Can] *see* oxycodone *on page 626*

oxymetazoline (oks i met AZ oh leen)

Sound-Alike/Look-Alike Issues

oxymetazoline may be confused with oxymetholone
Afrin® may be confused with aspirin
Visine® may be confused with Visken®

Synonyms oxymetazoline hydrochloride

U.S./Canadian Brand Names 4-Way® 12 Hour [US-OTC]; Afrin® Extra Moisturizing [US-OTC]; Afrin® Original [US-OTC]; Afrin® Severe Congestion [US-OTC]; Afrin® Sinus [US-OTC]; Claritin® Allergic Decongestant [Can]; Dristan® Long Lasting Nasal [Can]; Drixoral® Nasal [Can]; Duramist® Plus [US-OTC]; Duration® [US-OTC]; Genasal [US-OTC]; Neo-Synephrine® 12 Hour Extra Moisturizing [US-OTC]; Neo-Synephrine® 12 Hour [US-OTC]; NRS® [US-OTC]; Nōstrilla® [US-OTC]; Vicks Sinex® 12 Hour Ultrafine Mist [US-OTC]; Vicks Sinex® 12 Hour [US-OTC]; Visine® L.R. [US-OTC]

Therapeutic Category Adrenergic Agonist Agent

Use Adjunctive therapy of middle ear infections, associated with acute or chronic rhinitis, the common cold, sinusitis, hay fever, or other allergies

Ophthalmic: Relief of redness of eye due to minor eye irritations

Usual Dosage

Intranasal (therapy should not exceed 3 days): Children ≥6 years and Adults: 0.05% solution: Instill 2-3 sprays into each nostril twice daily

Ophthalmic: Children ≥6 years and Adults: 0.025% solution: Instill 1-2 drops in affected eye(s) every 6 hours as needed or as directed by healthcare provider

Dosage Forms

Solution, intranasal, as hydrochloride [spray]: 0.05% (15 mL, 30 mL)

Afrin® Extra Moisturizing: 0.05% (15 mL) [contains benzyl alcohol and glycerin; regular or no drip formula]
Afrin® Original: 0.05% (15 mL, 30 mL) [contains benzalkonium chloride]
Afrin® Original: 0.05% (15 mL) [contains benzyl alcohol and benzalkonium chloride; no drip formula]

Afrin® Severe Congestion: 0.05% (15 mL) [contains benzyl alcohol and menthol; regular or no drip formula]

Afrin® Sinus: 0.05% (15 mL) [contains benzyl alcohol, benzalkonium chloride, camphor, phenol; regular or no drip formula]

Duramist® Plus, Neo-Synephrine® 12 Hour, Nōstrilla®, Vicks Sinex® 12 Hour Ultrafine Mist, Vicks Sinex® 12 Hour, 4-Way® 12 Hour: 0.05% (15 mL) [contains benzalkonium chloride]

Duration®: 0.05% (30 mL) [contains benzalkonium chloride]

Genasal, NRS®: 0.05% (15 mL, 30 mL) [contains benzalkonium chloride]

Neo-Synephrine® 12 Hour Extra Moisturizing: 0.05% (15 mL) [contains glycerin]

Solution, ophthalmic, as hydrochloride (Visine® L.R.): 0.025% (15 mL, 30 mL) [contains benzalkonium chloride]

oxymetazoline hydrochloride *see* oxymetazoline *on previous page*

oxymetholone (oks i METH oh lone)

Sound-Alike/Look-Alike Issues

oxymetholone may be confused with oxymetazoline, oxymorphone

U.S./Canadian Brand Names Anadrol® [US]

Therapeutic Category Anabolic Steroid

Controlled Substance C-III

Use Treatment of anemias caused by deficient red cell production

Usual Dosage Children and Adults: Erythropoietic effects: Oral: 1-5 mg/kg/day in one daily dose; usual effective dose: 1-2 mg/kg/day; give for a minimum trial of 3-6 months because response may be delayed

Dosage Forms Tablet: 50 mg

oxymorphone (oks i MOR fone)

Sound-Alike/Look-Alike Issues

oxymorphone may be confused with oxymetholone

Synonyms oxymorphone hydrochloride

U.S./Canadian Brand Names Numorphan® [US]

Therapeutic Category Analgesic, Narcotic

Controlled Substance C-II

Use

Parenteral: Management of moderate-to-severe pain and preoperatively as a sedative and/or supplement to anesthesia

Oral, regular release: Management of moderate-to-severe pain

Oral, extended release: Management of moderate-to-severe pain in patients requiring around-the-clock opioid treatment for an extended period of time

Usual Dosage Adults: **Note:** Dosage must be individualized.

I.M., SubQ: Initial: 0.5 mg; may repeat with 1-1.5 mg every 4-6 hours as needed

I.V.: Initial: 0.5 mg every 4-6 hours

Oral:

Immediate release:

Opioid-naive: 10-20 mg every 4-6 hours as needed. Initial dosages as low as 5 mg may be considered in selected patients and/or patients with renal impairment. Dosage adjustment should be based on level of analgesia, side effects, and pain intensity. Initiation of therapy with initial dose >20 mg is **not** recommended.

Currently on stable dose of parenteral oxymorphone: ~10 times the daily parenteral requirement. The calculated amount should be divided and given in 4-6 equal doses.

Currently on other opioids: Use standard conversion chart to convert daily dose to oxymorphone equivalent. Generally start with 1/2 the calculated daily oxymorphone dosage and administered in divided doses every 4-6 hours.

Extended release (Opana® ER):

Opioid-naive: Initial: 5 mg every 12 hours. Supplemental doses of immediate-release oxymorphone may be used as "rescue" medication as dosage is titrated.

Note: Continued requirement for supplemental dosing may be used to titrate the dose of extended-release continuous therapy. Adjust therapy incrementally, by 5-10 mg every 12 hours at intervals of every 3-7 days. Ideally, basal dosage may be titrated to generally mild pain or no pain with the regular use of fewer than 2 supplemental doses per 24 hours.

Currently on stable dose of parenteral oxymorphone: Approximately 10 times the daily parenteral requirement. The calculated amount should be given in 2 divided doses (every 12 hours).

(Continued)

oxymorphone *(Continued)*

Currently on opioids: Use standard conversion chart to convert daily dose to oxymorphone equivalent. Generally start with 1/2 the calculated daily oxymorphone dosage. Divide daily dose in 2 (for every 12-hour dosing) and round down to nearest dosage form.

Conversion of stable dose of immediate-release oxymorphone to extended-release oxymorphone: Administer 1/2 of the daily dose of immediate-release oxymorphone (Opana®) as the extended-release formulation (Opana® ER) every 12 hours

Dosage Forms

Injection, solution, as hydrochloride:
Numorphan®: 1 mg (1 mL)
Tablet, as hydrochloride:
Opana®: 5 mg, 10 mg
Tablet, extended release, as hydrochloride:
Opana®: ER: 5 mg, 10 mg, 20 mg, 40 mg

oxymorphone hydrochloride *see* oxymorphone *on previous page*

oxytetracycline (oks i tet ra SYE kleen)

Sound-Alike/Look-Alike Issues

Terramycin® may be confused with Garamycin®

Synonyms oxytetracycline hydrochloride

U.S./Canadian Brand Names Terramycin® [Can]

Therapeutic Category Tetracycline Derivative

Use Treatment of susceptible bacterial infections; both gram-positive and gram-negative, as well as, *Rickettsia* and *Mycoplasma* organisms

Usual Dosage I.M.:

Children >8 years: 15-25 mg/kg/day (maximum: 250 mg/dose) in divided doses every 8-12 hours
Adults: 250 mg every 24 hours or 300 mg/day divided every 8-12 hours

Dosage Forms [DSC] = Discontinued product

Injection, solution:
Terramycin® I.M: 5% [50 mg/mL] (10 mL) [contains lidocaine hydrochloride 2%] [DSC]

oxytetracycline hydrochloride *see* oxytetracycline *on this page*

oxytocin (oks i TOE sin)

Sound-Alike/Look-Alike Issues

Pitocin® may be confused with Pitressin®

Synonyms pit

U.S./Canadian Brand Names Pitocin® [US/Can]; Syntocinon® [Can]

Therapeutic Category Oxytocic Agent

Use Induction of labor at term; control of postpartum bleeding; adjunctive therapy in management of abortion

Usual Dosage I.V. administration requires the use of an infusion pump. Adults:

Induction of labor: I.V.: 0.5-1 milliunits/minute; gradually increase dose in increments of 1-2 milliunits/minute until desired contraction pattern is established; dose may be decreased after desired frequency of contractions is reached and labor has progressed to 5-6 cm dilation. Infusion rates of 6 milliunits/minute provide oxytocin levels similar to those at spontaneous labor; rates of >9-10 milliunits/minute are rarely required.

Postpartum bleeding:
I.M.: Total dose of 10 units after delivery
I.V.: 10-40 units by I.V. infusion in 1000 mL of intravenous fluid at a rate sufficient to control uterine atony

Adjunctive treatment of abortion: I.V.: 10-20 milliunits/minute; maximum total dose: 30 units/12 hours

Dosage Forms

Injection, solution: 10 units/mL (1 mL, 10 mL)
Pitocin®: 10 units/mL (1 mL)

Oxytrol® [US/Can] *see* oxybutynin *on page 625*

Oysco 500 [US-OTC] *see* calcium carbonate *on page 135*

Oyst-Cal 500 [US-OTC] *see* calcium carbonate *on page 135*

P2E1 ***(Discontinued)***

P-V-Tussin® Syrup [US] *see* pseudoephedrine, hydrocodone, and chlorpheniramine *on page 716*

P-V Tussin Tablet [US] *see* hydrocodone and pseudoephedrine *on page 424*

P-071 *see* cetirizine *on page 167*

Pacerone® [US] *see* amiodarone *on page 43*

Pacis™ [Can] *see* BCG vaccine *on page 94*

paclitaxel (pac li TAKS el)

Sound-Alike/Look-Alike Issues

paclitaxel may be confused with docetaxel, paroxetine, Paxil®
paclitaxel (conventional) may be confused with paclitaxel (protein-bound)
Taxol® may be confused with Abraxane™, Paxil®, Taxotere®

Synonyms NSC-125973; NSC-673089

U.S./Canadian Brand Names Apo-Paclitaxel® [Can]; Onxol™ [US]; Taxol® [US/Can]

Therapeutic Category Antineoplastic Agent

Use Treatment of breast, lung (small-cell and nonsmall-cell), and ovarian cancers; treatment of AIDS-related Kaposi sarcoma (KS)

Usual Dosage Premedication with dexamethasone (20 mg orally or I.V. at 12 and 6 hours **or** 14 and 7 hours before the dose; reduce dexamethasone dose to 10 mg orally with advanced HIV disease), diphenhydramine (50 mg I.V. 30-60 minutes prior to the dose), and cimetidine, famotidine or ranitidine (I.V. 30-60 minutes prior to the dose) is recommended.

Adults: I.V.: Refer to individual protocols

Ovarian carcinoma: 135-175 mg/m² over 3 hours every 3 weeks **or**
135 mg/m² over 24 hours every 3 weeks **or**
50-80 mg/m² over 1-3 hours weekly **or**
1.4-4 mg/m²/day continuous infusion for 14 days every 4 weeks

Metastatic breast cancer: 175-250 mg/m² over 3 hours every 3 weeks **or**
50-80 mg/m² weekly **or**
1.4-4 mg/m²/day continuous infusion for 14 days every 4 weeks

Nonsmall-cell lung carcinoma: 135 mg/m² over 24 hours every 3 weeks

AIDS-related Kaposi sarcoma: 135 mg/m² over 3 hours every 3 weeks **or**
100 mg/m² over 3 hours every 2 weeks

Dosage modification for toxicity (solid tumors, including ovary, breast, and lung carcinoma): Courses of paclitaxel should not be repeated until the neutrophil count is ≥1500 cells/mm³ and the platelet count is ≥100,000 cells/mm³; reduce dosage by 20% for patients experiencing severe peripheral neuropathy or severe neutropenia (neutrophil <500 cells/mm³ for a week or longer)

Dosage modification for immunosuppression in advanced HIV disease: Paclitaxel should not be given to patients with HIV if the baseline or subsequent neutrophil count is <1000 cells/mm³. Additional modifications include: Reduce dosage of dexamethasone in premedication to 10 mg orally; reduce dosage by 20% in patients experiencing severe peripheral neuropathy or severe neutropenia (neutrophil <500 cells/mm³ for a week or longer); initiate concurrent hematopoietic growth factor (G-CSF) as clinically indicated

Dosage Forms

Injection, solution: 6 mg/mL (5 mL, 16.7 mL, 25 mL, 50 mL) [contains alcohol and purified Cremophor® EL (polyoxyethylated castor oil)]

Onxol™: 6 mg/mL (5 mL, 25 mL, 50 mL) [contains alcohol and purified Cremophor® EL (polyoxyethylated castor oil)]

Taxol®: 6 mg/mL (5 mL, 16.7 mL, 50 mL) [contains alcohol and purified Cremophor® EL (polyoxyethylated castor oil)]

paclitaxel (protein bound) (pac li TAKS el PROE teen bownd)

Sound-Alike/Look-Alike Issues

paclitaxel (protein bound) may be confused with paclitaxel (conventional)
Abraxane™ may be confused with Paxil®, Taxol®, Taxotere®

Synonyms BI-007; NAB-paclitaxel; protein-bound paclitaxel

U.S./Canadian Brand Names Abraxane™ [US]

Therapeutic Category Antineoplastic Agent, Antimicrotubular; Antineoplastic Agent, Natural Source (Plant) Derivative

Use Treatment of breast cancer (second-line)

Usual Dosage I.V.: Adults: Breast cancer: 260 mg/m² every 3 weeks

Dosage Forms Injection, powder for reconstitution: 100 mg [contains human albumin 900 mg]

Pain-A-Lay® [US-OTC] *see* phenol *on page 658*

Pain-Eze [US-OTC] *see* acetaminophen *on page 5*

Pain-Off [US-OTC] *see* acetaminophen, aspirin, and caffeine *on page 10*

Palafer® [Can] *see* ferrous fumarate *on page 342*

Palcaps [US] *see* pancrelipase *on page 634*

Palgic [US] *see* carbinoxamine *on page 148*

Palgic®-D [US] *see* carbinoxamine and pseudoephedrine *on page 149*

Palgic®-DS [US] *see* carbinoxamine and pseudoephedrine *on page 149*

palifermin (pal ee FER min)

Synonyms AMJ 9701; rHu-KGF

U.S./Canadian Brand Names Kepivance™ [US]

Therapeutic Category Keratinocyte Growth Factor

Use Decrease the incidence and severity of severe oral mucositis associated with hematologic malignancies in patients receiving myelotoxic therapy requiring hematopoietic stem cell support

Usual Dosage I.V.: Adults: 60 mcg/kg/day for 3 consecutive days before and after myelotoxic therapy; total of 6 doses

Note: Administer first 3 doses prior to myelotoxic therapy, with the 3rd dose given 24-48 hours before therapy begins. The last 3 doses should be administered after myelotoxic therapy, with the first of these doses after but on the same day of hematopoietic stem cell infusion and at least 4 days after the most recent dose of palifermin.

Dosage Forms Injection, powder for reconstitution [preservative free]: 6.25 mg [contains mannitol 50 mg, sucrose 25 mg]

palivizumab (pah li VIZ u mab)

Sound-Alike/Look-Alike Issues

Synagis® may be confused with Synalgos®-DC, Synvisc®

U.S./Canadian Brand Names Synagis® [US/Can]

Therapeutic Category Monoclonal Antibody

Use Prevention of serious lower respiratory tract disease caused by respiratory syncytial virus (RSV) in infants and children <2 years of age at high risk of RSV disease

Usual Dosage I.M.: Infants and Children: 15 mg/kg of body weight, monthly throughout RSV season (First dose administered prior to commencement of RSV season)

Dosage Forms [DSC] = Discontinued product

Injection, powder for reconstitution:

Synagis®: 50 mg, 100 mg [DSC]

Injection, solution [preservative free]:

Synagis®: 50 mg/0.5 mL (0.5 mL); 100 mg/mL (1 mL)

Palladone™ *(Discontinued)* *see* hydromorphone *on page 429*

Palmer's® Skin Success Acne [US-OTC] *see* benzoyl peroxide *on page 102*

Palmer's® Skin Success Acne Cleanser [US-OTC] *see* salicylic acid *on page 758*

Palmer's® Skin Success Eventone® Fade Cream [US-OTC] *see* hydroquinone *on page 430*

Palmitate-A® [US-OTC] *see* vitamin A *on page 874*

palonosetron (pal oh NOE se tron)

Sound-Alike/Look-Alike Issues

palonosetron may be confused with dolasetron, granisetron, ondansetron

Aloxi™ may be confused with oxaliplatin

Synonyms palonosetron hydrochloride; RS-25259; RS-25259-197

U.S./Canadian Brand Names Aloxi® [US]

Therapeutic Category Antiemetic; Selective 5-HT_3 Receptor Antagonist

Use Prevention of acute (within 24 hours) and delayed (2-5 days) chemotherapy-induced nausea and vomiting

Note: Not recommended for treatment of existing chemotherapy-induced emesis (CIE)

Usual Dosage I.V.: Adults:

Chemotherapy-induced nausea and vomiting: 0.25 mg 30 minutes prior to chemotherapy administration, day 1 of each cycle (doses should not be given more than once weekly)

Breakthrough: Palonosetron has not been shown to be effective in terminating nausea or vomiting once it occurs and should not be used for this purpose.

Dosage Forms
Injection, solution:
Aloxi®: 0.05 mg/mL (5 mL) [contains disodium edetate]

palonosetron hydrochloride *see* palonosetron *on previous page*

2-PAM *see* pralidoxime *on page 690*

Pamelor® [US] *see* nortriptyline *on page 600*

pamidronate (pa mi DROE nate)

Sound-Alike/Look-Alike Issues
Aredia® may be confused with Adriamycin

Synonyms pamidronate disodium

U.S./Canadian Brand Names Aredia® [US/Can]; Rhoxal-pamidronate [Can]

Therapeutic Category Bisphosphonate Derivative

Use Treatment of hypercalcemia associated with malignancy; treatment of osteolytic bone lesions associated with multiple myeloma or metastatic breast cancer; moderate to severe Paget disease of bone

Usual Dosage Drug must be diluted properly before administration and infused intravenously slowly. Due to risk of nephrotoxicity, doses should not exceed 90 mg. I.V.: Adults:
Hypercalcemia of malignancy:
Moderate cancer-related hypercalcemia (corrected serum calcium: 12-13.5 mg/dL): 60-90 mg, as a single dose
Severe cancer-related hypercalcemia (corrected serum calcium: >13.5 mg/dL): 90 mg, as a single dose
A period of 7 days should elapse before the use of second course; repeat infusions every 2-3 weeks have been suggested, however, could be administered every 2-3 months according to the degree and of severity of hypercalcemia and/or the type of malignancy.
Osteolytic bone lesions with multiple myeloma: 90 mg monthly
Osteolytic bone lesions with metastatic breast cancer: 90 mg repeated every 3-4 weeks
Paget disease: 30 mg for 3 consecutive days

Dosage Forms
Injection, powder for reconstitution, as disodium: 30 mg, 90 mg
Aredia®: 30 mg, 90 mg
Injection, solution: 3 mg/mL (10 mL); 6 mg/mL (10 mL); 9 mg/mL (10 mL)

pamidronate disodium *see* pamidronate *on this page*

Pamine® [US/Can] *see* methscopolamine *on page 543*

Pamine® Forte [US] *see* methscopolamine *on page 543*

p-aminoclonidine *see* apraclonidine *on page 71*

Pamix™ [US-OTC] *see* pyrantel pamoate *on page 719*

Pamprin IB® *(Discontinued)* *see* ibuprofen *on page 437*

Pamprin® Maximum Strength All Day Relief [US-OTC] *see* naproxen *on page 578*

Pan-2400™ [US-OTC] *see* pancreatin *on this page*

Panadol® *(Discontinued)* *see* acetaminophen *on page 5*

Panasal® 5/500 *(Discontinued)* *see* hydrocodone and aspirin *on page 422*

pan-B antibody *see* rituximab *on page 749*

Pancrease® [Can] *see* pancrelipase *on next page*

Pancrease® MT [US/Can] *see* pancrelipase *on next page*

pancreatin (PAN kree a tin)

Sound-Alike/Look-Alike Issues
pancreatin may be confused with Panretin®

U.S./Canadian Brand Names Hi-Vegi-Lip [US-OTC]; ku-zyme® [US]; kutrase® [US]; Lapase [Can]; Pan-2400™ [US-OTC]; Pancreatin 4X [US-OTC]; Pancreatin 8X [US-OTC]; Veg-Pancreatin 4X [US-OTC]

Therapeutic Category Enzyme

Use Relief of functional indigestion due to enzyme deficiency or imbalance

Usual Dosage Oral: Adults: Actual dose varies with condition of patient and is usually given with each meal or snack.
ku-zyme®: 1-2 capsules with each meal or snack
kutrase®: 1 capsule with each meal or snack
(Continued)

pancreatin *(Continued)*

Dosage Forms

Capsule: Lipase 8500 units, protease 50,000 units, amylase 50,000 units [pancreatin 500 mg]

Dygase, kutrase®: Lipase 2400 units, protease 30,000 units, amylase 30,000 units

ku-zyme®: Lipase 1200 units, protease 15,000 units, amylase 15,000 units

Lapase: Lipase 1200 units, protease 15,000 units, and amylase 15,000 units [contains tartrazine]

Pan-2400™: Lipase 9816 units, protease 60,214 units, amylase 75,900 units [pancreatin 2400 mg]

Tablet: Lipase 565 units, protease 8200 units, amylase 8200 units [pancreatin 325 mg]; lipase 2400 units, protease 30,000 units, amylase 30,000 units [pancreatin 1200 mg]

Hi-Vegi-Lip: Lipase 4800 units, protease 60,000 units, amylase 60,000 units [pancreatin 2400 mg; vegetable source]

Pancreatin 4X: Lipase 4800 units, protease 60,000 units, amylase 60,000 units [pancreatin 600 mg]

Pancreatin 8X: Lipase 14,400 units, protease 180,000 units, amylase 180,000 units [pancreatin 900 mg]

Veg-Pancreatin 4X: Lipase 5500 units, protease 690,000 units, amylase 690,000 units [pancreatin 690 mg; vegetable source]

Pancreatin 4X [US-OTC] *see* pancreatin *on previous page*

Pancreatin 8X [US-OTC] *see* pancreatin *on previous page*

Pancrecarb MS® [US] *see* pancrelipase *on this page*

pancrelipase (pan kre LYE pase)

Synonyms lipancreatin

U.S./Canadian Brand Names Cotazym® [Can]; Creon® 10 [Can]; Creon® 20 [Can]; Creon® 25 [Can]; Creon® 5 [Can]; Creon® [US]; ku-zyme® HP [US]; Lipram 4500 [US]; Lipram-CR [US]; Lipram-PN [US]; Lipram-UL [US]; Palcaps [US]; Pancrease® MT [US/Can]; Pancrease® [Can]; Pancrecarb MS® [US]; Pangestyme™ CN [US]; Pangestyme™ EC [US]; Pangestyme™ MT [US]; Pangestyme™ UL [US]; Panocaps MT [US]; Panocaps [US]; Panokase® 16 [US]; Panokase® [US]; Plaretase® 8000 [US]; Ultracaps MT [US]; Ultrase® MT [US/Can]; Ultrase® [US/Can]; Viokase® [US/Can]

Therapeutic Category Enzyme

Use Replacement therapy in symptomatic treatment of malabsorption syndrome caused by pancreatic insufficiency

Usual Dosage Oral:

Powder: Actual dose depends on the condition being treated and the digestive requirements of the patient

Children <1 year: Start with 1/8 teaspoonful with feedings

Adults: 0.7 g (1/4 teaspoonful) with meals

Capsules/tablets: The following dosage recommendations are only an approximation for initial dosages. The actual dosage will depend on the condition being treated and the digestive requirements of the individual patient. Adjust dose based on body weight and stool fat content. Total daily dose reflects ~3 meals/day and 2-3 snacks/day, with half the mealtime dose given with a snack. Older patients may need less units/kg due to increased weight, but decreased ingestion of fat/kg. Maximum dose: 2500 units of lipase/kg/meal (10,000 units of lipase/kg/day)

Children:

<1 year: 2000 units of lipase with meals

1-6 years: 4000-8000 units of lipase with meals and 4000 units with snacks

7-12 years: 4000-12,000 units of lipase with meals and snacks

Adults: 4000-48,000 units of lipase with meals and with snacks

Occluded feeding tubes: One tablet of Viokase® crushed with one 325 mg tablet of sodium bicarbonate (to activate the Viokase®) in 5 mL of water can be instilled into the nasogastric tube and clamped for 5 minutes; then, flushed with 50 mL of tap water

Dosage Forms [DSC] = Discontinued product

Capsule:

ku-zyme® HP: Lipase 8000 units, protease 30,000 units, and amylase 30,000 units

Capsule, delayed release, enteric coated granules:

Pangestyme™ CN-10: Lipase 10,000 units, protease 37,500 units, amylase 33,200 units

Pangestyme™ CN-20: Lipase 20,000 units, protease 75,000 units, amylase 66,400 units

Pangestyme™ EC: Lipase 4500 units, protease 25,000 units, and amylase 20,000 units

Pangestyme™ MT16: Lipase 16,000 units, protease 48,000 units, and amylase 48,000 units

Pangestyme™ UL 12: Lipase 12,000 units, protease 39,000 units, and amylase 39,000 units

Pangestyme™ UL 18: Lipase 18,000 units, protease 58,500 units, and amylase 58,500 units

Pangestyme™ UL 20: Lipase 20,000 units, protease 65,000 units, and amylase 65,000 units

Capsule, delayed release, enteric coated microspheres: Lipase 4500 units, protease 25,000 units, and amylase 20,000 units

Creon® 5: Lipase 5000 units, protease 18,750 units, and amylase 16,600 units
Creon® 10, Palcaps 10: Lipase 10,000 units, protease 37,500 units, and amylase 33,200 units
Creon® 20, Palcaps 20: Lipase 20,000 units, protease 75,000 units, and amylase 66,400 units
Lipram 4500, Panocaps: Lipase 4500 units, protease 25,000 units, and amylase 20,000 units
Lipram-CR5: Lipase 5000 units, protease 18,750 units, and amylase 16,600 units [DSC]
Lipram-CR10: Lipase 10,000 units, protease 37,500 units, and amylase 33,200 units
Lipram-CR20: Lipase 20,000 units, protease 75,000 units, and amylase 66,400 units
Lipram-PN10: Lipase 10,000 units, protease 30,000 units, and amylase 30,000 units
Lipram-PN16, Panocap MT 16: Lipase 16,000 units, protease 48,000 units, and amylase 48,000 units
Lipram-PN20, Panocap MT 20: Lipase 20,000 units, protease 44,000 units, and amylase 56,000 units
Lipram-UL12: Lipase 12,000 units, protease 39,000 units, and amylase 39,000 units [DSC]
Lipram-UL18: Lipase 18,000 units, protease 58,500 units, and amylase 58,500 units [DSC]
Lipram-UL20, Ultracaps MT 20: Lipase 20,000 units, protease 65,000 units, and amylase 65,000 units
Pancrecarb MS-4®: Lipase 4000 units, protease 25,000 units, and amylase 25,000 units [buffered]
Pancrecarb MS-8®: Lipase 8000 units, protease 45,000 units, and amylase 40,000 units [buffered]

Capsule, enteric coated microspheres:
Pancrease® [DSC], Ultrase®: Lipase 4500 units, protease 25,000 units, and amylase 20,000 units

Capsule, enteric coated microtablets:
Pancrease® MT 4: Lipase 4000 units, protease 12,000 units, and amylase 12,000 units
Pancrease® MT 10: Lipase 10,000 units, protease 30,000 units, and amylase 30,000 units
Pancrease® MT 16: Lipase 16,000 units, protease 48,000 units, and amylase 48,000 units
Pancrease® MT 20: Lipase 20,000 units, protease 44,000 units, and amylase 56,000 units

Capsule, enteric coated minitablets:
Ultrase® MT12: Lipase 12,000 units, protease 39,000 units, and amylase 39,000 units
Ultrase® MT18: Lipase 18,000 units, protease 58,500 units, and amylase 58,500 units
Ultrase® MT20: Lipase 20,000 units, protease 65,000 units, and amylase 65,000 units

Powder (Viokase®): Lipase 16,800 units, protease 70,000 units, and amylase 70,000 units per 0.7 g (227 g)

Tablet: Lipase 8000 units, protease 30,000 units, and amylase 30,000 units
Panokase®: Lipase 8000 units, protease 30,000 units, and amylase 30,000 units
Panokase® 16: Lipase 16,000 units, protease 60,000 units, and amylase 60,000 units
Plaretase™ 8000: Lipase 8000 units, protease 30,000 units, and amylase 30,000 units
Viokase® 8: Lipase 8000 units, protease 30,000 units, and amylase 30,000 units
Viokase® 16: Lipase 16,000 units, protease 60,000 units, and amylase 60,000 units

pancuronium (pan kyoo ROE nee um)

Sound-Alike/Look-Alike Issues
pancuronium may be confused with pipecuronium

Synonyms pancuronium bromide

Therapeutic Category Skeletal Muscle Relaxant

Use Adjunct to general anesthesia to facilitate endotracheal intubation and to relax skeletal muscles during surgery; to facilitate mechanical ventilation in ICU patients; does not relieve pain or produce sedation

Drug of choice for neuromuscular blockade except in patients with renal failure, hepatic failure, or cardiovascular instability or in situations not suited for pancuronium's long duration of action

Usual Dosage Administer I.V.; dose to effect; doses will vary due to interpatient variability; use ideal body weight for obese patients

Surgery:

Neonates <1 month:

Test dose: 0.02 mg/kg to measure responsiveness

Initial: 0.03 mg/kg/dose repeated twice at 5- to 10-minute intervals as needed; maintenance: 0.03-0.09 mg/kg/dose every 30 minutes to 4 hours as needed

Infants >1 month, Children, and Adults: Initial: 0.06-0.1 mg/kg or 0.05 mg/kg after initial dose of succinylcholine for intubation; maintenance dose: 0.01 mg/kg 60-100 minutes after initial dose and then 0.01 mg/kg every 25-60 minutes

Pretreatment/priming: 10% of intubating dose given 3-5 minutes before initial dose

ICU: 0.05-0.1 mg/kg bolus followed by 0.8-1.7 mcg/kg/minute once initial recovery from bolus observed or 0.1-0.2 mg/kg every 1-3 hours

Dosage Forms Injection, solution, as bromide: 1 mg/mL (10 mL); 2 mg/mL (2 mL, 5 mL) [may contain benzyl alcohol]

pancuronium bromide *see* pancuronium *on this page*

Pandel® [US] *see* hydrocortisone (topical) *on page 428*

Panectyl® [Can] *see* trimeprazine *(Canada only) on page 850*
Pangestyme™ CN [US] *see* pancrelipase *on page 634*
Pangestyme™ EC [US] *see* pancrelipase *on page 634*
Pangestyme™ MT [US] *see* pancrelipase *on page 634*
Pangestyme™ UL [US] *see* pancrelipase *on page 634*
Panglobulin® NF [US] *see* immune globulin (intravenous) *on page 444*
Panhematin® [US] *see* hemin *on page 408*
Panixine DisperDose™ *(Discontinued)* *see* cephalexin *on page 166*
Panlor® DC [US] *see* acetaminophen, caffeine, and dihydrocodeine *on page 10*
Panlor® SS [US] *see* acetaminophen, caffeine, and dihydrocodeine *on page 10*
PanMist®-JR [US] *see* guaifenesin and pseudoephedrine *on page 398*
PanMist®-LA [US] *see* guaifenesin and pseudoephedrine *on page 398*
PanMist®-S [US] *see* guaifenesin and pseudoephedrine *on page 398*
Panocaps [US] *see* pancrelipase *on page 634*
Panocaps MT [US] *see* pancrelipase *on page 634*
Panokase® [US] *see* pancrelipase *on page 634*
Panokase® 16 [US] *see* pancrelipase *on page 634*
PanOxyl® [US/Can] *see* benzoyl peroxide *on page 102*
PanOxyl®-AQ [US] *see* benzoyl peroxide *on page 102*
PanOxyl® Aqua Gel [US] *see* benzoyl peroxide *on page 102*
PanOxyl® Bar [US-OTC] *see* benzoyl peroxide *on page 102*
Panretin® [US/Can] *see* alitretinoin *on page 29*
Panscol® Lotion *(Discontinued)* *see* salicylic acid *on page 758*
Panscol® Ointment *(Discontinued)* *see* salicylic acid *on page 758*
Panthoderm® [US-OTC] *see* dexpanthenol *on page 242*
Panto™ IV [Can] *see* pantoprazole *on this page*
Panto-250 [US] *see* pantothenic acid *on next page*
Pantoloc® [Can] *see* pantoprazole *on this page*
Pantopon® *(Discontinued)*

pantoprazole (pan TOE pra zole)

Sound-Alike/Look-Alike Issues

Protonix® may be confused with Lotronex®, Lovenox®, protamine

U.S./Canadian Brand Names Pantoloc® [Can]; Panto™ IV [Can]; Protonix® [US/Can]

Therapeutic Category Proton Pump Inhibitor

Use

Oral: Treatment and maintenance of healing of erosive esophagitis associated with GERD; reduction in relapse rates of daytime and nighttime heartburn symptoms in GERD; hypersecretory disorders associated with Zollinger-Ellison syndrome or other neoplastic disorders

I.V.: Short-term treatment (7-10 days) of patients with gastroesophageal reflux disease (GERD) and a history of erosive esophagitis; hypersecretory disorders associated with Zollinger-Ellison syndrome or other neoplastic disorders

Usual Dosage Adults:

Oral:

Erosive esophagitis associated with GERD:

Treatment: 40 mg once daily for up to 8 weeks; an additional 8 weeks may be used in patients who have not healed after an 8-week course

Maintenance of healing: 40 mg once daily

Note: Lower doses (20 mg once daily) have been used successfully in mild GERD treatment and maintenance of healing

Hypersecretory disorders (including Zollinger-Ellison): Initial: 40 mg twice daily; adjust dose based on patient needs; doses up to 240 mg/day have been administered

I.V.:

Erosive esophagitis associated with GERD: 40 mg once daily for 7-10 days

Hypersecretory disorders: 80 mg twice daily; adjust dose based on acid output measurements; 160-240 mg/day in divided doses has been used for a limited period (up to 7 days)

Dosage Forms Note: Strength expressed as base

Injection, powder for reconstitution, as sodium:

Protonix®: 40 mg [contains edetate sodium 1 mg]

Tablet, delayed release, as sodium:

Protonix®: 20 mg, 40 mg

pantothenic acid (pan toe THEN ik AS id)

Synonyms calcium pantothenate; vitamin B_5

U.S./Canadian Brand Names Panto-250 [US]

Therapeutic Category Vitamin, Water Soluble

Use Pantothenic acid deficiency

Usual Dosage Adults: Oral: Recommended daily dose 4-7 mg/day

Dosage Forms

Capsule:

Panto-250: 250 mg [contains calcium 23 mg]

Liquid: 200 mg/5 mL (240 mL)

Tablet: 100 mg, 200 mg, 250 mg, 500 mg

Tablet, sustained release: 500 mg

pantothenyl alcohol *see* dexpanthenol *on page 242*

papain and urea (pa PAY in & yoor EE a)

U.S./Canadian Brand Names Accuzyme® [US]; Allanzyme 650 [US]; Allanzyme [US]; Ethezyme™ 830 [US]; Ethezyme™ [US]; Gladase® [US]; Kovia® [US]

Therapeutic Category Enzyme, Topical Debridement; Topical Skin Product

Use Debridement of necrotic tissue and liquefaction of slough in acute and chronic lesions such as pressure ulcers, varicose and diabetic ulcers, burns, postoperative wounds, pilonidal cyst wounds, carbuncles, and miscellaneous traumatic or infected wounds

Usual Dosage Topical: Adults: Apply with each dressing change. Daily or twice daily dressing changes are preferred, but may be every 2-3 days. Cover with dressing following application.

Ointment: Apply 1/8-inch thickness over the wound with clean applicator.

Spray: Completely cover the wound site so that the wound is not visible.

Dosage Forms

Ointment, topical:

Accuzyme®: Papain 6.5 x 10^5 units/g and urea 10% (6 g, 30 g)

Allanzyme 650: Papain 6.5 x 10^5 units/g and urea 10% (30 g)

Ethezyme™: Papain 1.1 x 10^6 units and urea 10% (30 g)

Ethezyme™ 830: Papain 8.3 x 10^5 units/g and urea 10% (30 g)

Gladase®: Papain 8.3 x 10^5 units/g and urea 10% (6 g, 30 g)

Kovia®: Papain 8.3 x 10^5 units/g and urea 10% (3.5 g) [single-dose packet]; 30 g

Spray, topical:

Accuzyme®, Allanzyme: Papain 6.5 x 10^5 units/g and urea 10% (33 mL)

papaverine (pa PAV er een)

Synonyms papaverine hydrochloride

U.S./Canadian Brand Names Para-Time S.R.® [US]

Therapeutic Category Vasodilator

Use Oral: Relief of peripheral and cerebral ischemia associated with arterial spasm and myocardial ischemia complicated by arrhythmias

Usual Dosage

I.M., I.V.:

Children: 6 mg/kg/day in 4 divided doses

Adults: 30-65 mg (rarely up to 120 mg); may repeat every 3 hours

Oral, sustained release: Adults: 150-300 mg every 12 hours; in difficult cases: 150 mg every 8 hours

Dosage Forms

Capsule, sustained release, as hydrochloride: 150 mg

Para-Time SR®: 150 mg

Injection, solution, as hydrochloride: 30 mg/mL (2 mL, 10 mL)

papaverine hydrochloride *see* papaverine *on this page*

papillomavirus (Types 6, 11, 16, 18) recombinant vaccine

(pap ih LO ma VYE rus typs six e LEV en SIX teen aye teen ree KOM be nant vak SEEN)

Synonyms HPV vaccine; papillomavirus vaccine, recombinant; quadrivalent human papillomavirus vaccine

U.S./Canadian Brand Names Gardasil® [US]

Therapeutic Category Vaccine

Use Prevention of cervical cancer, genital warts, cervical adenocarcinoma *in situ*, and vulvar, vaginal, or cervical intraepithelial neoplasia caused by human papillomavirus (HPV) types 6, 11, 16, 18

Usual Dosage I.M.: Females: Children ≥9 years and Adults ≤26 years: 0.5 mL followed by 0.5 mL at 2 and 6 months after initial dose

Dosage Forms

Injection, suspension [preservative free]:

Gardasil®: HPV 6 L1 protein 20 mcg, HPV 11 L1 protein 40 mcg, HPV 16 L1 protein 40 mcg, and HPV 18 L1 protein 20 mcg per 0.5 mL (0.5 mL) [contains polysorbate 80; packaged in vials or prefilled syringe]

papillomavirus vaccine, recombinant *see* papillomavirus (Types 6, 11, 16, 18) recombinant vaccine *on this page*

para-aminosalicylate sodium *see* aminosalicylic acid *on page 43*

parabromdylamine *see* brompheniramine *on page 118*

paracetamol *see* acetaminophen *on page 5*

Paraflex® *(Discontinued)* *see* chlorzoxazone *on page 185*

Parafon Forte® [Can] *see* chlorzoxazone *on page 185*

Parafon Forte® *(Discontinued)* *see* chlorzoxazone *on page 185*

Paraplatin® [US] *see* carboplatin *on page 151*

Paraplatin-AQ [Can] *see* carboplatin *on page 151*

parathyroid hormone (1-34) *see* teriparatide *on page 812*

Para-Time S.R.® [US] *see* papaverine *on previous page*

Parcopa™ [US] *see* levodopa and carbidopa *on page 489*

Paredrine® *(Discontinued)*

paregoric

(par e GOR ik)

Sound-Alike/Look-Alike Issues

camphorated tincture of opium is an error-prone synonym (mistaken as opium tincture)

paregoric may be confused with Percogesic®

Therapeutic Category Analgesic, Narcotic

Controlled Substance C-III

Use Treatment of diarrhea or relief of pain; neonatal opiate withdrawal

Usual Dosage Oral:

Neonatal opiate withdrawal: 3-6 drops every 3-6 hours as needed, or initially 0.2 mL every 3 hours; increase dosage by approximately 0.05 mL every 3 hours until withdrawal symptoms are controlled; it is rare to exceed 0.7 mL/dose. Stabilize withdrawal symptoms for 3-5 days, then gradually decrease dosage over a 2- to 4-week period.

Children: 0.25-0.5 mL/kg 1-4 times/day

Adults: 5-10 mL 1-4 times/day

Dosage Forms Liquid, oral: Morphine equivalent 2 mg/5 mL (473 mL) [equivalent to opium 20 mg powder; contains alcohol 45% and benzoic acid]

parenteral nutrition *see* total parenteral nutrition *on page 838*

Parepectolin® *(Discontinued)*

paricalcitol

(pah ri KAL si tole)

U.S./Canadian Brand Names Zemplar® [US/Can]

Therapeutic Category Vitamin D Analog

Use

I.V.: Prevention and treatment of secondary hyperparathyroidism associated with stage 5 chronic kidney disease (CKD)

Oral: Prevention and treatment of secondary hyperparathyroidism associated with stage 3 and 4 CKD

Usual Dosage Note: If hypercalcemia or Ca x P >75 is observed, reduce or interrupt dosing until parameters are normalized.

Secondary hyperparathyroidism associated with chronic renal failure (stage 5 CKD): Children ≥5 years and Adults: I.V.: 0.04-0.1 mcg/kg (2.8-7 mcg) given as a bolus dose no more frequently than every other day at any time during dialysis; dose may be increased by 2-4 mcg every 2-4 weeks; doses as high as 0.24 mcg/kg (16.8 mcg) have been administered safely; the dose of paricalcitol should be adjusted based on serum intact PTH (iPTH) levels, as follows:
Same or increasing iPTH level: Increase paricalcitol dose
iPTH level decreased by <30%: Increase paricalcitol dose
iPTH level decreased by >30% and <60%: Maintain paricalcitol dose
iPTH level decrease by >60%: Decrease paricalcitol dose
iPTH level 1.5-3 times upper limit of normal: Maintain paricalcitol dose

Secondary hyperparathyroidism associated with stage 3 and 4 CKD: Adults: Oral: Initial dose based on baseline iPTH:
iPTH ≤500 pg/mL: 1 mcg/day or 2 mcg 3 times/week
iPTH >500 pg/mL: 2 mcg/day or 4 mcg 3 times/week

Dosage adjustment based on iPTH level relative to baseline, adjust dose at 2-4 week intervals:
iPTH same or increased: Increase paricalcitol dose by 1 mcg/day or 2 mcg 3 times/week
iPTH decreased by <30%: Increase paricalcitol dose by 1 mcg/day or 2 mcg 3 times//week
iPTH decreased by ≥30% or ≤60%: Maintain paricalcitol dose
iPTH decreased by >60%: Decrease paricalcitol dose by 1 mcg/day* or 2 mcg 3 times/week
iPTH <60 pg/mL: Decrease paricalcitol dose by 1 mcg/day* or 2 mcg 3 times/week
*If patient is taking the lowest dose on a once-daily regimen, but further dose reduction is needed, decrease dose to 1 mcg 3 times/week. If further dose reduction is required, withhold drug as needed and restart at a lower dose. If applicable, calcium-phosphate binder dosing may also be adjusted or withheld, or switch to noncalcium-based binder

Dosage Forms
Capsule, gelatin: 1 mcg, 2 mcg, 4 mcg [contains alcohol and coconut or palm kernel oil]
Injection, solution: 2 mcg/mL (1 mL); 5 mcg/mL (1 mL, 2 mL) [contains alcohol 20% v/v and propylene glycol 30% v/v]

Pariet® [Can] *see* rabeprazole *on page 727*

pariprazole *see* rabeprazole *on page 727*

Parlodel® [US/Can] *see* bromocriptine *on page 117*

Parnate® [US/Can] *see* tranylcypromine *on page 843*

paromomycin (par oh moe MYE sin)

Synonyms paromomycin sulfate
U.S./Canadian Brand Names Humatin® [US/Can]
Therapeutic Category Amebicide
Use Treatment of acute and chronic intestinal amebiasis; hepatic coma
Usual Dosage Oral:
Intestinal amebiasis: Children and Adults: 25-35 mg/kg/day in 3 divided doses for 5-10 days
Dientamoeba fragilis: Children and Adults: 25-30 mg/kg/day in 3 divided doses for 7 days
Tapeworm (fish, dog, bovine, porcine):
Children: 11 mg/kg every 15 minutes for 4 doses
Adults: 1 g every 15 minutes for 4 doses
Hepatic coma: Adults: 4 g/day in 2-4 divided doses for 5-6 days
Dwarf tapeworm: Children and Adults: 45 mg/kg/dose every day for 5-7 days
Dosage Forms Capsule: 250 mg

paromomycin sulfate *see* paromomycin *on this page*

paroxetine (pa ROKS e teen)

Sound-Alike/Look-Alike Issues
paroxetine may be confused with paclitaxel, pyridoxine
Paxil® may be confused with Doxil®, paclitaxel, Plavix®, Taxol®
Synonyms paroxetine hydrochloride; paroxetine mesylate
U.S./Canadian Brand Names Apo-Paroxetine® [Can]; CO Paroxetine [Can]; Gen-Paroxetine [Can]; Novo-Paroxetine [Can]; Paxil CR® [US/Can]; Paxil® [US/Can]; Pexeva® [US]; PMS-Paroxetine [Can]; ratio-Paroxetine [Can]; Rhoxal-paroxetine [Can]
(Continued)

paroxetine *(Continued)*

Therapeutic Category Antidepressant, Selective Serotonin Reuptake Inhibitor

Use Treatment of depression in adults; treatment of panic disorder with or without agoraphobia; obsessive-compulsive disorder (OCD) in adults; social anxiety disorder (social phobia); generalized anxiety disorder (GAD); post-traumatic stress disorder (PTSD)

Paxil CR®: Treatment of depression; panic disorder; premenstrual dysphoric disorder (PMDD); social anxiety disorder (social phobia)

Usual Dosage Oral: Adults:

Depression:

Paxil®, Pexeva®: Initial: 20 mg once daily, preferably in the morning; increase if needed by 10 mg/day increments at intervals of at least 1 week; maximum dose: 50 mg/day

Paxil CR®: Initial: 25 mg once daily; increase if needed by 12.5 mg/day increments at intervals of at least 1 week; maximum dose: 62.5 mg/day

GAD (Paxil®): Initial: 20 mg once daily, preferably in the morning; doses of 20-50 mg/day were used in clinical trials, however, no greater benefit was seen with doses >20 mg. If dose is increased, adjust in increments of 10 mg/day at 1-week intervals.

OCD (Paxil®, Pexeva™): Initial: 20 mg once daily, preferably in the morning; increase if needed by 10 mg/day increments at intervals of at least 1 week; recommended dose: 40 mg/day; range: 20-60 mg/day; maximum dose: 60 mg/day

Panic disorder:

Paxil®, Pexeva®: Initial: 10 mg once daily, preferably in the morning; increase if needed by 10 mg/day increments at intervals of at least 1 week; recommended dose: 40 mg/day; range: 10-60 mg/day; maximum dose: 60 mg/day

Paxil CR®: Initial: 12.5 mg once daily; increase if needed by 12.5 mg/day at intervals of at least 1 week; maximum dose: 75 mg/day

PMDD (Paxil CR®): Initial: 12.5 mg once daily in the morning; may be increased to 25 mg/day; dosing changes should occur at intervals of at least 1 week. May be given daily throughout the menstrual cycle or limited to the luteal phase.

PTSD (Paxil®): Initial: 20 mg once daily, preferably in the morning; increase if needed by 10 mg/day increments at intervals of at least 1 week; range: 20-50 mg. Limited data suggest doses of 40 mg/day were not more efficacious than 20 mg/day.

Social anxiety disorder:

Paxil®: Initial: 20 mg once daily, preferably in the morning; recommended dose: 20 mg/day; range: 20-60 mg/day; doses >20 mg may not have additional benefit

Paxil CR®: Initial: 12.5 mg once daily, preferably in the morning; may be increased by 12.5 mg/day at intervals of at least 1 week; maximum dose: 37.5 mg/day

Note: Upon discontinuation of paroxetine therapy, gradually taper dose:

Paxil®: 10 mg/day at weekly intervals; when 20 mg/day dose is reached, continue for 1 week before treatment is discontinued. Some patients may need to be titrated to 10 mg/day for 1 week before discontinuation.

Paxil CR®: Patients receiving 37.5 mg/day in clinical trials had their dose decreased by 12.5 mg/day to a dose of 25 mg/day and remained at a dose of 25 mg/day for 1 week before treatment was discontinued.

Dosage Forms Note: Available as paroxetine hydrochloride or mesylate; mg strength refers to paroxetine

Suspension, oral, as hydrochloride:

Paxil®: 10 mg/5 mL (250 mL) [orange flavor]

Tablet, as hydrochloride: 10 mg, 20 mg, 30 mg, 40 mg

Paxil®: 10 mg, 20 mg, 30 mg, 40 mg

Tablet, as mesylate:

Paxil®: 10 mg, 20 mg, 30 mg, 40 mg

Tablet, controlled release, as hydrochloride:

Paxil CR®: 12.5 mg, 25 mg, 37.5 mg

paroxetine hydrochloride *see* paroxetine *on previous page*

paroxetine mesylate *see* paroxetine *on previous page*

Partuss® LA *(Discontinued)*

Parvolex® [Can] *see* acetylcysteine *on page 15*

PAS *see* aminosalicylic acid *on page 43*

Paser® [US] *see* aminosalicylic acid *on page 43*

Patanol® [US/Can] *see* olopatadine *on page 614*

Pathilon® *(Discontinued)*

Pathocil® [Can] *see* dicloxacillin *on page 251*

Pathocil® ***(Discontinued)*** *see* dicloxacillin *on page 251*

Pavabid® ***(Discontinued)*** *see* papaverine *on page 637*

Pavatine® ***(Discontinued)***

Pavulon® ***(Discontinued)*** *see* pancuronium *on page 635*

Paxene® ***(Discontinued)*** *see* paclitaxel *on page 631*

Paxil® [US/Can] *see* paroxetine *on page 639*

Paxil CR® [US/Can] *see* paroxetine *on page 639*

PCE® [US/Can] *see* erythromycin *on page 303*

PCEC *see* rabies virus vaccine *on page 728*

PCM [US] *see* chlorpheniramine, phenylephrine, and methscopolamine *on page 180*

PCM Allergy [US] *see* chlorpheniramine, phenylephrine, and methscopolamine *on page 180*

PCV7 *see* pneumococcal conjugate vaccine (7-valent) *on page 675*

pectin and kaolin *see* kaolin and pectin *on page 470*

pectin, gelatin, and methylcellulose *see* gelatin, pectin, and methylcellulose *on page 377*

Pedameth® ***(Discontinued)***

Pediacare® Children's Long Acting Cough Plus Cold [US-OTC] *see* pseudoephedrine and dextromethorphan *on page 714*

PediaCare® Children's Medicated Freezer Pops Long Acting Cough [US-OTC] *see* dextromethorphan *on page 245*

PediaCare® Cold and Allergy ***(Discontinued)*** *see* chlorpheniramine and pseudoephedrine *on page 177*

PediaCare® Decongestant Infants [US-OTC] *see* pseudoephedrine *on page 712*

Pediacare® Infants' Decongestant & Cough [US-OTC] *see* pseudoephedrine and dextromethorphan *on page 714*

PediaCare® Infants' Long-Acting Cough [US-OTC] *see* dextromethorphan *on page 245*

PediaCare® Multi-Symptom Cold [US-OTC] *see* chlorpheniramine, pseudoephedrine, and dextromethorphan *on page 182*

PediaCare® NightRest Cough and Cold [US-OTC] *see* chlorpheniramine, pseudoephedrine, and dextromethorphan *on page 182*

Pediacof® ***(Discontinued)*** *see* chlorpheniramine, phenylephrine, codeine, and potassium iodide *on page 182*

Pediaflor® ***(Discontinued)*** *see* fluoride *on page 354*

PediaHist DM [US] *see* brompheniramine, pseudoephedrine, and dextromethorphan *on page 120*

Pedialyte® [US-OTC] *see* nutritional formula, enteral/oral *on page 608*

PediaPatch Transdermal Patch ***(Discontinued)*** *see* salicylic acid *on page 758*

Pediapred® [US/Can] *see* prednisolone (systemic) *on page 695*

Pedia-Profen™ ***(Discontinued)*** *see* ibuprofen *on page 437*

Pedia Relief Cough and Cold [US-OTC] *see* pseudoephedrine and dextromethorphan *on page 714*

Pedia Relief Infants [US-OTC] *see* pseudoephedrine and dextromethorphan *on page 714*

Pediarix™ [US] *see* diphtheria, tetanus toxoids, acellular pertussis, hepatitis B (recombinant), and poliovirus (inactivated) vaccine *on page 265*

Pediatex™ 12 ***(Discontinued)*** *see* carbinoxamine *on page 148*

Pediatex™-D ***(Discontinued)*** *see* carbinoxamine and pseudoephedrine *on page 149*

Pediatex™ ***(Discontinued)*** *see* carbinoxamine *on page 148*

Pediatex™ DM ***(Discontinued)*** *see* carbinoxamine, pseudoephedrine, and dextromethorphan *on page 150*

Pediatex™ HC [US] *see* pseudoephedrine, hydrocodone, and chlorpheniramine *on page 716*

Pediatric Digoxin CSD [Can] *see* digoxin *on page 254*

Pediatric Triban® *(Discontinued)*

Pediatrix [Can] *see* acetaminophen *on page 5*

Pediazole® [US/Can] *see* erythromycin and sulfisoxazole *on page 305*

Pedi-Boro® [US-OTC] *see* aluminum sulfate and calcium acetate *on page 38*

Pedi-Dri® [US] *see* nystatin *on page 609*

PediOtic® [US] *see* neomycin, polymyxin B, and hydrocortisone *on page 584*

Pedisilk® [US-OTC] *see* salicylic acid *on page 758*

Pedtrace-4® [US] *see* trace metals *on page 839*

PedvaxHIB® [US/Can] *see Haemophilus* B conjugate vaccine *on page 405*

PEG *see* polyethylene glycol 3350 *on page 678*

PEG-L-asparaginase *see* pegaspargase *on this page*

pegademase (bovine) (peg A de mase BOE vine)

U.S./Canadian Brand Names Adagen® [US/Can]

Therapeutic Category Enzyme

Use **Orphan drug:** Enzyme replacement therapy for adenosine deaminase (ADA) deficiency in patients with severe combined immunodeficiency disease (SCID) who can not benefit from bone marrow transplant; not a cure for SCID, unlike bone marrow transplants, injections must be used the rest of the child's life, therefore is not really an alternative

Usual Dosage Children: I.M.: Dose given every 7 days, 10 units/kg the first dose, 15 units/kg the second dose, and 20 units/kg the third dose; maintenance dose: 20 units/kg/week is recommended depending on patient's ADA level; maximum single dose: 30 units/kg

Dosage Forms

Injection, solution [preservative free]:

Adagen®: 250 units/mL (1.5 mL)

Peganone® [US/Can] *see* ethotoin *on page 328*

pegaptanib (peg AP ta nib)

Synonyms EYE001; pegaptanib sodium

U.S./Canadian Brand Names Macugen® [US/Can]

Therapeutic Category Ophthalmic Agent; Vaccine, Recombinant

Use Treatment of neovascular (wet) age-related macular degeneration (AMD)

Usual Dosage Intravitreous injection: Adults: AMD: 0.3 mg into affected eye every 6 weeks

Dosage Forms Injection, solution [preservative free]: 0.3 mg/90 µL (90 µL) [prefilled syringe]

pegaptanib sodium *see* pegaptanib *on this page*

pegaspargase (peg AS par jase)

Sound-Alike/Look-Alike Issues

pegaspargase may be confused with asparaginase

Synonyms NSC-644954; PEG-L-asparaginase

U.S./Canadian Brand Names Oncaspar® [US]

Therapeutic Category Antineoplastic Agent

Use Treatment of acute lymphocytic leukemia (ALL); treatment of ALL with previous hypersensitivity to native L-asparaginase

Usual Dosage Usually administered as part of a combination chemotherapy regimen.

I.M. administration is **preferred** over I.V. administration due to lower incidence of hepatotoxicity, coagulopathy, gastrointestinal and renal disorders with I.M. administration.

Children: I.M., I.V.:

Body surface area <0.6 m^2: 82.5 int. units/kg every 14 days

Body surface area ≥0.6 m^2: 2500 int. units/m^2 every 14 days

Adults: I.M., I.V.: 2500 int. units/m^2 every 14 days

Hemodialysis: Significant drug removal is unlikely based on physiochemical characteristics

Peritoneal dialysis: Significant drug removal is unlikely based on physiochemical characteristics

Dosage Forms

Injection, solution [preservative free]:

Oncaspar®: 750 units/mL (5 mL)

Pegasys® [US/Can] *see* peginterferon alfa-2a *on this page*

Pegasys® RBV [Can] *see* peginterferon alfa-2b and ribavirin *(Canada only) on next page*

Pegetron™ [Can] *see* peginterferon alfa-2b and ribavirin *(Canada only) on next page*

pegfilgrastim (peg fil GRA stim)

Sound-Alike/Look-Alike Issues

Neulasta® may be confused with Neumega®

Synonyms G-CSF (PEG conjugate); granulocyte colony stimulating factor (PEG conjugate)

U.S./Canadian Brand Names Neulasta® [US/Can]

Therapeutic Category Colony-Stimulating Factor

Use Decrease the incidence of infection, by stimulation of granulocyte production, in patients with nonmyeloid malignancies receiving myelosuppressive therapy associated with a significant risk of febrile neutropenia

Usual Dosage SubQ: Adolescents >45 kg and Adults: 6 mg once per chemotherapy cycle; do not administer in the period between 14 days before and 24 hours after administration of cytotoxic chemotherapy; do not use in infants, children, and smaller adolescents weighing <45 kg

Dosage Forms Injection, solution [preservative free]: 10 mg/mL (0.6 mL) [prefilled syringe]

peginterferon alfa-2a (peg in ter FEER on AL fa too aye)

Synonyms interferon alfa-2a (PEG conjugate); pegylated interferon alfa-2a

U.S./Canadian Brand Names Pegasys® [US/Can]

Therapeutic Category Interferon

Use Treatment of chronic hepatitis C (CHC), alone or in combination with ribavirin, in patients with compensated liver disease and histological evidence of cirrhosis (Child-Pugh class A) and patients with clinically-stable HIV disease; treatment of patients with HBeAg positive and HBeAg negative chronic hepatitis B with compensated liver disease and evidence of viral replication and liver inflammation

Usual Dosage SubQ: Adults:

Chronic hepatitis C (monoinfection or coinfection with HIV):

Monotherapy: 180 mcg once weekly for 48 weeks

Combination therapy with ribavirin: Recommended dosage: 180 mcg once/week with ribavirin (Copegus®)

Duration of therapy: Monoinfection (based on genotype):

Genotype 1,4: 48 weeks

Genotype 2,3: 24 weeks

Duration of therapy: Coinfection with HIV: 48 weeks

Chronic hepatitis B: 180 mcg once weekly for 48 weeks

Dose modifications for adverse reactions/toxicity:

For moderate-to-severe adverse reactions: Initial: 135 mcg/week; may need decreased to 90 mcg/week in some cases

Based on hematologic parameters:

ANC <750/mm^3: 135 mcg/week

ANC <500/mm^3: Suspend therapy until >1000/mm^3, then restart at 90 mcg/week and monitor

Platelet count <50,000/mm^3: 90 mcg/week

Platelet count <25,000/mm^3: Discontinue therapy

Depression (severity based on DSM-IV criteria):

Mild depression: No dosage adjustment required; evaluate once weekly by visit/phone call. If depression remains stable, continue weekly visits. If depression improves, resume normal visit schedule

Moderate depression: Decrease interferon dose to 90-135 mcg once/week; evaluate once weekly with an office visit at least every other week. If depression remains stable, consider psychiatric evaluation and continue with reduced dosing. If symptoms improve and remain stable for 4 weeks, resume normal visit schedule; continue reduced dosing or return to normal dose.

Severe depression: Discontinue interferon permanently. Obtain immediate psychiatric consultation. Discontinue ribavirin if using concurrently.

Dosage Forms

Injection solution:

Pegasys®:

180 mcg/0.5 mL (0.5 mL) [prefilled syringe; contains benzyl alcohol and polysorbate 80; packaged with needles and alcohol swabs]

180 mcg/mL (1 mL) [vial; contains benzyl alcohol and polysorbate 80]

peginterferon alfa-2b (peg in ter FEER on AL fa too bee)

Synonyms interferon alfa-2b (PEG conjugate); pegylated interferon alfa-2b

U.S./Canadian Brand Names PEG-Intron® [US/Can]

Therapeutic Category Interferon

Use Treatment of chronic hepatitis C (as monotherapy or in combination with ribavirin) in adult patients who have never received interferon alpha and have compensated liver disease

Usual Dosage SubQ:

Children: Safety and efficacy have not been established

Adults: Chronic hepatitis C: Administer dose once weekly; **Note:** Usual duration is for 1 year; after 24 weeks of treatment, if serum HCV RNA is not below the limit of detection of the assay, consider discontinuation:

Monotherapy: Initial:
- ≤45 kg: 40 mcg
- 46-56 kg: 50 mcg
- 57-72 kg: 64 mcg
- 73-88 kg: 80 mcg
- 89-106 kg: 96 mcg
- 107-136 kg: 120 mcg
- 137-160 kg: 150 mcg

Combination therapy with ribavirin (400 mg twice daily): Initial: 1.5 mcg/kg/week
- <40 kg: 50 mcg
- 40-50 kg: 64 mcg
- 51-60 kg: 80 mcg
- 61-75 kg: 96 mcg
- 76-85 kg: 120 mcg
- >85 kg: 150 mcg

Dosage adjustment if serious adverse event occurs: Depression (severity based upon DSM-IV criteria):

Mild depression: No dosage adjustment required; evaluate once weekly by visit/phone call. If depression remains stable, continue weekly visits. If depression improves, resume normal visit schedule.

Moderate depression: Decrease interferon dose by 50%; evaluate once weekly with an office visit at least every other week. If depression remains stable, consider psychiatric evaluation and continue with reduced dosing. If symptoms improve and remain stable for 4 weeks, resume normal visit schedule; continue reduced dosing or return to normal dose.

Severe depression: Discontinue interferon and ribavirin permanently. Obtain immediate psychiatric consultation.

Dosage Forms

Injection, powder for reconstitution [prefilled syringe]:

PEG-Intron® Redipen®: 50 mcg, 80 mcg, 120 mcg, 150 mcg [contains polysorbate 80 and sucrose; packaged with alcohol swabs and needle for injection]

Injection, powder for reconstitution [vial]:

PEG-Intron®: 50 mcg, 80 mcg, 120 mcg, 150 mcg [contains polysorbate 80 and sucrose; packaged with SWFI, alcohol swabs, and syringes]

peginterferon alfa-2b and ribavirin *(Canada only)*

(peg in ter FEER on AL fa too bee & rye ba VYE rin)

Synonyms ribavirin and peginterferon alfa-2b

U.S./Canadian Brand Names Pegasys® RBV [Can]; Pegetron™ [Can]

Therapeutic Category Antiviral Agent; Interferon

Use Combination therapy for the treatment of chronic hepatitis C in patients with compensated liver disease

Usual Dosage Chronic hepatitis C:

Recommended dosage of combination therapy:

Intron® A: SubQ: 1.5 mcg/kg/week

and

Rebetol®: Oral:
- ≤64 kg: 800 mg/day (two 200 mg capsules in the morning and two 200 mg capsules in the evening)
- 64-84 kg: 1000 mg/day (two 200 mg capsules in the morning and three 200 mg capsules in the evening)
- ≥85 kg: 1200 mg/day (three 200 mg capsules in the morning and three 200 mg capsules in the evening)

Recommended duration of therapy: 1 year. Consider discontinuing therapy in any patient not achieving HCV-RNA below the limit of assay detection by 24 weeks.

Dosage Forms Combination package:

Injection, powder for reconstitution (Peginterferon alfa-2b): 50 mcg/0.5 mL

Capsules: Ribavirin (Rebetol®): 200 mg (56s)

Injection, powder for reconstitution (Peginterferon alfa-2b): 80 mcg/0.5 mL
Capsules: Ribavirin (Rebetol®): 200 mg (56s)

Injection, powder for reconstitution (Peginterferon alfa-2b): 100 mcg/0.5 mL
Capsules: Ribavirin (Rebetol®): 200 mg (70s)

Injection, powder for reconstitution (Peginterferon alfa-2b): 120 mcg/0.5 mL
Capsules: Ribavirin (Rebetol®): 200 mg (70s)

Injection, powder for reconstitution (Peginterferon alfa-2b): 150 mcg/0.5 mL
Capsules: Ribavirin (Rebetol®): 200 mg (84s)

PEG-Intron® [US/Can] *see* peginterferon alfa-2b *on previous page*

PegLyte® [Can] *see* polyethylene glycol-electrolyte solution *on page 679*

pegvisomant (peg VI soe mant)

Synonyms B2036-PEG

U.S./Canadian Brand Names Somavert® [US]

Therapeutic Category Growth Hormone Receptor Antagonist

Use Treatment of acromegaly in patients resistant to or unable to tolerate other therapies

Usual Dosage SubQ: Adults: Initial loading dose: 40 mg; maintenance dose: 10 mg once daily; doses may be adjusted by 5 mg in 4- to 6-week intervals based on IGF-I concentrations (maximum dose: 30 mg/day)

Dosage Forms Injection, powder for reconstitution [preservative free]: 10 mg, 15 mg, 20 mg [vial stopper contains latex; packaged with SWFI]

pegylated interferon alfa-2a *see* peginterferon alfa-2a *on page 643*

pegylated interferon alfa-2b *see* peginterferon alfa-2b *on previous page*

pemetrexed (pem e TREKS ed)

Synonyms LY231514; MTA; multitargeted antifolate; NSC-698037; pemetrexed disodium

U.S./Canadian Brand Names Alimta® [US/Can]

Therapeutic Category Antineoplastic Agent, Antimetabolite; Antineoplastic Agent, Antimetabolite (Antifolate)

Use Treatment of malignant pleural mesothelioma in combination with cisplatin; treatment of nonsmall cell lung cancer

Usual Dosage I.V.: Adults: Refer to individual protocols:

Nonsmall cell lung cancer: 500 mg/m^2 on day 1 of each 21-day cycle

Malignant pleural mesothelioma: 500 mg/m^2 on day 1 of each 21-day cycle (in combination with cisplatin)

Note: Start vitamin supplements 1 week before initial dose of pemetrexed. Folic acid 350-1000 mcg/day orally (continuing for 21 days after last dose of pemetrexed) and vitamin B_{12} 1000 mcg I.M. every 9 weeks. Dexamethasone 4 mg twice daily can be started the day before therapy, and continued the day of and the day after to minimize cutaneous reactions.

Dosage Forms

Injection, powder for reconstitution:

Alimta®: 500 mg

pemetrexed disodium *see* pemetrexed *on this page*

pemirolast (pe MIR oh last)

U.S./Canadian Brand Names Alamast® [US/Can]

Therapeutic Category Mast Cell Stabilizer; Ophthalmic Agent, Miscellaneous

Use Prevention of itching of the eye due to allergic conjunctivitis

Usual Dosage Children >3 years and Adults: 1-2 drops instilled in affected eye(s) 4 times/day

Dosage Forms Solution, ophthalmic, as potassium: 0.1% (10 mL) [contains lauralkonium chloride]

pemoline ***(Discontinued)***

penbutolol (pen BYOO toe lole)

Sound-Alike/Look-Alike Issues

Levatol® may be confused with Lipitor®

(Continued)

penbutolol *(Continued)*

Synonyms penbutolol sulfate

U.S./Canadian Brand Names Levatol® [US/Can]

Therapeutic Category Beta-Adrenergic Blocker

Use Treatment of mild to moderate arterial hypertension

Usual Dosage Adults: Oral: Initial: 20 mg once daily, full effect of a 20 or 40 mg dose is seen by the end of a 2-week period, doses of 40-80 mg have been tolerated but have shown little additional antihypertensive effects; usual dose range (JNC 7): 10-40 mg once daily

Dosage Forms Tablet, as sulfate: 20 mg

penbutolol sulfate *see* penbutolol *on previous page*

penciclovir (pen SYE kloe veer)

Sound-Alike/Look-Alike Issues

Denavir® may be confused with indinavir

U.S./Canadian Brand Names Denavir® [US]

Therapeutic Category Antiviral Agent

Use Topical treatment of herpes simplex labialis (cold sores)

Usual Dosage Children ≥12 years and Adults: Topical: Apply cream at the first sign or symptom of cold sore (eg, tingling, swelling); apply every 2 hours during waking hours for 4 days

Dosage Forms Cream: 1% (1.5 g)

Pendo-5 ASA [Can] *see* mesalamine *on page 533*

Penetrex® *(Discontinued)*

penicillamine (pen i SIL a meen)

Sound-Alike/Look-Alike Issues

penicillamine may be confused with penicillin

Depen® may be confused with Endal®

Synonyms β,β-dimethylcysteine; D-3-mercaptovaline; D-penicillamine

U.S./Canadian Brand Names Cuprimine® [US/Can]; Depen® [US/Can]

Therapeutic Category Chelating Agent

Use Treatment of Wilson disease, cystinuria; adjunctive treatment of rheumatoid arthritis

Usual Dosage Oral:

Rheumatoid arthritis:

Adults: 125-250 mg/day, may increase dose at 1- to 3-month intervals up to 1-1.5 g/day; maximum in older adults: 750 mg/day

Wilson disease (doses titrated to maintain urinary copper excretion >2 mg/day); decrease dose for surgery and during last trimester of pregnancy

Children <12 years: 20 mg/kg/day in 2-3 divided doses, round off to the nearest 250 mg dose; maximum 1 g/day

Adults: 250 mg 4 times/day (maximum in older adults: 750 mg/day)

Cystinuria: **Note:** Adjust dose to limit cystine excretion to 100-200 mg/day (<100 mg/day with history of stone formation)

Children: 30 mg/kg/day in 4 divided doses

Adults: 1-4 g/day in divided doses every 6 hours; usual dose: 2 g/day

Dosage Forms [DSC] = Discontinued product

Capsule (Cuprimine®): 125 mg [DSC], 250 mg

Tablet (Depen®): 250 mg

penicillin G benzathine (pen i SIL in jee BENZ a theen)

Sound-Alike/Look-Alike Issues

penicillin may be confused with penicillamine

Bicillin® may be confused with Wycillin®

Bicillin® C-R (penicillin G benzathine and penicillin G procaine) may be confused with Bicillin® L-A (penicillin G benzathine). Penicillin G benzathine is the only product currently approved for the treatment of syphilis. Administration of penicillin G benzathine and penicillin G procaine combination instead of Bicillin® L-A may result in inadequate treatment response.

Synonyms benzathine benzylpenicillin; benzathine penicillin G; benzylpenicillin benzathine

U.S./Canadian Brand Names Bicillin® L-A [US]

Therapeutic Category Penicillin

Use Active against some gram-positive organisms, few gram-negative organisms such as *Neisseria gonorrhoeae*, and some anaerobes and spirochetes; used in the treatment of syphilis; used only for the treatment of mild to moderately severe infections caused by organisms susceptible to low concentrations of penicillin G or for prophylaxis of infections caused by these organisms

Usual Dosage **Note:** Administer undiluted injection; higher doses result in more sustained rather than higher levels. Use a penicillin G benzathine-penicillin G procaine combination to achieve early peak levels in acute infections.

Usual dosage range:

Children: I.M.: 25,000-50,000 units/kg as a single dose (maximum: 2.4 million units)

Adults: I.M.: 1.2-2.4 million units as a single dose

Indication-specific dosing:

Neonates >1200 g: I.M.:

Congenital syphilis (asymptomatic): 50,000 units/kg as a single dose

Infants and Children: I.M.:

Group A streptococcal upper respiratory infection: 25,000-50,000 units/kg as a single dose (maximum: 1.2 million units)

Prophylaxis of recurrent rheumatic fever: 25,000-50,000 units/kg every 3-4 weeks (maximum: 1.2 million units/dose)

Syphilis:

Early: 50,000 units/kg as a single injection (maximum: 2.4 million units)

More than 1-year duration: 50,000 units/kg every week for 3 doses (maximum: 2.4 million units/dose)

Adults: I.M.:

Group A streptococcal upper respiratory infection: 1.2 million units as a single dose

Prophylaxis of recurrent rheumatic fever: 1.2 million units every 3-4 weeks or 600,000 units twice monthly

Syphilis:

Early: 2.4 million units as a single dose in 2 injection sites

More than 1-year duration: 2.4 million units in 2 injection sites once weekly for 3 doses

Neurosyphilis: Not indicated as single-drug therapy, but may be given once weekly for 3 weeks following I.V. treatment; refer to penicillin G parenteral/aqueous monograph for dosing

Dosage Forms Injection, suspension [prefilled syringe]: 600,000 units/mL (1 mL, 2 mL, 4 mL)

penicillin G benzathine and penicillin G procaine

(pen i SIL in jee BENZ a theen & pen i SIL in jee PROE kane)

Sound-Alike/Look-Alike Issues

penicillin may be confused with penicillamine

Bicillin® may be confused with Wycillin®

Bicillin® C-R (penicillin G benzathine and penicillin G procaine) may be confused with Bicillin® L-A (penicillin G benzathine). Penicillin G benzathine is the only product currently approved for the treatment of syphilis. Administration of penicillin G benzathine and penicillin G procaine combination instead of Bicillin® L-A may result in inadequate treatment response.

Synonyms penicillin G procaine and benzathine combined

U.S./Canadian Brand Names Bicillin® C-R 900/300 [US]; Bicillin® C-R [US]

Therapeutic Category Penicillin

Use May be used in specific situations in the treatment of streptococcal infections

Usual Dosage

Usual dosage range and indication-specific dosing:

Streptococcal infections:

Children: I.M.:

<14 kg: 600,000 units in a single dose

14-27 kg: 900,000 units to 1.2 million units in a single dose

Children >27 kg and Adults: 2.4 million units in a single dose

Dosage Forms Injection, suspension [prefilled syringe]:

Bicillin® C-R:

600,000 units: Penicillin G benzathine 300,000 units and penicillin G procaine 300,000 units per 1 mL (1 mL)

1,200,000 units: Penicillin G benzathine 600,000 units and penicillin G procaine 600,000 units per 2 mL (2 mL)

2,400,000 units: Penicillin G benzathine 1,200,000 units and penicillin G procaine 1,200,000 units per 4 mL (4 mL)

(Continued)

penicillin G benzathine and penicillin G procaine *(Continued)*

Bicillin® C-R 900/300: 1,200,000 units: Penicillin G benzathine 900,000 units and penicillin G procaine 300,000 units per 2 mL (2 mL)

penicillin G (parenteral/aqueous) (pen i SIL in jee, pa REN ter al, AYE kwee us)

Sound-Alike/Look-Alike Issues
penicillin may be confused with penicillamine

Synonyms benzylpenicillin potassium; benzylpenicillin sodium; crystalline penicillin; penicillin G potassium; penicillin G sodium

U.S./Canadian Brand Names Pfizerpen® [US/Can]

Therapeutic Category Penicillin

Use Active against some gram-positive organisms, generally not *Staphylococcus aureus*; some gram-negative organisms such as *Neisseria gonorrhoeae*, and some anaerobes and spirochetes

Usual Dosage

Usual dosage range:

Neonates: I.M., I.V.:

<7 days, <2000 g: 25,000-50,000 units/kg every 12 hours
<7 days, >2000 g: 25,000-50,000 units/kg every 8 hours
>7 days, <2000 g: 25,000-50,000 units/kg every 8 hours
>7 days, >2000 g: 25,000-50,000 units/kg every 6 hours

Infants and Children: I.M., I.V.: 250,000 to 400,000 units/kg/day in divided doses every 4-6 hours (maximum dose: 24 million units/day)

Adults: I.M., I.V.: 2-24 million units/day in divided doses every 4 hours depending on sensitivity of the organism and severity of the infection

Indication-specific dosing:

Infants and Children:

Gonococcal:

Disseminated or ophthalmia: I.V.: 100,000 units/kg/day in 2 divided doses (>1 week of age: 4 divided doses)

Meningitis: I.V.: 150,000 units/kg in 2 divided doses (>1 week of age: 4 divided doses)

Mild-to-moderate infections: I.M., I.V.: 25,000-50,000 units/kg/day in 4 divided doses

Severe infections: I.M., I.V.: 250,000-400,000 units/kg/day in divided doses every 4-6 hours (maximum dose: 24 million units/day)

Syphilis (congenital):

Neonates:

≤7 days: 50,000 units/kg I.V. every 12 hours for a total of 10 days
>7 days: 50,000 units/kg I.V. every 8 hours for a total of 10 days

Infants: I.V.: 50,000 units/kg every 4-6 hours for 10 days

Adults:

***Actinomyces* species:** I.V.: 10-20 million units/day divided every 4-6 hours for 4-6 weeks

Anthrax (cutaneous): I.V.: 2 million units every 3 hours for 5-7 days

Clostridium perfringens: I.V.: 24 million units/day divided every 4-6 hours with clindamycin

Corynebacterium diphtheriae: I.V.: 25,000-50,000 units/kg to maximum 1.2 million units every 12 hours, until oral therapy tolerated

Erysipelas: I.V.: 1-2 million units every 4-6 hours

Erysipelothrix: I.V.: 2-4 million units every 4 hours

Fascial space infections: I.V.: 2-4 million units every 4-6 hours with metronidazole

Leptospirosis: I.V.: 1.5 million units every 6 hours for 7 days

Listeria: I.V.: 300,000 units/kg/day every 4 hours

Lyme disease (meningitis): I.V.: 20 million units/day in divided doses

Neurosyphilis: I.M., I.V.: 18-24 million units/day in divided doses every 4 hours (or by continuous infusion) for 10-14 days

Streptococcus:

Brain abscess: I.V.: 20-24 million units/day in divided doses with metronidazole

Endocarditis or osteomyelitis: I.V.: 3-4 million units every 4 hours for at least 4 weeks

Meningitis: I.V.: 3-4 million units every 4 hours for 2-3 weeks

Pregnancy (prophylaxis GBS): I.V.: 5-6 million units x 1 dose, then 2.5-3 million units every 4 hours until delivery

Skin and soft tissue: I.V.: 3-4 million units every 4 hours for 10 days

Toxic shock: I.V.: 24 million units/day in divided doses with clindamycin

Streptococcal pneumonia:

Meningitis: I.V.: 2-4 million units every 2-4 hours

Nonmeningitis: I.V.: 2-3 million units every 4 hours

Whipple disease: I.V.: 2 million units every 4 hours (with streptomycin) for 10-14 days, followed by oral trimethoprim/sulfamethoxazole or doxycycline for 1 year

Dosage Forms

Infusion, as potassium [premixed iso-osmotic dextrose solution, frozen]: 1 million units (50 mL), 2 million units (50 mL), 3 million units (50 mL) [contains sodium 1.02 mEq and potassium 1.7 mEq per 1 million units]

Injection, powder for reconstitution, as potassium (Pfizerpen®): 5 million units, 20 million units [contains sodium 6.8 mg (0.3 mEq) and potassium 65.6 mg (1.68 mEq) per 1 million units]

Injection, powder for reconstitution, as sodium: 5 million units [contains sodium 1.68 mEq per 1 million units]

penicillin G potassium *see* penicillin G (parenteral/aqueous) *on previous page*

penicillin G procaine (pen i SIL in jee PROE kane)

Sound-Alike/Look-Alike Issues

penicillin G procaine may be confused with penicillin V potassium

Wycillin® may be confused with Bicillin®

Synonyms APPG; aqueous procaine penicillin G; procaine benzylpenicillin; procaine penicillin G

U.S./Canadian Brand Names Pfizerpen-AS® [Can]; Wycillin® [Can]

Therapeutic Category Penicillin

Use Moderately severe infections due to *Treponema pallidum* and other penicillin G-sensitive microorganisms that are susceptible to low, but prolonged serum penicillin concentrations; anthrax due to *Bacillus anthracis* (postexposure) to reduce the incidence or progression of disease following exposure to aerolized *Bacillus anthracis*

Usual Dosage

Usual dosage range:

Infants and Children: I.M.: 25,000-50,000 units/kg/day in divided doses 1-2 times/day; (maximum: 4.8 million units/day)

Adults: I.M.: 0.6-4.8 million units/day in divided doses every 12-24 hours

Indication-specific dosing:

Children: I.M.:

Anthrax, inhalational (postexposure prophylaxis): 25,000 units/kg every 12 hours (maximum: 1,200,000 units every 12 hours); see "Note" in Adults dosing

Syphilis (congenital): 50,000 units/kg/day for 10 days; if more than 1 day of therapy is missed, the entire course should be restarted

Adults: I.M.:

Anthrax:

Inhalational (postexposure prophylaxis): 1,200,000 units every 12 hours

Note: Overall treatment duration should be 60 days. Available safety data suggest continued administration of penicillin G procaine for longer than 2 weeks may incur additional risk for adverse reactions. Clinicians may consider switching to effective alternative treatment for completion of therapy beyond 2 weeks.

Cutaneous (treatment): 600,000-1,200,000 units/day; alternative therapy is recommended in severe cutaneous or other forms of anthrax infection

Endocarditis caused by susceptible viridans *Streptococcus* (when used in conjunction with an aminoglycoside): 1.2 million units every 6 hours for 2-4 weeks

Gonorrhea (uncomplicated): 4.8 million units as a single dose divided in 2 sites given 30 minutes after probenecid 1 g orally

Neurosyphilis: 2.4 million units/day with 500 mg probenecid by mouth 4 times/day for 10-14 days; **Note: Penicillin G aqueous I.V. is the preferred agent**

Whipple's disease: 1.2 million units/day (with streptomycin) for 10-14 days, followed by oral trimethoprim/sulfamethoxazole or doxycycline for 1 year

Dosage Forms Injection, suspension: 600,000 units/mL (1 mL, 2 mL)

penicillin G procaine and benzathine combined *see* penicillin G benzathine and penicillin G procaine *on page 647*

penicillin G sodium *see* penicillin G (parenteral/aqueous) *on previous page*

penicillin V potassium (pen i SIL in vee poe TASS ee um)

Sound-Alike/Look-Alike Issues

penicillin V procaine may be confused with penicillin G potassium

(Continued)

penicillin V potassium *(Continued)*

Synonyms pen VK; phenoxymethyl penicillin

U.S./Canadian Brand Names Apo-Pen VK® [Can]; Novo-Pen-VK [Can]; Nu-Pen-VK [Can]; Veetids® [US]

Therapeutic Category Penicillin

Use Treatment of infections caused by susceptible organisms involving the respiratory tract, otitis media, sinusitis, skin, and urinary tract; prophylaxis in rheumatic fever

Usual Dosage

Usual dosage range:

Children <12 years: Oral: 25-50 mg/kg/day in divided doses every 6-8 hours (maximum dose: 3 g/day)

Children ≥12 years and Adults: Oral: 125-500 mg every 6-8 hours

Indication-specific dosing:

Children: Oral:

Pharyngitis (streptococcal): 250 mg 2-3 times/day for 10 days

Prophylaxis of pneumococcal infections:

Children <5 years: 125 mg twice daily

Children ≥5 years: 250 mg twice daily

Prophylaxis of recurrent rheumatic fever:

Children <5 years: 125 mg twice daily

Children ≥5 years: 250 mg twice daily

Adults: Oral:

Acintomycosis:

Mild: 2-4 g/day in 4 divided doses for 8 weeks

Surgical: 2-4 g/day in 4 divided doses for 6-12 months (after I.V. penicillin G therapy of 4-6 weeks)

Erysipelas: 500 mg 4 times/day

Pharyngitis (streptococcal): 500 mg 3-4 times/day for 10 days

Prophylaxis of pneumococcal or recurrent rheumatic fever infections: 250 mg twice daily

Dosage Forms Note: 250 mg = 400,000 units

Powder for oral solution: 125 mg/5 mL (100 mL, 200 mL); 250 mg/5 mL (100 mL, 200 mL)

Tablet: 250 mg, 500 mg

penicilloyl-polylysine *see* benzylpenicilloyl-polylysine *on page 105*

Penlac® [US/Can] *see* ciclopirox *on page 187*

Pennsaid® [Can] *see* diclofenac *on page 250*

Pentacarinat® Injection *(Discontinued)* *see* pentamidine *on this page*

pentahydrate *see* sodium thiosulfate *on page 783*

Pentam-300® [US] *see* pentamidine *on this page*

pentamidine (pen TAM i deen)

Synonyms pentamidine isethionate

U.S./Canadian Brand Names NebuPent® [US]; Pentam-300® [US]

Therapeutic Category Antiprotozoal

Use Treatment and prevention of pneumonia caused by *Pneumocystis carinii* (PCP)

Usual Dosage

Children:

Treatment of PCP pneumonia: I.M., I.V. (I.V. preferred): 4 mg/kg/day once daily for 10-14 days

Prevention of PCP pneumonia:

I.M., I.V.: 4 mg/kg monthly or every 2 weeks

Inhalation (aerosolized pentamidine in children ≥5 years): 300 mg/dose given every 3-4 weeks via Respirgard® II inhaler (8 mg/kg dose has also been used in children <5 years)

Adults:

Treatment: I.M., I.V. (I.V. preferred): 4 mg/kg/day once daily for 14-21 days

Prevention: Inhalation: 300 mg every 4 weeks via Respirgard® II nebulizer

Dosage Forms

Injection, powder for reconstitution, as isethionate (Pentam-300®): 300 mg

Powder for nebulization, as isethionate (NebuPent®): 300 mg

pentamidine isethionate *see* pentamidine *on this page*

Pentamycetin® [Can] *see* chloramphenicol *on page 172*

Pentasa® [US/Can] *see* mesalamine *on page 533*

Pentaspan® [US/Can] *see* pentastarch *on next page*

pentastarch (PEN ta starch)

U.S./Canadian Brand Names Pentaspan® [US/Can]

Therapeutic Category Blood Modifiers

Use Orphan drug: Adjunct in leukapheresis to improve harvesting and increase yield of leukocytes by centrifugal means

Usual Dosage 250-700 mL to which citrate anticoagulant has been added is administered by adding to the input line of the centrifugation apparatus at a ratio of 1:8-1:13 to venous whole blood

Dosage Forms Infusion [premixed in NS]: 10% (500 mL)

Penta-Triamterene HCTZ [Can] *see* hydrochlorothiazide and triamterene *on page 420*

pentavalent human-bovine reassortant rotavirus vaccine *see* rotavirus vaccine *on page 755*

pentazocine (pen TAZ oh seen)

Synonyms naloxone hydrochloride and pentazocine hydrochloride; pentazocine hydrochloride; pentazocine hydrochloride and naloxone hydrochloride; pentazocine lactate

U.S./Canadian Brand Names Talwin® NX [US]; Talwin® [US/Can]

Therapeutic Category Analgesic, Narcotic

Controlled Substance C-IV

Use Relief of moderate to severe pain; has also been used as a sedative prior to surgery and as a supplement to surgical anesthesia

Usual Dosage

Preoperative/preanesthetic: Children 1-16 years: I.M.: 0.5 mg/kg

Analgesia:

Children: I.M.:

5-8 years: 15 mg

8-14 years: 30 mg

Children >12 years and Adults: Oral: 50 mg every 3-4 hours; may increase to 100 mg/dose if needed, but should not exceed 600 mg/day

Adults:

I.M., SubQ: 30-60 mg every 3-4 hours; do not exceed 60 mg/dose (maximum: 360 mg/day)

Dosage Forms

Injection, solution:

Talwin®: 30 mg/mL (1 mL, 10 mL) [10 mL size contains sodium bisulfite]

Tablet: Pentazocine 50 mg and naloxone 0.5 mg

Talwin® NX: Pentazocine 50 mg and naloxone 0.5 mg

pentazocine and acetaminophen (pen TAZ oh seen & a seet a MIN oh fen)

Sound-Alike/Look-Alike Issues

Talacen® may be confused with Tegison®, Timoptic®, Tinactin®

Synonyms acetaminophen and pentazocine; pentazocine hydrochloride and acetaminophen

U.S./Canadian Brand Names Talacen® [US]

Therapeutic Category Analgesic Combination (Opioid)

Controlled Substance C-IV

Use Relief of mild to moderate pain

Usual Dosage Oral: Adults: Analgesic: 1 caplet every 4 hours, up to a maximum of 6 caplets

Dosage Forms

Caplet:

Talacen®: Pentazocine 25 mg and acetaminophen 650 mg [contains sodium metabisulfite]

Tablet: Pentazocine 25 mg and acetaminophen 650 mg

pentazocine hydrochloride *see* pentazocine *on this page*

pentazocine hydrochloride and acetaminophen *see* pentazocine and acetaminophen *on this page*

pentazocine hydrochloride and naloxone hydrochloride *see* pentazocine *on this page*

pentazocine lactate *see* pentazocine *on this page*

pentetate calcium trisodium *see* diethylene triamine penta-acetic acid *on page 252*

pentetate zinc trisodium *see* diethylene triamine penta-acetic acid *on page 252*

Penthrane® ***(Discontinued)***

pentobarbital (pen toe BAR bi tal)

Sound-Alike/Look-Alike Issues
pentobarbital may be confused with phenobarbital
Nembutal® may be confused with Myambutol®

Synonyms pentobarbital sodium

U.S./Canadian Brand Names Nembutal® [US]

Therapeutic Category Barbiturate

Controlled Substance C-II

Use Sedative/hypnotic; preanesthetic; high-dose barbiturate coma for treatment of increased intracranial pressure or status epilepticus unresponsive to other therapy

Usual Dosage
Children:
Hypnotic: I.M.: 2-6 mg/kg; maximum: 100 mg/dose
Preoperative/preprocedure sedation: ≥6 months:
Note: Limited information is available for infants <6 months of age.
I.M.: 2-6 mg/kg; maximum: 100 mg/dose
I.V.: 1-3 mg/kg to a maximum of 100 mg until asleep
Conscious sedation prior to a procedure: Children 5-12 years: I.V.: 2 mg/kg 5-10 minutes before procedures, may repeat one time
Adolescents: Conscious sedation: I.V.: 100 mg prior to a procedure
Children and Adults: Barbiturate coma in head injury patients: I.V.: Loading dose: 5-10 mg/kg given slowly over 1-2 hours; monitor blood pressure and respiratory rate; Maintenance infusion: Initial: 1 mg/kg/hour; may increase to 2-3 mg/kg/hour; maintain burst suppression on EEG
Status epilepticus: I.V.: **Note**: Intubation required; monitor hemodynamics
Children: Loading dose: 5-15 mg/kg given slowly over 1-2 hours; maintenance infusion: 0.5-5 mg/kg/hour
Adults: Loading dose: 2-15 mg/kg given slowly over 1-2 hours; maintenance infusion: 0.5-3 mg/kg/hour
Adults:
Hypnotic:
I.M.: 150-200 mg
I.V.: Initial: 100 mg, may repeat every 1-3 minutes up to 200-500 mg total dose
Preoperative sedation: I.M.: 150-200 mg

Dosage Forms Injection, solution, as sodium: 50 mg/mL (20 mL, 50 mL) [contains alcohol 10% and propylene glycol 40%]

pentobarbital sodium *see* pentobarbital *on this page*

pentosan polysulfate sodium (PEN toe san pol i SUL fate SOW dee um)

Sound-Alike/Look-Alike Issues
pentosan may be confused with pentostatin
Elmiron® may be confused with Imuran®

Synonyms PPS

U.S./Canadian Brand Names Elmiron® [US/Can]

Therapeutic Category Analgesic, Urinary

Use **Orphan drug:** Relief of bladder pain or discomfort due to interstitial cystitis

Usual Dosage Adults: Oral: 100 mg 3 times/day taken with water 1 hour before or 2 hours after meals

Patients should be evaluated at 3 months and may be continued an additional 3 months if there has been no improvement and if there are no therapy-limiting side effects. **The risks and benefits of continued use beyond 6 months in patients who have not responded is not yet known**.

Dosage Forms Capsule: 100 mg

pentostatin (pen toe STAT in)

Sound-Alike/Look-Alike Issues
pentostatin may be confused with pentosan

Synonyms CL-825; co-vidarabine; dCF; deoxycoformycin; NSC-218321; 2′-deoxycoformycin

U.S./Canadian Brand Names Nipent® [US/Can]

Therapeutic Category Antineoplastic Agent

Use Treatment of hairy cell leukemia; non-Hodgkin lymphoma, cutaneous T-cell lymphoma

Usual Dosage Refractory hairy cell leukemia: Adults (refer to individual protocols):
4 mg/m^2 every other week **or**
4 mg/m^2 weekly for 3 weeks, then every 2 weeks **or**
5 mg/m^2 daily for 3 days every 3 weeks

Dosage Forms
Injection, powder for reconstitution [preservative free]:
Nipent®: 10 mg

Pentothal® [US/Can] *see* thiopental *on page 822*

Pentothal® Sodium Rectal Suspension *(Discontinued)* *see* thiopental *on page 822*

pentoxifylline (pen toks IF I lin)

Sound-Alike/Look-Alike Issues
pentoxifylline may be confused with tamoxifen
Trental® may be confused with Bentyl®, Tegretol®, Trandate®

Synonyms oxpentifylline

U.S./Canadian Brand Names Albert® Pentoxifylline [Can]; Apo-Pentoxifylline SR® [Can]; Nu-Pentoxifylline SR [Can]; Pentoxil® [US]; ratio-Pentoxifylline [Can]; Trental® [US/Can]

Therapeutic Category Blood Viscosity Reducer Agent

Use Treatment of intermittent claudication on the basis of chronic occlusive arterial disease of the limbs; may improve function and symptoms, but not intended to replace more definitive therapy

Usual Dosage Adults: Oral: 400 mg 3 times/day with meals; maximal therapeutic benefit may take 2-4 weeks to develop; recommended to maintain therapy for at least 8 weeks. May reduce to 400 mg twice daily if GI or CNS side effects occur.

Dosage Forms
Tablet, controlled release:
Trental®: 400 mg
Tablet, extended release: 400 mg
Pentoxil®: 400 mg

Pentoxil® [US] *see* pentoxifylline *on this page*

Pen.Vee® K *(Discontinued)* *see* penicillin V potassium *on page 649*

pen VK *see* penicillin V potassium *on page 649*

Pepcid® [US/Can] *see* famotidine *on page 335*

Pepcid® AC [US-OTC/Can] *see* famotidine *on page 335*

Pepcid® Complete [US-OTC/Can] *see* famotidine, calcium carbonate, and magnesium hydroxide *on page 336*

Pepcid® I.V. [Can] *see* famotidine *on page 335*

Pepcid RPD® *(Discontinued)* *see* famotidine *on page 335*

Pepto-Bismol® [US-OTC] *see* bismuth subsalicylate *on page 112*

Pepto-Bismol® Maximum Strength [US-OTC] *see* bismuth subsalicylate *on page 112*

Pepto® Diarrhea Control *(Discontinued)* *see* loperamide *on page 503*

Perchloracap® [US] *see* radiological/contrast media (ionic) *on page 728*

Percocet® [US/Can] *see* oxycodone and acetaminophen *on page 627*

Percocet®-Demi [Can] *see* oxycodone and acetaminophen *on page 627*

Percodan® [US/Can] *see* oxycodone and aspirin *on page 628*

Percodan®-Demi *(Discontinued)* *see* oxycodone and aspirin *on page 628*

Percogesic® [US-OTC] *see* acetaminophen and phenyltoloxamine *on page 8*

Percogesic® Extra Strength [US-OTC] *see* acetaminophen and diphenhydramine *on page 7*

Percolone® *(Discontinued)* *see* oxycodone *on page 626*

Perdiem® Overnight Relief [US-OTC] *see* senna *on page 767*

Perfectoderm® Gel *(Discontinued)* *see* benzoyl peroxide *on page 102*

perflutren lipid microspheres (per FLOO tren LIP id MIKE roe sfeers)

U.S./Canadian Brand Names Definity® [US/Can]

Therapeutic Category Diagnostic Agent

Use Opacification of left ventricular chamber and improvement of delineation of the left ventricular endocardial border in patients with suboptimal echocardiograms
(Continued)

perflutren lipid microspheres *(Continued)*

Usual Dosage Adults: Dose should be given following baseline noncontrast echocardiography. Imaging should begin immediately following dose and compared to noncontrast image. Mechanical index for the ultrasound device should be set at ≤0.8.

I.V. bolus: 10 µL/kg of activated product, followed by 10 mL saline flush. May repeat in 30 minutes if needed (maximum dose: 2 bolus infusions).

I.V. infusion: Initial: 4 mL/minute of prepared infusion; titrate to achieve optimal image; maximum rate: 10 mL/minute (maximum dose: 1 intravenous infusion).

Dosage Forms Injection, solution [preservative free]: OFP 6.52 mg/mL and lipid blend 0.75 mg/mL (2 mL) [following activation, forms a suspension containing perflutren lipid microspheres 1.2 x 10^{10}/mL and OFP 1.1 mg/mL]

pergolide (PER go lide)

Sound-Alike/Look-Alike Issues

Permax® may be confused with Bumex®, Pentrax®, Pernox®

Synonyms pergolide mesylate

U.S./Canadian Brand Names Permax® [US/Can]

Therapeutic Category Anti-Parkinson Agent; Dopaminergic Agent (Anti-Parkinson); Ergot Alkaloid and Derivative

Use Adjunctive treatment to levodopa/carbidopa in the management of Parkinson disease

Usual Dosage When adding pergolide to levodopa/carbidopa, the dose of the latter can usually and should be decreased. Patients no longer responsive to bromocriptine may benefit by being switched to pergolide.

Oral: Adults: Parkinson disease: Start with 0.05 mg/day for 2 days, then increase dosage by 0.1 or 0.15 mg/day every 3 days over next 12 days, increase dose by 0.25 mg/day every 3 days until optimal therapeutic dose is achieved, up to 5 mg/day maximum; usual dosage range: 2-3 mg/day in 3 divided doses

Dosage Forms

Tablet [scored]: 0.05 mg, 0.25 mg, 1 mg

Permax®: 0.05 mg, 0.25 mg, 1 mg

pergolide mesylate *see* pergolide *on this page*

Pergonal® ***(Discontinued)*** *see* menotropins *on page 528*

Periactin® ***(Discontinued)*** *see* cyproheptadine *on page 223*

Peri-Colace® ***(reformulation)*** **[US-OTC]** *see* docusate and senna *on page 271*

pericyazine *(Canada only)* (per ee CYE ah zeen)

U.S./Canadian Brand Names Neuleptil® [Can]

Therapeutic Category Phenothiazine Derivative

Use As adjunctive medication in some psychotic patients, for the control of residual prevailing hostility, impulsiveness and aggressiveness

Usual Dosage Oral:

Children >5 years: 2.5-10 mg in the morning and 5-30 mg in the evening. In general, lower dosage should be used on initiation and gradually increased based on effect and tolerance.

Adults: 5-20 mg in the morning followed by 10-40 mg in the evening. In dividing doses, it is suggested that the larger dose should be administered in the evening. In general, lower dosage should be used on initiation and gradually increased based on effect and tolerance.

Dosage Forms

Capsule: 5 mg, 10 mg, 20 mg

Drops, oral: 10 mg/mL (100 mL)

Peridex® [US] *see* chlorhexidine gluconate *on page 173*

Peridol [Can] *see* haloperidol *on page 406*

perindopril and indapamide *(Canada only)* (per IN doe pril & in DAP a mide)

U.S./Canadian Brand Names Coversyl® Plus [Can]; Preterax® [Can]

Therapeutic Category Miscellaneous Product

Use Hypertension

Usual Dosage Adults: Oral: One tablet daily

Dosage Forms Tablet: Perindopril 2 mg and indapamide 0.625 mg

perindopril erbumine (per IN doe pril er BYOO meen)

U.S./Canadian Brand Names Aceon® [US]; Coversyl® [Can]

Therapeutic Category Miscellaneous Product

Use Treatment of essential hypertension; reduction of cardiovascular mortality or nonfatal myocardial infarction in patients with stable coronary artery disease

Usual Dosage Oral: Adults:

Essential hypertension: Initial: 4 mg/day but may be titrated to response; usual range: 4-8 mg/day (may be given in 2 divided doses); increase at 1- to 2-week intervals (maximum: 16 mg/day)

Concomitant therapy with diuretics: To reduce the risk of hypotension, discontinue diuretic, if possible, 2-3 days prior to initiating perindopril. If unable to stop diuretic, initiate perindopril at 2-4 mg/day and monitor blood pressure closely for the first 2 weeks of therapy, and after any dose adjustment of perindopril or diuretic.

Stable coronary artery disease: Initial: 4 mg once daily for 2 weeks; increase as tolerated to 8 mg once daily.

Dosage Forms Tablet: 2 mg, 4 mg, 8 mg

PerioChip® [US] *see* chlorhexidine gluconate *on page 173*

PerioGard® [US] *see* chlorhexidine gluconate *on page 173*

PerioMed™ [US] *see* fluoride *on page 354*

Periostat® [US/Can] *see* doxycycline *on page 278*

Permax® [US/Can] *see* pergolide *on previous page*

permethrin (per METH rin)

U.S./Canadian Brand Names A200® Lice [US-OTC]; Acticin® [US]; Elimite® [US]; Kwellada-P™ [Can]; Nix® [US-OTC/Can]; Rid® Spray [US-OTC]

Therapeutic Category Scabicides/Pediculicides

Use Single-application treatment of infestation with *Pediculus humanus capitis* (head louse) and its nits or *Sarcoptes scabiei* (scabies); indicated for prophylactic use during epidemics of lice

Usual Dosage Topical:

Head lice: Children >2 months and Adults: After hair has been washed with shampoo, rinsed with water, and towel dried, apply a sufficient volume of topical liquid (lotion or cream rinse) to saturate the hair and scalp. Leave on hair for 10 minutes before rinsing off with water; remove remaining nits; may repeat in 1 week if lice or nits still present.

Scabies: Apply cream from head to toe; leave on for 8-14 hours before washing off with water; for infants, also apply on the hairline, neck, scalp, temple, and forehead; may reapply in 1 week if live mites appear

Permethrin 5% cream was shown to be safe and effective when applied to an infant <1 month of age with neonatal scabies; time of application was limited to 6 hours before rinsing with soap and water

Dosage Forms

Cream, topical (Acticin®, Elimite®): 5% (60 g) [contains coconut oil]

Lotion, topical: 1% (59 mL)

Liquid, topical [creme rinse formulation] (Nix®): 1% (60 mL) [contains isopropyl alcohol 20%]

Solution, spray [for bedding and furniture]:

- A200® Lice: 0.5% (180 mL)
- Nix®: 0.25% (148 mL)
- Rid®: 0.5% (150 mL)

Permitil® Oral *(Discontinued)* *see* fluphenazine *on page 358*

Peroxin A5® *(Discontinued)* *see* benzoyl peroxide *on page 102*

Peroxin A10® *(Discontinued)* *see* benzoyl peroxide *on page 102*

perphenazine (per FEN a zeen)

Sound-Alike/Look-Alike Issues

Trilafon® may be confused with Tri-Levlen®

U.S./Canadian Brand Names Apo-Perphenazine® [Can]

Therapeutic Category Phenothiazine Derivative

Use Treatment of schizophrenia; nausea and vomiting

Usual Dosage Oral:

Children:

Schizophrenia/psychoses:

- 1-6 years: 4-6 mg/day in divided doses
- 6-12 years: 6 mg/day in divided doses
- >12 years: 4-16 mg 2-4 times/day

(Continued)

perphenazine *(Continued)*

Adults:

Schizophrenia/psychoses: 4-16 mg 2-4 times/day not to exceed 64 mg/day

Nausea/vomiting: 8-16 mg/day in divided doses up to 24 mg/day

Dosage Forms Tablet: 2 mg, 4 mg, 8 mg, 16 mg

perphenazine and amitriptyline hydrochloride *see* amitriptyline and perphenazine *on page 45*

Persa-Gel® *(Discontinued)* *see* benzoyl peroxide *on page 102*

Persantine® [US/Can] *see* dipyridamole *on page 267*

Pertussin® CS *(Discontinued)* *see* dextromethorphan *on page 245*

Pertussin® ES *(Discontinued)* *see* dextromethorphan *on page 245*

pethidine hydrochloride *see* meperidine *on page 529*

Pexeva® [US] *see* paroxetine *on page 639*

Pexicam® [Can] *see* piroxicam *on page 671*

PFA *see* foscarnet *on page 369*

Pfizerpen® [US/Can] *see* penicillin G (parenteral/aqueous) *on page 648*

Pfizerpen-AS® [Can] *see* penicillin G procaine *on page 649*

PGE_1 *see* alprostadil *on page 32*

PGE_2 *see* dinoprostone *on page 260*

PGI_2 *see* epoprostenol *on page 299*

PGX *see* epoprostenol *on page 299*

Phanasin [US-OTC] *see* guaifenesin *on page 392*

Phanasin® Diabetic Choice [US-OTC] *see* guaifenesin *on page 392*

Phanatuss® DM [US-OTC] *see* guaifenesin and dextromethorphan *on page 394*

Pharmaflur® [US] *see* fluoride *on page 354*

Pharmaflur® 1.1 [US] *see* fluoride *on page 354*

Pharmorubicin® [Can] *see* epirubicin *on page 297*

Phazyme® [Can] *see* simethicone *on page 772*

Phazyme® *(Discontinued)* *see* simethicone *on page 772*

Phazyme® Quick Dissolve [US-OTC] *see* simethicone *on page 772*

Phazyme® Ultra Strength [US-OTC] *see* simethicone *on page 772*

Phenabid DM® [US] *see* chlorpheniramine, phenylephrine, and dextromethorphan *on page 179*

Phenadex® Senior *(Discontinued)* *see* guaifenesin and dextromethorphan *on page 394*

Phenadoz™ [US] *see* promethazine *on page 703*

Phenagesic [US-OTC] *see* acetaminophen and phenyltoloxamine *on page 8*

Phenameth® DM *(Discontinued)* *see* promethazine and dextromethorphan *on page 704*

Phenaphen® *(Discontinued)* *see* acetaminophen *on page 5*

Phenaseptic [US-OTC] *see* phenol *on page 658*

PhenaVent™ [US] *see* guaifenesin and phenylephrine *on page 396*

PhenaVent™ D [US] *see* guaifenesin and phenylephrine *on page 396*

PhenaVent™ Ped [US] *see* guaifenesin and phenylephrine *on page 396*

Phenazine® Injection *(Discontinued)* *see* promethazine *on page 703*

Phenazo™ [Can] *see* phenazopyridine *on this page*

phenazopyridine (fen az oh PEER i deen)

Sound-Alike/Look-Alike Issues

Pyridium® may be confused with Dyrenium®, Perdiem®, pyridoxine, pyrithione

Synonyms phenazopyridine hydrochloride; phenylazo diamino pyridine hydrochloride

U.S./Canadian Brand Names AZO-Gesic® [US-OTC]; AZO-Standard® [US-OTC]; Baridium® [US-OTC]; Phenazo™ [Can]; Pyridium® [US]; ReAzo [US-OTC]; Uristat® [US-OTC]; UTI Relief® [US-OTC]

Therapeutic Category Analgesic, Urinary

Use Symptomatic relief of urinary burning, itching, frequency and urgency in association with urinary tract infection or following urologic procedures

Usual Dosage Oral:

Children: 12 mg/kg/day in 3 divided doses administered after meals for 2 days

Adults: 100-200 mg 3 times/day after meals for 2 days when used concomitantly with an antibacterial agent

Dosage Forms

Tablet, as hydrochloride: 100 mg, 200 mg

AZO-Gesic®, AZO-Standard®, Uristat®: 95 mg

Baridium®: 97.2 mg

ReAzo: 95 mg

Pyridium®: 100 mg, 200 mg

UTI Relief®: 97.2 mg

phenazopyridine hydrochloride *see* phenazopyridine *on previous page*

phendimetrazine (fen dye ME tra zeen)

Sound-Alike/Look-Alike Issues

Bontril PDM® may be confused with Bentyl®

Synonyms phendimetrazine tartrate

U.S./Canadian Brand Names Bontril® PDM [US]; Bontril® Slow-Release [US]; Bontril® [Can]; Melfiat® [US]; Plegine® [Can]; Statobex® [Can]

Therapeutic Category Anorexiant

Controlled Substance C-III

Use Appetite suppressant during the first few weeks of dieting to help establish new eating habits; its effectiveness lasts only for short periods (3-12 weeks)

Usual Dosage Adults: Oral:

Tablet: 35 mg 2 or 3 times daily, 1 hour before meals

Capsule, timed release: 105 mg once daily in the morning before breakfast

Dosage Forms [DSC] = Discontinued product

Capsule, slow release, as tartrate: 105 mg

Bontril® Slow Release: 105 mg

Capsule, sustained release, as tartrate:

Melfiat®: 105 mg [DSC]

Tablet, as tartrate: 35 mg

Bontril PDM®: 35 mg

phendimetrazine tartrate *see* phendimetrazine *on this page*

Phendry® Oral *(Discontinued)* *see* diphenhydramine *on page 261*

phenelzine (FEN el zeen)

Sound-Alike/Look-Alike Issues

phenelzine may be confused with phenytoin

Nardil® may be confused with Norinyl®

Synonyms phenelzine sulfate

U.S./Canadian Brand Names Nardil® [US/Can]

Therapeutic Category Antidepressant, Monoamine Oxidase Inhibitor

Use Symptomatic treatment of atypical, nonendogenous, or neurotic depression

Usual Dosage Oral: Adults: Depression: 15 mg 3 times/day; may increase to 60-90 mg/day during early phase of treatment, then reduce dose for maintenance therapy slowly after maximum benefit is obtained; takes 2-4 weeks for a significant response to occur

Dosage Forms Tablet: 15 mg

phenelzine sulfate *see* phenelzine *on this page*

Phenerbel-S® *(Discontinued)*

Phenergan® [US/Can] *see* promethazine *on page 703*

Phenergan® VC With Codeine *(Discontinued)* *see* promethazine, phenylephrine, and codeine *on page 705*

Phenergan® With Dextromethorphan *(Discontinued)* *see* promethazine and dextromethorphan *on page 704*

pheniramine and naphazoline *see* naphazoline and pheniramine *on page 578*

phenobarbital (fee noe BAR bi tal)

Sound-Alike/Look-Alike Issues
phenobarbital may be confused with pentobarbital
Luminal® may be confused with Tuinal®

Synonyms phenobarbital sodium; phenobarbitone; phenylethylmalonylurea

U.S./Canadian Brand Names Luminal® Sodium [US]; PMS-Phenobarbital [Can]

Therapeutic Category Anticonvulsant; Barbiturate

Controlled Substance C-IV

Use Management of generalized tonic-clonic (grand mal) and partial seizures; sedative

Usual Dosage
Children:
Sedation: Oral: 2 mg/kg 3 times/day
Hypnotic: I.M., I.V., SubQ: 3-5 mg/kg at bedtime
Preoperative sedation: Oral, I.M., I.V.: 1-3 mg/kg 1-1.5 hours before procedure
Adults:
Sedation: Oral, I.M.: 30-120 mg/day in 2-3 divided doses
Hypnotic: Oral, I.M., I.V., SubQ: 100-320 mg at bedtime
Preoperative sedation: I.M.: 100-200 mg 1-1.5 hours before procedure
Anticonvulsant: Status epilepticus: **Loading dose:** I.V.:
Infants and Children: 10-20 mg/kg in a single or divided dose; in select patients may administer additional 5 mg/kg/dose every 15-30 minutes until seizure is controlled or a total dose of 40 mg/kg is reached
Adults: 300-800 mg initially followed by 120-240 mg/dose at 20-minute intervals until seizures are controlled or a total dose of 1-2 g
Anticonvulsant maintenance dose: Oral, I.V.:
Infants: 5-8 mg/kg/day in 1-2 divided doses
Children:
1-5 years: 6-8 mg/kg/day in 1-2 divided doses
5-12 years: 4-6 mg/kg/day in 1-2 divided doses
Children >12 years and Adults: 1-3 mg/kg/day in divided doses or 50-100 mg 2-3 times/day

Dosage Forms
Elixir: 20 mg/5 mL (473 mL) [contains alcohol]
Injection, solution, as sodium: 65 mg/mL (1 mL); 130 mg/mL (1 mL) [contains alcohol and propylene glycol]
Luminal® Sodium: 60 mg/mL (1 mL); 130 mg/mL (1 mL) [contains alcohol 10% and propylene glycol]
Tablet: 15 mg, 30 mg, 32 mg, 60 mg, 65 mg, 100 mg

phenobarbital, belladonna, and ergotamine tartrate *see* belladonna, phenobarbital, and ergotamine *on page 96*

phenobarbital, hyoscyamine, atropine, and scopolamine *see* hyoscyamine, atropine, scopolamine, and phenobarbital *on page 435*

phenobarbital sodium *see* phenobarbital *on this page*

phenobarbitone *see* phenobarbital *on this page*

phenol (FEE nol)

Sound-Alike/Look-Alike Issues
Cēpastat® may be confused with Capastat®

Synonyms carbolic acid

U.S./Canadian Brand Names Cepastat® Extra Strength [US-OTC]; Cepastat® [US-OTC]; Cheracol® [US-OTC]; Chloraseptic® Gargle [US-OTC]; Chloraseptic® Mouth Pain [US-OTC]; Chloraseptic® Rinse [US-OTC]; Chloraseptic® Spray for Kids [US-OTC]; Chloraseptic® Spray [US-OTC]; P & S™ Liquid Phenol [Can]; Pain-A-Lay® [US-OTC]; Phenaseptic [US-OTC]; Phenol EZ® [US-OTC]; Ulcerease® [US-OTC]

Therapeutic Category Pharmaceutical Aid

Use Relief of sore throat pain, mouth, gum, and throat irritations; antiseptic; topical anesthetic

Usual Dosage Oral:
Sore throat:
Children 2-12 years:
Chloraseptic®: Three sprays onto throat or affected area; may repeat every 2 hours
Chloraseptic® for Kids: Five sprays onto throat or affected area; may repeat every 2 hours

Children >3 years (Ulcerease®): Refer to adult dosing.
Children 6-12 years:
Cepastat®: Up to 1 lozenge every 2 hours as needed (maximum: 18 lozenges/24 hours)
Cepastat® Extra Strength: Up to 1 lozenge every 2 hours as needed (maximum: 10 lozenges/24 hours)
Pain-A-Lay® Gargle: Using gauze pad, apply 10 mL to affected area, or gargle or swish for 15 seconds, then expectorate
Children ≥12 years and Adults:
Cepastat® Extra Strength, Cēpastat®: Up to 2 lozenges every 2 hours as needed
Cheracol®, Pain-A-Lay® Spray: Spray directly in throat; rinse for 15 seconds then expectorate; may repeat every 2 hours
Chloraseptic®: Five sprays onto throat or affected area; may repeat every 2 hours
Chloraseptic® Gargle, Chloraseptic® Mouth Pain, Pain-A-Lay® Gargle, Ulcerease®: Gargle or swish for 15 seconds, then expectorate; may repeat every 2 hours
Topical: Antiseptic: Adults: Castellani Paint Modified: Apply small amount to affected area 1-3 times/day

Dosage Forms
Liquid, oral (Ulcerease®): 0.6% (180 mL) [contains glycerin; sugar free]
Lozenge:
Cēpastat®: 14.5 mg (18s) [contains eucalyptus oil and menthol; sugar free; cherry flavor]
Cēpastat® Extra Strength: 29 mg (18s) [contains eucalyptus oil and menthol; sugar free; eucalyptus flavor]
Solution, oral:
Chloraseptic® [gargle]: 1.4% (296 mL) [cool mint flavor]
Chloraseptic® [rinse]: 1.4% (240 mL) [cinnamon flavor]
Pain-A-Lay®: 1.4% (240 mL) [gargle; contains tartrazine]
Solution, oral spray: 1.4% (180 mL)
Chloraseptic®: 1.4% (180 mL) [cherry flavor]
Chloraseptic® for Kids: 0.5% (177 mL) [grape flavor]
Chloraseptic® Mouth Pain Spray: 1.4% (30 mL) [cherry blast or cool mint flavor]
Pain-A-Lay®: 1.4% (180 mL) [contains tartrazine]
Solution, topical: Phenol 1.5%, alcohol 13%, basic fuchsin, resorcinol, acetone (30 mL, 480 mL)

phenol and camphor *see* camphor and phenol *on page 141*

Phenol EZ® [US-OTC] *see* phenol *on previous page*

Phenoxine® ***(Discontinued)***

phenoxybenzamine (fen oks ee BEN za meen)

Synonyms phenoxybenzamine hydrochloride
U.S./Canadian Brand Names Dibenzyline® [US/Can]
Therapeutic Category Alpha-Adrenergic Blocking Agent
Use Symptomatic management of pheochromocytoma; treatment of hypertensive crisis caused by sympathomimetic amines
Usual Dosage Oral:
Children: Initial: 0.2 mg/kg (maximum: 10 mg) once daily, increase by 0.2 mg/kg increments; usual maintenance dose: 0.4-1.2 mg/kg/day every 6-8 hours, higher doses may be necessary
Adults: Initial: 10 mg twice daily, increase by 10 mg every other day until optimum dose is achieved; usual range: 20-40 mg 2-3 times/day
Dosage Forms Capsule, as hydrochloride: 10 mg [contains benzyl alcohol]

phenoxybenzamine hydrochloride *see* phenoxybenzamine *on this page*

phenoxymethyl penicillin *see* penicillin V potassium *on page 649*

phentermine (FEN ter meen)

Sound-Alike/Look-Alike Issues
phentermine may be confused with phentolamine, phenytoin
Ionamin® may be confused with Imodium®
Synonyms phentermine hydrochloride
U.S./Canadian Brand Names Adipex-P® [US]; Ionamin® [US/Can]
Therapeutic Category Anorexiant
Controlled Substance C-IV
Use Short-term adjunct in a regimen of weight reduction based on exercise, behavioral modification, and caloric reduction in the management of exogenous obesity for patients with an initial body mass index ≥30 kg/m^2 or ≥27 kg/m^2 in the presence of other risk factors (diabetes, hypertension)
(Continued)

phentermine *(Continued)*

Usual Dosage Oral: Adults: Obesity: 8 mg 3 times/day 30 minutes before meals or food or 15-37.5 mg/day before breakfast or 10-14 hours before retiring

Dosage Forms

Capsule, as hydrochloride: 15 mg, 30 mg

Adipex-P®: 37.5 mg

Capsule, resin complex:

Ionamin®: 15 mg; 30 mg [DSC]

Tablet, as hydrochloride: 37.5 mg

Adipex-P®: 37.5 mg

phentermine hydrochloride *see* phentermine *on previous page*

phentolamine (fen TOLE a meen)

Sound-Alike/Look-Alike Issues

phentolamine may be confused with phentermine, Ventolin®

Synonyms phentolamine mesylate

U.S./Canadian Brand Names Regitine® [Can]; Rogitine® [Can]

Therapeutic Category Alpha-Adrenergic Blocking Agent; Diagnostic Agent

Use Diagnosis of pheochromocytoma and treatment of hypertension associated with pheochromocytoma or other forms of hypertension caused by excess sympathomimetic amines; as treatment of dermal necrosis after extravasation of drugs with alpha-adrenergic effects (norepinephrine, dopamine, epinephrine)

Usual Dosage

Treatment of alpha-adrenergic drug extravasation: SubQ:

Children: 0.1-0.2 mg/kg diluted in 10 mL 0.9% sodium chloride infiltrated into area of extravasation within 12 hours

Adults: Infiltrate area with small amount of solution made by diluting 5-10 mg in 10 mL 0.9% sodium chloride within 12 hours of extravasation; do not exceed 0.1-0.2 mg/kg or 5 mg total

If dose is effective, normal skin color should return to the blanched area within 1 hour

Diagnosis of pheochromocytoma: I.M., I.V.:

Children: 0.05-0.1 mg/kg/dose, maximum single dose: 5 mg

Adults: 5 mg

Surgery for pheochromocytoma: Hypertension: I.M., I.V.:

Children: 0.05-0.1 mg/kg/dose given 1-2 hours before procedure; repeat as needed every 2-4 hours until hypertension is controlled; maximum single dose: 5 mg

Adults: 5 mg given 1-2 hours before procedure and repeated as needed every 2-4 hours

Hypertensive crisis: Adults: 5-20 mg

Dosage Forms Injection, powder for reconstitution, as mesylate: 5 mg

phentolamine mesylate *see* phentolamine *on this page*

phenylalanine mustard *see* melphalan *on page 526*

phenylazo diamino pyridine hydrochloride *see* phenazopyridine *on page 656*

Phenyldrine® *(Discontinued)*

phenylephrine (fen il EF rin)

Sound-Alike/Look-Alike Issues

Mydfrin® may be confused with Midrin®

Synonyms phenylephrine hydrochloride; phenylephrine tannate

U.S./Canadian Brand Names AK-Dilate® [US]; Altafrin [US]; Anu-Med [US-OTC]; Dionephrine® [Can]; Formulation R™ [US-OTC]; Medicone® [US-OTC]; Mydfrin® [US/Can]; Neo-Synephrine® Extra Strength [US-OTC]; Neo-Synephrine® Mild [US-OTC]; Neo-Synephrine® Regular Strength [US-OTC]; Neo-Synephrine® [Can]; Nāsop™ [US]; Rectacaine [US-OTC]; Relief® [US-OTC]; Rhinall [US-OTC]; Sudafed PE™ [US-OTC]; Tronolane® Suppository [US-OTC]; Vicks® Sinex® Nasal Spray [US-OTC]; Vicks® Sinex® UltraFine Mist [US-OTC]

Therapeutic Category Adrenergic Agonist Agent

Use Treatment of hypotension, vascular failure in shock; as a vasoconstrictor in regional analgesia; as a mydriatic in ophthalmic procedures and treatment of wide-angle glaucoma; supraventricular tachycardia

For OTC use as symptomatic relief of nasal and nasopharyngeal mucosal congestion, treatment of hemorrhoids, relief of redness of the eye due to irritation

Usual Dosage

Hemorrhoids: Children ≥12 years and Adults: Rectal:

Cream/ointment: Apply to clean dry area, up to 4 times/day; may be used externally or inserted rectally using applicator.

Suppository: Insert 1 suppository rectally, up to 4 times/day

Hypotension/shock:

Children:

I.V. bolus: 5-20 mcg/kg/dose every 10-15 minutes as needed

I.V. infusion: 0.1-0.5 mcg/kg/minute

Adults:

I.V. bolus: 0.1-0.5 mg/dose every 10-15 minutes as needed (initial dose should not exceed 0.5 mg)

I.V. infusion: Initial dose: 100-180 mcg/minute; when blood pressure is stabilized, maintenance rate: 40-60 mcg/minute; rates up to 360 mcg/minute have been reported; dosing range: 0.4-9.1 mcg/kg/minute

Nasal decongestant:

Children:

2-6 years:

Intranasal: Instill 1 drop every 2-4 hours of 0.125% solution as needed. (**Note:** Therapy should not exceed 3 continuous days.)

Oral: Tannate salt (NāSop™ suspension): 1.87-3.75 mg every 12 hours

6-12 years:

Intranasal: Instill 1-2 sprays or instill 1-2 drops every 4 hours of 0.25% solution as needed. (**Note:** Therapy should not exceed 3 continuous days.)

Oral:

Hydrochloride salt: 10 mg every 4 hours

Tannate salt (NāSop™ suspension): 3.75-7.5 mg every 12 hours

Children >12 years and Adults:

Intranasal: Instill 1-2 sprays or instill 1-2 drops every 4 hours of 0.25% to 0.5% solution as needed; 1% solution may be used in adult in cases of extreme nasal congestion; do not use nasal solutions more than 3 days

Oral:

Hydrochloride salt: 10-20 mg every 4 hours

Tannate salt (NāSop™ suspension): 7.5-15 mg every 12 hours

Ocular procedures:

Infants <1 year: Instill 1 drop of 2.5% 15-30 minutes before procedures

Children and Adults: Instill 1 drop of 2.5% or 10% solution, may repeat in 10-60 minutes as needed

Ophthalmic irritation (OTC formulation for relief of eye redness): Adults: Instill 1-2 drops 0.12% solution into affected eye, up to 4 times/day; do not use for >72 hours

Paroxysmal supraventricular tachycardia: I.V.:

Children: 5-10 mcg/kg/dose over 20-30 seconds

Adults: 0.25-0.5 mg/dose over 20-30 seconds

Dosage Forms [DSC] = Discontinued product

Cream, rectal, as hydrochloride (Formulation R™): 0.25% (54 g) [contains sodium benzoate]

Injection, solution, as hydrochloride: 1% [10 mg/mL] (1 mL, 5 mL) [may contain sodium metabisulfite]

Neo-Synephrine®: 1% (1 mL) [contains sodium metabisulfite]

Ointment, rectal, as hydrochloride:

Formulation R™: 0.25% (30 g, 60 g) [contains benzoic acid]

Rectacaine: 0.25% (30 g) [contains shark liver oil]

Solution, intranasal drops, as hydrochloride:

Neo-Synephrine® Extra Strength: 1% (15 mL) [contains benzalkonium chloride]

Neo-Synephrine® Regular Strength: 0.5% (15 mL) [contains benzalkonium chloride]

Rhinall: 0.25% (30 mL) [contains benzalkonium chloride and sodium bisulfite]

Solution, intranasal spray, as hydrochloride:

Neo-Synephrine® Extra Strength: 1% (15 mL) [contains benzalkonium chloride]

Neo-Synephrine® Mild: 0.25% (15 mL) [contains benzalkonium chloride]

Neo-Synephrine® Regular Strength: 0.5% (15 mL) [contains benzalkonium chloride]

Rhinall: 0.25% (40 mL) [contains benzalkonium chloride and sodium bisulfite]

Vicks® Sinex®, Vicks® Sinex® UltraFine Mist: 0.5% (15 mL) [contains benzalkonium chloride]

Solution, ophthalmic, as hydrochloride: 2.5% (1 mL, 2 mL, 3 mL, 5 mL, 15 mL) [may contain sodium bisulfite]

AK-Dilate®: 2.5% (2 mL, 15 mL); 10% (5 mL)

Altrafrin: 0.12% (15 mL) [OTC]; 2.5% (5 mL, 15 mL) [RX; contains benzalkonium chloride]; 10% (5 mL) [RX; contains benzalkonium chloride]

Mydfrin®: 2.5% (3 mL, 5 mL) [contains sodium bisulfite]

Neo-Synephrine®: 2.5% (15 mL); 10% (5 mL) [contains benzalkonium chloride] [DSC]

(Continued)

phenylephrine *(Continued)*

Neo-Synephrine® Viscous: 10% (5 mL) [contains benzalkonium chloride] [DSC]
Suppository, rectal, as hydrochloride: 0.25% (12s)
Anu-Med, Tronolane®: 0.25% (12s)
Medicone®: 0.25% (18s, 24s)
Rectacaine: 0.25% (12s) [contains shark liver oil]
Suspension, oral, as tannate (NāSop™): 7.5 mg/5 mL (120 mL) [orange flavor]
Tablet, as hydrochloride (Sudafed PE™): 10 mg
Tablet, chewable, as hydrochloride:
AH-chew® D: 10 mg [DSC]
Tablet, orally dissolving, as hydrochloride (NāSop™): 10 mg [contains phenylalanine 4 mg/tablet; bubble gum flavor]

phenylephrine and chlorpheniramine *see* chlorpheniramine and phenylephrine *on page 176*

phenylephrine and cyclopentolate *see* cyclopentolate and phenylephrine *on page 220*

phenylephrine and promethazine *see* promethazine and phenylephrine *on page 705*

phenylephrine and pyrilamine (fen il EF rin & peer IL a meen)

Synonyms pyrilamine tannate and phenylephrine tannate

U.S./Canadian Brand Names AllanVan-S [US]; Pyrilafen Tannate-12™ [US]; Ry-T 12 [US]; Ryna-12 S™ [US]; Ryna-12™ [US]; V-Tann [US]; Viravan® [US]

Therapeutic Category Antihistamine; Antihistamine/Decongestant Combination; Sympathomimetic

Use Symptomatic relief of nasal congestion and discharge associated with the common cold, sinusitis, allergic rhinitis, and other respiratory tract conditions

Usual Dosage Oral: Relief of cough, congestion (Viravan®):
Children 2-6 years: 2.5 mL of the suspension or 1/2 tablet every 12 hours
Children 6-12 years: 5 mL of the suspension or 1/2 to 1 tablet every 12 hours
Children >12 years and Adults: 5-10 mL of the suspension or 1-2 tablets every 12 hours

Dosage Forms
Suspension:
AllanVan-S: Phenylephrine tannate 12.5 mg and pyrilamine tannate 30 mg per 5 mL (120 mL, 480 mL) [contains sodium benzoate; grape flavor]
Pyrilafen Tannate-12™: Phenylephrine tannate 5 mg and pyrilamine tannate 30 mg per 5 mL (120 mL, 480 mL) [strawberry-black currant flavor]
Ryna-12 S™: Phenylephrine tannate 5 mg and pyrilamine tannate 30 mg per 5 mL (120 mL) [contains benzoic acid; strawberry-currant flavor]
Ry-T 12: Phenylephrine tannate 5 mg and pyrilamine tannate 30 mg per 5 mL (120 mL, 480 mL)
Viravan®, V-Tann: Phenylephrine tannate 12.5 mg and pyrilamine tannate 30 mg per 5 mL (120 mL, 480 mL) [contains sodium benzoate; grape flavor]
Tablet (Ryna-12™): Phenylephrine tannate 25 mg and pyrilamine tannate 60 mg
Tablet, chewable (Viravan®): Phenylephrine tannate 25 mg and pyrilamine tannate 30 mg [dye free; grape flavor]

phenylephrine and scopolamine (fen il EF rin & skoe POL a meen)

Sound-Alike/Look-Alike Issues
Murocoll-2® may be confused with Murocel®

Synonyms scopolamine and phenylephrine

U.S./Canadian Brand Names Murocoll-2® [US]

Therapeutic Category Anticholinergic/Adrenergic Agonist

Use Mydriasis, cycloplegia, and to break posterior synechiae in iritis

Usual Dosage Ophthalmic: Instill 1-2 drops into eye(s); repeat in 5 minutes

Dosage Forms Solution, ophthalmic: Phenylephrine hydrochloride 10% and scopolamine hydrobromide 0.3% (5 mL) [contains benzalkonium chloride and sodium metabisulfite]

phenylephrine and zinc sulfate (fen il EF rin & zingk SUL fate)

Synonyms zinc sulfate and phenylephrine

U.S./Canadian Brand Names Zincfrin® [US-OTC/Can]

Therapeutic Category Adrenergic Agonist Agent

Use Soothe, moisturize, and remove redness due to minor eye irritation

Usual Dosage Ophthalmic: Instill 1-2 drops in eye(s) 2-4 times/day as needed

Dosage Forms Solution, ophthalmic: Phenylephrine hydrochloride 0.12% and zinc sulfate 0.25% (15 mL)

phenylephrine, chlorpheniramine, and carbetapentane *see* carbetapentane, phenylephrine, and chlorpheniramine *on page 147*

phenylephrine, chlorpheniramine, and dextromethorphan *see* chlorpheniramine, phenylephrine, and dextromethorphan *on page 179*

phenylephrine, chlorpheniramine, and phenyltoloxamine *see* chlorpheniramine, phenylephrine, and phenyltoloxamine *on page 181*

phenylephrine, chlorpheniramine, codeine, and potassium iodide *see* chlorpheniramine, phenylephrine, codeine, and potassium iodide *on page 182*

phenylephrine, diphenhydramine, and hydrocodone *see* hydrocodone, phenylephrine, and diphenhydramine *on page 425*

phenylephrine, ephedrine, chlorpheniramine, and carbetapentane *see* chlorpheniramine, ephedrine, phenylephrine, and carbetapentane *on page 178*

phenylephrine hydrochloride *see* phenylephrine *on page 660*

phenylephrine hydrochloride and guaifenesin *see* guaifenesin and phenylephrine *on page 396*

phenylephrine hydrochloride, guaifenesin, and dextromethorphan hydrobromide *see* guaifenesin, dextromethorphan, and phenylephrine *on page 400*

phenylephrine hydrochloride, hydrocodone bitartrate, and chlorpheniramine maleate *see* phenylephrine, hydrocodone, and chlorpheniramine *on this page*

phenylephrine, hydrocodone, and chlorpheniramine

(fen il EF rin, hye droe KOE done, & klor fen IR a meen)

Synonyms chlorpheniramine, phenylephrine, and hydrocodone; dihydrocodeine bitartrate, phenylephrine hydrochloride, and chlorpheniramine maleate; hydrocodone, phenylephrine, and chlorpheniramine; phenylephrine hydrochloride, hydrocodone bitartrate, and chlorpheniramine maleate

U.S./Canadian Brand Names Coughtuss [US]; Cytuss HC [US]; De-Chlor HC [US]; De-Chlor HD [US]; Endal® HD Plus [US]; H-C Tussive [US]; Histinex® HC [US]; Histussin® HC [US]; Hydro PC II Plus [US]; Hydro-PC II [US]; Hydron CP [US]; Maxi-Tuss HCX [US]; Maxi-Tuss HC® [US]; Mintuss HC [US]; Mintuss HD [US]; Mintuss MS [US]; Relacon-HC [US]; Rindal HD Plus [US]; Uni-Tricof HC [US]; Uni-Tuss HC [US]; Z-Cof HC [US]

Therapeutic Category Antihistamine; Antihistamine/Decongestant/Antitussive; Antitussive; Decongestant

Controlled Substance C-III

Use Symptomatic relief of cough and congestion associated with the common cold, sinusitis, or acute upper respiratory tract infections

Usual Dosage Oral:

Children 2-6 years: Z-Cof HC: 1.25-2.5 mL every 4-6 hours (maximum: 10 mL/24 hours)

Children 6-12 years:

- Endagen™-HD, Vanex-HD®: 5 mL 3-4 times/day (maximum: 20 mL/24 hours)
- Histinex® HC, Cytuss HC, Endal® HD Plus: 5 mL every 4 hours (maximum: 20 mL/24 hours)
- Maxi-Tuss HC®, Maxi-Tuss HCX: 2.5 mL every 4 hours (maximum: 15 mL/24 hours)
- Z-Cof HC: 2.5-5 mL every 4-6 hours as needed (maximum: 20 mL/24 hours)

Adults:

- Endagen™-HD, Vanex-HD®: 10 mL 3-4 times/day (maximum: 40 mL/24 hours)
- Histinex® HC, Cytuss HC, Endal® HD Plus: 10 mL every 4 hours (maximum: 40 mL/24 hours)
- Maxi-Tuss HC®, Maxi-Tuss HCX: 5 mL every 4 hours (maximum: 30 mL/24 hours)
- Z-Cof HC: 5-10 mL every 4-6 hours (maximum: 40 mL/24 hours)

Dosage Forms [DSC] = Discontinued product

Liquid: Phenylephrine hydrochloride 5 mg, hydrocodone bitartrate 5 mg, and chlorpheniramine maleate 2 mg per 5 mL (480 mL); phenylephrine hydrochloride 10 mg, hydrocodone bitartrate 2.5 mg, and chlorpheniramine maleate 4 mg per 5 mL (480 mL); phenylephrine hydrochloride 10 mg, hydrocodone bitartrate 5 mg, and chlorpheniramine maleate 2 mg per 5 mL (480 mL)

- Coughtuss: Phenylephrine hydrochloride 5 mg, hydrocodone bitartrate 5 mg, and chlorpheniramine maleate 2 mg per 5 mL (480 mL) [alcohol free, sugar free]
- De-Chlor HC: Phenylephrine hydrochloride 10 mg, hydrocodone bitartrate 2.5 mg, and chlorpheniramine maleate 2 mg per 5 mL (480 mL) [cherry flavor]
- De-Chlor HD: Phenylephrine hydrochloride 10 mg, hydrocodone bitartrate 2.5 mg, and chlorpheniramine maleate 4 mg per 5 mL (480 mL) [cherry flavor]
- Endal® HD Plus: Phenylephrine hydrochloride 7.5 mg, hydrocodone bitartrate 3.5 mg, and chlorpheniramine maleate 2 mg per 5 mL (480 mL) [alcohol free, sugar free; black raspberry flavor]

(Continued)

phenylephrine, hydrocodone, and chlorpheniramine *(Continued)*

Hydron CP: Phenylephrine hydrochloride 10 mg, hydrocodone bitartrate 5 mg, and chlorpheniramine maleate 2 mg per 5 mL (480 mL) [pineapple-orange flavor]

Hydro PC II Plus: Phenylephrine hydrochloride 7.5 mg, hydrocodone bitartrate 3.5 mg, and chlorpheniramine maleate 2 mg per 5 mL (480 mL) [strawberry flavor]

Maxi-Tuss HCX: Phenylephrine hydrochloride 12 mg, hydrocodone bitartrate 6 mg and chlorpheniramine maleate 2 mg per 5 mL (480 mL) [alcohol free, sugar free; contains aspartame; vanilla bean flavor]

Relacon-HC: Phenylephrine hydrochloride 10 mg, hydrocodone bitartrate 3.5 mg, and chlorpheniramine maleate 2.5 mg per 5 mL (480 mL) [raspberry flavor]

Uni-Tricof HC: Phenylephrine hydrochloride 5 mg, hydrocodone bitartrate 1.67 mg, and chlorpheniramine maleate 2 mg per 5 mL (480 mL) [strawberry flavor]

Vanex-HD®: Phenylephrine hydrochloride 5 mg, hydrocodone bitartrate 1.7 mg, and chlorpheniramine maleate 2 mg per 5 mL (480 mL) [dye free; cherry flavor] [DSC]

Z-Cof HC: Phenylephrine hydrochloride 10 mg, hydrocodone bitartrate 3.5 mg, and chlorpheniramine maleate 2.5 mg per 5 mL (480 mL) [alcohol free, sugar free; raspberry flavor]

Syrup:

Cytuss HC: Phenylephrine hydrochloride 5 mg, hydrocodone bitartrate 2.5 mg, and chlorpheniramine maleate 2 mg per 5 mL (480 mL) [peach flavor]

Endagen™-HD: Phenylephrine hydrochloride 5 mg, hydrocodone bitartrate 1.7 mg, and chlorpheniramine maleate 2 mg per 5 mL (480 mL) [cherry flavor] [DSC]

H-C Tussive: Phenylephrine hydrochloride 5 mg, hydrocodone bitartrate 2.5 mg, and chlorpheniramine maleate 2 mg per 5 mL (120 mL, 480 mL, 4000 mL) [orange-pineapple flavor]

Histinex® HC: Phenylephrine hydrochloride 5 mg, hydrocodone bitartrate 2.5 mg, and chlorpheniramine maleate 2 mg per 5 mL (480 mL, 960 mL) [alcohol free, sugar free; contains sodium benzoate]

Histussin® HC: Phenylephrine hydrochloride 5 mg, hydrocodone bitartrate 2.5 mg, and chlorpheniramine maleate 2 mg per 5 mL (480 mL) [alcohol free, sugar free; orange-pineapple flavor]

Hydro-PC II: Phenylephrine hydrochloride 7.5 mg, hydrocodone bitartrate 2 mg, and chlorpheniramine maleate 2 mg per 5 mL (480 mL) [strawberry flavor]

Maxi-Tuss HC®: Phenylephrine hydrochloride 10 mg, hydrocodone bitartrate 2.5 mg, and chlorpheniramine maleate 4 mg per 5 mL (480 mL) [orange flavor]

Mintuss HC: Phenylephrine hydrochloride 10 mg, hydrocodone bitartrate 2.5 mg, and chlorpheniramine maleate 2 mg per 5 mL (480 mL) [alcohol free; contains sodium benzoate; black cherry flavor]

Mintuss HD: Phenylephrine hydrochloride 10 mg, hydrocodone bitartrate 2.5 mg, and chlorpheniramine maleate 4 mg per 5 mL (480 mL) [alcohol free; contains sodium benzoate; cherry flavor]

Mintuss MS: Phenylephrine hydrochloride 10 mg, hydrocodone bitartrate 5 mg, and chlorpheniramine maleate 2 mg per 5 mL (480 mL) [alcohol free; contains sodium benzoate; orange flavor]

Rindal HD Plus: Phenylephrine hydrochloride 7.5 mg, hydrocodone bitartrate 3.5 mg, and chlorpheniramine maleate 2 mg per 5 mL (480 mL) [alcohol free, sugar free; contains sodium benzoate; black raspberry flavor]

Uni-Tuss HC: Phenylephrine hydrochloride 5 mg, hydrocodone bitartrate 1.67 mg, and chlorpheniramine maleate 2 mg per 5 mL (480 mL) [sugar free; orange flavor]

phenylephrine, hydrocodone, chlorpheniramine, acetaminophen, and caffeine *see* hydrocodone, chlorpheniramine, phenylephrine, acetaminophen, and caffeine *on page 424*

phenylephrine, promethazine, and codeine *see* promethazine, phenylephrine, and codeine *on page 705*

phenylephrine, pyrilamine, and dextromethorphan

(fen il EF rin, peer IL a meen, & deks troe meth OR fan)

Synonyms dextromethorphan tannate, pyrilamine tannate, and phenylephrine tannate; pyrilamine maleate, dextromethorphan hydrobromide, and phenylephrine hydrochloride

U.S./Canadian Brand Names AllanVan-DM [US]; Codal-DM [US-OTC]; Codimal® DM [US-OTC]; Coditussᴬ DM [US-OTC]; Tannate-V-DM [US]; Viravan®-DM [US]

Therapeutic Category Antihistamine; Antihistamine/Decongestant/Antitussive; Antitussive; Sympathomimetic

Use Symptomatic relief of cough, nasal congestion, and discharge associated with the common cold, sinusitis, allergic rhinitis, and other respiratory tract conditions

Usual Dosage Oral: Relief of cough, congestion:

Children 2-6 years (Viravan®-DM): 2.5 mL of the suspension or 1/2 tablet every 12 hours

Children 6-12 years:

Codimal® DM: 5 mL every 4 hours; maximum: 30 mL/24 hours

Viravan®-DM: 5 mL of the suspension or 1/2 to 1 tablet every 12 hours

Children >12 years and Adults:
Codimal® DM: 10 mL every 4 hours; maximum: 60 mL/24 hours
Viravan®-DM: 5-10 mL of the suspension or 1-2 tablets every 12 hours

Dosage Forms

Suspension:
AllanVan-DM, Tannate-V-DM, Viravan®-DM: Phenylephrine tannate 12.5 mg, pyrilamine tannate 30 mg, and dextromethorphan tannate 25 mg per 5 mL (480 mL) [contains sodium benzoate; grape flavor]

Syrup:
Codal-DM: Phenylephrine hydrochloride 5 mg, pyrilamine maleate 8.33 mg, and dextromethorphan hydrobromide 10 mg (480 mL) [cherry flavor]
Codimal® DM: Phenylephrine hydrochloride 5 mg, pyrilamine maleate 8.33 mg, and dextromethorphan hydrobromide 10 mg (120 mL, 480 mL) [alcohol free, dye free, sugar free; contains benzoic acid]
Codituss DM: Phenylephrine hydrochloride 5 mg, pyrilamine maleate 8.33 mg, and dextromethorphan hydrobromide 10 mg (120 mL, 480 mL) [alcohol free, dye free, sugar free; cherry punch flavor]

Tablet, chewable:
Viravan®-DM: Phenylephrine tannate 25 mg, pyrilamine tannate 30 mg, and dextromethorphan tannate 25 mg [dye free; grape flavor]

phenylephrine tannate *see* phenylephrine *on page 660*

phenylephrine tannate, chlorpheniramine tannate, and methscopolamine nitrate *see* chlorpheniramine, phenylephrine, and methscopolamine *on page 180*

phenylethylmalonylurea *see* phenobarbital *on page 658*

Phenylfenesin® L.A. *(Discontinued)*

Phenylgesic [US-OTC] *see* acetaminophen and phenyltoloxamine *on page 8*

phenyltoloxamine, chlorpheniramine, and phenylephrine *see* chlorpheniramine, phenylephrine, and phenyltoloxamine *on page 181*

phenyltoloxamine citrate and acetaminophen *see* acetaminophen and phenyltoloxamine *on page 8*

Phenytek™ [US] *see* phenytoin *on this page*

phenytoin (FEN i toyn)

Sound-Alike/Look-Alike Issues
phenytoin may be confused with phenelzine, phentermine
Dilantin® may be confused with Dilaudid®, diltiazem, Dipentum®

Synonyms diphenylhydantoin; DPH; phenytoin sodium; phenytoin sodium, extended; phenytoin sodium, prompt

U.S./Canadian Brand Names Dilantin® [US/Can]; Phenytek™ [US]

Therapeutic Category Antiarrhythmic Agent, Class I-B; Hydantoin

Use Management of generalized tonic-clonic (grand mal), complex partial seizures; prevention of seizures following head trauma/neurosurgery

Usual Dosage

Status epilepticus: I.V.:
Infants and Children: Loading dose: 15-20 mg/kg in a single or divided dose; maintenance dose: Initial: 5 mg/kg/day in 2 divided doses; usual doses:
6 months to 3 years: 8-10 mg/kg/day
4-6 years: 7.5-9 mg/kg/day
7-9 years: 7-8 mg/kg/day
10-16 years: 6-7 mg/kg/day, some patients may require every 8 hours dosing
Adults: Loading dose: Manufacturer recommends 10-15 mg/kg, however, 15-25 mg/kg has been used clinically; maintenance dose: 300 mg/day or 5-6 mg/kg/day in 3 divided doses or 1-2 divided doses using extended release

Anticonvulsant: Children and Adults: Oral:
Loading dose: 15-20 mg/kg; based on phenytoin serum concentrations and recent dosing history; administer oral loading dose in 3 divided doses given every 2-4 hours to decrease GI adverse effects and to ensure complete oral absorption; maintenance dose: same as I.V.
Neurosurgery (prophylactic): 100-200 mg at approximately 4-hour intervals during surgery and during the immediate postoperative period

Dosage Forms

Capsule, extended release, as sodium: 100 mg
Dilantin®: 30 mg [contains sodium benzoate], 100 mg
Phenytek™: 200 mg, 300 mg
(Continued)

phenytoin *(Continued)*

Capsule, prompt release, as sodium: 100 mg
Injection, solution, as sodium: 50 mg/mL (2 mL, 5 mL) [contains alcohol and propylene glycol]
Suspension, oral: 125 mg/5 mL (240 mL)
Dilantin®: 125 mg/5 mL (240 mL) [contains alcohol <0.6%, sodium benzoate; orange vanilla flavor]
Tablet, chewable:
Dilantin®: 50 mg

phenytoin sodium *see* phenytoin *on previous page*

phenytoin sodium, extended *see* phenytoin *on previous page*

phenytoin sodium, prompt *see* phenytoin *on previous page*

Pherazine® VC With Codeine *(Discontinued)* *see* promethazine, phenylephrine, and codeine *on page 705*

Pherazine® With Codeine *(Discontinued)* *see* promethazine and codeine *on page 704*

Pherazine® With DM *(Discontinued)* *see* promethazine and dextromethorphan *on page 704*

Phillips'® M-O [US-OTC] *see* magnesium hydroxide and mineral oil *on page 514*

Phillips'® Fibercaps [US-OTC] *see* polycarbophil *on page 678*

Phillips'® Milk of Magnesia [US-OTC] *see* magnesium hydroxide *on page 514*

Phillips'® Stool Softener Laxative [US-OTC] *see* docusate *on page 270*

pHisoHex® [US/Can] *see* hexachlorophene *on page 414*

PHL-Amoxicillin [Can] *see* amoxicillin *on page 47*

PHL-Citalopram [Can] *see* citalopram *on page 194*

PHL-Fenofibrate Supra [Can] *see* fenofibrate *on page 338*

PHL-Methimazole [Can] *see* methimazole *on page 539*

PHL-Sumatriptan [Can] *see* sumatriptan *on page 801*

PHL-Topiramate [Can] *see* topiramate *on page 836*

Phos-Flur® [US] *see* fluoride *on page 354*

Phos-Flur® Rinse [US-OTC] *see* fluoride *on page 354*

PhosLo® [US] *see* calcium acetate *on page 134*

Phos-NaK [US] *see* potassium phosphate and sodium phosphate *on page 688*

Phospha 250™ Neutral [US] *see* potassium phosphate and sodium phosphate *on page 688*

phosphate, potassium *see* potassium phosphate *on page 687*

Phospholine Iodide® [US] *see* echothiophate iodide *on page 285*

phosphonoformate *see* foscarnet *on page 369*

phosphonoformic acid *see* foscarnet *on page 369*

phosphorated carbohydrate solution *see* fructose, dextrose, and phosphoric acid *on page 371*

phosphoric acid, levulose and dextrose *see* fructose, dextrose, and phosphoric acid *on page 371*

Photofrin® [US/Can] *see* porfimer *on page 682*

Phoxal-timolol [Can] *see* timolol *on page 828*

Phrenilin® With Caffeine and Codeine [US] *see* butalbital, aspirin, caffeine, and codeine *on page 129*

***p*-hydroxyampicillin** *see* amoxicillin *on page 47*

Phyllocontin® [Can] *see* aminophylline *on page 42*

Phyllocontin®-350 [Can] *see* aminophylline *on page 42*

phylloquinone *see* phytonadione *on next page*

physostigmine (fye zoe STIG meen)

Sound-Alike/Look-Alike Issues

physostigmine may be confused with Prostigmin®, pyridostigmine

Synonyms eserine salicylate; physostigmine salicylate; physostigmine sulfate
U.S./Canadian Brand Names Eserine® [Can]; Isopto® Eserine [Can]
Therapeutic Category Cholinesterase Inhibitor
Use Reverse toxic CNS effects caused by anticholinergic drugs
Usual Dosage
Children: Anticholinergic drug overdose: Reserve for life-threatening situations only: I.V.: 0.01-0.03 mg/kg/dose (maximum: 0.5 mg/minute); may repeat after 5-10 minutes to a maximum total dose of 2 mg or until response occurs or adverse cholinergic effects occur
Adults: Anticholinergic drug overdose:
I.M., I.V., SubQ: 0.5-2 mg to start, repeat every 20 minutes until response occurs or adverse effect occurs
Repeat 1-4 mg every 30-60 minutes as life-threatening signs (arrhythmias, seizures, deep coma) recur; maximum I.V. rate: 1 mg/minute
Dosage Forms Injection, solution, as salicylate: 1 mg/mL (2 mL) [contains benzyl alcohol and sodium metabisulfite]

physostigmine salicylate *see* physostigmine *on previous page*
physostigmine sulfate *see* physostigmine *on previous page*
phytomenadione *see* phytonadione *on this page*

phytonadione (fye toe na DYE one)

Sound-Alike/Look-Alike Issues
Mephyton® may be confused with melphalan, methadone
Synonyms methylphytyl napthoquinone; phylloquinone; phytomenadione; vitamin K_1
U.S./Canadian Brand Names AquaMEPHYTON® [Can]; Konakion [Can]; Mephyton® [US/Can]
Therapeutic Category Vitamin, Fat Soluble
Use Prevention and treatment of hypoprothrombinemia caused by coumarin derivative-induced or other drug-induced vitamin K deficiency, hypoprothrombinemia caused by malabsorption or inability to synthesize vitamin K; hemorrhagic disease of the newborn
Usual Dosage SubQ is the preferred (per manufacturer) parenteral route; I.V. route should be restricted for emergency use only
Minimum daily requirement: Not well established
Infants: 1-5 mcg/kg/day
Adults: 0.03 mcg/kg/day
Hemorrhagic disease of the newborn:
Prophylaxis: I.M.: 0.5-1 mg within 1 hour of birth
Treatment: I.M., SubQ: 1-2 mg/dose/day
Oral anticoagulant overdose:
Infants and Children:
No bleeding, rapid reversal needed, patient **will require** further oral anticoagulant therapy: SubQ, I.V.: 0.5-2 mg
No bleeding, rapid reversal needed, patient **will not require** further oral anticoagulant therapy: SubQ, I.V.: 2-5 mg
Significant bleeding, not life-threatening: SubQ, I.V.: 0.5-2 mg
Significant bleeding, life-threatening: I.V.: 5 mg over 10-20 minutes
Adults: Oral, I.V., SubQ: 1-10 mg/dose depending on degree of INR elevation
Serious bleeding or major overdose: 10 mg I.V. (slow infusion); may repeat every 12 hours (have required doses up to 25 mg)
Vitamin K deficiency: Due to drugs, malabsorption, or decreased synthesis of vitamin K
Infants and Children:
Oral: 2.5-5 mg/24 hours
I.M., I.V., SubQ: 1-2 mg/dose as a single dose
Adults:
Oral: 5-25 mg/24 hours
I.M., I.V., SubQ: 10 mg
Dosage Forms
Injection, aqueous colloidal: 2 mg/mL (0.5 mL); 10 mg/mL (1 mL) [contains benzyl alcohol]
Tablet: 5 mg

α_1-PI *see* alpha$_1$-proteinase inhibitor *on page 31*
pidorubicin *see* epirubicin *on page 297*
pidorubicin hydrochloride *see* epirubicin *on page 297*
Pilagan® Ophthalmic *(Discontinued)* *see* pilocarpine *on next page*

pilocarpine (pye loe KAR peen)

Sound-Alike/Look-Alike Issues

Isopto® Carpine may be confused with Isopto® Carbachol

Salagen® may be confused with Salacid®, selegiline

Synonyms pilocarpine hydrochloride

U.S./Canadian Brand Names Diocarpine [Can]; Isopto® Carpine [US/Can]; Pilopine HS® [US/Can]; Salagen® [US/Can]

Therapeutic Category Cholinergic Agent

Use

Ophthalmic: Management of chronic simple glaucoma, chronic and acute angle-closure glaucoma

Oral: Symptomatic treatment of xerostomia caused by salivary gland hypofunction resulting from radiotherapy for cancer of the head and neck or Sjögren syndrome

Usual Dosage Adults:

Ophthalmic: Glaucoma:

Solution: Instill 1-2 drops up to 6 times/day; adjust the concentration and frequency as required to control elevated intraocular pressure

Gel: Instill 0.5" ribbon into lower conjunctival sac once daily at bedtime

Oral: Xerostomia:

Following head and neck cancer: 5 mg 3 times/day, titration up to 10 mg 3 times/day may be considered for patients who have not responded adequately; do not exceed 2 tablets/dose

Sjögren's syndrome: 5 mg 4 times/day

Dosage Forms

Gel, ophthalmic, as hydrochloride (Pilopine HS®): 4% (4 g) [contains benzalkonium chloride]

Solution, ophthalmic, as hydrochloride: 0.5% (15 mL); 1% (2 mL, 15 mL); 2% (2 mL, 15 mL); 3% (15 mL); 4% (2 mL, 15 mL); 6% (15 mL) [may contain benzalkonium chloride]

Isopto® Carpine: 1% (15 mL); 2% (15 mL); 4% (15 mL) [contains benzalkonium chloride]

Tablet, as hydrochloride: 5 mg

Salagen®: 5 mg, 7.5 mg

pilocarpine hydrochloride *see* pilocarpine *on this page*

Pilopine HS® [US/Can] *see* pilocarpine *on this page*

Pilostat® Ophthalmic *(Discontinued)* *see* pilocarpine *on this page*

Pima® [US] *see* potassium iodide *on page 686*

pimaricin *see* natamycin *on page 580*

pimecrolimus (pim e KROE li mus)

U.S./Canadian Brand Names Elidel® [US/Can]

Therapeutic Category Immunosuppressant Agent; Topical Skin Product

Use Short-term and intermittent long-term treatment of mild to moderate atopic dermatitis in patients not responsive to conventional therapy or when conventional therapy is not appropriate

Usual Dosage Children ≥2 years and Adults: Topical: Apply thin layer to affected area twice daily; rub in gently and completely. **Note:** Limit application to involved areas. Continue as long as signs and symptoms persist; discontinue if resolution occurs; re-evaluate if symptoms persist >6 weeks.

Dosage Forms Cream, topical: 1% (30 g, 60 g, 100 g)

pimozide (PI moe zide)

U.S./Canadian Brand Names Apo-Pimozide® [Can]; Orap® [US/Can]

Therapeutic Category Neuroleptic Agent

Use Suppression of severe motor and phonic tics in patients with Tourette disorder who have failed to respond satisfactorily to standard treatment

Usual Dosage Oral: **Note:** An ECG should be performed baseline and periodically thereafter, especially during dosage adjustment:

Children ≤12 years: Tourette disorder: Initial: 0.05 mg/kg preferably once at bedtime; may be increased every third day; usual range: 2-4 mg/day; do not exceed 10 mg/day (0.2 mg/kg/day)

Children >12 years and Adults: Tourette disorder: Initial: 1-2 mg/day in divided doses, then increase dosage as needed every other day; range is usually 7-16 mg/day, maximum dose: 10 mg/day or 0.2 mg/kg/day are not generally recommended

Note: Sudden unexpected deaths have occurred in patients taking doses >10 mg. Therefore, dosages exceeding 10 mg/day are generally not recommended.

Dosage Forms Tablet: 1 mg, 2 mg

Pin-X® [US-OTC] *see* pyrantel pamoate *on page 719*

pinaverium bromide *see* pinaverium *(Canada only)* *on this page*

pinaverium *(Canada only)* (pin ah VEER ee um)

Synonyms pinaverium bromide

U.S./Canadian Brand Names Dicetel® [Can]

Therapeutic Category Calcium Antagonist; Gastrointestinal Agent, Miscellaneous

Use Treatment and relief of symptoms associated with irritable bowel syndrome (IBS); treatment of symptoms related to functional disorders of the biliary tract

Usual Dosage Oral: Adults: 50 mg 3 times/day; in exceptional cases, the dosage may be increased up to 100 mg 3 times/day (maximum dose: 300 mg/day). Tablets should be taken with a full glass of water during a meal/snack.

Dosage Forms [CAN] = Canadian brand name

Tablet:

Dicetel® [CAN]: 50 mg, 100 mg [not available in the U.S.]

pindolol (PIN doe lole)

Sound-Alike/Look-Alike Issues

pindolol may be confused with Parlodel®, Plendil®

Visken® may be confused with Visine®

U.S./Canadian Brand Names Apo-Pindol® [Can]; Gen-Pindolol [Can]; Novo-Pindol [Can]; Nu-Pindol [Can]; PMS-Pindolol [Can]; Visken® [Can]

Therapeutic Category Beta-Adrenergic Blocker

Use Management of hypertension

Usual Dosage Oral: Adults:

Hypertension: Initial: 5 mg twice daily, increase as necessary by 10 mg/day every 3-4 weeks (maximum daily dose: 60 mg); usual dose range (JNC 7): 10-40 mg twice daily

Antidepressant augmentation: 2.5 mg 3 times/day

Dosage Forms Tablet: 5 mg, 10 mg

pink bismuth *see* bismuth subsalicylate *on page 112*

Pin-Rid® ***(Discontinued)*** *see* pyrantel pamoate *on page 719*

pioglitazone (pye oh GLI ta zone)

Sound-Alike/Look-Alike Issues

Actos® may be confused with Actidose®, Actonel®

U.S./Canadian Brand Names Actos® [US/Can]

Therapeutic Category Antidiabetic Agent; Thiazolidinedione Derivative

Use

Type 2 diabetes mellitus (noninsulin dependent, NIDDM), monotherapy: Adjunct to diet and exercise, to improve glycemic control

Type 2 diabetes mellitus (noninsulin dependent, NIDDM), combination therapy with sulfonylurea, metformin, or insulin: When diet, exercise, and a single agent alone does not result in adequate glycemic control

Usual Dosage Oral: Adults:

Monotherapy: Initial: 15-30 mg once daily; if response is inadequate, the dosage may be increased in increments up to 45 mg once daily; maximum recommended dose: 45 mg once daily

Combination therapy: Maximum recommended dose: 45 mg/day

With sulfonylureas: Initial: 15-30 mg once daily; dose of sulfonylurea should be reduced if the patient reports hypoglycemia

With metformin: Initial: 15-30 mg once daily; it is unlikely that the dose of metformin will need to be reduced due to hypoglycemia

With insulin: Initial: 15-30 mg once daily; dose of insulin should be reduced by 10% to 25% if the patient reports hypoglycemia or if the plasma glucose falls to <100 mg/dL.

Dosage adjustment in patients with CHF (NYHA Class II) in mono- or combination therapy: Initial: 15 mg once daily; may be increased after several months of treatment, with close attention to heart failure symptoms

Dosage Forms

Tablet:

Actos®: 15 mg, 30 mg, 45 mg

piperacillin (pi PER a sil in)

Synonyms piperacillin sodium

U.S./Canadian Brand Names Piperacillin for Injection, USP [Can]

Therapeutic Category Penicillin

Use Treatment of susceptible infections such as septicemia, acute and chronic respiratory tract infections, skin and soft tissue infections, and urinary tract infections due to susceptible strains of *Pseudomonas*, *Proteus*, and *Escherichia coli* and *Enterobacter*; active against some streptococci and some anaerobic bacteria; febrile neutropenia (as part of combination regimen)

Usual Dosage

Usual dosage range:

Neonates: I.M., I.V.: 100 mg/kg every 12 hours

Infants and Children: I.M., I.V.: 200-300 mg/kg/day in divided doses every 4-6 hours

Adults: I.M., I.V.: 2-4 g/dose every 4-6 hours (maximum: 24 g/day)

Indication-specific dosing:

Children: I.M., I.V.:

Cystic fibrosis: 350-500 mg/kg/day in divided doses every 4-6 hours

Adults:

Burn wound sepsis: I.V.: 4 g every 4 hours with vancomycin and amikacin

Cholangitis, acute: I.V.: 4 g every 6 hours

Keratitis *(Pseudomonas):* Ophthalmic: 6-12 mg/mL every 15-60 minutes around the clock for 24-72 hours, then slow reduction

Malignant otitis externa: I.V.: 4-6 g every 4-6 hours with tobramycin

Moderate infections: I.M., I.V.: 2-3 g/dose every 6-12 hours (maximum: 2 g I.M./site)

Prosthetic joint *(Pseudomonas):* I.V.: 3 g every 6 hours with aminoglycoside

***Pseudomonas* infections:** I.V.: 4 g every 4 hours

Severe infections: I.M., I.V.: 3-4 g/dose every 4-6 hours (maximum: 24 g/24 hours)

Urinary tract infections: I.V.: 2-3 g/dose every 6-12 hours

Uncomplicated gonorrhea: I.M.: 2 g in a single dose accompanied by 1 g probenecid 30 minutes prior to injection

Dosage Forms Injection, powder for reconstitution: 2 g, 3 g, 4 g, 40 g

piperacillin and tazobactam sodium (pi PER a sil in & ta zoe BAK tam SOW dee um)

Sound-Alike/Look-Alike Issues

Zosyn® may be confused with Zofran®, Zyvox™

Synonyms piperacillin sodium and tazobactam sodium; tazobactam and piperacillin

U.S./Canadian Brand Names Tazocin® [Can]; Zosyn® [US]

Therapeutic Category Penicillin

Use Treatment of moderate-to-severe infections caused by susceptible organisms, including infections of the lower respiratory tract (community-acquired pneumonia, nosocomial pneumonia); urinary tract; uncomplicated and complicated skin and skin structures; gynecologic (endometritis, pelvic inflammatory disease); bone and joint infections; intraabdominal infections (appendicitis with rupture/abscess, peritonitis); and septicemia. Tazobactam expands activity of piperacillin to include beta-lactamase producing strains of *S. aureus*, *H. influenzae*, *Bacteroides*, and other gram-negative bacteria.

Usual Dosage

Usual dosage range:

Adults: I.V.: 2.25-4.5 g every 6-8 hours; maximum: Piperacillin 18 g/day

Indication-specific dosing: I.V.:

Children: **Note:** Dosing based on piperacillin component:

Appendicitis, peritonitis:

2-9 months: 80 mg/kg every 8 hours

≥9 months and ≤40 kg: 100 mg/kg every 8 hours

>40 kg: refer to Adult dosing

Adults:

Diverticulitis, intraabdominal abscess, peritonitis: I.V.: 4.5 g every 8 hours or 3.375 g every 6 hours

Moderate infections: I.M.: 2.25 g every 6-8 hours; treatment should be continued for ≥7-10 days depending on severity of disease (**Note:** I.M. route not FDA-approved)

Pneumonia (nosocomial): I.V.: 4.5 g every 6 hours for 7-14 days (when used empirically, combination with an aminoglycoside is recommended; consider discontinuation of aminoglycoside if *P. aeruginosa* is not isolated)

Severe infections: I.V.: 4.5 g every 8 hours or 3.375 g every 6 hours for 7-10 days

Dosage Forms Note: 8:1 ratio of piperacillin sodium/tazobactam sodium

Infusion [premixed iso-osmotic solution, frozen]:

2.25 g: Piperacillin 2 g and tazobactam 0.25 g (50 mL) [contains sodium 5.58 mEq (128 mg) and EDTA]

3.375 g: Piperacillin 3 g and tazobactam 0.375 g (50 mL) [contains sodium 8.38 mEq (192 mg) and EDTA]
4.5 g: Piperacillin 4 g and tazobactam 0.5 g (50 mL) [contains sodium 11.17 mEq (256 mg) and EDTA]
Injection, powder for reconstitution:
2.25 g: Piperacillin 2 g and tazobactam 0.25 g [contains sodium 5.58 mEq (128 mg) and EDTA]
3.375 g: Piperacillin 3 g and tazobactam 0.375 g [contains sodium 8.38 mEq (192 mg) and EDTA]
4.5 g: Piperacillin 4 g and tazobactam 0.5 g [contains sodium 11.17 mEq (256 mg) and EDTA]
40.5 g: Piperacillin 36 g and tazobactam 4.5 g [contains sodium 100.4 mEq (2304 mg) and EDTA; bulk pharmacy vial]

Piperacillin for Injection, USP [Can] *see* piperacillin *on previous page*

piperacillin sodium *see* piperacillin *on previous page*

piperacillin sodium and tazobactam sodium *see* piperacillin and tazobactam sodium *on previous page*

piperazine estrone sulfate *see* estropipate *on page 314*

piperonyl butoxide and pyrethrins *see* pyrethrins and piperonyl butoxide *on page 720*

Pipracil® *(Discontinued)* *see* piperacillin *on previous page*

pirbuterol (peer BYOO ter ole)

Synonyms pirbuterol acetate

U.S./Canadian Brand Names Maxair™ Autohaler™ [US]

Therapeutic Category Adrenergic Agonist Agent

Use Prevention and treatment of reversible bronchospasm including asthma

Usual Dosage Children ≥12 years and Adults: 2 inhalations every 4-6 hours for prevention; two inhalations at an interval of at least 1-3 minutes, followed by a third inhalation in treatment of bronchospasm, not to exceed 12 inhalations/day

Dosage Forms Aerosol for oral inhalation, as acetate:
Maxair™ Autohaler™: 14 g [400 inhalations; contains chlorofluorocarbons]

pirbuterol acetate *see* pirbuterol *on this page*

piroxicam (peer OKS i kam)

U.S./Canadian Brand Names Apo-Piroxicam® [Can]; Feldene® [US]; Gen-Piroxicam [Can]; Novo-Pirocam [Can]; Nu-Pirox [Can]; Pexicam® [Can]

Therapeutic Category Analgesic, Nonnarcotic; Nonsteroidal Antiinflammatory Drug (NSAID)

Use Symptomatic treatment of acute and chronic rheumatoid arthritis and osteoarthritis

Usual Dosage Oral: Adults: 10-20 mg/day once daily; although associated with increase in GI adverse effects, doses >20 mg/day have been used (ie, 30-40 mg/day)

Dosage Forms Capsule: 10 mg, 20 mg

***p*-isobutylhydratropic acid** *see* ibuprofen *on page 437*

pit *see* oxytocin *on page 630*

Pitocin® [US/Can] *see* oxytocin *on page 630*

Pitressin® [US] *see* vasopressin *on page 868*

Pitrex [Can] *see* tolnaftate *on page 834*

pit viper antivenin *see* antivenin *(Crotalidae)* polyvalent *on page 63*

pivampicilin *see* pivampicillin *(Canada only) on this page*

pivampicillin *(Canada only)* (piv am pi SIL in)

Synonyms MK-191; pivampicilin

U.S./Canadian Brand Names Pondocillin® [Can]

Therapeutic Category Penicillin

Use Treatment of susceptible bacterial infections (nonbeta-lactamase-producing organisms); susceptible bacterial infections caused by streptococci, pneumococci, nonpenicillinase-producing staphylococci, *H. influenzae, N. gonorrhoeae, E. coli, P. mirabilis, Listeria, Salmonella, Shigella, Enterobacter*, and *Klebsiella*

Usual Dosage Oral:
Infants and Children: Bacterial infections: Oral suspension:
Infants <3 months: Use of pivampicillin in this age group should be avoided
Infants 3-12 months: Dosage range: 40-60 mg/kg/day in 2 divided doses
(Continued)

pivampicillin *(Canada only)* *(Continued)*

Children ≤10 years: Dosage range: 25-35 mg/kg/day, not to exceed recommended daily adult dose of 500 mg twice daily

Alternatively: Children:

1-3 years: 175 mg twice daily

4-6 years: 262.5 mg twice daily

7-10 years: 350 mg twice daily

Children >10 years and Adults: Usual dose: 500 mg (tablet) or 525 mg (suspension) twice daily; dosage may be doubled in severe infections

Gonococcal urethritis: 1.5 g as a single dose with 1 g probenecid concurrently

Dosage Forms [CAN] = Canadian brand name

Powder for oral suspension:

Pondocillin® [CAN]: 175 mg/5 mL (100 mL, 150 mL, 200 mL) [banana and vanilla flavors] not available in the U.S.]

Tablet:

Pondocillin® [CAN]: 500 mg [equivalent to 377 mg ampicillin] [not available in the U.S.]

pix carbonis *see* coal tar *on page 207*

pizotifen *(Canada only)* (pi ZOE ti fen)

Synonyms pizotifen malate

U.S./Canadian Brand Names Sandomigran DS® [Can]; Sandomigran® [Can]

Therapeutic Category Antimigraine Agent

Use Migraine prophylaxis

Usual Dosage Oral: Children ≥12 years and Adults: Migraine prophylaxis: Initial: 0.5 mg at bedtime; increase gradually to 0.5 mg 3 times/day; usual dosage range: 1-6 mg/day

Note: Therapeutic response may require several weeks of therapy. Do not discontinue abruptly (reduce gradually over 2-week period).

Dosage Forms [CAN] = Canadian brand name

Tablet:

Sandomigran® [CAN]: 0.5 mg [pizotifen malate 0.73 mg]

Tablet, double strength:

Sandomigran® DS [CAN]: 1 mg [pizotifen malate 1.46 mg]

pizotifen malate *see* pizotifen *(Canada only) on this page*

Plan B® [US/Can] *see* levonorgestrel *on page 491*

plantago seed *see* psyllium *on page 717*

plantain seed *see* psyllium *on page 717*

Plaquase® *(Discontinued)* *see* collagenase *on page 212*

Plaquenil® [US/Can] *see* hydroxychloroquine *on page 431*

Plaretase® 8000 [US] *see* pancrelipase *on page 634*

Plasbumin® [US] *see* albumin *on page 22*

Plasbumin®-5 [Can] *see* albumin *on page 22*

Plasbumin®-25 [Can] *see* albumin *on page 22*

Plasmanate® [US] *see* plasma protein fraction *on this page*

Plasma-Plex® *(Discontinued)* *see* plasma protein fraction *on this page*

plasma protein fraction (PLAS mah PROE teen FRAK shun)

U.S./Canadian Brand Names Plasmanate® [US]

Therapeutic Category Blood Product Derivative

Use Plasma volume expansion and maintenance of cardiac output in the treatment of certain types of shock or impending shock

Usual Dosage I.V.: 250-1500 mL/day

Dosage Forms Injection, solution [human]: 5% (50 mL, 250 mL) [contains sodium 145 mEq/L]

Plasmatein® *(Discontinued)* *see* plasma protein fraction *on this page*

Platinol®-AQ *(Discontinued)* *see* cisplatin *on page 193*

Plavix® [US/Can] *see* clopidogrel *on page 204*

Plegine® [Can] *see* phendimetrazine *on page 657*
Plegine® *(Discontinued)* *see* phendimetrazine *on page 657*
Plenaxis™ *(Discontinued)* *see* abarelix *on page 2*
Plendil® [US/Can] *see* felodipine *on page 338*
Pletal® [US/Can] *see* cilostazol *on page 188*
Plexion® [US] *see* sulfur and sulfacetamide *on page 800*
Plexion SCT® [US] *see* sulfur and sulfacetamide *on page 800*
Plexion TS® [US] *see* sulfur and sulfacetamide *on page 800*
PMPA *see* tenofovir *on page 810*
PMS-Alendronate [Can] *see* alendronate *on page 27*
PMS-Amantadine [Can] *see* amantadine *on page 38*
PMS-Amitriptyline [Can] *see* amitriptyline *on page 44*
PMS-Amoxicillin [Can] *see* amoxicillin *on page 47*
PMS-Anagrelide [Can] *see* anagrelide *on page 55*
PMS-Atenolol [Can] *see* atenolol *on page 80*
PMS-Azithromycin [Can] *see* azithromycin *on page 88*
PMS-Baclofen [Can] *see* baclofen *on page 91*
PMS-Benzydamine [Can] *see* benzydamine *(Canada only) on page 104*
PMS-Bethanechol [Can] *see* bethanechol *on page 109*
PMS-Bezafibrate [Can] *see* bezafibrate *(Canada only) on page 110*
PMS-Bicalutamide [Can] *see* bicalutamide *on page 110*
PMS-Brimonidine Tartrate [Can] *see* brimonidine *on page 116*
PMS-Bromocriptine [Can] *see* bromocriptine *on page 117*
PMS-Buspirone [Can] *see* buspirone *on page 127*
PMS-Butorphanol [Can] *see* butorphanol *on page 130*
PMS-Captopril [Can] *see* captopril *on page 143*
PMS-Carbamazepine [Can] *see* carbamazepine *on page 144*
PMS-Carvedilol [Can] *see* carvedilol *on page 154*
PMS-Cefaclor [Can] *see* cefaclor *on page 155*
PMS-Chloral Hydrate [Can] *see* chloral hydrate *on page 171*
PMS-Cholestyramine [Can] *see* cholestyramine resin *on page 186*
PMS-Cimetidine [Can] *see* cimetidine *on page 189*
PMS-Ciprofloxacin [Can] *see* ciprofloxacin *on page 190*
PMS-Citalopram [Can] *see* citalopram *on page 194*
PMS-Clobazam [Can] *see* clobazam *(Canada only) on page 200*
PMS-Clonazepam [Can] *see* clonazepam *on page 203*
PMS-Deferoxamine [Can] *see* deferoxamine *on page 233*
PMS-Desipramine [Can] *see* desipramine *on page 236*
PMS-Desonide [Can] *see* desonide *on page 238*
PMS-Dexamethasone [Can] *see* dexamethasone (systemic) *on page 239*
PMS-Diclofenac [Can] *see* diclofenac *on page 250*
PMS-Diclofenac SR [Can] *see* diclofenac *on page 250*
PMS-Diphenhydramine [Can] *see* diphenhydramine *on page 261*
PMS-Dipivefrin [Can] *see* dipivefrin *on page 267*
PMS-Docusate Calcium [Can] *see* docusate *on page 270*
PMS-Docusate Sodium [Can] *see* docusate *on page 270*
PMS-Erythromycin [Can] *see* erythromycin *on page 303*
PMS-Fenofibrate Micro [Can] *see* fenofibrate *on page 338*

PMS-Pravastatin [Can] *see* pravastatin *on page 692*

PMS-Procyclidine [Can] *see* procyclidine *on page 702*

PMS-Pseudoephedrine [Can] *see* pseudoephedrine *on page 712*

PMS-Ranitidine [Can] *see* ranitidine *on page 732*

PMS-Salbutamol [Can] *see* albuterol *on page 23*

PMS-Sertraline [Can] *see* sertraline *on page 769*

PMS-Simvastatin [Can] *see* simvastatin *on page 773*

PMS-Sodium Polystyrene Sulfonate [Can] *see* sodium polystyrene sulfonate *on page 783*

PMS-Sotalol [Can] *see* sotalol *on page 787*

PMS-Sucralate [Can] *see* sucralfate *on page 793*

PMS-Sumatriptan [Can] *see* sumatriptan *on page 801*

PMS-Temazepam [Can] *see* temazepam *on page 808*

PMS-Terazosin [Can] *see* terazosin *on page 810*

PMS-Theophylline [Can] *see* theophylline *on page 818*

PMS-Tiaprofenic [Can] *see* tiaprofenic acid *(Canada only) on page 826*

PMS-Timolol [Can] *see* timolol *on page 828*

PMS-Tobramycin [Can] *see* tobramycin *on page 831*

PMS-Topiramate [Can] *see* topiramate *on page 836*

PMS-Trazodone [Can] *see* trazodone *on page 843*

PMS-Trifluoperazine [Can] *see* trifluoperazine *on page 849*

PMS-Valproic Acid [Can] *see* valproic acid and derivatives *on page 864*

PMS-Valproic Acid E.C. [Can] *see* valproic acid and derivatives *on page 864*

PMS-Yohimbine [Can] *see* yohimbine *on page 883*

PMS-Zopiclone [Can] *see* zopiclone *(Canada only) on page 890*

PN *see* total parenteral nutrition *on page 838*

Pneumo 23™ [Can] *see* pneumococcal polysaccharide vaccine (polyvalent) *on next page*

pneumococcal 7-valent conjugate vaccine *see* pneumococcal conjugate vaccine (7-valent) *on this page*

pneumococcal conjugate vaccine (7-valent)

(noo moe KOK al KON ju gate vak SEEN, seven vay lent)

Sound-Alike/Look-Alike Issues

Prevnar® may be confused with PREVEN®

Synonyms diphtheria CRM_{197} protein; PCV7; pneumococcal 7-valent conjugate vaccine

U.S./Canadian Brand Names Prevnar® [US/Can]

Therapeutic Category Vaccine

Use Immunization of infants and toddlers against *Streptococcus pneumoniae* infection caused by serotypes included in the vaccine

Advisory Committee on Immunization Practices (ACIP) guidelines also recommend PCV7 for use in:

All children 2-23 months

Children ≥2-59 months with cochlear implants

Children ages 24-59 months with: Sickle cell disease (including other sickle cell hemoglobinopathies, asplenia, splenic dysfunction), HIV infection, immunocompromising conditions (congenital immunodeficiencies, renal failure, nephrotic syndrome, diseases associated with immunosuppressive or radiation therapy, solid organ transplant), chronic illnesses (cardiac disease, cerebrospinal fluid leaks, diabetes mellitus, pulmonary disease excluding asthma unless on high dose corticosteroids)

Consider use in all children 24-59 months with priority given to:

Children 24-35 months

Children 24-59 months who are of Alaska native, American Indian, or African-American descent

Children 24-59 months who attend group day care centers

Usual Dosage I.M.:

Infants: 2-6 months: 0.5 mL at approximately 2-month intervals for 3 consecutive doses, followed by a fourth dose of 0.5 mL at 12-15 months of age; first dose may be given as young as 6 weeks of age, but is typically given at 2 months of age. In case of a moderate shortage of vaccine, defer the fourth dose until

(Continued)

pneumococcal conjugate vaccine (7-valent) *(Continued)*

shortage is resolved; in case of a severe shortage of vaccine, defer third and fourth doses until shortage is resolved.

Previously Unvaccinated Older Infants and Children:

7-11 months: 0.5 mL for a total of 3 doses; 2 doses at least 4 weeks apart, followed by a third dose after the 1-year birthday (12-15 months), separated from the second dose by at least 2 months. In case of a severe shortage of vaccine, defer the third dose until shortage is resolved.

12-23 months: 0.5 mL for a total of 2 doses, separated by at least 2 months. In case of a severe shortage of vaccine, defer the second dose until shortage is resolved.

24-59 months:

Healthy Children: 0.5 mL as a single dose. In case of a severe shortage of vaccine, defer dosing until shortage is resolved.

Children with sickle cell disease, asplenia, HIV infection, chronic illness or immunocompromising conditions (not including bone marrow transplants - results pending; use PPV23 [pneumococcal polysaccharide vaccine, polyvalent] at 12- and 24-months until studies are complete): 0.5 mL for a total of 2 doses, separated by 2 months

Previously Vaccinated Children with a lapse in vaccine administration:

7-11 months: Previously received 1 or 2 doses PCV7: 0.5 mL dose at 7-11 months of age, followed by a second dose ≥2 months later at 12-15 months of age

12-23 months:

Previously received 1 dose before 12 months of age: 0.5 mL dose, followed by a second dose ≥2 months later

Previously received 2 doses before age 12 months: 0.5 mL dose ≥2 months after the most recent dose

24-59 months: Any incomplete schedule: 0.5 mL as a single dose; **Note:** Patients with chronic diseases or immunosuppressing conditions should receive 2 doses ≥2 months apart

Dosage Forms Injection, suspension: 2 mcg of each saccharide for serotypes 4, 9V, 14, 18C, 19F, and 23F, and 4 mcg of serotype 6B per 0.5 mL (0.5 mL) [contains 16 mcg total saccharide; also contains diphtheria CRM197 carrier protein ~20 mcg/0.5 mL and aluminum 0.125 mg/0.5 mL (as aluminum phosphate adjuvant); serotypes grown in soy peptone broth; vial stopper contains latex]

pneumococcal polysaccharide vaccine (polyvalent)

(noo moe KOK al pol i SAK a ride vak SEEN, pol i VAY lent)

Synonyms PPV23; 23PS; 23-valent pneumococcal polysaccharide vaccine

U.S./Canadian Brand Names Pneumo 23™ [Can]; Pneumovax® 23 [US/Can]

Therapeutic Category Vaccine, Inactivated Bacteria

Use Children ≥2 years of age and adults who are at increased risk of pneumococcal disease and its complications because of underlying health conditions (including patients with cochlear implants); routine use in older adults >50 years of age, including all those ≥65 years

Current Advisory Committee on Immunization Practices (ACIP) guidelines recommend **pneumococcal 7-valent conjugate vaccine (PCV7)** be used for children 2-23 months of age and, in certain situations, children up to 59 months of age

Usual Dosage I.M., SubQ:

Children >2 years and Adults: 0.5 mL

Previously vaccinated with PCV7 vaccine: Children ≥2 years and Adults:

With sickle cell disease, asplenia, immunocompromised or HIV infection: 0.5 mL at ≥2 years of age and ≥2 months after last dose of PCV7; revaccination with PPV23 should be given ≥5 years for children >10 years of age and every 3-5 years for children ≤10 years of age; revaccination should not be administered <3 years after the previous PPV23 dose

With chronic illness: 0.5 mL at ≥2 years of age and ≥2 months after last dose of PCV7; revaccination with PPV23 is not recommended

Following bone marrow transplant (use of PCV7 under study): Administer one dose PPV23 at 12- and 24-months following BMT

Revaccination should be considered:

1. If ≥6 years since initial vaccination has elapsed, or
2. In patients who received 14-valent pneumococcal vaccine and are at highest risk (asplenic) for fatal infection or
3. At ≥6 years in patients with nephrotic syndrome, renal failure, or transplant recipients, or
4. 3-5 years in children with nephrotic syndrome, asplenia, or sickle cell disease

Dosage Forms Injection, solution: 25 mcg each of 23 polysaccharide isolates/0.5 mL (0.5 mL, 2.5 mL)

Pneumomist® *(Discontinued)* *see* guaifenesin *on page 392*

Pneumotussin® [US] *see* hydrocodone and guaifenesin *on page 422*

Pneumovax® 23 [US/Can] *see* pneumococcal polysaccharide vaccine (polyvalent) *on previous page*

PNU-140690E *see* tipranavir *on page 830*

Pnu-Imune® 23 *(Discontinued)*

Pnu-Imune 23 Injection *(Discontinued)* *see* pneumococcal polysaccharide vaccine (polyvalent) *on previous page*

Podactin Cream [US-OTC] *see* miconazole *on page 553*

Podactin Powder [US-OTC] *see* tolnaftate *on page 834*

Pod-Ben-25® *(Discontinued)* *see* podophyllum resin *on this page*

Podocon-25® [US] *see* podophyllum resin *on this page*

Podofilm® [Can] *see* podophyllum resin *on this page*

podofilox (poe DOF il loks)

U.S./Canadian Brand Names Condyline™ [Can]; Condylox® [US]; Wartec® [Can]

Therapeutic Category Keratolytic Agent

Use Treatment of external genital warts

Usual Dosage Topical: Adults: Apply twice daily (morning and evening) for 3 consecutive days, then withhold use for 4 consecutive days; this cycle may be repeated up to 4 times until there is no visible wart tissue

Dosage Forms

Gel: 0.5% (3.5 g) [contains alcohol]

Solution, topical: 0.5% (3.5 mL) [contains alcohol]

Podofin® *(Discontinued)* *see* podophyllum resin *on this page*

podophyllin *see* podophyllum resin *on this page*

podophyllum resin (po DOF fil um REZ in)

Synonyms mandrake; may apple; podophyllin

U.S./Canadian Brand Names Podocon-25® [US]; Podofilm® [Can]

Therapeutic Category Keratolytic Agent

Use Topical treatment of benign growths including external genital and perianal warts, papillomas, fibroids; compound benzoin tincture generally is used as the medium for topical application

Usual Dosage Topical:

Children and Adults: 10% to 25% solution in compound benzoin tincture; apply drug to dry surface, use 1 drop at a time allowing drying between drops until area is covered; total volume should be limited to <0.5 mL per treatment session

Condylomata acuminatum: 25% solution is applied daily; use a 10% solution when applied to or near mucous membranes

Verrucae: 25% solution is applied 3-5 times/day directly to the wart

Dosage Forms Liquid, topical: 25% (15 mL) [in benzoin tincture]

Point-Two® *(Discontinued)* *see* fluoride *on page 354*

Poladex® *(Discontinued)* *see* dexchlorpheniramine *on page 241*

Polaramine® *(Discontinued)* *see* dexchlorpheniramine *on page 241*

poliovirus vaccine (inactivated) (POE lee oh VYE rus vak SEEN, in ak ti VAY ted)

Synonyms enhanced-potency inactivated poliovirus vaccine; IPV; salk vaccine

U.S./Canadian Brand Names IPOL® [US/Can]

Therapeutic Category Vaccine, Live Virus and Inactivated Virus

Use Active immunization against poliomyelitis caused by poliovirus types 1, 2 and 3. Routine immunization of adults in the United States is generally not recommended. Adults with previous wild poliovirus disease, who have never been immunized, or those who are incompletely immunized may receive inactivated poliovirus vaccine if they fall into one of the following categories:

- Travelers to regions or countries where poliomyelitis is endemic or epidemic
- Healthcare workers in close contact with patients who may be excreting poliovirus
- Laboratory workers handling specimens that may contain poliovirus
- Members of communities or specific population groups with diseases caused by wild poliovirus
- Incompletely vaccinated or unvaccinated adults in a household or with other close contact with children receiving oral poliovirus (may be at increased risk of vaccine associated paralytic poliomyelitis)

(Continued)

poliovirus vaccine (inactivated) *(Continued)*

Usual Dosage I.M., SubQ:

Children:

Primary immunization: Administer three 0.5 mL doses, preferably 8 or more weeks apart, at 2,4, and 6-18 months of age. First dose may be given as early as 6 weeks of age. Do not administer more frequently than 4 weeks apart.

Booster dose: 0.5 mL at 4-6 years of age

Adults:

Previously unvaccinated: Two 0.5 mL doses administered at 1- to 2-month intervals, followed by a third dose 6-12 months later. If <3 months, but at least 2 months are available before protection is needed, 3 doses may be administered at least 1 month apart. If administration must be completed within 1-2 months, give 2 doses at least 1 month apart. If <1 month is available, give 1 dose.

Incompletely vaccinated: Adults with at least 1 previous dose of OPV, <3 doses of IPV, or a combination of OPV and IPV equaling <3 doses, administer at least one 0.5 mL dose of IPV. Additional doses to complete the series may be given if time permits.

Completely vaccinated: One 0.5 mL dose

Dosage Forms

Injection, suspension:

IPOL®: Type 1 poliovirus 40 D antigen units, type 2 poliovirus 8 D antigen units, and type 3 poliovirus 32 D antigen units per 0.5 mL (5 mL) [contains 2-phenoxyethanol, formaldehyde, calf serum protein, neomycin, streptomycin, and polymyxin B; packaging contains natural latex rubber]

Polocaine® [US/Can] *see* mepivacaine *on page 530*

Polocaine® 2% and Levonordefrin 1:20,000 [Can] *see* mepivacaine and levonordefrin *on page 531*

Polocaine® Dental [US] *see* mepivacaine *on page 530*

Polocaine® MPF [US] *see* mepivacaine *on page 530*

polycarbophil (pol i KAR boe fil)

U.S./Canadian Brand Names Equalactin® [US-OTC]; Fiber-Lax® [US-OTC]; FiberCon® [US-OTC]; Konsyl® Fiber Tablets [US-OTC]; Phillips'® Fibercaps [US-OTC]

Therapeutic Category Gastrointestinal Agent, Miscellaneous; Laxative

Use Treatment of constipation or diarrhea

Usual Dosage Oral: General dosing guidelines (OTC labeling):

Children 6-12 years: 625 mg calcium polycarbophil 1-4 times/day

Children ≥12 years and Adults: 1250 mg calcium polycarbophil 1-4 times/day

Dosage Forms

Caplet:

FiberCon®: Calcium polycarbophil 625 mg [equivalent to polycarbophil 500 mg; contains calcium 122 mg/caplet]

Captab:

Fiber-Lax®: Calcium polycarbophil 625 mg [equivalent to polycarbophil 500 mg; contains calcium 170 mg/captab]

Tablet: Calcium polycarbophil 625 mg

Fiber-Tabs™: Calcium polycarbophil 625 mg [equivalent to polycarbophil 500 mg]

Konsyl® Fiber: Calcium polycarbophil 625 mg [equivalent to polycarbophil 500 mg; contains calcium 125 mg/tablet]

Tablet, chewable:

Equalactin®: Calcium polycarbophil 625 mg [equivalent to polycarbophil 500 mg; citrus flavor]

Polycitra® [US] *see* citric acid, sodium citrate, and potassium citrate *on page 195*

Polycitra®-K [US] *see* potassium citrate and citric acid *on page 686*

Polycitra®-LC [US] *see* citric acid, sodium citrate, and potassium citrate *on page 195*

Polycose® [US-OTC] *see* glucose polymers *on page 386*

Poly-Dex™ [US] *see* neomycin, polymyxin B, and dexamethasone *on page 584*

polyethylene glycol 3350 (pol i ETH i leen GLY kol 3350)

Sound-Alike/Look-Alike Issues

MiraLax™ may be confused with Mirapex®

Synonyms PEG

U.S./Canadian Brand Names GlycoLax™ [US]; MiraLax™ [US]

Therapeutic Category Laxative, Osmotic

Use Treatment of occasional constipation in adults

Usual Dosage Oral: Adults: Occasional constipation: 17 g of powder (~1 heaping tablespoon) dissolved in 8 oz of water, once daily; do not use for >2 weeks.

Dosage Forms

Powder, for oral solution: PEG 3350 17 g/packet (12s); PEG 3350 255 g (14 oz); PEG 3350 527 g (26 oz)

GlycoLax™: PEG 3350 17 g/packet (14s); PEG 3350 255 g (16 oz); PEG 3350 527 g (24 oz)

MiraLax™: PEG 3350 17 g/packet (12s); PEG 3350 255 g (14 oz); PEG 3350 527 g (26 oz)

polyethylene glycol-electrolyte solution

(pol i ETH i leen GLY kol ee LEK troe lite soe LOO shun)

Sound-Alike/Look-Alike Issues

GoLYTELY® may be confused with NuLYTELY®

NuLYTELY® may be confused with GoLYTELY®

Synonyms electrolyte lavage solution

U.S./Canadian Brand Names Colyte® [US/Can]; GoLYTELY® [US]; Klean-Prep® [Can]; NuLYTELY® [US]; PegLyte® [Can]; TriLyte™ [US]

Therapeutic Category Laxative

Use Bowel cleansing prior to GI examination or following toxic ingestion

Usual Dosage

Oral:

Children ≥6 months: Bowel cleansing prior to GI exam: 25-40 mL/kg/hour for 4-10 hours (until rectal effluent is clear). Ideally, patients should fast for ~3-4 hours prior to administration; absolutely no solid food for at least 2 hours before the solution is given. The solution may be given via nasogastric tube to patients who are unwilling or unable to drink the solution. Patients <2 years should be monitored closely.

Adults: Bowel cleansing prior to GI exam: 240 mL (8 oz) every 10 minutes, until 4 L are consumed or the rectal effluent is clear; rapid drinking of each portion is preferred to drinking small amounts continuously. Ideally, patients should fast for ~3-4 hours prior to administration; absolutely no solid food for at least 2 hours before the solution is given. The solution may be given via nasogastric tube to patients who are unwilling or unable to drink the solution.

Nasogastric tube:

Children ≥6 months: Bowel cleansing prior to GI exam: 25 mL/kg/hour until rectal effluent is clear. Ideally, patients should fast for ~3-4 hours prior to administration; absolutely no solid food for at least 2 hours before the solution is given.

Adults: Bowel cleansing prior to GI exam: 20-30 mL/minute (1.2-1.8 L/hour); the first bowel movement should occur ~1 hour after the start of administration. Ideally, patients should fast for ~3-4 hours prior to administration; absolutely no solid food for at least 2 hours before the solution is given.

Dosage Forms

Powder, for oral solution: PEG 3350 240 g, sodium sulfate 22.72 g, sodium bicarbonate 6.72 g, sodium chloride 5.84 g, and potassium chloride 2.98 g (4000 mL)

Colyte®:

PEG 3350 240 g, sodium sulfate 22.72 g, sodium bicarbonate 6.72 g, sodium chloride 5.84 g, and potassium chloride 2.98 g (4000 mL) [available with citrus berry, lemon lime, cherry, and pineapple flavor packets]

PEG 3350 227.1 g, sodium sulfate 21.5 g, sodium bicarbonate 6.36 g, sodium chloride 5.53 g, and potassium chloride 2.82 g (4000 mL) [regular and pineapple flavor]

GoLYTELY®:

Disposable jug: PEG 3350 236 g, sodium sulfate 22.74 g, sodium bicarbonate 6.74 g, sodium chloride 5.86 g, and potassium chloride 2.97 g (4000 mL) [regular and pineapple flavor]

Packets: PEG 3350 227.1 g, sodium sulfate 21.5 g, sodium bicarbonate 6.36 g, sodium chloride 5.53 g, and potassium chloride 2.82 g (4000 mL) [regular flavor]

MoviPrep®: Disposable jug: Pouch A: PEG 3350 100g, sodium sulfate 7.5 g, sodium chloride 2.69 g, potassium chloride 1.015 g; Pouch B: Ascorbic acid 4.7 g, sodium ascorbate 5.9 g (1000 mL) [contains phenylalanine 2.33 mg/treatment; lemon flavor; packaged with 2 of Pouch A and 2 of Pouch B in carton]

NuLYTELY®: PEG 3350 420 g, sodium bicarbonate 5.72 g, sodium chloride 11.2 g, and potassium chloride 1.48 (4000 mL) [cherry, lemon-lime, and orange flavors]

TriLyte™: PEG 3350 420 g, sodium bicarbonate 5.72 g, sodium chloride 11.2 g, and potassium chloride 1.48 (4000 mL) [supplied with flavor packets]

polyethylene glycol-electrolyte solution and bisacodyl

(pol i ETH i leen GLY kol ee LEK troe lite soe LOO shun & bis a KOE dil)

U.S./Canadian Brand Names HalfLytely® and Bisacodyl [US]

Therapeutic Category Laxative, Bowel Evacuant; Laxative, Stimulant

Use Bowel cleansing prior to GI examination

Usual Dosage Oral: Adults: Bowel cleansing:

Bisacodyl: 4 tablets as a single dose. After bowel movement or 6 hours (whichever occurs first), initiate polyethylene glycol-electrolyte solution

Polyethylene glycol-electrolyte solution: 8 ounces every 10 minutes until 2 L are consumed

Dosage Forms Kit (HalfLytely® and Bisacodyl) [each kit contains]:

Powder for oral solution (HalfLytely®): PEG 3350 210 g, sodium bicarbonate 2.86 g, sodium chloride 5.6 g, potassium chloride 0.74 g (2000 mL) [sulfate-free, regular, cherry, lemon-lime, orange flavor]

Tablet, delayed release (Bisacodyl): 5 mg (4s)

Polygam® S/D [US] *see* immune globulin (intravenous) *on page 444*

Poly-Histine-D® Capsule *(Discontinued)*

polymyxin B

(pol i MIKS in bee)

Synonyms polymyxin B sulfate

U.S./Canadian Brand Names Poly-Rx [US]

Therapeutic Category Antibiotic, Irrigation; Antibiotic, Miscellaneous

Use Treatment of acute infections caused by susceptible strains of *Pseudomonas aeruginosa*; used occasionally for gut decontamination; parenteral use of polymyxin B has mainly been replaced by less toxic antibiotics, reserved for life-threatening infections caused by organisms resistant to the preferred drugs (eg, pseudomonal meningitis - intrathecal administration)

Usual Dosage

Otic (in combination with other drugs): 1-2 drops, 3-4 times/day; should be used sparingly to avoid accumulation of excess debris

Infants <2 years:

- I.M.: Up to 40,000 units/kg/day divided every 6 hours (not routinely recommended due to pain at injection sites)
- I.V.: Up to 40,000 units/kg/day divided every 12 hours
- Intrathecal: 20,000 units/day for 3-4 days, then 25,000 units every other day for at least 2 weeks after CSF cultures are negative and CSF (glucose) has returned to within normal limits

Children ≥2 years and Adults:

- I.M.: 25,000-30,000 units/kg/day divided every 4-6 hours (not routinely recommended due to pain at injection sites)
- I.V.: 15,000-25,000 units/kg/day divided every 12 hours
- Intrathecal: 50,000 units/day for 3-4 days, then every other day for at least 2 weeks after CSF cultures are negative and CSF (glucose) has returned to within normal limits
- Total daily dose should not exceed 2,000,000 units/day
- Bladder irrigation: Continuous irrigant or rinse in the urinary bladder for up to 10 days using 20 mg (equal to 200,000 units) added to 1 L of normal saline; usually no more than 1 L of irrigant is used per day unless urine flow rate is high; administration rate is adjusted to patient's urine output
- Topical irrigation or topical solution: 500,000 units/L of normal saline; topical irrigation should not exceed 2 million units/day in adults
- Gut sterilization: Oral: 15,000-25,000 units/kg/day in divided doses every 6 hours
- *Clostridium difficile* enteritis: Oral: 25,000 units every 6 hours for 10 days
- Ophthalmic: A concentration of 0.1% to 0.25% is administered as 1-3 drops every hour, then increasing the interval as response indicates to 1-2 drops 4-6 times/day

Dosage Forms

Injection, powder for reconstitution: 500,000 units

Powder [for prescription compounding] (Poly-Rx): 100 million units (13 g)

polymyxin B and bacitracin *see* bacitracin and polymyxin B *on page 90*

polymyxin B and neomycin *see* neomycin and polymyxin B *on page 583*

polymyxin B and trimethoprim *see* trimethoprim and polymyxin B *on page 852*

polymyxin B, bacitracin, and neomycin *see* bacitracin, neomycin, and polymyxin B *on page 91*

polymyxin B, bacitracin, neomycin, and hydrocortisone *see* bacitracin, neomycin, polymyxin B, and hydrocortisone *on page 91*

polymyxin B, neomycin, and dexamethasone *see* neomycin, polymyxin B, and dexamethasone *on page 584*

polymyxin B, neomycin, and gramicidin *see* neomycin, polymyxin B, and gramicidin *on page 584*

polymyxin B, neomycin, and hydrocortisone *see* neomycin, polymyxin B, and hydrocortisone *on page 584*

polymyxin B, neomycin, and prednisolone *see* neomycin, polymyxin B, and prednisolone *on page 585*

polymyxin B, neomycin, bacitracin, and pramoxine *see* bacitracin, neomycin, polymyxin B, and pramoxine *on page 91*

polymyxin B sulfate *see* polymyxin B *on previous page*

Poly-Pred® [US] *see* neomycin, polymyxin B, and prednisolone *on page 585*

Poly-Rx [US] *see* polymyxin B *on previous page*

polysaccharide-iron complex (pol i SAK a ride-EYE ern KOM pleks)

Sound-Alike/Look-Alike Issues

Niferex® may be confused with Nephrox®

Synonyms iron-polysaccharide complex

U.S./Canadian Brand Names Ferrex 150 [US-OTC]; Hytinic® [US-OTC]; Niferex® 150 [US-OTC]; Niferex® [US-OTC]; Nu-Iron® 150 [US-OTC]

Therapeutic Category Electrolyte Supplement, Oral

Use Prevention and treatment of iron-deficiency anemias

Usual Dosage

Children ≥6 years: Tablets/elixir: 50-100 mg/day; may be given in divided doses

Adults:

Tablets/elixir: 50-100 mg twice daily

Capsules: 150-300 mg/day

Dosage Forms [DSC] = Discontinued product

Capsule (Ferrex 150, Fe-Tinic™ 150 [DSC], Hytinic®, Niferex® 150, Nu-Iron® 150): Elemental iron 150 mg

Elixir (Niferex®): Elemental iron 100 mg/5 mL (240 mL) [contains alcohol 10%]

Tablet (Niferex®): Elemental iron 50 mg

Polysporin® Ophthalmic [US] *see* bacitracin and polymyxin B *on page 90*

Polysporin® Topical [US-OTC] *see* bacitracin and polymyxin B *on page 90*

Polytapp® Allergy Dye-Free Medication [US-OTC] *see* brompheniramine *on page 118*

Polytar® [US-OTC] *see* coal tar *on page 207*

polythiazide and prazosin *see* prazosin and polythiazide *on page 693*

Polytrim® [US/Can] *see* trimethoprim and polymyxin B *on page 852*

Poly-Vi-Flor® [US] *see* vitamins (multiple/pediatric) *on page 878*

Poly-Vi-Flor® With Iron [US] *see* vitamins (multiple/pediatric) *on page 878*

polyvinyl alcohol *see* artificial tears *on page 75*

polyvinylpyrrolidone with iodine *see* povidone-iodine *on page 689*

Poly-Vi-Sol® [US-OTC] *see* vitamins (multiple/pediatric) *on page 878*

Poly-Vi-Sol® with Iron [US-OTC] *see* vitamins (multiple/pediatric) *on page 878*

Pondocillin® [Can] *see* pivampicillin *(Canada only) on page 671*

Ponstan® [Can] *see* mefenamic acid *on page 525*

Ponstel® [US] *see* mefenamic acid *on page 525*

Pontocaine® [US/Can] *see* tetracaine *on page 815*

Pontocaine® Niphanoid® [US] *see* tetracaine *on page 815*

Pontocaine® With Dextrose [US] *see* tetracaine and dextrose *on page 816*

poractant alfa (por AKT ant AL fa)

U.S./Canadian Brand Names Curosurf® [US/Can]

Therapeutic Category Lung Surfactant

Use **Orphan drug:** Treatment and prevention of respiratory distress syndrome (RDS) in premature infants

Usual Dosage Intratracheal use **only**: Premature infant with RDS: Initial dose is 2.5 mL/kg of birth weight. Up to 2 subsequent doses of 1.25 mL/kg birth weight can be administered at 12-hour intervals if needed in infants who continue to require mechanical ventilation and supplemental oxygen.

Dosage Forms Suspension for intratracheal instillation [preservative free; porcine derived]: 80 mg/mL (1.5 mL, 3 mL)

Porcelana® Sunscreen *(Discontinued)* *see* hydroquinone *on page 430*

porfimer (POR fi mer)

Synonyms CL-184116; dihematoporphyrin ether; porfimer sodium

U.S./Canadian Brand Names Photofrin® [US/Can]

Therapeutic Category Antineoplastic Agent

Use Adjunct to laser light therapy for obstructing esophageal cancer, obstructing endobronchial nonsmall cell lung cancer (NSCLC), ablation of high-grade dysplasia in Barrett esophagus

Usual Dosage I.V. (refer to individual protocols):

Children: Safety and efficacy have not been established

Adults: 2 mg/kg, followed by exposure to the appropriate laser light

Dosage Forms Injection, powder for reconstitution, as sodium: 75 mg

porfimer sodium *see* porfimer *on this page*

Portagen® [US-OTC] *see* nutritional formula, enteral/oral *on page 608*

Portia™ [US] *see* ethinyl estradiol and levonorgestrel *on page 320*

Post Peel Healing Balm [US-OTC] *see* hydrocortisone (topical) *on page 428*

Posture® [US-OTC] *see* calcium phosphate (tribasic) *on page 140*

Potasalan® *(Discontinued)* *see* potassium chloride *on page 684*

potassium acetate (poe TASS ee um AS e tate)

Therapeutic Category Electrolyte Supplement, Oral

Use Potassium deficiency; to avoid chloride when high concentration of potassium is needed, source of bicarbonate

Usual Dosage I.V. doses should be incorporated into the patient's maintenance I.V. fluids, intermittent I.V. potassium administration should be reserved for severe depletion situations and requires ECG monitoring; doses listed as mEq of potassium

Children:

Treatment of hypokalemia: I.V.: 2-5 mEq/kg/day

I.V. intermittent infusion (must be diluted prior to administration): 0.5-1 mEq/kg/dose (maximum: 30 mEq/dose) to infuse at 0.3-0.5 mEq/kg/hour (maximum: 1 mEq/kg/hour)

Note: Use caution in premature neonates; potassium acetate for injection contains aluminum.

Adults:

Treatment of hypokalemia: I.V.: 40-100 mEq/day

I.V. intermittent infusion (must be diluted prior to administration): 5-10 mEq/dose (maximum: 40 mEq/dose) to infuse over 2-3 hours (maximum: 40 mEq over 1 hour)

Note: Continuous cardiac monitor recommended for rates >0.5 mEq/hour

Potassium dosage/rate of infusion guidelines:

Serum potassium >2.5 mEq/L: Maximum infusion rate: 10 mEq/hour; maximum concentration: 40 mEq/L; maximum 24-hour dose: 200 mEq

Serum potassium <2.5 mEq/L: Maximum infusion rate: 40 mEq/hour; maximum concentration: 80 mEq/L; maximum 24-hour dose: 400 mEq

Dosage Forms Injection, solution: 2 mEq/mL (20 mL, 50 mL, 100 mL); 4 mEq/mL (50 mL) [contains aluminum ≤200 mcg/mL]

potassium acetate, potassium bicarbonate, and potassium citrate

(poe TASS ee um AS e tate, poe TASS ee um bye KAR bun ate, & poe TASS ee um SIT rate)

Synonyms potassium acetate, potassium citrate, and potassium bicarbonate; potassium bicarbonate, potassium acetate, and potassium citrate; potassium bicarbonate, potassium citrate, and potassium acetate; potassium citrate, potassium acetate, and potassium bicarbonate; potassium citrate, potassium bicarbonate, and potassium acetate

U.S./Canadian Brand Names Tri-K® [US]

Therapeutic Category Electrolyte Supplement, Oral

Use Treatment or prevention of hypokalemia

Usual Dosage Oral:

Children: 1-4 mEq/kg/24 hours in divided doses as required to maintain normal serum potassium

Adults:

Prevention: 16-24 mEq/day in 2-4 divided doses

Treatment: 40-100 mEq/day in 2-4 divided doses

Dosage Forms Solution, oral: Potassium 45 mEq/15 mL (480 mL) [from potassium acetate 1500 mg, potassium bicarbonate 1500 mg, and potassium citrate 1500 mg per 15 mL]

potassium acetate, potassium citrate, and potassium bicarbonate *see* potassium acetate, potassium bicarbonate, and potassium citrate *on previous page*

potassium acid phosphate (poe TASS ee um AS id FOS fate)

U.S./Canadian Brand Names K-Phos® Original [US]

Therapeutic Category Urinary Acidifying Agent

Use Acidifies urine and lowers urinary calcium concentration; reduces odor and rash caused by ammoniacal urine; increases the antibacterial activity of methenamine

Usual Dosage Adults: Oral: 1000 mg dissolved in 6-8 oz of water 4 times/day with meals and at bedtime; for best results, soak tablets in water for 2-5 minutes, then stir and swallow

Dosage Forms Tablet [scored]: 500 mg [phosphorus 114 mg and potassium 144 mg (3.7 mEq) per tablet; sodium free]

potassium bicarbonate (poe TASS ee um bye KAR bun ate)

Therapeutic Category Electrolyte Supplement, Oral

Use Potassium deficiency, hypokalemia

Usual Dosage Oral:

Children: 1-4 mEq/kg/day

Adults: 25 mEq 2-4 times/day

Dosage Forms Tablet for oral solution, effervescent: Potassium 25 mEq

potassium bicarbonate and potassium chloride

(poe TASS ee um bye KAR bun ate & poe TASS ee um KLOR ide)

Synonyms potassium bicarbonate and potassium chloride (effervescent)

U.S./Canadian Brand Names K-Lyte/Cl® [US]

Therapeutic Category Electrolyte Supplement, Oral

Use Treatment or prevention of hypokalemia

Usual Dosage Oral:

Children: 1-4 mEq/kg/24 hours in divided doses as required to maintain normal serum potassium

Adults:

Prevention: 16-24 mEq/day in 2-4 divided doses

Treatment: 40-100 mEq/day in 2-4 divided doses

Dosage Forms [DSC] = Discontinued product

Tablet for oral solution, effervescent:

K-Lyte/Cl®: Potassium chloride 25 mEq [potassium chloride 1.5 g and potassium bicarbonate 0.5 g; citrus or fruit punch flavor]

K-Lyte/Cl® 50: Potassium chloride 50 mEq [potassium chloride 2.24 g and potassium bicarbonate 2 g; citrus flavor] [DSC]

potassium bicarbonate and potassium chloride (effervescent) *see* potassium bicarbonate and potassium chloride *on this page*

potassium bicarbonate and potassium citrate

(poe TASS ee um bye KAR bun ate & poe TASS ee um SIT rate)

Sound-Alike/Look-Alike Issues

Klor-Con® may be confused with Klaron®, K-Lor®

(Continued)

potassium bicarbonate and potassium citrate *(Continued)*

Synonyms potassium bicarbonate and potassium citrate (effervescent)

U.S./Canadian Brand Names Effer-K™ [US]; K-Lyte® DS [US]; K-Lyte® [US]; Klor-Con®/EF [US]

Therapeutic Category Electrolyte Supplement, Oral

Use Treatment or prevention of hypokalemia

Usual Dosage Oral:

Children: 1-4 mEq/kg/24 hours in divided doses as required to maintain normal serum potassium

Adults:

- Prevention: 16-24 mEq/day in 2-4 divided doses
- Treatment: 40-100 mEq/day in 2-4 divided doses

Dosage Forms

Tablet, effervescent: Potassium 25 mEq

- Effer-K™: Potassium 25 mEq
- Klor-Con®/EF: Potassium 25 mEq [orange flavor]
- K-Lyte®: Potassium 25 mEq [orange flavor]
- K-Lyte® DS: Potassium 50 mEq [lime or orange flavor]

potassium bicarbonate and potassium citrate (effervescent) *see* potassium bicarbonate and potassium citrate *on previous page*

potassium bicarbonate, potassium acetate, and potassium citrate *see* potassium acetate, potassium bicarbonate, and potassium citrate *on page 682*

potassium bicarbonate, potassium citrate, and potassium acetate *see* potassium acetate, potassium bicarbonate, and potassium citrate *on page 682*

potassium chloride (poe TASS ee um KLOR ide)

Sound-Alike/Look-Alike Issues

- Kaon-Cl-10® may be confused with kaolin
- KCl may be confused with HCl
- K-Dur® may be confused with Cardura®, Imdur®
- K-Lor® may be confused with Kaochlor®, Klor-Con®
- Klor-Con® may be confused with Klaron®, K-Lor®
- Klotrix® may be confused with liotrix
- microK® may be confused with Micronase®

Synonyms KCl

U.S./Canadian Brand Names Apo-K® [Can]; K+ Potassium [US]; K-10® [Can]; K-Dur® 10 [US]; K-Dur® 20 [US]; K-Dur® [Can]; K-Lor® [US/Can]; K-Tab® [US]; Kaon-Cl-10® [US]; Kaon-Cl® 20 [US]; Kay Ciel® [US]; Klor-Con® 10 [US]; Klor-Con® 8 [US]; Klor-Con® M [US]; Klor-Con® [US]; Klor-Con®/25 [US]; Micro-K Extencaps® [Can]; microK® 10 [US]; microK® [US]; Roychlor® [Can]; Rum-K® [US]; Slo-Pot [Can]; Slow-K® [Can]

Therapeutic Category Electrolyte Supplement, Oral

Use Treatment or prevention of hypokalemia

Usual Dosage I.V. doses should be incorporated into the patient's maintenance I.V. fluids; intermittent I.V. potassium administration should be reserved for severe depletion situations in patients undergoing ECG monitoring.

Normal daily requirements: Oral, I.V.:

- Premature infants: 2-6 mEq/kg/24 hours
- Term infants 0-24 hours: 0-2 mEq/kg/24 hours
- Infants >24 hours: 1-2 mEq/kg/24 hours
- Children: 2-3 mEq/kg/day
- Adults: 40-80 mEq/day

Prevention during diuretic therapy: Oral:

- Children: 1-2 mEq/kg/day in 1-2 divided doses
- Adults: 20-40 mEq/day in 1-2 divided doses

Treatment of hypokalemia: Children:

- Oral: 1-2 mEq/kg initially, then as needed based on frequently obtained lab values. If deficits are severe or ongoing losses are great, I.V. route should be considered.
- I.V.: 1 mEq/kg over 1-2 hours initially, then repeated as needed based on frequently obtained lab values; severe depletion or ongoing losses may require >200% of normal limit needs
- I.V. intermittent infusion: Dose should not exceed 1 mEq/kg/hour, or 40 mEq/hour; if it exceeds 0.5 mEq/kg/hour, physician should be at bedside and patient should have continuous ECG monitoring; usual pediatric maximum: 3 mEq/kg/day or 40 mEq/m^2/day

Treatment of hypokalemia: Adults:
I.V. intermittent infusion: 5-10 mEq/hour (continuous cardiac monitor recommended for rates >5 mEq/hour), not to exceed 40 mEq/hour; usual adult maximum per 24 hours: 400 mEq/day.
Potassium dosage/rate of infusion guidelines:
Serum potassium >2.5 mEq/L: Maximum infusion rate: 10 mEq/hour; maximum concentration: 40 mEq/L; maximum 24-hour dose: 200 mEq
Serum potassium <2.5 mEq/L: Maximum infusion rate: 40 mEq/hour; maximum concentration: 80 mEq/L; maximum 24-hour dose: 400 mEq
Potassium >2.5 mEq/L:
Oral: 60-80 mEq/day plus additional amounts if needed
I.V.: 10 mEq over 1 hour with additional doses if needed
Potassium <2.5 mEq/L:
Oral: Up to 40-60 mEq initial dose, followed by further doses based on lab values
I.V.: Up to 40 mEq over 1 hour, with doses based on frequent lab monitoring; deficits at a plasma level of 2 mEq/L may be as high as 400-800 mEq of potassium

Dosage Forms [DSC] = Discontinued product
Capsule, extended release: 10 mEq [750 mg]
microK® [microencapsulated]: 8 mEq [600 mg]
microK® 10 [microencapsulated]: 10 mEq [750 mg]
Infusion [premixed in D_5W]: 20 mEq (1000 mL); 30 mEq (1000 mL); 40 mEq (1000 mL)
Infusion [premixed in D_5W and LR]: 20 mEq (1000 mL); 30 mEq (1000 mL); 40 mEq (1000 mL)
Infusion [premixed in D_5W and ¼NS]: 10 mEq (500 mL, 1000 mL); 20 mEq (250 mL, 500 mL, 1000 mL); 30 mEq (1000 mL); 40 mEq (1000 mL)
Infusion [premixed in D_5W and ½NS]: 10 mEq (500 mL, 1000 mL); 20 mEq (500 mL, 1000 mL); 30 mEq (1000 mL); 40 mEq (1000 mL)
Infusion [premixed in D_5 and NS]: 20 mEq (1000 mL); 40 mEq (1000 mL)
Infusion [premixed in D_5W and sodium chloride 0.3%]: 10 mEq (500 mL); 20 mEq (1000 mL); 30 mEq (1000 mL); 40 mEq (1000 mL)
Infusion [premixed in $D_{10}W$ and sodium chloride 0.2%]: 20 mEq (250 mL)
Infusion [premixed in NS]: 20 mEq (1000 mL); 40 mEq (1000 mL)
Infusion [premixed in SWFI; concentrate]: 10 mEq (50 mL, 100 mL); 20 mEq (50 mL, 100 mL); 30 mEq (100 mL); 40 mEq (100 mL)
Injection, solution [concentrate]: 2 mEq/mL (5 mL, 10 mL, 15 mL, 20 mL, 30 mL, 250 mL, 500 mL)
Powder, for oral solution: 20 mEq/packet (30s, 100s, 1000s)
K-Lor™: 20 mEq/packet (30s, 100s) [fruit flavor]
K+ Potassium: 20 mEq/packet (30s) [orange flavor]
Kay Ciel® 10%: 20 mEq/packet (30s, 100s) [sugar free]
Klor-Con®: 20 mEq/packet (30s, 100s) [sugar free; fruit flavor]
Klor-Con®/25: 25 mEq/packet (30s, 100s) [sugar free; fruit flavor]
Solution, oral: 20 mEq/15 mL (480 mL, 3840 mL); 40 mEq/15 mL (480 mL)
Kaon-Cl® 20: 40 mEq/15 mL (480 mL) [sugar free; contains alcohol; cherry flavor]
Kay Ciel®: 10%: 20 mEq/15 mL (480 mL) [sugar free; contains alcohol] [DSC]
Rum-K®: 20 mEq/10 mL (480 mL) [alcohol free, sugar free; butter/rum flavor]
Tablet, extended release: 8 mEq [600 mg]; 10 mEq [750 mg]; 20 mEq [1500 mg]
K-Dur® 10 [microencapsulated]: 10 mEq [750 mg]
K-Dur® 20 [microencapsulated]: 20 mEq [1500 mg; scored]
K-Tab®: 10 mEq [750 mg]
Kaon-Cl® 10: 10 mEq [750 mg]
Klor-Con® 8: 8 mEq [600 mg; wax matrix]
Klor-Con® 10: 10 mEq [750 mg; wax matrix]
Klor-Con® M10 [microencapsulated]: 10 mEq [750 mg]
Klor-Con® M15 [microencapsulated]: 15 mEq [1125 mg; scored]
Klor-Con® M20 [microencapsulated]: 20 mEq [1500 mg; scored]

potassium citrate (poe TASS ee um SIT rate)

Sound-Alike/Look-Alike Issues
Urocit®-K may be confused with Urised®

U.S./Canadian Brand Names K-Citra® [Can]; Urocit®-K [US]

Therapeutic Category Alkalinizing Agent

Use Prevention of uric acid nephrolithiasis; prevention of calcium renal stones in patients with hypocitraturia; urinary alkalinizer when sodium citrate is contraindicated

Usual Dosage Adults: Oral: 10-20 mEq 3 times/day with meals up to 100 mEq/day

Dosage Forms Tablet: 540 mg [5 mEq]; 1080 mg [10 mEq]

potassium citrate and citric acid (poe TASS ee um SIT rate & SI trik AS id)

Synonyms citric acid and potassium citrate

U.S./Canadian Brand Names Cytra-K [US]; Polycitra®-K [US]

Therapeutic Category Alkalinizing Agent

Use Treatment of metabolic acidosis; alkalinizing agent in conditions where long-term maintenance of an alkaline urine is desirable

Usual Dosage Urine alkalizing agent:

Children: Solution: 5-15 mL after meals and at bedtime; adjust dose based on urinary pH

Adults:

Powder: One packet dissolved in water after meals and at bedtime; adjust dose to urinary pH

Solution: 15-30 mL after meals and at bedtime; adjust dose based on urinary pH

Dosage Forms Note: Equivalent to potassium 2 mEq/mL and bicarbonate 2 mEq/mL

Powder:

Cytra-K: Potassium citrate 3300 mg and citric acid 1002 mg per packet (100s) [sugar free; fruit flavor]

Polycitra®-K: Potassium citrate 3300 mg and citric acid 1002 mg per packet (100s) [sugar free]

Solution:

Cytra-K: Potassium citrate 1100 mg and citric acid monohydrate 334 mg per 5 mL (480 mL) [alcohol free, sugar free; contains sodium benzoate; cherry flavor]

Polycitra®-K: Potassium citrate 1100 mg and citric acid monohydrate 334 mg per 5 mL (480 mL) [alcohol free, sugar free]

potassium citrate, citric acid, and sodium citrate *see* citric acid, sodium citrate, and potassium citrate *on page 195*

potassium citrate, potassium acetate, and potassium bicarbonate *see* potassium acetate, potassium bicarbonate, and potassium citrate *on page 682*

potassium citrate, potassium bicarbonate, and potassium acetate *see* potassium acetate, potassium bicarbonate, and potassium citrate *on page 682*

potassium gluconate (poe TASS ee um GLOO coe nate)

U.S./Canadian Brand Names Glu-K® [US-OTC]

Therapeutic Category Electrolyte Supplement, Oral

Use Treatment or prevention of hypokalemia

Usual Dosage Oral (doses listed as mEq of potassium):

Normal daily requirement:

Children: 2-3 mEq/kg/day

Adults: 40-80 mEq/day

Prevention of hypokalemia during diuretic therapy:

Children: 1-2 mEq/kg/day in 1-2 divided doses

Adults: 16-24 mEq/day in 1-2 divided doses

Treatment of hypokalemia:

Children: 2-5 mEq/kg/day in 2-4 divided doses

Adults: 40-100 mEq/day in 2-4 divided doses

Dosage Forms

Tablet: 500 mg, 610 mg

Glu-K®: 486 mg

Tablet, timed release: 595 mg

potassium iodide (poe TASS ee um EYE oh dide)

Sound-Alike/Look-Alike Issues

Potassium iodide products, including saturated solution of potassium iodide (SSKI®) may be confused with potassium iodide and iodine (Strong Iodide Solution or Lugol's solution)

Synonyms KI

U.S./Canadian Brand Names Iosat™ [US-OTC]; Pima® [US]; SSKI® [US]; ThyroSafe™ [US-OTC]; ThyroShield™ [US-OTC]

Therapeutic Category Antithyroid Agent; Expectorant

Use Expectorant for the symptomatic treatment of chronic pulmonary diseases complicated by mucous; reduce thyroid vascularity prior to thyroidectomy and management of thyrotoxic crisis; block thyroidal uptake of radioactive isotopes of iodine in a radiation emergency or other exposure to radioactive iodine

Usual Dosage Oral:

Adults: RDA: 150 mcg (iodine)

Expectorant:
Children (Pima®):
<3 years: 162 mg 3 times/day
>3 years: 325 mg 3 times/day
Adults:
Pima®: 325-650 mg 3 times/day
SSKI®: 300-600 mg 3-4 times/day
Preoperative thyroidectomy: Children and Adults: 50-250 mg (1-5 drops SSKI®) 3 times/day; administer for 10 days before surgery
Radiation protectant to radioactive isotopes of iodine (Pima®):
Children:
Infants up to 1 year: 65 mg once daily for 10 days; start 24 hours prior to exposure
>1 year: 130 mg once daily for 10 days; start 24 hours prior to exposure
Adults: 195 mg once daily for 10 days; start 24 hours prior to exposure 7
To reduce risk of thyroid cancer following nuclear accident (Iosat™, ThyroSafe™, ThyroShield™): Dosing should continue until risk of exposure has passed or other measures are implemented:
Children (see adult dose for children >68 kg):
Infants <1 month: 16.25 mg once daily
1 month to 3 years: 32.5 mg once daily
3-18 years: 65 mg once daily
Children >68 kg and Adults (including pregnant/lactating women): 130 mg once daily
Thyrotoxic crisis:
Infants <1 year: 150-250 mg (3-5 drops SSKI®) 3 times/day
Children and Adults: 300-500 mg (6-10 drops SSKI®) 3 times/day

Dosage Forms
Solution, oral:
SSKI®: 1 g/mL (30 mL, 240 mL) [contains sodium thiosulfate]
ThyroShield™: 65 mg/mL (30 mL) [black raspberry flavor]
Syrup (Pima®): 325 mg/5 mL (473 mL) [equivalent to iodide 249 mg/5 mL; black raspberry flavor]
Tablet:
Iosat™: 130 mg
ThyroSafe™: 65 mg [equivalent to iodine 50 mg]

potassium iodide, chlorpheniramine, phenylephrine, and codeine *see* chlorpheniramine, phenylephrine, codeine, and potassium iodide *on page 182*

potassium perchlorate *see* radiological/contrast media (ionic) *on page 728*

potassium phosphate (poe TASS ee um FOS fate)

Sound-Alike/Look-Alike Issues
Neutra-Phos®-K may be confused with K-Phos Neutral®

Synonyms phosphate, potassium

U.S./Canadian Brand Names Neutra-Phos®-K [US-OTC]

Therapeutic Category Electrolyte Supplement, Oral

Use Treatment and prevention of hypophosphatemia or hypokalemia

Usual Dosage I.V. doses should be incorporated into the patient's maintenance I.V. fluids; intermittent I.V. infusion should be reserved for severe depletion situations in patients undergoing continuous ECG monitoring. It is difficult to determine total body phosphorus deficit; the following dosages are empiric guidelines:

Normal requirements elemental phosphorus: Oral:
0-6 months: 240 mg
6-12 months: 360 mg
1-10 years: 800 mg
>10 years: 1200 mg
Pregnancy lactation: Additional 400 mg/day
Adults: 800 mg

Treatment: It is difficult to provide concrete guidelines for the treatment of severe hypophosphatemia because the extent of total body deficits and response to therapy are difficult to predict. Aggressive doses of phosphate may result in a transient serum elevation followed by redistribution into intracellular compartments or bone tissue. It is recommended that repletion of severe hypophosphatemia (<1 mg/dL in adults) be done I.V. because large doses of oral phosphate may cause diarrhea and intestinal absorption may be unreliable

(Continued)

potassium phosphate *(Continued)*

Pediatric I.V. phosphate repletion:

Children: 0.25-0.5 mmol/kg **administer over 4-6 hours and repeat if symptomatic hypophosphatemia persists**; to assess the need for further phosphate administration, obtain serum inorganic phosphate after administration of the first dose and base further doses on serum levels and clinical status

Adult I.V. phosphate repletion:

Initial dose: 0.08 mmol/kg if recent uncomplicated hypophosphatemia

Initial dose: 0.16 mmol/kg if prolonged hypophosphatemia with presumed total body deficits; increase dose by 25% to 50% if patient symptomatic with severe hypophosphatemia

Do not exceed 0.24 mmol/kg/dose; administer over 6-12 hours by I.V. infusion. Some investigators have used more rapid infusions.

With orders for I.V. phosphate, there is considerable confusion associated with the use of millimoles (mmol) versus milliequivalents (mEq) to express the phosphate requirement. Because inorganic phosphate exists as monobasic and dibasic anions, with the mixture of valences dependent on pH, ordering by mEq amounts is unreliable and may lead to large dosing errors. In addition, I.V. phosphate is available in the sodium and potassium salt; therefore, the content of these cations must be considered when ordering phosphate. The most reliable method of ordering I.V. phosphate is by millimoles, then specifying the potassium or sodium salt. For example, an order for 15 mmol of phosphate as potassium phosphate in one liter of normal saline. The dosing of phosphate should be 0.2-0.3 mmol/kg with a usual daily requirement of 30-60 mmol/day or 15 mmol of phosphate per liter of TPN or 15 mmol phosphate per 1000 calories of dextrose. Would also provide 22 mEq of potassium.

Maintenance:

I.V. solutions:

Children: 0.5-1.5 mmol/kg/24 hours I.V. or 2-3 mmol/kg/24 hours orally in divided doses

Adults: 15-30 mmol/24 hours I.V. or 50-150 mmol/24 hours orally in divided doses

Oral:

Children <4 years: 1 capsule (250 mg phosphorus/8 mmol) 4 times/day; dilute as instructed

Children >4 years and Adults: 1-2 capsules (250-500 mg phosphorus/8-16 mmol) 4 times/day; dilute as instructed

Dosage Forms

Injection, solution: Potassium 4.4 mEq and phosphorus 3 mmol per mL (5 mL, 15 mL, 50 mL) [equivalent to potassium 170 mg and phosphate 285 mg per mL]

Powder for oral solution [packet] (Neutra-Phos®-K): Monobasic potassium phosphate and dibasic potassium phosphate/packet (100s) [equivalent to elemental potassium 556 mg (14.2 mEq) and phosphorus 250 mg per packet; sodium and sugar free; fruit flavor]

potassium phosphate and sodium phosphate

(poe TASS ee um FOS fate & SOW dee um FOS fate)

Sound-Alike/Look-Alike Issues

K-Phos® Neutral may be confused with Neutra-Phos-K®

Synonyms sodium phosphate and potassium phosphate

U.S./Canadian Brand Names K-Phos® MF [US]; K-Phos® Neutral [US]; K-Phos® No. 2 [US]; Neutra-Phos® [US-OTC]; Phos-NaK [US]; Phospha 250™ Neutral [US]; Uro-KP-Neutral® [US]

Therapeutic Category Electrolyte Supplement, Oral

Use Treatment of conditions associated with excessive renal phosphate loss or inadequate GI absorption of phosphate; to acidify the urine to lower calcium concentrations; to increase the antibacterial activity of methenamine; reduce odor and rash caused by ammonia in urine

Usual Dosage All dosage forms to be mixed in 6-8 oz of water prior to administration

Children ≥4 years: Elemental phosphorus 250 mg 4 times/day after meals and at bedtime

Adults: Elemental phosphorus 250-500 mg 4 times/day after meals and at bedtime

Dosage Forms

Caplet:

Uro-KP-Neutral®: Sodium phosphate monobasic, dipotassium phosphate, and disodium phosphate [equivalent to elemental phosphorus 258 mg, sodium 262.4 mg (10.8 mEq), and potassium 49.4 mg (1.3 mEq)]

Powder, for oral solution:

Neutra-Phos®, Phos-NaK): Monobasic sodium, dibasic sodium, and potassium phosphate/packet (100s) [equivalent to elemental phosphorus 250 mg, sodium 164 mg (7.1 mEq), and potassium 278 mg (7.1 mEq) per packet]

Tablet:

K-Phos® MF: Potassium acid phosphate 155 mg and sodium acid phosphate 350 mg [equivalent to elemental phosphorus 125.6 mg, sodium 67 mg (2.9 mEq), and potassium 44.5 mg (1.1 mEq)]

K-Phos® Neutral: Dibasic sodium phosphate 852 mg, monobasic potassium phosphate 155 mg, and monobasic sodium phosphate 130 mg [equivalent to elemental phosphorus 250 mg, sodium 298 mg (13 mEq), and potassium 45 mg (1.1 mEq)]

K-Phos® No. 2: Potassium acid phosphate 305 mg and sodium acid phosphate 700 mg [equivalent to elemental phosphorus 250 mg, sodium 134 mg (5.8 mEq), and potassium 88 mg (2.3 mEq)]

Phospha 250™ Neutral: Dibasic sodium phosphate 852 mg, monobasic potassium phosphate 155 mg, and monobasic sodium phosphate 130 mg [equivalent to elemental phosphorus 250 mg, sodium 298 mg (13 mEq), and potassium 45 mg (1.1 mEq)]

Povidine™ [US-OTC] *see* povidone-iodine *on this page*

povidone-iodine (POE vi done EYE oh dyne)

Sound-Alike/Look-Alike Issues

Betadine® may be confused with Betagan®, betaine

Synonyms polyvinylpyrrolidone with iodine; PVP-I

U.S./Canadian Brand Names Betadine® Ophthalmic [US]; Betadine® [US-OTC/Can]; Minidyne® [US-OTC]; Operand® [US-OTC]; Povidine™ [US-OTC]; Proviodine [Can]; Summer's Eve® Medicated Douche [US-OTC]; Vagi-Gard® [US-OTC]

Therapeutic Category Antibacterial, Topical

Use External antiseptic with broad microbicidal spectrum for the prevention or treatment of topical infections associated with surgery, burns, minor cuts/scrapes; relief of minor vaginal irritation

Usual Dosage

Antiseptic: Apply topically to affected area as needed. Ophthalmic solution may be used to irrigate the eye or applied to area around the eye such as skin, eyelashes, or lid margins.

Surgical scrub: Topical: Apply solution to wet skin or hands, scrub for ~5 minutes, rinse; refer to product labeling for specific procedure-related instructions.

Vaginal irritation: Douche: Insert 0.3% solution vaginally once daily for 5-7 days

Dosage Forms [DSC] = Discontinued product

Gel, topical (Operand®): 10% (120 g)
Liquid, topical: 10% (30 mL)
Ointment, topical: 10% (1 g, 30 g)
- Betadine®: 10% (0.9 g, 3.7 g, 30 g) [DSC]
- Povidine™: 10% (30 g)

Pad [prep pads]: 10% (200s)
- Betadine® SwabAids: 10% (100s)

Scrub brush [solution impregnated]: 7.5% (30s)
Solution, ophthalmic (Betadine®): 5% (50 mL)
Solution, perineal (Operand®): 10% (240 mL) [concentrate]
Solution, topical: 10% (240 mL, 480 mL, 3840 mL)
- Betadine®: 10% (15 mL, 120 mL, 240 mL, 480 mL, 960 mL, 3840 mL)
- Minidyne®: 10% (15 mL)
- Operand®: 10% (60 mL, 120 mL, 240 mL, 480 mL, 960 mL, 3840 mL)

Solution, topical scrub:
- Betadine® Surgical Scrub: 7.5% (120 mL, 480 mL, 960 mL, 3840 mL)
- Betadine® Skin Cleanser: 7.5% (120 mL)
- Operand®: 7.5% (60 mL, 120 mL, 240 mL, 480 mL, 960 mL, 3840 mL)

Solution, topical spray:
- Betadine®: 5% (90 mL) [CFC free; contains dry natural rubber]
- Operand®: 10% (59 mL)

Solution, vaginal douche:
- Operand®: 10% (240 mL) [concentrate]
- Summer's Eve® Medicated Douche: 0.3% (135 mL)
- Vagi-Gard®: 10% (180 mL, 240 mL) [concentrate]

Solution, whirlpool (Operand®): 10% (3840 mL) [concentrate]
Swab [prep-swab ampul]: 10% (0.65 mL)
Swabsticks: 10% (25s, 50s)
- Betadine®: 10% (50s, 150s, 200s)

Swabsticks [gel saturated]: 10% (50s)
Swabsticks, topical scrub: 7.5% (25s, 50s)

PPD *see* tuberculin tests *on page 857*

PPI-149 *see* abarelix *on page 2*

PPL *see* benzylpenicilloyl-polylysine *on page 105*

PPS *see* pentosan polysulfate sodium *on page 652*

PPV23 *see* pneumococcal polysaccharide vaccine (polyvalent) *on page 676*

pralidoxime (pra li DOKS eem)

Sound-Alike/Look-Alike Issues

pralidoxime may be confused with pramoxine, pyridoxine

Protopam® may be confused with Proloprim®, protamine, Protropin®

Synonyms 2-PAM; pralidoxime chloride; 2-pyridine aldoxime methochloride

U.S./Canadian Brand Names Protopam® [US/Can]

Therapeutic Category Antidote

Use Reverse muscle paralysis caused by toxic exposure to organophosphate anticholinesterase pesticides and chemicals; control of overdose of anticholinesterase medications used to treat myasthenia gravis (ambenonium, neostigmine, pyridostigmine)

Usual Dosage

Organic phosphorus poisoning (use in conjunction with atropine; atropine effects should be established before pralidoxime is administered): I.V. (may be given I.M. or SubQ if I.V. is not feasible):

Children: 20-50 mg/kg/dose; repeat in 1-2 hours if muscle weakness has not been relieved, then at 8- to 12-hour intervals if cholinergic signs recur

Adults: 1-2 g; repeat in 1 hour if muscle weakness has not been relieved, then at 8- to 12-hour intervals if cholinergic signs recur. When the poison has been ingested, continued absorption from the lower bowel may require additional doses; patients should be titrated as long as signs of poisoning recur; dosing may need repeated every 3-8 hours.

Treatment of acetylcholinesterase inhibitor toxicity: Adults: I.V.: Initial: 1-2 g followed by increments of 250 mg every 5 minutes until response is observed

Infants and Children:

Prehospital ("in the field"): Mild-to-moderate symptoms: I.M.: 15 mg/kg; severe symptoms: 25 mg/kg

Hospital/emergency department: Mild-to-severe symptoms: I.V.: 15 mg/kg (up to 1 g)

Adults:

Prehospital ("in the field"): Mild-to-moderate symptoms: I.M.: 600 mg; severe symptoms: 1800 mg

Hospital/emergency department: Mild-to-severe symptoms: I.V.: 15 mg/kg (up to 1 g)

Frail patients:

Prehospital ("in the field"): Mild-to-moderate symptoms: I.M.: 10 mg/kg; severe symptoms: 25 mg/kg

Hospital/emergency department: Mild-to-severe symptoms: I.V.: 5-10 mg/kg

Dosage Forms Injection, powder for reconstitution, as chloride: 1 g

pralidoxime chloride *see* pralidoxime *on this page*

Pramet® FA *(Discontinued)*

Pramilet® FA *(Discontinued)*

pramipexole (pra mi PEKS ole)

Sound-Alike/Look-Alike Issues

Mirapex® may be confused with Mifeprex®, MiraLax™

U.S./Canadian Brand Names Mirapex® [US/Can]

Therapeutic Category Dopaminergic Agent (Anti-Parkinson)

Use Treatment of the signs and symptoms of idiopathic Parkinson disease

Usual Dosage Adults: Oral: Initial: 0.375 mg/day given in 3 divided doses, increase gradually by 0.125 mg/dose every 5-7 days; range: 1.5-4.5 mg/day

Dosage Forms Tablet, as dihydrochloride monohydrate: 0.125 mg, 0.25 mg, 0.5 mg, 1 mg, 1.5 mg

pramlintide (PRAM lin tide)

Synonyms pramlintide acetate

U.S./Canadian Brand Names Symlin® [US]

Therapeutic Category Antidiabetic Agent

Use

Adjunctive treatment with mealtime insulin in type 1 diabetes mellitus (insulin dependent, IDDM) patients who have failed to achieve desired glucose control despite optimal insulin therapy

Adjunctive treatment with mealtime insulin in type 2 diabetes mellitus (noninsulin dependent, NIDDM) patients who have failed to achieve desired glucose control despite optimal insulin therapy, with or without concurrent sulfonylurea and/or metformin

Usual Dosage SubQ: Adults: **Note:** When initiating pramlintide, reduce current insulin dose (including rapidly- and mixed-acting preparations) by 50% to avoid hypoglycemia.

Type 1 diabetes mellitus (insulin dependent, IDDM): Initial: 15 mcg immediately prior to meals; titrate in 15 mcg increments every 3 days (if no significant nausea occurs) to target dose of 30-60 mcg (consider discontinuation if intolerant of 30 mcg dose)

Type 2 diabetes mellitus (noninsulin dependent, NIDDM): Initial: 60 mcg immediately prior to meals; after 3-7 days, increase to 120 mcg prior to meals if no significant nausea occurs (if nausea occurs at 120 mcg dose, reduce to 60 mcg)

If pramlintide is discontinued for any reason, restart therapy with same initial titration protocol.

Dosage Forms Injection, solution: Pramlintide acetate 0.6 mg/mL (5 mL) [contains phenol-derivative metacresol]

pramlintide acetate *see* pramlintide *on previous page*

Pramosone® [US] *see* pramoxine and hydrocortisone *on this page*

Pramox® HC [Can] *see* pramoxine and hydrocortisone *on this page*

pramoxine (pra MOKS een)

Sound-Alike/Look-Alike Issues

pramoxine may be confused with pralidoxime

Anusol® may be confused with Anusol-HC®, Aplisol®, Aquasol®

Caladryl® may be confused with Benadryl®

Synonyms pramoxine hydrochloride

U.S./Canadian Brand Names Anusol® Ointment [US-OTC]; Caladryl® Clear [US-OTC]; CalaMycin® Cool and Clear [US-OTC]; Callergy Clear [US-OTC]; Curasore [US-OTC]; Itch-X® [US-OTC]; Prax® [US-OTC]; ProctoFoam® NS [US-OTC]; Sarna® Sensitive [US]; Tronolane® [US-OTC]; Tucks® Hemorrhoidal [US-OTC]

Therapeutic Category Local Anesthetic

Use Temporary relief of pain and itching associated with anogenital pruritus or irritation; dermatosis, minor burns, or hemorrhoids

Usual Dosage Adults: Topical: Apply as directed, usually every 3-4 hours to affected area (maximum adult dose: 200 mg)

Dosage Forms

Cream, topical, as hydrochloride:

Tronolane®: 1% (30 g, 60 g) [contains zinc oxide 5%]

Foam, aerosol, topical, as hydrochloride: 1% (15 g)

ProctoFoam® NS: 1% (15 g)

Gel, topical, as hydrochloride:

Itch-X®: 1% (35.4 g) [contains benzyl alcohol]

Liquid, topical, as hydrochloride:

Curasore®: 1% (15 mL) [contains ethyl alcohol; packaged with cotton applicators]

Lotion, topical, as hydrochloride:

Caladryl® Clear: 1% (177 mL) [contains zinc acetate 0.1%]

Callergy Clear: 1% (180 mL) [contains zinc acetate 0.1%]

Prax®: 1% (15 mL, 120 mL, 240 mL)

Sarna® Sensitive: 1% (222 mL)

Ointment, rectal, as hydrochloride:

Anusol®, Tucks® Hemorrhoidal: 1% (30 g) [contains zinc oxide 12.5% and mineral oil; Anusol® Ointment renamed Tucks® Hemorrhoidal]

Solution, topical spray, as hydrochloride:

CalaMycin® Cool and Clear: 1% (60 mL) [contains zinc acetate 0.1%]

Itch-X®: 1% (60 mL) [contains zinc oxide 1% and benzyl alcohol]

pramoxine and hydrocortisone (pra MOKS een & hye droe KOR ti sone)

Sound-Alike/Look-Alike Issues

pramosone® may be confused with predniSONE

Zone-A Forte® may be confused with Zonalon®

Synonyms hydrocortisone and pramoxine

U.S./Canadian Brand Names Analpram-HC® [US]; Enzone® [US]; Epifoam® [US]; Pramosone® [US]; Pramox® HC [Can]; ProctoFoam®-HC [US/Can]; Zone-A Forte® [US]; Zone-A® [US]

Therapeutic Category Anesthetic/Corticosteroid

Use Relief of inflammatory and pruritic manifestations of corticosteroid-responsive dermatoses

Usual Dosage Topical/rectal: Apply to affected areas 3-4 times/day

(Continued)

pramoxine and hydrocortisone *(Continued)*

Dosage Forms

Cream, topical:

Analpram-HC®: Pramoxine hydrochloride 1% and hydrocortisone acetate 1% (30 g); pramoxine hydrochloride 1% and hydrocortisone acetate 2.5% (30 g)

Enzone®: Pramoxine hydrochloride 1% and hydrocortisone acetate 1% (30 g)

Pramosone®: Pramoxine hydrochloride 1% and hydrocortisone acetate 1% (30 g, 60 g); pramoxine hydrochloride 1% and hydrocortisone acetate 2.5% (30 g, 60 g)

Foam, rectal (ProctoFoam®-HC): Pramoxine hydrochloride 1% and hydrocortisone acetate 1% (10 g)

Foam, topical (Epifoam®): Pramoxine hydrochloride 1% and hydrocortisone acetate 1% (10 g)

Lotion, topical:

Analpram-HC®: Pramoxine hydrochloride 1% and hydrocortisone 2.5% (60 mL)

Pramosone®: Pramoxine hydrochloride 1% and hydrocortisone 1% (60 mL, 120 mL, 240 mL); pramoxine hydrochloride 1% and hydrocortisone 2.5% (60 mL, 120 mL)

Zone-A®: Pramoxine hydrochloride 1% and hydrocortisone 1% (60 mL)

Zone-A Forte®: Pramoxine hydrochloride 1% and hydrocortisone 2.5% (60 mL)

Ointment, topical (Pramosone®): Pramoxine hydrochloride 1% and hydrocortisone 1% (30 g); pramoxine hydrochloride 1% and hydrocortisone 2.5% (30 g)

pramoxine hydrochloride *see* pramoxine *on previous page*

pramoxine, neomycin, bacitracin, and polymyxin B *see* bacitracin, neomycin, polymyxin B, and pramoxine *on page 91*

Prandase® [Can] *see* acarbose *on page 4*

Prandin® [US/Can] *see* repaglinide *on page 737*

Pravachol® [US/Can] *see* pravastatin *on this page*

pravastatin (prav a STAT in)

Sound-Alike/Look-Alike Issues

Pravachol® may be confused with Prevacid®, Prinivil®, propranolol

Synonyms pravastatin sodium

U.S./Canadian Brand Names Apo-Pravastatin® [Can]; CO Pravastatin [Can]; Novo-Pravastatin [Can]; PMS-Pravastatin [Can]; Pravachol® [US/Can]; ratio-Pravastatin [Can]; Riva-Pravastatin [Can]; Sandoz-Pravastatin [Can]

Therapeutic Category HMG-CoA Reductase Inhibitor

Use Use with dietary therapy for the following:

Primary prevention of coronary events: In hypercholesterolemic patients without established coronary heart disease to reduce cardiovascular morbidity (myocardial infarction, coronary revascularization procedures) and mortality.

Secondary prevention of cardiovascular events in patients with established coronary heart disease: To slow the progression of coronary atherosclerosis; to reduce cardiovascular morbidity (myocardial infarction, coronary vascular procedures) and to reduce mortality; to reduce the risk of stroke and transient ischemic attacks

Hyperlipidemias: Reduce elevations in total cholesterol, LDL-C, apolipoprotein B, and triglycerides (elevations of 1 or more components are present in Fredrickson type IIa, IIb, III, and IV hyperlipidemias)

Heterozygous familial hypercholesterolemia (HeFH): In pediatric patients, 8-18 years of age, with HeFH having LDL-C ≥190 mg/dL **or** LDL ≥160 mg/dL with positive family history of premature cardiovascular disease (CVD) or 2 or more CVD risk factors in the pediatric patient

Usual Dosage Oral: **Note:** Doses should be individualized according to the baseline LDL-cholesterol levels, the recommended goal of therapy, and patient response; adjustments should be made at intervals of 4 weeks or more; doses may need adjusted based on concomitant medications

Children: HeFH:

8-13 years: 20 mg/day

14-18 years: 40 mg/day

Dosage adjustment for pravastatin based on concomitant immunosuppressants (ie, cyclosporine): Refer to Adults dosing section

Adults: Hyperlipidemias, primary prevention of coronary events, secondary prevention of cardiovascular events: Initial: 40 mg once daily; titrate dosage to response; usual range: 10-80 mg; (maximum dose: 80 mg once daily)

Dosage adjustment for pravastatin based on concomitant immunosuppressants (ie, cyclosporine): Initial: 10 mg/day, titrate with caution (maximum dose: 20 mg/day)

Dosage Forms
Tablet, as sodium: 10 mg, 20 mg, 40 mg,
Pravachol®: 10 mg, 20 mg, 40 mg, 80 mg

pravastatin sodium *see* pravastatin *on previous page*

Prax® [US-OTC] *see* pramoxine *on page 691*

praziquantel (pray zi KWON tel)

U.S./Canadian Brand Names Biltricide® [US/Can]
Therapeutic Category Anthelmintic
Use All stages of schistosomiasis caused by all *Schistosoma* species pathogenic to humans; clonorchiasis and opisthorchiasis
Usual Dosage Children >4 years and Adults: Oral:
Schistosomiasis: 20 mg/kg/dose 2-3 times/day for 1 day at 4- to 6-hour intervals
Clonorchiasis/opisthorchiasis: 3 doses of 25 mg/kg as a 1-day treatment
Dosage Forms Tablet [tri-scored]: 600 mg

prazosin (PRAZ oh sin)

Sound-Alike/Look-Alike Issues
prazosin may be confused with prazepam, predniSONE
Synonyms furazosin; prazosin hydrochloride
U.S./Canadian Brand Names Apo-Prazo® [Can]; Minipress® [US/Can]; Novo-Prazin [Can]; Nu-Prazo [Can]
Therapeutic Category Alpha-Adrenergic Blocking Agent
Use Treatment of hypertension
Usual Dosage Oral:
Children: Initial: 5 mcg/kg/dose (to assess hypotensive effects); usual dosing interval: every 6 hours; increase dosage gradually up to maximum of 25 mcg/kg/dose every 6 hours
Adults:
Hypertension: Initial: 1 mg/dose 2-3 times/day; usual maintenance dose: 3-15 mg/day in divided doses 2-4 times/day; maximum daily dose: 20 mg
Hypertensive urgency: 10-20 mg once, may repeat in 30 minutes
Dosage Forms Capsule, as hydrochloride: 1 mg, 2 mg, 5 mg

prazosin and polythiazide (PRAZ oh sin & pol i THYE a zide)

Sound-Alike/Look-Alike Issues
Minizide® may be confused with Minocin®
Synonyms polythiazide and prazosin
U.S./Canadian Brand Names Minizide® [US]
Therapeutic Category Antihypertensive Agent, Combination
Use Management of mild-to-moderate hypertension
Usual Dosage Hypertension: Adults: Oral: Initial: One capsule 2-3 times/day. Maintenance: May be slowly increased to a total daily prazosin dose of 20 mg; polythiazide dose is 1-4 mg/day.
Dosage Forms Capsule:
Minizide® 1: Prazosin 1 mg and polythiazide 0.5 mg
Minizide® 2: Prazosin 2 mg and polythiazide 0.5 mg
Minizide® 5: Prazosin 5 mg and polythiazide 0.5 mg

prazosin hydrochloride *see* prazosin *on this page*

PreCare® [US] *see* vitamins (multiple/prenatal) *on page 879*

PreCare® Conceive™ [US] *see* vitamins (multiple/prenatal) *on page 879*

PreCare® Prenatal [US] *see* vitamins (multiple/prenatal) *on page 879*

Precedex™ [US/Can] *see* dexmedetomidine *on page 241*

Precose® [US] *see* acarbose *on page 4*

Pred Forte® [US/Can] *see* prednisolone (ophthalmic) *on next page*

Pred-G® [US] *see* prednisolone and gentamicin *on next page*

Pred Mild® [US/Can] *see* prednisolone (ophthalmic) *on next page*

prednicarbate (pred ni KAR bate)

Sound-Alike/Look-Alike Issues

Dermatop® may be confused with Dimetapp®

U.S./Canadian Brand Names Dermatop® [US/Can]

Therapeutic Category Corticosteroid, Topical

Use Relief of the inflammatory and pruritic manifestations of corticosteroid-responsive dermatoses (medium potency topical corticosteroid)

Usual Dosage Adults: Topical: Apply a thin film to affected area twice daily. Therapy should be discontinued when control is achieved; if no improvement is seen, reassessment of diagnosis may be necessary.

Dosage Forms

Cream: 0.1% (15 g, 60 g)

Ointment: 0.1% (15 g, 60 g)

Prednicen-M® *(Discontinued)* *see* prednisone *on next page*

prednisolone acetate *see* prednisolone (systemic) *on next page*

prednisolone acetate, ophthalmic *see* prednisolone (ophthalmic) *on this page*

prednisolone and gentamicin (pred NIS oh lone & jen ta MYE sin)

Synonyms gentamicin and prednisolone

U.S./Canadian Brand Names Pred-G® [US]

Therapeutic Category Antibiotic/Corticosteroid, Ophthalmic

Use Treatment of steroid responsive inflammatory conditions and superficial ocular infections due to microorganisms susceptible to gentamicin

Usual Dosage Ophthalmic: Children and Adults:

Ointment: Apply ½ inch ribbon in the conjunctival sac 1-3 times/day

Suspension: 1 drop 2-4 times/day; during the initial 24-48 hours, the dosing frequency may be increased if necessary up to 1 drop every hour

Dosage Forms

Ointment, ophthalmic: Prednisolone acetate 0.6% and gentamicin sulfate 0.3% (3.5 g)

Suspension, ophthalmic: Prednisolone acetate 1% and gentamicin sulfate 0.3% (2 mL, 5 mL, 10 mL) [contains benzalkonium chloride]

prednisolone and sulfacetamide *see* sulfacetamide and prednisolone *on page 796*

prednisolone, neomycin, and polymyxin B *see* neomycin, polymyxin B, and prednisolone *on page 585*

prednisolone (ophthalmic) (pred NISS oh lone op THAL mik)

Sound-Alike/Look-Alike Issues

prednisoLONE may be confused with predniSONE

Synonyms prednisolone acetate, ophthalmic; prednisolone sodium phosphate, ophthalmic

Tall-Man predniso**LONE** (ophthalmic)

U.S./Canadian Brand Names AK-Pred® [US]; Econopred® Plus [US]; Inflamase® Mild [Can]; Ophtho-Tate® [Can]; Pred Forte® [US/Can]; Pred Mild® [US/Can]

Therapeutic Category Adrenal Corticosteroid

Use Treatment of palpebral and bulbar conjunctivitis; corneal injury from chemical, radiation, thermal burns, or foreign body penetration

Usual Dosage Ophthalmic suspension/solution: Conjunctivitis, corneal injury: Children and Adults: Instill 1-2 drops into conjunctival sac every hour during day, every 2 hours at night until favorable response is obtained, then use 1 drop every 4 hours.

Dosage Forms

Solution, ophthalmic, as sodium phosphate: 1% (5 mL, 10 mL, 15 mL) [contains benzalkonium chloride]

AK-Pred®: 1% (5 mL, 15 mL) [contains benzalkonium chloride]

Suspension, ophthalmic, as acetate: 1% (5 mL, 10 mL, 15 mL) [contains benzalkonium chloride]

Econopred® Plus: 1% (5 mL, 10 mL) [contains benzalkonium chloride]

Pred Forte®: 1% (1 mL, 5 mL, 10 mL, 15 mL) [contains benzalkonium chloride and sodium bisulfite]

Pred Mild®: 0.12% (5 mL, 10 mL) [contains benzalkonium chloride and sodium bisulfite]

prednisolone sodium phosphate *see* prednisolone (systemic) *on next page*

prednisolone sodium phosphate, ophthalmic *see* prednisolone (ophthalmic) *on this page*

prednisolone (systemic) (pred NISS oh lone sis TEM ik)

Sound-Alike/Look-Alike Issues

prednisoLONE may be confused with predniSONE

Pediapred® may be confused with Pediazole®

Synonyms deltahydrocortisone; metacortandralone; prednisolone acetate; prednisolone sodium phosphate

Tall-Man predniso**LONE** (systemic)

U.S./Canadian Brand Names Bubbli-Pred™ [US]; Diopred® [Can]; Hydeltra T.B.A.® [Can]; Novo-Prednisolone [Can]; Orapred® [US]; Pediapred® [US/Can]; Prelone® [US]; Sab-Prenase [Can]

Therapeutic Category Adrenal Corticosteroid

Use Treatment of endocrine disorders, rheumatic disorders, collagen diseases, dermatologic diseases, allergic states, ophthalmic diseases, respiratory diseases, hematologic disorders, neoplastic diseases, edematous states, and gastrointestinal diseases; resolution of acute exacerbations of multiple sclerosis

Usual Dosage Dose depends upon condition being treated and response of patient; dosage for infants and children should be based on severity of the disease and response of the patient rather than on strict adherence to dosage indicated by age, weight, or body surface area. Consider alternate day therapy for long-term therapy. Discontinuation of long-term therapy requires gradual withdrawal by tapering the dose. Patients undergoing unusual stress while receiving corticosteroids, should receive increased doses prior to, during, and after the stressful situation.

Children: Oral:

- Acute asthma: 1-2 mg/kg/day in divided doses 1-2 times/day for 3-5 days
- Antiinflammatory or immunosuppressive dose: 0.1-2 mg/kg/day in divided doses 1-4 times/day
- Nephrotic syndrome:
  - Initial (first 3 episodes): 2 mg/kg/day **or** 60 mg/m²/day (maximum: 80 mg/day) in divided doses 3-4 times/day until urine is protein free for 3 consecutive days (maximum: 28 days); followed by 1-1.5 mg/kg/dose **or** 40 mg/m²/dose given every other day for 4 weeks
  - Maintenance (long-term maintenance dose for frequent relapses): 0.5-1 mg/kg/dose given every other day for 3-6 months

Adults: Oral:

- Usual range: 5-60 mg/day
- Multiple sclerosis: 200 mg/day for 1 week followed by 80 mg every other day for 1 month
- Rheumatoid arthritis: Initial: 5-7.5 mg/day; adjust dose as necessary

Dosage Forms

Solution, oral, as sodium phosphate: Prednisolone base 5 mg/5 mL (120 mL)

- Bubbli-Pred™: Prednisolone base 5 mg/5 mL (120 mL) [bubble gum flavor]
- Orapred®: 20 mg/5 mL (240 mL) [equivalent to prednisolone base 15 mg/5 mL; dye free; contains alcohol 2%, sodium benzoate; grape flavor]
- Pediapred®: 6.7 mg/5 mL (120 mL) [equivalent to prednisolone base 5 mg/5 mL; dye free; raspberry flavor]

Syrup, as base: 5 mg/5 mL (120 mL); 15 mg/5 mL (240 mL, 480 mL)

- Prelone®: 15 mg/5 mL (240 mL, 480 mL) [contains alcohol 5%, benzoic acid; cherry flavor]

Tablet, as base: 5 mg

prednisone (PRED ni sone)

Sound-Alike/Look-Alike Issues

predniSONE may be confused with methylPREDNISolone, Pramosone®, prazosin, prednisoLONE, Prilosec®, primidone, promethazine

Synonyms deltacortisone; deltadehydrocortisone

Tall-Man predni**SONE**

U.S./Canadian Brand Names Apo-Prednisone® [Can]; Novo-Prednisone [Can]; Prednisone Intensol™ [US]; Sterapred® DS [US]; Sterapred® [US]; Winpred™ [Can]

Therapeutic Category Adrenal Corticosteroid

Use Treatment of a variety of diseases including adrenocortical insufficiency, hypercalcemia, rheumatic, and collagen disorders; dermatologic, ocular, respiratory, gastrointestinal, and neoplastic diseases; organ transplantation and a variety of diseases including those of hematologic, allergic, inflammatory, and autoimmune in origin; not available in injectable form, prednisolone must be used

Usual Dosage Oral: Dose depends upon condition being treated and response of patient; dosage for infants and children should be based on severity of the disease and response of the patient rather than on strict adherence to dosage indicated by age, weight, or body surface area. Consider alternate day therapy for long-term therapy. Discontinuation of long-term therapy requires gradual withdrawal by tapering the dose.

Children:

- Antiinflammatory or immunosuppressive dose: 0.05-2 mg/kg/day divided 1-4 times/day

(Continued)

prednisone *(Continued)*

Acute asthma: 1-2 mg/kg/day in divided doses 1-2 times/day for 3-5 days
Alternatively (for 3- to 5-day "burst"):
<1 year: 10 mg every 12 hours
1-4 years: 20 mg every 12 hours
5-13 years: 30 mg every 12 hours
>13 years: 40 mg every 12 hours
Asthma long-term therapy (alternative dosing by age):
<1 year: 10 mg every other day
1-4 years: 20 mg every other day
5-13 years: 30 mg every other day
>13 years: 40 mg every other day
Nephrotic syndrome:
Initial (first 3 episodes): 2 mg/kg/day **or** 60 mg/m²/day (maximum: 80 mg/day) in divided doses 3-4 times/day until urine is protein free for 3 consecutive days (maximum: 28 days); followed by 1-1.5 mg/kg/dose **or** 40 mg/m²/dose given every other day for 4 weeks
Maintenance dose (long-term maintenance dose for frequent relapses): 0.5-1 mg/kg/dose given every other day for 3-6 months
Children and Adults: Physiologic replacement: 4-5 mg/m²/day
Children ≥5 years and Adults: Asthma:
Moderate persistent: Inhaled corticosteroid (medium dose) or inhaled corticosteroid (low-medium dose) with a long-acting bronchodilator
Severe persistent: Inhaled corticosteroid (high dose) and corticosteroid tablets or syrup long term: 2 mg/kg/day, generally not to exceed 60 mg/day
Adults:
Immunosuppression/chemotherapy adjunct: Range: 5-60 mg/day in divided doses 1-4 times/day
Allergic reaction (contact dermatitis):
Day 1: 30 mg divided as 10 mg before breakfast, 5 mg at lunch, 5 mg at dinner, 10 mg at bedtime
Day 2: 5 mg at breakfast, 5 mg at lunch, 5 mg at dinner, 10 mg at bedtime
Day 3: 5 mg 4 times/day (with meals and at bedtime)
Day 4: 5 mg 3 times/day (breakfast, lunch, bedtime)
Day 5: 5 mg 2 times/day (breakfast, bedtime)
Day 6: 5 mg before breakfast
Pneumocystis carinii pneumonia (PCP):
40 mg twice daily for 5 days **followed by**
40 mg once daily for 5 days **followed by**
20 mg once daily for 11 days or until antimicrobial regimen is completed
Thyrotoxicosis: Oral: 60 mg/day
Chemotherapy (refer to individual protocols): Oral: Range: 20 mg/day to 100 mg/m²/day
Rheumatoid arthritis: Oral: Use lowest possible daily dose (often ≤7.5 mg/day)
Idiopathic thrombocytopenia purpura (ITP): Oral: 60 mg daily for 4-6 weeks, gradually tapered over several weeks
Systemic lupus erythematosus (SLE): Oral:
Acute: 1-2 mg/kg/day in 2-3 divided doses
Maintenance: Reduce to lowest possible dose, usually <1 mg/kg/day as single dose (morning)

Dosage Forms
Solution, oral: 1 mg/mL (5 mL, 120 mL, 500 mL) [contains alcohol 5%, sodium benzoate; vanilla flavor]
Solution, oral concentrate (Prednisone Intensol™): 5 mg/mL (30 mL) [contains alcohol 30%]
Tablet: 1 mg, 2.5 mg, 5 mg, 10 mg, 20 mg, 50 mg
Sterapred®: 5 mg [supplied as 21 tablet 6-day unit-dose package or 48 tablet 12-day unit-dose package]
Sterapred® DS: 10 mg [supplied as 21 tablet 6-day unit-dose package or 48 tablet 12-day unit-dose package]

Prednisone Intensol™ [US] *see* prednisone *on previous page*
Prefest™ [US] *see* estradiol and norgestimate *on page 311*
Prefrin™ *(Discontinued)* *see* phenylephrine *on page 660*

pregabalin (pre GAB a lin)

Synonyms CI-1008; S-(+)-3-isobutylgaba
U.S./Canadian Brand Names Lyrica® [US/Can]
Therapeutic Category Analgesic, Miscellaneous; Anticonvulsant, Miscellaneous
Controlled Substance C-V

Use Management of pain associated with diabetic peripheral neuropathy; management of postherpetic neuralgia; adjunctive therapy for partial-onset seizure disorder in adults

Usual Dosage Oral: Adults:

Neuropathic pain (diabetes-associated): Initial: 150 mg/day in divided doses (50 mg 3 times/day); may be increased within 1 week based on tolerability and effect; maximum dose: 300 mg/day (dosages up to 600 mg/day were evaluated with no significant additional benefit and an increase in adverse effects)

Postherpetic neuralgia: Initial: 150 mg/day in divided doses (75 mg 2 times/day or 50 mg 3 times/day); may be increased to 300 mg/day within 1 week based on tolerability and effect; further titration (to 600 mg/day) after 2-4 weeks may be considered in patients who do not experience sufficient relief of pain provided they are able to tolerate pregabalin. Maximum dose: 600 mg/day

Partial-onset seizures (adjunctive therapy): Initial: 150 mg per day in divided doses (75 mg 2 times/day or 50 mg 3 times/day); may be increased based on tolerability and effect (optimal titration schedule has not been defined). Maximum dose: 600 mg/day

Discontinuing therapy: Pregabalin should not be abruptly discontinued; taper dosage over at least 1 week

Dosage Forms Capsule: 25 mg, 50 mg, 75 mg, 100 mg, 150 mg, 200 mg, 225 mg, 300 mg

Pregestimil® [US-OTC] *see* nutritional formula, enteral/oral *on page 608*

pregnenedione *see* progesterone *on page 703*

Pregnyl® [US] *see* chorionic gonadotropin (human) *on page 186*

Prelone® [US] *see* prednisolone (systemic) *on page 695*

Prelu-2® *(Discontinued)* *see* phendimetrazine *on page 657*

Premarin® [US/Can] *see* estrogens (conjugated/equine) *on page 312*

Premarin® With Methyltestosterone *(Discontinued)*

Premjact® [US-OTC] *see* lidocaine *on page 493*

Premphase® [US/Can] *see* estrogens (conjugated/equine) and medroxyprogesterone *on page 313*

Premplus® [Can] *see* estrogens (conjugated/equine) and medroxyprogesterone *on page 313*

Prempro™ [US/Can] *see* estrogens (conjugated/equine) and medroxyprogesterone *on page 313*

Prenatal 1-A-Day [US] *see* vitamins (multiple/prenatal) *on page 879*

Prenatal AD [US] *see* vitamins (multiple/prenatal) *on page 879*

Prenatal H [US] *see* vitamins (multiple/prenatal) *on page 879*

Prenatal MR 90 Fe™ [US] *see* vitamins (multiple/prenatal) *on page 879*

Prenatal MTR with Selenium [US] *see* vitamins (multiple/prenatal) *on page 879*

Prenatal Plus [US] *see* vitamins (multiple/prenatal) *on page 879*

Prenatal Rx 1 [US] *see* vitamins (multiple/prenatal) *on page 879*

Prenatal U [US] *see* vitamins (multiple/prenatal) *on page 879*

prenatal vitamins *see* vitamins (multiple/prenatal) *on page 879*

Prenatal Z [US] *see* vitamins (multiple/prenatal) *on page 879*

Prenate Elite™ [US] *see* vitamins (multiple/prenatal) *on page 879*

Prenate GT™ [US] *see* vitamins (multiple/prenatal) *on page 879*

Preparation H® Cleansing Pads [Can] *see* witch hazel *on page 881*

Preparation H® Hydrocortisone [US-OTC] *see* hydrocortisone (rectal) *on page 426*

Preparation H® Medicated Wipes [US-OTC] *see* witch hazel *on page 881*

Prepcat® [US] *see* radiological/contrast media (ionic) *on page 728*

Pre-Pen® *(Discontinued)* *see* benzylpenicilloyl-polylysine *on page 105*

Prepidil® [US/Can] *see* dinoprostone *on page 260*

Prescription Strength Desenex® *(Discontinued)* *see* miconazole *on page 553*

Preservative-Free Cosopt® [Can] *see* dorzolamide and timolol *on page 274*

PreserVision® AREDS [US-OTC] *see* vitamins (multiple/oral) *on page 878*

PreserVision® Lutein [US-OTC] *see* vitamins (multiple/oral) *on page 878*

Pressyn® [Can] *see* vasopressin *on page 868*

Pressyn® AR [Can] *see* vasopressin *on page 868*

Preterax® [Can] *see* perindopril and indapamide *(Canada only) on page 654*

Pretz® [US-OTC] *see* sodium chloride *on page 777*

Pretz-D® [US-OTC] *see* ephedrine *on page 294*

Prevacare® [US-OTC] *see* alcohol (ethyl) *on page 25*

Prevacid® [US/Can] *see* lansoprazole *on page 481*

Prevacid® NapraPAC™ [US] *see* lansoprazole and naproxen *on page 483*

Prevacid® SoluTab™ [US] *see* lansoprazole *on page 481*

Prevalite® [US] *see* cholestyramine resin *on page 186*

PREVEN® [US] *see* ethinyl estradiol and levonorgestrel *on page 320*

Prevex® B [Can] *see* betamethasone (topical) *on page 107*

Prevex® HC [Can] *see* hydrocortisone (topical) *on page 428*

PreviDent® [US] *see* fluoride *on page 354*

PreviDent® 5000 Plus™ [US] *see* fluoride *on page 354*

Previfem™ [US] *see* ethinyl estradiol and norgestimate *on page 325*

Prevnar® [US/Can] *see* pneumococcal conjugate vaccine (7-valent) *on page 675*

Prevpac® [US/Can] *see* lansoprazole, amoxicillin, and clarithromycin *on page 482*

Prezista™ [US] *see* darunavir *on page 231*

Prialt® [US] *see* ziconotide *on page 885*

Priftin® [US/Can] *see* rifapentine *on page 746*

prilocaine (PRIL oh kane)

Sound-Alike/Look-Alike Issues

prilocaine may be confused with Polocaine®, Prilosec®

U.S./Canadian Brand Names Citanest® Plain [US/Can]

Therapeutic Category Local Anesthetic

Usual Dosage

Children <10 years: Doses >40 mg (1 mL) as a 4% solution per procedure rarely needed

Children >10 years and Adults: Dental anesthesia, infiltration, or conduction block: Initial: 40-80 mg (1-2 mL) as a 4% solution; up to a maximum of 400 mg (10 mL) as a 4% solution within a 2-hour period. Manufacturer's maximum recommended dose is not more than 600 mg to normal healthy adults. The effective anesthetic dose varies with procedure, intensity of anesthesia needed, duration of anesthesia required and physical condition of the patient. Always use the lowest effective dose along with careful aspiration.

Note: Adult and children doses of prilocaine hydrochloride cited from USP Dispensing Information (USP DI), 17th ed, The United States Pharmacopeial Convention, Inc, Rockville, MD, 1997, 139.

Dosage Forms Injection, solution: Prilocaine hydrochloride 4% (1.8 mL) [prefilled cartridge]

prilocaine and lidocaine *see* lidocaine and prilocaine *on page 496*

Prilosec® [US] *see* omeprazole *on page 615*

Prilosec OTC™ [US-OTC] *see* omeprazole *on page 615*

primaclone *see* primidone *on next page*

Primacor® [US] *see* milrinone *on page 557*

primaquine (PRIM a kween)

Synonyms primaquine phosphate; prymaccone

Therapeutic Category Aminoquinoline (Antimalarial)

Use Treatment of malaria

Usual Dosage Oral: Dosage expressed as mg of base (15 mg base = 26.3 mg primaquine phosphate):

Treatment of malaria (decrease risk of delayed primary attacks and prevent relapse):

Children: 0.3 mg base/kg/day once daily for 14 days (not to exceed 15 mg/day) or 0.9 mg base/kg once weekly for 8 weeks not to exceed 45 mg base/week

Adults: 15 mg/day (base) once daily for 14 days or 45 mg base once weekly for 8 weeks

CDC treatment recommendations: Begin therapy during last 2 weeks of, or following a course of, suppression with chloroquine or a comparable drug

Note: A second course (30 mg/day) for 14 days may be required in patients with relapse. Higher initial doses (30 mg/day) have also been used following exposure in S.E. Asia or Somalia.

Dosage Forms Tablet, as phosphate: 26.3 mg [15 mg base]

primaquine phosphate *see* primaquine *on previous page*

Primatene® Mist [US-OTC] *see* epinephrine *on page 295*

Primaxin® [US/Can] *see* imipenem and cilastatin *on page 441*

Primaxin® I.V. [Can] *see* imipenem and cilastatin *on page 441*

primidone (PRI mi done)

Sound-Alike/Look-Alike Issues
primidone may be confused with predniSONE

Synonyms desoxyphenobarbital; primaclone

U.S./Canadian Brand Names Apo-Primidone® [Can]; Mysoline® [US]

Therapeutic Category Anticonvulsant; Barbiturate

Use Management of grand mal, psychomotor, and focal seizures

Usual Dosage Oral:

Children <8 years: Initial: 50-125 mg/day given at bedtime; increase by 50-125 mg/day increments every 3-7 days; usual dose: 10-25 mg/kg/day in divided doses 3-4 times/day

Children ≥8 years and Adults: Initial: 125-250 mg/day at bedtime; increase by 125-250 mg/day every 3-7 days; usual dose: 750-1500 mg/day in divided doses 3-4 times/day with maximum dosage of 2 g/day

Dosage Forms Tablet: 50 mg, 250 mg [generic tablet may contain sodium benzoate]

Dosage forms available in Canada: Tablet: 125 mg, 250 mg. **Note:** 50 mg tablet is **not** available in Canada.

Primsol® [US] *see* trimethoprim *on page 851*

Prinivil® [US/Can] *see* lisinopril *on page 500*

Prinzide® [US/Can] *see* lisinopril and hydrochlorothiazide *on page 501*

Priorix™ [Can] *see* measles, mumps, and rubella vaccines, combined *on page 520*

pristinamycin *see* quinupristin and dalfopristin *on page 727*

Privine® [US-OTC] *see* naphazoline *on page 577*

ProAir™ HFA [US] *see* albuterol *on page 23*

ProAmatine® [US] *see* midodrine *on page 556*

Pro-Banthine® *(Discontinued)* *see* propantheline *on page 706*

probenecid (proe BEN e sid)

Sound-Alike/Look-Alike Issues
probenecid may be confused with Procanbid®

U.S./Canadian Brand Names Benuryl™ [Can]

Therapeutic Category Uricosuric Agent

Use Prevention of hyperuricemia associated with gout or gouty arthritis; prolongation and elevation of beta-lactam plasma levels

Usual Dosage Oral:

Children:

- <2 years: Contraindicated
- 2-14 years: Prolong penicillin serum levels: Initial: 25 mg/kg, then 40 mg/kg/day given 4 times/day (maximum: 500 mg/dose)
- Gonorrhea: >45 kg: Refer to adult guidelines

Adults:

- Hyperuricemia with gout: 250 mg twice daily for one week; increase to 250-500 mg/day; may increase by 500 mg/month, if needed, to maximum of 2-3 g/day (dosages may be increased by 500 mg every 6 months if serum urate concentrations are controlled)
- Prolong penicillin serum levels: 500 mg 4 times/day
- Gonorrhea: CDC guidelines (alternative regimen): Probenecid 1 g orally with cefoxitin 2 g I.M.
- Pelvic inflammatory disease: CDC guidelines: Cefoxitin 2 g I.M. plus probenecid 1 g orally as a single dose
- Neurosyphilis: CDC guidelines (alternative regimen): Procaine penicillin 2.4 million units/day I.M. plus probenecid 500 mg 4 times/day; both administered for 10-14 days

Dosage Forms Tablet: 500 mg

probenecid and colchicine *see* colchicine and probenecid *on page 210*

Pro-Bionate® *(Discontinued)*

procainamide (pro KANE a mide)

Sound-Alike/Look-Alike Issues

Procanbid® may be confused with probenecid

Pronestyl® may be confused with Ponstel®

PCA is an error-prone abbreviation (mistaken as patient controlled analgesia)

Synonyms procainamide hydrochloride; procaine amide hydrochloride

U.S./Canadian Brand Names Apo-Procainamide® [Can]; Procainamide Hydrochloride Injection, USP [Can]; Procanbid® [US]; Procan® SR [Can]

Therapeutic Category Antiarrhythmic Agent, Class I-A

Use Treatment of ventricular tachycardia (VT), premature ventricular contractions, paroxysmal atrial tachycardia (PSVT), and atrial fibrillation (AF); prevent recurrence of ventricular tachycardia, paroxysmal supraventricular tachycardia, atrial fibrillation or flutter

Usual Dosage Must be titrated to patient's response

Children:

Oral: 15-50 mg/kg/24 hours divided every 3-6 hours

I.M.: 50 mg/kg/24 hours divided into doses of $^1/_8$ to $^1/_4$ every 3-6 hours in divided doses until oral therapy is possible

I.V. (infusion requires use of an infusion pump):

Load: 3-6 mg/kg/dose over 5 minutes not to exceed 100 mg/dose; may repeat every 5-10 minutes to maximum of 15 mg/kg/load

Maintenance as continuous I.V. infusion: 20-80 mcg/kg/minute; maximum: 2 g/24 hours

Possible VT (pulses and poor perfusion) [PALS 2005 Guidelines]: I.V.; I.O.: 15 mg/kg over 30-60 minutes

Adults:

Oral: Usual dose: 50 mg/kg/24 hours: maximum: 5 g/24 hours (**Note:** Twice-daily dosing approved for Procanbid®.)

Immediate release formulation: 250-500 mg/dose every 3-6 hours

Extended release formulation: 500 mg to 1 g every 6 hours; Procanbid®: 1000-2500 mg every 12 hours

I.M.: 0.5-1 g every 4-8 hours until oral therapy is possible

I.V. (infusion requires use of an infusion pump):

Loading dose: 15-18 mg/kg administered as slow infusion over 25-30 minutes **or** 100-200 mg/dose repeated every 5 minutes as needed to a total dose of 1 g. Reduce loading dose to 12 mg/kg in severe renal or cardiac impairment.

Maintenance dose: 1-4 mg/minute by continuous infusion. Maintenance infusions should be reduced by one-third in patients with moderate renal or cardiac impairment and by two-thirds in patients with severe renal or cardiac impairment.

ACLS guidelines: Infuse 20 mg/minute until arrhythmia is controlled, hypotension occurs, QRS complex widens by 50% of its original width, or total of 17 mg/kg is given.

Dosage Forms

Capsule, as hydrochloride: 250 mg, 500 mg

Injection, solution, as hydrochloride: 100 mg/mL (10 mL); 500 mg/mL (2 mL) [contains sodium metabisulfite]

Tablet, extended release, as hydrochloride: 500 mg, 750 mg, 1000 mg

Procanbid®: 500 mg, 1000 mg

procainamide hydrochloride *see* procainamide *on this page*

Procainamide Hydrochloride Injection, USP [Can] *see* procainamide *on this page*

procaine (PROE kane)

Synonyms procaine hydrochloride

U.S./Canadian Brand Names Novocain® [US]

Therapeutic Category Local Anesthetic

Use Produces spinal anesthesia and epidural and peripheral nerve block by injection and infiltration methods

Usual Dosage Dose varies with procedure, desired depth, and duration of anesthesia, desired muscle relaxation, vascularity of tissues, physical condition, and age of patient

Dosage Forms Injection, solution, as hydrochloride: 1% [10 mg/mL] (2 mL) [contains sodium bisulfite]; 10% (2 mL) [contains sodium bisulfite]

procaine amide hydrochloride *see* procainamide *on this page*

procaine benzylpenicillin *see* penicillin G procaine *on page 649*

procaine hydrochloride *see* procaine *on previous page*

procaine penicillin G *see* penicillin G procaine *on page 649*

Pro-Cal-Sof® *(Discontinued)* *see* docusate *on page 270*

Procanbid® [US] *see* procainamide *on previous page*

Procan® SR [Can] *see* procainamide *on previous page*

procarbazine (proe KAR ba zeen)

Sound-Alike/Look-Alike Issues

procarbazine may be confused with dacarbazine
Matulane® may be confused with Modane®

Synonyms benzmethyzin; N-methylhydrazine; NSC-77213; procarbazine hydrochloride

U.S./Canadian Brand Names Matulane® [US/Can]; Natulan® [Can]

Therapeutic Category Antineoplastic Agent

Use Treatment of Hodgkin disease

Usual Dosage Refer to individual protocols. Manufacturer states that the dose is based on patient's ideal weight if the patient is obese or has abnormal fluid retention. Other studies suggest that ideal body weight may not be necessary. Oral (may be given as a single daily dose or in 2-3 divided doses):

Children:
BMT aplastic anemia conditioning regimen: 12.5 mg/kg/day every other day for 4 doses
Hodgkin's disease: MOPP/IC-MOPP regimens: 100 mg/m^2/day for 14 days and repeated every 4 weeks
Neuroblastoma and medulloblastoma: Doses as high as 100-200 mg/m^2/day once daily have been used

Adults: Initial: 2-4 mg/kg/day in single or divided doses for 7 days then increase dose to 4-6 mg/kg/day until response is obtained or leukocyte count decreased <4000/mm^3 or the platelet count decreased <100,000/mm^3; maintenance: 1-2 mg/kg/day

Dosage Forms

Capsule, as hydrochloride:
Matulane®: 50 mg

procarbazine hydrochloride *see* procarbazine *on this page*

Procardia® [US/Can] *see* nifedipine *on page 592*

Procardia XL® [US] *see* nifedipine *on page 592*

procetofene *see* fenofibrate *on page 338*

Prochieve™ [US] *see* progesterone *on page 703*

prochlorperazine (proe klor PER a zeen)

Sound-Alike/Look-Alike Issues

prochlorperazine may be confused with chlorproMAZINE
Compazine® may be confused with Copaxone®, Coumadin®
CPZ (occasional abbreviation for Compazine®) is an error-prone abbreviation (mistaken as chlorpromazine)

Synonyms chlormeprazine; prochlorperazine edisylate; prochlorperazine maleate

U.S./Canadian Brand Names Apo-Prochlorperazine® [Can]; Compazine® [Can]; Compro™ [US]; Nu-Prochlor [Can]; Stemetil® [Can]

Therapeutic Category Phenothiazine Derivative

Use Management of nausea and vomiting; psychotic disorders including schizophrenia; anxiety

Usual Dosage

Antiemetic: Children (therapy >1 day usually not required): **Note:** Not recommended for use in children <9 kg or <2 years:

Oral, rectal: >9 kg: 0.4 mg/kg/24 hours in 3-4 divided doses; **or**
9-13 kg: 2.5 mg every 12-24 hours as needed; maximum: 7.5 mg/day
13.1-17 kg: 2.5 mg every 8-12 hours as needed; maximum: 10 mg/day
17.1-37 kg: 2.5 mg every 8 hours or 5 mg every 12 hours as needed; maximum: 15 mg/day

I.M.: 0.13 mg/kg/dose; change to oral as soon as possible

Antiemetic: Adults:
Oral (tablet): 5-10 mg 3-4 times/day; usual maximum: 40 mg/day; larger doses may rarely be required
I.M. (deep): 5-10 mg every 3-4 hours; usual maximum: 40 mg/day
I.V.: 2.5-10 mg; maximum 10 mg/dose or 40 mg/day; may repeat dose every 3-4 hours as needed
Rectal: 25 mg twice daily

Surgical nausea/vomiting: Adults: **Note:** Should not exceed 40 mg/day

(Continued)

prochlorperazine *(Continued)*

I.M.: 5-10 mg 1-2 hours before induction or to control symptoms during or after surgery; may repeat once if necessary

I.V. (administer slow IVP <5 mg/minute): 5-10 mg 15-30 minutes before induction or to control symptoms during or after surgery; may repeat once if necessary

Antipsychotic:

Children 2-12 years (not recommended in children <9 kg or <2 years):

Oral, rectal: 2.5 mg 2-3 times/day; do not give more than 10 mg the first day; increase dosage as needed to maximum daily dose of 20 mg for 2-5 years and 25 mg for 6-12 years

I.M.: 0.13 mg/kg/dose; change to oral as soon as possible

Adults:

Oral: 5-10 mg 3-4 times/day; titrate dose slowly every 2-3 days; doses up to 150 mg/day may be required in some patients for treatment of severe disturbances

I.M.: Initial: 10-20 mg; if necessary repeat initial dose every 1-4 hours to gain control; more than 3-4 doses are rarely needed. If parenteral administration is still required; give 10-20 mg every 4-6 hours; change to oral as soon as possible.

Nonpsychotic anxiety: Oral (tablet): Adults: Usual dose: 15-20 mg/day in divided doses; do not give doses >20 mg/day or for longer than 12 weeks

Dosage Forms

Injection, solution, as edisylate: 5 mg/mL (2 mL, 10 mL) [contains benzyl alcohol]

Suppository, rectal: 2.5 mg (12s), 5 mg (12s), 25 mg (12s) [may contain coconut and palm oil]

Compro™: 25 mg (12s) [contains coconut and palm oils]

Tablet, as maleate: 5 mg, 10 mg

prochlorperazine edisylate *see* prochlorperazine *on previous page*

prochlorperazine maleate *see* prochlorperazine *on previous page*

Procrit® [US] *see* epoetin alfa *on page 298*

Proctocort® [US] *see* hydrocortisone (rectal) *on page 426*

ProctoCream® HC [US] *see* hydrocortisone (rectal) *on page 426*

proctofene *see* fenofibrate *on page 338*

ProctoFoam®-HC [US/Can] *see* pramoxine and hydrocortisone *on page 691*

ProctoFoam® NS [US-OTC] *see* pramoxine *on page 691*

Procto-Kit™ [US] *see* hydrocortisone (rectal) *on page 426*

Procto-Pak™ [US] *see* hydrocortisone (rectal) *on page 426*

Proctosert [US] *see* hydrocortisone (rectal) *on page 426*

Proctosol-HC® [US] *see* hydrocortisone (rectal) *on page 426*

Proctozone-HC™ [US] *see* hydrocortisone (rectal) *on page 426*

procyclidine (proe SYE kli deen)

Sound-Alike/Look-Alike Issues

Kemadrin® may be confused with Coumadin®

Synonyms procyclidine hydrochloride

U.S./Canadian Brand Names Kemadrin® [US]; PMS-Procyclidine [Can]

Therapeutic Category Anti-Parkinson Agent; Anticholinergic Agent

Use Relieves symptoms of parkinsonian syndrome and drug-induced extrapyramidal symptoms

Usual Dosage Adults: Oral: 2.5 mg 3 times/day after meals; if tolerated, gradually increase dose, maximum of 20 mg/day if necessary

Dosage Forms Tablet, as hydrochloride [scored]: 5 mg

procyclidine hydrochloride *see* procyclidine *on this page*

Procytox® [Can] *see* cyclophosphamide *on page 220*

Profasi® HP [Can] *see* chorionic gonadotropin (human) *on page 186*

Profen II® [US] *see* guaifenesin and pseudoephedrine *on page 398*

Profen II DM® [US] *see* guaifenesin, pseudoephedrine, and dextromethorphan *on page 401*

Profen Forte® [US] *see* guaifenesin and pseudoephedrine *on page 398*

Profen Forte™ DM [US] *see* guaifenesin, pseudoephedrine, and dextromethorphan *on page 401*

Profen LA® ***(Discontinued)***

Profilnine® SD [US] *see* factor IX complex (human) *on page 334*

Proflavanol C™ [Can] *see* ascorbic acid *on page 76*

progesterone (proe JES ter one)

Sound-Alike/Look-Alike Issues

progesterone may be confused with medroxyPROGESTERone

Synonyms pregnenedione; progestin

U.S./Canadian Brand Names Crinone® [US/Can]; Prochieve™ [US]; Prometrium® [US/Can]

Therapeutic Category Progestin

Use

Oral: Prevention of endometrial hyperplasia in nonhysterectomized, postmenopausal women who are receiving conjugated estrogen tablets; secondary amenorrhea

I.M.: Amenorrhea; abnormal uterine bleeding due to hormonal imbalance

Intravaginal gel: Part of assisted reproductive technology (ART) for infertile women with progesterone deficiency; secondary amenorrhea

Usual Dosage Adults:

I.M.: Female:

Amenorrhea: 5-10 mg/day for 6-8 consecutive days

Functional uterine bleeding: 5-10 mg/day for 6 doses

Oral: Female:

Prevention of endometrial hyperplasia (in postmenopausal women with a uterus who are receiving daily conjugated estrogen tablets): 200 mg as a single daily dose every evening for 12 days sequentially per 28-day cycle

Amenorrhea: 400 mg every evening for 10 days

Intravaginal gel: Female:

ART in women who require progesterone supplementation: 90 mg (8% gel) once daily; if pregnancy occurs, may continue treatment for up to 10-12 weeks

ART in women with partial or complete ovarian failure: 90 mg (8% gel) intravaginally twice daily; if pregnancy occurs, may continue up to 10-12 weeks

Secondary amenorrhea: 45 mg (4% gel) intravaginally every other day for up to 6 doses; women who fail to respond may be increased to 90 mg (8% gel) every other day for up to 6 doses

Dosage Forms

Capsule (Prometrium®): 100 mg, 200 mg [contains peanut oil]

Gel, vaginal (Crinone®, Prochieve™): 4% (45 mg); 8% (90 mg) [contains palm oil; prefilled applicators]

Injection, oil: 50 mg/mL (10 mL) [contains benzyl alcohol 10%, sesame oil]

progestin *see* progesterone *on this page*

Proglycem® [US/Can] *see* diazoxide *on page 249*

Prograf® [US/Can] *see* tacrolimus *on page 803*

proguanil and atovaquone *see* atovaquone and proguanil *on page 82*

ProHance® [US] *see* radiological/contrast media (nonionic) *on page 730*

ProHIBiT® *(Discontinued)*

Prolastin® [US/Can] *see* alpha$_1$-proteinase inhibitor *on page 31*

Proleukin® [US/Can] *see* aldesleukin *on page 26*

Prolex™-D [US] *see* guaifenesin and phenylephrine *on page 396*

Prolixin Decanoate® [US] *see* fluphenazine *on page 358*

Prolixin® *(Discontinued)* *see* fluphenazine *on page 358*

Prolixin Enanthate® *(Discontinued)* *see* fluphenazine *on page 358*

Prolopa® [Can] *see* benserazide and levodopa *(Canada only)* *on page 98*

Proloprim® [US] *see* trimethoprim *on page 851*

Prometa® *(Discontinued)*

promethazine (proe METH a zeen)

Sound-Alike/Look-Alike Issues

promethazine may be confused with chlorproMAZINE, predniSONE, promazine

Phenergan® may be confused with Phenaphen®, Phrenilin®, Theragran®

(Continued)

promethazine *(Continued)*

Synonyms promethazine hydrochloride

U.S./Canadian Brand Names Phenadoz™ [US]; Phenergan® [US/Can]; Promethegan™ [US]

Therapeutic Category Antiemetic; Phenothiazine Derivative

Use Symptomatic treatment of various allergic conditions; antiemetic; motion sickness; sedative; postoperative pain (adjunctive therapy); anesthetic (adjunctive therapy); anaphylactic reactions (adjunctive therapy)

Usual Dosage

Children ≥2 years:

Allergic conditions: Oral, rectal: 0.1 mg/kg/dose (maximum: 12.5 mg) every 6 hours during the day and 0.5 mg/kg/dose (maximum: 25 mg) at bedtime as needed

Antiemetic: Oral, I.M., I.V., rectal: 0.25-1 mg/kg 4-6 times/day as needed (maximum: 25 mg/dose)

Motion sickness: Oral, rectal: 0.5 mg/kg/dose 30 minutes to 1 hour before departure, then every 12 hours as needed (maximum dose: 25 mg twice daily)

Sedation: Oral, I.M., I.V., rectal: 0.5-1 mg/kg/dose every 6 hours as needed (maximum: 50 mg/dose)

Adults:

Allergic conditions (including allergic reactions to blood or plasma):

Oral, rectal: 25 mg at bedtime **or** 12.5 mg before meals and at bedtime (range: 6.25-12.5 mg 3 times/day)

I.M., I.V.: 25 mg, may repeat in 2 hours when necessary; switch to oral route as soon as feasible

Antiemetic: Oral, I.M., I.V., rectal: 12.5-25 mg every 4-6 hours as needed

Motion sickness: Oral, rectal: 25 mg 30-60 minutes before departure, then every 12 hours as needed

Sedation: Oral, I.M., I.V., rectal: 12.5-50 mg/dose

Dosage Forms [DSC] = Discontinued product

Injection, solution, as hydrochloride: 25 mg/mL (1 mL); 50 mg/mL (1 mL)

Phenergan®: 25 mg/mL (1 mL); 50 mg/mL (1 mL) [contains sodium metabisulfite]

Suppository, rectal, as hydrochloride: 12.5 mg, 25 mg, 50 mg

Phenadoz™: 12.5 mg, 25 mg

Phenergan®: 25 mg, 50 mg [DSC]

Promethegan™: 12.5 mg, 25 mg, 50 mg

Syrup, as hydrochloride: 6.25 mg/5 mL (120 mL, 480 mL) [contains alcohol]

Tablet, as hydrochloride: 12.5 mg, 25 mg, 50 mg

Phenergan®: 25 mg [DSC]

promethazine and codeine (proe METH a zeen & KOE deen)

Sound-Alike/Look-Alike Issues

Phenergan® may be confused with Phenaphen®, Phrenilin®, Theragran®

Synonyms codeine and promethazine

Therapeutic Category Antihistamine/Antitussive

Controlled Substance C-V

Use Temporary relief of coughs and upper respiratory symptoms associated with allergy or the common cold

Usual Dosage Oral:

Children:

<2 years: Use of promethazine is contraindicated

2 to <6 years:

12 kg: 1.25-2.5 mL every 4-6 hours (maximum: 6 mL/24 hours)

14 kg: 1.25-2.5 mL every 4-6 hours (maximum: 7 mL/24 hours)

16 kg: 1.25-2.5 mL every 4-6 hours (maximum: 8 mL/24 hours)

18 kg: 1.25-2.5 mL every 4-6 hours (maximum: 9 mL/24 hours)

6-12 years: 2.5-5 mL every 4-6 hours (maximum: 30 mL/24 hours)

Adults: 5 mL every 4-6 hours (maximum 30 mL/24 hours)

Dosage Forms Syrup: Promethazine hydrochloride 6.25 mg and codeine phosphate 10 mg per 5 mL (120 mL, 473 mL) [contains alcohol]

promethazine and dextromethorphan (proe METH a zeen & deks troe meth OR fan)

Synonyms dextromethorphan and promethazine

Therapeutic Category Antihistamine/Antitussive

Use Temporary relief of coughs and upper respiratory symptoms associated with allergy or the common cold

Usual Dosage Oral:

Children:

2-6 years: 1.25-2.5 mL every 4-6 hours up to 10 mL in 24 hours

6-12 years: 2.5-5 mL every 4-6 hours up to 20 mL in 24 hours

Adults: 5 mL every 4-6 hours up to 30 mL in 24 hours

Dosage Forms Syrup: Promethazine hydrochloride 6.25 mg and dextromethorphan hydrobromide 15 mg per 5 mL (120 mL, 480 mL) [contains alcohol 7%]

promethazine and meperidine *see* meperidine and promethazine *on page 530*

promethazine and phenylephrine (proe METH a zeen & fen il EF rin)

Synonyms phenylephrine and promethazine

Therapeutic Category Antihistamine/Decongestant Combination

Use Temporary relief of upper respiratory symptoms associated with allergy or the common cold

Usual Dosage Oral:

Children:

2-6 years: 1.25-2.5 mL every 4-6 hours, not to exceed 7.5 mL in 24 hours

6-12 years: 2.5-5 mL every 4-6 hours, not to exceed 30 mL in 24 hours

Children >12 years and Adults: 5 mL every 4-6 hours, not to exceed 30 mL in 24 hours

Dosage Forms Syrup: Promethazine hydrochloride 6.25 mg and phenylephrine hydrochloride 5 mg per 5 mL (473 mL) [contains alcohol]

promethazine hydrochloride *see* promethazine *on page 703*

promethazine, phenylephrine, and codeine

(proe METH a zeen, fen il EF rin, & KOE deen)

Synonyms codeine, promethazine, and phenylephrine; phenylephrine, promethazine, and codeine

Therapeutic Category Antihistamine/Decongestant/Antitussive

Controlled Substance C-V

Use Temporary relief of coughs and upper respiratory symptoms including nasal congestion associated with allergy or the common cold

Usual Dosage Oral:

Children:

2 to <6 years:

12 kg: 1.25-2.5 mL every 4-6 hours, not to exceed 6 mL/24 hours

14 kg: 1.25-2.5 mL every 4-6 hours, not to exceed 7 mL/24 hours

16 kg: 1.25-2.5 mL every 4-6 hours, not to exceed 8 mL/24 hours

18 kg: 1.25-2.5 mL every 4-6 hours, not to exceed 9 mL/24 hours

6 to <12 years: 2.5-5 mL every 4-6 hours, not to exceed 30 mL/24 hours

Adults: 5 mL every 4-6 hours, not to exceed 30 mL/24 hours

Dosage Forms Syrup: Promethazine hydrochloride 6.25 mg, phenylephrine hydrochloride 5 mg, and codeine phosphate 10 mg per 5 mL (480 mL) [contains alcohol and sodium benzoate]

Promethegan™ [US] *see* promethazine *on page 703*

Promethist® With Codeine *(Discontinued)* *see* promethazine, phenylephrine, and codeine *on this page*

Prometh® VC Plain Liquid *(Discontinued)* *see* promethazine and phenylephrine *on this page*

Prometh® VC With Codeine *(Discontinued)* *see* promethazine, phenylephrine, and codeine *on this page*

Prometrium® [US/Can] *see* progesterone *on page 703*

Promit® [US] *see* dextran 1 *on page 243*

Pronap-100® [US] *see* propoxyphene and acetaminophen *on page 708*

Pronestyl® *(Discontinued)* *see* procainamide *on page 700*

Pronto® Complete Lice Killing Kit [US-OTC] *see* pyrethrins and piperonyl butoxide *on page 720*

Pronto® Lice Control [Can] *see* pyrethrins and piperonyl butoxide *on page 720*

Pronto® Plus Hair and Scalp Masque [US-OTC] *see* pyrethrins and piperonyl butoxide *on page 720*

Pronto® Plus Mousse [US-OTC] *see* pyrethrins and piperonyl butoxide *on page 720*

Pronto® Plus Warm Oil Treatment and Conditioner [US-OTC] *see* pyrethrins and piperonyl butoxide *on page 720*

Pronto® Plus with Natural Extracts and Oils [US-OTC] *see* pyrethrins and piperonyl butoxide *on page 720*

Propac™ [US-OTC] *see* nutritional formula, enteral/oral *on page 608*

Propacet® *(Discontinued)* *see* propoxyphene and acetaminophen *on page 708*

Propaderm® [Can] *see* beclomethasone *on page 95*

propafenone (pro PAF en one)

Synonyms propafenone hydrochloride

U.S./Canadian Brand Names Apo-Propafenone® [Can]; Rythmol® Gen-Propafenone [Can]; Rythmol® SR [US]; Rythmol® [US]

Therapeutic Category Antiarrhythmic Agent, Class I-C

Use Treatment of life-threatening ventricular arrhythmias

Rythmol® SR: Maintenance of normal sinus rhythm in patients with symptomatic atrial fibrillation

Usual Dosage Oral: Adults: **Note:** Patients who exhibit significant widening of QRS complex or second- or third-degree AV block may need dose reduction.

Immediate release tablet: Initial: 150 mg every 8 hours, increase at 3- to 4-day intervals up to 300 mg every 8 hours.

Extended release capsule: Initial: 225 mg every 12 hours; dosage increase may be made at a minimum of 5-day intervals; may increase to 325 mg every 12 hours; if further increase is necessary, may increase to 425 mg every 12 hours

Dosage Forms

Capsule, extended release, as hydrochloride (Rythmol® SR): 225 mg, 325 mg, 425 mg [contains soy lecithin]

Tablet, as hydrochloride (Rythmol®): 150 mg, 225 mg, 300 mg

propafenone hydrochloride *see* propafenone *on this page*

Propagest® *(Discontinued)*

propantheline (proe PAN the leen)

Synonyms propantheline bromide

Therapeutic Category Anticholinergic Agent

Use Adjunctive treatment of peptic ulcer, irritable bowel syndrome, pancreatitis, ureteral and urinary bladder spasm; reduce duodenal motility during diagnostic radiologic procedures

Usual Dosage Oral:

Antisecretory:

Children: 1-2 mg/kg/day in 3-4 divided doses

Adults: 15 mg 3 times/day before meals or food and 30 mg at bedtime

Antispasmodic:

Children: 2-3 mg/kg/day in divided doses every 4-6 hours and at bedtime

Adults: 15 mg 3 times/day before meals or food and 30 mg at bedtime

Dosage Forms Tablet, as bromide: 15 mg [contains lactose 23.2 mg]

propantheline bromide *see* propantheline *on this page*

Propa pH [US-OTC] *see* salicylic acid *on page 758*

proparacaine (proe PAR a kane)

Sound-Alike/Look-Alike Issues

proparacaine may be confused with propoxyphene

Synonyms proparacaine hydrochloride; proxymetacaine

U.S./Canadian Brand Names Alcaine® [US/Can]; Diocaine® [Can]; Ophthetic® [US]

Therapeutic Category Local Anesthetic

Use Anesthesia for tonometry, gonioscopy; suture removal from cornea; removal of corneal foreign body; cataract extraction, glaucoma surgery; short operative procedure involving the cornea and conjunctiva

Usual Dosage Children and Adults:

Ophthalmic surgery: Instill 1 drop of 0.5% solution in eye every 5-10 minutes for 5-7 doses

Tonometry, gonioscopy, suture removal: Instill 1-2 drops of 0.5% solution in eye just prior to procedure

Dosage Forms Solution, ophthalmic, as hydrochloride: 0.5% (15 mL) [contains benzalkonium chloride]

proparacaine and fluorescein (proe PAR a kane & FLURE e seen)

Synonyms fluorescein and proparacaine

U.S./Canadian Brand Names Flucaine® [US]; Fluoracaine® [US]

Therapeutic Category Diagnostic Agent; Local Anesthetic

Use Anesthesia for tonometry, gonioscopy; suture removal from cornea; removal of corneal foreign body; cataract extraction, glaucoma surgery

Usual Dosage

Ophthalmic surgery: Children and Adults: Instill 1 drop in each eye every 5-10 minutes for 5-7 doses

Tonometry, gonioscopy, suture removal: Adults: Instill 1-2 drops in each eye just prior to procedure

Dosage Forms Solution, ophthalmic: Proparacaine hydrochloride 0.5% and fluorescein sodium 0.25% (5 mL)

proparacaine hydrochloride *see* proparacaine *on previous page*

Propecia® [US/Can] *see* finasteride *on page 346*

Propine® [US] *see* dipivefrin *on page 267*

Proplex® T [US] *see* factor IX complex (human) *on page 334*

propofol (PROE po fole)

Sound-Alike/Look-Alike Issues

Diprivan® may be confused with Diflucan®, Ditropan®

U.S./Canadian Brand Names Diprivan® [US/Can]

Therapeutic Category General Anesthetic

Use Induction of anesthesia for inpatient or outpatient surgery in patients ≥3 years of age; maintenance of anesthesia for inpatient or outpatient surgery in patients >2 months of age; in adults, for the induction and maintenance of monitored anesthesia care sedation during diagnostic procedures; treatment of agitation in intubated, mechanically-ventilated ICU patients

Usual Dosage Dosage must be individualized based on total body weight and titrated to the desired clinical effect; wait at least 3-5 minutes between dosage adjustments to clinically assess drug effects; smaller doses are required when used with narcotics; the following are general dosing guidelines:

General anesthesia:

Induction: I.V.:

Children 3-16 years, ASA I or II: 2.5-3.5 mg/kg over 20-30 seconds; use a lower dose for children ASA III or IV

Adults, ASA I or II, <55 years: 2-2.5 mg/kg (~40 mg every 10 seconds until onset of induction)

Cardiac anesthesia: 0.5-1.5 mg/kg (~20 mg every 10 seconds until onset of induction)

Neurosurgical patients: 1-2 mg/kg (~20 mg every 10 seconds until onset of induction)

Maintenance: I.V. infusion:

Children 2 months to 16 years, ASA I or II: Initial: 200-300 mcg/kg/minute; decrease dose after 30 minutes if clinical signs of light anesthesia are absent; usual infusion rate: 125-150 mcg/kg/minute (range: 125-300 mcg/kg/minute; 7.5-18 mg/kg/hour); children ≤5 years may require larger infusion rates compared to older children

Adults, ASA I or II, <55 years: Initial: 150-200 mcg/kg/minute for 10-15 minutes; decrease by 30% to 50% during first 30 minutes of maintenance; usual infusion rate: 100-200 mcg/kg/minute (6-12 mg/kg/hour)

Cardiac anesthesia:

Low-dose propofol with primary opioid: 50-100 mcg/kg/minute (see manufacturer's labeling)

Primary propofol with secondary opioid: 100-150 mcg/kg/minute

Neurosurgical patients: 100-200 mcg/kg/minute (6-12 mg/kg/hour)

Maintenance: I.V. intermittent bolus: Adults, ASA I or II, <55 years: 20-50 mg increments as needed

Monitored anesthesia care sedation:

Initiation: Adults, ASA I or II, <55 years: Slow I.V. infusion: 100-150 mcg/kg/minute for 3-5 minutes **or** slow injection: 0.5 mg/kg over 3-5 minutes

Maintenance: Adults, ASA I or II, <55 years: I.V. infusion using variable rates (preferred over intermittent boluses): 25-75 mcg/kg/minute **or** incremental bolus doses: 10 mg or 20 mg

ICU sedation in intubated mechanically-ventilated patients: Avoid rapid bolus injection; individualize dose and titrate to response Continuous infusion: Initial: 0.3 mg/kg/hour (5 mcg/kg/min); increase by 0.3-0.6 mg/kg/hour (5-10 mcg/kg/min) every 5-10 minutes until desired sedation level is achieved; usual maintenance: 0.3-4.8 mg/kg/hour (5-80 mcg/kg/min) or higher; reduce dose by 80% in elderly, debilitated, and ASA III or IV patients; reduce dose after adequate sedation established and adjust to response (ie, evaluate frequently to use minimum dose for sedation). Some clinicians recommend daily interruption of infusion to perform clinical evaluation.

Dosage Forms

Injection, emulsion: 10 mg/mL (20 mL, 50 mL, 100 mL) [products may contain egg lecithin, and soybean oil; may contain benzyl alcohol, sodium benzoate, or sodium metabisulfite]

Diprivan®: 10 mg/mL (20 mL, 50 mL, 100 mL) [contains egg lecithin, soybean oil, and disodium edetate]

Propoxacet-N® ***(Discontinued)*** *see* propoxyphene and acetaminophen *on next page*

propoxyphene (proe POKS i feen)

Sound-Alike/Look-Alike Issues

propoxyphene may be confused with proparacaine

Darvon® may be confused with Devrom®, Diovan®

Darvon-N® may be confused with Darvocet-N®

Synonyms dextropropoxyphene; propoxyphene hydrochloride; propoxyphene napsylate

U.S./Canadian Brand Names 642® Tablet [Can]; Darvon-N® [US/Can]; Darvon® [US]

Therapeutic Category Analgesic, Narcotic

Controlled Substance C-IV

Use Management of mild to moderate pain

Usual Dosage Oral:

Children: Doses for children are not well established; doses of the hydrochloride of 2-3 mg/kg/day divided every 6 hours have been used

Adults:

Hydrochloride: 65 mg every 3-4 hours as needed for pain; maximum: 390 mg/day

Napsylate: 100 mg every 4 hours as needed for pain; maximum: 600 mg/day

Dosage Forms

Capsule, as hydrochloride (Darvon®): 65 mg

Tablet, as napsylate (Darvon-N®): 100 mg

propoxyphene and acetaminophen (proe POKS i feen & a seet a MIN oh fen)

Sound-Alike/Look-Alike Issues

Darvocet-N® may be confused with Darvon-N®

Synonyms acetaminophen and propoxyphene; propoxyphene hydrochloride and acetaminophen; propoxyphene napsylate and acetaminophen

U.S./Canadian Brand Names Balacet 325™ [US]; Darvocet A500™ [US]; Darvocet-N® 100 [US/Can]; Darvocet-N® 50 [US/Can]; Pronap-100® [US]

Therapeutic Category Analgesic, Narcotic

Controlled Substance C-IV

Use Management of mild to moderate pain

Usual Dosage Oral: Adults:

Darvocet A500™, Darvocet-N® 100: 1 tablet every 4 hours as needed; maximum: 600 mg propoxyphene napsylate/day

Darvocet-N® 50: 1-2 tablets every 4 hours as needed; maximum: 600 mg propoxyphene napsylate/day

Propoxyphene hydrochloride 65 mg and acetaminophen 650 mg: 1 tablet every 4 hours as needed; maximum: 390 mg/day propoxyphene hydrochloride, 4 g/day acetaminophen)

Note: Dosage of acetaminophen should not exceed 4 g/day (6 tablets of Darvocet-N® 100); possibly less in patients with ethanol

Dosage Forms

Tablet: Propoxyphene hydrochloride 65 mg and acetaminophen 650 mg, propoxyphene napsylate 100 mg, and acetaminophen 650 mg

Balacet 325™: Propoxyphene napsylate 100 mg and acetaminophen 325 mg

Darvocet A500™: Propoxyphene napsylate 100 mg and acetaminophen 500 mg [contains lactose]

Darvocet-N® 50: Propoxyphene napsylate 50 mg and acetaminophen 325 mg

Darvocet-N® 100, Pronap-100®: Propoxyphene napsylate 100 mg and acetaminophen 650 mg

propoxyphene, aspirin, and caffeine (proe POKS i feen, AS pir in, & KAF een)

Sound-Alike/Look-Alike Issues

Darvon® may be confused with Devrom®, Diovan®

Synonyms aspirin, caffeine, and propoxyphene; caffeine, propoxyphene, and aspirin; propoxyphene hydrochloride, aspirin, and caffeine

Therapeutic Category Analgesic Combination (Narcotic)

Controlled Substance C-IV

Use Treatment of mild-to-moderate pain

Usual Dosage Oral: Adults: Pain: One capsule (providing propoxyphene 65 mg) every 4 hours as needed; maximum propoxyphene 390 mg/day. This will also provide aspirin 389 mg and caffeine 32.4 mg per capsule.

Dosage Forms [DSC] = Discontinued product

Capsule (Darvon® Compound 65): Propoxyphene hydrochloride 65 mg, aspirin 389 mg, and caffeine 32.4 mg [DSC]

propoxyphene hydrochloride *see* propoxyphene *on this page*

propoxyphene hydrochloride and acetaminophen *see* propoxyphene and acetaminophen *on previous page*

propoxyphene hydrochloride, aspirin, and caffeine *see* propoxyphene, aspirin, and caffeine *on previous page*

propoxyphene napsylate *see* propoxyphene *on previous page*

propoxyphene napsylate and acetaminophen *see* propoxyphene and acetaminophen *on previous page*

propranolol (proe PRAN oh lole)

Sound-Alike/Look-Alike Issues

propranolol may be confused with Pravachol®, Propulsid®

Inderal® may be confused with Adderall®, Enduron®, Enduronyl®, Imdur®, Imuran®, Inderide®, Isordil®, Medrol®, Toradol®

Inderal® 40 may be confused with Enduronyl® Forte

Synonyms propranolol hydrochloride

U.S./Canadian Brand Names Apo-Propranolol® [Can]; Inderal® LA [US/Can]; Inderal® [US/Can]; InnoPran XL™ [US]; Novo-Pranol [Can]; Nu-Propranolol [Can]; Propranolol Hydrochloride Injection, USP [Can]

Therapeutic Category Antiarrhythmic Agent, Class II; Beta-Adrenergic Blocker

Use Management of hypertension; angina pectoris; pheochromocytoma; essential tremor; supraventricular arrhythmias (such as atrial fibrillation and flutter, AV nodal re-entrant tachycardias), ventricular tachycardias (catecholamine-induced arrhythmias, digoxin toxicity); prevention of myocardial infarction; migraine headache; symptomatic treatment of hypertrophic subaortic stenosis

Usual Dosage

Akathisia: Oral: Adults: 30-120 mg/day in 2-3 divided doses

Angina: Oral: Adults: 80-320 mg/day in doses divided 2-4 times/day

Long-acting formulation: Initial: 80 mg once daily; maximum dose: 320 mg once daily

Essential tremor: Oral: Adults: 20-40 mg twice daily initially; maintenance doses: usually 120-320 mg/day

Hypertension:

Oral:

Children: Initial: 0.5-1 mg/kg/day in divided doses every 6-12 hours; increase gradually every 5-7 days; maximum: 16 mg/kg/24 hours

Adults: Initial: 40 mg twice daily; increase dosage every 3-7 days; usual dose: ≤320 mg divided in 2-3 doses/day; maximum daily dose: 640 mg; usual dosage range (JNC 7): 40-160 mg/day in 2 divided doses

Long-acting formulation: Initial: 80 mg once daily; usual maintenance: 120-160 mg once daily; maximum daily dose: 640 mg; usual dosage range (JNC 7): 60-180 mg/day once daily

I.V.: Children: 0.01-0.05 mg/kg over 1 hour; maximum dose: 10 mg

Hypertrophic subaortic stenosis: Oral: Adults: 20-40 mg 3-4 times/day

Long-acting formulation: 80-160 mg once daily

Migraine headache prophylaxis: Oral:

Children: Initial: 2-4 mg/kg/day **or**

≤35 kg: 10-20 mg 3 times/day

>35 kg: 20-40 mg 3 times/day

Adults: Initial: 80 mg/day divided every 6-8 hours; increase by 20-40 mg/dose every 3-4 weeks to a maximum of 160-240 mg/day given in divided doses every 6-8 hours; if satisfactory response not achieved within 6 weeks of starting therapy, drug should be withdrawn gradually over several weeks

Long-acting formulation: Initial: 80 mg once daily; effective dose range: 160-240 mg once daily

Myocardial infarction prophylaxis: Oral: Adults: 180-240 mg/day in 3-4 divided doses

Pheochromocytoma: Oral: Adults: 30-60 mg/day in divided doses

Tachyarrhythmias:

Oral:

Children: Initial: 0.5-1 mg/kg/day in divided doses every 6-8 hours; titrate dosage upward every 3-7 days; usual dose: 2-6 mg/kg/day; higher doses may be needed; do not exceed 16 mg/kg/day or 60 mg/day

Adults: 10-30 mg/dose every 6-8 hours

I.V.:

Children: 0.01-0.1 mg/kg/dose slow IVP over 10 minutes; maximum dose: 1 mg for infants; 3 mg for children

Adults (in patients having nonfunctional GI tract): 1 mg/dose slow IVP; repeat every 5 minutes up to a total of 5 mg; titrate initial dose to desired response

(Continued)

propranolol *(Continued)*

Tetralogy spells: Children:

Oral: Palliation: Initial: 1 mg/kg/day every 6 hours; if ineffective, may increase dose after 1 week by 1 mg/kg/day to a maximum of 5 mg/kg/day; if patient becomes refractory, may increase slowly to a maximum of 10-15 mg/kg/day. Allow 24 hours between dosing changes.

I.V.: 0.01-0.2 mg/kg/dose infused over 10 minutes; maximum initial dose: 1 mg

Thyrotoxicosis:

Oral:

Children: 2 mg/kg/day, divided every 6-8 hours, titrate to effective dose

Adolescents and Adults: Oral: 10-40 mg/dose every 6 hours

I.V.: Adults: 1-3 mg/dose slow IVP as a single dose

Dosage Forms

Capsule, extended release, as hydrochloride (InnoPran XL™): 80 mg, 120 mg

Capsule, sustained release, as hydrochloride (Inderal® LA): 60 mg, 80 mg, 120 mg, 160 mg

Injection, solution, as hydrochloride: 1 mg/mL (1 mL)

Inderal®: 1 mg/mL (1 mL)

Solution, oral, as hydrochloride: 4 mg/mL (5 mL, 500 mL); 8 mg/mL (500 mL) [strawberry-mint flavor; contains alcohol 0.6%]

Tablet, as hydrochloride:

Inderal®: 10 mg, 20 mg, 40 mg, 60 mg, 80 mg

propranolol and hydrochlorothiazide (proe PRAN oh lole & hye droe klor oh THYE a zide)

Sound-Alike/Look-Alike Issues

Inderide® may be confused with Inderal®

Synonyms hydrochlorothiazide and propranolol

U.S./Canadian Brand Names Inderide® [US]

Therapeutic Category Antihypertensive Agent, Combination

Use Management of hypertension

Usual Dosage Oral: Adults: Hypertension: Dose is individualized; typical dosages of **hydrochlorothiazide**: 12.5-50 mg/day; initial dose of **propranolol**: 80 mg/day

Daily dose of tablet form should be divided into 2 daily doses; may be used to maximum dosage of up to 160 mg of propranolol; higher dosages would result in higher than optimal thiazide dosages.

Dosage Forms [DSC] = Discontinued product

Tablet: Propranolol hydrochloride 40 mg and hydrochlorothiazide 25 mg; propranolol hydrochloride 80 mg and hydrochlorothiazide 25 mg

Inderide®:

40/25: Propranolol hydrochloride 40 mg and hydrochlorothiazide 25 mg

80/25: Propranolol hydrochloride 80 mg and hydrochlorothiazide 25 mg [DSC]

propranolol hydrochloride *see* propranolol *on previous page*

Propranolol Hydrochloride Injection, USP [Can] *see* propranolol *on previous page*

Proprinal [US-OTC] *see* ibuprofen *on page 437*

Proprinal® Cold and Sinus [US-OTC] *see* pseudoephedrine and ibuprofen *on page 715*

Propulsid® [US] *see* cisapride *on page 192*

propylene glycol diacetate, acetic acid, and hydrocortisone *see* acetic acid, propylene glycol diacetate, and hydrocortisone *on page 15*

propylhexedrine (proe pil HEKS e dreen)

U.S./Canadian Brand Names Benzedrex® [US-OTC]

Therapeutic Category Adrenergic Agonist Agent

Use Topical nasal decongestant

Usual Dosage Nasal: Children 6-12 years and Adults: Two inhalations in each nostril, not more frequently than every 2 hours

Dosage Forms Inhaler, nasal: 0.4-0.5 mg/inhalation (1s) [total content 250 mg]

propyliodone *see* radiological/contrast media (ionic) *on page 728*

2-propylpentanoic acid *see* valproic acid and derivatives *on page 864*

propylthiouracil (proe pil thye oh YOOR a sil)

Sound-Alike/Look-Alike Issues

propylthiouracil may be confused with Purinethol®

PTU is an error-prone abbreviation (mistaken as mercaptopurine [Purinethol®; 6-MP])

U.S./Canadian Brand Names Propyl-Thyracil® [Can]

Therapeutic Category Antithyroid Agent

Use Palliative treatment of hyperthyroidism as an adjunct to ameliorate hyperthyroidism in preparation for surgical treatment or radioactive iodine therapy; management of thyrotoxic crisis

Usual Dosage Oral: Administer in 3 equally divided doses at approximately 8-hour intervals. Adjust dosage to maintain T_3, T_4, and TSH levels in normal range; elevated T_3 may be sole indicator of inadequate treatment. Elevated TSH indicates excessive antithyroid treatment.

Children: Initial: 5-7 mg/kg/day **or** 150-200 mg/m²/day in divided doses every 8 hours

or

6-10 years: 50-150 mg/day

>10 years: 150-300 mg/day

Maintenance: Determined by patient response **or** 1/3 to 2/3 of the initial dose in divided doses every 8-12 hours. This usually begins after 2 months on an effective initial dose.

Adults: Initial: 300 mg/day in divided doses every 8 hours. In patients with severe hyperthyroidism, very large goiters, or both, the initial dosage is usually 450 mg/day; an occasional patient will require 600-900 mg/day; maintenance: 100-150 mg/day in divided doses every 8-12 hours

Withdrawal of therapy: Therapy should be withdrawn gradually with evaluation of the patient every 4-6 weeks for the first 3 months then every 3 months for the first year after discontinuation of therapy to detect any reoccurrence of a hyperthyroid state.

Dosage Forms Tablet: 50 mg

Propyl-Thyracil® [Can] *see* propylthiouracil *on this page*

2-propylvaleric acid *see* valproic acid and derivatives *on page 864*

ProQuad® [US] *see* measles, mumps, rubella, and varicella virus vaccine *on page 521*

Proquin® XR [US] *see* ciprofloxacin *on page 190*

Proscar® [US/Can] *see* finasteride *on page 346*

ProSom® [US] *see* estazolam *on page 307*

prostacyclin *see* epoprostenol *on page 299*

prostacyclin PGI_2 *see* iloprost *on page 440*

prostaglandin E_1 *see* alprostadil *on page 32*

prostaglandin E_2 *see* dinoprostone *on page 260*

prostaglandin F_2 *see* carboprost tromethamine *on page 151*

ProStep® Patch *(Discontinued)* *see* nicotine *on page 591*

Prostigmin® [US/Can] *see* neostigmine *on page 585*

Prostin E_2® [US/Can] *see* dinoprostone *on page 260*

Prostin F_2 Alpha® *(Discontinued)*

Prostin® VR [Can] *see* alprostadil *on page 32*

Prostin VR Pediatric® [US] *see* alprostadil *on page 32*

protamine sulfate (PROE ta meen SUL fate)

Sound-Alike/Look-Alike Issues

protamine may be confused with ProAmatine®, protamine, Protopam®, Protropin®

Therapeutic Category Antidote

Use Treatment of heparin overdosage; neutralize heparin during surgery or dialysis procedures

Usual Dosage

Heparin neutralization: I.V.: Protamine dosage is determined by the dosage of heparin; 1 mg of protamine neutralizes 90 USP units of heparin (lung) and 115 USP units of heparin (intestinal); maximum dose: 50 mg

Heparin overdosage, following intravenous administration: I.V.: Since blood heparin concentrations decrease rapidly **after** administration, adjust the protamine dosage depending upon the duration of time since heparin administration.

Note: Excessive protamine doses may worsen bleeding potential.

Dosage Forms Injection, solution, as sulfate [preservative free]: 10 mg/mL (5 mL, 25 mL)

Protection Plus® [US-OTC] *see* alcohol (ethyl) *on page 25*

protein C (activated), human, recombinant *see* drotrecogin alfa *on page 282*

protein-bound paclitaxel *see* paclitaxel (protein bound) *on page 631*

Protenate® *(Discontinued)* *see* plasma protein fraction *on page 672*

Prothazine-DC® *(Discontinued)* *see* promethazine and codeine *on page 704*

prothrombin complex concentrate *see* factor IX complex (human) *on page 334*

Protilase® *(Discontinued)* *see* pancrelipase *on page 634*

Protonix® [US/Can] *see* pantoprazole *on page 636*

Protopam® [US/Can] *see* pralidoxime *on page 690*

Protopic® [US/Can] *see* tacrolimus *on page 803*

Protostat® Oral *(Discontinued)* *see* metronidazole *on page 551*

protriptyline (proe TRIP ti leen)

Synonyms protriptyline hydrochloride

U.S./Canadian Brand Names Vivactil® [US]

Therapeutic Category Antidepressant, Tricyclic (Secondary Amine)

Use Treatment of depression

Usual Dosage Oral:

Adolescents: 15-20 mg/day

Adults: 15-60 mg in 3-4 divided doses

Dosage Forms Tablet, as hydrochloride: 5 mg, 10 mg

protriptyline hydrochloride *see* protriptyline *on this page*

Protuss®-DM *(Discontinued)* *see* guaifenesin, pseudoephedrine, and dextromethorphan *on page 401*

Proventil® [US] *see* albuterol *on page 23*

Proventil® HFA [US] *see* albuterol *on page 23*

Proventil® Inhaler *(Discontinued)* *see* albuterol *on page 23*

Proventil® Solution *(Discontinued)* *see* albuterol *on page 23*

Proventil® Tablet *(Discontinued)* *see* albuterol *on page 23*

Provera® [US/Can] *see* medroxyprogesterone *on page 524*

Provera-Pak [Can] *see* medroxyprogesterone *on page 524*

Provigil® [US/Can] *see* modafinil *on page 562*

Proviodine [Can] *see* povidone-iodine *on page 689*

Provisc® [US] *see* hyaluronate and derivatives *on page 416*

Provocholine® [US/Can] *see* methacholine *on page 537*

proxymetacaine *see* proparacaine *on page 706*

Prozac® [US/Can] *see* fluoxetine *on page 357*

Prozac® Weekly™ [US] *see* fluoxetine *on page 357*

PRP-OMP *see Haemophilus* B conjugate vaccine *on page 405*

PRP-T *see Haemophilus* B conjugate vaccine *on page 405*

Prudoxin™ [US] *see* doxepin *on page 276*

prussian blue *see* ferric hexacyanoferrate *on page 342*

prymaccone *see* primaquine *on page 698*

23PS *see* pneumococcal polysaccharide vaccine (polyvalent) *on page 676*

PS-341 *see* bortezomib *on page 114*

pseudoephedrine (soo doe e FED rin)

Sound-Alike/Look-Alike Issues

Dimetapp® may be confused with Dermatop®, Dimetabs®, Dimetane®

Sudafed® may be confused with Sufenta®

Synonyms *d*-isoephedrine hydrochloride; pseudoephedrine hydrochloride; pseudoephedrine sulfate

U.S./Canadian Brand Names Balminil Decongestant [Can]; Benylin® D for Infants [Can]; Biofed [US-OTC]; Contact® Cold [US-OTC]; Contac® Cold 12 Hour Relief Non Drowsy [Can]; Dimetapp® 12-Hour Non-Drowsy Extentabs® [US-OTC]; Dimetapp® Decongestant Infant [US-OTC]; Drixoral® ND [Can]; ElixSure™ Congestion [US-OTC]; Eltor® [Can]; Genaphed® [US-OTC]; Kidkare Decongestant [US-OTC]; Kodet SE [US-OTC]; Oranyl [US-OTC]; PediaCare® Decongestant Infants [US-OTC]; PMS-Pseudoephedrine [Can]; Pseudofrin [Can]; Robidrine® [Can]; Silfedrine Children's [US-OTC]; Simply Stuffy™ [US-OTC]; Sudafed® 12 Hour [US-OTC]; Sudafed® 24 Hour [US-OTC]; Sudafed® Children's [US-OTC]; Sudafed® Decongestant [Can]; Sudafed® [US-OTC]; Sudo-Tab® [US-OTC]; Sudodrin [US-OTC]; SudoGest [US-OTC]

Therapeutic Category Adrenergic Agonist Agent

Use Temporary symptomatic relief of nasal congestion due to common cold, upper respiratory allergies, and sinusitis; also promotes nasal or sinus drainage

Usual Dosage Oral: General dosing guidelines:

Children:

<2 years: 4 mg/kg/day in divided doses every 6 hours

2-5 years: 15 mg every 4-6 hours; maximum: 60 mg/24 hours

6-12 years: 30 mg every 4-6 hours; maximum: 120 mg/24 hours

Adults: 30-60 mg every 4-6 hours, sustained release: 120 mg every 12 hours; maximum: 240 mg/24 hours

Dosage Forms [DSC] = Discontinued product

Caplet, extended release, as hydrochloride:

Contac® Cold [DSC], Sudafed® 12 Hour: 120 mg

Liquid, as hydrochloride: 30 mg/5 mL (120 mL, 480 mL)

Silfedrine Children's: 15 mg/5 mL (120 mL, 480 mL) [alcohol and sugar free; grape flavor]

Simply Stuffy™: 15 mg/5 mL (120 mL) [alcohol free; contains sodium benzoate; cherry berry flavor] [DSC]

Sudafed® Children's: 15 mg/5 mL (120 mL) [alcohol and sugar free; contains sodium benzoate; grape flavor]

Liquid, oral, as hydrochloride [drops]:

Dimetapp® Decongestant Infant Drops: 7.5 mg/0.8 mL (15 mL) [alcohol free; contains sodium benzoate; grape flavor]

Kidkare Decongestant: 7.5 mg/0.8 mL (30 mL) [alcohol free; contains benzoic acid and sodium benzoate; cherry flavor]

PediaCare® Decongestant: 7.5 mg/0.8 mL (15 mL) [alcohol free, dye free; contains benzoic acid, sodium benzoate; fruit flavor]

Syrup, as hydrochloride:

Biofed: 30 mg/5 mL (120 mL, 240 mL, 480 mL, 3840 mL) [alcohol free; contains sodium benzoate]

ElixSure™ Congestion: 15 mg/5 mL (120 mL) [grape bubble gum flavor]

Tablet, as hydrochloride: 30 mg, 60 mg

Genaphed®, Kodet SE, Oranyl, Sudafed®, Sudodrin, Sudo-Tab®: 30 mg

SudoGest: 30 mg, 60 mg

Tablet, chewable, as hydrochloride (Sudafed® Children's): 15 mg [sugar free; contains phenylalanine 0.78 mg/tablet; orange flavor]

Tablet, extended release, as hydrochloride:

Dimetapp® 12-Hour Non-Drowsy Extentabs®: 120 mg

Sudafed® 24 Hour: 240 mg

pseudoephedrine, acetaminophen, and chlorpheniramine *see* acetaminophen, chlorpheniramine, and pseudoephedrine *on page 11*

pseudoephedrine, acetaminophen, and dextromethorphan *see* acetaminophen, dextromethorphan, and pseudoephedrine *on page 12*

pseudoephedrine and acetaminophen *see* acetaminophen and pseudoephedrine *on page 9*

pseudoephedrine and brompheniramine *see* brompheniramine and pseudoephedrine *on page 118*

pseudoephedrine and carbetapentane *see* carbetapentane and pseudoephedrine *on page 146*

pseudoephedrine and carbinoxamine *see* carbinoxamine and pseudoephedrine *on page 149*

pseudoephedrine and chlorpheniramine *see* chlorpheniramine and pseudoephedrine *on page 177*

pseudoephedrine and dexbrompheniramine *see* dexbrompheniramine and pseudoephedrine *on page 241*

pseudoephedrine and dextromethorphan (soo doe e FED rin & deks troe meth OR fan)

Synonyms dextromethorphan and pseudoephedrine

U.S./Canadian Brand Names Balminil DM D [Can]; Benylin® DM-D [Can]; Dimetapp® Infant Decongestant Plus Cough [US-OTC]; Koffex DM-D [Can]; Novahistex® DM Decongestant [Can]; Novahistine® DM Decongestant [Can]; Pedia Relief Cough and Cold [US-OTC]; Pedia Relief Infants [US-OTC]; Pediacare® Children's Long Acting Cough Plus Cold [US-OTC]; Pediacare® Infants' Decongestant & Cough [US-OTC]; Robitussin® Childrens Cough & Cold [Can]; Robitussin® Maximum Strength Cough & Cold [US-OTC]; Robitussin® Pediatric Cough & Cold [US-OTC]; Sudafed® Children's Cold & Cough [US-OTC]; SudoGest Children's [US-OTC]; Triaminic® Cough & Nasal Congestion [US-OTC]; Triaminic® Cough [US-OTC]; Vicks® 44D Cough & Head Congestion [US-OTC]

Therapeutic Category Antitussive/Decongestant

Use Temporary symptomatic relief of nasal congestion and cough due to common cold, hay fever, upper respiratory allergies

Usual Dosage Relief of nasal congestion and cough: Oral:

General dosing guidelines base on pseudoephedrine component:
- Children 2-6 years: 15 mg every 4-6 hours (maximum: 60 mg/24 hours)
- Children 6-12 years: 30 mg every 4-6 hours (maximum: 120 mg/24 hours)
- Children ≥12 years and Adults: 60 mg every 4-6 hours (maximum: 240 mg/24 hours)

Product-specific dosing:
- Children 2-3 years (PediaCare® Infants Decongestant & Cough): 1.6 mL every 4-6 hours (maximum: 6.4 mL/24 hours)
- Children 2-6 years:
  - Pediacare® Children's Long Acting Cough Plus Cold: One chewable tablet or 5 mL every 6-8 hours (maximum: 4 doses/24 hours)
  - Robitussin® Pediatric Cough & Cold, Triaminic® Cough and Nasal Congestion: 5 mL every 6 hours (maximum: 20 mL/24 hours)
  - Sudafed® Children's Cold & Cough: 5 mL every 4 hours (maximum: 20 mL/24 hours)
  - Triaminic® Cough: 5 mL every 4-6 hours (maximum: 20 mL/24 hours)
- Children 6-12 years:
  - Pediacare® Children's Long Acting Cough Plus Cold: Two chewable tablets or 10 mL every 6-8 hours (maximum: 4 doses/24 hours)
  - Robitussin® Pediatric Cough & Cold, Triaminic® Cough and Nasal Congestion: 10 mL every 6 hours (maximum: 40 mL/24 hours)
  - Sudafed® Children's Cold & Cough: 10 mL every 4 hours (maximum: 40 mL/24 hours)
  - Triaminic Cough: 10 mL every 4-6 hours (maximum: 40 mL/24 hours)
  - Vicks® 44D Cough & Head Congestion: 7.5 mL every 6 hours (maximum: 30 mL/24 hours)
- Children ≥12 years and Adults:
  - Robitussin® Maximum Strength Cough & Cold: 10 mL every 6 hours as needed (maximum: 40 mL/24 hours)
  - Sudafed® Children's Cold & Cough: 20 mL every 4 hours (maximum: 80 mL/24 hours)
  - Vicks® 44D Cough & Head Congestion: 15 mL every 6 hours (maximum: 60 mL/24 hours)

Dosage Forms

Liquid: Pseudoephedrine hydrochloride 15 mg and dextromethorphan hydrobromide 7.5 mg per 5 mL (120 mL)
- PediaCare® Children's Long Acting Cough Plus Cold: Pseudoephedrine hydrochloride 15 mg and dextromethorphan hydrobromide 7.5 mg per 5 mL (120 mL) [alcohol free; contains sodium benzoate; grape flavor]
- Sudafed® Children's Cold & Cough: Pseudoephedrine hydrochloride 15 mg and dextromethorphan hydrobromide 5 mg per 5 mL (120 mL) [alcohol free, sugar free; contains sodium benzoate; cherry berry flavor]
- Triaminic® Cough: Pseudoephedrine hydrochloride 15 mg and dextromethorphan hydrobromide 5 mg per 5 mL (120 mL, 150 mL) [alcohol free; contains benzoic acid, sodium 20 mg/5 mL; berry flavor]
- Triaminic® Cough & Nasal Congestion: Pseudoephedrine hydrochloride 15 mg and dextromethorphan hydrobromide 7.5 mg per 5 mL (120 mL) [alcohol free; contains benzoic acid, sodium 7 mg/5 mL; orange strawberry flavor]
- Vicks® 44D Cough & Head Congestion: Pseudoephedrine hydrochloride 20 mg and dextromethorphan hydrobromide 10 mg per 5 mL (120 mL, 240 mL) [contains alcohol 5%, sodium 10.3 mg/5 mL and sodium benzoate; cherry flavor]

Liquid, oral drops:
- Dimetapp® Infant Decongestant Plus Cough: Pseudoephedrine hydrochloride 7.5 mg and dextromethorphan hydrobromide 2.5 mg per 0.8 mL (15 mL) [alcohol free, sugar free; grape flavor]
- PediaCare® Infants' Decongestant & Cough: Pseudoephedrine hydrochloride 7.5 mg and dextromethorphan hydrobromide 2.5 mg per 0.8 mL (15 mL) [alcohol free; contains sodium benzoate; cherry flavor]

Pedia Relief Infants: Pseudoephedrine hydrochloride 7.5 mg and dextromethorphan hydrobromide 2.5 mg per 0.8 mL (15 mL) [cherry flavor]

Syrup:

Pedia Relief Cough and Cold: Pseudoephedrine hydrochloride 15 mg and dextromethorphan hydrobromide 7.5 mg per 5 mL (120 mL) [cherry flavor]

Robitussin® Maximum Strength Cough & Cold: Pseudoephedrine hydrochloride 30 mg and dextromethorphan hydrobromide 15 mg per 5 mL (120 mL, 240 mL) [contains alcohol 1.4% and sodium benzoate]

Robitussin® Pediatric Cough & Cold: Pseudoephedrine hydrochloride 15 mg and dextromethorphan hydrobromide 7.5 mg per 5 mL (120 mL, 240 mL) [alcohol free; contains sodium benzoate; fruit punch flavor]

SudoGest Children's: Pseudoephedrine hydrochloride 15 mg and dextromethorphan hydrobromide 5 mg per 5 mL (120 mL)

Tablet, chewable (PediaCare® Children's Long Acting Cough Plus Cold): Pseudoephedrine hydrochloride 15 mg and dextromethorphan hydrobromide 7.5 mg [contains phenylalanine 5 mg per tablet; grape flavor]

pseudoephedrine and diphenhydramine *see* diphenhydramine and pseudoephedrine *on page 263*

pseudoephedrine and fexofenadine *see* fexofenadine and pseudoephedrine *on page 344*

pseudoephedrine and guaifenesin *see* guaifenesin and pseudoephedrine *on page 398*

pseudoephedrine and hydrocodone *see* hydrocodone and pseudoephedrine *on page 424*

pseudoephedrine and ibuprofen (soo doe e FED rin & eye byoo PROE fen)

Synonyms ibuprofen and pseudoephedrine

U.S./Canadian Brand Names Advil® Cold & Sinus [US-OTC/Can]; Advil® Cold, Children's [US-OTC]; Children's Advil® Cold [Can]; Dristan® Sinus [US-OTC]; Motrin® Cold and Sinus [US-OTC]; Motrin® Cold, Children's [US-OTC]; Proprinal® Cold and Sinus [US-OTC]; Sudafed® Sinus Advance [Can]

Therapeutic Category Decongestant/Analgesic

Use For temporary relief of cold, sinus and flu symptoms (including nasal congestion, headache, sore throat, minor body aches and pains, and fever)

Usual Dosage OTC labeling: Oral:

Children: Ibuprofen 100 mg and pseudoephedrine 15 mg per 5 mL: May repeat dose every 6 hours (maximum: 4 doses/24 hours); dose should be based on weight when possible. Contact healthcare provider if symptoms have not improved within 3 days (2 days if treating sore throat accompanied by fever).

2-5 years or 11 to <22 kg (24-47 pounds): 5 mL

6-11 years or 22-43 kg (48-95 pounds): 10 mL

Children ≥12 years and Adults: Ibuprofen 200 mg and pseudoephedrine 30 mg per dose: One dose every 4-6 hours as needed; may increase to 2 doses if necessary (maximum: 6 doses/24 hours). Contact healthcare provider if symptoms have not improved within 7 days when treating cold symptoms or within 3 days when treating fever.

Dosage Forms

Caplet (Advil® Cold and Sinus, Dristan® Sinus, Motrin® Cold and Sinus, Proprinal® Cold and Sinus): Pseudoephedrine hydrochloride 30 mg and ibuprofen 200 mg

Capsule, liquid filled (Advil® Cold and Sinus): Pseudoephedrine hydrochloride 30 mg and ibuprofen 200 mg [solubilized ibuprofen as free acid and potassium salt; contains coconut oil]

Suspension:

Advil® Cold, Children's: Pseudoephedrine hydrochloride 15 mg and ibuprofen 100 mg per 5 mL (120 mL) [alcohol free; contains sodium benzoate; grape flavor]

Motrin® Cold, Children's: Pseudoephedrine hydrochloride 15 mg and ibuprofen 100 mg per 5 mL (120 mL) [contains sodium benzoate; berry, dye free berry, and grape flavors]

Tablet (Advil® Cold and Sinus): Pseudoephedrine hydrochloride 30 mg and ibuprofen 200 mg

pseudoephedrine and loratadine *see* loratadine and pseudoephedrine *on page 505*

pseudoephedrine and triprolidine *see* triprolidine and pseudoephedrine *on page 853*

pseudoephedrine, carbinoxamine, and dextromethorphan *see* carbinoxamine, pseudoephedrine, and dextromethorphan *on page 150*

pseudoephedrine, chlorpheniramine, and acetaminophen *see* acetaminophen, chlorpheniramine, and pseudoephedrine *on page 11*

pseudoephedrine, chlorpheniramine, and codeine *see* chlorpheniramine, pseudoephedrine, and codeine *on page 182*

pseudoephedrine, chlorpheniramine, and dextromethorphan *see* chlorpheniramine, pseudoephedrine, and dextromethorphan *on page 182*

pseudoephedrine, chlorpheniramine, and ibuprofen *see* ibuprofen, pseudoephedrine, and chlorpheniramine *on page 439*

pseudoephedrine, codeine, and triprolidine *see* triprolidine, pseudoephedrine, and codeine *(Canada only) on page 853*

pseudoephedrine, dextromethorphan, and acetaminophen *see* acetaminophen, dextromethorphan, and pseudoephedrine *on page 12*

pseudoephedrine, dextromethorphan, and carbinoxamine *see* carbinoxamine, pseudoephedrine, and dextromethorphan *on page 150*

pseudoephedrine, dextromethorphan, and guaifenesin *see* guaifenesin, pseudoephedrine, and dextromethorphan *on page 401*

pseudoephedrine, guaifenesin, and codeine *see* guaifenesin, pseudoephedrine, and codeine *on page 401*

pseudoephedrine hydrochloride *see* pseudoephedrine *on page 712*

pseudoephedrine hydrochloride and acrivastine *see* acrivastine and pseudoephedrine *on page 17*

pseudoephedrine hydrochloride and cetirizine hydrochloride *see* cetirizine and pseudoephedrine *on page 168*

pseudoephedrine hydrochloride, hydrocodone bitartrate, and chlorpheniramine maleate *see* pseudoephedrine, hydrocodone, and chlorpheniramine *on this page*

pseudoephedrine, hydrocodone, and carbinoxamine *see* hydrocodone, carbinoxamine, and pseudoephedrine *on page 424*

pseudoephedrine, hydrocodone, and chlorpheniramine

(soo doe e FED rin, hye droe KOE done, & klor fen IR a meen)

Synonyms chlorpheniramine, pseudoephedrine, and hydrocodone; hydrocodone, chlorpheniramine, and pseudoephedrine; pseudoephedrine hydrochloride, hydrocodone bitartrate, and chlorpheniramine maleate

U.S./Canadian Brand Names Atuss® HD [US]; Coldcough HC [US]; Cordron-HC [US]; Detuss [US]; Histinex® PV [US]; Hydro-Tussin™ HC [US]; Hydron PSC [US]; Hyphed [US]; P-V-Tussin® Syrup [US]; Pediatex™ HC [US]; Q-V Tussin [US]; Vasophrinic DH [Can]

Therapeutic Category Antihistamine; Antihistamine/Decongestant/Antitussive; Antitussive; Decongestant

Controlled Substance C-III

Use Temporary relief of cough, congestion, and sneezing due to colds, respiratory infections, or hay fever

Usual Dosage Oral:

Children:

2-6 years:

Hydro-Tussin™ HC: 1.25-2.5 mL every 4-6 hours; do not exceed 4 doses in 24 hours

Histinex® PV, Pediatex™ HC, P-V-Tussin®: 2.5 mL every 4-6 hours; do not exceed 4 doses in 24 hours

6-12 years:

Histinex® PV, Pediatex™ HC, P-V-Tussin®, Tussend®: 5 mL or 1/2 tablet every 4-6 hours; do not exceed 4 doses in 24 hours

Hydro-Tussin™ HC: 2.5-5 mL or 1/2 tablet every 4-6 hours; do not exceed 4 doses in 24 hours

Children >12 years and Adults:

Histinex® PV, Pediatex™ HC, P-V-Tussin®, Tussend®: 10 mL or 1 tablet every 4-6 hours; do not exceed 4 doses in 24 hours

Hydro-Tussin™ HC: 5-10 mL or 1 tablet every 4-6 hours; do not exceed 4 doses in 24 hours

Dosage Forms

Capsule, variable release:

Atuss® HD: Pseudoephedrine hydrochloride 30 mg [sustained release], hydrocodone bitartrate 5 mg [immediate release], and chlorpheniramine maleate 2 mg [sustained release]

Liquid:

Cordron-HC: Pseudoephedrine hydrochloride 20 mg, hydrocodone bitartrate 1.67 mg, and chlorpheniramine maleate 2.5 mg per 5 mL (480 mL) [vanilla mint flavor]

Detuss: Pseudoephedrine hydrochloride 30 mg, hydrocodone bitartrate 5 mg, and chlorpheniramine maleate 2 mg per 5 mL (480 mL) [alcohol free; vanilla flavor]

Hydron PSC: Pseudoephedrine hydrochloride 30 mg, hydrocodone bitartrate 5 mg, and chlorpheniramine maleate 2 mg per 5 mL (480 mL) [vanilla flavor]

Pediatex™ HC: Pseudoephedrine hydrochloride 20 mg, hydrocodone bitartrate 1.67 mg, and chlorpheniramine maleate 2.5 mg per 5 mL (480 mL) [alcohol free, sugar free; vanilla mint flavor]

Syrup:

Coldcough HC: Pseudoephedrine hydrochloride 15 mg, hydrocodone bitartrate 3 mg, and chlorpheniramine maleate 2 mg per 5 mL (480 mL) [alcohol free, dye free, sugar free; grape flavor]

Histinex® PV: Pseudoephedrine hydrochloride 30 mg, hydrocodone bitartrate 2.5 mg, and chlorpheniramine maleate 2 mg per 5 mL (480 mL) [alcohol free, sugar free; apricot flavor]

Hydro-Tussin™ HC: Pseudoephedrine hydrochloride 15 mg, hydrocodone bitartrate 3 mg, and chlorpheniramine maleate 2 mg per 5 mL (480 mL) [alcohol free, dye free, sugar free]

Hyphed: Pseudoephedrine hydrochloride 30 mg, hydrocodone bitartrate 2.5 mg, and chlorpheniramine maleate 2 mg per 5 mL (480 mL) [contains alcohol 5%; raspberry flavor]

P-V-Tussin®, Q-V Tussin, Tussend® [DSC]: Pseudoephedrine hydrochloride 30 mg, hydrocodone bitartrate 2.5 mg, and chlorpheniramine maleate 2 mg per 5 mL (480 mL) [contains alcohol 5%; banana flavor]

Tablet [scored]:

Tussend®: Pseudoephedrine hydrochloride 60 mg, hydrocodone bitartrate 5 mg, and chlorpheniramine maleate 4 mg [DSC]

pseudoephedrine, hydrocodone, and guaifenesin *see* hydrocodone, pseudoephedrine, and guaifenesin *on page 425*

pseudoephedrine sulfate *see* pseudoephedrine *on page 712*

pseudoephedrine tannate, dextromethorphan tannate, and brompheniramine tannate *see* brompheniramine, pseudoephedrine, and dextromethorphan *on page 120*

pseudoephedrine, triprolidine, and codeine *see* triprolidine, pseudoephedrine, and codeine *(Canada only) on page 853*

Pseudofrin [Can] *see* pseudoephedrine *on page 712*

Pseudo-Gest Plus® Tablet *(Discontinued)* *see* chlorpheniramine and pseudoephedrine *on page 177*

Pseudo GG TR [US] *see* guaifenesin and pseudoephedrine *on page 398*

Pseudo Max DMX [US] *see* guaifenesin, pseudoephedrine, and dextromethorphan *on page 401*

pseudomonic acid A *see* mupirocin *on page 569*

Pseudovent™ [US] *see* guaifenesin and pseudoephedrine *on page 398*

Pseudovent™ 400 [US] *see* guaifenesin and pseudoephedrine *on page 398*

Pseudovent™ DM [US] *see* guaifenesin, pseudoephedrine, and dextromethorphan *on page 401*

Pseudovent™-Ped [US] *see* guaifenesin and pseudoephedrine *on page 398*

P & S™ Liquid Phenol [Can] *see* phenol *on page 658*

Psorcon® [Can] *see* diflorasone *on page 253*

Psorcon® *(Discontinued)* *see* diflorasone *on page 253*

Psorcon® e™ [US] *see* diflorasone *on page 253*

Psoriatec™ [US] *see* anthralin *on page 58*

PsoriGel® *(Discontinued)* *see* coal tar *on page 207*

Psorion® Topical *(Discontinued)*

psyllium (SIL i yum)

Sound-Alike/Look-Alike Issues

Fiberall® may be confused with Feverall®
Hydrocil® may be confused with Hydrocet®
Modane® may be confused with Matulane®, Moban®
Perdiem® may be confused with Pyridium®

Synonyms plantago seed; plantain seed; psyllium hydrophilic mucilloid

U.S./Canadian Brand Names Fiberall® [US]; Fibro-Lax [US-OTC]; Fibro-XL [US-OTC]; Genfiber® [US-OTC]; Hydrocil® Instant [US-OTC]; Konsyl-D® [US-OTC]; Konsyl® Easy Mix [US-OTC]; Konsyl® Orange [US-OTC]; Konsyl® [US-OTC]; Metamucil® Plus Calcium [US-OTC]; Metamucil® Smooth Texture [US-OTC]; Metamucil® [US-OTC/Can]; Modane® Bulk [US-OTC]; Natural Fiber Therapy [US-OTC]; Reguloid® [US-OTC]; Serutan® [US-OTC]

(Continued)

psyllium *(Continued)*

Therapeutic Category Laxative

Use Treatment of chronic atonic or spastic constipation and in constipation associated with rectal disorders; management of irritable bowel syndrome; labeled for OTC use as fiber supplement, treatment of constipation

Usual Dosage Oral (administer at least 2 hours before or after other drugs):

Children 6-11 years: Approximately ½ adult dosage

Children ≥12 years and Adults: Take 1 dose up to 3 times/day; all doses should be followed with 8 oz of water or liquid

Capsule: 4 capsules/dose (range: 2-6); swallow capsules one at a time

Powder: 1 rounded tablespoonful/dose (1 teaspoonful/dose for many sugar free or select concentrated products) mixed in 8 oz liquid

Tablet: 1 tablet/dose

Wafer: 2 wafers/dose

Dosage Forms

Capsule:

Fibro XL: 675 mg

Metamucil®: 0.52 g [contains potassium 5 mg/capsule; provides 3 g dietary fiber 2.4 g per 6 capsules]

Metamucil® Plus Calcium: 0.42 g [contains potassium 6 mg/capsule; provides dietary fiber 2.1 g and calcium 300 mg per 5 capsules]

Granules (Serutan®): 2.5 g/teaspoon (510 g) [contains sodium benzoate]

Powder: 3.4 g/dose (390 g, 570 g)

Bulk-K: 4.725 g/dose (392 g)

Fiberall®: 3.5 g/dose (454 g) [sugar free; contains phenylalanine; orange flavor]

Fibro-Lax: 4.725 g /dose (140 g, 392g)

Genfiber®: 3.4 g/dose (397 g, 595 g) [regular flavor]

Genfiber®: 3.5 g/dose (283 g) [sugar free; orange flavor]

Hydrocil® Instant: 3.5 g/dose (3.7 g unit-dose packets, 300 g) [sugar free]

Konsyl®: 6 g/dose (6 g unit-dose packets, 300 g, 450 g) [sugar free; contains sodium 4.1 mg/dose; regular flavor]

Konsyl-D®: 3.4 g/dose (6.5 g unit-dose packets, 325 g, 397 g, 500 g) [contains sodium 2.3 mg/dose and dextrose]

Konsyl® Easy Mix: 6 g/dose (6 g unit-dose packets, 250 g) [sugar free; contains sodium 4.4 mg/dose]

Konsyl® Orange: 3.4 g/dose (12 g unit-dose packets, 538 g) [contains sodium 2.3 mg/dose and sucrose; orange flavor]

Konsyl® Orange: 3.4 g/dose (425 g) [sugar free; contains sodium 2.3 mg/dose; orange flavor]

Metamucil®: 3.4 g/dose:

(390 g, 570 g, 870 g) [contains sodium 3 mg and potassium 30 mg per dose; regular flavor]

(570 g, 870 g, 1254 g) [contains sodium 5 mg and potassium 30 mg per dose; orange flavor]

Metamucil® Smooth Texture: 3.4 g/dose:

(unit-dose packets, 609 g, 912 g, 1446 g) [contains sodium 5 mg and potassium 30 mg per dose; orange flavor]

(300 g, 450 g, 690 g) [contains sodium 4 mg and potassium 30 mg per dose; regular flavor]

(unit-dose packets, 183 g, 300 g, 450 g, 699 g, 1104 g) [sugar free; contains phenylalanine 25 mg, sodium 5 mg, and potassium 30 mg per dose; orange flavor]

Modane® Bulk: 3.4 g/dose (390 g) [contains dextrose; flavor free]

Natural Fiber Therapy: 3.4 g/dose (369 g, 539 g) [natural and orange flavors]

Reguloid®: 3.4 g/dose (300 g, 450 g) [sugar free; regular or orange flavors]; (390 g, 570g) [regular or orange flavors]

Wafers (Metamucil®): 3.4 g/dose (24s) [one dose = 2 wafers; contains sodium 20 mg and potassium 60 mg per dose; apple crisp and cinnamon spice flavors]

psyllium hydrophilic mucilloid *see* psyllium *on previous page*

P.T.E.-4® [US] *see* trace metals *on page 839*

P.T.E.-5® [US] *see* trace metals *on page 839*

pteroylglutamic acid *see* folic acid *on page 364*

Pulmicort® [Can] *see* budesonide *on page 122*

Pulmicort Respules® [US] *see* budesonide *on page 122*

Pulmicort Turbuhaler® [US] *see* budesonide *on page 122*

Pulmophylline [Can] *see* theophylline *on page 818*

Pulmozyme® [US/Can] *see* dornase alfa *on page 274*

Puralube® Tears [US-OTC] *see* artificial tears *on page 75*

Purell® [US-OTC] *see* alcohol (ethyl) *on page 25*

Purell® 2 in 1 [US-OTC] *see* alcohol (ethyl) *on page 25*

Purell® with Aloe [US-OTC] *see* alcohol (ethyl) *on page 25*

Purge® [US-OTC] *see* castor oil *on page 155*

Puri-Clens™ [US-OTC] *see* methylbenzethonium chloride *on page 544*

purified chick embryo cell *see* rabies virus vaccine *on page 728*

Purinethol® [US/Can] *see* mercaptopurine *on page 532*

PVP-I *see* povidone-iodine *on page 689*

pyrantel pamoate (pi RAN tel PAM oh ate)

U.S./Canadian Brand Names Combantrin™ [Can]; Pamix™ [US-OTC]; Pin-X® [US-OTC]; Reese's® Pinworm Medicine [US-OTC]

Therapeutic Category Anthelmintic

Use Treatment of pinworms (*Enterobius vermicularis*) and roundworms (*Ascaris lumbricoides*)

Usual Dosage Children and Adults (purgation is not required prior to use): Oral: Roundworm, pinworm, or trichostrongyliasis: 11 mg/kg administered as a single dose; maximum dose: 1 g. (**Note:** For pinworm infection, dosage should be repeated in 2 weeks and all family members should be treated).

Dosage Forms

Suspension, oral as pamoate:

Pamix™: 144 mg/mL (30 mL, 60 mL, 240 mL) [equivalent to pyrantel base 50 mg/mL; contains sodium benzoate]

Pin-X®: 144 mg/mL (30 mL, 60 mL) [equivalent to pyrantel base 50 mg/mL; contains sodium benzoate; caramel flavor]

Reese's® Pinworm Medicine: 144 mg/mL (30 mL) [equivalent to pyrantel base 50 mg/mL]

Tablet, as pamoate (Reese's® Pinworm Medicine): 180 mg [equivalent to pyrantel base 62.5 mg/tablet]

pyrazinamide (peer a ZIN a mide)

Synonyms pyrazinoic acid amide

U.S./Canadian Brand Names Tebrazid™ [Can]

Therapeutic Category Antitubercular Agent

Use Adjunctive treatment of tuberculosis in combination with other antituberculosis agents

Usual Dosage Oral: Treatment of tuberculosis:

Note: Used as part of a multidrug regimen. Treatment regimens consist of an initial 2-month phase, followed by a continuation phase of 4 or 7 additional months; frequency of dosing may differ depending on phase of therapy.

Children:

Daily therapy: 15-30 mg/kg/day (maximum: 2 g/day)

Twice weekly directly observed therapy (DOT): 50 mg/kg/dose (maximum: 4 g/dose)

Adults (dosing is based on lean body weight):

Daily therapy: 15-30 mg/kg/day

40-55 kg: 1000 mg

56-75 kg: 1500 mg

76-90 kg: 2000 mg (maximum dose regardless of weight)

Twice weekly directly observed therapy (DOT): 50 mg/kg

40-55 kg: 2000 mg

56-75 kg: 3000 mg

76-90 kg: 4000 mg (maximum dose regardless of weight)

Three times/week DOT: 25-30 mg/kg (maximum: 2.5 g)

40-55 kg: 1500 mg

56-75 kg: 2500 mg

76-90 kg: 3000 mg (maximum dose regardless of weight)

Dosage Forms Tablet: 500 mg

pyrazinamide, rifampin, and isoniazid *see* rifampin, isoniazid, and pyrazinamide *on page 745*

pyrazinoic acid amide *see* pyrazinamide *on this page*

pyrethrins and piperonyl butoxide (pye RE thrins & pi PER oh nil byo TOKS ide)

Synonyms piperonyl butoxide and pyrethrins

U.S./Canadian Brand Names A-200® Maximum Strength [US-OTC]; Lice-Aid [US-OTC]; Licide® [US-OTC]; Pronto® Complete Lice Killing Kit [US-OTC]; Pronto® Lice Control [Can]; Pronto® Plus Hair and Scalp Masque [US-OTC]; Pronto® Plus Mousse [US-OTC]; Pronto® Plus Warm Oil Treatment and Conditioner [US-OTC]; Pronto® Plus with Natural Extracts and Oils [US-OTC]; Pyrinyl Plus® [US-OTC]; R & C™ II [Can]; R & C™ Shampoo/Conditioner [Can]; RID® Maximum Strength [US-OTC]; RID® Mousse [Can]; Tisit® Blue Gel [US-OTC]; Tisit® [US-OTC]

Therapeutic Category Scabicides/Pediculicides

Use Treatment of *Pediculus humanus* infestations (head lice, body lice, pubic lice and their eggs)

Usual Dosage Application of pyrethrins:

Topical products:

Apply enough solution to completely wet infested area, including hair

Allow to remain on area for 10 minutes

Wash and rinse with large amounts of warm water.

Use fine-toothed comb to remove lice and eggs from hair

Shampoo hair to restore body and luster

Treatment may be repeated if necessary once in a 24-hour period

Repeat treatment in 7-10 days to kill newly hatched lice

Note: Keep out of eyes when rinsing hair; protect eyes with a washcloth or towel

Solution for furniture, bedding: Spray on entire area to be treated; allow to dry before use. Intended for use on items which cannot be laundered or dry cleaned. **Not for use on humans or animals.**

Dosage Forms

Cream, topical (Pronto® Plus Hair and Scalp Masque): Pyrethrins 0.33% and piperonyl butoxide 4% (60 g) [green cream shampoo; contains coconut and sesame oil; apple herb scent; packaged with nit removal comb]

Foam, topical [mousse] (RID® Maximum Strength): Pyrethrins 0.33% and piperonyl butoxide 4% (156 g) [packaged with nit removal comb]

Gel (Tisit® Blue Gel): Pyrethrins 0.33% and piperonyl butoxide 3% (30 g)

Liquid, topical (Tisit®): Pyrethrins 0.33% and piperonyl butoxide 2% (60 mL, 120 mL) [packaged with nit removal comb]

Oil, topical (Pronto® Plus Warm Oil Treatment and Conditioner): Pyrethrins 0.33% and piperonyl butoxide 4% (36 mL) [fruity herbal scent; packaged with nit removal comb]

Shampoo: Pyrethrins 0.33% and piperonyl butoxide 4% (60 mL, 120 mL)

A-200® Maximum Strength: Pyrethrins 0.33% and piperonyl butoxide 4% (60 mL, 120 mL) [contains benzyl alcohol; packaged with nit removal comb]

Lice-Aid: Pyrethrins 0.33% and piperonyl butoxide 4% (120 mL)

Licide®: Pyrethrins 0.33% and piperonyl butoxide 4% (120 mL) [packaged with nit removal comb; also available in a kit containing shampoo, household spray and nit removal comb]

Pronto® Complete Lice Killing Kit: Pyrethrins 0.33% and piperonyl butoxide 4% (120 mL) [contains benzyl alcohol; packaged in a kit containing shampoo, creme rinse, hair separators, nit removal comb, magnifying glass, and furniture spray]

Pronto® Plus Mousse: Pyrethrins 0.33% and piperonyl butoxide 4% (120 mL) [blue mousse shampoo; contains vitamin E; packaged with nit removal comb]

Pronto® Plus with Natural Extracts and Oils: Pyrethrins 0.33% and piperonyl butoxide 4% (60 mL) [orange scent; packaged with metal nit removal comb; also available in a kit packaged with lice/egg remover and household spray]

Pyrinyl Plus®: Pyrethrins 0.33% and piperonyl butoxide 4% (60 mL) [contains benzyl alcohol; packaged with nit removal comb]

RID® Maximum Strength: Pyrethrins 0.33% and piperonyl butoxide 4% (60 mL, 120 mL, 180 mL, 240 mL) [packaged with nit removal comb; also available in a kit containing shampoo, gel, and furniture spray]

Tisit®: Pyrethrins 0.33% and piperonyl butoxide 3% (60 mL, 120 mL) [also available in a kit containing shampoo, nit removal comb, and furniture spray]

Solution, spray [for furniture, garments, bedding; not for human or animal use] (Tisit®): Pyrethrins 0.4% and piperonyl butoxide 2% (150 mL)

2-pyridine aldoxime methochloride *see* pralidoxime *on page 690*

Pyridium® [US] *see* phenazopyridine *on page 656*

pyridostigmine (peer id oh STIG meen)

Sound-Alike/Look-Alike Issues

pyridostigmine may be confused with physostigmine

Mestinon® may be confused with Metatensin®

Regonol® may be confused with Reglan®, Renagel®

Synonyms pyridostigmine bromide

U.S./Canadian Brand Names Mestinon® Timespan® [US]; Mestinon® [US/Can]; Mestinon®-SR [Can]; Regonol® [US]

Therapeutic Category Cholinergic Agent

Use Symptomatic treatment of myasthenia gravis; antidote for nondepolarizing neuromuscular blockers

Military use: Pretreatment for Soman nerve gas exposure

Usual Dosage

Myasthenia gravis:

Oral:

Children: 7 mg/kg/24 hours divided into 5-6 doses

Adults: Highly individualized dosing ranges: 60-1500 mg/day, usually 600 mg/day divided into 5-6 doses, spaced to provide maximum relief

Sustained release formulation: Highly individualized dosing ranges: 180-540 mg once or twice daily (doses separated by at least 6 hours); **Note:** Most clinicians reserve sustained release dosage form for bedtime dose only.

I.M., slow I.V. push:

Children: 0.05-0.15 mg/kg/dose

Adults: To supplement oral dosage pre- and postoperatively during labor and postpartum, during myasthenic crisis, or when oral therapy is impractical: ~1/30th of oral dose; observe patient closely for cholinergic reactions

or

I.V. infusion: Initial: 2 mg/hour with gradual titration in increments of 0.5-1 mg/hour, up to a maximum rate of 4 mg/hour

Pretreatment for Soman nerve gas exposure (military use): Oral: Adults: 30 mg every 8 hours beginning several hours prior to exposure; discontinue at first sign of nerve agent exposure, then begin atropine and pralidoxime

Reversal of nondepolarizing muscle relaxants: **Note:** Atropine sulfate (0.6-1.2 mg) I.V. immediately prior to pyridostigmine to minimize side effects: I.V.:

Children: Dosing range: 0.1-0.25 mg/kg/dose*

Adults: 0.1-0.25 mg/kg/dose; 10-20 mg is usually sufficient*

*Full recovery usually occurs ≤15 minutes, but ≥30 minutes may be required

Dosage Forms

Injection, solution, as bromide:

Mestinon®: 5 mg/mL (2 mL)

Regonol®: 5 mg/mL (2 mL) [contains benzyl alcohol]

Syrup, as bromide (Mestinon®): 60 mg/5 mL (480 mL) [raspberry flavor; contains alcohol 5%, sodium benzoate]

Tablet, as bromide (Mestinon®): 60 mg

Tablet, sustained release, as bromide (Mestinon® Timespan®): 180 mg

pyridostigmine bromide *see* pyridostigmine *on previous page*

pyridoxine (peer i DOKS een)

Sound-Alike/Look-Alike Issues

pyridoxine may be confused with paroxetine, pralidoxime, Pyridium®

Synonyms pyridoxine hydrochloride; vitamin B_6

U.S./Canadian Brand Names Aminoxin® [US-OTC]

Therapeutic Category Vitamin, Water Soluble

Use Prevention and treatment of vitamin B_6 deficiency, pyridoxine-dependent seizures in infants; adjunct to treatment of acute toxicity from isoniazid, cycloserine, or hydrazine overdose

Usual Dosage

Recommended daily allowance (RDA):

Children:

1-3 years: 0.9 mg

4-6 years: 1.3 mg

7-10 years: 1.6 mg

Adults:

Male: 1.7-2.0 mg

Female: 1.4-1.6 mg

Pyridoxine-dependent Infants:

Oral: 2-100 mg/day

I.M., I.V., SubQ: 10-100 mg

(Continued)

pyridoxine *(Continued)*

Dietary deficiency: Oral:
Children: 5-25 mg/24 hours for 3 weeks, then 1.5-2.5 mg/day in multiple vitamin product
Adults: 10-20 mg/day for 3 weeks
Drug-induced neuritis (eg, isoniazid, hydralazine, penicillamine, cycloserine): Oral:
Children:
Treatment: 10-50 mg/24 hours
Prophylaxis: 1-2 mg/kg/24 hours
Adults:
Treatment: 100-200 mg/24 hours
Prophylaxis: 25-100 mg/24 hours
Treatment of seizures and/or coma from acute isoniazid toxicity, a dose of pyridoxine hydrochloride equal to the amount of INH ingested can be given I.M./I.V. in divided doses together with other anticonvulsants; if the amount INH ingested is not known, administer 5 g I.V. pyridoxine
Treatment of acute hydrazine toxicity, a pyridoxine dose of 25 mg/kg in divided doses I.M./I.V. has been used

Dosage Forms
Capsule, as hydrochloride: 250 mg
Injection, solution, as hydrochloride: 100 mg/mL (1 mL)
Tablet, as hydrochloride: 25 mg, 50 mg, 100 mg, 200 mg, 250 mg, 500 mg
Tablet, enteric coated, as hydrochloride (Aminoxin®): 20 mg

pyridoxine and doxylamine *see* doxylamine and pyridoxine *(Canada only)* *on page 280*

pyridoxine, folic acid, and cyanocobalamin *see* folic acid, cyanocobalamin, and pyridoxine *on page 365*

pyridoxine hydrochloride *see* pyridoxine *on previous page*

Pyrilafen Tannate-12™ [US] *see* phenylephrine and pyrilamine *on page 662*

pyrilamine maleate, dextromethorphan hydrobromide, and phenylephrine hydrochloride *see* phenylephrine, pyrilamine, and dextromethorphan *on page 664*

pyrilamine tannate and phenylephrine tannate *see* phenylephrine and pyrilamine *on page 662*

pyrimethamine (peer i METH a meen)

Sound-Alike/Look-Alike Issues
Daraprim® may be confused with Dantrium®, Daranide®

U.S./Canadian Brand Names Daraprim® [US/Can]

Therapeutic Category Folic Acid Antagonist (Antimalarial)

Use Prophylaxis of malaria due to susceptible strains of plasmodia; used in conjunction with quinine and sulfadiazine for the treatment of uncomplicated attacks of chloroquine-resistant *P. falciparum* malaria; used in conjunction with fast-acting schizonticide to initiate transmission control and suppression cure; synergistic combination with sulfonamide in treatment of toxoplasmosis

Usual Dosage
Malaria chemoprophylaxis (for areas where chloroquine-resistant *P. falciparum* exists): Begin prophylaxis 2 weeks before entering endemic area:
Children: 0.5 mg/kg once weekly; not to exceed 25 mg/dose
or
Children:
<4 years: 6.25 mg once weekly
4-10 years: 12.5 mg once weekly
Children >10 years and Adults: 25 mg once weekly
Dosage should be continued for all age groups for at least 6-10 weeks after leaving endemic areas
Chloroquine-resistant *P. falciparum* malaria (when used in conjunction with quinine and sulfadiazine):
Children:
<10 kg: 6.25 mg/day once daily for 3 days
10-20 kg: 12.5 mg/day once daily for 3 days
20-40 kg: 25 mg/day once daily for 3 days
Adults: 25 mg twice daily for 3 days
Toxoplasmosis:
Infants (congenital toxoplasmosis): Oral: 1 mg/kg once daily for 6 months with sulfadiazine then every other month with sulfa, alternating with spiramycin.
Children: Loading dose: 2 mg/kg/day divided into 2 equal daily doses for 1-3 days (maximum: 100 mg/day) followed by 1 mg/kg/day divided into 2 doses for 4 weeks; maximum: 25 mg/day

With sulfadiazine or trisulfapyrimidines: 2 mg/kg/day divided every 12 hours for 3 days, followed by 1 mg/kg/day once daily or divided twice daily for 4 weeks given with trisulfapyrimidines or sulfadiazine

Adults: 50-75 mg/day together with 1-4 g of a sulfonamide for 1-3 weeks depending on patient's tolerance and response, then reduce dose by 50% and continue for 4-5 weeks **or** 25-50 mg/day for 3-4 weeks

Prophylaxis for first episode of *Toxoplasma gondii*:

Children ≥1 month of age: 1 mg/kg/day once daily with dapsone, plus oral folinic acid 5 mg every 3 days

Adolescents and Adults: 50 mg once weekly with dapsone, plus oral folinic acid 25 mg once weekly

Prophylaxis to prevent recurrence of *Toxoplasma gondii*:

Children ≥1 month of age: 1 mg/kg/day once daily given with sulfadiazine or clindamycin, plus oral folinic acid 5 mg every 3 days

Adolescents and Adults: 25-50 mg once daily in combination with sulfadiazine or clindamycin, plus oral folinic acid 10-25 mg daily; atovaquone plus oral folinic acid has also been used in combination with pyrimethamine.

Dosage Forms Tablet: 25 mg

pyrimethamine and sulfadoxine *see* sulfadoxine and pyrimethamine *on page 797*

Pyrinyl Plus® [US-OTC] *see* pyrethrins and piperonyl butoxide *on page 720*

pyrithione zinc (peer i THYE one zingk)

Sound-Alike/Look-Alike Issues

pyrithione may be confused with Pyridium®

U.S./Canadian Brand Names BetaMed [US-OTC]; DermaZinc™ [US-OTC]; DHS™ Zinc [US-OTC]; Head & Shoulders® Citrus Breeze [US-OTC]; Head & Shoulders® Classic Clean 2-In-1 [US-OTC]; Head & Shoulders® Classic Clean [US-OTC]; Head & Shoulders® Dry Scalp Care [US-OTC]; Head & Shoulders® Extra Volume [US-OTC]; Head & Shoulders® Leave-in Treatment [US-OTC]; Head & Shoulders® Refresh [US-OTC]; Head & Shoulders® Sensitive Care [US-OTC]; Head & Shoulders® Smooth & Silky 2-In-1 [US-OTC]; Skin Care™ [US-OTC]; Zincon® [US-OTC]; ZNP® Bar [US-OTC]

Therapeutic Category Antiseborrheic Agent, Topical

Use Relieves the itching, irritation and scalp flaking associated with dandruff and/or seborrheal dermatitis

Usual Dosage Adults: Products should be used at least twice weekly for best results, but may be used with each washing.

Bar: May be used on body and or scalp; wet area, massage in, and rinse.

Shampoo: Should be applied to wet hair and massaged into scalp; rinse. May be followed with conditioner

Dosage Forms

Conditioner, topical:

DermaZinc™: 0.25% (120 g)

Head & Shoulders® Dry Scalp Care: 0.5% (400 mL)

Head & Shoulders® Extra Volume: 0.5% (200 mL, 400 mL)

Lotion, topical:

Head & Shoulders® Leave-in Treatment: 0.1% (200 mL)

Skin Care™: 0.25% (120 mL) [pump spray]

Shampoo, topical:

BetaMed: 2% (480 mL) [dye free]

DermaZinc™: 2% (240 mL)

DHS™ Zinc: 2% (240 mL, 360 mL)

Head & Shoulders® Citrus Breeze: 1% (400 mL, 700 mL)

Head & Shoulders® Classic Clean: 1% (50 mL, 200 mL, 400 mL, 700 mL, 1000 mL, 1200 mL)

Head & Shoulders® Dry Scalp Care: 1% (400 mL, 700 mL, 1200 mL)

Head & Shoulders® Extra Volume: 1% (400 mL, 700 mL)

Head & Shoulders® Refresh: 1% (400 mL, 700 mL, 1200 mL)

Head & Shoulders® Sensitive Care: 1% (400 mL, 700 mL, 1200 mL)

Zincon®: 1% (120 mL, 240 mL)

Shampoo, topical [with conditioner]:

Head & Shoulders® Classic Clean 2-in-1: 1% (200 mL, 400 mL, 700 mL)

Head & Shoulders® Dry Scalp Care: 0.5% (400 mL, 700 mL)

Head & Shoulders® Smooth and Silky 2-in-1: 1% (400 mL)

Soap, topical (ZNP®): 2% (119 g) [bar]

Solution, topical (DermaZinc™): 0.25% (120 mL) [spray/drops]

Q-V Tussin [US] *see* pseudoephedrine, hydrocodone, and chlorpheniramine *on page 716*

Q-Bid DM [US] *see* guaifenesin and dextromethorphan *on page 394*

QDALL® [US] *see* chlorpheniramine and pseudoephedrine *on page 177*

QDALL® AR [US] *see* chlorpheniramine *on page 175*

Q-Dryl [US-OTC] *see* diphenhydramine *on page 261*

Q-Naftate [US-OTC] *see* tolnaftate *on page 834*

Q-Tapp DM [OTC] *see* brompheniramine, pseudoephedrine, and dextromethorphan *on page 120*

Q-Tussin [US-OTC] *see* guaifenesin *on page 392*

Q-Tussin DM [US-OTC] *see* guaifenesin and dextromethorphan *on page 394*

quadrivalent human papillomavirus vaccine *see* papillomavirus (Types 6, 11, 16, 18) recombinant vaccine *on page 638*

quaternium-18 bentonite *see* bentoquatam *on page 98*

quazepam (KWAZ e pam)

Sound-Alike/Look-Alike Issues
quazepam may be confused with oxazepam

U.S./Canadian Brand Names Doral® [US/Can]

Therapeutic Category Benzodiazepine

Controlled Substance C-IV

Use Treatment of insomnia

Usual Dosage Adults: Oral: Initial: 15 mg at bedtime, in some patients the dose may be reduced to 7.5 mg after a few nights

Dosage Forms Tablet: 7.5 mg, 15 mg

Quelicin® [US/Can] *see* succinylcholine *on page 793*

Queltuss® *(Discontinued)* *see* guaifenesin and dextromethorphan *on page 394*

Quenalin [US-OTC] *see* diphenhydramine *on page 261*

Questran® [US] *see* cholestyramine resin *on page 186*

Questran® Light [US] *see* cholestyramine resin *on page 186*

Questran® Light Sugar Free [Can] *see* cholestyramine resin *on page 186*

quetiapine (kwe TYE a peen)

Sound-Alike/Look-Alike Issues
Seroquel® may be confused with Serentil®, Serzone®, Sinequan®

Synonyms quetiapine fumarate

U.S./Canadian Brand Names Seroquel® [US/Can]

Therapeutic Category Antipsychotic Agent

Use Treatment of schizophrenia; treatment of acute manic episodes associated with bipolar disorder (as monotherapy or in combination with lithium or valproate)

Usual Dosage Oral: Adults:

Schizophrenia/psychoses: Initial: 25 mg twice daily; increase in increments of 25-50 mg 2-3 times/day on the second and third day, if tolerated, to a target dose of 300-400 mg in 2-3 divided doses by day 4. Make further adjustments as needed at intervals of at least 2 days in adjustments of 25-50 mg twice daily. Usual maintenance range: 300-800 mg/day

Mania: Initial: 50 mg twice daily on day 1, increase dose in increments of 100 mg/day to 200 mg twice daily on day 4; may increase to a target dose of 800 mg/day by day 6 at increments of ≤200 mg/day. Usual dosage range: 400-800 mg/day

Note: Dose reductions should be attempted periodically to establish lowest effective dose in patients with psychosis or to establish need to continue treating agitated symptoms in demented older adults. Patients being restarted after 1 week of no drug need to be titrated as above.

Dosage Forms

Tablet, as fumarate:
Seroquel®: 25 mg, 50 mg, 100 mg, 200 mg, 300 mg, 400 mg

quetiapine fumarate *see* quetiapine *on this page*

Quibron® *(Discontinued)* *see* theophylline and guaifenesin *on page 820*

Quiess® Injection *(Discontinued)* *see* hydroxyzine *on page 433*

Quinaglute® Dura-Tabs® *(Discontinued)* *see* quinidine *on next page*

quinagolide *(Discontinued)*

Quinalan® *(Discontinued)* *see* quinidine *on next page*

quinalbarbitone sodium *see* secobarbital *on page 766*

quinapril (KWIN a pril)

Sound-Alike/Look-Alike Issues

Accupril® may be confused with Accolate®, Accutane®, AcipHex®, Monopril®

Synonyms quinapril hydrochloride

U.S./Canadian Brand Names Accupril® [US/Can]

Therapeutic Category Angiotensin-Converting Enzyme (ACE) Inhibitor

Use Management of hypertension; treatment of congestive heart failure

Usual Dosage

Adults: Oral:

Hypertension: Initial: 10-20 mg once daily, adjust according to blood pressure response at peak and trough blood levels; initial dose may be reduced to 5 mg in patients receiving diuretic therapy if the diuretic is continued; usual dose range (JNC 7): 10-40 mg once daily

Congestive heart failure or post-MI: Initial: 5 mg once or twice daily, titrated at weekly intervals to 20-40 mg daily in 2 divided doses; target dose (heart failure): 20 mg twice daily (ACC/AHA 2005 Heart Failure Guidelines)

Dosage Forms

Tablet: 5 mg, 10 mg, 20 mg, 40 mg

Accupril®: 5 mg, 10 mg, 20 mg, 40 mg

quinapril and hydrochlorothiazide (KWIN a pril & hye droe klor oh THYE a zide)

Synonyms hydrochlorothiazide and quinapril

U.S./Canadian Brand Names Accuretic® [US/Can]; Quinaretic [US]

Therapeutic Category Antihypertensive Agent, Combination

Use Treatment of hypertension (not for initial therapy)

Usual Dosage Oral:

Children: Safety and efficacy have not been established.

Adults: Initial:

Patients who have failed quinapril monotherapy:

Quinapril 10 mg/hydrochlorothiazide 12.5 mg **or**

Quinapril 20 mg/hydrochlorothiazide 12.5 mg once daily

Patients with adequate blood pressure control on hydrochlorothiazide 25 mg/day, but significant potassium loss:

Quinapril 10 mg/hydrochlorothiazide 12.5 mg **or**

Quinapril 20 mg/hydrochlorothiazide 12.5 mg once daily

Note: Clinical trials of quinapril/hydrochlorothiazide combinations used quinapril doses of 2.5-40 mg/day and hydrochlorothiazide doses of 6.25-25 mg/day.

Dosage Forms Tablet:

10/12.5: Quinapril 10 mg and hydrochlorothiazide 12.5 mg

20/12.5: Quinapril 20 mg and hydrochlorothiazide 12.5 mg

20/25: Quinapril 20 mg and hydrochlorothiazide 25 mg

quinapril hydrochloride *see* quinapril *on this page*

Quinaretic [US] *see* quinapril and hydrochlorothiazide *on this page*

Quinate® [Can] *see* quinidine *on this page*

quinidine (KWIN i deen)

Sound-Alike/Look-Alike Issues

quinidine may be confused with clonidine, quinine, Quinora®

Synonyms quinidine gluconate; quinidine polygalacturonate; quinidine sulfate

U.S./Canadian Brand Names Apo-Quinidine® [Can]; BioQuin® Durules™ [Can]; Novo-Quinidin [Can]; Quinate® [Can]

Therapeutic Category Antiarrhythmic Agent, Class I-A

Use Prophylaxis after cardioversion of atrial fibrillation and/or flutter to maintain normal sinus rhythm; prevent recurrence of paroxysmal supraventricular tachycardia, paroxysmal AV junctional rhythm, paroxysmal ventricular tachycardia, paroxysmal atrial fibrillation, and atrial or ventricular premature contractions; has activity against *Plasmodium falciparum* malaria

Usual Dosage **Dosage expressed in terms of the salt: 267 mg of quinidine gluconate = 200 mg of quinidine sulfate.**

Children: Test dose for idiosyncratic reaction (sulfate, oral or gluconate, I.M.): 2 mg/kg or 60 mg/m^2

(Continued)

quinidine *(Continued)*

Oral (quinidine sulfate): 15-60 mg/kg/day in 4-5 divided doses or 6 mg/kg every 4-6 hours; usual 30 mg/kg/day or 900 mg/m²/day given in 5 daily doses

I.V. **not** recommended (quinidine gluconate): 2-10 mg/kg/dose given at a rate ≤10 mg/minute every 3-6 hours as needed

Adults: Test dose: Oral, I.M.: 200 mg administered several hours before full dosage (to determine possibility of idiosyncratic reaction)

Oral (for malaria):

Sulfate: 100-600 mg/dose every 4-6 hours; begin at 200 mg/dose and titrate to desired effect (maximum daily dose: 3-4 g)

Gluconate: 324-972 mg every 8-12 hours

I.M.: 400 mg/dose every 2-6 hours; initial dose: 600 mg (gluconate)

I.V.: 200-400 mg/dose diluted and given at a rate ≤10 mg/minute; may require as much as 500-750 mg

Dosage Forms

Injection, solution, as gluconate: 80 mg/mL (10 mL) [equivalent to quinidine base 50 mg/mL]

Tablet, as sulfate: 200 mg, 300 mg

Tablet, extended release, as gluconate: 324 mg [equivalent to quinidine base 202 mg]

Tablet, extended release, as sulfate: 300 mg [equivalent to quinidine base 249 mg]

quinidine gluconate *see* quinidine *on previous page*

quinidine polygalacturonate *see* quinidine *on previous page*

quinidine sulfate *see* quinidine *on previous page*

quinine (KWYE nine)

Sound-Alike/Look-Alike Issues

quinine may be confused with quinidine

Synonyms quinine sulfate

U.S./Canadian Brand Names Apo-Quinine® [Can]; Novo-Quinine [Can]; Quinine-Odan™ [Can]

Therapeutic Category Antimalarial Agent

Use In conjunction with other antimalarial agents, treatment of uncomplicated chloroquine-resistant *P. falciparum* malaria

Usual Dosage Oral:

Children:

Treatment of chloroquine-resistant malaria: 25-30 mg/kg/day in divided doses every 8 hours for 3-7 days with tetracycline (consider risk versus benefit in children <8 years of age)

Babesiosis: 25 mg/kg/day divided every 8 hours for 7 days

Adults:

Treatment of chloroquine-resistant malaria: 650 mg every 8 hours for 3-7 days with tetracycline

Suppression of malaria: 325 mg twice daily and continued for 6 weeks after exposure

Babesiosis: 650 mg every 6-8 hours for 7 days

Leg cramps: 200-300 mg at bedtime

Dosage Forms

Capsule, as sulfate: 200 mg, 325 mg

Qualaquin™: 324 mg

Tablet, as sulfate: 260 mg

Quinine-Odan™ [Can] *see* quinine *on this page*

quinine sulfate *see* quinine *on this page*

quinol *see* hydroquinone *on page 430*

Quinora® ***(Discontinued)*** *see* quinidine *on previous page*

Quintabs [US-OTC] *see* vitamins (multiple/oral) *on page 878*

Quintabs-M [US-OTC] *see* vitamins (multiple/oral) *on page 878*

Quintasa® [Can] *see* mesalamine *on page 533*

quinupristin and dalfopristin (kwi NYOO pris tin & dal FOE pris tin)

Synonyms pristinamycin; RP-59500

U.S./Canadian Brand Names Synercid® [US/Can]

Therapeutic Category Antibiotic, Streptogramin

Use Treatment of serious or life-threatening infections associated with vancomycin-resistant *Enterococcus faecium* bacteremia; treatment of complicated skin and skin structure infections caused by methcillin-susceptible *Staphylococcus aureus* or *Streptococcus pyogenes*

Has been studied in the treatment of a variety of infections caused by *Enterococcus faecium* (not *E. fecalis*) including vancomycin-resistant strains. May also be effective in the treatment of serious infections caused by *Staphylococcus* species including those resistant to methicillin.

Usual Dosage I.V.:

Children (limited information): Dosages similar to adult dosing have been used in the treatment of complicated skin/soft tissue infections and infections caused by vancomycin-resistant *Enterococcus faecium*

CNS shunt infection due to vancomycin-resistant *Enterococcus faecium*: 7.5 mg/kg/dose every 8 hours; concurrent intrathecal doses of 1-2 mg/day have been administered for up to 68 days

Adults:

Vancomycin-resistant *Enterococcus faecium*: 7.5 mg/kg every 8 hours

Complicated skin and skin structure infection: 7.5 mg/kg every 12 hours

Dosage Forms Injection, powder for reconstitution:

500 mg: Quinupristin 150 mg and dalfopristin 350 mg

600 mg: Quinupristin 180 mg and dalfopristin 420 mg

Quixin™ [US] *see* levofloxacin *on page 490*

QVAR® [US/Can] *see* beclomethasone *on page 95*

R 14-15 *see* erlotinib *on page 302*

R & C™ II [Can] *see* pyrethrins and piperonyl butoxide *on page 720*

R & C® Lice *(Discontinued)* *see* permethrin *on page 655*

R & C™ Shampoo/Conditioner [Can] *see* pyrethrins and piperonyl butoxide *on page 720*

R-3827 *see* abarelix *on page 2*

RabAvert® [US/Can] *see* rabies virus vaccine *on next page*

rabeprazole (ra BEP ra zole)

Sound-Alike/Look-Alike Issues

rabeprazole may be confused with aripiprazole

AcipHex® may be confused with Acephen®, Accupril®, Aricept®

Synonyms pariprazole

U.S./Canadian Brand Names AcipHex® [US/Can]; Pariet® [Can]

Therapeutic Category Gastric Acid Secretion Inhibitor

Use Short-term (4-8 weeks) treatment and maintenance of erosive or ulcerative gastroesophageal reflux disease (GERD); symptomatic GERD; short-term (up to 4 weeks) treatment of duodenal ulcers; long-term treatment of pathological hypersecretory conditions, including Zollinger-Ellison syndrome; *H. pylori* eradication (in combination with amoxicillin and clarithromycin)

Usual Dosage Oral: Adults >18 years:

GERD: 20 mg once daily for 4-8 weeks; maintenance: 20 mg once daily

Duodenal ulcer: 20 mg/day before breakfast for 4 weeks

H. pylori eradication: 20 mg twice daily for 7 days; to be administered with amoxicillin 1000 mg and clarithromycin 500 mg, also given twice daily for 7 days.

Hypersecretory conditions: 60 mg once daily; dose may need to be adjusted as necessary. Doses as high as 100 mg once daily and 60 mg twice daily have been used.

Dosage Forms Tablet, delayed release, enteric coated, as sodium: 20 mg

rabies immune globulin (human) (RAY beez i MYUN GLOB yoo lin, HYU man)

Synonyms RIG

U.S./Canadian Brand Names BayRab® [Can]; HyperRAB™ S/D [US]; Imogam® Rabies Pasteurized [Can]; Imogam® Rabies-HT [US]

Therapeutic Category Immune Globulin

Use Part of postexposure prophylaxis of persons with rabies exposure who lack a history of pre-exposure or postexposure prophylaxis with rabies vaccine or a recently documented neutralizing antibody response to previous rabies vaccination; although it is preferable to administer RIG with the first dose of vaccine, it can be given up to 8 days after vaccination

(Continued)

rabies immune globulin (human) *(Continued)*

Usual Dosage Children and Adults: I.M.: 20 units/kg in a single dose (RIG should always be administered as part of rabies vaccine (HDCV)) regimen (as soon as possible after the first dose of vaccine, up to 8 days); infiltrate 1/2 of the dose locally around the wound; administer the remainder I.M.

Note: Persons known to have an adequate titer or who have been completely immunized with rabies vaccine should not receive RIG, only booster doses of HDCV

Dosage Forms Injection, solution:

BayRab® [DSC], HyperRAB™ S/D: 150 int. units/mL (2 mL, 10 mL) [solvent/detergent treated]

Imogam® Rabies-HT: 150 int. units/mL (2 mL, 10 mL) [heat treated]

rabies virus vaccine (RAY beez VYE rus vak SEEN)

Synonyms HDCV; human diploid cell cultures rabies vaccine; PCEC; purified chick embryo cell

U.S./Canadian Brand Names Imovax® Rabies [US/Can]; RabAvert® [US/Can]

Therapeutic Category Vaccine, Inactivated Virus

Use Pre-exposure immunization: Vaccinate persons with greater than usual risk due to occupation or avocation including veterinarians, rangers, animal handlers, certain laboratory workers, and persons living in or visiting countries for longer than 1 month where rabies is a constant threat.

Postexposure prophylaxis: If a bite from a carrier animal is unprovoked, if it is not captured and rabies is present in that species and area, administer rabies immune globulin (RIG) and the vaccine as indicated

Usual Dosage

Pre-exposure prophylaxis: 1 mL I.M. on days 0, 7, and 21 to 28. **Note:** Prolonging the interval between doses does not interfere with immunity achieved after the concluding dose of the basic series.

Postexposure prophylaxis: All postexposure treatment should begin with immediate cleansing of the wound with soap and water

Persons not previously immunized as above: I.M.: 5 doses (1 mL each) on days 0, 3, 7, 14, 28. In addition, patients should receive rabies immune globulin 20 units/kg body weight, half infiltrated at bite site if possible, remainder I.M.)

Persons who have previously received postexposure prophylaxis with rabies vaccine, received a recommended I.M. pre-exposure series of rabies vaccine or have a previously documented rabies antibody titer considered adequate: 1 mL of either vaccine I.M. only on days 0 and 3; do not administer RIG

Booster (for occupational or other continuing risk): 1 mL I.M. every 2-5 years or based on antibody titers

Dosage Forms Injection, powder for reconstitution:

Imovax® Rabies: 2.5 int. units [HDCV; grown in human diploid cell culture; contains albumin <100 mg, neomycin <150 mcg]

RabAvert®: 2.5 int. units [PCEC; grown in chicken fibroblasts; contains amphotericin <2 ng, chlortetracycline <20 ng, and neomycin <1 mcg]

racepinephrine *see* epinephrine *on page 295*

Radiogardase™ [US] *see* ferric hexacyanoferrate *on page 342*

radiological/contrast media (ionic) (ray deo LOG ik al/KON trast MEE dia eye ON ik)

Synonyms barium sulfate; diatrizoate meglumine; diatrizoate meglumine and diatrizoate sodium; diatrizoate meglumine and iodipamide meglumine; diatrizoate sodium; ethiodized oil; gadopentetate dimeglumine; iocetamic acid; iodamide meglumine; iodipamide meglumine; iopanoic acid; iothalamate meglumine and iothalamate sodium; iothalamate sodium; ipodate calcium; ipodate sodium; isosulfan blue; potassium perchlorate; propyliodone; tyropanoate sodium

U.S./Canadian Brand Names Anatrast® [US]; Angio Conray® [US]; Angiovist® [US]; Bar-Test® [US]; Baricon® [US]; Baro-CAT® [US]; Barobag® [US]; Baroflave® [US]; Barosperse® [US]; Cholebrine® [US]; Cholografin® Meglumine [US]; Conray® [US]; Cystografin® [US]; Dionosil Oily® [US]; Enecat® [US]; Entrobar® [US]; Epi-C® [US]; Ethiodol® [US]; Flo-Coat® [US]; Gastrografin® [US]; HD 200 Plus® [US]; HD 85® [US]; Hexabrix™ [US]; Hypaque-Cysto® [US]; Hypaque® Meglumine [US]; Hypaque® Sodium [US]; Liquid Barosperse® [US]; Liquipake® [US]; Lymphazurin® [US/Can]; Magnevist® [US/Can]; MD-Gastroview® [US]; Oragrafin® Calcium [US]; Oragrafin® Sodium [US]; Perchloracap® [US]; Prepcat® [US]; Reno-M-30® [US]; Reno-M-60® [US]; Reno-M-DIP® [US]; Renovue®-65 [US]; Renovue®-DIP [US]; Sinografin® [US]; Telepaque® [US]; Tomocat® [US]; Tonopaque® [US]; Urovist Cysto® [US]; Urovist® Meglumine [US]; Urovist® Sodium 300 [US]; Vascoray® [US]

Therapeutic Category Radiopaque Agents

Use Enhance visualization of structures during radiologic procedures

Usual Dosage Varies with procedure

Dosage Forms [DSC] = Discontinued product

Oral cholecystographic agents:

Iocetamic acid: Tablet (Cholebrine®): 750 mg
Iopanoic acid: Tablet (Telepaque®): 500 mg
Ipodate calcium: Granules for oral suspension (Oragrafin® Calcium): 3 g
Ipodate sodium: Capsule (Bilivist®, Oragrafin® Sodium): 500 mg
Tyropanoate sodium: Capsule (Bilopaque®): 750 mg [DSC]

GI contrast agents: **Barium sulfate**:

Paste (Anatrast®): 100% (500 g)
Powder:
- Baroflave®: 100%
- Baricon®, HD 200 Plus®: 98%
- Barosperse®, Tonopaque®: 95%

Suspension:
- Baro-CAT®, Prepcat®: 1.5%
- Enecat®, Tomocat®: 5%
- Entrobar®: 50%
- Liquid Barasperse®: 60%
- HD 85®: 85%
- Barobag®: 97%
- Flo-Coat®, Liquipake®: 100%
- Epi-C®: 150%

Tablet (Bar-Test®): 650 mg

Parenteral agents: Injection:

Diatrizoate meglumine:
- Hypaque® Meglumine
- Reno-M-DIP®
- Urovist® Meglumine
- Angiovist® 282
- Hypaque® Meglumine
- Reno-M-60®

Diatrizoate sodium:
- Hypaque® Sodium
- Urovist® Sodium 300

Gadopentetate dimeglumine: Magnevist®

Iodamide meglumine:
- Renovue®-DIP
- Renovue®-65

Iodipamide meglumine: Cholografin® meglumine

Iothalamate meglumine:
- Conray® 30
- Conray® 43
- Conray®

Iothalamate sodium:
- Angio Conray®
- Conray® 325
- Conray® 400

Diatrizoate meglumine and diatrizoate sodium:
- Angiovist® 292
- Angiovist® 370
- Hypaque-76®
- Hypaque-M®, 75%
- Hypaque-M®, 90%
- MD-60®
- MD-76®
- Renografin-60®
- Renografin-76®
- Renovist® II
- Renovist®

Iothalamate meglumine and iothalamate sodium:
- Vascoray®
- Hexabrix™

(Continued)

radiological/contrast media (ionic) *(Continued)*

Miscellaneous agents (**NOT** for intravascular use, for instillation into various cavities):

Diatrizoate meglumine: Urogenital solution, sterile:

Crystografin®
Crystografin® Dilute
Hypaque-Cysto®
Reno-M-30®
Urovist Cysto®

Diatrizoate meglumine and diatrizoate sodium: Solution, oral or rectal:

Gastrografin®
MD-Gastroview®

Diatrizoate sodium:

Solution, oral or rectal (Hypaque® sodium oral)
Solution, urogenital (Hypaque® sodium 20%)

Iothalamate meglumine: Solution, urogenital:

Cysto-Conray®
Cysto-Conray® II

Diatrizoate meglumine and iodipamide meglumine:

Injection, urogenital for intrauterine instillation (Sinografin®)

Ethiodized oil: Injection (Ethiodol®)

Propyliodone: Suspension (Dionosil Oily®)

Isosulfan blue: Injection (Lymphazurin® 1%)

Potassium perchlorate: Capsule (Perchloracap®): 200 mg

radiological/contrast media (nonionic)

(ray deo LOG ik al/KON trast MEE dia non eye ON ik)

Sound-Alike/Look-Alike Issues

Optiray® may be confused with Optivar™

Synonyms gadoteridol; iohexol; iopamidol; ioversol; metrizamide

U.S./Canadian Brand Names Isovue® [US]; Omnipaque® [US]; Optiray® [US]; ProHance® [US]

Therapeutic Category Radiopaque Agents

Use Enhance visualization of structures during radiologic procedures

Usual Dosage Dose varies with procedure

Dosage Forms [DSC] = Discontinued product

Injection, solution:

Gadoteridol (ProHance®): 279.3 mg/mL (15 mL, 30 mL, 50 mL) [single use vial]; 279.3 mg/mL (20 mL) [prefilled syringe]

Iohexol (Omnipaque®): 140 mg/mL, 180 mg/mL, 210 mg/mL, 240 mg/mL, 300 mg/mL, 350 mg/mL

Iopamidol:

Isovue-128®
Isovue-200®
Isovue-300®
Isovue-370®
Isovue-M 200®
Isovue-M 300®

Ioversol:

Optiray® 160
Optiray® 240
Optiray® 320

Metrizamide: Amipaque® [DSC]

rAHF *see* antihemophilic factor (recombinant) *on page 59*

R-albuterol *see* levalbuterol *on page 487*

Ralix [US] *see* chlorpheniramine, phenylephrine, and methscopolamine *on page 180*

raloxifene (ral OKS i feen)

Sound-Alike/Look-Alike Issues

Evista® may be confused with Avinza™

Synonyms keoxifene hydrochloride; NSC-706725; raloxifene hydrochloride
U.S./Canadian Brand Names Evista® [US/Can]
Therapeutic Category Selective Estrogen Receptor Modulator (SERM)
Use Prevention and treatment of osteoporosis in postmenopausal women
Usual Dosage Adults: Female: Oral:
Osteoporosis: 60 mg/day
Dosage Forms
Tablet, as hydrochloride:
Evista®: 60 mg

raloxifene hydrochloride *see* raloxifene *on previous page*

raltitrexed *(Canada only)* (ral ti TREX ed)

Synonyms ICI-D1694; NSC-639186; raltitrexed disodium; ZD1694
U.S./Canadian Brand Names Tomudex® [Can]
Therapeutic Category Antineoplastic Agent
Use Treatment of advanced colorectal neoplasms
Usual Dosage Refer to individual protocols.
I.V.: 3 mg/m^2 every 3 weeks
Dosage Forms Injection, powder for reconstitution, as disodium: 2 mg

raltitrexed disodium *see* raltitrexed *(Canada only) on this page*

ramelteon (ra MEL tee on)

Sound-Alike/Look-Alike Issues
Rozerem™ may be confused with Razadyne™
Synonyms TAK-375
U.S./Canadian Brand Names Rozerem™ [US]
Therapeutic Category Hypnotic, Nonbenzodiazepine
Use Treatment of insomnia characterized by difficulty with sleep onset
Usual Dosage Oral: Adults: One 8 mg tablet within 30 minutes of bedtime
Dosage Forms Tablet: 8 mg

ramipril (RA mi pril)

Sound-Alike/Look-Alike Issues
ramipril may be confused with enalapril, Monopril®
Altace® may be confused with alteplase, Amaryl®, Amerge®, Artane®
U.S./Canadian Brand Names Altace® [US/Can]
Therapeutic Category Angiotensin-Converting Enzyme (ACE) Inhibitor
Use Treatment of hypertension, alone or in combination with thiazide diuretics; treatment of left ventricular dysfunction after myocardial infarction; to reduce risk of heart attack, stroke, and death in patients at increased risk for these problems
Usual Dosage Adults: Oral:
Hypertension: 2.5-5 mg once daily, maximum: 20 mg/day
Reduction in risk of MI, stroke, and death from cardiovascular causes: Initial: 2.5 mg once daily for 1 week, then 5 mg once daily for the next 3 weeks, then increase as tolerated to 10 mg once daily (may be given as divided dose)
Heart failure postmyocardial infarction: Initial: 2.5 mg twice daily titrated upward, if possible, to 5 mg twice daily.
Note: The dose of any concomitant diuretic should be reduced. If the diuretic cannot be discontinued, initiate therapy with 1.25 mg. After the initial dose, the patient should be monitored carefully until blood pressure has stabilized.
Dosage Forms Capsule: 1.25 mg, 2.5 mg, 5 mg, 10 mg

RAN™-Carvedilol [Can] *see* carvedilol *on page 154*
RAN™-Ciprofloxacin [Can] *see* ciprofloxacin *on page 190*
RAN™-Citalopram [Can] *see* citalopram *on page 194*
RAN™-Domperidone [Can] *see* domperidone *(Canada only) on page 273*
Ranexa™ [US] *see* ranolazine *on page 733*

ranibizumab (ra ni BIZ oo mab)

Synonyms rhuFabV2

U.S./Canadian Brand Names Lucentis™ [US]

Therapeutic Category Monoclonal Antibody; Ophthalmic Agent; Vascular Endothelial Growth Factor (VEGF) Inhibitor

Use Treatment of neovascular (wet) age-related macular degeneration (AMD)

Usual Dosage Ophthalmic: Adults: AMD: Intravitreal injection: 0.5 mg once a month. Although not as effective, frequency may be reduced after the first 4 injections to once every 3 months if monthly injections are not feasible. Dosing every 3 months will lead to an ~5 letter (1 line) loss of visual acuity over 9 months, as compared to monthly dosing.

Dosage Forms

Injection, solution [preservative free]:

Lucentis™: 10 mg/mL (0.05 mL)

Raniclor™ [US] *see* cefaclor *on page 155*

ranitidine (ra NI ti deen)

Sound-Alike/Look-Alike Issues

ranitidine may be confused with amantadine, rimantadine

Zantac® may be confused with Xanax®, Zarontin®, Zofran®, Zyrtec®

Synonyms ranitidine hydrochloride

U.S./Canadian Brand Names Alti-Ranitidine [Can]; Apo-Ranitidine® [Can]; BCI-Ranitidine [Can]; CO Ranitidine [Can]; Gen-Ranidine [Can]; Novo-Ranidine [Can]; Nu-Ranit [Can]; PMS-Ranitidine [Can]; Ranitidine Injection, USP [Can]; Rhoxal-ranitidine [Can]; Sandoz-Ranitidine [Can]; Zantac 150™ [US-OTC]; Zantac 75® [US-OTC/Can]; Zantac® EFFERdose® [US]; Zantac® [US/Can]

Therapeutic Category Histamine H_2 Antagonist

Use

Zantac®: Short-term and maintenance therapy of duodenal ulcer, gastric ulcer, gastroesophageal reflux, active benign ulcer, erosive esophagitis, and pathological hypersecretory conditions; as part of a multidrug regimen for *H. pylori* eradication to reduce the risk of duodenal ulcer recurrence

Zantac® 75 [OTC]: Relief of heartburn, acid indigestion, and sour stomach

Usual Dosage

Children 1 month to 16 years:

Duodenal and gastric ulcer:

Oral:

Treatment: 2-4 mg/kg/day divided twice daily; maximum treatment dose: 300 mg/day

Maintenance: 2-4 mg/kg once daily; maximum maintenance dose: 150 mg/day

I.V.: 2-4 mg/kg/day divided every 6-8 hours; maximum: 150 mg/day

GERD and erosive esophagitis:

Oral: 5-10 mg/kg/day divided twice daily; maximum: GERD: 300 mg/day, erosive esophagitis: 600 mg/day

I.V.: 2-4 mg/kg/day divided every 6-8 hours; maximum: 150 mg/day **or as an alternative**

Continuous infusion: Initial: 1 mg/kg/dose for one dose followed by infusion of 0.08-0.17 mg/kg/hour or 2-4 mg/kg/day

Children ≥12 years: Prevention of heartburn: Oral: Zantac® 75 [OTC]: 75 mg 30-60 minutes before eating food or drinking beverages which cause heartburn; maximum: 150 mg/24 hours; do not use for more than 14 days

Adults:

Duodenal ulcer: Oral: Treatment: 150 mg twice daily, or 300 mg once daily after the evening meal or at bedtime; maintenance: 150 mg once daily at bedtime

Helicobacter pylori eradication: 150 mg twice daily; requires combination therapy

Pathological hypersecretory conditions:

Oral: 150 mg twice daily; adjust dose or frequency as clinically indicated; doses of up to 6 g/day have been used

I.V.: Continuous infusion for Zollinger-Ellison: 1 mg/kg/hour; measure gastric acid output at 4 hours, if >10 mEq or if patient is symptomatic, increase dose in increments of 0.5 mg/kg/hour; doses of up to 2.5 mg/kg/hour have been used

Gastric ulcer, benign: Oral: 150 mg twice daily; maintenance: 150 mg once daily at bedtime

Erosive esophagitis: Oral: Treatment: 150 mg 4 times/day; maintenance: 150 mg twice daily

Prevention of heartburn: Oral: Zantac® 75 [OTC]: 75 mg 30-60 minutes before eating food or drinking beverages which cause heartburn; maximum: 150 mg in 24 hours; do not use for more than 14 days

Patients not able to take oral medication:
I.M.: 50 mg every 6-8 hours
I.V.: Intermittent bolus or infusion: 50 mg every 6-8 hours
Continuous I.V. infusion: 6.25 mg/hour

Dosage Forms
Capsule 150 mg, 300 mg
Infusion [premixed in NaCl 0.45%; preservative free]:
Zantac®: 50 mg (50 mL)
Injection, solution: 25 mg/mL (2 mL, 6 mL)
Zantac®: 25 mg/mL (2 mL, 6 mL, 40 mL) [contains phenol 0.5% as preservative]
Syrup: 15 mg/mL (10 mL) [contains alcohol 7.5%; peppermint flavor]
Zantac®: 15 mg/mL (473 mL) [contains alcohol 7.5%; peppermint flavor]
Tablet: 75 mg [OTC], 150 mg, 300 mg
Zantac®: 150 mg, 300 mg
Zantac 75®: 75 mg
Zantac 150™: 150 mg
Tablet, effervescent:
Zantac® EFFERdose®: 25 mg [contains sodium 1.33 mEq/tablet, phenylalanine 2.81 mg/tablet, and sodium benzoate]; 150 mg [contains sodium 7.96 mEq/tablet, phenylalanine 16.84 mg/tablet, and sodium benzoate]

ranitidine hydrochloride *see* ranitidine *on previous page*

Ranitidine Injection, USP [Can] *see* ranitidine *on previous page*

RAN™-Lovastatin [Can] *see* lovastatin *on page 508*

RAN™-Metformin [Can] *see* metformin *on page 535*

ranolazine (ra NOE la zeen)

U.S./Canadian Brand Names Ranexa™ [US]
Therapeutic Category Cardiovascular Agent, Miscellaneous
Use Treatment of chronic angina in combination with amlodipine, beta-blockers, or nitrates
Usual Dosage Oral: Chronic angina: Adults: Initial: 500 mg twice daily; maximum recommended dose: 1000 mg twice daily
Dosage Forms Tablet, extended release: 500 mg

RAN™-Zopiclone [Can] *see* zopiclone *(Canada only) on page 890*

Rapamune® [US/Can] *see* sirolimus *on page 774*

Raphon [US-OTC] *see* epinephrine *on page 295*

Raplon® ***(Discontinued)***

Raptiva® [US] *see* efalizumab *on page 288*

rasagiline (ra SA ji leen)

Sound-Alike/Look-Alike Issues
Azilect® may be confused with Aricept®
Synonyms AGN 1135; rasagiline mesylate; TVP-1012
U.S./Canadian Brand Names Azilect® [US]
Therapeutic Category Anti-Parkinson Agent, MAO Type B Inhibitor
Use Initial monotherapy or as adjunct to levodopa in the treatment of idiopathic Parkinson disease
Usual Dosage Oral: Adults: Parkinson disease:
Monotherapy: 1 mg once daily
Adjunctive therapy with levodopa: Initial: 0.5 mg once daily; may increase to 1 mg once daily based on response and tolerability

Dosage Forms
Tablet, as mesylate:
Azilect®: 0.5 mg, 1 mg

rasagiline mesylate *see* rasagiline *on this page*

rasburicase (ras BYOOR i kayse)

U.S./Canadian Brand Names Elitek™ [US]; Fasturtec® [Can]

Therapeutic Category Enzyme

Use Initial management of uric acid levels in pediatric patients with leukemia, lymphoma, and solid tumor malignancies receiving anticancer therapy expected to result in tumor lysis and elevation of plasma uric acid

Usual Dosage I.V.:

Children: Management of uric acid levels: 0.15 mg/kg or 0.2 mg/kg once daily for 5 days (manufacturer-recommended duration); begin chemotherapy 4-24 hours after the first dose

Limited data suggest that a single prechemotherapy dose (versus multiple-day administration) may be sufficiently efficacious. Monitoring electrolytes, hydration status, and uric acid concentrations are necessary to identify the need for additional doses. Other clinical manifestations of tumor lysis syndrome (eg, hyperphosphatemia, hypocalcemia, and hyperkalemia) may occur.

Adults: Refer to pediatric dosing; insufficient data collected in adult/geriatric patients to determine response to treatment

Dosage Forms Injection, powder for reconstitution: 1.5 mg [packaged with three 1 mL ampuls of diluent]

ratio-Aclavulanate [Can] *see* amoxicillin and clavulanate potassium *on page 49*

ratio-Acyclovir [Can] *see* acyclovir *on page 18*

ratio-Alendronate [Can] *see* alendronate *on page 27*

ratio-Amcinonide [Can] *see* amcinonide *on page 39*

ratio-Azithromycin [Can] *see* azithromycin *on page 88*

ratio-Benzydamine [Can] *see* benzydamine *(Canada only) on page 104*

ratio-Bicalutamide [Can] *see* bicalutamide *on page 110*

ratio-Brimonidine [Can] *see* brimonidine *on page 116*

ratio-Carvedilol [Can] *see* carvedilol *on page 154*

ratio-Cefuroxime [Can] *see* cefuroxime *on page 163*

ratio-Ciprofloxacin [Can] *see* ciprofloxacin *on page 190*

ratio-Citalopram [Can] *see* citalopram *on page 194*

ratio-Clarithromycin [Can] *see* clarithromycin *on page 195*

ratio-Clobazam [Can] *see* clobazam *(Canada only) on page 200*

ratio-Cotridin [Can] *see* triprolidine, pseudoephedrine, and codeine *(Canada only) on page 853*

ratio-Diltiazem CD [Can] *see* diltiazem *on page 257*

ratio-Domperidone [Can] *see* domperidone *(Canada only) on page 273*

ratio-Emtec [Can] *see* acetaminophen and codeine *on page 6*

ratio-Fenofibrate MC [Can] *see* fenofibrate *on page 338*

ratio-Fosinopril [Can] *see* fosinopril *on page 369*

ratio-Glimepiride [Can] *see* glimepiride *on page 384*

ratio-Glyburide [Can] *see* glyburide *on page 387*

ratio-Inspra-Sal [Can] *see* albuterol *on page 23*

ratio-Ketorolac [Can] *see* ketorolac *on page 472*

ratio-Lamotrigine [Can] *see* lamotrigine *on page 480*

ratio-Lenoltec [Can] *see* acetaminophen and codeine *on page 6*

ratio-Lovastatin [Can] *see* lovastatin *on page 508*

ratio-Magnesium [Can] *see* magnesium glucoheptonate *on page 513*

ratio-Metformin [Can] *see* metformin *on page 535*

ratio-Methotrexate [Can] *see* methotrexate *on page 540*

ratio-Mirtazapine [Can] *see* mirtazapine *on page 559*

ratio-Mometasone [Can] *see* mometasone furoate *on page 563*

ratio-Morphine SR [Can] *see* morphine sulfate *on page 565*

Ratio-Orciprenaline® [Can] *see* metaproterenol *on page 535*

ratio-Paroxetine [Can] *see* paroxetine *on page 639*

Refresh Tears® [US-OTC/Can] *see* carboxymethylcellulose *on page 151*
Regitine® [Can] *see* phentolamine *on page 660*
Regitine® *(Discontinued)* *see* phentolamine *on page 660*
Reglan® [US] *see* metoclopramide *on page 549*
Reglan® Syrup *(Discontinued)* *see* metoclopramide *on page 549*
Regonol® [US] *see* pyridostigmine *on page 720*
Regranex® [US/Can] *see* becaplermin *on page 95*
Regular Iletin® II *(Discontinued)*
regular insulin *see* insulin regular *on page 453*
Regulax SS® *(Discontinued)* *see* docusate *on page 270*
Regulex® [Can] *see* docusate *on page 270*
Reguloid® [US-OTC] *see* psyllium *on page 717*
Rejuva-A® [Can] *see* tretinoin (topical) *on page 844*
Relacon-DM NR [US] *see* guaifenesin, pseudoephedrine, and dextromethorphan *on page 401*
Relacon-HC [US] *see* phenylephrine, hydrocodone, and chlorpheniramine *on page 663*
Relafen® [Can] *see* nabumetone *on page 572*
Relafen® *(Discontinued)* *see* nabumetone *on page 572*
Relenza® [US/Can] *see* zanamivir *on page 884*
Relief® [US-OTC] *see* phenylephrine *on page 660*
Relief® Ophthalmic Solution *(Discontinued)* *see* phenylephrine *on page 660*
Relpax® [US/Can] *see* eletriptan *on page 289*
Remeron® [US/Can] *see* mirtazapine *on page 559*
Remeron® RD [Can] *see* mirtazapine *on page 559*
Remeron SolTab® [US] *see* mirtazapine *on page 559*
Reme-T™ [US-OTC] *see* coal tar *on page 207*
Remicade® [US/Can] *see* infliximab *on page 447*

remifentanil (rem i FEN ta nil)

Sound-Alike/Look-Alike Issues
remifentanil may be confused with alfentanil

Synonyms GI87084B

U.S./Canadian Brand Names Ultiva® [US/Can]

Therapeutic Category Analgesic, Narcotic

Controlled Substance C-II

Use Analgesic for use during the induction and maintenance of general anesthesia; for continued analgesia into the immediate postoperative period; analgesic component of monitored anesthesia

Usual Dosage I.V. continuous infusion: Dose should be based on ideal body weight (IBW) in obese patients (>30% over IBW).

Children birth to 2 months: Maintenance of anesthesia with nitrous oxide (70%): 0.4 mcg/kg/minute (range: 0.4-1 mcg/kg/minute); supplemental bolus dose of 1 mcg/kg may be administered, smaller bolus dose may be required with potent inhalation agents, potent neuraxial anesthesia, significant comorbidities, significant fluid shifts, or without atropine pretreatment. Clearance in neonates is highly variable; dose should be carefully titrated.

Children 1-12 years: Maintenance of anesthesia with halothane, sevoflurane or isoflurane: 0.25 mcg/kg/minute (range 0.05-1.3 mcg/kg/minute); supplemental bolus dose of 1 mcg/kg may be administered every 2-5 minutes. Consider increasing concomitant anesthetics with infusion rate >1 mcg/kg/minute. Infusion rate can be titrated upward in increments up to 50% or titrated downward in decrements of 25% to 50%. May titrate every 2-5 minutes.

Adults:

Induction of anesthesia: 0.5-1 mcg/kg/minute; if endotracheal intubation is to occur in <8 minutes, an initial dose of 1 mcg/kg may be given over 30-60 seconds

Coronary bypass surgery: 1 mcg/kg/minute

Maintenance of anesthesia: **Note:** Supplemental bolus dose of 1 mcg/kg may be administered every 2-5 minutes. Consider increasing concomitant anesthetics with infusion rate >1 mcg/kg/minute. Infusion rate can be titrated upward in increments of 25% to 100% or downward in decrements of 25% to 50%. May titrate every 2-5 minutes.

With nitrous oxide (66%): 0.4 mcg/kg/minute (range: 0.1-2 mcg/kg/minute)

With isoflurane: 0.25 mcg/kg/minute (range: 0.05-2 mcg/kg/minute)

With propofol: 0.25 mcg/kg/minute (range: 0.05-2 mcg/kg/minute)

Coronary bypass surgery: 1 mcg/kg/minute (range: 0.125-4 mcg/kg/minute); supplemental dose: 0.5-1 mcg/kg

Continuation as an analgesic in immediate postoperative period: 0.1 mcg/kg/minute (range: 0.025-0.2 mcg/kg/minute). Infusion rate may be adjusted every 5 minutes in increments of 0.025 mcg/kg/minute. Bolus doses are not recommended. Infusion rates >0.2 mcg/kg/minute are associated with respiratory depression.

Coronary bypass surgery, continuation as an analgesic into the ICU: 1 mcg/kg/minute (range: 0.05-1 mcg/kg/minute)

Analgesic component of monitored anesthesia care: **Note:** Supplemental oxygen is recommended:

Single I.V. dose given 90 seconds prior to local anesthetic:

Remifentanil alone: 1 mcg/kg over 30-60 seconds

With midazolam: 0.5 mcg/kg over 30-60 seconds

Continuous infusion beginning 5 minutes prior to local anesthetic:

Remifentanil alone: 0.1 mcg/kg minute

With midazolam: 0.05 mcg/kg/minute

Continuous infusion given after local anesthetic:

Remifentanil alone: 0.05 mcg/kg/minute (range: 0.025-0.2 mcg/kg/minute)

With midazolam: 0.025 mcg/kg/minute (range: 0.025-0.2 mcg/kg/minute)

Note: Following local or anesthetic block, infusion rate should be decreased to 0.05 mcg/kg/minute; rate adjustments of 0.025 mcg/kg/minute may be done at 5-minute intervals

Dosage Forms Injection, powder for reconstitution: 1 mg, 2 mg, 5 mg [contains glycine 15 mg]

Reminyl® [Can] *see* galantamine *on page 374*

Reminyl® *(Discontinued)* *see* galantamine *on page 374*

Reminyl® ER [Can] *see* galantamine *on page 374*

Remodulin® [US/Can] *see* treprostinil *on page 844*

Renacidin® [US] *see* citric acid, magnesium carbonate, and glucono-delta-lactone *on page 194*

Renagel® [US/Can] *see* sevelamer *on page 770*

Renedil® [Can] *see* felodipine *on page 338*

Reno-M-30® [US] *see* radiological/contrast media (ionic) *on page 728*

Reno-M-60® [US] *see* radiological/contrast media (ionic) *on page 728*

Reno-M-DIP® [US] *see* radiological/contrast media (ionic) *on page 728*

Renografin-60® *(Discontinued)* *see* radiological/contrast media (ionic) *on page 728*

Renografin-76® *(Discontinued)* *see* radiological/contrast media (ionic) *on page 728*

Renoquid® *(Discontinued)*

Renova® [US] *see* tretinoin (topical) *on page 844*

Renovist® II *(Discontinued)* *see* radiological/contrast media (ionic) *on page 728*

Renovist® *(Discontinued)* *see* radiological/contrast media (ionic) *on page 728*

Renovue®-65 [US] *see* radiological/contrast media (ionic) *on page 728*

Renovue®-DIP [US] *see* radiological/contrast media (ionic) *on page 728*

ReoPro® [US/Can] *see* abciximab *on page 3*

repaglinide (re PAG li nide)

Sound-Alike/Look-Alike Issues

Prandin® may be confused with Avandia®

U.S./Canadian Brand Names GlucoNorm® [Can]; Prandin® [US/Can]

Therapeutic Category Hypoglycemic Agent, Oral

Use Management of type 2 diabetes mellitus (noninsulin-dependent, NIDDM); may be used in combination with metformin or thiazolidinediones

Usual Dosage Adults: Oral: Should be taken within 15 minutes of the meal, but time may vary from immediately preceding the meal to as long as 30 minutes before the meal

(Continued)

repaglinide *(Continued)*

Initial: For patients not previously treated or whose Hb A_{1c} is <8%, the starting dose is 0.5 mg. For patients previously treated with blood glucose-lowering agents whose Hb A_{1c} is ≥8%, the initial dose is 1 or 2 mg before each meal.

Dose adjustment: Determine dosing adjustments by blood glucose response, usually fasting blood glucose. Double the preprandial dose up to 4 mg until satisfactory blood glucose response is achieved. At least 1 week should elapse to assess response after each dose adjustment.

Dose range: 0.5-4 mg taken with meals. Repaglinide may be dosed preprandial 2, 3 or 4 times/day in response to changes in the patient's meal pattern. Maximum recommended daily dose: 16 mg.

Patients receiving other oral hypoglycemic agents: When repaglinide is used to replace therapy with other oral hypoglycemic agents, it may be started the day after the final dose is given. Observe patients carefully for hypoglycemia because of potential overlapping of drug effects. When transferred from longer half-life sulfonylureas (eg, chlorpropamide), close monitoring may be indicated for up to ≥1 week.

Combination therapy: If repaglinide monotherapy does not result in adequate glycemic control, metformin or a thiazolidinedione may be added. Or, if metformin or thiazolidinedione therapy does not provide adequate control, repaglinide may be added. The starting dose and dose adjustments for combination therapy are the same as repaglinide monotherapy. Carefully adjust the dose of each drug to determine the minimal dose required to achieve the desired pharmacologic effect. Failure to do so could result in an increase in the incidence of hypoglycemic episodes. Use appropriate monitoring of FPG and Hb A_{1c} measurements to ensure that the patient is not subjected to excessive drug exposure or increased probability of secondary drug failure. If glucose is not achieved after a suitable trial of combination therapy, consider discontinuing these drugs and using insulin.

Dosage Forms

Tablet:

Prandin®: 0.5 mg, 1 mg, 2 mg

Repan® [US] *see* butalbital, acetaminophen, and caffeine *on page 129*

Replace [US-OTC] *see* vitamins (multiple/oral) *on page 878*

Replace with Iron [US-OTC] *see* vitamins (multiple/oral) *on page 878*

Repliva 21/7™ [US] *see* vitamins (multiple/oral) *on page 878*

Reposans-10® Oral *(Discontinued)* *see* chlordiazepoxide *on page 172*

Reprexain™ [US] *see* hydrocodone and ibuprofen *on page 424*

Repronex® [US/Can] *see* menotropins *on page 528*

Requip® [US/Can] *see* ropinirole *on page 753*

Resa® *(Discontinued)* *see* reserpine *on this page*

Rescon® MX [US] *see* chlorpheniramine, phenylephrine, and methscopolamine *on page 180*

Rescon DM [US-OTC] *see* chlorpheniramine, pseudoephedrine, and dextromethorphan *on page 182*

Rescon GG [US] *see* guaifenesin and phenylephrine *on page 396*

Rescon-Jr [US] *see* chlorpheniramine and phenylephrine *on page 176*

Rescriptor® [US/Can] *see* delavirdine *on page 234*

Rescula® *(Discontinued)*

Resectisol® [US] *see* mannitol *on page 518*

reserpine (re SER peen)

Sound-Alike/Look-Alike Issues

reserpine may be confused with Risperdal®, risperidone

Therapeutic Category Rauwolfia Alkaloid

Use Management of mild-to-moderate hypertension; treatment of agitated psychotic states (schizophrenia)

Usual Dosage Note: When used for management of hypertension, full antihypertensive effects may take as long as 3 weeks.

Oral:

Children: Hypertension: 0.01-0.02 mg/kg/24 hours divided every 12 hours; maximum dose: 0.25 mg/day (not recommended in children)

Adults:

Hypertension:

Manufacturer's labeling: Initial: 0.5 mg/day for 1-2 weeks; maintenance: 0.1-0.25 mg/day

Note: Clinically, the need for a "loading" period (as recommended by the manufacturer) is not well supported, and alternative dosing is preferred.

Usual dose range (JNC 7): 0.05-0.25 mg once daily; 0.1 mg every other day may be given to achieve 0.05 mg once daily

Schizophrenia: Dosing recommendations vary; initial dose recommendations generally range from 0.05-0.25 mg (manufacturer recommends 0.5 mg once daily initially in schizophrenia). May be increased in increments of 0.1-0.25 mg.

Dosage Forms Tablet: 0.1 mg, 0.25 mg

Respa-DM® [US] *see* guaifenesin and dextromethorphan *on page 394*

Respa-GF® ***(Discontinued)*** *see* guaifenesin *on page 392*

Respaire®-60 SR [US] *see* guaifenesin and pseudoephedrine *on page 398*

Respaire®-120 SR [US] *see* guaifenesin and pseudoephedrine *on page 398*

Respbid® ***(Discontinued)*** *see* theophylline *on page 818*

Respi-Tann™ [US] *see* carbetapentane and pseudoephedrine *on page 146*

Resporal® ***(Discontinued)*** *see* dexbrompheniramine and pseudoephedrine *on page 241*

Restall® ***(Discontinued)*** *see* hydroxyzine *on page 433*

Restasis® [US] *see* cyclosporine *on page 221*

Restoril® [US/Can] *see* temazepam *on page 808*

Restylane® [US] *see* hyaluronate and derivatives *on page 416*

Retavase® [US/Can] *see* reteplase *on this page*

reteplase (RE ta plase)

Synonyms recombinant plasminogen activator; r-PA

U.S./Canadian Brand Names Retavase® [US/Can]

Therapeutic Category Fibrinolytic Agent

Use Management of acute myocardial infarction (AMI); improvement of ventricular function; reduction of the incidence of CHF and the reduction of mortality following AMI

Usual Dosage Adults: 10 units I.V. over 2 minutes, followed by a second dose 30 minutes later of 10 units I.V. over 2 minutes

Withhold second dose if serious bleeding or anaphylaxis occurs

Dosage Forms Injection, powder for reconstitution [preservative free]: 10.4 units [equivalent to reteplase 18.1 mg; contains sucrose and polysorbate 80; packaged with sterile water for injection]

Retin-A® [US/Can] *see* tretinoin (topical) *on page 844*

Retin-A® Micro [US/Can] *see* tretinoin (topical) *on page 844*

retinoic acid *see* tretinoin (topical) *on page 844*

Retinova® [Can] *see* tretinoin (topical) *on page 844*

Retisert™ [US] *see* fluocinolone *on page 352*

Retrovir® [US/Can] *see* zidovudine *on page 886*

Revatio™ [US] *see* sildenafil *on page 771*

Reversol® [US] *see* edrophonium *on page 287*

Revex® [US] *see* nalmefene *on page 575*

ReVia® [US/Can] *see* naltrexone *on page 577*

Revitalose C-1000® [Can] *see* ascorbic acid *on page 76*

Revlimid® [US] *see* lenalidomide *on page 484*

Rexigen Forte® ***(Discontinued)*** *see* phendimetrazine *on page 657*

Reyataz® [US/Can] *see* atazanavir *on page 80*

Rezulin® ***(Discontinued)***

rFVIIa *see* factor VIIa (recombinant) *on page 333*

R-Gel® ***(Discontinued)*** *see* capsaicin *on page 142*

R-Gene® [US] *see* arginine *on page 73*

rGM-CSF *see* sargramostim *on page 763*

rhASB *see* galsulfase *on page 374*

r-hCG *see* chorionic gonadotropin (recombinant) *on page 187*

Rheaban® *(Discontinued)* *see* attapulgite *on page 84*

Rheomacrodex® *(Discontinued)* *see* dextran *on page 243*

Rheumatrex® [US] *see* methotrexate *on page 540*

rhGAA *see* alglucosidase alfa *on page 28*

r-h α-GAL *see* agalsidase beta *on page 21*

RhIG *see* Rh_o(D) immune globulin *on this page*

rhIGF-1 *see* mecasermin *on page 522*

rhIGF-1/rhIGFBP-3 *see* mecasermin *on page 522*

rhIL-11 *see* oprelvekin *on page 618*

Rhinalar® [Can] *see* flunisolide *on page 352*

Rhinall [US-OTC] *see* phenylephrine *on page 660*

Rhinocort® Aqua® [US] *see* budesonide *on page 122*

Rhinocort® Nasal Inhaler *(Discontinued)* *see* budesonide *on page 122*

Rhinocort® Turbuhaler® [Can] *see* budesonide *on page 122*

RhinoFlex™ [US] *see* acetaminophen and phenyltoloxamine *on page 8*

RhinoFlex 650 [US] *see* acetaminophen and phenyltoloxamine *on page 8*

r-hLH *see* lutropin alfa *on page 510*

Rho(D) immune globulin (human) *see* Rh_o(D) immune globulin *on this page*

Rho®-Clonazepam [Can] *see* clonazepam *on page 203*

Rhodacine® [Can] *see* indomethacin *on page 446*

Rh_o(D) immune globulin (ar aych oh (dee) i MYUN GLOB yoo lin)

Synonyms RhIG; Rho(D) immune globulin (human); RhoIGIV; RhoIVIM

U.S./Canadian Brand Names BayRho-D® Full-Dose [Can]; HyperRHO™ S/D Full Dose [US]; HyperRHO™ S/D Mini Dose [US]; MICRhoGAM® [US]; RhoGAM® [US]; Rhophylac® [US]; WinRho® SDF [US]

Therapeutic Category Immune Globulin

Use

Suppression of Rh isoimmunization: Use in the following situations when an Rh_o(D)-negative individual is exposed to Rh_o(D)-positive blood: During delivery of an Rh_o(D)-positive infant; abortion; amniocentesis; chorionic villus sampling; ruptured tubal pregnancy; abdominal trauma; transplacental hemorrhage. Used when the mother is Rh_o(D) negative, the father of the child is either Rh_o(D) positive or Rh_o(D) unknown, the baby is either Rh_o(D) positive or Rh_o(D) unknown.

Transfusion: Suppression of Rh isoimmunization in Rh_o(D)-negative female children and female adults in their childbearing years transfused with Rh_o(D) antigen-positive RBCs or blood components containing Rh_o(D) antigen-positive RBCs

Treatment of idiopathic thrombocytopenic purpura (ITP): Used in the following nonsplenectomized Rh_o(D) positive individuals: Children with acute or chronic ITP, adults with chronic ITP, children and adults with ITP secondary to HIV infection

Usual Dosage

ITP: Children and Adults: WinRho® SDF: I.V.:

Initial: 50 mcg/kg as a single injection, or can be given as a divided dose on separate days. If hemoglobin is <10 g/dL: Dose should be reduced to 25-40 mcg/kg.

Subsequent dosing: 25-60 mcg/kg can be used if required to elevate platelet count

Maintenance dosing if patient **did respond** to initial dosing: 25-60 mcg/kg based on platelet and hemoglobin levels:

Maintenance dosing if patient **did not respond** to initial dosing:

Hemoglobin 8-10 g/dL: Redose between 25-40 mcg/kg

Hemoglobin >10 g/dL: Redose between 50-60 mcg/kg

Hemoglobin <8 g/dL: Use with caution

Rh_o(D) suppression: Adults: **Note:** One "full dose" (300 mcg) provides enough antibody to prevent Rh sensitization if the volume of RBC entering the circulation is ≤15 mL. When >15 mL is suspected, a fetal red cell count should be performed to determine the appropriate dose.

Pregnancy:

Antepartum prophylaxis: In general, dose is given at 28 weeks. If given early in pregnancy, administer every 12 weeks to ensure adequate levels of passively acquired anti-Rh

BayRho-D® Full Dose, HyperRHO™ S/D Full Dose, RhoGAM®: I.M.: 300 mcg

Rhophylac®, WinRho® SDF: I.M., I.V.: 300 mcg

Postpartum prophylaxis: In general, dose is administered as soon as possible after delivery, preferably within 72 hours. Can be given up to 28 days following delivery

BayRho-D® Full Dose, HyperRHO™ S/D Full Dose, RhoGAM®: I.M.: 300 mcg

Rhophylac®: I.M., I.V.: 300 mcg

WinRho® SDF: I.M., I.V.: 120 mcg

Threatened abortion, any time during pregnancy (with continuation of pregnancy):

BayRho-D® Full Dose, HyperRHO™ S/D Full Dose, RhoGAM®: I.M.: 300 mcg; administer as soon as possible

Rhophylac®, WinRho® SDF: I.M., I.V.: 300 mcg; administer as soon as possible

Abortion, miscarriage, termination of ectopic pregnancy:

BayRho-D®, RhoGAM®: I.M.: ≥13 weeks gestation: 300 mcg.

BayRho-D® Mini Dose, HyperRHO™ S/D Mini Dose, MICRhoGAM®: <13 weeks gestation: I.M.: 50 mcg

Rhophylac®: I.M., I.V.: 300 mcg

WinRho® SDF: I.M., I.V.: After 34 weeks gestation: 120 mcg; administer immediately or within 72 hours

Amniocentesis, chorionic villus sampling:

BayRho-D®, HyperRHO™ S/D Full Dose, RhoGAM®: I.M.: At 15-18 weeks gestation or during the 3rd trimester: 300 mcg. If dose is given between 13-18 weeks, repeat at 26-28 weeks and within 72 hours of delivery.

Rhophylac®: I.M., I.V.: 300 mcg

WinRho® SDF: I.M., I.V.: Before 34 weeks gestation: 300 mcg; administer immediately, repeat dose every 12 weeks during pregnancy; After 34 weeks gestation: 120 mcg, administered immediately or within 72 hours

Abdominal trauma, manipulation:

BayRho-D®, HyperRHO™ S/D Full Dose, RhoGAM®: I.M.: 2nd or 3rd trimester: 300 mcg. If dose is given between 13-18 weeks, repeat at 26-28 weeks and within 72 hours of delivery

WinRho® SDF: I.M./I.V.: After 34 weeks gestation: 120 mcg; administer immediately or within 72 hours

Transfusion:

Children and Adults: WinRho® SDF: Administer within 72 hours after exposure of incompatible blood transfusions or massive fetal hemorrhage.

I.V.: Calculate dose as follows; administer 600 mcg every 8 hours until the total dose is administered:

Exposure to $Rh_o(D)$ positive whole blood: 9 mcg/mL blood

Exposure to $Rh_o(D)$ positive red blood cells: 18 mcg/mL cells

I.M.: Calculate dose as follows; administer 1200 mcg every 12 hours until the total dose is administered:

Exposure to $Rh_o(D)$ positive whole blood: 12 mcg/mL blood

Exposure to $Rh_o(D)$ positive red blood cells: 24 mcg/mL cells

Adults:

BayRho-D®, HyperRHO™ S/D Full Dose, RhoGAM®: I.M.: Multiply the volume of Rh positive whole blood administered by the hematocrit of the donor unit to equal the volume of RBCs transfused. The volume of RBCs is then divided by 15 mL, providing the number of 300 mcg doses (vials/syringes) to administer. If the dose calculated results in a fraction, round up to the next higher whole 300 mcg dose (vial/syringe).

Rhophylac®: I.M., I.V.: 20 mcg/2 mL transfused blood or 20 mcg/mL erythrocyte concentrate

Dosage Forms [DSC] = Discontinued product

Injection, solution [preservative free]:

BayRho-D® Full-Dose [DSC], HyperRHO™ S/D Full Dose, RhoGAM®: 300 mcg [for I.M. use only]

BayRho-D® Mini-Dose [DSC], HyperRHO™ S/D Mini Dose, MICRhoGAM®: 50 mcg [for I.M. use only]

Rhophylac®: 300 mcg/2 mL (2 mL) [1500 int. units; for I.M. or I.V. use]

WinRho® SDF:

120 mcg/~0.5 mL (~0.5 mL) [600 int. units; contains maltose and polysorbate 80; for I.M. or I.V. use]

300 mcg/~1.3 mL (~1.3 mL) [1500 int. units; contains maltose and polysorbate 80; for I.M. or I.V. use]

500 mcg/~2.2 mL (~2.2 mL) [2500 int. units; contains maltose and polysorbate 80; for I.M. or I.V. use]

1000 mcg/~4.4 mL (~4.4 mL) [5000 int. units; contains maltose and polysorbate 80; for I.M. or I.V. use]

3000 mcg/~13 mL (~13 mL) [15,000 int. units; contains maltose and polysorbate 80; for I.M. or I.V. use]

Injection, powder for reconstitution [preservative free] (WinRho® SDF):

120 mcg [600 int. units; for I.M. or I.V. use] [DSC]

300 mcg [1500 int. units; for I.M. or I.V. use] [DSC]

1000 mcg [5000 int. units; for I.M. or I.V. use] [DSC]

Rhodis™ [Can] *see* ketoprofen *on page 472*

Rhodis-EC™ [Can] *see* ketoprofen *on page 472*
Rhodis SR™ [Can] *see* ketoprofen *on page 472*
RhoGAM® [US] *see* Rh_o(D) immune globulin *on page 740*
RhoIGIV *see* Rh_o(D) immune globulin *on page 740*
RhoIVIM *see* Rh_o(D) immune globulin *on page 740*
Rho®-Loperamine [Can] *see* loperamide *on page 503*
Rho®-Metformin [Can] *see* metformin *on page 535*
Rho-Nitro [Can] *see* nitroglycerin *on page 595*
Rhophylac® [US] *see* Rh_o(D) immune globulin *on page 740*
Rho®-Sotalol [Can] *see* sotalol *on page 787*
Rhotral [Can] *see* acebutolol *on page 4*
Rhotrimine® [Can] *see* trimipramine *on page 852*
Rhovane® [Can] *see* zopiclone *(Canada only) on page 890*
Rhoxal-acebutolol [Can] *see* acebutolol *on page 4*
Rhoxal-amiodarone [Can] *see* amiodarone *on page 43*
Rhoxal-anagrelide [Can] *see* anagrelide *on page 55*
Rhoxal-atenolol [Can] *see* atenolol *on page 80*
Rhoxal-ciprofloxacin [Can] *see* ciprofloxacin *on page 190*
Rhoxal-citalopram [Can] *see* citalopram *on page 194*
Rhoxal-cyclosporine [Can] *see* cyclosporine *on page 221*
Rhoxal-diltiazem CD [Can] *see* diltiazem *on page 257*
Rhoxal-diltiazem SR [Can] *see* diltiazem *on page 257*
Rhoxal-diltiazem T [Can] *see* diltiazem *on page 257*
Rhoxal-fluoxetine [Can] *see* fluoxetine *on page 357*
Rhoxal-fluvoxamine [Can] *see* fluvoxamine *on page 364*
Rhoxal-gliclazide [Can] *see* gliclazide *(Canada only) on page 384*
Rhoxal-glimepiride [Can] *see* glimepiride *on page 384*
Rhoxal-minocycline [Can] *see* minocycline *on page 558*
Rhoxal-mirtazapine [Can] *see* mirtazapine *on page 559*
Rhoxal-mirtazapine FC [Can] *see* mirtazapine *on page 559*
Rhoxal-nabumetone [Can] *see* nabumetone *on page 572*
Rhoxal-orphendrine [Can] *see* orphenadrine *on page 620*
Rhoxal-pamidronate [Can] *see* pamidronate *on page 633*
Rhoxal-paroxetine [Can] *see* paroxetine *on page 639*
Rhoxal-ranitidine [Can] *see* ranitidine *on page 732*
Rhoxal-salbutamol [Can] *see* albuterol *on page 23*
Rhoxal-Sertraline [Can] *see* sertraline *on page 769*
Rhoxal-sumatriptan [Can] *see* sumatriptan *on page 801*
Rhoxal-ticlopidine [Can] *see* ticlopidine *on page 827*
Rhoxal-topiramate [Can] *see* topiramate *on page 836*
Rhoxal-valproic [Can] *see* valproic acid and derivatives *on page 864*
Rhoxal-zopiclone [Can] *see* zopiclone *(Canada only) on page 890*
rhPTH(1-34) *see* teriparatide *on page 812*
rHuEPO-α *see* epoetin alfa *on page 298*
rhuFabV2 *see* ranibizumab *on page 732*
rHu-KGF *see* palifermin *on page 632*
Rhulicaine® ***(Discontinued)*** *see* benzocaine *on page 99*
rhuMAb-E25 *see* omalizumab *on page 615*

rhuMAb-VEGF *see* bevacizumab *on page 109*
Ribasphere™ [US] *see* ribavirin *on this page*

ribavirin (rye ba VYE rin)

Sound-Alike/Look-Alike Issues
ribavirin may be confused with riboflavin

Synonyms RTCA; tribavirin

U.S./Canadian Brand Names Copegus® [US]; Rebetol® [US]; Ribasphere™ [US]; Virazole® [US/Can]

Therapeutic Category Antiviral Agent

Use

Inhalation: Treatment of patients with respiratory syncytial virus (RSV) infections; specially indicated for treatment of severe lower respiratory tract RSV infections in patients with an underlying compromising condition (prematurity, bronchopulmonary dysplasia and other chronic lung conditions, congenital heart disease, immunodeficiency, immunosuppression), and recent transplant recipients

Oral capsule:

In combination with interferon alfa-2b (Intron® A) injection for the treatment of chronic hepatitis C in patients with compensated liver disease who have relapsed after alpha interferon therapy or were previously untreated with alpha interferons

In combination with peginterferon alfa-2b (PEG-Intron®) injection for the treatment of chronic hepatitis C in patients with compensated liver disease who were previously untreated with alpha interferons

Oral solution: In combination with interferon alfa 2b (Intron® A) injection for the treatment of chronic hepatitis C in patients ≥3 years of age with compensated liver disease who were previously untreated with alpha interferons or patients ≥18 years of age who have relapsed after alpha interferon therapy

Oral tablet: In combination with peginterferon alfa-2a (Pegasys®) injection for the treatment of chronic hepatitis C in patients with compensated liver disease who were previously untreated with alpha interferons (includes patients with histological evidence of cirrhosis [Child-Pugh class A] and patients with clinically-stable HIV disease)

Usual Dosage

Aerosol inhalation: Infants and children: Use with Viratek® small particle aerosol generator (SPAG-2) at a concentration of 20 mg/mL (6 g reconstituted with 300 mL of sterile water without preservatives). Continuous aerosol administration: 12-18 hours/day for 3 days, up to 7 days in length

Oral capsule or solution: Children ≥3 years: Chronic hepatitis C (in combination with interferon alfa-2b):

Rebetol®: Oral: **Note:** Oral solution should be used in children 3-5 years of age, children ≤25 kg, or those unable to swallow capsules.

Capsule/solution: 15 mg/kg/day in 2 divided doses (morning and evening)

Capsule dosing recommendations:

25-36 kg: 400 mg/day (200 mg morning and evening)
37-49 kg: 600 mg/day (200 mg in the morning and two 200 mg capsules in the evening)
50-61 kg: 800 mg/day (two 200 mg capsules morning and evening)
>61 kg: Refer to Adults dosing

Note: Duration of therapy is 48 weeks in pediatric patients with genotype 1 and 24 weeks in patients with genotype 2,3. Discontinue treatment in any patient if HCV-RNA is not below the limit of detection of the assay after 24 weeks of therapy.

Note: Also refer to interferon alfa-2b/ribavirin combination pack monograph.

Oral capsule (Rebetol®, Ribasphere™): Adults:

Chronic hepatitis C (in combination with interferon alfa-2b):

≤75 kg: 400 mg in the morning, then 600 mg in the evening
>75 kg: 600 mg in the morning, then 600 mg in the evening

Note: If HCV-RNA is undetectable at 24 weeks, duration of therapy is 48 weeks. In patients who relapse following interferon therapy, duration of dual therapy is 24 weeks.

Note: Also refer to interferon alfa-2b/ribavirin combination pack monograph.

Chronic hepatitis C (in combination with peginterferon alfa-2b): 400 mg twice daily; duration of therapy is 1 year; after 24 weeks of treatment, if serum HCV-RNA is not below the limit of detection of the assay, consider discontinuation.

Oral tablet (Copegus®, in combination with peginterferon alfa-2b): Adults: Chronic hepatitis C:

Monoinfection, genotype 1,4:

<75kg: 1000 mg/day in 2 divided doses for 48 weeks
≥75kg: 1200 mg/day in 2 divided doses for 48 weeks

Monoinfection, genotype 2,3: 800 mg/day in 2 divided doses for 24 weeks

Coinfection with HIV: 800 mg/day in 2 divided doses for 48 weeks

Note: Also refer to peginterferon alfa-2a monograph.

Dosage Forms

Capsule: 200 mg

Rebetol®, Ribasphere™: 200 mg

(Continued)

ribavirin *(Continued)*

Powder for solution, inhalation [for aerosol administration]:
Virazole®: 6 g [reconstituted product provides 20 mg/mL]
Solution, oral:
Rebetol®: 40 mg/mL (100 mL) [contains sodium benzoate; bubble-gum flavor]
Tablet: 200 mg
Copegus®: 200 mg
Tablet [dose pack]:
RibaPak™: 400 mg (14s), 600 mg (14s)

ribavirin and interferon alfa-2b combination pack *see* interferon alfa-2b and ribavirin *on page 455*

ribavirin and peginterferon alfa-2b *see* peginterferon alfa-2b and ribavirin *(Canada only) on page 644*

Ribo-100 [US] *see* riboflavin *on this page*

riboflavin (RYE boe flay vin)

Sound-Alike/Look-Alike Issues
riboflavin may be confused with ribavirin
Synonyms lactoflavin; vitamin B_2; vitamin G
U.S./Canadian Brand Names Ribo-100 [US]
Therapeutic Category Vitamin, Water Soluble
Use Prevention of riboflavin deficiency and treatment of ariboflavinosis
Usual Dosage Oral:
Riboflavin deficiency:
Children: 2.5-10 mg/day in divided doses
Adults: 5-30 mg/day in divided doses
Recommended daily allowance:
Children: 0.4-1.8 mg
Adults: 1.2-1.7 mg
Dosage Forms
Tablet: 25 mg, 50 mg, 100 mg
Ribo-100: 100 mg

Rid-A-Pain Dental Drops [US-OTC] *see* benzocaine *on page 99*

Ridaura® [US/Can] *see* auranofin *on page 85*

RID® *(Discontinued)* *see* pyrethrins and piperonyl butoxide *on page 720*

RID® Maximum Strength [US-OTC] *see* pyrethrins and piperonyl butoxide *on page 720*

RID® Mousse [Can] *see* pyrethrins and piperonyl butoxide *on page 720*

Rid® Spray [US-OTC] *see* permethrin *on page 655*

rifabutin (rif a BYOO tin)

Sound-Alike/Look-Alike Issues
rifabutin may be confused with rifampin
Synonyms ansamycin
U.S./Canadian Brand Names Mycobutin® [US/Can]
Therapeutic Category Antibiotic, Miscellaneous
Use Prevention of disseminated *Mycobacterium avium* complex (MAC) in patients with advanced HIV infection
Usual Dosage Oral:
Children >1 year: Prophylaxis: 5 mg/kg daily; higher dosages have been used in limited trials
Adults: Prophylaxis: 300 mg once daily (alone or in combination with azithromycin)
Dosage Forms Capsule: 150 mg

Rifadin® [US/Can] *see* rifampin *on next page*

Rifamate® [US/Can] *see* rifampin and isoniazid *on next page*

rifampicin *see* rifampin *on next page*

rifampin (rif AM pin)

Sound-Alike/Look-Alike Issues

rifampin may be confused with rifabutin, Rifamate®, rifapentine, rifaximin

Rifadin® may be confused with Ritalin®

Rimactane® may be confused with rimantadine

Synonyms rifampicin

U.S./Canadian Brand Names Rifadin® [US/Can]; Rofact™ [Can]

Therapeutic Category Antibiotic, Miscellaneous

Use Management of active tuberculosis in combination with other agents; elimination of meningococci from the nasopharynx in asymptomatic carriers

Usual Dosage Oral (I.V. infusion dose is the same as for the oral route):

Tuberculosis therapy (drug susceptible): Note: A four-drug regimen (isoniazid, rifampin, pyrazinamide, and ethambutol) is preferred for the initial, empiric treatment of TB. When the drug susceptibility results are available, the regimen should be altered as appropriate.

Infants and Children <12 years:

Daily therapy: 10-20 mg/kg/day usually as a single dose (maximum: 600 mg/day)

Twice weekly directly observed therapy (DOT): 10-20 mg/kg (maximum: 600 mg)

Adults:

Daily therapy: 10 mg/kg/day (maximum: 600 mg/day)

Twice weekly directly observed therapy (DOT): 10 mg/kg (maximum: 600 mg); 3 times/week: 10 mg/kg (maximum: 600 mg)

Latent tuberculosis infection (LTBI): As an alternative to isoniazid:

Children: 10-20 mg/kg/day (maximum: 600 mg/day) for 6 months

Adults: 10 mg/kg/day (maximum: 600 mg/day) for 4 months. **Note:** Combination with pyrazinamide should not generally be offered (*MMWR*, Aug 8, 2003).

Meningococcal meningitis prophylaxis:

Infants <1 month: 10 mg/kg/day in divided doses every 12 hours for 2 days

Infants ≥1 month and Children: 20 mg/kg/day in divided doses every 12 hours for 2 days (maximum: 600 mg/dose)

Meningitis *(Pneumococcus* or *Staphylococcus):* I.V.: Adults: 600 mg once daily

Adults: 600 mg every 12 hours for 2 days

Dosage Forms

Capsule: 150 mg, 300 mg

Injection, powder for reconstitution: 600 mg

rifampin and isoniazid (rif AM pin & eye soe NYE a zid)

Sound-Alike/Look-Alike Issues

Rifamate® may be confused with rifampin

Synonyms isoniazid and rifampin

U.S./Canadian Brand Names IsonaRif™ [US]; Rifamate® [US/Can]

Therapeutic Category Antibiotic, Miscellaneous

Use Management of active tuberculosis; see individual agents for additional information

Usual Dosage Oral: 2 capsules/day

Dosage Forms

Capsule:

IsonaRif™, Rifamate®: 300/150: Rifampin 300 mg and isoniazid 150 mg

rifampin, isoniazid, and pyrazinamide

(rif AM pin, eye soe NYE a zid, & peer a ZIN a mide)

Synonyms isoniazid, rifampin, and pyrazinamide; pyrazinamide, rifampin, and isoniazid

U.S./Canadian Brand Names Rifater® [US/Can]

Therapeutic Category Antibiotic, Miscellaneous

Use Initial phase, short-course treatment of pulmonary tuberculosis; see individual agents for additional information

Usual Dosage Adults: Oral: Patients weighing:

≤44 kg: 4 tablets

45-54 kg: 5 tablets

≥55 kg: 6 tablets

Doses should be administered in a single daily dose

Dosage Forms Tablet: Rifampin 120 mg, isoniazid 50 mg, and pyrazinamide 300 mg

rifapentine (rif a PEN teen)

Sound-Alike/Look-Alike Issues
rifapentine may be confused with rifampin

U.S./Canadian Brand Names Priftin® [US/Can]

Therapeutic Category Antitubercular Agent

Use Treatment of pulmonary tuberculosis; rifapentine must always be used in conjunction with at least one other antituberculosis drug to which the isolate is susceptible; it may also be necessary to add a third agent (either streptomycin or ethambutol) until susceptibility is known.

Usual Dosage
Children: No dosing information available
Adults: **Rifapentine should not be used alone**; initial phase should include a 3- to 4-drug regimen
Intensive phase (initial 2 months) of short-term therapy: 600 mg (four 150 mg tablets) given twice weekly (with an interval of not less than 72 hours between doses); following the intensive phase, treatment should continue with rifapentine 600 mg once weekly for 4 months in combination with INH or appropriate agent for susceptible organisms

Dosage Forms Tablet: 150 mg

Rifater® [US/Can] *see* rifampin, isoniazid, and pyrazinamide *on previous page*

rifaximin (rif AX i min)

Sound-Alike/Look-Alike Issues
rifaximin may be confused with rifampin

U.S./Canadian Brand Names Xifaxan™ [US]

Therapeutic Category Antibiotic, Miscellaneous

Use Treatment of travelers' diarrhea caused by noninvasive strains of *E. coli*

Usual Dosage Oral: Children ≥12 years and Adults: Traveler's diarrhea: 200 mg 3 times/day for 3 days

Dosage Forms Tablet: 200 mg

rIFN-A *see* interferon alfa-2a *on page 454*

rIFN beta-1a *see* interferon beta-1a *on page 457*

rIFN beta-1b *see* interferon beta-1b *on page 457*

RIG *see* rabies immune globulin (human) *on page 727*

rIL-11 *see* oprelvekin *on page 618*

Rilutek® [US/Can] *see* riluzole *on this page*

riluzole (RIL yoo zole)

Synonyms 2-amino-6-trifluoromethoxy-benzothiazole; RP-54274

U.S./Canadian Brand Names Rilutek® [US/Can]

Therapeutic Category Miscellaneous Product

Use Treatment of amyotrophic lateral sclerosis (ALS); riluzole can extend survival or time to tracheostomy

Usual Dosage Adults: Oral: 50 mg every 12 hours; no increased benefit can be expected from higher daily doses, but adverse events are increased

Dosage adjustment in smoking: Cigarette smoking is known to induce CYP1A2; patients who smoke cigarettes would be expected to eliminate riluzole faster. There is no information, however, on the effect of, or need for, dosage adjustment in these patients.

Dosage adjustment in special populations: Females and Japanese patients may possess a lower metabolic capacity to eliminate riluzole compared with male and Caucasian subjects, respectively

Dosage Forms Tablet: 50 mg

rimantadine (ri MAN ta deen)

Sound-Alike/Look-Alike Issues
rimantadine may be confused with amantadine, ranitidine, Rimactane®
Flumadine® may be confused with fludarabine, flunisolide, flutamide

Synonyms rimantadine hydrochloride

U.S./Canadian Brand Names Flumadine® [US/Can]

Therapeutic Category Antiviral Agent

Use Prophylaxis (adults and children >1 year of age) and treatment (adults) of influenza A viral infection (per manufacturer labeling; also refer to current CDC guidelines for recommendations during current flu season)

Usual Dosage Oral:
Prophylaxis:
Children 1-10 years: 5 mg/kg/day; maximum: 150 mg/day
Children >10 years and Adults: 100 mg twice daily
Treatment: Adults: 100 mg twice daily

Dosage Forms
Syrup, as hydrochloride:
Flumadine®: 50 mg/5 mL (240 mL) [raspberry flavor]
Tablet, as hydrochloride: 100 mg
Flumadine®: 100 mg

rimantadine hydrochloride *see* rimantadine *on previous page*

rimexolone (ri MEKS oh lone)

Sound-Alike/Look-Alike Issues
Vexol® may be confused with VoSol®

U.S./Canadian Brand Names Vexol® [US/Can]

Therapeutic Category Adrenal Corticosteroid

Use Treatment of inflammation after ocular surgery and the treatment of anterior uveitis

Usual Dosage Adults: Ophthalmic: Instill 1 drop in conjunctival sac 2-4 times/day up to every 4 hours; may use every 1-2 hours during first 1-2 days

Dosage Forms Suspension, ophthalmic: 1% (5 mL, 10 mL) [contains benzalkonium chloride]

Rimso®-50 [US/Can] *see* dimethyl sulfoxide *on page 260*

Rindal HD Plus [US] *see* phenylephrine, hydrocodone, and chlorpheniramine *on page 663*

Riobin® ***(Discontinued)*** *see* riboflavin *on page 744*

Riomet™ [US] *see* metformin *on page 535*

Riopan® Plus ***(Discontinued)*** *see* magaldrate and simethicone *on page 511*

Riopan® Plus Double Strength ***(Discontinued)*** *see* magaldrate and simethicone *on page 511*

Riphenidate [Can] *see* methylphenidate *on page 546*

risedronate (ris ED roe nate)

Synonyms risedronate sodium

U.S./Canadian Brand Names Actonel® [US/Can]

Therapeutic Category Bisphosphonate Derivative

Use Paget disease of the bone; treatment and prevention of glucocorticoid-induced osteoporosis; treatment and prevention of osteoporosis in postmenopausal women

Usual Dosage Oral: Adults:
Paget's disease of bone: 30 mg once daily for 2 months
Retreatment may be considered (following post-treatment observation of at least 2 months) if relapse occurs, or if treatment fails to normalize serum alkaline phosphatase. For retreatment, the dose and duration of therapy are the same as for initial treatment. No data are available on more than one course of retreatment.
Osteoporosis (postmenopausal) prevention and treatment: 5 mg once daily or 35 mg once weekly
Osteoporosis (male) treatment: 35 mg once weekly
Osteoporosis (glucocorticoid-induced) prevention and treatment: 5 mg once daily

Dosage Forms
Tablet, as sodium:
Actonel®: 5 mg, 30 mg, 35 mg

risedronate and calcium (ris ED roe nate & KAL see um)

Synonyms calcium and risedronate; risedronate sodium and calcium carbonate

U.S./Canadian Brand Names Actonel® and Calcium [US]

Therapeutic Category Bisphosphonate Derivative; Calcium Salt

Use Treatment and prevention of osteoporosis in postmenopausal women

Usual Dosage
Oral: Adults: Osteoporosis in postmenopausal females:
Risedronate: 35 mg once weekly on day 1 of 7-day treatment cycle
Calcium carbonate: 1250 mg (elemental calcium 500 mg) once daily on days 2 through 7 of 7-day treatment cycle
(Continued)

risedronate and calcium *(Continued)*

Dosage Forms Combination package [each package contains]:

Tablet (Actonel®): Risedronate 35 mg (4s)

Tablet: Calcium carbonate 1250 mg (24s) [equivalent to elemental calcium 500 mg]

risedronate sodium *see* risedronate *on previous page*

risedronate sodium and calcium carbonate *see* risedronate and calcium *on previous page*

Risperdal® [US/Can] *see* risperidone *on this page*

Risperdal® M-Tab® [US/Can] *see* risperidone *on this page*

Risperdal® Consta™ [US/Can] *see* risperidone *on this page*

risperidone (ris PER i done)

Sound-Alike/Look-Alike Issues

risperidone may be confused with reserpine

Risperdal® may be confused with lisinopril, reserpine

U.S./Canadian Brand Names Apo-Risperidone® [Can]; Risperdal® Consta™ [US/Can]; Risperdal® M-Tab® [US/Can]; Risperdal® [US/Can]

Therapeutic Category Antipsychotic Agent, Benzisoxazole

Use Treatment of schizophrenia; treatment of acute mania or mixed episodes associated with bipolar I disorder (as monotherapy or in combination with lithium or valproate)

Usual Dosage

Oral: Adults:

Schizophrenia:

Initial: 1 mg twice daily; may be increased to 2 mg/day to a target dose of 6 mg/day; usual range: 4-8 mg/day; may be given as a single daily dose once maintenance dose is achieved; daily dosages >6 mg do not appear to confer any additional benefit, and the incidence of extrapyramidal symptoms is higher than with lower doses. Further dose adjustments should be made in increments/decrements of 1-2 mg/day on a weekly basis. Dose range studied in clinical trials: 4-16 mg/day.

Maintenance: Target dose: 4 mg once daily (range 2-8 mg/day)

Bipolar mania:

Initial: 2-3 mg once daily; if needed, adjust dose by 1 mg/day in intervals ≥24 hours; dosing range: 1-6 mg/day

Maintenance: No dosing recommendation available for treatment >3 weeks duration.

I.M.: Adults: Schizophrenia (Risperdal® Consta™): 25 mg every 2 weeks; some patients may benefit from larger doses; maximum dose not to exceed 50 mg every 2 weeks. Dosage adjustments should not be made more frequently than every 4 weeks.

Note: Oral risperidone (or other antipsychotic) should be administered with the initial injection of Risperdal® Consta™ and continued for 3 weeks (then discontinued) to maintain adequate therapeutic plasma concentrations prior to main release phase of risperidone from injection site. When switching from depot administration to a short-acting formulation, administer short-acting agent in place of the next regularly-scheduled depot injection.

Dosage Forms

Injection, microspheres for reconstitution, extended release (Risperdal® Consta™): 25 mg, 37.5 mg, 50 mg [supplied in a dose-pack containing vial with active ingredient in microsphere formulation, prefilled syringe with diluent, needle-free vial access device, and safety needle]

Solution, oral: 1 mg/mL (30 mL) [contains benzoic acid]

Tablet: 0.25 mg, 0.5 mg, 1 mg, 2 mg, 3 mg, 4 mg

Tablet, orally disintegrating (Risperdal® M-Tabs™): 0.5 mg [contains phenylalanine 0.42 mg]; 1 mg [contains phenylalanine 0.28 mg]; 2 mg [contains phenylalanine 0.56 mg]; 3 mg [contains phenylalanine 0.63 mg]; 4 mg [contains phenylalanine 0.84 mg]

Ritalin® [US/Can] *see* methylphenidate *on page 546*

Ritalin® LA [US] *see* methylphenidate *on page 546*

Ritalin-SR® [US/Can] *see* methylphenidate *on page 546*

ritonavir (ri TOE na veer)

Sound-Alike/Look-Alike Issues

ritonavir may be confused with Retrovir®

Norvir® may be confused with Norvasc®

U.S./Canadian Brand Names Norvir® SEC [Can]; Norvir® [US/Can]

Therapeutic Category Antiviral Agent

Use Treatment of HIV infection; should always be used as part of a multidrug regimen (at least three antiretroviral agents); may be used as a pharmacokinetic "booster" for other protease inhibitors

Usual Dosage Treatment of HIV infection: Oral:

Children >1 month: 350-400 mg/m^2 twice daily (maximum dose: 600 mg twice daily). Initiate dose at 250 mg/m^2 twice daily; titrate dose upward every 2-3 days by 50 mg/m^2 twice daily.

Adults: 600 mg twice daily; dose escalation tends to avoid nausea that many patients experience upon initiation of full dosing. Escalate the dose as follows: 300 mg twice daily for 1 day, 400 mg twice daily for 2 days, 500 mg twice daily for 1 day, then 600 mg twice daily. Ritonavir may be better tolerated when used in combination with other antiretrovirals by initiating the drug alone and subsequently adding the second agent within 2 weeks.

Pharmacokinetic "booster" in combination with other protease inhibitors: 100-400 mg/day

Refer to individual monographs; specific dosage recommendations often require adjustment of both agents.

Note: Dosage adjustments for ritonavir when administered in combination therapy:

Amprenavir: Adjustments necessary for each agent:

Amprenavir 1200 mg with ritonavir 200 mg once daily **or**

Amprenavir 600 mg with ritonavir 100 mg twice daily

Amprenavir plus efavirenz (3-drug regimen): Amprenavir 1200 mg twice daily plus ritonavir 200 mg twice daily plus efavirenz at standard dose

Indinavir: Adjustments necessary for both agents:

Indinavir 800 mg twice daily plus ritonavir 100-200 mg twice daily **or**

Indinavir 400 mg twice daily plus ritonavir 400 mg twice daily

Nelfinavir or saquinavir: Ritonavir 400 mg twice daily

Rifabutin: Decrease rifabutin dose to 150 mg every other day

Saquinavir: Ritonavir 400 mg twice daily

Dosage Forms

Capsule: 100 mg [contains ethanol and polyoxyl 35 castor oil]

Solution: 80 mg/mL (240 mL) [contains ethanol and polyoxyl 35 castor oil; peppermint and caramel flavor]

ritonavir and lopinavir *see* lopinavir and ritonavir *on page 504*

Rituxan® [US/Can] *see* rituximab *on this page*

rituximab (ri TUK si mab)

Sound-Alike/Look-Alike Issues

Rituxan® may be confused with Remicade®

Synonyms anti-CD20 monoclonal antibody; C2B8; C2B8 monoclonal antibody; IDEC-C2B8; NSC-687451; pan-B antibody

U.S./Canadian Brand Names Rituxan® [US/Can]

Therapeutic Category Antineoplastic Agent

Use Treatment of relapsed or refractory CD20 positive, B-cell non-Hodgkin lymphoma

Usual Dosage Note: Pretreatment with acetaminophen and diphenhydramine is recommended.

Adults: I.V. infusion (refer to individual protocols):

NHL: 375 mg/m^2 once weekly for 4 or 8 doses

or

100 mg/m^2 I.V. day 1, then 375 mg/m^2 3 times/week for 11 doses has also been reported (cycles may be repeated in patients with refractory or relapsed disease)

Retreatment following disease progression: 375 mg/m^2 once weekly for 4 doses

Diffuse large B-cell NHL: 375 mg/m^2 given on day 1 of each chemotherapy cycle for up to 8 doses; chemotherapy may be CHOP or other anthracycline-based regimen

Rheumatoid arthritis: 1000 mg on days 1 and 15 in combination with methotrexate; premedication with a corticosteroid (eg, methylprednisolone 100 mg I.V.) prior to each rituximab dose is recommended. In clinical trials, patients received oral corticosteroids on a tapering schedule from baseline through day 16.

Combination therapy with ibritumomab: 250 mg/m^2 I.V. day 1; repeat in 7-9 days with ibritumomab (also see ibritumomab monograph)

Dosage Forms Injection, solution [preservative free]: 10 mg/mL (10 mL, 50 mL)

Riva-Alendronate [Can] *see* alendronate *on page 27*

Riva-Atenolol [Can] *see* atenolol *on page 80*

Riva-Cloxacillin [Can] *see* cloxacillin *on page 206*

Riva-Diclofenac [Can] *see* diclofenac *on page 250*

Riva-Diclofenac-K [Can] *see* diclofenac *on page 250*

Riva-Dicyclomine [Can] *see* dicyclomine *on page 251*

Riva-Famotidine [Can] *see* famotidine *on page 335*

Riva-Fluconazole [Can] *see* fluconazole *on page 349*

Riva-Loperamine [Can] *see* loperamide *on page 503*

Riva-Lorazepam [Can] *see* lorazepam *on page 506*

Riva-Lovastatin [Can] *see* lovastatin *on page 508*

Riva-Mirtazapine [Can] *see* mirtazapine *on page 559*

Riva-Naproxen [Can] *see* naproxen *on page 578*

Rivanase AQ [Can] *see* beclomethasone *on page 95*

Riva-Norfloxacin [Can] *see* norfloxacin *on page 599*

Riva-Oxazepam [Can] *see* oxazepam *on page 623*

Riva-Pravastatin [Can] *see* pravastatin *on page 692*

Riva-Rosinopril [Can] *see* fosinopril *on page 369*

Riva-Simvastatin [Can] *see* simvastatin *on page 773*

Rivasol [Can] *see* zinc sulfate *on page 888*

Riva-Sotalol [Can] *see* sotalol *on page 787*

rivastigmine (ri va STIG meen)

Synonyms ENA 713; rivastigmine tartrate; SDZ ENA 713

U.S./Canadian Brand Names Exelon® [US/Can]

Therapeutic Category Acetylcholinesterase Inhibitor; Cholinergic Agent

Use Mild to moderate dementia from Alzheimer disease

Usual Dosage Note: Exelon® oral solution and capsules are bioequivalent.

Adults: Oral:

Mild-to-moderate Alzheimer's dementia: Initial: 1.5 mg twice daily; may increase by 3 mg/day (1.5 mg/dose) every 2 weeks based on tolerability (maximum recommended dose: 6 mg twice daily)

Note: If GI adverse events occur, discontinue treatment for several doses then restart at the same or next lower dosage level; antiemetics have been used to control GI symptoms. If treatment is interrupted for longer than several days, restart the treatment at the lowest dose and titrate as previously described.

Mild-to-moderate Parkinson-related dementia: Initial: 1.5 mg twice daily; may increase by 3 mg/day (1.5 mg/dose) every 4 weeks based on tolerability (maximum recommended dose: 6 mg twice daily)

Dosage Forms

Capsule:

Exelon®: 1.5 mg, 3 mg, 4.5 mg, 6 mg

Solution, oral:

Exelon®: 2 mg/mL (120 mL) [contains sodium benzoate]

rivastigmine tartrate *see* rivastigmine *on this page*

Riva-Sumatriptan [Can] *see* sumatriptan *on page 801*

Riva-Verapamil SR [Can] *see* verapamil *on page 870*

Riva-Zide [Can] *see* hydrochlorothiazide and triamterene *on page 420*

Riva-Zopiclone [Can] *see* zopiclone *(Canada only) on page 890*

Rivotril® [Can] *see* clonazepam *on page 203*

rizatriptan (rye za TRIP tan)

Synonyms MK462

U.S./Canadian Brand Names Maxalt RPD™ [Can]; Maxalt-MLT® [US]; Maxalt® [US/Can]

Therapeutic Category Antimigraine Agent; Serotonin Agonist

Use Acute treatment of migraine with or without aura

Usual Dosage Note: In patients with risk factors for coronary artery disease, following adequate evaluation to establish the absence of coronary artery disease, the initial dose should be administered in a setting where response may be evaluated (physician's office or similarly staffed setting). ECG monitoring may be considered.

Oral: 5-10 mg, repeat after 2 hours if significant relief is not attained; maximum: 30 mg in a 24-hour period (use 5 mg dose in patients receiving propranolol with a maximum of 15 mg in 24 hours)

Note: For orally-disintegrating tablets (Maxalt-MLT®): Patient should be instructed to place tablet on tongue and allow to dissolve. Dissolved tablet will be swallowed with saliva.

Dosage Forms

Tablet, as benzoate (Maxalt®): 5 mg, 10 mg

Tablet, orally disintegrating, as benzoate (Maxalt-MLT®): 5 mg [contains phenylalanine 1.05 mg/tablet; peppermint flavor]; 10 mg [contains phenylalanine 2.1 mg/tablet; peppermint flavor]

rLFN-α2 *see* interferon alfa-2b *on page 454*

RMS® [US] *see* morphine sulfate *on page 565*

Ro 5488 *see* tretinoin (oral) *on page 844*

Robafen® AC [US] *see* guaifenesin and codeine *on page 393*

Robafen® CF *(Discontinued)*

Robafen DM [US-OTC] *see* guaifenesin and dextromethorphan *on page 394*

Robaxin® [US/Can] *see* methocarbamol *on page 539*

Robidrine® [Can] *see* pseudoephedrine *on page 712*

Robinul® [US] *see* glycopyrrolate *on page 389*

Robinul® Forte [US] *see* glycopyrrolate *on page 389*

Robitussin® [US-OTC/Can] *see* guaifenesin *on page 392*

Robitussin® A-C *(Discontinued)* *see* guaifenesin and codeine *on page 393*

Robitussin® Childrens Cough & Cold [Can] *see* pseudoephedrine and dextromethorphan *on page 714*

Robitussin® Cough and Cold® [US-OTC/Can] *see* guaifenesin, pseudoephedrine, and dextromethorphan *on page 401*

Robitussin® Cough and Cold CF [US-OTC] *see* guaifenesin, pseudoephedrine, and dextromethorphan *on page 401*

Robitussin® Cough and Cold Infant [US-OTC] *see* guaifenesin, pseudoephedrine, and dextromethorphan *on page 401*

Robitussin® Cough and Congestion [US-OTC] *see* guaifenesin and dextromethorphan *on page 394*

Robitussin® CoughGels™ [US-OTC] *see* dextromethorphan *on page 245*

Robitussin®-DAC *(Discontinued)* *see* guaifenesin, pseudoephedrine, and codeine *on page 401*

Robitussin® DM [US-OTC/Can] *see* guaifenesin and dextromethorphan *on page 394*

Robitussin® DM Infant [US-OTC] *see* guaifenesin and dextromethorphan *on page 394*

Robitussin® Honey Cough [US-OTC] *see* dextromethorphan *on page 245*

Robitussin® Maximum Strength Cough [US-OTC] *see* dextromethorphan *on page 245*

Robitussin® Maximum Strength Cough & Cold [US-OTC] *see* pseudoephedrine and dextromethorphan *on page 714*

Robitussin-PE® [US-OTC] *see* guaifenesin and pseudoephedrine *on page 398*

Robitussin® Pediatric Cough [US-OTC] *see* dextromethorphan *on page 245*

Robitussin® Pediatric Cough & Cold [US-OTC] *see* pseudoephedrine and dextromethorphan *on page 714*

Robitussin® Pediatric Night Relief [US-OTC] *see* chlorpheniramine, pseudoephedrine, and dextromethorphan *on page 182*

Robitussin® Severe Congestion [US-OTC] *see* guaifenesin and pseudoephedrine *on page 398*

Robitussin® Sugar Free Cough [US-OTC] *see* guaifenesin and dextromethorphan *on page 394*

Rocaltrol® [US/Can] *see* calcitriol *on page 134*

Rocephin® [US/Can] *see* ceftriaxone *on page 162*

rocuronium (roe kyoor OH nee um)

Sound-Alike/Look-Alike Issues

Zemuron® may be confused with Remeron®

(Continued)

rocuronium *(Continued)*

Synonyms ORG 946; rocuronium bromide

U.S./Canadian Brand Names Zemuron® [US/Can]

Therapeutic Category Skeletal Muscle Relaxant

Use Adjunct to general anesthesia to facilitate both rapid sequence and routine endotracheal intubation and to relax skeletal muscles during surgery; to facilitate mechanical ventilation in ICU patients; does not relieve pain or produce sedation

Usual Dosage Administer I.V.; dose to effect; doses will vary due to interpatient variability; use ideal body weight for obese patients

Children:

Initial: 0.6 mg/kg under halothane anesthesia produce excellent to good intubating conditions within 1 minute and will provide a median time of 41 minutes of clinical relaxation in children 3 months to 1 year of age, and 27 minutes in children 1-12 years

Maintenance: 0.075-0.125 mg/kg administered upon return of T_1 to 25% of control provides clinical relaxation for 7-10 minutes

Adults:

Tracheal intubation: I.V.:

Initial: 0.6 mg/kg is expected to provide approximately 31 minutes of clinical relaxation under opioid/nitrous oxide/oxygen anesthesia with neuromuscular block sufficient for intubation attained in 1-2 minutes; lower doses (0.45 mg/kg) may be used to provide 22 minutes of clinical relaxation with median time to neuromuscular block of 1-3 minutes; maximum blockade is achieved in <4 minutes

Maximum: 0.9-1.2 mg/kg may be given during surgery under opioid/nitrous oxide/oxygen anesthesia without adverse cardiovascular effects and is expected to provide 58-67 minutes of clinical relaxation; neuromuscular blockade sufficient for intubation is achieved in <2 minutes with maximum blockade in <3 minutes

Maintenance: 0.1, 0.15, and 0.2 mg/kg administered at 25% recovery of control T_1 (defined as 3 twitches of train-of-four) provides a median of 12, 17, and 24 minutes of clinical duration under anesthesia

Rapid sequence intubation: 0.6-1.2 mg/kg in appropriately premedicated and anesthetized patients with excellent or good intubating conditions within 2 minutes

Continuous infusion: Initial: 0.01-0.012 mg/kg/minute only after early evidence of spontaneous recovery of neuromuscular function is evident; infusion rates have ranged from 4-16 mcg/kg/minute

ICU: 10 mcg/kg/minute; adjust dose to maintain appropriate degree of neuromuscular blockade (eg, 1 or 2 twitches on train-of-four)

Dosage Forms Injection, solution, as bromide: 10 mg/mL (5 mL, 10 mL)

rocuronium bromide *see* rocuronium *on previous page*

Rofact™ [Can] *see* rifampin *on page 745*

Roferon-A® [US/Can] *see* interferon alfa-2a *on page 454*

Rogaine® [Can] *see* minoxidil *on page 559*

Rogaine® Extra Strength for Men [US-OTC] *see* minoxidil *on page 559*

Rogaine® for Men [US-OTC] *see* minoxidil *on page 559*

Rogaine® for Women [US-OTC] *see* minoxidil *on page 559*

Rogitine® [Can] *see* phentolamine *on page 660*

Rolaids® [US-OTC] *see* calcium carbonate and magnesium hydroxide *on page 136*

Rolaids® Extra Strength [US-OTC] *see* calcium carbonate and magnesium hydroxide *on page 136*

Rolaids® Softchews [US-OTC] *see* calcium carbonate *on page 135*

Rolatuss® Plain Liquid *(Discontinued)* *see* chlorpheniramine and phenylephrine *on page 176*

Romazicon® [US/Can] *see* flumazenil *on page 351*

Romilar® AC [US] *see* guaifenesin and codeine *on page 393*

Romycin® [US] *see* erythromycin *on page 303*

Rondec® *[reformulation]* [US] *see* chlorpheniramine and phenylephrine *on page 176*

Rondec®-DM *[reformulation]* [US] *see* chlorpheniramine, phenylephrine, and dextromethorphan *on page 179*

Rondec®-DM Drops *(Discontinued)* *see* carbinoxamine, pseudoephedrine, and dextromethorphan *on page 150*

Rondec®-DM Syrup *(Discontinued)* *see* brompheniramine, pseudoephedrine, and dextromethorphan *on page 120*

Rondec® Drops *(Discontinued)* *see* carbinoxamine and pseudoephedrine *on page 149*

Rondec® Syrup *(Discontinued)* *see* brompheniramine and pseudoephedrine *on page 118*

Rondec® Tablets [US] *see* carbinoxamine and pseudoephedrine *on page 149*

Rondec-TR® [US] *see* carbinoxamine and pseudoephedrine *on page 149*

Rondomycin® Capsule *(Discontinued)*

ropinirole (roe PIN i role)

Sound-Alike/Look-Alike Issues
ropinirole may be confused with ropivacaine

Synonyms ropinirole hydrochloride

U.S./Canadian Brand Names Requip® [US/Can]

Therapeutic Category Anti-Parkinson Agent

Use Treatment of idiopathic Parkinson disease; in patients with early Parkinson disease who were not receiving concomitant levodopa therapy as well as in patients with advanced disease on concomitant levodopa; treatment of moderate-to-severe primary restless legs syndrome (RLS)

Usual Dosage Oral: Adults:

Parkinson disease: The dosage should be increased to achieve a maximum therapeutic effect, balanced against the principal side effects of nausea, dizziness, somnolence and dyskinesia. Recommended starting dose is 0.25 mg 3 times/day; based on individual patient response, the dosage should be titrated with weekly increments as described below:

- Week 1: 0.25 mg 3 times/day; total daily dose: 0.75 mg
- Week 2: 0.5 mg 3 times/day; total daily dose: 1.5 mg
- Week 3: 0.75 mg 3 times/day; total daily dose: 2.25 mg
- Week 4: 1 mg 3 times/day; total daily dose: 3 mg

Note: After week 4, if necessary, daily dosage may be increased by 1.5 mg per day on a weekly basis up to a dose of 9 mg/day, and then by up to 3 mg/day weekly to a total of 24 mg/day

Parkinson disease discontinuation taper: Ropinirole should be gradually tapered over 7 days as follows: reduce frequency of administration from 3 times daily to twice daily for 4 days, then reduce to once daily for remaining 3 days.

Restless Legs Syndrome: Initial: 0.25 mg once daily 1-3 hours before bedtime. Dose may be increased after 2 days to 0.5 mg daily, and after 7 days to 1 mg daily. Dose may be further titrated upward in 0.5 mg increments every week until reaching a daily dose of 3 mg during week 6. If symptoms persist or reappear, the daily dose may be increased to a maximum of 4 mg beginning week 7.

Note: Doses up to 4 mg per day may be discontinued without tapering.

Dosage Forms

Combination package:
Requip® [starter kit; contents per each administration card]: Tablet: 0.25 mg (2s), 0.5 mg (5s), 1 mg (7s)

Tablet:
Requip®: 0.25 mg, 0.5 mg, 1 mg, 2 mg, 3 mg, 4 mg, 5 mg

ropinirole hydrochloride *see* ropinirole *on this page*

ropivacaine (roe PIV a kane)

Sound-Alike/Look-Alike Issues
ropivacaine may be confused with bupivacaine, ropinirole

Synonyms ropivacaine hydrochloride

U.S./Canadian Brand Names Naropin® [US/Can]

Therapeutic Category Local Anesthetic

Use Local anesthetic for use in surgery, postoperative pain management, and obstetrical procedures when local or regional anesthesia is needed

Usual Dosage Dose varies with procedure, onset and depth of anesthesia desired, vascularity of tissues, duration of anesthesia, and condition of patient: Adults:

Surgical anesthesia:
Lumbar epidural: 15-30 mL of 0.5% to 1% solution
Lumbar epidural block for cesarean section:
20-30 mL dose of 0.5% solution
15-20 mL dose of 0.75% solution
Thoracic epidural block: 5-15 mL dose of 0.5% to 0.75% solution
Major nerve block:
35-50 mL dose of 0.5% solution (175-250 mg)
10-40 mL dose of 0.75% solution (75-300 mg)

(Continued)

ropivacaine *(Continued)*

Field block: 1-40 mL dose of 0.5% solution (5-200 mg)

Labor pain management: Lumbar epidural: Initial: 10-20 mL 0.2% solution; continuous infusion dose: 6-14 mL/hour of 0.2% solution with incremental injections of 10-15 mL/hour of 0.2% solution

Postoperative pain management:

Lumbar or thoracic epidural: Continuous infusion dose: 6-14 mL/hour of 0.2% solution

Infiltration/minor nerve block:

1-100 mL dose of 0.2% solution

1-40 mL dose of 0.5% solution

Dosage Forms

Infusion, as hydrochloride:

Naropin®: 2 mg/mL (100 mL, 200 mL)

Injection, solution, as hydrochloride [preservative free]:

Naropin®: 2 mg/mL (10 mL, 20 mL); 5 mg/mL (20 mL, 30 mL); 7.5 mg/mL (20 mL); 10 mg/mL (10 mL, 20 mL)

ropivacaine hydrochloride *see* ropivacaine *on previous page*

Rosac® [US] *see* sulfur and sulfacetamide *on page 800*

Rosanil® [US] *see* sulfur and sulfacetamide *on page 800*

rosiglitazone (roh si GLI ta zone)

Sound-Alike/Look-Alike Issues

Avandia® may be confused with Avalide®, Coumadin®, Prandin®

U.S./Canadian Brand Names Avandia® [US/Can]

Therapeutic Category Hypoglycemic Agent, Oral; Thiazolidinedione Derivative

Use Type 2 diabetes mellitus (noninsulin dependent, NIDDM):

Monotherapy: Improve glycemic control as an adjunct to diet and exercise

Combination therapy: In combination with a sulfonylurea, metformin, or insulin, or sulfonylurea plus metformin when diet, exercise, and a single agent do not result in adequate glycemic control

Usual Dosage Oral: Adults: **Note:** All patients should be initiated at the lowest recommended dose.

Monotherapy: Initial: 4 mg daily as a single daily dose or in divided doses twice daily. If response is inadequate after 8-12 weeks of treatment, the dosage may be increased to 8 mg daily as a single daily dose or in divided doses twice daily. In clinical trials, the 4 mg twice-daily regimen resulted in the greatest reduction in fasting plasma glucose and Hb A_{1c}.

Combination therapy: When adding rosiglitazone to existing therapy, continue current dose(s) of previous agents:

With sulfonylureas or metformin (or sulfonylurea plus metformin): Initial: 4 mg daily as a single daily dose or in divided doses twice daily. If response is inadequate after 8-12 weeks of treatment, the dosage may be increased to 8 mg daily as a single daily dose or in divided doses twice daily. Reduce dose of sulfonylurea if hypoglycemia occurs. It is unlikely that the dose of metformin will need to be reduced to hypoglycemia.

With insulin: Initial: 4 mg daily as a single daily dose or in divided doses twice daily. Dose of insulin should be reduced by 10% to 25% if the patient reports hypoglycemia or if the plasma glucose falls to <100 mg/dL. Doses of rosiglitazone >4 mg/day are not indicated in combination with insulin.

Dosage Forms Tablet: 2 mg, 4 mg, 8 mg

rosiglitazone and metformin (roh si GLI ta zone & met FOR min)

Synonyms metformin and rosiglitazone; metformin hydrochloride and rosiglitazone maleate; rosiglitazone maleate and metformin hydrochloride

U.S./Canadian Brand Names Avandamet™ [US/Can]

Therapeutic Category Antidiabetic Agent (Biguanide); Antidiabetic Agent (Thiazolidinedione)

Use Management of type 2 diabetes mellitus (noninsulin-dependent, NIDDM) in patients who are already treated with the combination of rosiglitazone and metformin, or who are not adequately controlled on metformin alone. Used as an adjunct to diet and exercise to lower the blood glucose when hyperglycemia cannot be controlled satisfactorily by diet and exercise alone

Usual Dosage Oral:

Adults: Type 2 diabetes mellitus: Daily dose should be divided and given with meals:

First-line therapy (drug-naive patients): Initial: Rosiglitazone 2 mg and metformin 500 mg once or twice daily; may increase by 2 mg/500 mg per day after 4 weeks to a maximum of 8 mg/2000 mg per day.

Second-line therapy:

Patients inadequately controlled on **metformin alone**: Initial dose: Rosiglitazone 4 mg/day plus current dose of metformin

Patients inadequately controlled on **rosiglitazone alone**: Initial dose: Metformin 1000 mg/day plus current dose of rosiglitazone

Note: When switching from combination rosiglitazone and metformin as separate tablets: Use current dose

Dose adjustment: Doses may be increased as increments of rosiglitazone 4 mg and/or metformin 500 mg, up to the maximum dose; doses should be titrated gradually.

After a change in the metformin dosage, titration can be done after 1-2 weeks

After a change in the rosiglitazone dosage, titration can be done after 8-12 weeks

Maximum dose: Rosiglitazone 8 mg/metformin 2000 mg daily

Dosage Forms

Tablet:

Avandamet®: 1/500: Rosiglitazone 1 mg and metformin hydrochloride 500 mg

Avandamet®: 2/500: Rosiglitazone 2 mg and metformin hydrochloride 500 mg

Avandamet®: 4/500: Rosiglitazone 4 mg and metformin hydrochloride 500 mg

Avandamet®: 2/1000: Rosiglitazone 2 mg and metformin hydrochloride 1000 mg

Avandamet®: 4/1000: Rosiglitazone 4 mg and metformin hydrochloride 1000 mg

rosiglitazone maleate and metformin hydrochloride *see* rosiglitazone and metformin *on previous page*

Rosula® [US] *see* sulfur and sulfacetamide *on page 800*

rosuvastatin (roe soo va STAT in)

Synonyms rosuvastatin calcium

U.S./Canadian Brand Names Crestor® [US/Can]

Therapeutic Category Antilipemic Agent, HMG-CoA Reductase Inhibitor

Use Used with dietary therapy for hyperlipidemias to reduce elevations in total cholesterol (TC), LDL-C, apolipoprotein B, and triglycerides (TG) in patients with primary hypercholesterolemia (elevations of 1 or more components are present in Fredrickson type IIa, IIb, and IV hyperlipidemias); treatment of homozygous familial hypercholesterolemia (FH)

Usual Dosage Adults: Oral:

Heterozygous familial and nonfamilial hypercholesterolemia; mixed dyslipidemia:

Initial dose:

General dosing: 10 mg once daily (20 mg in patients with severe hypercholesterolemia)

Conservative dosing: Patients requiring less aggressive treatment or predisposed to myopathy (including patients of Asian descent): 5 mg once daily

Titration: After 2 weeks, may be increased by 5-10 mg once daily; dosing range: 5-40 mg/day (maximum dose: 40 mg once daily)

Note: The 40 mg dose should be reserved for patients who have not achieved goal cholesterol levels on a dose of 20 mg/day, including patients switched from another HMG-CoA reductase inhibitor.

Homozygous FH: Initial: 20 mg once daily (maximum dose: 40 mg/day)

Dosage adjustment with concomitant medications:

Cyclosporine: Rosuvastatin dose should not exceed 5 mg/day

Gemfibrozil: Rosuvastatin dose should not exceed 10 mg/day

Dosage adjustment for persistent, unexplained proteinuria while on 40 mg/day: Reduce dose and evaluate causes

Dosage Forms Tablet, as calcium: 5 mg, 10 mg, 20 mg, 40 mg

rosuvastatin calcium *see* rosuvastatin *on this page*

RotaShield® ***(Discontinued)***

RotaTeq® [US] *see* rotavirus vaccine *on this page*

rotavirus vaccine (ROE ta vye rus vak SEEN)

Synonyms pentavalent human-bovine reassortant rotavirus vaccine; rotavirus vaccine, pentavalent

U.S./Canadian Brand Names RotaTeq® [US]

Therapeutic Category Vaccine

Use Prevention of rotavirus gastroenteritis in infants and children

Usual Dosage Oral: Children 6-32 weeks: Three 2 mL doses, the first given at 6-12 weeks of age, followed by subsequent doses at 4- to 10-week intervals. Routine administration of the first dose at >12 weeks of age is not recommended (insufficient data). Administer all doses by 32 weeks of age. Infants who have had rotavirus gastroenteritis before getting the full course of vaccine should still initiate or complete the 3-dose schedule; initial infection provides only partial immunity.

(Continued)

rotavirus vaccine *(Continued)*

Dosage Forms

Suspension, oral [preservative free]:

RotaTeq®: G1 ≥2.2 10^6 infectious units, G2 ≥2.8 10^6 infectious units, G3 ≥2.2 10^6 infectious units, G4 ≥2.0 10^6 infectious units, and P1 [8] ≥2.3 10^6 infectious units (2 mL) [bovine and human derived; available in a prefilled, ready-to-use dosing tube]

rotavirus vaccine, pentavalent *see* rotavirus vaccine *on previous page*

Rowasa® [US/Can] *see* mesalamine *on page 533*

Roxanol™ [US] *see* morphine sulfate *on page 565*

Roxanol 100™ [US] *see* morphine sulfate *on page 565*

Roxanol SR™ Oral *(Discontinued)* *see* morphine sulfate *on page 565*

Roxanol™-T *(Discontinued)* *see* morphine sulfate *on page 565*

Roxicet™ [US] *see* oxycodone and acetaminophen *on page 627*

Roxicet™ 5/500 [US] *see* oxycodone and acetaminophen *on page 627*

Roxicodone® [US] *see* oxycodone *on page 626*

Roxiprin® *(Discontinued)* *see* oxycodone and aspirin *on page 628*

Roychlor® [Can] *see* potassium chloride *on page 684*

Rozerem™ [US] *see* ramelteon *on page 731*

RP-6976 *see* docetaxel *on page 269*

RP-54274 *see* riluzole *on page 746*

RP-59500 *see* quinupristin and dalfopristin *on page 727*

r-PA *see* reteplase *on page 739*

rPDGF-BB *see* becaplermin *on page 95*

RS-25259 *see* palonosetron *on page 632*

RS-25259-197 *see* palonosetron *on page 632*

R-Tanna [US] *see* chlorpheniramine and phenylephrine *on page 176*

RTCA *see* ribavirin *on page 743*

RU 0211 *see* lubiprostone *on page 509*

RU-486 *see* mifepristone *on page 556*

RU-23908 *see* nilutamide *on page 593*

RU-38486 *see* mifepristone *on page 556*

rubella, measles and mumps vaccines, combined *see* measles, mumps, and rubella vaccines, combined *on page 520*

rubella, varicella, measles, and mumps vaccine *see* measles, mumps, rubella, and varicella virus vaccine *on page 521*

rubella virus vaccine (live) (rue BEL a VYE rus vak SEEN, live)

Sound-Alike/Look-Alike Issues

Meruvax® II may be confused with Attenuvax®

Synonyms German measles vaccine

U.S./Canadian Brand Names Meruvax® II [US]

Therapeutic Category Vaccine, Live Virus

Use Selective active immunization against rubella; vaccination is routinely recommended for persons from 12 months of age to puberty. All adults, both male and female, lacking documentation of live vaccine on or after first birthday, or laboratory evidence of immunity (particularly women of childbearing age and young adults who work in or congregate in hospitals, colleges, and on military bases) should be vaccinated. Susceptible travelers should be vaccinated.

Note: Trivalent measles - mumps - rubella (MMR) vaccine is the preferred immunizing agent for most children and many adults.

Usual Dosage Children ≥12 months and Adults: SubQ: 0.5 mL in outer aspect of upper arm; children vaccinated before 12 months of age should be revaccinated. Recommended age for primary immunization is 12-15 months; revaccination with MMR-II is recommended prior to elementary school.

Dosage Forms Injection, powder for reconstitution [single dose]: 1000 $TCID_{50}$ (Wistar RA 27/3 Strain) [contains gelatin, human albumin, and neomycin]

rubeola vaccine *see* measles virus vaccine (live) *on page 521*

Rubex® [US] *see* doxorubicin *on page 277*

rubidomycin hydrochloride *see* daunorubicin hydrochloride *on page 232*

Rubramin-PC® *(Discontinued)* *see* cyanocobalamin *on page 219*

Rulox [US-OTC] *see* aluminum hydroxide and magnesium hydroxide *on page 36*

Rulox No. 1 *(Discontinued)* *see* aluminum hydroxide and magnesium hydroxide *on page 36*

Rum-K® [US] *see* potassium chloride *on page 684*

Ru-Tuss DM [US] *see* guaifenesin, pseudoephedrine, and dextromethorphan *on page 401*

Ru-Tuss® Liquid *(Discontinued)* *see* chlorpheniramine and phenylephrine *on page 176*

Ru-Vert-M® *(Discontinued)* *see* meclizine *on page 522*

Rylosol [Can] *see* sotalol *on page 787*

Rymed® *(Discontinued)* *see* guaifenesin and pseudoephedrine *on page 398*

Rymed-TR® *(Discontinued)*

Ryna-12™ [US] *see* phenylephrine and pyrilamine *on page 662*

Ryna-12 S™ [US] *see* phenylephrine and pyrilamine *on page 662*

Ryna-C® *(Discontinued)* *see* chlorpheniramine, pseudoephedrine, and codeine *on page 182*

Ryna® *(Discontinued)* *see* chlorpheniramine, pseudoephedrine, and codeine *on page 182*

Rynatan® [US] *see* chlorpheniramine and phenylephrine *on page 176*

Rynatan® Pediatric Suspension [US] *see* chlorpheniramine and phenylephrine *on page 176*

Rynatuss® [US] *see* chlorpheniramine, ephedrine, phenylephrine, and carbetapentane *on page 178*

Rynatuss® Pediatric [US] *see* chlorpheniramine, ephedrine, phenylephrine, and carbetapentane *on page 178*

Ry-T 12 [US] *see* phenylephrine and pyrilamine *on page 662*

Rythmodan® [Can] *see* disopyramide *on page 268*

Rythmodan®-LA [Can] *see* disopyramide *on page 268*

Rythmol® [US] *see* propafenone *on page 706*

Rythmol® Gen-Propafenone [Can] *see* propafenone *on page 706*

Rythmol® SR [US] *see* propafenone *on page 706*

Rēv-Eyes™ [US] *see* dapiprazole *on page 229*

S2® [US-OTC] *see* epinephrine *on page 295*

S-(+)-3-isobutylgaba *see* pregabalin *on page 696*

SAB-Dimenhydrinate [Can] *see* dimenhydrinate *on page 258*

SAB-Gentamicin [Can] *see* gentamicin *on page 381*

Sab-Prenase [Can] *see* prednisolone (systemic) *on page 695*

Sabril® [Can] *see* vigabatrin *(Canada only) on page 872*

SAB-Trifluridine [Can] *see* trifluridine *on page 849*

sacrosidase (sak ROE si dase)

U.S./Canadian Brand Names Sucraid® [US/Can]

Therapeutic Category Enzyme

Use Orphan drug: Oral replacement therapy in sucrase deficiency, as seen in congenital sucrase-isomaltase deficiency (CSID)

Usual Dosage Oral:

Infants ≥5 months and Children <15 kg: 8500 int. units (1 mL) per meal or snack

Children >15 kg and Adults: 17,000 int. units (2 mL) per meal or snack

Doses should be diluted with 2-4 oz of water, milk, or formula with each meal or snack. Approximately one-half of the dose may be taken before, and the remainder of a dose taken at the completion of each meal or snack.

Dosage Forms Solution, oral: 8500 int. units per mL (118 mL)

Safe Tussin® [US-OTC] *see* guaifenesin and dextromethorphan *on page 394*

Saizen® [US/Can] *see* somatropin *on page 785*

SalAc® [US-OTC] *see* salicylic acid *on this page*

Sal-Acid® [US-OTC] *see* salicylic acid *on this page*

Salacid® Ointment *(Discontinued)* *see* salicylic acid *on this page*

Salactic® [US-OTC] *see* salicylic acid *on this page*

Salagen® [US/Can] *see* pilocarpine *on page 668*

Salazopyrin® [Can] *see* sulfasalazine *on page 799*

Salazopyrin En-Tabs® [Can] *see* sulfasalazine *on page 799*

Salbu-2 [Can] *see* albuterol *on page 23*

Salbu-4 [Can] *see* albuterol *on page 23*

salbutamol *see* albuterol *on page 23*

salbutamol and ipratropium *see* ipratropium and albuterol *on page 460*

Saleto-200® *(Discontinued)* *see* ibuprofen *on page 437*

Saleto-400® *(Discontinued)* *see* ibuprofen *on page 437*

Salflex® [Can] *see* salsalate *on page 761*

Salgesic® *(Discontinued)* *see* salsalate *on page 761*

salicylazosulfapyridine *see* sulfasalazine *on page 799*

salicylic acid (sal i SIL ik AS id)

U.S./Canadian Brand Names Compound W® One Step Wart Remover [US-OTC]; Compound W® [US-OTC]; DHS™ Sal [US-OTC]; Dr. Scholl's® Callus Remover [US-OTC]; Dr. Scholl's® Clear Away [US-OTC]; DuoFilm® [US-OTC/Can]; Duoforte® 27 [Can]; Freezone® [US-OTC]; Fung-O® [US-OTC]; Gordofilm® [US-OTC]; Hydrisalic™ [US-OTC]; Ionil® Plus [US-OTC]; Ionil® [US-OTC]; Keralyt® [US-OTC]; LupiCare™ Dandruff [US-OTC]; LupiCare™ II Psoriasis [US-OTC]; LupiCare™ Psoriasis [US-OTC]; Mediplast® [US-OTC]; MG217 Sal-Acid® [US-OTC]; Mosco® Corn and Callus Remover [US-OTC]; NeoCeuticals™ Acne Spot Treatment [US-OTC]; Neutrogena® Acne Wash [US-OTC]; Neutrogena® Body Clear™ [US-OTC]; Neutrogena® Clear Pore Shine Control [US-OTC]; Neutrogena® Clear Pore [US-OTC]; Neutrogena® Healthy Scalp [US-OTC]; Neutrogena® Maximum Strength T/Sal® [US-OTC]; Neutrogena® On The Spot® Acne Patch [US-OTC]; Occlusal®-HP [US-OTC/Can]; Oxy Balance® Deep Pore [US-OTC]; Oxy Balance® [US-OTC]; Palmer's® Skin Success Acne Cleanser [US-OTC]; Pedisilk® [US-OTC]; Propa pH [US-OTC]; Sal-Acid® [US-OTC]; Sal-Plant® [US-OTC]; Salactic® [US-OTC]; SalAc® [US-OTC]; Sebcur® [Can]; Soluver® Plus [Can]; Soluver® [Can]; Stri-dex® Body Focus [US-OTC]; Stri-dex® Facewipes To Go™ [US-OTC]; Stri-dex® Maximum Strength [US-OTC]; Stri-dex® [US-OTC]; Tinamed® [US-OTC]; Tiseb® [US-OTC]; Trans-Plantar® [Can]; Trans-Ver-Sal® [US-OTC/Can]; Wart-Off® Maximum Strength [US-OTC]; Zapzyt® Acne Wash [US-OTC]; Zapzyt® Pore Treatment [US-OTC]

Therapeutic Category Keratolytic Agent

Use Topically for its keratolytic effect in controlling seborrheic dermatitis or psoriasis of body and scalp, dandruff, and other scaling dermatoses; also used to remove warts, corns, and calluses; acne

Usual Dosage Children and Adults (consult specific product labeling for use in children <12 years):

Acne:

Cream, cloth, foam, or liquid cleansers (2%): Use to cleanse skin once or twice daily. Massage gently into skin, work into lather and rinse thoroughly. Cloths should be wet with water prior to using and disposed of (not flushed) after use.

Gel (0.5% or 2%): Apply small amount to face in the morning or evening; if peeling occurs, may be used every other day. Some products may be labeled for OTC use up to 3 or 4 times per day. Apply to clean, dry skin

Pads (0.5% or 2%): Use pad to cover affected area with thin layer of salicylic acid one to three times a day. Apply to clean, dry skin. Do not leave pad on skin.

Patch (2%): At bedtime, after washing face, allow skin to dry at least 5 minutes. Apply patch directly over pimple being treated. Remove in the morning.

Shower/bath gels or soap (2%): Use once daily in shower or bath to massage over skin prone to acne. Rinse well.

Callus, corns, or warts:

Gel or liquid (17%): Apply to each wart and allow to dry. May repeat once or twice daily, up to 12 weeks. Apply to clean dry area.

Gel (6%): Apply to affected area once daily, generally used at night and rinsed off in the morning.

Plaster or transdermal patch (40%): Apply directly over affected area, leave in place for 48 hours. Some products may be cut to fit area or secured with adhesive strips. May repeat procedure for up to 12 weeks. Apply to clean, dry skin

Transdermal patch (15%): Apply directly over affected area at bedtime, leave in place overnight and remove in the morning. Patch should be trimmed to cover affected area. May repeat daily for up to 12 weeks.

Dandruff, psoriasis, or seborrheic dermatitis:

Cream (2.5%): Apply to affected area 3-4 times daily. Apply to clean, dry skin. Some products may be left in place overnight.

Ointment (3%): Apply to scales or plaques on skin up to 4 times per day (not for scalp or face)

Shampoo (1.8% to 3%): Massage into wet hair or affected area; leave in place for several minutes; rinse thoroughly. Labeled for OTC use 2-3 times a week, or as directed by healthcare provider. Some products may be left in place overnight.

Dosage Forms [DSC] = Discontinued product

Cream:
- LupiCare™ Dandruff, LupiCare™ Psoriasis: 2.5% (120 g, 240 g) [contains alcohol]
- LupiCare™ II Psoriasis: 2.5% (60 g, 240 g) [contains alcohol]
- Neutrogena® Acne Wash: 2% (200 mL) [contains alcohol]

Cloths (Neutrogena® Acne Wash): 2% (30s) [disposable cloths]

Foam:
- Neutrogena® Acne Wash: 2% (150 mL) [foaming cleanser]
- SalAc®: 2% (100 g)

Gel: 17% (15 g)
- Compound W®: 17% (7 g) [contains alcohol]
- DuoPlant® [DSC]: 17% (15 g)
- Hydrisalic™: 6% (28 g) [contains alcohol and propylene glycol]
- Keralyt®: 6% (30 g) [contains alcohol and propylene glycol]
- NeoCeuticals™ Acne Spot Treatment: 2% (15 g) [contains alcohol]
- Neutrogena® Clear Pore: 2% (60 g) [contains alcohol]
- Neutrogena® Clear Pore Shine Control: 0.5% (10 g)
- Oxy Balance®: 2% (240 mL) [shower gel]
- Sal-Plant®: 17% (14 g) [contains alcohol]
- Stri-dex® Body Focus™: 2% (300 mL)
- Zapzyt® Acne Wash: 2% (190 g) [alcohol free]
- Zapzyt® Pore Treatment: 2% (23 g) [alcohol free]

Liquid, topical:
- Compound W®: 17% (9 mL) [contains alcohol]
- DuoFilm®: 17% (15 mL) [contains alcohol]
- Freezone®: 17.6% (9.3 mL) [contains alcohol]
- Fung-O®: 17% (15 mL)
- Gordofilm®: 16.7% (15 mL)
- Mosco® Corn and Callus Remover: 17.6% (10 mL)
- NeoCeuticals™ Acne Spot Treatment: 2% (60 mL) [contains alcohol]
- Neutrogena® Acne Wash: 2% (180 mL) [contains tartrazine]
- Neutrogena® Body Clear™ [body scrub with microbeads]: 2% (250 mL) [contains tartrazine]
- Neutrogena® Body Clear™ [body wash]: 2% (250 mL) [contains tartrazine]
- Occlusal®-HP: 17% (10 mL)
- Palmer's® Skin Success Acne Cleanser: 0.5% (240 mL)
- Pedisilk®: 17% (15 mL)
- Propa pH: 2% (80 mL) [alcohol free; contains aloe vera]
- SalAc®: 2% (180 mL)
- Salactic®: 17% (15 mL) [contains alcohol]
- Tinamed®: 17% (15 mL)
- Wart-Off®: 17% (13 mL) [contains alcohol]

Ointment (MG217 Sal-Acid®): 3% (56 g) [contains vitamin E]

Pads:
- Oxy Balance®, Oxy Balance® Deep Pore: 0.5% (55s, 90s) [contains alcohol]
- Stri-dex®: 0.5% (55s)
- Stri-dex® Facewipes To Go™: 0.5% (32s) [contains alcohol]
- Stri-dex® Maximum Strength: 2% (32s, 55s, 90s)

(Continued)

salicylic acid *(Continued)*

Patch, transdermal:
- Compound W® One Step Wart Remover: 40% (12s, 14s)
- Dr. Scholl's® Callus Remover: 40% (4s)
- Dr. Scholl's® Clear Away: 40% (14s, 16s, 18s, 24s)
- DuoFilm®: 40% (18s)
- Neutrogena® On The Spot® Acne Patch: 2% (27s)
- Trans-Ver-Sal®: 15% [6 mm PediaPatch, 12 mm AdultPatch, 20 mm PlantarPatch] (10s, 12s, 15s, 25s, 40s)

Plaster:
- Mediplast®: 40% (25s)
- Sal-Acid®: 40% (14s)
- Tinamed®: 40% (24s)

Shampoo:
- DHS™ Sal: 3% (120 mL)
- Ionil®: 2% (240 mL, 480 mL, 960 mL)
- Ionil® Plus: 2% (240 mL) [conditioning shampoo]
- LupiCare™ Dandruff, LupiCare™ Psoriasis: 2% (120 mL, 240 mL)
- Neutrogena® Healthy Scalp: 1.8% (90 mL, 180 mL)
- Neutrogena® Maximum Strength T/Sal®: 3% (135 mL)
- Tiseb®: 2% (240 mL)

Soap: 2% (114 g)

salicylic acid and coal tar *see* coal tar and salicylic acid *on page 208*

salicylsalicylic acid *see* salsalate *on next page*

SalineX® [US-OTC] *see* sodium chloride *on page 777*

Salivart® [US-OTC] *see* saliva substitute *on this page*

saliva substitute (sa LYE va SUB stee tute)

U.S./Canadian Brand Names Entertainer's Secret® [US-OTC]; Moi-Stir® [US-OTC]; Mouthkote® [US-OTC]; Saliva Substitute™ [US-OTC]; Salivart® [US-OTC]; Salix® [US-OTC]

Therapeutic Category Gastrointestinal Agent, Miscellaneous

Use Relief of dry mouth and throat in xerostomia

Usual Dosage Use as needed

Dosage Forms [DSC] = Discontinued product

Liquid:
- Numoisyn™: Water, sorbitol, linseed extract, *Chondrus crispus*, methylparaben, sodium benzoate, potassium sorbate, dipotassium phosphate, propylparaben (300 mL)

Lozenge:
- Numoisyn™: Sorbitol 0.3 g/lozenge, polyethylene glycol, malic acid, sodium citrate, calcium phosphate dibasic, hydrogenated cottonseed oil, citric acid, magnesium stearate, silicon dioxide (100s)
- SalivaSure™: Xylitol, citric acid, apple acid, sodium citrate dihydrate, sodium carboxymethylcellulose, dibasic calcium phosphate, silica colloidal, magnesium stearate, stearic acid (90s)

Solution, oral:
- Caphosol: Dibasic sodium phosphate 0.032%, monobasic sodium phosphate 0.009%, calcium chloride 0.052%, sodium chloride 0.569%, purified water (30 mL) [packaged in two 15 mL ampuls when mixed together provide one 30 mL dose]
- Entertainer's Secret®: Sodium carboxymethylcellulose, aloe vera gel, glycerin (60 mL) [honey-apple flavor]
- Saliva Substitute®: Sorbitol, sodium carboxymethylcellulose, methylparaben (120 mL)

Spray, oral:
- Moi-Stir®: Water, sorbitol, sodium carboxymethylcellulose, methylparaben, propylparaben, potassium chloride, dibasic sodium phosphate, calcium chloride, magnesium chloride, sodium chloride (120 mL)
- Mouthkote®: Water, xylitol, sorbitol, yerba santa, citric acid, ascorbic acid, sodium saccharin, sodium benzoate (5 mL, 60 mL, 240 mL) [lemon-lime flavor]
- Salivart®: Water, sodium carboxymethylcellulose, sorbitol, sodium chloride, potassium chloride, calcium chloride, magnesium chloride, potassium phosphate (70 mL)

Swabsticks, oral:
- Moi-Stir®: Water, sorbitol, sodium carboxymethylcellulose, methylparaben, propylparaben, potassium chloride, dibasic sodium phosphate, calcium chloride, magnesium chloride, sodium chloride (300s) [DSC]

Saliva Substitute™ [US-OTC] *see* saliva substitute *on this page*

Salix® [US-OTC] *see* saliva substitute *on previous page*

salk vaccine *see* poliovirus vaccine (inactivated) *on page 677*

salmeterol (sal ME te role)

Sound-Alike/Look-Alike Issues
salmeterol may be confused with Salbutamol
Serevent® may be confused with Serentil®

Synonyms salmeterol xinafoate

U.S./Canadian Brand Names Serevent® Diskus® [US]; Serevent® [Can]

Therapeutic Category Adrenergic Agonist Agent

Use Maintenance treatment of asthma and in prevention of bronchospasm with reversible obstructive airway disease, including patients with symptoms of nocturnal asthma; prevention of exercise-induced bronchospasm; maintenance treatment of bronchospasm associated with COPD

Usual Dosage Inhalation, powder (Serevent® Diskus®):
Asthma, maintenance and prevention: Children ≥4 years and Adults: One inhalation (50 mcg) twice daily (~12 hours apart); maximum: 1 inhalation twice daily
Exercise-induced asthma, prevention: Children ≥4 years and Adults: One inhalation (50 mcg) at least 30 minutes prior to exercise; additional doses should not be used for 12 hours; should not be used in individuals already receiving salmeterol twice daily
COPD (maintenance treatment of associated bronchospasm): Adults: One inhalation (50 mcg) twice daily (~12 hours apart); maximum: 1 inhalation twice daily

Dosage Forms Powder for oral inhalation: 50 mcg (28s, 60s) [delivers 50 mcg/inhalation; contains lactose]

salmeterol and fluticasone *see* fluticasone and salmeterol *on page 360*

salmeterol xinafoate *see* salmeterol *on this page*

Salmonella typhi Vi capsular polysaccharide vaccine *(Canada only)*

(sal mo NEL la TI fi vi CAP su lar po le SAK ar ide VAK seen)

U.S./Canadian Brand Names Typherix™ [Can]

Therapeutic Category Vaccine

Use For active immunization against typhoid fever in persons 2 years of age and older.

Usual Dosage One dose administered I.M. ensures protection for at least 3 years. The vaccine must be given at least 2 weeks prior to travel to endemic areas.

Dosage Forms Injection: Vi polysaccharide vaccine of *S. typhi* 25 mcg (0.5 mL)

Salmonine® ***(Discontinued)*** *see* calcitonin *on page 133*

Salofalk® [Can] *see* mesalamine *on page 533*

Sal-Plant® [US-OTC] *see* salicylic acid *on page 758*

salsalate (SAL sa late)

Sound-Alike/Look-Alike Issues
salsalate may be confused with sucralfate, sulfasalazine

Synonyms disalicylic acid; salicylsalicylic acid

U.S./Canadian Brand Names Amigesic® [US/Can]; Salflex® [Can]

Therapeutic Category Analgesic, Nonnarcotic; Antipyretic; Nonsteroidal Antiinflammatory Drug (NSAID)

Use Treatment of minor pain or fever; arthritis

Usual Dosage Adults: Oral: 3 g/day in 2-3 divided doses

Dosage Forms
Tablet: 500 mg, 750 mg
Amigesic®: 500 mg, 750 mg

Salsitab® ***(Discontinued)*** *see* salsalate *on this page*

salt *see* sodium chloride *on page 777*

salt poor albumin *see* albumin *on page 22*

Sal-Tropine™ [US] *see* atropine *on page 83*

Sanctura™ [US] *see* trospium *on page 856*

Sandimmune® [US] *see* cyclosporine *on page 221*

Sandimmune® I.V. [Can] *see* cyclosporine *on page 221*

Sandomigran® [Can] *see* pizotifen *(Canada only)* *on page 672*

Sans Acne® [Can] *see* erythromycin *on page 303*

Santyl® [US] *see* collagenase *on page 212*

saquinavir (sa KWIN a veer)

Sound-Alike/Look-Alike Issues

saquinavir may be confused with Sinequan®
Fortovase® may be confused with Invirase®
Invirase® may be confused with Fortovase®

Synonyms saquinavir mesylate

U.S./Canadian Brand Names Fortovase® [Can]; Invirase® [US/Can]

Therapeutic Category Antiviral Agent

Use Treatment of HIV infection; used in combination with at least two other antiretroviral agents

Usual Dosage Oral: Children ≥16 years and Adults: **Note:** Fortovase® and Invirase® are not bioequivalent and should not be used interchangeably; only Fortovase® should be used to initiate therapy:

Unboosted regimen: Fortovase®: 1200 mg (six 200 mg capsules) 3 times/day or 1600 mg twice daily within 2 hours after a meal in combination with a nucleoside analog

Note: Saquinavir hard-gel capsules (Invirase®) should not be used in "unboosted regimens."

Ritonavir-boosted regimens:

Fortovase®: 1000 mg (five 200 mg capsules) twice daily in combination with ritonavir 100 mg twice daily

Invirase®: 1000 mg (five 200 mg capsules or two 500 mg tablets) twice daily given in combination with ritonavir 100 mg twice daily. This combination should be given together and within 2 hours after a full meal in combination with a nucleoside analog.

Dosage Forms Note: Strength expressed as base; [DSC] = Discontinued product

Capsule, as mesylate:
Invirase®: 200 mg [contains lactose 63.3 mg/capsule]

Capsule, soft gelatin, as base:
Fortovase®: 200 mg [DSC]

Tablet, as mesylate:
Invirase®: 500 mg

saquinavir mesylate *see* saquinavir *on this page*

Sarafem® [US] *see* fluoxetine *on page 357*

sargramostim (sar GRAM oh stim)

Sound-Alike/Look-Alike Issues

Leukine® may be confused with Leukeran®

Synonyms GM-CSF; granulocyte-macrophage colony stimulating factor; rGM-CSF

U.S./Canadian Brand Names Leukine® [US/Can]

Therapeutic Category Colony-Stimulating Factor

Use

Myeloid reconstitution after autologous bone marrow transplantation: Non-Hodgkin lymphoma (NHL), acute lymphoblastic leukemia (ALL), Hodgkin lymphoma, metastatic breast cancer

Myeloid reconstitution after allogeneic bone marrow transplantation

Peripheral stem cell transplantation: Metastatic breast cancer, non-Hodgkin lymphoma, Hodgkin lymphoma, multiple myeloma

Orphan drug:

Acute myelogenous leukemia (AML) following induction chemotherapy in older adults to shorten time to neutrophil recovery and to reduce the incidence of severe and life-threatening infections and infections resulting in death

Bone marrow transplant (allogeneic or autologous) failure or engraftment delay

Safety and efficacy of GM-CSF given simultaneously with cytotoxic chemotherapy have not been established. Concurrent treatment may increase myelosuppression.

Usual Dosage

Children and Adults: I.V. infusion over ≥2 hours or SubQ: **Rounding the dose to the nearest vial size enhances patient convenience and reduces costs without clinical detriment**

Myeloid reconstitution after peripheral stem cell, allogeneic or autologous bone marrow transplant:

I.V.: 250 mcg/m²/day for 21 days to begin 2-4 hours after the marrow infusion or ≥24 hours after chemotherapy or 12 hours after last dose of radiotherapy

If a severe adverse reaction occurs, reduce or temporarily discontinue the dose until the reaction abates

If blast cells appear or progression of the underlying disease occurs, disrupt treatment

Interrupt or reduce the dose by half if ANC is >20,000 cells/mm³

Patients should not receive sargramostim until the postmarrow infusion ANC is <500 cells/mm³

(Continued)

sargramostim *(Continued)*

Neutrophil recovery following chemotherapy in AML: I.V.: 250 mcg/m^2/day over a 4-hour period starting approximately day 11 or 4 days following the completion of induction chemotherapy, if day 10 bone marrow is hypoblastic with <5% blasts

If a second cycle of chemotherapy is necessary, administer ~4 days after the completion of chemotherapy if the bone marrow is hypoblastic with <5% blasts

Continue sargramostim until ANC is >1500 cells/mm^3 for consecutive days or a maximum of 42 days

Discontinue sargramostim immediately if leukemic regrowth occurs

If a severe adverse reaction occurs, reduce the dose by 50% or temporarily discontinue the dose until the reaction abates

Mobilization of peripheral blood progenitor cells: I.V.: 250 mcg/m^2/day over 24 hours or SubQ once daily

Continue the same dose through the period of PBPC collection

The optimal schedule for PBPC collection has not been established (usually begun by day 5 and performed daily until protocol specified targets are achieved)

If WBC >50,000 cells/mm^3, reduce the dose by 50%

If adequate numbers of progenitor cells are not collected, consider other mobilization therapy

Postperipheral blood progenitor cell transplantation: I.V.: 250 mcg/m^2/day or SubQ once daily beginning immediately following infusion of progenitor cells and continuing until ANC is >1500 for 3 consecutive days is attained

BMT failure or engraftment delay: I.V.: 250 mcg/m^2/day for 14 days

The dose can be repeated after 7 days off therapy if engraftment has not occurred

If engraftment still has not occurred, a third course of 500 mcg/m^2/day for 14 days may be tried after another 7 days off therapy; if there is still no improvement, it is unlikely that further dose escalation will be beneficial

If a severe adverse reaction occurs, reduce or temporarily discontinue the dose until the reaction abates

If blast cells appear or disease progression occurs, discontinue treatment

Dosage Forms

Injection, powder for reconstitution:

Leukine®: 250 mcg [contains sucrose 10 mg/mL]

Injection, solution:

Leukine®: 500 mcg/mL (1 mL) [contains benzyl alcohol, disodium edetate, and sucrose 10 mg/mL]

Sarna® HC [Can] *see* hydrocortisone (topical) *on page 428*

Sarna® Sensitive [US] *see* pramoxine *on page 691*

Sarnol®-HC [US-OTC] *see* hydrocortisone (topical) *on page 428*

Sativex® [Can] *see* tetrahydrocannabinol and cannabidiol *(Canada only) on page 816*

SB-265805 *see* gemifloxacin *on page 379*

SC 33428 *see* idarubicin *on page 439*

SCH 13521 *see* flutamide *on page 360*

S-citalopram *see* escitalopram *on page 306*

Scleromate® [US] *see* morrhuate sodium *on page 567*

Scopace™ [US] *see* scopolamine derivatives *on this page*

scopolamine and phenylephrine *see* phenylephrine and scopolamine *on page 662*

scopolamine butylbromide *see* scopolamine derivatives *on this page*

scopolamine derivatives (skoe POL a meen dah RIV ah tives)

Synonyms hyoscine butylbromide; hyoscine hydrobromide; scopolamine butylbromide; scopolamine hydrobromide

U.S./Canadian Brand Names Buscopan® [Can]; Isopto® Hyoscine [US]; Scopace™ [US]; Transderm Scōp® [US]; Transderm-V® [Can]

Therapeutic Category Anticholinergic Agent

Use

Scopolamine hydrobromide:

Injection: Preoperative medication to produce amnesia, sedation, and decrease salivary and respiratory secretions

Ophthalmic: Produce cycloplegia and mydriasis; treatment of iridocyclitis

Oral: Symptomatic treatment of postencephalitic parkinsonism and paralysis agitans; inhibits excessive motility and hypertonus of the genitourinary or gastrointestinal tract in such conditions as the irritable colon syndrome, mild dysentery, diverticulitis, pylorospasm, and cardiospasm

Transdermal: Prevention of nausea/vomiting associated with anesthesia or opiate analgesia; prevention of motion sickness

Scopolamine butylbromide:

Oral/injection: Treatment of smooth muscle spasm of the genitourinary or gastrointestinal tract; injection may also be used to prior to radiological/diagnostic procedures to prevent spasm

Usual Dosage Note: Scopolamine (hyoscine) hydrobromide should not be interchanged with scopolamine butylbromide formulations. Dosages are not equivalent.

Scopolamine hydrobromide:

Preoperative:

Children: I.M., SubQ: 6 mcg/kg/dose (maximum: 0.3 mg/dose) every 6-8 hours

Adults:

I.M., I.V., SubQ: 0.3-0.65 mg; may be repeated every 4-6 hours

Transdermal patch: Apply 2.5 cm^2 patch to hairless area behind ear the night before surgery or 1 hour prior to cesarean section (the patch should be applied no sooner than 1 hour before surgery for best results and removed 24 hours after surgery)

Motion sickness: Transdermal: Adults: Apply 1 disc behind the ear at least 4 hours prior to exposure and every 3 days as needed; effective if applied as soon as 2-3 hours before anticipated need, best if 12 hours before

Refraction: Ophthalmic:

Children: Instill 1 drop of 0.25% to eye(s) twice daily for 2 days before procedure

Adults: Instill 1-2 drops of 0.25% to eye(s) 1 hour before procedure

Iridocyclitis: Ophthalmic:

Children: Instill 1 drop of 0.25% to eye(s) up to 3 times/day

Adults: Instill 1-2 drops of 0.25% to eye(s) up to 4 times/day

Parkinsonism, spasticity, motion sickness: Oral: 0.4-0.8 mg as a range; the dosage may be cautiously increased in parkinsonism and spastic states.

Scopolamine butylbromide:

Gastrointestinal/genitourinary spasm (Buscopan® [CAN]; not available in the U.S.): Adults:

Oral: 10-20 mg daily (1-2 tablets); maximum: 6 tablets/day

I.M., I.V., SubQ: 10-20 mg; maximum: 100 mg/day. Intramuscular injections should be administered 10-15 minutes prior to radiological/diagnostic procedures

Dosage Forms [CAN] = Canadian brand name

Injection, solution, as hydrobromide: 0.4 mg/mL (1 mL)

Injection, solution, as hyoscine-N-butylbromide:

Buscopan® [CAN]: 20 mg/mL [not available in U.S.]

Solution, ophthalmic, as hydrobromide:

Isopto® Hyoscine: 0.25% (5 mL, 15 mL) [contains benzalkonium chloride]

Tablet, as hyoscine-N-butylbromide:

Buscopan® [CAN]: 10 mg [not available in U.S.]

Tablet, soluble, as hydrobromide:

Maldemar™, Scopace™: 0.4 mg

Transdermal system:

Transderm Scōp®: 1.5 mg (4s, 10s, 24s) [releases ~1 mg over 72 hours]

scopolamine hydrobromide *see* scopolamine derivatives *on previous page*

scopolamine, hyoscyamine, atropine, and phenobarbital *see* hyoscyamine, atropine, scopolamine, and phenobarbital *on page 435*

Scot-Tussin DM® Cough Chasers [US-OTC] *see* dextromethorphan *on page 245*

Scot-Tussin® Expectorant [US-OTC] *see* guaifenesin *on page 392*

Scot-Tussin® Senior [US-OTC] *see* guaifenesin and dextromethorphan *on page 394*

SDZ ENA 713 *see* rivastigmine *on page 750*

Seasonale® [US] *see* ethinyl estradiol and levonorgestrel *on page 320*

Seasonique™ [US] *see* ethinyl estradiol and levonorgestrel *on page 320*

Seba-Gel™ [US] *see* benzoyl peroxide *on page 102*

Sebcur® [Can] *see* salicylic acid *on page 758*

Sebcur/T® [Can] *see* coal tar and salicylic acid *on page 208*

Sebizon® *(Discontinued)* *see* sulfacetamide *on page 795*

secobarbital (see koe BAR bi tal)

Sound-Alike/Look-Alike Issues

Seconal® may be confused with Sectral®

Synonyms quinalbarbitone sodium; secobarbital sodium

U.S./Canadian Brand Names Seconal® [US]

Therapeutic Category Barbiturate

Controlled Substance C-II

Use Preanesthetic agent; short-term treatment of insomnia

Usual Dosage Oral:

Children:

Preoperative sedation: 2-6 mg/kg (maximum dose: 100 mg/dose) 1-2 hours before procedure

Sedation: 6 mg/kg/day divided every 8 hours

Adults:

Hypnotic: Usual: 100 mg/dose at bedtime; range 100-200 mg/dose

Preoperative sedation: 100-300 mg 1-2 hours before procedure

Dosage Forms Capsule, as sodium: 100 mg

secobarbital sodium *see* secobarbital *on this page*

Seconal® [US] *see* secobarbital *on this page*

Secran® *(Discontinued)*

SecreFlo™ [US] *see* secretin *on this page*

secretin (SEE kre tin)

Synonyms secretin, human; secretin, porcine

U.S./Canadian Brand Names SecreFlo™ [US]

Therapeutic Category Diagnostic Agent

Use Secretin-stimulation testing to aid in diagnosis of pancreatic exocrine dysfunction; diagnosis of gastrinoma (Zollinger-Ellison syndrome); facilitation of ERCP visualization

Usual Dosage I.V.: Adults: **Note:** A test dose of 0.2 mcg (0.1 mL) is injected to test for possible allergy. Dosing may be completed if no reaction occurs after 1 minute.

Diagnosis of pancreatic dysfunction, facilitation of ERCP: 0.2 mcg/kg over 1 minute

Diagnosis of gastrinoma: 0.4 mcg/kg over 1 minute

Dosage Forms

Injection, powder for reconstitution [human]:

ChiRhoStim™: 16 mcg

Injection, powder for reconstitution [porcine]:

SecreFlo™: 16 mcg

secretin, human *see* secretin *on this page*

secretin, porcine *see* secretin *on this page*

Sectral® [US/Can] *see* acebutolol *on page 4*

Secura® Antifungal [US-OTC] *see* miconazole *on page 553*

Selax® [Can] *see* docusate *on page 270*

Select™ 1/35 [Can] *see* ethinyl estradiol and norethindrone *on page 323*

selegiline (se LE ji leen)

Sound-Alike/Look-Alike Issues

selegiline may be confused with Salagen®, Serentil®, sertraline, Serzone®, Stelazine®

Eldepryl® may be confused with Elavil®, enalapril

Synonyms deprenyl; L-deprenyl; selegiline hydrochloride

U.S./Canadian Brand Names Apo-Selegiline® [Can]; Eldepryl® [US]; Emsam® [US]; Gen-Selegiline [Can]; Novo-Selegiline [Can]; Nu-Selegiline [Can]; Zelapar™ [US]

Therapeutic Category Anti-Parkinson Agent; Dopaminergic Agent (Anti-Parkinson)

Use Adjunct in the management of parkinsonian patients in which levodopa/carbidopa therapy is deteriorating (oral products); treatment of major depressive disorder (transdermal product)

Usual Dosage Adults:

Capsule/tablet: Parkinson disease: 5 mg twice daily with breakfast and lunch or 10 mg in the morning

Orally disintegrating tablet (Zelapar™): Parkinson disease: Initial 1.25 mg daily for at least 6 weeks; may increase to 2.5 mg daily based on clinical response (maximum: 2.5 mg daily)

Transdermal (Emsam®): Depression: Initial: 6 mg/24 hours once daily; may titrate based on clinical response in increments of 3 mg/day every 2 weeks up to a maximum of 12 mg/24 hours

Dosage Forms

Capsule, as hydrochloride: 5 mg

Eldepryl®: 5 mg

Tablet, as hydrochloride: 5 mg

Tablet, orally-disintegrating:

Zelapar™: 1.25 mg [contains phenylalanine 1.25 mg/tablet]

Transdermal system [once-daily patch]:

Emsam®: 6 mg/24 hours (30s); 9 mg/24 hours (30s); 12 mg/24 hours (30s)

selegiline hydrochloride *see* selegiline *on previous page*

selenium *see* trace metals *on page 839*

selenium sulfide (se LEE nee um SUL fide)

U.S./Canadian Brand Names Head & Shoulders® Intensive Treatment [US-OTC]; Selsun Blue® 2-in-1 Treatment [US-OTC]; Selsun Blue® Balanced Treatment [US-OTC]; Selsun Blue® Medicated Treatment [US-OTC]; Selsun Blue® Moisturizing Treatment [US-OTC]; Selsun® [US]; Versel® [Can]

Therapeutic Category Antiseborrheic Agent, Topical

Use Treatment of itching and flaking of the scalp associated with dandruff, to control scalp seborrheic dermatitis; treatment of tinea versicolor

Usual Dosage Topical:

Dandruff, seborrhea: Massage 5-10 mL into wet scalp, leave on scalp 2-3 minutes, rinse thoroughly

Tinea versicolor: Apply the 2.5% lotion to affected area and lather with small amounts of water; leave on skin for 10 minutes, then rinse thoroughly; apply every day for 7 days

Dosage Forms [DSC] = Discontinued product

Lotion, topical: 2.5% (120 mL)

Shampoo, topical: 1% (210 mL)

Exsel® [DSC], Selsun®: 2.5% (120 mL)

Head & Shoulders® Intensive Treatment: 1% (400 mL)

Selsun Blue® Balanced Treatment, Selsun Blue® Medicated Treatment, Selsun Blue® Moisturizing Treatment, Selsun Blue® 2-in-1 Treatment: 1% (120 mL, 210 mL, 330 mL)

Selepen® [US] *see* trace metals *on page 839*

Selpak® *(Discontinued)* *see* selegiline *on previous page*

Selsun® [US] *see* selenium sulfide *on this page*

Selsun Blue® 2-in-1 Treatment [US-OTC] *see* selenium sulfide *on this page*

Selsun Blue® Balanced Treatment [US-OTC] *see* selenium sulfide *on this page*

Selsun Blue® Medicated Treatment [US-OTC] *see* selenium sulfide *on this page*

Selsun Blue® Moisturizing Treatment [US-OTC] *see* selenium sulfide *on this page*

Selsun Gold® for Women *(Discontinued)* *see* selenium sulfide *on this page*

Semprex®-D [US] *see* acrivastine and pseudoephedrine *on page 17*

Senexon® [US-OTC] *see* senna *on this page*

senna (SEN na)

Sound-Alike/Look-Alike Issues

Senexon® may be confused with Cenestin®

Senokot® may be confused with Depakote®

U.S./Canadian Brand Names Black Draught Tablets [US-OTC]; Evac-U-Gen [US-OTC]; ex-lax® Maximum Strength [US-OTC]; ex-lax® [US-OTC]; Fletcher's® Castoria® [US-OTC]; Perdiem® Overnight Relief [US-OTC]; Senexon® [US-OTC]; Senna-Gen® [US-OTC]; Sennatural™ [US-OTC]; Senokot® [US-OTC]; Uni-Senna [US-OTC]

Therapeutic Category Laxative

Use Short-term treatment of constipation; evacuate the colon for bowel or rectal examinations

Usual Dosage Oral:

Bowel evacuation: OTC labeling: Children ≥12 years and Adults: Usual dose: Sennosides 130 mg (X-Prep® 75 mL) between 2-4 PM the afternoon of the day prior to procedure

(Continued)

senna *(Continued)*

Constipation: OTC ranges:
Children:
2-6 years:
Sennosides: Initial: 3.75 mg once daily (maximum: 15 mg/day, divided twice daily)
Senna concentrate: 33.3 mg/mL: 5-10 mL up to twice daily
6-12 years:
Sennosides: Initial: 8.6 mg once daily (maximum: 50 mg/day, divided twice daily)
Senna concentrate: 33.3 mg/mL: 10-30 mL up to twice daily
Children ≥12 years and Adults: Sennosides 15 mg once daily (maximum: 70-100 mg/day, divided twice daily)

Dosage Forms [DSC] = Discontinued product
Granules (Senokot®): Sennosides 15 mg/teaspoon (60 g, 180 g, 360 g) [cocoa flavor] [DSC]
Liquid:
Senexon: Sennosides 8.8 mg/5 mL (240 mL)
X-Prep®: Sennosides 8.8 mg/5 mL (75 mL) [alcohol free; contains sugar 50 g/75 mL; available individually or in a kit] [DSC]
Liquid concentrate (Fletcher's® Castoria®): Senna concentrate 33.3 mg/mL (75 mL) [alcohol free; contains sodium benzoate; root beer flavor]
Syrup (Uni-Senna): Sennosides 8.8 mg/5 mL (240 mL) [contains alcohol; butterscotch flavor]
Tablet: Sennosides 8.6 mg, 15 mg, 25 mg
ex-lax®: Sennosides USP 15 mg
ex-lax® Maximum Strength: Sennosides USP 25 mg
Perdiem® Overnight Relief: Sennosides USP 15 mg
Sennatural™, Senokot®, Senexon®, Senna-Gen®, Uni-Senna: Sennosides 8.6 mg
Tablet, chewable:
ex-lax®: Sennosides USP 15 mg [chocolate flavor]
Evac-U-Gen: Sennosides 10 mg

senna and docusate *see* docusate and senna *on page 271*

Senna-Gen® [US-OTC] *see* senna *on previous page*

senna-S *see* docusate and senna *on page 271*

Sennatural™ [US-OTC] *see* senna *on previous page*

Senokot® [US-OTC] *see* senna *on previous page*

Senokot-S® [US-OTC] *see* docusate and senna *on page 271*

Sensipar™ [US] *see* cinacalcet *on page 189*

Sensorcaine® [US/Can] *see* bupivacaine *on page 124*

Sensorcaine®-MPF [US] *see* bupivacaine *on page 124*

Sensorcaine®-MPF with Epinephrine [US] *see* bupivacaine and epinephrine *on page 124*

Sensorcaine® with Epinephrine [US/Can] *see* bupivacaine and epinephrine *on page 124*

Septanest® N [Can] *see* articaine and epinephrine *on page 75*

Septanest® SP [Can] *see* articaine and epinephrine *on page 75*

Septa® Topical Ointment *(Discontinued)* *see* bacitracin, neomycin, and polymyxin B *on page 91*

Septisol® *(Discontinued)* *see* hexachlorophene *on page 414*

Septocaine® [US] *see* articaine and epinephrine *on page 75*

Septra® [US] *see* sulfamethoxazole and trimethoprim *on page 797*

Septra® DS [US] *see* sulfamethoxazole and trimethoprim *on page 797*

Septra® Injection [Can] *see* sulfamethoxazole and trimethoprim *on page 797*

Serax® [US] *see* oxazepam *on page 623*

Serc® [Can] *see* betahistine *(Canada only) on page 106*

Serevent® [Can] *see* salmeterol *on page 761*

Serevent® *(Discontinued)* *see* salmeterol *on page 761*

Serevent® Diskus® [US] *see* salmeterol *on page 761*

sermorelin acetate (ser moe REL in AS e tate)

U.S./Canadian Brand Names Geref® Diagnostic [US]

Therapeutic Category Diagnostic Agent

Use

Geref® Diagnostic: For evaluation of the ability of the pituitary gland to secrete growth hormone (GH)

Usual Dosage Children and Adults: Diagnostic: I.V.: 1 mcg/kg as a single dose in the morning following an overnight fast

Note: Response to diagnostic test may be decreased in patients >40 years

Dosage Forms Injection, powder for reconstitution, as acetate: 50 mcg [packaged with diluent]

Seromycin® [US] *see* cycloserine *on page 221*

Serophene® [US/Can] *see* clomiphene *on page 202*

Seroquel® [US/Can] *see* quetiapine *on page 724*

Serostim® [US/Can] *see* somatropin *on page 785*

Serpalan® *(Discontinued)* *see* reserpine *on page 738*

Serpatabs® *(Discontinued)* *see* reserpine *on page 738*

sertaconazole (ser ta KOE na zole)

Synonyms sertaconazole nitrate

U.S./Canadian Brand Names Ertaczo™ [US]

Therapeutic Category Antifungal Agent, Topical

Use Topical treatment of tinea pedis (athlete's foot)

Usual Dosage Topical: Children ≥12 years and Adults: Apply between toes and to surrounding healthy skin twice daily for 4 weeks

Dosage Forms Cream, topical, as nitrate: 2% (30 g)

sertaconazole nitrate *see* sertaconazole *on this page*

sertraline (SER tra leen)

Sound-Alike/Look-Alike Issues

sertraline may be confused with selegiline, Serentil®

Zoloft® may be confused with Zocor®

Synonyms sertraline hydrochloride

U.S./Canadian Brand Names Apo-Sertraline® [Can]; Gen-Sertraline [Can]; GMD-Sertraline [Can]; Novo-Sertraline [Can]; Nu-Sertraline [Can]; PMS-Sertraline [Can]; ratio-Sertraline [Can]; Rhoxal-Sertraline [Can]; Sandoz-Sertraline [Can]; Zoloft® [US/Can]

Therapeutic Category Antidepressant, Selective Serotonin Reuptake Inhibitor

Use Treatment of major depression; obsessive-compulsive disorder (OCD); panic disorder; post-traumatic stress disorder (PTSD); premenstrual dysphoric disorder (PMDD); social anxiety disorder

Usual Dosage Oral:

Children and Adolescents: OCD:

6-12 years: Initial: 25 mg once daily

13-17 years: Initial: 50 mg once daily

Note: May increase daily dose, at intervals of not less than 1 week, to a maximum of 200 mg/day. If somnolence is noted, give at bedtime.

Adults:

Depression/OCD: Oral: Initial: 50 mg/day (see "Note" above)

Panic disorder, PTSD, social anxiety disorder: Initial: 25 mg once daily; increase to 50 mg once daily after 1 week (see "Note" above)

PMDD: 50 mg/day either daily throughout menstrual cycle **or** limited to the luteal phase of menstrual cycle, depending on physician assessment. Patients not responding to 50 mg/day may benefit from dose increases (50 mg increments per menstrual cycle) up to 150 mg/day when dosing throughout menstrual cycle **or** up to 100 mg day when dosing during luteal phase only. If a 100 mg/day dose has been established with luteal phase dosing, a 50 mg/day titration step for 3 days should be utilized at the beginning of each luteal phase dosing period.

Dosage Forms Note: Available as sertraline hydrochloride; mg strength refers to sertraline

Solution, oral [concentrate]: 20 mg/mL (60 mL)

Zoloft®: 20 mg/mL (60 mL) [contains alcohol 12%; dropper contains dry natural rubber]

Tablet: 25 mg, 50 mg, 100 mg

Zoloft®: 25 mg, 50 mg, 100 mg

sertraline hydrochloride *see* sertraline *on previous page*

Serutan® [US-OTC] *see* psyllium *on page 717*

Serzone® *(Discontinued)* *see* nefazodone *on page 581*

sevelamer (se VEL a mer)

Sound-Alike/Look-Alike Issues

Renagel® may be confused with Reglan®, Regonol®

Synonyms sevelamer hydrochloride

U.S./Canadian Brand Names Renagel® [US/Can]

Therapeutic Category Phosphate Binder

Use Reduction of serum phosphorous in patients with chronic kidney disease on hemodialysis

Usual Dosage

Adults: Oral: Patients not taking a phosphate binder: 800-1600 mg 3 times/day with meals; the initial dose may be based on serum phosphorous levels:

>5.5 mg/dL to <7.5 mg/dL: 800 mg 3 times/day

≥7.5 mg/dL to <9.0 mg/dL: 1200-1600 mg 3 times/day

≥9.0 mg/dL: 1600 mg 3 times/day

Maintenance dose adjustment based on serum phosphorous concentration (goal of lowering to <5.5 mg/dL; maximum daily dose studied was equivalent to 13 g/day):

>5.5 mg/dL: Increase by 1 tablet per meal every 2 weeks

3.5-5.5 mg/dL: Maintain current dose

<3.5 mg/dL: Decrease by 1 tablet per meal

Dosage adjustment when switching between phosphate binder products: 667 mg of calcium acetate is equivalent to 800 mg sevelamer

Dosage Forms Tablet, as hydrochloride: 400 mg, 800 mg

sevelamer hydrochloride *see* sevelamer *on this page*

sevoflurane (see voe FLOO rane)

Sound-Alike/Look-Alike Issues

Ultane® may be confused with Ultram®

U.S./Canadian Brand Names Sevorane™ [Can]; Ultane® [US]

Therapeutic Category General Anesthetic

Use Induction and maintenance of general anesthesia

Usual Dosage Minimum alveolar concentration (MAC), the concentration that abolishes movement in response to a noxious stimulus (surgical incision) in 50% of patients, is 2.6% (25 years of age) for sevoflurane. Surgical levels of anesthesia are generally achieved with concentrations from 0.5% to 3%; the concentration at which amnesia and loss of awareness occur is 0.6%.

Minimum alveolar concentrations (MAC) values for surgical levels of anesthesia:

0 to 1 month old full-term neonates: Sevoflurane in oxygen: 3.3%

1 to <6 months: Sevoflurane in oxygen: 3%

6 months to <3 years:

Sevoflurane in oxygen: 2.8%

Sevoflurane in 60% N_2O/40% oxygen: 2%

3-12 years: Sevoflurane in oxygen: 2.5%

25 years:

Sevoflurane in oxygen: 2.6%

Sevoflurane in 65% N_2O/35% oxygen: 1.4%

40 years:

Sevoflurane in oxygen: 2.1%

Sevoflurane in 65% N_2O/35% oxygen: 1.1%

60 years:

Sevoflurane in oxygen: 1.7%

Sevoflurane in 65% N_2O/35% oxygen: 0.9%

80 years:

Sevoflurane in oxygen: 1.4%

Sevoflurane in 65% N_2O/35% oxygen: 0.7%

Dosage Forms Liquid for inhalation: 100% (250 mL)

Sevorane™ [Can] *see* sevoflurane *on this page*

shingles vaccine *see* zoster vaccine *on page 891*

Shur-Seal® *(Discontinued)* *see* nonoxynol 9 *on page 597*

Sibelium® [Can] *see* flunarizine *(Canada only) on page 351*

sibutramine (si BYOO tra meen)

Synonyms sibutramine hydrochloride monohydrate

U.S./Canadian Brand Names Meridia® [US/Can]

Therapeutic Category Anorexiant

Controlled Substance C-IV

Use Management of obesity, including weight loss and maintenance of weight loss; should be used in conjunction with a reduced-calorie diet

Usual Dosage Adults ≥16 years: Initial: 10 mg once daily; after 4 weeks may titrate up to 15 mg once daily as needed and tolerated (may be used for up to 2 years, per manufacturer labeling)

Dosage Forms Capsule, as hydrochloride: 5 mg, 10 mg, 15 mg

sibutramine hydrochloride monohydrate *see* sibutramine *on this page*

Silace [US-OTC] *see* docusate *on page 270*

Siladryl® Allergy [US-OTC] *see* diphenhydramine *on page 261*

Siladryl® DAS [US-OTC] *see* diphenhydramine *on page 261*

Silafed® [US-OTC] *see* triprolidine and pseudoephedrine *on page 853*

Silain® *(Discontinued)* *see* simethicone *on next page*

Silaminic® Expectorant *(Discontinued)*

Silapap® Children's [US-OTC] *see* acetaminophen *on page 5*

Silapap® Infants [US-OTC] *see* acetaminophen *on page 5*

Sildec *(Discontinued)* *see* carbinoxamine and pseudoephedrine *on page 149*

Sildec-DM *(Discontinued)* *see* carbinoxamine, pseudoephedrine, and dextromethorphan *on page 150*

sildenafil (sil DEN a fil)

Sound-Alike/Look-Alike Issues

Viagra® may be confused with Allegra®, Vaniqa™

Synonyms UK92480

U.S./Canadian Brand Names Revatio™ [US]; Viagra® [US/Can]

Therapeutic Category Phosphodiesterase (Type 5) Enzyme Inhibitor

Use Treatment of erectile dysfunction; treatment of pulmonary arterial hypertension

Usual Dosage Adults: Oral:

Erectile dysfunction (Viagra®): For most patients, the recommended dose is 25-50 mg taken as needed, approximately 1 hour before sexual activity. However, sildenafil may be taken anywhere from 30 minutes to 4 hours before sexual activity. Based on effectiveness and tolerance, the dose may be increased to a maximum recommended dose of 100 mg or decreased to 25 mg. The maximum recommended dosing frequency is once daily.

Pulmonary arterial hypertension (Revatio™): 20 mg 3 times/day, taken 4-6 hours apart

Dosage considerations for patients stable on alpha blockers: Viagra®: Initial 25 mg

Dosage adjustment for concomitant use of potent CYP34A inhibitors:

Revatio™:

Erythromycin, saquinavir: No dosage adjustment

Itraconazole, ketoconazole, ritonavir: Not recommended

Viagra®:

Erythromycin, itraconazole, ketoconazole, saquinavir: Starting dose of 25 mg should be considered

Ritonavir: Maximum: 25 mg every 48 hours

Dosage Forms Tablet:

Revatio™: 20 mg

Viagra®: 25 mg, 50 mg, 100 mg

Sildicon-E® *(Discontinued)*

Silexin® [US-OTC] *see* guaifenesin and dextromethorphan *on page 394*

Silfedrine Children's [US-OTC] *see* pseudoephedrine *on page 712*

Silphen® [US-OTC] *see* diphenhydramine *on page 261*

Silphen DM® [US-OTC] *see* dextromethorphan *on page 245*

Sil-Tex [US] *see* guaifenesin and phenylephrine *on page 396*

Siltussin-CF® ***(Discontinued)***

Siltussin DAS [US-OTC] *see* guaifenesin *on page 392*

Siltussin DM [US-OTC] *see* guaifenesin and dextromethorphan *on page 394*

Siltussin DM DAS [US-OTC] *see* guaifenesin and dextromethorphan *on page 394*

Siltussin SA [US-OTC] *see* guaifenesin *on page 392*

Silvadene® [US] *see* silver sulfadiazine *on this page*

silver nitrate (SIL ver NYE trate)

Synonyms $AgNO_3$

Therapeutic Category Topical Skin Product

Use Cauterization of wounds and sluggish ulcers, removal of granulation tissue and warts; aseptic prophylaxis of burns

Usual Dosage Children and Adults:

Sticks: Apply to mucous membranes and other moist skin surfaces only on area to be treated 2-3 times/week for 2-3 weeks

Topical solution: Apply a cotton applicator dipped in solution on the affected area 2-3 times/week for 2-3 weeks

Dosage Forms

Applicator sticks, topical: Silver nitrate 75% and potassium nitrate 25% (6", 12", 18")

Solution, topical: 10% (30 mL); 25% (30 mL); 50% (30 mL)

silver sulfadiazine (SIL ver sul fa DYE a zeen)

U.S./Canadian Brand Names Flamazine® [Can]; Silvadene® [US]; SSD® AF [US]; SSD® [US]; Thermazene® [US]

Therapeutic Category Antibacterial, Topical

Use Prevention and treatment of infection in second and third degree burns

Usual Dosage Children and Adults: Topical: Apply once or twice daily with a sterile-gloved hand; apply to a thickness of $^1/_{16}$"; burned area should be covered with cream at all times

Dosage Forms

Cream, topical: 1% (25 g, 50 mg, 85 g, 400 g)

Silvadene®, Thermazene®: 1% (20 g, 50 g, 85 g, 400 g, 1000 g)

SSD®: 1% (25 g, 50 g, 85 g, 400 g)

SSD® AF: 1% (50 g, 400 g)

simethicone (sye METH i kone)

Sound-Alike/Look-Alike Issues

simethicone may be confused with cimetidine

Mylanta® may be confused with Mynatal®

Mylicon® may be confused with Modicon®, Myleran®

Phazyme® may be confused with Pherazine®

Synonyms activated dimethicone; activated methylpolysiloxane

U.S./Canadian Brand Names Equalizer Gas Relief [US-OTC]; Gas-X® Extra Strength [US-OTC]; Gas-X® Maximum Strength [US-OTC]; Gas-X® [US-OTC]; GasAid [US-OTC]; Genasyme® [US-OTC]; Infantaire Gas Drops [US-OTC]; Mylanta® Gas Maximum Strength [US-OTC]; Mylanta® Gas [US-OTC]; Mylicon® Infants [US-OTC]; Ovol® [Can]; Phazyme® Quick Dissolve [US-OTC]; Phazyme® Ultra Strength [US-OTC]; Phazyme® [Can]

Therapeutic Category Antiflatulent

Use Relieves flatulence and functional gastric bloating, and postoperative gas pains

Usual Dosage Oral:

Infants: 20 mg 4 times/day

Children <12 years: 40 mg 4 times/day

Children >12 years and Adults: 40-120 mg after meals and at bedtime as needed, not to exceed 500 mg/day

Dosage Forms

Softgels: 125 mg

GasAid, Gas-X® Extra Strength, Mylanta® Gas Maximum Strength: 125 mg

Gas-X® Maximum Strength: 166 mg

Phazyme® Ultra Strength: 180 mg

Suspension, oral drops: 40 mg/0.6 mL (30 mL)

Equalizer Gas Relief, Genasyme®, Infantaire Gas: 40 mg/0.6 mL (30 mL)
Mylicon® Infants: 40 mg/0.6 mL (15 mL, 30 mL) [alcohol free; contains sodium benzoate; available in a nonstaining formula]
Tablet, chewable: 80 mg, 125 mg
Gas-X®: 80 mg [sodium free; peppermint crème or cherry crème flavor]
Gas-X® Extra Strength: 125 mg [peppermint crème or cherry crème flavor]
Genasyme®: 80 mg
Mylanta® Gas: 80 mg [mint flavor]
Mylanta® Gas Maximum Strength: 125 mg [cherry and mint flavors]
Phazyme® Quick Dissolve: 125 mg [contains phenylalanine 0.4 mg per tablet; mint flavor]

simethicone, aluminum hydroxide, and magnesium hydroxide *see* aluminum hydroxide, magnesium hydroxide, and simethicone *on page 37*

simethicone and calcium carbonate *see* calcium carbonate and simethicone *on page 137*

simethicone and magaldrate *see* magaldrate and simethicone *on page 511*

Simply Cough® [US-OTC] *see* dextromethorphan *on page 245*

Simply Saline® [US-OTC] *see* sodium chloride *on page 777*

Simply Saline® Baby [US-OTC] *see* sodium chloride *on page 777*

Simply Saline® Nasal Moist® [US-OTC] *see* sodium chloride *on page 777*

Simply Sleep® [US-OTC/Can] *see* diphenhydramine *on page 261*

Simply Stuffy™ [US-OTC] *see* pseudoephedrine *on page 712*

Simulect® [US/Can] *see* basiliximab *on page 93*

simvastatin (sim va STAT in)

Sound-Alike/Look-Alike Issues
Zocor® may be confused with Cozaar®, Yocon®, Zoloft®

U.S./Canadian Brand Names Apo-Simvastatin® [Can]; BCI-Simvastatin [Can]; CO Simvastatin [Can]; Gen-Simvastatin [Can]; Novo-Simvastatin [Can]; PMS-Simvastatin [Can]; ratio-Simvastatin [Can]; Riva-Simvastatin [Can]; Sandoz-Simvastatin [Can]; Taro-Simvastatin [Can]; Zocor® [US/Can]

Therapeutic Category HMG-CoA Reductase Inhibitor

Use Used with dietary therapy for the following:
Secondary prevention of cardiovascular events in hypercholesterolemic patients with established coronary heart disease (CHD) or at high risk for CHD: To reduce cardiovascular morbidity (myocardial infarction, coronary revascularization procedures) and mortality; to reduce the risk of stroke and transient ischemic attacks
Hyperlipidemias: To reduce elevations in total cholesterol, LDL-C, apolipoprotein B, and triglycerides in patients with primary hypercholesterolemia (elevations of 1 or more components are present in Fredrickson type IIa, IIb, III, and IV hyperlipidemias); treatment of homozygous familial hypercholesterolemia
Heterozygous familial hypercholesterolemia (HeFH): In adolescent patients (10-17 years of age, females >1 year postmenarche) with HeFH having LDL-C ≥190 mg/dL **or** LDL ≥160 mg/dL with positive family history of premature cardiovascular disease (CVD), or 2 or more CVD risk factors in the adolescent patient

Usual Dosage Oral: **Note:** Doses should be individualized according to the baseline LDL-cholesterol levels, the recommended goal of therapy, and the patient's response; adjustments should be made at intervals of 4 weeks or more; doses may need adjusted based on concomitant medications
Children 10-17 years (females >1 year postmenarche): HeFH: 10 mg once daily in the evening; range: 10-40 mg/day (maximum: 40 mg/day)
Dosage adjustment for simvastatin with concomitant cyclosporine, danazol, fibrates, niacin, amiodarone, or verapamil: Refer to drug-specific dosing in Adults dosing section
Adults:
Homozygous familial hypercholesterolemia: 40 mg once daily in the evening **or** 80 mg/day (given as 20 mg, 20 mg, and 40 mg evening dose)
Prevention of cardiovascular events, hyperlipidemias: 20-40 mg once daily in the evening; range: 5-80 mg/day
Patients requiring only moderate reduction of LDL-cholesterol may be started at 10 mg once daily
Patients requiring reduction of >45% in low-density lipoprotein (LDL) cholesterol may be started at 40 mg once daily in the evening
Patients with CHD or at high risk for CHD: Dosing should be started at 40 mg once daily in the evening; simvastatin may be started simultaneously with diet
(Continued)

simvastatin *(Continued)*

Dosage Forms

Tablet: 5 mg, 10 mg, 20 mg, 40 mg

Zocor®: 5 mg, 10 mg, 20 mg, 40 mg, 80 mg

Sina-12X [US] *see* guaifenesin and phenylephrine *on page 396*

sincalide (SIN ka lide)

Synonyms C8-CCK; OP-CCK

U.S./Canadian Brand Names Kinevac® [US]

Therapeutic Category Diagnostic Agent

Use Postevacuation cholecystography; gallbladder bile sampling; stimulate pancreatic secretion for analysis; accelerate the transit of barium through the small bowel

Usual Dosage Adults:

Contraction of gallbladder:

I.V.: 0.02 mcg/kg over 30-60 seconds; may repeat in 15 minutes with a 0.04 mcg/kg dose

Infusion: 0.12 mcg/kg in 100 mL of NS; administer over 50 minutes

I.M.: 0.1 mcg/kg

Pancreatic function: I.V.: 0.02 mcg/kg over 30 minutes

Accelerate barium transit through small bowel:

I.V.: 0.04 mcg/kg over 30-60 seconds; if movement of barium has not occurred in 30 minutes, may repeat dose

Infusion: 0.12 mcg/kg in 30 mL of NS; administer over 30 minutes

Dosage Forms Injection, powder for reconstitution: 5 mcg [contains sodium metabisulfitel]

Sine-Aid® IB *(Discontinued)* *see* pseudoephedrine and ibuprofen *on page 715*

Sinemet® [US/Can] *see* levodopa and carbidopa *on page 489*

Sinemet® CR [US/Can] *see* levodopa and carbidopa *on page 489*

Sinequan® [Can] *see* doxepin *on page 276*

Sinequan® *(Discontinued)* *see* doxepin *on page 276*

Singulair® [US/Can] *see* montelukast *on page 565*

Sinografin® [US] *see* radiological/contrast media (ionic) *on page 728*

Sinubid® *(Discontinued)*

Sinufed® Timecelles® *(Discontinued)* *see* guaifenesin and pseudoephedrine *on page 398*

Sinumed® *(Discontinued)* *see* acetaminophen, chlorpheniramine, and pseudoephedrine *on page 11*

Sinumist®-SR Capsulets® *(Discontinued)* *see* guaifenesin *on page 392*

Sinus-Relief® [US-OTC] *see* acetaminophen and pseudoephedrine *on page 9*

Sinutab® Non Drowsy [Can] *see* acetaminophen and pseudoephedrine *on page 9*

Sinutab® Sinus [US-OTC] *see* acetaminophen and pseudoephedrine *on page 9*

Sinutab® Sinus & Allergy [Can] *see* acetaminophen, chlorpheniramine, and pseudoephedrine *on page 11*

Sinutab® Sinus Allergy Maximum Strength [US-OTC] *see* acetaminophen, chlorpheniramine, and pseudoephedrine *on page 11*

SINUtuss® DM [US] *see* guaifenesin, dextromethorphan, and phenylephrine *on page 400*

SINUvent® PE [US] *see* guaifenesin and phenylephrine *on page 396*

Sirdalud® *(Discontinued)* *see* tizanidine *on page 831*

sirolimus (sir OH li mus)

U.S./Canadian Brand Names Rapamune® [US/Can]

Therapeutic Category Immunosuppressant Agent

Use Prophylaxis of organ rejection in patients receiving renal transplants, in combination with corticosteroids and cyclosporine (cyclosporine may be withdrawn in low-to-moderate immunological risk patients after 2-4 months, in conjunction with an increase in sirolimus dosage)

Usual Dosage

Oral:

Combination therapy with cyclosporine: Doses should be taken 4 hours after cyclosporine, and should be taken consistently either with or without food.

Children ≥13 years and Adults: Dosing by body weight:

<40 kg: Loading dose: Loading dose: 3 mg/m^2 on day 1, followed by maintenance dosing of 1 mg/m^2 once daily

≥40 kg: Loading dose: 6 mg on day 1; maintenance: 2 mg once daily

Maintenance therapy after withdrawal of cyclosporine: Following 2-4 months of combined therapy, withdrawal of cyclosporine may be considered in low-to-moderate risk patients. Cyclosporine withdrawal in not recommended in high immunological risk patients. Cyclosporine should be discontinued over 4-8 weeks, and a necessary increase in the dosage of sirolimus (up to fourfold) should be anticipated due to removal of metabolic inhibition by cyclosporine and to maintain adequate immunosuppressive effects.

Sirolimus dosages should be adjusted to maintain trough concentrations of 16-24 ng/mL for 1 year after transplant. Dosage should be adjusted at intervals of 7-14 days to account for the long half-life of sirolimus.

Dosage adjustments: New sirolimus dose **equals** current dose **multiplied by** (target concentration/current concentration). **Note:** If large dose increase is required, consider loading dose calculated as:

Loading dose **equals** (new maintenance dose **minus** current maintenance dose) **multiplied by** 3

Loading doses >40 mg may be administered over 2 days. Serum concentrations should not be used as the sole basis for dosage adjustment (monitor clinical signs/symptoms, tissue biopsy, and laboratory parameters).

Dosage Forms

Solution, oral [bottle]: 1 mg/mL (60 mL) [contains ethanol 1.5% to 2.5%; packaged with oral syringes and a carrying case]

Tablet: 1 mg, 2 mg

smallpox vaccine (SMAL poks vak SEEN)

Synonyms dried smallpox vaccine; vaccinia vaccine

U.S./Canadian Brand Names Dryvax® [US]

Therapeutic Category Vaccine

Use Active immunization against vaccinia virus, the causative agent of smallpox in persons determined to be at risk for smallpox infection. The ACIP recommends vaccination of laboratory workers at risk of exposure from cultures or contaminated animals which may be a source of vaccinia or related Orthopoxviruses capable of causing infections in humans (monkeypox, cowpox, or variola). The ACIP also recommends that consideration be given for vaccination in healthcare workers having contact with clinical specimens, contaminated material, or patients receiving vaccinia or recombinant vaccinia viruses. Revaccination is recommended every 10 years. The Armed Forces recommend vaccination of certain personnel categories. Recommendations for use in response to bioterrorism are regularly updated by the CDC, and may be found at www.cdc.gov.

Usual Dosage Not for I.M., I.V., or SubQ injection: Vaccination by scarification (multiple-puncture technique) only: **Note:** A trace of blood should appear at vaccination site after 15-20 seconds; if no trace of blood is visible, an additional 3 insertions should be made using the same needle, without reinserting the needle into the vaccine bottle.

Adults (children ≥12 months in emergency conditions only):

Primary vaccination: Use a single drop of vaccine suspension and 2 or 3 needle punctures (using the same needle) into the superficial skin

Revaccination: Use a single drop of vaccine suspension and 15 needle punctures (using the same needle) into the superficial skin

Dosage Forms Injection, powder for reconstitution [calf liver source]: ~100 million vaccinia virions per mL following reconstitution [contains polymyxin B, neomycin, dihydrostreptomycin sulfate, and chlortetracycline (trace amounts); packed with diluent, venting needle, and 100 bifurcated needles; vial stopper contains latex]

smelling salts *see* ammonia spirit (aromatic) *on page 46*

SMZ-TMP *see* sulfamethoxazole and trimethoprim *on page 797*

snake (pit vipers) antivenin *see* antivenin *(Crotalidae)* polyvalent *on page 63*

Snaplets-EX® ***(Discontinued)***

(+)-(*S*)-*N*-methyl-γ-(1-naphthyloxy)-2-thiophenepropylamine hydrochloride *see* duloxetine *on page 283*

sodium 2-mercaptoethane sulfonate *see* mesna *on page 534*

sodium 4-hydroxybutyrate *see* sodium oxybate *on page 780*

sodium *L*-triiodothyronine *see* liothyronine *on page 498*

sodium acetate (SOW dee um AS e tate)

Therapeutic Category Alkalinizing Agent; Electrolyte Supplement, Oral

Use Sodium source in large volume I.V. fluids to prevent or correct hyponatremia in patients with restricted intake; used to counter acidosis through conversion to bicarbonate

Usual Dosage Sodium acetate is metabolized to bicarbonate on an equimolar basis outside the liver; administer in large volume I.V. fluids as a sodium source. Refer to sodium bicarbonate monograph.

Maintenance electrolyte requirements of sodium in parenteral nutrition solutions:

Daily requirements: 3-4 mEq/kg/24 hours or 25-40 mEq/1000 kcal/24 hours

Maximum: 100-150 mEq/24 hours

Dosage Forms Injection, solution: 2 mEq/mL (20 mL, 50 mL, 100 mL); 4 mEq/mL (50 mL, 100 mL)

sodium acid carbonate *see* sodium bicarbonate *on this page*

sodium benzoate and caffeine *see* caffeine *on page 132*

sodium benzoate and sodium phenylacetate *see* sodium phenylacetate and sodium benzoate *on page 780*

sodium bicarbonate (SOW dee um bye KAR bun ate)

Synonyms baking soda; $NaHCO_3$; sodium acid carbonate; sodium hydrogen carbonate

U.S./Canadian Brand Names Brioschi® [US-OTC]; Neut® [US]

Therapeutic Category Alkalinizing Agent; Antacid; Electrolyte Supplement, Oral

Use Management of metabolic acidosis; gastric hyperacidity; as an alkalinization agent for the urine; treatment of hyperkalemia; management of overdose of certain drugs, including tricyclic antidepressants and aspirin

Usual Dosage

Cardiac arrest: **Routine use of $NaHCO_3$ is not recommended and should be given only after adequate alveolar ventilation has been established and effective cardiac compressions are provided**

Infants and Children: I.V.: 0.5-1 mEq/kg/dose repeated every 10 minutes or as indicated by arterial blood gases; rate of infusion should not exceed 10 mEq/minute; neonates and children <2 years of age should receive 4.2% (0.5 mEq/mL) solution

Adults: I.V.: Initial: 1 mEq/kg/dose one time; maintenance: 0.5 mEq/kg/dose every 10 minutes or as indicated by arterial blood gases

Metabolic acidosis: Infants, Children, and Adults: Dosage should be based on the following formula if blood gases and pH measurements are available:

HCO_3^-(mEq) = 0.3 x weight (kg) x base deficit (mEq/L)

Administer 1/2 dose initially, then remaining 1/2 dose over the next 24 hours; monitor pH, serum HCO_3^-, and clinical status

Note: If acid-base status is not available: Dose for older Children and Adults: 2-5 mEq/kg I.V. infusion over 4-8 hours; subsequent doses should be based on patient's acid-base status

Chronic renal failure: Oral: Initiate when plasma HCO_3^- <15 mEq/L

Children: 1-3 mEq/kg/day

Adults: Start with 20-36 mEq/day in divided doses, titrate to bicarbonate level of 18-20 mEq/L

Hyperkalemia: Adults: I.V.: 1 mEq/kg over 5 minutes

Renal tubular acidosis: Oral:

Distal:

Children: 2-3 mEq/kg/day

Adults: 0.5-2 mEq/kg/day in 4-5 divided doses

Proximal: Children and Adults: Initial: 5-10 mEq/kg/day; maintenance: Increase as required to maintain serum bicarbonate in the normal range

Urine alkalinization: Oral:

Children: 1-10 mEq (84-840 mg)/kg/day in divided doses every 4-6 hours; dose should be titrated to desired urinary pH

Adults: Initial: 48 mEq (4 g), then 12-24 mEq (1-2 g) every 4 hours; dose should be titrated to desired urinary pH; doses up to 16 g/day (200 mEq) in patients <60 years and 8 g (100 mEq) in patients >60 years

Antacid: Adults: Oral: 325 mg to 2 g 1-4 times/day

Dosage Forms

Granules, effervescent (Brioschi®): 2.69 g/packet (6 g) [unit-dose packets; contains sodium 770 mg/packet; lemon flavor]; 2.69 g/capful (120 g, 240 g) [contains sodium 770 mg/capful; lemon flavor]

Infusion [premixed in sterile water]: 5% (500 mL)

Injection, solution:

4.2% [42 mg/mL = 5 mEq/10 mL] (10 mL)

7.5% [75 mg/mL = 8.92 mEq/10 mL] (50 mL)

8.4% [84 mg/mL = 10 mEq/10 mL] (10 mL, 50 mL)

Neut®: 4% [40 mg/mL = 2.4 mEq/5 mL] (5 mL)

Powder: Sodium bicarbonate USP (120 g, 480 g) [contains sodium 30 mEq per 1/2 teaspoon]

Tablet: 325 mg [3.8 mEq]; 650 mg [7.6 mEq]

sodium cellulose phosphate *see* cellulose sodium phosphate *on page 165*

sodium chloride (SOW dee um KLOR ide)

Synonyms NaCl; normal saline; salt

U.S./Canadian Brand Names 4-Way® Saline Moisturizing Mist [US-OTC]; Altachlore [US-OTC]; Altamist [US-OTC]; Ayr® Baby Saline [US-OTC]; Ayr® Saline No-Drip [US-OTC]; Ayr® Saline [US-OTC]; Breathe Right® Saline [US-OTC]; Broncho Saline® [US-OTC]; Deep Sea [US-OTC]; Entsol® [US-OTC]; Muro 128® [US-OTC]; Mycinaire™ [US-OTC]; Na-Zone® [US-OTC]; Nasal Moist® [US-OTC]; NaSal™ [US-OTC]; Ocean® for Kids [US-OTC]; Ocean® [US-OTC]; Pretz® [US-OTC]; SalineX® [US-OTC]; Simply Saline® Baby [US-OTC]; Simply Saline® Nasal Moist® [US-OTC]; Simply Saline® [US-OTC]; Syrex [US]; Wound Wash Saline™ [US-OTC]

Therapeutic Category Electrolyte Supplement, Oral; Lubricant, Ocular

Use

Parenteral: Restores sodium ion in patients with restricted oral intake (especially hyponatremia states or low salt syndrome). In general, parenteral saline uses:

Bacteriostatic sodium chloride: Dilution or dissolving drugs for I.M., I.V., or SubQ injections

Concentrated sodium chloride: Additive for parenteral fluid therapy

Hypertonic sodium chloride: For severe hyponatremia and hypochloremia

Hypotonic sodium chloride: Hydrating solution

(Continued)

sodium chloride *(Continued)*

Normal saline: Restores water/sodium losses

Pharmaceutical aid/diluent for infusion of compatible drug additives

Ophthalmic: Reduces corneal edema

Inhalation: Restores moisture to pulmonary system; loosens and thins congestion caused by colds or allergies; diluent for bronchodilator solutions that require dilution before inhalation

Intranasal: Restores moisture to nasal membranes

Irrigation: Wound cleansing, irrigation, and flushing

Usual Dosage

Children: I.V.: Hypertonic solutions (>0.9%) should only be used for the initial treatment of acute serious symptomatic hyponatremia; maintenance: 3-4 mEq/kg/day; maximum: 100-150 mEq/day; dosage varies widely depending on clinical condition

Replacement: Determined by laboratory determinations mEq

Sodium deficiency (mEq/kg) = [% dehydration (L/kg)/100 x 70 (mEq/L)] + [0.6 (L/kg) x (140 - serum sodium) (mEq/L)]

Children ≥2 years and Adults:

Intranasal: 2-3 sprays in each nostril as needed

Irrigation: Spray affected area

Children and Adults: Inhalation: Bronchodilator diluent: 1-3 sprays (1-3 mL) to dilute bronchodilator solution in nebulizer prior to administration

Adults:

GU irrigant: 1-3 L/day by intermittent irrigation

Replacement I.V.: Determined by laboratory determinations mEq

Sodium deficiency (mEq/kg) = [% dehydration (L/kg)/100 x 70 (mEq/L)] + [0.6 (L/kg) x (140 - serum sodium) (mEq/L)]

To correct acute, serious hyponatremia: mEq sodium = [desired sodium (mEq/L) - actual sodium (mEq/L)] x [0.6 x wt (kg)]; for acute correction use 125 mEq/L as the desired serum sodium; acutely correct serum sodium in 5 mEq/L/dose increments; more gradual correction in increments of 10 mEq/L/day is indicated in the asymptomatic patient

Chloride maintenance electrolyte requirement in parenteral nutrition: 2-4 mEq/kg/24 hours or 25-40 mEq/1000 kcals/24 hours; maximum: 100-150 mEq/24 hours

Sodium maintenance electrolyte requirement in parenteral nutrition: 3-4 mEq/kg/24 hours or 25-40 mEq/1000 kcals/24 hours; maximum: 100-150 mEq/24 hours.

Ophthalmic:

Ointment: Apply once daily or more often

Solution: Instill 1-2 drops into affected eye(s) every 3-4 hours

Dosage Forms

Gel, intranasal:

Ayr® Saline No-Drip: 0.5% (22 mL) [spray gel; contains benzalkonium chloride, benzyl alcohol and soybean oil]

Ayr® Saline: 0.5% (14 g) [contains soybean oil]

Entsol®: 3% (20 g) [contains aloe, benzalkonium chloride, and vitamin E]

Simply Saline® Nasal Moist®: 0.65% (30 g)

Injection, solution [preservative free]: 0.9% (2 mL, 5 mL, 10 mL, 20 mL, 100 mL)

Injection, solution [preservative free, prefilled I.V. flush syringe]: 0.9% (2 mL, 2.5 mL, 3 mL, 5 mL, 10 mL)

Injection, solution: 0.45% (25 mL, 50 mL, 100 mL, 250 mL, 500 mL, 1000 mL); 0.9% (3 mL, 5 mL, 10 mL, 20 mL, 25 mL, 30 mL, 50 mL, 100 mL, 150 mL, 250 mL, 500 mL, 1000 mL); 3% (500 mL); 5% (500 mL)

Syrex: 0.9% (2.5 mL, 5 mL, 10 mL) [prefilled syringe]

Injection, solution [bacteriostatic]: 0.9% (10 mL, 20 mL, 30 mL) [contains benzyl alcohol]

Injection, solution [concentrate]: 14.6% (2.5 mEq/mL) (20 mL, 40 mL); 23.4% (4 mEq/mL) (30 mL, 100 mL, 200 mL, 250 mL)

Ointment, ophthalmic: 5% (3.5 g)

Altachlore, Muro 128®: 5% (3.5 g)

Powder for nasal solution (Entsol®): 3% (10.5 g)

Solution for inhalation: 0.45% (3 mL, 5 mL); 0.9% (3 mL, 5 mL, 15 mL); 3% (15 mL); 10% (15 mL)

Broncho® Saline: 0.9% (90 mL, 240 mL) [for dilution of bronchodilator solutions]

Solution, intranasal: 0.65% (45 mL)

Altamist: 0.65% (60 mL) [spray; contains benzalkonium chloride]

Ayr® Baby Saline: 0.65% (30 mL) [spray/drops; contains benzalkonium chloride]

Ayr® Saline: 0.65% (50 mL) [drops; contains benzalkonium chloride]

Ayr® Saline: 0.65% (50 mL) [mist, contains benzalkonium chloride]

Breathe Right® Saline: 0.65% (44 mL) [spray; contains benzalkonium chloride]

Deep Sea: 0.65% (45 mL) [spray; contains benzalkonium chloride]

Entsol® Mist: 3% (30 mL) [spray; contains benzalkonium chloride]
Entsol® [preservative free]: 3% (100 mL) [spray]
Entsol® [preservative free]: 3% (240 mL) [nasal wash]
Mycinaire™: 0.65% (30 mL) [mist; contains benzalkonium chloride]
Na-Zone®: 0.65% (60 mL) [spray; contains benzalkonium chloride]
NaSal™: 0.65% (15 mL) [drops; contains benzalkonium chloride], (30 mL) [spray; contains benzalkonium chloride]
Nasal Moist®: 0.65% (45 mL) [spray]
Ocean®: 0.65% (45 mL) [mist/spray/drops; contains benzalkonium chloride]; (473 mL) [refill bottle; contains benzalkonium chloride]
Ocean® for Kids: 0.65% (37.5 mL) [drops/spray/stream; contains benzalkonium chloride]
Pretz®: 0.75% (50 mL) [spray; contains benzalkonium chloride and yerba santa]; (240 mL) [irrigation; contains benzalkonium chloride and yerba santa]; (960 mL) [refill bottle; contains benzalkonium chloride and yerba santa]
SalineX®: 0.4% (15 mL) [drops]; (50 mL) [spray]
Simply Saline®: 0.9% (44 mL, 90 mL) [mist]
Simply Saline® Baby: 0.9% (45 mL) [mist]
4-Way® Saline Moisturizing Mist: 0.74% (30 mL) [alcohol free; contains benzalkonium chloride, eucalyptol, and menthol]
Solution for irrigation: 0.45% (1500 mL, 2000 mL); 0.9% (250 mL, 500 mL, 1000 mL, 1500 mL, 2000 mL, 3000 mL, 4000 mL, 5000 mL)
Wound Wash Saline™: 0.9% (90 mL, 210 mL)
Solution, ophthalmic: 5% (15 mL)
Altachlore: 5% (15 mL, 30 mL)
Muro 128®: 2% (15 mL); 5% (15 mL, 30 mL)

sodium citrate, citric acid, and potassium citrate *see* citric acid, sodium citrate, and potassium citrate *on page 195*

sodium edetate *see* edetate disodium *on page 287*

sodium etidronate *see* etidronate disodium *on page 329*

sodium ferric gluconate *see* ferric gluconate *on page 342*

sodium fluoride *see* fluoride *on page 354*

sodium fusidate *see* fusidic acid *(Canada only) on page 373*

sodium hyaluronate *see* hyaluronate and derivatives *on page 416*

sodium hyaluronate and chrondroitin sulfate *see* chondroitin sulfate and sodium hyaluronate *on page 186*

sodium hydrogen carbonate *see* sodium bicarbonate *on page 776*

sodium hypochlorite solution (SOW dee um hye poe KLOR ite soe LOO shun)

Synonyms modified Dakin's solution
U.S./Canadian Brand Names Dakin's Solution [US]; Di-Dak-Sol [US]
Therapeutic Category Disinfectant
Use Treatment of athlete's foot (0.5%); wound irrigation (0.5%); disinfection of utensils and equipment (5%)
Usual Dosage Topical irrigation
Dosage Forms Solution, topical:
Dakin's: 0.25% (480 mL); 0.5% (480 mL, 3840 mL)
Di-Dak-Sol: 0.0125% (480 mL)

sodium hyposulfate *see* sodium thiosulfate *on page 783*

sodium lactate (SOW dee um LAK tate)

Therapeutic Category Alkalinizing Agent
Use Source of bicarbonate for prevention and treatment of mild to moderate metabolic acidosis
Usual Dosage Dosage depends on degree of acidosis
Dosage Forms Injection, solution: 560 mg/mL [sodium 5 mEq and lactate 5 mEq per mL] (10 mL)

sodium nafcillin *see* nafcillin *on page 574*

sodium nitrite, sodium thiosulfate, and amyl nitrite

(SOW dee um NYE trite, SOW dee um thye oh SUL fate, & AM il NYE trite)

Synonyms amyl nitrite, sodium thiosulfate, and sodium nitrite; cyanide antidote kit; sodium thiosulfate, sodium nitrite, and amyl nitrite

U.S./Canadian Brand Names Cyanide Antidote Package [US]

Therapeutic Category Antidote

Use Treatment of cyanide poisoning

Usual Dosage Cyanide poisoning:

Children: 0.3 mL ampul of amyl nitrite is crushed every minute and vapor is inhaled for 15-30 seconds until an I.V. sodium nitrite infusion is available. Following administration of sodium nitrite I.V. 6-8 mL/m² (~0.2 mL/kg, maximum: 10 mL), inject sodium thiosulfate I.V. 7 g/m² (maximum 12.5 g) over ~10 minutes, if needed; injection of both may be repeated at ½ the original dose.

Adults: 0.3 mL ampul of amyl nitrite is crushed every minute and vapor is inhaled for 15-30 seconds until an I.V. sodium nitrite infusion is available. Following administration of 300 mg I.V. sodium nitrite, inject 12.5 g sodium thiosulfate I.V. (over ~10 minutes), if needed; injection of both may be repeated at ½ the original dose.

Dosage Forms Kit [each kit contains] (Cyanide Antidote Package):

Injection, solution:

Sodium nitrite 300 mg/10 mL (2)

Sodium thiosulfate 12.5 g/50 mL (2)

Inhalant: Amyl nitrite 0.3 mL (12)

[kit also includes disposable syringes, stomach tube, tourniquet, and instructions]

sodium nitroferricyanide *see* nitroprusside *on page 596*

sodium nitroprusside *see* nitroprusside *on page 596*

sodium oxybate (SOW dee um ox i BATE)

Synonyms gamma hydroxybutyric acid; GHB; 4-hydroxybutyrate; sodium 4-hydroxybutyrate

U.S./Canadian Brand Names Xyrem® [US/Can]

Therapeutic Category Central Nervous System Depressant

Controlled Substance C-I (illicit use); C-III (medical use)

Use Treatment of cataplexy and daytime sleepiness in patients with narcolepsy

Usual Dosage Oral: Children ≥16 years and Adults: Narcolepsy: Initial: 4.5 g/day, in 2 equal doses; first dose to be given at bedtime after the patient is in bed, and second dose to be given 2.5-4 hours later. Dose may be increased or adjusted in 2-week intervals; average dose: 6-9 g/day (maximum: 9 g/day)

Dosage Forms Solution, oral: 500 mg/mL (180 mL) [supplied in a kit containing two dosing cups and measuring device]

sodium PAS *see* aminosalicylic acid *on page 43*

sodium-PCA and lactic acid *see* lactic acid *on page 477*

sodium phenylacetate and sodium benzoate

(SOW dee um fen il AS e tate & SOW dee um BENZ oh ate)

Synonyms NAPA and NABZ; sodium benzoate and sodium phenylacetate

U.S./Canadian Brand Names Ammonul® [US]

Therapeutic Category Ammonium Detoxicant

Use Adjunct to treatment of acute hyperammonemia and encephalopathy in patients with urea cycle disorders involving partial or complete deficiencies of carbamyl-phosphate synthetase (CPS), ornithine transcarbamoylase (OTC), argininosuccinate lysase (ASL), or argininosuccinate synthetase (ASS); for use with hemodialysis in acute neonatal hyperammonemic coma, moderate-to-severe hyperammonemic encephalopathy and hyperammonemia which fails to respond to initial therapy

Usual Dosage Administer as a loading dose over 90-120 minutes, followed by an equivalent maintenance infusion given over 24 hours. Dosage based on weight and specific enzyme deficiency; therapy should continue until ammonia levels are in normal range.

≤20 kg:

CPS and OTC deficiency: Ammonul® 2.5 mL/kg and arginine 10% 2 mL/kg (provides sodium phenylacetate 250 mg/kg, sodium benzoate 250 mg/kg, and arginine hydrochloride 200 mg/kg).

ASS and ASL deficiency: Ammonul® 2.5 mL/kg and arginine 10% 6 mL/kg (provides sodium phenylacetate 250 mg/kg, sodium benzoate 250 mg/kg, and arginine hydrochloride 600 mg/kg)

Note: Pending a specific diagnosis in infants, the bolus and maintenance dose of arginine should be 6 mL/kg. If ASS or ASL are excluded as diagnostic possibilities, reduce dose of arginine to 2 mL/kg/day.

>20 kg:

CPS and OTC deficiency: Ammonul® 55 mL/m^2 and arginine 10% 2 mL/kg (provides sodium phenylacetate 5.5 g/m^2, sodium benzoate 5.5 g/m^2, and arginine hydrochloride 200 mg/kg)

ASS and ASL deficiency: Ammonul® 55 mL/m^2 and arginine 10% 6 mL/kg (provides sodium phenylacetate 5.5 g/m^2, sodium benzoate 5.5 g/m^2, and arginine hydrochloride 600 mg/kg)

Dosage Forms Injection, solution: Sodium phenylacetate 100 mg and sodium benzoate 100 mg per mL (50 mL)

sodium phenylbutyrate (SOW dee um fen il BYOO ti rate)

Synonyms ammonapse

U.S./Canadian Brand Names Buphenyl® [US]

Therapeutic Category Miscellaneous Product

Use **Orphan drug:** Adjunctive therapy in the chronic management of patients with urea cycle disorder involving deficiencies of carbamoylphosphate synthetase, ornithine transcarbamylase, or argininosuccinic acid synthetase

Usual Dosage Oral:

Powder: Patients weighing <20 kg: 450-600 mg/kg/day or 9.9-13 g/m^2/day, administered in equally divided amounts with each meal or feeding, four to six times daily; safety and efficacy of doses >20 g/day has not been established

Tablet: Children >20 kg and Adults: 450-600 mg/kg/day or 9.9-13 g/m^2/day, administered in equally divided amounts with each meal; safety and efficacy of doses >20 g/day have not been established

Dosage Forms

Powder, for oral solution: 3 g/level teaspoon (250 g) [contains sodium 125 mg/g; packaged with measuring device]

Tablet: 500 mg [contains sodium 124 mg/g]

sodium phosphate and potassium phosphate *see* potassium phosphate and sodium phosphate *on page 688*

sodium phosphates (SOW dee um FOS fates)

U.S./Canadian Brand Names Fleet Enema® [Can]; Fleet® Accu-Prep® [US-OTC]; Fleet® Enema [US-OTC]; Fleet® Phospho-Soda® Oral Laxative [Can]; Fleet® Phospho-Soda® [US-OTC]; OsmoPrep™ [US]; Visicol® [US]

Therapeutic Category Electrolyte Supplement, Oral; Laxative

Use

Oral, rectal: Short-term treatment of constipation and to evacuate the colon for rectal and bowel exams

I.V.: Source of phosphate in large volume I.V. fluids and parenteral nutrition; treatment and prevention of hypophosphatemia

Usual Dosage

Normal requirements elemental phosphorus: Oral:

0-6 months: Adequate intake: 100 mg/day
6-12 months: Adequate intake: 275 mg/day
1-3 years: RDA: 460 mg
4-8 years: RDA: 500 mg
9-18 years: RDA: 1250 mg
≥19 years: RDA: 700 mg

Hypophosphatemia: It is difficult to provide concrete guidelines for the treatment of severe hypophosphatemia because the extent of total body deficits and response to therapy are difficult to predict. Aggressive doses of phosphate may result in a transient serum elevation followed by redistribution into intracellular compartments or bone tissue. Intermittent I.V. infusion should be reserved for severe depletion situations (<1 mg/dL in adults); large doses of oral phosphate may cause diarrhea and intestinal absorption may be unreliable. I.V. solutions should be infused slowly. Use caution when mixing with calcium and magnesium, precipitate may form. The following dosages are empiric guidelines. **Note:** 1 mmol phosphate = 31 mg phosphorus; 1 mg phosphorus = 0.032 mmol phosphate

Hypophosphatemia treatment: Doses listed as mmol of phosphate:

Intermittent I.V. infusion: Acute repletion or replacement:

Children:

Low dose: 0.08 mmol/kg over 6 hours; use if losses are recent and uncomplicated

Intermediate dose: 0.16-0.24 mmol/kg over 4-6 hours; use if serum phosphorus level 0.5-1 mg/dL

High dose: 0.36 mmol/kg over 6 hours; use if serum phosphorus <0.5 mg/dL

Adults: Varying dosages: 0.15-0.3 mmol/kg/dose over 12 hours; may repeat as needed to achieve desired serum level **or**

15 mmol/dose over 2 hours; use if serum phosphorus <2 mg/dL **or**

(Continued)

sodium phosphates *(Continued)*

Low dose: 0.16 mmol/kg over 4-6 hours; use if serum phosphorus level 2.3-3 mg/dL
Intermediate dose: 0.32 mmol/kg over 4-6 hours; use if serum phosphorus level 1.6-2.2 mg/dL
High dose: 0.64 mmol/kg over 8-12 hours; use if serum phosphorus <1.5 mg/dL

Oral: Adults: 0.5-1 g elemental phosphorus 2-3 times/day may be used when serum phosphorus level is 1-2.5 mg/dL

Maintenance: Doses listed as mmol of phosphate:

Children:
Oral: 2-3 mmol/kg/day in divided doses
I.V.: 0.5-1.5 mmol/kg/day

Adults:
Oral: 50-150 mmol/day in divided doses
I.V.: 50-70 mmol/day

Laxative (Fleet®): Rectal:
Children 2-<5 years: One-half contents of one 2.25 oz pediatric enema
Children 5-12 years: Contents of one 2.25 oz pediatric enema, may repeat
Children ≥12 years and Adults: Contents of one 4.5 oz enema as a single dose, may repeat

Laxative (Fleet® Phospho-Soda®): Oral: Take on an empty stomach; dilute dose with 8 ounces cool water, then follow dose with 8 ounces water; **do not repeat dose within 24 hours**
Children 5-9 years: 7.5 mL as a single dose; maximum daily dose: 7.5 mL
Children 10-12 years: 15 mL as a single dose; maximum daily dose: 15 mL
Children ≥12 years and Adults: 15 mL as a single dose; maximum daily dose: 45 mL

Bowel cleansing prior to colonoscopy: Adults: **Note:** Each dose should be taken with a minimum of 8 ounces of clear liquids. Do not repeat treatment within 7 days. Do not use additional agents, especially sodium phosphate products.

Fleet® Phospho-Soda®: Oral: Prior to procedure (timing of doses determined by prescriber): One dose is equal to 45 mL (2 doses are recommended): Each dose is diluted as follows:
Mix 45 mL with 120 mL clear liquid; drink, then follow with at least 240 mL of clear liquid; **or**
Mix 15 mL with 240 mL clear liquid; drink, then follow with 240 mL clear liquid; repeat every 10 minutes for a total of 45 mL

Visicol™: Oral: Adults: A total of 40 tablets divided as follows:
Evening before colonoscopy: 3 tablets every 15 minutes for 6 doses, then 2 additional tablets in 15 minutes (total of 20 tablets)
3-5 hours prior to colonoscopy: 3 tablets every 15 minutes for 6 doses, then 2 additional tablets in 15 minutes (total of 20 tablets)

OsmoPrep™: A total of 32 tablets divided as follows:
Evening before colonoscopy: 4 tablets every 15 minutes for 5 doses (total of 20 tablets)
3-5 hours prior to colonoscopy: 4 tablets every 15 minutes for 3 doses (total of 12 tablets)

Dosage Forms

Kit:
Fleet® Accu-Prep®:
Solution, oral (Fleet® Phosph-Soda®): Monobasic sodium phosphate monohydrate 2.4 g and dibasic sodium phosphate heptahydrate 0.9 g per 5 mL (15 mL) [contains contains sodium 556 mg/5 mL, phosphate 62.25 mEq/5 mL and sodium benzoate; kit contains six 15 mL unit-dose containers (equal to two 45 mL doses)]
Pads, anorectal (Fleet® Relief™): Pramoxine hydrochloride 1% and glycerin 12% (4s)

Injection, solution [preservative free]: Phosphorus 3 mmol and sodium 4 mEq per mL (5 mL, 15 mL, 50 mL)

Solution, oral:
Fleet® Phospho-Soda®: Monobasic sodium phosphate monohydrate 2.4 g and dibasic sodium phosphate heptahydrate 0.9 g per 5 mL (45 mL) [sugar free; contains sodium 556 mg/5 mL, sodium benzoate, and phosphate 62.25 mEq/5 mL; unflavored or ginger-lemon flavor]

Solution, rectal [enema]: Monobasic sodium phosphate 19 g and dibasic sodium phosphate 7 g per 118 mL delivered dose (135 mL)
Fleet® Enema: Monobasic sodium phosphate 19 g and dibasic sodium phosphate 7 g per 118 mL delivered dose (135 mL)
Fleet® Enema for Children: Monobasic sodium phosphate 9.5 g and dibasic sodium phosphate 3.5 g per 59 mL delivered dose (68 mL)

Tablet, oral:
OsmoPrep™: Sodium phosphate monobasic monohydrate 1.102 g and sodium phosphate dibasic anhydrous 0.398 g [sodium phosphate 1.5 g per tablet; gluten free]
Visicol®: Sodium phosphate monobasic monohydrate 1.102 g and sodium phosphate dibasic anhydrous 0.398 g [sodium phosphate 1.5 g per tablet]

sodium polystyrene sulfonate (SOW dee um pol ee STYE reen SUL fon ate)

Sound-Alike/Look-Alike Issues

Kayexalate® may be confused with Kaopectate®

U.S./Canadian Brand Names Kayexalate® [US/Can]; Kionex™ [US]; PMS-Sodium Polystyrene Sulfonate [Can]; SPS® [US]

Therapeutic Category Antidote

Use Treatment of hyperkalemia

Usual Dosage

Children:

Oral: 1 g/kg/dose every 6 hours

Rectal: 1 g/kg/dose every 2-6 hours (In small children and infants, employ lower doses by using the practical exchange ratio of 1 mEq K^+/g of resin as the basis for calculation)

Adults: Hyperkalemia:

Oral: 15 g (60 mL) 1-4 times/day

Rectal: 30-50 g every 6 hours

Dosage Forms

Powder for suspension, oral/rectal:

Kayexalate®: 15 g/4 level teaspoons (480 g) [contains sodium 100 mg (4.1 mEq)/g]

Kionex™: 15 g/4 level teaspoons (454 g) [contains sodium 100 mg (4.1 mEq)/g]

Suspension, oral/rectal: 15 g/60 mL (60 mL, 120 mL, 200 mL, 500 mL) [contains sodium 1500 mg (65 mEq)/60 mL, sorbitol, and alcohol 0.1%; cherry/caramel flavor]

SPS®: 15 g/60 mL (60 mL, 120 mL, 480 mL) [contains alcohol 0.3%, sodium 1500 mg (65 mEq)/60 mL, and sorbitol; cherry flavor]

sodium sulfacetamide *see* sulfacetamide *on page 795*

sodium sulfacetamide and sulfur *see* sulfur and sulfacetamide *on page 800*

sodium tetradecyl (SOW dee um tetra DEK il)

Synonyms sodium tetradecyl sulfate

U.S./Canadian Brand Names Sotradecol® [US]; Trombovar® [Can]

Therapeutic Category Sclerosing Agent

Use Treatment of small, uncomplicated varicose veins of the lower extremities

Usual Dosage I.V.: Test dose: 0.5 mL given several hours prior to administration of larger dose; 0.5-2 mL (preferred maximum: 1 mL) in each vein, maximum: 10 mL per treatment session; 3% solution reserved for large varices

Dosage Forms Injection, as sulfate: 1% [10 mg/mL] (2 mL) [contains benzyl alcohol]; 3% [30 mg/mL] (2 mL) [contains benzyl alcohol]

sodium tetradecyl sulfate *see* sodium tetradecyl *on this page*

sodium thiosulfate (SOW dee um thye oh SUL fate)

Synonyms disodium thiosulfate pentahydrate; pentahydrate; sodium hyposulfate; sodium thiosulphate; thiosulfuric acid disodium salt

U.S./Canadian Brand Names Versiclear™ [US]

Therapeutic Category Antidote; Antifungal Agent

Use

Parenteral: Used alone or with sodium nitrite or amyl nitrite in cyanide poisoning; reduce the risk of nephrotoxicity associated with cisplatin therapy

Topical: Treatment of tinea versicolor

Usual Dosage

Cyanide and nitroprusside antidote: I.V.:

Children <25 kg: 50 mg/kg after receiving 4.5-10 mg/kg sodium nitrite; a half dose of each may be repeated if necessary

Children >25 kg and Adults: 12.5 g after 300 mg of sodium nitrite; a half dose of each may be repeated if necessary

Cyanide poisoning: I.V.: Dose should be based on determination as with nitrite, at rate of 2.5-5 mL/minute to maximum of 50 mL.

Cisplatin rescue should be given before or during cisplatin administration: I.V. infusion (in sterile water): 12 g/m^2 over 6 hours or 9 g/m^2 I.V. push followed by 1.2 g/m^2 continuous infusion for 6 hours

Tinea versicolor: Children and Adults: Topical: 20% to 25% solution: Apply a thin layer to affected areas twice daily

(Continued)

sodium thiosulfate *(Continued)*

Dosage Forms

Injection, solution [preservative free]: 100 mg/mL (10 mL); 250 mg/mL (50 mL)

Lotion: Sodium thiosulfate 25% and salicylic acid 1% (120 mL) [contains isopropyl alcohol 10%]

sodium thiosulfate, sodium nitrite, and amyl nitrite *see* sodium nitrite, sodium thiosulfate, and amyl nitrite *on page 780*

sodium thiosulphate *see* sodium thiosulfate *on previous page*

Soflax™ [Can] *see* docusate *on page 270*

Sofra-Tulle® [Can] *see* framycetin *(Canada only) on page 370*

Solagé™ [US/Can] *see* mequinol and tretinoin *on page 532*

Solaquin® [US-OTC/Can] *see* hydroquinone *on page 430*

Solaquin Forte® [US] *see* hydroquinone *on page 430*

Solaraze® [US] *see* diclofenac *on page 250*

Solarcaine® Aloe Extra Burn Relief [US-OTC] *see* lidocaine *on page 493*

Solfoton® *(Discontinued)* *see* phenobarbital *on page 658*

Solia™ [US] *see* ethinyl estradiol and desogestrel *on page 317*

solifenacin (sol i FEN a sin)

Synonyms solifenacin succinate

U.S./Canadian Brand Names VESIcare® [US]

Therapeutic Category Anticholinergic Agent

Use Treatment of overactive bladder with symptoms of urinary frequency, urgency, or urge incontinence

Usual Dosage Oral:

Children: Use is not recommended.

Adults: 5 mg/day; if tolerated, may increase to 10 mg/day

Dosage Forms Tablet: 5 mg, 10 mg

solifenacin succinate *see* solifenacin *on this page*

Solodyn™ [US] *see* minocycline *on page 558*

Soltamox™ [US] *see* tamoxifen *on page 804*

soluble fluorescein *see* fluorescein sodium *on page 354*

Solu-Cortef® [US/Can] *see* hydrocortisone (systemic) *on page 427*

Solugel® [Can] *see* benzoyl peroxide *on page 102*

Solu-Medrol® [US/Can] *see* methylprednisolone *on page 547*

Soluver® [Can] *see* salicylic acid *on page 758*

Soluver® Plus [Can] *see* salicylic acid *on page 758*

Soluvite-F [US] *see* vitamins (multiple/pediatric) *on page 878*

Soma® [US/Can] *see* carisoprodol *on page 152*

Soma® Compound [US] *see* carisoprodol and aspirin *on page 152*

Soma® Compound w/Codeine [US] *see* carisoprodol, aspirin, and codeine *on page 152*

somatostatin *(Canada only)* (soe mat oh STA tin)

U.S./Canadian Brand Names Stilamin® [Can]

Therapeutic Category Variceal Bleeding (Acute) Agent

Use For the symptomatic treatment of acute bleeding from esophageal varices. Other treatment options for long-term management of the condition may be considered if necessary, once initial control has been established.

Usual Dosage Slow 250 mcg I.V. bolus injection over 3 to 5 minutes, followed by a continuous infusion at a rate of 250 mcg/hour until bleeding from the varices has stopped (usually within 12 to 24 hours). Once bleeding has been controlled, it is recommended that the infusion be continued for at least another 48 to 72 hours, or out to a maximum of 120 hours to prevent recurrent bleeding.

Dosage Forms Injection: 250 mcg, 3 mg

somatrem *see* somatropin *on next page*

somatropin (soe ma TROE pin)

Sound-Alike/Look-Alike Issues

somatropin may be confused with somatrem, sumatriptan
somatrem may be confused with somatropin

Synonyms hGH; human growth hormone; somatrem

U.S./Canadian Brand Names Genotropin Miniquick® [US]; Genotropin® [US]; Humatrope® [US/Can]; Norditropin® NordiFlex® [US]; Norditropin® [US]; Nutropin AQ® [US]; Nutropine® [Can]; Nutropin® AQ [Can]; Nutropin® [US]; Omnitrope™ [US]; Saizen® [US/Can]; Serostim® [US/Can]; Tev-Tropin™ [US]; Zorbtive™ [US]

Therapeutic Category Growth Hormone

Use

Children:

Long-term treatment of growth failure due to inadequate endogenous growth hormone secretion (Genotropin®, Humatrope®, Norditropin®, Nutropin®, Nutropin AQ®, Omnitrope™, Saizen®, Tev-Tropin™)

Long-term treatment of short stature associated with Turner syndrome (Genotropin®, Humatrope®, Nutropin®, Nutropin AQ®)

Treatment of Prader-Willi syndrome (Genotropin®)

Treatment of growth failure associated with chronic renal insufficiency (CRI) up until the time of renal transplantation (Nutropin®, Nutropin AQ®)

Long-term treatment of growth failure in children born small for gestational age who fail to manifest catch-up growth by 2 years of age (Genotropin®)

Long-term treatment of idiopathic short stature (nongrowth hormone-deficient short stature) defined by height standard deviation score (SDS) less than or equal to -2.25 and growth rate not likely to attain normal adult height (Humatrope®, Nutropin®, Nutropin AQ®)

Adults:

AIDS-wasting or cachexia with concomitant antiviral therapy (Serostim®)

Replacement of endogenous growth hormone in patients with adult growth hormone deficiency who meet both of the following criteria (Genotropin®, Humatrope®, Norditropin®, Nutropin®, Nutropin AQ®, Omnitrope™, Saizen®):

Biochemical diagnosis of adult growth hormone deficiency by means of a subnormal response to a standard growth hormone stimulation test (peak growth hormone ≤5 mcg/L)

and

Adult-onset: Patients who have adult growth hormone deficiency whether alone or with multiple hormone deficiencies (hypopituitarism) as a result of pituitary disease, hypothalamic disease, surgery, radiation therapy, or trauma

or

Childhood-onset: Patients who were growth hormone deficient during childhood, confirmed as an adult before replacement therapy is initiated

Treatment of short-bowel syndrome (Zorbtive™)

Usual Dosage

Children (individualize dose):

Growth hormone deficiency:

Genotropin®, Omnitrope™: SubQ: Weekly dosage: 0.16-0.24 mg/kg divided into 6-7 doses

Humatrope®: I.M., SubQ: Weekly dosage: 0.18 mg/kg; maximum replacement dose: 0.3 mg/kg/week; dosing should be divided into equal doses given 3 times/week on alternating days, 6 times/week, or daily

Norditropin®: SubQ: 0.024-0.034 mg/kg/day, 6-7 times/week

Nutropin®, Nutropin® AQ: SubQ: Weekly dosage: 0.3 mg/kg divided into daily doses; pubertal patients: ≤0.7 mg/kg/week divided daily

Tev-Tropin™: SubQ: Up to 0.1 mg/kg administered 3 times/week

Saizen®: I.M., SubQ: 0.06 mg/kg/dose administered 3 times/week

Note: Therapy should be discontinued when patient has reached satisfactory adult height, when epiphyses have fused, or when the patient ceases to respond. Growth of 5 cm/year or more is expected, if growth rate does not exceed 2.5 cm in a 6-month period, double the dose for the next 6 months; if there is still no satisfactory response, discontinue therapy

Chronic renal insufficiency (CRI): Nutropin®, Nutropin® AQ: SubQ: Weekly dosage: 0.35 mg/kg divided into daily injections; continue until the time of renal transplantation

Dosage recommendations in patients treated for CRI who require dialysis:

Hemodialysis: Administer dose at night prior to bedtime or at least 3-4 hours after hemodialysis to prevent hematoma formation from heparin

CCPD: Administer dose in the morning following dialysis

CAPD: Administer dose in the evening at the time of overnight exchange

(Continued)

somatropin *(Continued)*

Turner syndrome:

Genotropin®: SubQ: Weekly dosage: 0.33 mg/kg divided into 6-7 doses

Humatrope®, Nutropin®, Nutropin® AQ: SubQ: Weekly dosage: ≤0.375 mg/kg divided into equal doses 3-7 times per week

Prader-Willi syndrome: Genotropin®: SubQ: Weekly dosage: 0.24 mg/kg divided into 6-7 doses

Small for gestational age: Genotropin®: SubQ: Weekly dosage: 0.48 mg/kg divided into 6-7 doses

Idiopathic short stature:

Humatrope®: SubQ: Weekly dosage: 0.37 mg/kg divided into equal doses 6-7 times per week

Nutropin®, Nutropin AQ®: SubQ: Weekly dosage: Up to 0.3 mg/kg divided into daily doses

Adults:

Growth hormone deficiency: To minimize adverse events in older or overweight patients, reduced dosages may be necessary. During therapy, dosage should be decreased if required by the occurrence of side effects or excessive IGF-I levels.

Norditropin®: SubQ: Initial dose ≤0.004 mg/kg/day; after 6 weeks of therapy, may increase dose to 0.016 mg/kg/day

Nutropin®, Nutropin® AQ: SubQ: ≤0.006 mg/kg/day; dose may be increased according to individual requirements, up to a maximum of 0.025 mg/kg/day in patients <35 years of age, or up to a maximum of 0.0125 mg/kg/day in patients ≥35 years of age

Humatrope®: SubQ: ≤0.006 mg/kg/day; dose may be increased according to individual requirements, up to a maximum of 0.0125 mg/kg/day

Genotropin®, Omnitrope™: SubQ: Weekly dosage: ≤0.04 mg/kg divided into 6-7 doses; dose may be increased at 4- to 8-week intervals according to individual requirements, to a maximum of 0.08 mg/kg/week

Saizen®: SubQ: ≤0.005 mg/kg/day; dose may be increased to not more than 0.01 mg/kg/day after 4 weeks, based on individual requirements.

AIDS-wasting or cachexia:

Serostim®: SubQ: Dose should be given once daily at bedtime; patients who continue to lose weight after 2 weeks should be re-evaluated for opportunistic infections or other clinical events; rotate injection sites to avoid lipodystrophy

Daily dose based on body weight:

<35 kg: 0.1 mg/kg

35-45 kg: 4 mg

45-55 kg: 5 mg

>55 kg: 6 mg

Short-bowel syndrome (Zorbtive™): SubQ: 0.1 mg/kg once daily for 4 weeks (maximum: 8 mg/day)

Fluid retention (moderate) or arthralgias: Treat symptomatically or reduce dose by 50%

Severe toxicity: Discontinue therapy for up to 5 days; when symptoms resolve, restart at 50% of dose. If severe toxicity recurs or does not disappear within 5 days after discontinuation, permanently discontinue treatment.

Dosage Forms

Injection, powder for reconstitution [rDNA origin]:

Genotropin®: 5.8 mg [15 units/mL; delivers 5 mg/mL]; 13.8 mg [36 int units/mL; delivers 12 mg/mL]

Genotropin Miniquick® [preservative free]: 0.2 mg, 0.4 mg, 0.6 mg, 0.8 mg, 1 mg, 1.2 mg, 1.4 mg, 1.6 mg, 1.8 mg, 2 mg [each strength delivers 0.25 mL]

Humatrope®: 5 mg [~15 int. units], 6 mg [18 int. units], 12 mg [36 int. units], 24 mg [72 int. units]

Nutropin®: 5 mg [~15 int. units; packaged with diluent containing benzyl alcohol]; 10 mg [~30 int. units; packaged with diluent containing benzyl alcohol]

Omnitrope™: 1.5 mg [~4.5 int. units; packaged with preservative free diluent]; 5.8 mg [~17.4 int. units; packaged with diluent containing benzyl alcohol]

Tev-Tropin™: 5 mg [15 int. units/mL; packaged with diluent containing benzyl alcohol]

Saizen®: 5 mg [~15 int. units; contains sucrose 34.2 mg; packaged with diluent containing benzyl alcohol]; 8.8 mg [~26.4 int. units; contains sucrose 60.2 mg; packaged with diluent containing benzyl alcohol]

Serostim®: 4 mg [12 int. units; contains sucrose 27.3 mg]; 5 mg [15 int. units; contains sucrose 34.2 mg]; 6 mg [18 int. units; contains sucrose 41 mg]

Zorbtive™: 8.8 mg [~26.4 int. units; contains sucrose 60.19 mg; packaged with diluent containing benzyl alcohol]

Injection, solution [rDNA origin]:

Norditropin®: 5 mg/1.5 mL (1.5 mL); 15 mg/1.5 mL (1.5 mL) [cartridge]

Norditropin® NordiFlex®: 5 mg/1.5 mL (1.5 mL); 15 mg/1.5 mL (1.5 mL) [prefilled pen]

Nutropin AQ®: 5 mg/mL (2 mL) [~15 int. units/mL; vial or cartridge]

Somavert® [US] *see* pegvisomant *on page 645*

Sominex® [US-OTC] *see* diphenhydramine *on page 261*

Sominex® Maximum Strength [US-OTC] *see* diphenhydramine *on page 261*

Somnote™ [US] *see* chloral hydrate *on page 171*

Som Pam [Can] *see* flurazepam *on page 359*

Sonata® [US/Can] *see* zaleplon *on page 884*

sorafenib (sor AF e nib)

Synonyms BAY 43-9006; sorafenib tosylate

U.S./Canadian Brand Names Nexavar® [US]

Therapeutic Category Antineoplastic Agent, Tyrosine Kinase Inhibitor; Vascular Endothelial Growth Factor (VEGF) Inhibitor

Use Treatment of advanced renal cell cancer

Usual Dosage Oral: Adults: Advanced renal cell carcinoma: 400 mg twice daily

Dosage Forms Tablet, as tosylate: 200 mg

sorafenib tosylate *see* sorafenib *on this page*

sorbitol (SOR bi tole)

Therapeutic Category Genitourinary Irrigant; Laxative

Use Genitourinary irrigant in transurethral prostatic resection or other transurethral resection or other transurethral surgical procedures; diuretic; humectant; sweetening agent; hyperosmotic laxative; facilitate the passage of sodium polystyrene sulfonate through the intestinal tract

Usual Dosage Hyperosmotic laxative (as single dose, at infrequent intervals):

Children 2-11 years:

Oral: 2 mL/kg (as 70% solution)

Rectal enema: 30-60 mL as 25% to 30% solution

Children >12 years and Adults:

Oral: 30-150 mL (as 70% solution)

Rectal enema: 120 mL as 25% to 30% solution

Adjunct to sodium polystyrene sulfonate: 15 mL as 70% solution orally until diarrhea occurs (10-20 mL/2 hours) or 20-100 mL as an oral vehicle for the sodium polystyrene sulfonate resin

When administered with charcoal:

Oral:

Children: 4.3 mL/kg of 35% sorbitol with 1 g/kg of activated charcoal

Adults: 4.3 mL/kg of 70% sorbitol with 1 g/kg of activated charcoal every 4 hours until first stool containing charcoal is passed

Topical: 3% to 3.3% as transurethral surgical procedure irrigation

Dosage Forms

Solution, genitourinary irrigation: 3% (3000 mL, 5000 mL); 3.3% (2000 mL, 4000 mL)

Solution, oral: 70% (30 mL, 480 mL, 3840 mL)

Sorbitrate® *(Discontinued)* *see* isosorbide dinitrate *on page 465*

Soriatane® [US/Can] *see* acitretin *on page 16*

Sorine® [US] *see* sotalol *on this page*

Sotacor® [Can] *see* sotalol *on this page*

sotalol (SOE ta lole)

Sound-Alike/Look-Alike Issues

sotalol may be confused with Stadol®

Betapace® may be confused with Betapace AF®

Betapace AF® may be confused with Betapace®

Synonyms sotalol hydrochloride

U.S./Canadian Brand Names Alti-Sotalol [Can]; Apo-Sotalol® [Can]; Betapace AF® [US/Can]; Betapace® [US]; CO Sotalol [Can]; Gen-Sotalol [Can]; Lin-Sotalol [Can]; Novo-Sotalol [Can]; Nu-Sotalol [Can]; PMS-Sotalol [Can]; Rho®-Sotalol [Can]; Riva-Sotalol [Can]; Rylosol [Can]; Sorine® [US]; Sotacor® [Can]

Therapeutic Category Antiarrhythmic Agent, Class II; Antiarrhythmic Agent, Class III; Beta-Adrenergic Blocker, Nonselective

Use Treatment of documented ventricular arrhythmias (ie, sustained ventricular tachycardia), that in the judgment of the physician are life-threatening; maintenance of normal sinus rhythm in patients with

(Continued)

sotalol *(Continued)*

symptomatic atrial fibrillation and atrial flutter who are currently in sinus rhythm. Manufacturer states substitutions should not be made for Betapace AF® since Betapace AF® is distributed with a patient package insert specific for atrial fibrillation/flutter.

Usual Dosage Sotalol should be initiated and doses increased in a hospital with facilities for cardiac rhythm monitoring and assessment. Proarrhythmic events can occur after initiation of therapy and with each upward dosage adjustment.

Children: Oral: The safety and efficacy of sotalol in children have not been established

Note: Dosing per manufacturer, based on pediatric pharmacokinetic data; wait at least 36 hours between dosage adjustments to allow monitoring of QT intervals

≤2 years: Dosage should be adjusted (decreased) by plotting of the child's age on a logarithmic scale; refer to manufacturer's package labeling.

>2 years: Initial: 90 mg/m^2/day in 3 divided doses; may be incrementally increased to a maximum of 180 mg/m^2/day

Adults: Oral:

Ventricular arrhythmias (Betapace®, Sorine®):

Initial: 80 mg twice daily

Dose may be increased gradually to 240-320 mg/day; allow 3 days between dosing increments in order to attain steady-state plasma concentrations and to allow monitoring of QT intervals

Most patients respond to a total daily dose of 160-320 mg/day in 2-3 divided doses.

Some patients, with life-threatening refractory ventricular arrhythmias, may require doses as high as 480-640 mg/day; however, these doses should only be prescribed when the potential benefit outweighs the increased of adverse events.

Atrial fibrillation or atrial flutter (Betapace AF®): Initial: 80 mg twice daily

If the initial dose does not reduce the frequency of relapses of atrial fibrillation/flutter and is tolerated without excessive QT prolongation (not >520 msec) after 3 days, the dose may be increased to 120 mg twice daily. This may be further increased to 160 mg twice daily if response is inadequate and QT prolongation is not excessive.

Dosage Forms

Tablet, as hydrochloride: 80 mg, 80 mg [AF], 120 mg, 120 mg [AF], 160 mg, 160 mg [AF], 240 mg

Betapace® [light blue]: 80 mg, 120 mg, 160 mg, 240 mg

Betapace AF® [white]: 80 mg, 120 mg, 160 mg

Sorine® [white]: 80 mg, 120 mg, 160 mg, 240 mg

sotalol hydrochloride *see* sotalol *on previous page*

Sotradecol® [US] *see* sodium tetradecyl *on page 783*

Sotret® [US] *see* isotretinoin *on page 466*

Soyacal® ***(Discontinued)*** *see* fat emulsion *on page 336*

Soyalac® [US-OTC] *see* nutritional formula, enteral/oral *on page 608*

SPA *see* albumin *on page 22*

Spacol ***(Discontinued)*** *see* hyoscyamine *on page 434*

Spacol T/S ***(Discontinued)*** *see* hyoscyamine *on page 434*

Span-FF® ***(Discontinued)*** *see* ferrous fumarate *on page 342*

Spasmolin® ***(Discontinued)*** *see* hyoscyamine, atropine, scopolamine, and phenobarbital *on page 435*

SPD417 *see* carbamazepine *on page 144*

Spectazole® [US/Can] *see* econazole *on page 286*

Spec-T® ***(Discontinued)*** *see* benzocaine *on page 99*

spectinomycin (spek ti noe MYE sin)

Sound-Alike/Look-Alike Issues

Trobicin® may be confused with tobramycin

Synonyms spectinomycin hydrochloride

Therapeutic Category Antibiotic, Miscellaneous

Use Treatment of uncomplicated gonorrhea

Usual Dosage I.M.:

Children:

<45 kg: 40 mg/kg/dose 1 time (ceftriaxone preferred)

≥45 kg: Refer to adult dosing.

Children >8 years who are allergic to PCNS/cephalosporins may be treated with oral tetracycline

Adults:

Uncomplicated urethral, cervical, pharyngeal, or rectal gonorrhea: 2 g deep I.M. or 4 g where antibiotic resistance is prevalent 1 time; 4 g (10 mL) dose should be given as two 5 mL injections, followed by adequate chlamydial treatment (doxycycline 100 mg twice daily for 7 days)

Disseminated gonococcal infection: 2 g every 12 hours

Dosage Forms

Injection, powder for reconstitution, as hydrochloride:

Trobicin®: 2 g [diluent contains benzyl alcohol] [DSC]

spectinomycin hydrochloride *see* spectinomycin *on previous page*

Spectracef™ [US] *see* cefditoren *on page 157*

Spectrocin Plus™ [US-OTC] *see* bacitracin, neomycin, polymyxin B, and pramoxine *on page 91*

SPI 0211 *see* lubiprostone *on page 509*

Spiriva® [US/Can] *see* tiotropium *on page 830*

Spironazide® ***(Discontinued)*** *see* hydrochlorothiazide and spironolactone *on page 420*

spironolactone (speer on oh LAK tone)

Sound-Alike/Look-Alike Issues

Aldactone® may be confused with Aldactazide®

U.S./Canadian Brand Names Aldactone® [US/Can]; Novo-Spiroton [Can]

Therapeutic Category Diuretic, Potassium Sparing

Use Management of edema associated with excessive aldosterone excretion; hypertension; congestive heart failure; primary hyperaldosteronism; hypokalemia; cirrhosis of liver accompanied by edema or ascites

Usual Dosage To reduce delay in onset of effect, a loading dose of 2 or 3 times the daily dose may be administered on the first day of therapy. Adults: Oral:

Edema, hypokalemia: 25-200 mg/day in 1-2 divided doses

Hypertension (JNC 7): 25-50 mg/day in 1-2 divided doses

Diagnosis of primary aldosteronism: 100-400 mg/day in 1-2 divided doses

CHF, severe (with ACE inhibitor and a loop diuretic ± digoxin): 12.5-25 mg/day; maximum daily dose: 50 mg (higher doses may occasionallly be used). In the RALES trial, 25 mg every other day was the lowest maintenance dose possible.

Note: If potassium >5.4 mEq/L, consider dosage reduction.

Dosage Forms Tablet: 25 mg, 50 mg, 100 mg

spironolactone and hydrochlorothiazide *see* hydrochlorothiazide and spironolactone *on page 420*

Spirozide® ***(Discontinued)*** *see* hydrochlorothiazide and spironolactone *on page 420*

Sporanox® [US/Can] *see* itraconazole *on page 467*

Sportscreme® [US-OTC] *see* trolamine *on page 855*

Sprintec™ [US] *see* ethinyl estradiol and norgestimate *on page 325*

Sprycel™ [US] *see* dasatinib *on page 231*

SPS® [US] *see* sodium polystyrene sulfonate *on page 783*

SRC® Expectorant ***(Discontinued)*** *see* hydrocodone, pseudoephedrine, and guaifenesin *on page 425*

SSD® [US] *see* silver sulfadiazine *on page 772*

SSD® AF [US] *see* silver sulfadiazine *on page 772*

SSKI® [US] *see* potassium iodide *on page 686*

S.T. 37® [US-OTC] *see* hexylresorcinol *on page 414*

Stadol® [US] *see* butorphanol *on page 130*

Stadol® NS ***(Discontinued)*** *see* butorphanol *on page 130*

Staflex [US] *see* acetaminophen and phenyltoloxamine *on page 8*

Stagesic® [US] *see* hydrocodone and acetaminophen *on page 420*

Stalevo™ [US] *see* levodopa, carbidopa, and entacapone *on page 489*

StanGard® [US] *see* fluoride *on page 354*

StanGard® Perio [US] *see* fluoride *on page 354*

stannous fluoride *see* fluoride *on page 354*

stanozolol (stan OH zoe lole)

U.S./Canadian Brand Names Winstrol® [US]

Therapeutic Category Anabolic Steroid

Controlled Substance C-III

Use Prophylactic use against hereditary angioedema

Usual Dosage

Children: Acute attacks:

<6 years: 1 mg/day

6-12 years: 2 mg/day

Adults: Oral: Initial: 2 mg 3 times/day, may then reduce to a maintenance dose of 2 mg/day or 2 mg every other day after 1-3 months

Dosage Forms Tablet: 2 mg

Starlix® [US/Can] *see* nateglinide *on page 580*

Starnoc® [Can] *see* zaleplon *on page 884*

Statex® [Can] *see* morphine sulfate *on page 565*

Staticin® *(Discontinued)* *see* erythromycin *on page 303*

Statobex® [Can] *see* phendimetrazine *on page 657*

stavudine (STAV yoo deen)

Sound-Alike/Look-Alike Issues

Zerit® may be confused with Ziac®

Synonyms d4T

U.S./Canadian Brand Names Zerit® [US/Can]

Therapeutic Category Antiviral Agent

Use Treatment of HIV infection in combination with other antiretroviral agents

Usual Dosage Oral:

Newborns (Birth to 13 days): 0.5 mg/kg every 12 hours

Children:

>14 days and <30 kg: 1 mg/kg every 12 hours

≥30 kg: Refer to Adults dosing

Adults:

≥60 kg: 40 mg every 12 hours

<60 kg: 30 mg every 12 hours

Dosage Forms

Capsule: 15 mg, 20 mg, 30 mg, 40 mg

Powder, for oral solution: 1 mg/mL (200 mL) [dye free; fruit flavor]

Stelazine® *(Discontinued)* *see* trifluoperazine *on page 849*

Stemetil® [Can] *see* prochlorperazine *on page 701*

Sterapred® [US] *see* prednisone *on page 695*

Sterapred® DS [US] *see* prednisone *on page 695*

STI571 *see* imatinib *on page 441*

Stilamin® [Can] *see* somatostatin *(Canada only) on page 784*

Stimate™ [US] *see* desmopressin acetate *on page 237*

Sting-Kill [US-OTC] *see* benzocaine *on page 99*

St. Joseph® Adult Aspirin [US-OTC] *see* aspirin *on page 77*

St. Joseph® Cough Suppressant *(Discontinued)* *see* dextromethorphan *on page 245*

St. Joseph® Measured Dose Nasal Solution *(Discontinued)* *see* phenylephrine *on page 660*

Stop® [US] *see* fluoride *on page 354*

Strattera® [US/Can] *see* atomoxetine *on page 81*

Streptase® [US/Can] *see* streptokinase *on next page*

streptokinase (strep toe KYE nase)

Synonyms SK

U.S./Canadian Brand Names Streptase® [US/Can]

Therapeutic Category Fibrinolytic Agent

Use Thrombolytic agent used in treatment of recent severe or massive deep vein thrombosis, pulmonary emboli, myocardial infarction, and occluded arteriovenous cannulas

Usual Dosage I.V.:

Children: Safety and efficacy have not been not established. Limited studies have used 3500-4000 units/kg over 30 minutes followed by 1000-1500 units/kg/hour.

Clotted catheter: I.V.: **Note:** Not recommended due to possibility of allergic reactions with repeated doses: 10,000-25,000 units diluted in NS to a final volume equivalent to catheter volume; instill into catheter and leave in place for 1 hour, then aspirate contents out of catheter and flush catheter with normal saline.

Adults: Antibodies to streptokinase remain for at least 3-6 months after initial dose: Administration requires the use of an infusion pump.

An intradermal skin test of 100 units has been suggested to predict allergic response to streptokinase. If a positive reaction is not seen after 15-20 minutes, a therapeutic dose may be administered.

Guidelines for acute myocardial infarction (AMI): 1.5 million units over 60 minutes

Administration:

Dilute two 750,000 unit vials of streptokinase with 5 mL dextrose 5% in water (D_5W) each, gently swirl to dissolve.

Add this dose of the 1.5 million units to 150 mL D_5W.

This should be infused over 60 minutes; an in-line filter ≥0.45 micron should be used.

Monitor for the first few hours for signs of anaphylaxis or allergic reaction. **Infusion should be slowed if blood pressure falls by 25 mm Hg or terminated if asthmatic symptoms appear.**

Following completion of streptokinase, initiate heparin, if directed, when aPTT returns to less than 2 times the upper limit of control; do not use a bolus, but initiate infusion adjusted to a target aPTT of 1.5-2 times the upper limit of control. If prolonged (>48 hours) heparin is required, infusion may be switched to subcutaneous therapy.

Guidelines for acute pulmonary embolism (APE): 3 million unit dose over 24 hours

Administration:

Dilute four 750,000 unit vials of streptokinase with 5 mL dextrose 5% in water (D_5W) each, gently swirl to dissolve.

Add this dose of 3 million units to 250 mL D_5W, an in-line filter ≥0.45 micron should be used.

Administer 250,000 units (23 mL) over 30 minutes followed by 100,000 units/hour (9 mL/hour) for 24 hours.

Monitor for the first few hours for signs of anaphylaxis or allergic reaction. **Infusion should be slowed if blood pressure is lowered by 25 mm Hg or if asthmatic symptoms appear.**

Begin heparin 1000 units/hour about 3-4 hours after completion of streptokinase infusion or when PTT is <100 seconds.

Monitor PT, PTT, and fibrinogen levels during therapy.

Thromboses: 250,000 units to start, then 100,000 units/hour for 24-72 hours depending on location.

Cannula occlusion: 250,000 units into cannula, clamp for 2 hours, then aspirate contents and flush with normal saline

Dosage Forms [DSC] = Discontinued product

Injection, powder for reconstitution: 250,000 int. units; 750,000 int. units; 1,500,000 int. units [DSC]

streptomycin (strep toe MYE sin)

Sound-Alike/Look-Alike Issues

streptomycin may be confused with streptozocin

Synonyms streptomycin sulfate

Therapeutic Category Antibiotic, Aminoglycoside; Antitubercular Agent

Use Part of combination therapy of active tuberculosis; used in combination with other agents for treatment of streptococcal or enterococcal endocarditis, mycobacterial infections, plague, tularemia, and brucellosis

Usual Dosage Note: For I.M. administration; I.V. use is not recommended

Usual dosage range:

Children: 20-40 mg/kg/day (maximum: 1 g)

Adults: 15-30 mg/kg/day or 1-2 g/day

Indication-specific dosing:

Children: **Tuberculosis:** I.M.:

Daily therapy: 20-40 mg/kg/day (maximum: 1 g/day)

Directly observed therapy (DOT): Twice weekly: 25-30 mg/kg (maximum: 1.5 g)

Directly observed therapy DOT: 3 times/week: 25-30 mg/kg (maximum: 1.5 g)

(Continued)

streptomycin *(Continued)*

Adults: I.M.:

Brucellosis: 1 g/day for 14-21 days (with doxycycline, 100 mg twice daily for 6 weeks)

Endocarditis:

Enterococcal: 1 g every 12 hours for 2 weeks, 500 mg every 12 hours for 4 weeks in combination with penicillin

Streptococcal: 1 g every 12 hours for 1 week, 500 mg every 12 hours for 1 week

***Mycobacterium avium* complex:** Adjunct therapy (with macrolide, rifamycin, and ethambutol): 15 mg/kg 3 times/week for first 2-3 months for severe disease

Plague: 15 mg/kg (or 1 g) every 12 hours until the patient is afebrile for at least 3 days

Tuberculosis:

Daily therapy: 15 mg/kg/day (maximum: 1 g)

Directly observed therapy (DOT): Twice weekly: 25-30 mg/kg (maximum: 1.5 g)

Directly observed therapy DOT: 3 times/week: 25-30 mg/kg (maximum: 1.5 g)

Tularemia: 10-15 mg/kg every 12 hours (maximum: 2 g/day) for 7-10 days or until patient is afebrile for 5-7 days

Dosage Forms Injection, powder for reconstitution: 1 g

streptomycin sulfate *see* streptomycin *on previous page*

streptozocin (strep toe ZOE sin)

Sound-Alike/Look-Alike Issues

streptozocin may be confused with streptomycin

Synonyms NSC-85998

U.S./Canadian Brand Names Zanosar® [US/Can]

Therapeutic Category Antineoplastic Agent

Use Treatment of metastatic islet cell carcinoma of the pancreas, carcinoid tumor and syndrome, Hodgkin disease, palliative treatment of colorectal cancer

Usual Dosage I.V. (refer to individual protocols): Children and Adults:

Single agent therapy: 1-1.5 g/m^2 weekly for 6 weeks followed by a 4-week rest period

Combination therapy: 0.5-1 g/m^2 for 5 consecutive days followed by a 4- to 6-week rest period

Dosage Forms Injection, powder for reconstitution: 1 g

Stresstabs® B-Complex [US-OTC] *see* vitamin B complex combinations *on page 876*

Stresstabs® B-Complex + Iron [US-OTC] *see* vitamin B complex combinations *on page 876*

Stresstabs® B-Complex + Zinc [US-OTC] *see* vitamin B complex combinations *on page 876*

Striant® [US] *see* testosterone *on page 812*

Stri-dex® [US-OTC] *see* salicylic acid *on page 758*

Stri-dex® Body Focus [US-OTC] *see* salicylic acid *on page 758*

Stri-dex® Facewipes To Go™ [US-OTC] *see* salicylic acid *on page 758*

Stri-dex® Maximum Strength [US-OTC] *see* salicylic acid *on page 758*

Strifon Forte® [Can] *see* chlorzoxazone *on page 185*

Stromectol® [US] *see* ivermectin *on page 468*

StrongStart™ [US] *see* vitamins (multiple/prenatal) *on page 879*

strontium-89 chloride *see* strontium-89 *on this page*

strontium-89 (STRON shee um atey nine)

Synonyms strontium-89 chloride

U.S./Canadian Brand Names Metastron® [US/Can]

Therapeutic Category Radiopharmaceutical

Use Relief of bone pain in patients with skeletal metastases

Usual Dosage Adults: I.V.: 148 megabecquerel (4 millicurie) administered by slow I.V. injection over 1-2 minutes or 1.5-2.2 megabecquerel (40-60 microcurie)/kg; repeated doses are generally not recommended at intervals <90 days; measure the patient dose by a suitable radioactivity calibration system immediately prior to administration

Dosage Forms Injection, solution, as chloride [preservative free]: 10.9-22.6 mg/mL [148 megabecquerel, 4 millicurie] (10 mL)

Strovite® Forte [US] *see* vitamins (multiple/oral) *on page 878*

Stuartnatal® Plus 3™ [OTC] *(Discontinued)* *see* vitamins (multiple/prenatal) *on page 879*

Stuart Prenatal® [US-OTC] *see* vitamins (multiple/prenatal) *on page 879*

SU11248 *see* sunitinib *on page 801*

Sublimaze® [US] *see* fentanyl *on page 340*

Suboxone® [US] *see* buprenorphine and naloxone *on page 126*

Subutex® [US/Can] *see* buprenorphine *on page 125*

succimer (SUKS si mer)

Synonyms DMSA

U.S./Canadian Brand Names Chemet® [US/Can]

Therapeutic Category Chelating Agent

Use **Orphan drug:** Treatment of lead poisoning in children with blood levels >45 mcg/dL. It is not indicated for prophylaxis of lead poisoning in a lead-containing environment. Following oral administration, succimer is generally well tolerated and produces a linear dose-dependent reduction in serum lead concentrations. This agent appears to offer advantages over existing lead chelating agents.

Usual Dosage Children and Adults: Oral: 10 mg/kg/dose every 8 hours for 5 days followed by 10 mg/kg/dose every 12 hours for 14 days

Dosage Forms Capsule: 100 mg

succinylcholine (suks in il KOE leen)

Synonyms succinylcholine chloride; suxamethonium chloride

U.S./Canadian Brand Names Quelicin® [US/Can]

Therapeutic Category Skeletal Muscle Relaxant

Use Adjunct to general anesthesia to facilitate both rapid sequence and routine endotracheal intubation and to relax skeletal muscles during surgery; to reduce the intensity of muscle contractions of pharmacologically- or electrically-induced convulsions; does not relieve pain or produce sedation

Usual Dosage I.M., I.V.: Dose to effect; doses will vary due to interpatient variability; use ideal body weight for obese patients

I.M.: 2.5-4 mg/kg, total dose should not exceed 150 mg

I.V.:

Children: Initial: 1-2 mg/kg; maintenance: 0.3-0.6 mg/kg every 5-10 minutes as needed; because of the risk of malignant hyperthermia, use of continuous infusions is not recommended in infants and children

Adults: 1-1.5 mg/kg, up to 150 mg total dose

Maintenance: 0.04-0.07 mg/kg every 5-10 minutes as needed

Continuous infusion: 10-100 mcg/kg/minute (or 0.5-10 mg/minute); dilute to concentration of 1-2 mg/mL in D_5W or NS

Note: Initial dose of succinylcholine must be increased when nondepolarizing agent pretreatment used because of the antagonism between succinylcholine and nondepolarizing neuromuscular blocking agents

Dosage Forms Injection, solution, as chloride: 20 mg/mL (5 mL, 10 mL); 50 mg/mL (10 mL); 100 mg/mL (10 mL)

succinylcholine chloride *see* succinylcholine *on this page*

Sucraid® [US/Can] *see* sacrosidase *on page 757*

sucralfate (soo KRAL fate)

Sound-Alike/Look-Alike Issues

sucralfate may be confused with salsalate

Carafate® may be confused with Cafergot®

Synonyms aluminum sucrose sulfate, basic

U.S./Canadian Brand Names Carafate® [US]; Novo-Sucralate [Can]; Nu-Sucralate [Can]; PMS-Sucralate [Can]; Sulcrate® Suspension Plus [Can]; Sulcrate® [Can]

Therapeutic Category Gastrointestinal Agent, Gastric or Duodenal Ulcer Treatment

Use Short-term management of duodenal ulcers; maintenance of duodenal ulcers

Usual Dosage Oral:

Children: Dose not established, doses of 40-80 mg/kg/day divided every 6 hours have been used

Adults:

Stress ulcer prophylaxis: 1 g 4 times/day

Stress ulcer treatment: 1 g every 4 hours

(Continued)

sucralfate *(Continued)*

Duodenal ulcer:

Treatment: 1 g 4 times/day on an empty stomach and at bedtime for 4-8 weeks, or alternatively 2 g twice daily; treatment is recommended for 4-8 weeks in adults

Maintenance: Prophylaxis: 1 g twice daily

Dosage Forms

Suspension, oral: 1 g/10 mL (10 mL)

Carafate®: 1 g/10 mL (420 mL)

Tablet: 1 g

Carafate®: 1 g

Sucrets® [US-OTC] *see* dyclonine *on page 284*

Sucrets® Cough Calmers *(Discontinued)* *see* dextromethorphan *on page 245*

Sucrets® Original [US-OTC] *see* hexylresorcinol *on page 414*

Sudafed® [US-OTC] *see* pseudoephedrine *on page 712*

Sudafed® 12 Hour [US-OTC] *see* pseudoephedrine *on page 712*

Sudafed® 24 Hour [US-OTC] *see* pseudoephedrine *on page 712*

Sudafed® Children's [US-OTC] *see* pseudoephedrine *on page 712*

Sudafed® Children's Cold & Cough [US-OTC] *see* pseudoephedrine and dextromethorphan *on page 714*

Sudafed® Cold & Cough Extra Strength [Can] *see* acetaminophen, dextromethorphan, and pseudoephedrine *on page 12*

Sudafed® Decongestant [Can] *see* pseudoephedrine *on page 712*

Sudafed® Head Cold and Sinus Extra Strength [Can] *see* acetaminophen and pseudoephedrine *on page 9*

Sudafed® Non-Drying Sinus [US-OTC] *see* guaifenesin and pseudoephedrine *on page 398*

Sudafed PE™ [US-OTC] *see* phenylephrine *on page 660*

Sudafed® Severe Cold [US-OTC] *see* acetaminophen, dextromethorphan, and pseudoephedrine *on page 12*

Sudafed® Sinus Advance [Can] *see* pseudoephedrine and ibuprofen *on page 715*

Sudafed® Sinus & Allergy [US-OTC] *see* chlorpheniramine and pseudoephedrine *on page 177*

Sudafed® Sinus and Cold [US-OTC] *see* acetaminophen and pseudoephedrine *on page 9*

Sudafed® Sinus Headache [US-OTC] *see* acetaminophen and pseudoephedrine *on page 9*

Sudafed® Sinus Nighttime [US-OTC] *see* triprolidine and pseudoephedrine *on page 853*

Sudal® 12 [US] *see* chlorpheniramine and pseudoephedrine *on page 177*

Sudex® *(Discontinued)* *see* guaifenesin and pseudoephedrine *on page 398*

Sudodrin [US-OTC] *see* pseudoephedrine *on page 712*

SudoGest [US-OTC] *see* pseudoephedrine *on page 712*

SudoGest Children's [US-OTC] *see* pseudoephedrine and dextromethorphan *on page 714*

SudoGest Sinus [US-OTC] *see* acetaminophen and pseudoephedrine *on page 9*

Sudo-Tab® [US-OTC] *see* pseudoephedrine *on page 712*

Sufedrin® *(Discontinued)* *see* pseudoephedrine *on page 712*

Sufenta® [US/Can] *see* sufentanil *on this page*

sufentanil (soo FEN ta nil)

Sound-Alike/Look-Alike Issues

sufentanil may be confused with alfentanil, fentanyl

Sufenta® may be confused with Alfenta®, Sudafed®, Survanta®

Synonyms sufentanil citrate

U.S./Canadian Brand Names Sufenta® [US/Can]

Therapeutic Category Analgesic, Narcotic; General Anesthetic

Controlled Substance C-II

Use Analgesic supplement in maintenance of balanced general anesthesia

Usual Dosage

Children 2-12 years: 10-25 mcg/kg (10-15 mcg/kg most common dose) with 100% O_2, maintenance: up to 1-2 mcg/kg total dose

Adults: Dose should be based on body weight. **Note:** In obese patients (ie, >20% above ideal body weight), use lean body weight to determine dosage.

1-2 mcg/kg with N_2O/O_2 for endotracheal intubation; maintenance: 10-25 mcg as needed

2-8 mcg/kg with N_2O/O_2 more complicated major surgical procedures; maintenance: 10-50 mcg as needed

8-30 mcg/kg with 100% O_2 and muscle relaxant produces sleep; at doses ≥8 mcg/kg maintains a deep level of anesthesia; maintenance: 10-50 mcg as needed

Dosage Forms Injection, solution [preservative free]: 50 mcg/mL (1 mL, 2 mL, 5 mL)

sufentanil citrate *see* sufentanil *on previous page*

Sular® [US] *see* nisoldipine *on page 593*

sulbactam and ampicillin *see* ampicillin and sulbactam *on page 54*

sulconazole (sul KON a zole)

Synonyms sulconazole nitrate

U.S./Canadian Brand Names Exelderm® [US/Can]

Therapeutic Category Antifungal Agent

Use Treatment of superficial fungal infections of the skin, including tinea cruris (jock itch), tinea corporis (ringworm), tinea versicolor, and possibly tinea pedis (athlete's foot, cream only)

Usual Dosage Adults: Topical: Apply a small amount to the affected area and gently massage once or twice daily for 3 weeks (tinea cruris, tinea corporis, tinea versicolor) to 4 weeks (tinea pedis).

Dosage Forms

Cream, as nitrate: 1% (15 g, 30 g, 60 g)

Solution, topical, as nitrate: 1% (30 mL)

sulconazole nitrate *see* sulconazole *on this page*

Sulcrate® [Can] *see* sucralfate *on page 793*

Sulcrate® Suspension Plus [Can] *see* sucralfate *on page 793*

sulfabenzamide, sulfacetamide, and sulfathiazole

(sul fa BENZ a mide, sul fa SEE ta mide, & sul fa THYE a zole)

Synonyms triple sulfa

U.S./Canadian Brand Names V.V.S.® [US]

Therapeutic Category Antibiotic, Vaginal

Use Treatment of *Haemophilus vaginalis* vaginitis

Usual Dosage Intravaginal: Adults: Female: Cream: Insert one applicatorful into vagina twice daily for 4-6 days; dosage may then be decreased to ½ to ¼ of an applicatorful twice daily

Dosage Forms Cream, vaginal: Sulfabenzamide 3.7%, sulfacetamide 2.86%, and sulfathiazole 3.42% (78 g with applicator)

sulfacetamide (sul fa SEE ta mide)

Sound-Alike/Look-Alike Issues

Bleph®-10 may be confused with Blephamide®

Klaron® may be confused with Klor-Con®

Synonyms sodium sulfacetamide; sulfacetamide sodium

U.S./Canadian Brand Names Bleph®-10 [US]; Carmol® Scalp [US]; Cetamide™ [Can]; Diosulf™ [Can]; Klaron® [US]; Ovace™ [US]

Therapeutic Category Antibiotic, Ophthalmic

Use

Ophthalmic: Treatment and prophylaxis of conjunctivitis due to susceptible organisms; corneal ulcers; adjunctive treatment with systemic sulfonamides for therapy of trachoma

Dermatologic: Scaling dermatosis (seborrheic); bacterial infections of the skin; acne vulgaris

Usual Dosage

Children >2 months and Adults: Ophthalmic:

Ointment: Apply to lower conjunctival sac 1-4 times/day and at bedtime

Solution: Instill 1-2 drops several times daily up to every 2-3 hours in lower conjunctival sac during waking hours and less frequently at night; increase dosing interval as condition responds. Usual duration of treatment: 7-10 days

(Continued)

sulfacetamide *(Continued)*

Trachoma: Instill 2 drops into the conjunctival sac every 2 hours; must be used in conjunction with systemic therapy

Children >12 years and Adults: Topical:

Acne: Apply thin film to affected area twice daily

Seborrheic dermatitis: Apply at bedtime and allow to remain overnight; in severe cases, may apply twice daily. Duration of therapy is usually 8-10 applications; dosing interval may be increased as eruption subsides. Applications once or twice weekly, or every other week may be used to prevent eruptions.

Secondary cutaneous bacterial infections: Apply 2-4 times/day until infection clears

Dosage Forms [DSC] = Discontinued product

Cream, topical, as sodium (Ovace™): 10% (30 g, 60 g)

Foam, topical, as sodium (Ovace™): 10% (50 g, 100 g)

Gel, topical, as sodium (Ovace™): 10% (30 g, 60 g)

Lotion, as sodium:

Carmol® Scalp: 10% (85 g) [contains urea 10%]

Klaron®: 10% (120 mL) [contains sodium metabisulfite]

Ovace™: 10% (180 mL, 360 mL)

Ointment, ophthalmic, as sodium: 10% (3.5 g)

Solution, ophthalmic, as sodium: 10% (15 mL)

Bleph®-10: 10% (5 mL; 15 mL [DSC]) [contains benzalkonium chloride]

sulfacetamide and prednisolone (sul fa SEE ta mide & pred NIS oh lone)

Sound-Alike/Look-Alike Issues

Blephamide® may be confused with Bleph®-10

Vasocidin® may be confused with Vasodilan®

Synonyms prednisolone and sulfacetamide

U.S./Canadian Brand Names Blephamide® [US/Can]; Dioptimyd® [Can]

Therapeutic Category Antibiotic/Corticosteroid, Ophthalmic

Use Steroid-responsive inflammatory ocular conditions where infection is present or there is a risk of infection; ophthalmic suspension may be used as an otic preparation

Usual Dosage Children >2 months and Adults: Ophthalmic:

Ointment: Apply to lower conjunctival sac 1-4 times/day

Solution, suspension: Instill 1-3 drops every 2-3 hours while awake

Dosage Forms

Ointment, ophthalmic (Blephamide®): Sulfacetamide sodium 10% and prednisolone acetate 0.2% (3.5 g)

Solution, ophthalmic: Sulfacetamide sodium 10% and prednisolone sodium phosphate 0.25% (5 mL, 10 mL)

Suspension, ophthalmic (Blephamide®): Sulfacetamide sodium 10% and prednisolone acetate 0.2% (5 mL, 10 mL) [contains benzalkonium chloride]

sulfacetamide and sulfur *see* sulfur and sulfacetamide *on page 800*

sulfacetamide sodium *see* sulfacetamide *on previous page*

sulfacetamide sodium and fluorometholone

(sul fa SEE ta mide SOW dee um & flure oh METH oh lone)

Synonyms fluorometholone and sulfacetamide

U.S./Canadian Brand Names FML-S® [US]

Therapeutic Category Antibiotic/Corticosteroid, Ophthalmic

Use Steroid-responsive inflammatory ocular conditions where infection is present or there is a risk of infection

Usual Dosage Ophthalmic: Children >2 years and Adults: Instill 1 drop into affected eye(s) 4 times/day

Note: Dose may be decreased but should not be discontinued prematurely; re-evaluation should occur if improvement is not seen within 2 days; in chronic conditions, dosing frequency should be gradually decreased prior to discontinuing treatment

Dosage Forms Suspension, ophthalmic: Sulfacetamide sodium 10% and fluorometholone 0.1% (5 mL, 10 mL) [contains benzalkonium chloride]

Sulfacet-R® [US/Can] *see* sulfur and sulfacetamide *on page 800*

sulfadiazine (sul fa DYE a zeen)

Sound-Alike/Look-Alike Issues

sulfaDIAZINE may be confused with sulfasalazine, sulfiSOXAZOLE

Tall-Man sulfa**DIAZINE**

Therapeutic Category Sulfonamide

Use Treatment of urinary tract infections and nocardiosis; adjunctive treatment in toxoplasmosis; uncomplicated attack of malaria

Usual Dosage Oral:

Asymptomatic meningococcal carriers:

Infants 1-12 months: 500 mg once daily for 2 days

Children 1-12 years: 500 mg twice daily for 2 days

Adults: 1 g twice daily for 2 days

Congenital toxoplasmosis:

Newborns and Children <2 months: 100 mg/kg/day divided every 6 hours in conjunction with pyrimethamine 1 mg/kg/day once daily and supplemental folinic acid 5 mg every 3 days for 6 months

Children >2 months: 25-50 mg/kg/dose 4 times/day

Nocardiosis: 4-8 g/day for a minimum of 6 weeks

Toxoplasmosis:

Children >2 months: Loading dose: 75 mg/kg; maintenance dose: 120-150 mg/kg/day, maximum dose: 6 g/day; divided every 4-6 hours in conjunction with pyrimethamine 2 mg/kg/day divided every 12 hours for 3 days followed by 1 mg/kg/day once daily with supplemental folinic acid

Adults: 2-6 g/day in divided doses every 6 hours in conjunction with pyrimethamine 50-75 mg/day and with supplemental folinic acid

Dosage Forms Tablet: 500 mg

sulfadoxine and pyrimethamine (sul fa DOKS een & peer i METH a meen)

Synonyms pyrimethamine and sulfadoxine

U.S./Canadian Brand Names Fansidar® [US]

Therapeutic Category Antimalarial Agent

Use Treatment of *Plasmodium falciparum* malaria in patients in whom chloroquine resistance is suspected; malaria prophylaxis for travelers to areas where chloroquine-resistant malaria is endemic

Usual Dosage Children and Adults: Oral:

Treatment of acute attack of malaria: A single dose of the following number of Fansidar® tablets is used in sequence with quinine or alone:

2-11 months: 1/4 tablet

1-3 years: 1/2 tablet

4-8 years: 1 tablet

9-14 years: 2 tablets

>14 years: 3 tablets

Malaria prophylaxis: A single dose should be carried for self-treatment in the event of febrile illness when medical attention is not immediately available:

2-11 months: 1/4 tablet

1-3 years: 1/2 tablet

4-8 years: 1 tablet

9-14 years: 2 tablets

>14 years and Adults: 3 tablets

Dosage Forms Tablet: Sulfadoxine 500 mg and pyrimethamine 25 mg

Sulfa-Gyn® *(Discontinued)* *see* sulfabenzamide, sulfacetamide, and sulfathiazole *on page 795*

Sulfamethoprim® *(Discontinued)*

sulfamethoxazole and trimethoprim (sul fa meth OKS a zole & trye METH oh prim)

Sound-Alike/Look-Alike Issues

Bactrim™ may be confused with bacitracin, Bactine®

co-trimoxazole may be confused with clotrimazole

Septra® may be confused with Ceptaz®, Sectral®, Septa®

Synonyms co-trimoxazole; SMZ-TMP; sulfatrim; TMP-SMZ; trimethoprim and sulfamethoxazole

U.S./Canadian Brand Names Apo-Sulfatrim® DS [Can]; Apo-Sulfatrim® Pediatric [Can]; Apo-Sulfatrim® [Can]; Bactrim™ DS [US]; Bactrim™ [US]; Novo-Trimel D.S. [Can]; Novo-Trimel [Can]; Nu-Cotrimox [Can]; Septra® DS [US]; Septra® Injection [Can]; Septra® [US]

Therapeutic Category Sulfonamide

Use

Oral treatment of urinary tract infections due to *E. coli, Klebsiella* and *Enterobacter* sp, *M. morganii, P. mirabilis* and *P. vulgaris*; acute otitis media in children; acute exacerbations of chronic bronchitis in adults due to susceptible strains of *H. influenzae* or *S. pneumoniae*; treatment and prophylaxis of *Pneumocystis*

(Continued)

sulfamethoxazole and trimethoprim *(Continued)*

carinii pneumonitis (PCP); traveler's diarrhea due to enterotoxigenic *E. coli*; treatment of enteritis caused by *Shigella flexneri* or *Shigella sonnei*

I.V. treatment or severe or complicated infections when oral therapy is not feasible, for documented PCP, empiric treatment of PCP in immune compromised patients; treatment of documented or suspected shigellosis, typhoid fever, *Nocardia asteroides* infection, or other infections caused by susceptible bacteria

Usual Dosage Dosage recommendations are based on the trimethoprim component. Double-strength tablets are equivalent to sulfamethoxazole 800 mg and trimethoprim 160 mg.

Children >2 months:

General dosing guidelines:

Mild-to-moderate infections: Oral: 8-12 mg TMP/kg/day in divided doses every 12 hours

Serious infection:

Oral: 20 mg TMP/kg/day in divided doses every 6 hours

I.V.: 8-12 mg TMP/kg/day in divided doses every 6 hours

Acute otitis media: Oral: 8 mg TMP/kg/day in divided doses every 12 hours for 10 days

Urinary tract infection:

Treatment:

Oral: 6-12 mg TMP/kg/day in divided doses every 12 hours

I.V.: 8-10 mg TMP/kg/day in divided doses every 6, 8, or 12 hours for up to 4 days with serious infections

Prophylaxis: Oral: 2 mg TMP/kg/dose daily or 5 mg TMP/kg/dose twice weekly

Pneumocystis:

Treatment: Oral, I.V.: 15-20 mg TMP/kg/day in divided doses every 6-8 hours

Prophylaxis: Oral, 150 mg TMP/m²/day in divided doses every 12 hours for 3 days/week; dose should not exceed trimethoprim 320 mg and sulfamethoxazole 1600 mg daily

Alternative prophylaxis dosing schedules include:

150 mg TMP/m²/day as a single daily dose 3 times/week on consecutive days

or

150 mg TMP/m²/day in divided doses every 12 hours administered 7 days/week

or

150 mg TMP/m²/day in divided doses every 12 hours administered 3 times/week on alternate days

Shigellosis:

Oral: 8 mg TMP/kg/day in divided doses every 12 hours for 5 days

I.V.: 8-10 mg TMP/kg/day in divided doses every 6, 8, or 12 hours for up to 5 days

Adults:

Urinary tract infection:

Oral: One double-strength tablet every 12 hours

Duration of therapy: Uncomplicated: 3-5 days; Complicated: 7-10 days

Pyelonephritis: 14 days

Prostatitis: Acute: 2 weeks; Chronic: 2-3 months

I.V.: 8-10 mg TMP/kg/day in divided doses every 6, 8, or 12 hours for up to 14 days with severe infections

Chronic bronchitis: Oral: One double-strength tablet every 12 hours for 10-14 days

Meningitis (bacterial): I.V.: 10-20 mg TMP/kg/day in divided doses every 6-12 hours

Shigellosis:

Oral: One double strength tablet every 12 hours for 5 days

I.V.: 8-10 mg TMP/kg/day in divided doses every 6, 8, or 12 hours for up to 5 days

Travelers' diarrhea: Oral: One double strength tablet every 12 hours for 5 days

Sepsis: I.V.: 20 TMP/kg/day divided every 6 hours

Pneumocystis carinii:

Prophylaxis: Oral: 1 double strength tablet daily or 3 times/week

Treatment: Oral, I.V.: 15-20 mg TMP/kg/day in 3-4 divided doses

Dosage Forms Note: The 5:1 ratio (SMX:TMP) remains constant in all dosage forms.

Injection, solution: Sulfamethoxazole 80 mg and trimethoprim 16 mg per mL (5 mL, 10 mL, 30 mL) [contains propylene glycol ~400 mg/mL, alcohol, benzyl alcohol, and sodium metabisulfite]

Suspension, oral: Sulfamethoxazole 200 mg and trimethoprim 40 mg per 5 mL (480 mL) [contains alcohol]

Septra®: Sulfamethoxazole 200 mg and trimethoprim 40 mg per 5 mL (480 mL) [contains alcohol 0.26% and sodium benzoate; cherry and grape flavors] [DSC]

Tablet: Sulfamethoxazole 400 mg and trimethoprim 80 mg

Bactrim™: Sulfamethoxazole 400 mg and trimethoprim 80 mg [contains sodium benzoate]

Septra®: Sulfamethoxazole 400 mg and trimethoprim 80 mg

Tablet, double strength: Sulfamethoxazole 800 mg and trimethoprim 160 mg

Bactrim™ DS: Sulfamethoxazole 800 mg and trimethoprim 160 mg [contains sodium benzoate]

Septra® DS: Sulfamethoxazole 800 mg and trimethoprim 160 mg

Sulfamylon® [US] *see* mafenide *on page 511*

sulfasalazine (sul fa SAL a zeen)

Sound-Alike/Look-Alike Issues

sulfasalazine may be confused with salsalate, sulfaDIAZINE, sulfiSOXAZOLE

Azulfidine® may be confused with Augmentin®, azathioprine

Synonyms salicylazosulfapyridine

U.S./Canadian Brand Names Alti-Sulfasalazine [Can]; Azulfidine® EN-tabs® [US]; Azulfidine® [US]; Salazopyrin En-Tabs® [Can]; Salazopyrin® [Can]; Sulfazine EC [US]; Sulfazine [US]

Therapeutic Category 5-Aminosalicylic Acid Derivative

Use Management of ulcerative colitis; enteric coated tablets are also used for rheumatoid arthritis (including juvenile rheumatoid arthritis) in patients who inadequately respond to analgesics and NSAIDs

Usual Dosage Oral:

Children ≥2 years: Ulcerative colitis: Initial: 40-60 mg/kg/day in 3-6 divided doses; maintenance dose: 20-30 mg/kg/day in 4 divided doses

Children ≥6 years: Juvenile rheumatoid arthritis: Enteric coated tablet: 30-50 mg/kg/day in 2 divided doses; Initial: Begin with 1/4 to 1/3 of expected maintenance dose; increase weekly; maximum: 2 g/day typically

Adults:

Ulcerative colitis: Initial: 1 g 3-4 times/day, 2 g/day maintenance in divided doses; may initiate therapy with 0.5-1 g/day

Rheumatoid arthritis: Enteric coated tablet: Initial: 0.5-1 g/day; increase weekly to maintenance dose of 2 g/day in 2 divided doses; maximum: 3 g/day (if response to 2 g/day is inadequate after 12 weeks of treatment)

Dosage Forms

Tablet (Azulfidine®, Sulfazine): 500 mg

Tablet, delayed release, enteric coated (Azulfidine® EN-tabs®, Sulfazine EC): 500 mg

sulfatrim *see* sulfamethoxazole and trimethoprim *on page 797*

Sulfa-Trip® ***(Discontinued)*** *see* sulfabenzamide, sulfacetamide, and sulfathiazole *on page 795*

Sulfazine [US] *see* sulfasalazine *on this page*

Sulfazine EC [US] *see* sulfasalazine *on this page*

sulfinpyrazone (sul fin PEER a zone)

U.S./Canadian Brand Names Apo-Sulfinpyrazone® [Can]; Nu-Sulfinpyrazone [Can]

Therapeutic Category Uricosuric Agent

Use Treatment of chronic gouty arthritis and intermittent gouty arthritis

Usual Dosage Adults: Oral: 100-200 mg twice daily; maximum daily dose: 800 mg

Dosage Forms Tablet: 100 mg

sulfisoxazole (sul fi SOKS a zole)

Sound-Alike/Look-Alike Issues

sulfiSOXAZOLE may be confused with sulfaDIAZINE, sulfamethoxazole, sulfasalazine

Gantrisin® may be confused with Gastrosed™

Synonyms sulfisoxazole acetyl; sulphafurazole

Tall-Man sulfi**SOXAZOLE**

U.S./Canadian Brand Names Gantrisin® [US]; Novo-Soxazole [Can]; Sulfizole® [Can]

Therapeutic Category Sulfonamide

Use Treatment of urinary tract infections, otitis media, *Chlamydia*; nocardiosis

Usual Dosage Oral: Not for use in patients <2 months of age:

Children >2 months: Initial: 75 mg/kg, followed by 120-150 mg/kg/day in divided doses every 4-6 hours; not to exceed 6 g/day

Adults: Initial: 2-4 g, then 4-8 g/day in divided doses every 4-6 hours

Dosage Forms

Suspension, oral, pediatric, as acetyl (Gantrisin®): 500 mg/5 mL (480 mL) [contains alcohol 0.3%; raspberry flavor]

Tablet: 500 mg

sulfisoxazole acetyl *see* sulfisoxazole *on this page*

sulfisoxazole and erythromycin *see* erythromycin and sulfisoxazole *on page 305*

Sulfizole® [Can] *see* sulfisoxazole *on this page*

sulfur and sulfacetamide (SUL fur & sul fa SEE ta mide)

Synonyms sodium sulfacetamide and sulfur; sulfacetamide and sulfur; sulfur and sulfacetamide sodium

U.S./Canadian Brand Names AVAR™ Green [US]; AVAR™ [US]; AVAR™-e Green [US]; AVAR™-e [US]; Clenia™ [US]; Plexion SCT® [US]; Plexion TS® [US]; Plexion® [US]; Rosac® [US]; Rosanil® [US]; Rosula® [US]; Sulfacet-R® [US/Can]; Zetacet® [US]

Therapeutic Category Antiseborrheic Agent, Topical

Use Aid in the treatment of acne vulgaris, acne rosacea, and seborrheic dermatitis

Usual Dosage Topical: Children ≥12 years and Adults: Apply in a thin film 1-3 times/day. Cleansing products should be used 1-2 times/day.

Dosage Forms [DSC] = Discontinued product

Cleanser, topical:

AVAR™ : Sulfur 5% and sulfacetamide sodium 10% (228 g)

Plexion®: Sulfur 5% and sulfacetamide sodium 10% (170 g, 340 g)

Rosanil®: Sulfur 5% and sulfacetamide sodium 10% (170 g) [DSC]

Rosula®: Sulfur 5% and sulfacetamide sodium 10% (355 mL) [contains urea 10%]

Cream, topical:

AVAR™-e: Sulfur 5% and sulfacetamide sodium 10% (45 g) [contains benzyl alcohol]

AVAR™-e Green: Sulfur 5% and sulfacetamide sodium 10% (45 g) [contains benzyl alcohol; color corrective cream]

Clenia™: Sulfur 5% and sulfacetamide sodium 10% (28 g)

Plexion SCT®: Sulfur 5% and sulfacetamide sodium 10% (120 g) [contains benzyl alcohol]

Rosac®: Sulfur 5% and sulfacetamide sodium 10% (45 g) [contains benzyl alcohol and sunscreen}

Suphera™: Sulfur 5% and sulfacetamide sodium 10% (113 g)

Gel, topical:

AVAR™: Sulfur 5% and sulfacetamide sodium 10% (45 g) [contains benzyl alcohol]

AVAR™ Green: Sulfur 5% and sulfacetamide sodium 10% (45 g) [contains benzyl alcohol; color corrective gel]

Rosula®: Sulfur 5% and sulfacetamide sodium 10% (45 mL) [contains urea 10% and benzyl alcohol]

Lotion, topical: Sulfur 5% and sulfacetamide sodium 10% (25 g, 30 g, 45 g, 60 g)

Sulfacet-R®: Sulfur 5% and sulfacetamide sodium 10% (25 g) [contains sodium metabisulfate; available with tint or tint-free formulations]

Zetacet®: Sulfur 5% and sulfacetamide sodium 10% (25 g) [contains sodium metabisulfite]

Pad [cleansing cloth] (Plexion®): Sulfur 5% and sulfacetamide sodium 10% (30s) [contains aloe vera]

Suspension, topical:

Plexion® TS: Sulfur 5% and sulfacetamide sodium 10% (30 g) [contains benzyl alcohol]

Zetacet®: Sulfur 5% and sulfacetamide sodium 10% (30 g) [contains benzyl alcohol]

Wash, topical: Sulfur 5% and sulfacetamide sodium 10% (170 g, 340 g)

Clenia™: Sulfur 5% and sulfacetamide sodium 10% (170 g, 340 g)

Zetacet®: Sulfur 5% and sulfacetamide sodium 10% (170 g, 340 g)

sulfur and sulfacetamide sodium *see* sulfur and sulfacetamide *on this page*

sulindac (SUL in dak)

Sound-Alike/Look-Alike Issues

Clinoril® may be confused with Cleocin®, Clozaril®, Oruvail®

U.S./Canadian Brand Names Apo-Sulin® [Can]; Clinoril® [US]; Novo-Sundac [Can]; Nu-Sundac [Can]

Therapeutic Category Analgesic, Nonnarcotic; Nonsteroidal Antiinflammatory Drug (NSAID)

Use Management of inflammatory disease, osteoarthritis, rheumatoid disorders, acute gouty arthritis, ankylosing spondylitis, bursitis/tendonitis of shoulder

Usual Dosage Oral:

Children: Dose not established

Adults: **Note:** Maximum daily dose: 400 mg

Osteoarthritis, rheumatoid arthritis, ankylosing spondylitis: 150 mg twice/daily

Bursitis/tendonitis: 200 mg twice daily; usual treatment: 7-14 days

Acute gouty arthritis: 200 mg twice daily; usual treatment: 7 days

Dosage Forms

Tablet: 150 mg, 200 mg

Clinoril®: 200 mg

sulphafurazole *see* sulfisoxazole *on previous page*

Sultrin™ *(Discontinued)* *see* sulfabenzamide, sulfacetamide, and sulfathiazole *on page 795*

sumatriptan (soo ma TRIP tan)

Sound-Alike/Look-Alike Issues
sumatriptan may be confused with somatropin, zolmitriptan

Synonyms sumatriptan succinate

U.S./Canadian Brand Names Apo-Sumatriptan® [Can]; CO Sumatriptan [Can]; Dom-Sumatriptan [Can]; Gen-Sumatriptan [Can]; Imitrex® DF [Can]; Imitrex® Nasal Spray [Can]; Imitrex® [US/Can]; Novo-Sumatriptan [Can]; PHL-Sumatriptan [Can]; PMS-Sumatriptan [Can]; ratio-Sumatriptan [Can]; Rhoxal-sumatriptan [Can]; Riva-Sumatriptan [Can]; Sandoz-Sumatriptan [Can]; Sumatryx [Can]

Therapeutic Category Antimigraine Agent

Use
Oral, SubQ: Acute treatment of migraine with or without aura
SubQ: Acute treatment of cluster headache episodes

Usual Dosage Adults:
Oral: A single dose of 25 mg, 50 mg, or 100 mg (taken with fluids). If a satisfactory response has not been obtained at 2 hours, a second dose may be administered. Results from clinical trials show that initial doses of 50 mg and 100 mg are more effective than doses of 25 mg, and that 100 mg doses do not provide a greater effect than 50 mg and may have increased incidence of side effects. Although doses of up to 300 mg/day have been studied, the total daily dose should not exceed 200 mg. The safety of treating an average of >4 headaches in a 30-day period have not been established.
Intranasal: A single dose of 5 mg, 10 mg, or 20 mg administered in one nostril. A 10 mg dose may be achieved by administering a single 5 mg dose in each nostril. If headache returns, the dose may be repeated once after 2 hours, not to exceed a total daily dose of 40 mg. The safety of treating an average of >4 headaches in a 30-day period has not been established.
SubQ: 6 mg; a second injection may be administered at least 1 hour after the initial dose, but not more than 2 injections in a 24-hour period. If side effects are dose-limiting, lower doses may be used.

Dosage Forms **Note:** Strength expressed as sumatriptan base
Injection, solution, as succinate: 8 mg/mL (0.5 mL) [disposable cartridge for use with STATdose System®]; 12 mg/mL (0.5 mL) [disposable cartridge for use with STATdose System® or vial]
Solution, intranasal spray: 5 mg (100 µL unit dose spray device); 20 mg (100 µL unit dose spray device)
Tablet, as succinate: 25 mg, 50 mg, 100 mg

sumatriptan succinate *see* sumatriptan *on this page*

Sumatryx [Can] *see* sumatriptan *on this page*

Summer's Eve® Medicated Douche [US-OTC] *see* povidone-iodine *on page 689*

Summer's Eve® SpecialCare™ Medicated Anti-Itch Cream [US-OTC] *see* hydrocortisone (topical) *on page 428*

Sumycin® [US] *see* tetracycline *on page 816*

Sun-Benz® [Can] *see* benzydamine *(Canada only) on page 104*

sunitinib (su NIT e nib)

Synonyms NSC736511; SU11248; sunitinib maleate

U.S./Canadian Brand Names Sutent® [US]

Therapeutic Category Antineoplastic Agent, Tyrosine Kinase Inhibitor; Vascular Endothelial Growth Factor (VEGF) Inhibitor

Use Treatment of gastrointestinal stromal tumor (GIST) following failure of or intolerance to imatinib; treatment of advanced renal cell cancer (RCC)

Usual Dosage Oral: Adults: Gastrointestinal stromal tumor, renal cell cancer: 50 mg once daily for 4 weeks of a 6-week treatment cycle (4 weeks on, 2 weeks off). **Note:** Dose increase or reduction should be done in increments of 12.5 mg; individualize based on safety and tolerability.

Dosage Forms Capsule: 12.5 mg, 25 mg, 50 mg

sunitinib maleate *see* sunitinib *on this page*

Supartz™ [US] *see* hyaluronate and derivatives *on page 416*

Superdophilus® [US-OTC] *see* Lactobacillus *on page 477*

Supeudol® [Can] *see* oxycodone *on page 626*

Suplasyn® [Can] *see* hyaluronate and derivatives *on page 416*

Suppress® *(Discontinued)* *see* dextromethorphan *on page 245*

Suprane® [US/Can] *see* desflurane *on page 236*

Surbex-T® [US-OTC] *see* vitamin B complex combinations *on page 876*

Sureprin 81™ [US-OTC] *see* aspirin *on page 77*
Surfak® [US-OTC] *see* docusate *on page 270*
Surgam® [Can] *see* tiaprofenic acid *(Canada only) on page 826*
Surgam® SR [Can] *see* tiaprofenic acid *(Canada only) on page 826*
Surgicel® [US] *see* cellulose, oxidized regenerated *on page 165*
Surgicel® Fibrillar [US] *see* cellulose, oxidized regenerated *on page 165*
Surgicel® NuKnit [US] *see* cellulose, oxidized regenerated *on page 165*
Surmontil® [US] *see* trimipramine *on page 852*
Survanta® [US/Can] *see* beractant *on page 105*
Sus-Phrine® ***(Discontinued)*** *see* epinephrine *on page 295*
Sustaire® ***(Discontinued)*** *see* theophylline *on page 818*
Sustiva® [US/Can] *see* efavirenz *on page 288*
Sutent® [US] *see* sunitinib *on previous page*
Su-Tuss DM [US] *see* guaifenesin and dextromethorphan *on page 394*
Su-Tuss®-HD [US] *see* hydrocodone, pseudoephedrine, and guaifenesin *on page 425*
suxamethonium chloride *see* succinylcholine *on page 793*
Sween Cream® [US-OTC] *see* vitamin A and vitamin D *on page 876*
Symadine® ***(Discontinued)***
Symax SL [US] *see* hyoscyamine *on page 434*
Symax SR [US] *see* hyoscyamine *on page 434*
Symbicort® [Can] *see* budesonide and formoterol *(Canada only) on page 123*
Symbyax™ [US] *see* olanzapine and fluoxetine *on page 613*
Symlin® [US] *see* pramlintide *on page 690*
Symmetrel® [US/Can] *see* amantadine *on page 38*
synacthen *see* cosyntropin *on page 216*
Synagis® [US/Can] *see* palivizumab *on page 632*
Synalar® [US/Can] *see* fluocinolone *on page 352*
Synalar-HP® Topical ***(Discontinued)*** *see* fluocinolone *on page 352*
Synalgos®-DC [US] *see* dihydrocodeine, aspirin, and caffeine *on page 256*
Synarel® [US/Can] *see* nafarelin *on page 573*
Syn-Diltiazem® [Can] *see* diltiazem *on page 257*
Synemol® Topical ***(Discontinued)*** *see* fluocinolone *on page 352*
Synercid® [US/Can] *see* quinupristin and dalfopristin *on page 727*
Synphasic® [Can] *see* ethinyl estradiol and norethindrone *on page 323*
Syntest D.S. [US] *see* estrogens (esterified) and methyltestosterone *on page 314*
Syntest H.S. [US] *see* estrogens (esterified) and methyltestosterone *on page 314*
Synthroid® [US/Can] *see* levothyroxine *on page 491*
Syntocinon® [Can] *see* oxytocin *on page 630*
Synvisc® [US] *see* hyaluronate and derivatives *on page 416*
Syprine® [US/Can] *see* trientine *on page 848*
Syrex [US] *see* sodium chloride *on page 777*
SyringeAvitene™ [US] *see* collagen hemostat *on page 212*
syrup of ipecac *see* ipecac syrup *on page 459*
Sytobex® ***(Discontinued)*** *see* cyanocobalamin *on page 219*
T_3/T_4 liotrix *see* liotrix *on page 499*
T_4 *see* levothyroxine *on page 491*
T-20 *see* enfuvirtide *on page 293*
642® Tablet [Can] *see* propoxyphene *on page 708*

Tabloid® [US] *see* thioguanine *on page 822*

Tac™-40 Injection *(Discontinued)*

Taclonex® [US] *see* calcipotriene and betamethasone *on page 133*

tacrine (TAK reen)

Sound-Alike/Look-Alike Issues

Cognex® may be confused with Corgard®

Synonyms tacrine hydrochloride; tetrahydroaminoacrine; THA

U.S./Canadian Brand Names Cognex® [US]

Therapeutic Category Acetylcholinesterase Inhibitor; Cholinergic Agent

Use Treatment of mild to moderate dementia of the Alzheimer type

Usual Dosage Adults: Initial: 10 mg 4 times/day; may increase by 40 mg/day adjusted every 6 weeks; maximum: 160 mg/day; best administered separate from meal times.

Dose adjustment based upon transaminase elevations:

ALT ≤3 times ULN*: Continue titration

ALT >3 to ≤5 times ULN*: Decrease dose by 40 mg/day, resume when ALT returns to normal

ALT >5 times ULN*: Stop treatment, may rechallenge upon return of ALT to normal

*ULN = upper limit of normal

Patients with clinical jaundice confirmed by elevated total bilirubin (>3 mg/dL) should not be rechallenged with tacrine

Dosage Forms Capsule, as hydrochloride: 10 mg, 20 mg, 30 mg, 40 mg

tacrine hydrochloride *see* tacrine *on this page*

tacrolimus (ta KROE li mus)

Sound-Alike/Look-Alike Issues

Prograf® may be confused with Gengraf®

Synonyms FK506

U.S./Canadian Brand Names Prograf® [US/Can]; Protopic® [US/Can]

Therapeutic Category Immunosuppressant Agent

Use

Oral/injection: Potent immunosuppressive drug used in heart, kidney, or liver transplant recipients

Topical: Moderate-to-severe atopic dermatitis in patients not responsive to conventional therapy or when conventional therapy is not appropriate

Usual Dosage

Oral:

Children: **Notes:** Patients without pre-existing renal or hepatic dysfunction have required (and tolerated) higher doses than adults to achieve similar blood concentrations. It is recommended that therapy be initiated at high end of the recommended adult I.V. and oral dosing ranges; dosage adjustments may be required. If switching from I.V. to oral, the oral dose should be started 8-12 hours after stopping the infusion. Adjunctive therapy with corticosteroids is recommended early post-transplant.

Liver transplant: Initial dose: 0.15-0.20 mg/kg/day in 2 divided doses, given every 12 hours; begin oral dose no sooner than 6 hours post-transplant

Adults: **Notes:** If switching from I.V. to oral, the oral dose should be started 8-12 hours after stopping the infusion. Adjunctive therapy with corticosteroids is recommended early post-transplant.

Heart transplant: Initial dose: 0.075 mg/kg/day in 2 divided doses, given every 12 hours; begin oral dose no sooner than 6 hours post-transplant

Kidney transplant: Initial dose: 0.2 mg/kg/day in 2 divided doses, given every 12 hours; initial dose may be given within 24 hours of transplant, but should be delayed until renal function has recovered; African-American patients may require larger doses to maintain trough concentration

Liver transplant: Initial dose: 0.1-0.15 mg/kg/day in 2 divided doses, given every 12 hours; begin oral dose no sooner than 6 hours post-transplant

I.V.: Children and Adults: **Note:** I.V. route should only be used in patients not able to take oral medications and continued only until oral medication can be tolerated; anaphylaxis has been reported. Begin no sooner than 6 hours post-transplant; adjunctive therapy with corticosteroids is recommended.

Heart transplant: Initial dose: 0.01 mg/kg/day as a continuous infusion

Kidney, liver transplant: Initial dose: 0.03-0.05 mg/kg/day as a continuous infusion

Prevention of graft-vs-host disease: 0.03 mg/kg/day as continuous infusion

Topical: Children ≥2 years and Adults: Atopic dermatitis (moderate to severe): Apply minimum amount of 0.03% or 0.1% ointment to affected area twice daily; rub in gently and completely. Discontinue use when

(Continued)

tacrolimus *(Continued)*

symptoms have cleared. If no improvement within 6 weeks, patients should be re-examined to confirm diagnosis.

Dosage Forms

Capsule (Prograf®): 0.5 mg, 1 mg, 5 mg

Injection, solution (Prograf®): 5 mg/mL (1 mL) [contains dehydrated alcohol 80% and polyoxyl 60 hydrogenated castor oil]

Ointment, topical (Protopic®): 0.03% (30 g, 60 g, 100 g); 0.1% (30 g, 60 g, 100 g)

tadalafil (tah DA la fil)

Synonyms GF196960

U.S./Canadian Brand Names Cialis® [US/Can]

Therapeutic Category Phosphodiesterase (Type 5) Enzyme Inhibitor

Use Treatment of erectile dysfunction

Usual Dosage Oral: Adults: Erectile dysfunction: 10 mg prior to anticipated sexual activity (dosing range: 5-20 mg); to be given as one single dose and not given more than once daily. **Note:** Erectile function may be improved for up to 36 hours following a single dose; adjust dose.

Dosing adjustment with concomitant medications:

Alpha$_1$-blockers: If stabilized on either alpha blockers or tadalafil therapy, initiate new therapy with the other agent at the lowest possible dose.

CYP3A4 inhibitors: Dose reduction of tadalafil is recommended with strong CYP3A4 inhibitors. The dose of tadalafil should not exceed 10 mg, and tadalafil should not be taken more frequently than once every 72 hours. Examples of such inhibitors include amprenavir, atazanavir, clarithromycin, conivaptan, delavirdine, diclofenac, fosamprenavir, imatinib, indinavir, isoniazid, itraconazole, ketoconazole, miconazole, nefazodone, nelfinavir, nicardipine, propofol, quinidine, ritonavir, and telithromycin.

Dosage Forms Tablet: 5 mg, 10 mg, 20 mg

Tagamet® [US] *see* cimetidine *on page 189*

Tagamet® 800 mg *(Discontinued)* *see* cimetidine *on page 189*

Tagamet® HB [Can] *see* cimetidine *on page 189*

Tagamet® HB 200 [US-OTC] *see* cimetidine *on page 189*

TAK-375 *see* ramelteon *on page 731*

Talacen® [US] *see* pentazocine and acetaminophen *on page 651*

Talwin® [US/Can] *see* pentazocine *on page 651*

Talwin® NX [US] *see* pentazocine *on page 651*

TAM *see* tamoxifen *on this page*

Tambocor™ [US/Can] *see* flecainide *on page 347*

Tamiflu® [US/Can] *see* oseltamivir *on page 621*

Tamofen® [Can] *see* tamoxifen *on this page*

tamoxifen (ta MOKS i fen)

Sound-Alike/Look-Alike Issues

tamoxifen may be confused with pentoxifylline, Tambocor™

Synonyms ICI-46474; NSC-180973; TAM; tamoxifen citrate

U.S./Canadian Brand Names Apo-Tamox® [Can]; Gen-Tamoxifen [Can]; Nolvadex® [Can]; Nolvadex®-D [Can]; Novo-Tamoxifen [Can]; Soltamox™ [US]; Tamofen® [Can]

Therapeutic Category Antineoplastic Agent

Use Palliative or adjunctive treatment of advanced breast cancer; reduce the incidence of breast cancer in women at high risk; reduce risk of invasive breast cancer in women with ductal carcinoma *in situ* (DCIS); metastatic female and male breast cancer

Usual Dosage Adults: Oral (refer to individual protocols):

Breast cancer:

Metastatic (males and females) or adjuvant therapy (females): 20-40 mg/day; daily doses >20 mg should be given in 2 divided doses (morning and evening)

Prevention (high-risk females): 20 mg/day for 5 years

DCIS (females): 20 mg once daily for 5 years

Note: Higher dosages (up to 700 mg/day) have been investigated for use in modulation of multidrug resistance (MDR), but are not routinely used in clinical practice

Dosage Forms
Solution, oral:
Soltamox™: 10 mg/5 mL (150 mL) [licorice flavor]
Tablet: 10 mg, 20 mg
Nolvadex®: 10 mg, 20 mg [DSC]

tamoxifen citrate *see* tamoxifen *on previous page*

tamsulosin (tam SOO loe sin)

Sound-Alike/Look-Alike Issues
Flomax® may be confused with Fosamax®, Volmax®

Synonyms tamsulosin hydrochloride

U.S./Canadian Brand Names Flomax® CR [Can]; Flomax® [US/Can]

Therapeutic Category Alpha-Adrenergic Blocking Agent

Use Treatment of signs and symptoms of benign prostatic hyperplasia (BPH)

Usual Dosage Oral: Adults: 0.4 mg once daily ~30 minutes after the same meal each day; dose may be increased after 2-4 weeks to 0.8 mg once daily in patients who fail to respond. If therapy is interrupted for several days, restart with 0.4 mg once daily.

Dosage Forms Capsule, as hydrochloride: 0.4 mg

tamsulosin hydrochloride *see* tamsulosin *on this page*
Tanac® [US-OTC] *see* benzocaine *on page 99*
Tanafed® *(Discontinued)* *see* chlorpheniramine and pseudoephedrine *on page 177*
Tanafed DMX™ [US] *see* chlorpheniramine, pseudoephedrine, and dextromethorphan *on page 182*
Tannate-V-DM [US] *see* phenylephrine, pyrilamine, and dextromethorphan *on page 664*
Tannate 12 S [US] *see* carbetapentane and chlorpheniramine *on page 146*
Tannic-12 [US] *see* carbetapentane and chlorpheniramine *on page 146*
Tannic-12 S [US] *see* carbetapentane and chlorpheniramine *on page 146*
Tannihist-12 RF [US] *see* carbetapentane and chlorpheniramine *on page 146*
Tanta-Orciprenaline® [Can] *see* metaproterenol *on page 535*
Tantum® [Can] *see* benzydamine *(Canada only) on page 104*
TAP-144 *see* leuprolide *on page 486*
Tapazole® [US/Can] *see* methimazole *on page 539*
Tarabine® PFS *(Discontinued)* *see* cytarabine *on page 224*
Tarceva® [US/Can] *see* erlotinib *on page 302*
Targel® [Can] *see* coal tar *on page 207*
Targretin® [US/Can] *see* bexarotene *on page 109*
Tarka® [US/Can] *see* trandolapril and verapamil *on page 842*
Taro-Amcinonide [Can] *see* amcinonide *on page 39*
Taro-Carbamazepine Chewable [Can] *see* carbamazepine *on page 144*
Taro-Ciprofloxacin [Can] *see* ciprofloxacin *on page 190*
Taro-Clindamycin [Can] *see* clindamycin *on page 198*
Taro-Clobetasol [Can] *see* clobetasol *on page 200*
Taro-Desoximetasone [Can] *see* desoximetasone *on page 238*
Taro-Mometasone [Can] *see* mometasone furoate *on page 563*
Taro-Simvastatin [Can] *see* simvastatin *on page 773*
Taro-Sone® [Can] *see* betamethasone (topical) *on page 107*
Taro-Warfarin [Can] *see* warfarin *on page 881*
Tarsum® [US-OTC] *see* coal tar and salicylic acid *on page 208*
Tasmar® [US] *see* tolcapone *on page 834*
Tavist® Allergy [US-OTC] *see* clemastine *on page 197*
Tavist® ND [US-OTC] *see* loratadine *on page 505*

Taxol® [US/Can] *see* paclitaxel *on page 631*

Taxotere® [US/Can] *see* docetaxel *on page 269*

tazarotene (taz AR oh teen)

U.S./Canadian Brand Names Avage™ [US]; Tazorac® [US/Can]

Therapeutic Category Keratolytic Agent

Use Topical treatment of facial acne vulgaris; topical treatment of stable plaque psoriasis of up to 20% body surface area involvement; mitigation (palliation) of facial skin wrinkling, facial mottled hyper-/hypopigmentation, and benign facial lentigines

Usual Dosage Topical: **Note:** In patients experiencing excessive pruritus, burning, skin redness, or peeling, discontinue until integrity of the skin is restored, or reduce dosing to an interval the patient is able to tolerate.

Children ≥12 years and Adults:

Acne: Tazorac® cream/gel 0.1%: Cleanse the face gently. After the skin is dry, apply a thin film of tazarotene (2 mg/cm^2) once daily, in the evening, to the skin where the acne lesions appear; use enough to cover the entire affected area

Psoriasis: Tazorac® gel 0.05% or 0.1%: Apply once daily, in the evening, to psoriatic lesions using enough (2 mg/cm^2) to cover only the lesion with a thin film to no more than 20% of body surface area. If a bath or shower is taken prior to application, dry the skin before applying. Unaffected skin may be more susceptible to irritation, avoid application to these areas.

Children ≥17 years and Adults: Palliation of fine facial wrinkles, facial mottled hyper/hypopigmentation, benign facial lentigines: Avage™: Apply a pea-sized amount once daily to clean dry face at bedtime; lightly cover entire face including eyelids if desired. Emollients or moisturizers may be applied before or after; if applied before tazarotene, ensure cream or lotion has absorbed into the skin and has dried completely.

Adults: Psoriasis: Tazorac® cream 0.05% or 0.1%: Apply once daily, in the evening, to psoriatic lesions using enough (2 mg/cm^2) to cover only the lesion with a thin film to no more than 20% of body surface area. If a bath or shower is taken prior to application, dry the skin before applying. Unaffected skin may be more susceptible to irritation, avoid application to these areas.

Dosage Forms

Cream:

Avage™: 0.1% (30 g) [contains benzyl alcohol]

Tazorac®: 0.05% (30 g, 60 g); 0.1% (30 g, 60 g) [contains benzyl alcohol]

Gel (Tazorac®): 0.05% (30 g, 100 g); 0.1% (30 g, 100 g) [contains benzyl alcohol]

Tazicef® [US] *see* ceftazidime *on page 161*

tazobactam and piperacillin *see* piperacillin and tazobactam sodium *on page 670*

Tazocin® [Can] *see* piperacillin and tazobactam sodium *on page 670*

Tazorac® [US/Can] *see* tazarotene *on this page*

Taztia XT™ [US] *see* diltiazem *on page 257*

3TC® [Can] *see* lamivudine *on page 479*

3TC *see* lamivudine *on page 479*

3TC, abacavir, and zidovudine *see* abacavir, lamivudine, and zidovudine *on page 2*

T-cell growth factor *see* aldesleukin *on page 26*

TCGF *see* aldesleukin *on page 26*

TCN *see* tetracycline *on page 816*

Td *see* diphtheria and tetanus toxoid *on page 264*

Tdap *see* diphtheria, tetanus toxoids, and acellular pertussis vaccine *on page 265*

TDF *see* tenofovir *on page 810*

Teardrops® [Can] *see* artificial tears *on page 75*

Tear Drop® Solution *(Discontinued)* *see* artificial tears *on page 75*

TearGard® Ophthalmic Solution *(Discontinued)* *see* artificial tears *on page 75*

Teargen® [US-OTC] *see* artificial tears *on page 75*

Teargen® II [US-OTC] *see* artificial tears *on page 75*

Tearisol® [US-OTC] *see* artificial tears *on page 75*

Tearisol® [US-OTC] *see* hydroxypropyl methylcellulose *on page 432*

Tears Again® [US-OTC] *see* artificial tears *on page 75*

Tears Again® MC [US-OTC] *see* hydroxypropyl methylcellulose *on page 432*

Tears Again® Gel Drops™ [US-OTC] *see* carboxymethylcellulose *on page 151*

Tears Again® Night and Day™ [US-OTC] *see* carboxymethylcellulose *on page 151*

Tears Naturale® [US-OTC] *see* artificial tears *on page 75*

Tears Naturale® II [US-OTC] *see* artificial tears *on page 75*

Tears Naturale® Free [US-OTC] *see* artificial tears *on page 75*

Tears Plus® [US-OTC] *see* artificial tears *on page 75*

Tears Renewed® [US-OTC] *see* artificial tears *on page 75*

TEAS *see* trolamine *on page 855*

Tebamide™ [US] *see* trimethobenzamide *on page 851*

Tebrazid™ [Can] *see* pyrazinamide *on page 719*

Tecnal C 1/2 [Can] *see* butalbital, aspirin, caffeine, and codeine *on page 129*

Tecnal C 1/4 [Can] *see* butalbital, aspirin, caffeine, and codeine *on page 129*

tegaserod (teg a SER od)

Synonyms HTF919; tegaserod maleate

U.S./Canadian Brand Names Zelnorm® [US/Can]

Therapeutic Category Serotonin 5-HT_4 Receptor Agonist

Use Short-term treatment of constipation-predominate irritable bowel syndrome (IBS) in women; treatment of chronic idiopathic constipation

Usual Dosage Oral: Adults:

IBS with constipation (females): 6 mg twice daily, before meals, for 4-6 weeks; may consider continuing treatment for an additional 4-6 weeks in patients who respond initially

Chronic idiopathic constipation: 6 mg twice daily, before meals; the need for continued therapy should be reassessed periodically

Dosage Forms Tablet: 2 mg, 6 mg

tegaserod maleate *see* tegaserod *on this page*

Tega-Vert® Oral *(Discontinued)* *see* dimenhydrinate *on page 258*

Tegretol® [US/Can] *see* carbamazepine *on page 144*

Tegretol®-XR [US] *see* carbamazepine *on page 144*

Telachlor® Oral *(Discontinued)* *see* chlorpheniramine *on page 175*

Teladar® Topical *(Discontinued)*

Teldrin® HBP [US-OTC] *see* chlorpheniramine *on page 175*

Teldrin® Oral *(Discontinued)* *see* chlorpheniramine *on page 175*

Telepaque® [US] *see* radiological/contrast media (ionic) *on page 728*

telithromycin (tel ith roe MYE sin)

Synonyms HMR 3647

U.S./Canadian Brand Names Ketek® [US/Can]

Therapeutic Category Antibiotic, Ketolide

Use Treatment of community-acquired pneumonia (mild-to-moderate) caused by susceptible strains of *Streptococcus pneumoniae* (including multidrug-resistant isolates), *Haemophilus influenzae*, *Chlamydia pneumoniae*, *Moraxella catarrhalis*, and *Mycoplasma pneumoniae*; treatment of bacterial exacerbation of chronic bronchitis caused by susceptible strains of *S. pneumoniae*, *H. influenzae* and *Moraxella catarrhalis*; treatment of acute bacterial sinusitis caused by *Streptococcus pneumoniae*, *Haemophilus influenzae*, *Moraxella catarrhalis*, and *Staphylococcus aureus*

Usual Dosage Oral: Adults:

Acute exacerbation of chronic bronchitis, acute bacterial sinusitis: 800 mg once daily for 5 days

Community-acquired pneumonia: 800 mg once daily for 7-10 days

Dosage Forms

Tablet:

Ketek®: 300 mg [not available in Canada], 400 mg

Ketek Pak™ [blister pack]: 400 mg (10s) [packaged as 10 tablets/card; 2 tablets/blister]

telmisartan (tel mi SAR tan)

U.S./Canadian Brand Names Micardis® [US/Can]

Therapeutic Category Angiotensin II Receptor Antagonist

Use Treatment of hypertension; may be used alone or in combination with other antihypertensive agents

Usual Dosage Adults: Oral: Initial: 40 mg once daily; usual maintenance dose range: 20-80 mg/day. Patients with volume depletion should be initiated on the lower dosage with close supervision.

Dosage Forms Tablet: 20 mg, 40 mg, 80 mg

telmisartan and hydrochlorothiazide (tel mi SAR tan & hye droe klor oh THYE a zide)

Synonyms hydrochlorothiazide and telmisartan

U.S./Canadian Brand Names Micardis® HCT [US]; Micardis® Plus [Can]

Therapeutic Category Antihypertensive Agent, Combination

Use Treatment of hypertension; combination product should not be used for initial therapy

Usual Dosage Adults: Oral: Replacement therapy: Combination product can be substituted for individual titrated agents. Initiation of combination therapy when monotherapy has failed to achieve desired effects:

Patients currently on telmisartan: Initial dose if blood pressure is not currently controlled on monotherapy of 80 mg telmisartan: Telmisartan 80 mg/hydrochlorothiazide 12.5 mg once daily; may titrate up to telmisartan 160 mg/hydrochlorothiazide 25 mg if needed

Patients currently on HCTZ: Initial dose if blood pressure is not currently controlled on monotherapy of 25 mg once daily: Telmisartan 80 mg/hydrochlorothiazide 12.5 mg once daily or telmisartan 80 mg/hydrochlorothiazide 25 mg once daily; may titrate up to telmisartan 160 mg/hydrochlorothiazide 25 mg if blood pressure remains uncontrolled after 2-4 weeks of therapy. Patients who develop hypokalemia may be switched to telmisartan 80 mg/hydrochlorothiazide 12.5 mg.

Dosage Forms [CAN]: Canadian brand name

Tablet:

Micardis® HCT [available in U.S.]:

40/12.5: Telmisartan 40 mg and hydrochlorothiazide 12.5 mg

80/12.5: Telmisartan 80 mg and hydrochlorothiazide 12.5 mg

80/25: Telmisartan 80 mg and hydrochlorothiazide 25 mg

Micardis® Plus [CAN]: 80/25: Telmisartan 80 mg and hydrochlorothiazide 25 mg [Not available in U.S.]

Telzir® [Can] *see* fosamprenavir *on page 368*

temazepam (te MAZ e pam)

Sound-Alike/Look-Alike Issues

temazepam may be confused with flurazepam, lorazepam

Restoril® may be confused with Vistaril®, Zestril®

U.S./Canadian Brand Names Apo-Temazepam® [Can]; CO Temazepam [Can]; Gen-Temazepam [Can]; Novo-Temazepam [Can]; Nu-Temazepam [Can]; PMS-Temazepam [Can]; ratio-Temazepam [Can]; Restoril® [US/Can]

Therapeutic Category Benzodiazepine

Controlled Substance C-IV

Use Short-term treatment of insomnia

Usual Dosage Oral: Adults: 15-30 mg at bedtime

Dosage Forms

Capsule: 15 mg, 30 mg

Restoril®: 7.5 mg, 15 mg, 30 mg

Temodal™ [Can] *see* temozolomide *on this page*

Temodar® [US/Can] *see* temozolomide *on this page*

Temovate® [US] *see* clobetasol *on page 200*

Temovate E® [US] *see* clobetasol *on page 200*

temozolomide (te moe ZOE loe mide)

Synonyms NSC-362856; TMZ

U.S./Canadian Brand Names Temodal™ [Can]; Temodar® [US/Can]

Therapeutic Category Antineoplastic Agent, Alkylating Agent

Use Treatment of adult patients with refractory (first relapse) anaplastic astrocytoma who have experienced disease progression on nitrosourea and procarbazine; newly-diagnosed glioblastoma multiforme

Usual Dosage Oral (refer to individual protocols): Adults:

Anaplastic astrocytoma (refractory): Initial dose: 150 mg/m²/day for 5 days; repeat every 28 days. Subsequent doses of 100-200 mg/m²/day; based upon hematologic tolerance. This monthly-cycle regimen may be preceded by a 6- to 7-week regimen of 75 mg/m²/day.

ANC <1000/mm³ or platelets <50,000/mm³ on day 22 or day 29 (day 1 of next cycle): Postpone therapy until ANC >1500/mm³ and platelets >100,000/mm³; reduce dose by 50 mg/m²/day for subsequent cycle

ANC 1000-1500/mm³ or platelets 50,000-100,000/mm³ on day 22 or day 29 (day 1 of next cycle): Postpone therapy until ANC >1500/mm³ and platelets >100,000/mm³; maintain initial dose

ANC >1500/mm³ and platelets >100,000/mm³ on day 22 or day 29 (day 1 of next cycle): Increase dose to or maintain dose at 200 mg/m²/day for 5 days for subsequent cycle

Glioblastoma multiforme (high-grade glioma):

Concomitant phase: 75 mg/m²/day for 42 days with radiotherapy (60Gy administered in 30 fractions). **Note:** PCP prophylaxis is required during concomitant phase and should continue in patients who develop lymphocytopenia until recovery (common toxicity criteria [CTC] ≤1). Obtain weekly CBC.

ANC ≥1500/mm³, platelet count ≥100,000/mm³, and nonhematologic CTC ≤grade 1 (excludes alopecia, nausea/vomiting): Temodar® 75 mg/m²/day may be continued throughout the 42-day concomitant period up to 49 days

Dosage modification:

ANC ≥500/mm³ but <1500/mm³ **or** platelet count ≥10,000/mm³ but <100,000/mm³ **or** nonhematologic CTC grade 2 (excludes alopecia, nausea/vomiting): Interrupt therapy

ANC <500/mm³ **or** platelet count <10,000/mm³ **or** nonhematologic CTC grade 3/4 (excludes alopecia, nausea/vomiting): Discontinue therapy

Maintenance phase (consists of 6 treatment cycles): Begin 4 weeks after concomitant phase completion. **Note:** Each subsequent cycle is 28 days (consisting of 5 days of drug treatment followed by 23 days without treatment). Draw CBC within 48 hours of day 22; hold next cycle and do weekly CBC until ANC >1500/mm³ and platelet count >100,000/mm³; dosing modification should be based on lowest blood counts and worst nonhematologic toxicity during the previous cycle.

Cycle 1: 150 mg/m²/day for 5 days

Dosage modification for next cycle:

ANC <1000/mm³, platelet count <50,000/mm³, or nonhematologic CTC grade 3 (excludes for alopecia, nausea/vomiting) during previous cycle: Decrease dose by 50 mg/m²/day for 5 days, unless dose has already been lowered to 100 mg/m²/day, then discontinue therapy.

If dose reduction <100 mg/m²/day is required or nonhematologic CTC grade 4 (excludes for alopecia, nausea/vomiting), or if the same grade 3 nonhematologic toxicity occurs after dose reduction: Discontinue therapy

Cycle 2: 200 mg/m²/day for 5 days unless prior toxicity, then refer to Dosage Modifications under "Cycle 1" and give adjusted dose for 5 days

Cycles 3-6: Continue with previous cycle's dose for 5 days unless toxicity has occurred then, refer to Dosage Modifications under "Cycle 1" and give adjusted dose for 5 days

Dosage Forms Capsule: 5 mg, 20 mg, 100 mg, 250 mg

Tempra® [Can] *see* acetaminophen *on page 5*

Tempra® *(Discontinued)* *see* acetaminophen *on page 5*

tenecteplase (ten EK te plase)

Sound-Alike/Look-Alike Issues

TNKase™ may be confused with t-PA

TNK (occasional abbreviation for TNKase™) is an error-prone abbreviation (mistaken as TPA)

U.S./Canadian Brand Names TNKase™ [US/Can]

Therapeutic Category Thrombolytic Agent

Use Thrombolytic agent used in the management of acute myocardial infarction for the lysis of thrombi in the coronary vasculature to restore perfusion and reduce mortality.

Usual Dosage I.V.:

Adult: Recommended total dose should not exceed 50 mg and is based on patient's weight; administer as a bolus over 5 seconds

If patient's weight:

<60 kg, dose: 30 mg

≥60 to <70 kg, dose: 35 mg

≥70 to <80 kg, dose: 40 mg

≥80 to <90 kg, dose: 45 mg

≥90 kg, dose: 50 mg

All patients received 150-325 mg of aspirin as soon as possible and then daily. Intravenous heparin was initiated as soon as possible and aPTT was maintained between 50-70 seconds.

Dosage Forms Injection, powder for reconstitution, recombinant: 50 mg [packaged with diluent and syringe]

Tenex® [US/Can] *see* guanfacine *on page 403*

teniposide (ten i POE side)

Sound-Alike/Look-Alike Issues
teniposide may be confused with etoposide

Synonyms EPT; VM-26

U.S./Canadian Brand Names Vumon® [US/Can]

Therapeutic Category Antineoplastic Agent

Use Treatment of acute lymphocytic leukemia, small-cell lung cancer

Usual Dosage I.V.:

Children: 130 mg/m^2/week, increasing to 150 mg/m^2 after 3 weeks and up to 180 mg/m^2 after 6 weeks

Acute lymphoblastic leukemia (ALL): 165 mg/m^2 twice weekly for 8-9 doses **or** 250 mg/m^2 weekly for 4-8 weeks

Adults: 50-180 mg/m^2 once or twice weekly for 4-6 weeks or 20-60 mg/m^2/day for 5 days

Small cell lung cancer: 80-90 mg/m^2/day for 5 days every 4-6 weeks

Dosage Forms Injection, solution: 10 mg/mL (5 mL) [contains benzyl alcohol, dehydrated alcohol, and polyoxyethylated castor oil]

Ten-K® *(Discontinued)* *see* potassium chloride *on page 684*

tenofovir (te NOE fo veer)

Synonyms PMPA; TDF; tenofovir disoproxil fumarate

U.S./Canadian Brand Names Viread® [US/Can]

Therapeutic Category Antiretroviral Agent, Reverse Transcriptase Inhibitor (Nucleotide)

Use Management of HIV infections in combination with at least two other antiretroviral agents

Usual Dosage Oral: Adults: HIV infection: 300 mg once daily

Dosage Forms Tablet, as disoproxil fumarate: 300 mg [equivalent to 245 mg tenofovir disoproxil]

tenofovir and emtricitabine *see* emtricitabine and tenofovir *on page 290*

tenofovir disoproxil fumarate *see* tenofovir *on this page*

Tenolin [Can] *see* atenolol *on page 80*

Tenoretic® [US/Can] *see* atenolol and chlorthalidone *on page 80*

Tenormin® [US/Can] *see* atenolol *on page 80*

Tenuate® [Can] *see* diethylpropion *on page 253*

Tenuate® Dospan® [Can] *see* diethylpropion *on page 253*

Tequin® [Can] *see* gatifloxacin *on page 376*

Tequin® *(Discontinued)* *see* gatifloxacin *on page 376*

Tera-Gel™ [US-OTC] *see* coal tar *on page 207*

Terazol® [Can] *see* terconazole *on next page*

Terazol® 3 [US] *see* terconazole *on next page*

Terazol® 7 [US] *see* terconazole *on next page*

terazosin (ter AY zoe sin)

U.S./Canadian Brand Names Alti-Terazosin [Can]; Apo-Terazosin® [Can]; Hytrin® [US/Can]; Novo-Terazosin [Can]; Nu-Terazosin [Can]; PMS-Terazosin [Can]

Therapeutic Category Alpha-Adrenergic Blocking Agent

Use Management of mild to moderate hypertension; alone or in combination with other agents such as diuretics or beta-blockers; benign prostate hyperplasia (BPH)

Usual Dosage Oral: Adults:

Hypertension: Initial: 1 mg at bedtime; slowly increase dose to achieve desired blood pressure, up to 20 mg/day; usual dose range (JNC 7): 1-20 mg once daily

Dosage reduction may be needed when adding a diuretic or other antihypertensive agent; if drug is discontinued for greater than several days, consider beginning with initial dose and retitrate as needed; dosage may be given on a twice daily regimen if response is diminished at 24 hours and hypotensive is observed at 2-4 hours following a dose

Benign prostatic hyperplasia: Initial: 1 mg at bedtime, increasing as needed; most patients require 10 mg day; if no response after 4-6 weeks of 10 mg/day, may increase to 20 mg/day

Dosage Forms Capsule: 1 mg, 2 mg, 5 mg, 10 mg

terbinafine (oral) (TER bin a feen OR al)

U.S./Canadian Brand Names Lamisil® Oral [US/Can]

Therapeutic Category Antifungal Agent

Use Treatment of onychomycosis infections of the toenail or fingernail

Usual Dosage Adults: Oral:

Fingernail onychomycosis: 250 mg once daily for 6 weeks

Toenail onychomycosis: 250 mg once daily for 12 weeks

Dosage Forms Tablet: 250 mg

terbinafine (topical) (TER bin a feen TOP i kal)

U.S./Canadian Brand Names Lamisil® Topical [US/Can]

Therapeutic Category Antifungal Agent

Use Topical antifungal for the treatment of tinea pedis (athlete's foot), tinea cruris (jock itch), and tinea corporis (ring worm); tinea versicolor (lotion)

Usual Dosage Adults: Topical:

Athlete's foot: Apply to affected area twice daily for at least 1 week, not to exceed 4 weeks

Ringworm and jock itch: Apply to affected area once or twice daily for at least 1 week, not to exceed 4 weeks

Dosage Forms

Cream: 1% (15 g, 30 g)

Lotion: 1%

terbutaline (ter BYOO ta leen)

Sound-Alike/Look-Alike Issues

terbutaline may be confused with terbinafine, TOLBUTamide

U.S./Canadian Brand Names Brethine® [US]; Bricanyl® [Can]

Therapeutic Category Adrenergic Agonist Agent

Use Bronchodilator in reversible airway obstruction and bronchial asthma

Usual Dosage

Children <12 years: Bronchoconstriction:

Oral: Initial: 0.05 mg/kg/dose 3 times/day, increased gradually as required; maximum: 0.15 mg/kg/dose 3-4 times/day or a total of 5 mg/24 hours

SubQ: 0.005-0.01 mg/kg/dose to a maximum of 0.3 mg/dose; may repeat in 15-20 minutes

Children ≥6 years and Adults: Bronchospasm (acute): Inhalation (Bricanyl® [CAN] MDI: 500 mcg/puff, *not labeled for use in the U.S.*): One puff as needed; may repeat with 1 inhalation (after 5 minutes); more than 6 inhalations should not be necessary in any 24 hour period. **Note:** If a previously effective dosage regimen fails to provide the usual relief, or the effects of a dose last for >3 hours, medical advice should be sought immediately; this is a sign of seriously worsening asthma that requires reassessment of therapy.

Children >12 years and Adults: Bronchoconstriction:

Oral:

12-15 years: 2.5 mg every 6 hours 3 times/day; not to exceed 7.5 mg in 24 hours

>15 years: 5 mg/dose every 6 hours 3 times/day; if side effects occur, reduce dose to 2.5 mg every 6 hours; not to exceed 15 mg in 24 hours

SubQ: 0.25 mg/dose; may repeat in 15-30 minutes (maximum: 0.5 mg/4-hour period)

Dosage Forms

Injection, solution, as sulfate: 1 mg/mL (1 mL)

Tablet, as sulfate: 2.5 mg, 5 mg

Additional dosage forms available in Canada: Powder for oral inhalation (Bricanyl® Turbuhaler): 500 mcg/actuation [50 or 200 metered doses]

terconazole (ter KONE a zole)

Sound-Alike/Look-Alike Issues

terconazole may be confused with tioconazole

Synonyms triaconazole

U.S./Canadian Brand Names Terazol® 3 [US]; Terazol® 7 [US]; Terazol® [Can]

Therapeutic Category Antifungal Agent

Use Local treatment of vulvovaginal candidiasis

Usual Dosage Adults: Female:

Terazol® 3 vaginal cream: Insert 1 applicatorful intravaginally at bedtime for 3 consecutive days

Terazol® 7 vaginal cream: Insert 1 applicatorful intravaginally at bedtime for 7 consecutive days

(Continued)

terconazole *(Continued)*

Terazol® 3 vaginal suppository: Insert 1 suppository intravaginally at bedtime for 3 consecutive days

Dosage Forms

Cream, vaginal:

Terazol® 7: 0.4% (45 g) [packaged with measured-dose applicator]

Terazol® 3: 0.8% (20 g) [packaged with measured-dose applicator]

Suppository, vaginal (Terazol® 3): 80 mg (3s) [may contain coconut and/or palm kernel oil]

Terfluzine [Can] *see* trifluoperazine *on page 849*

teriparatide (ter i PAR a tide)

Synonyms parathyroid hormone (1-34); recombinant human parathyroid hormone (1-34); rhPTH(1-34)

U.S./Canadian Brand Names Forteo™ [US/Can]

Therapeutic Category Diagnostic Agent

Use Treatment of osteoporosis in postmenopausal women at high risk of fracture; treatment of primary or hypogonadal osteoporosis in men at high risk of fracture

Usual Dosage SubQ: Adults: 20 mcg once daily; **Note:** Initial administration should occur under circumstances in which the patient may sit or lie down, in the event of orthostasis.

Dosage Forms Injection, solution: 250 mcg/mL (3 mL) [prefilled syringe, delivers teriparatide 20 mcg/dose]

terpin hydrate ***(Discontinued)***

Terra-Cortril® Ophthalmic Suspension ***(Discontinued)***

Terramycin® [Can] *see* oxytetracycline *on page 630*

Terramycin® I.M. ***(Discontinued)*** *see* oxytetracycline *on page 630*

Terramycin® Oral ***(Discontinued)*** *see* oxytetracycline *on page 630*

Terrell™ [US] *see* isoflurane *on page 463*

Tesamone® Injection ***(Discontinued)*** *see* testosterone *on this page*

Teslac® [US/Can] *see* testolactone *on this page*

TESPA *see* thiotepa *on page 823*

Tessalon® [US/Can] *see* benzonatate *on page 102*

Testim® [US] *see* testosterone *on this page*

Testoderm® ***(Discontinued)*** *see* testosterone *on this page*

Testoderm® TTS ***(Discontinued)*** *see* testosterone *on this page*

Testoderm® With Adhesive ***(Discontinued)*** *see* testosterone *on this page*

testolactone (tes toe LAK tone)

Sound-Alike/Look-Alike Issues

testolactone may be confused with testosterone

U.S./Canadian Brand Names Teslac® [US/Can]

Therapeutic Category Androgen

Controlled Substance C-III

Use Palliative treatment of advanced or disseminated breast carcinoma

Usual Dosage Adults: Female: Oral: 250 mg 4 times/day for at least 3 months; desired response may take as long as 3 months

Dosage Forms Tablet: 50 mg

Testomar® ***(Discontinued)*** *see* yohimbine *on page 883*

Testopel® [US] *see* testosterone *on this page*

Testopel® Pellet ***(Discontinued)*** *see* testosterone *on this page*

testosterone (tes TOS ter one)

Sound-Alike/Look-Alike Issues

testosterone may be confused with testolactone

Testoderm® may be confused with Estraderm®

Synonyms testosterone cypionate; testosterone enanthate

U.S./Canadian Brand Names Andriol® [Can]; Androderm® [US/Can]; AndroGel® [US/Can]; Andropository [Can]; Delatestryl® [US/Can]; Depotest® 100 [Can]; Depo®-Testosterone [US]; Everone® 200 [Can]; First®

Testosterone MC [US]; First® Testosterone [US]; Striant® [US]; Testim® [US]; Testopel® [US]; Virilon® IM [Can]

Therapeutic Category Androgen

Controlled Substance C-III

Use

Injection: Androgen replacement therapy in the treatment of delayed male puberty; male hypogonadism (primary or hypogonadotropic); inoperable female breast cancer (enanthate only)

Pellet: Androgen replacement therapy in the treatment of delayed male puberty; male hypogonadism (primary or hypogonadotropic)

Buccal, topical: Male hypogonadism (primary or hypogonadotropic)

Capsule (not available in U.S.): Management of congenital or acquired primary hypogonadism and hypogonadotropic hypogonadism; development and maintainenance of secondary sexual characteristics in males with testosterone deficiency; stimulation of puberty in carefully selected males with clearly delayed puberty not secondary to a pathological disorder; replacement therapy in syndromes with symptoms of deficiency or absence of endogenous testosterone; replacement therapy in impotence or for male climacteric symptoms when the conditions are due to a measured or documented androgen deficiency

Usual Dosage

Adolescents: I.M.:

Male hypogonadism:

Initiation of pubertal growth: 40-50 mg/m^2/dose (cypionate or enanthate ester) monthly until the growth rate falls to prepubertal levels

Terminal growth phase: 100 mg/m^2/dose (cypionate or enanthate ester) monthly until growth ceases

Maintenance virilizing dose: 100 mg/m^2/dose (cypionate or enanthate ester) twice monthly

Delayed male puberty: 40-50 mg/m^2/dose monthly (cypionate or enanthate ester) for 6 months

Adolescents and Adults:

Pellet (for subcutaneous implantation): Delayed male puberty, male hypogonadism: 150-450 mg every 3-6 months

Oral: Hypogonadism or hypogonadotropic hypogonadism:

Buccal: 30 mg twice daily (every 12 hours) applied to the gum region above the incisor tooth

Capsule (Andriol®; not available in U.S.): Initial: 120-160 mg/day in 2 divided doses for 2-3 weeks; adjust according to individual response; usual maintenance dose: 40-120 mg/day (in divided doses)

Adults:

I.M.:

Female: Inoperable breast cancer: Testosterone enanthate: 200-400 mg every 2-4 weeks

Male: Long-acting formulations: Testosterone enanthate (in oil)/testosterone cypionate (in oil):

Hypogonadism: 50-400 mg every 2-4 weeks

Delayed puberty: 50-200 mg every 2-4 weeks for a limited duration

Transdermal: Primary male hypogonadism **or** hypogonadotropic hypogonadism:

Androderm®: Initial: Apply 5 mg/day once nightly to clean, dry area on the back, abdomen, upper arms, or thighs (do **not** apply to scrotum); dosing range: 2.5-7.5 mg/day; in nonvirilized patients, dose may be initiated at 2.5 mg/day

AndroGel®, Testim®: 5 g (to deliver 50 mg of testosterone with 5 mg systemically absorbed) applied once daily (preferably in the morning) to clean, dry, intact skin of the shoulder and upper arms. AndroGel® may also be applied to the abdomen. Dosage may be increased to a maximum of 10 g (100 mg). **Do not apply testosterone gel to the genitals.**

Dosage Forms [CAN] = Canadian brand name

Capsule, gelatin, as deconate (Andriol™ [CAN]): 40 mg (10s) [not available in U.S.]

Gel, topical:

AndroGel®:

1.25 g/actuation (75 g) [1% metered-dose pump; delivers 5 g/4 actuations; provides 60 1.25 g actuations; contains ethanol]

2.5 g (30s) [1% unit dose packets; contains ethanol]

5 g (30s) [1% unit dose packets; contains ethanol]

Testim®: 5 g (30s) [1% unit-dose tube; contains ethanol]

Injection, in oil, as cypionate: 200 mg/mL (10 mL)

Depo®-Testosterone: 100 mg/mL (10 mL); 200 mg/mL (1 mL, 10 mL) [contains benzyl alcohol, benzyl benzoate, and cottonseed oil]

Injection, in oil, as enanthate: 200 mg/mL (5 mL)

Delatestryl®: 200 mg/mL (1 mL) [prefilled syringe; contains sesame oil]; (5 mL) [multidose vial; contains sesame oil]

Kit [for prescription compounding testosterone 2%; kits also contain mixing jar and stirrer]:

First® Testosterone:

Injection, in oil: Testosterone propionate 100 mg/mL (12 mL) [contains sesame oil and benzyl alcohol]

Ointment: White petroleum (48 g)

(Continued)

testosterone *(Continued)*

First® Testosterone MC:

Injection, in oil: Testosterone propionate 100 mg/mL (12 mL) [contains sesame oil and benzyl alcohol]

Cream: Moisturizing cream (48 g)

Mucoadhesive, for buccal application [buccal system] (Striant®): 30 mg (10s)

Pellet, for subcutaneous implantation (Testopel®): 75 mg (1 pellet/vial)

Transdermal system (Androderm®): 2.5 mg/day (60s); 5 mg/day (30s) [contains ethanol]

testosterone cypionate *see* testosterone *on page 812*

testosterone enanthate *see* testosterone *on page 812*

Testred® [US] *see* methyltestosterone *on page 548*

tetanus and diphtheria toxoid *see* diphtheria and tetanus toxoid *on page 264*

tetanus immune globulin (human) (TET a nus i MYUN GLOB yoo lin HYU man)

Synonyms TIG

U.S./Canadian Brand Names BayTet™ [Can]; HyperTET™ S/D [US]

Therapeutic Category Immune Globulin

Use Passive immunization against tetanus; tetanus immune globulin is preferred over tetanus antitoxin for treatment of active tetanus; part of the management of an unclean, wound in a person whose history of previous receipt of tetanus toxoid is unknown or who has received less than three doses of tetanus toxoid

Usual Dosage I.M.:

Prophylaxis of tetanus:

Children: 4 units/kg; some recommend administering 250 units to small children

Adults: 250 units

Treatment of tetanus:

Children: 500-3000 units; some should infiltrate locally around the wound

Adults: 3000-6000 units

Dosage Forms

Injection, solution [preservative free]:

BayTet™[DSC], HyperTET™ S/D: 250 units/mL (1 mL) [prefilled syringe]

tetanus toxoid (adsorbed) (TET a nus TOKS oyd, ad SORBED)

Sound-Alike/Look-Alike Issues

Tetanus toxoid products may be confused with influenza virus vaccine and tuberculin products. Medication errors have occurred when tetanus toxoid products have been inadvertently administered instead of tuberculin skin tests (PPD) and influenza virus vaccine. These products are refrigerated and often stored in close proximity to each other.

Therapeutic Category Toxoid

Use Active immunization against tetanus when combination antigen preparations are not indicated. **Note:** Tetanus and diphtheria toxoids for adult use (Td) is the preferred immunizing agent for most adults and for children after their seventh birthday. Young children should receive trivalent DTaP (diphtheria/tetanus/acellular pertussis), as part of their childhood immunization program, unless pertussis is contraindicated, then TD is warranted.

Usual Dosage Children ≥7 years and Adults: I.M.:

Primary immunization: 0.5 mL; repeat 0.5 mL at 4-8 weeks after first dose and at 6-12 months after second dose

Routine booster dose: Recommended every 10 years

Note: In most patients, Td is the recommended product for primary immunization, booster doses, and tetanus immunization in wound management (refer to diphtheria and tetanus toxoid monograph)

Dosage Forms Injection, suspension: Tetanus 5 Lf units per 0.5 mL (0.5 mL) [contains trace amounts of thimerosal]; (5 mL) [contains thimerosal; vial stopper contains latex]

tetanus toxoid (fluid) (TET a nus TOKS oyd FLOO id)

Sound-Alike/Look-Alike Issues

Tetanus toxoid products may be confused with influenza virus vaccine and tuberculin products. Medication errors have occurred when tetanus toxoid products have been inadvertently administered instead of tuberculin skin tests (PPD) and influenza virus vaccine. These products are refrigerated and often stored in close proximity to each other.

Synonyms tetanus toxoid plain

Therapeutic Category Toxoid

Use Indicated as booster dose in the active immunization against tetanus in the rare adult or child who is allergic to the aluminum adjuvant (a product containing adsorbed tetanus toxoid is preferred); not indicated for primary immunization

Usual Dosage

Primary immunization: Not indicated for this use.

Booster doses: I.M., SubQ: 0.5 mL every 10 years

Dosage Forms Injection, solution: Tetanus 4 Lf units per 0.5 mL (7.5 mL) [contains thimerosal; vial stopper contains dry natural latex rubber]

tetanus toxoid plain *see* tetanus toxoid (fluid) *on previous page*

tetanus toxoid, reduced diphtheria toxoid, and acellular pertussis, adsorbed *see* diphtheria, tetanus toxoids, and acellular pertussis vaccine *on page 265*

tetrabenazine *(Canada only)* (tet ra BEN a zeen)

U.S./Canadian Brand Names Nitoman™ [Can]

Therapeutic Category Monoamine Depleting Agent

Use Treatment of hyperkinetic movement disorders, including Huntington chorea, hemiballismus, senile chorea, Tourette syndrome, and tardive dyskinesia

Usual Dosage Oral:

Children (limited data): Consider initiation at 1/2 recommended adult dosage; must be titrated slowly to individualize dosage

Adults: Initial: 12.5 mg twice daily (may be given 3 times/day); may be increased by 12.5 mg/day every 3-5 days; should be titrated slowly to maximal tolerated and effective dose (dose is individualized)

Usual maximum tolerated dosage: 25 mg 3 times/day; maximum recommended dose: 200 mg/day

Note: If there is no improvement at the maximum tolerated dose after 7 days, improvement is unlikely; discontinuation should be considered.

Dosage Forms Tablet: 25 mg

tetracaine (TET ra kane)

Synonyms amethocaine hydrochloride; tetracaine hydrochloride

U.S./Canadian Brand Names Ametop™ [Can]; Pontocaine® Niphanoid® [US]; Pontocaine® [US/Can]

Therapeutic Category Local Anesthetic

Use Spinal anesthesia; local anesthesia in the eye for various diagnostic and examination purposes; topically applied to nose and throat for various diagnostic procedures

Usual Dosage Adults:

Ophthalmic: Short-term anesthesia of the eye: 0.5% solution: Instill 1-2 drops; prolonged use (especially for at-home self-medication) is not recommended

Injection: Spinal anesthesia: **Note:** Dosage varies with the anesthetic procedure, the degree of anesthesia required, and the individual patient response; it is administered by subarachnoid injection for spinal anesthesia.

Perineal anesthesia: 5 mg

Perineal and lower extremities: 10 mg

Anesthesia extending up to costal margin: 15 mg; doses up to 20 mg may be given, but are reserved for exceptional cases

Low spinal anesthesia (saddle block): 2-5 mg

Topical mucous membranes (rhinolaryngology): Used as a 0.25% or 0.5% solution by direct application or nebulization; total dose should not exceed 20 mg

Dosage Forms [DSC] = Discontinued product

Injection, solution, as hydrochloride [preservative free] (Pontocaine®): 1% [10 mg/mL] (2 mL) [contains sodium bisulfite]

Injection, solution, as hydrochloride [premixed in dextrose 6%] (Pontocaine®): 0.3% [3 mg/mL] (5 mL) [DSC]

Injection, powder for reconstitution, as hydrochloride [preservative free] (Pontocaine® Niphanoid®): 20 mg

Solution, ophthalmic, as hydrochloride: 0.5% [5 mg/mL] (15 mL)

Solution, topical, as hydrochloride (Pontocaine®): 2% [20 mg/mL] (30 mL, 118 mL) [for rhinolaryngology]

tetracaine and dextrose (TET ra kane & DEKS trose)

Synonyms dextrose and tetracaine

U.S./Canadian Brand Names Pontocaine® With Dextrose [US]

Therapeutic Category Local Anesthetic

Use Spinal anesthesia (saddle block)

Usual Dosage Dose varies with procedure, depth of anesthesia, duration desired and physical condition of patient

Dosage Forms Injection, as hydrochloride [premixed in dextrose 6%]: Tetracaine hydrochloride 0.3% and dextrose 6% (5 mL)

tetracaine hydrochloride *see* tetracaine *on previous page*

tetracaine hydrochloride, benzocaine, butyl aminobenzoate, and benzalkonium chloride *see* benzocaine, butyl aminobenzoate, tetracaine, and benzalkonium chloride *on page 101*

Tetracap® *(Discontinued)* *see* tetracycline *on this page*

tetracosactide *see* cosyntropin *on page 216*

tetracycline (tet ra SYE kleen)

Sound-Alike/Look-Alike Issues

tetracycline may be confused with tetradecyl sulfate

achromycin may be confused with actinomycin, Adriamycin PFS®

Synonyms achromycin; TCN; tetracycline hydrochloride

U.S./Canadian Brand Names Apo-Tetra® [Can]; Nu-Tetra [Can]; Sumycin® [US]

Therapeutic Category Antibiotic, Ophthalmic; Antibiotic, Topical; Tetracycline Derivative

Use Treatment of susceptible bacterial infections of both gram-positive and gram-negative organisms; also infections due to *Mycoplasma*, *Chlamydia*, and *Rickettsia*; indicated for acne, exacerbations of chronic bronchitis, and treatment of gonorrhea and syphilis in patients that are allergic to penicillin; as part of a multidrug regimen for *H. pylori* eradication to reduce the risk of duodenal ulcer recurrence

Usual Dosage

Usual dosage range:

Children >8 years: Oral: 25-50 mg/kg/day in divided doses every 6 hours

Adults: Oral: 250-500 mg/dose every 6 hours

Indication-specific dosing:

Adults: Oral:

Acne: 250-500 twice daily

Chronic bronchitis, acute exacerbation: 500 mg 4 times/day

Erlichiosis: 500 mg 4 times/day for 7-14 days

Peptic ulcer disease: Eradication of *Helicobacter pylori*: 500 mg 2-4 times/day depending on regimen; requires combination therapy with at least one other antibiotic and an acid-suppressing agent (proton pump inhibitor or H_2 blocker)

Periodontitis: 250 mg every 6 hours until improvement (usually 10 days)

Vibrio cholerae: 500 mg 4 times/day for 3 days

Dosage Forms

Capsule, as hydrochloride: 250 mg, 500 mg

Suspension, oral, as hydrochloride (Sumycin®): 125 mg/5 mL (480 mL) [contains sodium benzoate and sodium metabisulfite; fruit flavor]

Tablet, as hydrochloride (Sumycin®): 250 mg, 500 mg

tetracycline hydrochloride *see* tetracycline *on this page*

tetracycline, metronidazole, and bismuth subsalicylate *see* bismuth subsalicylate, metronidazole, and tetracycline *on page 112*

tetrahydroaminoacrine *see* tacrine *on page 803*

tetrahydrocannabinol *see* dronabinol *on page 281*

tetrahydrocannabinol and cannabidiol *(Canada only)*

(TET ra hye droe can NAB e nol & can nab e DYE ol)

Synonyms cannabidiol and tetrahydrocannabinol; delta-9-tetrahydrocannabinol and cannabinol; GW-1000-02; THC and CBD

U.S./Canadian Brand Names Sativex® [Can]

Therapeutic Category Analgesic, Miscellaneous

Controlled Substance CDSA-II

Use Adjunctive treatment of neuropathic pain in multiple sclerosis

Usual Dosage

Note: For buccal use only; spray should be directed below the tongue or on the inside of the cheeks (the site should be varied); avoid direction to the pharynx.

Buccal spray:

Initial: One spray every 4 hours to a maximum of 4 sprays.

Titration and individualization: Dosage is self-titrated by the patient. The mean daily dosage after titration in clinical trials was 5 actuations per day. Dosage should be adjusted as necessary, based on effect and tolerance. Sprays should be evenly distributed over the course of the day during initial titration. If adverse reactions, including intoxication-type symptoms, are noted the dosage should be suspended until resolution of the symptoms; a dosage reduction or extension of the interval between doses may be used to avoid a recurrence of symptoms. Retitration may be required in the event of adverse reactions and/or worsening of symptoms.

Dosage Forms

Aerosol, buccal spray (Sativex®): Delta-9 tetrahydrocannabinol 27 mg/mL and cannabidiol 25 mg/mL (5.5 mL) [delivers 100 microliters/spray; 51 metered sprays; contains ethanol 50%, peppermint oil, and propylene glycol]

tetrahydrozoline (tet ra hye DROZ a leen)

Sound-Alike/Look-Alike Issues

Visine® may be confused with Visken®

Synonyms tetrahydrozoline hydrochloride; tetryzoline

U.S./Canadian Brand Names Eye-Sine™ [US-OTC]; Geneye® [US-OTC]; Murine® Tears Plus [US-OTC]; Optigene® 3 [US-OTC]; Tyzine® Pediatric [US]; Tyzine® [US]; Visine® Advanced Relief [US-OTC]; Visine® Original [US-OTC]

Therapeutic Category Adrenergic Agonist Agent

Use Symptomatic relief of nasal congestion and conjunctival congestion

Usual Dosage

Nasal congestion: Intranasal:

Children 2-6 years: Instill 2-3 drops of 0.05% solution every 4-6 hours as needed, no more frequent than every 3 hours

Children >6 years and Adults: Instill 2-4 drops or 3-4 sprays of 0.1% solution every 3-4 hours as needed, no more frequent than every 3 hours

Conjunctival congestion: Ophthalmic: Adults: Instill 1-2 drops in each eye 2-4 times/day

Dosage Forms

Solution, intranasal, as hydrochloride:

Tyzine®: 0.1% (15 mL) [spray bottle; contains benzalkonium chloride]; (30 mL) [dropper bottle; contains benzalkonium chloride]

Tyzine® Pediatric: 0.05% (15 mL) [spray bottle; contains benzalkonium chloride]

Solution, ophthalmic, as hydrochloride: 0.05% (15 mL)

Eye-Sine™, Geneye®, Optigene® 3: 0.05% (15 mL) [may contain benzalkonium chloride]

Murine® Tears Plus: 0.05% (15 mL, 30 mL) [contains benzalkonium chloride]

Visine® Advanced Relief: 0.05% (30 mL) [contains benzalkonium chloride and polyethylene glycol]

Visine® Original: 0.05% (15 mL, 30 mL) [contains benzalkonium chloride; 15 mL size also available with dropper]

tetrahydrozoline hydrochloride *see* tetrahydrozoline *on this page*

Tetramune® *(Discontinued)*

Tetrasine® Extra Ophthalmic *(Discontinued)* *see* tetrahydrozoline *on this page*

Tetrasine® Ophthalmic *(Discontinued)* *see* tetrahydrozoline *on this page*

Tetra Tannate Pediatric [US] *see* chlorpheniramine, ephedrine, phenylephrine, and carbetapentane *on page 178*

tetryzoline *see* tetrahydrozoline *on this page*

Teveten® [US/Can] *see* eprosartan *on page 299*

Teveten® HCT [US/Can] *see* eprosartan and hydrochlorothiazide *on page 300*

Teveten® Plus [Can] *see* eprosartan and hydrochlorothiazide *on page 300*

Tev-Tropin™ [US] *see* somatropin *on page 785*

Texacort® [US] *see* hydrocortisone (topical) *on page 428*

TG *see* thioguanine *on page 822*

T-Gen® *(Discontinued)* *see* trimethobenzamide *on page 851*

THA *see* tacrine *on page 803*

thalidomide (tha LI doe mide)

Sound-Alike/Look-Alike Issues

thalidomide may be confused with flutamide

Synonyms NSC-66847

U.S./Canadian Brand Names Thalomid® [US/Can]

Therapeutic Category Immunosuppressant Agent

Use Treatment of multiple myeloma (in combination with dexamethasone); treatment and maintenance of cutaneous manifestations of erythema nodosum leprosum (ENL)

Usual Dosage Oral:

Multiple myeloma: 200 mg once daily (with dexamethasone 40 mg daily on days 1-4, 9-12, and 17-20 of a 28-day treatment cycle)

Cutaneous ENL:

Initial: 100-300 mg/day taken once daily at bedtime with water (at least 1 hour after evening meal)

Patients weighing <50 kg: Initiate at lower end of the dosing range

Severe cutaneous reaction or patients previously requiring high dose may be initiated at 400 mg/day; doses may be divided, but taken 1 hour after meals

Maintenance: Dosing should continue until active reaction subsides (usually at least 2 weeks), then tapered in 50 mg decrements every 2-4 weeks

Patients who flare during tapering or with a history or requiring prolonged maintenance should be maintained on the minimum dosage necessary to control the reaction. Efforts to taper should be repeated every 3-6 months, in increments of 50 mg every 2-4 weeks.

Dosage Forms

Capsule:

Thalomid®: 50 mg, 100 mg, 200 mg

Thalitone® [US] *see* chlorthalidone *on page 185*

Thalomid® [US/Can] *see* thalidomide *on this page*

THAM® [US] *see* tromethamine *on page 855*

THC *see* dronabinol *on page 281*

THC and CBD *see* tetrahydrocannabinol and cannabidiol *(Canada only)* *on page 816*

Theo-X® *(Discontinued)* *see* theophylline *on this page*

Theo-24® [US] *see* theophylline *on this page*

Theobid® *(Discontinued)* *see* theophylline *on this page*

TheoCap™ [US] *see* theophylline *on this page*

Theochron® [US] *see* theophylline *on this page*

Theochron® SR [Can] *see* theophylline *on this page*

Theoclear-80® *(Discontinued)* *see* theophylline *on this page*

Theoclear®-L.A. *(Discontinued)* *see* theophylline *on this page*

Theo-Dur® (all products) *(Discontinued)* *see* theophylline *on this page*

Theolair™ [Can] *see* theophylline *on this page*

Theolair-SR® *(Discontinued)* *see* theophylline *on this page*

Theolate *(Discontinued)* *see* theophylline and guaifenesin *on page 820*

theophylline (thee OFF i lin)

Sound-Alike/Look-Alike Issues

Theolair™ may be confused with Thiola®, Thyrolar®

Synonyms theophylline anhydrous

U.S./Canadian Brand Names Apo-Theo LA® [Can]; Elixophyllin® [US]; Novo-Theophyl SR [Can]; PMS-Theophylline [Can]; Pulmophylline [Can]; ratio-Theo-Bronc [Can]; Theo-24® [US]; TheoCap™ [US]; Theochron® SR [Can]; Theochron® [US]; Theolair™ [Can]; Uniphyl® SRT [Can]; Uniphyl® [US]

Therapeutic Category Theophylline Derivative

Use Treatment of symptoms and reversible airway obstruction due to chronic asthma, chronic bronchitis, or COPD

Usual Dosage Use ideal body weight for obese patients

I.V.: Initial: Maintenance infusion rates:
Children:
6 weeks to 6 months: 0.5 mg/kg/hour
6 months to 1 year: 0.6-0.7 mg/kg/hour
Children >1 year and Adults:
Acute bronchospasm: Approximate I.V. theophylline dosage for treatment of acute bronchospasm: **Note:** Equivalent hydrousaminophylline dosage is indicated in parentheses.

Infants 6 weeks to 6 months: 0.5 mg/kg/hour for next 12 hours
Children 6 months to 1 year: 0.6-0.7 mg/kg/hour for next 12 hours
Children 1-9 years: 0.95 mg/kg/hour (1.2 mg/kg/hour) for next 12 hours; 0.79 mg/kg/hour (1 mg/kg/hour) after 12 hours
Children 9-16 years and young adult smokers: 0.79 mg/kg/hour (1 mg/kg/hour) for next 12 hours;0.63 mg/kg/hour (0.8 mg/kg/hour) after 12 hours
Healthy, nonsmoking adults: 0.55 mg/kg/hour (0.7 mg/kg/hour) for next 12 hours; 0.39 mg/kg/hour (0.5 mg/kg/hour) after 12 hours
Older patients and patients with corpulmonale: 0.47 mg/kg/hour (0.6 mg/kg/hour) for next 12 hours;0.24 mg/kg/hour (0.3 mg/kg/hour) after 12 hours
Patients with congestive heart failure or liver failure: 0.39 mg/kg/hour (0.5 mg/kg/hour) for next 12 hours; 0.08-0.16 mg/kg/hour (0.1-0.2 mg/kg/hour) after 12 hours

Approximate I.V. maintenance dosages are based upon continuous infusions; bolus dosing (often used in children <6 months of age) may be determined by multiplying the hourly infusion rate by 24 hours and dividing by the desired number of doses/day. See the following: Maintenance dose for acute symptoms:

Premature infant or newborn to 6 weeks (for apnea/bradycardia):
Oral theophylline: 4 mg/kg/day
I.V. aminophylline: 5 mg/kg/day
6 weeks to 6 months:
Oral theophylline: 10 mg/kg/day
I.V. aminophylline: 12 mg/kg/day or continuous I.V. infusion[1]
Infants 6 months to 1 year:
Oral theophylline: 12-18 mg/kg/day
I.V. aminophylline: 15 mg/kg/day or continuous I.V. infusion[1]
Children 1-9 years:
Oral theophylline: 20-24 mg/kg/day
I.V. aminophylline: 1 mg/kg/hour
Children 9-12 years, and adolescent daily smokers of cigarettes or marijuana, and otherwise healthy adult smokers <50 years:
Oral theophylline: 16 mg/kg/day
I.V. aminophylline: 0.9 mg/kg/hour
Adolescents 12-16 years (nonsmokers):
Oral theophylline: 13 mg/kg/day
I.V. aminophylline: 0.7 mg/kg/hour
Otherwise healthy nonsmoking adults:
Oral theophylline: 10 mg/kg/day (not to exceed 900 mg/day)
I.V. aminophylline: 0.5 mg/kg/hour
Cardiac decompensation, corpulmonale, and/or liver dysfunction:
Oral theophylline: 5 mg/kg/day (not to exceed 400 mg/day)
I.V. aminophylline: 0.25 mg/kg/hour
[1]For continuous I.V. infusion, divide total daily dose by 24 = mg/kg/hour.

Oral theophylline dosage for bronchial asthma (by age):
<1 year:
Initial 3 days and second 3 days: 0.2 x (age in weeks) + 5 = mg/kg/24 hours of theophylline
Steady-state maintenance: 0.3 x (age in weeks) + 8 = mg/kg/24 hours of theophylline
1-9 years:
Initial 3 days: 16 mg/kg/24 hours of theophylline, up to a maximum of 400 mg/24 hours
Second 3 days: 20 mg/kg/24 hours of theophylline
Steady-state maintenance: 22 mg/kg/24 hours of theophylline
9-12 years:
Initial 3 days: 16 mg/kg/24 hours of theophylline, up to a maximum of 400 mg/24 hours
Second 3 days: 16 mg/kg/24 hours of theophylline, up to a maximum of 600 mg/24 hours
Steady-state maintenance: 20 mg/kg/24 hours of theophylline, up to a maximum of 800 mg/24 hours
(Continued)

theophylline *(Continued)*

12-16 years:
Initial 3 days: 16 mg/kg/24 hours of theophylline, up to a maximum of 400 mg/24 hours
Second 3 days: 16 mg/kg/24 hours of theophylline, up to a maximum of 600 mg/24 hours
Steady-state maintenance: 18 mg/kg/24 hours of theophylline, up to a maximum of 900 mg/24 hours
Adults:
Initial 3 days: 400 mg/24 hours
Second 3 days: 600 mg/24 hours
Steady-state maintenance: 900 mg/24 hours
Increasing dose: The dosage may be increased in approximately 25% increments at 2- to 3-day intervals so long as the drug is tolerated or until the maximum dose is reached
Maintenance dose: In children and healthy adults, a slow-release product can be used; the total daily dose can be divided every 8-12 hours

Dosage Forms
Capsule, extended release: 100 mg, 125 mg, 200 mg, 300 mg
TheoCap™: 125 mg, 200 mg, 300 mg [12 hour]
Theo-24®: 100 mg, 200 mg, 300 mg, 400 mg [24 hours]
Elixir:
Elixophyllin®: 80 mg/15 mL (480 mL) [contains alcohol 20%; fruit flavor]
Infusion [premixed in D_5W]: 200 mg (50 mL, 100 mL); 400 mg (100 mL, 250 mL, 500 mL); 800 mg (250 mL, 500 mL, 1000 mL)
Tablet, controlled release:
Uniphyl®: 400 mg, 600 mg [24 hours; contains cetostearyl alcohol]
Tablet, extended release: 100 mg, 200 mg, 300 mg, 450 mg
Theochron®: 100 mg, 200 mg, 300 mg, 450 mg [12-24 hours]
Tablet, immediate release:
Quibron®-T: 300 mg [DSC]
Tablet, sustained release:
Quibron®-T/SR: 300 mg [8-12 hours] [DSC]

theophylline and guaifenesin (thee OFF i lin & gwye FEN e sin)

Synonyms guaifenesin and theophylline
U.S./Canadian Brand Names Elixophyllin-GG® [US]
Therapeutic Category Theophylline Derivative
Use Symptomatic treatment of bronchospasm associated with bronchial asthma, chronic bronchitis, and pulmonary emphysema
Usual Dosage Adults: Oral: 16 mg/kg/day or 400 mg theophylline/day, in divided doses, every 6-8 hours
Dosage Forms [DSC] = Discontinued product
Capsule:
Quibron®: Theophylline 150 mg and guaifenesin 90 mg [DSC]
Liquid:
Elixophyllin-GG®: Theophylline 100 mg and guaifenesin 100 mg per 15 mL (240 mL, 480 mL) [alcohol free, dye free, sugar free; cherry-berry flavor]

theophylline anhydrous *see* theophylline *on page 818*
theophylline ethylenediamine *see* aminophylline *on page 42*
Theo-Sav® *(Discontinued)* *see* theophylline *on page 818*
Theospan®-SR *(Discontinued)* *see* theophylline *on page 818*
Theostat-80® *(Discontinued)* *see* theophylline *on page 818*
Theovent® *(Discontinued)* *see* theophylline *on page 818*
Therabid® *(Discontinued)*
TheraCys® [US] *see* BCG vaccine *on page 94*
Thera-Flu® Cold and Sore Throat Night Time [US-OTC] *see* acetaminophen, chlorpheniramine, and pseudoephedrine *on page 11*
Thera-Flur® *(Discontinued)* *see* fluoride *on page 354*
Thera-Flur-N® [US] *see* fluoride *on page 354*
Thera-Flu® Severe Cold Non-Drowsy *(Discontinued)* *see* acetaminophen, dextromethorphan, and pseudoephedrine *on page 12*
Theragran-M® Advanced Formula *(Discontinued)* *see* vitamins (multiple/oral) *on page 878*

Theragran® Heart Right™ *(Discontinued)* *see* vitamins (multiple/oral) *on page 878*

Theramycin Z® [US] *see* erythromycin *on page 303*

TheraPatch® Warm *(Discontinued)* *see* capsaicin *on page 142*

therapeutic multivitamins *see* vitamins (multiple/oral) *on page 878*

Theratears® [US] *see* carboxymethylcellulose *on page 151*

Thermazene® [US] *see* silver sulfadiazine *on page 772*

thiabendazole (thye a BEN da zole)

Synonyms tiabendazole

U.S./Canadian Brand Names Mintezol® [US]

Therapeutic Category Anthelmintic

Use Treatment of strongyloidiasis, cutaneous larva migrans, visceral larva migrans, dracunculiasis, trichinosis, and mixed helminthic infections

Usual Dosage Purgation is not required prior to use; drinking of fruit juice aids in expulsion of worms by removing the mucous to which the intestinal tapeworms attach themselves.

Children and Adults:

Oral: 50 mg/kg/day divided every 12 hours (if >68 kg: 1.5 g/dose); maximum dose: 3 g/day

Treatment duration:

Strongyloidiasis, ascariasis, uncinariasis: For 2 consecutive days

Cutaneous larva migrans: For 2 consecutive days; if active lesions are still present 2 days after completion, a second course of treatment is recommended.

Visceral larva migrans: For 7 consecutive days

Trichinosis: For 2-4 consecutive days; optimal dosage not established

Dracunculosis: 50-75 mg/kg/day divided every 12 hours for 3 days

Dosage Forms [DSC] = Discontinued product

Suspension, oral: 500 mg/5 mL (120 mL) [DSC]

Tablet, chewable: 500 mg [orange flavor]

thiamazole *see* methimazole *on page 539*

thiamine (THYE a min)

Sound-Alike/Look-Alike Issues

thiamine may be confused with Tenormin®, Thorazine®

Synonyms aneurine hydrochloride; thiamine hydrochloride; thiaminium chloride hydrochloride; vitamin B_1

U.S./Canadian Brand Names Betaxin® [Can]

Therapeutic Category Vitamin, Water Soluble

Use Treatment of thiamine deficiency including beriberi, Wernicke encephalopathy syndrome, and peripheral neuritis associated with pellagra, alcoholic patients with altered sensorium; various genetic metabolic disorders

Usual Dosage

Recommended daily allowance:

<6 months: 0.3 mg

6 months to 1 year: 0.4 mg

1-3 years: 0.7 mg

4-6 years: 0.9 mg

7-10 years: 1 mg

11-14 years: 1.1-1.3 mg

>14 years: 1-1.5 mg

Thiamine deficiency (beriberi):

Children: 10-25 mg/dose I.M. or I.V. daily (if critically ill), or 10-50 mg/dose orally every day for 2 weeks, then 5-10 mg/dose orally daily for 1 month

Adults: 5-30 mg/dose I.M. or I.V. 3 times/day (if critically ill); then orally 5-30 mg/day in single or divided doses 3 times/day for 1 month

Wernicke's encephalopathy: Adults: Initial: 100 mg I.V., then 50-100 mg/day I.M. or I.V. until consuming a regular, balanced diet

Dietary supplement (depends on caloric or carbohydrate content of the diet):

Infants: 0.3-0.5 mg/day

Children: 0.5-1 mg/day

Adults: 1-2 mg/day

Note: The above doses can be found in multivitamin preparations

Metabolic disorders: Oral: Adults: 10-20 mg/day (dosages up to 4 g/day in divided doses have been used)

(Continued)

thiamine *(Continued)*

Dosage Forms

Injection, solution, as hydrochloride: 100 mg/mL (2 mL)
Tablet, as hydrochloride: 50 mg, 100 mg, 250 mg, 500 mg

thiamine hydrochloride *see* thiamine *on previous page*

thiaminium chloride hydrochloride *see* thiamine *on previous page*

thimerosal (thye MER oh sal)

U.S./Canadian Brand Names Mersol® [US-OTC]; Merthiolate® [US-OTC]
Therapeutic Category Antibacterial, Topical
Use Organomercurial antiseptic with sustained bacteriostatic and fungistatic activity
Usual Dosage Apply 1-3 times/day
Dosage Forms

Solution, topical (Merthiolate®): 0.1% [1 mg/mL = 1:1000] (30 mL)
Solution, topical spray (Merthiolate®): 0.1% [1 mg/mL = 1:1000] (60 g)
Tincture, topical (Mersol®): 0.1% [1 mg/mL = 1:1000] (120 mL, 480 mL, 4000 mL)

thioguanine (thye oh GWAH neen)

Sound-Alike/Look-Alike Issues

6-thioguanine and 6-TG are error-prone abbreviations (associated with six-fold overdoses of thioguanine)

Synonyms 2-amino-6-mercaptopurine; NSC-752; TG; tioguanine
U.S./Canadian Brand Names Lanvis® [Can]; Tabloid® [US]
Therapeutic Category Antineoplastic Agent
Use Treatment of acute myelogenous (nonlymphocytic) leukemia; treatment of chronic myelogenous leukemia and granulocytic leukemia
Usual Dosage Total daily dose can be given at one time.

Oral (refer to individual protocols):

Infants and Children <3 years: Combination drug therapy for acute nonlymphocytic leukemia: 3.3 mg/kg/day in divided doses twice daily for 4 days

Children and Adults: 2-3 mg/kg/day calculated to nearest 20 mg or 75-200 mg/m^2/day in 1-2 divided doses for 5-7 days or until remission is attained

Dosage Forms

Injection, powder for reconstitution: 75 mg [investigational in U.S.]
Tablet [scored]: 40 mg

Thiola® [US/Can] *see* tiopronin *on page 830*

thiopental (thye oh PEN tal)

Synonyms thiopental sodium
U.S./Canadian Brand Names Pentothal® [US/Can]
Therapeutic Category Barbiturate
Controlled Substance C-III
Use Induction of anesthesia; adjunct for intubation in head injury patients; control of convulsive states; treatment of elevated intracranial pressure
Usual Dosage I.V.:

Induction anesthesia:
Infants: 5-8 mg/kg
Children 1-12 years: 5-6 mg/kg
Adults: 3-5 mg/kg

Maintenance anesthesia:
Children: 1 mg/kg as needed
Adults: 25-100 mg as needed

Increased intracranial pressure: Children and Adults: 1.5-5 mg/kg/dose; repeat as needed to control intracranial pressure

Seizures:
Children: 2-3 mg/kg/dose; repeat as needed
Adults: 75-250 mg/dose; repeat as needed

Dosage Forms Injection, powder for reconstitution, as sodium: 250 mg, 400 mg, 500 mg, 1 g

thiopental sodium *see* thiopental *on this page*

thiophosphoramide *see* thiotepa *on next page*

Thioplex® ***(Discontinued)*** *see* thiotepa *on this page*

thioproperazine *(Canada only)* (thye oh pro PER a zeen)

U.S./Canadian Brand Names Majeptil® [Can]

Therapeutic Category Neuroleptic Agent

Use All types of acute and chronic schizophrenia, including those which did not respond to the usual neuroleptics; manic syndromes.

Usual Dosage Initial treatment: Adults: It is recommended to start treatment at a low dosage of about 5 mg/day in a single dose or in divided doses. This initial dosage is gradually increased by the same amount every 2-3 days until the usual effective dosage of 30-40 mg/day is reached. In some cases, higher dosages of 90 mg or more per day, are necessary to control the psychotic manifestations.

Children >10 years of age: Start treatment with a daily dosage of 1-3 mg following the method of treatment described for adults

Maintenance therapy: Adults and Children: Dosage should be reduced gradually to the lowest effective level, which may be as low as a few mg per day and maintained as long as necessary

Dosage Forms Tablet, as mesylate: 10 mg

thioridazine (thye oh RID a zeen)

Sound-Alike/Look-Alike Issues

thioridazine may be confused with thiothixene, Thorazine®

Mellaril® may be confused with Elavil®, Mebaral®

Synonyms thioridazine hydrochloride

U.S./Canadian Brand Names Mellaril® [Can]

Therapeutic Category Phenothiazine Derivative

Use Management of schizophrenic patients who fail to respond adequately to treatment with other antipsychotic drugs, either because of insufficient effectiveness or the inability to achieve an effective dose due to intolerable adverse effects from those medications

Usual Dosage Oral:

Children >2-12 years: Range: 0.5-3 mg/kg/day in 2-3 divided doses; usual: 1 mg/kg/day; maximum: 3 mg/kg/day

Behavior problems: Initial: 10 mg 2-3 times/day, increase gradually

Severe psychoses: Initial: 25 mg 2-3 times/day, increase gradually

Children >12 years and Adults:

Schizophrenia/psychoses: Initial: 50-100 mg 3 times/day with gradual increments as needed and tolerated; maximum: 800 mg/day in 2-4 divided doses

Depressive disorders/dementia: Initial: 25 mg 3 times/day; maintenance dose: 20-200 mg/day

Dosage Forms Tablet, as hydrochloride: 10 mg, 15 mg, 25 mg, 50 mg, 100 mg, 150 mg, 200 mg

thioridazine hydrochloride *see* thioridazine *on this page*

thiosulfuric acid disodium salt *see* sodium thiosulfate *on page 783*

thiotepa (thye oh TEP a)

Synonyms TESPA; thiophosphoramide; triethylenethiophosphoramide; TSPA

Therapeutic Category Antineoplastic Agent

Use Treatment of superficial tumors of the bladder; palliative treatment of adenocarcinoma of breast or ovary; lymphomas and sarcomas; controlling intracavitary effusions caused by metastatic tumors; I.T. use: CNS leukemia/lymphoma, CNS metastases

Usual Dosage Refer to individual protocols.

Children: Sarcomas: I.V.: 25-65 mg/m^2 as a single dose every 21 days

Adults:

I.M., I.V., SubQ: 30-60 mg/m^2 once weekly

I.V.: 0.3-0.4 mg/kg by rapid I.V. administration every 1-4 weeks, **or** 0.2 mg/kg or 6-8 mg/m^2/day for 4-5 days every 2-4 weeks

High-dose therapy for bone marrow transplant: I.V.: 500 mg/m^2, up to 900 mg/m^2

I.M.: 15-30 mg in various schedules have been given

Intracavitary: 0.6-0.8 mg/kg or 30-60 mg weekly

Intrapericardial: 15-30 mg

Intrathecal: 10-15 mg or 5-11.5 mg/m^2

Dosage Forms Injection, powder for reconstitution: 15 mg, 30 mg

thiothixene (thye oh THIKS een)

Sound-Alike/Look-Alike Issues

thiothixene may be confused with thioridazine

Navane® may be confused with Norvasc®, Nubain®

Synonyms tiotixene

U.S./Canadian Brand Names Navane® [US/Can]

Therapeutic Category Thioxanthene Derivative

Use Management of schizophrenia

Usual Dosage Oral: Children >12 years and Adults:

Mild to moderate psychosis: 2 mg 3 times/day, up to 20-30 mg/day; more severe psychosis: Initial: 5 mg 2 times/day, may increase gradually, if necessary; maximum: 60 mg/day

Rapid tranquilization of the agitated patient (administered every 30-60 minutes): 5-10 mg; average total dose for tranquilization: 15-30 mg

Dosage Forms [DSC] = Discontinued product

Capsule: 1 mg, 2 mg, 5 mg, 10 mg

Navane®: 1 mg [DSC], 2 mg, 5 mg, 10 mg, 20 mg

thonzonium, neomycin, colistin, and hydrocortisone *see* neomycin, colistin, hydrocortisone, and thonzonium *on page 583*

Thorazine® *(Discontinued)* *see* chlorpromazine *on page 184*

Thorets [US-OTC] *see* benzocaine *on page 99*

Thrombate III® [US/Can] *see* antithrombin III *on page 62*

Thrombinar® *(Discontinued)* *see* thrombin (topical) *on this page*

Thrombin-JMI® [US] *see* thrombin (topical) *on this page*

thrombin (topical) (THROM bin, TOP i kal)

U.S./Canadian Brand Names Thrombin-JMI® [US]

Therapeutic Category Hemostatic Agent

Use Hemostasis whenever minor bleeding from capillaries and small venules is accessible

Usual Dosage Use 1000-2000 units/mL of solution where bleeding is profuse; apply powder directly to the site of bleeding or on oozing surfaces; use 100 units/mL for bleeding from skin or mucosal surfaces

Dosage Forms Powder for reconstitution, topical:

Thrombin-JMI®: 5000 units, 20,000 units [packaged with diluent]

Thrombin-JMI® Spray Kit: 20,000 units [packaged with diluent and spray pump]

Thrombin-JMI® Syringe Spray Kit: 20,000 units [packaged with diluent, spray tip, and syringe]

Thrombostat® *(Discontinued)* *see* thrombin (topical) *on this page*

thymocyte stimulating factor *see* aldesleukin *on page 26*

Thymoglobulin® [US] *see* antithymocyte globulin (rabbit) *on page 63*

Thyrar® *(Discontinued)* *see* thyroid *on this page*

Thyro-Block® *(Discontinued)* *see* potassium iodide *on page 686*

Thyrogen® [US/Can] *see* thyrotropin alpha *on next page*

thyroid (THYE roid)

Synonyms desiccated thyroid; thyroid extract; thyroid USP

U.S./Canadian Brand Names Armour® Thyroid [US]; Nature-Throid® NT [US]; Westhroid® [US]

Therapeutic Category Thyroid Product

Use Replacement or supplemental therapy in hypothyroidism; pituitary TSH suppressants (thyroid nodules, thyroiditis, multinodular goiter, thyroid cancer), thyrotoxicosis, diagnostic suppression tests

Usual Dosage Oral:

Children: Recommended pediatric dosage for congenital hypothyroidism:

0-6 months: 15-30 mg/day; 4.8-6 mg/kg/day

6-12 months: 30-45 mg/day; 3.6-4.8 mg/kg/day

1-5 years: 45-60 mg/day; 3-3.6 mg/kg/day

6-12 years: 60-90 mg/day; 2.4-3 mg/kg/day

>12 years: >90 mg/day; 1.2-1.8 mg/kg/day

Adults: Initial: 15-30 mg; increase with 15 mg increments every 2-4 weeks; use 15 mg in patients with cardiovascular disease or myxedema. Maintenance dose: Usually 60-120 mg/day; monitor TSH and clinical symptoms.

Thyroid cancer: Requires larger amounts than replacement therapy

Dosage Forms

Tablet: 30 mg, 32.5 mg, 60 mg, 65 mg, 90 mg, 120 mg, 130 mg, 180 mg, 240 mg, 300 mg

Armour® Thyroid: 15 mg, 30 mg, 60 mg, 90 mg, 120 mg, 180 mg, 240 mg, 300 mg

Nature-Throid® NT, Westhroid®: 32.5 mg, 65 mg, 130 mg, 195 mg

thyroid extract *see* thyroid *on previous page*

Thyroid Strong® *(Discontinued)* *see* thyroid *on previous page*

thyroid USP *see* thyroid *on previous page*

Thyrolar® [US/Can] *see* liotrix *on page 499*

ThyroSafe™ [US-OTC] *see* potassium iodide *on page 686*

ThyroShield™ [US-OTC] *see* potassium iodide *on page 686*

thyrotropin alpha (thye roe TROH pin AL fa)

Sound-Alike/Look-Alike Issues

Thyrogen® may be confused with Thyrolar®

Synonyms human thyroid stimulating hormone; TSH

U.S./Canadian Brand Names Thyrogen® [US/Can]

Therapeutic Category Diagnostic Agent

Use As an adjunctive diagnostic tool for serum thyroglobulin (Tg) testing with or without radioiodine imaging in the follow-up of patients with well-differentiated thyroid cancer

Potential clinical use:

1. Patients with an undetectable Tg on thyroid hormone suppressive therapy to exclude the diagnosis of residual or recurrent thyroid cancer
2. Patients requiring serum Tg testing and radioiodine imaging who are unwilling to undergo thyroid hormone withdrawal testing and whose treating physician believes that use of a less sensitive test is justified
3. Patients who are either unable to mount an adequate endogenous TSH response to thyroid hormone withdrawal or in whom withdrawal is medically contraindicated

Usual Dosage Children >16 years and Adults: I.M.: 0.9 mg every 24 hours for 2 doses or every 72 hours for 3 doses

For radioiodine imaging, radioiodine administration should be given 24 hours following the final Thyrogen® injection. Scanning should be performed 48 hours after radioiodine administration (72 hours after the final injection of Thyrogen®).

For serum testing, serum Tg should be obtained 72 hours after final injection of Thyrogen®.

Dosage Forms Injection, powder for reconstitution: Four-vial kit: 1.1 mg [supplied as two vials of Thyrogen® and two 10 mL vials of SWFI]

tiabendazole *see* thiabendazole *on page 821*

tiagabine (tye AG a been)

Sound-Alike/Look-Alike Issues

tiagabine may be confused with tizanidine

Synonyms tiagabine hydrochloride

U.S./Canadian Brand Names Gabitril® [US/Can]

Therapeutic Category Anticonvulsant

Use Adjunctive therapy in adults and children ≥12 years of age in the treatment of partial seizures

Usual Dosage Oral (administer with food):

Patients receiving enzyme-inducing AED regimens:

Children 12-18 years: 4 mg once daily for 1 week; may increase to 8 mg daily in 2 divided doses for 1 week; then may increase by 4-8 mg weekly to response or up to 32 mg daily in 2-4 divided doses

Adults: 4 mg once daily for 1 week; may increase by 4-8 mg weekly to response or up to 56 mg daily in 2-4 divided doses; usual maintenance: 32-56 mg/day

Patients **not** receiving enzyme-inducing AED regimens: The estimated plasma concentrations of tiagabine in patients not taking enzyme-inducing medications is twice that of patients receiving enzyme-inducing AEDs. Lower doses are required; slower titration may be necessary.

Dosage Forms Tablet, as hydrochloride: 2 mg, 4 mg, 6 mg, 8 mg, 10 mg, 12 mg, 16 mg

tiagabine hydrochloride *see* tiagabine *on this page*

Tiamate® *(Discontinued)* *see* diltiazem *on page 257*

Tiamol® [Can] *see* fluocinonide *on page 353*

Tiaprofenic-200 [Can] *see* tiaprofenic acid *(Canada only)* *on this page*

Tiaprofenic-300 [Can] *see* tiaprofenic acid *(Canada only)* *on this page*

tiaprofenic acid *(Canada only)* (tye ah PRO fen ik AS id)

U.S./Canadian Brand Names Albert® Tiafen [Can]; Apo-Tiaprofenic® [Can]; Dom-Tiaprofenic® [Can]; Novo-Tiaprofenic [Can]; Nu-Tiaprofenic [Can]; PMS-Tiaprofenic [Can]; Surgam® SR [Can]; Surgam® [Can]; Tiaprofenic-200 [Can]; Tiaprofenic-300 [Can]

Therapeutic Category Nonsteroidal Antiinflammatory Drug (NSAID)

Use Relief of signs and symptoms of rheumatoid arthritis and osteoarthritis (degenerative joint disease)

Usual Dosage Oral: Adults:

Rheumatoid arthritis:

Tablet: Usual initial and maintenance dose: 600 mg/day in 3 divided doses; some patients may do well on 300 mg twice daily; maximum daily dose: 600 mg

Sustained release capsule: Initial and maintenance dose: 2 sustained release capsules of 300 mg once daily; Surgam® SR capsules should be swallowed whole

Osteoarthritis:

Tablet: Usual initial and maintenance dose: 600 mg/day in 2 or 3 divided doses; in rare instances patients may be maintained on 300 mg/day in divided doses; maximum daily dose: 600 mg

Sustained release capsule: Initial and maintenance dose: 2 sustained release capsules of 300 mg once daily; Surgam® SR capsules should be swallowed whole

Dosage Forms

Capsule, sustained release: 300 mg

Tablet: 200 mg, 300 mg

Tiazac® [US/Can] *see* diltiazem *on page 257*

Tiazac® XC [Can] *see* diltiazem *on page 257*

Ticar® [US] *see* ticarcillin *on this page*

ticarcillin (tye kar SIL in)

Sound-Alike/Look-Alike Issues

Ticar® may be confused with Tigan®

Synonyms ticarcillin disodium

U.S./Canadian Brand Names Ticar® [US]

Therapeutic Category Penicillin

Use Treatment of susceptible infections such as septicemia, acute and chronic respiratory tract infections, skin and soft tissue infections, and urinary tract infections due to susceptible strains of *Pseudomonas*, and other gram-negative bacteria

Usual Dosage Note: Ticarcillin is generally given I.V., I.M. injection is only for the treatment of uncomplicated urinary tract infections and dose should not exceed 2 g/injection when administered I.M.

Usual dosage range:

Neonates: I.M., I.V.:

Postnatal age <7 days:

<2000 g: 75 mg/kg/dose every 12 hours

>2000 g: 75 mg/kg/dose every 8 hours

Postnatal age >7 days:

<1200 g: 75 mg/kg/dose every 12 hours

1200-2000 g: 75 mg/kg/dose every 8 hours

>2000 g: 75 mg/kg/dose every 6 hours

Infants and Children:

I.M.: 50-100 mg/kg/day in divided doses every 6-8 hours

I.V.: 50-300 mg/kg/day in divided doses every 4-8 hours (maximum dose: 24 g/day)

Adults: I.M., I.V.: 1-4 g every 4-6 hours

Indication-specific dosing:

Infants and Children:

Cystic fibrosis (acute pulmonary exacerbations): I.V.: 100 mg/kg every 6 hours

Systemic infection: I.V.: 200-300 mg/kg/day in divided doses every 4-6 hours

Urinary tract infections: I.M., I.V.: 50-100 mg/kg/day in divided doses every 6-8 hours

Adults:

Otitis externa (malignant): I.V.: 3 g every 4 hours with tobramycin

***Pseudomonas* infections:** I.V.: 3 g every 4 hours

Dosage Forms Injection, powder for reconstitution, as disodium: 3 g

ticarcillin and clavulanate potassium (tye kar SIL in & klav yoo LAN ate poe TASS ee um)

Synonyms ticarcillin and clavulanic acid

U.S./Canadian Brand Names Timentin® [US/Can]

Therapeutic Category Penicillin

Use Treatment of infections of lower respiratory tract, urinary tract, skin and skin structures, bone and joint, and septicemia caused by susceptible organisms. Clavulanate expands activity of ticarcillin to include beta-lactamase producing strains of *S. aureus*, *H. influenzae*, *Bacteroides* species, and some other gram-negative bacilli

Usual Dosage

Usual dosage range:

Children and Adults <60 kg: I.V.: 75-300 mg of ticarcillin component/kg/day in divided doses every 4-6 hours

Children ≥60 kg and Adults: I.V.: 3.1 g (ticarcillin 3 g plus clavulanic acid 0.1 g) every 4-6 hours (maximum: 24 g/day)

Indication-specific dosing:

Children: I.V.:

Bite wounds (animal): 200 mg/kg/day in divided doses

Neutropenic fever: 75 mg/kg every 6 hours (maximum 3.1 g)

Pneumonia (nosocomial): 300 mg/kg/day in 4 divided doses (maximum: 18-24 g/day)

Children ≥60 kg and Adults: I.V.:

Amnionitis, cholangitis, diverticulitis, endometritis, epididymo-orchitis, mastoiditis, orbital cellulitis, peritonitis, pneumonia (aspiration): 3.1 g every 6 hours

Liver abscess, parafascial space infections, septic thrombophlebitis: 3.1 g every 4 hours

***Pseudomonas* infections:** 3.1 g every 4 hours

Urinary tract infections: 3.1 g every 6-8 hours

Dosage Forms

Infusion [premixed, frozen]: Ticarcillin 3 g and clavulanic acid 0.1 g (100 mL) [contains sodium 4.51 mEq and potassium 0.15 mEq per g]

Injection, powder for reconstitution: Ticarcillin 3 g and clavulanic acid 0.1 g (3.1 g, 31 g) [contains sodium 4.51 mEq and potassium 0.15 mEq per g]

ticarcillin and clavulanic acid *see* ticarcillin and clavulanate potassium *on this page*

ticarcillin disodium *see* ticarcillin *on previous page*

TICE® BCG [US] *see* BCG vaccine *on page 94*

Ticlid® [US/Can] *see* ticlopidine *on this page*

ticlopidine (tye KLOE pi deen)

Synonyms ticlopidine hydrochloride

U.S./Canadian Brand Names Alti-Ticlopidine [Can]; Apo-Ticlopidine® [Can]; Gen-Ticlopidine [Can]; Novo-Ticlopidine [Can]; Nu-Ticlopidine [Can]; Rhoxal-ticlopidine [Can]; Sandoz-Ticlopidine [Can]; Ticlid® [US/Can]

Therapeutic Category Antiplatelet Agent

Use Platelet aggregation inhibitor that reduces the risk of thrombotic stroke in patients who have had a stroke or stroke precursors. **Note:** Due to its association with life-threatening hematologic disorders, ticlopidine should be reserved for patients who are intolerant to aspirin, or who have failed aspirin therapy. Adjunctive therapy (with aspirin) following successful coronary stent implantation to reduce the incidence of subacute stent thrombosis.

Usual Dosage Oral: Adults:

Stroke prevention: 250 mg twice daily with food

Coronary artery stenting (initiate after successful implantation): 250 mg twice daily with food (in combination with antiplatelet doses of aspirin) for up to 30 days

Dosage Forms Tablet, as hydrochloride: 250 mg

ticlopidine hydrochloride *see* ticlopidine *on this page*

Ticon® *(Discontinued)* *see* trimethobenzamide *on page 851*

TIG *see* tetanus immune globulin (human) *on page 814*

Tigan® [US/Can] *see* trimethobenzamide *on page 851*

tigecycline (tye ge SYE kleen)

Synonyms GAR-936

U.S./Canadian Brand Names Tygacil™ [US]

Therapeutic Category Antibiotic, Glycylcycline

Use Treatment of complicated skin and skin structure infections caused by susceptible organisms, including methicillin-resistant *Staphylococcus aureus* and vancomycin-sensitive *Enterococcus faecalis*; treatment of complicated intraabdominal infections

Usual Dosage I.V.: Adults:

Initial: 100 mg as a single dose

Maintenance dose: 50 mg every 12 hours

Recommended duration of therapy: Intraabdominal infections or complicated skin/skin structure infections: 5-14 days.

Dosage Forms Injection, powder for reconstitution: 50 mg

Tikosyn™ [US/Can] *see* dofetilide *on page 271*

Tilade® [US/Can] *see* nedocromil (inhalation) *on page 581*

tiludronate (tye LOO droe nate)

Synonyms tiludronate disodium

U.S./Canadian Brand Names Skelid® [US]

Therapeutic Category Bisphosphonate Derivative

Use Treatment of Paget disease of the bone in patients who have a level of serum alkaline phosphatase (SAP) at least twice the upper limit of normal, or who are symptomatic, or who are at risk for future complications of their disease

Usual Dosage Tiludronate should be taken with 6-8 oz of plain water and not taken within 2 hours of food

Adults: Oral: 400 mg (2 tablets of tiludronic acid) daily for a period of 3 months; allow an interval of 3 months to assess response

Dosage Forms Tablet, tiludronic acid: 200 mg [equivalent to 240 mg tiludronate disodium]

tiludronate disodium *see* tiludronate *on this page*

Tim-AK [Can] *see* timolol *on this page*

Timecelles® *(Discontinued)* *see* ascorbic acid *on page 76*

Timentin® [US/Can] *see* ticarcillin and clavulanate potassium *on previous page*

timolol (TIM oh lol)

Sound-Alike/Look-Alike Issues

timolol may be confused with atenolol, Tylenol®

Timoptic® may be confused with Talacen®, Viroptic®

Synonyms timolol hemihydrate; timolol maleate

U.S./Canadian Brand Names Alti-Timolol [Can]; Apo-Timol® [Can]; Apo-Timop® [Can]; Betimol® [US]; Blocadren® [US]; Gen-Timolol [Can]; Istalol™ [US]; Nu-Timolol [Can]; Phoxal-timolol [Can]; PMS-Timolol [Can]; Sandoz-Timolol [Can]; Tim-AK [Can]; Timoptic-XE® [US/Can]; Timoptic® in OcuDose® [US]; Timoptic® [US/Can]

Therapeutic Category Beta-Adrenergic Blocker

Use

Ophthalmic: Treatment of elevated intraocular pressure such as glaucoma or ocular hypertension

Oral: Treatment of hypertension and angina; to reduce mortality following myocardial infarction; prophylaxis of migraine

Usual Dosage

Ophthalmic:

Children and Adults:

Solution: Initial: Instill 1 drop (0.25% solution) into affected eye(s) twice daily; increase to 0.5% solution if response not adequate; decrease to 1 drop/day if controlled; do not exceed 1 drop twice daily of 0.5% solution

Gel-forming solution (Timoptic-XE®): Instill 1 drop (either 0.25% or 0.5% solution) once daily

Adults: Solution (Istalol®): Instill 1 drop (0.5% solution) once daily in the morning

Oral: Adults:

Hypertension: Initial: 10 mg twice daily, increase gradually every 7 days, usual dosage: 20-40 mg/day in 2 divided doses; maximum: 60 mg/day

Prevention of myocardial infarction: 10 mg twice daily initiated within 1-4 weeks after infarction

Migraine headache: Initial: 10 mg twice daily, increase to maximum of 30 mg/day

Dosage Forms Note: Unless otherwise specified, strength expressed as base.

Gel-forming solution, ophthalmic, as maleate: 0.25% (5 mL); 0.5% (2.5 mL, 5 mL)

Timoptic-XE®: 0.25% (5 mL); 0.5% (5 mL)

Solution, ophthalmic, as hemihydrate:

Betimol®: 0.25% (5 mL, 10 mL, 15 mL); 0.5% (5 mL, 10 mL, 15 mL) [contains benzalkonium chloride]

Solution, ophthalmic, as maleate: 0.25% (5 mL, 10 mL, 15 mL); 0.5% (5 mL, 10 mL, 15 mL) [contains benzalkonium chloride]

Istalol™: 0.5% (10 mL) [contains benzalkonium chloride and potassium sorbate]

Timoptic®: 0.25% (5 mL); 0.5% (5 mL, 10 mL) [contains benzalkonium chloride]

Solution, ophthalmic, as maleate [preservative free]:

Timoptic® in OcuDose®: 0.25% (0.2 mL); 0.5% (0.2 mL) [single use]

Tablet, as maleate: 5 mg, 10 mg, 20 mg [strength expressed as salt]

Blocadren®: 20 mg [strength expressed as salt]

timolol and dorzolamide *see* dorzolamide and timolol *on page 274*

timolol hemihydrate *see* timolol *on previous page*

timolol maleate *see* timolol *on previous page*

Timoptic® [US/Can] *see* timolol *on previous page*

Timoptic® in OcuDose® [US] *see* timolol *on previous page*

Timoptic-XE® [US/Can] *see* timolol *on previous page*

Tinactin® Antifungal [US-OTC] *see* tolnaftate *on page 834*

Tinactin® Antifungal Jock Itch [US-OTC] *see* tolnaftate *on page 834*

Tinaderm [US-OTC] *see* tolnaftate *on page 834*

Tinamed® [US-OTC] *see* salicylic acid *on page 758*

TinBen® *(Discontinued)* *see* benzoin *on page 102*

Tindamax™ [US] *see* tinidazole *on this page*

tine test *see* tuberculin tests *on page 857*

Ting® Cream [US-OTC] *see* tolnaftate *on page 834*

tinidazole (tye NI da zole)

U.S./Canadian Brand Names Tindamax™ [US]

Therapeutic Category Amebicide; Antibiotic, Miscellaneous; Antiprotozoal, Nitroimidazole

Use Treatment of trichomoniasis caused by *T. vaginalis*; treatment of giardiasis caused by *G. duodenalis* (*G. lamblia*); treatment of intestinal amebiasis and amebic liver abscess caused by *E. histolytica*

Usual Dosage Oral:

Children >3 years:

Amebiasis, intestinal: 50 mg/kg/day for 3 days (maximum dose: 2 g/day)

Amebiasis, liver abscess: 50 mg/kg/day for 3-5 days (maximum dose: 2 g/day)

Giardiasis: 50 mg/kg as a single dose (maximum dose: 2 g)

Adults:

Amebiasis, intestinal: 2 g/day for 3 days

Amebiasis, liver abscess: 2 g/day for 3-5 days

Giardiasis: 2 g as a single dose

Trichomoniasis: Oral: 2 g as a single dose; sexual partners should be treated at the same time

Dosage Forms Tablet [scored]: 250 mg, 500 mg

Tinver® *(Discontinued)* *see* sodium thiosulfate *on page 783*

tinzaparin (tin ZA pa rin)

Synonyms tinzaparin sodium

U.S./Canadian Brand Names Innohep® [US/Can]

Therapeutic Category Anticoagulant (Other)

Use Treatment of acute symptomatic deep vein thrombosis, with or without pulmonary embolism, in conjunction with warfarin sodium

Usual Dosage SubQ:

Adults: 175 anti-Xa int. units/kg of body weight once daily. Warfarin sodium should be started when appropriate. Administer tinzaparin for at least 6 days and until patient is adequately anticoagulated with warfarin.

(Continued)

tinzaparin *(Continued)*

Note: To calculate the volume of solution to administer per dose: Volume to be administered (mL) = patient weight (kg) x 0.00875 mL/kg (may be rounded off to the nearest 0.05 mL)

Dosage Forms Injection, solution, as sodium: 20,000 anti-Xa int. units/mL (2 mL) [contains benzyl alcohol and sodium metabisulfite]

tinzaparin sodium *see* tinzaparin *on previous page*

tioconazole (tye oh KONE a zole)

Sound-Alike/Look-Alike Issues
tioconazole may be confused with terconazole

U.S./Canadian Brand Names 1-Day™ [US-OTC]; Vagistat®-1 [US-OTC]

Therapeutic Category Antifungal Agent

Use Local treatment of vulvovaginal candidiasis

Usual Dosage Adults: Vaginal: Insert 1 applicatorful in vagina, just prior to bedtime, as a single dose

Dosage Forms Ointment, vaginal: 6.5% (4.6 g) [with applicator]

tioguanine *see* thioguanine *on page 822*

tiopronin (tye oh PROE nin)

Sound-Alike/Look-Alike Issues
Thiola® may be confused with Theolair™

U.S./Canadian Brand Names Thiola® [US/Can]

Therapeutic Category Urinary Tract Product

Use Prevention of kidney stone (cystine) formation in patients with severe homozygous cystinuric who have urinary cystine >500 mg/day who are resistant to treatment with high fluid intake, alkali, and diet modification, or who have had adverse reactions to penicillamine

Usual Dosage Adults: Initial dose is 800 mg/day, average dose is 1000 mg/day

Dosage Forms Tablet: 100 mg

tiotixene *see* thiothixene *on page 824*

tiotropium (ty oh TRO pee um)

Sound-Alike/Look-Alike Issues
Spiriva® may be confused with Inspra™

Synonyms tiotropium bromide monohydrate

U.S./Canadian Brand Names Spiriva® [US/Can]

Therapeutic Category Anticholinergic Agent

Use Maintenance treatment of bronchospasm associated with COPD (bronchitis and emphysema)

Usual Dosage Oral inhalation: Adults: Contents of 1 capsule (18 mcg) inhaled once daily using HandiHaler® device

Dosage Forms Powder for oral inhalation [capsule]: 18 mcg/capsule [contains lactose; packaged in 6s or 30s with HandiHaler® device]

tiotropium bromide monohydrate *see* tiotropium *on this page*

tipranavir (tip RA na veer)

Synonyms PNU-140690E; TPV

U.S./Canadian Brand Names Aptivus® [US/Can]

Therapeutic Category Antiretroviral Agent, Protease Inhibitor

Use Treatment of HIV-1 infections in combination with ritonavir and other antiretroviral agents; limited to highly treatment-experienced or multiprotease inhibitor-resistant patients.

Usual Dosage Oral: Adults: 500 mg twice daily with a high-fat meal. **Note:** Coadministration with ritonavir (200 mg twice daily) is required.

Dosage Forms Capsule, gelatin: 250 mg [contains dehydrated ethanol 7% per capsule]

TipTapToe *(Discontinued)* *see* tolnaftate *on page 834*

tirofiban (tye roe FYE ban)

Sound-Alike/Look-Alike Issues
Aggrastat® may be confused with Aggrenox®, argatroban

Synonyms MK383; tirofiban hydrochloride

U.S./Canadian Brand Names Aggrastat® [US/Can]

Therapeutic Category Antiplatelet Agent

Use In combination with heparin, is indicated for the treatment of acute coronary syndrome, including patients who are to be managed medically and those undergoing PTCA or atherectomy. In this setting, it has been shown to decrease the rate of a combined endpoint of death, new myocardial infarction or refractory ischemia/repeat cardiac procedure.

Usual Dosage Adults: I.V.: Initial rate of 0.4 mcg/kg/minute for 30 minutes and then continued at 0.1 mcg/kg/minute; dosing should be continued through angiography and for 12-24 hours after angioplasty or atherectomy.

Dosage Forms

Infusion [premixed in sodium chloride]: 50 mcg/mL (100 mL, 250 mL)

Injection, solution: 250 mcg/mL (50 mL)

tirofiban hydrochloride *see* tirofiban *on previous page*

Tiseb® [US-OTC] *see* salicylic acid *on page 758*

Tisit® [US-OTC] *see* pyrethrins and piperonyl butoxide *on page 720*

Tisit® Blue Gel [US-OTC] *see* pyrethrins and piperonyl butoxide *on page 720*

Tisseel® VH [US/Can] *see* fibrin sealant kit *on page 345*

Titralac™ [US-OTC] *see* calcium carbonate *on page 135*

Titralac™ Extra Strength [US-OTC] *see* calcium carbonate *on page 135*

Titralac® Plus [US-OTC] *see* calcium carbonate and simethicone *on page 137*

Ti-U-Lac® H [Can] *see* urea and hydrocortisone *on page 861*

tizanidine (tye ZAN i deen)

Sound-Alike/Look-Alike Issues

tizanidine may be confused with tiagabine

U.S./Canadian Brand Names Apo-Tizanidine® [Can]; Gen-Tizanidine [Can]; Zanaflex® [US/Can]

Therapeutic Category Alpha$_2$-Adrenergic Agonist Agent

Use Skeletal muscle relaxant used for treatment of muscle spasticity

Usual Dosage Adults: 2-4 mg 3 times/day

Usual initial dose: 4 mg, may increase by 2-4 mg as needed for satisfactory reduction of muscle tone every 6-8 hours to a maximum of three doses in any 24 hour period

Maximum dose: 36 mg/day

Dosage Forms

Capsule:

Zanaflex®: 2 mg, 4 mg, 6 mg

Tablet: 2 mg, 4 mg

Zanaflex®: 2 mg [DSC], 4 mg

TMC-114 *see* darunavir *on page 231*

TMP *see* trimethoprim *on page 851*

TMP-SMZ *see* sulfamethoxazole and trimethoprim *on page 797*

TMZ *see* temozolomide *on page 808*

T.N. Dickinson's® Hazelets [US-OTC] *see* witch hazel *on page 881*

TNKase™ [US/Can] *see* tenecteplase *on page 809*

TOBI® [US/Can] *see* tobramycin *on this page*

TobraDex® [US/Can] *see* tobramycin and dexamethasone *on page 833*

tobramycin (toe bra MYE sin)

Sound-Alike/Look-Alike Issues

tobramycin may be confused with Trobicin®

AKTob® may be confused with AK-Trol®

Nebcin® may be confused with Inapsine®, Naprosyn®, Nubain®

Tobrex® may be confused with TobraDex®

Synonyms tobramycin sulfate

U.S./Canadian Brand Names AKTob® [US]; PMS-Tobramycin [Can]; Sandoz-Tobramycin [Can]; TOBI® [US/Can]; Tobramycin Injection, USP [Can]; Tobrex® [US/Can]

(Continued)

tobramycin *(Continued)*

Therapeutic Category Aminoglycoside (Antibiotic); Antibiotic, Ophthalmic

Use Treatment of documented or suspected infections caused by susceptible gram-negative bacilli including *Pseudomonas aeruginosa*; topically used to treat superficial ophthalmic infections caused by susceptible bacteria. Tobramycin solution for inhalation is indicated for the management of cystic fibrosis patients (>6 years of age) with *Pseudomonas aeruginosa*.

Usual Dosage Note: Dosage individualization is **critical** because of the low therapeutic index.

Use of ideal body weight (IBW) for determining the mg/kg/dose appears to be more accurate than dosing on the basis of total body weight (TBW). In morbid obesity, dosage requirement may best be estimated using a dosing weight of IBW + 0.4 (TBW - IBW).

Initial and periodic plasma drug levels (eg, peak and trough with conventional dosing) should be determined, particularly in critically-ill patients with serious infections or in disease states known to significantly alter aminoglycoside pharmacokinetics (eg, cystic fibrosis, burns, or major surgery).

Usual dosage range:

Infants and Children <5 years: I.M., I.V.: 2.5 mg/kg/dose every 8 hours

Children ≥5 years: I.M., I.V.: 2-2.5 mg/kg/dose every 8 hours

Note: Higher individual doses and/or more frequent intervals (eg, every 6 hours) may be required in selected clinical situations (cystic fibrosis) or serum levels document the need.

Children and Adults:

Inhalation:

Children: 40-80 mg 2-3 times/day

Adults: 60-80 mg 3 times/day

High-dose regimen: Children ≥6 years and Adults: 300 mg every 12 hours (do not administer doses <6 hours apart); administer in repeated cycles of 28 days on drug followed by 28 days off drug

Intrathecal: 4-8 mg/day

Ophthalmic: Children ≥2 months and Adults:

Ointment: Instill½' (1.25 cm) 2-3 times/day every 3-4 hours

Solution: Instill 1-2 drops every 2-4 hours, up to 2 drops every hour for severe infections

Topical: Apply 3-4 times/day to affected area

Adults: I.M., I.V.:

Conventional: 1-2.5 mg/kg/dose every 8-12 hours; to ensure adequate peak concentrations early in therapy, higher initial dosage may be considered in selected patients when extracellular water is increased (edema, septic shock, postsurgical, and/or trauma)

Once-daily: 4-7 mg/kg/dose once daily; some clinicians recommend this approach for all patients with normal renal function; this dose is at least as efficacious with similar, if not less, toxicity than conventional dosing.

Indication-specific dosing:

Neonates: I.M., I.V.:

Meningitis:

0-7 days: <2000 g: 2.5 mg/kg every 18-24 hours; >2000 g: 2.5 mg/kg every 12 hours

8-28 days: <2000 g: 2.5 mg/kg every 8-12 hours; >2000 g: 2.5 mg/kg every 8 hours

Children:

Cystic fibrosis:

I.M., I.V.: 2.5-3.3 mg/kg every 6-8 hours; **Note:** Some patients may require larger or more frequent doses if serum levels document the need (eg, cystic fibrosis or febrile granulocytopenic patients).

Inhalation:

Standard aerosolized tobramycin: 40-80 mg 2-3 times/day

High-dose regimen (TOBI®): Children ≥6 years: See adult dosing.

Adults: I.M., I.V.:

Brucellosis: 240 mg (I.M.) daily or 5 mg/kg (I.V.) daily for 7 days; either regimen recommended in combination with doxycycline

Cholangitis: 4-6 mg/kg once daily with ampicillin

Diverticulitis, complicated: 1.5-2 mg/kg every 8 hours (with ampicillin and metronidazole)

Endocarditis prophylaxis (dental, oral, upper respiratory procedures, GI/GU procedures): 1.5 mg/kg with ampicillin (50 mg/kg) 30 minutes prior to procedure

Endocarditis or synergy (for gram-positive infections): 1 mg/kg every 8 hours (with ampicillin)

Meningitis *(Enterococcus or Pseudomonas aeruginosa):* I.V.: Loading dose: 2 mg/kg, then 1.7 mg/kg/dose every 8 hours (administered with another bacteriocidal drug)

Pelvic inflammatory disease: Loading dose: 2 mg/kg, then 1.5 mg/kg every 8 hours **or** 4.5 mg/kg once daily

Plague *(Yersinia pestis):* Treatment: 5 mg/kg/day, followed by postexposure prophylaxis with doxycycline

Pneumonia, hospital- or ventilator-associated: 7 mg/kg/day (with antipseudomonal beta-lactam or carbapenem)
Tularemia: 5 mg/kg/day divided every 8 hours for 1-2 weeks
Urinary tract infection: 1.5 mg/kg/dose every 8 hours

Dosage Forms
Infusion [premixed in NS]: 60 mg (50 mL); 80 mg (100 mL)
Injection, powder for reconstitution: 1.2 g
Injection, solution: 10 mg/mL (2 mL, 8 mL); 40 mg/mL (2 mL, 30 mL, 50 mL) [may contain sodium metabisulfite]
Ointment, ophthalmic (Tobrex®): 0.3% (3.5 g)
Solution for nebulization [preservative free] (TOBI®): 60 mg/mL (5 mL)
Solution, ophthalmic (AKTob®, Tobrex®): 0.3% (5 mL) [contains benzalkonium chloride]

tobramycin and dexamethasone (toe bra MYE sin & deks a METH a sone)

Sound-Alike/Look-Alike Issues
TobraDex® may be confused with Tobrex®
Synonyms dexamethasone and tobramycin
U.S./Canadian Brand Names TobraDex® [US/Can]
Therapeutic Category Antibiotic/Corticosteroid, Ophthalmic
Use Treatment of external ocular infection caused by susceptible gram-negative bacteria and steroid responsive inflammatory conditions of the palpebral and bulbar conjunctiva, lid, cornea, and anterior segment of the globe
Usual Dosage Children and Adults: Ophthalmic: Instill 1-2 drops of solution every 4 hours; apply ointment 2-3 times/day; for severe infections apply ointment every 3-4 hours, or solution 2 drops every 30-60 minutes initially, then reduce to less frequent intervals
Dosage Forms
Ointment, ophthalmic: Tobramycin 0.3% and dexamethasone 0.1% (3.5 g)
Suspension, ophthalmic: Tobramycin 0.3% and dexamethasone 0.1% (2.5 mL, 5 mL, 10 mL) [contains benzalkonium chloride]

Tobramycin Injection, USP [Can] *see* tobramycin *on page 831*

tobramycin sulfate *see* tobramycin *on page 831*

Tobrex® [US/Can] *see* tobramycin *on page 831*

tocophersolan ***(Discontinued)***

Today® Sponge [US-OTC] *see* nonoxynol 9 *on page 597*

Tofranil® [US/Can] *see* imipramine *on page 442*

Tofranil-PM® [US] *see* imipramine *on page 442*

tolazamide (tole AZ a mide)

Sound-Alike/Look-Alike Issues
TOLAZamide may be confused with tolazoline, TOLBUTamide
Tolinase® may be confused with Orinase®
Tall-Man TOLAZamide
U.S./Canadian Brand Names Tolinase® [Can]
Therapeutic Category Antidiabetic Agent, Oral
Use Adjunct to diet for the management of mild to moderately severe, stable, type 2 diabetes mellitus (noninsulin dependent, NIDDM)
Usual Dosage Oral (doses >1000 mg/day normally do not improve diabetic control):
Adults:
Initial: 100-250 mg/day with breakfast or the first main meal of the day
Fasting blood sugar <200 mg/dL: 100 mg/day
Fasting blood sugar >200 mg/dL: 250 mg/day
Patient is malnourished, underweight, elderly, or not eating properly: 100 mg/day
Adjust dose in increments of 100-250 mg/day at weekly intervals to response. If >500 mg/day is required, give in divided doses twice daily; maximum daily dose: 1 g (doses >1 g/day are not likely to improve control)
Conversion from insulin to tolazamide
10 units day = 100 mg/day
20-40 units/day = 250 mg/day
>40 units/day = 250 mg/day and 50% of insulin dose
Doses >500 mg/day should be given in 2 divided doses
(Continued)

tolazamide *(Continued)*

Dosage Forms [DSC] = Discontinued product
Tablet: 100 mg, 250 mg, 500 mg
Tolinase® [DSC]: 100 mg, 250 mg

tolbutamide (tole BYOO ta mide)

Sound-Alike/Look-Alike Issues
TOLBUTamide may be confused with terbutaline, TOLAZamide
Orinase® may be confused with Orabase®, Ornex®, Tolinase®
Synonyms tolbutamide sodium
Tall-Man TOLBUTamide
U.S./Canadian Brand Names Apo-Tolbutamide® [Can]
Therapeutic Category Antidiabetic Agent, Oral
Use Adjunct to diet for the management of mild to moderately severe, stable, type 2 diabetes mellitus (noninsulin dependent, NIDDM)
Usual Dosage Divided doses may improve gastrointestinal tolerance
Adults: Oral: Initial: 1-2 g/day as a single dose in the morning or in divided doses throughout the day. Total doses may be taken in the morning; however, divided doses may allow increased gastrointestinal tolerance. Maintenance dose: 0.25-3 g/day; however, a maintenance dose >2 g/day is seldom required.
Dosage Forms Tablet: 500 mg

tolbutamide sodium *see* tolbutamide *on this page*

tolcapone (TOLE ka pone)

U.S./Canadian Brand Names Tasmar® [US]
Therapeutic Category Anti-Parkinson Agent
Use Adjunct to levodopa and carbidopa for the treatment of signs and symptoms of idiopathic Parkinson disease
Usual Dosage Oral: Adults: Initial: 100 mg 3 times/day; may increase as tolerated to 200 mg 3 times/day; levodopa dose may need to be decreased upon initiation of tolcapone (average reduction in clinical trials was 30%)
Note: If clinical improvement is not observed after 3 weeks of therapy (regardless of dose), tolcapone treatment should be discontinued.
Dosage Forms Tablet: 100 mg, 200 mg

Tolectin® [US] *see* tolmetin *on this page*

Tolectin® DS *(Discontinued)* *see* tolmetin *on this page*

Tolinase® [Can] *see* tolazamide *on previous page*

Tolinase® *(Discontinued)* *see* tolazamide *on previous page*

tolmetin (TOLE met in)

Synonyms tolmetin sodium
U.S./Canadian Brand Names Tolectin® [US]
Therapeutic Category Analgesic, Nonnarcotic; Nonsteroidal Antiinflammatory Drug (NSAID)
Use Treatment of rheumatoid arthritis and osteoarthritis, juvenile rheumatoid arthritis
Usual Dosage Oral:
Children ≥2 years:
Antiinflammatory: Initial: 20 mg/kg/day in 3 divided doses, then 15-30 mg/kg/day in 3 divided doses
Analgesic: 5-7 mg/kg/dose every 6-8 hours
Adults: 400 mg 3 times/day; usual dose: 600 mg to 1.8 g/day; maximum: 2 g/day
Dosage Forms
Capsule: 400 mg
Tablet: 200 mg, 600 mg
Tolectin®: 600 mg [contains sodium 54 mg (2.35 mEq)]

tolmetin sodium *see* tolmetin *on this page*

tolnaftate (tole NAF tate)

Sound-Alike/Look-Alike Issues
tolnaftate may be confused with Tornalate®
Tinactin® may be confused with Talacen®

U.S./Canadian Brand Names Blis-To-Sol® [US-OTC]; Fungi-Guard [US-OTC]; Gold Bond® Antifungal [US-OTC]; Pitrex [Can]; Podactin Powder [US-OTC]; Q-Naftate [US-OTC]; Tinactin® Antifungal Jock Itch [US-OTC]; Tinactin® Antifungal [US-OTC]; Tinaderm [US-OTC]; Ting® Cream [US-OTC]

Therapeutic Category Antifungal Agent

Use Treatment of tinea pedis, tinea cruris, tinea corporis

Usual Dosage Children ≥2 years and Adults: Topical: Wash and dry affected area; spray aerosol or apply 1-3 drops of solution or a small amount of cream, or powder and rub into the affected areas 2 times/day

Note: May use for up to 4 weeks for tinea pedis or tinea corporis, and up to 2 weeks for tinea cruris

Dosage Forms [DSC] = Discontinued product

Aerosol, liquid, topical:
- Aftate®: 1% (120 mL) [contains alcohol] [DSC]
- Tinactin® Antifungal: 1% (60 mL, 150 mL) [contains alcohol]

Aerosol, powder, topical:
- Aftate®: 1% (105 g) [contains alcohol] [DSC]
- Tinactin® Antifungal: 1% (133 g) [contains alcohol]
- Tinactin® Antifungal Jock Itch: 1% (100 g, 133 g) [contains alcohol]

Cream, topical: 1% (15 g, 30 g)
- Fungi-Guard, Tinactin® Antifungal Jock Itch, Ting®: 1% (15 g)
- Q-Naftate, Tinactin® Antifungal: 1% (15 g, 30 g)

Liquid, topical:
- Blis-To-Sol®: 1% (30 mL, 55 mL)
- Fungi-Guard: 1% (30 mL) [contains vitamin E and aloe; brush applicator provided]

Powder, topical: 1% (45 g)
- Podactin: 1% (45 g)
- Tinactin® Antifungal: 1% (108 g)

Solution, topical: 1% (10 mL)
- Tinaderm: 1% (10 mL)

Swab, topical [liquid-filled swabstick]: 1% (36s)
- Gold Bond® Antifungal: 1% (24s)

tolterodine (tole TER oh deen)

Sound-Alike/Look-Alike Issues

Detrol® may be confused with Ditropan®

Synonyms tolterodine tartrate

U.S./Canadian Brand Names Detrol® LA [US/Can]; Detrol® [US/Can]; Unidet® [Can]

Therapeutic Category Anticholinergic Agent

Use Treatment of patients with an overactive bladder with symptoms of urinary frequency, urgency, or urge incontinence

Usual Dosage Oral: Adults: Treatment of overactive bladder:

Immediate release tablet: 2 mg twice daily; the dose may be lowered to 1 mg twice daily based on individual response and tolerability

Dosing adjustment in patients concurrently taking CYP3A4 inhibitors: 1 mg twice daily

Extended release capsule: 4 mg once a day; dose may be lowered to 2 mg daily based on individual response and tolerability

Dosing adjustment in patients concurrently taking CYP3A4 inhibitors: 2 mg daily

Dosage Forms

Capsule, extended release, as tartrate (Detrol® LA): 2 mg, 4 mg

Tablet, as tartrate (Detrol®): 1 mg, 2 mg

tolterodine tartrate *see* tolterodine *on this page*

Tomocat® [US] *see* radiological/contrast media (ionic) *on page 728*

tomoxetine *see* atomoxetine *on page 81*

Tomudex® [Can] *see* raltitrexed *(Canada only) on page 731*

Tomycine® ***(Discontinued)*** *see* tobramycin *on page 831*

Tonocard® ***(Discontinued)***

Tonopaque® [US] *see* radiological/contrast media (ionic) *on page 728*

Topamax® [US/Can] *see* topiramate *on next page*

Topamax® 200 mg Tablet ***(Discontinued)*** *see* topiramate *on next page*

Topicaine® [US-OTC] *see* lidocaine *on page 493*

Topicort® [US/Can] *see* desoximetasone *on page 238*

Topicort®-LP [US] *see* desoximetasone *on page 238*

Topicycline® Topical *(Discontinued)* *see* tetracycline *on page 816*

Topilene® [Can] *see* betamethasone (topical) *on page 107*

topiramate (toe PYRE a mate)

Sound-Alike/Look-Alike Issues

Topamax® may be confused with Toprol-XL®

U.S./Canadian Brand Names Dom-Topiramate [Can]; Gen-Topiramate [Can]; Novo-Topiramate [Can]; PHL-Topiramate [Can]; PMS-Topiramate [Can]; ratio-Topiramate [Can]; Rhoxal-topiramate [Can]; Sandoz-Topiramate [Can]; Topamax® [US/Can]

Therapeutic Category Anticonvulsant

Use Monotherapy or adjunctive therapy for partial onset seizures and primary generalized tonic-clonic seizures; adjunctive treatment of seizures associated with Lennox-Gastaut syndrome; prophylaxis of migraine headache

Usual Dosage Oral: **Note:** Do not abruptly discontinue therapy; taper dosage gradually to prevent rebound seizure.

Monotherapy: Children ≥10 years and Adults: Partial onset seizure and primary generalized tonic-clonic seizure: Initial: 25 mg twice daily; may increase weekly by 50 mg/day up to 100 mg twice daily (week 4 dose); thereafter, may further increase weekly by 100 mg/day up to the recommended maximum of 200 mg twice daily.

Adjunctive therapy:

Children 2-16 years:

Partial onset seizure or seizure associated with Lennox-Gastaut syndrome: Initial dose titration should begin at 25 mg (or less, based on a range of 1-3 mg/kg/day) nightly for the first week; dosage may be increased in increments of 1-3 mg/kg/day (administered in 2 divided doses) at 1- or 2-week intervals to a total daily dose of 5-9 mg/kg/day

Primary generalized tonic-clonic seizure: Use initial dose listed above, but use slower initial titration rate; titrate to recommended maintenance dose by the end of 8 weeks

Adolescents ≥17 years and Adults:

Partial onset seizures: Initial: 25-50 mg/day (given in 2 divided doses) for 1 week; increase at weekly intervals by 25-50 mg/day until response; usual maintenance dose: 100-200 mg twice daily. Doses >1600 mg/day have not been studied.

Primary generalized tonic-clonic seizures: Use initial dose as listed above for partial onset seizures, but use slower initial titration rate; titrate upwards to recommended dose by the end of 8 weeks; usual maintenance dose: 200 mg twice daily. Doses >1600 mg/day have not been studied.

Adults: Migraine prophylaxis: Initial: 25 mg/day (in the evening), titrated at weekly intervals in 25 mg increments, up to the recommended total daily dose of 100 mg/day given in 2 divided doses

Dosage Forms

Capsule, sprinkle: 15 mg, 25 mg

Tablet: 25 mg, 50 mg, 100 mg, 200 mg

Topisone® [Can] *see* betamethasone (topical) *on page 107*

TOPO *see* topotecan *on this page*

Toposar® [US] *see* etoposide *on page 330*

topotecan (toe poe TEE kan)

Sound-Alike/Look-Alike Issues

Hycamtin® may be confused with Hycomine®

Synonyms hycamptamine; NSC-609699; SK and F 104864; SKF 104864; SKF 104864-A; TOPO; topotecan hydrochloride; TPT

U.S./Canadian Brand Names Hycamtin® [US/Can]

Therapeutic Category Antineoplastic Agent

Use Treatment of ovarian cancer and small cell lung cancer; cervical cancer (in combination with cisplatin)

Usual Dosage Adults (refer to individual protocols):

Metastatic ovarian cancer and small cell lung cancer: IVPB: 1.5 mg/m^2/day for 5 days; repeated every 21 days (baseline neutrophil count should be >1500/mm^3 and platelet count should be >100,000/mm^3)

Cervical cancer: IVPB: 0.75 mg/m^2/day for 3 days (followed by cisplatin 50 mg/m^2 on day 1 only, [with hydration]); repeated every 21 days (baseline neutrophil count should be >1500/mm^3 and platelet count should be >100,000/mm^3)

Dosage Forms
Injection, powder for reconstitution, as hydrochloride:
Hycamtin®: 4 mg [base]

topotecan hydrochloride *see* topotecan *on previous page*

Toprol-XL® [US/Can] *see* metoprolol *on page 550*

Topsyn® [Can] *see* fluocinonide *on page 353*

Toradol® [US/Can] *see* ketorolac *on page 472*

Toradol® IM [Can] *see* ketorolac *on page 472*

toremifene (tore EM I feen)

Synonyms FC1157a; toremifene citrate
U.S./Canadian Brand Names Fareston® [US/Can]
Therapeutic Category Antineoplastic Agent
Use Treatment of advanced breast cancer; management of desmoid tumors and endometrial carcinoma
Usual Dosage Refer to individual protocols.
Adults: Oral: 60 mg once daily, generally continued until disease progression is observed
Dosage Forms Tablet: 60 mg

toremifene citrate *see* toremifene *on this page*

torsemide (TORE se mide)

Sound-Alike/Look-Alike Issues
torsemide may be confused with furosemide
Demadex® may be confused with Denorex®
U.S./Canadian Brand Names Demadex® [US]
Therapeutic Category Diuretic, Loop
Use Management of edema associated with congestive heart failure and hepatic or renal disease; used alone or in combination with antihypertensives in treatment of hypertension; I.V. form is indicated when rapid onset is desired
Usual Dosage Adults: Oral, I.V.:
Congestive heart failure: 10-20 mg once daily; may increase gradually for chronic treatment by doubling dose until the diuretic response is apparent (for acute treatment, I.V. dose may be repeated every 2 hours with double the dose as needed). **Note:** ACC/AHA 2005 guidelines for chronic heart failure recommend a maximum daily oral dose of 200 mg; maximum single I.V. dose of 100-200 mg
Continuous I.V. infusion: 20 mg I.V. load then 5-20 mg/hour
Chronic renal failure: 20 mg once daily; increase as described above
Hepatic cirrhosis: 5-10 mg once daily with an aldosterone antagonist or a potassium-sparing diuretic; increase as described above
Hypertension: 2.5-5 mg once daily; increase to 10 mg after 4-6 weeks if an adequate hypotensive response is not apparent; if still not effective, an additional antihypertensive agent may be added
Dosage Forms
Injection, solution: 10 mg/mL (2 mL, 5 mL)
Tablet: 5 mg, 10 mg, 20 mg, 100 mg

tositumomab I-131 *see* tositumomab and iodine I 131 tositumomab *on this page*

tositumomab and iodine I 131 tositumomab

(toe si TYOO mo mab & EYE oh dyne eye one THUR tee one toe si TYOO mo mab)
Synonyms anti-CD20-murine monoclonal antibody I-131; B1; B1 antibody; 131 I anti-B1 antibody; 131 I-anti-B1 monoclonal antibody; iodine I 131 tositumomab and tositumomab; tositumomab I-131
U.S./Canadian Brand Names Bexxar® [US]
Therapeutic Category Antineoplastic Agent, Monoclonal Antibody; Radiopharmaceutical
Use Treatment of relapsed or refractory CD20 positive, low-grade, follicular, or transformed non-Hodgkin lymphoma
Usual Dosage I.V.: Adults: Dosing consists of four components administered in 2 steps. Thyroid protective agents (SSKI, Lugol's solution or potassium iodide), acetaminophen and diphenhydramine should be given prior to or with treatment.
Step 1: Dosimetric step (Day 0):
Tositumomab 450 mg in NS 50 mL administered over 60 minutes
Iodine I 131 tositumomab (containing I-131 5.0 mCi and tositumomab 35 mg) in NS 30 mL administered over 20 minutes
(Continued)

tositumomab and iodine I 131 tositumomab *(Continued)*

Note: Whole body dosimetry and biodistribution should be determined on Day 0; days 2, 3, or 4; and day 6 or 7 prior to administration of Step 2. If biodistribution is not acceptable, do not administer the therapeutic step. On day 6 or 7, calculate the patient specific activity of iodine I 131 tositumomab to deliver 75 cGy TBD or 65 cGy TBD (in mCi).

Step 2: Therapeutic step (Day 7):

Tositumomab 450 mg in NS 50 mL administered over 60 minutes

Iodine I 131 tositumomab:

Platelets ≥150,000/mm^3: Iodine I 131 calculated to deliver 75 cGy total body irradiation and tositumomab 35 mg over 20 minutes

Platelets ≥100,000/mm^3 and <150,000/mm^3: Iodine I 131 calculated to deliver 65 cGy total body irradiation and tositumomab 35 mg over 20 minutes

Dosage Forms Note: Not all components are shipped from the same facility. When ordering, ensure that all will arrive on the same day.

Kit [dosimetric package]: Tositumomab 225 mg/16.1 mL [2 vials], tositumomab 35 mg/2.5 mL [1 vial], and iodine I 131 tositumomab 0.1 mg/mL and 0.61mCi/mL (20 mL) [1 vial]

Kit [therapeutic package]: Tositumomab 225 mg/16.1 mL [2 vials], tositumomab 35 mg/2.5 mL [1 vial], and iodine I 131 tositumomab 1.1 mg/mL and 5.6 mCi/mL (20 mL) [1 or 2 vials]

Totacillin® *(Discontinued)* *see* ampicillin *on page 53*

total parenteral nutrition (TOE tal par EN ter al noo TRISH un)

Synonyms hyperal; hyperalimentation; parenteral nutrition; PN; TPN

Therapeutic Category Caloric Agent; Intravenous Nutritional Therapy

Use Infusion of nutrient solutions into the bloodstream to support nutritional needs during a time when patient is unable to absorb nutrients via the gastrointestinal tract, cannot take adequate nutrition orally or enterally, or have had (or are expected to have) inadequate oral intake for 7-14 days

Usual Dosage PN is a highly-individualized therapy. The following general guidelines may be used in the estimation of needs. Electrolytes, vitamins, and trace minerals should be added to TPN mixtures based on patients individualized needs.

Neonates: I.V.: **Note:** When indicated for premature neonates, start on day 1 of life if possible.

Total calories:

Term: 85-105 kcal/kg/day

Preterm (stable): 90-120 kcal/kg/day

Fluid:

<1.5 kg: 130-150 mL/kg/day

1.5-2 kg: 110-130 mL/kg/day

2-10 kg: 100 mL/kg/day

Carbohydrate (dextrose): 40% to 50 % of caloric intake; advance as tolerated

Term: Initial: 6-8 mg/kg/minute; goal: 10-14 mg/kg/minute

Premature: Initial: 6 mg/kg/minute; goal: 10-13 mg/kg/minute

Protein (amino acids):

Term: Initial: 2.5 g/kg/day; goal: 3 g/kg/day

Extremely (<1000 g) and very (<1500 g) low-birth-weight (stable): Initial: 1-1.5 g/kg/day; goal: 3.5-3.85 g/kg/day to promote utero growth rates.

Sepsis, hypoxia: Initial: 1 g/kg/day; goal: 3-3.85 g/kg/day

Fat:

Term: Initial: 0.5-1 g/kg/day (maximum: 3 g/kg/day); administer over 24 hours

Preterm: Initial: 0.25-0.5 g/kg/day (maximum: 3 g/kg/day or 1 g/kg/day if on phototherapy); administer over 24 hours

Note: Monitor triglycerides while receiving intralipids. If triglycerides >200 mg/dL, stop infusion and restart at 0.5-1g/kg/day

Heparin: 1 unit/mL of parenteral nutrition fluids should be added to enhance clearance of lipid emulsions

Children: I.V.: **Note:** Give within 5-7 days if unable to meet needs orally or with enteral nutrition:

Total calories:

<6 months: 85-105 kcal/kg/day

6-12 months: 80-100 kcal/kg/day

1-7 years: 75-90 kcal/kg/day

7-12 years: 50-75 kcal/kg/day

12-18 years: 30-50 kcal/kg/day

Fluid:

2-10 kg: 100 mL/kg

>10-20 kg: 1000 mL for 10 kg plus 50 mL/kg for each kg >10
>20 kg: 1500 mL for 10 kg plus 20 mL/kg for each kg >20

Carbohydrate (dextrose): 40% to 50% of caloric intake
<1 year: Initial: 6-8 mg/kg/minute; goal: 10-14 mg/kg/minute
1-10 years: Initial: 10% to 12.5%; daily increase: 5% increments (maximum: 15 mg/kg/minute)
>10 years: Initial: 10% to 15%; daily increase: 5% increments (maximum: 8.5 mg/kg/minute)

Protein (amino acids):
1-12 months: Initial: 2-3 g/kg/day; daily increase: 1 g/kg/day (maximum: 3 g/kg/day)
1-10 years: Initial: 1-2 g/kg/day; daily increase: 1 g/kg/day (maximum: 2-2.5 g/kg/day)
>10 years: Initial: 0.8-1.5 g/kg/day; daily increase: 1 g/kg/day (maximum: 1.5-2 g/kg/day)

Fat: Initial: 1 g/kg/day; daily increase: 1 g/kg/day (maximum: 3 g/kg/day); **Note:** Monitor triglycerides while receiving intralipids.

Adults: I.V.:

Total calories: Calculate using Harris-Benedict equation or based on stress level as indicated below:

Harris-Benedict Equation (BEE):
Females: 655.1 + [(9.56 x W) + (1.85 x H) - (4.68 x A)]
Males: 66.47 + [(13.75 x W) + (5 x H) - (6.76 x A)]
Then multiply BEE x (activity factor) x (stress factor)
W = weight in kg; H = height in cm; A = age in years
Activity factor = 1.2 sedentary, 1.3 normal activity, 1.4 active, 1.5 very active
Stress factor = 1.5 for trauma, stressed, or surgical patients and underweight (to promote weight gain); 2.0 for severe burn patients

Stress level:
Normal/mild stress level: 20-25 kcal/kg/day
Moderate stress level: 25-30 kcal/kg/day
Severe stress level: 30-40 kcal/kg/day
Pregnant women in second or third trimester: Add an additional 300 kcal/day

Fluid: mL/day = 30-40 mL/kg

Carbohydrate (dextrose):
5 g/kg/day or 3.5 mg/kg/minute (maximum rate: 4-7 mg/kg/minute)
Minimum recommended amount: 400 calories/day or 100 g/day

Protein (amino acids):
Maintenance: 0.8-1 g/kg/day
Normal/mild stress level: 1-1.2 g/kg/day
Moderate stress level: 1.2-1.5 g/kg/day
Severe stress level: 1.5-2 g/kg/day
Burn patients (severe): Increase protein until significant wound healing achieved
Solid organ transplant: Perioperative: 1.5-2 g/kg/day

Dosage Forms No commercially-available dosage forms; TPN is compounded from optimal combinations of macronutrients (water, protein, dextrose, and lipids) and micronutrients (electrolytes, trace elements, and vitamins) to meet the specific nutritional requirements of a patient.

Touro® CC [US] *see* guaifenesin, pseudoephedrine, and dextromethorphan *on page 401*

Touro® CC-LD [US] *see* guaifenesin, pseudoephedrine, and dextromethorphan *on page 401*

Touro™ Allergy [US] *see* brompheniramine and pseudoephedrine *on page 118*

Touro® DM [US] *see* guaifenesin and dextromethorphan *on page 394*

Touro Ex® *(Discontinued)* *see* guaifenesin *on page 392*

Touro LA® [US] *see* guaifenesin and pseudoephedrine *on page 398*

tPA *see* alteplase *on page 34*

TPN *see* total parenteral nutrition *on previous page*

TPT *see* topotecan *on page 836*

TPV *see* tipranavir *on page 830*

tRA *see* tretinoin (oral) *on page 844*

trace metals (trase MET als)

Synonyms chromium; copper; iodine; manganese; molybdenum; neonatal trace metals; selenium; zinc

U.S./Canadian Brand Names Iodopen® [US]; M.T.E.-4® [US]; M.T.E.-5® [US]; M.T.E.-6® [US]; M.T.E.-7® [US]; Molypen® [US]; Multitrace™-4 Neonatal [US]; Multitrace™-4 Pediatric [US]; Multitrace™-4 [US]; Multitrace™-5 [US]; Neotrace-4® [US]; P.T.E.-4® [US]; P.T.E.-5® [US]; Pedtrace-4® [US]; Selepen® [US]
(Continued)

trace metals *(Continued)*

Therapeutic Category Trace Element

Use Prevention and correction of trace metal deficiencies

Usual Dosage Recommended daily parenteral dosage:

Chromium:[1]
- Infants: 0.2 mcg/kg
- Children: 0.2 mcg/kg (maximum: 5 mcg)
- Adults: 10-15 mcg

Copper:[2]
- Infants: 20 mcg/kg
- Children: 20 mcg/kg (maximum: 300 mcg)
- Adults: 0.5-1.5 mg

Manganese:[2,3]
- Infants: 1 mcg/kg
- Children: 1 mcg/kg (maximum: 50 mcg)
- Adults: 150-800 mcg

Molybdenum:[1,4]
- Infants: 0.25 mcg/kg
- Children: 0.25 mcg/kg (maximum: 5 mcg)
- Adults: 20-120 mcg

Selenium:[1,4]
- Infants: 2 mcg/kg
- Children: 2 mcg/kg (maximum: 30 mcg)
- Adults: 20-40 mcg

Zinc:
- Infants, preterm: 400 mcg/kg
- Infants, term <3 months: 250 mcg/kg
- Infants, term >3 months: 100 mcg/kg
- Children: 50 mcg/kg (maximum: 5 mg)
- Adults: 2.5-4 mg

[1]Omit in patients with renal dysfunction.

[2]Omit in patients with obstructive jaundice.

[3]Current available commercial products are not in appropriate ratios to maintain this recommendation; doses of up to 10 mcg/kg have been used.

[4]Indicated for use in long-term parenteral nutrition patients.

Dosage Forms

Injection, solution [combination products]:

- M.T.E.-4®: Chromium 4 mcg, copper 0.4 mg, manganese 0.1 mg, and zinc 1 mg per mL (3 mL, 10 mL, 30 mL) [30 mL contains benzyl alcohol]
- M.T.E.-4® Concentrate: Chromium 10 mcg, copper 1 mg, manganese 0.5 mg, and zinc 5 mg per mL (1 mL, 10 mL) [10 mL contains benzyl alcohol]
- M.T.E.-5® [preservative free]: Chromium 4 mcg, copper 0.4 mg, manganese 0.1 mg, selenium 20 mcg, and zinc 1 mg per mL (10 mL)
- M.T.E.-5® Concentrate: Chromium 10 mcg, copper 1 mg, manganese 0.5 mg, selenium 60 mcg, and zinc 5 mg per mL (1 mL, 10 mL) [10 mL contains benzyl alcohol]
- M.T.E.-6® [preservative free]: Chromium 4 mcg, copper 0.4 mg, iodide 25 mcg, manganese 0.1 mg, selenium 20 mcg, and zinc 1 mg per mL (10 mL)
- M.T.E.-6® Concentrate: Chromium 10 mcg, copper 1 mg, iodide 75 mcg, manganese 0.5 mg, selenium 60 mcg, and zinc 5 mg per mL (10 mL) [contains benzyl alcohol]
- M.T.E.-7® [preservative free]: Chromium 4 mcg, copper 0.4 mg, iodide 25 mcg, manganese 0.1 mg, molybdenum 25 mcg, selenium 20 mcg, and zinc 1 mg per mL (10 mL)
- Multitrace™-4: Chromium 4 mcg, copper 0.4 mg, manganese 0.1 mg, and zinc 1 mg per mL (10 mL) [contains benzyl alcohol]
- Multitrace™-4 Neonatal: Chromium 0.85 mcg, copper 0.1 mg, manganese 0.025 mg, and zinc 1.5 mg per mL (2 mL)
- Multitrace™-4 Pediatric: Chromium 1 mcg, copper 0.1 mg, manganese 0.025 mg, and zinc 1 mg per mL (3 mL)
- Multitrace™-4 Concentrate: Chromium 10 mcg, copper 1 mg, manganese 0.5 mg, and zinc 5 mg per mL (1 mL, 10 mL) [10 mL contains benzyl alcohol]
- Multitrace™-5: Chromium 4 mcg, copper 0.4 mg, manganese 0.1 mg, selenium 20 mcg, and zinc 1 mg per mL (10 mL) [contains benzyl alcohol]
- Multitrace™-5 Concentrate: Chromium 10 mcg, copper 1 mg, manganese 0.5 mg, selenium 60 mcg, and zinc 5 mg per mL (1 mL, 10 mL) [10 mL contains benzyl alcohol]

Neotrace-4® [preservative free]: Chromium 0.85 mcg, copper 0.1 mg, manganese 0.025 mg, and zinc 1.5 mg per mL (2 mL)
Pedtrace-4® [preservative free]: Chromium 0.85 mcg, copper 0.1 mg, manganese 0.025 mg, and zinc 0.5 mg per mL (3 mL, 10 mL)
P.T.E.-4® [preservative free]: Chromium 1 mcg, copper 0.1 mg, manganese 0.025 mg, and zinc 1 mg per mL (3 mL)
P.T.E.-5® [preservative free]: Chromium 1 mcg, copper 0.1 mg, manganese 0.025 mg, selenium 15 mcg, and zinc 1 mg per mL (3 mL)
Trace elements pediatric: Chromium 1 mcg, copper 0.1 mg, manganese 0.03 mg, and zinc 0.5 mg per mL (10 mL) [contains benzyl alcohol]
Injection, solution [elemental equivalence]:
Chromium, as chromic chloride (hexahydrate) [preservative free]: 0.0205 mg/mL [0.004 mg/mL] (10 mL)
Copper, as cupric chloride: 1.07 mg/mL [0.4 mg/mL] (10 mL)
Iodine, as iodine sodium (Iodopen®): 0.118 mg/mL [0.1 mg/mL] (10 mL)
Manganese:
As chloride: 0.36 mg/mL [0.1 mg/mL] (10 mL)
As sulfate [preservative free]: 0.31 mg/mL [0.1 mg/mL] (10 mL)
Molybdenum, as ammonium molybdate (tetrahydrate) (Molypen®): 46 mcg/mL [25 mcg/mL] (10 mL)
Selenium, as selenious acid: 0.0654 mg/mL [0.04 mg/mL] (10 mL)
Selepen®: 0.0654 mg/mL [0.04 mg/mL] (10 mL, 30 mL) [30 mL contains benzyl alcohol]
Zinc:
As chloride: 2.09 mg/mL [1 mg/mL] (10 mL, 50 mL)
As sulfate, anhydrous [preservative free]: 2.46 mg/mL [1 mg/mL] (10 mL)
As sulfate, anhydrous, concentrate [preservative free]: 12.32 mg/mL [5 mg/mL] (5 mL)

Tracleer® [US/Can] *see* bosentan *on page 115*

Tracrium® [US] *see* atracurium *on page 82*

Tramacet [Can] *see* acetaminophen and tramadol *on page 10*

tramadol (TRA ma dole)

Sound-Alike/Look-Alike Issues
tramadol may be confused with Toradol®, Trandate®, Voltaren®
Ultram® may be confused with Ultane®, Voltaren®

Synonyms tramadol hydrochloride

U.S./Canadian Brand Names Ultram® ER [US]; Ultram® [US/Can]

Therapeutic Category Analgesic, Nonnarcotic

Use Relief of moderate to moderately-severe pain

Usual Dosage Adults: Moderate-to-severe chronic pain: Oral:
Immediate release formulation: 50-100 mg every 4-6 hours (not to exceed 400 mg/day)
For patients not requiring rapid onset of effect, tolerability may be improved by starting dose at 25 mg/day and titrating dose by 25 mg every 3 days, until reaching 25 mg 4 times/day. Dose may then be increased by 50 mg every 3 days as tolerated, to reach dose of 50 mg 4 times/day.
Extended release formulation: 100 mg once daily; titrate every 5 days (maximum: 300 mg/day)

Dosage Forms
Tablet, as hydrochloride: 50 mg
Ultram®: 50 mg
Tablet, extended release, as hydrochloride:
Ultram® ER: 100 mg, 200 mg, 300 mg

tramadol hydrochloride *see* tramadol *on this page*

tramadol hydrochloride and acetaminophen *see* acetaminophen and tramadol *on page 10*

Trandate® [US/Can] *see* labetalol *on page 475*

trandolapril (tran DOE la pril)

U.S./Canadian Brand Names Mavik® [US/Can]

Therapeutic Category Angiotensin-Converting Enzyme (ACE) Inhibitor

Use Management of hypertension alone or in combination with other antihypertensive agents; treatment of left ventricular dysfunction after myocardial infarction

Usual Dosage Adults: Oral:
Hypertension: Initial dose in patients not receiving a diuretic: 1 mg/day (2 mg/day in black patients). Adjust dosage according to the blood pressure response. Make dosage adjustments at intervals of ≥1 week. Most patients have required dosages of 2-4 mg/day. There is a little experience with doses >8 mg/day.
(Continued)

trandolapril *(Continued)*

Patients inadequately treated with once daily dosing at 4 mg may be treated with twice daily dosing. If blood pressure is not adequately controlled with trandolapril monotherapy, a diuretic may be added.

Usual dose range (JNC 7): 1-4 mg once daily

Heart failure postmyocardial infarction or left ventricular dysfunction postmyocardial infarction: Initial: 1 mg/day; titrate patients (as tolerated) towards the target dose of 4 mg/day. If a 4 mg dose is not tolerated, patients can continue therapy with the greatest tolerated dose.

Dosage Forms Tablet: 1 mg, 2 mg, 4 mg

trandolapril and verapamil (tran DOE la pril & ver AP a mil)

Synonyms verapamil and trandolapril

U.S./Canadian Brand Names Tarka® [US/Can]

Therapeutic Category Antihypertensive Agent, Combination

Use Combination drug for the treatment of hypertension, however, not indicated for initial treatment of hypertension; replacement therapy in patients receiving separate dosage forms (for patient convenience); when monotherapy with one component fails to achieve desired antihypertensive effect, or when dose-limiting adverse effects limit upward titration of monotherapy

Usual Dosage Dose is individualized.

Dosage Forms Tablet, variable release:

1/240: Trandolapril 1 mg [immediate release] and verapamil hydrochloride 240 mg [sustained release]
2/180: Trandolapril 2 mg [immediate release] and verapamil hydrochloride 180 mg [sustained release]
2/240: Trandolapril 2 mg [immediate release] and verapamil hydrochloride 240 mg [sustained release]
4/240: Trandolapril 4 mg [immediate release] and verapamil hydrochloride 240 mg [sustained release]

tranexamic acid (tran eks AM ik AS id)

Sound-Alike/Look-Alike Issues

Cyklokapron® may be confused with cycloSPORINE

U.S./Canadian Brand Names Cyklokapron® [US/Can]; Tranexamic Acid Injection BP [Can]

Therapeutic Category Antihemophilic Agent

Use Short-term use (2-8 days) in hemophilia patients during and following tooth extraction to reduce or prevent hemorrhage

Usual Dosage Children and Adults: I.V.: 10 mg/kg immediately before surgery, then 25 mg/kg/dose orally 3-4 times/day for 2-8 days

Alternatively:

Oral: 25 mg/kg 3-4 times/day beginning 1 day prior to surgery
I.V.: 10 mg/kg 3-4 times/day in patients who are unable to take oral

Dosage Forms

Injection, solution: 100 mg/mL (10 mL)
Tablet: 500 mg [Not marketed in U.S.; available from manufacturer for select cases]

Tranexamic Acid Injection BP [Can] *see* tranexamic acid *on this page*

transamine sulphate *see* tranylcypromine *on next page*

Transderm-V® [Can] *see* scopolamine derivatives *on page 764*

Transdermal-NTG® Patch *(Discontinued)* *see* nitroglycerin *on page 595*

Transderm-Nitro® [Can] *see* nitroglycerin *on page 595*

Transderm Scōp® [US] *see* scopolamine derivatives *on page 764*

Trans-Plantar® [Can] *see* salicylic acid *on page 758*

Trans-Plantar® Transdermal Patch *(Discontinued)* *see* salicylic acid *on page 758*

***trans*-retinoic acid** *see* tretinoin (topical) *on page 844*

Trans-Ver-Sal® [US-OTC/Can] *see* salicylic acid *on page 758*

Tranxene® SD™ [US] *see* clorazepate *on page 205*

Tranxene® SD™-Half Strength [US] *see* clorazepate *on page 205*

Tranxene® T-Tab® [US] *see* clorazepate *on page 205*

tranylcypromine (tran il SIP roe meen)

Synonyms transamine sulphate; tranylcypromine sulfate

U.S./Canadian Brand Names Parnate® [US/Can]

Therapeutic Category Antidepressant, Monoamine Oxidase Inhibitor

Use Treatment of major depressive episode without melancholia

Usual Dosage Adults: Oral: 10 mg twice daily, increase by 10 mg increments at 1- to 3-week intervals; maximum: 60 mg/day; usual effective dose: 30 mg/day

Dosage Forms Tablet: 10 mg

tranylcypromine sulfate *see* tranylcypromine *on this page*

Trasicor® [Can] *see* oxprenolol *(Canada only) on page 625*

trastuzumab (tras TU zoo mab)

U.S./Canadian Brand Names Herceptin® [US/Can]

Therapeutic Category Antineoplastic Agent

Use Treatment of metastatic breast cancer whose tumors overexpress the HER-2/*neu* protein

Usual Dosage I.V. infusion: Adults:

Initial loading dose: 4 mg/kg intravenous infusion over 90 minutes

Maintenance dose: 2 mg/kg intravenous infusion over 90 minutes (can be administered over 30 minutes if prior infusions are well tolerated) weekly until disease progression

Dosage Forms Injection, powder for reconstitution: 440 mg [packaged with bacteriostatic water for injection; diluent contains benzyl alcohol]

Trasylol® [US/Can] *see* aprotinin *on page 71*

Travatan® [US/Can] *see* travoprost *on this page*

travoprost (TRA voe prost)

Sound-Alike/Look-Alike Issues

Travatan® may be confused with Xalatan®

U.S./Canadian Brand Names Travatan® [US/Can]

Therapeutic Category Prostaglandin, Ophthalmic

Use Reduction of elevated intraocular pressure in patients with open-angle glaucoma or ocular hypertension who are intolerant of the other IOP-lowering medications or insufficiently responsive (failed to achieve target IOP determined after multiple measurements over time) to another IOP-lowering medication

Usual Dosage Ophthalmic: Adults: Glaucoma (open angle) or ocular hypertension: Instill 1 drop into affected eye(s) once daily in the evening; do not exceed once-daily dosing (may decrease IOP-lowering effect). If used with other topical ophthalmic agents, separate administration by at least 5 minutes.

Dosage Forms Solution, ophthalmic: 0.004% (2.5 mL, 5 mL) [contains benzalkonium chloride]

trazodone (TRAZ oh done)

Sound-Alike/Look-Alike Issues

Desyrel® may be confused with Demerol®, Delsym®, Zestril®

Synonyms trazodone hydrochloride

U.S./Canadian Brand Names Alti-Trazodone [Can]; Apo-Trazodone D® [Can]; Apo-Trazodone® [Can]; Desyrel® [US/Can]; Gen-Trazodone [Can]; Novo-Trazodone [Can]; Nu-Trazodone [Can]; PMS-Trazodone [Can]; ratio-Trazodone [Can]; Trazorel® [Can]

Therapeutic Category Antidepressant, Triazolopyridine

Use Treatment of depression

Usual Dosage Oral: Therapeutic effects may take up to 6 weeks to occur; therapy is normally maintained for 6-12 months after optimum response is reached to prevent recurrence of depression

Adults: Depression: Initial: 150 mg/day in 3 divided doses (may increase by 50 mg/day every 3-7 days); maximum: 600 mg/day

Dosage Forms [DSC] = Discontinued product

Tablet: 50 mg, 100 mg, 150 mg, 300 mg

Desyrel®: 50 mg, 100 mg, 150 mg, 300 mg [DSC]

trazodone hydrochloride *see* trazodone *on this page*

Trazorel® [Can] *see* trazodone *on this page*

Trecator® [US/Can] *see* ethionamide *on page 328*

Trelstar™ [Can] *see* triptorelin *on page 854*

Trelstar™ Depot [US/Can] *see* triptorelin *on page 854*

Trelstar™ LA [US/Can] *see* triptorelin *on page 854*

Trendar® *(Discontinued)* *see* ibuprofen *on page 437*

Trental® [US/Can] *see* pentoxifylline *on page 653*

treprostinil (tre PROST in il)

Synonyms treprostinil sodium

U.S./Canadian Brand Names Remodulin® [US/Can]

Therapeutic Category Vasodilator

Use Treatment of pulmonary arterial hypertension (PAH) in patients with NYHA Class II-IV symptoms to decrease exercise-associated symptoms; to diminish clinical deterioration when transitioning from epoprostenol (I.V.)

Usual Dosage SubQ or I.V. infusion: Adults: PAH: Initial: 1.25 ng/kg/minute continuous; if dose cannot be tolerated, reduce to 0.625 ng/kg/minute. Increase at rate not >1.25 ng/kg/minute per week for first 4 weeks, and not >2.5 ng/kg/minute per week for remainder of therapy. Limited experience with doses >40 ng/kg/minute.

Note: Dose must be carefully and individually titrated (symptom improvement with minimal adverse effects). Avoid abrupt withdrawal.

Dosage Forms Injection, solution: 1 mg/mL (20 mL) [contains sodium chloride 5.3 mg/mL]; 2.5 mg/mL (20 mL) [contains sodium chloride 5.3 mg/mL]; 5 mg/mL (20 mL) [contains sodium chloride 5.3 mg/mL]; 10 mg/mL (20 mL) [contains sodium chloride 4 mg/mL]

treprostinil sodium *see* treprostinil *on this page*

tretinoin and mequinol *see* mequinol and tretinoin *on page 532*

tretinoin, fluocinolone acetonide, and hydroquinone *see* fluocinolone, hydroquinone, and tretinoin *on page 353*

tretinoin (oral) (TRET i noyn, oral)

Sound-Alike/Look-Alike Issues

tretinoin may be confused with trientine

Synonyms all-*trans*-retinoic acid; ATRA; NSC-122758; Ro 5488; tRA

U.S./Canadian Brand Names Vesanoid® [US/Can]

Therapeutic Category Antineoplastic Agent

Use Induction of remission in patients with acute promyelocytic leukemia (APL), French American British (FAB) classification M3 (including the M3 variant)

Usual Dosage Oral: Children and Adults:

Remission induction: 45 mg/m²/day in 2-3 divided doses for up to 30 days after complete remission (maximum duration of treatment: 90 days)

Remission maintenance: 45-200 mg/m²/day in 2-3 divided doses for up to 12 months.

Dosage Forms Capsule: 10 mg [contains soybean oil and parabens]

tretinoin (topical) (TRET i noyn TOP i kal)

Sound-Alike/Look-Alike Issues

tretinoin may be confused with trientine

Synonyms retinoic acid; *trans*-retinoic acid; vitamin A acid

U.S./Canadian Brand Names Avita® [US]; Rejuva-A® [Can]; Renova® [US]; Retin-A® Micro [US/Can]; Retin-A® [US/Can]; Retinova® [Can]

Therapeutic Category Retinoic Acid Derivative

Use Treatment of acne vulgaris; photodamaged skin; palliation of fine wrinkles, mottled hyperpigmentation, and tactile roughness of facial skin as part of a comprehensive skin care and sun avoidance program

Usual Dosage Topical:

Children >12 years and Adults: Acne vulgaris: Begin therapy with a weaker formulation of tretinoin (0.025% cream, 0.04% microsphere gel, or 0.01% gel) and increase the concentration as tolerated; apply once daily to acne lesions before retiring or on alternate days; if stinging or irritation develop, decrease frequency of application

Adults ≥18: Palliation of fine wrinkles, mottled hyperpigmentation, and tactile roughness of facial skin: Pea-sized amount of the 0.02% or 0.05% cream applied to entire face once daily in the evening

Dosage Forms

Cream, topical: 0.025% (20 g, 45 g); 0.05% (20 g, 45 g); 0.1% (20 g, 45 g)

Altinac™: 0.025% (20 g, 45 g); 0.05% (20 g, 45 g); 0.1% (20 g, 45 g)

Avita®: 0.025% (20 g, 45 g)
Renova®: 0.02% (40 g); 0.05% (40 g, 60 g)
Retin-A®: 0.025% (20 g, 45 g); 0.05% (20 g, 45 g); 0.1% (20 g, 45 g)
Gel, topical: 0.025% (15 g, 45 g)
Avita®: 0.025% (15 g, 45 g)
Retin-A®: 0.01% (15 g, 45 g); 0.025% (15 g, 45 g)
Retin-A® Micro [microsphere gel]: 0.04% (20 g, 45 g); 0.1% (20 g, 45 g)
Liquid, topical (Retin-A®): 0.05% (28 mL)

Trexall™ [US] *see* methotrexate *on page 540*

triacetin (trye a SEE tin)

Sound-Alike/Look-Alike Issues
triacetin may be confused with Triacin®

Synonyms glycerol triacetate

U.S./Canadian Brand Names Myco-Nail [US-OTC]

Therapeutic Category Antifungal Agent

Use Fungistat for athlete's foot and other superficial fungal infections

Usual Dosage Apply twice daily, cleanse areas with dilute alcohol or mild soap and water before application; continue treatment for 7 days after symptoms have disappeared

Dosage Forms Liquid, topical: 25% (30 mL)

Triacin-C® ***(Discontinued)*** *see* triprolidine, pseudoephedrine, and codeine *(Canada only) on page 853*

triaconazole *see* terconazole *on page 811*

Triaderm [Can] *see* triamcinolone (topical) *on next page*

Triafed® ***(Discontinued)*** *see* triprolidine and pseudoephedrine *on page 853*

triamcinolone acetonide, parenteral *see* triamcinolone (systemic) *on next page*

triamcinolone and nystatin *see* nystatin and triamcinolone *on page 610*

triamcinolone diacetate, oral *see* triamcinolone (systemic) *on next page*

triamcinolone diacetate, parenteral *see* triamcinolone (systemic) *on next page*

triamcinolone hexacetonide *see* triamcinolone (systemic) *on next page*

triamcinolone (inhalation, nasal) (trye am SIN oh lone in hil LA shun, NAY sal)

Sound-Alike/Look-Alike Issues
Nasacort® may be confused with NasalCrom®

U.S./Canadian Brand Names Nasacort® AQ [US/Can]; Nasacort® HFA [US]; Tri-Nasal® [US/Can]

Therapeutic Category Adrenal Corticosteroid

Use Nasal inhalation: Management of seasonal and perennial allergic rhinitis in patients ≥6 years of age

Usual Dosage Intranasal: Perennial allergic rhinitis, seasonal allergic rhinitis:
Nasal spray:
Children 6-11 years: 110 mcg/day as 1 spray in each nostril once daily.
Children ≥12 years and Adults: 220 mcg/day as 2 sprays in each nostril once daily
Nasal inhaler:
Children 6-11 years: Initial: 220 mcg/day as 2 sprays in each nostril once daily
Children ≥12 years and Adults: Initial: 220 mcg/day as 2 sprays in each nostril once daily; may increase dose to 440 mcg/day (given once daily or divided and given 2 or 4 times/day)

Dosage Forms
Aerosol for nasal inhalation, as acetonide [CFC free] (Nasacort® [HFA]): 55 mcg/inhalation (9.3 g) [100 doses]
Solution, spray for nasal inhalation, as acetonide (Tri-Nasal®): 50 mcg/inhalation (15 mL) [120 doses]
Suspension, spray for nasal inhalation, as acetonide (Nasacort® AQ): 55 mcg/inhalation (16.5 g) [120 doses]

triamcinolone (inhalation, oral) (trye am SIN oh lone in hil LA shun, OR al)

Sound-Alike/Look-Alike Issues
TAC (occasional abbreviation for triamcinolone) is an error-prone abbreviation (mistaken as tetracaine-adrenaline-cocaine)
(Continued)

triamcinolone (inhalation, oral) *(Continued)*

U.S./Canadian Brand Names Azmacort® [US]

Therapeutic Category Adrenal Corticosteroid

Use Oral inhalation: Control of bronchial asthma and related bronchospastic conditions

Usual Dosage Oral inhalation: Asthma:

Children 6-12 years: 100-200 mcg 3-4 times/day **or** 200-400 mcg twice daily; maximum dose: 1200 mg/day

Children >12 years and Adults: 200 mcg 3-4 times/day **or** 400 mcg twice daily; maximum dose: 1600 mcg/day

Dosage Forms Aerosol for oral inhalation, as acetonide (Azmacort®): 100 mcg per actuation (20 g) [240 actuations]

triamcinolone, oral *see* triamcinolone (systemic) *on this page*

triamcinolone (systemic) (trye am SIN oh lone sis TEM ik)

Sound-Alike/Look-Alike Issues

Kenalog® may be confused with Ketalar®

Synonyms triamcinolone acetonide, parenteral; triamcinolone diacetate, oral; triamcinolone diacetate, parenteral; triamcinolone hexacetonide; triamcinolone, oral

U.S./Canadian Brand Names Aristocort® [US/Can]; Aristospan® [US/Can]; Kenalog-10® [US]; Kenalog-40® [US]; Kenalog® [US/Can]; Oracort [Can]

Therapeutic Category Adrenal Corticosteroid

Use Systemic: Adrenocortical insufficiency, rheumatic disorders, allergic states, respiratory diseases, systemic lupus erythematosus (SLE), and other diseases requiring antiinflammatory or immunosuppressive effects

Usual Dosage The lowest possible dose should be used to control the condition; when dose reduction is possible, the dose should be reduced gradually. Parenteral dose is usually 1/3 to 1/2 the oral dose given every 12 hours. In life-threatening situations, parenteral doses larger than the oral dose may be needed.

Injection:

Acetonide:

Intra-articular, intrabursal, tendon sheaths: Adults: Initial: Smaller joints: 2.5-5 mg, larger joints: 5-15 mg

Intradermal: Adults: Initial: 1 mg

I.M.: Range: 2.5-60 mg/day

Children 6-12 years: Initial: 40 mg

Children >12 years and Adults: Initial: 60 mg

Hexacetonide: Adults:

Intralesional, sublesional: Up to 0.5 mg/square inch of affected skin

Intra-articular: Range: 2-20 mg

Oral: Adults:

Acute rheumatic carditis: Initial: 20-60 mg/day; reduce dose during maintenance therapy

Acute seasonal or perennial allergic rhinitis: 8-12 mg/day

Adrenocortical insufficiency: Range 4-12 mg/day

Bronchial asthma: 8-16 mg/day

Dermatological disorders, contact/atopic dermatitis: Initial: 8-16 mg/day

Ophthalmic disorders: 12-40 mg/day

Rheumatic disorders: Range: 8-16 mg/day

SLE: Initial: 20-32 mg/day, some patients may need initial doses ≥48 mg; reduce dose during maintenance therapy

Dosage Forms

Injection, suspension, as acetonide:

Kenalog-10®: 10 mg/mL (5 mL) [contains benzyl alcohol; not for I.V. or I.M. use]

Kenalog-40®: 40 mg/mL (1 mL, 5 mL, 10 mL) [contains benzyl alcohol; not for I.V. or intradermal use]

Injection, suspension, as hexacetonide (Aristospan®): 5 mg/mL (5 mL); 20 mg/mL (1 mL, 5 mL) [contains benzyl alcohol; not for I.V. use]

Tablet (Aristocort®): 4 mg [contains lactose and sodium benzoate]

triamcinolone (topical) (trye am SIN oh lone TOP i kal)

Sound-Alike/Look-Alike Issues

Kenalog® may be confused with Ketalar®

U.S./Canadian Brand Names Aristocort® A [US]; Kenalog® in Orabase [Can]; Kenalog® [US/Can]; Triaderm [Can]; Triderm® [US]

Therapeutic Category Corticosteroid, Topical

Use

Oral topical: Adjunctive treatment and temporary relief of symptoms associated with oral inflammatory lesions and ulcerative lesions resulting from trauma

Topical: Inflammatory dermatoses responsive to steroids

Usual Dosage

Oral topical: Oral inflammatory lesions/ulcers: Press a small dab (about 1/4 inch) to the lesion until a thin film develops. A larger quantity may be required for coverage of some lesions. For optimal results use only enough to coat the lesion with a thin film; do not rub in.

Topical:

Cream, Ointment: Apply thin film to affected areas 2-4 times/day

Spray: Apply to affected area 3-4 times/day

Dosage Forms

Cream, as acetonide: 0.025% (15 g, 80 g, 454 g); 0.1% (15 g, 80 g, 454 g, 2270 g); 0.5% (15 g)

Aristocort® A: 0.025% (15 g, 60 g); 0.1% (15 g, 60 g); 0.5% (15 g) [contains benzyl alcohol]

Triderm®: 0.1% (30 g, 85 g)

Lotion, as acetonide: 0.025% (60 mL); 0.1% (60 mL)

Ointment, topical, as acetonide: 0.025% (15g, 80 g, 454 g); 0.1% (15 g, 80 g, 454 g); 0.5% (15 g)

Aristocort® A: 0.1% (15 g, 60 g)

Paste, oral, topical, as acetonide: 0.1% (5 g)

Triaminic® Allerchews™ [US-OTC] *see* loratadine *on page 505*

Triaminic® Cold and Allergy [US-OTC/Can] *see* chlorpheniramine and pseudoephedrine *on page 177*

Triaminic® Cold and Cough [US-OTC] *see* chlorpheniramine, pseudoephedrine, and dextromethorphan *on page 182*

Triaminic® Cough [US-OTC] *see* pseudoephedrine and dextromethorphan *on page 714*

Triaminic® Cough and Sore Throat Formula [US-OTC] *see* acetaminophen, dextromethorphan, and pseudoephedrine *on page 12*

Triaminic® Cough & Nasal Congestion [US-OTC] *see* pseudoephedrine and dextromethorphan *on page 714*

Triaminic® Expectorant *(Discontinued)*

Triaminic® Night Time Cough and Cold [US-OTC] *see* chlorpheniramine, pseudoephedrine, and dextromethorphan *on page 182*

Triaminic® Thin Strips™ Cough and Runny Nose [US-OTC] *see* diphenhydramine *on page 261*

Triaminic® Thin Strips™ Long Acting Cough [US-OTC] *see* dextromethorphan *on page 245*

Triamonide® Injection *(Discontinued)*

triamterene (trye AM ter een)

Sound-Alike/Look-Alike Issues

triamterene may be confused with trimipramine

Dyrenium® may be confused with Pyridium®

U.S./Canadian Brand Names Dyrenium® [US]

Therapeutic Category Diuretic, Potassium Sparing

Use Alone or in combination with other diuretics in treatment of edema and hypertension; decreases potassium excretion caused by kaliuretic diuretics

Usual Dosage Adults: Oral: 100-300 mg/day in 1-2 divided doses; maximum dose: 300 mg/day; usual dosage range (JNC 7): 50-100 mg/day

Dosage Forms Capsule: 50 mg, 100 mg [contains benzyl alcohol]

triamterene and hydrochlorothiazide *see* hydrochlorothiazide and triamterene *on page 420*

Triapin® *(Discontinued)*

Triatec-8 [Can] *see* acetaminophen and codeine *on page 6*

Triatec-8 Strong [Can] *see* acetaminophen and codeine *on page 6*

Triatec-30 [Can] *see* acetaminophen and codeine *on page 6*

Triavil® *(Discontinued)* *see* amitriptyline and perphenazine *on page 45*

Triaz® [US] *see* benzoyl peroxide *on page 102*

Triaz® Cleanser [US] *see* benzoyl peroxide *on page 102*

triazolam (trye AY zoe lam)

Sound-Alike/Look-Alike Issues

triazolam may be confused with alprazolam

Halcion® may be confused with halcinonide, Haldol®, Healon®

U.S./Canadian Brand Names Apo-Triazo® [Can]; Gen-Triazolam [Can]; Halcion® [US/Can]

Therapeutic Category Benzodiazepine

Controlled Substance C-IV

Use Short-term treatment of insomnia

Usual Dosage Oral (onset of action is rapid, patient should be in bed when taking medication):

Children <18 years: Dosage not established

Adults:

Hypnotic: 0.125-0.25 mg at bedtime (maximum dose: 0.5 mg/day)

Preprocedure sedation (dental): 0.25 mg taken the evening before oral surgery; or 0.25 mg 1 hour before procedure

Dosage Forms Tablet: 0.125 mg, 0.25 mg [contains sodium benzoate]

tribavirin *see* ribavirin *on page 743*

tricalcium phosphate *see* calcium phosphate (tribasic) *on page 140*

Tricardio B [US] *see* folic acid, cyanocobalamin, and pyridoxine *on page 365*

Tri-Chlor® [US] *see* trichloroacetic acid *on this page*

Trichlor Fresh Pac™ [US] *see* trichloroacetic acid *on this page*

trichloroacetaldehyde monohydrate *see* chloral hydrate *on page 171*

trichloroacetic acid (trye klor oh a SEE tik AS id)

U.S./Canadian Brand Names Tri-Chlor® [US]; Trichlor Fresh Pac™ [US]

Therapeutic Category Keratolytic Agent

Use Chemical used in compounding agents for the treatment of warts, skin resurfacing (chemical peels)

Usual Dosage Topical: Apply to verruca, cover with bandage for 5-6 days, remove verruca, reapply as needed

Dosage Forms

Liquid (Tri-Chlor®): 80% (15 mL)

Powder for reconstitution, topical (Trichlor Fresh Pac™): 10% (28 mL); 15% (28 mL); 20% (28 mL); 25% (28 mL); 30% (28 mL); 35% (28 mL); 40% (28 mL); 50% (28 mL) [supplied with diluent]

trichloromonofluoromethane and dichlorodifluoromethane *see* dichlorodifluoromethane and trichloromonofluoromethane *on page 250*

Trichophyton skin test (trye koe FYE ton skin test)

Therapeutic Category Diagnostic Agent

Use Assess cell-mediated immunity

Usual Dosage 0.1 mL intradermally, examine reaction site in 24-48 hours; induration of ≥5 mm in diameter is a positive reaction

Dosage Forms Injection, solution: 1:500 (1 mL)

Tri-Clear® Expectorant *(Discontinued)*

TriCor® [US/Can] *see* fenofibrate *on page 338*

tricosal *see* choline magnesium trisalicylate *on page 186*

Tri-Cyclen® [Can] *see* ethinyl estradiol and norgestimate *on page 325*

Tri-Cyclen® Lo [Can] *see* ethinyl estradiol and norgestimate *on page 325*

Triderm® [US] *see* triamcinolone (topical) *on page 846*

Tridesilon® [US] *see* desonide *on page 238*

Tridil® Injection *(Discontinued)* *see* nitroglycerin *on page 595*

trientine (TRYE en teen)

Sound-Alike/Look-Alike Issues

trientine may be confused with Trental®, tretinoin

Synonyms trientine hydrochloride
U.S./Canadian Brand Names Syprine® [US/Can]
Therapeutic Category Chelating Agent
Use Treatment of Wilson disease in patients intolerant to penicillamine
Usual Dosage Oral (administer on an empty stomach):
Children <12 years: 500-750 mg/day in divided doses 2-4 times/day; maximum: 1.5 g/day
Adults: 750-1250 mg/day in divided doses 2-4 times/day; maximum dose: 2 g/day
Dosage Forms Capsule, as hydrochloride: 250 mg

trientine hydrochloride *see* trientine *on previous page*

triethanolamine polypeptide oleate-condensate

(trye eth a NOLE a meen pol i PEP tide OH lee ate-KON den sate)
U.S./Canadian Brand Names Cerumenex® [Can]
Therapeutic Category Otic Agent, Ceruminolytic
Use Removal of ear wax (cerumen)
Usual Dosage Children and Adults: Otic: Fill ear canal, insert cotton plug; allow to remain 15-30 minutes; flush ear with lukewarm water as a single treatment; if a second application is needed for unusually hard impactions, repeat the procedure
Dosage Forms [DSC] = Discontinued product
Solution, otic: 10% (6 mL, 12 mL) [DSC]

triethanolamine salicylate *see* trolamine *on page 855*
triethylenethiophosphoramide *see* thiotepa *on page 823*
Trifed-C® *(Discontinued)* *see* triprolidine, pseudoephedrine, and codeine *(Canada only)* *on page 853*

trifluoperazine (trye floo oh PER a zeen)

Sound-Alike/Look-Alike Issues
trifluoperazine may be confused with triflupromazine, trihexyphenidyl
Stelazine® may be confused with selegiline
Synonyms trifluoperazine hydrochloride
U.S./Canadian Brand Names Apo-Trifluoperazine® [Can]; Novo-Trifluzine [Can]; PMS-Trifluoperazine [Can]; Terfluzine [Can]
Therapeutic Category Phenothiazine Derivative
Use Treatment of schizophrenia
Usual Dosage Oral:
Children 6-12 years: Schizophrenia/psychoses: Hospitalized or well-supervised patients: Initial: 1 mg 1-2 times/day, gradually increase until symptoms are controlled or adverse effects become troublesome; maximum: 15 mg/day
Adults:
Schizophrenia/psychoses:
Outpatients: 1-2 mg twice daily
Hospitalized or well-supervised patients: Initial: 2-5 mg twice daily with optimum response in the 15-20 mg/day range; do not exceed 40 mg/day
Nonpsychotic anxiety: 1-2 mg twice daily; maximum: 6 mg/day; therapy for anxiety should not exceed 12 weeks; do not exceed 6 mg/day for longer than 12 weeks when treating anxiety; agitation, jitteriness, or insomnia may be confused with original neurotic or psychotic symptoms
Dosage Forms Tablet: 1 mg, 2 mg, 5 mg, 10 mg

trifluoperazine hydrochloride *see* trifluoperazine *on this page*
trifluorothymidine *see* trifluridine *on this page*

trifluridine (trye FLURE i deen)

Sound-Alike/Look-Alike Issues
Viroptic® may be confused with Timoptic®
Synonyms F_3T; trifluorothymidine
U.S./Canadian Brand Names SAB-Trifluridine [Can]; Sandoz-Trifluridine [Can]; Viroptic® [US/Can]
Therapeutic Category Antiviral Agent
Use Treatment of primary keratoconjunctivitis and recurrent epithelial keratitis caused by herpes simplex virus types I and II
(Continued)

trifluridine *(Continued)*

Usual Dosage Adults: Instill 1 drop into affected eye every 2 hours while awake, to a maximum of 9 drops/day, until reepithelialization of corneal ulcer occurs; then use 1 drop every 4 hours for another 7 days; do **not** exceed 21 days of treatment; if improvement has not taken place in 7-14 days, consider another form of therapy

Dosage Forms Solution, ophthalmic: 1% (7.5 mL)

Triglide™ [US] *see* fenofibrate *on page 338*

triglycerides, medium chain *see* medium chain triglycerides *on page 524*

trihexyphenidyl (trye heks ee FEN i dil)

Sound-Alike/Look-Alike Issues

trihexyphenidyl may be confused with trifluoperazine

Artane® may be confused with Altace®, Anturane®, Aramine®

Synonyms benzhexol hydrochloride; trihexyphenidyl hydrochloride

U.S./Canadian Brand Names Apo-Trihex® [Can]

Therapeutic Category Anti-Parkinson Agent; Anticholinergic Agent

Use Adjunctive treatment of Parkinson disease; treatment of drug-induced extrapyramidal symptoms

Usual Dosage Adults: Oral: Initial: 1-2 mg/day, increase by 2 mg increments at intervals of 3-5 days; usual dose: 5-15 mg/day in 3-4 divided doses

Dosage Forms

Elixir, as hydrochloride: 2 mg/5 mL (480 mL)

Tablet, as hydrochloride: 2 mg, 5 mg

trihexyphenidyl hydrochloride *see* trihexyphenidyl *on this page*

TriHIBit® [US] *see* diphtheria, tetanus toxoids, and acellular pertussis vaccine and *Haemophilus influenzae* b conjugate vaccine *on page 266*

Tri-K® [US] *see* potassium acetate, potassium bicarbonate, and potassium citrate *on page 682*

Trikacide [Can] *see* metronidazole *on page 551*

TRIKOF-D® ***(Discontinued)***

Tri-Kort® Injection ***(Discontinued)***

Trilafon® ***(Discontinued)*** *see* perphenazine *on page 655*

Trileptal® [US/Can] *see* oxcarbazepine *on page 624*

Tri-Levlen® [US] *see* ethinyl estradiol and levonorgestrel *on page 320*

Trilisate® ***(Discontinued)*** *see* choline magnesium trisalicylate *on page 186*

Trilog® Injection ***(Discontinued)***

Trilone® Injection ***(Discontinued)***

Tri-Luma™ [US] *see* fluocinolone, hydroquinone, and tretinoin *on page 353*

TriLyte™ [US] *see* polyethylene glycol-electrolyte solution *on page 679*

Trimazide® ***(Discontinued)*** *see* trimethobenzamide *on next page*

trimebutine *(Canada only)* (trye me BYOO teen)

Synonyms trimebutine maleate

U.S./Canadian Brand Names Apo-Trimebutine® [Can]; Modulon® [Can]

Therapeutic Category Antispasmodic Agent, Gastrointestinal

Use Treatment and relief of symptoms associated with irritable bowel syndrome (IBS) (spastic colon). In postoperative paralytic ileus in order to accelerate the resumption of the intestinal transit following abdominal surgery.

Usual Dosage Children ≥12 years and Adults: Oral: 200 mg 3 times/day before meals

Dosage Forms Tablet, as maleate: 100 mg, 200 mg

trimebutine maleate *see* trimebutine *(Canada only) on this page*

trimeprazine *(Canada only)* (trye MEP re zeen)

U.S./Canadian Brand Names Panectyl® [Can]

Therapeutic Category Antihistamine

Use Perennial and seasonal allergic rhinitis and other allergic symptoms including urticaria

Usual Dosage Oral:

Children:

6 months to 3 years: 1.25 mg at bedtime or 3 times/day if needed

>3 years: 2.5 mg at bedtime or 3 times/day if needed

>6 years: Sustained release: 5 mg/day

Adults: 2.5 mg 4 times/day (5 mg every 12-hour sustained release)

Dosage Forms Tablet, as tartrate: 2.5 mg, 5 mg

trimethobenzamide (trye meth oh BEN za mide)

Sound-Alike/Look-Alike Issues

Tigan® may be confused with Tiazac®, Ticar®

Synonyms trimethobenzamide hydrochloride

U.S./Canadian Brand Names Tebamide™ [US]; Tigan® [US/Can]

Therapeutic Category Anticholinergic Agent; Antiemetic

Use Treatment of nausea and vomiting

Usual Dosage Rectal use is contraindicated in neonates and premature infants

Children:

<14 kg: Rectal: 100 mg 3-4 times/day

14-40 kg: Rectal: 100-200 mg 3-4 times/day

>40 kg:

Oral: 300 mg 3-4 times/day

Rectal: 200 mg 3-4 times/day

Adults:

Oral: 300 mg 3-4 times/day

I.M., rectal: 200 mg 3-4 times/day

Postoperative nausea and vomiting (PONV): I.M.: 200 mg, followed 1 hour later by a second 200 mg dose

Dosage Forms

Capsule, as hydrochloride (Tigan®): 300 mg

Injection, solution, as hydrochloride: 100 mg/mL (2 mL)

Tigan®: 100 mg/mL (2 mL [preservative free], 20 mL)

Suppository, rectal, as hydrochloride: 100 mg, 200 mg

Tebamide™: 100 mg, 200 mg [contains benzocaine]

Tigan®, Trimazide [DSC]: 200 mg [contains benzocaine]

trimethobenzamide hydrochloride *see* trimethobenzamide *on this page*

trimethoprim (trye METH oh prim)

Sound-Alike/Look-Alike Issues

trimethoprim may be confused with trimethaphan

Proloprim® may be confused with Prolixin®, Protropin®

Synonyms TMP

U.S./Canadian Brand Names Apo-Trimethoprim® [Can]; Primsol® [US]; Proloprim® [US]

Therapeutic Category Antibiotic, Miscellaneous

Use Treatment of urinary tract infections due to susceptible strains of *E. coli*, *P. mirabilis*, *K. pneumoniae*, *Enterobacter* sp and coagulase-negative *Staphylococcus* including *S. saprophyticus*; acute otitis media in children; acute exacerbations of chronic bronchitis in adults; in combination with other agents for treatment of toxoplasmosis, *Pneumocystis carinii*; treatment of superficial ocular infections involving the conjunctiva and cornea

Usual Dosage Oral:

Children: 4 mg/kg/day in divided doses every 12 hours

Adults: 100 mg every 12 hours or 200 mg every 24 hours for 10 days; longer treatment periods may be necessary for prostatitis (ie, 4-16 weeks); in the treatment of *Pneumocystis carinii* pneumonia; dose may be as high as 15-20 mg/kg/day in 3-4 divided doses

Dosage Forms [DSC] = Discontinued product

Solution, oral (Primsol®): 50 mg (base)/5 mL (480 mL) [contains sodium benzoate; bubble gum flavor]

Tablet: 100 mg

Proloprim®: 100 mg, 200 mg [DSC]

trimethoprim and polymyxin B (trye METH oh prim & pol i MIKS in bee)

Synonyms polymyxin B and trimethoprim

U.S./Canadian Brand Names PMS-Polytrimethoprim [Can]; Polytrim® [US/Can]

Therapeutic Category Antibiotic, Ophthalmic

Use Treatment of surface ocular bacterial conjunctivitis and blepharoconjunctivitis

Usual Dosage Instill 1-2 drops in eye(s) every 4-6 hours

Dosage Forms Solution, ophthalmic: Trimethoprim 1 mg and polymyxin B sulfate 10,000 units per mL (10 mL) [contains benzalkonium chloride]

trimethoprim and sulfamethoxazole *see* sulfamethoxazole and trimethoprim *on page 797*

trimetrexate (tri me TREKS ate)

Synonyms NSC-352122; trimetrexate glucuronate

U.S./Canadian Brand Names NeuTrexin® [US]

Therapeutic Category Antibiotic, Miscellaneous

Use Alternative therapy for the treatment of moderate-to-severe *Pneumocystis jiroveci* pneumonia (PCP) in immunocompromised patients, including patients with acquired immunodeficiency syndrome (AIDS), who are intolerant of, or are refractory to, sulfamethoxazole/trimethoprim therapy or for whom sulfamethoxazole/trimethoprim and pentamidine are contraindicated

Usual Dosage Note: Concurrent leucovorin 20 mg/m^2 every 6 hours must be administered daily (oral or I.V.) during treatment and for 72 hours past the last dose of trimetrexate glucuronate.

Adults: I.V.:

Pneumocystis jiroveci pneumonia (PCP): 45 mg/m^2 once daily for 21 days; **alternative dosing based on weight:**

<50 kg: Trimetrexate 1.5 mg/kg/day; leucovorin 0.6 mg/kg 4 times/day

50-80 kg: Trimetrexate 1.2 mg/kg/day; leucovorin 0.5 mg/kg/4 times/day

>80 kg: Trimetrexate 1 mg/kg/day; leucovorin 0.5 mg/kg/4 times/day

Note: Oral doses of leucovorin should be rounded up to the next higher 25 mg increment.

Dosage Forms Injection, powder for reconstitution [preservative free]: 25 mg, 200 mg

trimetrexate glucuronate *see* trimetrexate *on this page*

trimipramine (trye MI pra meen)

Sound-Alike/Look-Alike Issues

trimipramine may be confused with triamterene, trimeprazine

Synonyms trimipramine maleate

U.S./Canadian Brand Names Apo-Trimip® [Can]; Nu-Trimipramine [Can]; Rhotrimine® [Can]; Surmontil® [US]

Therapeutic Category Antidepressant, Tricyclic (Tertiary Amine)

Use Treatment of depression

Usual Dosage Oral: Adults: 50-150 mg/day as a single bedtime dose up to a maximum of 200 mg/day outpatient and 300 mg/day inpatient

Dosage Forms Capsule: 25 mg, 50 mg, 100 mg

trimipramine maleate *see* trimipramine *on this page*

Trimox® *(Discontinued)* *see* amoxicillin *on page 47*

Trimpex® *(Discontinued)* *see* trimethoprim *on previous page*

Tri-Nasal® [US/Can] *see* triamcinolone (inhalation, nasal) *on page 845*

Trinate [US] *see* vitamins (multiple/prenatal) *on page 879*

TriNessa™ [US] *see* ethinyl estradiol and norgestimate *on page 325*

Trinipatch® 0.2 [Can] *see* nitroglycerin *on page 595*

Trinipatch® 0.4 [Can] *see* nitroglycerin *on page 595*

Trinipatch® 0.6 [Can] *see* nitroglycerin *on page 595*

Tri-Norinyl® [US] *see* ethinyl estradiol and norethindrone *on page 323*

Trinsicon® [US] *see* vitamin B complex combinations *on page 876*

Triofed® Syrup *(Discontinued)* *see* triprolidine and pseudoephedrine *on next page*

Triostat® [US] *see* liothyronine *on page 498*

Tripedia® [US] *see* diphtheria, tetanus toxoids, and acellular pertussis vaccine *on page 265*

Triphasil® [US/Can] *see* ethinyl estradiol and levonorgestrel *on page 320*

Triphenyl® Expectorant *(Discontinued)*

triple antibiotic *see* bacitracin, neomycin, and polymyxin B *on page 91*

triple sulfa *see* sulfabenzamide, sulfacetamide, and sulfathiazole *on page 795*

Triposed® Syrup *(Discontinued)* *see* triprolidine and pseudoephedrine *on this page*

Tri-Previfem™ [US] *see* ethinyl estradiol and norgestimate *on page 325*

triprolidine and pseudoephedrine (trye PROE li deen & soo doe e FED rin)

Sound-Alike/Look-Alike Issues

Aprodine® may be confused with Aphrodyne®

Synonyms pseudoephedrine and triprolidine

U.S./Canadian Brand Names Actifed® Cold and Allergy [US-OTC]; Actifed® [Can]; Allerfrim® [US-OTC]; Aphedrid™ [US-OTC]; Aprodine® [US-OTC]; Genac® [US-OTC]; Silafed® [US-OTC]; Sudafed® Sinus Nighttime [US-OTC]; Tri-Sudo® [US-OTC]

Therapeutic Category Antihistamine/Decongestant Combination

Use Temporary relief of nasal congestion, decongest sinus openings, running nose, sneezing, itching of nose or throat and itchy, watery eyes due to common cold, hay fever, or other upper respiratory allergies

Usual Dosage Oral:

Children:

Syrup:

4 months to 2 years: 1.25 mL 3-4 times/day

2-4 years: 2.5 mL 3-4 times/day

4-6 years: 3.75 mL 3-4 times/day

6-12 years: 5 mL every 4-6 hours; do not exceed 4 doses in 24 hours

Tablet: $^{1}/_{2}$ every 4-6 hours; do not exceed 4 doses in 24 hours

Children >12 years and Adults:

Syrup: 10 mL every 4-6 hours; do not exceed 4 doses in 24 hours

Tablet: 1 every 4-6 hours; do not exceed 4 doses in 24 hours

Dosage Forms

Syrup: Triprolidine hydrochloride 1.25 mg and pseudoephedrine hydrochloride 30 mg per 5 mL (120 mL)

Allerfrim®: Triprolidine hydrochloride 1.25 mg and pseudoephedrine hydrochloride 30 mg per 5 mL (120 mL, 480 mL) [contains sodium benzoate]

Aprodine®: Triprolidine hydrochloride 1.25 mg and pseudoephedrine hydrochloride 30 mg per 5 mL (120 mL)

Silafed®: Triprolidine hydrochloride 1.25 mg and pseudoephedrine hydrochloride 30 mg per 5 mL (120 mL, 240 mL)

Tablet (Actifed® Cold and Allergy, Allerfrim®, Aphedrid™, Aprodine®, Genac®, Tri-Sudo®): Triprolidine hydrochloride 2.5 mg and pseudoephedrine hydrochloride 60 mg

triprolidine, codeine, and pseudoephedrine *see* triprolidine, pseudoephedrine, and codeine *(Canada only)* *on this page*

triprolidine, pseudoephedrine, and codeine *(Canada only)*

(trye PROE li deen, soo doe e FED rin, & KOE deen)

Sound-Alike/Look-Alike Issues

Triacin-C® may be confused with triacetin

Synonyms codeine, pseudoephedrine, and triprolidine; codeine, triprolidine, and pseudoephedrine; pseudoephedrine, codeine, and triprolidine; pseudoephedrine, triprolidine, and codeine; triprolidine, codeine, and pseudoephedrine

U.S./Canadian Brand Names CoActifed® [Can]; Covan® [Can]; ratio-Cotridin [Can]

Therapeutic Category Antihistamine/Decongestant/Antitussive

Controlled Substance C-V (CDSA-I)

Use Symptomatic relief of upper respiratory symptoms and cough

Usual Dosage Oral:

Children:

2-6 years: 2.5 mL 4 times/day

7-12 years: 5 mL 4 times/day **or** $^{1}/_{2}$ tablet 4 times/day

Children >12 years and Adults: 10 mL 4 times/day **or** 1 tablet 4 times/day

(Continued)

triprolidine, pseudoephedrine, and codeine *(Canada only)* (Continued)

Dosage Forms

Syrup:

Triprolidine hydrochloride 1.25 mg, pseudoephedrine hydrochloride 30 mg, and codeine phosphate 10 mg per 5 mL [contains alcohol 4.3%]

CoActifed®, CoVan®, ratio-Cotridin: Triprolidine hydrochloride 2 mg, pseudoephedrine hydrochloride 30 mg, and codeine phosphate 10 mg per 5 mL [available in Canada; not available in U.S.]

Tablet (CoActifed®): Triprolidine hydrochloride 4 mg, pseudoephedrine hydrochloride 60 mg, and codeine phosphate 20 mg (50s) [available in Canada; not available in U.S.]

Tri-Pseudo® *(Discontinued)* *see* triprolidine and pseudoephedrine *on previous page*

TripTone® *(Discontinued)* *see* dimenhydrinate *on page 258*

triptoraline *see* triptorelin *on this page*

triptorelin (trip toe REL in)

Synonyms AY-25650; CL-118,532; D-Trp(6)-LHRH; triptoraline; triptorelin pamoate; tryptoreline

U.S./Canadian Brand Names Trelstar™ Depot [US/Can]; Trelstar™ LA [US/Can]; Trelstar™ [Can]

Therapeutic Category Luteinizing Hormone-Releasing Hormone Analog

Use Palliative treatment of advanced prostate cancer as an alternative to orchiectomy or estrogen administration

Usual Dosage I.M.: Adults: Prostate cancer:

Trelstar™ Depot: 3.75 mg once every 28 days

Trelstar™ LA: 11.25 mg once every 84 days

Dosage Forms Injection, powder for reconstitution, as pamoate [also available packaged with Debioclip™ (prefilled syringe containing sterile water)]:

Trelstar™ Depot: 3.75 mg

Trelstar™ LA: 11.25 mg

triptorelin pamoate *see* triptorelin *on this page*

Triquilar® [Can] *see* ethinyl estradiol and levonorgestrel *on page 320*

tris buffer *see* tromethamine *on next page*

Trisenox® [US] *see* arsenic trioxide *on page 74*

tris(hydroxymethyl)aminomethane *see* tromethamine *on next page*

trisodium calcium diethylenetriaminepentaacetate (Ca-DTPA) *see* diethylene triamine pentaacetic acid *on page 252*

Tri-Sprintec™ [US] *see* ethinyl estradiol and norgestimate *on page 325*

Tri-Statin® II Topical *(Discontinued)* *see* nystatin and triamcinolone *on page 610*

Tristoject® Injection *(Discontinued)*

Trisudex® *(Discontinued)* *see* triprolidine and pseudoephedrine *on previous page*

Tri-Sudo® [US-OTC] *see* triprolidine and pseudoephedrine *on previous page*

Tri-Tannate Plus® *(Discontinued)* *see* chlorpheniramine, ephedrine, phenylephrine, and carbetapentane *on page 178*

TriTuss® [US] *see* guaifenesin, dextromethorphan, and phenylephrine *on page 400*

TriTuss® ER [US] *see* guaifenesin, dextromethorphan, and phenylephrine *on page 400*

Trivagizole-3® [Can] *see* clotrimazole *on page 205*

Trivagizole-3® *(Discontinued)* *see* clotrimazole *on page 205*

trivalent inactivated influenza vaccine (TIV) *see* influenza virus vaccine *on page 448*

Tri-Vent™ DM [US] *see* guaifenesin, pseudoephedrine, and dextromethorphan *on page 401*

Tri-Vent™ DPC [US] *see* chlorpheniramine, phenylephrine, and dextromethorphan *on page 179*

Tri-Vent™ HC [US] *see* hydrocodone, carbinoxamine, and pseudoephedrine *on page 424*

Tri-Vi-Flor® [US] *see* vitamins (multiple/pediatric) *on page 878*

Tri-Vi-Flor® with Iron [US] *see* vitamins (multiple/pediatric) *on page 878*

Tri-Vi-Sol® [US-OTC] *see* vitamins (multiple/pediatric) *on page 878*

Tri-Vi-Sol® with Iron [US-OTC] *see* vitamins (multiple/pediatric) *on page 878*

Trivora® [US] *see* ethinyl estradiol and levonorgestrel *on page 320*

Trizivir® [US] *see* abacavir, lamivudine, and zidovudine *on page 2*

Trobicin® *(Discontinued)* *see* spectinomycin *on page 788*

Trocaine® [US-OTC] *see* benzocaine *on page 99*

Trocal® *(Discontinued)* *see* dextromethorphan *on page 245*

trolamine (TROLE a meen)

Sound-Alike/Look-Alike Issues

Myoflex® may be confused with Mycelex®

Synonyms TEAS; triethanolamine salicylate

U.S./Canadian Brand Names Antiphlogistine Rub A-535 No Odour [Can]; Aspercreme® [US-OTC]; Flex-Power [US-OTC]; Mobisyl® [US-OTC]; Myoflex® [US-OTC/Can]; Sportscreme® [US-OTC]

Therapeutic Category Analgesic, Topical

Use Relief of pain of muscular aches, rheumatism, neuralgia, sprains, arthritis on intact skin

Usual Dosage Topical: Apply to area as needed

Dosage Forms

Cream, topical: 10% (90 g)

Aspercreme®: 10% (5 g, 35 g, 142 g) [odorless]

Flex-Power: 10% (113 g) [clean or light scent; contains sodium metabisulfite and tartrazine]

Mobisyl®: 10% (100 g, 227 g) [odorless; contains sweet almond oil]

Myoflex®: 10% (60 g, 120 g) [odorless]

Sportscreme®: 10% (40 g, 90 g) [odorless fresh scent; contains tartrazine]

Lotion, topical:

Aspercreme®: 10% (180 mL) [odorless]

Patch, topical:

Aspercreme®: 10% (5s) [odorless]

Trombovar® [Can] *see* sodium tetradecyl *on page 783*

tromethamine (troe METH a meen)

Sound-Alike/Look-Alike Issues

tromethamine may be confused with TrophAmine®

Synonyms tris buffer; tris(hydroxymethyl)aminomethane

U.S./Canadian Brand Names THAM® [US]

Therapeutic Category Alkalinizing Agent

Use Correction of metabolic acidosis associated with cardiac bypass surgery or cardiac arrest; to correct excess acidity of stored blood that is preserved with acid citrate dextrose (ACD); indicated in infants needing alkalinization after receiving maximum sodium bicarbonate (8-10 mEq/kg/24 hours)

Usual Dosage

Neonates and Infants: Metabolic acidosis associated with RDS: Initial: Approximately 1 mL/kg for each pH unit below 7.4; additional dosess determined by changes in PaO_2, pH, and pCO_2; **Note:** Although THAM® solution does not raise pCO_2 when treating metabolic acidosis with concurrent respiratory acidosis, bicarbonate may be preferred because the osmotic effects of THAM® are greater.

Adults: Dose depends on buffer base deficit; when deficit is known: tromethamine (mL of 0.3 M solution) = body weight (kg) x base deficit (mEq/L); when base deficit is not known: 3-6 mL/kg/dose I.V. (1-2 mEq/kg/dose)

Metabolic acidosis with cardiac arrest:

I.V.: 3.5-6 mL/kg (1-2 mEq/kg/dose) into large peripheral vein; 500-1000 mL if needed in adults

I.V. continuous drip: Infuse slowly by syringe pump over 3-6 hours

Acidosis associated with cardiac bypass surgery: Average dose: 9 mL/kg (2.7 mEq/kg); 500 mL is adequate for most adults; maximum dose: 500 mg/kg in ≤1 hour

Excess acidity of acid citrate dextrose priming blood: 14-70 mL of 0.3 molar solution added to each 500 mL of blood

Dosage Forms

Injection, solution:

THAM®: 18 g [0.3 molar] (500 mL)

Tronolane® [US-OTC] *see* pramoxine *on page 691*

Tronolane® Suppository [US-OTC] *see* phenylephrine *on page 660*

Tropicacyl® [US] *see* tropicamide *on next page*

tropicamide (troe PIK a mide)

Synonyms bistropamide

U.S./Canadian Brand Names Diotrope® [Can]; Mydral™ [US]; Mydriacyl® [US/Can]; Tropicacyl® [US]

Therapeutic Category Anticholinergic Agent

Use Short-acting mydriatic used in diagnostic procedures; as well as preoperatively and postoperatively; treatment of some cases of acute iritis, iridocyclitis, and keratitis

Usual Dosage Ophthalmic: Children and Adults (individuals with heavily pigmented eyes may require larger doses):

Cycloplegia: Instill 1-2 drops (1%); may repeat in 5 minutes

Exam must be performed within 30 minutes after the repeat dose; if the patient is not examined within 20-30 minutes, instill an additional drop

Mydriasis: Instill 1-2 drops (0.5%) 15-20 minutes before exam; may repeat every 30 minutes as needed

Dosage Forms

Solution, ophthalmic: 0.5% (15 mL); 1% (2 mL, 15 mL) [contains benzalkonium chloride]

Mydriacyl®: 1% (3 mL, 15 mL) [contains benzalkonium chloride]

Mydral™, Tropicacyl®: 0.5% (15 mL); 1% (15 mL) [contains benzalkonium chloride]

Trosec [Can] *see* trospium *on this page*

trospium (TROSE pee um)

Synonyms trospium chloride

U.S./Canadian Brand Names Sanctura™ [US]; Trosec [Can]

Therapeutic Category Anticholinergic Agent

Use Treatment of overactive bladder with symptoms of urgency, incontinence, and urinary frequency

Usual Dosage Oral: Adults: 20 mg twice daily

Dosage Forms

Tablet, as chloride:

Sanctura™: 20 mg

trospium chloride *see* trospium *on this page*

Trovan® ***(Discontinued)***

Truphylline® ***(Discontinued)*** *see* aminophylline *on page 42*

Trusopt® [US/Can] *see* dorzolamide *on page 274*

Truvada® [US/Can] *see* emtricitabine and tenofovir *on page 290*

trypsin, balsam peru, and castor oil (TRIP sin, BAL sam pe RUE, & KAS tor oyl)

Sound-Alike/Look-Alike Issues

Granulex® may be confused with Regranex®

Synonyms balsam peru, trypsin, and castor oil; castor oil, trypsin, and balsam peru

U.S./Canadian Brand Names Granulex® [US]; Optase™ [US]; Xenaderm™ [US]

Therapeutic Category Protectant, Topical

Use Treatment of decubitus ulcers, varicose ulcers, debridement of eschar, dehiscent wounds and sunburn; promote wound healing; reduce odor from necrotic wounds

Usual Dosage Topical: Apply a minimum of twice daily or as often as necessary

Dosage Forms

Aerosol, topical: Trypsin 0.12 mg, balsam Peru 87 mg, and castor oil 788 mg per gram (120 g)

Granulex®: Trypsin 0.12 mg, balsam Peru 87 mg, and castor oil 788 mg per gram (60 g, 120 g)

Gel, topical:

Optase™: Trypsin 0.12 mg, balsam Peru 87 mg, and castor oil 788 mg per gram (95 g)

Ointment, topical:

Xenaderm™: Trypsin 90 USP units, balsam Peru 87 mg, and castor oil 788 mg per gram (30 g, 60 g)

tryptoreline *see* triptorelin *on page 854*

Trysul® ***(Discontinued)*** *see* sulfabenzamide, sulfacetamide, and sulfathiazole *on page 795*

TSH *see* thyrotropin alpha *on page 825*

TSPA *see* thiotepa *on page 823*

TST *see* tuberculin tests *on next page*

T-Stat® ***(Discontinued)*** *see* erythromycin *on page 303*

tuberculin purified protein derivative *see* tuberculin tests *on next page*

tuberculin skin test *see* tuberculin tests *on this page*

tuberculin tests (too BER kyoo lin tests)

Sound-Alike/Look-Alike Issues

Aplisol® may be confused with Anusol®, A.P.L.®, Aplitest®, Atropisol®

Tuberculin products may be confused with tetanus toxoid products and influenza virus vaccine. Medication errors have occurred when tuberculin skin tests (PPD) have been inadvertently administered instead of tetanus toxoid products and influenza virus vaccine. These products are refrigerated and often stored in close proximity to each other.

Synonyms mantoux; PPD; tine test; TST; tuberculin purified protein derivative; tuberculin skin test

U.S./Canadian Brand Names Aplisol® [US]; Tubersol® [US]

Therapeutic Category Diagnostic Agent

Use Skin test in diagnosis of tuberculosis, cell-mediated immunodeficiencies

Usual Dosage Children and Adults: Intradermal: 0.1 mL about 4" below elbow; use 1/4" to 1/2" or 26- or 27-gauge needle; significant reactions are ≥5 mm in diameter

Interpretation of induration of tuberculin skin test injections: Positive: ≥10 mm; inconclusive: 5-9 mm; negative: <5 mm

Interpretation of induration of Tine test injections: Positive: >2 mm and vesiculation present; inconclusive: <2 mm (give patient Mantoux test of 5 TU/0.1 mL - base decisions on results of Mantoux test); negative: <2 mm or erythema of any size (no need for retesting unless person is a contact of a patient with tuberculosis or there is clinical evidence suggestive of the disease)

Dosage Forms Injection, solution: 5 TU/0.1 mL (1 mL, 5 mL)

Tubersol® [US] *see* tuberculin tests *on this page*

Tucks® [US-OTC] *see* witch hazel *on page 881*

Tucks® Anti-Itch [US-OTC] *see* hydrocortisone (topical) *on page 428*

Tucks® Hemorrhoidal [US-OTC] *see* pramoxine *on page 691*

Tums® [US-OTC] *see* calcium carbonate *on page 135*

Tums® E-X [US-OTC] *see* calcium carbonate *on page 135*

Tums® Extra Strength Sugar Free [US-OTC] *see* calcium carbonate *on page 135*

Tums® Smoothies™ [US-OTC] *see* calcium carbonate *on page 135*

Tums® Ultra [US-OTC] *see* calcium carbonate *on page 135*

Tusal® *(Discontinued)*

Tusibron® *(Discontinued)* *see* guaifenesin *on page 392*

Tusibron-DM® *(Discontinued)* *see* guaifenesin and dextromethorphan *on page 394*

Tusnel Pediatric® [US] *see* guaifenesin, pseudoephedrine, and dextromethorphan *on page 401*

Tussafed® *(Discontinued)* *see* carbinoxamine, pseudoephedrine, and dextromethorphan *on page 150*

Tussafin® Expectorant *(Discontinued)* *see* hydrocodone, pseudoephedrine, and guaifenesin *on page 425*

Tussend® Expectorant *(Discontinued)* *see* hydrocodone, pseudoephedrine, and guaifenesin *on page 425*

Tussend® Syrup *(Discontinued)* *see* pseudoephedrine, hydrocodone, and chlorpheniramine *on page 716*

Tussend® Tablet *(Discontinued)* *see* pseudoephedrine, hydrocodone, and chlorpheniramine *on page 716*

Tussi-12® [US] *see* carbetapentane and chlorpheniramine *on page 146*

Tussi-12 S™ [US] *see* carbetapentane and chlorpheniramine *on page 146*

Tussigon® [US] *see* hydrocodone and homatropine *on page 423*

Tussin [US-OTC] *see* guaifenesin *on page 392*

TussiNate™ [US] *see* hydrocodone, phenylephrine, and diphenhydramine *on page 425*

Tussionex® [US] *see* hydrocodone and chlorpheniramine *on page 422*

Tussi-Organidin® DM NR *(Discontinued)* *see* guaifenesin and dextromethorphan *on page 394*

Tussi-Organidin® NR [US] *see* guaifenesin and codeine *on page 393*

Tussi-Organidin® S-NR [US] *see* guaifenesin and codeine *on page 393*

Tussizone-12 RF™ [US] *see* carbetapentane and chlorpheniramine *on page 146*
Tuss-LA® *(Discontinued)* *see* guaifenesin and pseudoephedrine *on page 398*
T-Vites [US-OTC] *see* vitamins (multiple/oral) *on page 878*
TVP-1012 *see* rasagiline *on page 733*
Twelve Resin-K [US] *see* cyanocobalamin *on page 219*
Twilite® [US-OTC] *see* diphenhydramine *on page 261*
Twinject™ [US] *see* epinephrine *on page 295*
Twin-K® *(Discontinued)*
Twinrix® [US/Can] *see* hepatitis A inactivated and hepatitis B (recombinant) vaccine *on page 410*
Two-Dyne® *(Discontinued)*
Tycolene [US-OTC] *see* acetaminophen *on page 5*
Tycolene Maximum Strength [US-OTC] *see* acetaminophen *on page 5*
Tygacil™ [US] *see* tigecycline *on page 828*
Tylenol® [US-OTC/Can] *see* acetaminophen *on page 5*
Tylenol® 8 Hour [US-OTC] *see* acetaminophen *on page 5*
Tylenol® Allergy Complete [US-OTC] *see* acetaminophen, chlorpheniramine, and pseudoephedrine *on page 11*
Tylenol® Allergy Sinus [Can] *see* acetaminophen, chlorpheniramine, and pseudoephedrine *on page 11*
Tylenol® Allergy Sinus *(Discontinued)* *see* acetaminophen, chlorpheniramine, and pseudoephedrine *on page 11*
Tylenol® Arthritis Pain [US-OTC] *see* acetaminophen *on page 5*
Tylenol® Children's [US-OTC] *see* acetaminophen *on page 5*
Tylenol® Children's Plus Cold Nighttime [US-OTC] *see* acetaminophen, chlorpheniramine, and pseudoephedrine *on page 11*
Tylenol® Children's with Flavor Creator [US-OTC] *see* acetaminophen *on page 5*
Tylenol® Cold Day Non-Drowsy [US-OTC] *see* acetaminophen, dextromethorphan, and pseudoephedrine *on page 12*
Tylenol® Cold Daytime [Can] *see* acetaminophen, dextromethorphan, and pseudoephedrine *on page 12*
Tylenol® Cold, Infants [US-OTC] *see* acetaminophen and pseudoephedrine *on page 9*
Tylenol® Decongestant [Can] *see* acetaminophen and pseudoephedrine *on page 9*
Tylenol® Elixir with Codeine [Can] *see* acetaminophen and codeine *on page 6*
Tylenol® Extra Strength [US-OTC] *see* acetaminophen *on page 5*
Tylenol® Flu Non-Drowsy Maximum Strength [US-OTC] *see* acetaminophen, dextromethorphan, and pseudoephedrine *on page 12*
Tylenol® Infants [US-OTC] *see* acetaminophen *on page 5*
Tylenol® Junior [US-OTC] *see* acetaminophen *on page 5*
Tylenol® No. 1 [Can] *see* acetaminophen and codeine *on page 6*
Tylenol® No. 1 Forte [Can] *see* acetaminophen and codeine *on page 6*
Tylenol® No. 2 with Codeine [Can] *see* acetaminophen and codeine *on page 6*
Tylenol® No. 3 with Codeine [Can] *see* acetaminophen and codeine *on page 6*
Tylenol® No. 4 with Codeine [Can] *see* acetaminophen and codeine *on page 6*
Tylenol® PM [US-OTC] *see* acetaminophen and diphenhydramine *on page 7*
Tylenol® Severe Allergy [US-OTC] *see* acetaminophen and diphenhydramine *on page 7*
Tylenol® Sinus [Can] *see* acetaminophen and pseudoephedrine *on page 9*
Tylenol® Sinus, Children's [US-OTC] *see* acetaminophen and pseudoephedrine *on page 9*
Tylenol® Sinus Day Non-Drowsy [US-OTC] *see* acetaminophen and pseudoephedrine *on page 9*
Tylenol® With Codeine [US] *see* acetaminophen and codeine *on page 6*

Tylenol® with Codeine (Elixir) ***(Discontinued)*** *see* acetaminophen and codeine *on page 6*

Tylox® [US] *see* oxycodone and acetaminophen *on page 627*

Typherix™ [Can] *see Salmonella typhi* Vi capsular polysaccharide vaccine *(Canada only) on page 761*

Typhim Vi® [US] *see* typhoid vaccine *on this page*

typhoid vaccine (TYE foid vak SEEN)

Synonyms typhoid vaccine live oral Ty21a

U.S./Canadian Brand Names Typhim Vi® [US]; Vivotif Berna® [US]

Therapeutic Category Vaccine, Inactivated Bacteria

Use Typhoid vaccine: Live, attenuated Ty21a typhoid vaccine should not be administered to immunocompromised persons, including those known to be infected with HIV. Parenteral inactivated vaccine is a theoretically safer alternative for this group.

Parenteral: Promotes active immunity to typhoid fever for patients intimately exposed to a typhoid carrier or foreign travel to a typhoid fever endemic area

Oral: For immunization of children >6 years of age and adults who expect intimate exposure of or household contact with typhoid fever, travelers to areas of world with risk of exposure to typhoid fever, and workers in microbiology laboratories with expected frequent contact with *S. typhi*

Usual Dosage Immunization:

Oral: Children ≥6 years and Adults:

Primary immunization: One capsule on alternate days (day 1, 3, 5, and 7) for a total of 4 doses; all doses should be complete at least 1 week prior to potential exposure

Booster immunization: Repeat full course of primary immunization every 5 years

I.M. (Typhim Vi®): Children ≥2 years and Adults: 0.5 mL given at least 2 weeks prior to expected exposure

Reimmunization: 0.5 mL; optimal schedule has not been established; a single dose every 2 years is currently recommended for repeated or continued exposure

Dosage Forms

Capsule, enteric coated (Vivotif Berna®): Viable *S. typhi* Ty21a colony-forming units 2-6 x 10^9 and nonviable *S. typhi* Ty21a colony-forming units 5-50 x 10^9 [contains lactose]

Injection, solution (Typhim Vi®): Purified Vi capsular polysaccharide 25 mcg/0.5 mL (0.5 mL, 10 mL)

typhoid vaccine live oral Ty21a *see* typhoid vaccine *on this page*

Tyrodone® Liquid ***(Discontinued)*** *see* hydrocodone and pseudoephedrine *on page 424*

tyropanoate sodium *see* radiological/contrast media (ionic) *on page 728*

Tysabri® [US] *see* natalizumab *on page 580*

Tyzine® [US] *see* tetrahydrozoline *on page 817*

Tyzine® Pediatric [US] *see* tetrahydrozoline *on page 817*

506U78 *see* nelarabine *on page 582*

U-90152S *see* delavirdine *on page 234*

UAA® [US] *see* methenamine, phenyl salicylate, atropine, hyoscyamine, benzoic acid, and methylene blue *on page 539*

UAD Otic® ***(Discontinued)*** *see* neomycin, polymyxin B, and hydrocortisone *on page 584*

UCB-P071 *see* cetirizine *on page 167*

UK-88,525 *see* darifenacin *on page 231*

UK92480 *see* sildenafil *on page 771*

UK109496 *see* voriconazole *on page 880*

Ulcerease® [US-OTC] *see* phenol *on page 658*

Ulcidine [Can] *see* famotidine *on page 335*

ULR-LA® ***(Discontinued)***

Ultane® [US] *see* sevoflurane *on page 770*

Ultiva® [US/Can] *see* remifentanil *on page 736*

Ultracaine® D-S [Can] *see* articaine and epinephrine *on page 75*

Ultracaine® D-S Forte [Can] *see* articaine and epinephrine *on page 75*

Ultracaps MT [US] *see* pancrelipase *on page 634*

Ultracet™ [US] *see* acetaminophen and tramadol *on page 10*

Ultra Freeda Iron Free [US-OTC] *see* vitamins (multiple/oral) *on page 878*

Ultra Freeda with Iron [US-OTC] *see* vitamins (multiple/oral) *on page 878*

Ultram® [US/Can] *see* tramadol *on page 841*

Ultram® ER [US] *see* tramadol *on page 841*

Ultra Mide® [US-OTC] *see* urea *on next page*

UltraMide 25™ [Can] *see* urea *on next page*

Ultramop™ [Can] *see* methoxsalen *on page 542*

Ultra NatalCare® [US] *see* vitamins (multiple/prenatal) *on page 879*

Ultraprin [US-OTC] *see* ibuprofen *on page 437*

Ultraquin™ [Can] *see* hydroquinone *on page 430*

Ultrase® [US/Can] *see* pancrelipase *on page 634*

Ultrase® MT [US/Can] *see* pancrelipase *on page 634*

Ultra Tears® [US-OTC] *see* artificial tears *on page 75*

Ultravate® [US/Can] *see* halobetasol *on page 406*

Umecta® [US] *see* urea *on next page*

Unasyn® [US/Can] *see* ampicillin and sulbactam *on page 54*

undecylenic acid and derivatives (un de sil EN ik AS id & dah RIV ah tivs)

Synonyms zinc undecylenate

U.S./Canadian Brand Names Fungi-Nail® [US-OTC]

Therapeutic Category Antifungal Agent

Use Treatment of athlete's foot (tinea pedis); ringworm (except nails and scalp)

Usual Dosage Children and Adults: Topical: Apply twice daily to affected area for 4 weeks; apply to clean, dry area

Dosage Forms Solution, topical: Undecylenic acid 25% (29.57 mL)

Unguentine® ***(Discontinued)*** *see* benzocaine *on page 99*

Uni-Bent® Cough Syrup ***(Discontinued)*** *see* diphenhydramine *on page 261*

Unicap M® [US-OTC] *see* vitamins (multiple/oral) *on page 878*

Unicap Sr® [US-OTC] *see* vitamins (multiple/oral) *on page 878*

Unicap T™ [US-OTC] *see* vitamins (multiple/oral) *on page 878*

Unidet® [Can] *see* tolterodine *on page 835*

Uni-Dur® ***(Discontinued)*** *see* theophylline *on page 818*

Unipen® [Can] *see* nafcillin *on page 574*

Uniphyl® [US] *see* theophylline *on page 818*

Uniphyl® SRT [Can] *see* theophylline *on page 818*

Uni-Pro® ***(Discontinued)*** *see* ibuprofen *on page 437*

Uniretic® [US/Can] *see* moexipril and hydrochlorothiazide *on page 563*

Uni-Senna [US-OTC] *see* senna *on page 767*

Unisom®-2 [Can] *see* doxylamine *on page 280*

Unisom® Maximum Strength SleepGels® [US-OTC] *see* diphenhydramine *on page 261*

Unisom® SleepTabs® [US-OTC] *see* doxylamine *on page 280*

Unithroid® [US] *see* levothyroxine *on page 491*

Uni-Tricof HC [US] *see* phenylephrine, hydrocodone, and chlorpheniramine *on page 663*

Unitrol® ***(Discontinued)***

Uni-Tuss HC [US] *see* phenylephrine, hydrocodone, and chlorpheniramine *on page 663*

Uni-tussin® ***(Discontinued)*** *see* guaifenesin *on page 392*

Uni-tussin® DM ***(Discontinued)*** *see* guaifenesin and dextromethorphan *on page 394*

Univasc® [US] *see* moexipril *on page 562*

unna's boot *see* zinc gelatin *on page 887*

unna's paste *see* zinc gelatin *on page 887*

Urabeth® *(Discontinued)* *see* bethanechol *on page 109*

Urasal® [Can] *see* methenamine *on page 538*

urea (yoor EE a)

Synonyms carbamide

U.S./Canadian Brand Names Amino-Cerv™ [US]; Aquacare® [US-OTC]; Aquaphilic® With Carbamide [US-OTC]; Carmol® 10 [US-OTC]; Carmol® 20 [US-OTC]; Carmol® 40 [US]; Carmol® Deep Cleaning [US]; Cerovel™ [US]; DPM™ [US-OTC]; Gormel® [US-OTC]; Keralac™ Nailstik [US]; Keralac™ [US]; Lanaphilic® [US-OTC]; Nutraplus® [US-OTC]; Rea-Lo® [US-OTC]; Ultra Mide® [US-OTC]; UltraMide 25™ [Can]; Umecta® [US]; Ureacin® [US-OTC]; Uremol® [Can]; Urisec® [Can]; Vanamide™ [US]

Therapeutic Category Diuretic, Osmotic; Topical Skin Product

Use

Topical: Keratolytic agent to soften nails or skin; OTC: Moisturizer for dry, rough skin
Vaginal: Treatment of cervicitis

Usual Dosage Adults:

Hyperkeratotic conditions, dry skin: Topical: Apply 1-3 times/day
Cervicitis: Vaginal: Insert 1 applicatorful in vagina at bedtime for 2-4 weeks

Dosage Forms

Cream: 40% (30 g, 85 g, 199 g)
- Aquacare®: 10% (75 g)
- Carmol® 20: 20% (90 g)
- Carmol® 40: 40% (30 g, 90 g, 210 g)
- Cerovel™: 40% (133 g)
- DPM™: 20% (118 g) [contains menthol and peppermint oil]
- Gormel®: 20% (75 g, 120 g, 454 g, 2270 g)
- Keralac™: 50% (142 g, 255 g) [contains lactic acid, vitamin E, and zinc]
- Nutraplus®: 10% (90 g, 454 g)
- Rea-Lo®: 30% (60 g, 240 g)
- Ureacin®-20: 20% (120 g)
- Vanamide™: 40% (85 g, 199 g)

Cream, vaginal (Amino-Cerv™): 8.34% [83.4 mg/g] (82.5 g)

Emulsion, topical (Umecta®): 40% (120 mL, 480 mL)

Gel: 40% (15 mL)
- Carmol® 40: 40% (15 mL)
- Cerovel™: 40% (25 mL)
- Keralac™: 50% (18 mL) [contains lactic acid and zinc]

Lotion: 40% (240 mL)
- Aquacare®: 10% (240 mL)
- Carmol® 10: 10% (180 mL)
- Carmol® 40: 40% (240 mL)
- Cerovel™: 40% (325 mL)
- Keralac™: 35% (207 mL, 325 mL) [contains lactic acid, vitamin E, and zinc]
- Nutraplus®: 10% (240 mL, 480 mL)
- Ultra Mide®: 25% (120 mL, 240 mL)
- Ureacin®-10: 10% (240 mL)

Ointment:
- Aquaphilic® with Carbamide: 10% (180 g, 480 g); 20% (480 g)
- Keralac™: 50% (90 g)
- Lanaphilic®: 10% (454 g); 20% (454 g)

Shampoo (Carmol® Deep Cleaning): 10% (240 mL)

Solution, topical (Keralac™ Nailstick): 50% (2.4 mL)

Suspension, topical (Umecta®): 40% (18 mL) [nail film with applicator], (300 mL)

urea and hydrocortisone (yoor EE a & hye droe KOR ti sone)

Synonyms hydrocortisone and urea

U.S./Canadian Brand Names Carmol-HC® [US]; Ti-U-Lac® H [Can]; Uremol® HC [Can]

Therapeutic Category Corticosteroid, Topical

Use Inflammation of corticosteroid-responsive dermatoses

Usual Dosage Apply thin film and rub in well 1-4 times/day. Therapy should be discontinued when control is achieved; if no improvement is seen, reassessment of diagnosis may be necessary.

(Continued)

urea and hydrocortisone *(Continued)*

Dosage Forms Cream: Urea 10% and hydrocortisone acetate 1% (30 g) [in water soluble vanishing cream base]

Ureacin® [US-OTC] *see* urea *on previous page*

urea peroxide *see* carbamide peroxide *on page 145*

Urecholine® [US] *see* bethanechol *on page 109*

Urelle® [US] *see* methenamine, phenyl salicylate, atropine, hyoscyamine, benzoic acid, and methylene blue *on page 539*

Uremol® [Can] *see* urea *on previous page*

Uremol® HC [Can] *see* urea and hydrocortisone *on previous page*

Urex® [US/Can] *see* methenamine *on page 538*

Uridon Modified® [US] *see* methenamine, phenyl salicylate, atropine, hyoscyamine, benzoic acid, and methylene blue *on page 539*

Urisec® [Can] *see* urea *on previous page*

Urised® [US] *see* methenamine, phenyl salicylate, atropine, hyoscyamine, benzoic acid, and methylene blue *on page 539*

Urispas® [US/Can] *see* flavoxate *on page 347*

Uristat® [US-OTC] *see* phenazopyridine *on page 656*

Uritin® [US] *see* methenamine, phenyl salicylate, atropine, hyoscyamine, benzoic acid, and methylene blue *on page 539*

Urocit®-K [US] *see* potassium citrate *on page 685*

Urodine® *(Discontinued)* *see* phenazopyridine *on page 656*

Uro-KP-Neutral® [US] *see* potassium phosphate and sodium phosphate *on page 688*

Urolene Blue® [US] *see* methylene blue *on page 545*

Uro-Mag® [US-OTC] *see* magnesium oxide *on page 515*

Uromax® [Can] *see* oxybutynin *on page 625*

Uromitexan [Can] *see* mesna *on page 534*

Uroplus® DS *(Discontinued)*

Uroplus® SS *(Discontinued)*

Urovist Cysto® [US] *see* radiological/contrast media (ionic) *on page 728*

Urovist® Meglumine [US] *see* radiological/contrast media (ionic) *on page 728*

Urovist® Sodium 300 [US] *see* radiological/contrast media (ionic) *on page 728*

Uroxatral™ [US] *see* alfuzosin *on page 28*

Urso® [Can] *see* ursodiol *on this page*

Urso 250™ [US] *see* ursodiol *on this page*

ursodeoxycholic acid *see* ursodiol *on this page*

ursodiol (ur soe DYE ol)

Synonyms ursodeoxycholic acid

U.S./Canadian Brand Names Actigall® [US]; Urso 250™ [US]; Urso Forte™ [US]; Urso® DS [Can]; Urso® [Can]

Therapeutic Category Gallstone Dissolution Agent

Use Actigall®: Gallbladder stone dissolution; prevention of gallstones in obese patients experiencing rapid weight loss; Urso®: Primary biliary cirrhosis

Usual Dosage Adults: Oral:

Gallstone dissolution: 8-10 mg/kg/day in 2-3 divided doses; use beyond 24 months is not established; obtain ultrasound images at 6-month intervals for the first year of therapy; 30% of patients have stone recurrence after dissolution

Gallstone prevention: 300 mg twice daily

Primary biliary cirrhosis: 13-15 mg/kg/day in 2-4 divided doses (with food)

Dosage Forms

Capsule (Actigall®): 300 mg

Tablet:
Urso 250™: 250 mg
Urso Forte™: 500 mg

Urso® DS [Can] *see* ursodiol *on previous page*
Urso Forte™ [US] *see* ursodiol *on previous page*
UTI Relief® [US-OTC] *see* phenazopyridine *on page 656*
Utradol™ [Can] *see* etodolac *on page 329*
Uvadex® [US/Can] *see* methoxsalen *on page 542*
vaccinia vaccine *see* smallpox vaccine *on page 776*
Vagifem® [US/Can] *see* estradiol *on page 308*
Vagi-Gard® [US-OTC] *see* povidone-iodine *on page 689*
Vagistat®-1 [US-OTC] *see* tioconazole *on page 830*
Vagitrol® ***(Discontinued)***

valacyclovir (val ay SYE kloe veer)

Sound-Alike/Look-Alike Issues
valacyclovir may be confused with valganciclovir
Valtrex® may be confused with Valcyte™
Synonyms valacyclovir hydrochloride
U.S./Canadian Brand Names Valtrex® [US/Can]
Therapeutic Category Antiviral Agent
Use Treatment of herpes zoster (shingles) in immunocompetent patients; treatment of first-episode genital herpes; episodic treatment of recurrent genital herpes; suppression of recurrent genital herpes and reduction of heterosexual transmission of genital herpes in immunocompetent patients; suppression of genital herpes in HIV-infected individuals; treatment of herpes labialis (cold sores)
Usual Dosage Oral:
Adolescents and Adults: Herpes labialis (cold sores): 2 g twice daily for 1 day (separate doses by ~12 hours)
Adults:
Herpes zoster (shingles): 1 g 3 times/day for 7 days
Genital herpes:
Initial episode: 1 g twice daily for 10 days
Recurrent episode: 500 mg twice daily for 3 days
Reduction of transmission: 500 mg once daily (source partner)
Suppressive therapy:
Immunocompetent patients: 1000 mg once daily (500 mg once daily in patients with <9 recurrences per year)
HIV-infected patients (CD4 ≥100 cells/mm^3): 500 mg twice daily
Dosage Forms Caplet: 500 mg, 1000 mg

valacyclovir hydrochloride *see* valacyclovir *on this page*
Valcyte™ [US/Can] *see* valganciclovir *on this page*
23-valent pneumococcal polysaccharide vaccine *see* pneumococcal polysaccharide vaccine (polyvalent) *on page 676*

valganciclovir (val gan SYE kloh veer)

Sound-Alike/Look-Alike Issues
valganciclovir may be confused with valacyclovir
Valcyte™ may be confused with Valium®, Valtrex®
Synonyms valganciclovir hydrochloride
U.S./Canadian Brand Names Valcyte™ [US/Can]
Therapeutic Category Antiviral Agent
Use Treatment of cytomegalovirus (CMV) retinitis in patients with acquired immunodeficiency syndrome (AIDS); prevention of CMV disease in high-risk patients (donor CMV positive/recipient CMV negative) undergoing kidney, heart, or kidney/pancreas transplantation
Usual Dosage Oral: Adults:
CMV retinitis:
Induction: 900 mg twice daily for 21 days (with food)
(Continued)

valganciclovir *(Continued)*

Maintenance: Following induction treatment, or for patients with inactive CMV retinitis who require maintenance therapy: Recommended dose: 900 mg once daily (with food)

Prevention of CMV disease following transplantation: 900 mg once daily (with food) beginning within 10 days of transplantation; continue therapy until 100 days post-transplantation

Dosage Forms Tablet, as hydrochloride: 450 mg [valganciclovir hydrochloride 496.3 mg equivalent to valganciclovir 450 mg]

valganciclovir hydrochloride *see* valganciclovir *on previous page*

Valisone® Scalp Lotion [Can] *see* betamethasone (topical) *on page 107*

Valisone® Topical *(Discontinued)*

Valium® [US/Can] *see* diazepam *on page 248*

Valorin [US-OTC] *see* acetaminophen *on page 5*

Valorin Extra [US-OTC] *see* acetaminophen *on page 5*

valproate semisodium *see* valproic acid and derivatives *on this page*

valproate sodium *see* valproic acid and derivatives *on this page*

valproic acid *see* valproic acid and derivatives *on this page*

valproic acid and derivatives (val PROE ik AS id & dah RIV ah tives)

Sound-Alike/Look-Alike Issues

Depakene® may be confused with Depakote®

Depakote® may be confused with Depakene®, Depakote® ER, Senokot®

Synonyms dipropylacetic acid; divalproex sodium; DPA; 2-propylpentanoic acid; 2-propylvaleric acid; valproate semisodium; valproate sodium; valproic acid

U.S./Canadian Brand Names Alti-Divalproex [Can]; Apo-Divalproex® [Can]; Apo-Valproic® [Can]; Depacon® [US]; Depakene® [US/Can]; Depakote® Delayed Release [US]; Depakote® ER [US]; Depakote® Sprinkle® [US]; Epival® I.V. [Can]; Gen-Divalproex [Can]; Novo-Divalproex [Can]; Nu-Divalproex [Can]; PMS-Valproic Acid E.C. [Can]; PMS-Valproic Acid [Can]; Rhoxal-valproic [Can]; Sandoz-Valporic [Can]

Therapeutic Category Anticonvulsant

Use Monotherapy and adjunctive therapy in the treatment of patients with complex partial seizures; monotherapy and adjunctive therapy of simple and complex absence seizures; adjunctive therapy patients with multiple seizure types that include absence seizures; treatment of acute or mixed manic episodes associated with bipolar disorder; migraine prophylaxis

Mania associated with bipolar disorder (Depakote®)

Migraine prophylaxis (Depakote®, Depakote® ER)

Usual Dosage

Seizures:

Children ≥10 years and Adults:

Oral: Initial: 10-15 mg/kg/day in 1-3 divided doses; increase by 5-10 mg/kg/day at weekly intervals until therapeutic levels are achieved; maintenance: 30-60 mg/kg/day. Adult usual dose: 1000-2500 mg/day. **Note:** Regular release and delayed release formulations are usually given in 2-4 divided doses/day, extended release formulation (Depakote® ER) is usually given once daily. Conversion to Depakote® ER from a stable dose of Depakote® may require an increase in the total daily dose between 8% and 20% to maintain similar serum concentrations.

Children receiving more than one anticonvulsant (ie, polytherapy) may require doses up to 100 mg/kg/day in 3-4 divided doses

I.V.: Administer as a 60-minute infusion (≤20 mg/minute) with the same frequency as oral products; switch patient to oral products as soon as possible. Alternatively, rapid infusions have been given: ≤15 mg/kg over 5-10 minutes (1.5-3 mg/kg/minute).

Mania: Adults: Oral: 750-1500 mg/day in divided doses; dose should be adjusted as rapidly as possible to desired clinical effect; a loading dose of 20 mg/kg may be used; maximum recommended dosage: 60 mg/kg/day

Extended release tablets: Initial: 25 mg/kg/day given once daily; dose should be adjusted as rapidly as possible to desired clinical effect; maximum recommended dose: 60 mg/kg/day.

Migraine prophylaxis: Adults: Oral:

Extended release tablets: 500 mg once daily for 7 days, then increase to 1000 mg once daily; adjust dose based on patient response; usual dosage range 500-1000 mg/day

Delayed release tablets: 250 mg twice daily; adjust dose based on patient response, up to 1000 mg/day

Dosage Forms Note: Strength expressed as valproic acid
Capsule, as valproic acid (Depakene®): 250 mg
Capsule, sprinkles, as divalproex sodium (Depakote® Sprinkle®): 125 mg
Injection, solution, as valproate sodium (Depacon®): 100 mg/mL (5 mL) [contains edetate disodium]
Syrup, as valproic acid: 250 mg/5 mL (480 mL)
Depakene®: 250 mg/5 mL (480 mL)
Tablet, delayed release, as divalproex sodium (Depakote®): 125 mg, 250 mg, 500 mg
Tablet, extended release, as divalproex sodium (Depakote® ER): 250 mg, 500 mg

valsartan (val SAR tan)

Sound-Alike/Look-Alike Issues
valsartan may be confused with losartan, Valstar™
Diovan® may be confused with Darvon®, Dioval®, Zyban®
U.S./Canadian Brand Names Diovan® [US/Can]
Therapeutic Category Angiotensin II Receptor Antagonist
Use Alone or in combination with other antihypertensive agents in the treatment of essential hypertension; treatment of heart failure (NYHA Class II-IV); reduction of cardiovascular mortality in patients with left ventricular dysfunction postmyocardial infarction
Usual Dosage Adults: Oral:
Hypertension: Initial: 80 mg or 160 mg once daily (in patients who are not volume depleted); dose may be increased to achieve desired effect; maximum recommended dose: 320 mg/day
Heart failure: Initial: 40 mg twice daily; titrate dose to 80-160 mg twice daily, as tolerated; maximum daily dose: 320 mg
Left ventricular dysfunction after MI: Initial: 20 mg twice daily; titrate dose to target of 160 mg twice daily as tolerated; may initiate ≥12 hours following MI
Dosage Forms Tablet: 40 mg, 80 mg, 160 mg, 320 mg

valsartan and hydrochlorothiazide (val SAR tan & hye droe klor oh THYE a zide)

Sound-Alike/Look-Alike Issues
Diovan® may be confused with Darvon®, Dioval®, Zyban®
Synonyms hydrochlorothiazide and valsartan
U.S./Canadian Brand Names Diovan HCT® [US/Can]
Therapeutic Category Antihypertensive Agent, Combination
Use Treatment of hypertension (not indicated for initial therapy)
Usual Dosage Oral: Adults: Dose is individualized (combination substituted for individual components); dose may be titrated after 3-4 weeks of therapy.
Usual recommended starting dose of valsartan: 80 mg or 160 mg once daily (maximum: 320 mg/day) when used as monotherapy in patients who are not volume depleted
Usual recommended starting dose of hydrochlorothiazide: 12.5-25 mg once daily (maximum: 25 mg/day)
Dosage Forms Tablet:
Diovan HCT® 80 mg/12.5 mg: Valsartan 80 mg and hydrochlorothiazide 12.5 mg
Diovan HCT®160 mg/12.5 mg: Valsartan 160 mg and hydrochlorothiazide 12.5 mg
Diovan HCT®160 mg/25 mg: Valsartan 160 mg and hydrochlorothiazide 25 mg
Diovan HCT®320 mg/12.5 mg: Valsartan 320 mg and hydrochlorothiazide 12.5 mg
Diovan HCT®320 mg/25 mg: Valsartan 320 mg and hydrochlorothiazide 25 mg

Valstar® *(Discontinued)*

Valtrex® [US/Can] *see* valacyclovir *on page 863*

Vamate® Oral *(Discontinued)* *see* hydroxyzine *on page 433*

Vanamide™ [US] *see* urea *on page 861*

Vanatrip® *(Discontinued)* *see* amitriptyline *on page 44*

Vancenase® AQ 84 mcg *(Discontinued)* *see* beclomethasone *on page 95*

Vancenase® Pockethaler® *(Discontinued)* *see* beclomethasone *on page 95*

Vanceril® AEM [Can] *see* beclomethasone *on page 95*

Vanceril® *(Discontinued)* *see* beclomethasone *on page 95*

Vancocin® [US/Can] *see* vancomycin *on this page*

vancomycin (van koe MYE sin)

Sound-Alike/Look-Alike Issues
vancomycin may be confused with vecuronium
(Continued)

vancomycin *(Continued)*

I.V. vancomycin may be confused with Invanz®

Synonyms vancomycin hydrochloride

U.S./Canadian Brand Names Vancocin® [US/Can]

Therapeutic Category Antibiotic, Miscellaneous

Use Treatment of patients with infections caused by staphylococcal species and streptococcal species; used orally for staphylococcal enterocolitis or for antibiotic-associated pseudomembranous colitis produced by *C. difficile*

Usual Dosage Initial dosage recommendation:

Neonates: I.V.:

Postnatal age ≤7 days:

<1200 g: 15 mg/kg/dose every 24 hours

1200-2000 g: 10 mg/kg/dose every 12 hours

>2000 g: 15 mg/kg/dose every 12 hours

Postnatal age >7 days:

<1200 g: 15 mg/kg/dose every 24 hours

≥1200 g: 10 mg/kg/dose every 8 hours

Infants >1 month and Children: I.V.:

40 mg/kg/day in divided doses every 6 hours

Prophylaxis for bacterial endocarditis:

Dental, oral, or upper respiratory tract surgery: 20 mg/kg 1 hour prior to the procedure

GI/GU procedure: 20 mg/kg plus gentamicin 2 mg/kg 1 hour prior to surgery

Infants >1 month and Children with staphylococcal central nervous system infection: I.V.: 60 mg/kg/day in divided doses every 6 hours

Adults: I.V.:

With normal renal function: 1 g **or** 10-15 mg/kg/dose every 12 hours

Hospital-acquired pneumonia (HAP): 15 mg/kg/dose every 12 hours (American Thoracic Society/ATS guidelines)

Meningitis (*Pneumococcus* or *Staphylococcus*): 30-45 mg/kg/day in divided doses every 8-12 hours **or** 500-750 mg every 6 hours (with third-generation cephalosporin for PCN-resistant *Streptococcus pneumoniae*); maximum dose: 2-3 g/day

Prophylaxis for bacterial endocarditis:

Dental, oral, or upper respiratory tract surgery: 1 g 1 hour before surgery

GI/GU procedure: 1 g plus 1.5 mg/kg gentamicin 1 hour prior to surgery

Antibiotic lock technique (for catheter infections): 2 mg/mL in SWI/NS or D_5W; instill 3-5 mL into catheter port as a flush solution instead of heparin lock (**Note:** Do not mix with any other solutions)

Intrathecal: Vancomycin is available as a powder for injection and may be diluted to 1-5 mg/mL concentration in preservative-free 0.9% sodium chloride for administration into the CSF

Neonates: 5-10 mg/day

Children: 5-20 mg/day

Adults: Up to 20 mg/day

Oral: Pseudomembranous colitis produced by *C. difficile*:

Neonates: 10 mg/kg/day in divided doses

Children: 40 mg/kg/day in divided doses, added to fluids

Adults: 125 mg 4 times/day for 10 days

Dosage Forms

Capsule (Vancocin®): 125 mg, 250 mg

Infusion [premixed in iso-osmotic dextrose] (Vancocin®): 500 mg (100 mL); 1 g (200 mL)

Injection, powder for reconstitution: 500 mg, 1 g, 5 g, 10 g

vancomycin hydrochloride *see* vancomycin *on previous page*

Vandazole™ [US] *see* metronidazole *on page 551*

Vanex Forte™-D *(Discontinued)* *see* chlorpheniramine, phenylephrine, and methscopolamine *on page 180*

Vanex-HD® *(Discontinued)* *see* phenylephrine, hydrocodone, and chlorpheniramine *on page 663*

Vaniqa™ [US/Can] *see* eflornithine *on page 288*

Vanos™ [US] *see* fluocinonide *on page 353*

Vanoxide® *(Discontinued)* *see* benzoyl peroxide *on page 102*

Vanoxide-HC® [US/Can] *see* benzoyl peroxide and hydrocortisone *on page 104*

Vanquish® Extra Strength Pain Reliever [US-OTC] *see* acetaminophen, aspirin, and caffeine *on page 10*

Vansil™ *(Discontinued)*

Vantin® [US/Can] *see* cefpodoxime *on page 160*

Vaponefrin® *(Discontinued)* *see* epinephrine *on page 295*

Vaprisol® [US] *see* conivaptan *on page 213*

VAQTA® [US/Can] *see* hepatitis A vaccine *on page 410*

vardenafil (var DEN a fil)

Sound-Alike/Look-Alike Issues

Levitra® may be confused with Lexiva™

Synonyms vardenafil hydrochloride

U.S./Canadian Brand Names Levitra® [US/Can]

Therapeutic Category Phosphodiesterase (Type 5) Enzyme Inhibitor

Use Treatment of erectile dysfunction

Usual Dosage Oral: Adults: Erectile dysfunction: 10 mg 60 minutes prior to sexual activity; dosing range: 5-20 mg; to be given as one single dose and not given more than once daily

Dosing adjustment with concomitant medications:

Alpha blocker (dose should be stable at time of vardenafil initiation): Initial vardenafil dose: 5 mg/24 hours; if an alpha blocker is added to vardenafil therapy, it should be initiated at the smallest possible dose, and titrated carefully.

Erythromycin: Maximum vardenafil dose: 5 mg/24 hours

Indinavir: Maximum vardenafil dose: 2.5 mg/24 hours

Itraconazole:

200 mg/day: Maximum vardenafil dose: 5 mg/24 hours

400 mg/day: Maximum vardenafil dose: 2.5 mg/24 hours

Ketoconazole:

200 mg/day: Maximum vardenafil dose: 5 mg/24 hours

400 mg/day: Maximum vardenafil dose: 2.5 mg/24 hours

Ritonavir: Maximum vardenafil dose: 2.5 mg/72 hours

Dosage Forms Tablet: 2.5 mg, 5 mg, 10 mg, 20 mg

vardenafil hydrochloride *see* vardenafil *on this page*

varenicline (var e NI kleen)

Synonyms varenicline tartrate

U.S./Canadian Brand Names Chantix™ [US]

Therapeutic Category Partial Nicotine Agonist

Use Treatment to aid in smoking cessation

Usual Dosage Oral: Adults:

Initial:

Days 1-3: 0.5 mg once daily

Days 4-7: 0.5 mg twice daily

Maintenance (week 2-12): 1 mg twice daily

Note: Start 1 week before target quit date. Patients who cannot tolerate adverse events may require temporary reduction in dose. If patient successfully quits smoking during the 12 weeks, may continue for another 12 weeks to help maintain success. If not successful in first 12 weeks, then stop medication and reassess factors contributing to failure.

Dosage Forms

Tablet, as tartrate:

Chantix™: 0.5 mg, 1 mg

varenicline tartrate *see* varenicline *on this page*

varicella, measles, mumps, and rubella vaccine *see* measles, mumps, rubella, and varicella virus vaccine *on page 521*

varicella virus vaccine (var i SEL a VYE rus vak SEEN)

Sound-Alike/Look-Alike Issues

varicella virus vaccine has been given in error (instead of the indicated varicella immune globulin) to pregnant women exposed to varicella

(Continued)

varicella virus vaccine *(Continued)*

Synonyms chicken pox vaccine; varicella-zoster virus (VZV) vaccine (varicella); VZV vaccine (varicella)

U.S./Canadian Brand Names Varilrix® [Can]; Varivax® III [Can]; Varivax® [US]

Therapeutic Category Vaccine, Live Virus

Use Immunization against varicella in children ≥12 months of age and adults

Usual Dosage SubQ:

Children 12 months to 12 years: 0.5 mL; a second dose may be administered ≥3 months later

Children ≥13 years to Adults: 2 doses of 0.5 mL separated by 4-8 weeks

Dosage Forms [CAN] = Canadian brand name

Injection, powder for reconstitution [preservative free]:

Varivax®: 1350 plaque-forming units (PFU) [contains gelatin and trace amounts of neomycin; packaged with diluent]

Varivax® III [CAN]: 1350 plaque-forming units (PFU) [contains gelatin and trace amounts of neomycin; packaged with diluent; not available in U.S.]

Injection, powder for reconstitution (Valrilix® [CAN]): $10^{3.3}$ plaque-forming units (PFU) [contains albumin and gelatin; packaged with diluent; not available in U.S.]

varicella-zoster virus (VZV) vaccine (varicella) *see* varicella virus vaccine *on previous page*

varicella-zoster (VZV) vaccine (zoster) *see* zoster vaccine *on page 891*

Varilrix® [Can] *see* varicella virus vaccine *on previous page*

Varivax® [US] *see* varicella virus vaccine *on previous page*

Varivax® III [Can] *see* varicella virus vaccine *on previous page*

Vascoray® [US] *see* radiological/contrast media (ionic) *on page 728*

Vaseretic® [US/Can] *see* enalapril and hydrochlorothiazide *on page 292*

VasoClear® *(Discontinued)* *see* naphazoline *on page 577*

Vasocon® [Can] *see* naphazoline *on page 577*

Vasocon®-A *(Discontinued)*

Vasocon Regular® Ophthalmic *(Discontinued)* *see* naphazoline *on page 577*

Vasodilan® *(Discontinued)* *see* isoxsuprine *on page 466*

Vasophrinic DH [Can] *see* pseudoephedrine, hydrocodone, and chlorpheniramine *on page 716*

vasopressin (vay soe PRES in)

Sound-Alike/Look-Alike Issues

Pitressin® may be confused with Pitocin®

Synonyms ADH; antidiuretic hormone; 8-arginine vasopressin

U.S./Canadian Brand Names Pitressin® [US]; Pressyn® AR [Can]; Pressyn® [Can]

Therapeutic Category Hormone, Posterior Pituitary

Use Treatment of diabetes insipidus; prevention and treatment of postoperative abdominal distention; differential diagnosis of diabetes insipidus

Usual Dosage

Diabetes insipidus (highly variable dosage; titrated based on serum and urine sodium and osmolality in addition to fluid balance and urine output):

I.M., SubQ:

Children: 2.5-10 units 2-4 times/day as needed

Adults: 5-10 units 2-4 times/day as needed (dosage range 5-60 units/day)

Continuous I.V. infusion: Children and Adults: 0.5 milliunit/kg/hour (0.0005 unit/kg/hour); double dosage as needed every 30 minutes to a maximum of 0.01 unit/kg/hour

Intranasal: Administer on cotton pledget, as nasal spray, or by dropper

Abdominal distention: Adults: I.M.: 5 units stat, 10 units every 3-4 hours

Dosage Forms

Injection, solution: 20 units/mL (0.5 mL, 1 mL, 10 mL)

Pitressin®: 20 units/mL (1 mL)

Vasotec® [US/Can] *see* enalapril *on page 291*

Vaxigrip® [Can] *see* influenza virus vaccine *on page 448*

VCF™ [US-OTC] *see* nonoxynol 9 *on page 597*

VCR *see* vincristine *on page 873*

Vectrin® *(Discontinued)* *see* minocycline *on page 558*

vecuronium (vek ue ROE nee um)

Sound-Alike/Look-Alike Issues

vecuronium may be confused with vancomycin

Norcuron® may be confused with Narcan®

Synonyms ORG NC 45

Therapeutic Category Skeletal Muscle Relaxant

Use Adjunct to general anesthesia to facilitate endotracheal intubation and to relax skeletal muscles during surgery; to facilitate mechanical ventilation in ICU patients; does not relieve pain or produce sedation

Usual Dosage Administer I.V.; dose to effect; doses will vary due to interpatient variability; use ideal body weight for obese patients

Surgery:

Neonates: 0.1 mg/kg/dose; maintenance: 0.03-0.15 mg/kg every 1-2 hours as needed

Infants >7 weeks to 1 year: Initial: 0.08-0.1 mg/kg/dose; maintenance: 0.05-0.1 mg/kg every 60 minutes as needed

Children >1 year and Adults: Initial: 0.08-0.1 mg/kg or 0.04-0.06 mg/kg after initial dose of succinylcholine for intubation; maintenance: 0.01-0.015 mg/kg 25-40 minutes after initial dose, then 0.01-0.015 mg/kg every 12-15 minutes (higher doses will allow less frequent maintenance doses); may be administered as a continuous infusion at 0.8-2 mcg/kg/minute

Pretreatment/priming: Adults: 10% of intubating dose given 3-5 minutes before initial dose

ICU: Adults: 0.05-0.1 mg/kg bolus followed by 0.8-1.7 mcg/kg/minute once initial recovery from bolus observed or 0.1-0.2 mg/kg/dose every 1 hour

Note: Children (1-10 years) may require slightly higher initial doses and slightly more frequent supplementation; infants >7 weeks to 1 year may be more sensitive to vecuronium and have a longer recovery time

Dosage Forms Injection, powder for reconstitution, as bromide: 10 mg, 20 mg [may be supplied with diluent containing benzyl alcohol]

Veetids® [US] *see* penicillin V potassium *on page 649*

Veg-Pancreatin 4X [US-OTC] *see* pancreatin *on page 633*

Velban® *(Discontinued)* *see* vinblastine *on page 873*

Velcade® [US/Can] *see* bortezomib *on page 114*

Velivet™ [US] *see* ethinyl estradiol and desogestrel *on page 317*

Velosulin® BR (Buffered) *(Discontinued)*

venlafaxine (ven la FAX een)

U.S./Canadian Brand Names Effexor® XR [US/Can]; Effexor® [US]

Therapeutic Category Antidepressant, Phenethylamine

Use Treatment of major depressive disorder; generalized anxiety disorder (GAD), social anxiety disorder (social phobia); panic disorder

Usual Dosage Oral: Adults:

Depression:

Immediate-release tablets: 75 mg/day, administered in 2 or 3 divided doses, taken with food; dose may be increased in 75 mg/day increments at intervals of at least 4 days, up to 225-375 mg/day

Extended-release capsules: 75 mg once daily taken with food; for some new patients, it may be desirable to start at 37.5 mg/day for 4-7 days before increasing to 75 mg once daily; dose may be increased by up to 75 mg/day increments every 4 days as tolerated, up to a maximum of 225 mg/day

GAD, social anxiety disorder: Extended-release capsules: 75 mg once daily taken with food; for some new patients, it may be desirable to start at 37.5 mg/day for 4-7 days before increasing to 75 mg once daily; dose may be increased by up to 75 mg/day increments every 4 days as tolerated, up to a maximum of 225 mg/day

Panic disorder: Extended-release capsules: 37.5 mg once daily for 1 week; may increase to 75 mg daily, with subsequent weekly increases of 75 mg/day up to a maximum of 225 mg/day.

Note: When discontinuing this medication after more than 1 week of treatment, it is generally recommended that the dose be tapered. If venlafaxine is used for 6 weeks or longer, the dose should be tapered over 2 weeks when discontinuing its use.

Dosage Forms

Capsule, extended release:

Effexor® XR: 37.5 mg, 75 mg, 150 mg

Tablet: 25 mg, 37.5 mg, 50 mg, 75 mg, 100 mg

Effexor®: 25 mg, 37.5 mg, 50 mg, 75 mg, 100 mg

Venofer® [US/Can] *see* iron sucrose *on page 463*

Venoglobulin®-I *(Discontinued)* *see* immune globulin (intravenous) *on page 444*

Venoglobulin®-S *(Discontinued)* *see* immune globulin (intravenous) *on page 444*

Ventavis™ [US] *see* iloprost *on page 440*

Ventolin® [Can] *see* albuterol *on page 23*

Ventolin® *(Discontinued)* *see* albuterol *on page 23*

Ventolin® Diskus [Can] *see* albuterol *on page 23*

Ventolin® HFA [US/Can] *see* albuterol *on page 23*

Ventolin® Inhaler Aerosol *(Discontinued)* *see* albuterol *on page 23*

Ventrodisk [Can] *see* albuterol *on page 23*

VePesid® [US/Can] *see* etoposide *on page 330*

Veracolate [US-OTC] *see* bisacodyl *on page 111*

verapamil (ver AP a mil)

Sound-Alike/Look-Alike Issues

verapamil may be confused with Verelan®
Calan® may be confused with Colace®
Covera-HS® may be confused with Provera®
Isoptin® may be confused with Isopto® Tears
Verelan® may be confused with verapamil, Virilon®, Voltaren®

Synonyms iproveratril hydrochloride; verapamil hydrochloride

U.S./Canadian Brand Names Alti-Verapamil [Can]; Apo-Verap® SR [Can]; Apo-Verap® [Can]; Calan® SR [US]; Calan® [US/Can]; Chronovera® [Can]; Covera-HS® [US/Can]; Covera® [Can]; Gen-Verapamil SR [Can]; Gen-Verapamil [Can]; Isoptin® SR [US/Can]; Novo-Veramil SR [Can]; Nu-Verap [Can]; Riva-Verapamil SR [Can]; Verapamil Hydrochloride Injection, USP [Can]; Verelan® PM [US]; Verelan® [US]

Therapeutic Category Antiarrhythmic Agent, Class IV; Calcium Channel Blocker

Use Orally for treatment of angina pectoris (vasospastic, chronic stable, unstable) and hypertension; I.V. for supraventricular tachyarrhythmias (PSVT, atrial fibrillation, atrial flutter)

Usual Dosage

Children: SVT:
- I.V.:
  - <1 year: 0.1-0.2 mg/kg over 2 minutes; repeat every 30 minutes as needed
  - 1-15 years: 0.1-0.3 mg/kg over 2 minutes; maximum: 5 mg/dose, may repeat dose in 15 minutes if adequate response not achieved; maximum for second dose: 10 mg/dose
- Oral (dose not well established):
  - 1-5 years: 4-8 mg/kg/day in 3 divided doses **or** 40-80 mg every 8 hours
  - >5 years: 80 mg every 6-8 hours

Adults:
- SVT: I.V.: 2.5-5 mg (over 2 minutes); second dose of 5-10 mg (~0.15 mg/kg) may be given 15-30 minutes after the initial dose if patient tolerates, but does not respond to initial dose; maximum total dose: 20 mg
- Angina: Oral: Initial dose: 80-120 mg 3 times/day (elderly or small stature: 40 mg 3 times/day); range: 240-480 mg/day in 3-4 divided doses
- Hypertension: Oral:
  - Immediate release: 80 mg 3 times/day; usual dose range (JNC 7): 80-320 mg/day in 2 divided doses
  - Sustained release: 240 mg/day; usual dose range (JNC 7): 120-360 mg/day in 1-2 divided doses; 120 mg/day in the elderly or small patients (no evidence of additional benefit in doses >360 mg/day).
  - Extended release:
    - Covera-HS®: Usual dose range (JNC 7): 120-360 mg once daily (once-daily dosing is recommended at bedtime)
    - Verelan® PM: Usual dose range: 200-400 mg once daily at bedtime

Dosage Forms

Caplet, sustained release: 120 mg, 180 mg, 240 mg
- Calan® SR: 120 mg, 180 mg, 240 mg

Capsule, extended release, controlled onset, as hydrochloride:
- Verelan® PM: 100 mg, 200 mg, 300 mg

Capsule, sustained release, as hydrochloride: 120 mg, 180 mg, 240 mg, 360 mg
- Verelan®: 120 mg, 180 mg, 240 mg, 360 mg

Injection, solution, as hydrochloride: 2.5 mg/mL (2 mL, 4 mL)

Tablet, as hydrochloride: 80 mg, 120 mg

Calan®: 40 mg, 80 mg, 120 mg
Tablet, extended release: 120 mg, 180 mg, 240 mg
Tablet, extended release, controlled onset, as hydrochloride:
Covera-HS®: 180 mg, 240 mg
Tablet, sustained release, as hydrochloride: 120 mg, 180 mg, 240 mg
Isoptin® SR: 120 mg, 180 mg, 240 mg

verapamil and trandolapril *see* trandolapril and verapamil *on page 842*

verapamil hydrochloride *see* verapamil *on previous page*

Verapamil Hydrochloride Injection, USP [Can] *see* verapamil *on previous page*

Verazinc® Oral *(Discontinued)* *see* zinc sulfate *on page 888*

Verelan® [US] *see* verapamil *on previous page*

Verelan® PM [US] *see* verapamil *on previous page*

Vergogel® Gel *(Discontinued)* *see* salicylic acid *on page 758*

Vergon® *(Discontinued)* *see* meclizine *on page 522*

Vermox® [Can] *see* mebendazole *on page 521*

Vermox® *(Discontinued)* *see* mebendazole *on page 521*

Versed® *(Discontinued)* *see* midazolam *on page 555*

Versel® [Can] *see* selenium sulfide *on page 767*

Versiclear™ [US] *see* sodium thiosulfate *on page 783*

verteporfin (ver te POR fin)

U.S./Canadian Brand Names Visudyne® [US/Can]

Therapeutic Category Ophthalmic Agent

Use Treatment of predominantly classic subfoveal choroidal neovascularization due to macular degeneration, presumed ocular histoplasmosis, or pathologic myopia

Usual Dosage Therapy is a two-step process; first the infusion of verteporfin, then the activation of verteporfin with a nonthermal diode laser.

Adults: I.V.: 6 mg/m^2 body surface area

Note: Treatment in more than one eye: Patients who have lesions in both eyes should be evaluated and treatment should first be done to the more aggressive lesion. Following safe and acceptable treatment, the second eye can be treated one week later. Patients who have had previous verteporfin therapy, with an acceptable safety profile, may then have both eyes treated concurrently. Treat the more aggressive lesion followed immediately with the second eye. The light treatment to the second eye should begin no later than 20 minutes from the start of the infusion.

Dosage Forms Injection, powder for reconstitution: 15 mg [contains egg phosphatidylglycerol]

Verukan® Solution *(Discontinued)* *see* salicylic acid *on page 758*

Vesanoid® [US/Can] *see* tretinoin (oral) *on page 844*

VESIcare® [US] *see* solifenacin *on page 784*

Vexol® [US/Can] *see* rimexolone *on page 747*

VFEND® [US/Can] *see* voriconazole *on page 880*

Viactiv® Multivitamin [US-OTC] *see* vitamins (multiple/oral) *on page 878*

Viadur® [US/Can] *see* leuprolide *on page 486*

Viagra® [US/Can] *see* sildenafil *on page 771*

Vibramycin® [US] *see* doxycycline *on page 278*

Vibramycin® I.V. *(Discontinued)* *see* doxycycline *on page 278*

Vibra-Tabs® [US/Can] *see* doxycycline *on page 278*

Vicks® 44® Cough Relief [US-OTC] *see* dextromethorphan *on page 245*

Vicks® 44D Cough & Head Congestion [US-OTC] *see* pseudoephedrine and dextromethorphan *on page 714*

Vicks® 44E [US-OTC] *see* guaifenesin and dextromethorphan *on page 394*

Vicks® 44® Non-Drowsy Cold & Cough Liqui-Caps *(Discontinued)* *see* pseudoephedrine and dextromethorphan *on page 714*

Vicks® Casero™ [US-OTC] *see* guaifenesin *on page 392*

Vicks® Children's Chloraseptic® *(Discontinued)* *see* benzocaine *on page 99*

Vicks® Children's NyQuil® [US-OTC] *see* chlorpheniramine, pseudoephedrine, and dextromethorphan *on page 182*

Vicks® Chloraseptic® Sore Throat *(Discontinued)* *see* benzocaine *on page 99*

Vicks® DayQuil® Multi-Symptom Cold and Flu [US-OTC] *see* acetaminophen, dextromethorphan, and pseudoephedrine *on page 12*

Vicks® DayQuil® Sinus Pressure & Congestion Relief *(Discontinued)*

Vicks® Formula 44® *(Discontinued)* *see* dextromethorphan *on page 245*

Vicks® Formula 44® Pediatric Formula *(Discontinued)* *see* dextromethorphan *on page 245*

Vicks® Pediatric 44®m [US-OTC] *see* chlorpheniramine, pseudoephedrine, and dextromethorphan *on page 182*

Vicks® Pediatric Formula 44E [US-OTC] *see* guaifenesin and dextromethorphan *on page 394*

Vicks Sinex® 12 Hour [US-OTC] *see* oxymetazoline *on page 628*

Vicks Sinex® 12 Hour Ultrafine Mist [US-OTC] *see* oxymetazoline *on page 628*

Vicks® Sinex® Nasal Spray [US-OTC] *see* phenylephrine *on page 660*

Vicks® Sinex® UltraFine Mist [US-OTC] *see* phenylephrine *on page 660*

Vicodin® [US] *see* hydrocodone and acetaminophen *on page 420*

Vicodin® ES [US] *see* hydrocodone and acetaminophen *on page 420*

Vicodin® HP [US] *see* hydrocodone and acetaminophen *on page 420*

Vicon Forte® [US] *see* vitamins (multiple/oral) *on page 878*

Vicoprofen® [US/Can] *see* hydrocodone and ibuprofen *on page 424*

Vi-Daylin® ADC *(Discontinued)* *see* vitamins (multiple/pediatric) *on page 878*

Vi-Daylin® ADC + Iron *(Discontinued)* *see* vitamins (multiple/pediatric) *on page 878*

Vi-Daylin® Drops *(Discontinued)* *see* vitamins (multiple/pediatric) *on page 878*

Vi-Daylin®/F ADC *(Discontinued)* *see* vitamins (multiple/pediatric) *on page 878*

Vi-Daylin®/F ADC + Iron *(Discontinued)* *see* vitamins (multiple/pediatric) *on page 878*

Vi-Daylin®/F *(Discontinued)* *see* vitamins (multiple/pediatric) *on page 878*

Vi-Daylin®/F + Iron *(Discontinued)* *see* vitamins (multiple/pediatric) *on page 878*

Vi-Daylin® + Iron Drops *(Discontinued)* *see* vitamins (multiple/pediatric) *on page 878*

Vi-Daylin® + Iron Liquid *(Discontinued)* *see* vitamins (multiple/oral) *on page 878*

Vi-Daylin® Liquid *(Discontinued)* *see* vitamins (multiple/oral) *on page 878*

Vidaza™ [US] *see* azacitidine *on page 86*

Videx® [US/Can] *see* didanosine *on page 252*

Videx® EC [US/Can] *see* didanosine *on page 252*

vigabatrin *(Canada only)* (vye GA ba trin)

U.S./Canadian Brand Names Sabril® [Can]

Therapeutic Category Anticonvulsant

Use Active management of partial or secondary generalized seizures not controlled by usual treatments; treatment of infantile spasms

Usual Dosage Oral:

Children: **Note:** Administer daily dose in 2 divided doses, especially in the higher dosage ranges:

Adjunctive treatment of seizures: Initial: 40 mg/kg/day; maintenance dosages based on patient weight:

10-15 kg: 0.5-1 g/day

16-30 kg: 1-1.5 g/day

31-50 kg: 1.5-3 g/day

>50 kg: 2-3 g/day

Infantile spasms: 50-100 mg/kg/day, depending on severity of symptoms; higher doses (up to 150 mg/kg/day) have been used in some cases.

Adults: Adjunctive treatment of seizures: Initial: 1 g/day (severe manifestations may require 2 g/day); dose may be given as a single daily dose or divided into 2 equal doses. Increase daily dose by 0.5 g based on response and tolerability. Optimal dose range: 2-3 g/day (maximum dose: 3 g/day)

Dosage Forms
Powder for oral suspension [sachets]: 0.5 g [contains povidone]
Tablet: 500 mg

Vigamox™ [US/Can] *see* moxifloxacin *on page 568*

vinblastine (vin BLAS teen)

Sound-Alike/Look-Alike Issues
vinBLAStine may be confused with vinCRIStine, vinorelbine
Synonyms NSC-49842; vinblastine sulfate; VLB
Tall-Man vin**BLAS**tine
Therapeutic Category Antineoplastic Agent
Use Treatment of Hodgkin and non-Hodgkin lymphoma, testicular, lung, head and neck, breast, and renal carcinomas, Mycosis fungoides, Kaposi sarcoma, histiocytosis, choriocarcinoma, and idiopathic thrombocytopenic purpura
Usual Dosage Refer to individual protocols.
Children and Adults: I.V.: 4-20 mg/m^2 (0.1-0.5 mg/kg) every 7-10 days **or** 5-day continuous infusion of 1.5-2 mg/m^2/day **or** 0.1-0.5 mg/kg/week
Dosage Forms
Injection, powder for reconstitution, as sulfate: 10 mg
Injection, solution, as sulfate: 1 mg/mL (10 mL) [contains benzyl alcohol]

vinblastine sulfate *see* vinblastine *on this page*

Vincasar PFS® [US/Can] *see* vincristine *on this page*

vincristine (vin KRIS teen)

Sound-Alike/Look-Alike Issues
vinCRIStine may be confused with vinBLAStine
Oncovin® may be confused with Ancobon®
Synonyms LCR; leurocristine sulfate; NSC-67574; VCR; vincristine sulfate
Tall-Man vin**CRIS**tine
U.S./Canadian Brand Names Vincasar PFS® [US/Can]
Therapeutic Category Antineoplastic Agent
Use Treatment of leukemias, Hodgkin disease, non-Hodgkin lymphomas, Wilms tumor, neuroblastoma, rhabdomyosarcoma
Usual Dosage Note: Doses are often capped at 2 mg; however, this may reduce the efficacy of the therapy and may not be advisable. Refer to individual protocols; orders for single doses >2.5 mg or >5 mg/treatment cycle should be verified with the specific treatment regimen and/or an experienced oncologist prior to dispensing. I.V.:

Children ≤10 kg or BSA <1 m^2: Initial therapy: 0.05 mg/kg once weekly then titrate dose
Children >10 kg or BSA ≥1 m^2: 1-2 mg/m^2, may repeat once weekly for 3-6 weeks; maximum single dose: 2 mg
Neuroblastoma: I.V. continuous infusion with doxorubicin: 1 mg/m^2/day for 72 hours
Adults: 0.4-1.4 mg/m^2, may repeat every week **or**
0.4-0.5 mg/day continuous infusion for 4 days every 4 weeks **or**
0.25-0.5 mg/m^2/day for 5 days every 4 weeks
Dosage Forms Injection, solution, as sulfate: 1 mg/mL (1 mL, 2 mL)

vincristine sulfate *see* vincristine *on this page*

vinorelbine (vi NOR el been)

Sound-Alike/Look-Alike Issues
vinorelbine may be confused with vinBLAStine
Synonyms dihydroxydeoxynorvinkaleukoblastine; NVB; vinorelbine tartrate
U.S./Canadian Brand Names Navelbine® [US/Can]; Vinorelbine Injection, USP [Can]; Vinorelbine Tartrate for Injection [Can]
Therapeutic Category Antineoplastic Agent
Use Treatment of nonsmall-cell lung cancer
Usual Dosage Refer to individual protocols.
Adults: I.V.:
Single-agent therapy: 30 mg/m^2 every 7 days
(Continued)

vinorelbine *(Continued)*

Combination therapy with cisplatin: 25 mg/m^2 every 7 days (with cisplatin 100 mg/m^2 every 4 weeks); **Alternatively:** 30 mg/m^2 in combination with cisplatin 120 mg/m^2 on days 1 and 29, then every 6 weeks

Dosage Forms Injection, solution [preservative free]: 10 mg/mL (1 mL, 5 mL)

Vinorelbine Injection, USP [Can] *see* vinorelbine *on previous page*

vinorelbine tartrate *see* vinorelbine *on previous page*

Vinorelbine Tartrate for Injection [Can] *see* vinorelbine *on previous page*

Viokase® [US/Can] *see* pancrelipase *on page 634*

viosterol *see* ergocalciferol *on page 301*

Vioxx® *(Discontinued)*

Viracept® [US/Can] *see* nelfinavir *on page 582*

Viramune® [US/Can] *see* nevirapine *on page 587*

Viravan® [US] *see* phenylephrine and pyrilamine *on page 662*

Viravan®-DM [US] *see* phenylephrine, pyrilamine, and dextromethorphan *on page 664*

Virazole® [US/Can] *see* ribavirin *on page 743*

Viread® [US/Can] *see* tenofovir *on page 810*

Virilon® [US] *see* methyltestosterone *on page 548*

Virilon® IM [Can] *see* testosterone *on page 812*

Viroptic® [US/Can] *see* trifluridine *on page 849*

Viscoat® [US] *see* chondroitin sulfate and sodium hyaluronate *on page 186*

Visicol® [US] *see* sodium phosphates *on page 781*

Visine-A™ [US-OTC] *see* naphazoline and pheniramine *on page 578*

Visine® Advanced Allergy [Can] *see* naphazoline and pheniramine *on page 578*

Visine® Advanced Relief [US-OTC] *see* tetrahydrozoline *on page 817*

Visine® L.R. [US-OTC] *see* oxymetazoline *on page 628*

Visine® Original [US-OTC] *see* tetrahydrozoline *on page 817*

Visken® [Can] *see* pindolol *on page 669*

Visken® *(Discontinued)* *see* pindolol *on page 669*

Vistacon-50® Injection *(Discontinued)* *see* hydroxyzine *on page 433*

Vistaquel® Injection *(Discontinued)* *see* hydroxyzine *on page 433*

Vistaril® [US/Can] *see* hydroxyzine *on page 433*

Vistazine® Injection *(Discontinued)* *see* hydroxyzine *on page 433*

Vistide® [US] *see* cidofovir *on page 188*

Visudyne® [US/Can] *see* verteporfin *on page 871*

Vita-C® [US-OTC] *see* ascorbic acid *on page 76*

Vitaball® [US-OTC] *see* vitamins (multiple/pediatric) *on page 878*

Vitaball® Wild 'N Fruity [US-OTC] *see* vitamins (multiple/pediatric) *on page 878*

VitaCarn® Oral *(Discontinued)* *see* levocarnitine *on page 488*

Vitacon Forte [US] *see* vitamins (multiple/oral) *on page 878*

Vital HN® [US-OTC] *see* nutritional formula, enteral/oral *on page 608*

vitamin C *see* ascorbic acid *on page 76*

vitamin D_2 *see* ergocalciferol *on page 301*

vitamin D_3 *see* alendronate and cholecalciferol *on page 27*

vitamin A (VYE ta min aye)

Sound-Alike/Look-Alike Issues

Aquasol® may be confused with Anusol®

Synonyms oleovitamin A

U.S./Canadian Brand Names Aquasol A® [US]; Palmitate-A® [US-OTC]

Therapeutic Category Vitamin, Fat Soluble

Use Treatment and prevention of vitamin A deficiency; parenteral (I.M.) route is indicated when oral administration is not feasible or when absorption is insufficient (malabsorption syndrome)

Usual Dosage

RDA:

- <1 year: 375 mcg
- 1-3 years: 400 mcg
- 4-6 years: 500 mcg*
- 7-10 years: 700 mcg*
- >10 years: 800-1000 mcg*
- Male: 1000 mcg
- Female: 800 mcg
- * mcg retinol equivalent (0.3 mcg retinol = 1 unit vitamin A)

Vitamin A supplementation in measles (recommendation of the World Health Organization): Children: Oral: Administer as a single dose; repeat the next day and at 4 weeks for children with ophthalmologic evidence of vitamin A deficiency:

- 6 months to 1 year: 100,000 units
- >1 year: 200,000 units

Note: Use of vitamin A in measles is recommended only for patients 6 months to 2 years of age hospitalized with measles and its complications **or** patients >6 months of age who have any of the following risk factors and who are not already receiving vitamin A: immunodeficiency, ophthalmologic evidence of vitamin A deficiency including night blindness, Bitot spots or evidence of xerophthalmia, impaired intestinal absorption, moderate to severe malnutrition including that associated with eating disorders, or recent immigration from areas where high mortality rates from measles have been observed

Note: Monitor patients closely; dosages >25,000 units/kg have been associated with toxicity

Severe deficiency with xerophthalmia: Oral:

- Children 1-8 years: 5000-10,000 units/kg/day for 5 days or until recovery occurs
- Children >8 years and Adults: 500,000 units/day for 3 days, then 50,000 units/day for 14 days, then 10,000-20,000 units/day for 2 months

Deficiency (without corneal changes): Oral:

- Infants <1 year: 100,000 units every 4-6 months
- Children 1-8 years: 200,000 units every 4-6 months
- Children >8 years and Adults: 100,000 units/day for 3 days then 50,000 units/day for 14 days

Deficiency: I.M.: **Note:** I.M. route is indicated when oral administration is not feasible or when absorption is insufficient (malabsorption syndrome):

- Infants: 7500-15,000 units/day for 10 days
- Children 1-8 years: 17,500-35,000 units/day for 10 days
- Children >8 years and Adults: 100,000 units/day for 3 days, followed by 50,000 units/day for 2 weeks

Note: Follow-up therapy with an oral therapeutic multivitamin (containing additional vitamin A) is recommended:

- Low Birth Weight Infants: Additional vitamin A is recommended, however, no dosage amount has been established
- Children ≤8 years: 5000-10,000 units/day
- Children >8 years and Adults: 10,000-20,000 units/day

Malabsorption syndrome (prophylaxis): Children >8 years and Adults: Oral: 10,000-50,000 units/day of water miscible product

Dietary supplement: Oral:

- Infants up to 6 months: 1500 units/day
- Children:
  - 6 months to 3 years: 1500-2000 units/day
  - 4-6 years: 2500 units/day
  - 7-10 years: 3300-3500 units/day
- Children >10 years and Adults: 4000-5000 units/day

Dosage Forms

Capsule [softgel]: 10,000 units; 25,000 units

Injection, solution (Aquasol A®): 50,000 units/mL (2 mL) [contains polysorbate 80]

Tablet (Palmitate-A®): 5000 units, 15,000 units

vitamin A acid *see* tretinoin (topical) *on page 844*

vitamin A and vitamin D (VYE ta min aye & VYE ta min dee)

Synonyms cod liver oil

U.S./Canadian Brand Names A and D® Original [US-OTC]; Baza® Clear [US-OTC]; Sween Cream® [US-OTC]

Therapeutic Category Protectant, Topical

Use Temporary relief of discomfort due to chapped skin, diaper rash, minor burns, abrasions, as well as irritations associated with ostomy skin care

Usual Dosage Topical: Apply locally with gentle massage as needed

Dosage Forms

Capsule, softgel: Vitamin A 1250 int. units and vitamin D 135 int. units; vitamin A 1250 int. units and vitamin D 130 int. units; vitamin A 5,000 int. units and vitamin D 400 int. units; vitamin A 10,000 int. units and vitamin D 400 int. units; vitamin A 10,000 int. units and vitamin D 5000 int. units; vitamin A 25,000 int. units and vitamin D 1000 int. units

Cream:

Sween Cream®: 2 g, 85 g, 184 g, 339 g [original]

Sween Cream®: 57 g, 142 g [fresh scent]

Sween Cream®: 57 g [fragrance free]

Ointment: 0.9 g, 5 g, 60 g, 120 g, 454 g [in lanolin-petrolatum base]

A and D® Original: 45 g, 120 g, 454 g

Baza® Clear: 50 g, 150 g, 240 g

Tablet: Vitamin A 10,000 int. units and vitamin D 400 int. units

vitamin B_1 *see* thiamine *on page 821*

vitamin B_2 *see* riboflavin *on page 744*

vitamin B_3 *see* niacin *on page 588*

vitamin B_3 *see* niacinamide *on page 589*

vitamin B_5 *see* pantothenic acid *on page 637*

vitamin B_6 *see* pyridoxine *on page 721*

vitamin B_{12} *see* cyanocobalamin *on page 219*

vitamin B complex combinations (VYE ta min bee KOM pleks kom bi NAY shuns)

Sound-Alike/Look-Alike Issues

Nephrocaps® may be confused with Nephro-Calci®

Surbex® may be confused with Sebex®, Suprax®, Surfak®

Synonyms B complex combinations; B vitamin combinations

U.S./Canadian Brand Names Allbee® C-800 + Iron [US-OTC]; Allbee® C-800 [US-OTC]; Allbee® with C [US-OTC]; Apatate® [US-OTC]; DiatxFe™ [US]; Diatx™ [US]; Gevrabon® [US-OTC]; NephPlex® Rx [US]; Nephro-Vite® Rx [US]; Nephro-Vite® [US]; Nephrocaps® [US]; Nephron FA® [US]; Stresstabs® B-Complex + Iron [US-OTC]; Stresstabs® B-Complex + Zinc [US-OTC]; Stresstabs® B-Complex [US-OTC]; Surbex-T® [US-OTC]; Trinsicon® [US]; Z-Bec® [US-OTC]

Therapeutic Category Vitamin, Water Soluble

Use Supplement for use in the wasting syndrome in chronic renal failure, uremia, impaired metabolic functions of the kidney, dialysis; labeled for OTC use as a dietary supplement

Usual Dosage Oral: Adults:

Dietary supplement: One tablet daily

Apatate® liquid: One teaspoonful daily, 1 hour prior to mid-day meal

Gevrabon® liquid: Two tablespoonsful (30 mL) once daily; shake well before use

Renal patients: One tablet or capsule daily between meals; take after treatment if on dialysis

Nephron FA®: Two tablets once daily, between meals

Dosage Forms Content varies depending on product used. For more detailed information on ingredients in these and other multivitamins, please refer to Vitamin Products on page 1010.

vitamin E (VYE ta min ee)

Sound-Alike/Look-Alike Issues

Aquasol E® may be confused with Anusol®

Synonyms *d*-alpha tocopherol; *dl*-alpha tocopherol

U.S./Canadian Brand Names Alph-E [US-OTC]; Alph-E-Mixed [US-OTC]; Aquasol E® [US-OTC]; Aquavit-E® [US-OTC]; d-Alpha-Gems™ [US-OTC]; E-Gems Elite® [US-OTC]; E-Gems Plus® [US-OTC]; E-Gems® [US-OTC]; Ester-E™ [US-OTC]; Gamma E-Gems® [US-OTC]; Gamma-E Plus [US-OTC]; High Gamma Vitamin E Complete™ [US-OTC]; Key-E® Kaps [US-OTC]; Key-E® [US-OTC]

Therapeutic Category Vitamin, Fat Soluble; Vitamin, Topical

Use Dietary supplement

Usual Dosage Vitamin E may be expressed as alpha-tocopherol equivalents (ATE), which refer to the biologically active (R) stereoisomer content. Oral:

Recommended daily allowance (RDA):

Infants (adequate intake; RDA not establshed):

≤6 months: 4 mg

7-12 months: 6 mg

Children:

1-3 years: 6 mg; upper limit of intake should not exceed 200 mg/day

4-8 years: 7 mg; upper limit of intake should not exceed 300 mg/day

9-13 years: 11 mg; upper limit of intake should not exceed 600 mg/day

14-18 years: 15 mg; upper limit of intake should not exceed 800 mg/day

Adults: 15 mg; upper limit of intake should not exceed 1000 mg/day

Pregnant female:

≤18 years: 15 mg; upper level of intake should not exceed 800 mg/day

19-50 years: 15 mg; upper level of intake should not exceed 1000 mg/day

Lactating female:

≤18 years: 19 mg; upper level of intake should not exceed 800 mg/day

19-50 years: 19 mg; upper level of intake should not exceed 1000 mg/day

Vitamin E deficiency:

Children (with malabsorption syndrome): 1 unit/kg/day of water miscible vitamin E (to raise plasma tocopherol concentrations to the normal range within 2 months and to maintain normal plasma concentrations)

Adults: 60-75 units/day

Prevention of vitamin E deficiency: Adults: 30 units/day

Cystic fibrosis, beta-thalassemia, sickle cell anemia may require higher daily maintenance doses:

Children:

Cystic fibrosis: 100-400 units/day

Beta-thalassemia: 750 units/day

Adults: Sickle cell: 450 units/day

Dosage Forms

Capsule: 400 int. units, 1000 int. units

Key-E® Kaps: 200 int. units, 400 int. units

Capsule, softgel: 200 int. units, 400 int. units, 600 int. units, 1000 int. units

Alph-E: 200 int. units, 400 int. units

Alph-E-Mixed: 200 int. units [contains mixed tocopherols]; 400 int. units [contains mixed tocopherols], 1000 int. units [sugar free; contains mixed tocopherols]

Aqua Gem E®: 200 units, 400 units

d-Alpha-Gems™: 400 int. units [derived from soybean oil]

E-Gems®: 30 int. units, 100 int. units, 200 int. units, 400 int. units, 600 int. units, 800 int. units, 1000 int. units, 1200 int. units [derived from soybean oil]

E-Gems Plus®: 200 int. units, 400 int. units, 800 int. units [contains mixed tocopherols]

E-Gems Elite®: 400 int. units [contains mixed tocopherols]

Ester-E™: 400 int. units

Gamma E-Gems®: 90 int. units [also contains mixed tocopherols]

Gamma-E Plus: 200 int. units [contains soybean oil]

High Gamma Vitamin E Complete™: 200 int. units [contains soybean oil, mixed tocopherols]

Cream: 50 int. units/g (60 g), 100 int. units/g (60 g), 1000 int. units/120 g (120 g), 30,000 int. units/57 g (57 g)

Key-E®: 30 int. units/g (60 g, 120 g, 600 g)

Lip balm (E-Gem® Lip Care): 1000 int. units/tube [contains vitamin A and aloe]

Oil, oral/topical: 100 int. units/0.25 mL (60 mL, 75 mL); 1150 units/0.25 mL (30 mL, 60 mL, 120 mL); 28,000 int. units/30 mL (30 mL)

Alph-E: 28,000 int. units/30 mL (30 mL) [topical]

E-Gems®: 100 units/10 drops (15 mL, 60 mL)

Ointment, topical (Key-E®): 30 units/g (60 g, 120 g, 480 g)

Powder (Key-E®): 700 int. units per 1/4 teaspoon (15 g, 75 g, 1000 g) [derived from soybean oil]

Solution, oral drops: 15 int. units/0.3 mL (30 mL)

Aquasol E®: 15 int. units/0.3 mL (12 mL, 30 mL) [latex free]

Aquavit-E: 15 int. units/0.3 mL (30 mL) [butterscotch flavor]

Suppository, rectal/vaginal (Key-E®): 30 int. units (12s, 24s) [contains coconut oil]

Tablet: 100 int. units, 200 int. units, 400 int. units, 500 int. units

Key-E®: 200 int. units, 400 int. units

vitamin G *see* riboflavin *on page 744*

vitamin K$_1$ *see* phytonadione *on page 667*

vitamins (multiple/injectable) (VYE ta mins, MUL ti pul/in JEK ti bal)

U.S./Canadian Brand Names Infuvite® Adult [US]; Infuvite® Pediatric [US]; M.V.I. Adult™ [US]; M.V.I® Pediatric [US]

Therapeutic Category Vitamin

Use Nutritional supplement in patients receiving parenteral nutrition or requiring intravenous administration

Usual Dosage I.V.: Not for direct infusion

Children: ≥3 kg to 11 years: Pediatric formulation: 5 mL/day added to TPN or ≥100 mL of appropriate solution

Children >11 years and Adults: Adult formulation: 10 mL/day added to TPN or ≥500 mL of appropriate solution

Dosage Forms Content varies depending on product used. For more detailed information on ingredients in these and other multivitamins, please refer to Vitamin Products on page 1010.

vitamins (multiple/oral) (VYE ta mins, MUL ti pul/OR al)

Sound-Alike/Look-Alike Issues

Theragran® may be confused with Phenergan®

Synonyms multiple vitamins; therapeutic multivitamins; vitamins, multiple (oral); vitamins, multiple (therapeutic); vitamins, multiple with iron

U.S./Canadian Brand Names Centrum® Performance™ [US-OTC]; Centrum® Silver® [US-OTC]; Centrum® [US-OTC]; FemTabs® [US]; Geriation [US-OTC]; Geritol Complete® [US-OTC]; Geritol Extend® [US-OTC]; Geritol® Tonic [US-OTC]; Glutofac®-MX [US]; Glutofac®-ZX [US]; Gynovite® Plus [US-OTC]; Hemocyte Plus® [US]; Hi-Kovite [US-OTC] ; Iberet® [US-OTC]; Iberet®-500 [US-OTC]; Monocaps [US-OTC]; Multiret Folic 500 [US]; Ocuvite® Extra® [US-OTC]; Ocuvite® Lutein [US-OTC]; Ocuvite® [US-OTC]; Olay® Vitamins Complete Women's 50+[US-OTC]; Olay® Vitamins Complete Women's [US-OTC]; Olay® Vitamins Even Complexion [US-OTC]; One-A-Day® 50 Plus Formula [US-OTC]; One-A-Day® Active Formula [US-OTC]; One-A-Day® Carb Smart [US-OTC]; One-A-Day® Cholesterol Plus™ [US-OTC]; One-A-Day® Essential Formula [US-OTC]; One-A-Day® Maximum Formula [US-OTC]; One-A-Day® Men's Formula [US-OTC]; One-A-Day® Today [US-OTC]; One-A-Day® Weight Smart [US-OTC] ; One-A-Day® Women's Formula [US-OTC]; Optivite® P.M.T. [US-OTC]; PreserVision® AREDS [US-OTC]; PreserVision® Lutein [US-OTC]; Quintabs [US-OTC]; Quintabs-M [US-OTC]; Replace with Iron [US-OTC]; Replace [US-OTC]; Repliva 21/7™ [US]; Strovite® Forte [US]; T-Vites [US-OTC]; Ultra Freeda Iron Free [US-OTC]; Ultra Freeda with Iron [US-OTC]; Unicap M® [US-OTC]; Unicap Sr® [US-OTC]; Unicap T™ [US-OTC]; Viactiv® Multivitamin [US-OTC]; Vicon Forte® [US]; Vitacon Forte [US]; Xtramins [US-OTC]

Therapeutic Category Vitamin

Use Prevention/treatment of vitamin and mineral deficiencies; labeled for OTC use as a dietary supplement

Usual Dosage Oral: Adults: Daily dose of adult preparations varies by product. Generally, 1 tablet or capsule or 5-15 mL of liquid per day. Consult package labeling. Prescription doses may be higher for burn or cystic fibrosis patients.

Dosage Forms Content varies depending on product used. For more detailed information on ingredients in these and other multivitamins, please refer to Vitamin Products on page 1010.

vitamins, multiple (oral) *see* vitamins (multiple/oral) *on this page*

vitamins (multiple/pediatric) (VYE ta mins, MUL ti pul/pe de AT rik)

Synonyms children's vitamins; multivitamins/fluoride

U.S./Canadian Brand Names ADEKs [US-OTC]; Centrum® Kids Jimmy Neutron® Complete [US-OTC]; Centrum® Kids Jimmy Neutron® Extra C [US-OTC]; Centrum® Kids Rugrats™ Complete [US-OTC]; Centrum® Kids Rugrats™ Extra C [US-OTC]; Centrum® Kids Rugrats™ Extra Calcium [US-OTC]; Flintstones® Complete [US-OTC]; Flintstones® Plus Calcium [US-OTC]; Flintstones® Plus Extra C [US-OTC]; Flintstones® Plus Iron [US-OTC]; My First Flintstones® [US-OTC]; One-A-Day® Kids Bugs Bunny and Friends Complete [US-OTC]; One-A-Day® Kids Bugs Bunny and Friends Plus Extra C [US-OTC]; One-A-Day® Kids Extreme Sports [US-OTC]; One-A-Day® Kids Scooby-Doo! Complete [US-OTC]; One-A-Day® Kids Scooby-Doo! Fizzy Vites [US-OTC]; One-A-Day® Kids Scooby-Doo! Plus Calcium [US-OTC]; Poly-Vi-Flor® With Iron [US]; Poly-Vi-Flor® [US]; Poly-Vi-Sol® with Iron [US-OTC]; Poly-Vi-Sol® [US-OTC]; Soluvite-F [US]; Tri-Vi-Flor® with Iron [US]; Tri-Vi-Flor® [US]; Tri-Vi-Sol® with Iron [US-OTC]; Tri-Vi-Sol® [US-OTC]; Vitaball® Wild 'N Fruity [US-OTC]; Vitaball® [US-OTC]

Therapeutic Category Vitamin

Use Prevention/treatment of vitamin deficiency; products containing fluoride are used to prevent dental caries; labeled for OTC use as a dietary supplement

Usual Dosage Daily dose varies by product; refer to package insert for specific product labeling

Dosage Forms Content varies depending on product used. For more detailed information on ingredients in these and other multivitamins, please refer to Vitamin Products on page 1010.

vitamins (multiple/prenatal) (VYE ta mins, MUL ti pul/pree NAY tal)

Sound-Alike/Look-Alike Issues

Niferex® may be confused with Nephrox®

PreCare® may be confused with Precose®

Synonyms prenatal vitamins

U.S./Canadian Brand Names A-Free Prenatal [US]; Advanced NatalCare® [US]; Aminate Fe-90 [US]; Cal-Nate™ [US]; Chromagen® OB [US]; Citracal® Prenatal Rx [US]; Duet® [US]; Duet™ DHA [US]; KPN Prenatal [US]; NataChew™ [US]; NataFort® [US]; NatalCare® GlossTabs™ [US]; NatalCare® PIC Forte [US]; NatalCare® PIC [US]; NatalCare® Plus [US]; NatalCare® Rx [US]; NatalCare® Three [US]; NataTab™ CFe [US]; NataTab™ FA [US]; NataTab™ Rx [US]; Natelle® Prefer [US]; Natelle® [US]; Natelle®-ez [US]; Nestabs® CBF [US]; Nestabs® FA [US]; Nestabs® RX [US]; Niferex®-PN Forte [US]; Niferex®-PN [US]; NutriNate® [US]; OB-20 [US]; Obegyn® [US]; PreCare® Conceive™ [US]; PreCare® Prenatal [US]; PreCare® [US]; Prenatal 1-A-Day [US]; Prenatal AD [US]; Prenatal H [US]; Prenatal MR 90 Fe™ [US]; Prenatal MTR with Selenium [US]; Prenatal Plus [US]; Prenatal Rx 1 [US]; Prenatal U [US]; Prenatal Z [US]; Prenate Elite™ [US]; Prenate GT™ [US]; StrongStart™ [US]; Stuart Prenatal® [US-OTC]; Trinate [US]; Ultra NatalCare® [US]

Therapeutic Category Vitamin

Use Nutritional supplement for use prior to conception, during pregnancy, and postnatal (in lactating and nonlactating women)

Usual Dosage Oral: Adults:

Capsule, tablet: One daily

Powder: 4 teaspoonfuls/day; given once daily or in divided doses; mix 1 teaspoonful in 1 ounce of water

Dosage Forms Content varies depending on product used. For more detailed information on ingredients in these and other multivitamins, please refer to Vitamin Products on page 1010.

vitamins, multiple (therapeutic) *see* vitamins (multiple/oral) *on previous page*

vitamins, multiple with iron *see* vitamins (multiple/oral) *on previous page*

Vitaneed™ [US-OTC] *see* nutritional formula, enteral/oral *on page 608*

Vitelle™ Irospan® *(Discontinued)* *see* ferrous sulfate and ascorbic acid *on page 343*

Vitrase® [US] *see* hyaluronidase *on page 417*

Vitrasert® [US/Can] *see* ganciclovir *on page 375*

Vitravene™ [Can] *see* fomivirsen *(Canada only) on page 366*

Vitravene™ *(Discontinued)* *see* fomivirsen *(Canada only) on page 366*

Vitrax® [US] *see* hyaluronate and derivatives *on page 416*

Vitussin [US] *see* hydrocodone and guaifenesin *on page 422*

Vivactil® [US] *see* protriptyline *on page 712*

Viva-Drops® [US-OTC] *see* artificial tears *on page 75*

Vivarin® [US-OTC] *see* caffeine *on page 132*

Vivelle® [US] *see* estradiol *on page 308*

Vivelle-Dot® [US] *see* estradiol *on page 308*

Vivitrol™ [US] *see* naltrexone *on page 577*

Vivonex® [US-OTC] *see* nutritional formula, enteral/oral *on page 608*

Vivonex® T.E.N. [US-OTC] *see* nutritional formula, enteral/oral *on page 608*

Vivotif Berna® [US] *see* typhoid vaccine *on page 859*

VLB *see* vinblastine *on page 873*

VM-26 *see* teniposide *on page 810*

Volmax® *(Discontinued)* *see* albuterol *on page 23*

Voltaren® [US/Can] *see* diclofenac *on page 250*

Voltaren Ophtha® [Can] *see* diclofenac *on page 250*

Voltaren Ophthalmic® [US] *see* diclofenac *on page 250*

Voltaren Rapide® [Can] *see* diclofenac *on page 250*

Voltaren®-XR [US] *see* diclofenac *on page 250*

Voluven® [Can] *see* hetastarch *on page 413*

voriconazole (vor i KOE na zole)

Synonyms UK109496

U.S./Canadian Brand Names VFEND® [US/Can]

Therapeutic Category Antifungal Agent

Use Treatment of invasive aspergillosis; treatment of esophageal candidiasis; treatment of candidemia (in nonneutropenic patients); treatment of *Candida* deep tissue infections; treatment of serious fungal infections caused by *Scedosporium apiospermum* and *Fusarium* spp (including *Fusarium solani*) in patients intolerant of, or refractory to, other therapy

Usual Dosage

Usual dosage ranges:

Children <12 years: Dosage not established

Children ≥12 years and Adults:

Oral: 100-300 mg every 12 hours

I.V.: 6 mg/kg every 12 hours for 2 doses; followed by maintenance dose of 4 mg/kg every 12 hours

Indication-specific dosing: Children ≥12 years and Adults:

Aspergillosis (invasive) and other serious fungal infections: I.V.: Initial: Loading dose: 6 mg/kg every 12 hours for 2 doses; followed by maintenance dose of 4 mg/kg every 12 hours

Candidemia and other deep tissue *Candida* infections: I.V.: Initial: Loading dose 6 mg/kg every 12 hours for 2 doses; followed by maintenance dose of 3-4 mg/kg every 12 hours

Note: Conversion to oral dosing:

Patients <40 kg: 100 mg every 12 hours; increase to 150 mg every 12 hours in patients who fail to respond adequately

Patients ≥40 kg: 200 mg every 12 hours; increase to 300 mg every 12 hours in patients who fail to respond adequately

Endophthalmitis, fungal: I.V.: 6 mg/kg every 12 hours for 2 doses, then 200 mg orally twice daily

Esophageal candidiasis: Oral:

Patients <40 kg: 100 mg every 12 hours

Patients ≥40 kg: 200 mg every 12 hours

Note: Treatment should continue for a minimum of 14 days, and for at least 7 days following resolution of symptoms.

Dosage adjustment in patients unable to tolerate treatment:

I.V.: Dose may be reduced to 3 mg/kg every 12 hours

Oral: Dose may be reduced in 50 mg increments to a minimum dosage of 200 mg every 12 hours in patients weighing ≥40 kg (100 mg every 12 hours in patients <40 kg)

Dosage adjustment in patients receiving concomitant phenytoin:

I.V.: Increase maintenance dosage to 5 mg/kg every 12 hours

Oral: Increase dose from 200 mg to 400 mg every 12 hours in patients ≥40 kg (100 mg to 200 mg every 12 hours in patients <40 kg)

Dosage adjustment in patients receiving concomitant cyclosporine: Reduce cyclosporine dose by $^1/_2$ and monitor closely.

Dosage Forms

Injection, powder for reconstitution: 200 mg [contains SBECD 3200 mg]

Powder for oral suspension: 200 mg/5 mL (70 mL) [contains sodium benzoate and sucrose; orange flavor]

Tablet: 50 mg, 200 mg [contains lactose]

VoSol® *(Discontinued)* *see* acetic acid *on page 14*

VoSol® HC [US] *see* acetic acid, propylene glycol diacetate, and hydrocortisone *on page 15*

VoSpire ER® [US] *see* albuterol *on page 23*

VP-16 *see* etoposide *on page 330*

VP-16-213 *see* etoposide *on page 330*

V-Tann [US] *see* phenylephrine and pyrilamine *on page 662*

Vumon® [US/Can] *see* teniposide *on page 810*

V.V.S.® [US] *see* sulfabenzamide, sulfacetamide, and sulfathiazole *on page 795*

Vytone® [US] *see* iodoquinol and hydrocortisone *on page 459*

Vytorin™ [US] *see* ezetimibe and simvastatin *on page 332*

VZV vaccine (varicella) *see* varicella virus vaccine *on page 867*

VZV vaccine (zoster) *see* zoster vaccine *on page 891*

warfarin (WAR far in)

Sound-Alike/Look-Alike Issues

Coumadin® may be confused with Avandia®, Cardura®, Compazine®, Kemadrin®

Synonyms warfarin sodium

U.S./Canadian Brand Names Apo-Warfarin® [Can]; Coumadin® [US/Can]; Gen-Warfarin [Can]; Jantoven™ [US]; Novo-Warfarin [Can]; Taro-Warfarin [Can]

Therapeutic Category Anticoagulant (Other)

Use Prophylaxis and treatment of venous thrombosis, pulmonary embolism and thromboembolic disorders; atrial fibrillation with risk of embolism and as an adjunct in the prophylaxis of systemic embolism after myocardial infarction

Usual Dosage

Oral:

Infants and Children: 0.05-0.34 mg/kg/day; infants <12 months of age may require doses at or near the high end of this range; consistent anticoagulation may be difficult to maintain in children <5 years of age

Adults: Initial dosing must be individualized. Consider the patient (hepatic function, cardiac function, age, nutritional status, concurrent therapy, risk of bleeding) in addition to prior dose response (if available) and the clinical situation. Start 5-10 mg daily for 2 days. Adjust dose according to INR results; usual maintenance dose ranges from 2-10 mg daily (individual patients may require loading and maintenance doses outside these general guidelines).

Note: Lower starting doses may be required for patients with hepatic impairment, poor nutrition, CHF, elderly, high risk of bleeding, or patients that are debilitated. Higher initial doses may be reasonable in selected patients (ie, receiving enzyme-inducing agents and with low risk of bleeding).

I.V. (administer as a slow bolus injection): 2-5 mg/day

Dosage Forms

Injection, powder for reconstitution, as sodium:

Coumadin®: 5 mg

Tablet, as sodium: 1 mg, 2 mg, 2.5 mg, 3 mg, 4 mg, 5 mg, 6 mg, 7.5 mg, 10 mg

Coumadin®, Jantoven™: 1 mg, 2 mg, 2.5 mg, 3 mg, 4 mg, 5 mg, 6 mg, 7.5 mg, 10 mg

warfarin sodium *see* warfarin *on this page*

Wartec® [Can] *see* podofilox *on page 677*

Wart-Off® Maximum Strength [US-OTC] *see* salicylic acid *on page 758*

4-Way® 12 Hour [US-OTC] *see* oxymetazoline *on page 628*

4-Way® Saline Moisturizing Mist [US-OTC] *see* sodium chloride *on page 777*

WelChol® [US/Can] *see* colesevelam *on page 211*

Wellbutrin® [US/Can] *see* bupropion *on page 126*

Wellbutrin XL™ [US/Can] *see* bupropion *on page 126*

Wellbutrin SR® [US] *see* bupropion *on page 126*

Wellcovorin® *(Discontinued)* *see* leucovorin *on page 485*

Westcort® [US/Can] *see* hydrocortisone (topical) *on page 428*

Westhroid® [US] *see* thyroid *on page 824*

40 Winks® *(Discontinued)* *see* diphenhydramine *on page 261*

Winpred™ [Can] *see* prednisone *on page 695*

WinRho SD® *(Discontinued)*

WinRho® SDF [US] *see* Rh_o(D) immune globulin *on page 740*

Winstrol® [US] *see* stanozolol *on page 790*

witch hazel (witch HAY zel)

Synonyms hamamelis water

U.S./Canadian Brand Names Dickinson's® Witch Hazel [US-OTC]; Preparation H® Cleansing Pads [Can]; Preparation H® Medicated Wipes [US-OTC]; T.N. Dickinson's® Hazelets [US-OTC]; Tucks® [US-OTC]

(Continued)

witch hazel *(Continued)*

Therapeutic Category Astringent

Use After-stool wipe to remove most causes of local irritation; temporary management of vulvitis, pruritus ani and vulva; help relieve the discomfort of simple hemorrhoids, anorectal surgical wounds, and episiotomies

Usual Dosage Apply to anorectal area as needed

Dosage Forms

Liquid, topical: 100% (120 mL, 480 mL)

Dickinson's® Witch Hazel: 100% (60 mL, 240 mL, 480 mL)

Pads: 50% (100s)

Dickinson's® Witch Hazel: 50% (20s) [towelettes]; (50s) [contains aloe]; (100s) [hemorrhoidal]

Preparation H® Medicated Wipes: 50% (8s, 48s) [contains aloe]

T.N. Dickinson's® Hazelets: 50% (50s) [contains aloe]; (60s)

Tucks®: 50% (12s, 40s, 100s)

Wolfina® ***(Discontinued)***

Wound Wash Saline™ [US-OTC] *see* sodium chloride *on page 777*

WR-2721 *see* amifostine *on page 40*

WR-139007 *see* dacarbazine *on page 226*

WR-139013 *see* chlorambucil *on page 171*

WR-139021 *see* carmustine *on page 153*

Wycillin® [Can] *see* penicillin G procaine *on page 649*

Wycillin ***(Discontinued)*** *see* penicillin G procaine *on page 649*

Wydase® ***(Discontinued)*** *see* hyaluronidase *on page 417*

Wygesic® ***(Discontinued)*** *see* propoxyphene and acetaminophen *on page 708*

Wymox® ***(Discontinued)*** *see* amoxicillin *on page 47*

Wytensin® [Can] *see* guanabenz *on page 403*

Wytensin® ***(Discontinued)*** *see* guanabenz *on page 403*

Xalatan® [US/Can] *see* latanoprost *on page 483*

Xanax® [US/Can] *see* alprazolam *on page 32*

Xanax TS™ [Can] *see* alprazolam *on page 32*

Xanax XR® [US] *see* alprazolam *on page 32*

Xatral [Can] *see* alfuzosin *on page 28*

Xeloda® [US/Can] *see* capecitabine *on page 142*

Xenaderm™ [US] *see* trypsin, balsam peru, and castor oil *on page 856*

Xenical® [US/Can] *see* orlistat *on page 620*

Xerac AC™ [US] *see* aluminum chloride hexahydrate *on page 35*

Xibrom™ [US] *see* bromfenac *on page 117*

Xifaxan™ [US] *see* rifaximin *on page 746*

Xigris® [US/Can] *see* drotrecogin alfa *on page 282*

XiraTuss [US] *see* carbetapentane, phenylephrine, and chlorpheniramine *on page 147*

Xolair® [US/Can] *see* omalizumab *on page 615*

Xopenex® [US/Can] *see* levalbuterol *on page 487*

Xopenex HFA™ [US] *see* levalbuterol *on page 487*

XPECT™ [US-OTC] *see* guaifenesin *on page 392*

X-Prep® ***(Discontinued)*** *see* senna *on page 767*

X-Seb T® Pearl [US-OTC] *see* coal tar and salicylic acid *on page 208*

X-Seb T® Plus [US-OTC] *see* coal tar and salicylic acid *on page 208*

Xtramins [US-OTC] *see* vitamins (multiple/oral) *on page 878*

Xylocaine® [US/Can] *see* lidocaine *on page 493*

Xylocaine® MPF [US] *see* lidocaine *on page 493*

Xylocaine® MPF With Epinephrine [US] *see* lidocaine and epinephrine *on page 495*

Xylocaine® Viscous [US] *see* lidocaine *on page 493*

Xylocaine® With Epinephrine [US/Can] *see* lidocaine and epinephrine *on page 495*

Xylocard® [Can] *see* lidocaine *on page 493*

Xyrem® [US/Can] *see* sodium oxybate *on page 780*

Y-90 zevalin *see* ibritumomab *on page 437*

Yasmin® [US/Can] *see* ethinyl estradiol and drospirenone *on page 318*

Yaz [US] *see* ethinyl estradiol and drospirenone *on page 318*

yellow fever vaccine (YEL oh FEE ver vak SEEN)

U.S./Canadian Brand Names YF-VAX® [US/Can]

Therapeutic Category Vaccine, Live Virus

Use Induction of active immunity against yellow fever virus, primarily among persons traveling or living in areas where yellow fever infection exists

Usual Dosage Children ≥9 months and Adults: SubQ: One dose (0.5 mL) ≥10 days before travel; Booster: Every 10 years

Dosage Forms Injection, powder for reconstitution [17D-204 strain]: ≥4.74 Log_{10} plaque-forming units (PFU) per 0.5 mL dose [single-dose or 5-dose vial; produced in chicken embryos; packaged with diluent; vial stopper contains latex]

YF-VAX® [US/Can] *see* yellow fever vaccine *on this page*

YM087 *see* conivaptan *on page 213*

YM-08310 *see* amifostine *on page 40*

Yocon® [US/Can] *see* yohimbine *on this page*

Yodoxin® [US] *see* iodoquinol *on page 459*

yohimbine (yo HIM bine)

Sound-Alike/Look-Alike Issues

Aphrodyne® may be confused with Aprodine®

Yocon® may be confused with Zocor®

Synonyms yohimbine hydrochloride

U.S./Canadian Brand Names Aphrodyne® [US]; PMS-Yohimbine [Can]; Yocon® [US/Can]

Therapeutic Category Miscellaneous Product

Usual Dosage Adults: Oral:

Male erectile impotence: 5.4 mg tablet 3 times/day have been used. If side effects occur, reduce to 1/2 tablet (2.7 mg) 3 times/day followed by gradual increases to 1 tablet 3 times/day. Results of therapy >10 weeks are not known.

Orthostatic hypotension: Doses of 12.5 mg/day have been utilized; however, more research is necessary

Dosage Forms Tablet, as hydrochloride: 5.4 mg

yohimbine hydrochloride *see* yohimbine *on this page*

Yohimex™ *(Discontinued)* *see* yohimbine *on this page*

Yutopar® Injection *(Discontinued)*

Z4942 *see* ifosfamide *on page 440*

Zaditen® [Can] *see* ketotifen *on page 473*

Zaditor™ [US/Can] *see* ketotifen *on page 473*

zafirlukast (za FIR loo kast)

Sound-Alike/Look-Alike Issues

Accolate® may be confused with Accupril®, Accutane®, Aclovate®

Synonyms ICI-204,219

U.S./Canadian Brand Names Accolate® [US/Can]

Therapeutic Category Leukotriene Receptor Antagonist

Use Prophylaxis and chronic treatment of asthma in adults and children ≥5 years of age

Usual Dosage Oral:

Children <5 years: Safety and effectiveness have not been established

Children 5-11 years: 10 mg twice daily

Children ≥12 years and Adults: 20 mg twice daily

Dosage Forms Tablet: 10 mg, 20 mg

Zagam® *(Discontinued)*

zalcitabine (zal SITE a been)

Synonyms ddC; dideoxycytidine

U.S./Canadian Brand Names Hivid® [US/Can]

Therapeutic Category Antiviral Agent

Use In combination with at least two other antiretrovirals in the treatment of patients with HIV infection; it is not recommended that zalcitabine be given in combination with didanosine, stavudine, or lamivudine due to overlapping toxicities, virologic interactions, or lack of clinical data

Usual Dosage Oral: Adolescents and Adults: 0.75 mg 3 times/day

Dosage Forms [DSC] = Discontinued product

Tablet:

Hivid®: 0.375 mg [DSC], 0.75 mg

zaleplon (ZAL e plon)

U.S./Canadian Brand Names Sonata® [US/Can]; Starnoc® [Can]

Therapeutic Category Hypnotic, Nonbenzodiazepine (Pyrazolopyrimidine)

Controlled Substance C-IV

Use Short-term (7-10 days) treatment of insomnia (has been demonstrated to be effective for up to 5 weeks in controlled trial)

Usual Dosage Oral: Adults: 10 mg at bedtime (range: 5-20 mg); has been used for up to 5 weeks of treatment in controlled trial setting

Dosage Forms Capsule: 5 mg, 10 mg [contains tartrazine]

Zanaflex® [US/Can] *see* tizanidine *on page 831*

zanamivir (za NA mi veer)

U.S./Canadian Brand Names Relenza® [US/Can]

Therapeutic Category Antiviral Agent, Inhalation Therapy

Use Treatment of uncomplicated acute illness due to influenza virus A and B; treatment should only be initiated in patients who have been symptomatic for no more than 2 days. Prophylaxis against influenza virus A and B

Usual Dosage Oral inhalation:

Children ≥5 years and Adults: Prophylaxis (household setting): Two inhalations (10 mg) once daily for 10 days. Begin within 1 1/2 days following onset of signs or symptoms of index case.

Children ≥7 years and Adults: Treatment: Two inhalations (10 mg total) twice daily for 5 days. Doses on first day should be separated by at least 2 hours; on subsequent days, doses should be spaced by ~12 hours. Begin within 2 days of signs or symptoms.

Adolescents and Adults: Prophylaxis (community outbreak): Two inhalations (10 mg) once daily for 28 days. Begin within 5 days of outbreak.

Dosage Forms Powder for oral inhalation: 5 mg/blister (20s) [4 blisters per Rotadisk® foil pack, 5 Rotadisk® per package; packaged with Diskhaler® inhalation device; contains lactose]

Zanosar® [US/Can] *see* streptozocin *on page 792*

Zantac® [US/Can] *see* ranitidine *on page 732*

Zantac 75® [US-OTC/Can] *see* ranitidine *on page 732*

Zantac 150™ [US-OTC] *see* ranitidine *on page 732*

Zantac® EFFERdose® [US] *see* ranitidine *on page 732*

Zantryl® *(Discontinued)* *see* phentermine *on page 659*

Zapzyt® [US-OTC] *see* benzoyl peroxide *on page 102*

Zapzyt® Acne Wash [US-OTC] *see* salicylic acid *on page 758*

Zapzyt® Pore Treatment [US-OTC] *see* salicylic acid *on page 758*

Zarontin® [US/Can] *see* ethosuximide *on page 328*

Zaroxolyn® [US/Can] *see* metolazone *on page 549*

Zartan® *(Discontinued)* *see* cephalexin *on page 166*

Zavesca® [US/Can] *see* miglustat *on page 557*

Z-Bec® [US-OTC] *see* vitamin B complex combinations *on page 876*

Z-chlopenthixol *see* zuclopenthixol *(Canada only) on page 891*

Z-Cof™ DM [US] *see* guaifenesin, pseudoephedrine, and dextromethorphan *on page 401*

Z-Cof HC [US] *see* phenylephrine, hydrocodone, and chlorpheniramine *on page 663*

Z-Cof LA™ [US] *see* guaifenesin and dextromethorphan *on page 394*

ZD1033 *see* anastrozole *on page 56*

ZD1694 *see* raltitrexed *(Canada only) on page 731*

ZD1839 *see* gefitinib *on page 377*

ZDV *see* zidovudine *on next page*

ZDV, abacavir, and lamivudine *see* abacavir, lamivudine, and zidovudine *on page 2*

Zeasorb®-AF [US-OTC] *see* miconazole *on page 553*

Zebeta® [US/Can] *see* bisoprolol *on page 113*

Zebutal™ [US] *see* butalbital, acetaminophen, and caffeine *on page 129*

Zefazone® ***(Discontinued)***

Zelapar™ [US] *see* selegiline *on page 766*

zeldox *see* ziprasidone *on page 888*

Zelnorm® [US/Can] *see* tegaserod *on page 807*

Zemaira® [US] *see* alpha$_1$-proteinase inhibitor *on page 31*

Zemplar® [US/Can] *see* paricalcitol *on page 638*

Zemuron® [US/Can] *see* rocuronium *on page 751*

Zenapax® [US/Can] *see* daclizumab *on page 226*

zeneca 182,780 *see* fulvestrant *on page 372*

Zephiran® [US-OTC] *see* benzalkonium chloride *on page 99*

Zephrex® [US] *see* guaifenesin and pseudoephedrine *on page 398*

Zephrex LA® [US] *see* guaifenesin and pseudoephedrine *on page 398*

Zerit® [US/Can] *see* stavudine *on page 790*

ZerLor™ [US] *see* acetaminophen, caffeine, and dihydrocodeine *on page 10*

Zestoretic® [US/Can] *see* lisinopril and hydrochlorothiazide *on page 501*

Zestril® [US/Can] *see* lisinopril *on page 500*

Zetacet® [US] *see* sulfur and sulfacetamide *on page 800*

Zetar® [US-OTC] *see* coal tar *on page 207*

Zetia™ [US] *see* ezetimibe *on page 332*

Zevalin® [US] *see* ibritumomab *on page 437*

Ziac® [US/Can] *see* bisoprolol and hydrochlorothiazide *on page 113*

Ziagen® [US/Can] *see* abacavir *on page 2*

ziconotide (zi KOE no tide)

U.S./Canadian Brand Names Prialt® [US]

Therapeutic Category Analgesic, Nonnarcotic; Calcium Channel Blocker, N-Type

Use Management of severe chronic pain in patients requiring intrathecal (I.T.) therapy and are intolerant or refractory to other therapies

Usual Dosage I.T.: Adults: Chronic pain: Initial dose: 2.4 mcg/day (0.1 mcg/hour)

Dose may be titrated by ≤2.4 mcg/day (0.1 mcg/hour) at intervals ≥2-3 times/week to a maximum dose of 19.2 mcg/day (0.8 mcg/hour) by day 21; average dose at day 21: 6.9 mcg/day (0.29 mcg/hour). A faster titration should be used only if the urgent need for analgesia outweighs the possible risk to patient safety.

Dosage Forms Injection, solution, as acetate [preservative free]: 25 mcg/mL (20 mL); 100 mcg/mL (1 mL, 2 mL, 5 mL)

zidovudine (zye DOE vyoo deen)

Sound-Alike/Look-Alike Issues

azidothymidine may be confused with azathioprine, aztreonam

Retrovir® may be confused with ritonavir

AZT is an error-prone abbreviation (mistaken as azathioprine, aztreonam)

Synonyms azidothymidine; compound S; ZDV

U.S./Canadian Brand Names Apo-Zidovudine® [Can]; AZT™ [Can]; Retrovir® [US/Can]

Therapeutic Category Antiviral Agent

Use Treatment of HIV infection in combination with at least two other antiretroviral agents; prevention of maternal/fetal HIV transmission as monotherapy

Usual Dosage

Prevention of maternal-fetal HIV transmission:

Neonatal: **Note:** Dosing should begin 8-12 hours after birth and continue for the first 6 weeks of life.

Oral:

Full-term infants: 2 mg/kg/dose every 6 hours

Infants ≥30 weeks and <35 weeks gestation at birth: 2 mg/kg/dose every 12 hours; at 2 weeks of age, advance to 2 mg/kg/dose every 8 hours

Infants <30 weeks gestation at birth: 2 mg/kg/dose every 12 hours; at 4 weeks of age, advance to 2 mg/kg/dose every 8 hours

I.V.: Infants unable to receive oral dosing:

Full term: 1.5 mg/kg/dose every 6 hours

Infants ≥30 weeks and <35 weeks gestation at birth: 1.5 mg/kg/dose every 12 hours; at 2 weeks of age, advance to 1.5 mg/kg/dose every 8 hours

Infants <30 weeks gestation at birth: 1.5 mg/kg/dose every 12 hours; at 4 weeks of age, advance to 1.5 mg/kg/dose every 8 hours

Maternal: Oral (per AIDSinfo guidelines): 100 mg 5 times/day **or** 200 mg 3 times/day **or** 300 mg twice daily. Begin at 14-34 weeks gestation and continue until start of labor.

During labor and delivery, administer zidovudine I.V. at 2 mg/kg as loading dose followed by a continuous I.V. infusion of 1 mg/kg/hour until the umbilical cord is clamped

Treatment of HIV infection:

Children 6 weeks to 12 years:

Oral: 160 mg/m^2/dose every 8 hours (maximum: 200 mg every 8 hours); some Working Group members use a dose of 180 mg/m^2 to 240 mg/m^2 every 12 hours when using in drug combinations with other antiretroviral compounds, but data on this dosing in children is limited

I.V. continuous infusion: 20 mg/m^2/hour

I.V. intermittent infusion: 120 mg/m^2/dose every 6 hours

Adults:

Oral: 300 mg twice daily or 200 mg 3 times/day

I.V.: 1 mg/kg/dose administered every 4 hours around-the-clock (5-6 doses/day)

Dosage Forms

Capsule:

Retrovir®: 100 mg

Injection, solution [preservative free]:

Retrovir®: 10 mg/mL (20 mL)

Syrup:

Retrovir®: 50 mg/5 mL (240 mL) [contains sodium benzoate; strawberry flavor]

Tablet: 300 mg

Retrovir®: 300 mg

zidovudine, abacavir, and lamivudine *see* abacavir, lamivudine, and zidovudine *on page 2*

zidovudine and lamivudine (zye DOE vyoo deen & la MI vyoo deen)

Sound-Alike/Look-Alike Issues

Combivir® may be confused with Combivent®, Epivir®

AZT is an error-prone abbreviation (mistaken as azathioprine, aztreonam)

Synonyms lamivudine and zidovudine

U.S./Canadian Brand Names Combivir® [US/Can]

Therapeutic Category Antiviral Agent

Use Treatment of HIV infection when therapy is warranted based on clinical and/or immunological evidence of disease progression. Combivir® given twice daily, provides an alternative regimen to lamivudine 150 mg twice daily plus zidovudine 600 mg/day in divided doses; this drug form reduces capsule/tablet intake for these two drugs to 2 per day instead of up to 8.

Usual Dosage Children >12 years and Adults: Oral: One tablet twice daily

Note: Because this is a fixed-dose combination product, avoid use in patients requiring dosage reduction including children <12 years of age, renally impaired patients with a creatinine clearance ≤50 mL/minute, patients with low body weight (<50 kg or 110 pounds), or those experiencing dose-limiting adverse effects.

Dosage Forms Tablet: Zidovudine 300 mg and lamivudine 150 mg

Zilactin® [Can] *see* lidocaine *on page 493*

Zilactin-L® [US-OTC] *see* lidocaine *on page 493*

Zilactin®-B [US-OTC/Can] *see* benzocaine *on page 99*

Zilactin Baby® [Can] *see* benzocaine *on page 99*

Zilactin Toothache and Gum Pain® [US-OTC] *see* benzocaine *on page 99*

Zinacef® [US/Can] *see* cefuroxime *on page 163*

zinc *see* trace metals *on page 839*

Zincate® [US] *see* zinc sulfate *on next page*

zinc chloride (zink KLOR ide)

Therapeutic Category Trace Element

Use Cofactor for replacement therapy to different enzymes helps maintain normal growth rates, normal skin hydration and senses of taste and smell

Usual Dosage Clinical response may not occur for up to 6-8 weeks

Supplemental to I.V. solutions:

- Premature Infants <1500 g, up to 3 kg: 300 mcg/kg/day
- Full-term Infants and Children ≤5 years: 100 mcg/kg/day
- Adults:
  - Stable with fluid loss from small bowel: 12.2 mg zinc/liter TPN or 17.1 mg zinc/kg (added to 1000 mL I.V. fluids) of stool or ileostomy output
  - Metabolically stable: 2.5-4 mg/day, add 2 mg/day for acute catabolic states

Dosage Forms Injection, solution: 1 mg/mL (10 mL, 50 mL)

zinc diethylenetriaminepentaacetate (Zn-DTPA) *see* diethylene triamine penta-acetic acid *on page 252*

Zincfrin® [US-OTC/Can] *see* phenylephrine and zinc sulfate *on page 662*

zinc gelatin (zink JEL ah tin)

Synonyms dome paste bandage; unna's boot; unna's paste; zinc gelatin boot

U.S./Canadian Brand Names Gelucast® [US]

Therapeutic Category Protectant, Topical

Use As a protectant and to support varicosities and similar lesions of the lower limbs

Usual Dosage Apply externally as an occlusive boot

Dosage Forms Bandage: 3" x 10 yards; 4" x 10 yards

zinc gelatin boot *see* zinc gelatin *on this page*

Zincofax® [Can] *see* zinc oxide *on this page*

Zincon® [US-OTC] *see* pyrithione zinc *on page 723*

zinc oxide (zink OKS ide)

Synonyms base ointment; lassar's zinc paste

U.S./Canadian Brand Names Ammens® Medicated Deodorant [US-OTC]; Balmex® [US-OTC]; Boudreaux's® Butt Paste [US-OTC]; Critic-Aid Skin Care® [US-OTC]; Desitin® Creamy [US-OTC]; Desitin® [US-OTC]; Zincofax® [Can]

Therapeutic Category Topical Skin Product

Use Protective coating for mild skin irritations and abrasions, soothing and protective ointment to promote healing of chapped skin, diaper rash

Usual Dosage Infants, Children, and Adults: Topical: Apply as required for affected areas several times daily

Dosage Forms

Cream:

- Balmex®: 11.3% (60 g, 120 g, 480 g) [contains aloe and vitamin E]

Ointment, topical: 20% (30 g, 60 g, 480 g); 40% (120 g)

- Desitin®: 40% (30 g, 60 g, 90 g, 120 g, 270 g, 480 g) [contains cod liver oil and lanolin]
- Desitin® Creamy: 10% (60 g, 120 g)

(Continued)

zinc oxide *(Continued)*

Paste, topical:

Boudreaux's® Butt Paste: 16% (30 g, 60 g, 120 g, 480 g) [contains castor oil, boric acid, mineral oil, and Peruvian balsam]

Critic-Aid Skin Care®: 20% (71 g, 170 g)

Powder, topical (Ammens® Medicated Deodorant): 9.1% (187.5 g, 330 g) [original and shower fresh scent]

zinc sulfate (zink SUL fate)

Sound-Alike/Look-Alike Issues

$ZnSO_4$ is an error-prone abbreviation (mistaken as morphine sulfate)

U.S./Canadian Brand Names Anuzinc [Can]; Orazinc® [US-OTC]; Rivasol [Can]; Zincate® [US]

Therapeutic Category Electrolyte Supplement, Oral

Use Zinc supplement (oral and parenteral); may improve wound healing in those who are deficient

Usual Dosage

RDA: Oral:

- Birth to 6 months: 3 mg elemental zinc/day
- 6-12 months: 5 mg elemental zinc/day
- 1-10 years: 10 mg elemental zinc/day
- ≥11 years: 15 mg elemental zinc/day

Zinc deficiency: Oral:

- Infants and Children: 0.5-1 mg elemental zinc/kg/day divided 1-3 times/day; somewhat larger quantities may be needed if there is impaired intestinal absorption or an excessive loss of zinc
- Adults: 110-220 mg zinc sulfate (25-50 mg elemental zinc)/dose 3 times/day

Parenteral TPN: I.V.:

- Infants (premature, birth weight <1500 g up to 3 kg): 300 mcg/kg/day
- Infants (full-term) and Children ≤5 years: 100 mcg/kg/day
- Adults:
  - Acute metabolic states: 4.5-6 mg/day
  - Metabolically stable: 2.5-4 mg/day
  - Stable with fluid loss from the small bowel: 12.2 mg zinc/L of TPN solution, or an additional 17.1 mg zinc (added to 1000 mL I.V. fluids) per kg of stool or ileostomy output

Dosage Forms

Capsule (Orazinc®, Zincate®): 220 mg [elemental zinc 50 mg]

Injection, solution [preservative free]: 1 mg elemental zinc/mL (10 mL); 5 mg elemental zinc/mL (5 mL)

Tablet (Orazinc®): 110 mg [elemental zinc 25 mg]

zinc sulfate and phenylephrine *see* phenylephrine and zinc sulfate *on page 662*

zinc undecylenate *see* undecylenic acid and derivatives *on page 860*

Zinecard® [US/Can] *see* dexrazoxane *on page 242*

ziprasidone (zi PRAS i done)

Synonyms zeldox; ziprasidone hydrochloride; ziprasidone mesylate

U.S./Canadian Brand Names Geodon® [US]

Therapeutic Category Antipsychotic Agent

Use Treatment of schizophrenia; treatment of acute manic or mixed episodes associated with bipolar disorder with or without psychosis; acute agitation in patients with schizophrenia

Usual Dosage Adults:

Bipolar mania: Oral: Initial: 40 mg twice daily (with food)

Adjustment: May increase to 60 or 80 mg twice daily on second day of treatment; average dose 40-80 mg twice daily

Schizophrenia: Oral: Initial: 20 mg twice daily (with food)

Adjustment: Increases (if indicated) should be made no more frequently than every 2 days; ordinarily patients should be observed for improvement over several weeks before adjusting the dose

Maintenance: Range 20-100 mg twice daily; however, dosages >80 mg twice daily are generally not recommended

Acute agitation (schizophrenia): I.M.: 10 mg every 2 hours **or** 20 mg every 4 hours; maximum: 40 mg/day; oral therapy should replace I.M. administration as soon as possible

Dosage Forms

Capsule, as hydrochloride: 20 mg, 40 mg, 60 mg, 80 mg

Injection, powder for reconstitution, as mesylate: 20 mg

ziprasidone hydrochloride *see* ziprasidone *on this page*

ziprasidone mesylate *see* ziprasidone *on previous page*

Zithromax® [US/Can] *see* azithromycin *on page 88*

Zithromax® TRI-PAK™ *see* azithromycin *on page 88*

Zithromax® Z-PAK® *see* azithromycin *on page 88*

ZM-182,780 *see* fulvestrant *on page 372*

Zmax™ [US] *see* azithromycin *on page 88*

Zn-DTPA *see* diethylene triamine penta-acetic acid *on page 252*

ZNP® Bar [US-OTC] *see* pyrithione zinc *on page 723*

Zocor® [US/Can] *see* simvastatin *on page 773*

Zoderm® [US] *see* benzoyl peroxide *on page 102*

Zofran® [US/Can] *see* ondansetron *on page 616*

Zofran® ODT [US/Can] *see* ondansetron *on page 616*

Zoladex® [US/Can] *see* goserelin *on page 391*

Zoladex® LA [Can] *see* goserelin *on page 391*

zoledronate *see* zoledronic acid *on this page*

zoledronic acid (zoe le DRON ik AS id)

Synonyms CGP-42446; NSC-721517; zoledronate

U.S./Canadian Brand Names Aclasta® [Can]; Zometa® [US/Can]

Therapeutic Category Bisphosphonate Derivative

Use Treatment of hypercalcemia of malignancy, multiple myeloma, bone metastases of solid tumors

Usual Dosage I.V.: Adults:

Hypercalcemia of malignancy (albumin-corrected serum calcium ≥12 mg/dL): 4 mg (maximum) given as a single dose. Wait at least 7 days before considering retreatment. Dosage adjustment may be needed in patients with decreased renal function following treatment.

Multiple myeloma or metastatic bone lesions from solid tumors: 4 mg every 3-4 weeks

Note: Patients should receive a daily calcium supplement and multivitamin containing vitamin D

Paget's disease (Aclasta®, not available in U.S.): 5 mg infused over at least 15 minutes. **Note:** Data concerning retreatment is not available.

Dosage Forms [CAN] = Canadian brand name

Infusion, solution [premixed]:

Aclasta® [CAN]: 5 mg (100 mL) [not available in U.S.]

Injection, solution:

Zometa®: 4 mg/5 mL (5 mL) [as monohydrate 4.264 mg]

Zolicef® *(Discontinued)* *see* cefazolin *on page 156*

zolmitriptan (zohl mi TRIP tan)

Sound-Alike/Look-Alike Issues

zolmitriptan may be confused with sumatriptan

Synonyms 311C90

U.S./Canadian Brand Names Zomig-ZMT™ [US]; Zomig® Nasal Spray [Can]; Zomig® Rapimelt [Can]; Zomig® [US/Can]

Therapeutic Category Antimigraine Agent; Serotonin Agonist

Use Acute treatment of migraine with or without aura

Usual Dosage Oral:

Children: Safety and efficacy have not been established

Adults: Migraine:

Tablet: Initial: ≤2.5 mg at the onset of migraine headache; may break 2.5 mg tablet in half

Orally-disintegrating tablet: Initial: 2.5 mg at the onset of migraine headache

Nasal spray: Initial: 1 spray (5 mg) at the onset of migraine headache

Note: Use the lowest possible dose to minimize adverse events. If the headache returns, the dose may be repeated after 2 hours; do not exceed 10 mg within a 24-hour period. Controlled trials have not established the effectiveness of a second dose if the initial one was ineffective

Dosage Forms

Solution, nasal spray [single dose] (Zomig®): 5 mg/0.1 mL (0.1 mL)

Tablet (Zomig®): 2.5 mg, 5 mg

(Continued)

zolmitriptan *(Continued)*

Tablet, orally disintegrating (Zomig-ZMT™): 2.5 mg [contains phenylalanine 2.81 mg/tablet; orange flavor]; 5 mg [contains phenylalanine 5.62 mg/tablet; orange flavor]

Zoloft® [US/Can] *see* sertraline *on page 769*

zolpidem (zole PI dem)

Sound-Alike/Look-Alike Issues
Ambien® may be confused with Ambi 10®

Synonyms zolpidem tartrate

U.S./Canadian Brand Names Ambien CR™ [US]; Ambien® [US]

Therapeutic Category Hypnotic, Nonbarbiturate

Controlled Substance C-IV

Use Short-term treatment of insomnia (sleep onset and/or sleep maintenance)

Usual Dosage Oral:
Ambien®: 10 mg immediately before bedtime; maximum dose: 10 mg
Ambien CR™: 12.5 mg immediately before bedtime

Dosage Forms [DSC] = Discontinued product
Tablet, as tartrate:
Ambien®: 5 mg, 10 mg
Ambien® PAK™ [dose pack]: 5 mg (30s); 10 mg (30s) [DSC]
Tablet, extended release, as tartrate (Ambien CR™): 6.25 mg, 12.5 mg

zolpidem tartrate *see* zolpidem *on this page*
Zometa® [US/Can] *see* zoledronic acid *on previous page*
Zomig® [US/Can] *see* zolmitriptan *on previous page*
Zomig® Nasal Spray [Can] *see* zolmitriptan *on previous page*
Zomig® Rapimelt [Can] *see* zolmitriptan *on previous page*
Zomig-ZMT™ [US] *see* zolmitriptan *on previous page*
Zomorph® [Can] *see* morphine sulfate *on page 565*
Zonalon® [US/Can] *see* doxepin *on page 276*
Zone-A® [US] *see* pramoxine and hydrocortisone *on page 691*
Zone-A Forte® [US] *see* pramoxine and hydrocortisone *on page 691*
Zonegran® [US/Can] *see* zonisamide *on this page*

zonisamide (zoe NIS a mide)

U.S./Canadian Brand Names Zonegran® [US/Can]

Therapeutic Category Anticonvulsant, Sulfonamide

Use Adjunct treatment of partial seizures in children >16 years of age and adults with epilepsy

Usual Dosage Oral: Children >16 years and Adults: Adjunctive treatment of partial seizures: Initial: 100 mg/day; dose may be increased to 200 mg/day after 2 weeks. Further dosage increases to 300 mg/day and 400 mg/day can then be made with a minimum of 2 weeks between adjustments, in order to reach steady state at each dosage level. Doses of up to 600 mg/day have been studied, however, there is no evidence of increased response with doses above 400 mg/day.

Dosage Forms [DSC] = Discontinued product
Capsule: 25 mg, 50 mg, 100 mg
Zonegran®: 25 mg, 50 mg [DSC], 100 mg

zopiclone *(Canada only)* (ZOE pi clone)

U.S./Canadian Brand Names Alti-Zopiclone [Can]; Apo-Zopiclone® [Can]; CO Zopiclone [Can]; Gen-Zopiclone [Can]; Imovane® [Can]; Novo-Zopiclone [Can]; Nu-Zopiclone [Can]; PMS-Zopiclone [Can]; RAN™-Zopiclone [Can]; Rhovane® [Can]; Rhoxal-zopiclone [Can]; Riva-Zopiclone [Can]; Sandoz-Zopiclone [Can]

Therapeutic Category Hypnotic

Use Symptomatic relief of transient and short-term insomnia

Usual Dosage Administer just before bedtime: Oral: Adults: 5-7.5 mg
Patients with chronic respiratory insufficiency: 3.75 mg; may increase up to 7.5 mg with caution in appropriate cases

Dosage Forms Tablet: 5 mg, 7.5 mg

Zorbtive™ [US] *see* somatropin *on page 785*

Zorcaine™ [US] *see* articaine and epinephrine *on page 75*

ZORprin® [US] *see* aspirin *on page 77*

Zostavax® [US] *see* zoster vaccine *on this page*

zoster vaccine (ZOS ter vak SEEN)

Synonyms shingles vaccine; varicella-zoster (VZV) vaccine (zoster); VZV vaccine (zoster)

U.S./Canadian Brand Names Zostavax® [US]

Therapeutic Category Vaccine

Use Prevention of herpes zoster (shingles) in patients ≥60 years of age

Usual Dosage SubQ: Adults ≥65 years: 0.65 mL administered as a single dose; there is no data to support readministration of the vaccine

Dosage Forms

Injection, powder for reconstitution [preservative free]

Zostavax®: 19,400 plaque-forming units (PFU) [contains gelatin, sucrose, and trace amounts of neomycin]

Zostrix® [US-OTC/Can] *see* capsaicin *on page 142*

Zostrix®-HP [US-OTC/Can] *see* capsaicin *on page 142*

Zosyn® [US] *see* piperacillin and tazobactam sodium *on page 670*

Zovia™ [US] *see* ethinyl estradiol and ethynodiol diacetate *on page 319*

Zovirax® [US/Can] *see* acyclovir *on page 18*

Ztuss™ Tablet [US] *see* hydrocodone, pseudoephedrine, and guaifenesin *on page 425*

zuclopenthixol acetate *see* zuclopenthixol *(Canada only) on this page*

zuclopenthixol *(Canada only)* (zoo kloe pen THIX ol)

Synonyms Z-chlopenthixol; zuclopenthixol acetate; zuclopenthixol decanoate; zuclopenthixol dihydrochloride

U.S./Canadian Brand Names Clopixol-Acuphase® [Can]; Clopixol® Depot [Can]; Clopixol® [Can]

Therapeutic Category Antipsychotic Agent

Use Management of schizophrenia; acetate injection is intended for short-term acute treatment; decanoate injection is for long-term management; dihydrochloride tablets may be used in either phase

Usual Dosage Adults:

Oral: Zuclopenthixol dihydrochloride: Initial: 20-30 mg/day in 2-3 divided doses; usual maintenance dose: 20-40 mg/day; maximum daily dose: 100 mg

I.M.:

Zuclopenthixol acetate: 50-150 mg; may be repeated in 2-3 days; no more than 4 injections should be given in the course of treatment; maximum dose during course of treatment: 400 mg (maximum treatment period: 2 weeks)

Transfer of patients from I.M. acetate (Acuphase®) to oral (tablets):

50 mg = 20 mg daily

100 mg = 40 mg daily

150 mg = 60 mg daily

Zuclopenthixol decanoate: 100 mg by deep I.M. injection; additional I.M. doses of 100-200 mg may be given over the following 1-4 weeks; maximum weekly dose: 600 mg; usual maintenance dose: 150-300 mg every 2 weeks

Transfer of patients from oral (tablets) to I.M. decanoate (depot):

≤20 mg daily = 100 mg every 2 weeks

25-40 mg daily = 200 mg every 2 weeks

50-75 mg daily = 300 mg every 2 weeks

>75 mg/day = 400 mg every 2 weeks

Transfer of patients from I.M. acetate (Acuphase®) to I.M. decanoate (depot):

50 mg every 2-3 days = 100 mg every 2 weeks

100 mg every 2-3 days = 200 mg every 2 weeks

150 mg every 2-3 days = 300 mg every 2 weeks

Dosage Forms [CAN] = Canadian brand name

Injection, as acetate:

Clopixol Acuphase® [CAN]: 50 mg/mL [zuclopenthixol 42.5 mg/mL] (1 mL, 2 mL) [not available in the U.S.]

Injection, as decanoate:

Clopixol® Depot [CAN]: 200 mg/mL [zuclopenthixol 144.4 mg/mL] (10 mL) [not available in the U.S.]

Tablet, as dihydrochloride:

Clopixol® [CAN]: 10 mg, 25 mg, 40 mg [not available in the U.S.]

(Continued)

zuclopenthixol decanoate *see* zuclopenthixol *(Canada only) on previous page*

zuclopenthixol dihydrochloride *see* zuclopenthixol *(Canada only) on previous page*

Zyban® [US/Can] *see* bupropion *on page 126*

Zydone® [US] *see* hydrocodone and acetaminophen *on page 420*

Zyloprim® [US/Can] *see* allopurinol *on page 30*

Zymar™ [US/Can] *see* gatifloxacin *on page 376*

Zymase® *(Discontinued)* *see* pancrelipase *on page 634*

Zyprexa® [US/Can] *see* olanzapine *on page 613*

Zyprexa® Zydis® [US/Can] *see* olanzapine *on page 613*

Zyrtec® [US] *see* cetirizine *on page 167*

Zyrtec-D 12 Hour™ [US] *see* cetirizine and pseudoephedrine *on page 168*

Zyvox™ [US] *see* linezolid *on page 498*

Zyvoxam® [Can] *see* linezolid *on page 498*

APPENDIX

ABBREVIATIONS & SYMBOLS COMMONLY USED IN MEDICAL ORDERS

Abbreviation	From	Meaning
<		less than
>		greater than
≤		less than or equal to
≥		greater than or equal to
$\overline{aa}$, aa	ana	of each
AA		Alcoholics Anonymous
ABG		arterial blood gases
ac	ante cibum	before meals or food
ACA		Adult Children of Alcoholics
ACLS		advanced cardiac life support
ad	ad	to, up to
a.d.	aurio dextra	right ear
ADHD		attention-deficit/hyperactivity disorder
ADLs		activities of daily living
ad lib	ad libitum	at pleasure
AIDS		acquired immune deficiency syndrome
AIMS		Abnormal Involuntary Movement Scale
a.l.	aurio laeva	left ear
ALS		amyotrophic lateral sclerosis
AM	ante meridiem	morning
AMA		against medical advice
amp		ampul
amt		amount
aq	aqua	water
aq. dest.	aqua destillata	distilled water
ARC		AIDS-related complex
ARDS		adult respiratory distress syndrome
ARF		acute renal failure
a.s.	aurio sinister	left ear
ASAP		as soon as possible
a.u.	aures utrae	each ear
AUC		area under the curve
BDI		Beck Depression Inventory
bid	bis in die	twice daily
BLS		basic life support
bm		bowel movement
BMI		body mass index
bp		blood pressure
BPH		benign prostatic hyperplasia
BPRS		Brief Psychiatric Rating Scale
BSA		body surface area
c	cong	a gallon
$\bar{c}$	cum	with
CA		cancer
CABG		coronary artery bypass graft
CAD		coronary artery disease
cal		calorie
cap	capsula	capsule
CBT		cognitive behavioral therapy
cc		cubic centimeter
CCL		creatinine clearance
CF		cystic fibrosis
CGI		Clinical Global Impression
CIE		chemotherapy-induced emesis
CIV		continuous I.V. infusion
cm		centimeter
CNS		central nervous system
comp	compositus	compound
cont		continue
COPD		chronic obstructive pulmonary disease
CRF		chronic renal failure
CT		computed tomography

(continued)

Abbreviation	From	Meaning
d	dies	day
DBP		diastolic blood pressure
d/c		discontinue
dil	dilue	dilute
disp	dispensa	dispense
div	divide	divide
DOE		dyspnea on exertion
DSC		discontinued
DSM-IV		Diagnostic and Statistical Manual
DTs		delirium tremens
dtd	dentur tales doses	give of such a dose
DVT		deep vein thrombosis
Dx		diagnosis
ECG		electrocardiogram
ECT		electroconvulsive therapy
EEG		electroencephalogram
elix, el	elixir	elixir
emp		as directed
EPS		extrapyramidal side effects
ESRD		end stage renal disease
et	et	and
EtOH		alcohol
ex aq		in water
f, ft	fac, fiat, fiant	make, let be made
FDA		Food and Drug Administration
FMS		fibromyalgia syndrome
g	gramma	gram
GA		Gamblers Anonymous
GABA		gamma-aminobutyric acid
GAD		generalized anxiety disorder
GAF		Global Assessment of Functioning Scale
GERD		gastroesophageal reflux disease
GFR		glomerular filtration rate
GITS		gastrointestinal therapeutic system
gr	granum	grain
gtt	gutta	a drop
GVHD		graft versus host disease
h	hora	hour
HAM-A		Hamilton Anxiety Scale
HAM-D		Hamilton Depression Scale
hs	hora somni	at bedtime
HSV		herpes simplex virus
HTN		hypertension
IBD		inflammatory bowel disease
IBS		irritable bowel syndrome
ICH		intracranial hemorrhage
IHSS		idiopathic hypertrophic subaortic stenosis
I.M.		intramuscular
IOP		intraocular pressure
IU		international unit
I.V.		intravenous
kcal		kilocalorie
kg		kilogram
KIU		kallikrein inhibitor unit
L		liter
LAMM		L-α-acetyl methadol
liq	liquor	a liquor, solution
LVH		left ventricular hypertrophy
M	misce	mix; Molar
MADRS		Montgomery Asbery Depression Rating Scale
MAOIs		monoamine oxidase inhibitors
mcg		microgram
MDEA		3.4-methylene-dioxy amphetamine
m. dict	more dictor	as directed
MDMA		3,4-methylene-dioxy methamphetamine

(continued)

Abbreviation	From	Meaning
mEq		milliequivalent
mg		milligram
mixt	mixtura	a mixture
mL		milliliter
mm		millimeter
mM		millimolar
MMSE		Mini-Mental State Examination
MPPP		l-methyl-4-proprionoxy-4-phenyl pyridine
MR		mental retardation
MRI		magnetic resonance image
MS		multiple sclerosis
NF		National Formulary
NKA		no known allergies
NMS		neuroleptic malignant syndrome
no.	numerus	number
noc	nocturnal	in the night
non rep	non repetatur	do not repeat, no refills
NPO		nothing by mouth
NSAID		nonsteroidal antiinflammatory drug
NV		nausea and vomiting
O, Oct	octarius	a pint
OA		osteoarthritis
OCD		obsessive-compulsive disorder
o.d.	oculus dexter	right eye
o.l.	oculus laevus	left eye
o.s.	oculus sinister	left eye
o.u.	oculo uterque	each eye
PANSS		Positive and Negative Symptom Scale
PAT		paroxysmal artrial tachycardia
pc, post cib	post cibos	after meals
PCP		phencyclidine
PD		Parkinson disease
PE		pulmonary embolus
per		through or by
PID		pelvic inflammatory disease
PM	post meridiem	afternoon or evening
P.O.	per os	by mouth
PONV		postoperative nausea and vomiting
P.R.	per rectum	rectally
prn	pro re nata	as needed
PSVT		paroxysmal supraventricular tachycardia
PTA		prior to admission
PTSD		post-traumatic stress disorder
PUD		peptic ulcer disease
pulv	pulvis	a powder
PVD		peripheral vascular disease
q		every
qad	quoque alternis die	every other day
qd		every day, daily
qh	quiaque hora	every hour
qid	quater in die	four times a day
qod		every other day
qs	quantum sufficiat	a sufficient quantity
qs ad		a sufficient quantity to make
qty		quantity
qv	quam volueris	as much as you wish
RA		rheumatoid arthritis
REM		rapid eye movement
Rx	recipe	take, a recipe
rep	repetatur	let it be repeated
$\overline{s}$	sine	without
sa	secundum artem	according to art
SAH		subarachnoid hemorrhage
sat	sataratus	saturated
SBE		subacute bacterial endocarditis

(continued)

Abbreviation	From	Meaning
SBP		systolic blood pressure
SIADH		syndrome of inappropriate antidiuretic hormone secretion
sig	signa	label, or let it be printed
SL		sublingual
SLE		systemic lupus erythematosus
SOB		shortness of breath
sol	solutio	solution
solv		dissolve
$\overline{ss}$, ss	semis	one-half
sos	si opus sit	if there is need
SSKI		saturated solution of potassium iodide
SSRIs		selective serotonin reuptake inhibitors
stat	statim	at once, immediately
STD		sexually transmitted disease
SubQ		subcutaneous
supp	suppositorium	suppository
SVT		supraventricular tachycardia
Sx		symptom
syr	syrupus	syrup
tab	tabella	tablet
tal		such
TCA		tricyclic antidepressant
TD		tardive dyskinesia
tid	ter in die	three times a day
TKO		to keep open
TPN		total parenteral nutrition
tr, tinct	tincture	tincture
trit		triturate
tsp		teaspoonful
Tx		treatment
u.d., ut dict		as directed
ULN		upper limits of normal
ung	unguentum	ointment
URI		upper respiratory infection
USAN		United States Adopted Names
USP		United States Pharmacopeia
UTI		urinary tract infection
v.o.		verbal order
VTE		venous thromboembolism
VZV		varicella zoster virus
w.a.		while awake
x3		3 times
x4		4 times
YBOC		Yale Brown Obsessive-Compulsive Scale
YMRS		Young Mania Rating Scale

NORMAL LABORATORY VALUES FOR ADULTS

Automated Chemistry (CHEMISTRY A)

Test	Values	Remarks
SERUM / PLASMA		
Acetone	Negative	
Albumin	3.2-5 g/dL	
Alcohol, ethyl	Negative	
Aldolase	1.2-7.6 IU/L	
Ammonia	20-70 mcg/dL	Specimen to be placed on ice as soon as collected
Amylase	30-110 units/L	
Bilirubin, direct	0-0.3 mg/dL	
Bilirubin, total	0.1-1.2 mg/dL	
Calcium	8.6-10.3 mg/dL	
Calcium, ionized	2.24-2.46 mEq/L	
Chloride	95-108 mEq/L	
Cholesterol, total	≤200 mg/dL	Fasted blood required --- normal value affected by dietary habits This reference range is for a general adult population
HDL cholesterol	40-60 mg/dL	Fasted blood required --- normal value affected by dietary habits
LDL cholesterol	<160 mg/dL	If triglyceride is >400 mg/dL, LDL cannot be calculated accurately (Friedewald equation). Target LDL-C depends on patient's risk factors.
CO_2	23-30 mEq/L	
Creatine kinase (CK) isoenzymes		
CK-BB	0%	
CK-MB (cardiac)	0%-3.9%	
CK-MM (muscle)	96%-100%	

CK-MB levels must be both ≥4% and 10 IU/L to meet diagnostic criteria for CK-MB positive result consistent with myocardial injury.

Test	Values	Remarks
Creatine phosphokinase (CPK)	8-150 IU/L	
Creatinine	0.5-1.4 mg/dL	
Ferritin	13-300 ng/mL	
Folate	3.6-20 ng/dL	
GGT (gamma-glutamyltranspeptidase)		
male	11-63 IU/L	
female	8-35 IU/L	
GLDH	To be determined	
Glucose (preprandial)	<115 mg/dL	Goals different for diabetics
Glucose, fasting	60-110 mg/dL	Goals different for diabetics
Glucose, nonfasting (2-h postprandial)	<120 mg/dL	Goals different for diabetics
Hemoglobin A_{1c}	<8	
Hemoglobin, plasma free	<2.5 mg/100 mL	
Hemoglobin, total glycosolated (Hb A_1)	4%-8%	
Iron	65-150 mcg/dL	
Iron binding capacity, total (TIBC)	250-420 mcg/dL	
Lactic acid	0.7-2.1 mEq/L	Specimen to be kept on ice and sent to lab as soon as possible
Lactate dehydrogenase (LDH)	56-194 IU/L	
Lactate dehydrogenase (LDH) isoenzymes		
LD_1	20%-34%	
LD_2	29%-41%	
LD_3	15%-25%	
LD_4	1%-12%	
LD_5	1%-15%	

Test	Values	Remarks
Flipped LD_1/LD_2 ratios (>1 may be consistent with myocardial injury) particularly when considered in combination with a recent CK-MB positive result		
Lipase	23-208 units/L	
Magnesium	1.6-2.5 mg/dL	Increased by slight hemolysis
Osmolality	289-308 mOsm/kg	
Phosphatase, alkaline		
adults 25-60 y	33-131 IU/L	
adults 61 y or older	51-153 IU/L	
infancy-adolescence	Values range up to 3-5 times higher than adults	
Phosphate, inorganic	2.8-4.2 mg/dL	
Potassium	3.5-5.2 mEq/L	Increased by slight hemolysis
Prealbumin	>15 mg/dL	
Protein, total	6.5-7.9 g/dL	
SGOT (AST)	<35 IU/L (20-48)	
SGPT (ALT) (10-35)	<35 IU/L	
Sodium	134-149 mEq/L	
Thyroid stimulating hormone (TSH)		
adult ≤20 y	0.7-6.4 mIU/L	
21-54 y	0.4-4.2 mIU/L	
55-87 y	0.5-8.9 mIU/L	
Transferrin	>200 mg/dL	
Triglycerides	45-155 mg/dL	Fasted blood required
Troponin I	<1.5 ng/mL	
Urea nitrogen (BUN)	7-20 mg/dL	
Uric acid		
male	2-8 mg/dL	
female	2-7.5 mg/dL	

APPENDIX

Test	Values	Remarks
CEREBROSPINAL FLUID		
Glucose	50-70 mg/dL	
Protein	15-45 mg/dL	CSF obtained by lumbar puncture
Note: Bloody specimen gives erroneously high value due to contamination with blood proteins		
URINE		
(24-hour specimen is required for all these tests unless specified)		
Amylase	32-641 units/L	The value is in units/L and **not** calculated for total volume
Amylase, fluid (random samples)		Interpretation of value left for physician, depends on the nature of fluid
Calcium	Depends upon dietary intake	
Creatine		
male	150 mg/24 h	Higher value on children and during pregnancy
female	250 mg/24 h	
Creatinine	1000-2000 mg/24 h	
Creatinine clearance (endogenous)		
male female	85-125 mL/min 75-115 mL/min	A blood sample must accompany urine specimen
Glucose	1 g/24 h	
5-hydroxyindoleacetic acid	2-8 mg/24 h	
Iron	0.15 mg/24 h	Acid washed container required
Magnesium	146-209 mg/24 h	
Osmolality	500-800 mOsm/kg	With normal fluid intake
Oxalate	10-40 mg/24 h	
Phosphate	400-1300 mg/24 h	
Potassium	25-120 mEq/24 h	Varies with diet; the interpretation of urine electrolytes and osmolality should be left for the physician
Sodium	40-220 mEq/24 h	
Porphobilinogen, qualitative	Negative	
Porphyrins, qualitative	Negative	
Proteins	0.05-0.1 g/24 h	
Salicylate	Negative	
Urea clearance	60-95 mL/min	A blood sample must accompany specimen
Urea N	10-40 g/24 h	Dependent on protein intake
Uric acid	250-750 mg/24 h	Dependent on diet and therapy
Urobilinogen	0.5-3.5 mg/24 h	For qualitative determination on random urine, send sample to urinalysis section in Hematology Lab
Xylose absorption test		
children	16%-33% of ingested xylose	
FECES		
Fat, 3-day collection	<5 g/d	Value depends on fat intake of 100 g/d for 3 days preceding and during collection
GASTRIC ACIDITY		
Acidity, total, 12 h	10-60 mEq/L	Titrated at pH 7

BLOOD GASES

	Arterial	Capillary	Venous
pH	7.35-7.45	7.35-7.45	7.32-7.42
pCO_2 (mm Hg)	35-45	35-45	38-52
pO_2 (mm Hg)	70-100	60-80	24-48
HCO_3 (mEq/L)	19-25	19-25	19-25
TCO_2 (mEq/L)	19-29	19-29	23-33
O_2 saturation (%)	90-95	90-95	40-70
Base excess (mEq/L)	-5 to +5	-5 to +5	-5 to +5

HEMATOLOGY

Complete Blood Count

Age	Hgb (g/dL)	Hct (%)	MCV (fL)	MCH (pg)	MCHC (%)	RBC (mill/mm^3)	RDW	PLTS (x 10^3/mm^3)
0-3 d	15.0-20.0	45-61	95-115	31-37	29-37	4.0-5.9	<18.0	250-450
1-2 wk	12.5-18.5	39-57	86-110	28-36	28-38	3.6-5.5	<17.0	250-450
1-6 mo	10.0-13.0	29-42	74-96	25-35	30-36	3.1-4.3	<16.5	300-700
7 mo - 2 y	10.5-13.0	33-38	70-84	23-30	31-37	3.7-4.9	<16.0	250-600
2-5 y	11.5-13.0	34-39	75-87	24-30	31-37	3.9-5.0	<15.0	250-550
5-8 y	11.5-14.5	35-42	77-95	25-33	31-37	4.0-4.9	<15.0	250-550
13-18 y	12.0-15.2	36-47	78-96	25-35	31-37	4.5-5.1	<14.5	150-450
Adult male	13.5-16.5	41-50	80-100	26-34	31-37	4.5-5.5	<14.5	150-450
Adult female	12.0-15.0	36-44	80-100	26-34	31-37	4.0-4.9	<14.5	150-450

WBC and Diff

Age	WBC (x $10^3/mm^3$)	Segs	Bands	Eos	Basos	Lymphs	Atypical Lymphs	Monos	# of NRBCs
0-3 d	9.0-35.0	32-62	10-18	0-2	0-1	19-29	0-8	5-7	0-2
1-2 wk	5.0-20.0	14-34	6-14	0-2	0-1	36-45	0-8	6-10	0
1-6 mo	6.0-17.5	13-33	4-12	0-3	0-1	41-71	0-8	4-7	0
7 mo - 2 y	6.0-17.0	15-35	5-11	0-3	0-1	45-76	0-8	3-6	0
2-5 y	5.5-15.5	23-45	5-11	0-3	0-1	35-65	0-8	3-6	0
5-8 y	5.0-14.5	32-54	5-11	0-3	0-1	28-48	0-8	3-6	0
13-18 y	4.5-13.0	34-64	5-11	0-3	0-1	25-45	0-8	3-6	0
Adults	4.5-11.0	35-66	5-11	0-3	0-1	24-44	0-8	3-6	0

Erythrocyte Sedimentation Rates and Reticulocyte Counts

Sedimentation rate, Westergren

Children	0-20 mm/hour
Adult male	0-15 mm/hour
Adult female	0-20 mm/hour

Sedimentation rate, Wintrobe

Children	0-13 mm/hour
Adult male	0-10 mm/hour
Adult female	0-15 mm/hour

Reticulocyte count

Newborns	2%-6%
1-6 mo	0%-2.8%
Adults	0.5%-1.5%

NORMAL LABORATORY VALUES FOR CHILDREN

CHEMISTRY		Normal Values
Albumin	0-1 y	2.0-4.0 g/dL
	1 y - adult	3.5-5.5 g/dL
Ammonia	Newborns	90-150 mcg/dL
	Children	40-120 mcg/dL
	Adults	18-54 mcg/dL
Amylase	Newborns	0-60 units/L
	Adults	30-110 units/L
Bilirubin, conjugated, direct	Newborns	<1.5 mg/dL
	1 mo - adult	0-0.5 mg/dL
Bilirubin, total	0-3 d	2.0-10.0 mg/dL
	1 mo - adult	0-1.5 mg/dL
Bilirubin, unconjugated, indirect		0.6-10.5 mg/dL
Calcium	Newborns	7.0-12.0 mg/dL
	0-2 y	8.8-11.2 mg/dL
	2 y - adult	9.0-11.0 mg/dL
Calcium, ionized, whole blood		4.4-5.4 mg/dL
Carbon dioxide, total		23-33 mEq/L
Chloride		95-105 mEq/L
Cholesterol	Newborns	45-170 mg/dL
	0-1 y	65-175 mg/dL
	1-20 y	120-230 mg/dL
Creatinine	0-1 y	≤0.6 mg/dL
	1 y - adult	0.5-1.5 mg/dL
Glucose	Newborns	30-90 mg/dL
	0-2 y	60-105 mg/dL
	Children to Adults	70-110 mg/dL
Iron	Newborns	110-270 mcg/dL
	Infants	30-70 mcg/dL
	Children	55-120 mcg/dL
	Adults	70-180 mcg/dL
Iron binding	Newborns	59-175 mcg/dL
	Infants	100-400 mcg/dL
	Adults	250-400 mcg/dL
Lactic acid, lactate		2-20 mg/dL
Lead, whole blood		<10 mcg/dL
Lipase	Children	20-140 units/L
	Adults	0-190 units/L
Magnesium		1.5-2.5 mEq/L
Osmolality, serum		275-296 mOsm/kg
Osmolality, urine		50-1400 mOsm/kg

CHEMISTRY		Normal Values
Phosphorus	Newborns	4.2-9.0 mg/dL
	6 wk to 19 mo	3.8-6.7 mg/dL
	19 mo to 3 y	2.9-5.9 mg/dL
	3-15 y	3.6-5.6 mg/dL
	>15 y	2.5-5.0 mg/dL
Potassium, plasma	Newborns	4.5-7.2 mEq/L
	2 d - 3 mo	4.0-6.2 mEq/L
	3 mo - 1 y	3.7-5.6 mEq/L
	1-16 y	3.5-5.0 mEq/L
Protein, total	0-2 y	4.2-7.4 g/dL
	>2 y	6.0-8.0 g/dL
Sodium		136-145 mEq/L
Triglycerides	Infants	0-171 mg/dL
	Children	20-130 mg/dL
	Adults	30-200 mg/dL
Urea nitrogen, blood	0-2 y	4-15 mg/dL
	2 y - adult	5-20 mg/dL
Uric acid	Male	3.0-7.0 mg/dL
	Female	2.0-6.0 mg/dL

ENZYMES

Alanine aminotransferase (ALT) (SGPT)	0-2 mo	8-78 units/L
	>2 mo	8-36 units/L
Alkaline phosphatase (ALKP)	Newborns	60-130 units/L
	0-16 y	85-400 units/L
	>16 y	30-115 units/L
Aspartate aminotransferase (AST) (SGOT)	Infants	18-74 units/L
	Children	15-46 units/L
	Adults	5-35 units/L
Creatine kinase (CK)	Infants	20-200 units/L
	Children	10-90 units/L
	Adult Male	0-206 units/L
	Adult Female	0-175 units/L
Lactate dehydrogenase (LDH)	Newborns	290-501 units/L
	1 mo - 2 y	110-144 units/L
	>16 y	60-170 units/L

BLOOD GASES

	Arterial	Capillary	Venous
pH	7.35-7.45	7.35-7.45	7.32-7.42
pCO_2 (mm Hg)	35-45	35-45	38-52
pO_2 (mm Hg)	70-100	60-80	24-48
HCO_3 (mEq/L)	19-25	19-25	19-25
TCO_2 (mEq/L)	19-29	19-29	23-33
O_2 saturation (%)	90-95	90-95	40-70
Base excess (mEq/L)	-5 to +5	-5 to +5	-5 to +5

THYROID FUNCTION TESTS

T_4 (thyroxine)	1-7 d	10.1-20.9 mcg/dL
	8-14 d	9.8-16.6 mcg/dL
	1 mo - 1 y	5.5-16.0 mcg/dL
	>1 y	4.0-12.0 mcg/dL
FTI	1-3 d	9.3-26.6
	1-4 wk	7.6-20.8
	1-4 mo	7.4-17.9
	4-12 mo	5.1-14.5
	1-6 y	5.7-13.3
	>6 y	4.8-14.0
T_3 by RIA	Newborns	100-470 ng/dL
	1-5 y	100-260 ng/dL
	5-10 y	90-240 ng/dL
	10 y - adult	70-210 ng/dL
T_3 uptake		35%-45%
TSH	Cord	3-22 µIU/mL
	1-3 d	<40 µIU/mL
	3-7 d	<25 µIU/mL
	>7 d	0-10 µIU/mL

APOTHECARY/METRIC CONVERSIONS

Approximate Liquid Measures

Basic equivalent: 1 fluid ounce = 30 mL

Examples:

1 gallon . . . . . 3800 mL
1 quart . . . . 960 mL
1 pint . . . . 480 mL
8 fluid oz . . . . . . 240 mL

4 fluid oz . . . . 120 mL
15 minims . . . . 1 mL
10 minims . . . . 0.6 mL

1 gallon . . . . . . 128 fluid ounces
1 quart . . . . 32 fluid ounces
1 pint . . . . 16 fluid ounces

Approximate Household Equivalents

1 teaspoonful . . . . 5 mL

1 tablespoonful . . . 15 mL

Weights

Basic equivalents:

1 oz = 30 g

15 gr = 1 g

Examples:

4 oz . . . . 120 g
2 oz . . . . 60 g
10 gr . . . . 600 mg
7 $^1/_2$ gr . . . . 500 mg
16 oz . . . . 1 pound

1 gr . . . . 60 mg
$^1/_{100}$ gr . . . . 600 mcg
$^1/_{150}$ gr . . . . 400 mcg
$^1/_{200}$ gr . . . . 300 mcg

Metric Conversions

Basic equivalents:

1 g . . . . 1000 mg

1 mg . . . . 1000 mcg

Examples:

5 g . . . . 5000 mg
0.5 g . . . . 500 mg
0.05 g . . . . 50 mg

5 mg . . . . 5000 mcg
0.5 mg . . . . 500 mcg
0.05 mg . . . . 50 mcg

Exact Equivalents

1 g = 15.43 grains
1 milliliter (mL) = 16.23 minims
1 minim = 0.06 milliliter
1 gr = 64.8 milligrams
1 pint (pt) = 473.2 milliliters
1 oz = 28.35 grams
1 lb = 453.6 grams
1 kg = 2.2 pounds
1 qt = 946.4 milliliters

0.1 mg = $^1/_{600}$ gr
0.12 mg = $^1/_{500}$ gr
0.15 mg = $^1/_{400}$ gr
0.2 mg = $^1/_{300}$ gr
0.3 mg = $^1/_{200}$ gr
0.4 mg = $^1/_{150}$ gr
0.5 mg = $^1/_{120}$ gr
0.6 mg = $^1/_{100}$ gr
0.8 mg = $^1/_{80}$ gr
1 mg = $^1/_{65}$ gr

Solids*

$^1/_4$ grain = 15 mg
$^1/_2$ grain = 30 mg
1 grain = 60 mg
1$^1/_2$ grains = 90 mg
5 grains = 300 mg
10 grains = 600 mg

*Use exact equivalents for compounding and calculations requiring a high degree of accuracy.

POUNDS/KILOGRAMS CONVERSION

1 pound = 0.45359 kilograms
1 kilogram = 2.2 pounds

lb	=	kg	lb	=	kg	lb	=	kg
1		0.45	70		31.75	140		63.50
5		2.27	75		34.02	145		65.77
10		4.54	80		36.29	150		68.04
15		6.80	85		38.56	155		70.31
20		9.07	90		40.82	160		72.58
25		11.34	95		43.09	165		74.84
30		13.61	100		45.36	170		77.11
35		15.88	105		47.63	175		79.38
40		18.14	110		49.90	180		81.65
45		20.41	115		52.16	185		83.92
50		22.68	120		54.43	190		86.18
55		24.95	125		56.70	195		88.45
60		27.22	130		58.91	200		90.72
65		29.48	135		61.24			

TEMPERATURE CONVERSION

Centigrade to Fahrenheit = (°C x 9/5) + 32 = °F
Fahrenheit to Centigrade = (°F - 32) x 5/9 = °C

°C	=	°F	°C	=	°F	°C	=	°F
100.0		212.0	39.0		102.2	36.8		98.2
50.0		122.0	38.8		101.8	36.6		97.9
41.0		105.8	38.6		101.5	36.4		97.5
40.8		105.4	38.4		101.1	36.2		97.2
40.6		105.1	38.2		100.8	36.0		96.8
40.4		104.7	38.0		100.4	35.8		96.4
40.2		104.4	37.8		100.1	35.6		96.1
40.0		104.0	37.6		99.7	35.4		95.7
39.8		103.6	37.4		99.3	35.2		95.4
39.6		103.3	37.2		99.0	35.0		95.0
39.4		102.9	37.0		98.6	0		32.0
39.2		102.6						

ACQUIRED IMMUNODEFICIENCY SYNDROME (AIDS) — LAB TESTS AND APPROVED DRUGS FOR HIV INFECTION AND AIDS-RELATED CONDITIONS

This list of tests is not intended in any way to suggest patterns of physician's orders, nor is it complete. These tests may support possible clinical diagnoses or rule out other diagnostic possibilities. Each laboratory test relevant to AIDS is listed and weighted. Two symbols (**) indicate that the test is diagnostic, that is, documents the diagnosis if the expected is found. A single symbol (*) indicates a test frequently used in the diagnosis or management of the disease. The other listed tests are useful on a selective basis with consideration of clinical factors and specific aspects of the case.

Acid-Fast Stain
Acid-Fast Stain, Modified, *Nocardia* Species
Antimicrobial Susceptibility Testing, Fungi
Antimicrobial Susceptibility Testing, Mycobacteria
Arthropod Identification
Babesiosis Serological Test
Bacteremia Detection, Buffy Coat Micromethod
Bacterial Culture, Blood
Bacterial Culture, Bronchoscopy Specimen
Bacterial Culture, Sputum
Bacterial Culture, Stool
Bacterial Culture, Throat
Bacterial Culture, Urine, Clean Catch
$Beta_2$-Microglobulin
Blood and Fluid Precautions, Specimen Collection
Bronchial Washings Cytology
Bronchoalveolar Lavage Cytology
Brushings Cytology
Candida Antigen
Candidiasis Serologic Test
Cat Scratch Disease Serology
CD4/CD8 Enumeration
Cerebrospinal Fluid Cytology
Cryptococcal Antigen Titer
Cryptosporidium Diagnostic Procedures
Cytomegalic Inclusion Disease Cytology
Cytomegalovirus Antibody
Cytomegalovirus Antigen Detection
Cytomegalovirus Culture
Cytomegalovirus DNA Detection
Darkfield Examination, Syphilis
Electron Microscopy
Folic Acid, Serum
Fungal Culture, Biopsy or Body Fluid
Fungal Culture, Blood
Fungal Culture, Cerebrospinal Fluid
Fungal Culture, Sputum
Fungal Culture, Stool
Fungal Culture, Urine
Hemoglobin A_2
Hepatitis B Surface Antigen
Herpes Cytology
Herpes Simplex Virus Antigen Detection
Herpes Simplex Virus Culture
Histopathology
Histoplasmosis Antibody
Histoplasmosis Antigen
**HIV-1/HIV-2 Serology
HTLV-I/II Antibody
*Human Immunodeficiency Virus Culture
*Human Immunodeficiency Virus DNA Amplification

India Ink Preparation
Inhibitor, Lupus, Phospholipid Type
KOH Preparation
Leishmaniasis Serological Test
Leukocyte Immunophenotyping
Lymphocyte Transformation Test
Microsporidia Diagnostic Procedures
Mycobacteria by DNA Probe
Mycobacterial Culture, Biopsy or Body Fluid
Mycobacterial Culture, Cerebrospinal Fluid
Mycobacterial Culture, Cutaneous and Subcutaneous Tissue
Mycobacterial Culture, Sputum
Mycobacterial Culture, Stool
Neisseria gonorrhoeae Culture and Smear
Nocardia Culture
Ova and Parasites, Stool
*p24 Antigen
Platelet Count
Pneumocystis carinii Preparation
Pneumocystis Immunofluorescence
Polymerase Chain Reaction
Red Blood Cell Indices
Risks of Transfusion
Skin Biopsy
Sputum Cytology
Toxoplasmosis Serology
VDRL, Serum
Viral Culture
Viral Culture, Blood
Viral Culture, Body Fluid
Viral Culture, Central Nervous System Symptoms
Viral Culture, Dermatological Symptoms
Viral Culture, Tissue
Virus, Direct Detection by Fluorescent Antibody
White Blood Count

CURRENTLY APPROVED ANTIRETROVIRAL DRUGS

Antiretroviral Drugs

Generic Name	Synonyms	Brand Name
FUSION INHIBITOR		
enfuvirtide	T-20	Fuzeon®
NONNUCLEOSIDE REVERSE TRANSCRIPTASE INHIBITORS (NNRTIs)		
delavidine		Rescriptor®
efavirenz		Sustiva®
nevirapine		Viramune®
NUCLEOTIDE ANALOG REVERSE TRANSCRIPTASE INHIBITORS (NtARTIs)		
adefovir	bis-POM PMPA	Preveon®
tenofovir		Viread®
PROTEASE INHIBITORS (PI)		
amprenavir		Agenerase®
atazanavir		Reyataz®
fosamprenavir		Lexiva®
indinavir		Crixivan®
lopinavir		----
nelfinavir		Viracept®
ritonavir		Norvir®
saquinavir		Fortovase®
tipranavir		Aptivus®
REVERSE TRANSCRIPTASE INHIBITORS (RTIs)		
abacavir	ABC	Ziagen®
didanosine	ddI	Videx®
emtricitabine	FTC	Emtriva®
lamivudine	3TC	Epivir®
stavudine	d4T	Zerit®
zalcitabine	ddC	Hivid®
zidovudine	AZT, ZDV, azidothymidine	Retrovir®
COMBINATION PRODUCTS		
Combivir® = AZT + 3TC		
Trizivir® = abacavir (ABC) + AZT + 3TC		
Kaletra® = lopinavir + ritonavir		
Epzicom® = ABC + 3TC		
Truvada® = emtricitabine + tenofovir		
Tripla® = efavirenz + emtricitabine + tenofovir		

DRUGS USED TO TREAT COMPLICATIONS OF HIV / AIDS

Brand Name	Generic Name (Synonym)	Use
Abelcet®, Ambisome®	amphotericin B, ABLC	Antifungal for aspergillosis
Bactrim®, Septra®	sulfamethoxazole and trimethoprim, SMZ/TMP	Antiprotozoal antibiotic for *Pneumocystis carinii* pneumonia treatment and prevention
Biaxin®	clarithromycin	Antibiotic for *Mycobacterium avium* prevention and treatment
Cytovene®	ganciclovir, DHPG	Antiviral for CMV retinitis
DaunoXome®	daunorubicin citrate (liposomal)	Chemotherapy for Kaposi sarcoma
Diflucan®	fluconazole	Antifungal for candidiasis, crytococcal meningitis
Doxil®	doxorubicin (liposomal)	Chemotherapy for Kaposi sarcoma
Eraxis™	anidulafungin	Antifungal (intravenous), used to treat *Candida* infections in the esophagus (candidiasis), blood stream (candidemia), and other forms of *Candida* infections, including abdominal abscesses and peritonitis (inflammation of the lining of the abdominal cavity)
Famvir®	famciclovir	Antiviral for herpes
Foscarnet®	foscavir	Antiviral for herpes, CMV retinitis
Gamimune® N	immune globulin, gamma globulin, IGIV	Immune booster to prevent bacterial infections in children
Intron® A	interferon alfa-2b	Karposi sarcoma, hepatitis C
Marinol®	dronabinol	Treat appetite loss
Megace®	megestrol acetate	Treat appetite and weight loss
Mepron®	atovaquone	Antiprotozoal antibiotic for *Pneumocystis carinii* pneumonia treatment and prevention
Mycobutin®	rifabutin	Antimycobacterial antibiotic for *Mycobacterium avium* prevention
NebuPent®	pentamidine	Antiprotozoal antibiotic for *Pneumocystis carinii* pneumonia prevention
Neutrexin®	trimetrexate glucuronate and leucovorin	Antiprotozoal antibiotic for *Pneumocystis carinii* pneumonia treatment
Panretin® Gel	alitretinoin gel 0.1%	AIDS-related Karposi sarcoma
Procrit®, Epogen®	erythropoetin, EPO	Treat anemia related to AZT therapy
Roferon-A®	interferon alfa-2a	Karposi sarcoma and hepatitis C
Serostim®	somatropin rDNA	Treat weight loss
Sporanox®	itraconazole	Antifungal for blastomycosis, histoplasmosis, aspergillosis, and candidiasis
Taxol®	paclitaxel	Karposi sarcoma
Valcyte™	valganciclovir	Antiviral for CMV retinitis
VFEND®	voriconazole	Antifungal for invasive aspergillosis and serious fungal infections due to *Fusarium sporotrichoides and Scedosporium apiospermum*, and Esophageal Candidiasis
Vistide®	cidofovir, HPMPC	Antiviral for CMV retinitis
Vitrasert® Implant	ganciclovir insert	Antiviral for CMV retinitis
Vitravene® Intravitreal Injectable	fomivirsen sodium injection	Antiviral for CMV retinitis
Zithromax®	azithromycin	Antibiotic for *Mycobacterium avium*

CHEMOTHERAPY REGIMENS

5 + 2

Use: Leukemia, acute myeloid (induction)

Regimen:

Cytarabine: I.V.: 100-200 mg/m^2/day continuous infusion days 1-5 [total dose/cycle = 500-1000 mg/m^2]

with

Daunorubicin: I.V.: 45 mg/m^2/day days 1 and 2 [total dose/cycle = 90 mg/m^2]

or

Mitoxantrone: I.V.: 12 mg/m^2/day days 1 and 2 [total dose/cycle = 24 mg/m^2]

7 + 3 (Daunorubicin)

Use: Leukemia, acute myeloid (induction)

Regimen:

Cytarabine: I.V.: 100 mg/m^2/day continuous infusion days 1-7 [total dose/cycle = 700 mg/m^2]

Daunorubicin: I.V.: 45 mg/m^2/day days 1-3 [total dose/cycle = 135 mg/m^2]

Administer one cycle only

7 + 3 (Idarubicin)

Use: Leukemia, acute myeloid (induction)

Regimen:

Cytarabine: I.V.: 100-200 mg/m^2/day continuous infusion days 1-7 [total dose/cycle = 700-1400 mg/m^2]

Idarubicin: I.V.: 12 mg/m^2/day days 1-3 [total dose/cycle = 36 mg/m^2]

Administer one cycle only

7 + 3 (Mitoxantrone)

Use: Leukemia, acute myeloid (induction)

Regimen:

Cytarabine: I.V.: 100-200 mg/m^2/day continuous infusion days 1-7 [total dose/cycle = 700-1400 mg/m^2]

Mitoxantrone: I.V.: 12 mg/m^2/day days 1-3 [total dose/cycle = 36 mg/m^2]

Administer one cycle only

7 + 3 + 7

Use: Leukemia, acute myeloid

Regimen:

Cytarabine: I.V.: 100 mg/m^2/day continuous infusion days 1-7 [total dose/cycle = 700 mg/m^2]

Daunorubicin: I.V.: 50 mg/m^2/day days 1-3 [total dose/cycle = 150 mg/m^2]

Etoposide: I.V.: 75 mg/m^2/day days 1-7 [total dose/cycle = 525 mg/m^2]

Repeat cycle every 21 days; up to 3 cycles may be given based on individual response

8 in 1 (Brain Tumors)

Use: Brain tumors

Regimen: Note: Multiple variations are listed below.

Variation 1:

Methylprednisolone: I.V.: 300 mg/m^2 every 6 hours day 1 (3 doses) [total dose/cycle = 900 mg/m^2]

Vincristine: I.V.: 1.5 mg/m^2 (maximum 2 mg) day 1 [total dose/cycle = 1.5 mg/m^2]

Lomustine: Oral: 75 mg/m^2 day 1 [total dose/cycle = 75 mg/m^2]

Procarbazine: Oral: 75 mg/m^2 day 1; 1 hour after methylprednisolone and vincristine [total dose/cycle = 75 mg/m^2]

Hydroxyurea: Oral: 3000 mg/m^2 day 1; 2 hours after methylprednisolone and vincristine [total dose/cycle = 3000 mg/m^2]

Cisplatin: I.V.: 90 mg/m^2 day 1; 3 hours after methylprednisolone and vincristine [total dose/cycle = 90 mg/m^2]

Cytarabine: I.V.: 300 mg/m^2 day 1; 9 hours after methylprednisolone and vincristine [total dose/cycle = 300 mg/m^2]

Dacarbazine: I.V.: 150 mg/m^2 day 1; 12 hours after methylprednisolone and vincristine [total dose/cycle = 150 mg/m^2]

Repeat cycle every 14 days

Variation 2:

Methylprednisolone: I.V.: 300 mg/m^2 every 6 hours day 1 (3 doses) [total dose/cycle = 900 mg/m^2]

Vincristine: I.V.: 1.5 mg/m^2 (maximum 2 mg) day 1 [total dose/cycle = 1.5 mg/m^2]

Lomustine: Oral: 75 mg/m^2 day 1 [total dose/cycle = 75 mg/m^2]

Procarbazine: Oral: 75 mg/m^2 day 1; 1 hour after methylprednisolone and vincristine [total dose/cycle = 75 mg/m^2]

Hydroxyurea: Oral: 3000 mg/m^2 day 1; 2 hours after methylprednisolone and vincristine [total dose/cycle = 3000 mg/m^2]

Cisplatin: I.V.: 60 mg/m^2 day 1; 3 hours after methylprednisolone and vincristine [total dose/cycle = 60 mg/m^2]

Cytarabine: I.V.: 300 mg/m^2 day 1; 9 hours after methylprednisolone and vincristine [total dose/cycle = 300 mg/m^2]

Cyclophosphamide: I.V.: 300 mg/m^2 day 1; 12 hours after methylprednisolone and vincristine [total dose/cycle = 300 mg/m^2]

Repeat cycle every 14 days

8 in 1 (Retinoblastoma)

Use: Retinoblastoma

Regimen:

Vincristine: I.V.: 1.5 mg/m^2 day 1 [total dose/cycle = 1.5 mg/m^2]

Methylprednisolone: I.V.: 300 mg/m^2 day 1 [total dose/cycle = 300 mg/m^2]

Lomustine: Oral: 75 mg/m^2 day 1 [total dose/cycle = 75 mg/m^2]

Procarbazine: Oral: 75 mg/m^2 day 1 [total dose/cycle = 75 mg/m^2]

Hydroxyurea: Oral: 1500 mg/m^2 day 1 [total dose/cycle = 1500 mg/m^2]

Cisplatin: I.V.: 60 mg/m^2 day 1 [total dose/cycle = 60 mg/m^2]

Cytarabine: I.V.: 300 mg/m^2 day 1 [total dose/cycle = 300 mg/m^2]

Repeat cycle every 28 days

AAV (DD)

Use: Wilms Tumor

Regimen:

Dactinomycin: I.V.: 15 mcg/kg/day days 1-5 of weeks 0, 13, 26, 39, 52, 65 [total dose/cycle = 450 mcg/kg]

Doxorubicin: I.V.: 20 mg/m^2/day days 1-3 of weeks 6, 19, 32, 45, 58 [total dose/cycle = 300 mg/m^2]

Vincristine: I.V.: 1.5 mg/m^2 day 1 of weeks 0-10, 13, 14, 26, 27, 39, 40, 52, 53, 65, 66 [total dose/cycle = 31.5 mg/m^2]

ABVD

Use: Lymphoma, Hodgkin disease

Regimen:

Doxorubicin: I.V.: 25 mg/m^2/day days 1 and 15 [total dose/cycle = 50 mg/m^2]

Bleomycin: I.V.: 10 units/m^2/day days 1 and 15 [total dose/cycle = 20 units/m^2]

Vinblastine: I.V.: 6 mg/m^2/day days 1 and 15 [total dose/cycle = 12 mg/m^2]

Dacarbazine: I.V.: 375 mg/m^2/day days 1 and 15 [total dose/cycle = 750 mg/m^2]

Repeat cycle every 28 days

AC

Use: Breast cancer

Regimen: Note: Multiple variations are listed below.

Variation 1:

Doxorubicin: I.V.: 60 mg/m^2 day 1 [total dose/cycle = 60 mg/m^2]

Cyclophosphamide: I.V.: 600 mg/m^2 day 1 [total dose/cycle = 600 mg/m^2]

Repeat cycle every 21 days

Variation 2:

Doxorubicin: I.V.: 60 mg/m^2 day 1 [total dose/cycle = 60 mg/m^2]

Cyclophosphamide: I.V.: 600 mg/m^2 day 1 [total dose/cycle = 600 mg/m^2]

Filgrastim: SubQ: 5 mcg/kg for 7-10 days, beginning day 3 [total dose/cycle = 35-50 mcg/kg]

Repeat cycle every 14 days

ACAV (J)

Use: Wilms tumor

Regimen:

Dactinomycin: I.V.: 15 mcg/kg/day days 1-5 of weeks 0, 13, 26, 39, 52, 65
[total dose/cycle = 450 mcg/kg]

Cyclophosphamide: I.V.: 10 mg/kg/day days 1-3 of weeks 0, 6, 13, 19, 26, 32, 39, 45, 52, 58, 65
[total dose/cycle = 330 mg/kg]

Doxorubicin: I.V.: 20 mg/m^2/day days 1-3 of weeks 6, 19, 32, 45, 58
[total dose/cycle = 300 mg/m^2]

Vincristine: I.V.: 1.5 mg/m^2 day 1 of weeks 0-10, 13, 14, 19, 20, 26, 27, 32, 33, 39, 40, 45, 52, 53, 56, 57, 65, 66
[total dose/cycle = 42 mg/m^2]

AD

Use: Soft tissue sarcoma

Regimen:

Doxorubicin: I.V.: 60 mg/m^2/day day 1 [total dose/cycle = 60 mg/m^2]

Dacarbazine: I.V.: 250 mg/m^2 days 1-5 [total dose/cycle = 1250 mg/m^2]

Repeat cycle every 21 days

AP

Use: Endometrial Cancer

Regimen:

Doxorubicin: I.V.: 60 mg/m^2 day 1 [total dose/cycle = 60 mg/m^2]

Cisplatin: I.V.: 60 mg/m^2 day 1 [total dose/cycle = 60 mg/m^2]

Repeat cycle every 21 days

AV (EE)

Use: Wilms Tumor

Regimen:

Dactinomycin: I.V.: 15 mcg/kg/day days 1-5 of weeks 0, 5, 13, 26 [total dose/cycle = 300 mcg/kg]

Vincristine: I.V.: 1.5 mg/m^2/dose day 1 of weeks 0-10, 13, 14, 16, 17
[total dose/cycle = 22.5 mg/m^2]

AV (K)

Use: Wilms tumor

Regimen:

Dactinomycin: I.V.: 15 mcg/kg/day days 1-5 of weeks 0, 5, 13, 22, 31, 40, 49, 58
[total dose/cycle = 600 mcg/kg]

Vincristine: I.V.: 1.5 mg/m^2/dose day 1 of weeks 0-10, 15-20, 24-29, 33-38, 42-47, 51-56, 60-65
[total dose/cycle = 70.5 mg/m^2]

AV (L)

Use: Wilms tumor

Regimen:

Dactinomycin: I.V.: 15 mcg/kg/day days 1-5 of weeks 0 and 5 [total dose/cycle = 450 mcg/kg]

Vincristine: I.V.: 1.5 mg/m^2 day 1 of weeks 0-10 [total dose/cycle = 16.5 mg/m^2]

AV (Wilms tumor)

Use: Wilms tumor

Regimen:

Dactinomycin: I.V.: 15 mcg/kg/day days 1-5 of weeks 0, 13, 26, 39, 52, 65
[total dose/cycle = 450 mcg/kg]

Vincristine: I.V.: 1.5 mg/m^2/dose day 1 of weeks 0-8, 13, 14, 26, 27, 39, 40, 52, 53, 65, 66
[total dose/cycle = 28.5 mg/m^2]

AVD

Use: Wilms tumor

Regimen:

Dactinomycin: I.V.: 15 mcg/kg/day days 1-5 of weeks 0, 13, 26, 39, 52, 65
[total dose/cycle = 450 mcg/kg]

Doxorubicin: I.V.: 20 mg/m^2/day days 1-3 of weeks 6, 19, 32, 45, 58
[total dose/cycle = 300 mg/m^2]

Vincristine: I.V.: 1.5 mg/m^2 day 1 of weeks 0-8, 13, 14, 26, 27, 39, 40, 52, 53, 65, 66
[total dose/cycle = 28.5 mg/m^2]

BEACOPP

Use: Lymphoma, Hodgkin disease

Regimen:

Bleomycin: I.V.: 10 units/m^2 day 8 [total dose/cycle = 10 units/m^2]

Etoposide: I.V.: 100 mg/m^2/day days 1-3 [total dose/cycle = 300 mg/m^2]

Doxorubicin: I.V.: 25 mg/m^2 day 1 [total dose/cycle = 25 mg/m^2]

Cyclophosphamide: I.V.: 650 mg/m^2 day 1 [total dose/cycle = 650 mg/m^2]

Vincristine: I.V.: 1.4 mg/m^2 (maximum 2 mg) day 1 [total dose/cycle = 1.4 mg/m^2]

Procarbazine: Oral: 100 mg/m^2/day days 1-7 [total dose/cycle = 700 mg/m^2]

Prednisone: Oral: 40 mg/m^2/day days 1-14 [total dose/cycle = 560 mg/m^2]

Filgrastim: SubQ: 300-480 mcg daily from day 8 until leukocytes >2000 cells/mm^3 for 3 days

Repeat cycle every 21 days

BEP (Ovarian)

Use: Ovarian cancer

Regimen:

Bleomycin: I.V.: 20 units/m^2 day 1 [total dose/cycle = 20 units/m^2]

Etoposide: I.V.: 75 mg/m^2/day days 1-5 [total dose/cycle = 375 mg/m^2]

Cisplatin: I.V.: 20 mg/m^2/day days 1-5 [total dose/cycle = 100 mg/m^2]

Repeat cycle every 3 weeks

BEP (Ovarian, Testicular)

Use: Ovarian cancer; Testicular cancer
Regimen:
Bleomycin: I.V.: 30 units/day days 2, 9, 16 [total dose/cycle = 90 units]
Etoposide: I.V.: 100 mg/m^2/day days 1-5 [total dose/cycle = 500 mg/m^2]
or 120 mg/m^2/day days 1-3 [total dose/cycle = 360 mg/m^2]
Cisplatin: I.V.: 20 mg/m^2/day days 1-5 [total dose/cycle = 100 mg/m^2]
Repeat cycle every 21 days

BEP (Testicular)

Use: Testicular cancer
Regimen: Note: Multiple variations are listed below.
Variation 1:
Bleomycin: I.V.: 30 units/day days 2, 9, 16 [total dose/cycle = 90 units]
Etoposide: I.V.: 100 mg/m^2/day days 1-5 [total dose/cycle = 500 mg/m^2]
Cisplatin: I.V.: 20 mg/m^2/day days 1-5 [total dose/cycle = 100 mg/m^2]
Repeat cycle every 21 days
Variation 2:
Bleomycin: I.V.: 30 units once weekly [total dose/cycle = 90 units]
Etoposide: I.V.: 120 mg/m^2/day days 1, 3, 5 [total dose/cycle = 360 mg/m^2]
Cisplatin: I.V.: 20 mg/m^2/day days 1-5 [total dose/cycle = 100 mg/m^2]
Repeat cycle every 21 days
Variation 3:
Bleomycin: I.V.: 30 units/day days 1, 8, 15 [total dose/cycle = 90 units]
Etoposide: I.V.: 165 mg/m^2/day days 1-3 [total dose/cycle = 495 mg/m^2]
Cisplatin: I.V.: 50 mg/m^2/day days 1, 2 [total dose/cycle = 100 mg/m^2]
Repeat cycle every 21 days

Bicalutamide + LHRH-A

Use: Prostate Cancer
Regimen:
Bicalutamide: Oral: 50 mg/day [total dose/cycle = 50 mg] **with**
Goserelin acetate: SubQ: 3.6 mg day 1 [total dose/cycle = 3.6 mg] **or**
Leuprolide depot: I.M.: 7.5 mg day 1 [total dose/cycle = 7.5 mg]
Repeat cycle every 28 days

BOLD

Use: Melanoma
Regimen:
Dacarbazine: I.V.: 200 mg/m^2/day days 1-5 [total dose/cycle = 1000 mg/m^2]
Vincristine: I.V.: 1 mg/m^2/day days 1 and 4 [total dose/cycle = 2 mg/m^2]
Bleomycin: I.V.: 15 units/day days 2 and 5 [total dose/cycle = 30 units]
Lomustine: Oral: 80 mg day 1 [total dose/cycle = 80 mg]
Repeat cycle every 4 weeks

CA

Use: Leukemia, acute myeloid
Regimen:
Cytarabine: I.V.: 3000 mg/m^2 every 12 hours days 1 and 2 (4 doses)
[total dose/cycle = 12,000 mg/m^2]
Asparaginase: I.M.: 6000 units/m^2 at hour 42 [total dose/cycle = 6000 units/m^2]
Repeat cycle every 7 days for 2 or 3 cycles

CABO

Use: Head and neck cancer
Regimen:
Cisplatin: I.V.: 50 mg/m^2 day 4 [total dose/cycle = 50 mg/m^2]
Methotrexate: I.V.: 40 mg/m^2/day days 1 and 15 [total dose/cycle = 80 mg/m^2]
Bleomycin: I.V.: 10 units/day days 1, 8, and 15 [total dose/cycle = 30 units]
Vincristine: I.V.: 2 mg/day days 1, 8, and 15 [total dose/cycle = 6 mg]
Repeat cycle every 21 days

CAD/MOPP/ABV

Use: Lymphoma, Hodgkin disease

Regimen:

CAD:

Lomustine: Oral: 100 mg/m^2 day 1 [total dose/cycle = 100 mg/m^2]
Melphalan: Oral: 6 mg/m^2/day days 1-4 [total dose/cycle = 24 mg/m^2]
Vindesine: I.V.: 3 mg/m^2/day days 1 and 8 [total dose/cycle = 6 mg/m^2]

MOPP:

Mechlorethamine: I.V.: 6 mg/m^2/day days 1 and 8 [total dose/cycle = 12 mg/m^2]
Vincristine: I.V.: 1.4 mg/m^2/day days 1 and 8 [total dose/cycle = 2.8 mg/m^2]
Procarbazine: Oral: 100 mg/m^2/day days 1-14 [total dose/cycle = 1400 mg/m^2]
Prednisone: Oral: 40 mg/m^2/day days 1-14 [total dose/cycle = 560 mg/m^2]

ABV:

Doxorubicin: I.V.: 25 mg/m^2/day days 1 and 14 [total dose/cycle = 50 mg/m^2]
Bleomycin: SubQ: 6 units/m^2/day days 1 and 14 [total dose/cycle = 12 units/m^2]
Vinblastine: I.V.: 2 mg/m^2 continuous infusion days 4-12 and 18-26 [total dose/cycle = 36 mg/m^2]

CAD is administered first, then MOPP begins on day 29 or day 37 following CAD. ABV is administered on day 29 following MOPP; CAD recycles on day 29 following ABV.

CAF

Use: Breast cancer

Regimen: Note: Multiple variations are listed below.

Variation 1:

Cyclophosphamide: Oral: 100 mg/m^2/day days 1-14 [total dose/cycle = 1400 mg/m^2]
Doxorubicin: I.V.: 30 mg/m^2/day days 1 and 8 [total dose/cycle = 60 mg/m^2]
Fluorouracil: I.V.: 500 mg/m^2/day days 1 and 8 [total dose/cycle = 1000 mg/m^2]
Repeat cycle every 28 days

Variation 2:

Cyclophosphamide: Oral: 100 mg/m^2/day days 1-14 [total dose/cycle = 1400 mg/m^2]
Doxorubicin: I.V.: 25 mg/m^2/day days 1 and 8 [total dose/cycle = 50 mg/m^2]
Fluorouracil: I.V.: 500 mg/m^2/day days 1 and 8 [total dose/cycle = 1000 mg/m^2]
Repeat cycle every 28 days

CAP

Use: Bladder Cancer

Regimen:

Cyclophosphamide: I.V.: 400 mg/m^2 day 1 [total dose = 400 mg/m^2]
Doxorubicin: I.V.: 40 mg/m^2 day 1 [total dose = 40 mg/m^2]
Cisplatin: I.V.: 60 mg/m^2 day 1 [total dose = 60 mg/m^2]
Repeat cycle every 21 days

Carbo-Tax (Adenocarcinoma)

Use: Adenocarcinoma, unknown primary

Regimen:

Paclitaxel: I.V.: 135 mg/m^2 infused over 24 hours day 1 [total dose = 135 mg/m^2]

followed by:

Carboplatin: I.V.: Target AUC 7.5 [total dose = AUC = 7.5]
Repeat cycle every 21 days

Carbo-Tax (Nonsmall-Cell Lung Cancer)

Use: Lung cancer, nonsmall-cell

Regimen:

Paclitaxel: I.V.: 135-215 mg/m^2 infused over 24 hours day 1 [total dose/cycle = 135-215 mg/m^2] **or**
175 mg/m^2 infused over 3 hours day 1 [total dose/cycle = 175 mg/m^2] **followed by:**
Carboplatin: I.V.: Target AUC 7.5 [total dose/cycle = AUC = 7.5]
Repeat cycle every 21 days

Carbo-Tax (Ovarian Cancer)

Use: Ovarian cancer
Regimen: Note: Multiple variations are listed below.

Variation 1:
Paclitaxel: I.V.: 135 mg/m^2 infused over 24 hours day 1 [total dose/cycle = 135 mg/m^2] **or**
175 mg/m^2 over 3 hours day 1 [total dose/cycle = 175 mg/m^2]
followed by:
Carboplatin: I.V.: Target AUC 5 [total dose/cycle = AUC = 5]
Repeat cycle every 21 days

Variation 2:
Paclitaxel: I.V.: 175 mg/m^2 day 1 [total dose/cycle = 175 mg/m^2]
Carboplatin: I.V.: AUC 7.5 day 1 [total dose/cycle = AUC = 7.5]
Repeat cycle every 21 days

Variation 3:
Paclitaxel: I.V.: 185 mg/m^2 day 1 [total dose/cycle = 185 mg/m^2]
Carboplatin: I.V.: AUC 6 day 1 [total dose/cycle = AUC = 6]
Repeat cycle every 21 days

CaT (Nonsmall-Cell Lung Cancer)

Use: Lung cancer, nonsmall-cell
Regimen: Note: Multiple variations are listed below.

Variation 1:
Paclitaxel: I.V.: 175 mg/m^2 day 1 [total dose/cycle = 175 mg/m^2] **or**
135 mg/m^2 continuous infusion day 1 [total dose/cycle = 135 mg/m^2]
Carboplatin: I.V.: AUC 7.5 day 1 or 2 [total dose/cycle = AUC = 7.5]
Repeat cycle every 21 days

Variation 2:
Paclitaxel: I.V.: 225 mg/m^2 day 1 [total dose/cycle = 225 mg/m^2]
Carboplatin: I.V.: AUC 6 day 1 [total dose/cycle = AUC = 6]
Repeat cycle every 21 days

CaT (Ovarian Cancer)

Use: Ovarian cancer
Regimen:
Paclitaxel: I.V.: 175 mg/m^2 day 1 [total dose/cycle = 175 mg/m^2] **or**
135 mg/m^2 continuous infusion day 1 [total dose/cycle = 135 mg/m^2]
Carboplatin: I.V.: AUC 7.5 day 1 or 2 [total dose/cycle = AUC = 7.5]
Repeat cycle every 21 days

CAVE

Use: Lung cancer, small-cell
Regimen:
Cyclophosphamide: I.V.: 750 mg/m^2 day 1 [total dose/cycle = 750 mg/m^2]
Doxorubicin: I.V.: 50 mg/m^2 day 1 [total dose/cycle = 50 mg/m^2]
Vincristine: I.V.: 1.4 mg/m^2 (maximum 2 mg) day 1 [total dose/cycle = 1.4 mg/m^2]
Etoposide: I.V.: 60-100 mg/m^2/day days 1-3 [total dose/cycle = 180-300 mg/m^2]
Repeat cycle every 21 days

CAV-P/VP

Use: Neuroblastomas
Regimen:

Course 1, 2, 4, 6:
Cyclophosphamide: I.V.: 70 mg/kg/day days 1 and 2 [total dose/cycle = 140 mg/kg]
Doxorubicin: I.V.: 25 mg/m^2/day continuous infusion days 1-3 [total dose/cycle = 75 mg/m^2]
Vincristine: I.V.: 0.033 mg/kg/day continuous infusion days 1-3 [total dose/cycle = .099 mg/kg]
Vincristine: I.V.: 1.5 mg/m^2 day 9

Course 3, 5, 7:
Etoposide: I.V.: 200 mg/m^2/day days 1-3 [total dose/cycle = 600 mg/m^2]
Cisplatin: I.V.: 50 mg/m^2/day days 1-4 [total dose/cycle = 200 mg/m^2]

CC

Use: Ovarian cancer

Regimen:

Carboplatin: I.V.: Target AUC 5-7.5 day 1 [total dose/cycle = AUC = 5-7.5]

Cyclophosphamide: I.V.: 600 mg/m^2 day 1 [total dose/cycle = 600 mg/m^2]

Repeat cycle every 28 days

CCCDE (Retinoblastoma)

Use: Retinoblastoma

Regimen:

Cyclophosphamide: I.V.: 150 mg/m^2/day days 1-7 [total dose/cycle = 1050 mg/m^2]

Cyclophosphamide: Oral: 150 mg/m^2/day days 22-28, 43-49 [total dose/cycle = 2100 mg/m^2]

Doxorubicin: I.V.: 35 mg/m^2/day days 10 and 52 [total dose/cycle = 70 mg/m^2]

Cisplatin: I.V.: 90 mg/m^2/day days 8, 50, 71 [total dose/cycle = 270 mg/m^2]

Etoposide: I.V.: 150 mg/m^2/day continuous infusion days 29-31, 73-75 [total dose/cycle = 900 mg/m^2]

CCDDT (Neuroblastomas)

Use: Neuroblastomas

Regimen:

Cyclophosphamide: I.V.: 40 mg/kg/day days 1 and 2 [total dose/cycle = 80 mg/kg]

Cisplatin: I.V.: 20 mg/m^2/day days 1-5 [total dose/cycle = 100 mg/m^2]

Teniposide: I.V.: 100 mg/m^2 day 7 [total dose/cycle = 100 mg/m^2]

Doxorubicin: I.V.: 60 mg/m^2 day 1 [total dose/cycle = 60 mg/m^2]

Dacarbazine: I.V.: 250 mg/m^2/day days 1-5 [total dose/cycle = 1250 mg/m^2]

Repeat cycle every 21-28 days

CCDT (Melanoma)

Use: Melanoma

Regimen:

Dacarbazine: I.V.: 220 mg/m^2/day days 1-3, every 21-28 days [total dose/cycle = 660 mg/m^2]

Carmustine: I.V.: 150 mg/m^2 day 1, every 42-56 days [total dose/cycle = 150 mg/m^2]

Cisplatin: I.V.: 25 mg/m^2/day days 1-3, every 21-28 days [total dose/cycle = 75 mg/m^2]

Tamoxifen: Oral: 20 mg/day (use of tamoxifen is optional)

CCT (Neuroblastomas)

Use: Neuroblastomas

Regimen:

Cyclophosphamide: I.V.: 40 mg/kg/day days 1 and 2 [total dose/cycle = 80 mg/kg]

Cisplatin: I.V.: 20 mg/m^2/day days 22-26 [total dose/cycle = 100 mg/m^2]

Teniposide: I.V.: 100 mg/m^2 day 28 [total dose/cycle = 100 mg/m^2]

Repeat every 42 days for 3 cycles

CDDP/VP-16

Use: Brain tumors

Regimen:

Cisplatin: I.V.: 90 mg/m^2 day 1 [total dose/cycle = 90 mg/m^2]

Etoposide: I.V.: 150 mg/m^2/day days 3 and 4 [total dose/cycle = 300 mg/m^2]

Repeat cycle every 21 days

CE (Neuroblastomas)

Use: Neuroblastomas

Regimen:

Carboplatin: I.V.: 500 mg/m^2/day days 1 and 2 [total dose/cycle = 1000 mg/m^2]

Etoposide: I.V.: 100 mg/m^2/day days 1-3 [total dose/cycle = 300 mg/m^2]

Repeat cycle every 21-28 days

CE (Retinoblastoma)

Use: Retinoblastoma
Regimen:
Etoposide: I.V.: 100 mg/m^2/day days 1-5 [total dose/cycle = 500 mg/m^2]
Carboplatin: I.V.: 160 mg/m^2/day days 1-5 [total dose/cycle = 800 mg/m^2]
Repeat cycle every 21 days

CE-CAdO

Use: Neuroblastomas
Regimen:
Carboplatin: I.V.: 160 mg/m^2/day days 1-5 [total dose/cycle = 800 mg/m^2]
Etoposide: I.V.: 100 mg/m^2/day days 1-5 [total dose/cycle = 500 mg/m^2] **or**
Carboplatin: I.V.: 200 mg/m^2/day days 1-3 [total dose/cycle = 600 mg/m^2]
Etoposide: I.V.: 150 mg/m^2/day days 1-3 [total dose/cycle = 450 mg/m^2] **and**
Cyclophosphamide: I.V.: 300 mg/m^2/day days 1-5 [total dose/cycle = 1500 mg/m^2]
Doxorubicin: I.V.: 60 mg/m^2 day 5 [total dose/cycle = 60 mg/m^2]
Vincristine: I.V.: 1.5 mg/m^2/day days 1 and 5 [total dose/cycle = 3 mg/m^2]
Repeat cycle every 21 days

CEF

Use: Breast cancer
Regimen:
Cyclophosphamide: Oral: 75 mg/m^2/day days 1-14 [total dose/cycle = 1050 mg/m^2]
Epirubicin: I.V.: 60 mg/m^2/day days 1 and 8 [total dose/cycle = 120 mg/m^2]
Fluorouracil: I.V.: 500 mg/m^2/day days 1 and 8 [total dose/cycle = 1000 mg/m^2]
Repeat cycle every 28 days

CEPP(B)

Use: Lymphoma, non-Hodgkin
Regimen:
Cyclophosphamide: I.V.: 600-650 mg/m^2/day days 1-8 [total dose/cycle = 1200-1300 mg/m^2]
Etoposide: I.V.: 70-85 mg/m^2/day days 1-3 [total dose/cycle = 210-255 mg/m^2]
Procarbazine: Oral: 60 mg/m^2/day days 1-10 [total dose/cycle = 600 mg/m^2]
Prednisone: Oral: 60 mg/m^2/day days 1-10 [total dose/cycle = 600 mg/m^2]
Bleomycin: I.V.: 15 units/m^2/day days 1 and 15 (bleomycin is sometimes omitted) [total dose/cycle = 30 units/m^2]
Repeat cycle every 28 days

CEV

Use: Rhabdomyosarcoma
Regimen:
Carboplatin: I.V.: 500 mg/m^2 day 1 [total dose/cycle = 500 mg/m^2]
Epirubicin: I.V.: 150 mg/m^2 day 1 [total dose/cycle = 150 mg/m^2]
Vincristine: I.V.: 1.5 mg/m^2/day days 1 and 7 [total dose/cycle = 3 mg/m^2]
Repeat cycle every 21 days

CF

Use: Head and neck cancer
Regimen: Note: Multiple variations are listed below.
Variation 1:
Cisplatin: I.V.: 100 mg/m^2 day 1 [total dose/cycle = 100 mg/m^2]
Fluorouracil: I.V.: 1000 mg/m^2/day continuous infusion days 1-4 [total dose/cycle = 4000 mg/m^2] **or** days 1-5 [total dose/cycle = 5000 mg/m^2]
Repeat cycle every 21-28 days
Variation 2:
Carboplatin: I.V.: 400 mg/m^2 day 1
Fluorouracil: I.V.: 1000 mg/m^2 continuous infusion days 1-4 or days 1-5
Repeat cycle every 21-28 days

CHAMOCA

Use: Gestational trophoblastic tumor
Regimen:

Hydroxyurea: Oral: 500 mg every 6 hours for 4 doses, day 1 (start at 6 AM)
[total dose/cycle = 2000 mg]
Dactinomycin: I.V.: 0.2 mg/day days 1-3 (give at 7 PM) [total dose/cycle = 0.6 mg]
followed by 0.5 mg/day days 4 and 5 (give at 7 PM) [total dose/cycle = 1 mg]
Cyclophosphamide: I.V.: 500 mg/m^2/day days 3 and 8 (give at 7 PM)
[total dose/cycle = 1000 mg/m^2]
Vincristine: I.V.: 1 mg/m^2 (maximum 2 mg) day 2 (give at 7 AM) [total dose/cycle = 1 mg/m^2]
Methotrexate: I.V. push: 100 mg/m^2 day 2 (give at 7 PM) [total dose/cycle = 100 mg/m^2]
followed by 200 mg/m^2 over 12 hours day 2 [total dose/cycle = 200 mg/m^2]
Leucovorin: I.M.: 14 mg/day every 6 hours for 6 doses days 3-5 (begin at 7 PM on day 3)
[total dose/cycle = 84 mg]
Doxorubicin: I.V.: 30 mg/m^2 day 8 (give at 7 PM) [total dose/cycle = 30 mg/m^2]
Repeat cycle every 18 days or as toxicity permits

ChlVPP

Use: Lymphoma, Hodgkin disease
Regimen:

Chlorambucil: Oral: 6 mg/m^2/day (maximum 10 mg) days 1-14 [total dose/cycle = 84 mg/m^2]
Vinblastine: I.V.: 6 mg/m^2/day (maximum 10 mg) days 1 and 8 [total dose/cycle = 12 mg/m^2]
Procarbazine: Oral: 100 mg/m^2/day (maximum 150 mg) days 1-14
[total dose/cycle = 1400 mg/m^2]
Prednisone: Oral: 40-50 mg/m^2/day days 1-14 [total dose/cycle = 560-700 mg]
Repeat cycle every 28 days

CHL + PRED

Use: Leukemia, chronic lymphocytic
Regimen:

Chlorambucil: Oral: 0.4 mg/kg/day for 1 day every other week; increase initial dose of 0.4 mg/kg by 0.1 mg/kg every 2 weeks until toxicity or disease control is achieved
Prednisone: Oral: 100 mg/day for 2 days every other week

CHOP

Use: Lymphoma, non-Hodgkin
Regimen: Note: Multiple variations are listed below.

Variation 1:
Cyclophosphamide: I.V.: 750 mg/m^2 day 1 [total dose/cycle = 750 mg/m^2]
Doxorubicin: I.V.: 50 mg/m^2 day 1 [total dose/cycle = 50 mg/m^2]
Vincristine: I.V.: 1.4 mg/m^2 (maximum 2 mg) day 1 [total dose/cycle = 1.4 mg/m^2]
Prednisone: Oral: 100 mg/day days 1-5 [total dose/cycle = 500 mg]
or 50 mg/m^2/day days 1-5 [total dose/cycle = 250 mg/m^2]
or 100 mg/m^2/day days 1-5 [total dose/cycle = 500 mg/m^2]
Repeat cycle every 21 days

Variation 2:
Cyclophosphamide: I.V.: 750 mg/m^2 day 1 [total dose/cycle = 750 mg/m^2]
Doxorubicin: I.V.: 50 mg/m^2 day 1 [total dose/cycle = 50 mg/m^2]
Vincristine: I.V.: 2 mg day 1 [total dose/cycle = 2 mg]
Prednisone: Oral: 75 mg/day days 1-5 [total dose/cycle = 375 mg]
Repeat cycle every 21 days

Variation 3:
Cyclophosphamide: I.V.: 750 mg/m^2/day days 1 and 8 [total dose/cycle = 1500 mg/m^2]
Doxorubicin: I.V.: 25 mg/m^2/day days 1 and 8 [total dose/cycle = 50 mg/m^2]
Vincristine: I.V.: 1.4 mg/m^2/day (maximum 2 mg) days 1 and 8 [total dose/cycle = 2.8 mg/m^2]
Prednisone: Oral: 50 mg/m^2/day days 1-8 [total dose/cycle = 400 mg/m^2]
Repeat cycle every 28 days

Variation 4 (mini-CHOP):
Cyclophosphamide: I.V.: 250 mg/m^2/day days 1, 8, 15 [total dose/cycle = 750 mg/m^2]
Doxorubicin: I.V.: 16.7 mg/m^2/day days 1, 8, 15 [total dose/cycle = 50.1 mg/m^2]
Vincristine: I.V.: 0.67 mg/day days 1, 8, 15 [total dose/cycle = 2.01 mg]
Prednisone: Oral: 75 mg/day days 1-5 [total dose/cycle = 375 mg]
Repeat cycle every 21 days

CI (Neuroblastomas)

Use: Neuroblastomas

Regimen:

Ifosfamide: I.V.: 1500 mg/m^2/day days 1-3 [total dose/cycle = 4500 mg/m^2]

Carboplatin: I.V.: 400 mg/m^2 day 4 [total dose/cycle = 400 mg/m^2]

Repeat cycle every 21-28 days

CISCA

Use: Bladder cancer

Regimen:

Cyclophosphamide: I.V.: 650 mg/m^2 day 1 [total dose = 650 mg/m^2]

Doxorubicin: I.V.: 50 mg/m^2 day 1 [total dose = 50 mg/m^2]

Cisplatin: I.V.: 100 mg/m^2 day 2 [total dose = 100 mg/m^2]

Repeat cycle every 21-28 days

Cisplatin-Docetaxel

Use: Bladder cancer

Regimen:

Cisplatin: I.V.: 30 mg/m^2 day 1 [total dose/cycle = 30 mg/m^2]

Docetaxel: I.V.: 40 mg/m^2 day 4 [total dose/cycle = 40 mg/m^2]

Repeat cycle weekly for 8 weeks

Cisplatin-Fluorouracil

Use: Cervical cancer

Regimen: Note: Multiple variations are listed below.

Variation 1:

Cisplatin: I.V.: 75 mg/m^2 day 1 [total dose/cycle = 75 mg/m^2]

Fluorouracil: I.V.: 1000 mg/m^2/day continuous infusion days 1-4 (96 hours) [total dose/cycle = 4000 mg/m^2]

Repeat cycle every 21 days

Variation 2:

Cisplatin: I.V.: 50 mg/m^2 day 1 starting 4 hours before radiotherapy [total dose/cycle = 50 mg/m^2]

Fluorouracil: I.V.: 1000 mg/m^2/day continuous infusion days 2-5 (96 hours) [total dose/cycle = 4000 mg/m^2]

Repeat cycle every 28 days

Cisplatin + Pemetrexed

Use: Malignant pleural mesothelioma

Regimen:

Pemetrexed: I.V.: 500 mg/m^2 infused over 10 minutes day 1 [total dose/cycle = 500 mg/m^2]

Cisplatin: I.V.: 75 mg/m^2 infused over 2 hours (start 30 minutes after pemetrexed) [total dose/cycle = 75 mg/m^2]

Repeat cycle every 21 days

Cisplatin-Vinorelbine

Use: Cervical cancer

Regimen:

Cisplatin: I.V.: 80 mg/m^2 day 1 [total dose/cycle = 80 mg/m^2]

Vinorelbine: I.V.: 25 mg/m^2/day days 1 and 8 [total dose/cycle = 50 mg/m^2]

Repeat cycle every 21 days

CMF

Use: Breast cancer

Regimen: Note: Multiple variations are listed below.

Variation 1:

Methotrexate: I.V.: 40 mg/m^2/day days 1 and 8 [total dose/cycle = 80 mg/m^2]
Fluorouracil: I.V.: 600 mg/m^2/day days 1 and 8 [total dose/cycle = 1200 mg/m^2]
Cyclophosphamide: Oral: 100 mg/m^2/day days 1-14 [total dose/cycle = 1400 mg/m^2]
Repeat cycle every 28 days

Variation 2 (older than 60 years):

Methotrexate: I.V.: 30 mg/m^2 days 1 and 8 [total dose/cycle = 60 mg/m^2]
Fluorouracil: I.V.: 400 mg/m^2 days 1 and 8 [total dose/cycle = 800 mg/m^2]
Cyclophosphamide: Oral: 100 mg/m^2 days 1-14 [total dose/cycle = 1400 mg/m^2]
Repeat cycle every 28 days

CMF-IV

Use: Breast cancer

Regimen:

Cyclophosphamide: I.V.: 600 mg/m^2 day 1 [total dose/cycle = 600 mg/m^2]
Methotrexate: I.V.: 40 mg/m^2 day 1 [total dose/cycle = 40 mg/m^2]
Fluorouracil: I.V.: 600 mg/m^2 day 1 [total dose/cycle = 600 mg/m^2]
Repeat cycle every 21 or 28 days

CMV

Use: Bladder cancer

Regimen:

Cisplatin: I.V.: 100 mg/m^2 infused over 4 hours (start 12 hours after methotrexate) day 2 [total dose = 100 mg/m^2]
Methotrexate: I.V.: 30 mg/m^2/day days 1 and 8 [total dose = 60 mg/m^2]
Vinblastine: I.V.: 4 mg/m^2/day days 1 and 8 [total dose = 8 mg/m^2]
Repeat cycle every 21 days

CNF

Use: Breast cancer

Regimen: Note: Multiple variations are listed below.

Variation 1:

Cyclophosphamide: I.V: 500 mg/m^2 day 1 [total dose/cycle = 500 mg/m^2]
Mitoxantrone: I.V.: 10 mg/m^2 day 1 [total dose/cycle = 10 mg/m^2]
Fluorouracil: I.V.: 500 mg/m^2 day 1 [total dose/cycle = 500 mg/m^2]
Repeat cycle every 21 days

Variation 2:

Cyclophosphamide: I.V.: 500-600 mg/m^2 day 1 [total dose/cycle = 500-600 mg/m^2]
Fluorouracil: I.V.: 500-600 mg/m^2 day 1 [total dose/cycle = 500-600 mg/m^2]
Mitoxantrone: I.V.: 10-12 mg/m^2 day 1 [total dose/cycle = 10-12 mg/m^2]
Repeat cycle every 21 days

CNOP

Use: Lymphoma, non-Hodgkin

Regimen:

Cyclophosphamide: I.V.: 750 mg/m^2 day 1 [total dose/cycle = 750 mg/m^2]
Mitoxantrone: I.V.: 10 mg/m^2 day 1 [total dose/cycle = 10 mg/m^2]
Vincristine: I.V.: 1.4 mg/m^2 day 1 [total dose/cycle = 1.4 mg/m^2]
Prednisone: Oral: 50 mg/m^2/day days 1-5 [total dose/cycle = 250 mg/m^2]
Repeat cycle every 21 days

CO

Use: Retinoblastoma

Regimen:

Cyclophosphamide: I.V.: 10 mg/kg/day days 1-3 [total dose/cycle = 30 mg/kg]
Vincristine: I.V.: 1.5 mg/m^2 day 1 [total dose/cycle = 1.5 mg/m^2]
Repeat cycle every 21 days

CODOX-M

Use: Lymphoma, non-Hodgkin

Regimen:

Cytarabine: I.T.: 70 mg/day days 1 and 3 [total dose/cycle = 140 mg]
Cyclophosphamide: I.V.: 800 mg/m^2 day 1, then 200 mg/m^2 days 2-5
[total dose/cycle = 1600 mg/m^2]
Vincristine: I.V.: 1.5 mg/m^2/day days 1, 8, 15 [total dose/cycle = 4.5 mg/m^2]
Doxorubicin: I.V.: 40 mg/m^2 day 1 [total dose/cycle = 40 mg/m^2]
Methotrexate:
I.T.: 12 mg day 15 [total dose/cycle = 12 mg]
I.V.: 1200 mg/m^2 loading dose then 240 mg/m^2/hour for 23 hours day 10
[total dose/cycle = 6720 mg/m^2]
Leucovorin: I.V.: 192 mg/m^2 day 11 then 6 mg/m^2 every 6 hours until MTX level <10^{-8}M
Sargramostim: SubQ: 7.5 mcg/kg day 13 until ANC >1000 cells/mm^3 [total dose/cycle = ANC = >1000 cells/mm^3]
Repeat cycle when ANC >1000 cells/mm^3

COMLA

Use: Lymphoma, non-Hodgkin

Regimen:

Cyclophosphamide: I.V.: 1500 mg/m^2 day 1 [total dose/cycle = 1500 mg/m^2]
Vincristine: I.V.: 1.4 mg/m^2/day (maximum 2 mg) days 1, 8, 15 [total dose/cycle = 4.2 mg/m^2]
Methotrexate: I.V.: 120 mg/m^2/day days 22, 29, 36, 43, 50, 57, 64, 71
[total dose/cycle = 960 mg/m^2]
Leucovorin: Oral: 25 mg/m^2 every 6 hours for 4 doses (beginning 24 hours after each methotrexate dose)
[total dose/cycle = 800 mg/m^2]
Cytarabine: I.V.: 300 mg/m^2/day days 22, 29, 36, 43, 50, 57, 64, 71
[total dose/cycle = 2400 mg/m^2]
Repeat cycle every 85 days

COMP

Use: Lymphoma, Hodgkin disease; Lymphoma, non-Hodgkin disease

Regimen:

Cyclophosphamide: I.V.: 1200 mg/m^2 day 1, cycle 1 [total dose/cycle = 1200 mg/m^2]
followed by 1000 mg/m^2 day 1 on subsequent cycles [total dose/cycle = 1000 mg/m^2]
Vincristine: I.V.: 2 mg/m^2/day (maximum 2 mg) days 3, 10, 17, 24, cycle 1
[total dose/cycle = 8 mg/m^2] **followed by** 1.5 mg/m^2/day days 1 and 4, on subsequent cycles
[total dose/cycle = 3 mg/m^2]
Methotrexate: I.V.: 300 mg/m^2 day 12 [total dose/cycle = 300 mg/m^2]
Prednisone: Oral: 60 mg/m^2/day (maximum 60 mg) days 3-30 then taper for 7 days, cycle 1
[total dose/cycle = 1620 mg/m^2 + taper dose over 7 days]
followed by 60 mg/m^2 (maximum 60 mg) days 1-5, on subsequent cycles [total dose/cycle = 300 mg/m^2]

Maintenance cycles repeat every 28 days

COP-BLAM

Use: Lymphoma, non-Hodgkin

Regimen:

Cyclophosphamide: I.V.: 400 mg/m^2 day 1 [total dose/cycle = 400 mg/m^2]
Vincristine: I.V.: 1 mg/m^2 day 1 [total dose/cycle = 1 mg/m^2]
Prednisone: Oral: 40 mg/m^2/day days 1-10 [total dose/cycle = 400 mg/m^2]
Bleomycin: I.V.: 15 mg day 14 [total dose/cycle = 15 mg]
Doxorubicin: I.V.: 40 mg/m^2 day 1 [total dose/cycle = 40 mg/m^2]
Procarbazine: Oral: 100 mg/m^2/day days 1-10 [total dose/cycle = 1000 mg/m^2]

COPE or Baby Brain I

Use: Brain tumors

Regimen:

Cycle A:
Vincristine: I.V.: 0.065 mg/kg/day (maximum 1.5 mg) days 1, 8 [total dose/cycle = 0.13 mg/kg]
Cyclophosphamide: I.V.: 65 mg/kg day 1 [total dose/cycle = 65 mg/kg]
Cycle B:
Cisplatin: I.V.: 4 mg/kg day 1 [total dose/cycle = 4 mg/kg]
Etoposide: I.V.: 6.5 mg/kg/day days 3, 4 [total dose/cycle = 13 mg/kg]
Repeat cycle every 28 days in the following sequence: AABAAB

COPP (C MOPP)

Use: Lymphoma, non-Hodgkin

Regimen:

Cyclophosphamide: I.V.: 450-650 mg/m^2/day days 1 and 8 [total dose/cycle = 900-1300 mg/m^2]

Vincristine: I.V.: 1.4-2 mg/m^2/day (maximum 2 mg) days 1 and 8 [total dose/cycle = 2.8-4 mg/m^2]

Procarbazine: Oral: 100 mg/m^2/day days 1-14 [total dose/cycle = 1400 mg/m^2]

Prednisone: Oral: 40 mg/m^2/day days 1-14 [total dose/cycle = 560 mg/m^2]

Repeat cycle every 28 days

CP (Leukemia)

Use: Leukemia, chronic lymphocytic

Regimen:

Chlorambucil: Oral: 30 mg/m^2 day 1 [total dose/cycle = 30 mg/m^2]

Prednisone: Oral: 80 mg/day days 1-5 [total dose/cycle = 400 mg]

Repeat cycle every 14 days

CP (Ovarian Cancer)

Use: Ovarian cancer

Regimen:

Cyclophosphamide: I.V.: 750 mg/m^2 day 1 [total dose/cycle = 750 mg/m^2]

Cisplatin: I.V.: 75 mg/m^2 day 1 [total dose/cycle = 75 mg/m^2]

Repeat cycle every 21 days

CT

Use: Ovarian cancer

Regimen:

Cisplatin: I.V.: 75 mg/m^2 day 2 [total dose/cycle = 75 mg/m^2]

Paclitaxel: I.V.: 135 mg/m^2 continuous infusion day 1 [total dose/cycle = 135 mg/m^2]

Repeat cycle every 21 days

CV

Use: Retinoblastoma

Regimen:

Cyclophosphamide: I.V.: 300 mg/m^2 [total dose/cycle = 300 mg/m^2]

Vincristine: I.V.: 1.5 mg/m^2 [total dose/cycle = 1.5 mg/m^2]

Repeat weekly for 6 weeks

followed by:

Cyclophosphamide: I.V.: 200 mg/m^2 [total dose/cycle = 200 mg/m^2]

Vincristine: I.V.: 1.5 mg/m^2 [total dose/cycle = 1.5 mg/m^2]

Repeat weekly for 42 weeks

CVD

Use: Melanoma

Regimen:

Cisplatin: I.V.: 20 mg/m^2/day days 2-5 [total dose/cycle = 80 mg/m^2]

Vinblastine: I.V.: 1.6 mg/m^2/day days 1-5 [total dose/cycle = 8 mg/m^2]

Dacarbazine: I.V.: 800 mg/m^2 day 1 [total dose/cycle = 800 mg/m^2]

Repeat cycle every 21 days

CVP (Leukemia)

Use: Leukemia, chronic lymphocytic

Regimen: Note: Multiple variations are listed below.

Variation 1:

Cyclophosphamide: Oral: 400 or 300 mg/m^2/day days 1-5 [total dose/cycle = 2000 or 1500 mg/m^2]

Vincristine: I.V.: 1.4 mg/m^2 (maximum 2 mg) day 1 [total dose/cycle = 1.4 mg/m^2]

Prednisone: Oral: 100 mg/m^2/day days 1-5 [total dose/cycle = 500 mg/m^2]

Repeat cycle every 21 days

Variation 2:

Cyclophosphamide: I.V.: 800 mg/m^2 day 1 [total dose/cycle = 800 mg/m^2]

Vincristine: I.V.: 1.4 mg/m^2 (maximum 2 mg) day 1 [total dose/cycle = 1.4 mg/m^2]

Prednisone: Oral: 100 mg/m^2/day days 1-5 [total dose/cycle = 500 mg/m^2]

Repeat cycle every 21 days

CVP (Lymphoma, non-Hodgkin)

Use: Lymphoma, non-Hodgkin

Regimen:

Cyclophosphamide: Oral: 400 mg/m^2/day days 1-5 [total dose/cycle = 2000 mg/m^2]

Vincristine: I.V.: 1.4 mg/m^2 day 1 [total dose/cycle = 1.4 mg/m^2]

Prednisone: Oral: 100 mg/m^2/day days 1-5 [total dose/cycle = 500 mg/m^2]

Repeat cycle every 21 days

Cyclophosphamide + Doxorubicin

Use: Prostate cancer

Regimen:

Doxorubicin: I.V.: 40 mg/m^2 day 1 [total dose/cycle = 40 mg/m^2]

Cyclophosphamide: I.V.: 800-2000 mg/m^2 day 1 [total dose/cycle = 800-2000 mg/m^2]

Filgrastim: SubQ: 5 mcg/kg/day days 2-10 (or until ANC >10,000 cells/µL) [total dose/cycle = 45 mcg/kg or ANC >10,000 cells/µL]

Repeat cycle every 21 days

Cyclophosphamide + Estramustine

Use: Prostate cancer

Regimen:

Cyclophosphamide: Oral: 2 mg/kg/day days 1-14 [total dose/cycle = 28 mg/kg]

Estramustine: Oral: 10 mg/kg/day days 1-14 [total dose/cycle = 140 mg/kg]

Repeat cycle every 28 days

Cyclophosphamide + Etoposide

Use: Prostate cancer

Regimen:

Cyclophosphamide: Oral: 100 mg/day days 1-14 [total dose/cycle = 1400 mg]

Etoposide: Oral: 50 mg/day days 1-14 [total dose/cycle = 700 mg]

Repeat cycle every 28 days

Cyclophosphamide + Vincristine + Dexamethasone

Use: Prostate cancer

Regimen:

Cyclophosphamide: Oral: 250 mg/day days 1-14 [total dose/cycle = 3500 mg]

Vincristine: I.V.: 1 mg/day days 1, 8, and 15 [total dose/cycle = 3 mg]

Dexamethasone: Oral: 0.75 mg twice daily days 1-14 [total dose/cycle = 21 mg]

Repeat cycle every 28 days

CYVADIC

Use: Sarcoma

Regimen:

Cyclophosphamide: I.V.: 500 mg/m^2 day 1 [total dose/cycle = 500 mg/m^2]

Vincristine: I.V.: 1.4 mg/m^2/day days 1 and 5 [total dose/cycle = 2.8 mg/m^2]

Doxorubicin: I.V.: 50 mg/m^2 day 1 [total dose/cycle = 50 mg/m^2]

Dacarbazine: I.V.: 250 mg/m^2/day days 1-5 [total dose/cycle = 1250 mg/m^2]

Repeat cycle every 21 days

DA

Use: Leukemia, acute myeloid (induction)

Regimen: Induction:

Daunorubicin: I.V.: 45 mg/m^2/day days 1-3 [total dose/cycle = 135 mg/m^2]

Cytarabine: I.V.: 100 mg/m^2/day continuous infusion days 1-7 [total dose/cycle = 700 mg/m^2]

Dacarbazine-Carboplatin-Aldesleukin-Interferon

Use: Melanoma

Regimen:

Dacarbazine: I.V.: 750 mg/m^2/day days 1 and 22 [total dose/cycle = 1500 mg/m^2]

Carboplatin: I.V.: 400 mg/m^2/day days 1 and 22 [total dose/cycle = 800 mg/m^2]

Aldesleukin: SubQ: 4,800,000 units every 8 hours days 36 and 57 [total dose/cycle = 14,400,000 units]

then 4,800,000 units every 12 hours days 37 and 58 [total dose/cycle = 9,600,000 units]

then 4,800,000 units/day days 38 to 40, 43 to 47, 50 to 54, 59 to 61, 65 to 68, 71 to 75 [total dose/cycle = 86,400,000 units]

Interferon alpha-2a: SubQ: 6,000,000 units days 38, 40, 43, 45, 47, 50, 52, 54, 59, 61, 64, 66, 68, 71, 73, and 75 [total dose/cycle = 96,000,000 units]

Repeat cycle every 78 days for 3 cycles

Dacarbazine/Tamoxifen

Use: Melanoma

Regimen:

Dacarbazine: I.V.: 250 mg/m^2/day days 1-5, every 21 days [total dose/cycle = 1250 mg/m^2]

Tamoxifen: Oral: 20 mg/day (use of tamoxifen is optional) [total dose/cycle = 20 mg]

Dartmouth Regimen

Use: Melanoma

Regimen:

Tamoxifen: Oral: 10 mg twice daily starting 1 week prior to chemotherapy and continuing indefinitely

Carmustine: I.V.: 150 mg/m^2 day 1 (every other cycle) [total dose/cycle = 150 mg/m^2]

Cisplatin: I.V.: 25 mg/m^2/day days 1-3 [total dose/cycle = 75 mg/m^2]

Dacarbazine: I.V.: 220 mg/m^2/day days 1-3 [total dose/cycle = 660 mg/m^2]

Repeat cycle every 21 days

DAT

Use: Leukemia, acute myeloid (induction)

Regimen: Induction:

Daunorubicin: I.V. bolus: 45 mg/m^2/day days 1-3 [total dose/cycle = 135 mg/m^2]

Cytarabine: I.V. bolus: 200 mg/m^2 [total dose/cycle = 200 mg/m^2]

Thioguanine: Oral: 100 mg/m^2/day days 1-7 [total dose/cycle = 700 mg/m^2]

DAV

Use: Leukemia, acute myeloid

Regimen:

Daunorubicin: I.V.: 60 mg/m^2/day days 3-5 [total dose/cycle = 180 mg/m^2]

Cytarabine: I.V.: 100 mg/m^2/day continuous infusion days 1-2 [total dose/cycle = 200 mg/m^2] **followed by** 100 mg/m^2 every 12 hours days 3-8 (12 doses) [total dose/cycle = 1200 mg/m^2]

Etoposide: I.V.: 150 mg/m^2/day days 6-8 [total dose/cycle = 450 mg/m^2]

Administer one cycle only

DHAP

Use: Lymphoma, non-Hodgkin

Regimen: Note: Multiple variations are listed below.

Variation 1:

Dexamethasone: I.V. or Oral: 40 mg/day days 1-4 [total dose/cycle = 160 mg]

Cisplatin: I.V.: 100 mg/m^2 day 1 [total dose/cycle = 100 mg/m^2]

Cytarabine: I.V.: 2000 mg/m^2 every 12 hours for 2 doses day 2 (begins at the end of the cisplatin infusion) [total dose/cycle = 4000 mg/m^2]

Repeat cycle every 3-4 weeks for 6-10 cycles (salvage therapy) or 1-2 cycles (mobilization prior to high-dose therapy with peripheral hematopoietic progenitor cell support)

Variation 2:

Dexamethasone: I.V. or Oral: 40 mg/day days 1-4 [total dose/cycle = 160 mg]

Oxaliplatin: I.V.: 130 mg/m^2 day 1 [total dose/cycle = 130 mg/m^2]

Cytarabine: I.V.: 2000 mg/m^2 every 12 hours for 2 doses day 2 [total dose/cycle = 4000 mg/m^2]

Repeat cycle every 3 weeks

Docetaxel-Cisplatin

Use: Lung cancer, nonsmall-cell

Regimen:

Docetaxel: I.V.: 75 mg/m^2 day 1 [total dose/cycle = 75 mg/m^2]

Cisplatin: I.V.: 75 mg/m^2 day 1 [total dose/cycle = 75 mg/m^2]

Repeat cycle every 21 days

Doxorubicin + Ketoconazole

Use: Prostate cancer

Regimen:

Doxorubicin: I.V.: 20 mg/m^2 continuous infusion day 1 [total dose/cycle = 20 mg/m^2]

Ketoconazole: Oral: 400 mg 3 times/day days 1-7 [total dose/cycle = 8400 mg]

Repeat cycle every 7 days

Doxorubicin + Ketoconazole/Estramustine + Vinblastine

Use: Prostate cancer

Regimen:

Doxorubicin: I.V.: 20 mg/m^2/day days 1, 15, and 29 [total dose/cycle = 60 mg/m^2]

Ketoconazole: Oral: 400 mg 3 times/day days 1-7, 15-21, and 29-35 [total dose/cycle = 25,200 mg]

Estramustine: Oral: 140 mg 3 times/day days 8-14, 22-28, and 36-42 [total dose/cycle = 8820 mg]

Vinblastine: I.V.: 5 mg/m^2/day days 8, 22, and 36 [total dose/cycle = 15 mg/m^2]

Repeat cycle every 8 weeks

DTPACE

Use: Multiple myeloma

Regimen:

Dexamethasone: Oral: 40 mg/day days 1-4 [total dose/cycle = 160 mg]

Thalidomide: Oral: 400 mg/day [total dose/cycle = 11,200-16,800 mg]

Cisplatin: I.V.: 10 mg/m^2/day continuous infusion days 1-4 [total dose/cycle = 40 mg/m^2]

Doxorubicin: I.V.: 10 mg/m^2/day continuous infusion days 1-4 [total dose/cycle = 40 mg/m^2]

Cyclophosphamide: I.V.: 400 mg/m^2 continuous infusion days 1-4 [total dose/cycle = 1600 mg/m^2]

Etoposide: I.V.: 40 mg/m^2 continuous infusion days 1-4 [total dose/cycle = 160 mg/m^2]

Repeat cycle every 4-6 weeks

DVD

Use: Multiple myeloma

Regimen:

Doxorubicin, liposomal: I.V.: 40 mg/m^2 day 1 [total dose/cycle = 40 mg/m^2]

Vincristine: I.V.: 2 mg day 1 [total dose/cycle = 2 mg]

Dexamethasone: Oral or I.V.: 40 mg/day days 1-4 [total dose/cycle = 160 mg]

Repeat cycle every 4 weeks

DVP

Use: Leukemia, acute lymphocytic

Regimen: Induction:

Daunorubicin: I.V.: 25 mg/m^2/day days 1, 8, and 15 [total dose/cycle = 75 mg/m^2]

Vincristine: I.V.: 1.5 mg/m^2/day (maximum 2 mg) days 1, 8, 15, and 22 [total dose/cycle = 6 mg/m^2]

Prednisone: Oral: 60 mg/m^2/day days 1-28 then taper over next 14 days [total dose/cycle = 1680 mg/m^2 + taper over next 14 days]

Administer single cycle; used in conjunction with intrathecal chemotherapy

EAP

Use: Gastric cancer

Regimen:

Etoposide: I.V.: 120 mg/m^2/day days 4-6 [total dose/cycle = 360 mg/m^2]

Doxorubicin: I.V.: 20 mg/m^2/day days 1 and 7 [total dose/cycle = 40 mg/m^2]

Cisplatin: I.V.: 40 mg/m^2/day days 2 and 8 [total dose/cycle = 80 mg/m^2]

Repeat cycle every 28 days

ECF

Use: Gastric cancer

Regimen:

Epirubicin: I.V.: 50 mg/m^2 day 1 [total dose/cycle = 50 mg/m^2]

Cisplatin: I.V.: 60 mg/m^2 day 1 [total dose/cycle = 60 mg/m^2]

Repeat cycle every 3 weeks

Fluorouracil: I.V.: 200 mg/m^2/day continuous infusion for up to 6 months [total dose/cycle = 36,000 mg/m^2]

EC (Nonsmall-Cell Lung Cancer)

Use: Lung cancer, nonsmall-cell

Regimen:

Etoposide: I.V.: 120 mg/m^2/day days 1-3 [total dose/cycle = 360 mg/m^2]

Carboplatin: I.V.: AUC 6 day 1 [total dose/cycle = AUC = 6]

Repeat cycle every 21-28 days

EC (Small-Cell Lung Cancer)

Use: Lung cancer, small-cell

Regimen: Note: Multiple variations are listed below.

Variation 1:

Etoposide: I.V.: 100-120 mg/m^2/day days 1-3 [total dose/cycle = 300-360 mg/m^2]

Carboplatin: I.V.: 325-400 mg/m^2 day 1 [total dose/cycle = 325-400 mg/m^2]

Repeat cycle every 28 days

Variation 2:

Etoposide: I.V.: 120 mg/m^2/day days 1-3 [total dose/cycle = 360 mg/m^2]

Carboplatin: I.V.: AUC 6 day 1 [total dose/cycle = AUC = 6]

Repeat cycle every 21-28 days

EE

Use: Wilms tumor

Regimen:

Dactinomycin: I.V.: 15 mcg/kg/day days 1-5 of weeks 0, 5, 13, 24 [total dose/cycle = 300 mcg/kg]

Vincristine: I.V.: 1.5 mg/m^2 day 1 of weeks 1-10, 13, 14, 24, 25 [total dose/cycle = 21 mg/m^2]

EE-4A

Use: Wilms tumor

Regimen:

Dactinomycin: I.V.: 45 mcg/kg day 1 of weeks 0, 3, 6, 9, 12, 15, 18 [total dose/cycle = 315 mcg/kg]

Vincristine: I.V.: 2 mg/m^2 day 1 of weeks 1-10, 12, 15, 18 [total dose/cycle = 26 mg/m^2]

ELF

Use: Gastric cancer

Regimen:

Leucovorin calcium: I.V.: 300 mg/m^2/day days 1-3, [total dose/cycle = 900 mg/m^2] **followed by:**

Etoposide: I.V.: 120 mg/m^2/day days 1-3, [total dose/cycle = 360 mg/m^2] **followed by:**

Fluorouracil: I.V.: 500 mg/m^2/day days 1-3 [total dose/cycle = 1500 mg/m^2]

Repeat cycle every 21-28 days

EMA 86

Use: Leukemia, acute myeloid

Regimen:

Mitoxantrone: I.V.: 12 mg/m^2/day days 1-3 [total dose/cycle = 36 mg/m^2]

Etoposide: I.V.: 200 mg/m^2/day continuous infusion days 8-10 [total dose/cycle = 600 mg/m^2]

Cytarabine: I.V.: 500 mg/m^2/day continuous infusion days 1-3 and 8-10 [total dose/cycle = 3000 mg/m^2]

Administer one cycle only

EMA/CO

Use: Gestational trophoblastic tumor

Regimen:

Etoposide: I.V.: 100 mg/m^2/day days 1 and 2 [total dose/cycle = 200 mg/m^2]

Methotrexate: I.V.: 300 mg/m^2 infused over 12 hours day 1 [total dose/cycle = 300 mg/m^2]

Dactinomycin: I.V. push: 0.5 mg/day days 1 and 2 [total dose/cycle = 1 mg]

Leucovorin: Oral, I.M.: 15 mg twice daily for 2 days (start 24 hours after the start of methotrexate) days 2, 3 [total dose/cycle = 60 mg]

Alternate weekly with:

Cyclophosphamide: I.V.: 600 mg/m^2 infused over 30 minutes day 1 [total dose/cycle = 600 mg/m^2]

Vincristine: I.V. push: 0.8 mg/m^2 (maximum 2 mg) day 1 [total dose/cycle = 0.8 mg/m^2]

EP (Adenocarcinoma)

Use: Adenocarcinoma, unknown primary
Regimen:
Cisplatin: I.V.: 60-100 mg/m^2 day 1 [total dose = 60-100 mg/m^2]
Etoposide: I.V.: 80-100 mg/m^2/day days 1-3 [total dose = 240-300 mg/m^2]
Repeat cycle every 21 days

EP (Nonsmall-Cell Lung Cancer)

Use: Lung cancer, nonsmall-cell
Regimen:
Etoposide: I.V.: 80-120 mg/m^2/day days 1-3 [total dose/cycle = 240-360 mg/m^2]
Cisplatin: I.V.: 80-100 mg/m^2 day 1 [total dose/cycle = 80-100 mg/m^2]
Repeat cycle every 21-28 days

EP (Small-Cell Lung Cancer)

Use: Lung cancer, small-cell
Regimen: Note: Multiple variations are listed below.
Variation 1:
Etoposide: I.V.: 100 mg/m^2/day days 1-3 [total dose/cycle = 300 mg/m^2]
Cisplatin: I.V.: 100 mg/m^2 day 1 [total dose/cycle = 100 mg/m^2]
Repeat cycle every 21 days
Variation 2:
Etoposide: I.V.: 80 mg/m^2/day days 1-3 [total dose/cycle = 240 mg/m^2]
Cisplatin: I.V.: 80 mg/m^2 day 1 [total dose/cycle = 80 mg/m^2]
Repeat cycle every 21-28 days

EP (Testicular Cancer)

Use: Testicular cancer
Regimen: Note: Multiple variations are listed below.
Variation 1:
Etoposide: I.V.: 100 mg/m^2/day days 1-5 [total dose/cycle = 500 mg/m^2]
Cisplatin: I.V.: 20 mg/m^2/day days 1-5 [total dose/cycle = 100 mg/m^2]
Repeat cycle every 21 days
Variation 2:
Etoposide: I.V.: 120 mg/m^2/day days 1-3 [total dose/cycle = 360 mg/m^2]
Cisplatin: I.V.: 20 mg/m^2/day days 1-5 [total dose/cycle = 100 mg/m^2]
Repeat cycle every 3 or 4 weeks
Variation 3:
Etoposide: I.V.: 120 mg/m^2/day days 1, 3, and 5 [total dose/cycle = 360 mg/m^2]
Cisplatin: I.V.: 20 mg/m^2/day days 1-5 [total dose/cycle = 100 mg/m^2]
Repeat cycle every 3 or 4 weeks

EP/EMA

Use: Gestational trophoblastic tumor
Regimen:
Etoposide: I.V.: 150 mg/m^2 day 1 [total dose/cycle = 150 mg/m^2]
Cisplatin: I.V.: 25 mg/m^2 infused over 4 hours for 3 consecutive doses, day 1 [total dose/cycle = 75 mg/m^2]
Alternate weekly with:
Etoposide: I.V.: 100 mg/m^2 day 1 [total dose/cycle = 100 mg/m^2]
Methotrexate: I.V.: 300 mg/m^2 infused over 12 hours day 1 [total dose/cycle = 300 mg/m^2]
Dactinomycin: I.V. push: 0.5 mg day 1 [total dose/cycle = 0.5 mg]
Leucovorin: Oral, I.M.: 15 mg twice daily for 2 days (start 24 hours after the start of methotrexate) days 2, 3 [total dose/cycle = 60 mg]

EP/PE

Use: Lung cancer, nonsmall-cell
Regimen:
Etoposide: I.V.: 120 mg/m^2/day days 1-3 [total dose/cycle = 360 mg/m^2]
Cisplatin: I.V.: 60-120 mg/m^2 day 1 [total dose/cycle = 60-120 mg/m^2]
Repeat cycle every 21-28 days

EPOCH

Use: Lymphoma, non-Hodgkin

Regimen:

Etoposide: I.V.: 50 mg/m^2/day continuous infusion days 1-4 [total dose/cycle = 200 mg/m^2]
Vincristine: I.V.: 0.4 mg/m^2/day continuous infusion days 1-4 [total dose/cycle = 1.6 mg/m^2]
Doxorubicin: I.V.: 10 mg/m^2/day continuous infusion days 1-4 [total dose/cycle = 40 mg/m^2]
Cyclophosphamide: I.V.: 750 mg/m^2 day 6 [total dose/cycle = 750 mg/m^2]
Prednisone: Oral: 60 mg/m^2/day days 1-6 [total dose/cycle = 360 mg/m^2]
Repeat cycle every 21 days

ESHAP

Use: Lymphoma, non-Hodgkin

Regimen: Note: Multiple variations are listed below.

Variation 1:
Etoposide: I.V.: 40 mg/m^2/day days 1-4 [total dose/cycle = 160 mg/m^2]
Methylprednisolone: I.V.: 500 mg/day days 1-5 [total dose/cycle = 2500 mg]
Cytarabine: I.V.: 2000 mg/m^2 day 1 [total dose/cycle = 2000 mg/m^2]
Cisplatin: I.V.: 25 mg/m^2/day continuous infusion days 1-4 [total dose/cycle = 100 mg/m^2]
Repeat cycle every 21-28 days

Variation 2:
Etoposide: I.V.: 40 mg/m^2/day days 1-4 [total dose/cycle = 160 mg/m^2]
Methylprednisolone: I.V.: 500 mg/day days 1-5 [total dose/cycle = 2500 mg]
Cytarabine: I.V.: 2000 mg/m^2 day 5 [total dose/cycle = 2000 mg/m^2]
Cisplatin: I.V.: 25 mg/m^2/day continuous infusion days 1-4 [total dose/cycle = 100 mg/m^2]
Repeat cycle every 21-28 days

Variation 3:
Etoposide: I.V.: 60 mg/m^2/day days 1-4 [total dose/cycle = 240 mg/m^2]
Methylprednisolone: I.V.: 500 mg/day days 1-4 [total dose/cycle = 2000 mg]
Cytarabine: I.V.: 2000 mg/m^2 day 5 [total dose/cycle = 2000 mg/m^2]
Cisplatin: I.V.: 25 mg/m^2/day continuous infusion days 1-4 [total dose/cycle = 100 mg/m^2]
Repeat cycle every 21 days

Estramustine + Docetaxel

Use: Prostate cancer

Regimen: Note: Multiple variations are listed below.

Variation 1:
Docetaxel: I.V.: 20-80 mg/m^2 day 2 [total dose/cycle = 20-80 mg/m^2]
Estramustine: Oral: 280 mg 3 times/day days 1-5 [total dose/cycle = 4200 mg]
Repeat cycle every 21 days

Variation 2:
Docetaxel: I.V.: 20-80 mg/m^2 day 2 [total dose/cycle = 20-80 mg/m^2]
Estramustine: Oral: 14 mg/kg/day days 1-21 [total dose/cycle = 294 mg/kg]
Repeat cycle every 21 days

Variation 3:
Docetaxel: I.V.: 35 mg/m^2/day days 2 and 9 [total dose/cycle = 70 mg/m^2]
Estramustine: Oral: 420 mg 3 times/day for 4 doses, then 280 mg 3 times/day for 5 doses days 1, 2, 3, 8, 9, and 10 [total dose/cycle = 6160 mg]
Repeat cycle every 21 days

Estramustine + Docetaxel + Carboplatin

Use: Prostate cancer

Regimen:

Docetaxel: I.V.: 70 mg/m^2 day 2 [total dose/cycle = 70 mg/m^2]
Estramustine: Oral: 280 mg 3 times/day days 1-5 [total dose/cycle = 4200 mg]
Carboplatin: I.V.: Target AUC 5 day 2 [total dose/cycle = AUC = 5]
Repeat cycle every 3 weeks

Estramustine + Docetaxel + Hydrocortisone

Use: Prostate cancer

Regimen:

Docetaxel: I.V.: 70 mg/m^2 day 2 [total dose/cycle = 70 mg/m^2]
Estramustine: Oral: 10 mg/kg/day days 1-5 [total dose/cycle = 50 mg/kg]
Hydrocortisone: Oral: 40 mg daily [total dose/cycle = 840 mg]
Repeat cycle every 3 weeks

Estramustine + Etoposide

Use: Prostate cancer

Regimen: Note: Multiple variations are listed below.

Variation 1:
Estramustine: Oral: 15 mg/kg/day days 1-21 [total dose/cycle = 315 mg/kg]
Etoposide: Oral: 50 mg/m^2/day days 1-21 [total dose/cycle = 1050 mg/m^2]
Repeat cycle every 4 weeks

Variation 2:
Estramustine: Oral: 10 mg/kg/day days 1-21 [total dose/cycle = 210 mg/kg]
Etoposide: Oral: 50 mg/m^2/day days 1-21 [total dose/cycle = 1050 mg/m^2]
Repeat cycle every 4 weeks

Variation 3:
Estramustine: Oral: 140 mg 3 times/day days 1-21 [total dose/cycle = 8820 mg]
Etoposide: Oral: 50 mg/m^2/day days 1-21 [total dose/cycle = 1050 mg/m^2]
Repeat cycle every 4 weeks

Estramustine + Vinorelbine

Use: Prostate cancer

Regimen: Note: Multiple variations are listed below.

Variation 1:
Estramustine: Oral: 140 mg 3 times/day days 1-14 [total dose/cycle = 5880 mg]
Vinorelbine: I.V.: 25 mg/m^2/day days 1 and 8 [total dose/cycle = 50 mg/m^2]
Repeat cycle every 21 days

Variation 2:
Estramustine: Oral: 280 mg 3 times/day days 1-3
Vinorelbine: I.V.: 15 or 20 mg/m^2 day 2
Give weekly for 8 weeks, then every other week

EV

Use: Prostate cancer

Regimen: Note: Multiple variations are listed below.

Variation 1:
Estramustine: Oral: 10 mg/kg/day days 1-42
[total dose/cycle = 420 mg/kg]
Vinblastine: I.V.: 4 mg/m^2/day days 1, 8, 15, 22, 29, and 36
[total dose/cycle = 24 mg/m^2]
Repeat cycle every 8 weeks

Variation 2:
Estramustine: Oral: 600 mg/m^2/day days 1-42
[total dose/cycle = 25,200 mg/m^2]
Vinblastine: I.V.: 4 mg/m^2/day days 1, 8, 15, 22, 29, and 36 [total dose/cycle = 24 mg/m^2]
Repeat cycle every 8 weeks

EVA

Use: Lymphoma, Hodgkin disease

Regimen:

Etoposide: I.V.: 100 mg/m^2/day days 1-3 [total dose/cycle = 300 mg/m^2]
Vinblastine: I.V.: 6 mg/m^2 day 1 [total dose/cycle = 6 mg/m^2]
Doxorubicin: I.V.: 50 mg/m^2 day 1 [total dose/cycle = 50 mg/m^2]
Repeat cycle every 28 days

FAC

Use: Breast cancer

Regimen: Note: Multiple variations are listed below.

Variation 1:

Fluorouracil: I.V.: 500 mg/m^2/day days 1 and 8 [total dose/cycle = 1000 mg/m^2]
or 500 mg/m^2 day 1 [total dose/cycle = 500 mg/m^2]
Doxorubicin: I.V.: 50 mg/m^2 day 1 [total dose/cycle = 50 mg/m^2]
Cyclophosphamide: I.V.: 500 mg/m^2 day 1 [total dose/cycle = 500 mg/m^2]
Repeat cycle every 21-28 days

Variation 2:

Fluorouracil: I.V.: 200 mg/m^2/day days 1-3 [total dose/cycle = 600 mg/m^2]
Doxorubicin: I.V.: 40 mg/m^2 day 1 [total dose/cycle = 40 mg/m^2]
Cyclophosphamide: I.V.: 400 mg/m^2 day 1 [total dose/cycle = 400 mg/m^2]
Repeat cycle every 28 days

Variation 3:

Fluorouracil: I.V.: 400 mg/m^2/day days 1 and 8 [total dose/cycle = 800 mg/m^2]
Doxorubicin: I.V.: 40 mg/m^2 day 1 [total dose/cycle = 40 mg/m^2]
Cyclophosphamide: I.V.: 400 mg/m^2 day 1 [total dose/cycle = 400 mg/m^2]
Repeat cycle every 28 days

Variation 4:

Fluorouracil: I.V.: 600 mg/m^2/day days 1 and 8 [total dose/cycle = 1200 mg/m^2]
Doxorubicin: I.V.: 60 mg/m^2 day 1 [total dose/cycle = 60 mg/m^2]
Cyclophosphamide: I.V.: 600 mg/m^2 day 1 [total dose/cycle = 600 mg/m^2]
Repeat cycle every 28 days

Variation 5:

Fluorouracil: I.V.: 300 mg/m^2/day days 1 and 8 [total dose/cycle = 600 mg/m^2]
Doxorubicin: I.V.: 30 mg/m^2 day 1 [total dose/cycle = 30 mg/m^2]
Cyclophosphamide: I.V.: 300 mg/m^2 day 1 [total dose/cycle = 300 mg/m^2]
Repeat cycle every 28 days

FAM

Use: Gastric cancer; Pancreatic cancer

Regimen:

Fluorouracil: I.V.: 600 mg/m^2/day days 1, 8, 29, 36 [total dose/cycle = 2400 mg/m^2]
Doxorubicin: I.V.: 30 mg/m^2/day days 1 and 29 [total dose/cycle = 60 mg/m^2]
Mitomycin C: I.V.: 10 mg/m^2 day 1 [total dose/cycle = 10 mg/m^2]
Repeat cycle every 8 weeks

FAMTX

Use: Gastric cancer

Regimen: Note: Multiple variations are listed below.

Variation 1:

Methotrexate: I.V.: 1500 mg/m^2 day 1 [total dose/cycle = 1500 mg/m^2]
Fluorouracil: I.V.: 1500 mg/m^2 (1 hour after methotrexate) day 1 [total dose/cycle = 1500 mg/m^2]
Leucovorin: Oral: 15 mg/m^2 every 6 hours for 48 hours (start 24 hours after methotrexate) day 2 [total dose/cycle = 120 mg/m^2]
Doxorubicin: I.V.: 30 mg/m^2 day 15 [total dose/cycle = 30 mg/m^2]
Repeat cycle every 28 days

Variation 2:

Methotrexate: I.V.: 1500 mg/m^2 day 1 [total dose/cycle = 1500 mg/m^2]
Fluorouracil: I.V.: 1500 mg/m^2 day 1 [total dose/cycle = 1500 mg/m^2]
Leucovorin: Oral: 15 mg/m^2 every 6 hours for 8 doses (start 24 hours after methotrexate) [total dose/cycle = 90 mg/m^2]
followed by 30 mg/m^2 every 6 hours for 8 more doses if 24-hour methotrexate level ≥2.5 mol/L (start 24 hours after methotrexate) [total dose/cycle = 360 mg/m^2]
Doxorubicin: I.V.: 30 mg/m^2 day 15 [total dose/cycle = 30 mg/m^2]
Repeat cycle every 28 days

F-CL

Use: Colorectal cancer

Regimen: Note: Multiple variations are listed below.

Variation 1 (Mayo Regimen):

Fluorouracil: I.V.: 425 mg/m^2/day days 1-5 [total dose/cycle = 2125 mg/m^2]
Leucovorin: I.V.: 20 mg/m^2/day days 1-5 [total dose/cycle = 100 mg/m^2]
Repeat cycle every 28 days

F-CL *(continued)*

Variation 2:
Fluorouracil: I.V.: 400 mg/m^2/day days 1-5 [total dose/cycle = 2000 mg/m^2]
Leucovorin: I.V.: 20 mg/m^2/day days 1-5 [total dose/cycle = 100 mg/m^2]
Repeat cycle every 28 days
Variation 3:
Fluorouracil: I.V.: 500 mg/m^2 day 1 [total dose/cycle = 500 mg/m^2]
Leucovorin: I.V.: 20 mg/m^2 (2-hour infusion) day 1
[total dose/cycle = 20 mg/m^2] **or** 500 mg/m^2 (2-hour infusion) day 1 [total dose/cycle = 500 mg/m^2]
Repeat cycle weekly
Variation 4:
Fluorouracil: I.V.: 600 mg/m^2 weekly for 6 weeks [total dose/cycle = 3600 mg/m^2]
Leucovorin: I.V.: 500 mg/m^2 (3-hour infusion) weekly for 6 weeks [total dose/cycle = 3000 mg/m^2]
Repeat cycle every 8 weeks
Variation 5:
Fluorouracil: I.V.: 600 mg/m^2 weekly for 6 weeks [total dose/cycle = 3600 mg/m^2]
Leucovorin: I.V.: 500 mg/m^2 weekly for 6 weeks [total dose/cycle = 3000 mg/m^2]
Repeat cycle every 8 weeks
Variation 6:
Fluorouracil: I.V.: 600 mg/m^2 weekly
Leucovorin: I.V.: 500 mg/m^2 (2-hour infusion) weekly
Repeat cycle weekly
Variation 7:
Fluorouracil: I.V.: 2600 mg/m^2 continuous infusion day 1 [total dose/cycle = 2600 mg/m^2]
Leucovorin: I.V.: 500 mg/m^2 continuous infusion day 1 [total dose/cycle = 500 mg/m^2]
Repeat cycle weekly
Variation 8:
Fluorouracil: I.V.: 2600 mg/m^2 continuous infusion day 1 [total dose/cycle = 2600 mg/m^2]
Leucovorin: I.V.: 300 mg/m^2 (maximum 500 mg) continuous infusion day 1
[total dose/cycle = 300 mg/m^2]
Repeat cycle weekly
Variation 9:
Fluorouracil: I.V.: 2600 mg/m^2 continuous infusion once weekly for 6 weeks
[total dose/cycle = 15,600 mg/m^2]
Leucovorin: I.V.: 500 mg/m^2 weekly for 6 weeks [total dose/cycle = 3000 mg/m^2]
Repeat cycle every 8 weeks
Variation 10:
Fluorouracil: I.V.: 2300 mg/m^2 continuous infusion day 1 [total dose/cycle = 2300 mg/m^2]
Leucovorin: I.V.: 50 mg/m^2 continuous infusion day 1 [total dose/cycle = 50 mg/m^2]
Repeat cycle weekly
Variation 11:
Fluorouracil: I.V.: 200 mg/m^2/day continuous infusion days 1-14 [total dose/cycle = 2800 mg/m^2]
Leucovorin: I.V.: 5 mg/m^2/day days 1-14 [total dose/cycle = 70 mg/m^2]
Repeat cycle every 28 days
Variation 12:
Fluorouracil: I.V.: 200 mg/m^2 continuous infusion daily for 4 weeks
followed by (starting week 5): 200 mg/m^2 continuous infusion days 1-21
[total dose/cycle = 4200 mg/m^2]
Leucovorin: I.V.: 20 mg/m^2/day days 1, 8, and 15 [total dose/cycle = 60 mg/m^2]
Repeat cycle every 4 weeks

FEC

Use: Breast cancer
Regimen:
Fluorouracil: I.V.: 500 mg/m^2 day 1 [total dose/cycle = 500 mg/m^2]
Cyclophosphamide: I.V.: 500 mg/m^2 day 1 [total dose/cycle = 500 mg/m^2]
Epirubicin: I.V.: 100 mg/m^2 day 1 [total dose/cycle = 100 mg/m^2]
Repeat cycle every 21 days

FIS-HAM

Use: Leukemia, acute lymphocytic; Leukemia, acute myeloid
Regimen:
Fludarabine: I.V.: 15 mg/m^2/day every 12 hours days 1, 2, 8, and 9 [total dose/cycle = 120 mg/m^2]
Cytarabine: I.V.: 750 mg/m^2/day every 3 hours days 1, 2, 8, and 9 [total dose/cycle = 24,000 mg/m^2]
Mitoxantrone: I.V.: 10 mg/m^2/day days 3, 4, 10, and 11 [total dose/cycle = 40 mg/m^2]

FL

Use: Prostate cancer

Regimen: Note: Multiple variations are listed below.

Variation 1:

Flutamide: Oral: 250 mg every 8 hours [total dose/cycle = 21,000 mg]

Leuprolide acetate: SubQ: 1 mg/day [total dose/cycle = 28 mg]

Repeat cycle every 28 days

Variation 2:

Flutamide: Oral: 250 mg every 8 hours [total dose/cycle = 67,500 mg]

Leuprolide acetate depot: I.M.: 22.5 mg day 1 [total dose/cycle = 22.5 mg]

Repeat cycle every 3 months

FLAG

Use: Leukemia, acute myeloid

Regimen:

Fludarabine: I.V.: 30 mg/m^2/day days 1-5 [total dose/cycle = 150 mg/m^2]

Cytarabine: I.V.: 2 g/m^2/day days 1-5 (3.5 hours after end of fludarabine infusion) [total dose/cycle = 10 g/m^2]

Filgrastim: SubQ: 5 mcg/kg day 1 [total dose/cycle = 5 mcg/kg] **followed by** 300 mcg daily until ANC >500-1000 cells/mcL postnadir [total dose/cycle = 40-7800 mcg/kg]

Repeat cycle every 3-4 weeks

FLe

Use: Colorectal cancer

Regimen:

Fluorouracil: I.V.: 450 mg/m^2/day for 5 days, [total dose/cycle = 2250 mg/m^2]

then after a pause of 4 weeks: 450 mg/m^2/week for 48 weeks [total dose/cycle = 21.6 g/m^2]

Levamisole: Oral: 50 mg 3 times/day for 3 days, repeated every 2 weeks for 1 year [total dose/cycle = 11.7 g/m^2]

Fludarabine-Rituximab

Use: Leukemia, chronic lymphocytic

Regimen:

Rituximab: I.V.: 375 mg/m^2/day days 1 and 4 (cycle 1); [total dose/cycle 1 = 750 mg/m^2] day 1 (cycles 2-6) [total dose/cycle = 375 mg/m^2]

Fludarabine: I.V.: 25 mg/m^2/day days 1-5 [total dose/cycle = 125 mg/m^2]

Repeat cycle every 4 weeks

FOIL

Use: Colorectal cancer

Regimen:

Irinotecan: I.V.: 175 mg/m^2 day 1 [total dose/cycle = 175 mg/m^2]

Oxaliplatin: I.V.: 100 mg/m^2 day 1 [total dose/cycle = 100 mg/m^2]

Leucovorin: I.V.: 200 mg/m^2 day 1 [total dose/cycle = 200 mg/m^2]

Fluorouracil: I.V.: 3800 mg/m^2/day continuous infusion days 1 and 2 [total dose/cycle = 7600 mg/m^2]

Repeat cycle every 14 days

FOLFOX 1

Use: Colorectal cancer

Regimen:

Oxaliplatin: I.V.: 130 mg/m^2 day 1 (every other cycle) [total dose/cycle = 130 mg/m^2]

Leucovorin: I.V.: 500 mg/m^2/day days 1 and 2 [total dose/cycle = 1000 mg/m^2]

Fluorouracil: I.V.: 1.5-2 g/m^2/day continuous infusion days 1 and 2 [total dose/cycle = 3-4 g/m^2]

Repeat cycle every 14 days

FOLFOX 2

Use: Colorectal cancer

Regimen:

Oxaliplatin: I.V.: 100 mg/m^2 day 1 [total dose/cycle = 100 mg/m^2]

Leucovorin: I.V.: 500 mg/m^2/day days 1 and 2 [total dose/cycle = 1000 mg/m^2]

Fluorouracil: I.V.: 1.5-2 g/m^2/day continuous infusion days 1 and 2 [total dose/cycle = 3-4 g/m^2]

Repeat cycle every 14 days

FOLFOX 3

Use: Colorectal cancer

Regimen:

Oxaliplatin: I.V.: 85 mg/m^2 day 1 [total dose/cycle = 85 mg/m^2]

Leucovorin: I.V.: 500 mg/m^2/day days 1 and 2 [total dose/cycle = 1000 mg/m^2]

Fluorouracil: I.V.: 1.5-2 g/m^2/day continuous infusion days 1 and 2 [total dose/cycle = 3-4 g/m^2]

Repeat cycle every 14 days

FOLFOX 4

Use: Colorectal cancer

Regimen:

Oxaliplatin: I.V.: 85 mg/m^2 day 1 [total dose/cycle = 85 mg/m^2]

Leucovorin: I.V.: 200 mg/m^2/day days 1 and 2 [total dose/cycle = 400 mg/m^2]

Fluorouracil: I.V. bolus: 400 mg/m^2/day days 1 and 2
[total dose/cycle = 800 mg/m^2] **followed by** 600 mg/m^2 CIVI (over 22-hour) days 1 and 2
[total dose/cycle = 1200 mg/m^2]

Note: Bolus fluorouracil and CIVI are both given on each day.

Repeat cycle every 14 days

FOLFOX 6

Use: Colorectal cancer

Regimen:

Oxaliplatin: I.V.: 100 mg/m^2 day 1 [total dose/cycle = 100 mg/m^2]

Leucovorin: I.V.: 400 mg/m^2 day 1 [total dose/cycle = 400 mg/m^2]

Fluorouracil: I.V. bolus: 400 mg/m^2 day 1 [total dose/cycle = 400 mg/m^2] **followed by** 2.4-3 g/m^2 CIVI (46 hours) continuous infusion extending over days 1 and 2 [total dose/cycle = 2.4-3 g/m^2]

Repeat cycle every 14 days

FOLFOX 7

Use: Colorectal cancer

Regimen:

Oxaliplatin: I.V.: 130 mg/m^2 day 1 [total dose/cycle = 130 mg/m^2]

Leucovorin: I.V.: 400 mg/m^2 day 1 [total dose/cycle = 400 mg/m^2]

Fluorouracil: I.V. bolus: 400 mg/m^2 day 1
[total dose/cycle = 400 mg/m^2] **followed by** 2.4 g/m^2 CIVI (46 hours) continuous infusion extending over days 1 and 2 [total dose/cycle = 2.4 g/m^2]

Repeat cycle every 14 days

FU HURT

Use: Head and neck cancer

Regimen:

Hydroxyurea: Oral: 1000 mg every 12 hours for 11 doses days 0-5 [total dose/cycle = 11,000 mg]

Fluorouracil: I.V.: 800 mg/m^2/day continuous infusion (start AM after admission) days 1-5
[total dose/cycle = 4000 mg/m^2]

Paclitaxel: I.V.: 5-25 mg/m^2/day continuous infusion days 1-5 [total dose/cycle = 25-125 mg/m^2]

Filgrastim: SubQ: 5 mcg/kg/day days 6-12 (start ≥12 hours after completion of fluorouracil infusion)

5-7 cycles may be administered

FU/LV/CPT-11

Use: Colorectal cancer

Regimen: Note: Multiple variations are listed below.

Variation: 1:

Irinotecan: I.V.: 350 mg/m^2 day 1 [total dose/cycle = 350 mg/m^2]
Leucovorin: I.V.: 20 mg/m^2/day days 22-26 [total dose/cycle = 100 mg/m^2]
Fluorouracil: I.V.: 425 mg/m^2/day days 22-26 [total dose/cycle = 2125 mg/m^2]
Repeat cycle every 6 weeks

Variation: 2:

Irinotecan: I.V.: 80 mg/m^2 day 1 [total dose/cycle = 80 mg/m^2]
Fluorouracil: I.V.: 2300 mg/m^2 continuous infusion day 1 [total dose/cycle = 2300 mg/m^2]
Leucovorin: I.V.: 500 mg/m^2 day 1 [total dose/cycle = 500 mg/m^2]
Repeat cycle weekly **or**
Irinotecan: I.V.: 180 mg/m^2 day 1 [total dose/cycle = 180 mg/m^2]
Leucovorin: I.V.: 200 mg/m^2/day days 1 and 2 [total dose/cycle = 400 mg/m^2]
Fluorouracil: I.V.: 400 mg/m^2/day days 1 and 2 [total dose/cycle = 800 mg/m^2]
followed by 600 mg/m^2/day continuous infusion days 1 and 2 [total dose/cycle = 1200 mg/m^2]
Repeat cycle every 2 weeks

Variation 3:

Irinotecan: I.V.: 175 mg/m^2 day 1 [total dose/cycle = 175 mg/m^2]
Leucovorin: I.V.: 250 mg/m^2 day 2 [total dose/cycle = 250 mg/m^2]
Fluorouracil: I.V.: 950 mg/m^2 day 2 [total dose/cycle = 950 mg/m^2] **or**
Irinotecan: I.V.: 200 mg/m^2 day 1 [total dose/cycle = 200 mg/m^2]
Leucovorin: I.V.: 250 mg/m^2 day 2 [total dose/cycle = 250 mg/m^2]
Fluorouracil: I.V.: 850 mg/m^2 day 2 [total dose/cycle = 850 mg/m^2]
Repeat cycle every other week

FU/LV/CPT-11 (Saltz Regimen)

Use: Colorectal cancer

Regimen:

Fluorouracil: I.V.: 500 mg/m^2/day days 1, 8, 15, and 22 [total dose/cycle = 2000 mg/m^2]
Leucovorin: I.V.: 20 mg/m^2/day days 1, 8, 15, and 22 [total dose/cycle = 80 mg/m^2]
Irinotecan: I.V.: 125 mg/m^2/day days 1, 8, 15, and 22 [total dose/cycle = 500 mg/m^2]
Repeat cycle every 42 days

FUP

Use: Gastric cancer

Regimen:

Fluorouracil: I.V.: 1000 mg/m^2/day continuous infusion days 1-5 [total dose/cycle = 5000 mg/m^2]
Cisplatin: I.V.: 100 mg/m^2 day 2 [total dose/cycle = 100 mg/m^2]
Repeat cycle every 28 days

FZ

Use: Prostate cancer

Regimen: Note: Multiple variations are listed below.

Variation 1:

Flutamide: Oral: 250 mg every 8 hours [total dose/cycle = 21,000 mg]
Goserelin acetate: SubQ: 3.6 mg day 1 [total dose/cycle = 3.6 mg]
Repeat cycle every 28 days

Variation 2:

Flutamide: Oral: 250 mg every 8 hours [total dose/cycle = 67,500 mg]
Goserelin acetate: SubQ: 10.8 mg day 1 [total dose/cycle = 10.8 mg]
Repeat cycle every 3 months

GC

Use: Lung cancer, nonsmall-cell

Regimen:

Gemcitabine: I.V.: 1000 mg/m^2/day days 1, 8, 15 [total dose/cycle = 3000 mg/m^2]
Cisplatin: I.V.: 100 mg/m^2 day 1 **or** 2 **or** 15 [total dose/cycle = 100 mg/m^2]
Repeat cycle every 28 days for 2-6 cycles

Gemcitabine/Capecitabine

Use: Pancreatic cancer

Regimen:

Gemcitabine: I.V.: 1000 mg/m^2/day days 1 and 8 [total dose/cycle = 2000 mg/m^2]
Capecitabine: Oral: 650 mg/m^2 twice daily days 1-14 [total dose/cycle = 18,200 mg/m^2]
Repeat cycle every 21 days

Gemcitabine-Carboplatin

Use: Lung cancer, nonsmall-cell

Regimen:

Gemcitabine: I.V.: 1000 or 1100 mg/m^2/day days 1 and 8
[total dose/cycle = 2000 or 2200 mg/m^2]
Carboplatin: I.V.: AUC 5 day 8 [total dose/cycle = AUC = 5]
Repeat cycle every 28 days

Gemcitabine-Cis

Use: Lung cancer, nonsmall-cell

Regimen: Note: Multiple variations are listed below.

Variation 1:
Gemcitabine: I.V.: 1000-1200 mg/m^2/day days 1, 8, 15 [total dose/cycle = 3000-3600 mg/m^2]
Cisplatin: I.V.: 100 mg/m^2 day 2 **or** 15 [total dose/cycle = 100 mg/m^2]
Repeat cycle every 28 days

Variation 2:
Gemcitabine: I.V.: 1000-1200 mg/m^2/day 1, 8, 15 [total dose/cycle = 3000-3600 mg/m^2]
Cisplatin: I.V.: 100 mg/m^2 day 1 **or** 2 **or** 15 [total dose/cycle = 100 mg/m^2]
Repeat cycle every 28 days

Gemcitabine-Cisplatin

Use: Bladder cancer

Regimen:

Gemcitabine: I.V.: 1000 mg/m^2/day days 1, 8, 15 [total dose/cycle = 3000 mg/m^2]
Cisplatin: I.V.: 70 mg/m^2 day 2 [total dose/cycle = 70 mg/m^2]
Repeat cycle every 28 days for 6 cycles

Gemcitabine-Docetaxel

Use: Bony sarcoma; Soft tissue sarcoma

Regimen:

Gemcitabine: I.V.: 675 mg/m^2/day days 1 and 8 [total dose/cycle = 1350 mg/m^2]
Docetaxel: I.V.: 100 mg/m^2 day 8 [total dose/cycle = 100 mg/m^2]
Repeat cycle every 21 days

Gemcitabine/Irinotecan

Use: Pancreatic cancer

Regimen:

Gemcitabine: I.V.: 1000 mg/m^2/day days 1 and 8 [total dose/cycle = 2000 mg/m^2]
Irinotecan: I.V.: 100 mg/m^2/day days 1 and 8 [total dose/cycle = 200 mg/m^2]
Repeat cycle every 21 days

Gemcitabine-Paclitaxel

Use: Ovarian cancer

Regimen:

Paclitaxel: I.V.: 80 mg/m^2 infused over 60 minutes days 1, 8, and 15
[total dose/cycle = 240 mg/m^2]
Gemcitabine: I.V.: 1000 mg/m^2/day (start at end of paclitaxel infusion) days 1, 8, and 15
[total dose/cycle = 3000 mg/m^2]
Repeat cycle every 4 weeks

Gemcitabine-Vinorelbine

Use: Lung cancer, nonsmall-cell

Regimen: Note: Multiple variations are listed below.

Variation 1:

Gemcitabine: I.V.: 1200 mg/m^2/day days 1 and 8 [total dose/cycle = 2400 mg/m^2]

Vinorelbine: I.V.: 30 mg/m^2/day days 1 and 8 [total dose/cycle = 60 mg/m^2]

Repeat cycle every 21 days for 6 cycles

Variation 2:

Gemcitabine: I.V.: 1000 mg/m^2/day days 1, 8, and 15 [total dose/cycle = 3000 mg/m^2]

Vinorelbine: I.V.: 20 mg/m^2/day days 1, 8, and 15 [total dose/cycle = 60 mg/m^2]

Repeat cycle every 28 days for 6 cycles

GEMOX

Use: Biliary adenocarcinoma

Regimen:

Gemcitabine: I.V.: 1000 mg/m^2 day 1 [total dose/cycle = 1000 mg/m^2]

Oxaliplatin: I.V.: 100 mg/m^2 day 2 [total dose/cycle = 100 mg/m^2]

Repeat cycle every 2 weeks

HDMTX (Osteosarcoma)

Use: Osteosarcoma

Regimen:

Methotrexate: I.V.: 12 g/m^2/week for 2-12 weeks [total dose/cycle = 24-144 g/m^2]

Leucovorin calcium rescue: Oral, I.V.: 15 mg/m^2 every 6 hours (beginning 30 hours after the beginning of the 4-hour methotrexate infusion) for 10 doses; **serum methotrexate levels must be monitored** [total dose/cycle = 150 mg/m^2]

HIPE-IVAD

Use: Neuroblastomas

Regimen:

Cisplatin: I.V.: 40 mg/m^2/day days 1-5 [total dose/cycle = 200 mg/m^2]

Etoposide: I.V.: 100 mg/m^2/day days 1-5 [total dose/cycle = 500 mg/m^2]

Ifosfamide: I.V.: 3 g/m^2/day days 21-23 [total dose/cycle = 9 g/m^2]

Mesna: I.V.: 3 g/m^2/day continuous infusion days 21-23 [total dose/cycle = 9 g/m^2]

Vincristine: I.V.: 1.5 mg/m^2 day 21 [total dose/cycle = 1.5 mg/m^2]

Doxorubicin: I.V.: 60 mg/m^2 day 23 [total dose/cycle = 60 mg/m^2]

Repeat cycle every 28 days

Hyper-CVAD

Use: Leukemia, acute myeloid

Regimen:

Course 1, 3, 5, and 7:

Cyclophosphamide: I.V.: 300 mg/m^2/day every 12 hours days 1-3 [total dose/cycle = 900 mg/m^2]

Mesna: I.V.: 3600 mg/m^2/day continuous infusion days 1-3 [total dose/cycle = 10,800 mg/m^2]

Methotrexate: I.T.: 12 mg day 2 [total dose/cycle = 12 mg]

Vincristine: I.V.: 2 mg/day days 4 and 11 [total dose/cycle = 4 mg]

Doxorubicin: I.V.: 50 mg/m^2 day 4 [total dose/cycle = 50 mg/m^2]

Cytarabine: I.T.: 100 mg day 8 [total dose/cycle = 100 mg]

Dexamethasone: Oral or I.V.: 40 mg/day days 1-4 and 11-14 [total dose/cycle = 320 mg]

Course 2, 4, 6, and 8:

Methotrexate: I.V.: 200 mg/m^2 day 1
[total dose/cycle = 200 mg/m^2] **followed by** 800 mg/m^2 continuous infusion day 1
[total dose/cycle = 800 mg/m^2]

Cytarabine: I.V.: 3 g/m^2 every 12 hours days 2 and 3 [total dose/cycle = 12 g/m^2]

Methotrexate: I.T.: 12 mg day 2 [total dose/cycle = 12 mg]

Leucovorin: I.V.: 15 mg every 6 hours days 3 and 4 [total dose/cycle = 120 mg]

Methylprednisolone: I.V.: 50 mg twice daily days 1-3 [total dose/cycle = 300 mg]

Cytarabine: I.T.: 100 mg day 8 [total dose/cycle = 100 mg]

Cycles are given when WBC is ≥3000 mm^3, Plt ≥60,000 mm^3

ICE (Lymphoma, non-Hodgkin)

Use: Lymphoma, non-Hodgkin

Regimen:

Etoposide: I.V.: 100 mg/m^2/day days 1-3 [total dose/cycle = 300 mg/m^2]
Carboplatin: I.V.: AUC 5 day 2 (maximum 800 mg) [total dose/cycle = AUC = 5]
Ifosfamide: I.V.: 5 g/m^2 continuous infusion day 2 [total dose/cycle = 5 g/m^2]
Mesna: I.V.: 5 g/m^2 continuous infusion day 2 [total dose/cycle = 5 g/m^2]
Repeat cycle every 2 weeks

ICE (Sarcoma)

Use: Osteosarcoma; Soft tissue sarcoma

Regimen:

Ifosfamide: I.V.: 1250-1500 mg/m^2/day days 1-3 [total dose/cycle = 3750-4500 mg/m^2]
Carboplatin: I.V.: 300-635 mg/m^2 day 3 [total dose/cycle = 300-635 mg/m^2]
Etopside: I.V.: 80-100 mg/m^2/day days 1-3 [total dose/cycle = 240-300 mg/m^2]
Mesna: I.V.: 1250 mg/m^2/day days 1-3 [total dose/cycle = 3750 mg/m^2]
or 20% of ifosfamide dose before, 4 and 8 hours after each ifosfamide infusion
[total dose/cycle = 60% of ifosfamide dose]
Repeat cycle every 21-28 days

ICE-T

Use: Soft tissue sarcoma

Regimen:

Ifosfamide: I.V.: 1250 mg/m^2/day days 1, 2, and 3 [total dose/cycle = 3750 mg/m^2]
Carboplatin: I.V.: 300 mg/m^2 day 1 [total dose/cycle = 300 mg/m^2]
Etopside: I.V.: 80 mg/m^2/day days 1, 2, and 3 [total dose/cycle = 240 mg/m^2]
Paclitaxel: I.V.: 175 mg/m^2 day 4 [total dose/cycle = 175 mg/m^2]
Mesna: I.V.: 20% of ifosfamide dose before
followed by: Oral: 40% of ifosfamide dose 4 and 8 hours after ifosfamide
[total dose/cycle = 100% of ifosfamide dose] **or**
Mesna: I.V.: 1250 mg/m^2/day days 1, 2, and 3 [total dose/cycle = 3750 mg/m^2]
Repeat cycle every 28 days

Idarubicin, Cytarabine, Etoposide (ICE Protocol)

Use: Leukemia, acute myeloid

Regimen:

Idarubicin: I.V.: 6 mg/m^2/day days 1-5 [total dose/cycle = 30 mg/m^2]
Cytarabine: I.V.: 600 mg/m^2/day days 1-5 [total dose/cycle = 3000 mg/m^2]
Etoposide: I.V.: 150 mg/m^2/day days 1-3 [total dose/cycle = 450 mg/m^2]
Administer one cycle only

Idarubicin, Cytarabine, Etoposide (IDA-Based BF12)

Use: Leukemia, acute myeloid

Regimen: Induction:

Idarubicin: I.V.: 5 mg/m^2/day days 1-5 [total dose/cycle = 25 mg/m^2]
Cytarabine: I.V.: 2000 mg/m^2 every 12 hours days 1-5 (10 doses)
[total dose/cycle = 20,000 mg/m^2]
Etoposide: I.V.: 100 mg/m^2/day days 1-5 [total dose/cycle = 500 mg/m^2]
Second cycle may be given based on individual respone; time between cycles not specified

IE

Use: Soft tissue sarcoma

Regimen:

Etoposide: I.V.: 100 mg/m^2/day days 1-3 [total dose/cycle = 300 mg/m^2]
Ifosfamide: I.V.: 2500 mg/m^2/day days 1-3 [total dose/cycle = 7500 mg/m^2]
Mesna: I.V.: 20% of ifosfamide dose prior to and at 4-, 8-, and 12 hours after ifosfamide administration
[total dose/cycle = 80% ifosfamide dose]
Repeat cycle every 28 days

IL-2 + IFN

Use: Melanoma

Regimen:

Cisplatin: I.V.: 20 mg/m²/day days 1-4 [total dose/cycle = 80 mg/m²]

Vinblastine: I.V.: 1.6 mg/m²/day days 1-4 [total dose/cycle = 6.4 mg/m²]

Dacarbazine: I.V.: 800 mg/m² day 1 [total dose/cycle = 800 mg/m²]

Aldesleukin: I.V.: 9 million units/m²/day continuous infusion days 1-4 [total dose/cycle = 36 million units/m²]

Interferon alfa-2b: SubQ: 5 million units/m²/day days 1-5, 7, 9, 11, 13 [total dose/cycle = 45 million units/m²]

Repeat cycle every 21 days

IMVP-16

Use: Lymphoma, non-Hodgkin

Regimen:

Ifosfamide: I.V.: 4 g/m² continuous infusion over 24 hours day 1 [total dose/cycle = 4 g/m²]

Mesna: I.V.: 800 mg/m² bolus prior to ifosfamide, then 4 g/m² continuous infusion over 12 hours concurrent with ifosfamide; then 2.4 g/m² continuous infusion over 12 hours after ifosfamide infusion day 1 [total dose/cycle = 7.2 g/m²]

Methotrexate: I.V.: 30 mg/m²/day days 3 and 10 [total dose/cycle = 60 mg/m²]

Etoposide: I.V.: 100 mg/m²/day days 1-3 [total dose/cycle = 300 mg/m²]

Repeat cycle every 21-28 days

Interleukin 2-Interferon Alfa 2

Use: Renal cell cancer

Regimen:

Weeks 1 and 4:

Aldesleukin: SubQ: 20 million units/m² 3 times weekly [total dose/cycle = 120 million units/m²]

Interferon alfa: SubQ: 6 million units/m² once weekly [total dose/cycle = 12 million units/m²]

Weeks 2, 3, 5, and 6:

Aldesleukin: SubQ: 5 million units/m² 3 times weekly [total dose/cycle = 60 million units/m²]

Interferon alfa: SubQ: 6 million units/m² 3 times weekly [total dose/cycle = 72 million units/m²]

Repeat cycle every 56 days

Interleukin 2-Interferon Alfa 2-Fluorouracil

Use: Renal cell cancer

Regimen:

Weeks 1 and 4:

Aldesleukin: SubQ: 20 million units/m² 3 times weekly [total dose/cycle = 120 million units/m²]

Interferon alfa: SubQ: 6 million units/m² once weekly [total dose/cycle = 12 million units/m²]

Weeks 2 and 3:

Aldesleukin: SubQ: 5 million units/m² 3 times weekly [total dose/cycle = 30 million units/m²]

Weeks 5-8:

Interferon alfa: SubQ: 9 million units/m² 3 times weekly [total dose/cycle = 108 million units/m²]

Fluorouracil: I.V.: 750 mg/m² once weekly [total dose/cycle = 3000 mg/m²]

Repeat cycle every 56 days

IPA

Use: Hepatoblastoma

Regimen:

Ifosfamide: I.V.: 500 mg/m² day 1 [total dose/cycle = 500 mg/m²] **followed by** 1000 mg/m²/day continuous infusion days 1-3 [total dose/cycle = 3000 mg/m²]

Cisplatin: I.V.: 20 mg/m²/day days 4-8 [total dose/cycle = 100 mg/m²]

Doxorubicin: I.V.: 30 mg/m²/day continuous infusion days 9 and 10 [total dose/cycle = 60 mg/m²]

Repeat cycle every 21 days

Irinotecan/Cisplatin

Use: Esophageal cancer

Regimen:

Cisplatin: I.V.: 30 mg/m^2/day days 1, 8, 15 and 22 [total dose/cycle = 120 mg/m^2]
Irinotecan: I.V.: 65 mg/m^2/day days 1, 8, 15 and 22 [total dose/cycle = 260 mg/m^2]
Repeat cycle every 6 weeks

IVAC

Use: Lymphoma, non-Hodgkin

Regimen:

Ifosfamide: I.V.: 1500 mg/m^2/day days 1-5 [total dose/cycle = 7500 mg/m^2]
Etoposide: I.V.: 60 mg/m^2/day days 1-5 [total dose/cycle = 300 mg/m^2]
Cytarabine: I.V.: 2 g/m^2 every 12 hours days 1 and 2 [total dose/cycle = 8 g/m^2]
Mesna: I.V.: 360 mg/m^2 every 3 hours days 1-5 [total dose/cycle = 14,400 mg/m^2]
Methotrexate: I.T.: 12 mg day 5 [total dose/cycle = 12 mg]
Sargramostim: SubQ: 7.5 mcg/kg day 7 until ANC >1000 cells/mm^3
Repeat when ANC >1000 cells/mm^3

Larson Regimen

Use: Leukemia, acute lymphocytic

Regimen: Induction:

Cyclophosphamide: I.V.: 1200 mg/m^2 day 1 [total dose/cycle = 1200 mg/m^2]
Daunorubicin: I.V.: 45 mg/m^2/day days 1-3 [total dose/cycle = 135 mg/m^2]
Vincristine: I.V.: 2 mg/day days 1, 8, 15, and 22 [total dose/cycle = 8 mg]
Prednisone: Oral or I.V.: 60 mg/m^2/day days 1-21 [total dose/cycle = 1260 mg/m^2]
Asparaginase: SubQ: 6000 units/m^2/day days 5, 8, 11, 15, 18, and 22
[total dose/cycle = 36,000 units/m^2]
Administer one cycle only

Linker Protocol

Use: Leukemia, acute lymphocytic

Regimen:

Remission induction:
Daunorubicin: I.V.: 50 mg/m^2/day days 1-3 [total dose/cycle = 150 mg/m^2]
Vincristine: I.V.: 2 mg/day days 1, 8, 15, and 22 [total dose/cycle = 8 mg]
Prednisone: Oral: 60 mg/m^2/day days 1-28 [total dose/cycle = 1680 mg/m^2]
Asparaginase: I.M.: 6000 units/m^2/day days 17-28 [total dose/cycle = 72,000 units/m^2]
If residual leukemia in bone marrow on day 14:
Daunorubicin: I.V.: 50 mg/m^2 day 15 [total dose/cycle = 50 mg/m^2]
If residual leukemia in bone marrow on day 28:
Daunorubicin: I.V.: 50 mg/m^2 days 29 and 30 [total dose/cycle = 100 mg/m^2]
Vincristine: I.V.: 2 mg/day days 29 and 36 [total dose/cycle = 4 mg]
Prednisone: Oral: 60 mg/m^2/day days 29-42 [total dose/cycle = 840 mg/m^2]
Asparaginase: I.M.: 6000 units/m^2/day days 29-35 [total dose/cycle = 42,000 units/m^2]
Consolidation therapy:
Treatment A (cycles 1, 3, 5, and 7)
Daunorubicin: I.V.: 50 mg/m^2/day days 1 and 2 [total dose/cycle = 100 mg/m^2]
Vincristine: I.V.: 2 mg/day days 1 and 8 [total dose/cycle = 4 mg]
Prednisone: Oral: 60 mg/m^2/day days 1-14 [total dose/cycle = 840 mg/m^2]
Asparaginase: I.M.: 12,000 units/m^2/day days 2, 4, 7, 9, 11, and 14
[total dose/cycle = 72,000 units/m^2]
Treatment B (cycles 2, 4, 6, and 8)
Teniposide: I.V.: 165 mg/m^2/day days 1, 4, 8, and 11 [total dose/cycle = 660 mg/m^2]
Cytarabine: I.V.: 300 mg/m^2/day days 1, 4, 8, and 11 [total dose/cycle = 1200 mg/m^2]
Treatment C (cycle 9)
Methotrexate: I.V.: 690 mg/m^2 continuous infusion day 1 (over 42 hours)
[total dose/cycle = 690 mg/m^2]
Leucovorin: I.V.: 15 mg/m^2 every 6 hours for 12 doses (start at end of methotrexate infusion)
[total dose/cycle = 180 mg/m^2]
Administer remission induction regimen for one cycle only. Repeat consolidation cycle every 28 days

LOPP

Use: Lymphoma, Hodgkin disease
Regimen:

Chlorambucil: Oral: 10 mg/day days 1-10 [total dose/cycle = 100 mg]
Vincristine: I.V.: 1.4 mg/m^2/day (maximum 2 mg) days 1 and 8 [total dose/cycle = 2.8 mg/m^2]
Procarbazine: Oral: 100 mg/m^2/day days 1-10 [total dose/cycle = 1000 mg/m^2]
Prednisone: Oral: 25 mg/m^2/day (maximum 60 mg) days 1-14
[total dose/cycle = 350 mg/m^2] **or**
Prednisolone: Oral: 25 mg/m^2/day (maximum 60 mg) days 1-14 [total dose/cycle = 350 mg/m^2]
Repeat cycle every 28 days

M-2

Use: Multiple myeloma
Regimen:

Vincristine: I.V.: 0.03 mg/kg (maximum 2 mg) day 1 [total dose/cycle = 0.03 mg/kg]
Carmustine: I.V.: 0.5 mg/kg day 1 [total dose/cycle = 0.5 mg/kg]
Cyclophosphamide: I.V.: 10 mg/kg day 1 [total dose/cycle = 10 mg/kg]
Melphalan: Oral: 0.25 mg/kg/day days 1-4 [total dose/cycle = 1 mg/kg] **or** 0.1 mg/kg/day days 1-7 or 1-10 [total dose/cycle = 0.7 or 1 mg/kg]
Prednisone: Oral: 1 mg/kg/day days 1-7
[total dose/cycle = 7 mg/kg]
Repeat cycle every 35-42 days

M-3

Use: Leukemia, acute promyelocytic
Regimen: Note: Multiple variations are listed below.

Induction:
Variation 1:
Tretinoin: Oral: 45 mg/m^2/day day 1 up to 90 days [total dose/cycle = 45-4050 mg/m^2]
≤20 years: 25 mg/m^2/day day 1 up to 90 days [total dose/cycle = 25-2250 mg/m^2]
Idarubicin: I.V.: 12 mg/m^2/day days 2, 4, 6, and 8 [total dose/cycle = 48 mg/m^2]
Consolidation:
Course 1:
Idarubicin: I.V.: 5 mg/m^2/day days 1-4 [total dose/cycle = 20 mg/m^2]
or 7 mg/m^2/day days 1-4 [total dose/cycle = 28 mg/m^2]
Tretinoin: Oral: 45 mg/m^2/day days 1-15 [total dose/cycle = 675 mg/m^2]
Course 2:
Mitoxantrone: I.V.: 10 mg/m^2/day days 1-5 [total dose/cycle = 50 mg/m^2]
or 10 mg/m^2/day days 1-5 [total dose/cycle = 50 mg/m^2]
Tretinoin: Oral: 45 mg/m^2/day days 1-15 [total dose/cycle = 675 mg/m^2]
Course 3:
Idarubicin: I.V.: 12 mg/m^2 on day 1 [total dose/cycle = 12 mg/m^2]
or 12 mg/m^2/day on days 1 and 2 [total dose/cycle = 24 mg/m^2]
Tretinoin: Oral: 45 mg/m^2/day days 1-15 [total dose/cycle = 675 mg/m^2]
Repeat course at one month intervals.
Maintenance:
Mercaptopurine: Oral: 50 mg/m^2 daily [total dose/cycle = 4.5 g/m^2]
Methotrexate: I.M.: 15 mg/m^2 weekly [total dose/cycle = 180 mg/m^2]
Tretinoin: Oral: 45 mg/m^2/day days 1-15 [total dose/cycle = 675 mg/m^2]
Repeat cycle every 3 months for 2 years
Variation 2:
Induction:
Tretinoin: Oral: 45 mg/m^2/day day 1 up to 90 days [total dose/cycle = 45-4050 mg/m^2]
≤15 years: 25 mg/m^2/day day 1 up to 90 days [total dose/cycle = 25-2250 mg/m^2]
Idarubicin: I.V.: 12 mg/m^2/day days 2, 4, 6, and 8 [total dose/cycle = 48 mg/m^2]
Consolidation:
Course 1:
Idarubicin: I.V.: 5 mg/m^2/day days 1-4 [total dose/cycle = 20 mg/m^2]
Course 2:
Mitoxantrone: I.V.: 10 mg/m^2/day days 1-5 [total dose/cycle = 50 mg/m^2]
Course 3:
Idarubicin: I.V.: 12 mg/m^2 day 1 [total dose/cycle = 12 mg/m^2]
Repeat course at one month intervals
Maintenance:
Mercaptopurine: Oral: 90 mg/m^2 daily [total dose/cycle = 8.1 g/m^2]
Methotrexate: I.M.: 15 mg/m^2 weekly [total dose/cycle = 60 mg/m^2]
Tretinoin: Oral: 45 mg/m^2/day days 1-15 [total dose/cycle = 675 mg/m^2]
Repeat cycle every 3 months for 2 years

MACOP-B

Use: Lymphoma, non-Hodgkin
Regimen:

Methotrexate: I.V.: 400 mg/m^2 weeks 2, 6, 10 [total dose/cycle = 1200 mg/m^2]
Doxorubicin: I.V.: 50 mg/m^2 weeks 1, 3, 5, 7, 9, 11 [total dose/cycle = 300 mg/m^2]
Cyclophosphamide: I.V.: 350 mg/m^2 weeks 1, 3, 5, 7, 9, 11 [total dose/cycle = 2100 mg/m^2]
Vincristine: I.V.: 1.4 mg/m^2 (maximum 2 mg) weeks 2, 4, 8, 10, 12 [total dose/cycle = 7 mg/m^2]
Bleomycin: I.V.: 10 units/m^2 weeks 4, 8, 12 [total dose/cycle = 30 units/m^2]
Prednisone: Oral: 75 mg/day for 12 weeks, taper over last 2 weeks
Leucovorin calcium: Oral: 15 mg/m^2 every 6 hours for 6 doses (beginning 24 hours after methotrexate) weeks 2, 6, 10 [total dose/cycle = 270 mg/m^2]
Sulfamethoxazole/trimethoprim (800 mg/160 mg): Oral: Tablet twice daily for 12 weeks
Ketoconazole: Oral: 200 mg/day
Administer one cycle

MAID

Use: Soft tissue sarcoma
Regimen:

Mesna: I.V.: 2500 mg/m^2/day continuous infusion days 1-4 [total dose/cycle = 10,000 mg/m^2]
Doxorubicin: I.V.: 20 mg/m^2/day continuous infusion days 1-3 [total dose/cycle = 60 mg/m^2]
Ifosfamide: I.V.: 2500 mg/m^2/day continuous infusion days 1-3 [total dose/cycle = 7500 mg/m^2]
Dacarbazine: I.V.: 300 mg/m^2/day continuous infusion days 1-3 [total dose/cycle = 900 mg/m^2]
Repeat cycle every 21-28 days

m-BACOD

Use: Lymphoma, non-Hodgkin
Regimen:

Methotrexate: I.V.: 200 mg/m^2/day days 8 and 15 [total dose/cycle = 400 mg/m^2]
Leucovorin calcium: Oral: 10 mg/m^2 every 6 hours for 8 doses (beginning 24 hours after each methotrexate dose) days 9 and 16 [total dose/cycle = 160 mg/m^2]
Bleomycin: I.V.: 4 units/m^2 day 1 [total dose/cycle = 4 units/m^2]
Doxorubicin: I.V.: 45 mg/m^2 day 1 [total dose/cycle = 45 mg/m^2]
Cyclophosphamide: I.V.: 600 mg/m^2 day 1 [total dose/cycle = 600 mg/m^2]
Vincristine: I.V.: 1 mg/m^2 day 1 [total dose/cycle = 1 mg/m^2]
Dexamethasone: Oral: 6 mg/m^2/day days 1-5 [total dose/cycle = 30 mg/m^2]
Repeat cycle every 21 days

MINE

Use: Lymphoma, non-Hodgkin
Regimen:

Mesna: I.V.: 1.33 g/m^2/day concurrent with ifosfamide dose, then 500 mg orally (4 hours after each ifosfamide infusion) days 1-3 [total dose/cycle = 3.99 g/m^2/1500 mg]
Ifosfamide: I.V.: 1.33 g/m^2/day days 1-3 [total dose/cycle = 3.99 mg/m^2]
Mitoxantrone: I.V.: 8 mg/m^2 day 1 [total dose/cycle = 8 mg/m^2]
Etoposide: I.V.: 65 mg/m^2/day days 1-3 [total dose/cycle = 195 mg/m^2]
Repeat cycle every 28 days

MINE-ESHAP

Use: Lymphoma, non-Hodgkin
Regimen:

Mesna: I.V.: 1.33 g/m^2 concurrent with ifosfamide dose, then 500 mg orally (4 hours after ifosfamide) days 1-3 [total dose/cycle = 3.99 g/m^2/1500 mg]
Ifosfamide: I.V.: 1.33 g/m^2/day days 1-3 [total dose/cycle = 3.99 mg/m^2]
Mitoxantrone: I.V.: 8 mg/m^2 day 1 [total dose/cycle = 8 mg/m^2]
Etoposide: I.V.: 65 mg/m^2/day days 1-3 [total dose/cycle = 195 mg/m^2]
Repeat cycle every 21 days for 6 cycles, followed by
3-6 cycles of ESHAP

mini-BEAM

Use: Lymphoma, Hodgkin disease
Regimen:

Carmustine: I.V.: 60 mg/m^2 day 1 [total dose/cycle = 60 mg/m^2]
Etoposide: I.V.: 75 mg/m^2/day days 2-5 [total dose/cycle = 300 mg/m^2]
Cytarabine: I.V.: 100 mg/m^2 every 12 hours days 2-5 (8 doses) [total dose/cycle = 800 mg/m^2]
Melphalan: I.V.: 30 mg/m^2 day 6 [total dose/cycle = 30 mg/m^2]
Repeat cycle every 4-6 weeks

Mitoxantrone + Hydrocortisone

Use: Prostate cancer
Regimen:

Mitoxantrone: I.V.: 14 mg/m^2 day 1 [total dose/cycle = 14 mg/m^2]
Hydrocortisone: Oral: 40 mg daily [total dose/cycle = 840 mg]
Repeat cycle every 3 weeks

MM

Use: Leukemia, acute lymphocytic (maintenance)
Regimen:

Mercaptopurine: Oral: 50-75 mg/m^2/day days 1-7 [total dose/cycle = 350-525 mg/m^2]
Methotrexate: Oral, I.V.: 20 mg/m^2 day 1 [total dose/cycle = 20 mg/m^2]
Repeat cycle every 7 days

MOP

Use: Brain tumors
Regimen:

Mechlorethamine: I.V.: 6 mg/m^2/day days 1 and 8 [total dose/cycle = 12 mg/m^2]
Vincristine: I.V.: 1.5 mg/m^2/day (maximum 2 mg) days 1 and 8 [total dose/cycle = 3 mg/m^2]
Procarbazine: Oral: 100 mg/m^2/day days 1-14 [total dose/cycle = 1400 mg/m^2]
Repeat cycle every 28 days

MOPP (Lymphoma, Hodgkin Disease)

Use: Lymphoma, Hodgkin disease
Regimen: Note: Multiple variations are listed below.

Variation 1:
Mechlorethamine: I.V.: 6 mg/m^2/day days 1 and 8 [total dose/cycle = 12 mg/m^2]
Vincristine: I.V.: 1.4 mg/m^2/day days 1 and 8 [total dose/cycle = 2.8 mg/m^2]
Procarbazine: Oral: 100 mg/m^2/day days 1-14 [total dose/cycle = 1400 mg/m^2]
Prednisone: Oral: 40 mg/m^2/day days 1-14 (cycles 1 and 4) [total dose/cycle = 560 mg/m^2]
Repeat cycle every 28 days for 6-8 cycles

Variation 2:
Mechlorethamine: I.V.: 6 mg/m^2/day (maximum 15 mg) days 1 and 8 [total dose/cycle = 12 mg/m^2]
Vincristine: I.V.: 1.4 mg/m^2/day (maximum 2 mg) days 1 and 8 [total dose/cycle = 2.8 mg/m^2]
Procarbazine: Oral: 100 mg/m^2/day days 1-10 [total dose/cycle = 1000 mg/m^2]
Prednisone: Oral: 25 mg/m^2/day (maximum 60 mg) days 1-14 [total dose/cycle = 350 mg/m^2] **or**
Prednisolone: Oral: 25 mg/m^2/day (maximum 60 mg) days 1-14 [total dose/cycle = 350 mg/m^2]
Repeat cycle every 28 days

Variation 3:

Mechlorethamine: I.V.: 6 mg/m^2/day days 1 and 8 [total dose/cycle = 12 mg/m^2]
Vincristine: I.V.: 1.4 mg/m^2/day days 1 and 8 [total dose/cycle = 2.8 mg/m^2]
Procarbazine: Oral: 50 mg day 1, 100 mg day 2, 100 mg/m^2/day days 3-14 [total dose/cycle = 150 mg / 1200 mg/m^2]
Prednisone: Oral: 40 mg/m^2/day days 1-14 [total dose/cycle = 560 mg/m^2]
Repeat cycle every 28 days

Variation 4:

Mechlorethamine: I.V.: 6 mg/m^2/day days 1 and 8 [total dose/cycle = 12 mg/m^2]
Vincristine: I.V.: 1.4 mg/m^2/day days 1 and 8 [total dose/cycle = 2.8 mg/m^2]
Procarbazine: Oral: 50 mg day 1, 100 mg day 2, 100 mg/m^2/day days 3-10 [total dose/cycle = 150 mg / 800 mg/m^2]
Prednisone: Oral: 40 mg/m^2/day days 1-14 [total dose/cycle = 560 mg/m^2]
Repeat cycle every 28 days

Variation 5:

Mechlorethamine: I.V.: 6 mg/m^2/day days 1 and 8 [total dose/cycle = 12 mg/m^2]
Vincristine: I.V.: 1.4 mg/m^2/day days 1 and 8 [total dose/cycle = 2.8 mg/m^2]
Procarbazine: Oral: 50 mg/m^2 day 1, then 100 mg/m^2/day days 2-14 [total dose/cycle = 1350 mg/m^2]
Prednisone: Oral: 40 mg/m^2/day days 1-14 [total dose/cycle = 560 mg/m^2]
Repeat cycle every 28 days

MOPP (Medulloblastoma)

Use: Brain tumors

Regimen:

Mechlorethamine: I.V.: 3 mg/m^2/day days 1 and 8 [total dose/cycle = 6 mg/m^2]
Vincristine: I.V.: 1.4 mg/m^2/day (maximum 2 mg) days 1 and 8 [total dose/cycle = 2.8 mg/m^2]
Prednisone: Oral: 40 mg/m^2/day days 1-10 [total dose/cycle = 400 mg/m^2]
Procarbazine: Oral: 50 mg day 1 [total dose = 50 mg] **followed by**
100 mg day 2 [total dose = 100 mg] **followed by**
100 mg/m^2/day days 3-10 [total dose = 800 mg/m^2]
Repeat cycle every 28 days

MOPP/ABV Hybrid

Use: Lymphoma, Hodgkin disease

Regimen:

Mechlorethamine: I.V.: 6 mg/m^2 day 1 [total dose/cycle = 6 mg/m^2]
Vincristine: I.V.: 1.4 mg/m^2 (maximum 2 mg) day 1 [total dose/cycle = 1.4 mg/m^2]
Procarbazine: Oral: 100 mg/m^2/day days 1-7 [total dose/cycle = 700 mg/m^2]
Prednisone: Oral: 40 mg/m^2/day days 1-14 [total dose/cycle = 560 mg/m^2]
Doxorubicin: I.V.: 35 mg/m^2 day 8 [total dose/cycle = 35 mg/m^2]
Bleomycin: I.V.: 10 units/m^2 day 8 [total dose/cycle = 10 units/m^2]
Vinblastine: I.V.: 6 mg/m^2 day 8 [total dose/cycle = 6 mg/m^2]
Repeat cycle every 28 days

MOPP/ABVD

Use: Lymphoma, Hodgkin disease

Regimen: Note: Multiple variations are listed below.

Variation 1:

Mechlorethamine: I.V.: 6 mg/m^2/day days 1 and 8 [total dose/cycle = 12 mg/m^2]
Vincristine: I.V.: 1.4 mg/m^2/day (maximum 2 mg) days 1 and 8 [total dose/cycle = 2.8 mg/m^2]
Procarbazine: I.V.: 100 mg/m^2/day days 1-14 [total dose/cycle = 1400 mg/m^2]
Prednisone: Oral: 40 mg/m^2/day days 1-14 (during cycles 1, 4, 7, and 10 only) [total dose/cycle = 560 mg/m^2]
Doxorubicin: Oral: 25 mg/m^2/day days 29 and 43 [total dose/cycle = 50 mg/m^2]
Bleomycin: I.V.: 10 units/m^2/day day 29 and 43 [total dose/cycle = 20 units/m^2]
Vinblastine: I.V.: 6 mg/m^2/day days 29 and 43 [total dose/cycle = 12 mg/m^2]
Dacarbazine: I.V.: 375 mg/m^2/day days 29 and 43 [total dose/cycle = 750 mg/m^2]
Repeat cycle every 56 days

MOPP/ABVD *(continued)*

Variation 2:
Mechlorethamine: I.V.: 6 mg/m^2/day days 1 and 8 [total dose/cycle = 12 mg/m^2]
Vincristine: I.V.: 1.4 mg/m^2/day (maximum 2 mg) days 1 and 8 [total dose/cycle = 2.8 mg/m^2]
Procarbazine: I.V.: 100 mg/m^2/day days 1-14 [total dose/cycle = 1400 mg/m^2]
Prednisone: Oral: 40 mg/m^2/day days 1-14 (during cycles 1 and 7 only)
[total dose/cycle = 560 mg/m^2]
Doxorubicin: Oral: 25 mg/m^2/day days 29 and 43 [total dose/cycle = 50 mg/m^2]
Bleomycin: I.V.: 10 units/m^2/day days 29 and 43 [total dose/cycle = 20 units/m^2]
Vinblastine: I.V.: 6 mg/m^2/day days 29 and 43 [total dose/cycle = 12 mg/m^2]
Dacarbazine: I.V.: 375 mg/m^2/day days 29 and 43 [total dose/cycle = 750 mg/m^2]
Repeat cycle every 56 days

Variation 3:
Mechlorethamine: I.V.: 6 mg/m^2/day days 1 and 8 [total dose/cycle = 12 mg/m^2]
Vincristine: I.V.: 1.4 mg/m^2/day (maximum 2 mg) days 1 and 8 [total dose/cycle = 2.8 mg/m^2]
Procarbazine: I.V.: 100 mg/m^2/day days 1-14 [total dose/cycle = 1400 mg/m^2]
Prednisone: Oral: 40 mg/m^2/day days 1-14 (every cycle) [total dose/cycle = 560 mg/m^2]
Doxorubicin: Oral: 25 mg/m^2/day days 29 and 43 [total dose/cycle = 50 mg/m^2]
Bleomycin: I.V.: 10 units/m^2/day days 29 and 43 [total dose/cycle = 20 units/m^2]
Vinblastine: I.V.: 6 mg/m^2/day days 29 and 43 [total dose/cycle = 12 mg/m^2]
Dacarbazine: I.V.: 375 mg/m^2/day days 29 and 43 [total dose/cycle = 750 mg/m^2]
Repeat cycle every 56 days

Variation 4:
MOPP Regimen:
Mechlorethamine: I.V.: 6 mg/m^2/day days 1 and 8 [total dose/cycle = 12 mg/m^2]
Vincristine: I.V.: 1.4 mg/m^2/day (maximum 2 mg) days 1 and 8 [total dose/cycle = 2.8 mg/m^2]
Procarbazine: I.V.: 100 mg/m^2/day days 1-14 [total dose/cycle = 1400 mg/m^2]
Prednisone: Oral: 25 mg/m^2/day days 1-14 [total dose/cycle = 350 mg/m^2]

ABVD Regimen:
Doxorubicin: Oral: 25 mg/m^2/day days 1 and 15 [total dose/cycle = 50 mg/m^2]
Bleomycin: I.V.: 6 units/m^2/day days 1 and 15 [total dose/cycle = 12 units/m^2]
Vinblastine: I.V.: 6 mg/m^2/day days 1 and 15 [total dose/cycle = 12 mg/m^2]
Dacarbazine: I.V.: 250 mg/m^2/day days 1 and 15 [total dose/cycle = 500 mg/m^2]
Each regimen cycle is 28 days. Administer regimens in alternating fashion as follows: 2 cycles of MOPP alternating with 2 cycles of ABVD for a total of 8 cycles

Variation 5 (pediatrics):
Mechlorethamine: I.V.: 6 mg/m^2/day days 1 and 8 [total dose/cycle = 12 mg/m^2]
Vincristine: I.V.: 1.4 mg/m^2/day days 1 and 8 [total dose/cycle = 2.8 mg/m^2]
Procarbazine: Oral: 100 mg/m^2/day days 1-14 [total dose/cycle = 1400 mg/m^2]
Prednisone: Oral: 40 mg/m^2/day days 1-14 [total dose/cycle = 560 mg/m^2]
Doxorubicin: Oral: 25 mg/m^2/day days 29 and 42 [total dose/cycle = 50 mg/m^2]
Bleomycin: I.V.: 10 units/m^2/day days 29 and 42 [total dose/cycle = 20 units/m^2]
Vinblastine: I.V.: 6 mg/m^2/day days 29 and 42 [total dose/cycle = 12 mg/m^2]
Dacarbazine: I.V.: 150 mg/m^2/day days 29-33 [total dose/cycle = 750 mg/m^2]
Repeat cycle evey 56 days for 4 cycles

Variation 6 (pediatrics):
Mechlorethamine: I.V.: 6 mg/m^2/day days 1 and 8 [total dose/cycle = 12 mg/m^2]
Vincristine: I.V.: 1.4 mg/m^2/day days 1 and 8 [total dose/cycle = 2.8 mg/m^2]
Procarbazine: Oral: 100 mg/m^2/day days 1-14 [total dose/cycle = 1400 mg/m^2]
Prednisone: Oral: 40 mg/m^2/day days 1-14 [total dose/cycle = 560 mg/m^2]
Doxorubicin: Oral: 25 mg/m^2/day days 29 and 42 [total dose/cycle = 50 mg/m^2]
Bleomycin: I.V.: 10 units/m^2/day days 29 and 42 [total dose/cycle = 20 units/m^2]
Vinblastine: I.V.: 6 mg/m^2/day days 29 and 42 [total dose/cycle = 12 mg/m^2]
Dacarbazine: I.V.: 375 mg/m^2/day days 29 and 43 [total dose/cycle = 750 mg/m^2]
Repeat cycle evey 56 days for 4 cycles

MP (Multiple Myeloma)

Use: Multiple myeloma

Regimen:

Melphalan: Oral: 8-10 mg/m^2/day days 1-4 [total dose/cycle = 32-40 mg/m^2]
Prednisone: Oral: 40-60 mg/m^2/day days 1-4 [total dose/cycle = 160-240 mg/m^2]
Repeat cycle every 28-42 days

MP (Prostate Cancer)

Use: Prostate cancer

Regimen:

Mitoxantrone: I.V.: 12 mg/m^2 day 1 [total dose/cycle = 12 mg/m^2]
Prednisone: Oral: 5 mg twice daily [total dose/cycle = 210 mg]
Repeat cycle every 21 days

MTX/6-MP/VP (Maintenance)

Use: Leukemia, acute lymphocytic

Regimen:

Methotrexate: Oral: 20 mg/m^2 weekly [total dose/cycle = 80 mg/m^2]
Mercaptopurine: Oral: 75 mg/m^2/day [total dose/cycle = 2250 mg/m^2]
Vincristine: I.V.: 1.5 mg/m^2 day 1 [total dose/cycle = 1.5 mg/m^2]
Prednisone: Oral: 40 mg/m^2/day days 1-5 [total dose/cycle = 200 mg/m^2]
Repeat monthly for 2-3 years

MTX-CDDPAdr

Use: Osteosarcoma

Regimen:

Cisplatin: I.V.: 75 mg/m^2 day 1 of cycles 1-7 [total dose/cycle = 75 mg/m^2]
then 120 mg/m^2 day 1 cycles 8-10 [total dose/cycle = 120 mg/m^2]
Doxorubicin: I.V.: 25 mg/m^2/day days 1-3 of cycles 1-7 [total dose/cycle = 75 mg/m^2]
Methotrexate: I.V.: 12 g/m^2/day days 21 and 28 [total dose/cycle = 24 g/m^2]
Leucovorin calcium rescue: I.V.: 20 mg/m^2 every 3 hours (beginning 16 hours after completion of methotrexate) for 8 doses, then orally every 6 hours for 8 doses [total dose/cycle = 640 mg/m^2]

MV

Use: Leukemia, acute myeloid

Regimen:

Mitoxantrone: I.V.: 10 mg/m^2/day days 1-5 [total dose/cycle = 50 mg/m^2]
Etoposide: I.V.: 100 mg/m^2/day days 1-5 [total dose/cycle = 500 mg/m^2]
Second cycle may be given based on individual respone; time between cycles not specified

M-VAC (Bladder Cancer)

Use: Bladder cancer

Regimen: Note: Multiple variations are listed below.

Variation 1:
Methotrexate: I.V.: 30 mg/m^2/day days 1, 15, 22 [total dose/cycle = 90 mg/m^2]
Vinblastine: I.V.: 3 mg/m^2/day days 2, 15, 22 [total dose/cycle = 9 mg/m^2]
Doxorubicin: I.V.: 30 mg/m^2 day 2 [total dose/cycle = 30 mg/m^2]
Cisplatin: I.V.: 70 mg/m^2 day 2 [total dose/cycle = 70 mg/m^2]
Repeat cycle every 4 weeks

Variation 2:
Methotrexate: I.V.: 40 or 50 mg/m^2/day days 1, 15, and 22 [total dose/cycle = 120 or 150 mg/m^2]
Vinblastine: I.V.: 4 or 5 mg/m^2/day days 2, 15, and 22 [total dose/cycle = 12 or 15 mg/m^2]
Doxorubicin: I.V.: 40 or 50 mg/m^2 day 2 [total dose/cycle = 40 or 50 mg/m^2]
Cisplatin: I.V.: 100 mg/m^2 day 2 [total dose/cycle = 100 mg/m^2]
Repeat cycle every 4 weeks

Variation 3:
Methotrexate: I.V.: 30 mg/m^2/day days 1, 15, and 22 [total dose/cycle = 90 mg/m^2]
Vinblastine: I.V.: 3 mg/m^2 day 2 [total dose/cycle = 3 mg/m^2]
Doxorubicin: I.V.: 30 mg/m^2 day 2 [total dose/cycle = 30 mg/m^2]
Cisplatin: I.V.: 70 mg/m^2 day 2 [total dose/cycle = 70 mg/m^2]
Repeat cycle every 4 weeks

M-VAC (Bladder Cancer) *(continued)*

Variation 4:
Methotrexate: I.V.: 60 mg/m^2 day 1 [total dose/cycle = 60 mg/m^2]
followed by 30 mg/m^2 day 16 [total dose/cycle = 30 mg/m^2]
Vinblastine: I.V.: 4 mg/m^2/day days 2 and 16 [total dose/cycle = 8 mg/m^2]
Doxorubicin: I.V.: 60 mg/m^2 day 2 [total dose/cycle = 60 mg/m^2]
Cisplatin: I.V.: 100 mg/m^2 day 2 [total dose/cycle = 100 mg/m^2]
Repeat cycle every 23 days
Variation 5:
Methotrexate: I.V.: 30 mg/m^2/day days 1, 16, and 23 [total dose/cycle = 90 mg/m^2]
Vinblastine: I.V.: 4 mg/m^2/day days 1, 16, and 23 [total dose/cycle = 12 mg/m^2]
Doxorubicin: I.V.: 60 mg/m^2 day 2 [total dose/cycle = 60 mg/m^2]
Cisplatin: I.V.: 100 mg/m^2 day 2 [total dose/cycle = 100 mg/m^2]
Repeat cycle every 23 days
Variation 6:
Methotrexate: I.V.: 30 or 35 mg/m^2 day 1 [total dose/cycle = 30 or 35 mg/m^2]
Vinblastine: I.V.: 3 or 3.5 mg/m^2 day 2 [total dose/cycle = 3 or 3.5 mg/m^2]
Doxorubicin: I.V.: 30 or 35 mg/m^2 day 2 [total dose/cycle = 30 or 35 mg/m^2]
Cisplatin: I.V.: 70 or 80 mg/m^2 day 2 [total dose/cycle = 70 or 80 mg/m^2]
Repeat cycle every 2 weeks
Variation 7:
Methotrexate: I.V.: 30 mg/m^2 day 1 [total dose/cycle = 30 mg/m^2]
Vinblastine: I.V.: 3 mg/m^2 day 2 [total dose/cycle = 3 mg/m^2]
Doxorubicin: I.V.: 30 mg/m^2 day 2 [total dose/cycle = 30 mg/m^2]
Cisplatin: I.V.: 70 mg/m^2 day 2 [total dose/cycle = 70 mg/m^2]
Repeat cycle every 14 days
Variation 8:
Methotrexate: I.V.: 30 mg/m^2/day days 1, 15, and 22 [total dose/cycle = 90 mg/m^2]
Vinblastine: I.V.: 3 mg/m^2/day days 1, 15, and 22 [total dose/cycle = 9 mg/m^2]
Doxorubicin: I.V.: 45 mg/m^2 day 2 [total dose/cycle = 45 mg/m^2]
Cisplatin: I.V.: 70 mg/m^2 day 2 [total dose/cycle = 70 mg/m^2]
Repeat cycle every 4 weeks
Variation 9:
Methotrexate: I.V.: 40 mg/m^2/day days 1 and 15 [total dose/cycle = 80 mg/m^2]
Vinblastine: I.V.: 4 mg/m^2/day days 1, 16, and 23 [total dose/cycle = 12 mg/m^2]
Doxorubicin: I.V.: 60 mg/m^2 day 2 [total dose/cycle = 60 mg/m^2]
Cisplatin: I.V.: 100 mg/m^2 day 2 [total dose/cycle = 100 mg/m^2]
Repeat cycle every 23 days
Variation 10:
Methotrexate: I.V.: 30 mg/m^2/day days 1, 15, and 22 [total dose/cycle = 90 mg/m^2]
Vinblastine: I.V.: 3 mg/m^2/day days 1, 16, and 22 [total dose/cycle = 9 mg/m^2]
Doxorubicin: I.V.: 30 mg/m^2 day 1 [total dose/cycle = 30 mg/m^2]
Cisplatin: I.V.: 70 mg/m^2 day 1 [total dose/cycle = 70 mg/m^2]
Repeat cycle every 4 weeks
Variation 11:
Methotrexate: I.V.: 30 mg/m^2/day days 1, 15, and 22 [total dose/cycle = 90 mg/m^2]
Vinblastine: I.V.: 3 mg/m^2/day days 2, 15, and 22 [total dose/cycle = 9 mg/m^2]
Doxorubicin: I.V.: 30 mg/m^2 day 2 [total dose/cycle = 30 mg/m^2]
Cisplatin: I.V.: 70 mg/m^2 day 2 [total dose/cycle = 70 mg/m^2]
Leucovorin: Oral: 15 mg every 6 hours for 4 doses, days 2, 16, and 23
[total dose/cycle = 180 mg]
Repeat cycle every 4 weeks
Variation 12:
Methotrexate: I.V.: 30 mg/m^2/day days 1 and 15 [total dose/cycle = 60 mg/m^2]
Vinblastine: I.V.: 3 mg/m^2/day days 2 and 15 [total dose/cycle = 6 mg/m^2]
Doxorubicin: I.V.: 30 or 40 mg/m^2 day 3 [total dose/cycle = 30 or 40 mg/m^2]
Cisplatin: I.V.: 70 mg/m^2 day 2 [total dose/cycle = 70 mg/m^2]
Repeat cycle every 4 weeks
Variation 13:
Methotrexate: I.V.: 30 mg/m^2/day days 1 and 15 [total dose/cycle = 60 mg/m^2]
Vinblastine: I.V.: 3 mg/m^2/day days 2 and 15 [total dose/cycle = 6 mg/m^2]
Doxorubicin: I.V.: 30 or 40 mg/m^2 day 2 [total dose/cycle = 30 or 40 mg/m^2]
Cisplatin: I.V.: 70 mg/m^2 day 2 [total dose/cycle = 70 mg/m^2]
Repeat cycle every 4 weeks

M-VAC (Breast Cancer)

Use: Breast cancer

Regimen:

Methotrexate: I.V.: 30 mg/m^2/day days 1, 15, and 22 [total dose/cycle = 90 mg/m^2]
Vinblastine: I.V.: 3 mg/m^2/day days 2, 15, and 22 [total dose/cycle = 9 mg/m^2]
Doxorubicin: I.V.: 30 mg/m^2 day 2 [total dose/cycle = 30 mg/m^2]
Cisplatin: I.V.: 70 mg/m^2 day 2 [total dose/cycle = 70 mg/m^2]
Leucovorin: Oral: 10 mg every 6 hours for 6 doses days 2, 16, and 23 [total dose/cycle = 180 mg]
Repeat cycle every 4 weeks

M-VAC (Cervical Cancer)

Use: Cervical cancer

Regimen:

Methotrexate: I.V.: 30 mg/m^2/day days 1, 15, and 22 [total dose/cycle = 90 mg/m^2]
Vinblastine: I.V.: 3 mg/m^2/day days 2, 15, and 22 [total dose/cycle = 9 mg/m^2]
Doxorubicin: I.V.: 30 mg/m^2 day 2 [total dose/cycle = 30 mg/m^2]
Cisplatin: I.V.: 70 mg/m^2 day 2 [total dose/cycle = 70 mg/m^2]
Repeat cycle every 4 weeks

M-VAC (Endometrial Cancer)

Use: Endometrial cancer

Regimen:

Methotrexate: I.V.: 30 mg/m^2/day days 1, 15, and 22 [total dose/cycle = 90 mg/m^2]
Vinblastine: I.V.: 3 mg/m^2/day days 2, 15, and 22 [total dose/cycle = 9 mg/m^2]
Doxorubicin: I.V.: 30 mg/m^2/day day 2 [total dose/cycle = 30 mg/m^2]
Cisplatin: I.V.: 70 mg/m^2/day day 2 [total dose/cycle = 70 mg/m^2]
Repeat cycle every 4 weeks

M-VAC (Head and Neck Cancer)

Use: Head and neck cancer

Regimen:

Methotrexate: I.V.: 30 mg/m^2/day days 1, 15, and 22 [total dose/cycle = 90 mg/m^2]
Vinblastine: I.V.: 3 mg/m^2/day days 2, 15, and 22 [total dose/cycle = 9 mg/m^2]
Doxorubicin: I.V.: 30 mg/m^2 day 2 [total dose/cycle = 30 mg/m^2]
Cisplatin: I.V.: 70 mg/m^2 day 2 [total dose/cycle = 70 mg/m^2]
Repeat cycle every 4 weeks

MVPP

Use: Lymphoma, Hodgkin disease

Regimen:

Mechlorethamine: I.V.: 6 mg/m^2/day days 1 and 8 [total dose/cycle = 12 mg/m^2]
Vinblastine: I.V.: 4 mg/m^2/day days 1 and 8 [total dose/cycle = 8 mg/m^2]
Procarbazine: Oral: 100 mg/m^2/day days 1-14 [total dose/cycle = 1400 mg/m^2]
Prednisone: Oral: 40 mg/m^2/day days 1-14 [total dose/cycle = 560 mg/m^2]
Repeat cycle every 4-6 weeks

N4SE Protocol

Use: Neuroblastomas

Regimen:

Vincristine: I.V.: 0.05 mg/kg/day days 1 and 2 [total dose/cycle = 0.1 mg/kg]
Doxorubicin: I.V.: 15 mg/m^2/day days 1 and 2 [total dose/cycle = 30 mg/m^2]
Cyclophosphamide: I.V.: 30 mg/kg/day days 1 and 2 [total dose/cycle = 60 mg/kg]
Fluorouracil: I.V.: 1 mg/kg/day days 3, 8, and 9 [total dose/cycle = 3 mg/kg]
Cytarabine: I.V.: 3 mg/kg/day days 3, 8, and 9 [total dose/cycle = 9 mg/kg]
Hydroxyurea: Oral: 40 mg/kg/day days 3, 8, and 9 [total dose/cycle = 120 mg/kg]
Repeat cycle every 21-28 days

N6 Protocol

Use: Neuroblastomas

Regimen:

Course 1, 2, 4, 6

Cyclophosphamide: I.V.: 70 mg/kg/day days 1 and 2 [total dose/cycle = 140 mg/kg]

Doxorubicin: I.V.: 25 mg/m^2/day continuous infusion days 1-3 [total dose/cycle = 75 mg/m^2]

Vincristine: I.V.: 0.033 mg/kg/day continuous infusion days 1-3 [total dose/cycle = 0.099 mg/kg]

Vincristine: I.V.: 1.5 mg/m^2 day 9 [total dose/cycle = 1.5 mg/m^2]

Course 3, 5, 7

Etoposide: I.V.: 200 mg/m^2/day days 1-3 [total dose/cycle = 600 mg/m^2]

Cisplatin: I.V.: 50 mg/m^2/day days 1-4 [total dose/cycle = 200 mg/m^2]

NFL

Use: Breast cancer

Regimen: Note: Multiple variations are listed below.

Variation 1:

Mitoxantrone: I.V.: 12 mg/m^2 day 1 [total dose/cycle = 12 mg/m^2]

Fluorouracil: I.V.: 350 mg/m^2/day days 1-3 [total dose/cycle = 1050 mg/m^2]

Leucovorin: I.V.: 300 mg/m^2/day days 1-3 [total dose/cycle = 900 mg/m^2]

Repeat cycle every 21 days

Variation 2:

Mitoxantrone: I.V.: 10 mg/m^2 day 1 [total dose/cycle = 10 mg/m^2]

Fluorouracil: I.V.: 1000 mg/m^2/day continuous infusion days 1-3 [total dose/cycle = 3000 mg/m^2]

Leucovorin: I.V.: 100 mg/m^2/day days 1-3 [total dose/cycle = 300 mg/m^2]

Repeat cycle every 21 days

OPA

Use: Lymphoma, Hodgkin disease

Regimen:

Vincristine: I.V.: 1.5 mg/m^2/day (maximum 2 mg) days 1, 8, and 15 [total dose/cycle = 4.5 mg/m^2]

Prednisone: Oral: 60 mg/m^2/day days 1-15 in 3 divided doses [total dose/cycle = 900 mg/m^2]

Doxorubicin: I.V.: 40 mg/m^2/day days 1 and 15 [total dose/cycle = 80 mg/m^2]

Second cycle may be given based on individual response; time between cycles not specified

OPEC

Use: Neuroblastomas

Regimen:

Vincristine: I.V.: 1.5 mg/m^2 day 1 [total dose/cycle = 1.5 mg/m^2]

Cyclophosphamide: I.V.: 600 mg/m^2 day 1 [total dose/cycle = 600 mg/m^2]

Cisplatin: I.V.: 100 mg/m^2 day 2 [total dose/cycle = 100 mg/m^2]

Teniposide: I.V.: 150 mg/m^2 day 4 [total dose/cycle = 150 mg/m^2]

Repeat cycle every 21 days

OPEC-D

Use: Neuroblastomas

Regimen:

Vincristine: I.V.: 1.5 mg/m^2 day 1 [total dose/cycle = 1.5 mg/m^2]

Cyclophosphamide: I.V.: 600 mg/m^2 day 1 [total dose/cycle = 600 mg/m^2]

Doxorubicin: I.V.: 40 mg/m^2 day 1 [total dose/cycle = 40 mg/m^2]

Cisplatin: I.V.: 100 mg/m^2 day 2 [total dose/cycle = 100 mg/m^2]

Teniposide: I.V.: 150 mg/m^2 day 4 [total dose/cycle = 150 mg/m^2]

Repeat cycle every 21 days

OPPA

Use: Lymphoma, Hodgkin disease

Regimen:

Vincristine: I.V.: 1.5 mg/m^2/day (maximum 2 mg) days 1, 8, and 15 [total dose/cycle = 4.5 mg/m^2]

Prednisone: Oral: 60 mg/m^2/day days 1-15 in 3 divided doses [total dose/cycle = 900 mg/m^2]

Doxorubicin: I.V.: 40 mg/m^2/day days 1 and 15 [total dose/cycle = 80 mg/m^2]

Procarbazine: Oral: 100 mg/m^2/day days 1-15 in 2 or 3 divided doses [total dose/cycle = 1500 mg/m^2]

Second cycle may be given based on individual response; time between cycles not specified

PAC (CAP)

Use: Ovarian cancer

Regimen:

Cisplatin: I.V.: 50 mg/m^2 day 1 [total dose/cycle = 50 mg/m^2]

Doxorubicin: I.V.: 50 mg/m^2 day 1 [total dose/cycle = 50 mg/m^2]

Cyclophosphamide: I.V.: 1000 mg/m^2 day 1 [total dose/cycle = 1000 mg/m^2]

Repeat cycle every 21 days for 8 cycles

PA-CI

Use: Hepatoblastoma

Regimen: Note: Multiple variations are listed below.

Variation 1:

Cisplatin: I.V.: 90 mg/m^2 day 1 [total dose/cycle = 90 mg/m^2]

Doxorubicin: I.V.: 20 mg/m^2/day continuous infusion days 2-5 [total dose/cycle = 80 mg/m^2]

Repeat cycle every 21 days

Variation 2:

Cisplatin: I.V.: 20 mg/m^2/day days 1-4 [total dose/cycle = 80 mg/m^2]

Doxorubicin: I.V.: 100 mg/m^2 continuous infusion day 1 [total dose/cycle = 100 mg/m^2]

Repeat cycle every 21-28 days

Paclitaxel, Carboplatin, Etoposide

Use: Adenocarcinoma, unknown primary

Regimen:

Paclitaxel: I.V.: 200 mg/m^2 infused over 1 hour day 1 [total dose/cycle = 200 mg/m^2] **followed by:**

Carboplatin: I.V.: Target AUC 6 [total dose/cycle = AUC = 6]

Etoposide: Oral: 50 mg/day, alternate with 100 mg/day, days 1-10 [total dose/cycle = 750 mg/day]

Repeat cycle every 21 days

Paclitaxel + Estramustine + Carboplatin

Use: Prostate cancer

Regimen:

Paclitaxel: I.V.: 100 mg/m^2 day 3 each week [total dose/cycle = 400 mg/m^2]

Estramustine: Oral: 10 mg/kg/day days 1-5 each week [total dose/cycle = 200 mg/kg]

Carboplatin: I.V.: Target AUC 6 day 3 [total dose/cycle = AUC = 6]

Repeat cycle every 28 days

Paclitaxel + Estramustine + Etoposide

Use: Prostate cancer

Regimen:

Paclitaxel: I.V.: 135 mg/m^2 day 2 [total dose/cycle = 135 mg/m^2]

Estramustine: Oral: 280 mg 3 times/day days 1-14 [total dose/cycle = 11,760 mg]

Etoposide: Oral: 100 mg/day days 1-14 [total dose/cycle = 1400 mg]

Repeat cycle every 21 days

Paclitaxel-Vinorelbine

Use: Breast cancer
Regimen:
Paclitaxel: I.V.: 135 mg/m^2 day 1 [total dose/cycle = 135 mg/m^2]
Vinorelbine: I.V.: 30 mg/m^2/day days 1 and 8 [total dose/cycle = 60 mg/m^2]
Repeat cycle every 28 days

PC (Bladder Cancer)

Use: Bladder cancer
Regimen:
Paclitaxel: I.V.: 200 mg/m^2 or 225 mg/m^2 day 1 [total dose/cycle = 200 or 225 mg/m^2]
Carboplatin: I.V.: AUC 5-6 day 1 [total dose/cycle = AUC = 5-6]
Repeat cycle every 21 days

PC (Nonsmall-Cell Lung Cancer)

Use: Lung cancer, nonsmall-cell
Regimen: Note: Multiple variations are listed below.
Variation 1:
Paclitaxel: I.V.: 175-225 mg/m^2 day 1 [total dose/cycle = 175-225 mg/m^2]
Carboplatin: I.V.: Target AUC 5-7 day 1 [total dose/cycle = AUC = 5-7]
Repeat cycle every 21 days for 2-8 cycles
Variation 2:
Paclitaxel: I.V.: 175 mg/m^2 day 1 [total dose/cycle = 175 mg/m^2]
Cisplatin: I.V.: 80 mg/m^2 day 1 [total dose/cycle = 80 mg/m^2]
Repeat cycle every 21 days
Variation 3:
Paclitaxel: I.V.: 135 mg/m^2 continuous infusion day 1 [total dose/cycle = 135 mg/m^2]
Carboplatin: I.V.: AUC 7.5 day 2 [total dose/cycle = AUC = 7.5]
Repeat cycle every 21 days
Variation 4:
Paclitaxel: I.V.: 135 mg/m^2 continuous infusion day 1 [total dose/cycle = 135 mg/m^2]
Cisplatin: I.V.: 75 mg/m^2 day 2 [total dose/cycle = 75 mg/m^2]
Repeat cycle every 21 days

PCV

Use: Brain tumors
Regimen:
Lomustine: Oral: 110 mg/m^2 day 1 [total dose/cycle = 110 mg/m^2]
Procarbazine: Oral: 60 mg/m^2/day days 8-21 [total dose/cycle = 840 mg/m^2]
Vincristine: I.V.: 1.4 mg/m^2/day (maximum 2 mg) days 8 and 29 [total dose/cycle = 2.8 mg/m^2]
Repeat cycle every 6-8 weeks

PE

Use: Prostate cancer
Regimen: Note: Multiple variations are listed below.
Variation 1:
Paclitaxel: I.V.: 30-35 mg/m^2/day continuous infusion (given in 2-3 divided doses daily) days 2-5 [total dose/cycle = 120-140 mg/m^2]
Estramustine: Oral: 600 mg/m^2/day days 1-21 [total dose/cycle = 12,600 mg/m^2]
Repeat cycle every 21 days
Variation 2:
Paclitaxel: I.V. 60-107 mg/m^2 infused over 3 hours weekly [total dose/cycle = 180-321 mg/m^2]
Estramustine: Oral: 280 mg twice daily 3 days/week [total dose/cycle = 5040 mg]
Variation 3:
Paclitaxel: I.V. 150 mg/m^2 weekly [total dose/cycle = 450 mg/m^2]
Estramustine: Oral: 280 mg 3 times/day 3 days/week [total dose/week = 7560 mg/m^2]
Variation 4:
Paclitaxel: I.V.: 100 mg/m^2/day days 1, 8, and 15 [total dose/cycle = 300 mg/m^2]
Estramustine: Oral: 280 mg 3 times/day days 1, 2, and 3 every week [total dose/cycle = 10,080 mg]
Repeat cycle every 4 weeks

PE-CAdO

Use: Neuroblastomas

Regimen:

Cisplatin: I.V.: 100 mg/m^2 day 1 [total dose/cycle = 100 mg/m^2]
Teniposide: I.V.: 160 mg/m^2 day 3 [total dose/cycle = 160 mg/m^2]
alternating with
Cyclophosphamide: I.V.: 300 mg/m^2/day days 1-5 [total dose/cycle = 1500 mg/m^2]
Doxorubicin: I.V.: 60 mg/m^2 day 5 [total dose/cycle = 60 mg/m^2]
Vincristine: I.V.: 1.5 mg/m^2/day days 1 and 5 [total dose/cycle = 3 mg/m^2]
Repeat cycle every 21 days

PFL (Colorectal Cancer)

Use: Colorectal cancer

Regimen:

Cisplatin: I.V.: 25 mg/m^2/day continuous infusion days 1-5 [total dose/cycle = 125 mg/m^2]
Fluorouracil: I.V.: 800 mg/m^2/day continuous infusion days 2-5 [total dose/cycle = 3200 mg/m^2]
Leucovorin calcium: I.V.: 500 mg/m^2/day continuous infusion days 1-5 [total dose/cycle = 2500 mg/m^2]
Repeat cycle every 28 days

PFL (Head and Neck Cancer)

Use: Head and neck cancer

Regimen: Note: Multiple variations are listed below.

Variation 1:
Cisplatin: I.V.: 25 mg/m^2/day continuous infusion days 1-5 [total dose/cycle = 125 mg/m^2]
Fluorouracil: I.V.: 800 mg/m^2/day continuous infusion days 2-6 [total dose/cycle = 4000 mg/m^2]
Leucovorin: I.V.: 500 mg/m^2/day continuous infusion days 1-6 [total dose/cycle = 3000 mg/m^2]
Repeat cycle every 28 days

Variation 2:
Cisplatin: I.V.: 100 mg/m^2 day 1 [total dose/cycle = 100 mg/m^2]
Fluorouracil: I.V.: 600-1000 mg/m^2/day continuous infusion days 1-5 [total dose/cycle = 3000-5000 mg/m^2]
Leucovorin: Oral: 50 mg/m^2 every 4-6 hours days 1-6 [total dose/cycle = 1200-1800 mg/m^2]
Repeat cycle every 21 days

PFL + IFN

Use: Head and neck cancer

Regimen:

Cisplatin: I.V.: 100 mg/m^2 day 1 [total dose/cycle = 100 mg/m^2]
Fluorouracil: I.V.: 640 mg/m^2/day continuous infusion days 1-5 [total dose/cycle = 3200 mg/m^2]
Leucovorin calcium: Oral: 100 mg every 4 hours days 1-5 [total dose/cycle = 3000 mg/m^2]
Interferon alfa-2b: SubQ: 2 x 10^6 units/m^2 days 1-6 [total dose/cycle = 12 x 10^6 units/m^2]

POC

Use: Brain tumors

Regimen:

Prednisone: Oral: 40 mg/m^2/day days 1-14 [total dose/cycle = 560 mg/m^2]
Vincristine: I.V.: 1.5 mg/m^2/day (maximum 2 mg) days 1, 8, and 15 [total dose/cycle = 4.5 mg/m^2]
Lomustine: Oral: 100 mg/m^2 day 1 [total dose/cycle = 100 mg/m^2]
Repeat cycle every 6 weeks

POG-8651

Use: Osteosarcoma

Regimen:

(Surgery at week 10)

Methotrexate: I.V.: 12 g/m^2 weeks 0, 1, 5, 6, 13, 14, 18, 19, 23, 24, 37, 38 [total dose/cycle = 144 g/m^2]

Leucovorin: (route not specified): 15 mg every 6 hours for 10 doses, weeks 0, 1, 5, 6, 13, 14, 18, 19, 23, 24, 37, 38 [total dose/cycle = 1800 mg]

Doxorubicin: I.V.: 37.5 mg/m^2/day day 1 and weeks 2, 7, 25, 28 and 30 mg/m^2 days 1, 2, 3, week 20 [total dose/cycle = 390 mg/m^2]

Cisplatin: I.V.: 60 mg/m^2/day days 1, 2, weeks 2, 7, 25, 28 [total dose/cycle = 480 mg/m^2]

Cyclophosphamide: I.V.: 600 mg/m^2/day days 1, 2, 3, weeks 15, 31, 34, 39, 42 [total dose/cycle = 9000 mg/m^2]

Bleomycin: I.V.: 15 units/m^2/day days 1, 2, 3, weeks 15, 31, 34, 39, 42 [total dose/cycle = 225 units/m^2]

Dactinomycin: I.V.: 0.6 mg/m^2/day days 1, 2, 3, weeks 15, 31, 34, 39, 42 [total dose/cycle = 9 mg/m^2]

OR

(Surgery at week 0)

Methotrexate: I.V.: 12 g/m^2 weeks 3, 4, 8, 9, 13, 14, 18, 19, 23, 24, 37, 38 [total dose/cycle = 144 g/m^2]

Leucovorin: (route not specified): 15 mg every 6 hours for 10 doses, weeks 3, 4, 8, 9, 13, 14, 18, 19, 23, 24, 37, 38 [total dose/cycle = 1800 mg]

Doxorubicin: I.V.: 37.5 mg/m^2/day days 1, 2, weeks 5, 10, 25, 28, and 30 mg/m^2 days 1, 2, 3, week 20 [total dose/cycle = 390 mg/m^2]

Cisplatin: I.V.: 60 mg/m^2/day days 1, 2, weeks, 5, 10, 25, 28 [total dose/cycle = 480 mg/m^2]

Cyclophosphamide: I.V.: 600 mg/m^2/day days 1, 2, 3, weeks 15, 31, 34, 39, 42 [total dose/cycle = 9000 mg/m^2]

Bleomycin: I.V.: 15 units/m^2/day days 1, 2, 3, weeks 15, 31, 34, 39, 42 [total dose/cycle = 225 mg/m^2]

Dactinomycin: I.V.: 0.6 mg/m^2/day days 1, 2, 3, weeks 15, 31, 34, 39, 42 [total dose/cycle = 9 mg/m^2]

POMP

Use: Leukemia, acute lymphocytic

Regimen: Maintenance:

Mercaptopurine: Oral: 50 mg 3 times a day [total dose/cycle = 4.5 g]

Methotrexate: Oral: 20 mg/m^2 once weekly [total dose/cycle = 80 mg/m^2]

Vincristine: I.V.: 2 mg day 1 [total dose/cycle = 2 mg]

Prednisone: Oral: 200 mg/day days 1-5 [total dose/cycle = 1000 mg]

Repeat cycle monthly for 2 years

Pro-MACE-CytaBOM

Use: Lymphoma, non-Hodgkin

Regimen:

Prednisone: Oral: 60 mg/m^2/day days 1-14 [total dose/cycle = 840 mg/m^2]

Doxorubicin: I.V.: 25 mg/m^2 day 1 [total dose/cycle = 25 mg/m^2]

Cyclophosphamide: I.V.: 650 mg/m^2 day 1 [total dose/cycle = 650 mg/m^2]

Etoposide: I.V.: 120 mg/m^2 day 1 [total dose/cycle = 120 mg/m^2]

Cytarabine: I.V.: 300 mg/m^2 day 8 [total dose/cycle = 300 mg/m^2]

Bleomycin: I.V.: 5 units/m^2 day 8 [total dose/cycle = 5 units/m^2]

Vincristine: I.V.: 1.4 mg/m^2 (maximum 2 mg) day 8 [total dose/cycle = 1.4 mg/m^2]

Methotrexate: I.V.: 120 mg/m^2 day 8 [total dose/cycle = 120 mg/m^2]

Leucovorin: Oral: 25 mg/m^2 every 6 hours for 4 doses (start 24 hours after methotrexate) day 9 [total dose/cycle = 100 mg/m^2]

Repeat cycle every 21 days

PV

Use: Breast cancer

Regimen: Note: Multiple variations are listed below.

Variation 1:

Paclitaxel: I.V.: 135 mg/m^2 day 1 [total dose/cycle = 135 mg/m^2]
Vinorelbine: I.V.: 30 mg/m^2 day 1 [total dose/cycle = 30 mg/m^2]
Repeat cycle every 21 days

Variation 2:

Paclitaxel: I.V.: 150 mg/m^2 day 1 [total dose/cycle = 150 mg/m^2]
Vinorelbine: I.V.: 25 mg/m^2 day 1 [total dose/cycle = 25 mg/m^2]
Repeat cycle every 21 days

PVA (POG 8602)

Use: Leukemia, acute lymphocytic

Regimen:

Induction:

Prednisone: Oral: 40 mg/m^2/day (maximum 60 mg) days 0-28 (given in 3 divided doses) [total dose/cycle = 1160 mg/m^2]
Vincristine: I.V.: 1.5 mg/m^2/day (maximum 2 mg) days 0, 7, 14, and 21 [total dose/cycle = 6 mg/m^2]
Asparaginase: I.M.: 6000 units/m^2 3 times per week for 2 weeks [total dose/cycle = 36,000/units/m^2]
Intrathecal therapy: Days 0 and 22
Administer one cycle only

CNS consolidation:

Mercaptopurine: Oral: 75 mg/m^2/day days 29-42 [total dose/cycle = 1050 mg/m^2]
Intrathecal therapy: Days 29 and 36
Administer one cycle only

Intensification:

Regimen A:

Methotrexate: I.V.: 1000 mg/m^2 continuous infusion day 1 [total dose/cycle = 1000 mg/m^2]
Cytarabine: I.V.: 1000 mg/m^2 continuous infusion day 1 (start 12 hours after methotrexate) [total dose/cycle = 1000 mg/m^2]
Leucovorin: I.M., I.V., or Oral: 30 mg/m^2 24 and 36 hours after the **start** of methotrexate [total dose/cycle = 60 mg/m^2]
followed by 3 mg/m^2 48, 60, and 72 hours after the **start** of methotrexate [total dose/cycle = 9 mg/m^2]
Intrathecal therapy: Weeks 9, 12, 15, and 18
Repeat cycle every 3 weeks for 6 cycles **or**

Regimen B:

Methotrexate: I.V.: 1000 mg/m^2 continuous infusion day 1 [total dose/cycle = 1000 mg/m^2]
Cytarabine: I.V.: 1000 mg/m^2 continuous infusion day 1 (start 12 hours after methotrexate) [total dose/cycle = 1000 mg/m^2]
Leucovorin: I.M., I.V., or Oral: 30 mg/m^2 24 and 36 hours after the **start** of methotrexate [total dose/cycle = 60 mg/m^2]
followed by 3 mg/m^2 48, 60, and 72 hours after the **start** of methotrexate [total dose/cycle = 9 mg/m^2]
Intrathecal therapy: Weeks 9, 12, 15, and 18
Repeat cycle every 12 weeks for 6 cycles

Maintenance:

Regimen A:

Methotrexate: I.M.: 20 mg/m^2 weekly [total dose/cycle = 2640 mg/m^2]
Mercaptopurine: Oral: 75 mg/m^2 daily [total dose/cycle = 69,300 mg/m^2]
Intrathecal therapy: Day 1 every 8 weeks for 10 doses
Weeks 25-156
Prednisone: Oral: 40 mg/m^2/day (maximum 60 mg) days 1-7 (given in 3 divided doses) [total dose/cycle = 280 mg/m^2]
Vincristine: I.V.: 1.5 mg/m^2/day (maximum 2 mg) days 1 and 8 [total dose/cycle = 3 mg/m^2]
Weeks 8, 17, 25, 41, 57, 73, 89, 105 **or**

Regimen B:

Methotrexate: I.M.: 20 mg/m^2 weekly for 7 weeks [total dose/cycle = 140 mg/m^2]
Mercaptopurine: Oral: 75 mg/m^2 daily for 7 weeks [total dose/cycle = 3675 mg/m^2]
Repeat cycle every 12 weeks for 4 cycles (begins weeks 22, 34, 46, 58, 70)
followed by
Methotrexate: I.M.: 20 mg/m^2 weekly [total dose/cycle = 1720 mg/m^2]
Mercaptopurine: Oral: 75 mg/m^2 daily [total dose/cycle = 45,150 mg/m^2]
Weeks 70-156

PVA (POG 8602) *(continued)*

Intrathecal therapy: Day 1 every 8 weeks for 10 doses
Weeks 25-156
Prednisone: Oral: 40 mg/m^2/day (maximum 60 mg) days 1-7 (given in 3 divided doses) [total dose/cycle = 280 mg/m^2]
Vincristine: I.V.: 1.5 mg/m^2/day (maximum 2 mg) days 1 and 8 [total dose/cycle = 3 mg/m^2]
Weeks 8, 17, 25, 41, 57, 73, 89, and 105

PVB

Use: Testicular cancer
Regimen: Note: Multiple variations are listed below.

Variation 1:
Cisplatin: I.V.: 20 mg/m^2/day days 1-5 [total dose/cycle = 100 mg/m^2]
Vinblastine: I.V.: 0.2 mg/m^2/day days 1 and 2 [total dose/cycle = 0.4 mg/kg]
Bleomycin: I.V.: 30 units/day days 2, 9, and 16 [total dose/cycle = 90 units]
Repeat cycle every 3 weeks

Variation 2:
Cisplatin: I.V.: 20 mg/m^2/day days 1-5 [total dose/cycle = 100 mg/m^2]
Vinblastine: I.V.: 0.15 mg/kg/day days 1 and 2 [total dose/cycle = 0.3 mg/kg]
Bleomycin: I.V.: 30 units days 2, 9, and 16 [total dose/cycle = 90 units]
Repeat cycle every 3 weeks

Variation 3:
Cisplatin: I.V.: 20 mg/m^2/day days 1-5 [total dose/cycle = 100 mg/m^2]
Vinblastine: I.V.: 6 mg/m^2/day days 1 and 2 [total dose/cycle = 12 mg/m^2]
Bleomycin: I.M.: 30 units days 2, 9, and 16 [total dose/cycle = 90 units]
Repeat cycle every 3 weeks

PVDA

Use: Leukemia, acute lymphocytic
Regimen: Induction:

Prednisone: Oral: 60 mg/m^2/day days 1-28 [total dose/cycle = 1680 mg/m^2]
Vincristine: I.V.: 1.5 mg/m^2/day days 1, 8, 15, and 22 [total dose/cycle = 6 mg/m^2]
Daunorubicin: I.V.: 25 mg/m^2/day days 1, 8, 15, and 22 [total dose/cycle = 100 mg/m^2]
Asparaginase: I.M., SubQ, or I.V.: 5000 units/m^2/day days 1-14 [total dose/cycle = 70,000 units/m^2]
Administer one cycle only; used in conjuction with intrathecal chemotherapy

R-CHOP

Use: Lymphoma, non-Hodgkin
Regimen:

Rituximab: I.V.: 375 mg/m^2 day 1 [total dose/cycle = 375 mg/m^2]
Cyclophosphamide: I.V.: 750 mg/m^2 day 1 [total dose/cycle = 750 mg/m^2]
Doxorubicin: I.V.: 50 mg/m^2 day 1 [total dose/cycle = 50 mg/m^2]
Vincristine: I.V.: 1.4 mg/m^2 (maximum 2 mg) day 1 [total dose/cycle = 1.4 mg/m^2]
Prednisone: Oral: 40 mg/m^2/day days 1-5 [total dose/cycle = 200 mg/m^2]
Repeat cycle every 21 days

R-CVP

Use: Lymphoma, non-Hodgkin
Regimen:

Rituximab: I.V.: 375 mg/m^2 day 1 [total dose/cycle = 375 mg/m^2]
Cyclophosphamide: I.V.: 750 mg/m^2 day 1 [total dose/cycle = 750 mg/m^2]
Vincristine: I.V.: 1.4 mg/m^2 day 1 [total dose/cycle = 1.4 mg/m^2]
Prednisolone: Oral: 40 mg/m^2/day days 1 to 5 [total dose/cycle = 200 mg/m^2]
Repeat cycle every 21 days

Regimen A1

Use: Neuroblastomas

Regimen:

Cyclophosphamide: I.V.: 1.2 g/m^2 day 1 [total dose/cycle = 1.2 g/m^2]
Vincristine: I.V.: 1.5 mg/m^2 day 1 [total dose/cycle = 1.5 mg/m^2]
Doxorubicin: I.V.: 40 mg/m^2 day 3 [total dose/cycle = 40 mg/m^2]
Cisplatin: I.V.: 90 mg/m^2 day 5 [total dose/cycle = 90 mg/m^2]
Repeat cycle every 28 days

Regimen A2

Use: Neuroblastomas

Regimen:

Cyclophosphamide: I.V.: 1.2 g/m^2 day 1 [total dose/cycle = 1.2 g/m^2]
Etoposide: I.V.: 100 mg/m^2/day days 1-5 [total dose/cycle = 500 mg/m^2]
Doxorubicin: I.V.: 40 mg/m^2 day 3 [total dose/cycle = 40 mg/m^2]
Cisplatin: I.V.: 90 mg/m^2 day 5 [total dose/cycle = 90 mg/m^2]
Repeat cycle every 28 days

Sequential Dox-CMF

Use: Breast cancer

Regimen:

Doxorubicin: I.V.: 75 mg/m^2 every 21 days for 4 cycles followed by 21- or 28-day CMF for 8 cycles

Stanford V

Use: Lymphoma, Hodgkin disease

Regimen:

Mechlorethamine: I.V.: 6 mg/m^2 day 1 [total dose/cycle = 6 mg/m^2]
Doxorubicin: I.V.: 25 mg/m^2/day days 1 and 15 [total dose/cycle = 50 mg/m^2]
Vinblastine: I.V.: 6 mg/m^2/day days 1 and 15 [total dose/cycle = 12 mg/m^2]
Vincristine: I.V.: 1.4 mg/m^2/day (maximum 2 mg) days 8 and 22 [total dose/cycle = 2.8 mg/m^2]
Bleomycin: I.V.: 5 units/m^2/day days 8 and 22 [total dose/cycle = 10 units/m^2]
Etoposide: I.V.: 60 mg/m^2/day days 15 and 16 [total dose/cycle = 120 mg/m^2]
Prednisone: Oral: 40 mg/m^2 every other day for 10 weeks
[total dose/cycle = 1400 mg/m^2] **followed by** tapering of dose by 10 mg every other day for next 14 days
Repeat cycle every 28 days

TAC

Use: Breast cancer

Regimen: Note: Multiple variations are listed below.

Variation 1:
Docetaxel: I.V.: 75 mg/m^2 day 1 [total dose/cycle = 75 mg/m^2]
Doxorubicin: I.V.: 50 mg/m^2 day 1 [total dose/cycle = 50 mg/m^2]
Cyclophosphamide: I.V.: 500 mg/m^2 day 1 [total dose/cycle = 500 mg/m^2]
Repeat cycle every 3 weeks

Variation 2:
Docetaxel: I.V.: 60 mg/m^2 day 1 [total dose/cycle = 60 mg/m^2]
Doxorubicin: I.V.: 60 mg/m^2 day 1 [total dose/cycle = 60 mg/m^2]
Cyclophosphamide: I.V.: 600 mg/m^2 day 1 [total dose/cycle = 600 mg/m^2]
Repeat cycle every 3 weeks

TAD

Use: Leukemia, acute myeloid

Regimen:

Daunorubicin: I.V.: 60 mg/m^2/day days 3-5 [total dose/cycle = 180 mg/m^2]
Cytarabine: I.V.: 100 mg/m^2/day continuous infusion days 1 and 2
[total dose/cycle = 200 mg/m^2] **followed by** 100 mg/m^2/day every 12 hours days 3-8
[total dose/cycle = 1200 mg/m^2]
Thioguanine: Oral: 100 mg/m^2/day every 12 hours days 3-9 [total dose/cycle = 1400 mg/m^2]
Administer one cycle only

Tamoxifen-Epirubicin

Use: Breast cancer

Regimen:

Tamoxifen: Oral: 20 mg daily [total dose/cycle = 560 mg]
Epirubicin: I.V.: 50 mg/m^2/day days 1 and 8 [total dose/cycle = 100 mg/m^2]
Repeat epirubicin cycle every 28 days for 6 cycles; continue tamoxifen for 4 years

TCF

Use: Esophageal cancer

Regimen:

Paclitaxel: I.V.: 175 mg/m^2 day 1 [total dose/cycle = 175 mg/m^2]
Cisplatin: I.V.: 20 mg/m^2/day days 1-5 [total dose/cycle = 100 mg/m^2]
Fluorouracil: I.V.: 750 mg/m^2/day continuous infusion days 1-5 [total dose/cycle = 3750 mg/m^2]
Repeat cycle every 28 days

Thalidomide + Dexamethasone

Use: Multiple myeloma

Regimen: Note: Multiple variations are listed below.

Variation 1:
Thalidomide: Oral: 100 mg/day days 1-28 [total dose/cycle = 2800 mg]
Dexamethasone: Oral: 40 mg/day days 1-4 [total dose/cycle = 160 mg]
Repeat cycle every 28 days

Variation 2:
Thalidomide: Oral: 200 mg/day days 1-14 cycle 1
followed by 400 mg/day days 15-28 cycle 1 [total dose/cycle = 8400 mg]
Thalidomide: Oral: 400 mg/day days 1-28 (subsequent cycles) [total dose/cycle = 11,200 mg]
Dexamethasone: Oral: 20 mg/m^2/day days 1-4, 9-12, and 17 to 20 cycle 1 (subsequent cycles) [total dose/cycle = 240 mg/m^2]
Dexamethasone: Oral: 20 mg/m^2/day days 1-4 (subsequent cycles) [total dose/cycle = 80 mg/m^2]
Repeat cycle every 28 days

Variation 3:
Thalidomide: Oral: 100 mg/day days 1-7, 150 mg/day days 8-14, 200 mg/day days 15-21, 250 mg/day days 22-28, and 300 mg/day days 29-35 (cycle 1) [total dose/cycle = 7000 mg]
Thalidomide: Oral: 300 mg/day days 1-35 (subsequent cycles) [total dose/cycle = 10,500 mg]
Dexamethasone: Oral: 20 mg/m^2/day days 1-4, 9-12, and 17-20 [total dose/cycle = 240 mg/m^2]
Repeat cycle every 35 days

Variation 4:
Thalidomide: Oral: 200 mg/day days 1-28 [total dose/cycle = 5600 mg]
Dexamethasone: Oral: 40 mg/day days 1-4, 9-12, and 17-20 (odd cycles) [total dose/cycle = 480 mg]
Dexamethasone: Oral: 40 mg/day days 1-4 (even cycles) [total dose/cycle = 160 mg]
Repeat cycle every 28 days

TIP

Use: Esophageal cancer; Head and neck cancer

Regimen:

Paclitaxel: I.V.: 175 mg/m^2 day 1 [total dose/cycle = 175 mg/m^2]
Ifosfamide: I.V.: 1000 mg/m^2/day days 1-3 [total dose/cycle = 3000 mg/m^2]
Mesna: I.V.: 400 mg/m^2/day before ifosfamide days 1-3 [total dose/cycle = 1200 mg/m^2]
followed by: 200 mg/m^2 4 hours after ifosfamide days 1-3 [total dose/cycle = 600 mg/m^2]
Cisplatin: I.V.: 60 mg/m^2 day 1 [total dose/cycle = 60 mg/m^2]
Repeat cycle every 21-28 days

Trastuzumab-Paclitaxel

Use: Breast cancer

Regimen:

Paclitaxel: I.V.: 175 mg/m^2 day 1 [total dose/cycle = 175 mg/m^2]
Trastuzumab: I.V.: 4 mg/kg (loading dose) day 1 cycle 1 [total dose/cycle = 4 mg/kg] **followed by**
Trastuzumab: I.V.: 2 mg/kg/day days 1, 8, and 15 [total dose/cycle = 6 mg/kg]
Repeat cycle every 21 days for at least 6 cycles

Tretinoin/Idarubicin

Use: Leukemia, acute promyelocytic

Regimen:

Variation 1: Induction:

Tretinoin: Oral: >20 years: 45 mg/m^2/day day 1 up to 90 days [total dose/cycle = 4050 mg/m^2]

Tretinoin Oral: ≤20 years: 25 mg/m^2/day day 1 up to 90 days [total dose/cycle = 2250 mg/m^2]

Idarubicin: I.V.: 12 mg/m^2/day days 2, 4, 6, and 8 [total dose/cycle = 48 mg/m^2]

Consolidation Course 1:

Idarubicin: I.V.: 5 mg/m^2/day days 1-4 [total dose/cycle = 20 mg/m^2] **or**

Idarubicin: I.V.: 7 mg/m^2/day days 1-4 [total dose/cycle = 28 mg/m^2]

Tretinoin: Oral: 45 mg/m^2/day days 1-15 [total dose/cycle = 675 mg/m^2]

Consolidation Course 2:

Mitoxantrone: I.V.: 10 mg/m^2/day days 1-5 [total dose/cycle = 50 mg/m^2]

Tretinoin: Oral: 45 mg/m^2/day days 1-15 [total dose/cycle = 675 mg/m^2]

Consolidation Course 3:

Idarubicin: I.V.: 12 mg/m^2 day 1 [total dose/cycle = 12 mg/m^2] **or**

Idarubicin: I.V.: 12 mg/m^2/day days 1-2 [total dose/cycle = 24 mg/m^2]

Tretinoin: Oral: 45 mg/m^2/day days 1-15 [total dose/cycle = 675 mg/m^2]

Given at 1 month intervals

Maintenance:

Mercaptopurine: Oral: 50 mg/m^2 daily [total dose/cycle = 4200 mg/m^2]

Methotrexate: I.M.: 15 mg/m^2 weekly [total dose/cycle = 180 mg/m^2]

Tretinoin: Oral: 45 mg/m^2/day days 1-15 [total dose/cycle = 675 mg/m^2]

Repeat every 3 months for 2 years

TVTG

Use: Leukemia, acute lymphocytic; Leukemia, acute myeloid

Regimen:

Topotecan: I.V.: 1 mg/m^2/day continuous infusion days 1-5 [total dose/cycle = 5 mg/m^2]

Vinorelbine: I.V.: 20 mg/m^2/day days 0, 7, 14, and 21 [total dose/cycle = 80 mg/m^2]

Thiotepa: I.V.: 15 mg/m^2 day 2 [total dose/cycle = 15 mg/m^2]

Gemcitabine: I.V.: 3600 mg/m^2 day 7 [total dose/cycle = 3600 mg/m^2]

Dexamethasone: Oral or I.V.: 45 mg/m^2/day days 7-14 (given in 3 divided doses) [total dose/cycle = 315 mg/m^2]

Repeat cycle when ANC >500 cells/mcL and platelet count >75,000 cells/mcL

VAC (Ovarian Cancer)

Use: Ovarian cancer

Regimen:

Vincristine: I.V.: 1.2-1.5 mg/m^2 (maximum 2 mg) weekly for 10-12 weeks [total dose/cycle = 12-15 mg/m^2 to 14.4-18]

or every 2 weeks for 12 doses [total dose/cycle = 14.4-18 mg/m^2]

Dactinomycin: I.V.: 0.3-0.4 mg/m^2/day days 1-5 [total dose/cycle = 1.5-2 mg/m^2]

Cyclophosphamide: I.V.: 150 mg/m^2/day days 1-5 [total dose/cycle = 750 mg/m^2]

Repeat every 28 days

VAC (Retinoblastoma)

Use: Retinoblastoma

Regimen:

Vincristine: I.V.: 1.5 mg/m^2 day 1 [total dose/cycle = 1.5 mg/m^2]

Dactinomycin: I.V.: 0.015 mg/kg/day days 1-5 [total dose/cycle = 0.075 mg/kg]

Cyclophosphamide: I.V.: 200 mg/m^2/day days 1-5 [total dose/cycle = 1000 mg/m^2]

VAC (Rhabdomyosarcoma)

Use: Rhabdomyosarcoma

Regimen:

Induction:

Vincristine: I.V. push: 1.5 mg/m^2 (maximum 2 mg) weekly for 12 weeks, then at week 16 [total dose/cycle = 19.5 mg/m^2]

Dactinomycin: I.V. push: 0.015 mg/kg/day (maximum 0.5 mg) days 1-5, repeat every 3 weeks for 3 cycles, then stop for 2 cycles; repeat at week 16

Cyclophosphamide: I.V.: 10 mg/kg/day days 1-3 (alternately: 2.2 g/m^2 day 1), repeat every 3 weeks for 5 cycles; then at week 16

Continuation:

Vincristine: I.V. push: 1.5 mg/m^2 (maximum 2 mg) weeks 20-25, 29-34, 38-43 [total dose/cycle = 27 mg/m^2]

Dactinomycin: I.V. push: 0.015 mg/kg (maximum 0.5 mg) weeks 20 and 23, 29 and 32, 38 and 41 [total dose/cycle = .18 mg/kg]

Cyclophosphamide: I.V.: 2.2 mg/m^2 weeks 20 and 23, 29 and 32, 38 and 41 [total dose/cycle = 26.4 g/m^2]

VAC Pulse

Use: Rhabdomyosarcoma

Regimen:

Vincristine: I.V.: 2 mg/m^2/dose (maximum 2 mg/dose) every 7 days for 12 weeks [total dose/cycle = 24 mg/m^2]

Dactinomycin: I.V.: 0.015 mg/kg/day (maximum 0.5 mg/day) days 1-5, weeks 1 and 13 [total dose/cycle = 0.15 mg/kg]

Cyclophosphamide: Oral, I.V.: 10 mg/kg/day for 7 days, repeat every 6 weeks

VAD

Use: Multiple myeloma

Regimen:

Vincristine: I.V.: 0.4 mg/day continuous infusion days 1-4 [total dose/cycle = 1.6 mg]

Doxorubicin: I.V.: 9 mg/m^2/day continuous infusion days 1-4 [total dose/cycle = 36 mg/m^2]

Dexamethasone: Oral: 40 mg/day days 1-4, 9-12, 17-20 [total dose/cycle = 480 mg]

Repeat cycle every 28-35 days

VAD/CVAD

Use: Leukemia, acute lymphocytic

Regimen:

Induction:

Vincristine: I.V.: 0.4 mg continuous infusion/day days 1-4 and 24-27 [total dose/cycle = 3.2 mg]

Doxorubicin: I.V.: 12 mg/m^2/day continuous infusion days 1-4 and 24-27 [total dose/cycle = 96 mg/m^2]

Dexamethasone: Oral: 40 mg/day days 1-4, 9-12 and 17-20 [total dose/cycle = 480 mg]

Cyclophosphamide: I.V.: 1 g/m^2 day 24 [total dose/cycle = 1 g/m^2]

Dexamethasone: Oral: 40 mg/day days 24-27, 32-35 and 40-43 [total dose/cycle = 480 mg]

Administer one cycle only

VATH

Use: Breast cancer

Regimen:

Vinblastine: I.V.: 4.5 mg/m^2 day 1 [total dose/cycle = 4.5 mg/m^2]

Doxorubicin: I.V.: 45 mg/m^2 day 1 [total dose/cycle = 45 mg/m^2]

Thiotepa: I.V.: 12 mg/m^2 day 1 [total dose/cycle = 12 mg/m^2]

Fluoxymesterone: Oral: 10 mg 3 times/day days 1-21 [total dose/cycle = 630 mg]

Repeat cycle every 21 days

VBAP

Use: Multiple myeloma

Regimen:

Vincristine: I.V.: 1 mg day 1 [total dose/cycle = 1 mg]
Carmustine: I.V.: 30 mg/m^2 day 1 [total dose/cycle = 30 mg/m^2]
Doxorubicin: I.V.: 30 mg/m^2 day 1 [total dose/cycle = 30 mg/m^2]
Prednisone: Oral: 100 mg/day days 1-4 [total dose/cycle = 400 mg]
Repeat cycle every 21 days

VBMCP

Use: Multiple myeloma

Regimen:

Vincristine: I.V.: 1.2 mg/m^2 (maximum 2 mg) day 1 [total dose/cycle = 1.2 mg/m^2]
Carmustine: I.V.: 20 mg/m^2 day 1 [total dose/cycle = 20 mg/m^2]
Melphalan: Oral: 8 mg/m^2/day days 1-4 [total dose/cycle = 32 mg/m^2]
Cyclophosphamide: I.V.: 400 mg/m^2 day 1 [total dose/cycle = 400 mg/m^2]
Prednisone: Oral: 40 mg/m^2/day days 1-7 (all cycles) [total dose/cycle = 280 mg/m^2]
followed by 20 mg/m^2/day days 8-14 (first 3 cycles only) [total dose/cycle = 140 mg/m^2]
Repeat cycle every 35 days

VBP (PVB)

Use: Testicular cancer

Regimen:

Vinblastine: I.V.: 6 mg/m^2/day days 1 and 2 [total dose/cycle = 12 mg/m^2]
Bleomycin: I.V.: 30 units/day days 1, 8, 15, (22) [total dose/cycle = 120 units]
Cisplatin: I.V.: 20 mg/m^2/day days 1-5 [total dose/cycle = 100 mg/m^2]
Repeat cycle every 21-28 days

VC

Use: Lung cancer, nonsmall-cell

Regimen: Note: Multiple variations are listed below.

Variation 1:

Vinorelbine: I.V.: 25 mg/m^2/day days 1, 8, 15, 22
Cisplatin: I.V.: 100 mg/m^2 day 1
Repeat cycle every 28 days for 2-8 cycles

Variation 2:

Vinorelbine: I.V.: 30 mg/m^2 weekly [total dose/cycle = 180 mg/m^2]
Cisplatin: I.V.: 120 mg/m^2/day days 1 and 29 (cycle 1); day 1 only on subsequent cycles [total dose/cycle = 240 mg/m^2]
Repeat cycle every 6 weeks

VCAP

Use: Multiple myeloma

Regimen:

Vincristine: I.V.: 1 mg day 1 [total dose/cycle = 1 mg]
Cyclophosphamide: Oral: 100 mg/m^2/day days 1-4 [total dose/cycle = 400 mg/m^2]
Doxorubicin: I.V.: 25 mg/m^2 day 2 [total dose/cycle = 25 mg/m^2]
Prednisone: Oral: 60 mg/m^2/day days 1-4 [total dose/cycle = 240 mg/m^2]
Repeat cycle every 28 days

Vinorelbine-Cis

Use: Lung cancer, nonsmall-cell

Regimen:

Vinorelbine: I.V.: 30 mg/m^2 every 7 days
Cisplatin: I.V.: 120 mg/m^2/day day 1 and 29, then every 6 weeks

Vinorelbine-Gemcitabine

Use: Lung cancer, nonsmall-cell
Regimen:
Vinorelbine: I.V.: 20 mg/m^2/day days 1, 8, and 15 [total dose/cycle = 60 mg/m^2]
Gemcitabine: I.V.: 800 mg/m^2/day days 1, 8, and 15 [total dose/cycle = 2400 mg/m^2]
Repeat cycle every 28 days

VIP (Etoposide) (Testicular Cancer)

Use: Testicular cancer
Regimen: Note: Multiple variations are listed below.
Variation 1:
Etoposide: I.V.: 75 mg/m^2/day days 1-5 [total dose/cycle = 375 mg/m^2]
Ifosfamide: I.V.: 1200 mg/m^2/day days 1-5 [total dose/cycle = 6000 mg/m^2]
Cisplatin: I.V.: 20 mg/m^2/day days 1-5 [total dose/cycle = 100 mg/m^2]
Repeat cycle every 21 days
Variation 2:
Etoposide: I.V.: 100 mg/m^2/day days 1-5 [total dose/cycle = 500 mg/m^2]
Ifosfamide: I.V.: 1200 mg/m^2/day days 1-5 [total dose/cycle = 6000 mg/m^2]
Cisplatin: I.V.: 20 mg/m^2/day days 1-5 [total dose/cycle = 100 mg/m^2]
Repeat cycle every 21 days
Variation 3:
Ifosfamide: I.V.: 2500 mg/m^2/day days 1 and 2 [total dose/cycle = 5000 mg/m^2]
Mesna: I.V.: 2400 mg/m^2/day days 1 and 2 [total dose/cycle = 4800 mg/m^2]
Etoposide: I.V.: 100 mg/m^2/day days 3, 4, and 5 [total dose/cycle = 300 mg/m^2]
Cisplatin: I.V.: 40 mg/m^2/day days 3, 4, and 5 [total dose/cycle = 120 mg/m^2]
Repeat cycle every 21 days
Variation 4:
Etoposide: I.V.: 75 mg/m^2/day days 1-5 [total dose/cycle = 375 mg/m^2]
Ifosfamide: I.V.: 1200 mg/m^2/day days 1-5 [total dose/cycle = 6000 mg/m^2]
Cisplatin: I.V.: 20 mg/m^2/day days 1-5 [total dose/cycle = 100 mg/m^2]
Mesna: I.V.: 400 mg/m^2, then 1200 mg/m^2 continuous infusion days 1-5
Repeat cycle every 21 days

VIP (Small-Cell Lung Cancer)

Use: Lung cancer, small-cell
Regimen:
Etoposide: I.V.: 75 mg/m^2/day days 1-4 [total dose/cycle = 300 mg/m^2] **or** 100 mg/m^2/day days 1-4
Ifosfamide: I.V.: 1200 mg/m^2/day days 1-4 [total dose/cycle = 4800 mg/m^2]
Cisplatin: I.V.: 20 mg/m^2/day days 1-4 [total dose/cycle = 80 mg/m^2]
Mesna: I.V.: 300 mg/m^2 day 1 [total dose/cycle = 300 mg/m^2] **followed by** 1200 mg/m^2/day continuous infusion days 1-4 [total dose/cycle = 4800 mg/m^2]
Repeat cycle every 21 days

VIP (Vinblastine) (Testicular Cancer)

Use: Testicular Cancer
Regimen: Note: Multiple variations are listed below.
Variation 1:
Vinblastine: I.V.: 0.11 mg/kg/day days 1 and 2 [total dose/cycle = 0.22 mg/kg]
Ifosfamide: I.V.: 1200 mg/m^2/day days 1-5 [total dose/cycle = 6000 mg/m^2]
Cisplatin: I.V.: 20 mg/m^2/day days 1-5 [total dose/cycle = 100 mg/m^2]
Repeat cycle every 21 days
Variation 2:
Vinblastine: I.V.: 6 mg/m^2/day days 1 and 2 [total dose/cycle = 12 mg/m^2]
Ifosfamide: I.V.: 1500 mg/m^2/day days 1-5 [total dose/cycle = 7500 mg/m^2]
Cisplatin: I.V.: 20 mg/m^2/day days 1-5 [total dose/cycle = 100 mg/m^2]
Repeat cycle every 21 days

VP (Small-Cell Lung Cancer)

Use: Lung cancer, small-cell
Regimen:
Etoposide: I.V.: 100 mg/m^2/day days 1-4 [total dose/cycle = 400 mg/m^2]
Cisplatin: I.V.: 20 mg/m^2/day days 1-4 [total dose/cycle = 80 mg/m^2]
Repeat cycle every 21 days

V-TAD

Use: Leukemia, acute myeloid

Regimen:

Induction:

Etoposide: I.V.: 50 mg/m^2/day days 1-3 [total dose/cycle = 150 mg/m^2]

Thioguanine: Oral: 75 mg/m^2/day every 12 hours days 1-5 [total dose/cycle = 750 mg/m^2]

Daunorubicin: I.V.: 20 mg/m^2/day days 1 and 2 [total dose/cycle = 40 mg/m^2]

Cytarabine: I.V.: 75 mg/m^2/day continuous infusion days 1-5 [total dose/cycle = 375 mg/m^2]

Up to 3 cycles may be given based on individual response; time between cycles not specified

XelOx

Use: Colorectal cancer

Regimen: Note: Multiple variations are listed below.

Variation 1:

Oxaliplatin: I.V.: 130 mg/m^2 day 1 [total dose/cycle = 130 mg/m^2]

Capecitabine: Oral: 2500 mg/m^2/day days 1-14 [total dose/cycle = 35,000 mg/m^2]

Repeat cycle every 21 days

Variation 2:

Oxaliplatin: I.V.: 85 mg/m^2/day day 1 [total dose/cycle = 85 mg/m^2]

Capecitabine: Oral: 3500 mg/m^2/day days 1-7 [total dose/cycle = 24,500 mg/m^2]

Repeat cycle every 14 days

Variation 3:

Oxaliplatin: I.V.: 50-80 mg/m^2/day days 1, 8, 22, and 29 [total dose/cycle = 200-320 mg/m^2]

Capecitabine: Oral: 1650 mg/m^2/day days 1-14 and 22-35 [total dose/cycle = 46,200 mg/m^2]

Variation 4:

Oxaliplatin: I.V.: 70 mg/m^2/day days 1 and 8 [total dose/cycle = 140 mg/m^2]

Capecitabine: Oral: 2000 mg/m^2/day days 1-14 [total dose/cycle = 28,000 mg/m^2]

Repeat cycle every 21 days

Variation 5:

Oxaliplatin: I.V.: 120 mg/m^2 day 1 [total dose/cycle = 120 mg/m^2]

Capecitabine: Oral: 2500 mg/m^2/day days 1-14 [total dose/cycle = 35,000 mg/m^2]

Repeat cycle every 21 days

Variation 6:

Oxaliplatin: I.V.: 85 mg/m^2 day 1 [total dose/cycle = 85 mg/m^2]

Capecitabine: Oral: 2500 mg/m^2/day days 1-7 [total dose/cycle = 17,500 mg/m^2] **or**

Capecitabine: Oral: 3000 mg/m^2/day days 1-7 [total dose/cycle = 21,000 mg/m^2] **or**

Capecitabine: Oral: 3500 mg/m^2/day days 1-7 [total dose/cycle = 24,500 mg/m^2] **or**

Capecitabine: Oral: 4000 mg/m^2/day days 1-7 [total dose/cycle = 28,000 mg/m^2]

Repeat cycle every 14 days

CHEMOTHERAPY REGIMEN INDEX

Adenocarcinoma, Unknown Primary

Brain

Neuroblastomas

Breast

Eye

Retinoblastoma

Gastrointestinal

Genitourinary

Genitourinary *(continued)*

Prostate Cancer

Bicalutamide + LHRH-A *on page 916*
Cyclophosphamide + Doxorubicin *on page 926*
Cyclophosphamide + Estramustine *on page 926*
Cyclophosphamide + Etoposide *on page 926*
Cyclophosphamide + Vincristine + Dexamethasone *on page 926*
Doxorubicin + Ketoconazole *on page 928*
Doxorubicin + Ketoconazole/Estramustine + Vinblastine *on page 928*
Estramustine + Docetaxel *on page 932*
Estramustine + Docetaxel + Carboplatin *on page 932*
Estramustine + Docetaxel + Hydrocortisone *on page 933*
Estramustine + Etoposide *on page 933*
Estramustine + Vinorelbine *on page 933*
EV *on page 933*
FL *on page 936*
FZ *on page 938*
Mitoxantrone + Hydrocortisone *on page 946*
MP (Prostate Cancer) *on page 949*
Paclitaxel + Estramustine + Carboplatin *on page 953*
Paclitaxel + Estramustine + Etoposide *on page 953*
PE *on page 954*

Renal Cell Cancer

Interleukin 2-Interferon Alfa 2 *on page 942*
Interleukin 2-Interferon Alfa 2-Fluorouracil *on page 942*

Testicular Cancer

BEP (Ovarian, Testicular) *on page 916*
BEP (Testicular) *on page 916*
EP (Testicular Cancer) *on page 931*
PVB *on page 958*
VBP (PVB) *on page 963*
VIP (Etoposide) (Testicular Cancer) *on page 964*
VIP (Vinblastine) (Testicular Cancer) *on page 964*

Wilms Tumor

AAV (DD) *on page 913*
ACAV (J) *on page 914*
AV (EE) *on page 914*
AV (K) *on page 915*
AV (L) *on page 915*
AV (Wilms tumor) *on page 915*
AVD *on page 915*
EE *on page 930*
EE-4A *on page 930*

Head and Neck Cancer

CABO *on page 916*
CF *on page 920*
FU HURT *on page 937*
M-VAC (Head and Neck Cancer) *on page 951*
PFL (Head and Neck Cancer) *on page 955*
PFL + IFN *on page 955*
TIP *on page 960*

Hematologic/Leukemia

Leukemia, Acute Lymphocytic

DVP *on page 929*
FIS-HAM *on page 935*
Larson Regimen *on page 943*
Linker Protocol *on page 943*
MM *on page 946*
MTX/6-MP/VP (Maintenance) *on page 949*
POMP *on page 956*
PVA (POG 8602) *on page 957*
PVDA *on page 958*
TVTG *on page 961*
VAD/CVAD *on page 962*

Hematologic/Leukemia *(continued)*

Lung

Lymphoid Tissue (Lymphoma)

Lymphoid Tissue (Lymphoma) *(continued)*

Malignant Pleural Mesothelioma

Myeloma

Sarcoma

Sarcoma *(continued)*

Soft Tissue Sarcoma

Skin

Melanoma

HERBS AND COMMON NATURAL AGENTS

The authors have chosen to include this list of natural products and their reported uses. Due to limited scientific evidence to support these uses, the information provided here is not intended as a cure for any disease, and should not be construed as curative or healing. In addition, the reader is strongly encouraged to seek other references that discuss this information in more detail, and that discuss important issues such as contraindications, warnings, precautions, adverse reactions, and interactions.

PROPOSED CLAIMS

Herb	Reported Uses
Acetyl-L-carnitine (ALC)	Alzheimer disease; depression; diabetic peripheral neuropathy; Parkinson disease
Adrenal extract	Depression; fatigue; stress; fibromylagia
Aloe (*Aloe supp*)	Gingivitis; healing agent for wounds, minor burns, and other minor skin irritations
Alpha-Lipoic acid	Diabetes, diabetic peripheral neuropathy; glaucoma; prevention of cataracts; prevention of neurologic disorders, including stroke; chemotherapy and radiation (adjunct); circulation; multiple sclerosis; hypertension
Androstenedione	Athletic performance (enhancement)
Aortic extract	Circulation structure, function, and integrity (arteries and veins); prevention of vascular disease including atherosclerosis, cerebral and peripheral arterial insufficiency, varicose veins, hemorrhoids, and vascular retinopathies such as macular degeneration
Arabinoxylane	Chemotherapy-induced leukopenia; immune system enhancement (antiviral and anticancer activity); HIV infection
Arginine	Cardiovascular disease; chronic heart failure; hypercholesterolemia; circulation; increases lean body mass; inflammatory bowel disease; immune support; male infertility; sexual vitality and enhancement; wound healing
Artichoke (*Cynara scolymus*)	Eczema and other dermatologic problems; hepatic protection/stimulation; hypercholesterolemia; bile flow; indigestion
Ashwagandha (*Withania somnifera*)	Adaptogen/tonic (promote wellness); chemotherapy and radiation (adjunct); stress, fatigue, nervous exhaustion
Astragalus (*Astragalus membranaceus*) [Milk Vetch]	Adaptogen/tonic (promote wellness); chemotherapy and radiation (adjunct); immune support; multiple sclerosis; otitis media; tissue oxygenation
Bacopa (*Bacopa monniera*)	Alzheimer disease/senility; memory enhancement and improvement of cognitive function
Beta-Carotene	Asthma; cervical dysplasia; coronary heart disease (risk reduction; in combination); immune support; photoprotection (erythropoietic protoporphyria); prevention of lung cancer
Betaine hydrochloride	Digestive aid (hypochlorhydria and achlorhydria); rosacea
Bifidobacterium bifidum (*bifidus*)	Crohn disease; diarrhea; gastrointestinal microflora recolonization (anaerobic); ulcerative colitis
Bilberry (*Vaccinium myrtillus*)	Diarrhea; hemorrhoids; ophthalmologic disorders (antioxidant) including myopia, diminished acuity, glaucoma; dark adaptation, macular degeneration, night blindness, diabetic retinopathy, cataracts; scleroderma; vascular disorders including varicose veins, capillary permeability/stability, phlebitis
Biotin (Vitamin H)	Brittle nails; diabetes; diabetic peripheral neuropathy; seborrheic dermatitis; uncombable hair syndrome
Bismuth	Ulcers
Bitter melon (*Momordica charantia*)	Antiviral; diabetes, including impaired glucose tolerance (IGT)
Black cohosh (*Cimicifuga racemosa*)	Arthritis; menopause symptoms (including vasomotor); premenstrual syndrome (PMS); mild depression
Bladderwrack (*Fucus vesiculosus*)	Fibrocystic breast disease; hypothyroidism; nutrient (rich source of iodine, potassium, magnesium, calcium, and iron)
Boron	Osteoarthritis; osteoporosis; rheumatoid arthritis
Boswellia (*Boswellia serrata*)	Antiinflammatory; arthritis; ulcerative colitis

(continued)

Herb	Reported Uses
Branched-chain amino acids (BCAAs)	Muscle development and lean body mass (increase)
Bromelain (*Anas comosus*)	Arthritis (antiinflammatory; proteolytic); cervical dysplasia; digestive enzyme; sinusitis
Bupleurum (*Bupleurum falcatum*)	Chronic inflammatory disease; fatigue; hepatic protection; systemic lupus erythematosus (SLE)
Calcium	Blood pressure regulation; cancer prevention; hypercholesterolemia; hypertension; kidney stones; poison ivy (topical; lactate form); premenstrual syndrome (PMS); pregnancy; prevention of osteoporosis
Calendula (*Calendula officinalis*)	Antibacterial, antifungal, antiviral, antiprotozoal; vulnerary; wound-healing (immune stimulant)
Caprylic acid	Antifungal/antiyeast; candidiasis; Crohn disease; dysbiosis
Carnitine	Athletic performance (enhancement); congestive heart failure (CHF); hypercholesterolemia; male infertility; weight loss
Cascara (*Rhamnus purshiana*)	Laxative
Cat's claw (*Uncaria tomentosa*)	Antiinflammatory; antimicrobial (antibacterial, antifungal, antiviral); antioxidant; cervical dysplasia; Crohn disease; diverticulitis; endometriosis; fibromyalgia; immune support; multiple sclerosis; rosacea; systemic lupus erythematosus (SLE)
Cayenne (*Capsicum annuum, Capsicum frutescens*)	Antiinflammatory and analgesic (topical); cardiovascular circulatory support; digestive stimulant
Chamomile, German (*Matricaria chamomilla, Matricaria recutita*)	Minor injury (topical antiinflammatory); carminative, antispasmodic; insomnia (mild sedative); anxiolytic; colic; diaper rash; indigestion; nausea/vomiting; oral health (as mouth rinse/gargle); stress/anxiety; teething; uterine tonic
Chasteberry (*Vitex agnus-castus*)	Acne vulgaris; cervical dysplasia; corpus luteum insufficiency; hyperprolactinemia and insufficient lactation; menopause; menorrhagia; menstrual disorders including amenorrhea, endometriosis, premenstrual syndrome (PMS); rosacea
Chitosan	Weight reduction
Chlorophyll	Antiinflammatory, antioxidant, and wound-healing properties; bacteriostatic; odor absorbent/suppressant (breath freshener, toothpaste, mouthwash, and deodorant); protectant
Chondroitin sulfate	Osteoarthritis
Chromium	Atherosclerosis; diabetes, type 1; diabetes, type 2; glaucoma; hypercholesterolemia; hypertriglyceridemia; hypothyroidism; premenstrual syndrome (PMS); weight loss
Clove (*Syzygium aromaticum*)	Antiseptic; analgesic (toothache and teething)
Coenzyme Q_{10}	Angina; cancer (preventive); chemotherapy (adjunct); chronic fatigue syndrome; congestive heart failure (CHF); fibromyalgia; gingivitis; hypercholesterolemia; hypertension; HMG-CoA reductase inhibitors may cause depletion of this nutraceutical; multiple sclerosis; muscular dystrophy; periodontal disease; weight loss
Coleus (*Coleus forskohlii*)	Asthma and allergies; eczema; hypertension and congestive heart failure (CHF); psoriasis
Collagen (Type II)	Arthritis (rheumatoid and osteo); burns (first- and second-degree); ulcers (pressure, venous stasis, diabetic); surgical and traumatic wounds; wound healing (topical)
Colostrum	Antiviral (mild); athletic performance (enhancement); diarrhea; immune support
Conjugated linoleic acid (CLA)	Muscle development and lean body mass (increase)
Copper	Anemia; osteoporosis; rheumatoid arthritis
Cordyceps (*Cordyceps sinensis*)	Adaptogen/tonic (promote wellness); antioxidant; chemotherapy and radiation (adjunct); endurance and stamina; fibromyalgia; hepatoprotection; lung, liver, and kidney function (general support); sexual vitality (males and females); tissue oxygenation; fatigue; immunomodulator
Cranberry (*Vaccinium macrocarpon*)	Nephrolithiasis (preventive); urinary tract infection, including prevention
Creatine	Enhancement of athletic performance (energy production and protein synthesis for muscle building)

(continued)

Herb	Reported Uses
Cyclo-hispro	Diabetes, type 2; hypoglycemia
Dandelion (*Taraxacum officinale*)	Leaf used as a diuretic; root used for disorders of bile secretion (choleretic), appetite stimulation, dyspepsia
Dehydroepiandrosterone (DHEA)	Antiaging; depression; diabetes, type 2; fatigue; lupus
Devil's claw (*Harpagophytum procumbens*)	Antiinflammatory; back pain; osteoarthritis, gout, and other inflammatory conditions
Docosahexaenoic acid (DHA)	Alzheimer disease; attention deficit disorder (ADD) and attention deficit hyperactivity disorder (ADHD); coronary heart disease (risk reduction); Crohn disease; diabetes; eczema; hypertension; hypertriglyceridemia; psoriasis; rheumatoid arthritis; stroke (risk reduction)
Dong quai (*Angelica sinensis*)	Anemia; energy enhancement (particularly in females); hypertension; menopause, dysmenorrhea, premenstrual syndrome (PMS), and amenorrhea; menorrhagia; phytoestrogen
Echinacea (*Echinacea purpurea, Echinacea angustifolia*)	Antibacterial (topical; boils, abscesses, tonsillitis, poison ivy); antiviral; arthritis (*E. augustifolia*); immune support (cold and other upper respiratory infections); otitis media
Elder (*Sambucus nigra, Sambucus canadensis*)	Berry used as an antiviral, antioxidant, and for influenza; flower used as an antiinflammatory, colds and influenza, diaphoretic, diuretic, fever, sinusitis, and sore throat
Evening primrose (*Oenothera biennis*)	Amenorrhea; attention deficit disorder (ADD); depression; diabetes; diabetic peripheral neuropathy; eczema, dermatitis, and psoriasis; endometriosis; fatigue; fibrocystic breast disease (FBD); hypercholesterolemia; irritable bowel syndrome; menorrhagia; multiple sclerosis; omega-6 fatty acid supplementation; premenstrual syndrome (PMS) and menopause; rheumatoid arthritis; rosacea; scleroderma
Eyebright (*Euphrasia officinalis*)	Eye fatigue; catarrh of the eyes
Fenugreek (*Trigonella foenum-graecum*)	Diabetes; hypercholesterolemia
Feverfew (*Tanacetum parthenium*)	Antiinflammatory, rheumatoid arthritis; migraine headache (preventive); muscle soreness
Fish oils	Acne vulgaris; asthma; cardiac death (sudden; preventive); cardiac support (general; proposed benefits); circulation; coronary heart disease (preventive); Crohn disease; diabetes; dysmenorrhea; eczema, psoriasis; fatigue; headache; heart disease and heart attack (risk reduction), including women; herpes simplex 2; hypertension; hypertriglyceridemia; memory enhancement; multiple sclerosis; premenstrual syndrome (PMS); rheumatoid arthritis; rosacea; scleroderma; stroke (risk reduction)
Flaxseed oil	Acne vulgaris; arthritis (rheumatoid); asthma; constipation; coronary heart disease (risk reduction); hemorrhoids; hypertension; multiple sclerosis; omega-3 essential fatty acid source (cell wall and cellular membrane structure; cholesterol transport and oxidation); premenstrual syndrome (PMS); prostaglandins production; psoriasis; stroke (risk reduction); systemic lupus erythematosus (SLE)
Folic acid	Alcoholism; anemia; atherosclerosis; cancer prevention (colon and breast); cervical dysplasia; coronary heart disease (risk reduction); coronary restenosis (rate reduction by decreasing plasma homocysteine levels); Crohn disease; dementia and Alzheimer disease (risk reduction); depression; gingivitis; osteoporosis; pregnancy (prevention of birth defects) and lactation; schizophrenia (risk reduction, by decreasing homocysteine levels); ulcer, aphthous
Garcinia (*Garcinia cambogia*)	Pancreatic function (supportive) and glucose regulation; weight loss
Garlic (*Allium sativum*)	Antimicrobial (bacterial and fungal); antioxidant (practitioners should be aware that aged garlic extracts have been reported to improve this benefit); coagulation (mild inhibitor of platelet-activating factor); hyperlipidemia; hypertension; immune support
Ginger (*Zingiber officinale*)	Antiemetic, for nausea and vomiting in pregnancy; motion sickness; antiinflammatory (musculoskeletal); diverticulitis; indigestion/heartburn; osteoarthritis
Ginkgo (*Ginkgo biloba*)	Alzheimer disease, dementia; asthma; depression; epilepsy; headaches; intermittent claudication; macular degeneration; memory enhancement; Parkinson disease; peripheral blood flow (cerebral vascular disease, peripheral vascular insufficiency, impotence, tinnitus, and depression); seizures; sexual dysfunction (antidepressant-induced)

(continued)

Herb	Reported Uses
Ginseng, Panax (*Panax ginseng*)	Adrenal tonic; diabetes; physical and mental performance, [energy enhancement], chemotherapy and radiation (adjunct); immune support
Ginseng, Siberian (*Eleutherococcus senticosus*)	Adaptogen/tonic (promote wellness); athletic performance (enhancement); stress (decreased fatigue); immune support
Glucosamine	Osteoarthritis and joint structure support; rheumatoid arthritis and other inflammatory conditions
Glutamine	Alcoholism; athletic performance (enhancement); cancer (adjunct); catabolic wasting; chemotherapy (prevention of adverse effects); fibromyalgia; HIV infection (adjunct); immune support; peptic ulcer disease; postsurgical healing; ulcerative colitis and other inflammatory bowel diseases
Glutathione	Hepatoprotection (alcohol-induced liver damage); immune support; peptic ulcer disease
Golden seal (*Hydrastis canadensis*)	Fever; gallbladder; mucous membrane tonifying (used in inflammation of mucosal membranes); gastritis; antimicrobial (antibacterial/antifungal); bronchitis, cystitis, and infectious diarrhea; sinusitis; sore throat; urinary tract infection (UTI)
Gotu kola (*Centella asiatica*)	Connective tissue (support); hemorrhoids (topical); macular degeneration; memory enhancement; psoriasis; venous insufficiency; wound healing (topical)
Grapefruit seed (*Citrus paradisi*)	Antifungal, antibacterial, antiparasitic; diarrhea; diverticulitis; eczema; endometriosis; irritable bowel syndrome (IBS); rosacea; sinusitis; sore throat; ulcerative colitis; urinary tract infection (UTI)
Grape seed (*Vitis vinifera*)	Allergies, antiinflammatory, asthma; antioxidant; circulation, platelet aggregation inhibitor, capillary fragility, arterial/venous insufficiency (intermittent claudification, varicose veins); gingivitis; glaucoma; macular degeneration; multiple sclerosis; Parkinson disease; scleroderma
Green tea (*Camellia sinensis*)	Antioxidant; cancer and cardiovascular disease (preventive); chemotherapy and radiation (adjunct); diarrhea; gingivitis; hypercholesterolemia; macular degeneration; platelet-aggregation inhibitor
Ground ivy (*Hedera helix*)	Croup; mucolytic; upper respiratory congestion and cough
Guggul (*Commiphora mukul*)	Hypercholesterolemia; hypothyroidism; osteoarthritis; weight loss
Gymnema (*Gymnema sylvestre*)	Diabetes, blood sugar regulation
Hawthorn (*Crataegus oxyacantha*)	Angina, hypotension, hypertension, peripheral vascular disease, tachycardia; cardiotonic; congestive heart failure
Hops (*Humulus lupulus*)	Sedative/hypnotic (mild)
Horse chestnut (*Aesculus hippocastanum*)	Scleroderma; venous insufficiency (varicose veins, hemorrhoids, deep venous thrombosis, lower extremity edema [oral and topical])
Horsetail (*Equisetum arvense*)	Diuretic; high mineral content (including silicic acid); bone and connective tissue strengthening, including osteoporosis
Huperzine A (*Huperzia serrata*)	Senile dementia and Alzheimer disease
Hydroxymethyl butyrate (HMB)	Athletic performance (enhancement)
5-Hydroxytryptophan (5-HTP)	Anxiety; depression; fibromyalgia; headache; migraine; sleep disorders, insomnia (stimulates the production of melatonin); weight loss
Inositol hexaphosphate (IP-6)	Cancer (preventive)
Iodine	Fibrocystic breast disease; goiter (preventive); hypothyroidism; mucolytic agent
Ipriflavone	Prevention of osteoporosis (men and women)
Iron	Anemia; menorrhagia; pregnancy; restless legs syndrome
Isoflavones (soy)	Benign prostatic hyperplasia (BPH); cancer (preventive); cervical dysplasia; chemotherapy (adjunct); endometriosis; hypercholesterolemia; menopausal symptoms; osteoarthritis; osteoporosis; premenstrual syndrome (PMS)
Kava kava (*Piper methysticum*)	Fibromyalgia; insomnia; anxiety/stress, skeletal muscle relaxation, postischemic episodes; muscle soreness
Lactobacillus acidophilus	Constipation; diarrhea (infantile); eczema (preventive); gastrointestinal microflora recolonization; hypercholesterolemia; immune support; lactose intolerance; vaginal candidiasis

(continued)

Herb	Reported Uses
Lavender (*Lavendula officinalis*)	Wound healing including minor burns (topical)
Lemon balm/Melissa (*Melissa officinalis*)	Antiviral (oral herpes virus); attention deficit hyperactivity disorder (ADHD); sedation (pediatrics); teething (topical)
Licorice (*Glycyrrhiza glabra*)	Adrenal insufficiency (licorice); Crohn disease; croup; expectorant and antitussive (licorice); gastrointestinal ulceration (DGL chewable products)
Liver extract	Liver tonic
Lutein	Cataracts; macular degeneration
Lycopene	Atherosclerosis; cancer (preventive; especially lung and prostate); macular degeneration
Lysine	Angina pectoris; herpes simplex; osteoporosis; ulcer, aphthous
Magnesium	Asthma; attention deficit hyperactivity disorder (ADHD); cardiovascular disease; circulation; colic (magnesium salt); congestive heart failure (CHF); diabetes; dysmenorrhea; epilepsy; fatigue; fibromyalgia (magnesium salt); gallbladder (magnesium salt); heart disease; hypertension; hypoglycemia; insomnia; kidney stones; migraine headache; mitral valve prolapse (MVP); muscle cramps; nervousness; osteoporosis; premenstrual syndrome (PMS); stress/anxiety; multiple sclerosis
Malic acid	Aluminum toxicity; fibromyalgia
Manganese	Diabetes; epilepsy; osteoporosis
Marshmallow (*Althaea officinalis*)	Cough; croup; mucilaginous, demulcent; peptic ulcer disease; sore throat
Mastic (*Pistacia lentiscus*)	*H. pylori* inhibitor; peptic ulcer disease
Melatonin	Insomnia; jet lag; oxidative stress in dialysis patients (preventive)
Methionine	Liver detoxification
Methyl sulfonyl methane (MSM)	Allergies; analgesic; arthritis (osteo and rheumatoid); interstitial cystitis; lupus
Milk thistle (*Silybum marianum*)	Antidote for poisoning by Death Cup mushroom; antioxidant (specifically hepatic cells), liver diseases including acute/chronic hepatitis, jaundice, and stimulation of bile secretion/cholagogue; chemotherapy and radiation (adjunct); constipation; eczema; gallbladder; halitosis; hepatoprotective, including drug toxicities (ie, phenothiazines, butyrophenones, ethanol, and acetaminophen); hyperthyroidism; psoriasis; rosacea
Modified citrus pectin (MCP)	Anticarcinogenic; hypercholesterolemia
Muira puama (*Ptychopetalum olacoides*)	Athletic performance (enhancement); sexual vitality (males)
N-Acetyl cysteine (NAC)	Acetaminophen toxicity; AIDS; asthma (mucolytic, antioxidant); bronchitis; cardioprotection (during chemotherapy); fatigue; glutathione production; heavy metal detoxification; hyperthyroidism; hypothyroidism; macular degeneration; multiple sclerosis; nephropathy (preventive); Parkinson disease; scleroderma; systemic lupus erythematosus (SLE)
Nicotinamide adenine dinucleotide (NADH)	Chronic fatigue; Parkinson disease; stamina and energy
Olive leaf (*Olea europaea*)	Acne vulgaris; antibacterial; antifungal, antiviral; Crohn disease; diabetes; diarrhea; diverticulitis; eczema; endometriosis; hypertension; multiple sclerosis; scleroderma; ulcerative colitis; urinary tract infection (UTI)
Pancreatic extract	Antiinflammatory; cancer (adjunct); celiac disease; digestive disturbances; food allergies; immune complex diseases
Para-Aminobenzoic acid (PABA)	Peyronie disease; scleroderma; vitiligo
Parsley (*Petroselinum crispum*)	Halitosis; antibacterial, antifungal
Passion flower (*Passiflora spp*)	Hyperthyroidism; insomnia (sedative)
Peppermint (*Mentha piperita*)	Carminative, spasmolytic; colic; indigestion; irritable bowel syndrome; motion sickness
Phenylalanine	Reward deficiency syndrome in addiction; analgesic; depression; vitiligo
Phosphatidyl choline (PC)	Alcohol-induced liver damage; Alzheimer disease; gallstones; hepatitis
Phosphatidyl serine (PS)	Alzheimer disease; depression; memory enhancement

(continued)

Herb	Reported Uses
Potassium	Cardiac arrhythmias; congestive heart failure (CHF); hypertension; kidney stones
Pregnenolone	Arthritis; hormone precursor (DHEA, cortisol, progesterone, estrogens, and testosterone); mental performance
Progesterone	Breast cancer (preventive); dysmenorrhea; endometriosis; menopause symptoms; osteoporosis; premenstrual syndromes (PMS)
Psyllium (*Plantago ovata, Plantago isphagula*)	Bulk-forming laxative (containing 10% to 30% mucilage); halitosis
Pygeum (*Pygeum africanum, Prunus africana*)	Benign prostatic hyperplasia (BPH)
Pyruvate	Athletic performance (enhancement); weight loss
Quercetin	Allergies; asthma; atherosclerosis; cataracts; peptic ulcer disease; sinusitis
Red clover (*Trifolium pratense*)	Endometriosis; liver and kidney detoxification (liquid extract); menopause symptoms (proprietary extract contains 4 phytoestrogens); menorrhagia
Red yeast rice (*Monascus purpureus*)	Hypercholesterolemia
Rehmannia (*Rehmannia glutinosa*)	Rheumatoid arthritis; systemic lupus erythematosus (SLE)
Reishi (*Ganoderma lucidum*)	Chemotherapy and radiation (adjunct); hypertension; seizure disorder; immune support; fatigue
SAMe (S-adenosyl methionine)	Cardiovascular disease; depression; fibromyalgia; headache; insomnia; liver disease; osteoarthritis; rheumatoid arthritis
Saw palmetto (*Serenoa repens*)	Benign prostatic hyperplasia (BPH)
Schisandra (*Schizandra chinensis*)	Adaptogen/tonic (to promote wellness); hepatic protection and detoxification; chemotherapy and radiation (adjunct); endurance, stamina, and work performance (enhancement); decreases fatigue
Selenium	Acne vulgaris (with vitamin E); AIDS; atherosclerosis; bronchial asthma; cancer (preventive); cardiomyopathy; cataracts; chemotherapy and radiation (adjunct); circulation; eczema; epilepsy; hemorrhoids; herpes simplex 1 and 2; hypothyroidism; macular degeneration; prostate cancer (preventive); ulcerative colitis
Senna (*Cassia senna*)	Laxative
Shark cartilage	Cancer; osteoarthritis, rheumatoid arthritis
Spleen extract	Chemotherapy and radiation (adjunct); cold/flu; fatigue; spleen function (supportive)
Stinging nettle (*Urtica dioica*)	Leaf used for allergic rhinitis, allergy and hay fever symptoms, uric acid excretion, and sinusitis; root used for benign prostatic hyperplasia (BPH)
St John's wort (*Hypericum perforatum*)	Antibacterial, antiinflammatory (topical: minor wounds, infections, bruises, muscle soreness, and sprains); mild to moderate depression, melancholia, stress and anxiety
Taurine	Congestive heart failure (CHF); diabetes; gallbladder; hypertension; seizure disorders
Tea tree (*Melaleuca alternifolia*)	**Not for ingestion**; acne vulgaris; antifungal, antibacterial; mouthwash for dental and oral health; burns, cuts, scrapes, insect bites
Thyme (*Thymus vulgaris*)	Antifungal; cough (upper respiratory origin); croup
Thymus extract	Fatigue; immune support; otitis media; sinusitis; systemic lupus erythematosus (SLE)
Thyroid extract	Fatigue; immune support; fibromyalgia
Tocotrienols	Cancer (preventive); heart disease; hypercholesterolemia; skin (supportive, protective)
Tribulus (*Tribulus terrestris*)	Athletic performance (enhancement), sexual vitality
Turmeric (*Curcuma longa*)	Antioxidant; antiinflammatory; antirheumatic; hypercholesterolemia; dysmenorrhea; muscle soreness
Tylophora (*Tylophora asthmatica*)	Allergies; asthma
Tyrosine	Alzheimer disease; depression; hypothyroidism; phenylketonuria (PKU); substance abuse
Uva-Ursi (*Arctostaphylos uva-ursi*)	Urinary tract infections and kidney stone prevention

(continued)

Herb	Reported Uses
Valerian (*Valeriana officinalis*)	Hyperthyroidism; insomnia (sedative/hypnotic); premenstrual syndrome (PMS), menopause; restless motor syndromes and muscle spasms
Vanadium	Diabetes, type 1; diabetes, type 2; hypoglycemia
Vinpocetine	Cognitive function; Alzheimer disease and senility
Vitamin A (Retinol)	Acne vulgaris; AIDS; cancer (preventive); cervical dysplasia; circulation; cold/flu; Crohn disease; diverticulitis; eczema; fibrocystic breast disease (FBD); glaucoma; hemorrhoids; measles; menorrhagia; night blindness; otitis media; premenstrual syndrome (PMS); psoriasis; rosacea; sore throat; ulcerative colitis; urinary tract infection (UTI)
Vitamin B_1 (Thiamine)	Alcoholism; Alzheimer disease; anemia (megaloblastic); congestive heart failure (CHF); diabetes; fibromyalgia; insomnia; neurological conditions (Bell palsy, trigeminal neuralgia, sciatica, sensory neuropathies); psychiatric illness
Vitamin B_2	Cataracts; depression; migraine
Vitamin B_3	Acne vulgaris (4% niacinamide topical gel); cataracts; coronary disease (preventive); diabetes, type 1; diabetes, type 2; hyperlipidemia (hypercholesterolemia, hypertriglyceridemia); impaired glucose tolerance; intermittent claudication; myocardial infarction (risk reduction); osteoarthritis; Raynaud syndrome; rheumatoid arthritis; schizophrenia; antioxidant
Vitamin B_5 (Pantothenic acid)	Adrenal support; allergies; arthritis; constipation; hyperlipidemia (pantethine, but not pantothenic acid, lowers cholesterol and triglycerides); rheumatoid arthritis; wound healing
Vitamin B_6 (Pyridoxine)	Arthritis; asthma; autism; cardiovascular disease; carpal tunnel syndrome; coronary heart disease (risk reduction); coronary restenosis (rate reduction by lowering plasma homocysteine levels); dementia and Alzheimer disease (risk reduction); depression (associated with oral contraceptives); diabetic peripheral neuropathy; epilepsy, B_6-dependant; headache; insomnia; kidney stones; monosodium glutamate (MSG) sensitivity; nausea and vomiting (in pregnancy); peptic ulcer disease; PMS
Vitamin B_{12} (Cobalamin)	AIDS; asthma; atherosclerosis (due to homocysteine elevation); coronary restenosis (rate reduction by lowering plasma homocysteine levels); Crohn disease; dementia and Alzheimer disease (risk reduction); depression; diabetic peripheral neuropathy; male infertility; memory loss; multiple sclerosis; pernicious anemia; sulfite sensitivity
Vitamin B complex-25	See individual B vitamins
Vitamin C	AIDS; allergies; antioxidant; asthma; atherosclerosis; cancer; cataracts; cervical dysplasia; circulation; cold; constipation; coronary heart disease (preventive, in patients laking lipid-lowering agents); Crohn disease; diabetes; diverticulitis; eczema; endometriosis; fatigue; fever; fibrocystic breast disease (FBD); fibromyalgia; gallbladder disease (risk reduction); gingivitis; glaucoma; herpes simplex virus 1 and 2; immune support; irritable bowel syndrome (IBS); multiple sclerosis; myocardial infarction (risk reduction); nitrate tolerance (preventive); osteoporosis; otitis media; Parkinson disease; peptic ulcer disease; psoriasis; reflex sympathetic dystrophy (preventive); sinusitis; sore throat; stress/anxiety; sunburn; ulcerative colitis; urinary tract infection (UTI); wound healing
Vitamin D	Crohn disease; epilepsy (during anticonvulsant therapy); hearing loss; osteoporosis; psoriasis; rickets; scleroderma
Vitamin E	Acne vulgaris (with selenium); Alzheimer disease; atherosclerosis; Benign prostatic hyperplasia (BPH); cancer (preventive); cataracts; cervical dysplasia; circulation; diabetes; dyslipidemias; eczema; endometriosis; epilepsy; fibrocystic breast disease (FBD); gallbladder; hemorrhoids; macular degeneration; multiple sclerosis; myocardial infarction (risk reduction); osteoarthritis; peptic ulcer disease; peripheral circulation; premenstrual syndrome (PMS); psoriasis; rheumatoid arthritis; scleroderma; sunburn; systemic lupus erythematosus; ulcerative colitis
Vitamin K	Osteoporosis; synthesis of blood clotting factors
White oak (*Quercus alba*)	Antiinflammatory (mild: throat and mouth as a soothing agent)
White willow (*Salix alba*)	Antipyretic; antiinflammatory
Wild yam (*Dioscorea villosa*)	Female vitality (conversion to progesterone in the body is poor)
Yohimbe (*Pausinystalia yohimbe*)	Sexual vitality (men and women); male erectile dysfunction
Zinc	Acne vulgaris; aphthous ulcers; benign prostatic hyperplasia (BPH); common cold; Crohn disease; diabetes; diaper rash; diverticulitis; gastric ulcer healing; immune support; macular degeneration; osteoporosis; otitis media; sexual vitality (men); skin conditions, eczema, psoriasis; sore throat; ulcerative colitis; wound healing

TOP 200 PRESCRIBED DRUGS*

Brand Name (if appropriate)	Generic Name	Rank
Accupril®	quinapril	118
----	acetaminophen and codeine	43
Aciphex®	rabeprazole	110
Actonel®	risedronate	81
Actos®	pioglitazone	79
----	acyclovir	158
Adderall XR™	dextroamphetamine and amphetamine	89
Advair™ Diskus®	fluticasone and salmeterol	34
----	albuterol (aerosol)	10
----	albuterol (nebulization solution)	108
Allegra®	fexofenadine	56
Allegra-D® 12 Hour	fexofenadine and pseudoephedrine	132
----	allopurinol	76
----	alprazolam	8
Altace®	ramipril	65
Amaryl®	glimepiride	127
Ambien®	zolpidem	19
----	amitriptyline	50
----	amoxicillin	3
----	amoxicillin and clavulanate potassium	33
Aricept®	donepezil	161
----	atenolol	6
----	atenolol chlorthalidone	199
Avalide®	irbesartan and hydrochlorothiazide	176
Avandia®	rosiglitazone	71
Avapro®	irbesartan	126
Aviane™	ethinyl estradiol and levonorgestrel	186
----	azithromycin	164
----	benazepril	124
Benicar®	olmesartan	146
Benicar HTC®	olmesartan and hydrochlorothiazide	171
----	benzonatate	180
----	betamethasone and clotrimazole	174
----	bisoprolol and hydrochlorothiazide	148
----	bupropion SR	179
----	buspirone	166
----	butalbital, acetaminophen, and caffeine	162
----	carisoprodol	74
Cartia® XT	diltiazem	183
Celebrex®	celecoxib	67
----	cephalexin	18
Cialis®	tadalafil	175
----	ciprofloxacin	53
----	citalopram	83
Clarinex®	desloratadine	149
----	clindamycin	119
----	clonazepam	39
----	clonidine	77

*NDC Health, "The Top 200 Prescriptions for 2005 by Number of U.S. Prescriptions Dispensed," Available at: http://www.rxlist.com/top200.htm

(continued)

Brand Name (if appropriate)	Generic Name	Rank
Combivent®	ipratropium and albuterol	123
Concerta™	methylphenidate	96
Coreg®	carvedilol	95
Coumadin®	warfarin	134
Cozaar®	losartan	93
Crestor®	rosuvastatin	102
Cymbalta®	duloxetine	143
----	cyclobenzaprine	49
Depakote®	valproic acid and derivatives	165
Detrol® LA	tolterodine	139
----	dextroamphetamine and amphetamine	188
----	diazepam	60
----	diclofenac	136
Digitek®	digoxin	111
----	digoxin	190
----	diltiazem CD	138
Diovan®	valsartan	58
Diovan HCT®	valsartan and hydrochlorothiazide	73
----	doxazosin	133
----	doxycycline	69
Effexor® XR	venlafaxine	36
----	enalapril	59
Endocet®	oxycodone and acetaminophen	197
----	estradiol	129
----	etodolac	198
Evista®	raloxifene	137
----	famotidine	189
----	fexofenadine	177
Flomax®	tamsulosin	101
Flonase®	fluticasone	47
----	fluconazole	62
----	fluoxetine	29
----	folic acid	91
Fosamax®	alendronate	35
----	furosemide	7
----	gabapentin	45
----	gemfibrozil	125
----	glipizide	135
----	glipizide ER	103
----	glyburide	87
----	glyburide and metformin	141
GlycoLax™	polyethylene glycol 3350	157
Humalog®	insulin lispro	184
----	hydrochlorothiazide	5
----	hydrochlorothiazide and triamterene	23
----	hydrocodone and acetaminophen	1
----	hydroxyzine	130
Hyzaar®	losartan and hydrochlorothiazide	116
----	ibuprofen	17
Imitrex®	sumatriptan	152
----	isosorbide mononitrate	85
Klor-Con®	potassium chloride	64
Lamictal®	lamotrigine	155

(continued)

Brand Name (if appropriate)	Generic Name	Rank
Lanoxin®	digoxin	187
Lantus®	insulin glargine	98
Levaquin®	levofloxacin	51
Levothroid®	levothyroxine	191
----	levothyroxine	12
Levoxyl®	levothyroxine	57
Lexapro®	escitalopram	16
Lipitor®	atorvastatin	2
----	lisinopril	4
----	lisinopril and hydrochlorothiazide	63
----	lorazepam	30
Lotrel®	amlodipine and benazepril	54
----	lovastatin	72
----	meclizine	140
----	metformin	14
----	metformin ER	115
----	methylprednisolone	78
----	methotrexate	168
----	metoclopramide	131
----	metoprolol	28
----	metronidazole	120
----	minocycline	151
----	mirtazapine	147
Mobic®	meloxicam	100
----	nabumetone	153
----	naproxen	61
Nasacort® AQ	triamcinolone	160
Nasonex®	mometasone	90
Nexium™	esomeprazole	22
Niaspan®	niacin	163
----	nifedipine ER	192
----	nitrofurantoin	144
Nitroquick®	nitroglycerin	195
----	nortriptyline	193
Norvasc®	amlodipine	11
----	omeprazole	106
Omnicef®	cefdinir	107
Ortho Evra®	ethinyl estradiol and norelgestromin	82
Ortho Tri-Cyclen®	ethinyl estradiol and norgestimate	178
Ortho Tri-Cyclen® Lo	ethinyl estradiol and norgestimate	104
----	oxycodone	150
----	oxycodone and acetaminophen	32
Oxycontin®	oxycodone	169
Patanol®	olopatadine	181
----	paroxetine	38
Paxil CR®	paroxetine	185
----	penicillin V potassium	86
----	phentermine	200
----	phenytoin	196
Plavix®	clopidogrel	31
----	potassium chloride	42
Pravachol®	pravastatin	80
----	prednisone	21
Premarin®	estrogens (conjugated)	46

(continued)

Brand Name (if appropriate)	Generic Name	Rank
Prevacid®	lansoprazole	27
----	promethazine	99
----	promethazine and codeine	145
----	propoxyphene and acetaminophen	24
----	propranolol	159
Protonix®	pantoprazole	41
----	quinine	182
----	ranitidine	55
Rhinocort® Aqua®	budesonide	170
Risperdal®	risperidone	109
Seroquel®	quetiapine	92
Singulair®	montelukast	26
Skelaxin®	metaxalone	173
----	spironolactone	112
----	sulfamethoxazole and trimethoprim	44
Strattera®	atomoxetine	142
Synthroid®	levothyroxine	13
----	temazepam	105
----	terazosin	172
Topamax®	topiramate	122
Toprol-XL®	metoprolol	9
----	tramadol	52
----	trazodone	48
----	triamcinin acetonide	121
TriCor®	fenofibrate	94
TriNessa™	ethinyl estradiol and norgestimate	128
Tri-Sprintec®	ethinyl estradiol and norgestimate	167
Tussionex®	hydrocodone and chlorpheniramine	194
Valtrex®	valacyclovir	113
----	verapamil	84
Viagra®	sildenafil	68
Vytorin™	ezetimibe and simvastatin	97
----	warfarin	37
Wellbutrin XL™	bupropion	66
Xalatan®	latanoprost	114
Yasmin® 28	ethinyl estradiol and drospirenone	75
Zetia™	ezetimibe	70
Zithromax® Z-Pak®	azithromycin	20
Zithromax® Tablets	azithromycin	117
Zithromax® Suspension	azithromycin	88
Zocor®	simvastatin	25
Zoloft®	sertraline	15
Zyprexa®	olanzapine	154
Zyrtec® Tablets	cetirizine	40
Zyrtec® Syrup	cetirizine	156

NEW DRUGS ADDED SINCE LAST EDITION

Brand Name	Generic Name	Use
Amitiza™	lubiprostone	A chloride channel activator for treatment of chronic idiopathic constipation
Azilect®	rasagiline	An MAO-B inhibitor for Parkinson disease
Chantix™	varenicline	A partial nicotinic receptor agonist for smoking cessation
Dacogen™	decitabine	Treatment of myelodysplastic syndromes
Erasis™	anidulafungin	An I.V. antifungal for treatment of *Candida* infection
Factive®	gemifloxacin	Bacterial sinusitis and community-acquired pneumonia
Gardasil®	papillomavirus (Types 6, 11, 16, 18) recombinant vaccine	Vaccine to prevent diseases caused by HPV (ie, cervical cancer, genital warts)
Lucentis™	ranibizumab	Treatment of "wet" age-related macular degeneration
Myozyme®	alglucosidase	Treatment of Pompe disease
Orencia®	abatacept	Rheumatoid arthritis
Prezista™	darunavir	A protease inhibitor used with ritonavir for advanced HIV disease
Ranexa™	ranolazine	An oral antianginal/anti-ischemic agent for treatment of chronic angina
Revlimid®	lenalidomide	Myelodysplastic syndromes
RotaTeq®	rotavirus vaccine	Oral vaccine to prevent rotavirus gastroenteritis in infants
Sprycel™	dasatinib	Treatment of leukemia
Sutent®	sunitinib	An oral tyrosine kinase inhibitor for stomach and kidney cancer
Vaprisol®	conivaptan	Hyponatremia
Zostavax®	zoster vaccine, live	Vaccine to prevent shingles in adults

PENDING DRUGS OR DRUGS IN CLINICAL TRIALS

Proposed Brand Name or Synonym	Generic Name	Use
Alvesco®	ciclesonide	Asthma
Certican®	everolimus	Prevention of rejection after transplants
Enterreg®	alvimopan	Postoperative ileus
Neurocrine®	indiplon	Insomnia
Nuvigal®	armodanfinil	Narcolepsy, sleepiness
Oxyprim®	oxypurinol	Hyperuricemia
Pargluva®	muraglitazar	Type 2 diabetes
Preos®	parathyroid hormone	Osteoporosis
Rasilez®	aliskiren	Hypertension
Retaane®	anecortave acetate	Macular degeneration
Riquent®	abetimus	Lupus
Sanvar IR®	vapreotide	Esophageal varices
Surfaxin®	lucinactant	Respiratory distress syndrome
Xcytrin®	motexafin gadolinium	Brain cancer

PHARMACEUTICAL MANUFACTURERS AND DISTRIBUTORS

AAI Development Services (aaiPharma)
2320 Scientific Park Drive
Wilmington, NC 28405
(800) 575-4224
www.aaiintl.com

aaiPharma
2320 Scientific Park Drive
Wilmington, NC 28405
(800) 575-4224
www.aaipharma.com

Abbott Laboratories (Pharmaceutical Products Division)
100 Abbott Park Road
Abbott Park, IL 60064-3500
(800) 222-6883
www.abbott.com

Actavis U.S.
200 Elmora Avenue
Elizabeth, NJ 07207
(800) 432-8534
www.actavis.us

Adams Respiratory Therapeutics
425 Main Street
Colonial Court
Chester, NJ 07930
(908) 879-1400
www.adamslabs.com

Advanced Medical Optics
1700 East Street Andrew Place
Santa Ana, CA 92705
(714) 247-8200
www.amo-inc.com

Advanced Vision Research
12 Alfred Street
Suite 200
Woburn, MA 01801
(800) 579-8327
www.theratears.com

Aero Pharmaceuticals, Inc
3848 FAU Boulevard
Suite 100
Boca Raton, FL 33431
(800) 223-6837
www.aeropharmaceuticals.com

Akorn, Inc
2500 Millbrook Drive
Buffalo Grove, IL 60089
(888) 519-8384
www.akorn.com

AkPharma, Inc
6840 Old Egg Harbor Road
Pleasantville, NJ 08232
(800) 994-4711
www.akpharma.com

Alcon Laboratories, Inc
6201 South Freeway
Fort Worth, TX 76134
(800) 451-3937
www.alconlabs.com

Allen & Hanburys
Five Moore Drive
Research Triangle Park, NC 27709
(800) 334-0089

ALLERDERM Laboratories
3400 East McDowell Road
Phoenix, AZ 85008-7899
(800) 365-6868
www.allerderm.com

Allergan, Inc
PO Box 19534
Irvine, CA 92623-9534
(800) 433-8871
www.allergan.com

Alliance Pharmaceutical, Inc
4660 LaJolla Village Drive
Suite 825
San Diego, CA 92122
(858) 410-5200
www.allp.com

Allscripts, LLC
2401 Commerce Avenue
Libertyville, IL 60048-4464
(800) 654-0889
www.allscripts.com

Almay, Inc
1501 Williamsboro Street
Oxford, NC 27565
(800) 992-5629
www.almay.com

Alpharma, Inc
One Executive Drive
Fort Lee, NJ 07024
(800) 645-4216
www.alpharma.com

Alpharma USPD, Inc (see Actavis U.S.)

Alpha Therapeutic (see Grifols)

Altaire Pharmaceuticals, Inc
PO Box 849
West Lane
Aquebogue, NY 11931
(800) 258-2471
www.otcdruggist.com

Alza Corp
1900 Charleston Road
PO Box 7210
Mountain View, CA 94039-7210
(650) 564-5000
www.alza.com

Amarin Pharmaceuticals, Inc
(see Valeant Pharmaceuticals)

Ambix Laboratories
55 West End Road
Totowa, NJ 07512
(973) 890-9002
www.ambixlabs.com

Amcon Laboratories
40 North Rock Hill Road
St Louis, MO 63119
(800) 255-6161
www.amcon-labs.com

American Lecithin Company
115 Hurley Road
Unit 2B
Oxford, CT 06478
(800) 364-4416
www.americanlecithin.com

American Medical Industries Health Products
330 East Third Street
Suite 2
Dell Rapids, SD 57022-1918
(605) 428-5501
www.ezhealthcare.com

American Pharmaceutical Partners, Inc (APP)
(See APP-Abraxis Pharmaceutical Products)

American Red Cross
2025 E Street Northwest
Washington, DC 20006
(202) 303-4498
www.redcross.org

American Regent Laboratories
One Luitpold Drive
Shirley, NY 11967
(800) 645-1706
www.americanregent.com

Amgen, Inc
One Amgen Center Drive
Thousand Oaks, CA 91320-1799
(800) 772-6436
www.amgen.com

AMSCO Scientific (see Steris Corp)

Amylin Pharmaceuticals, Inc
9360 Towne Centre Drive
Suite 110
San Diego, California 92121
(858) 552-2200
www.amylin.com

Andrew Jergens Company
2535 Spring Grove Avenue
Cincinnati, OH 45214-1773
(800) 742-8798
www.jergens.com

Andrx Corp
4955 Orange Drive
Davie, FL 33314
(954) 584-0300
www.andrx.com

Angelini Pharmaceuticals
50 Tice Boulevard
Woodcliff Lake, NJ 07677
(201) 476-9000
www.angelinipharmaceuticals.com

Antibodies, Inc
PO Box 1560
Davis, CA 95617
(800) 824-8540
www.antibodiesinc.com

Antigenics, Inc
630 Fifth Avenue
Suite 2100
New York, NY 10111
(212) 994-8200
www.antigenic.com

Apotex Corp
2400 North Commerce Parkway
Suite 400
Weston, FL 33326
(800) 706-5575
www.apotexcorp.com

Apothecary Products, Inc
11750 12th Avenue South
Burnsville, MN 55337-1295
(800) 328-2742
www.apothecaryproducts.com

Apothecon
PO Box 4500
Princeton, NJ 08543-4500
(800) 321-1335

Apothecus Pharmaceutical Corp
220 Townsend Square
Oyster Bay, NY 11771-1532
(800) 227-2393
www.apothecus.com

APP-Abraxis Pharmaceutical Products
1501 East Woodfield Road
Suite 300 East
Schaumburg, IL 60173-5837
(888) 386-1300
www.appdrugs.com

A P Pharma
123 Saginaw Drive
Redwood City, CA 94063
(650) 366-2626
www.appharma.com

Applied Genetics, Inc Dermatics
205 Buffalo Avenue
Freeport, NY 11520
(516) 868-9026
www.agiderm.com

Astellas Pharma U.S., Inc
Three Parkway North
Deerfield, IL 60015-2548
(800) 695-4321
www.astellas.com

AstraZeneca Pharmaceuticals, LP
1800 Concord Pike
PO Box 15437
Wilmington, DE 19850-5437
(800) 842-9920
www.astrazeneca-us.com

Atley Pharmaceuticals, Inc
10511 Old Ridge Road
Ashland, VA 23005
(804) 227-2250
www.atley.com

Aventis Behring
1020 First Avenue
PO Box 61501
King of Prussia, PA 19406-0901
(610) 878-4000
www.aventisbehring.com

Axcan Scandipharm, Inc
22 Inverness Center Parkway
Birmingham, AL 35242
(800) 472-2634
www.axcanscandipharm.com

AXM Pharma
7251 West Lake Mead Boulevard
Suite 300
Las Vegas, Nevada 89128
(702) 562-4155
www.axmpharma.com

Bajamar Chemical Company, Inc
9609 Dielman Rock Island
St Louis, MO 63132
(888) 242-3414
www.vesselvite.com

Banner
4100 Mendenhall Oaks Parkway
Suite 301
High Point, NC 27265
(336) 812-3442
www.banpharm.com

Barr Laboratories, Inc
2 Quaker Road
PO Box 2900
Pomona, NY 10970
(800) 222-0190
www.barrlabs.com

Bausch & Lomb Pharmaceuticals (BD)
8500 Hidden River Parkway
Tampa, FL 33637
(800) 323-0000
www.bausch.com

Bausch & Lomb Surgical, Inc
180 Via Verde
San Dimas, CA 91773
(800) 338-2020
www.bausch.com

Baxa Corp
13760 East Arapahoe Road
Englewood, CO 80112-3903
(800) 567-2292
www.baxa.com

Baxter Healthcare Corp
Corp Headquarters
One Baxter Parkway
Deerfield, IL 60015-4625
(800) 422-9837
www.baxter.com

Baxter Pharmaceutical Solutions
927 South Curry Pike
Bloomington, IN 47403
(800) 353-0887
www.baxterdrugdelivery.com

Bayer Corp
(Pharmaceutical Division)
400 Morgan Lane
West Haven, CT 06516-4175
(203) 812-2000
www.bayerus.com

Bayer Corp
(Consumer Care Division)
36 Columbia Road
PO Box 1910
Morristown, NJ 07962-1910
(800) 331-4536
www.bayercare.com

Bayer Corp
(Diagnostic Division)
511 Benedict Avenue
Tarrytown, NY 10591-5097
(914) 631-8000
www.bayerdiag.com

Bayer, Inc
77 Belfield Road
Etobicoke, Ontario, Canada M9W 1G6
(800) 268-1331
www.bayer.ca

B Braun Medical
824 Twelfth Avenue
Bethlehem, PA 18018
(800) 854-6851
www.bbraunusa.com

BD Medical Pharmaceutical Systems
One Becton Drive
Franklin Lakes, NJ 07417
(201) 847-4017
www.bd.com

BD Biosciences
2350 Qume Drive
San Jose, CA 95131-1807
(877) 232-8995
www.bdbiosciences.com

Beckman Coulter, Inc
4300 North Harbor Boulevard
PO Box 3100
Fullerton, CA 92834-3100
(800) 742-2345
www.beckman.com

Bedford Laboratories
300 Northfield Road
Bedford, OH 44146
(440) 232-3320
www.bedfordlabs.com

Beiersdorf, Inc
Wilton Corporate Center
187 Danbury Road
Wilton, CT 06897
(203) 563-5800
www.beiersdorf.com

Berlex Laboratories, Inc
340 Changebridge Road
PO Box 1000
Montville, NJ 07045-1000
(888) 237-5394
www.berlex.com

Berna Products Corp
4216 Ponce de Leon Boulevard
Coral Gables, FL 33146
(800) 533-5899
www.bernaproducts.com

Bertek Pharmaceuticals, Inc
781 Chestnut Ridge Road
Morgantown, WV 26505
(304) 285-6420
www.bertek.com

Beta Dermaceuticals, Inc
PO Box 691106
San Antonio, TX 78269-1106
(210) 349-9326
www.beta-derm.com

Beutlich Pharmaceuticals
1541 Shields Drive
Waukegan, IL 60085
(800) 238-8542
www.beutlich.com

B. F. Ascher & Company, Inc
15501 West 109th Street
Lenexa, KS 66219-1308
(800) 324-1880
www.bfascher.com

Biocraft Laboratories, Inc
(see Teva Pharmaceuticals USA)

BioCryst Pharmaceuticals, Inc
2190 Parkway Lake Drive
Birmingham, AL 35244
(205) 444-4600
www.biocryst.com

Biogen idec
14 Cambridge Center
Cambridge, MA 02142
(800) 262-4363
www.biogen.com

BioGenex
4600 Norris Canyon Road
San Ramon, CA 94583
(800) 421-4149
www.biogenex.net

Biomerica, Inc
1533 Monrovia Avenue
Newport Beach, CA 92663
(949) 645-2111
www.biomerica.com

Biomira USA, Inc
70 South Main Street
Suite B and C
Cranbury, NJ 08512
(877) 234-0444
www.biomira.com

Biopure Corp
11 Hurley Street
Cambridge, MA 02141
(617) 234-6500
www.biopure.com

BioScrip
10900 Red Circle Drive
Minnetonka, MN 55343
(800) 444-5951
www.bioscrip.com

Biospecifics Technologies Corp
35 Wilbur Street
Lynbrook, NY 11563
(516) 593-7000
www.biospecifics.com

BIO-TECH Pharmacal, Inc
PO Box 1992
Fayetteville, AR 72702
(800) 345-1199
www.bio-tech-pharm.com

Birchwood Laboratories, Inc
7900 Fuller Road
Eden Prairie, MN 55344-2195
(800) 328-6156
www.birchlabs.com

Blaine Pharmaceuticals
1717 Dixie Highway
Suite 700
Fort Wright, KY 41011
(800) 633-9353
www.blainepharma.com

Blairex Laboratories, Inc
1600 Brian Drive
PO Box 2127
Columbus, IN 47202-2127
(800) 252-4739
www.blairex.com

Blansett Pharmacal Company, Inc
PO Box 638
North Little Rock, AR 72115
(800) 816-9695
www.blansett.com

Blistex, Inc
1800 Swift Drive
Oak Brook, IL 60523-1574
(800) 837-1800
www.blistex.com

Block Drug Company, Inc
(see GlaxoSmithKline)

Bluco, Inc
28350 Schoolcraft
Livonia, MI 48150
(800) 832-4464
www.blucoinc.com

Boehringer Ingelheim Pharmaceuticals, Inc
900 Ridgebury Road
PO Box 368
Ridgefield, CT 06877-0368
(800) 542-6257
www.us.boehringer-ingelheim.com

Boehringer Mannheim (see Roche Pharmaceuticals)

Bone Care International
(see Genzyme Corp)

Bracco Diagnostics, Inc
107 College Road East
Princeton, NJ 08540
(800) 631-5245
www.bracco.com

Bradley Pharmaceuticals, Inc
383 Route 46 West
Fairfield, NJ 07004-2402
(973) 882-1505
www.bradpharm.com

Braintree Laboratories, Inc
PO Box 850929
Braintree, MA 02185-0929
(800) 874-6756
www.braintreeLabs.com

Breckenridge Pharmaceutical, Inc
1141 South Rogers Circle
Suite 3
Boca Raton, FL 33487
(800) 367-3395
www.breckenridgepharma.com

Bristol-Myers Squibb Company
(Pharmaceutical Division)
PO Box 4500
Princeton, NJ 08543-4500
(800) 631-5244
www.bms.com

Bristol-Myers Squibb OTC
1350 Liberty Avenue
Hillside, NJ 07205
(800) 468-7746
www.bms.com

Bryan Corp
4 Plympton Street
Woburn, MA 01801
(800) 343-7711
www.bryancorporation.com

Burroughs Wellcome Company
(see GlaxoSmithKline)

Calmoseptine, Inc
16602 Burke Lane
Huntington Beach, CA 92647
(800) 800-3405
www.calmoseptineointment.com

Capellon Pharmaceuticals, LTD
7509 Flagstone Street
Fort Worth, TX 76118
(817) 595-5820
www.capellon.com

Caraco Pharmaceutical Laboratories, LTD
1150 Elijah McCoy Drive
Detroit, MI 48202
(800) 818-4555
www.caraco.com

Cardinal Health, Inc
7000 Cardinal Place
Dublin, OH 43017
(800) 234-8701
www.cardinal.com

Cardinal Health, Inc
Nuclear Pharmacy Services
6464 Canoga Avenue
Woodland Hills, CA 91367
(818) 737-4000
www.cardinal.com/nps

Carma Laboratories, Inc
5801 West Airways Avenue
Franklin, WI 53132
(414) 421-7707
www.carma-labs.com

Carolina Medical Products Company
PO Box 147
Farmville, NC 27828
(800) 227-6637
www.carolinamedical.com

Carrington Laboratories
2001 Walnut Hill Lane
Irving, TX 73038
(972) 518-1300
www.carringtonlabs.com

C. B. Fleet Company, Inc
4615 Murray Place
PO Box 11349
Lynchburg, VA 24506
(800) 999-9711
www.cbfleet.com

CCA Industries, Inc
200 Murray Hill Parkway
East Rutherford, NJ 07073
(201) 330-1400
www.ccaindustries.com

Celgene Corp
7 Powder Horn Drive
Warren, NJ 07059
(732) 271-1001
www.celgene.com

Cellegy Pharmaceuticals, Inc
349 Oyster Point Boulevard
Suite 200
South San Francisco, CA 94080
(650) 616-2200
www.cellegy.com

Celltech Pharmaceuticals, Inc
755 Jefferson Road
Rochester, NY 14623
(800) 234-5535
www.celltechgroup.com

Centeon (see Aventis Behring)

Centers for Disease Control and Prevention
1600 Clifton Road
Atlanta, GA 30333
(800) 311-3435
www.cdc.gov

Centocor, Inc
800/850 Ridgeview Drive
Horsham, PA 19044
(610) 651-6000
www.centocor.com

Central Pharmaceuticals, Inc
(see Schwarz Pharma, Inc)

Cephalon, Inc
41 Moores Road
Frazer, PA 19355
(610) 344-0200
www.cephalon.com

Cetylite Industries, Inc
9051 River Road
Pennsauken, NJ 08110
(800) 257-7740
www.cetylite.com

Chesapeake Biological Laboratories, Inc
1111 South Paca Street
Baltimore, MD 21230
(410) 843-5000
www.cblinc.com

Chiron Corp
4560 Horton Street
Emeryville, CA 94608-2916
(510) 655-8730
www.chiron.com

Chronimed, Inc
(see BioScrip)

Chugai Pharma USA, LLC
One Crossroads Drive
Building A, 2nd Floor
Bedminister, NJ 07921-2688
(212) 759-8812
www.chugai-pharm.com

Ciba-Geigy Pharmaceuticals
(see Novartis Pharmaceuticals Corp)

CIBA Vision
11460 Johns Creek Parkway
Duluth, GA 30097
(678) 415-3937
www.cibavision.com

Circa Pharmaceuticals, Inc
(see Watson Laboratories, Inc)

Cirrus Healthcare Products, LLC
60 Main Street
PO Box 220
Cold Spring Harbor, NY 11724
(800) 327-6151
www.earplanes.com

CIS-US, Inc
10 DeAngelo Drive
Bedford, MA 01730
(800) 221-7554
www.cisusinc.com

Claragen, Inc
387 Technology Drive
College Park, MD 20742
(301) 405-8593
www.claragen.com

Clay-Park Labs, Inc (See Perrigo Company)

C & M Pharmacal, Inc
(see Genesis Pharmaceutical, Inc)

CNS, Inc
20 Troy Road
Whippany, NJ 07981
(800) 858-6673
www.cns.com

Colgate Oral Pharmaceuticals
One Colgate Way
Canton, MA 02021
(800) 226-5428
www.colgateprofessional.com

Colgate-Palmolive Company
300 Park Avenue
New York, NY 10022
(800) 468-6502
www.colgate.com

CollaGenex Pharmaceuticals, Inc
41 University Drive
Newtown, PA 18940
(888) 339-5678
www.collagenex.com

Columbia Laboratories, Inc
354 Eisenhower Parkway
Second Floor-Plaza 1
Livingston, NJ 07039
(973) 994-3999
www.columbialabs.com

Combe, Inc
1101 Westchester Avenue
White Plains, NY 10604
(800) 873-7400
www.combe.com

CompliMed Medical Research Group
1441 West Smith Road
Ferndale, WA 98248
(888) 977-8008
www.complimed.com

Conair Interplak Division
One Cummings Point Road
Stamford, CT 06902
(203) 351-9000
www.interplak.com

Connaught Labs (see Aventis Pasteur)

Connetics Corp
3160 Porter Drive
Palo Alto, CA 94304
(888) 969-2628
www.connetics.com

Contract Pharmacal Corp
135 Adams Avenue
Hauppauge, NY 11788
(631) 231-4610
www.contractpharmacal.com

ConvaTec
(Bristol-Myers Squibb Company)
PO Box 5254
Princeton, NJ 08543-5254
(800) 422-8811
www.convatec.com

CooperVision
370 Woodcliff Drive
Suite 200
Fairport, NY 14450
(800) 538-7850
www.coopervision.com

Corixa
1124 Columbia Street
Suite 200
Seattle, WA 98104
(206) 754-5711
www.corixa.com

C. R. Bard, Inc
8195 Industrial Boulevard
Covington, GA 30014
(800) 526-4455
www.bardmedical.com

Cumberland Pharmaceuticals, Inc
2525 West End Avenue
Suite 950
Nashville, TN 37203
(615) 255-0068
www.cumberlandpharma.com

Cyanotech Corp
73-4460 Queen Kaahamanu Highway
Suite 102
Kailua-Kona, HI 96740
(800) 395-1353
www.cyanotech.com

Cygnus, Inc
400 Penobscot Drive
Redwood City, CA 94063-4719
(650) 369-4300
www.cygn.com

CYNACON/OCuSOFT
5311 Avenue North
Rosenburg, TX 77471
(800) 233-5469
www.ocusoft.com

Cypress Pharmaceutical, Inc
135 Industrial Boulevard
Madison, MS 39110
(800) 856-4393
www.cypressrx.com

CYTOGEN Corp
650 College Road East
Suite 3100
Princeton, NJ 08540
(800) 833-3533
www.cytogen.com

CytRx Corp
11726 San Vicente Boulevard
Suite 650
Los Angeles, CA 90049
(310) 826-5648
www.cytrx.com

Daiichi Pharmaceutical Corp
11 Philips Parkway
Montvale, NJ 07645-1810
(877) 324-4244
www.daiichius.com

Danco Labs, LLC
PO Box 4816
New York, NY 10185
(877) 432-7596
www.earlyoptionpill.com

Dartmouth Pharmaceuticals
38 Church Avenue
Wareham, MA 02571
(800) 414-3566
www.ilovemynails.com

Davol, Inc
100 Sockanossett Crossroad
PO Box 8500
Cranston, RI 02920
(800) 556-6756
www.davol.com

Del Laboratories, Inc
726 EAB Plaza
Uniondale, NY 11553
(800) 952-5080
www.dellabs.com

Delmont Laboratories, Inc
715 Harvard Avenue
PO Box 269
Swarthmore, PA 19081
(800) 562-5541
www.delmont.com

Den-Mat Corp
2727 Skyway Drive
Santa Maria, CA 93455
(800) 445-0345
www.den-mat.com

Derma Sciences
214 Carnegie Center
Suite 100
Princeton, NJ 08540
(800) 825-4325
www.dermasciences.com

Dermik Laboratories
500 Arcola Road
PO Box 1200
Collegeville, PA 19426
(800) 340-7502
www.dermik.com

DeRoyal Industries, Inc
200 DeBusk Lane
Powell, TN 37849
(800) 337-6925
www.deroyal.com

DexGen Pharmaceuticals, Inc
PO Box 675
Manasquan, NJ 08736
(877) DEXGEN1
www.dexgen.com

Dey LP
2751 Napa Valley Corporate Drive
Napa, CA 94558
(800) 755-5560
www.deyinc.com

DiaPharma Group, Inc
8948 Beckett Road
West Chester, OH 45069
(800) 526-5224
www.diapharma.com

Diatide, Inc
9 Delta Drive
Londonderry, NH 03053
(603) 437-8970
www.diatide.com

Dickinson Brands, Inc
31 East High Street
East Hampton, CT 06424
(888) 860-2279
www.dickinsonbrands.com

Digestive Care, Inc
1120 Win Drive
Bethlehem, PA 18017-7059
(610) 882-5950
www.pancrecarb.com

Discovery Laboratories, Inc
350 South Main Street
Suite 307
Doylestown, PA 18901
(215) 340-4699
www.discoverylabs.com

Discus Dental, Inc
8550 Higuera Street
Culver City, CA 90232
(800) 422-9448
www.discusdental.com

Dista Products Company
(see Eli Lilly & Company)

Doak Dermatologics
383 Route 46 West
Fairfield, NJ 07004-2402
(800) 405-3625
www.bradpharm.com

Dow Hickam, Inc
(see Bertek Pharmaceuticals, Inc)

Dreir Pharmaceuticals, Inc
9602 North 122nd Place
Scottsdale, AZ 85259
(800) 541-4044
www.dreirpharmaceuticals.com

Dr Reddy's Laboratories, Inc
200 Somerset Corp Boulevard
Bridgewater, NJ 08807
(908) 203-4900
www.drreddys.com

DuPont Pharmaceuticals
Chestnut Run Plaza
974 Centre Road
Wilmington, DE 19805
(800) 474-2762
www.dupontpharma.com

Duramed Pharmaceuticals
5040 Duramed Drive
Cincinnati, OH 45213
(800) 543-8338
www.duramed.com

Dura Pharmaceuticals
(see Elan Pharmaceuticals)

Durex Consumer Products
3585 Engineering Drive
Suite 200
Norcross, GA 30092
(888) 566-3468
www.durex.com

Durham Pharmacal Corp
Route 145
Oak Hill, NY 12460
(888) 438-7426
www.cummingsadvertisingart.com/durham/index-dp2.htm

DUSA Pharmaceuticals, Inc
25 Upton Drive
Wilmington, MA 01887
(978) 657-7500
www.dusapharma.com

Eagle Vison, Inc
8500 Wolf Lake Drive
Suite 110
PO Box 34877
Memphis, TN 38133
(800) 222-7584
www.eaglevis.com

ECR Pharmaceuticals
PO Box 71600
Richmond, VA 23255
(804) 527-1950
www.ecrpharma.com

Edwards Lifesciences
One Edwards Way
Irvine, CA 92614
(949) 250-2500
www.edwards.com

E. Fougera & Company
60 Baylis Road
Melville, NY 11747
(800) 645-9833
www.fougera.com

Eisai, Inc
500 Frank W. Burr Boulevard
Teaneck, NJ 07666
(888) 793-4724
www.eisai.com

Elan Corp
800 Gateway Boulevard
South San Francisco, CA 94080
(650) 877-0900
www.elan.com

Eli Lilly & Company
Lilly Corporate Center
Indianapolis, IN 46285
(800) 545-5979
www.lilly.com

Elkins-Sinn, Inc
(see Wyeth Pharmaceuticals)

EMD Chemicals, Inc
480 South Democrat Road
Gibbstown, NJ 08027
(800) 222-0342
www.emdchemicals.com

Endo Pharmaceuticals
100 Endo Boulevard
Chadds Ford, PA 19317
(800) 462-3636
www.endo.com

EnviroDerm Pharmaceuticals, Inc
PO Box 32370
Louisville, KY 40232-2370
(800) 991-3376
www.enviroderm.com

Enzon, Inc
685 Route 202/206
Bridgewater, NJ 08807
(908) 541-8600
www.enzon.com

Eon Labs Manufacturing, Inc
227-15 North Conduit Avenue
Laurelton, NY 11413
(800) 526-0225
www.eonlabs.com

Epien Medical, Inc
4225 White Bear Parkway
Suite 600
St Paul, MN 55110-3389
(888) 884-4675
www.northernresearch.com

E. R. Squibb & Sons, Inc
(see Bristol-Myers Squibb Company)

Ethex Corp
10888 Metro Court
St Louis, MO 63043-2413
(800) 321-1705
www.ethex.com

Ethicon, Inc
(Johnson & Johnson)
US Route 22 West
PO Box 151
Somerville, NJ 08876-0151
(800) 255-2500
www.ethiconinc.com

Everett Laboratories, Inc
29 Spring Street
West Orange, NJ 07052
(973) 324-0200
www.everettlabs.com

E-Z-EM
717 Main Street
Westbury, NY 11590
(800) 544-4624
www.ezem.com

Female Health Company
515 North State Street
Suite 2225
Chicago, IL 60610
(312) 595-9123
www.femalehealth.com

Ferndale Laboratories, Inc
780 West Eight Mile Road
Ferndale, MI 48220
(800) 621-6003
www.ferndalelabs.com

Ferring Pharmaceuticals, Inc
400 Rella Boulevard
Suffern, NY 10901
(888) 337-7464
www.ferringusa.com

Fidia Pharmaceutical Corp
2000 K Street Northwest
Suite 700
Washington, DC 20006
(202) 371-9898
www.fidiapharma.com

First Horizon Pharmaceutical Corp
6195 Shiloh Road
Alpharetta, GA 30005
(770) 442-9707
www.horizonpharm.com

Fischer Pharmaceuticals, Inc
165 Gibraltar Court
Sunnyvale, CA 94089
(800) 782-0222
www.dr-fischer.com

Fisons Corp (see Celltech Pharmaceuticals, Inc)

Fleming & Company
1733 Gilsinn Lane
Fenton, MO 63026
(800) 343-0164
www.flemingcompany.com

Forest Laboratories, Inc
909 Third Avenue
New York, NY 10022
(800) 947-5227
www.frx.com

Freeda Vitamins, Inc
36 East 41st Street
New York, NY 10017
(800) 777-3737
www.freedavitamins.com

Fujisawa Healthcare, Inc
(see Astellas Pharma U.S., Inc)

Galderma Laboratories, Inc
14501 North Freeway
Fort Worth, TX 76177
(800) 582-8225
www.galdermausa.com

Gallipot, Inc
2020 Silver Bell Road
St Paul, MN 55122
(800) 423-6967
www.gallipot.com

Gambro Renal Products, USA
10810 West Collins Avenue
Lakewood, CO 80215-4498
(800) 525-2623
www.gambro.com

Gate Pharmaceuticals
PO Box 1090
North Wales, PA 19454-1090
(800) 292-4283
www.gatepharma.com

Gebauer Company
4444 East 153rd Street
Cleveland, OH 44128
(800) 321-9348
www.gebauerco.com

Geigy Pharmaceuticals
(see Novartis Pharmaceuticals Corp)

Genaissance Pharmaceuticals, Inc
Five Science Park
New Haven, CT 06511
(203) 773-1450
www.genaissance.com

GenDerm Corp (see Medicis Pharmaceutical Corp)

Gen-King (see Kinray)

Genentech, Inc
One DNA Way
South San Francisco, CA 94080-4990
(800) 551-2231
www.gene.com

General Injectables & Vaccines
US Highway 52 South
PO Box 9
Bastian, VA 24314-0009
(800) 521-7468
www.giv.com

General Nutrition, Inc
300 6th Avenue
Pittsburgh, PA 15222
(888) 462-2548
www.gnc.com

Genesis Nutrition
1816 Wall Street
Florence, SC 29501
(800) 451-7933
www.genesisnutrition.com

Genesis Pharmaceutical, Inc
1721 Maplelane Avenue
Hazel Park, MI 48030
(800) 459-8663
www.genesispharm.com

Geneva Pharmaceuticals, Inc
(see Sandoz, Inc)

GenPharm International, Inc
(see Medarex)

GensiaSicor Pharmaceuticals
(see SICOR Pharmaceuticals, Inc)

Genta, Inc
Two Connell Drive
Berkeley Heights, New Jersey 07922
(908) 286-9800
www.genta.com

GenVec, Inc
65 West Watkins Mill Road
Gaithersburg. MD 20878
(240) 632-0740
www.genvec.com

Genzyme Corp
500 Kendall Street
Cambridge, MA 02142
(800) 326-7002
www.genzyme.com

Geodesic MediTech, Inc
2921 Sandy Pointe No. 3
Del Mar, CA 92014
(888) 357-9399
www.geodesicmeditech.com

Gerber Products Company
445 State Street
Fremont, MI 49413-0001
(800) 443-7237
www.gerber.com

Geritrex Corp
144 Kingsbridge Road East
Mount Vernon, NY 10550
(800) 736-3437
www.geritrex.com

Geron Corp
230 Constitution Drive
Menlo Park, CA 94025
(650) 473-7700
www.geron.com

Gilead
333 Lakeside Drive
Foster City, CA 94404
(800) 445-3235
www.gilead.com

Glades Pharmaceuticals, LLC
6340 Sugarloaf Parkway
Duluth, GA 30097
(888) 445-2337
www.glades.com

GlaxoSmithKline
Five Moore Drive
PO Box 13398
Research Triangle Park, NC 27709
(888) 825-5249
www.gsk.com

GlaxoSmithKline
One Franklin Plaza
Philadelphia, PA 19102
(888) 825-5249
www.gsk.com

GlaxoSmithKline Consumer Healthcare
PO Box 1467
Pittsburgh, PA 15230
(412) 928-1000
www.gsk.com

GlaxoWellcome, Inc (see GlaxoSmithKline)

Glenwood, LLC
111 Cedar Lane
Englewood, NJ 07631
(800) 542-0772
www.glenwood-llc.com

Global Pharmaceuticals, Inc
3735 Castor Avenue
Philadelphia, PA 19124
(215) 289-2220
www.globalphar.com

Gordon Laboratories
6801 Ludlow Street
Upper Darby, PA 19082-2408
(800) 356-7870
www.gordonlabs.com

GF Health Products, Inc
2935 Northeast Parkway
Atlanta, GA 30360
(800) 347-5678
www.grahamfield.com

Grandpa Brands Company
1820 Airport Exchange Boulevard
Erlanger, KY 41018
(800) 684-1468
www.csdent.com

Green Turtle Bay Vitamin Company
56 High Street
Summit, NJ 07901
(800) 887-8535
www.energywave.com

Greer Laboratories, Inc
639 Nuway Circle
PO Box 800
Lenoir, NC 28645-0800
(800) 438-0088
www.greerlabs.com

Grifols
(Bioscience Division)
2410 Lillyvale Avenue
Los Angeles, CA 90032
(888) 474-3657
www.grifolsusa.com

Guilford Pharmaceuticals, Inc
6611 Tributary Street
Baltimore, MD 21224
(800) 453-3746
www.guilfordpharm.com

Gynetics
PO Box 8509
Somerville, NJ 08876
(800) 311-7378
www.gynetics.com

Halocarbon Products Corp
PO Box 661
River Edge, NJ 07661
(201) 262-8899
www.halocarbon.com

Hart Health & Safety
PO Box 94044
Seattle, WA 98124
(800) 234-4278
www.harthealth.com

Harvard Drug Group, LLC
31778 Enterprise Drive
Livonia, MI 48150
(800) 875-0123
www.harvarddrugs.com

Hauser Pharmaceutical, Inc
4401 East US Highway 30
Valparaiso, IN 46383
(800) 441-2309
www.hauserpharmaceutical.com

Hawthorn Pharmaceuticals, Inc
PO Box 2248
Madison, MS 39130
(888) 455-5253
www.hawthornrx.com

HDC Corp
628 Gibraltar Court
Milpitas, CA 95035
(800) 227-8162
www.hdccorp.com

HealthAsure, Inc
(Rainbow Light Nutritional Systems)
125 McPherson Street
Santa Cruz, CA 95060
(800) 635-1233
www.healthasure.com

Healthfirst Corp
22316 70th Avenue West
Unit A
Mountlake Terrace, WA 98043-2184
(425) 771-5733
www.healthfirst.com

Helix BioPharma Corp
305 Industrial Parkway South
Unit 3
Aurora, ON L4G 6X7
(905) 841-2300
www.helixbiopharma.com

Hemacare Corp
21101 Oxnard Street
Woodland HIlls, CA 91367
(877) 310-0717
www.hemacare.com

Hemagen Diagnostics, Inc
9033 Red Branch Road
Columbia, MD 21045
(800) 495-2180
www.hemagen.com

Hemispherx Biopharma, Inc
One Penn Center
1617 John F. Kennedy Boulevard
6th Floor
Philadelphia, PA 19103
(215) 988-0080
www.hemispherx.net

Henry Schein, Inc
135 Duryea Road
Melville, NY 11747
(631) 843-5500
www.henryschein.com

Hill Dermaceuticals, Inc
2650 South Mellonville Avenue
Sanford, FL 32773-9311
(800) 344-5707
www.hillderm.com

Hi-Tech Pharmacal, Inc
369 Bayview Avenue
Amityville, NY 11701
(800) 262-9010
www.hitechpharm.com

Hoechst-Marion Roussel, Inc (see Aventis)

Hoffmann-LaRoche
(see Roche Pharmaceuticals)

Hogil Pharmaceutical Corp
237 Mamaroneck Avenue
Suite 303
White Plains, NY 10605
(914) 681-1800
www.hogil.com

Hollister-Stier Laboratories, LLC
3525 North Regal Street
Spokane, WA 99207-5788
(800) 992-1120
www.hollister-stier.com

Home Access Health Corp
2401 West Hassell Road
Suite 1510
Hoffman Estates, IL 60195
(847) 781-2500
www.homeaccess.com

Hope Pharmaceuticals
8260 East Gelding Drive
Suite 104
Scottsdale, AZ 85260
(800) 755-9595
www.hopepharm.com

Horizon Diagnostics, Inc
2930 East Houston Street
San Antonio, TX 78202
(210) 222-2108
www.horizondiagnostics.com

Horizon Pharmaceutical Corp
(see First Horizon Pharmaceutical Corp)

Hospira, Inc
275 North Field Drive
Lake Forest, IL 60045
(800) 615-0187
www.hospira.com

Hyland Immuno
(Baxter)
550 North Brand Boulevard
Glendale, CA 91203
(800) 423-2090
http://baxdb1.baxter.com

Hyland Laboratories, Inc
(Standard Homeopathic Company)
210 West 131st Street
Los Angeles, CA 90061
(800) 624-9659
www.hylands.com

ICN Pharmaceuticals, Inc
(see Valeant Pharmaceuticals)

IDEC Pharmaceuticals
(see Bogen idec)

Ilex Oncology, Inc
(see Genzyme Corp)

Immune Response Corp
5931 Darwin Court
Carlsbad, CA 92008
(760) 431-7080
www.imnr.com

ImmunoGen, Inc
128 Sidney Street
Cambridge, MA 02139
(617) 995-2500
www.immunogen.com

Immunomedics, Inc
300 American Road
Morris Plains, NJ 07950
(973) 605-8200
www.immunomedics.com

IMPAX Laboratories, Inc
30831 Huntwood Avenue
Hayward, CA 94544
(510) 476-2000
www.impaxlabs.com

Incyte Corp
Experimental Station
Route 141 & Henry Clay Road
Building E336
Wilmington, DE 19880
(302) 498-6700
www.incyte.com

Indevus Pharmaceuticals, Inc
99 Hayden Avenue
Suite 200
Lexington, MA 02421
(781) 861-8444
www.interneuron.com

InKine Pharmaceutical Company, Inc
1787 Sentry Parkway
West Building 18
Suite 440
Blue Bell, PA 19422
(215) 283-6850
www.inkine.com

INO Therapeutics
6th State Route 173
Clinton, NJ 08809
(908) 238-6600
www.inotherapeutics.com

Inspire Pharmaceuticals, Inc
4222 Emperor Boulevard
Suite 200
Durham, NC 27703
(919) 941-9777
www.inspirepharm.com

Interferon Sciences, Inc
783 Jersey Avenue
New Brunswick, NJ 08901-3660
(888) 728-4372
www.interferonsciences.com

InterMune Pharmaceuticals, Inc
3280 Bayshore Boulevard
Brisbane, CA 94005
(415) 466-2200
www.intermune.com

International Medication Systems, Limited (IMS)
1886 Santa Anita Avenue
South El Monte, CA 91733
(800) 423-4136
www.ims-limited.com

IntraBiotics Pharmaceuticals, Inc
2483 East Bayshore Road
Suite 100
Palo Alto, CA 94303
(650) 526-6800
www.intrabiotics.com

Introgen Therapeutics, Inc
301 Congress Avenue
Suite 1850
Austin, TX 78701
(512) 708-9310
www.introgen.com

Inveresk
11000 Westen Parkway
Cary, NC 27513
(919) 460-9005
www.inveresk.com

Inverness Medical Innovations
51 Sawyer Road
Suite 200
Waltham, MA 02453-3448
(800) 899-7353
www.invernessmedical.com

Inwood Laboratories (Forest)
321 Prospect Street
Inwood, NY 11096
(800) 685-5227
www.frx.com

Iomed, Inc
2441 South 3850 West
Suite A
Salt Lake City, UT 84120
(800) 621-3347
www.iomed.com

IOP, Inc
3151 Airway Avenue
Costa Mesa, CA 92626
(800) 535-3545
www.iopinc.com

Isis Pharmaceuticals
2292 Faraday Avenue
Carlsbad, CA 92008
(760) 931-9200
www.isispharm.com

Ivax Pharmaceuticals, Inc
(see Teva Pharmaceuticals USA)

IVPCARE
7164 Technology Drive
Suite 100
Frisco, TX 75034
(800) 424-9002
www.ivpcare.com

Janssen Pharmaceutica Products, LP
1125 Trenton-Harbourton Road
PO Box 200
Titusville, NJ 08560-0200
(800) 526-7736
www.janssen.com

Jerome Stevens Pharmaceuticals, Inc
60 DaVinci Drive
Bohemia, NY 11716-2613
(631) 567-1113

Johnson & Johnson
One Johnson & Johnson Plaza
New Brunswick, NJ 08933
(732) 524-0400
www.jnj.com

Jones Pharma
(see King Pharmaceuticals, Inc)

J. R. Carlson Laboratories, Inc
15 College Drive
Arlington Heights, IL 60004-1985
(888) 234-5656
www.carlsonlabs.com

J. T. Baker, Inc (see Mallinckrodt Baker, Inc)

Kendall Healthcare Products
15 Hampshire Street
Mansfield, MA 02048
(800) 962-9888
www.kendallhq.com

Key Pharmaceuticals (see Schering-Plough Corp)

Kimberly-Clark/Ballard Medical Products
12050 Lone Peak Parkway
Draper, UT 84020
(800) 528-5591
www.kchealthcare.com

King Pharmaceuticals, Inc
501 Fifth Street
Bristol, TN 37620
(800) 776-3637
www.kingpharm.com

Kingswood Laboratories, Inc
10375 Hague Road
Indianapolis, IN 46256
(800) 968-7772
www.kingswood-labs.com

Kinray
152-35 10th Avenue
Whitestone, NY 11357
(800) 854-6729
www.kinray.com

Kirkman Laboratories, Inc
6400 Southwest Rosewood Street
Lake Oswego, OR 97035
(800) 245-8282
www.kirkmanlabs.com

KLI Corp
1119 Third Avenue Southwest
Carmel, IN 46032
(800) 308-7452
www.entertainers-secret.com

Knoll Pharmaceuticals Company
(see Abbott Laboratories)

Konsyl Pharmaceuticals, Inc
8050 Industrial Park Road
Easton, MD 21601
(800) 356-6795
www.konsyl.com

Kos Pharmaceuticals, Inc
One Cedar Brook Drive
Cranbury, New Jersey 08512-3618
(609) 495-0500
www.kospharm.com

Kramer Laboratories, Inc
8778 Southwest 8th Street
Miami, FL 33174
(800) 824-4894
www.kramerlabs.com

K. V. Pharmaceutical Company
2503 South Hanley Road
St Louis, MO 63144
(314) 645-6600
www.kvpharma.com

Lacrimedics, Inc
PO Box 1209
Eastsound, WA 98245
(800) 367-8327
www.lacrimedics.com

Lactaid, Inc
7050 Camp Hill Road
Fort Washington, PA 19034
(800) 522-8243
www.lactaid.com

Lannett Company, Inc
9000 State Road
Philadelphia, PA 19136
(800) 325-9994
www.lannett.com

LecTec Corp
5616 Lincoln Drive
Edina, MN 55436
(877) 587-2824
www.lectec.com

Lee Laboratories
1475 Athens Highway
Grayson, GA 30017
(770) 972-4450
www.leelabs.com

Lee Pharmaceuticals
1434 Santa Anita Avenue
South El Monte, CA 91733
(800) 950-5337
www.leepharmaceuticals.com

Leiner Health Products
901 East 233rd Street
Carson, CA 90745
(310) 835-8400
www.leiner.com

LifeScan, Inc
(Johnson & Johnson Company)
1000 Gibraltar Drive
Milpitas, CA 95035
(800) 227-8862
www.lifescan.com

LifeSign LLC
71 Veronica Avenue
PO Box 218
Somerset, NJ 08875-0218
(800) 526-2125
www.lifesignmed.com

Ligand Pharmaceuticals
10275 Science Center Drive
San Diego, CA 92121
(800) 526-2125
www.ligand.com

Lilly & Company (see Eli Lilly & Company)

Lincoln Diagnostics
PO Box 1128
Decatur, IL 62525
(217) 877-2531
www.lincolndiagnostics.com

LSI America Corp
4732 Twin Valley Drive
Austin, TX 78731-3537
(800) 720-5936
www.ondrox.com

Lyne Laboratories
10 Burke Drive
Brockton, MA 02301
(800) 525-0450
www.lyne.com

3M Pharmaceuticals
3M Center
Building 275-3W-01
PO Box 33275
St Paul, MN 55133
(800) 328-0255
3m.com/pharma

Magno-Humphries Laboratories
8800 Southwest Commercial Street
Tigard, OR 97223
(503) 684-5464
www.magno-humphries.com

Mallinckrodt Baker, Inc
222 Red School Lane
Phillipsburg, NJ 08865
(800) 582-2537
www.mallbaker.com

Mallinckrodt, Inc
(Corp Headquarters)
675 McDonnell Boulevard
Hazelwood, MO 63042
(314) 654-2000
www.mallinckrodt.com

Martec Pharmaceutical, Inc
1800 North Topping
Kansas City, MO 64120
(800) 822-6782
www.martec-kc.com

Martek Biosciences Corp
6480 Dobbin Road
Columbia, MD 21045
(410) 740-0081
www.martekbio.com

Mason Vitamins, Inc
5105 Northwest 159th Street
Miami Lakes, FL 33014-6370
(800) 327-6005
www.masonvitamins.com

Mayne Pharma (USA), Inc
650 From Road
(Mack-Cali Centre II)
Second Floor
Paramus, NJ 07652
(201) 225-5500
www.us.maynepharma.com

McGuff Company, Inc
3524 West Lake Center Drive
Santa Ana, CA 92704
(800) 854-7220
www.mcguffmedical.com

McNeil Consumer & Specialty Pharmaceuticals (Johnson & Johnson)
Camp Hill Road
Mail Stop 278
Fort Washington, PA 19034-2292
(800) 962-5357
www.jnj.com

Mead Johnson Laboratories
(see Bristol-Myers Squibb Company)

Medarex, Inc
707 State Road
Princeton, NJ 08540-1437
(609) 430-2880
www.medarex.com

Medco Lab, Inc
716 West 7th Street
Sioux City, IA 51103
(712) 255-8770
www.medcolab.com

Medeva Pharmaceuticals
(see Celltech Pharmaceuticals, Inc)

Medicis Pharmaceutical Corp
8125 North Hayden Road
Scottsdale, AZ 85258-2463
(800) 550-5115
www.medicis.com

Medi-Dose, Inc
70 Industrial Drive
Ivyland, PA 18974
(800) 523-8966
www.medidose.com

MedImmune, Inc
One MedImmune Way
Gaithersburg, MD 20878
(877) 633-4411
www.medimmune.com

Medisca, Inc
661 Route 3, Unit C
Plattsburgh, NY 12901
(800) 932-1039
www.medisca.com

MediSense, Inc (Abbott Laboratories)
4A Crosby Drive
Bedford, MA 01730
(800) 323-9100

Medix Pharmaceuticals Americas, Inc (MPA)
12505 Starkey Road
Suite M
Largo, FL 33773
(888) 242-3463
www.biafine.com

MedPointe Pharmaceuticals
265 Davidson Avenue
Suite 300
Somerset, NJ 08873-4120
(732) 564-2200
www.medpointeinc.com

Medtronic, Inc
710 Medtronic Parkway
Minneapolis, MN 55432-5604
(763) 514-4000
www.medtronic.com

Menicon America, Inc
1840 Gateway Drive
Second Floor
San Mateo, CA 94404
(800) MENICON
www.menicon.com

Mentholatum Company, Inc (Rohto Pharmaceutical Company)
707 Sterling Drive
Orchard Park, NY 14127
(800) 688-7660
www.mentholatum.com

Merck & Company
One Merck Drive
PO Box 100
Whitehouse Station, NJ 08889-0100
(800) 672-6372
www.merck.com

Mericon Industries, Inc
8819 North Pioneer Road
Peoria, IL 61615-1561
(800) 242-6464
www.mericon-industries.com

Meridian Medical Technologies (King Pharmaceuticals, Inc)
10240 Old Columbia Road
Columbia, MD 21046
(800) 638-8093
www.meridianmeds.com

Merit Pharmaceuticals
2611 San Fernando Road
Los Angeles, CA 90065
(800) 696-3748
www.meritpharm.com

Merz Pharmaceuticals
4215 Tudor Lane
Greensboro, NC 27410
(800) 334-0514
www.merzusa.com

Methapharm, Inc
11772 West Sample Road
Suite 101
Coral Springs, FL 33065
(800) 287-7686
www.methapharm.com

MGI Pharma, Inc
5775 West Old Shakopee Road
Suite 100
Bloomington, MN 55437-3174
(800) 562-5580
www.mgipharma.com

Mikart, Inc
1750 Chattahoochee Avenue
Atlanta, GA 30318
(404) 351-4510
www.mikart.com

Miles, Inc (see Bayer Corp)

Milex Products, Inc
4311 North Normandy
Chicago, IL 60634-1403
(800) 621-1278
www.milexproducts.com

Miller Pharmacal Group, Inc
350 Randy Road
Suite 2
Carol Stream, IL 60188-1831
(800) 323-2935
www.millerpharmacal.com

Mission Pharmacal Company
10999 IH-10 West
Suite 1000
San Antonio, TX 78230
(800) 531-3333
www.missionpharmacal.com

Monaghan Medical Corp
5 Latour Avenue
Suite 1600
PO Box 2805
Plattsburgh, NY 12901
(800) 833-9653
www.monaghanmed.com

Monarch Pharmaceuticals
(King Pharmaceuticals, Inc)
355 Beecham Street
Bristol, TN 37620
(800) 776-3637
www.monarchpharm.com

Monticello Drug Company
1604 Stockton Street
Jacksonville, FL 32204
(800) 735-0666
www.monticellocompanies.com

Moore Medical Corp
PO Box 1500
New Britain, CT 06050-1500
(800) 234-1464
www.mooremedical.com

Morton Grove Pharmaceuticals
6451 West Main Street
Morton Grove, IL 60053
(800) 346-6854
www.mgp-online.com

MotherSOY, Inc
424 South Kentucky Avenue
Evansville, IN 47714
(888) 769-0769
www.mothersoy.com

Mutual Pharmaceutical Company, Inc/United Research Laboratories
1100 Orthodox Street
Philadelphia, PA 19124
(800) 523-3684
www.urlmutual.com

Mylan Laboratories, Inc
1500 Corporate Drive
Suite 400
Canonsburg, PA 15317
(724) 514-1800
www.mylan.com

Mylan Pharmaceuticals, Inc
781 Chestnut Ridge Road
Morgantown, WV 26505
(800) 826-9526
www.mylanpharm.com

Nabi
(Corp Headquarters)
5800 Park of Commerce Boulevard Northwest
Boca Raton, FL 33487
(800) 642-8874
www.nabi.com

Nagase Pharmaceuticals
500 Fifth Avenue
Suite 840
New York, NY 10110
(212) 354-3140
www.nagase.com

Nastech Pharmaceutical Company, Inc
45 Adams Avenue
Hauppauge, NY 11788
(631) 273-0101
www.nastech.com

NATREN, Inc
3105 Willow Lane
Westlake Village, CA 91361
(800) 992-3323
www.natren.com

Natrol, Inc
21411 Prairie Street
Chatsworth, CA 91311
(800) 326-1520
www.natrol.com

Naturally Vitamins
(Marlyn Nutraceuticals, Inc)
4404 East Elwood
Phoenix, AZ 85040
(888) 766-4406
www.naturallyvitamins.com

Natures Bounty, Inc
(NBTY, Inc)
90 Orville Drive
Bohemia, NY 11716
(888) 465-6757
www.naturesbounty.com

Nature's Sunshine Products, Inc
75 East 1700 South
Provo, UT 84606
(800) 223-8225
www.nsponline.com

NeoPharm, Inc
150 Field Drive
Suite 195
Lake Forest, IL 60045
(847) 295-8678
www.neophrm.com

NeoRx Corp
300 Elliott Avenue West
Suite 500
Seattle, WA 98119-4007
(206) 281-7001
www.neorx.com

Nephron Pharmaceuticals Corp
4121 34th Street
Orlando, FL 32811
(800) 443-4313
www.nephronpharm.com

Nestle Clinical Nutrition
3 Parkway North
Suite 500
Deerfield, IL 60015
(800) 422-2752
www.nestleclinicalnutrition.com

NeuroGenesis/Matrix Tech, Inc
120 Park Avenue
League City, TX 77573
(800) 345-8912
www.neurogenesis.com

Neutrogena Corp
5760 West 96th Street
Los Angeles, CA 90045-5595
(800) 582-4048
www.neutrogena.com

NeXstar Pharmaceuticals, Inc
(see Gilead)

Niche Pharmaceuticals, Inc
209 North Oak Street
Roanoke, TX 76262
(800) 677-0355
www.niche-inc.com

Nnodum Pharmaceuticals (Zikspain)
PO Box 19725
Cincinnati, OH 45219
(800) 301-9457
www.zikspain.com

Nomax, Inc
40 North Rock Hill Road
St Louis, MO 63119
(314) 961-2500
www.nomax.com

Noramco, Inc (Johnson & Johnson)
1440 Olympic Drive
Athens, GA 30601
(706) 353-4400
www.noramco.com

Norstar Consumer Products Company, Inc
5517 95th Avenue
Kenosha, WI 53144
(262) 652-8505
www.norstarcpc.com

Northern Research Laboratories, Inc
(see Epien Medical, Inc)

Nova Factor, Inc
1620 Century Center Parkway
Suite 109
Memphis, TN 38134
(800) 235-8498
www.accredohealth.net/nova/

Novartis Pharmaceuticals Corp
One Health Plaza
East Hanover, NJ 07936-1080
(973) 781-8265
www.pharma.us.novartis.com

Noven Pharmaceuticals, Inc
11960 Southwest 144th Street
Miami, FL 33186
(305) 253-5099
www.noven.com

Novocol
(see Septodont, Inc)

Novo Nordisk Pharmaceuticals, Inc
100 College Road West
Princeton, NJ 08540
(800) 727-6500
www.novonordisk-us.com

Novopharm USA, Inc
165 East Commerce Drive
Suite 100
Schaumburg, IL 60173-5326
(800) 426-0769
www.novapharmusa.com

Numark Laboratories, Inc
164 Northfield Avenue
Edison, NJ 08837
(800) 338-8079
www.numarklabs.com

Nutraceutical Solutions, Inc
6704 Ranger Avenue
Corpus Christi, TX 78415
(800) 856-7040
www.eliquidsolutions.com

Nutramax Laboratories, Inc
2208 Lakeside Boulevard
Edgewood, MD 21040
(800) 925-5187
www.nutramaxlabs.com

NutriSoy International, Inc
(see MotherSOY, Inc)

Octamer, Inc
392 Cecilia Way
Tiburon, CA 94920
(415) 381-1602
www.octamer.com

Odyssey Pharmaceuticals, Inc
200 Park Avenue
PO Box 683
Florham Park, NJ 07932
(877) 427-9068
www.odysseypharm.com

Ohmeda Pharmaceuticals
(see Baxter Pharmaceutical Products, Inc)

Omnicell
1201 Charleston Road
Mountain View, CA 94043-1337
(800) 850-6664
www.omnicell.com

Omnii Products
1500 North Florida Mango Road
Suite 1
West Palm Beach, FL 33409
(800) 445-3386
www.omniiproducts.com

Onyx Pharmaceuticals, Inc
2100 Powell Street
Emeryville, CA 94608
(510) 597-6500
www.onyx-pharm.com

Optics Laboratory, Inc
9480 Telstar Avenue #3
El Monte, CA 91731
(626) 350-1926
www.opticslab.com

Optimox Corp
PO Box 3378
Torrance, CA 90510-3378
(800) 223-1601
www.optimox.com

Organogenesis, Inc
150 Dan Road
Canton, MA 02021
(781) 575-0775
(800) 631-1253
www.organogenesis.com

Organon, Inc
375 Mt Pleasant Avenue
West Orange, NJ 07052
(800) 631-1253
www.organon-usa.com

Orphan Medical, Inc
13911 Ridgedale Drive
Suite 250
Minnetonka, MN 55305
(888) 867-7426
www.orphan.com

Ortho Biotech Products, LP
430 Route 22 East
PO Box 6914
Bridgewater, NJ 08807-0914
(908) 541-4000
www.orthobiotech.com

Ortho-Clinical Diagnostics
(Johnson & Johnson)
100 Indigo Creek Drive
Rochester, NY 14626
(800) 828-6316
www.orthoclinical.com

Ortho-McNeil Pharmaceutical, Inc
1000 U.S. Route 202 South
Raritan, NJ 08869
(800) 682-6532
www.ortho-mcneil.com

Oscient Pharmaceuticals
1000 Winter Street
Suite 2200
Waltham, MA 02451
(781) 398-2300
www.oscient.com

Otsuka America Pharmaceutical, Inc
2440 Research Boulevard
Rockville, MD 20850
(800) 562-3974
www.otsuka.com

Ovation Pharmaceuticals, Inc
Four Parkway North
Deerfield, IL 60015
(847) 282-1000
www.ovationpharma.com

Oxford Pharmaceutical Services, Inc
One US Highway 46 West
Totowa, NJ 07512
(877) 284-9120
www.oxfordpharm.com

OXIS International, Inc
6040 North Cutter Circle
Suite 317
Portland, OR 97217
(503) 283-3911
www.oxis.com

Paddock Laboratories, Inc
3940 Quebec Avenue North
Minneapolis, MN 55427
(800) 328-5113
www.paddocklabs.com

PamLab LLC
(Pan American Laboratories, LLC)
PO Box 8950
Mandeville, LA 70470-8950
(888) 829-4097
www.panamericanlabs.com

Parke-Davis
(see Pfizer Pharmaceuticals Group PPG)

Parnell Pharmaceuticals
1525 Francisco Boulevard
San Rafael, CA 94901
(800) 457-4276
www.parnellpharm.com

Par Pharmaceutical, Inc
One Ram Ridge Road
Spring Valley, NY 10977
(800) 828-9393
www.parpharm.com

Pasteur Merieux Connaught USA
(see Sanofi Pasteur)

PDRx Pharmaceuticals, Inc
727 North Ann Arbor
Oklahoma City, OK 73127
(800) 299-7379
www.pdrx.com

Pediatric Pharmaceuticals, Inc
120 Wood Avenue South
Suite 300
Iselin, NJ 08830
(732) 603-7708
www.pediatricpharm.com

Pedinol Pharmacal, Inc
30 Banfi Plaza North
Farmingdale, NY 11735
(800) 733-4665
www.pedinol.com

Perrigo Company
515 Eastern Avenue
Allegan, MI 49010
(800) 827-2296
www.perrigo.com

Person & Covey, Inc
616 Allen Avenue
Glendale, CA 91201
(800) 423-2341
www.personandcovey.com

Pfizer Pharmaceuticals Group (PPG)
235 East 42nd Street
New York, NY 10017-5755
(800) 438-1985
www.pfizer.com

Pharma 21, Inc
1363 Shinly
Suite 100
Escondido, CA 92026
(760) 743-7441
www.pharma21.net

Pharmaceutical Formulations, Inc
PO Box 1904
Edison, NJ 08818-1904
(732) 985-7100
www.pfiotc.com

Pharmaceutical Specialties, Inc
PO Box 6298
Rochester, MN 55903-6298
(800) 325-8232
www.psico.com

Pharmacia Corp
(see Pfizer Pharmaceuticals Group (PPG))

Pharmakon Labs
6050 Jet Port Industrial Boulevard
Tampa, FL 33634
(800) 888-4045
www.pharmakonlabs.com

Pharmanex
75 West Center
Provo, UT 84601
(800) 487-1000
www.pharmanex.com

Pharmatek Laboratories, Inc
5626 Oberlin Drive
San Diego, CA 92121
(858) 587-8783
www.pharmatek.com

Pharmics, Inc
PO Box 27554
Salt Lake City, UT 84127
(801) 966-4138
www.pharmics.com

PhytoPharmica, Inc
825 Challenger Drive
Green Bay, WI 54311
(800) 553-2370
www.phytopharmica.com

Plantex USA, Inc
Two University Plaza
Suite 305
Hackensack, NJ 07601
(201) 343-4141
www.plantexusa.com

Playtex Company
74 Commerce Drive
Allendale, NJ 07401-1600
(800) 816-5742
www.playtex.com

PLIVA, Inc
72 Eagle Rock Avenue
East Hanover, NJ 07936
(973) 386-5566
www.plivainc.com

Plough, Inc
(see Schering-Plough Corp)

PolyMedica Corp
11 State Street
Woburn, MA 01801
(781) 933-2020
www.polymedica.com

Procter & Gamble Pharmaceuticals, Inc
One Proctor & Gamble Plaza
Cincinnati, OH 45201
(513) 983-1100
www.pg.com

ProCyte Corp
PO Box 808
Redmond, WA 98073-0808
(800) 848-3668
www.procyte.com

Protein Design Labs, Inc
34801 Campus Drive
Fremont, CA 94555
(510) 574-1400
www.pdl.com

Protein Sciences Corp
1000 Research Parkway
Meriden, CT 06450
(800) 488-7099
www.proteinsciences.com

Protherics, Inc
5214 Maryland Way
Suite 405
Brentwood, TN 37027
(615) 327-1027
www.protherics.com

Psychemedics Corp
1280 Massachusetts Avenue
Cambridge, MA 02138
(800) 628-8073
www.psychemedics.com

Purdue Pharma, LP
(The Purdue Frederick Company)
One Stamford Forum
201 Tresser Boulevard
Stamford, CT 06901-3431
(888) 726-7535
www.purduepharma.com

Purepac Pharmaceuticals Company
(see Actavis U.S.)

Puritan's Pride
1233 Montauk Highway
PO Box 9001
Oakdale, NY 11769-9001
(800) 645-1030
www.puritanspride.com

QLT, Inc
887 Great Northern Way
Vancouver, BC
Canada V5T 4T5
(800) 663-5486
www.qlt-pdt.com

Questcor Pharmaceuticals, Inc
3260 Whipple Road
Union City, CA 94587
(510) 400-0700
www.questcor.com

Quidel Corp
10165 McKellar Court
San Diego, CA 92121
(800) 874-1517
www.quidel.com

Ranbaxy Pharmaceuticals, Inc USA
600 College Road East
Princeton, NJ 08540
(888) 726-2299
www.ranbaxyusa.com

Reese Pharmaceutical Company, Inc
10617 Frank Avenue
Cleveland, OH 44106
(800) 321-7178
www.reesechemical.com

Regeneron Pharmaceuticals, Inc
777 Old Saw Mill River Road
Tarrytown, NY 10591
(914) 345-7400
www.regeneron.com

Remel, Inc
12076 Santa Fe Drive
PO Box 14428
Lenexa, KS 66215
(800) 255-6730
www.remelinc.com

Requa, Inc
540 Barnum Avenue
PO Box 2384
Bridgeport, CT 06608
(800) 321-1085
www.requa.com

Rexall Sundown, Inc
(Royal Numico, N.V.)
6111 Broken Sound Parkway Northwest
Boca Raton, FL 33487
(800) 327-0908
www.rexallsundown.com

Rhone-Poulenc Rorer Pharmaceuticals, Inc
500 Arcola Road
PO Box 1200
Collegeville, PA 19426-0998
(800) 340-7502

Richardson-Vicks, Inc
(see Procter & Gamble Pharmaceuticals, Inc)

Ricola, Inc
51 Gibraltar Drive
Morris Plains, NJ 07950
(973) 984-6811
www.ricolausa.com

R.I.D., Inc
(Bayer Consumer Care Division)
36 Columbia Road
PO Box 1910
Morristown, NJ 07962-1910
(800) 331-4536
www.licerid.com

Rite Aid Corp
PO Box 3165
Harrisburg, PA 17105
(800) 748-3243
www.riteaid.com

Roberts Pharmaceuticals Corp
(see Shire Pharmaceuticals)

Roche Pharmaceuticals
340 Kingsland Street
Nutley, NJ 07110
(800) 526-6367
www.rocheusa.com

Roerig
(see Pfizer Pharmaceuticals Group PPG)

Rorer (see Rhone-Poulenc Rorer Pharmaceuticals, Inc)

Ross Products Division
Abbott Labs
625 Cleveland Avenue
Columbus, OH 43215
(800) 986-8510
www.ross.com

Roxane Laboratories, Inc
PO Box 16532
Columbus, OH 43216
(800) 962-8364
www.roxane.com

R. P. Scherer, Inc
(see Cardinal Health, Inc)

RTI International
(Research Triangle Institute)
PO Box 12194
Research Triangle Park, NC 27709-2194
(919) 485-6000
www.rti.org

Salix Pharmaceuticals, Inc
1700 Perimeter Park Drive
Morrisville, NC 27560-8404
(919) 862-1000
www.salix.com

Sandoz, Inc
(Novartis Pharmaceuticals Corp)
506 Carnegie Center
Suite 400
Princeton, NJ 08540
(800) 525-8747
www.us.sandoz.com

SangStat, Inc
(see Genzyme Corp)

Sanofi-Aventis
300 Somerset Corporate Boulevard
Bridgewater, NJ 08807-2854
(800) 223-1062
www.sanofi-aventis.us

Sanofi Pasteur
Discovery Drive
Box 187
Swiftwater, PA 18370-0187
(570) 839-7187
www.sanofipasteur.com

Sanofi-Synthelabo, Inc
90 Park Avenue
New York, NY 10016
(800) 223-1062
www.sanofi-synthelabous.com

Santen, Inc
555 Gateway Drive
Napa, CA 94558
(707) 254-1750
www.santeninc.com

Savage Laboratories
(Altana Inc)
60 Baylis Road
Melville, NY 11747-2006
(800) 231-0206
www.savagelabs.com

Scandinavian Naturals
13 North 7th Street
Perkasie, PA 18944
(800) 288-2844
www.scandinaviannaturals.com

Scandipharm
(see Axcan Pharma, Inc)

Schaffer Laboratories
1058 North Allen Avenue
Pasadena, CA 91104
(800) 231-6725
www.schafferlabs.com

Schein Pharmaceutical, Inc
(see Watson Laboratories, Inc)

Schering-Plough Corp
(World Headquarters)
2000 Galloping Hill Road
Kenilworth, NJ 07033-0530
(908) 298-4000
www.schering-plough.com

Schwarz Pharma, Inc
6140 West Executive Drive
Mequon, WI 53092
(800) 558-5114
www.schwarzusa.com

SciClone Pharmaceuticals, Inc
901 Mariner's Island Boulevard
Suite 205
San Mateo, CA 94404
(650) 358-3456
www.sciclone.com

Scios
(Corp Headquarters)
6500 Paseo Padre Parkway
Freemont, CA 94555
(510) 248-2500
www.sciosinc.com

Sepracor
(Corp Headquarters)
84 Waterford Drive
Marlborough, MA 01752
(877) SEPRACOR
www.sepracor.com

Septodont, Inc
PO Box 11926
Wilmington, DE 19850
(800) 872-8305
www.septodontinc.com

Seres Laboratories, Inc
3331-B Industrial Drive
Santa Rosa, CA 95403
(707) 526-4526
www.sereslabs.com

Serono, Inc
One Technology Place
Rockland, MA 02370
(800) 283-8088
www.seronousa.com

Shaklee Corporation
(Corp Headquarters)
4747 Willow Road
Pleasanton, CA 94588
(925) 924-2000
www.shaklee.com

Sheffield Laboratories
(Faria Ltd LLC)
170 Broad Street
New London, CT 06320
(800) 442-4451
www.sheffield-labs.com

Sherwood Davis & Geck
(see Kendall Healthcare Products)

Sherwood Medical
(see Kendall Healthcare Products)

Shire Pharmaceuticals
725 Chesterbrook Boulevard
Wayne, PA 19087-5637
(484) 595-8800
www.shire.com

Shire Laboratories
1550 East Gude Drive
Rockville, MD 20850
(301) 838-2500
www.shirelabs.com

SHS North America
PO Box 117
Gaithersburg, MD 20884-0117
(800) 365-7354
www.SHSNA.com

SICOR Pharmaceuticals, Inc
(see Teva Pharmaceuticals USA)

Sigma-Tau, Inc
800 South Frederick Avenue
Suite 300
Gaithersburg, MD 20877
(800) 447-0169
www.sigma-tau.com

Silarx Pharmaceuticals, Inc
19 West Street
Spring Valley, NY 10977
(888) 974-5279
www.silarx.com

Sirius Laboratories, Inc
100 Fairway Drive
Suite 130
Vernon Hills, IL 60061
(866) 292-2108
www.siriuslabs.com

Sirna Therapeutics
185 Berry Street
Suite 6504
San Francisco, CA 94107
(415) 512-7624
www.sirna.com

SkyePharma US, Inc
10 East 63rd Street
New York, NY 10021
(212) 753-5780
www.skyepharma.com

Slim Fast Foods Company
PO Box 3625
West Palm Beach, FL 33402
(561) 833-9920
www.slim-fast.com

Smith & Nephew, Inc
150 Minuteman Road
Andover, MA 01810
(978) 749-1000
www.smithnephew.com

Snuva, Inc
715 South Boulevard
Oak Park, IL 60302
(708) 848-4783
www.snuva.com

Solvay Pharmaceuticals
901 Sawyer Road
Marietta, GA 30062
(800) 241-1643
www.solvaypharmaceuticals-us.com

Somerset Pharmaceuticals, Inc
2202 Northwest Shore Boulevard
Suite 450
Tampa, FL 33607
(800) 892-8889
www.somersetpharm.com

Sonus Pharmaceuticals
22026 20th Avenue Southeast
Bothell, Washington 98021
(425) 487-9500
www.sonuspharma.com

Spectrum Chemical Manufacturing Corp
14422 South San Pedro Street
Gardena, CA 90248-9985
(800) 813-1514
www.spectrumchemical.com

St Jude Medical, Inc
One Lillehei Plaza
St Paul, MN 55117-9983
(800) 328-9634
www.sjm.com

Stada Pharmaceuticals
5 Cedar Brook Drive
Cranbury, NJ 08512
(800) 542-6682
www.stadausa.com

Star Pharmaceuticals, Inc
1881 West State 84
Suite 101
Fort Lauderdale, FL 33315
(800) 845-7827
www.starpharm.com

Squibb (see Bristol-Myers Squibb Company)

Steris Corp
5960 Heisley Road
Mentor, OH 44060-1834
(440) 354-2600
www.americantable.com

Sterling Health
(see Bayer Corp Consumer Care Division)

Sterling Winthrop
(see Sanofi-Synthelabo, Inc)

Stiefel Laboratories, Inc
255 Alhambra Circle
Coral Gables, FL 33134
(800) 633-7647
www.stiefel.com

Stratus Pharmaceuticals, Inc
14377 Southwest 142nd Street
Miami, FL 33186
(800) 442-7882
www.stratuspharmaceuticals.com

SummaRx Laboratories
2940 FM 3028
Mineral Wells, TX 76067-9258
(800) 527-7319
www.summalabs.com

Summers Laboratories, Inc
103 G.P. Clement Drive
Collegeville, PA 19426-2044
(800) 533-7546
www.sumlab.com

Summit Pharmaceuticals
(see Novartis Pharmaceuticals Corp)

SuperGen, Inc
4140 Dublin Boulevard
Suite 200
Dublin, CA 94568
(925) 560-0100
www.supergen.com

Superior Pharmaceutical Company
1385 Kemper Meadow Drive
Cincinnati, OH 45240-1635
(800) 826-5035
www.superiorpharm.com

Swiss-American Products, Inc
4641 Nall Road
Dallas, TX 75244
(800) 633-8872
www.elta.net

Syncor
(see Cardinal Health, Inc)

Syntex Laboratories (see Roche Pharmaceuticals)

Takeda Pharmaceuticals North America, Inc
475 Half Day Road
Lincolnshire, IL 60069
(877) 582-5332
www.tpna.com

Tanox, Inc
10301 Stella Link
Houston, TX 77025-5445
(713) 578-4000
www.tanox.com

TAP Pharmaceutical Products, Inc
675 North Field Drive
Lake Forest, IL 60045
(800) 621-1020
www.tap.com

Targeted Genetics Corp
1100 Olive Way
Suite 100
Seattle, WA 98101
(206) 623-7612
www.targen.com

Taro Pharmaceuticals USA, Inc
5 Skyline Drive
Hawthorne, NY 10532
(800) 544-1449
www.tarousa.com

Tec Laboratories, Inc
7100 Tec Labs Way Southwest
Albany, OR 97321
(800) 482-4464
www.teclabsinc.com

Telluride Pharmaceutical Corp
300 Valley Road
Hillsborough, NJ 08844-4656
(908) 369-1800
www.tellpharm.com

Teva Pharmaceuticals USA
1090 Horsham Road
PO Box 1090
North Wales, PA 19454-1090
(888) 838-2872
www.tevapharmusa.com

The Key Company
1313 West Essex Avenue
St Louis, MO 63122
(800) 325-9592
www.thekeycompany.com

The Medicines Company
One Cambridge Center
Cambridge, MA 02142
(800) 264-4662
www.angiomax.com

Therasense
(see Abbott Laboratories)

Tishcon Corp
30 New York Avenue
Westbury, NY 11590-5910
(800) 848-8442
www.tishcon.com

Tom's of Maine, Inc
302 LaFayette Center
PO Box 710
Kennebunk, ME 04043
(800) 367-8667
www.tomsofmaine.com

Triton Consumer Products, Inc
561 West Golf Road
Arlington Heights, IL 60005-3904
(800) 942-2009
www.tritonconsumerproducts.com

Tweezerman International
2 Tri Harbor Court
Port Washington, NY 11050-4617
(800) 645-3340
www.tweezerman.com

TwinLab Corporation
150 Motor Parkway
Suite 210
Hauppauge, NY 11788
(800) 645-5626
www.twinlab.com

UAD Laboratories, Inc
(see Forest Laboratories, Inc)

UCB Pharmaceuticals, Inc
1950 Lake Park Drive
Smyrna, GA 30080
(800) 477-7877
www.ucb-pharma.com

UDL Laboratories, Inc
1718 Northrock Court
Rockford, IL 61103
(800) 848-0462
www.udllabs.com

Unimed Pharmaceuticals
(see Solvay Pharmaceuticals)

Unipath Diagnostics, Inc
51 Sawyer Road
Suite 200
Waltham, MA 02453
(781) 647-3900
www.unipath.com

United Guardian, Inc
230 Marcus Boulevard
PO Box 18050
Hauppauge, NY 11788
(800) 645-5566
www.u-g.com

Upjohn (see Pharmacia & Upjohn Company)

Upsher-Smith Laboratories, Inc
6701 Evenstad Drive
Maple Grove, MN 55369
(763) 315-2000
www.upsher-smith.com

UroCor Labs
800 Research Parkway
Oklahoma City, OK 73104
(800) 634-9330
www.urocor.com

Urologix
14405 21st Avenue North
Minneapolis, MN 55447
(800) 475-1403
www.urologix.com

USA Nutritionals, Inc
513 Commack Road
Deerpark, NY 11729
(631) 643-0600
www.USANutritionals.com

US DenTek
307 Excellence Way
Maryville, TN 37801
(800) 433-6835
www.usdentek.com

US Surgical
150 Glover Avenue
Norwalk, CT 06856
(800) 722-8772
www.ussurg.com

Valeant Pharmaceuticals International
Valeant Plaza
3300 Hyland Avenue
Costa Mesa, CA 92626
(800) 548-5100
www.valeant.com

Value in Pharmaceuticals
3000 Alt Boulevard
Grand Island, NY 14072
(800) 724-3784
www.vippharm.com

Vertex Pharmaceuticals, Inc
130 Waverly Street
Cambridge, MA 02139
(617) 444-6100
www.vpharm.com

VHA, Inc
220 East Las Colinas Boulevard
Irving, TX 75039
(800) 842-7587
www.vha.com

Vicks Health Care Products
(see Procter & Gamble Pharmaceuticals, Inc)

Vicks Pharmacy Products
(see Procter & Gamble Pharmaceuticals, Inc)

ViRexx Medical Corp
8223 Roper Road
Edmonton, Alberta Canada T6E 6S4
(780) 433-4411
www.virexx.com

VISION Pharmaceuticals, Inc
1022 North Main Street
PO Box 400
Mitchell, SD 57301
(800) 325-6789
www.visionpharm.com

VistaPharm
2224 Cahaba Valley Drive
Suite B3
Birmingham, AL 35242
(205) 981-1387
www.vistapharm.com

Vitaline Formulary
825 Challenger Drive
Green Bay, WI 54311
(800) 287-5972
www.vitalineformulary.com

Vitamin Research Products
4610 Arrowhead Drive
Carson City, NV 89706
(800) 877-2447
www.vrp.com

VIVUS, Inc
1172 Castro Street
Mountain View, CA 94040
(888) 345-MUSE
www.vivus.com

Walgreen Company
200 Wilmont Road
Dearfield, IL 60015
(847) 940-2500
www.walgreens.com

Wallace Pharmaceuticals
(see MedPointe Pharmaceuticals)

Wal-Mart Stores, Inc
702 Southwest 8th Street
Bentonville, AR 72716
(501) 273-4000
www.wal-mart.com

Wampole Laboratories
2 Research Way
Princeton, NJ 08540
(800) 257-9525
www.wampolelabs.com

Warner Chilcott Laboratories
100 Enterprise Drive
Rockaway, NJ 07866
(800) 424-5202
www.warnerchilcott.com

Watson Laboratories, Inc
311 Bonnie Circle
Corona, CA 92880
(800) 272-5525
www.watsonpharm.com

Wellements
3925 East Watkins Drive
Suite 200
Phoenix, AZ 85034
(800) 255-2690
www.mdlabs.com

Westwood-Squibb Pharmaceuticals (Bristol-Myers Squibb)
100 Forest Avenue
Buffalo, NY 14213
(800) 332-2056

W. F. Young, Inc
PO Box 1990
East Longmeadow, MA 01028-5990
(800) 628-9653
www.absorbine.com

Whitehall-Robins Healthcare
(see Wyeth Pharmaceuticals)

Winthrop Pharmaceuticals
(see Sanofi-Synthelabo, Inc)

Wisconsin Pharmacal Company (WPC Brands)
1 Pharmacal Way
Jackson, WI 53037
(800) 558-6614
www.pharmacalway.com

Women First Healthcare, Inc
5355 Mira Sorrento Place
Suite 700
San Diego, CA 92121
(858) 509-1171
www.womenfirst.com

Woodward Laboratories, Inc
125-B Columbia
Aliso Viejo, CA 92656-1458
(949) 362-4600
www.woodwardlabs.com

Wyeth Pharmaceuticals
5 Giralda Farms
Madison, NJ 07940
(800) 446-9824
www.wyeth.com

Xoma
2910 7th Street
Berkeley, CA 94710
(800) 544-9662
www.xoma.com

Xttrium Laboratories, Inc
415 West Pershing Road
Chicago, IL 60609
(877) 988-2721
www.adultrashcreme.com

Young Dental Manufacturing
13705 Shoreline Court East
Earth City, MO 63045
(800) 325-1881
www.youngdental.com

Zanfel Laboratories, Inc
Morton, IL 61550
(800) 401-4002
www.zanfel.com

Zeneca Pharmaceuticals
(see AstraZeneca Pharmaceuticals, LP)

Zenith Goldline Pharmaceuticals
(see Teva Pharmaceuticals USA)

Zila Pharmaceuticals, Inc
5227 North 7th Street
Phoenix, AZ 85014-2800
(800) 922-7887
www.zila.com

ZLB Behring
1020 First Avenue
PO Box 61501
King of Prussia, PA 19406
(610) 878-4000
www.zlbbehring.com

Zonagen, Inc
2408 Timberloch Place, B-1
The Woodlands, TX 77380
(281) 719-3400
www.zonagen.com

ZymeTx, Inc
655 Research Parkway
Suite 554
Oklahoma City, OK 73104
(888) 817-1314
www.zymetx.com

ZymoGenetics, Inc
1201 Eastlake Avenue East
Seattle, WA 98102-3702
(206) 442-6600
www.zymogenetics.com

VITAMIN PRODUCTS

Injectable Formulations

Product	A (int. units)	B_1 (mg)	B_2 (mg)	B_6 (mg)	B_{12} (mcg)	C (mg)	D (int. units)	E (int. units)	K (mcg)	Additional Information
Solution										
Infuvite® Adult (per 10 mL)	3300	6	3.6	6	5	200	200	10	150	Supplied as two 5 mL vials. Biotin 60 mcg, folic acid 600 mcg, niacinamide 40 mg, dexpanthenol 15 mg
Infuvite® Pediatric (per 5 mL)	2300	1.6	1.4	1	1	80	400	7	200	Supplied as one 4 mL vial and one 1 mL vial. Biotin 20 mcg, folic acid 140 mcg, niacinamide 17 mg, dexpanthenol 5 mg
M.V.I®-12 [DSC] (per 10 mL)	3300	3	3.6	4	12.5	100	200	10	---	Supplied as two 5 mL vials or a single 2-chambered 10 mL vial. Biotin 60 mcg, folic acid 400 mcg, niacinamide 40 mg, dexpanthenol 15 mg
M.V.I. Adult™ (per 10 mL)	3300	6	3.6	6	5	200	200	10	150	Supplied as two 5 mL vials or a single 2-chambered 10 mL vial. Also available in a pharmacy bulk package (two 50 mL vials). Biotin 60 mcg, folic acid 600 mcg, niacinamide 40 mg, dexpanthenol 15 mg
Powder for Reconstitution										
M.V.I.® Pediatric	2300	1.2	1.4	1	1	80	400	7	200	Biotin 20 mcg, folic acid 140 mcg, niacinamide 17 mg, dexpanthenol 5 mg, aluminum, polysorbate 80

Adult Formulations

Product	A (int. units)	B_1 (mg)	B_2 (mg)	B_6 (mg)	B_{12} (mcg)	C (mg)	D (int. units)	E (int. units)	Additional Information
Liquid									
Centrum® [OTC] (per 15 mL)	2500	1.5	1.7	2	6	60	400	30	Biotin 300 mcg, Cr 25 mcg, Fe 9 mg, iodine 150 mcg, Mn 2 mg, Mo 25 mg, niacin 20 mg, pantothenic acid 10 mg, Zn 3 mg; alcohol 5.4%, sodium benzoate (240 mL)
Geriation® [OTC] (per 30 mL)		5	2.5	1	1				Choline 100 mg, Fe 15 mg, iodine 100 mcg, Mg 2 mg, Mn 2 mg, niacinamide 50 mg, pantothenic acid 10 mg, Zn 2 mg; sherry flavor (480 mL)
Geritol® Tonic [OTC] (per 15 mL)		2.5	2.5	0.5					Chlorine bitartrate 50 mg, Fe 18 mg, methionine 25 mg, niacin 50 mg, pantothenic acid 2 mg; sugars 7 g, alcohol 12%, benzoic acid (120 mL, 360 mL)
Strovite® Forte (per 15 mL)	4000	15	17	20	20	300	400	30	Biotin 150 mcg, Cr 50 mcg, Cu 3 mg, Fe 10 mg, folic acid 1 mg, Mg 50 mg, Mn 5 mg, niacinamide 100 mg, pantothenic acid 25 mg, Se 55 mcg, Zn 15 mg; contains aspartame
Vi-Daylin® [OTC] [DSC] (per 5 mL)	2500	1.05	1.2	1.05	4.5	60	400	15	Niacin 13.5 mg; alcohol <0.5%, benzoic acid; lemon/orange flavor (240 mL, 480 mL)
Vi-Daylin® + Iron [OTC] [DSC] (per 5 mL)	2500	1.05	1.2	1.05	4.5	60	400	15	Fe 10 mg, niacin 13.5 mg; alcohol <0.5%, benzoic acid; lemon/orange flavor (240 mL, 480 mL)
Caplet									
Glutofac®-MX (per 1 light purple caplet and 1 dark purple caplet)					10				Ascorbic acid 100 mg, biotin 300 mcg, boron 150 mcg, Ca 425 mg, Cr 200 mcg, dioctyl sodium sulfosuccinate 10 mg, Fe 15 mg, folic acid 800 mcg, iodine 150 mcg, Mg 415 mg, Mn 5 mg, Mo 75 mcg, nickel 5 mcg, pantothenic acid 25 mg, phosphorus 130 mg, potassium 80 mg, Se 100 mcg, tin 10 mcg, vanadium 10 mcg, Zn 35 mg

(continued)

Product	A (int. units)	B_1 (mg)	B_2 (mg)	B_6 (mg)	B_{12} (mcg)	C (mg)	D (int. units)	E (int. units)	Additional Information
Glutofac®-ZX	5000	20	20	25	50	500	400	50	Biotin 200 mcg, Ca 66 mg, Cr 200 mcg, Cu 2.5 mg, niacinamide 100 mg, folic acid 1000 mcg, Mg 50 mg, Mn 5 mg, pantothenic acid 25 mg, Se 50 mcg, Zn 20 mg
Theragran® Heart Right™ [OTC] [DSC]	5000	3	3.4	16	30	120	400	400	Alpha-carotene, beta-carotene, biotin 30 mcg, Ca 55 mg, Cr 50 mcg, cryptoxanthin, Cu 1.5 mg, Fe 4 mg, folic acid as folate 0.6 mg, iodine 150 mcg, lutein, lycopene, Mg 150 mg, Mn 2 mg, Mo 75 mcg, niacin 20 mg, pantothenic acid 10 mg, Se 70 mcg, vitamin K 14 mcg, zeaxanthin, Zn 15 mg
Theragran-M® Advanced Formula [OTC] [DSC]	5000	3	3.4	6	12	90	400	60	Biotin 30 mcg, boron 150 mcg, Ca 40 mg, chloride 7.5 mg, Cr 50 mcg, Cu 2 mg, Fe 9 mg, folic acid 0.4 mg, iodine 150 mcg, Mg 100 mg, Mn 2 mg, Mo 75 mcg, niacin 20 mg, nickel 5 mcg, pantothenic acid 10 mg, phosphorus 31 mg, potassium 7.5 mg, Se 70 mcg, silicon 2 mg, tin 10 mcg, vanadium 10 mcg, vitamin K 28 mcg, Zn 15 mg
Capsule									
Hemocyte Plus®		10	6	5	15	200			Cu 0.8 mg, Fe 106 mg, folic acid 1 mg, Mg 6.9 mg, Mn 1.3 mg, niacinamide 30 mg, pantothenic acid 10 mg, Zn 18.2 mg
Multiret Folic 500		6	6	5	25	500			Calcium pantothenate 10 mg, Fe 525 mg (timed-release), niacinamide 30 mg
Ocuvite® Lutein						60		30	Cu 2 mg, lutein 6 mg, Zn 15 mg
Replace [OTC] (per 2 capsules)	5000	25	25	25	25	60	75	30	Betaine 20 mg, biotin 20 mcg, Ca 180 mg, choline 25 mg, Cr 50 mcg, Cu 0.1 mg, folic acid 400 mcg, inositol 25 mg, iodine 0.225 mg, lemon bioflavonoid complex 50 mg, Mg 90 mg, Mn 2.5 mg, Mo 20 mcg, niacin 40 mg, PABA 12.5 mg, pancreatin 50 mg, pantothenic acid 75 mg, potassium 20 mg, Se 50 mcg, Zn 10 mg

(continued)

Product	A (int. units)	B_1 (mg)	B_2 (mg)	B_6 (mg)	B_{12} (mcg)	C (mg)	D (int. units)	E (int. units)	Additional Information
Replace With Iron [OTC] (per 2 capsules)	5000	25	25	25	25	60	75	30	Betaine 20 mg, biotin 20 mcg, Ca 180 mg, choline 25 mg, Cr 50 mcg, Cu 0.1 mg, Fe 10 mg, folic acid 400 mcg, inositol 25 mg, iodine 0.225 mg, lemon bioflavonoid complex 50 mg, Mg 90 mg, Mn 2.5 mg, Mo 20 mcg, niacin 40 mg, PABA 12.5 mg, pancreatin 50 mg, pantothenic acid 75 mg, potassium 20 mg, Se 50 mcg, Zn 10 mg
Vicon Forte®	8000	10	5	2	10	150		50	Folic acid 1 mg, Mg 70 mg, Mn 4 mg, niacinamide 25 mg, Zn 80 mg
Vitacon Forte	8000	10	5	2	10	150		50	Folic acid 1 mg, Mg 70 mg, Mn 4 mg, niacinamide 25 mg, Zn 80 mg
Capsule, Softgel									
PreserVision® Lutein [OTC]						226		200	Cu 0.8 mg, lutein 5 mg, Zn 34.8 mg
PreserVision® AREDS [OTC]	14,320					226		200	Cu 0.8 mg, Zn 34.8 mg
Tablet									
Androvite® [OTC] (per 6 tablets)	2500	50	50	100	125	1000	400	400	Betaine 100 mg, boron 3 mg, Cr 200 mcg, Cu 2 mg, Fe 18 mg, folic acid 400 mcg, hesperidin 35 mg, inositol 36 mg, iodine 150 mcg, Mg 500 mg, Mn 10 mg, niacinamide 50 mg, PABA 25 mg, pancreatin 4X 75 mg, pantothenic acid 100 mg, rutin 25 mg, Se 200 mcg, Zn 50 mg
Centrum® [OTC]	3500	1.5	1.7	2	6	60	400	30	Biotin 30 mcg, boron 150 mcg, Ca 162 mg, chloride 72 mg, Cr 120 mcg, Cu 2 mg, Fe 18 mg, folic acid 0.4 mg, iodine 150 mcg, lutein 250 mcg, lycopene 300 mcg, Mg 100 mg, Mn 2 mg, Mo 75 mcg, niacin 20 mg, nickel 5 mcg, pantothenic acid 10 mg, phosphorus 109 mg, potassium 80 mg, Se 20 mcg, silicon 2 mg, tin 10 mcg, vanadium 10 mcg, vitamin K 25 mcg, Zn 15 mg

(continued)

Product	A (int. units)	B_1 (mg)	B_2 (mg)	B_6 (mg)	B_{12} (mcg)	C (mg)	D (int. units)	E (int. units)	Additional Information
Centrum® Carb Assist™ [OTC]	3500	4.5	5.1	6	18	120	400	60	Biotin 40 mcg, boron 60 mcg, Ca 100 mg, chloride 72 mg, Cr 120 mcg, Cu 2 mg, Fe 18 mg, folic acid 400 mcg, ginkgo biloba leaf 60 mg, ginseng root 50 mg, iodine 150 mcg, Mg 40 mg, Mo 75 mcg, niacin 40 mg, nickel 5 mcg, pantothenic acid 10 mg, phosphorus 48 mg, potassium 80 mg, Se 70 mcg, silicon 4 mg, tin 10 mcg, vanadium 10 mcg, vitamin K 25 mcg, Zn 15 mg
Centrum® Performance™ [OTC]	3500	4.5	5.1	6	18	120	400	60	Biotin 40 mcg, boron 60 mcg, chloride 72 mg, folic acid 0.4 mg, Ca 100 mg, Cr 120 mcg, Cu 2 mg, Fe 18 mg, ginkgo biloba leaf 60 mg, ginseng root 50 mg, iodine 150 mcg, Mg 40 mg, Mn 4 mg, Mo 75 mcg, niacin 40 mg, nickel 5 mcg, pantothenic acid 10 mg, phosphorus 48 mg, potassium 80 mg, Se 70 mcg, silicon 4 mg, tin 10 mcg, vanadium 10 mcg, vitamin K 25 mcg, Zn 15 mg
Centrum® Silver® [OTC]	3500	1.5	1.7	3	25	60	400	45	Biotin 30 mcg, boron 150 mcg, Ca 200 mg, chloride 72 mg, Cr 150 mcg, Cu 2 mg, folic acid 0.4 mg, iodine 150 mcg, lutein 250 mcg, lycopene 300 mcg, Mg 100 mg, Mn 2 mg, Mo 75 mcg, niacin 20 mg, nickel 5 mcg, pantothenic acid 10 mg, phosphorus 48 mg, potassium 80 mg, Se 20 mcg, silicon 2 mg, vanadium 10 mcg, vitamin K 10 mcg, Zn 15 mg
Diatx® ZN		1.5	1.5		2	60			Cu 1.5 mg, D-biotin 300 mcg, folic acid 5 mg, niacinamide 20 mg, pantothenic acid 10 mg, Zn 25 mg [gluten free, lactose free, sugar free, yeast free]
Freedavite [OTC]	5000	1.5	1.7	2	6	60	400	30	Biotin 30 mcg, Ca 20 mg, Cu 0.1 mg, Fe 1.8 mg, folic acid 400 mcg, iodine 75 mcg, Mg 8 mg, Mn 0.625 mg, niacinamide 20 mg, pantothenic acid 10 mg, Se 35 mcg, Zn 1.5 mg

(continued)

Product	A (int. units)	B_1 (mg)	B_2 (mg)	B_6 (mg)	B_{12} (mcg)	C (mg)	D (int. units)	E (int. units)	Additional Information
Geri-Freeda [OTC]	5000	15	15	15	15	150	400	15	Betaine 10 mg, biotin 15 mcg, Ca 50 mg, choline 10 mg, Cr 60 mcg, Cu 0.5 mg, folic acid 400 mcg, hesperidin 10 mg, inositol 25 mg, iodine 150 mcg, L-lysine 25 mg, Mg 25 mg, Mn 1 mg, niacinamide 50 mg, PABA 10 mg, pantothenic acid 15 mg, Se 35 mcg, Zn 7.5 mg
Geritol Complete® [OTC]	6100	1.5	1.7	2	6.7	57	400	30	Biotin 44 mcg, Ca 148 mg, chloride 20 mg, Cr 12 mcg, Cu 1.8 mg, Fe 16 mg, folic acid 0.38 mg, iodine 120 mcg, Mg 86 mg, Mn 2.4 mg, Mo 1 mcg, niacin 20 mg, pantothenic acid 13 mg, phosphorous 118 mg, potassium 36 mg, vitamin K 24 mcg, Zn 13.5 mg
Geritol Extend® [OTC]	3333	1.2	1.3	2	2.5	55	200	13	Ca 120 mg, Fe 9.5 mg, folic acid 0.2 mg, iodine 130 mcg, Mg 32 mg, niacin 15 mg, phosphorous 98 mg, Se 35 mcg, vitamin K 80 mcg, Zn 14 mg
Gynovite® Plus [OTC] (per 6 tablets)	5000	10	10	20	125	180	400	400	Betaine 100 mg, biotin 125 mcg, boron 3 mg, Ca 500 mg, Cr 200 mcg, Cu 2 mg, Fe 18 mg, folic acid 400 mcg, hesperidin 35 mg, inositol 50 mg, iodine 150 mcg, Mg 600 mg, Mn 10 mg, niacin 20 mg, PABA 25 mg, pancreatin 4X 93 mg, pantothenic acid 10 mg, rutin 25 mg, Se 200 mcg, Zn 15 mg
Hemocyte Plus®		10	6	5	15	200			Cu 0.8 mg, Fe 106 mg, folic acid 1 mg, Mg 6.9 mg, Mn 1.3 mg, niacinamide 30 mg, pantothenic acid 10 mg, Zn 18.2 mg
Hi-Kovite [OTC] (per contents of 1 vitamin tablet plus 1 mineral tablet)	5000	10	10	10	10	200	400	30	Bioflavonoids 10 mg, biotin 30 mcg, Ca 120 mg, Cu 0.5 mg, Fe 9 mg, folic acid 400 mcg, inositol 10 mg, iodine 9 mg, L-lysine 10 mg, Mg 60 mg, Mn 1 mg, niacinamide 100 mg, PABA 10 mg, pantothenic acid 10 mg, potassium 35 mg, Se 17.5 mg, Zn 7.5 mg

(continued)

Product	A (int. units)	B_1 (mg)	B_2 (mg)	B_6 (mg)	B_{12} (mcg)	C (mg)	D (int. units)	E (int. units)	Additional Information
Iberet®-500 [OTC]		4.96	5.4	3.7	22.5	500			Fe 95 mg (controlled release), niacin 27.2 mg, pantothenic acid 8.28 mg, sodium 65 mg
Iberet-Folic-500® [OTC]		6	6	5	25	500			Fe 105 mg (controlled release), folic acid 0.8 mg, niacinamide 30 mg, calcium pantothenate 10 mg
Monocaps [OTC]	5000	15	15	15	15	120	400	15	Biotin 15 mcg, Ca 50 mg, Cu 0.1 mg, Fe 14 mg, folic acid 400 mcg, iodine 150 mcg, lecithin 10 mg, L-lysine 10 mg, Mg 30 mg, Mn 1 mg, niacinamide 40 mg, PABA 10 mg, pantothenic acid 15 mg, Se 35 mcg, Zn 3.75 mg
Ocuvite® [OTC]	1000					200		60	Cu 2 mg, lutein 2 mg, Se 55 mcg, Zn 40 mg
Ocuvite® Extra [OTC]	1000		3			300		100	Cu 2 mg, L-glutathione 5 mg, lutein 2 mg, Mn 5 mg, niacinamide 40 mg, Se 55 mcg, Zn 40 mg
Olay® Vitamins Complete Women's [OTC]	5000	1.5	1.7	2	6	120	400	50	Biotin 30 mcg, boron 150 mcg, Ca 250 mg, chloride 36 mg, coenzyme Q_{10} 2 mg, Cr 120 mcg, Cu 5 mg, Fe 18 mg, folic acid 0.4 mg, iodine 150 mcg, lutein 250 mg, Mg 100 mg, Mn 2 mg, Mo 25 mcg, niacin 20 mg, nickel 5 mcg, pantothenic acid 10 mg, phosphorus 77 mg, potassium 40 mg, Se 25 mcg, silicon 2 mg, vanadium 10 mcg, Zn 15 mg
Olay® Vitamins Complete Women's 50+ [OTC]	5000	3	3.4	4	25	120	400	60	Biotin 30 mcg, boron 150 mcg, Ca 250 mg, chloride 72 mg, coenzyme Q_{10} 2 mg, Cr 120 mcg, Cu 5 mg, folic acid 0.4 mg, iodine 150 mcg, lutein 250 mg, Mg 120 mg, Mn 2 mg, Mo 25 mcg, niacin 20 mg, nickel 5 mcg, pantothenic acid 10 mg, phosphorus 48 mg, potassium 80 mg, Se 50 mcg, silicon 2 mg, vanadium 10 mcg, Zn 22 mg
Olay® Vitamins Even Complexion [OTC]	5000					120	100	60	Cu 2 mg, folic acid 200 mcg, Se 50 mcg, Zn 15 mg

(continued)

Product	A (int. units)	B_1 (mg)	B_2 (mg)	B_6 (mg)	B_{12} (mcg)	C (mg)	D (int. units)	E (int. units)	Additional Information
One-A-Day® 50 Plus Formula [OTC]	2500	4.5	3.4	6	25	120	400	33	Biotin 30 mcg, Ca 120 mg, chloride 34 mg, Cr 180 mcg, Cu 2 mg, folic acid 0.4 mg, iodine 150 mcg, Mg 100 mg, Mn 4 mg, Mo 90 mcg, niacin 20 mg, pantothenic acid 15 mg, potassium 37.5 mg, Se 105 mcg, vitamin K 20 mcg, Zn 22.5 mg
One-A-Day® Active Formula [OTC]	5000	4.5	5.1	6	18	120	400	60	American ginseng 55 mg, biotin 40 mcg, boron 150 mcg, Ca 110 mg, chloride 180 mg, Cr 100 mcg, Cu 2 mg, Fe 9 mg, folic acid 0.4 mg, iodine 150 mcg, Mg 40 mg, Mn 2 mg, Mo 25 mcg, niacin 40 mg, nickel 5 mcg, pantothenic acid 10 mg, phosphorus 48 mg, potassium 200 mg, Se 45 mcg, silicon 6 mg, tin 10 mcg, vanadium 10 mcg, vitamin K 25 mcg, Zn 15 mg
One-A-Day® Carb Smart [OTC]	2500	2.2	2.5	3	9	90	400	45	Biotin 450 mcg, Ca 200 mg, Cr 200 mcg, Cu 2 mg, folic acid 400 mcg, Mg 100 mg, Mn 2 mg, Mo 75 mg, niacin 25 mg, pantothenic acid 15 mg, phosphorous 154 mg, potassium 99 mg, Se 105 mcg, vitamin K 25 mcg, Zn 22.5 mg
One-A-Day® Cholesterol Plus™ [OTC]	2500	1.5	1.7	2	6	60	400	30	Biotin 50 mcg, Ca 100 mg, Cr 120 mcg, Cu 2 mg, folic acid 400 mcg, iodine 150 mg, Mg 100 mg, Mn 2 mg, Mo 75 mg, niacin 20 mg, pantothenic acid 10 mg, policosanol 10 mg, potassium 99 mg, Se 70 mcg, Zn 15 mg
One-A-Day® Essential Formula [OTC]	5000	1.5	1.7	2	6	60	400	30	Folic acid 0.4 mg, niacin 20 mg, pantothenic acid 10 mg
One-A-Day® Maximum Formula [OTC]	5000	1.5	1.7	2	6	60	400	30	Biotin 30 mcg, boron 150 mcg, Ca 210 mg, chloride 72 mg, Cr 120 mcg, Cu 2 mg, Fe 18 mg, folic acid 0.4 mg, iodine 150 mcg, lycopene 600 mcg, Mg 120 mg, Mn 2 mg, Mo 160 mcg, niacin 20 mg, nickel 5 mcg, pantothenic acid 5 mg, phosphorus 109 mg, potassium 100 mg, Se 105 mcg, silicon 2 mg, tin 10 mcg, vanadium 10 mcg, vitamin K 25 mcg, Zn 15 mg

(continued)

Product	A (int. units)	B_1 (mg)	B_2 (mg)	B_6 (mg)	B_{12} (mcg)	C (mg)	D (int. units)	E (int. units)	Additional Information
One-A-Day® Men's Formula [OTC]	3500	1.2	1.7	3	18	90	400	45	Biotin 30 mcg, chloride 34 mg, Cr 150 mcg, Cu 2 mg, folic acid 0.4 mg, iodine 150 mcg, Mg 100 mg, Mn 3.5 mg, Mo 42 mcg, niacin 16 mg, pantothenic acid 10 mg, potassium 37.5 mg, Se 87.5 mcg, vitamin K 20 mcg, Zn 15 mg
One-A-Day® Today [OTC]	3000	1.1	1.7	3	18	75	400	33	Biotin 30 mcg, Ca 240 mg, Cr 120 mcg, Cu 2 mg, folic acid 0.4 mg, Mg 120 mg, Mn 2 mg, niacin 14 mg, pantothenic acid 5 mg, potassium 100 mg, Se 70 mcg, soy extract 10 mg, vitamin K 20 mcg, Zn 15 mg
One-A-Day® Weight Smart [OTC]	2500	1.9	2.125	2.5	7.5	60	400	30	Ca 300 mg, Cr 200 mcg, Cu 2 mg, EGCG 32 mcg, Fe 18 mg, folic acid 400 mcg, Mg 50 mg, Mn 2 mg, niacin 25 mg, pantothenic acid 12.5 mg, Se 70 mcg, vitamin K 80 mcg, Zn 15 mg
One-A-Day® Women's Formula [OTC]	2500	1.5	1.7	2	6	60	400	30	Ca 450 mg, Fe 18 mg, folic acid 0.4 mg, Mg 50 mg, niacin 10 mg, pantothenic acid 5 mg, Zn 15 mg
Optivite® P.M.T. [OTC] (per 6 tablets)	125,000	25	25	300	60	1500	100	100	Betaine 100 mg, biotin 60 mcg, Ca 125 mg, choline 313 mg, citrus bioflavonioids 250 mg, Cr 100 mcg, Fe 15 mg, folic acid 200 mcg, inositol 24 mg, iodine 75 mcg, Mg 250 mg, Mn 10 mg, niacinamide 25 mg, PABA 25 mg, pancreatin 4X 93 mg, pantothenic acid 25 mg, potassium 48 mg, rutin 25 mg, Se 100 mcg, Zn 25 mg
PreserVision® AREDS [OTC]	14,320					226		200	Cu 0.8 mg, Zn 34.8 mg
Quintabs [OTC]	5000	30	30	30	30	300	400	50	Biotin 30 mcg, folic acid 400 mcg, niacinamide 100 mg, pantothenic acid 30 mg
Quintabs-M [OTC]	5000	30	30	30	30	300	400	50	Biotin 30 mcg, Ca 30 mg, Cu 0.2 mg, Fe 10 mg, folic acid 400 mcg, iodine 150 mcg, Mg 15 mg, Mn 2 mg, niacinamide 100 mg, PABA 10 mg, pantothenic acid 30 mg, Se 35 mcg, Zn 7.5 mg

(continued)

Product	A (int. units)	B_1 (mg)	B_2 (mg)	B_6 (mg)	B_{12} (mcg)	C (mg)	D (int. units)	E (int. units)	Additional Information
Repliva 21/7™					10	140 mg as ascorbic acid, 60 mg as calcium ascorbate, 0.8 mg as calcium threonate			Fe 70 mg as Ferrochel®, Fe 81 mg as fumarate, folic acid 1 mg, succinic acid 150 mg
T-Vites [OTC]		25	25	25	30	100	400		Biotin 30 mcg, folic acid 400 mcg, Mg 100 mg, Mn 0.5 mg, niacinamide 150 mg, pantothenic acid 25 mg, potassium 35 mg, Zn 3.75 mg
Ultra Freeda Iron Free [OTC] (per 3 tablets)	12,500	50	50	50	100	1000	400	200	Bioflavonoids 100 mg, biotin 300 mcg, Ca 250 mg, Cr 200 mcg, folic acid 800 mcg, Mg 100 mg, Mn 10 mg, Mo 12.5 mcg, niacinamide and niacin 100 mg, pantothenic acid 100 mg, potassium 35 mg, Se 100 mcg, Zn 22.5 mg
Ultra Freeda With Iron [OTC] (per 3 tablets)	5000	50	50	50	100	1000	400	200	Bioflavonoids 100 mg, biotin 300 mcg, Ca 250 mg, Cr 200 mcg, Fe 18 mg, folic acid 800 mcg, Mg 100 mg, Mn 10 mg, Mo 12.5 mcg, niacinamide and niacin 100 mg, pantothenic acid 100 mg, potassium 35 mg, Se 100 mcg, Zn 22.5 mg
Unicap Sr.® [OTC]	5000	1.2	1.4	2.2	3	60	200	15	Ca 100 mg, Cu 2 mg, Fe 10 mg, folic acid 400 mcg, iodine 150 mcg, Mg 30 mg, Mn 1 mg, niacin 16 mg, pantothenic acid 10 mg, phosphorus 77 mg, potassium 5 mg, Zn 15 mg
Unicap T® [OTC]	5000	10	10	6	18	500	400	30	Cu 2 mg, Fe 18 mg, folic acid 400 mcg, iodine 150 mcg, Mn 1 mg, niacin 100 mg, pantothenic acid 25 mg, potassium 5 mg, Se 10 mg, Zn 15 mg
Xtramins [OTC]	1000	5	2	5	10	50	100	10	Boron 1 mg, Ca 250 mg, Cr 40 mcg, Cu 0.5 mg, d-calcium pantothenate 5 mg, Fe 10 mg, folic acid 400 mcg, iodine 150 mcg, Mg 20 mg, Mn 2 mg, niacinamide 15 mg, PABA 5 mg, potassium 45 mg, Se 30 mcg, Zn 10 mg

(continued)

Product	A (int. units)	B_1 (mg)	B_2 (mg)	B_6 (mg)	B_{12} (mcg)	C (mg)	D (int. units)	E (int. units)	Additional Information
Tablet, Chewable									
Centrum® [OTC]	3500	1.5	1.7	2	6	60	400	30	Biotin 45 mcg, Ca 108 mg, Cr 20 mcg, Cu 2 mg, Fe 18 mg, folic acid 0.4 mg, iodine 150 mcg, Mg 40 mg, Mn 1 mg, Mo 20 mcg, niacin 20 mg, pantothenic acid 10 mg, phosphorus 50 mg, vitamin K 10 mcg, Zn 15 mg
Viactiv® Multivitamin [OTC] (softchews)	2500	1.5	1.7	2	6	60	400	33	Biotin 30 mcg, Ca 200 mg, folic acid 400 mcg, niacin 15 mg, pantothenic acid 10 mg; sodium 25 mg; milk chocolate flavor

Key: Ca = calcium, Cr = chromium, Cu = copper, Fe = iron, Mg = magnesium, Mn = manganese, Mo = molybdenum, Se = selenium, Zn = zinc.

Pediatric Formulations

Product	A (int. units)	B_1 (mg)	B_2 (mg)	B_6 (mg)	B_{12} (mcg)	C (mg)	D (int. units)	E (int. units)	Additional Information
Drops									
ADEKs [OTC] (per mL)	3170 (50% as beta-carotene)	0.5	0.6	0.6	4	45	400	40	Biotin 15 mcg, niacin 6 mg, pantothenic acid 3 mg, vitamin K 0.1 mg, Zn 5 mg; alcohol free, dye free (60 mL)
Poly-Vi-Flor® 0.25 mg (per mL)	1500	0.5	0.6	0.4	2	35	400	5	**Fluoride 0.25 mg**, niacin 8 mg; fruit flavor (50 mL)
Poly-Vi-Flor® 0.5 mg (per mL)	1500	0.5	0.6	0.4	2	35	400	5	**Fluoride 0.5 mg**, niacin 8 mg; fruit flavor (50 mL)
Poly-Vi-Flor® With Iron 0.25 mg (per mL)	1500	0.5	0.6	0.4		35	400	5	**Fluoride 0.25 mg**, iron 10 mg, niacin 8 mg; fruit flavor (50 mL)
Poly-Vi-Sol® [OTC] (per mL)	1500	0.5	0.6	0.4	2	35	400	5	Niacin 8 mg (50 mL)
Poly-Vi-Sol® With Iron [OTC] (per mL)	1500	0.5	0.6	0.4		35	400	5	Iron 10 mg, niacin 8 mg (50 mL)
Soluvite-F® (per 0.6 mL)	1500				35	400			**Fluoride 0.25 mg**; alcohol free, dye free, orange flavor (57 mL)
Tri-Vi-Flor® 0.25 mg (per mL)	1500					35	400		**Fluoride 0.25 mg**; fruit flavor (50 mL)
Tri-Vi-Flor® With Iron 0.25 mg (per mL)	1500					35	400		**Fluoride 0.25 mg**, iron 10 mg; fruit flavor (50 mL)
Tri-Vi-Sol® [OTC] (per mL)	1500					35	400		Fruit flavor (50 mL)
Tri-Vi-Sol® With Iron [OTC] (per mL)	1500					35	400		Iron 10 mg; fruit flavor (50 mL)
Vi-Daylin® [OTC] [DSC] (per mL)	1500	0.5	0.6	0.4	1.5	35	400	5	Niacin 8 mg; alcohol <0.5%, sugar free, fruit flavor (50 mL)
Vi-Daylin® + Iron [OTC] [DSC] (per mL)	1500	0.5	0.6	0.4		35	400	5	Iron 10 mg, niacin 8 mg; alcohol <0.5%, sugar free, fruit flavor (50 mL)
Vi-Daylin® ADC [OTC] [DSC] (per mL)	1500					35	400		Alcohol <0.5%, sugar free, fruit flavor (50 mL)

(continued)

Product	A (int. units)	B_1 (mg)	B_2 (mg)	B_6 (mg)	B_{12} (mcg)	C (mg)	D (int. units)	E (int. units)	Additional Information
Vi-Daylin® ADC + Iron [OTC] [DSC] (per mL)	1500					35	400		Iron 10 mg; benzoic acid, sugar free, fruit flavor (50 mL)
Vi-Daylin®/F [DSC] (per mL)	1500	0.5	0.6	0.4		35	400	5	**Fluoride 0.25 mg**, niacin 8 mg; alcohol <0.1%, benzoic acid, sugar free, fruit flavor (50 mL)
Vi-Daylin®/F + Iron [DSC] (per mL)	1500	0.5	0.6	0.4		35	400	5	**Fluoride 0.25 mg**, iron 10 mg, niacin 8 mg; alcohol <0.1%, benzoic acid, sugar free, fruit flavor (50 mL)
Vi-Daylin®/F ADC [DSC] (per mL)	1500					35	400		**Fluoride 0.25 mg**; sugar free, fruit flavor (50 mL)
Vi-Daylin®/F ADC + Iron [DSC] (per mL)	1500					35	400		**Fluoride 0.25 mg**, iron 10 mg; sugar free, fruit flavor (50 mL)
Gum									
Vitaball®	5000	1.5	1.7	2	6	60	400	30	Biotin 45 mcg, folic acid 400 mcg, niacinamide 20 mg, pantothenic acid 10 mg; bubble gum, cherry, grape, and watermelon (contains tartrazine) flavors
Vitaball® Wild 'N Fruity [OTC]	5000	1.5	1.7	2	6	240	400	30	Biotin 45 mcg, folic acid 400 mcg, niacinamide 20 mg, pantothenic acid 10 mg; berry, lemon (contains tartrazine), orange, and strawberry flavors
Tablet, Chewable									
ADEKs® [OTC]	9000 (60% as beta-carotene)	1.2	1.3	1.5	12	60	400	150	Biotin 50 mcg, folic acid 0.2 mg, niacin 10 mg, pantothenic acid 10 mg, vit K 150 mcg, Zn 7.5 mg; dye free
Centrum Kids® Jimmy Neutron™ Complete	5000	1.5	1.7	2	6	60	400	30	Biotin 45 mcg, Ca 108 mg, Cr 20 mcg, Cu 2 mg, Fe 18 mg, folic acid 0.4 mg, iodine 150 mcg, Mg 40 mg, Mn 1 mg, Mo 20 mcg, niacin 20 mg, pantothenic acid 10 mg, phosphorus 50 mg, vitamin K 10 mg, Zn 15 mg; **contains phenylalanine**; cherry, fruit punch, and orange flavors
Centrum Kids® Jimmy Neutron™ Extra C	5000	1.5	1.7	1	5	250	400	15	Ca 108 mg, Cu 0.5 mg, folic acid 0.3 mg, niacin 13.5 mg, phosphorus 50 mg, sodium 16 mg, Zn 4 mg; **contains phenylalanine**; cherry, fruit punch, and orange flavors
Centrum® Kids Rugrats™ Complete [OTC]	5000	1.5	1.7	2	6	60	400	30	Biotin 45 mcg, Ca 108 mg, Cr 20 mcg, Cu 2 mg, Fe 18 mg, folic acid 0.4 mg, iodine 150 mcg, Mg 40 mg, Mn 1 mg, Mo 20 mcg, niacin 20 mg, pantothenic acid 10 mg, phosphorus 50 mg, vitamin K 10 mg, Zn 15 mg; **contains phenylalanine**; cherry, fruit punch, and orange flavors

(continued)

Product	A (int. units)	B_1 (mg)	B_2 (mg)	B_6 (mg)	B_{12} (mcg)	C (mg)	D (int. units)	E (int. units)	Additional Information
Centrum® Kids Rugrats™ Extra C [OTC]	5000	1.5	1.7	1	5	250	400	15	Ca 108 mg, Cu 0.5 mg, folic acid 0.3 mg, niacin 13.5 mg, phosphorus 50 mg, sodium 15 mg, Zn 4 mg; **contains phenylalanine**; cherry, fruit punch, and orange flavors
Centrum® Kids Rugrats™ Extra Calcium [OTC]	5000	1.5	1.7	1	5	60	400	15	Ca 200 mg, Cu 0.5 mg, folic acid 0.3 mg, niacin 13.5 mg, phosphorus 50 mg, Zn 4 mg; **contains phenylalanine**; cherry, fruit punch, and orange flavors
Flintstones® Complete [OTC]	5000	1.5	1.7	2	6	60	400	30	Biotin 40 mcg, Ca 100 mg, Cu 2 mg, Fe 18 mg, folic acid 0.4 mg, iodine 150 mcg, Mg 20 mg, niacin 20 mg, pantothenic acid 10 mg, phosphorus 100 mg, Zn 15 mg; **phenylalanine 4.56 mg**; cherry, grape, and orange flavors
Flintstones® Plus Calcium [OTC]	2500	1.05	1.2	1.05	4.5	60	400	15	Ca 200 mg, folic acid 0.3 mg, niacin 13.5 mg; **phenylalanine <4 mg**; cherry, grape, and orange flavors
Flintstones® Plus Extra C [OTC]	2500	1.05	1.2	1.05	4.5	250	400	15	Folic acid 0.3 mg, niacin 13.5 mg; grape, orange, peach-apricot, raspberry, and strawberry flavors
Flintstones® Plus Iron [OTC]	2500	1.05	1.2	1.05	4.5	60	400	15	Fe 15 mg, folic acid 0.3 mg, niacin 13.5 mg; grape, orange, peach-apricot, raspberry, and strawberry flavors
My First Flintstones® [OTC]	2500	1.05	1.2	1.05	4.5	60	400	15	Folic acid 0.3 mg, niacin 13.5 mg; cherry, grape, and orange flavors
One-A-Day® Kids Bugs Bunny and Friends Complete [OTC]	3000	1.5	1.7	2	6	60	400	30	Biotin 40 mcg, Ca 100 mg, Cu 2 mg, Fe 18 mg, folic acid 0.4 mg, iodine 150 mcg, Mg 20 mg, niacin 15 mg, pantothenic acid 10 mg, phosphorus 100 mg, Zn 12 mg; **contains phenylalanine**; sugar free, fruity flavors
One-A-Day® Kids Bugs Bunny and Friends Plus Extra C [OTC]	2500	1.05	1.2	1.05	4.5	250	400	15	Folic acid 0.3 mg, niacin 13.5 mg, **contains phenylalanine**; sugar free, fruity flavors
One-A-Day® Kids Extreme Sports [OTC]	3000	1.5	1.7	2	6	60	400	30	Biotin 40 mcg, Ca 100 mg, Cu 2 mg, Fe 18 mg, folic acid 0.4 mg, iodine 150 mcg, Mg 20 mg, niacin 15 mg, pantothenic acid 10 mg, phosphorus 100 mg, Zn 12 mg; **contains phenylalanine**
One-A-Day® Kids Scooby-Doo! Complete [OTC]	3000	1.5	1.7	2	6	60	400	30	Biotin 40 mcg, Ca 100 mg, Cu 2 mg, Fe 18 mg, folic acid 0.4 mg, iodine 150 mcg, Mg 20 mg, niacin 15 mg, pantothenic acid 10 mg, phosphorus 100 mg, Zn 12 mg; **contains phenylalanine**; fruity flavors

(continued)

Product	A (int. units)	B_1 (mg)	B_2 (mg)	B_6 (mg)	B_{12} (mcg)	C (mg)	D (int. units)	E (int. units)	Additional Information
One-A-Day® Kids Scooby-Doo! Fizzy Vites [OTC]	1500	0.75	0.85	1	3	170	200	15	Biotin 20 mcg, Ca 50 mg, Cu 1 mg, Fe 9 mg, folic acid 0.2 mg, iodine 75 mcg, Mg 10 mg, niacin 7.5 mg, pantothenic acid 5 mg, phosphorus 50 mg, sodium 20 mg, Zn 6 mg; **contains phenylalanine**; crazy grape, orange pucker, and wild cherry flavors
One-A-Day® Kids Scooby-Doo! Plus Calcium [OTC]	2500	1.05	1.2	1.05	4.5	60	400	15	Ca 200 mg, folic acid 0.3 mg, niacin 13.5 mg; **contains phenylalanine**; fruity flavors
Poly-Vi-Flor® 0.25 mg	2500	1.05	1.2	1.05	4.5	60	400	15	Fluoride 0.25 mg, folic acid 0.3 mg, niacin 13.5 mg; fruity flavor
Poly-Vi-Flor® 0.5 mg	2500	1.05	1.2	1.05	4.5	60	400	15	Fluoride 0.5 mg, folic acid 0.3 mg, niacin 13.5 mg; fruity flavor
Poly-Vi-Flor® 1 mg	2500	1.05	1.2	1.05	4.5	60	400	15	Fluoride 1 mg, folic acid 0.3 mg, niacin 13.5 mg; fruity flavor
Poly-Vi-Flor® 0.25 mg With Iron	2500	1.05	1.2	1.05	4.5	60	400	15	Fluoride 0.25 mg, Cu 1 mg, folic acid 0.3 mg, iron 12 mg, niacin 13.5 mg, Zn 10 mg; fruity flavor
Poly-Vi-Flor® 0.5 mg With Iron	2500	1.05	1.2	1.05	4.5	60	400	15	Fluoride 0.5 mg, Cu 1 mg, folic acid 0.3 mg, iron 12 mg, niacin 13.5 mg, Zn 10 mg; fruity flavor

Key: Ca = calcium, Cr = chromium, Cu = copper, Fe = iron, Mg = magnesium, Mn = manganese, Mo = molybdenum, Se = selenium, Zn = zinc.

Prenatal Formulations

Product	A (int. units)	B_1 (mg)	B_2 (mg)	B_6 (mg)	B_{12} (mcg)	C (mg)	D (int. units)	E (int. units)	Additional Information
Caplet									
PreCare® Prenatal		3	3.4	50	12	50	6 mcg	3.5 mg	Ca 250 mg, Cu 2 mg, Fe 40 mg, folic acid 1 mg, Mg 50 mg, Zn 15 mg; dye free
StrongStart™	1000	3	3	20	12	100	400	30	Ca 200 mg, Fe 29 mg, folic acid 1 mg, niacinamide 15 mg, pantothenic acid 7 mg, Zn 20 mg; docusate sodium 25 mg
Capsule									
Chromagen OB®		1.6	1.8	20	12	60	400	30	Ca 200 mg, Cu 2 mg, Fe 28 mg, folic acid 1 mg, Mn 2 mg, niacinamide 5 mg, Zn 25 mg; docusate calcium 25 mg
Prenatal H		10	6	5	15	200			Cu 0.8 mg, Fe 106 mg, folic acid 1 mg, Mg 6.9 mg, Mn 1.3 mg, niacinamide 30 mg, pantothenic acid 10 mg, Zn 18.2 mg
Prenatal U		10	6	5	15	200			Cu 0.8 mg, Fe 106.5 mg, folic acid 1 mg, Mn 1.3 mg, niacinamide 30 mg, pantothenic acid 10 mg
Powder									
Obegyn® (per 4 level tsp/8.25 g)	2500 (as palmatate) 2500 (as beta-carotene)	1.7	2	10	12	120	400	60	Biotin 300 mcg, Ca 455 mg, Cu 2 mg, Fe 18 mg, folic acid 1 mg, iodine 150 mcg, Mg 150 mg, niacin 20 mg, pantothenic acid 10 mg, Zn 25 mg; **phenylalanine 84 mg/8.25 g**; orange flavor (495 g/60 doses)
Tablet									
A-Free Prenatal		2	2	1	2	33.3	133.3	10	Calcium 333.3 mg, biotin 10 mcg, Cu 0.1 mg, Fe 9 mg, folic acid 266.6 mcg, Mg 33.3 mg, Mn 0.1 mg, niacinamide 10 mg, pantothenic acid 5 mg, Zn 7.5 mg
Advanced NatalCare®	2700	3	3.4	20	12	120	400	30	Ca 200 mg, Cu 2 mg, Fe 90 mg, folic acid 1 mg, Mg 30 mg, niacinamide 20 mg, Zn 25 mg; docusate sodium 50 mg

(continued)

Product	A (int. units)	B_1 (mg)	B_2 (mg)	B_6 (mg)	B_{12} (mcg)	C (mg)	D (int. units)	E (int. units)	Additional Information
Aminate Fe-90	4000	3	3.4	20	12	120	400	30	Ca 250 mg, Cu 2 mg, Fe 90 mg, folic acid 1 mg, iodine 150 mcg, niacinamide 20 mg, Zn 25 mg; docusate sodium 50 mg
Cal-Nate™	2700	3	3.4	20		120	400	30	Ca 125 mg, Cu 2 mg, Fe 27 mg, folic acid 1 mg, iodine 150 mcg, niacinamide 20 mg, Zn 25 mg; docusate calcium 50 mg
Citracal® Prenatal Rx	2700	3	3.4	20		120	400	30	Ca 125 mg, Cu 2 mg, Fe 27 mg, folic acid 1 mg, iodine 150 mcg, niacinamide 20 mg, Zn 25 mg; docusate sodium 50 mg
Duet®	3000	1.8	4	25	12	120	400	30	Ca 200 mg, Cu 2 mg, Fe 29 mg, folic acid 1 mg, Mg 25 mg, niacinamide 20 mg, Zn 25 mg
KPN Prenatal	2666.6	2	2	1	2	33.3	133.3	10	Ca 333.3 mg, biotin 10 mcg, Cu 0.1 mg, Fe 9 mg, folic acid 266.6 mcg, Mg 33.3 mg, Mn 0.1 mg, niacinamide 10 mg, pantothenic acid 5 mg, Zn 7.5 mg
NatalCare® GlossTabs™	2700	3	3.4	20	12	120	400	10	Biotin 30 mcg, Ca 200 mg, Cu 2 mg, Fe 90 mg, folic acid 1 mg, Mg 30 mg, niacinamide 20 mg, pantothenic acid 6 mg, Zn 15 mg; docusate sodium 50 mg
NatalCare® PIC	4000	2.43	3	1.64	3	50	400		Ca 125 mg, folic acid 1 mg, niacinamide 10 mg, polysaccharide-iron complex 60 mg, Zn 18 mg
NatalCare® PIC Forte	5000	3	3.4	4	12	80	400	30	Ca 250 mg, Cu 2 mg, folic acid 1 mg, iodine 200 mcg, Mg 10 mg, niacinamide 20 mg, polysaccharide-iron complex 60 mg, Zn 25 mg
NatalCare® Plus	4000	1.84	3	10	12	120	400	22	Ca 200 mg, Cu 2 mg, Fe 27 mg, folic acid 1 mg, niacinamide 20 mg, Zn 25 mg
NatalCare® Rx	2000	0.75	0.8	2	1.25	40	200	7.5	Biotin 15 mcg, Ca 100 mg, Cu 1.5 mg, folate 0.5 mg, Fe 27 mg, Mg 50 mg, niacin 8.5 mg, pantothenic acid 3.75 mg, Zn 12.5 mg
NatalCare® Three	3000	1.8	4	25	12	120	400	22	Ca 200 mg, Cu 2 mg, Fe 28 mg, folic acid 1 mg, Mg 25 mg, niacinamide 20 mg, Zn 25 mg
NataFort®	1000	2	3	10	12	120	400	11	Fe 60 mg, folic acid 1 mg, niacinamide 20 mg
NataTab™ CFe	4000	3	3	3	8	120	400	30	Ca 200 mg, Fe 50 mg, folic acid 1 mg, iodine 150 mcg, niacin 20 mg, Zn 15 mg

(continued)

Product	A (int. units)	B_1 (mg)	B_2 (mg)	B_6 (mg)	B_{12} (mcg)	C (mg)	D (int. units)	E (int. units)	Additional Information
NataTab™ FA	4000	3	3	6	8	120	400	30	Ca 200 mg, Fe 29 mg, folic acid 1 mg, iodine 150 mcg, niacin 20 mg, Zn 15 mg
NataTab™ Rx	4000	3	3	3	8	120	400	30	Biotin 30 mcg, Ca 200 mg, Cu 3 mg, Fe 29 mg, folic acid 1 mg, iodine 150 mcg, Mg 100 mg, niacin 20 mg, pantothenic acid 7 mg, Zn 15 mg
Nestabs® CBF	4000	3	3	3	8	120	400	30	Ca 200 mg, Fe 50 mg, folic acid 1 mg, iodine 150 mcg, niacin 20 mg, Zn 15 mg
Nestabs® FA	4000	3	3	3	8	120	400	30	Ca 200 mg, Fe 29 mg, folic acid 1 mg, iodine 150 mcg, niacin 20 mg, Zn 15 mg
Nestabs® RX	4000	3	3	3	8	120	400	30	Biotin 30 mcg, Ca 200 mg, Cu 3 mg, Fe 29 mg, folic acid 1 mg, iodine 150 mcg, Mg 100 mg, niacin 20 mg, pantothenic acid 7 mg, Zn 15 mg
Niferex®-PN	4000	2.43	3	1.64	3	50	400		Ca 125 mg, folic acid 1 mg, niacinamide 10 mg, polysaccharide-iron complex 60 mg, Zn 18 mg
Niferex®-PN Forte	5000	3	3.4	4	12	80	400	30	Ca 250 mg, Cu 2 mg, folic acid 1 mg, iodine 200 mcg, Mg 10 mg, niacinamide 20 mg, polysaccharide-iron complex 60 mg, Zn 25 mg
OB-20	2000	43	0.5	2.5	2	30	100	15	Biotin 37.5 mcg, Ca 125 mg, Cr 6.25 mcg, Fe 12.5 mg, folic acid 2.5 mg, Mg 37.5 mg, Mn 1.25 mg, niacinamide 5 mg, pantothenic acid 2.5 mg, Se 6.25 mcg, Zn 6.2 mg
PreCare® Conceive™		3	3.4	50	12	60		30	Ca 200 mg, Cu 2 mg, Fe 30 mg, folic acid 1 mg, Mg 100 mg, niacinamide 20 mg, Zn 15 mg
Prenatal 1-A-Day	4000	2	3	3	10	100	400	15	Biotin 100 mcg, Ca 200 mg, Cu 2 mg, Fe 27 mg, folic acid 800 mcg, Mg 60 mg, Mn 2 mg, niacinamide 20 mg, pantothenic acid 10 mg, Zn 15 mg
Prenatal AD	2700	3	3.4	12	120	120	400	30	Ca 200 mg, Cu 2 mg, Fe 90 mg, folic acid 1 mg, Mg 30 mg, niacinamide 20 mg, Zn 25 mg; docusate sodium 50 mg
Prenatal MR 90 Fe™	4000	3	3.4	20	12	120	400	30	Ca 250 mg, Cu 2 mg, Fe 90 mg, folic acid 1 mg, iodine 150 mcg, niacinamide 20 mg, Zn 25 mg; docusate sodium 50 mg

(continued)

Product	A (int. units)	B_1 (mg)	B_2 (mg)	B_6 (mg)	B_{12} (mcg)	C (mg)	D (int. units)	E (int. units)	Additional Information
Prenatal MRT with Selenium	5000	3	3.4	10	12	120	400	30	Biotin 30 mcg, Ca 200 mg, Cr 25 mcg, Cu 2 mg, Fe 27 mg, folic acid 1 mg, iodine 150 mcg, Mg 25 mg, Mn 5 mg, Mo 25 mcg, niacinamide 20 mg, pantothenic acid 10 mg, Se 20 mcg, Zn 25 mg
Prenatal Plus	4000	1.8	3	10	12	120	400	22	Ca 200 mg, Cu 2 mg, Fe 27 mg, folic acid 1 mg, niacinamide 20 mg, Zn 25 mg
Prenatal Rx 1	4000	1.5	1.6	4	2.5	80	400	15	Biotin 30 mcg, Ca 200 mg, Cu 3 mg, Fe 60 mg, folic acid 1 mg, Mg 100 mg, niacinamide 17 mg, pantothenic acid 7 mg, Zn 25 mg
Prenatal Z	3000	1.5	1.6	2.2	2.2	70	400	10	Ca 200 mg, Fe 65 mg, folic acid 1 mg, iodine 175 mcg, Mg 100 mg, niacin 17 mg, Zn 15 mg
Prenate Elite™		3	3.4	20	12	120	400	10	Biotin 300 mcg, Ca 200 mg, Cu 2 mg, Fe 90 mg, folate 1 mg, Mg 30 mg, niacinamide 20 mg, pantothenic acid 6 mg, Zn 15 mg; docusate sodium 50 mg
Prenate GT™	2700	3	3.4	20	12	120	400	10	Biotin 30 mcg, Ca 200 mg, Cu 2 mg, Fe 90 mg, folic acid 1 mg, Mg 30 mg, niacinamide 20 mg, pantothenic acid 6 mg, Zn 15 mg; docusate sodium 50 mg
Stuartnatal® Plus 3™ [DSC]	3000	1.8	4	25	12	120	400	22	Ca 200 mg, Cu 2 mg, Fe 28 mg, folic acid 1 mg, Mg 25 mg, niacinamide 20 mg, Zn 25 mg
Stuart Prenatal®	4000	1.8	1.7	2.6	8	120	400	30	Ca 200 mg, Fe 28 mg, folic acid 0.8 mg, niacin 20 mg, Zn 25 mg
Trinate	3000	1.8	4	25	12	120	400	22	Ca 200 mg, Cu 2 mg, Fe 28 mg, folic acid 1 mg, Mg 25 mg, niacin 20 mg, Zn 25 mg

(continued)

Product	A (int. units)	B_1 (mg)	B_2 (mg)	B_6 (mg)	B_{12} (mcg)	C (mg)	D (int. units)	E (int. units)	Additional Information
Ultra NatalCare®	2700	3	3.4	20	12	120	400	30	Ca 200 mg, Cu 2 mg, Fe 90 mg, folic acid 1 mg, iodine 150 mcg, niacinamide 20 mg, Zn 25 mg; docusate sodium 50 mg
Tablet, Chewable									
Duet®	3000	1.8	4	25	12	120	400	30	Ca 100 mg, Cu 2 mg, Fe 29 mg, folic acid 1 mg, Mg 25 mg, niacinamide 20 mg, Zn 25 mg; **phenylalanine 15 mg/tablet**
NataChew™	1000	2	3	10	12	120	400	11	Fe 29 mg, folic acid 1 mg, niacinamide 20 mg; peanut extract, wild berry flavor
NutriNate®	1000	2	3	10	12	120	400	11	Fe 29 mg, folic acid 1 mg, niacinamide 20 mg; wild berry flavor
PreCare®				2		50	6 mcg	3.5 mg	Ca 250 mg, Cu 2 mg, Fe 40 mg, folic acid 1 mg, Mg 50 mg, Zn 15 mg
StrongStart™	1000	1	3	20	15	100	400	30	Ca 200 mg, Fe 29 mg, folic acid 1 mg, niacinamide 15 mg, pantothenic acid 7 mg, Zn 20 mg; **phenylalanine 6 mg/tablet**
Combination Package									
Duet™ DHA (tablet)	3000	1.8	4	25	12	120	400	30	Ca 200 mg, Cu 2 mg, Fe 29 mg, folic acid 1 mg, Mg 25 mg, niacinamide 20 mg, Zn 25 mg Packaged with capsules containing Omega-3 fatty acids ≥ DHA 200 mg

Key: Ca = calcium, Cr = chromium, Cu = copper, Fe = iron, Mg = magnesium, Mn = manganese, Mo = molybdenum, Se = selenium, Zn = zinc.

Vitamin B Complex Combinations

Product	B_1 (mg)	B_2 (mg)	B_6 (mg)	B_{12} (mcg)	C (mg)	E (int. units)	Additional Information
Caplet							
Allbee® with C [OTC]	15	10.2	5		300		Niacinamide 50 mg, pantothenic acid 10 mg
Allbee® C-800 [OTC]	15	17	25	12	800	45	Niacinamide 100 mg, pantothenic acid 25 mg
Allbee® C-800 + Iron [OTC]	15	17	25	12	800	45	Fe 27 mg, folic acid 0.4 mcg, niacinamide 100 mg, pantothenic acid 25 mg
Nephronex®	1.5	1.7	10	0.01	50		Biotin 300 mcg, nicotinic acid 20 mg, pantothenic acid 10 mg
Capsule							
Trinsicon® [DSC]				15			Fe 110 mg, folic acid 0.5 mg, liver-stomach concentrate (containing intrinsic factor and other vitamin B complex factors) 240 mg
Elixir							
Senilezol (per 30 mL)	2.5	2.5	1	5			Ca 5 mg, Fe 8 mg, niacin 10 mg [contain alcohol 15%]
Liquid							
Apatate® [OTC] (per 5 mL)	15		0.5	25			Cherry flavor (120 mL)
Gevrabon® [OTC] (per 30 mL)	5	2.5	1	1			Choline 10 mg, Fe 15 mg, iodine 100 mcg, Mg 2 mg, Mn 2 mg, niacinamide 60 mg, pantothenic acid 10 mg, Zn 2 mg; alcohol, benzoic acid; sherry wine flavor (480 mL)
Nephronex®	1.5	1.7	10	60			Biotin 300 mcg, folic acid 900 mcg, nicotinic acid 20 mg, pantothenic acid 10 mg
Softgel							
Nephrocaps®	1.5	1.7	10	6	100		Biotin 150 mcg, folic acid 1 mcg, niacinamide 20 mg, pantothenic acid 5 mg
Rhenaphro	1.5	1.7	10	6	100		Biotin 150 mcg, calcium pantothenate 5 mg, folic acid 1 mg, niacinamide 20 mg

(continued)

Product	B_1 (mg)	B_2 (mg)	B_6 (mg)	B_{12} (mcg)	C (mg)	E (int. units)	Additional Information
Syrup							
Vitafol (per 5 mL)				2	8.34		Fe 100 mg, folic acid 0.25 mg, niacinamide 13.3 mg [contains sodium benzoate; raspberry mint flavor]
Tablet							
DexFol™	1.5	1.5					Biotin 300 mcg, cobalamin 1 mg, folacin 5 mg, niacinamide 20 mg, pantothenic acid 10 mg, pyridoxine 50 mg, vitamin C 60 mg [dye, sugar, and lactose free]
Diatx™	1.5	1.5	50		60		Biotin 300 mcg, cobalamin 1 mg, folacin 5 mg, niacinamide 20 mg, pantothenic acid 10 mg [dye free, lactose free, sugar free]
Kobee [OTC]	10	10	10	10			Biotin 10 mcg, choline citrate 10 mg, folic acid 400 mcg, inositol 10 mg, niacinamide 50 mg, PABA 10 mg, pantothenic acid 10 mg
NephPlex® Rx	1.5	1.7	10	6	60		Biotin 300 mcg, folic acid 1 mg, niacinamide 20 mg, pantothenic acid 10 mg, zinc 12.5 mg
Nephro-Vite®	1.5	1.7	10	6	60		Biotin 300 mcg, folic acid 0.8 mcg, niacinamide 20 mg, pantothenic acid 10 mg
Nephro-Vite® Rx	1.5	1.7	10	6	60		Biotin 300 mcg, folic acid 1 mcg, niacinamide 20 mg, pantothenic acid 10 mg
Nephron FA®	1.5	1.7	10	6	40		Biotin 300 mcg, docusate sodium 75 mg, ferrous fumarate 200 mg, folic acid 1 mg, pantothenic acid 10 mg
Quin B Strong [OTC]	25	25	25	25			Biotin 25 mcg, folic acid 400 mg, niacinamide 100 mg, pantothenic acid 25 mg (in a base containing choline citrate, inositol, and PABA)
Rena-Vite [OTC]	1.5	1.7	10	6	60		Biotin 100 mcg, folic acid 800 mcg, niacin 20 mg, pantothenic acid 10 mg
Rena-Vite RX	1.5	1.7	10	6	60		Biotin 300 mcg, folate 1 mg, niacin 20 mg, pantothenic acid 10 mg
Stresstabs® High Potency Advanced [OTC]	10	10	5	12	250	30	Biotin 45 mcg, Ca 70 mg, Cu 3 mg, folic acid 400 mcg, Mg 25 mg, niacinamide 100 mg, patothenic acid 20 mg, phosphorus 30 mg, Zn 23.9 mg
Stresstabs® High Potency Energy [OTC]	10	10	5	12	300	30	Biotin 45 mcg, Ca 22 mg, Fe 4 mg, folic acid 400 mcg, niacinamide 100 mg, pantothenic acid 20 mg, phosphorus 15 mg

(continued)

Product	B_1 (mg)	B_2 (mg)	B_6 (mg)	B_{12} (mcg)	C (mg)	E (int. units)	Additional Information
Stresstabs® High Potency Weight [OTC]	10	10	5	12	300	30	Biotin 45 mcg, Ca 44 mg, chromium 200 mcg, folic acid 400 mcg, niacinamide 100 mg, pantothenic acid 20 mg, phosphorus 32 mg
Strovite	15	15	4	5	500		Folic acid 0.5 mg, niacinamide 100 mg, pantothenic acid 18 mg
Super Quints 50 [OTC]	50	50	50	50			Biotin 50 mcg, folic acid 50 mcg, niacinamide 50 mg, pantothenic acid 50 mg (in a base containing choline citrate, glutaminic acid, glutamine, glycine, inositol, lysine, and PABA)
Surbex-T® [OTC]	15	10	5	10	500		Ca 20 mg, niacinamide 100 mg
Z-Bec® [OTC]	15	10.2	10	6	600	45	Niacinamide 100 mg, pantothenic acid 25 mg, Zn 22.5 mg
Tablet, Chewable							
Apatate® [OTC] [DSC]	15		0.5	25			Cherry flavor

Key: Ca = calcium, Cr = chromium, Cu = copper, Fe = iron, Mg = magnesium, Mn = manganese, Mo = molybdenum, Se = selenium, Zn = zinc

INDICATION/THERAPEUTIC CATEGORY INDEX

Antibiotic, Miscellaneous

Antibiotic, Topical

General Anesthetic

ANESTHESIA (LOCAL)

Analgesic, Topical

Diagnostic Agent

Local Anesthetic

ANESTHESIA (OPHTHALMIC)

Diagnostic Agent

Local Anesthetic

ANGINA PECTORIS

Antiarrhythmic Agent, Class II

Antiarrhythmic Agent, Class IV

Antilipemic Agent, HMG-CoA Reductase Inhibitor

Antiplatelet Agent

Calcium Channel Blocker

Cardiovascular Agent, Miscellaneous

Vasodilator

ANGIOEDEMA (HEREDITARY)

Anabolic Steroid

Androgen

ANGIOGRAPHY (OPHTHALMIC)

Diagnostic Agent

ANTHRAX

Penicillin

Quinolone

Tetracycline Derivative

BROAD BETA DISEASE

Antihyperlipidemic Agent, Miscellaneous

BROMIDE INTOXICATION

Diuretic, Loop

BRONCHIECTASIS

Adrenergic Agonist Agent

Mucolytic Agent

BRONCHIOLITIS

Antiviral Agent

BRONCHITIS

Adrenergic Agonist Agent

Antibiotic, Cephalosporin

Antibiotic, Quinolone

Anticholinergic Agent

Antihistamine/Antitussive

Cephalosporin (Third Generation)

Mucolytic Agent

Theophylline Derivative

CACHEXIA

Antineoplastic Agent

CALCIUM CHANNEL BLOCKER TOXICITY

Electrolyte Supplement, Oral

CANCER

Antineoplastic Agent, Alkylating Agent

Antineoplastic Agent, Antimicrotubular

Antineoplastic Agent, Miscellaneous

Antineoplastic Agent, Natural Source (Plant) Derivative

Antineoplastic Agent, Tyrosine Kinase Inhibitor

Antineoplastic, Tyrosine Kinase Inhibitor

Vascular Endothelial Growth Factor (VEGF) Inhibitor

CANDIDIASIS

Antifungal Agent

Antihistamine/Decongestant Combination

Decongestant

Laxative, Osmotic

Laxative, Stimulant

Stool Softener

CONSTIPATION (CHRONIC IDIOPATHIC)

Gastrointestinal Agent, Miscellaneous

CONTRACEPTION

Contraceptive

Contraceptive, Implant (Progestin)

Contraceptive, Oral

Antitussive

Antitussive/Decongestant

Antitussive/Decongestant/Expectorant

Antitussive/Expectorant

DIABETES INSIPIDUS

Hormone, Posterior Pituitary

Vasopressin Analog, Synthetic

DIABETES MELLITUS, INSULIN-DEPENDENT (IDDM)

Antidiabetic Agent

Antidiabetic Agent, Insulin

DIABETES MELLITUS, NONINSULIN-DEPENDENT (NIDDM)

Antidiabetic Agent

DISCOID LUPUS ERYTHEMATOSUS (DLE)

Adrenal Corticosteroid

Aminoquinoline (Antimalarial)

Corticosteroid, Topical

DIVERTICULITIS

Amebicide

DRY EYES

Ophthalmic Agent, Miscellaneous

DRY MOUTH

Gastrointestinal Agent, Miscellaneous

DRY SKIN

Topical Skin Product

Vitamin, Topical

DUCTUS ARTERIOSUS (CLOSURE)

Nonsteroidal Antiinflammatory Drug (NSAID)

DUCTUS ARTERIOSUS (TEMPORARY MAINTENANCE OF PATENCY)

Prostaglandin

DUODENAL ULCER

Antacid

Antibiotic, Macrolide Combination

Antibiotic, Penicillin

Gastric Acid Secretion Inhibitor

EDEMA

Antihypertensive Agent, Combination

Diuretic, Combination

Diuretic, Loop

Contraceptive, Progestin Only

Hormone, Posterior Pituitary

Progestin

END-STAGE RENAL DISEASE (ESRD)

Phosphate Binder

ENURESIS

Antidepressant, Tricyclic (Tertiary Amine)

Antispasmodic Agent, Urinary

Vasopressin Analog, Synthetic

ENZYME DEFICIENCY

Enzyme

EPICONDYLITIS

Nonsteroidal Antiinflammatory Drug (NSAID)

EPIDERMAL GROWTH FACTOR RECEPTOR (EGFR)

Antineoplastic Agent, Monoclonal Antibody

Epidermal Growth Factor Receptor (EGFR) Inhibitor

EPILEPSY

Anticonvulsant

Anticonvulsant, Miscellaneous

FIBROCYSTIC BREAST DISEASE

Androgen

FIBROCYSTIC DISEASE

Vitamin, Fat Soluble

FIBROMYOSITIS

Antidepressant, Tricyclic (Tertiary Amine)

FUNGUS (DIAGNOSTIC)

Diagnostic Agent

GAG REFLEX SUPPRESSION

Local Anesthetic

GOITER

Thyroid Product

GOLD POISONING

Chelating Agent

GONOCOCCAL OPHTHALMIA NEONATORUM

Topical Skin Product

GONORRHEA

Antibiotic, Miscellaneous

Antibiotic, Quinolone

Antibiotic, Topical

Cephalosporin (Second Generation)

Cephalosporin (Third Generation)

Quinolone

Tetracycline Derivative

GOUT

Antigout Agent

Nonsteroidal Antiinflammatory Drug (NSAID)

HYDATIDIFORM MOLE (BENIGN)

Prostaglandin

HYPERACIDITY

Antacid

HYPERAMMONEMIA

Ammonium Detoxicant

HYPERCALCEMIA

Bisphosphonate Derivative

Chelating Agent

Polypeptide Hormone

HYPERLIPIDEMIA

Antihyperlipidemic Agent, Miscellaneous

Antilipemic Agent, HMG-CoA Reductase Inhibitor

Bile Acid Sequestrant

HMG-CoA Reductase Inhibitor

Vitamin, Water Soluble

HYPERMAGNESEMIA

Diuretic, Loop

Electrolyte Supplement, Oral

HYPERMENORRHEA (TREATMENT)

Contraceptive, Oral

Beta-Adrenergic Blocker

Beta Blocker, $Beta_1$ Selective

Calcium Channel Blocker

NAUSEA

Anticholinergic Agent

Antiemetic

Antihistamine

Antipsychotic Agent, Butyrophenone

Gastrointestinal Agent, Prokinetic

Phenothiazine Derivative

Selective 5-HT_3 Receptor Antagonist

Vitamin

NEISSERIA MENINGITIDIS

Vaccine, Live Bacteria

NEPHROLITHIASIS

Alkalinizing Agent

NEPHROPATHIC CYSTINOSIS

Urinary Tract Product

NEPHROTIC SYNDROME

Adrenal Corticosteroid

Antihypertensive Agent, Combination

Analgesic, Miscellaneous

Analgesic, Narcotic

Analgesic, Nonnarcotic

Analgesic, Opioid

Decongestant/Analgesic

Skeletal Muscle Relaxant

PAIN (ANOGENITAL)

Anesthetic/Corticosteroid

Local Anesthetic

PAIN (BONE)

Radiopharmaceutical

PAIN (DIABETIC NEUROPATHY NEURALGIA)

Analgesic, Topical

PAIN (LUMBAR PUNCTURE)

Analgesic, Topical

PAIN (MUSCLE)

Analgesic, Topical

PAIN (NEUROPATHIC)

Analgesic, Miscellaneous

PAIN (SKIN GRAFT HARVESTING)

Analgesic, Topical

PAIN (VENIPUNCTURE)

Analgesic, Topical

PANCREATIC EXOCRINE INSUFFICIENCY

Enzyme

PANCREATIC EXOCRINE INSUFFICIENCY (DIAGNOSTIC)

Diagnostic Agent

PROTEIN UTILIZATION

Dietary Supplement

PROTOZOAL INFECTIONS

Amebicide

Antibiotic, Miscellaneous

Antiprotozoal

PSEUDOGOUT

Antigout Agent

Nonsteroidal Antiinflammatory Drug (NSAID)

PSEUDOHYPOPARATHYROIDISM

Vitamin D Analog

PSORIASIS

Adrenal Corticosteroid

Antineoplastic Agent

Antipsoriatic Agent

Corticosteroid, Topical

Immunosuppressant Agent

Keratolytic Agent

Antibiotic/Corticosteroid, Topical

Antibiotic, Miscellaneous

Antibiotic, Topical

Antiprotozoal

Genitourinary Irrigant

Macrolide (Antibiotic)

Penicillin

Quinolone

Sulfonamide

Urinary Tract Product

URTICARIA

Antihistamine

2007

QUICK LOOK DRUG BOOK

Image Guide to Tablets and Capsules

The Quick Look Drug Book 2007 image insert displays actual color photographs of the most commonly prescribed tablets and capsules.

Drugs are listed alphabetically by generic name, and, where applicable, the trade name is listed. Dosages appear under each individual image.

Use the white scale at the bottom of each image to determine the actual size. The distance between each division on the scale is equivalent to 1/8 inch or 3.175 mm.

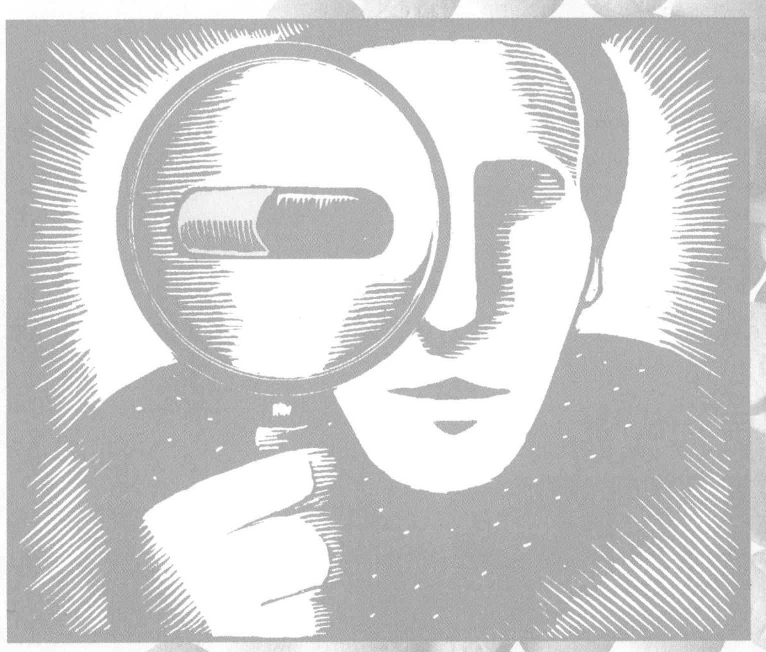

Acetaminophen and Codeine

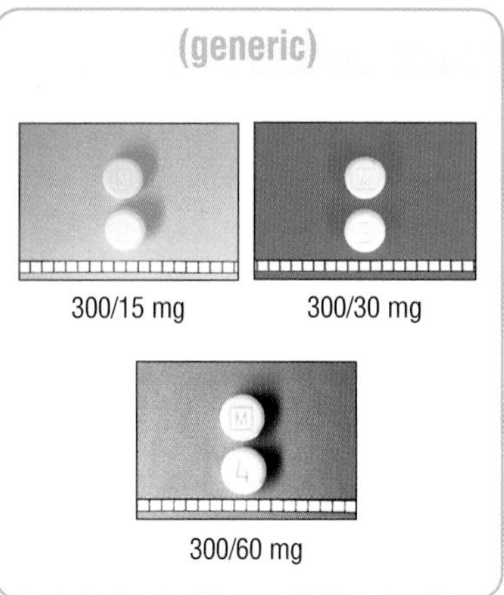

(generic)

300/15 mg 300/30 mg

300/60 mg

Acyclovir

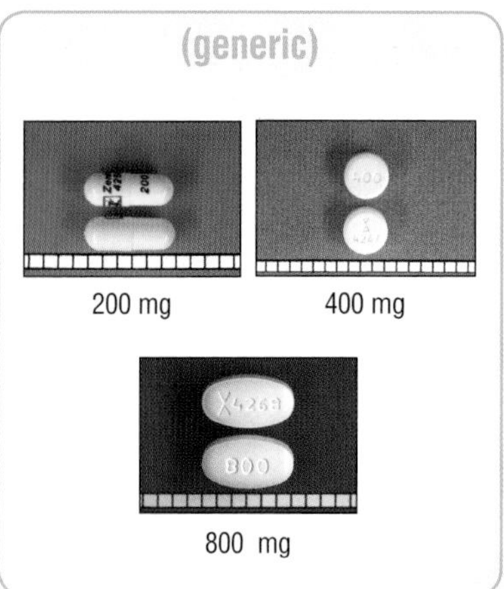

(generic)

200 mg 400 mg

800 mg

Alendronate

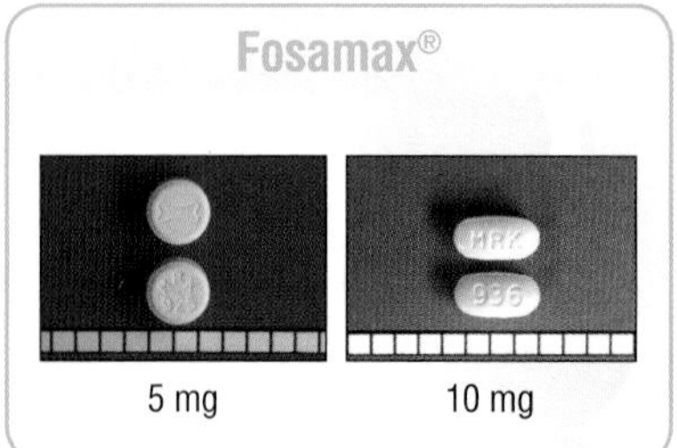

Fosamax®

5 mg 10 mg

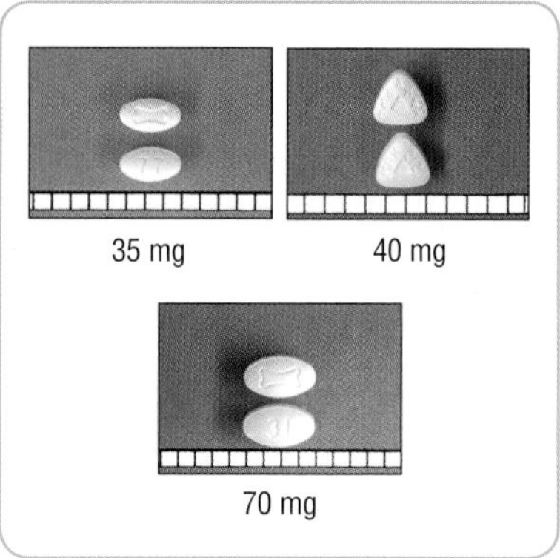

35 mg 40 mg

70 mg

Allopurinol

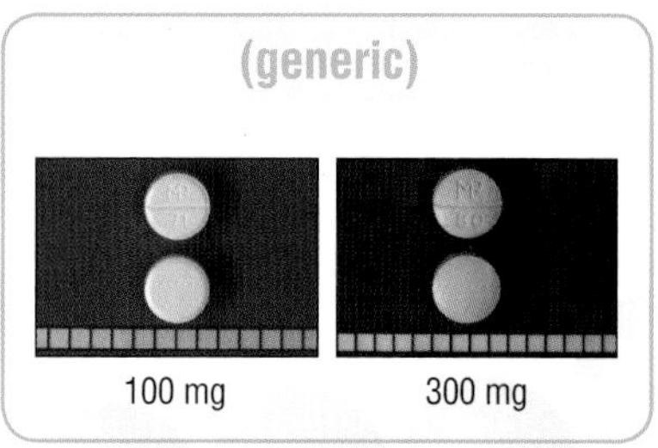

(generic)

100 mg 300 mg

Alprazolam

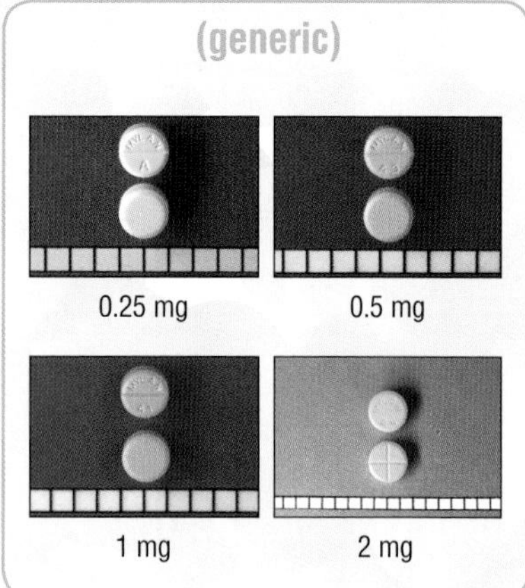

(generic)

0.25 mg 0.5 mg

1 mg 2 mg

Amitriptyline

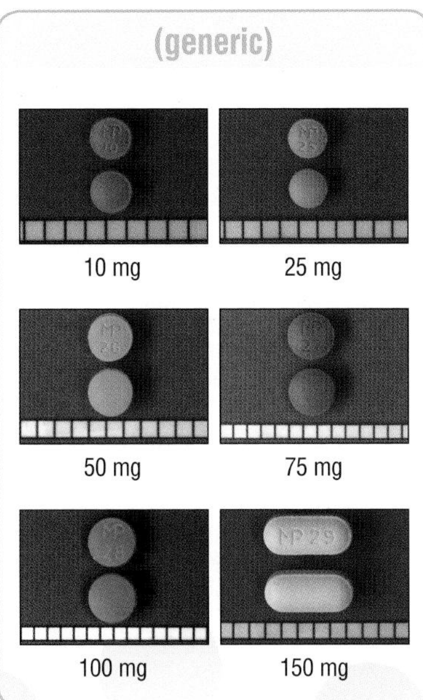

Amlodipine

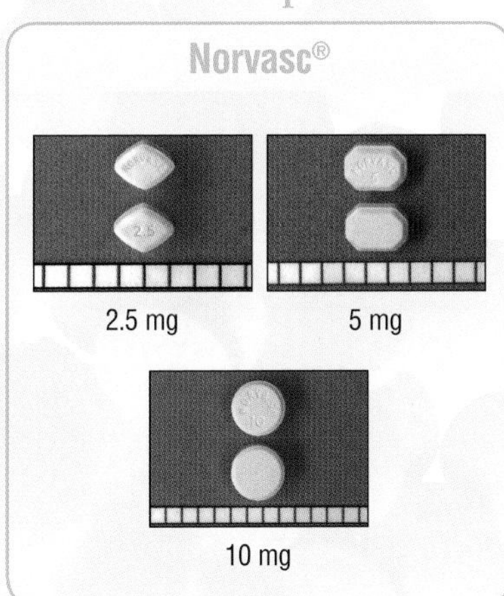

Amlodipine and Benazepril

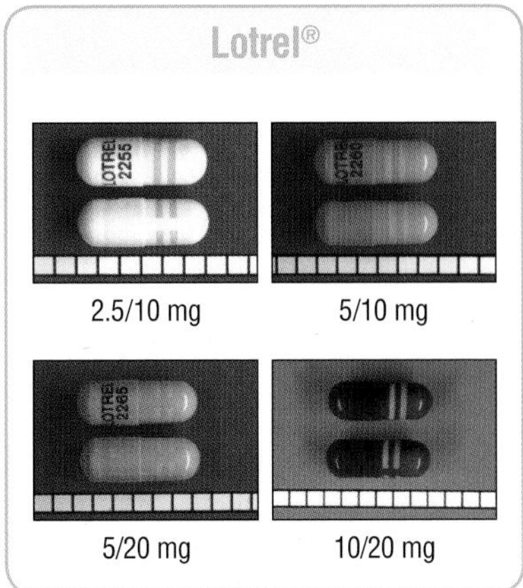

Amoxicillin

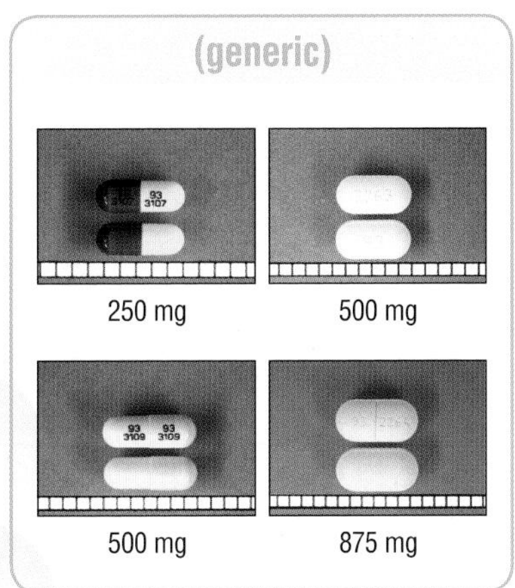

Amoxicillin and Clavulanate Potassium

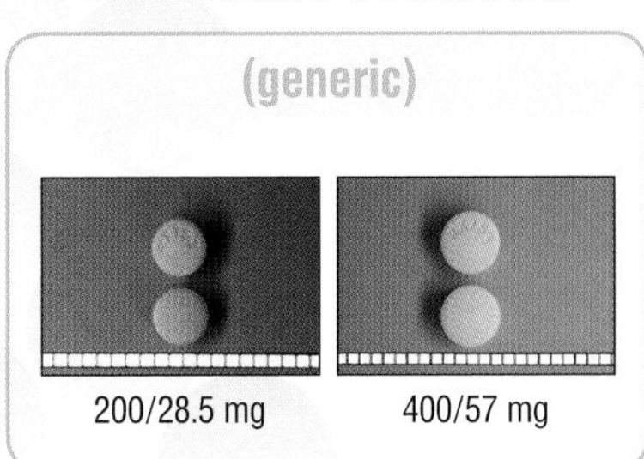

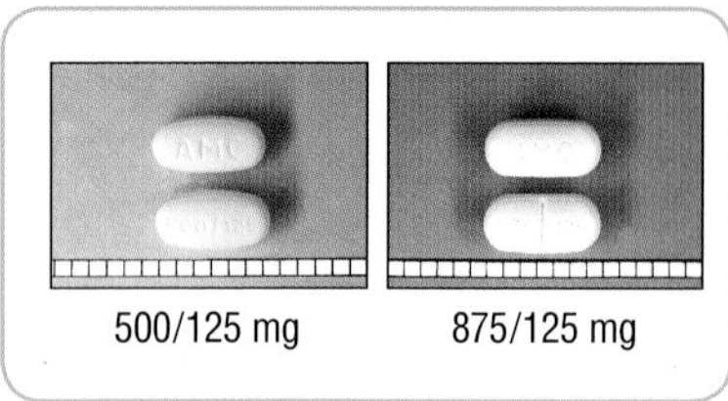

500/125 mg

875/125 mg

Atenolol

(generic)

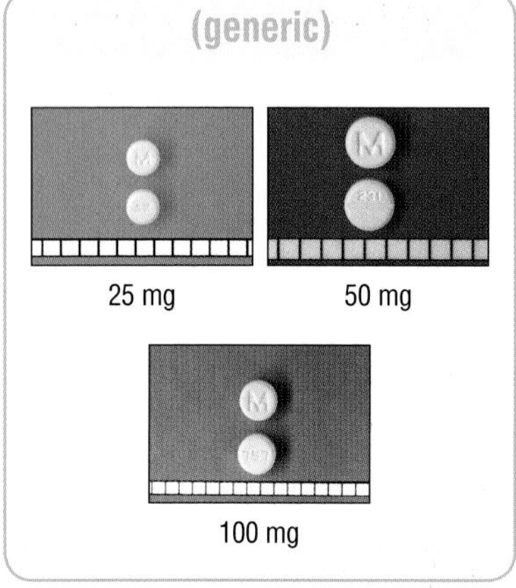

25 mg

50 mg

100 mg

Atenolol and Chlorthalidone

(generic)

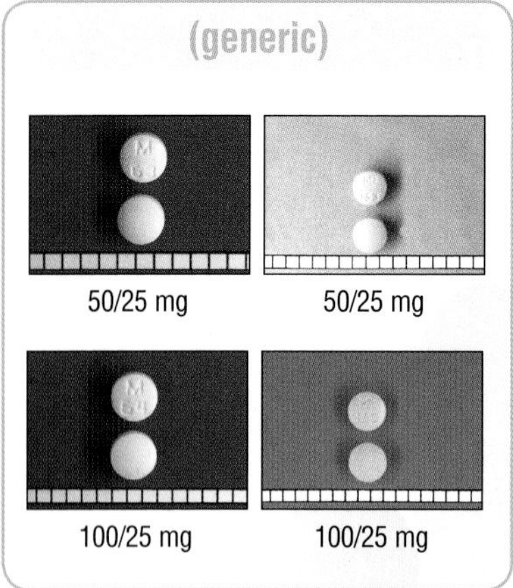

50/25 mg

50/25 mg

100/25 mg

100/25 mg

Atomoxetine

Strattera™

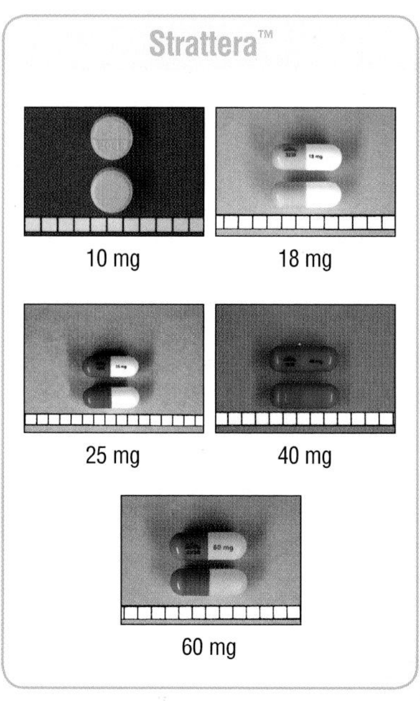

10 mg

18 mg

25 mg

40 mg

60 mg

Atorvastatin

Lipitor®

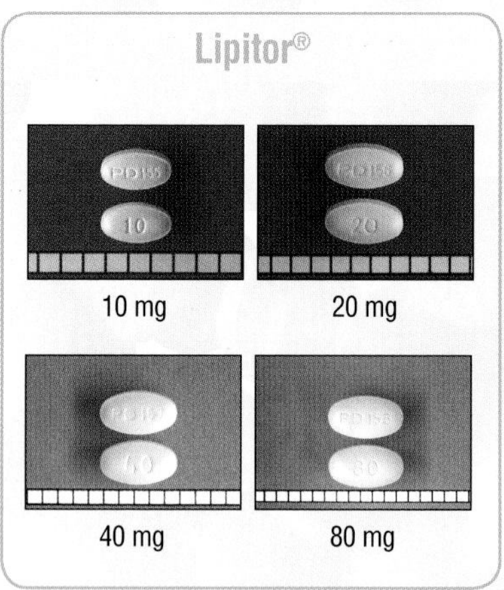

10 mg

20 mg

40 mg

80 mg

Azithromycin

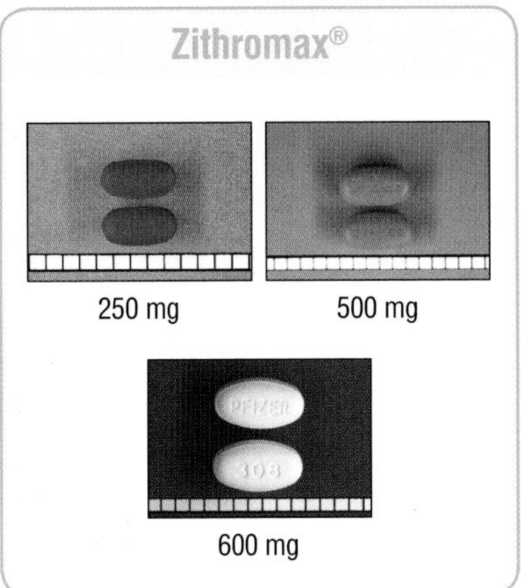

Benazepril

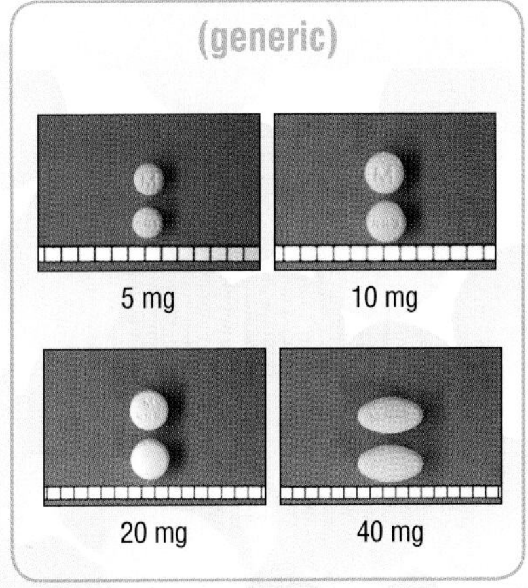

Benzonatate

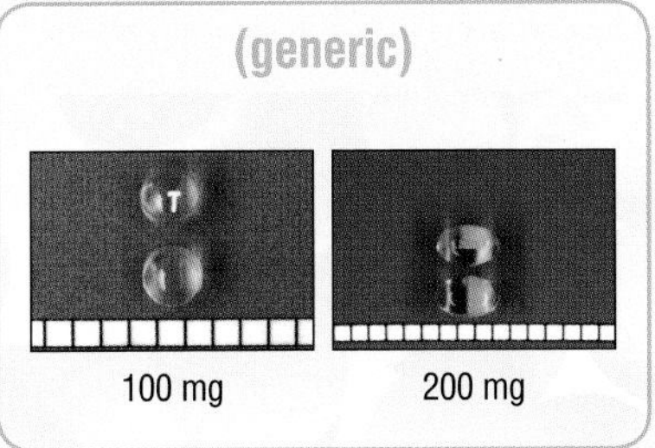

Bisoprolol and Hydrochlorothiazide

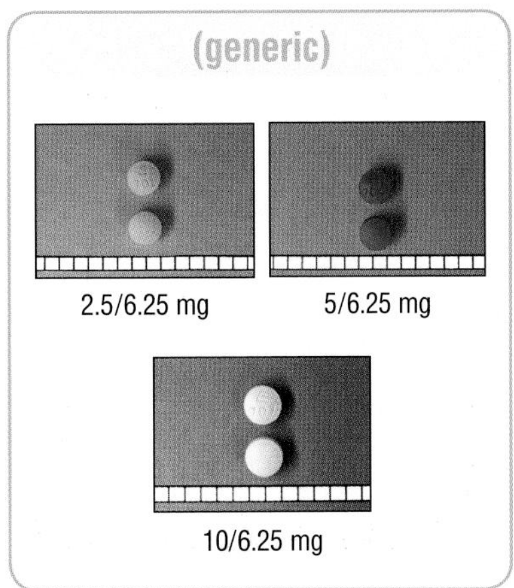

Bupropion

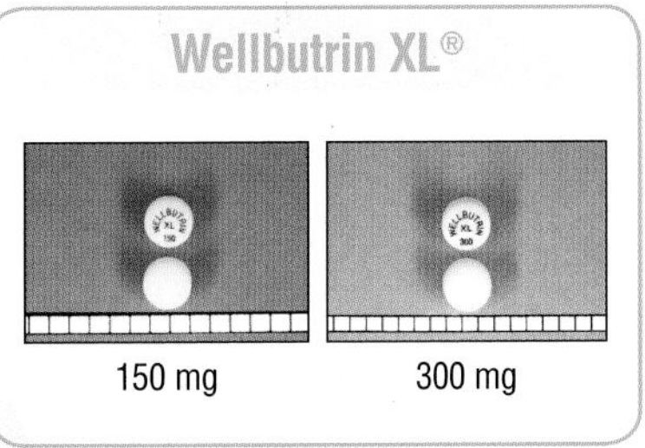

Buspirone

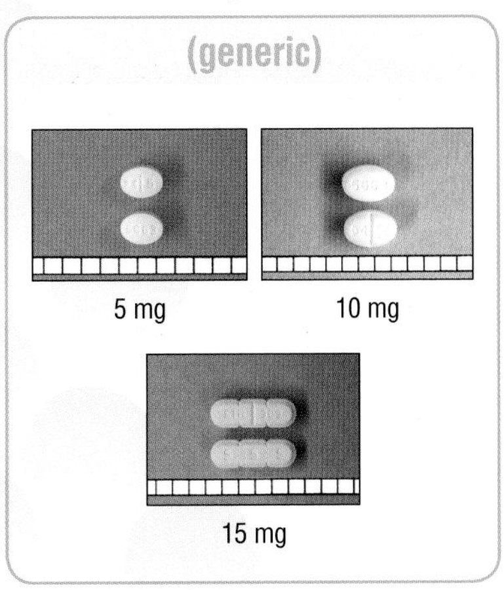

Butalbital Compound

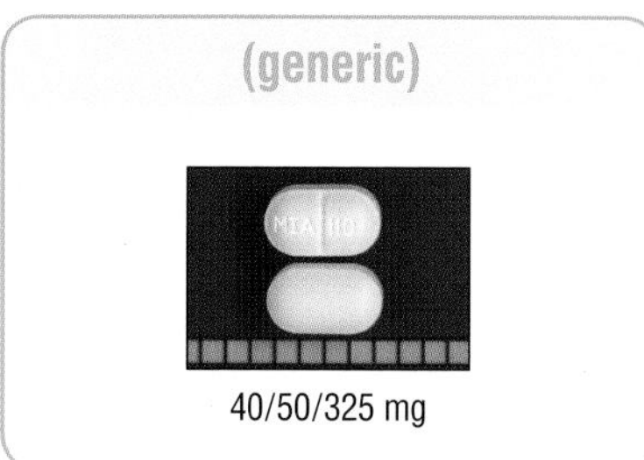

Carisoprodol

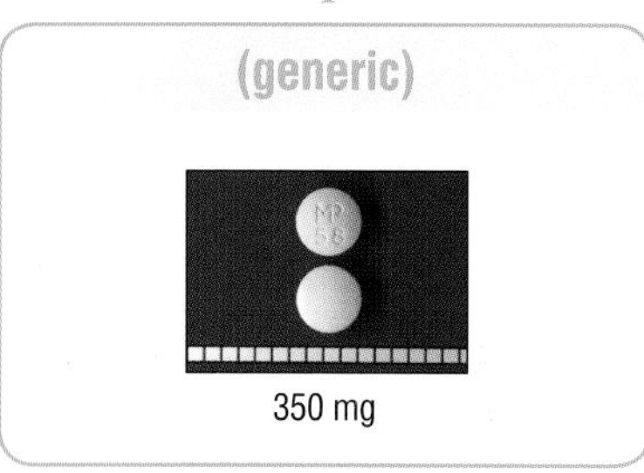

Carvedilol

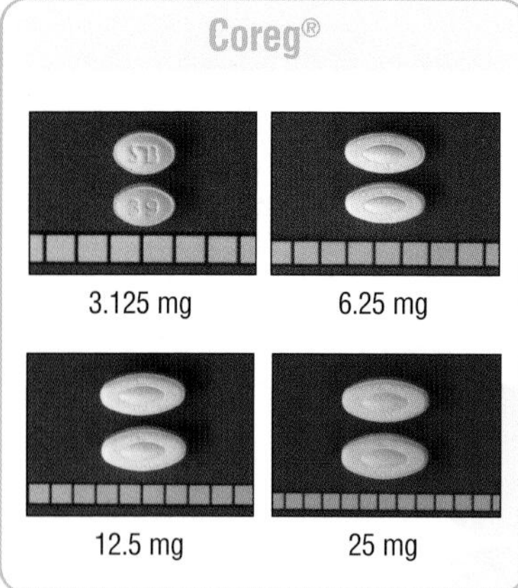

Cefdinir

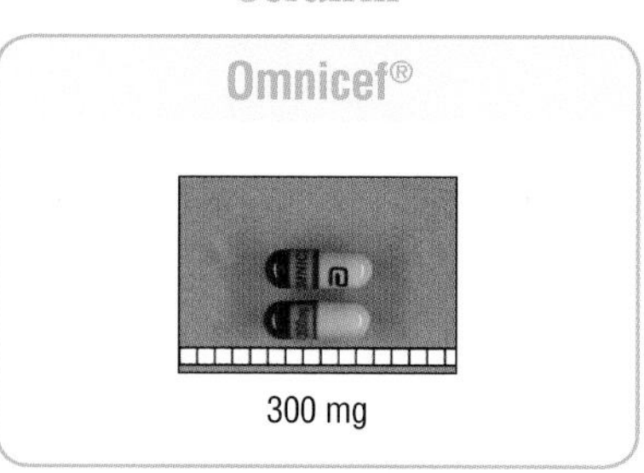

Celecoxib

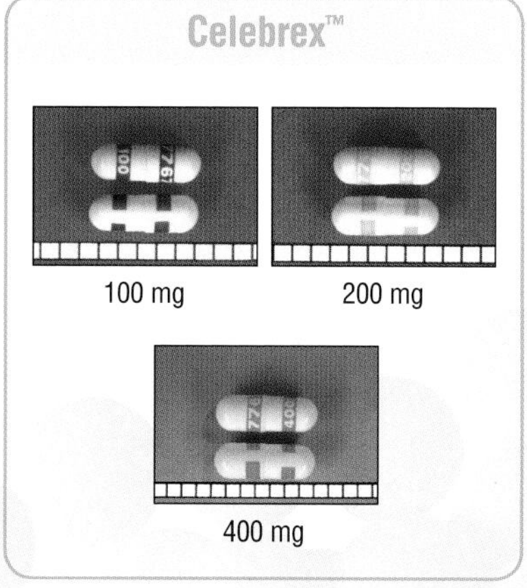

Cephalexin

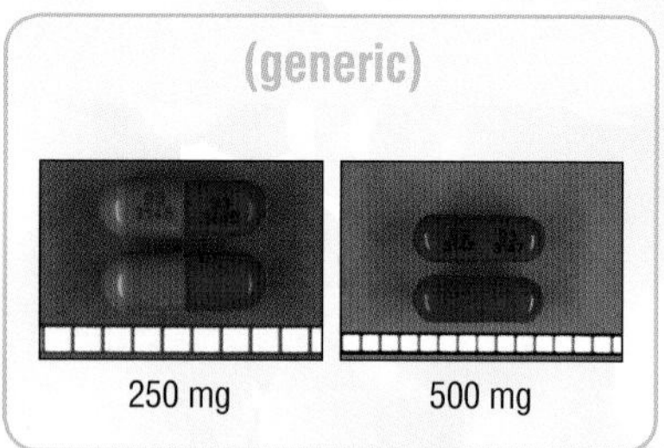

Cetirizine

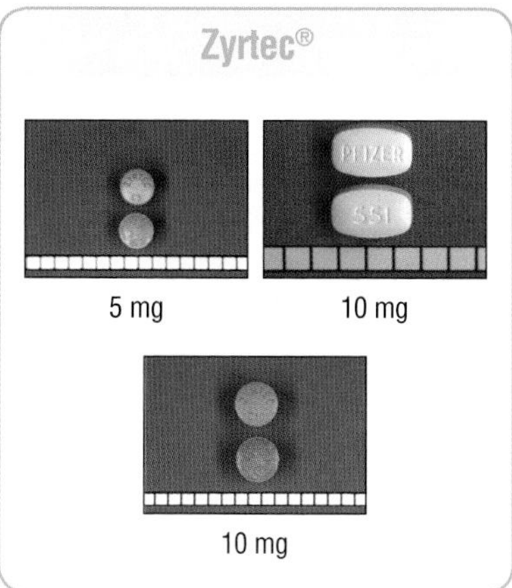

Ciprofloxacin

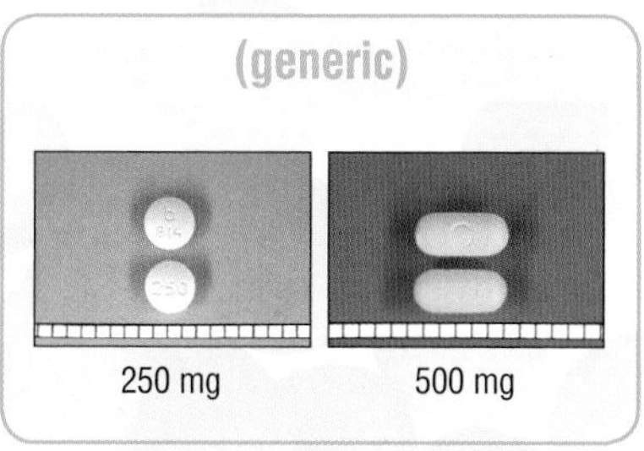

Citalopram

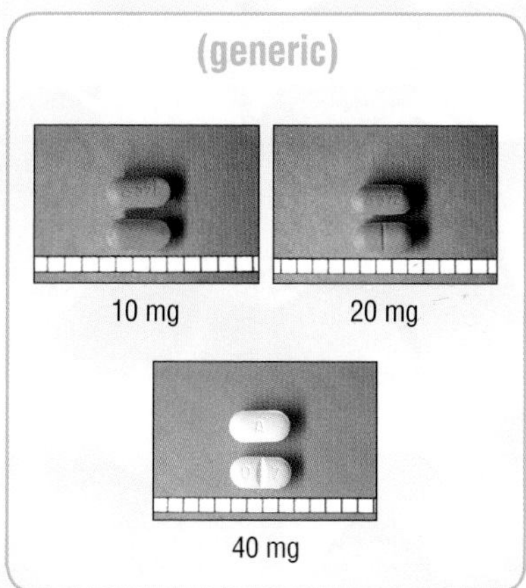

Clindamycin

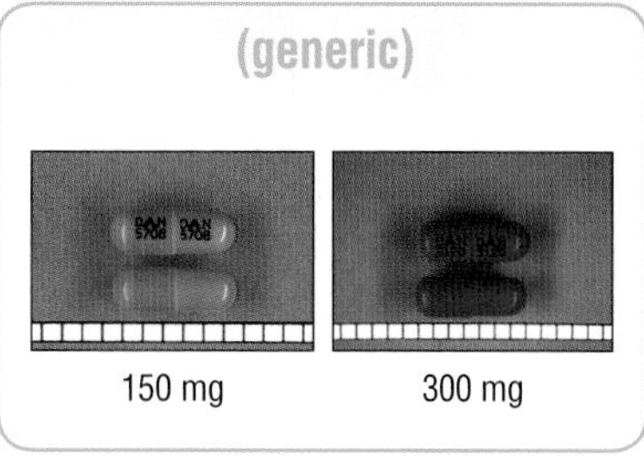

Clonazepam

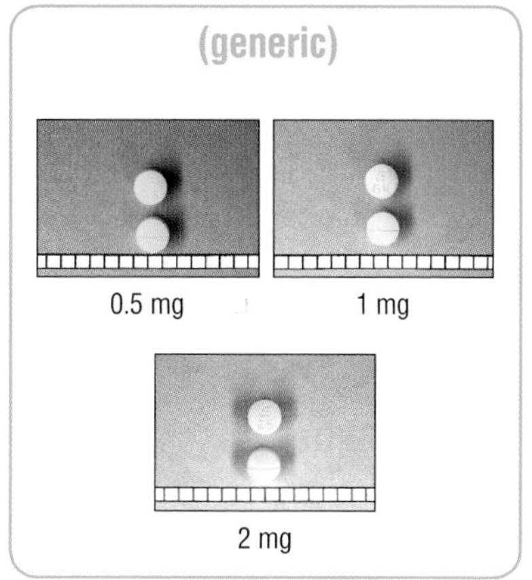

Clonidine

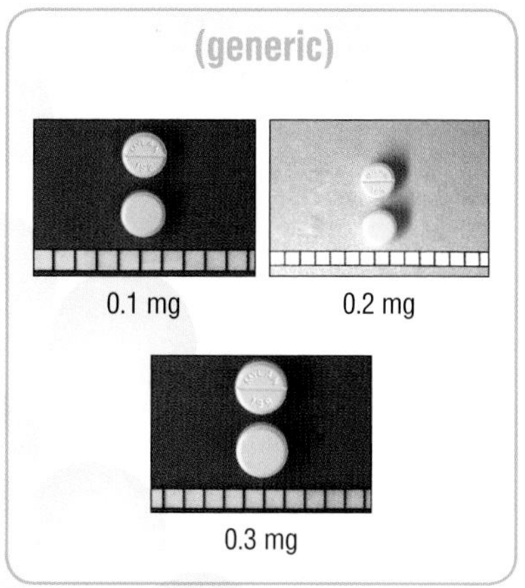

Clopidogrel

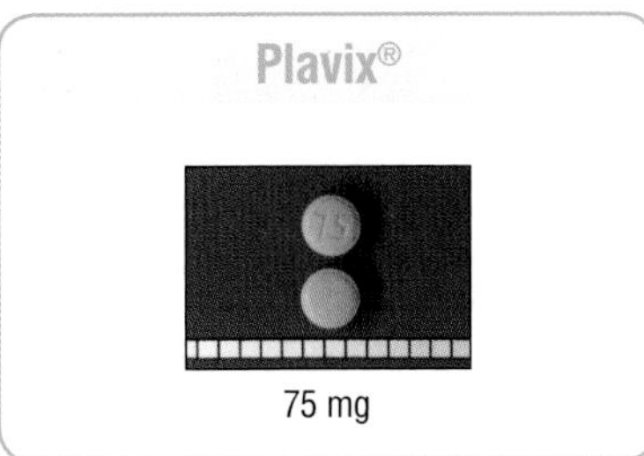
Plavix®

75 mg

Cyclobenzaprine

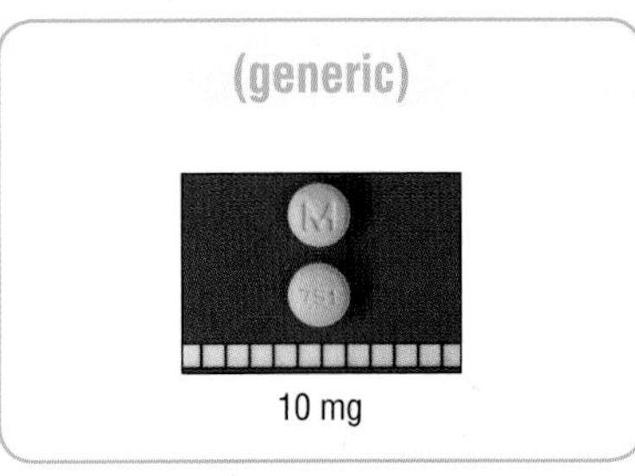
(generic)

10 mg

Desloratadine

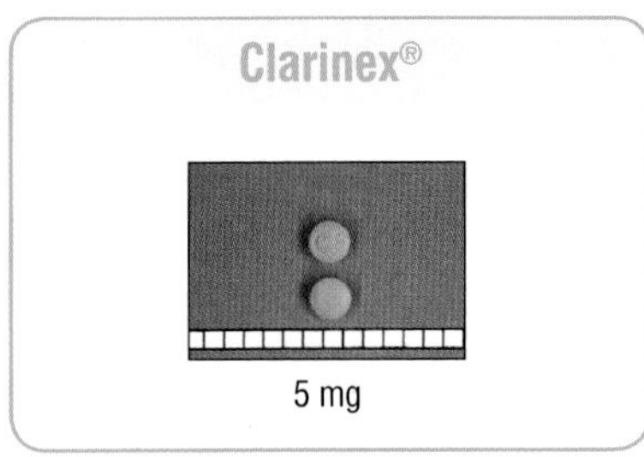
Clarinex®

5 mg

Dextroamphetamine and Amphetamine

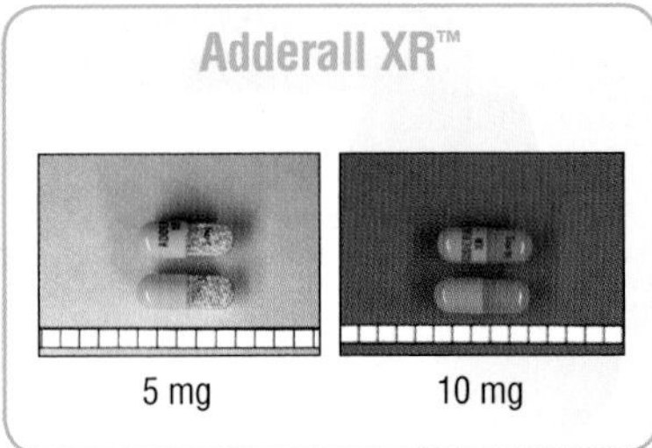
Adderall XR™

5 mg

10 mg

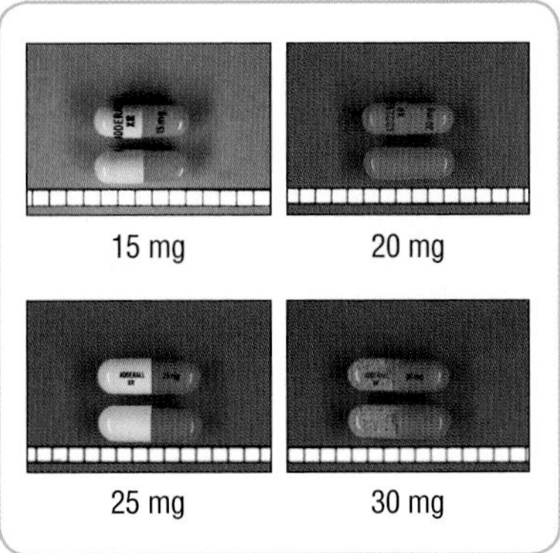
15 mg

20 mg

25 mg

30 mg

Diazepam

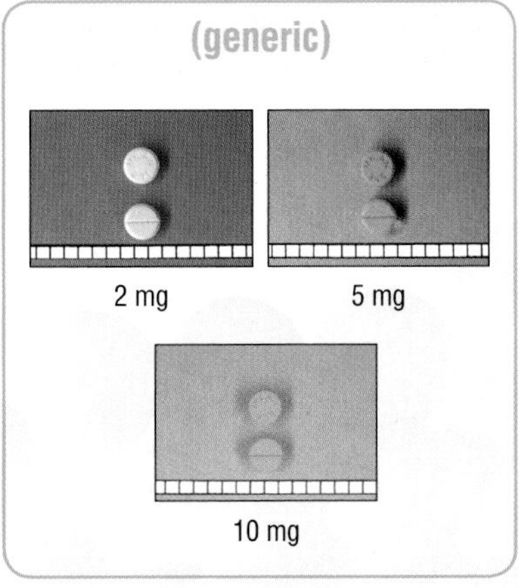
(generic)

2 mg

5 mg

10 mg

Diclofenac

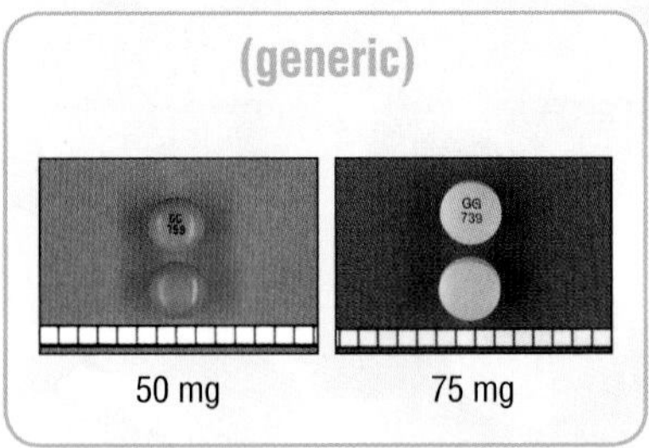

(generic)

50 mg

75 mg

Digoxin

Digitek®

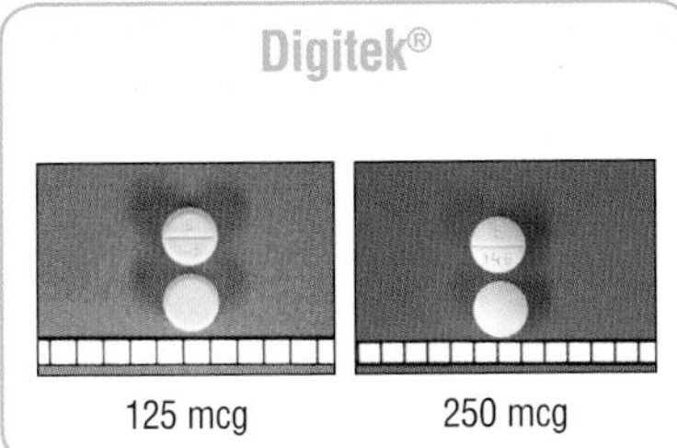

125 mcg | 250 mcg

Lanoxin®

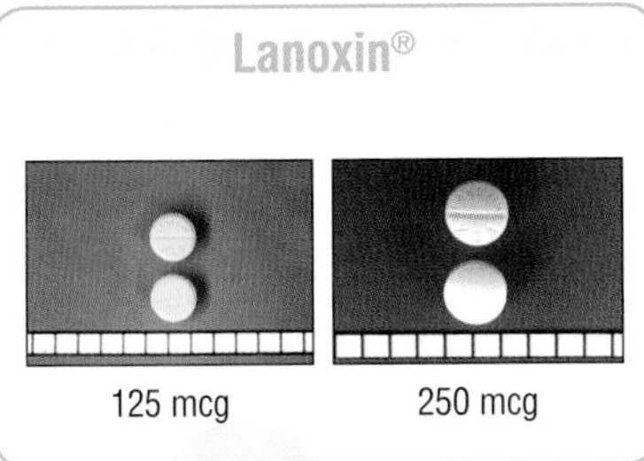

125 mcg | 250 mcg

Diltiazem

(generic)

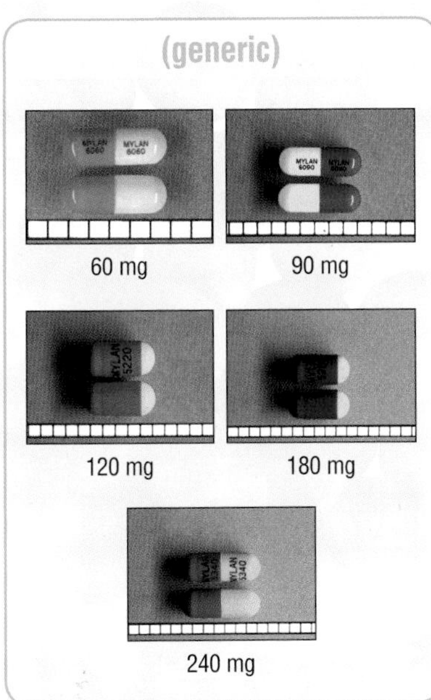

60 mg | 90 mg | 120 mg | 180 mg | 240 mg

Cartia XT™

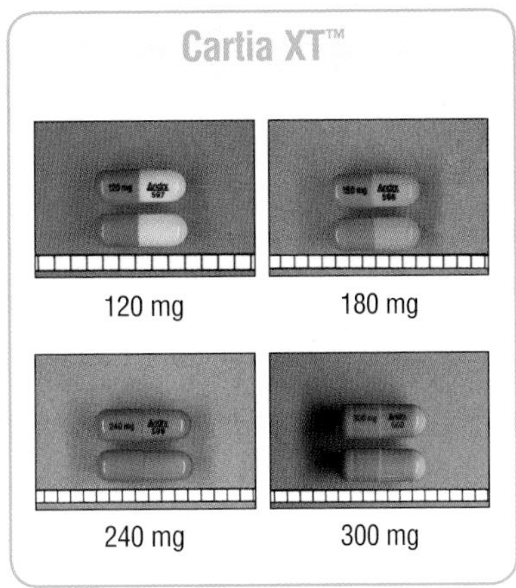

120 mg | 180 mg | 240 mg | 300 mg

Donepezil

Aricept®

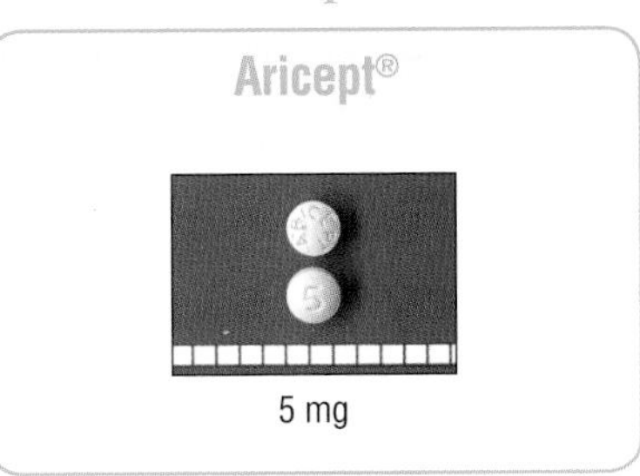

5 mg

Doxazosin

(generic)

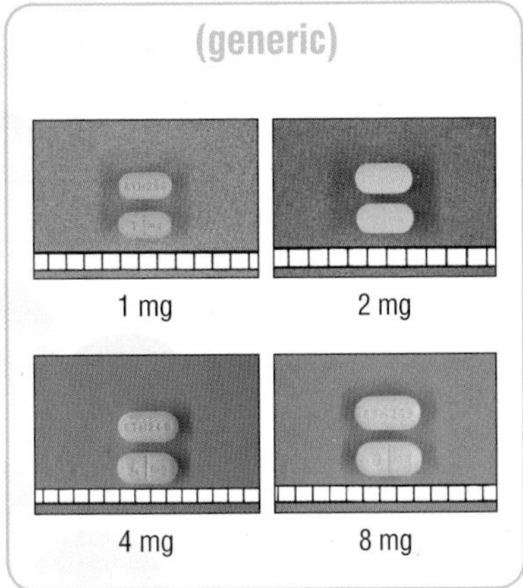

1 mg | 2 mg | 4 mg | 8 mg

Doxycycline

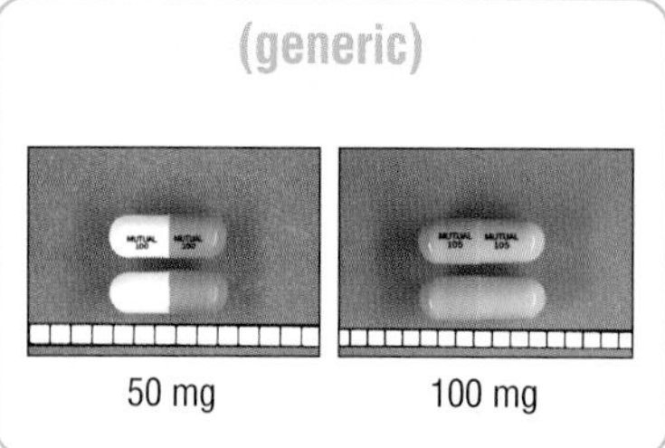

Duloxetine

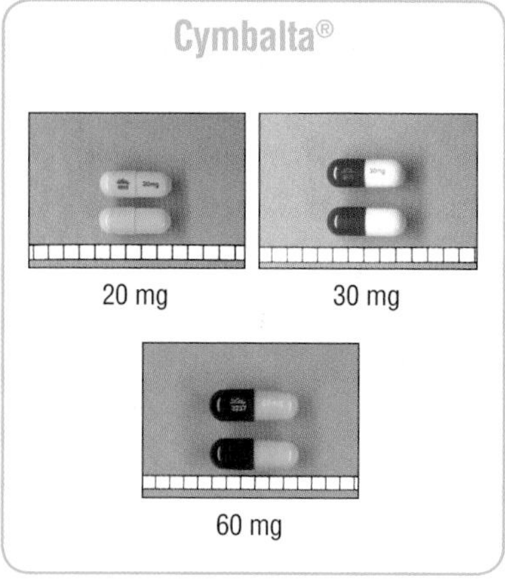

Enalapril

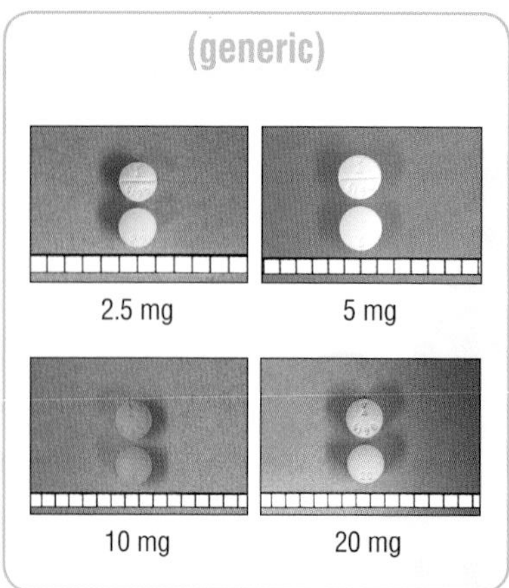

Escitalopram

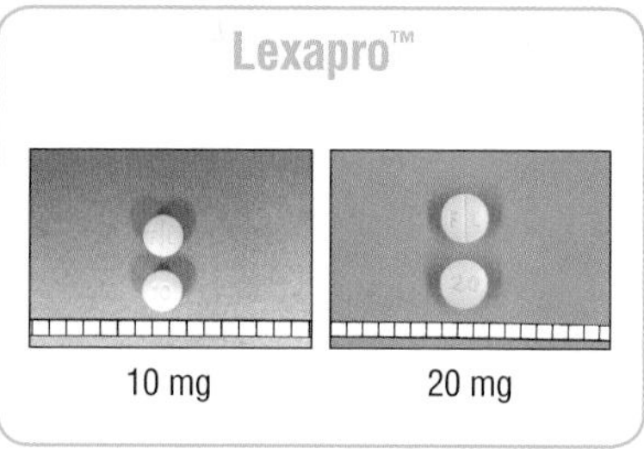

Estradiol

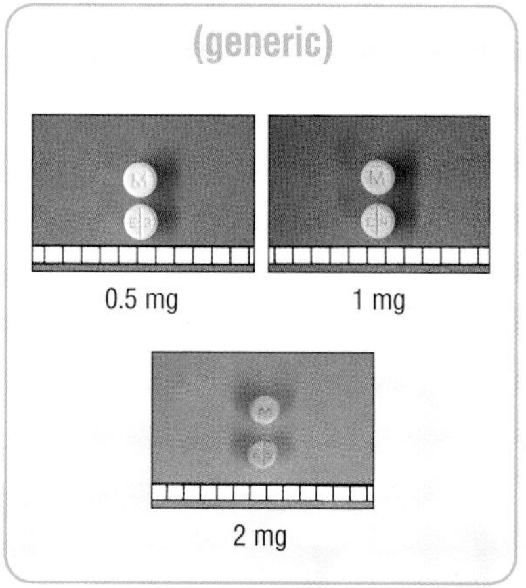

Estrogens (Conjugated/Equine)

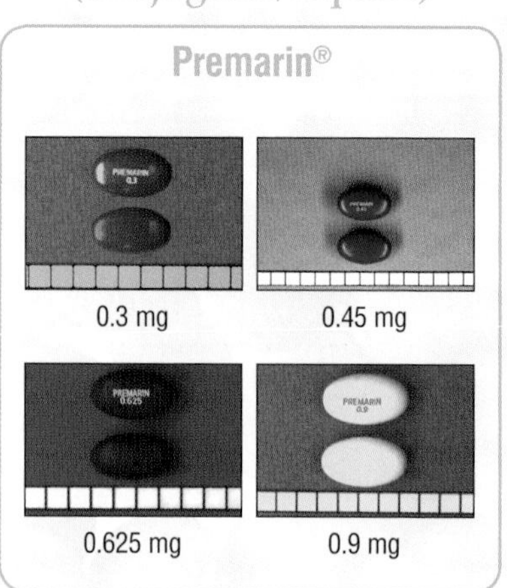

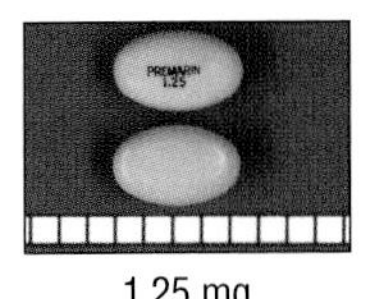

1.25 mg

Ethinyl Estradiol and Drospirenone

Yasmin®

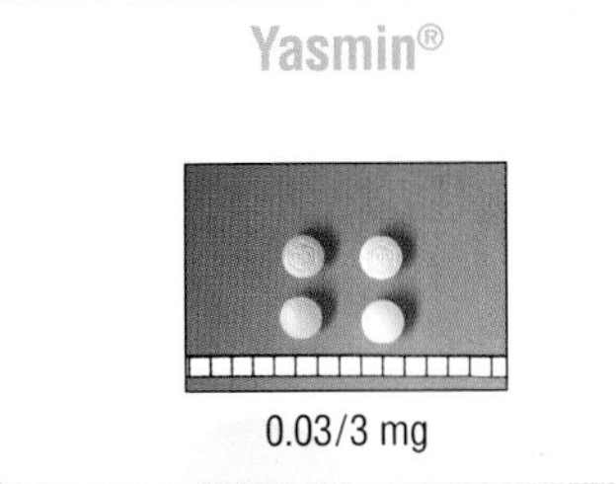

0.03/3 mg

Ethinyl Estradiol and Levonorgestrel

Aviane™ 28

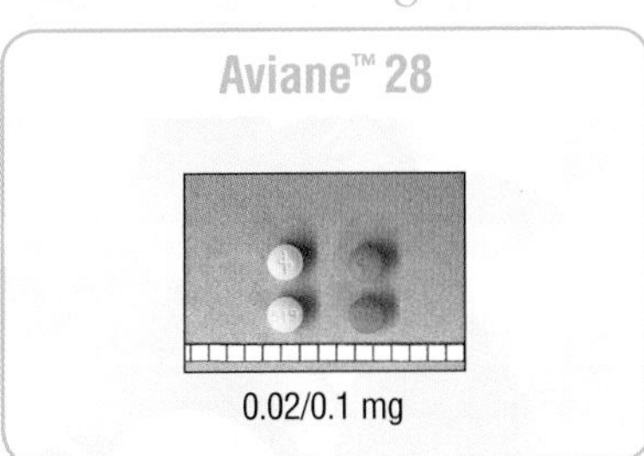

0.02/0.1 mg

Ethinyl Estradiol and Norgestimate

Ortho Tri-Cyclen® LO

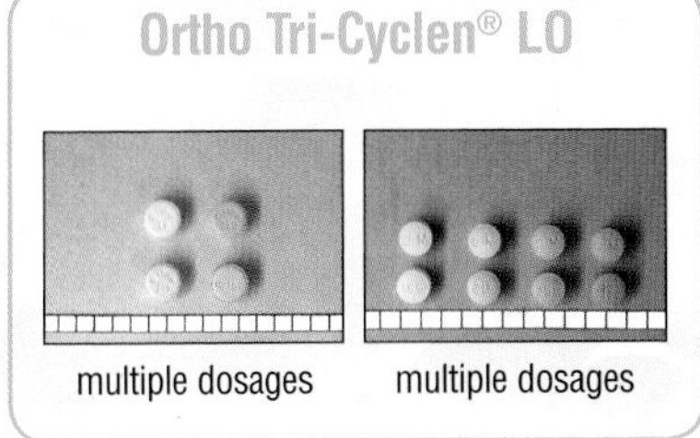

multiple dosages multiple dosages

Tri-Sprintec® 28

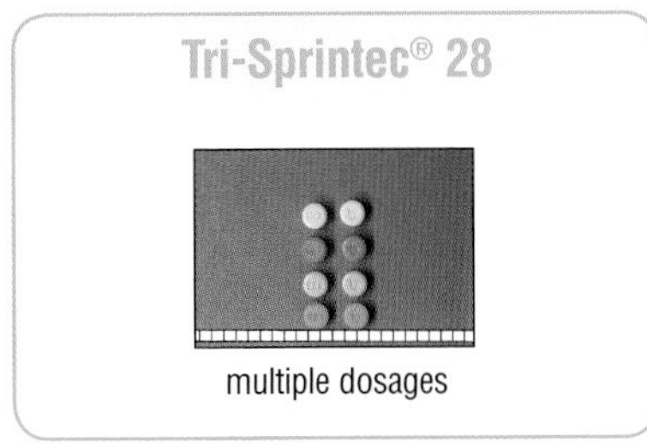

multiple dosages

Etodolac

(generic)

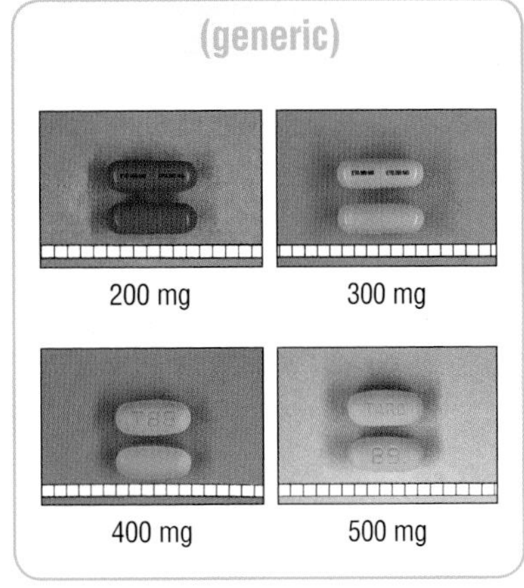

200 mg 300 mg

400 mg 500 mg

Ezetimibe

Zetia™

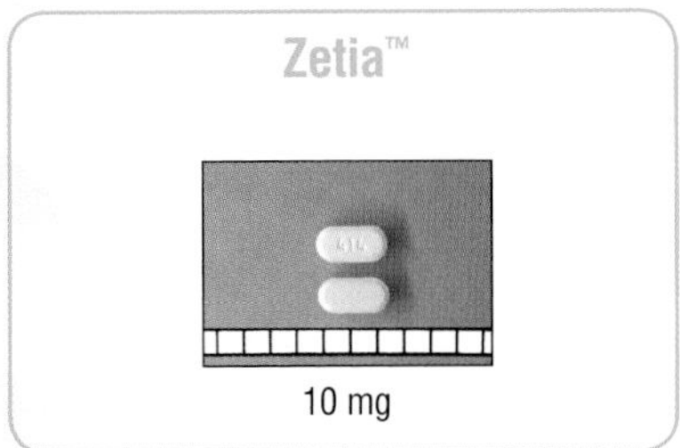

10 mg

Ezetimibe and Simvastatin

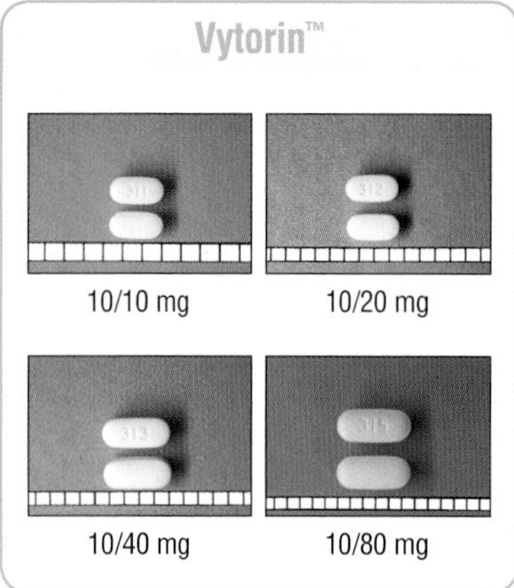

Famotidine

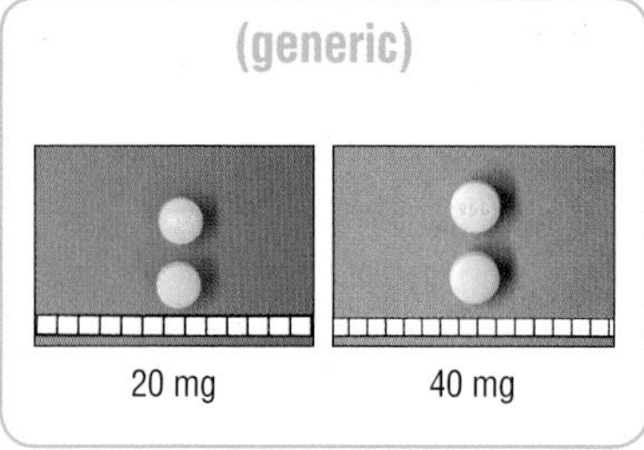

Fenofibrate

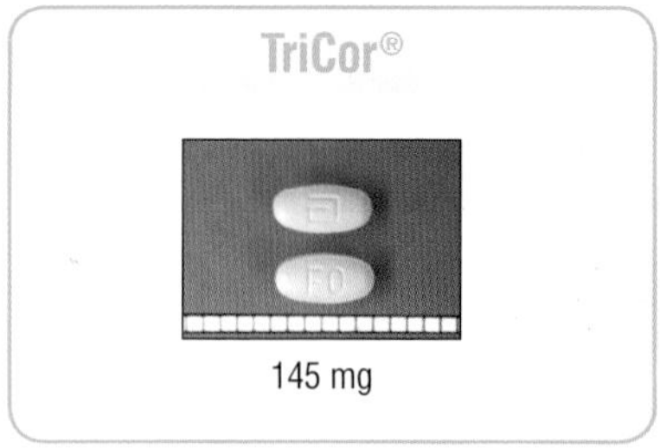

Fexofenadine

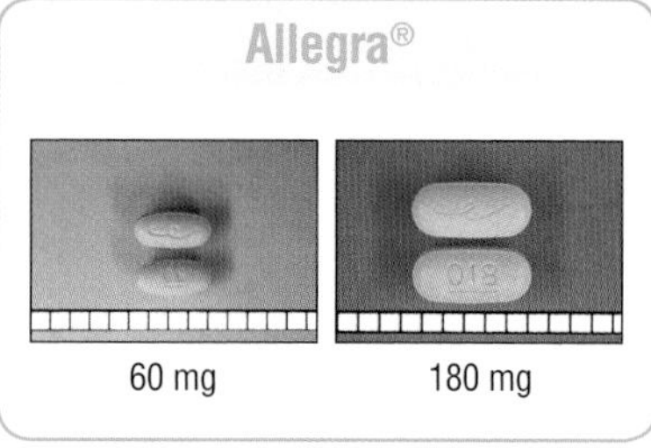

Fexofenadine and Pseudoephedrine

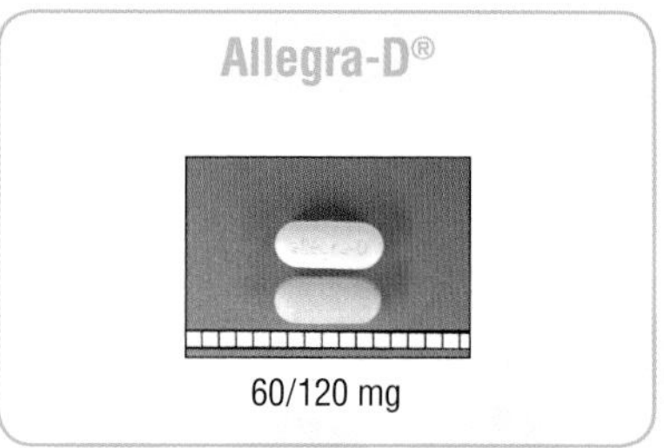

Fluoxetine

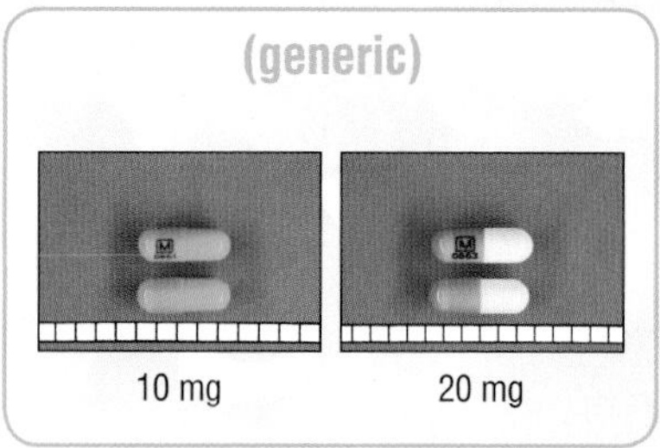

Folic Acid

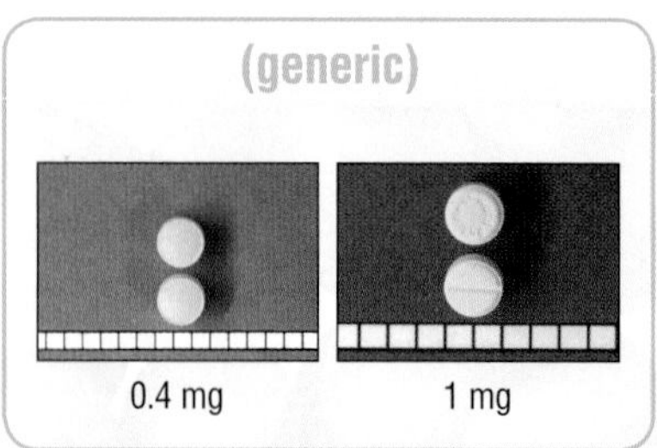

Furosemide

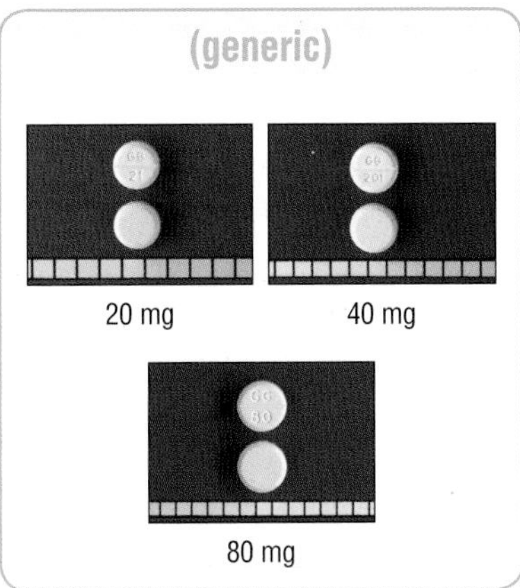

(generic)

20 mg | 40 mg | 80 mg

Gabapentin

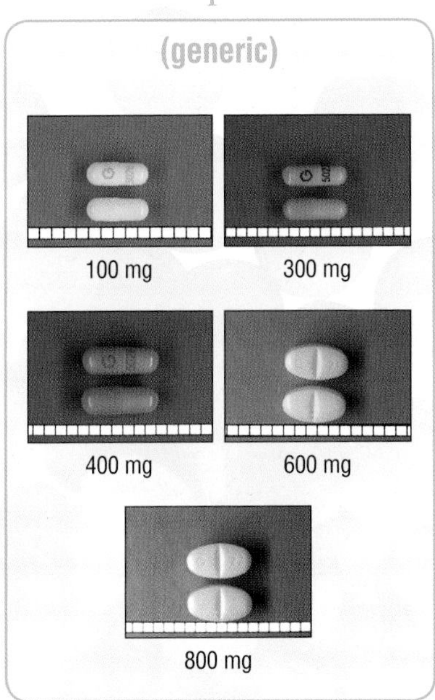

(generic)

100 mg | 300 mg | 400 mg | 600 mg | 800 mg

Gemfibrozil

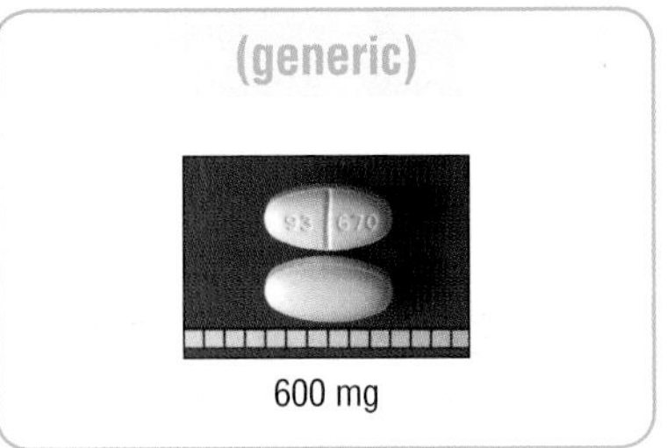

(generic)

600 mg

Glimepiride

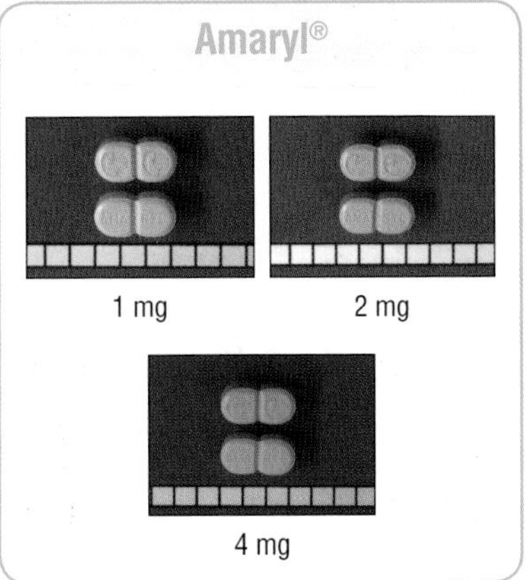

Amaryl®

1 mg | 2 mg | 4 mg

Glipizide

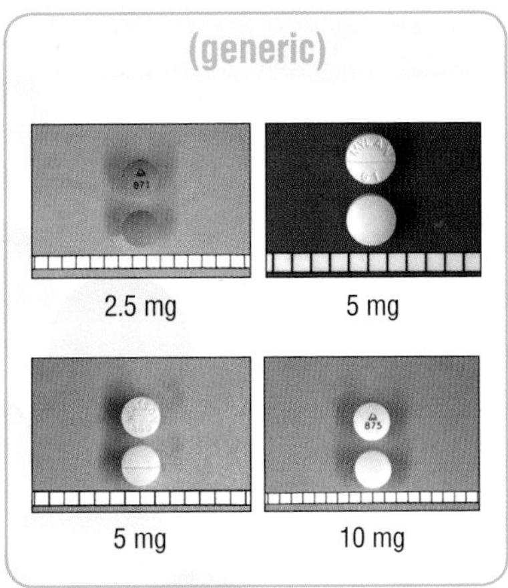

(generic)

2.5 mg | 5 mg | 5 mg | 10 mg

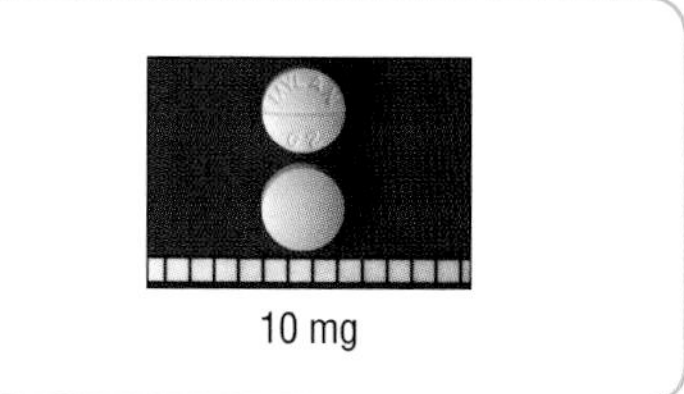

10 mg

Glyburide

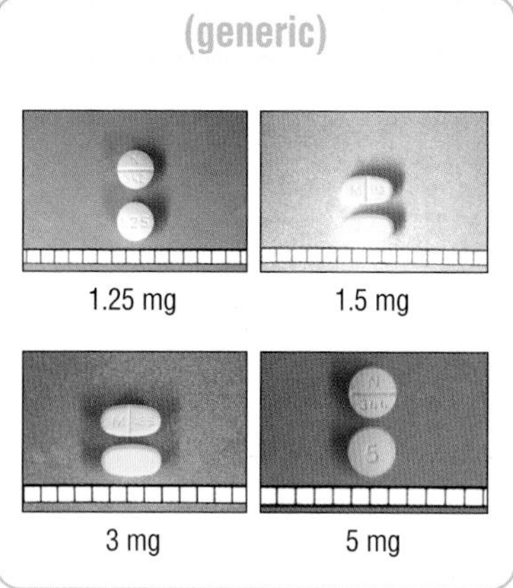

(generic)

1.25 mg 1.5 mg

3 mg 5 mg

Hydrochlorothiazide

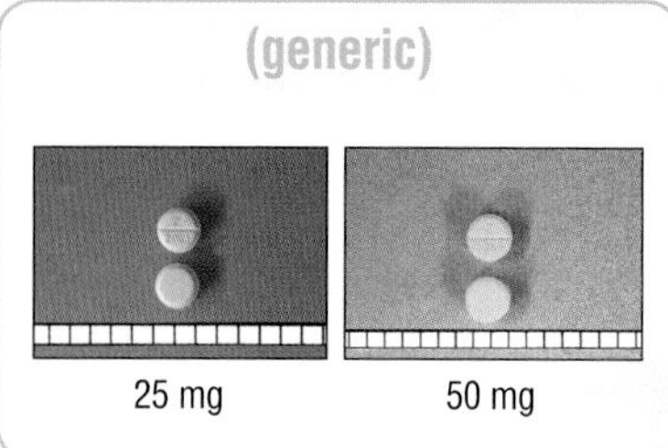

(generic)

25 mg 50 mg

Hydrochlorothiazide and Triamterene

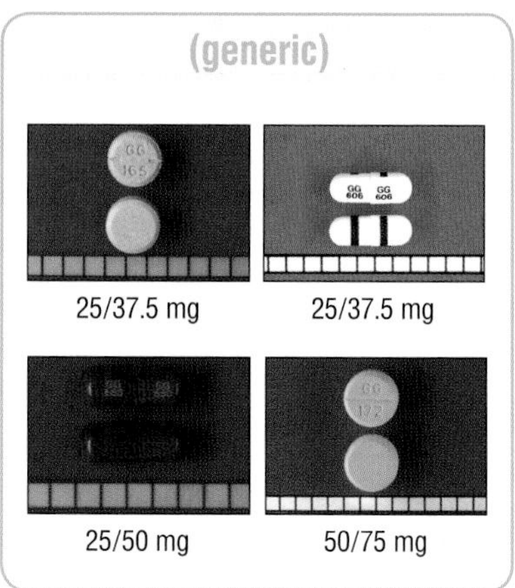

(generic)

25/37.5 mg 25/37.5 mg

25/50 mg 50/75 mg

Hydrocodone and Acetaminophen

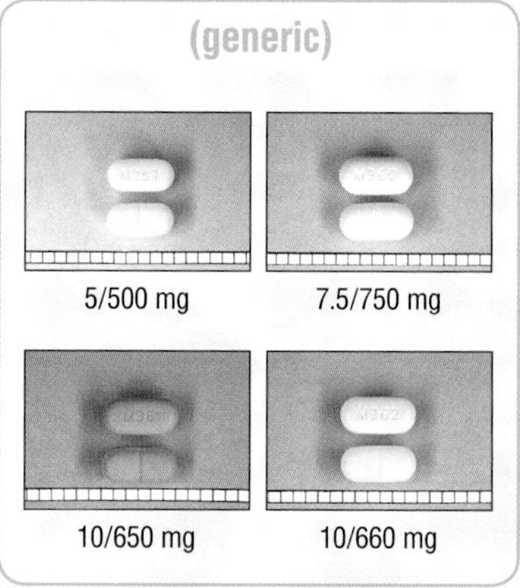

(generic)

5/500 mg 7.5/750 mg

10/650 mg 10/660 mg

Hydroxyzine

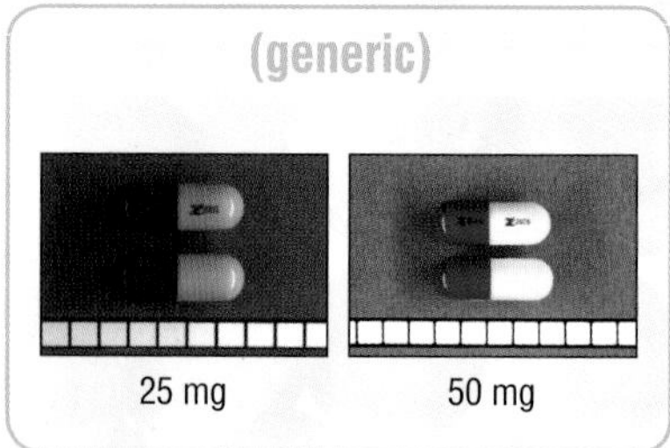

(generic)

25 mg 50 mg

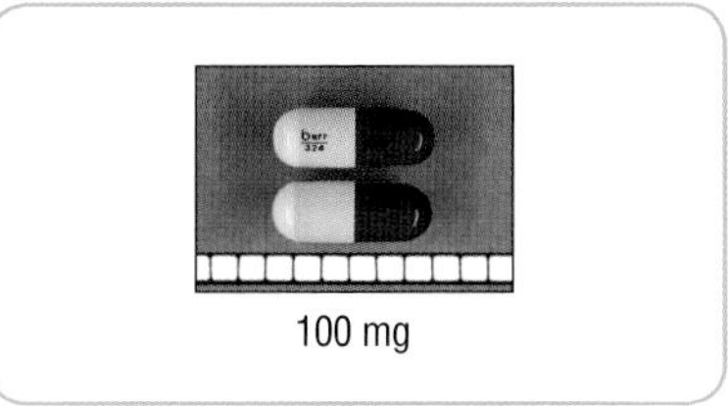

100 mg

Ibuprofen

(generic)

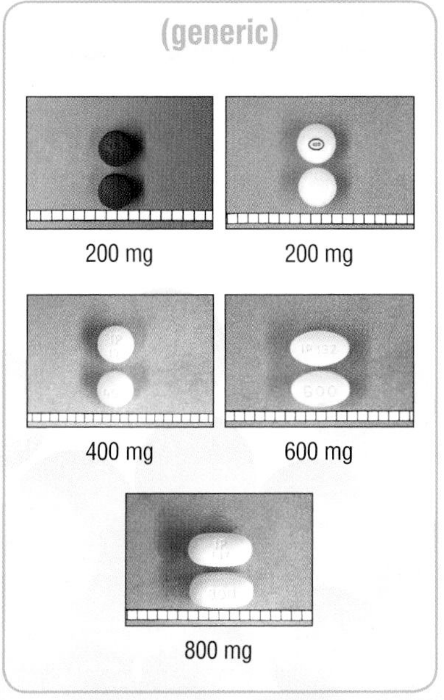

200 mg 200 mg

400 mg 600 mg

800 mg

Irbesartan

Avapro®

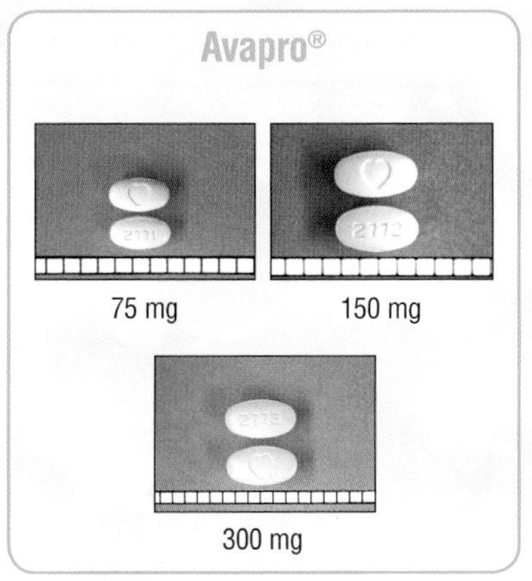

75 mg 150 mg

300 mg

Irbesartan and Hydrochlorothiazide

Avalide®

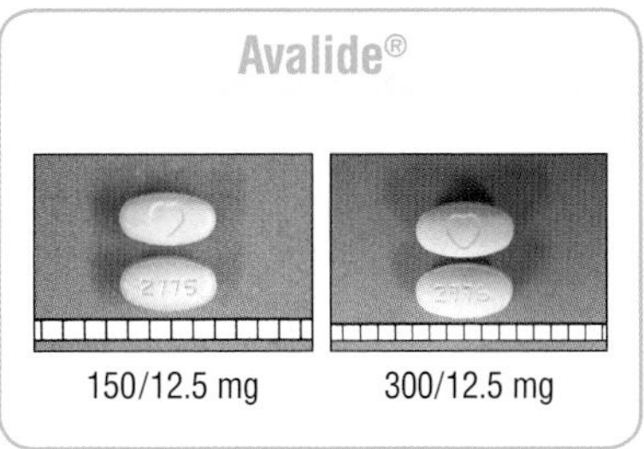

150/12.5 mg 300/12.5 mg

Isosorbide Mononitrate

(generic)

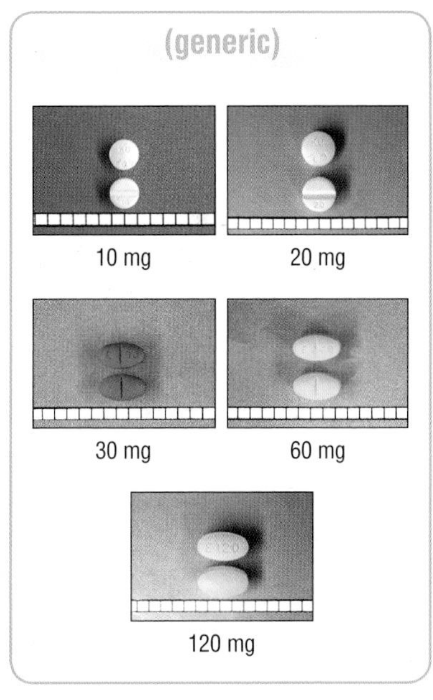

10 mg 20 mg

30 mg 60 mg

120 mg

Lamotrigine

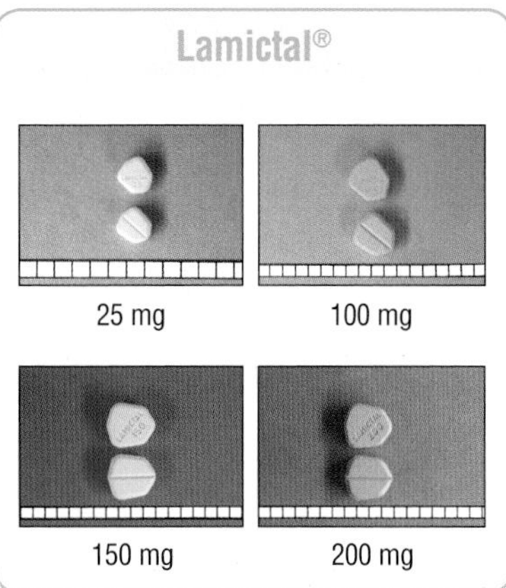

Lansoprazole

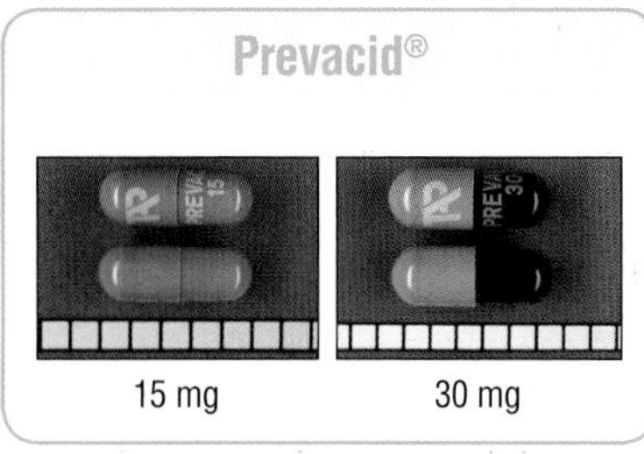

Levofloxacin

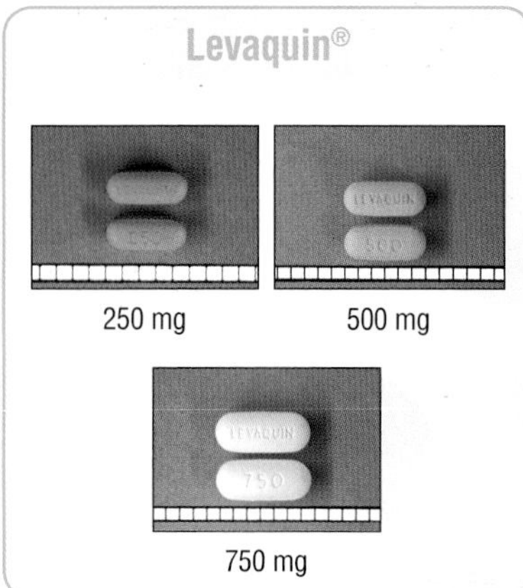

Levothyroxine

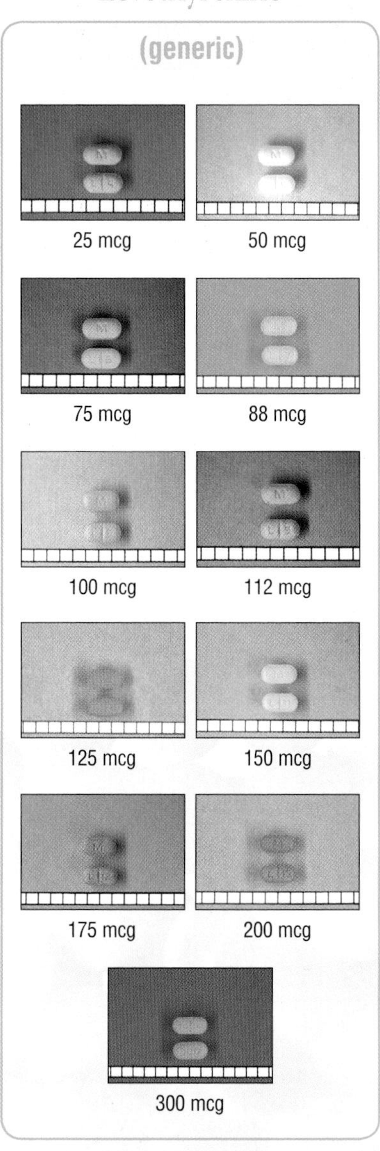

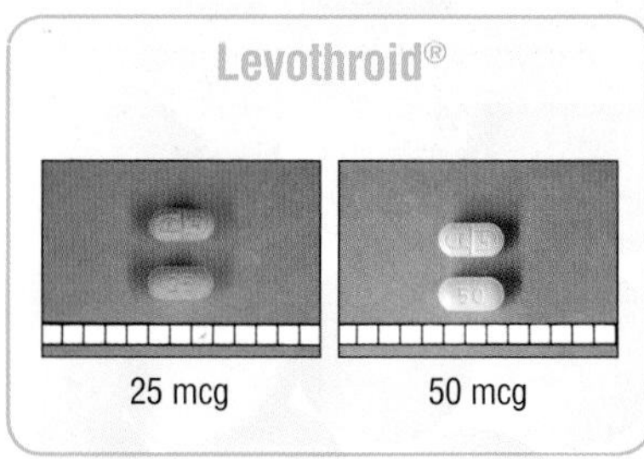

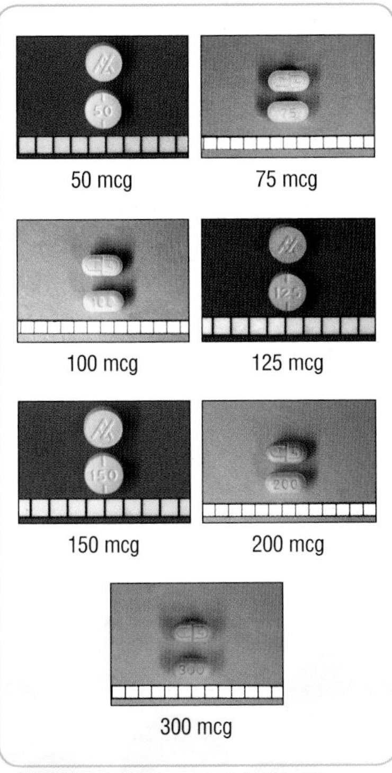

50 mcg 75 mcg
100 mcg 125 mcg
150 mcg 200 mcg
300 mcg

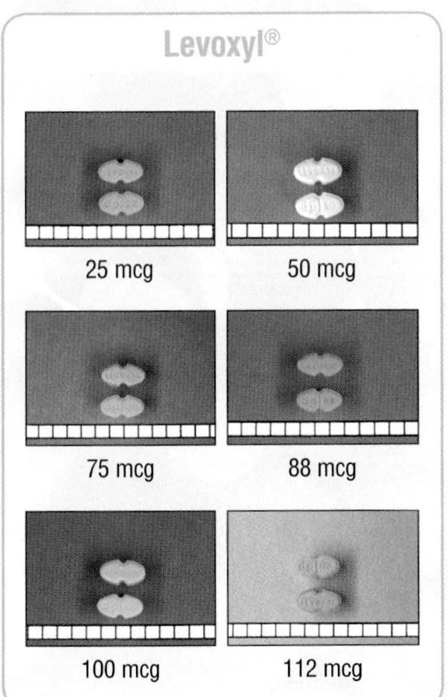

Levoxyl®

25 mcg 50 mcg
75 mcg 88 mcg
100 mcg 112 mcg

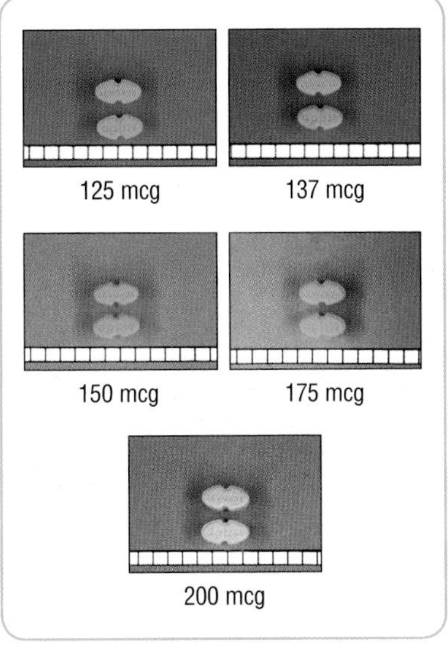

125 mcg 137 mcg
150 mcg 175 mcg
200 mcg

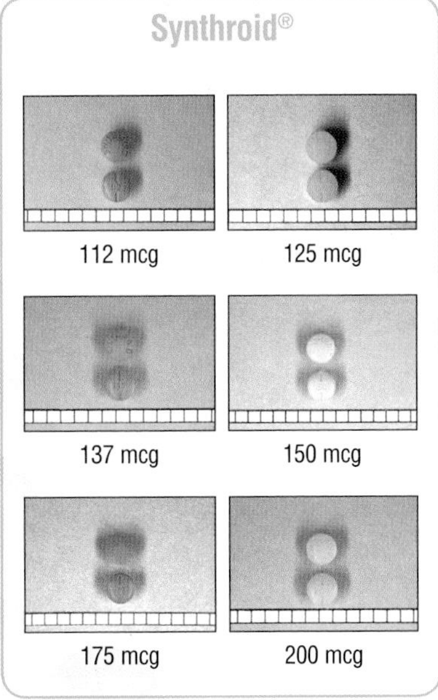

Synthroid®

112 mcg 125 mcg
137 mcg 150 mcg
175 mcg 200 mcg

Lisinopril

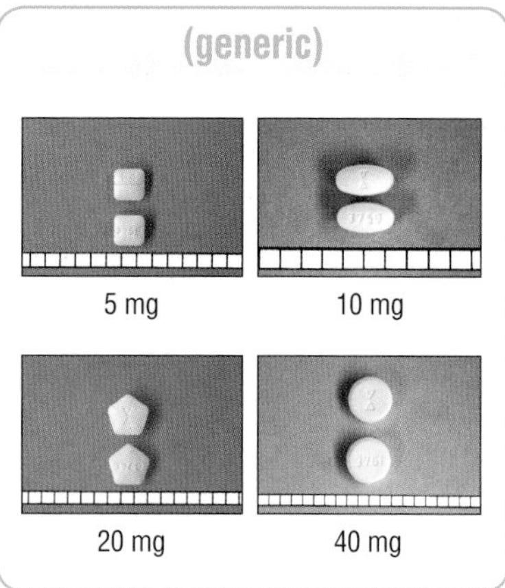
(generic)

5 mg 10 mg 20 mg 40 mg

Lisinopril and Hydrochlorothiazide

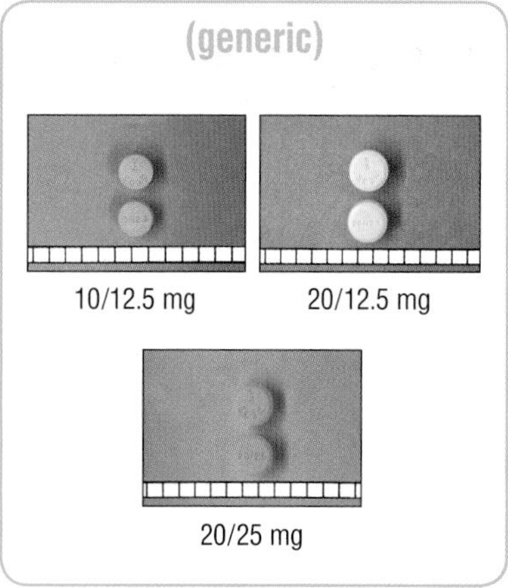
(generic)

10/12.5 mg 20/12.5 mg 20/25 mg

Lorazepam

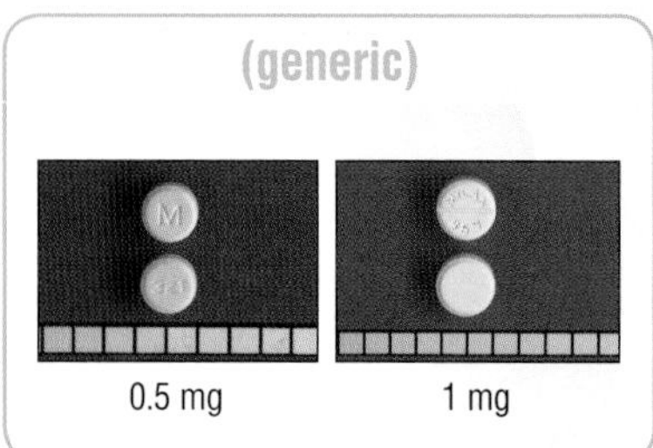
(generic)

0.5 mg 1 mg

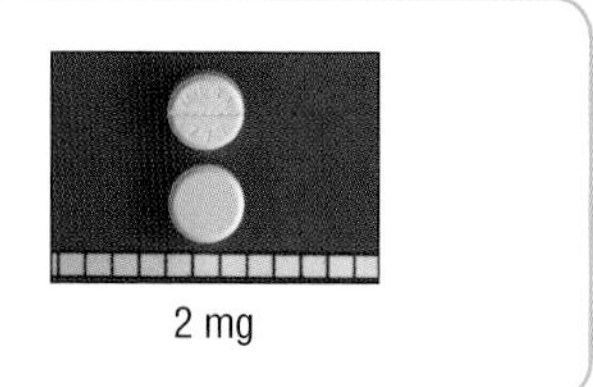
2 mg

Losartan

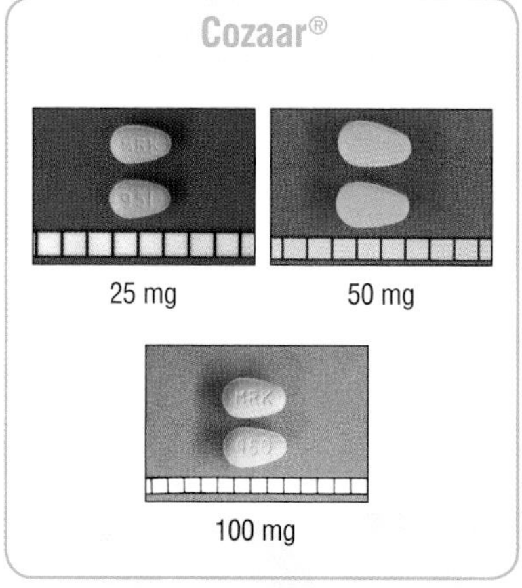
Cozaar®

25 mg 50 mg 100 mg

Losartan and Hydrochlorothiazide

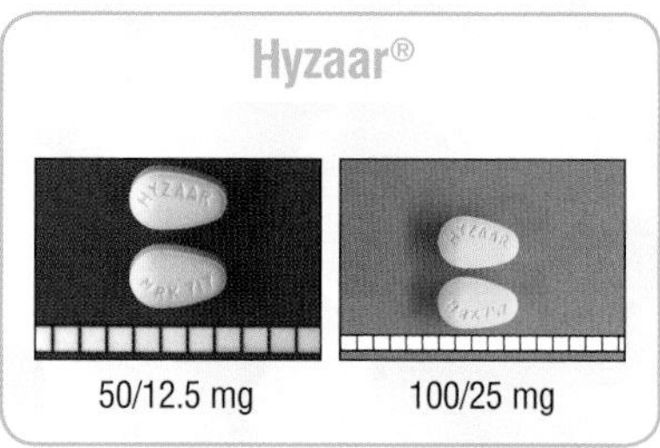
Hyzaar®

50/12.5 mg 100/25 mg

Lovastatin

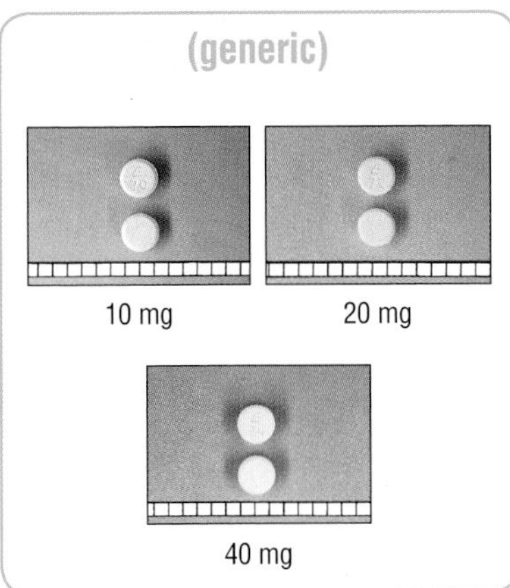
(generic)

10 mg 20 mg 40 mg

Meclizine

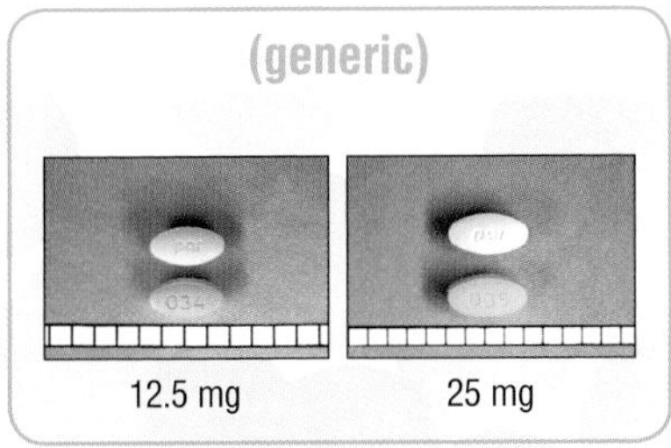
(generic)

12.5 mg 25 mg

Meloxicam

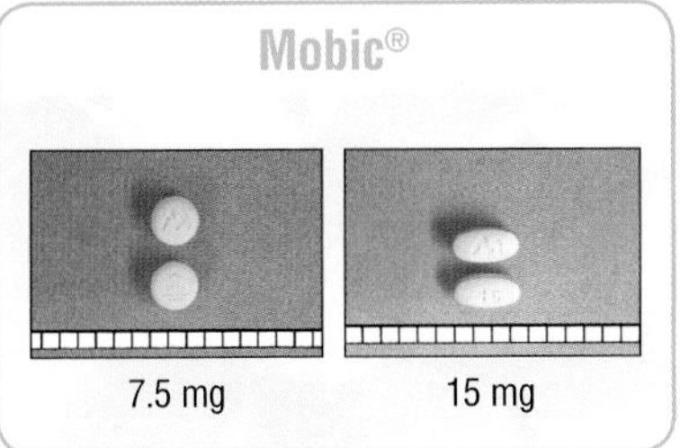
Mobic®

7.5 mg 15 mg

Metaxalone

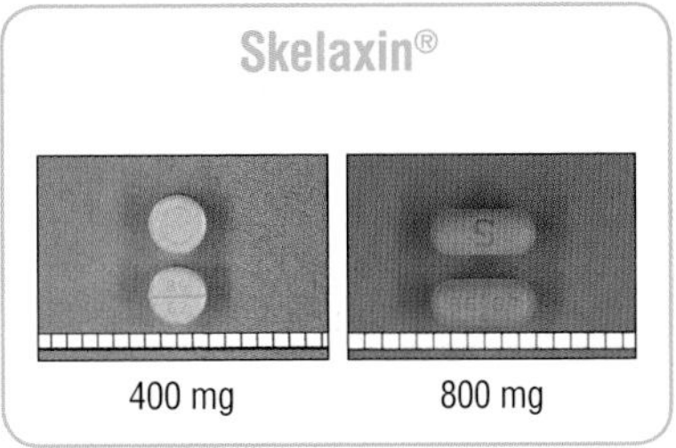
Skelaxin®

400 mg 800 mg

Metformin

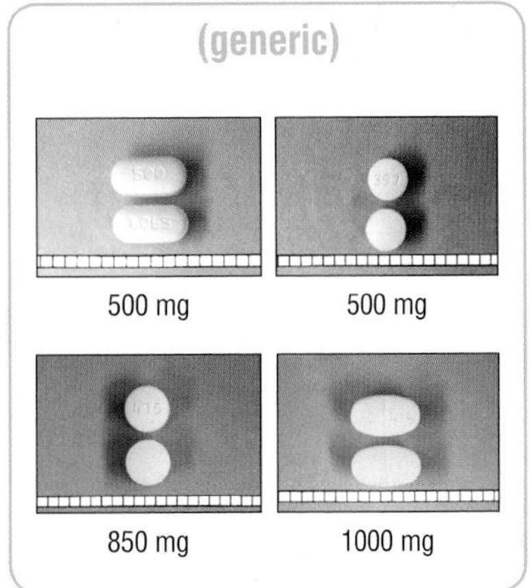
(generic)

500 mg 500 mg 850 mg 1000 mg

Methotrexate

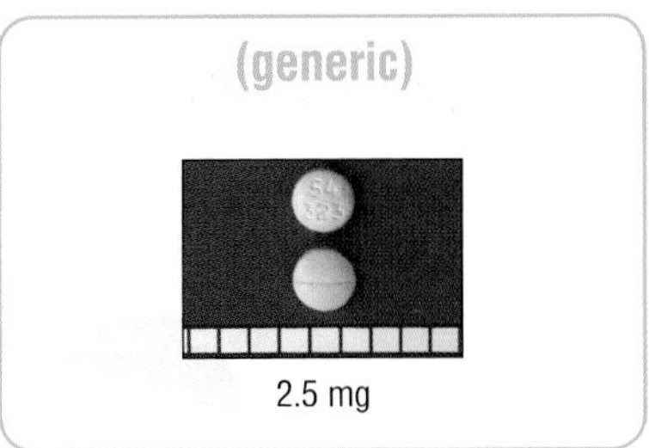
(generic)

2.5 mg

Methylphenidate

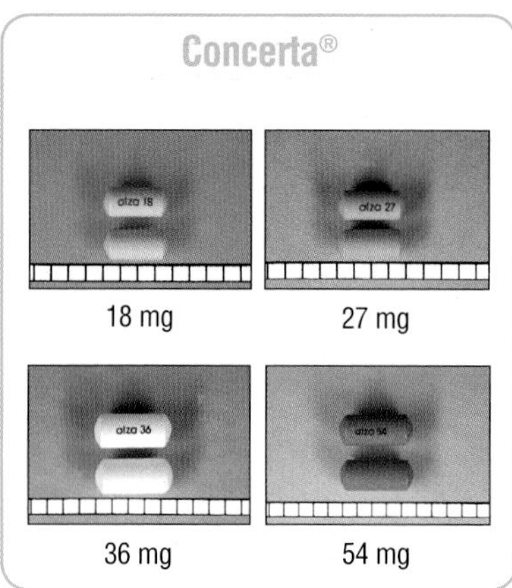

Concerta®

18 mg 27 mg

36 mg 54 mg

Methylprednisolone

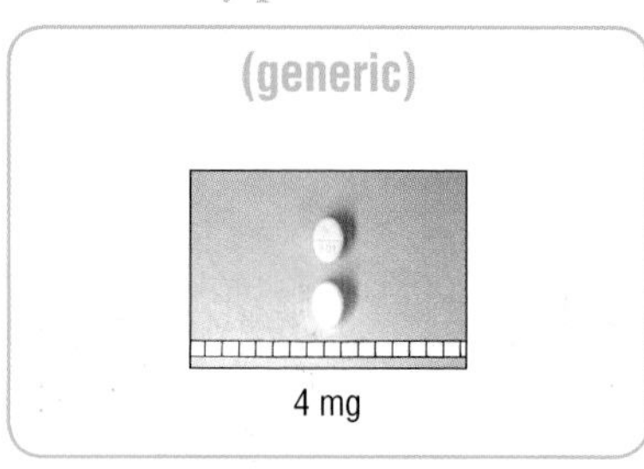

(generic)

4 mg

Metoclopramide

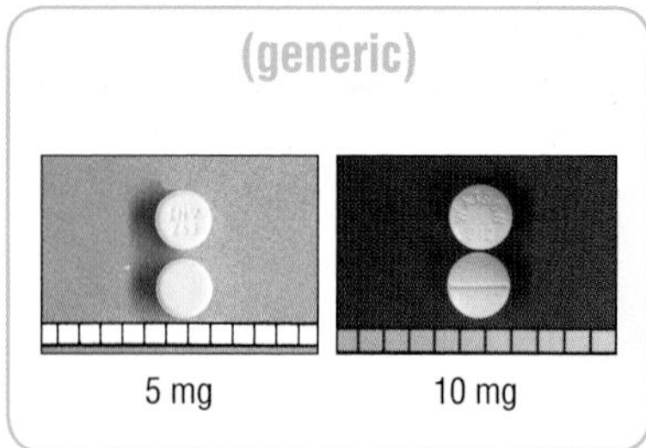

(generic)

5 mg 10 mg

Metoprolol

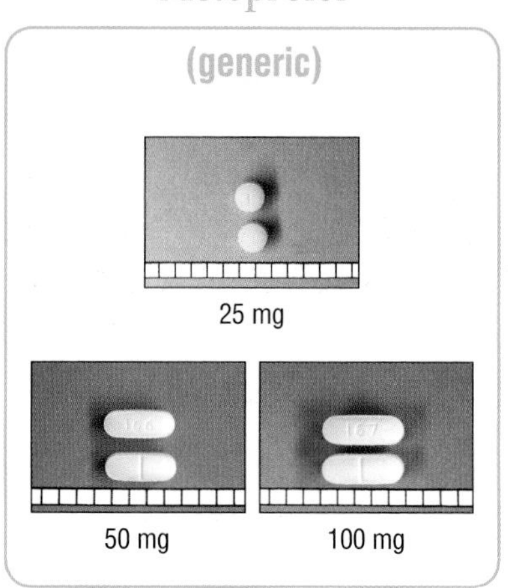

(generic)

25 mg

50 mg 100 mg

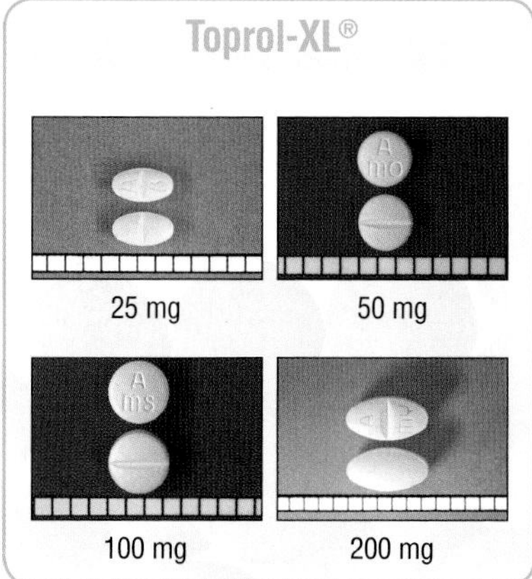

Toprol-XL®

25 mg 50 mg

100 mg 200 mg

Metronidazole

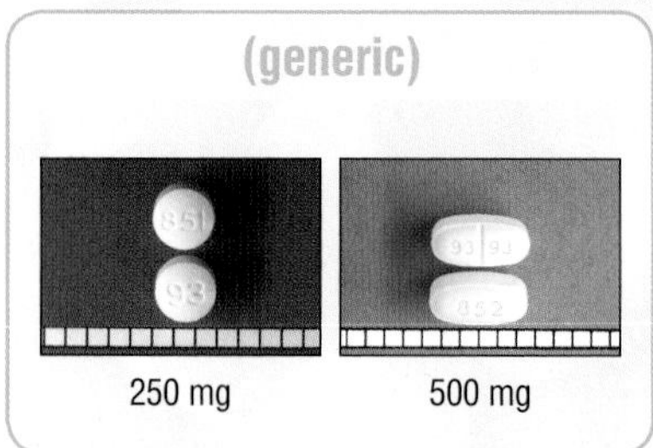

(generic)

250 mg 500 mg

Minocycline

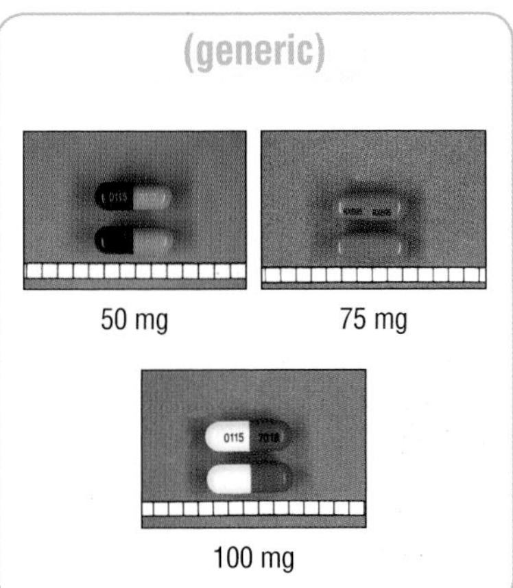
(generic)

50 mg 75 mg

100 mg

Mirtazapine

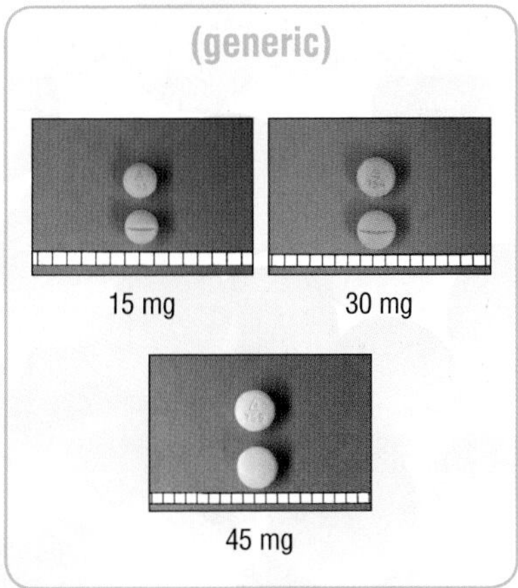
(generic)

15 mg 30 mg

45 mg

Montelukast

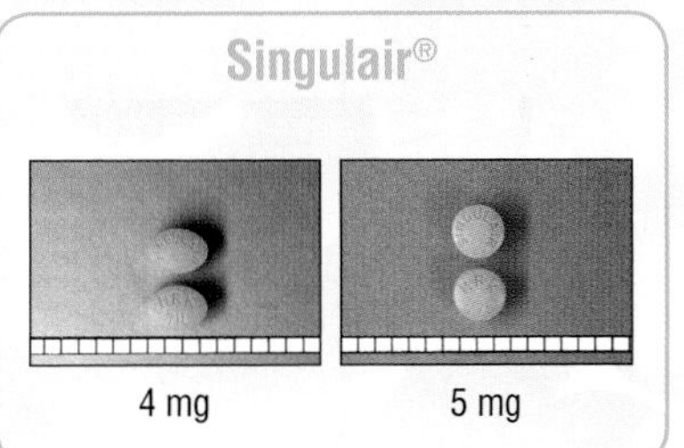
Singulair®

4 mg 5 mg

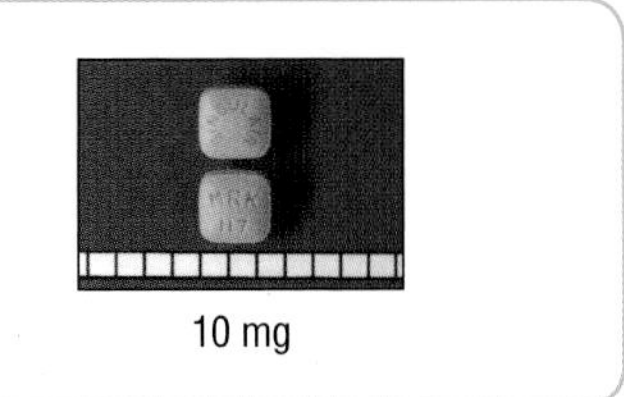
10 mg

Nabumetone

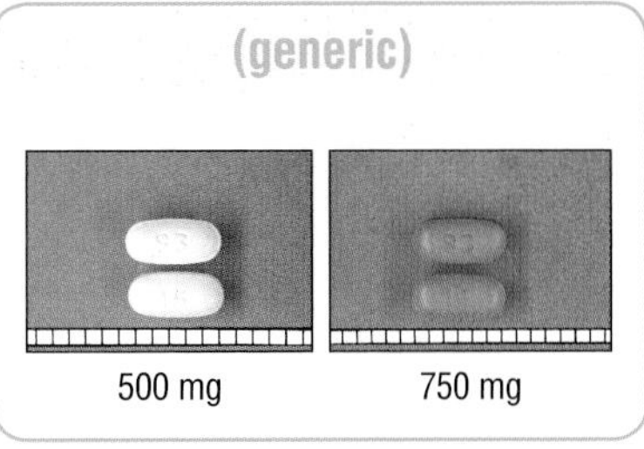
(generic)

500 mg 750 mg

Naproxen

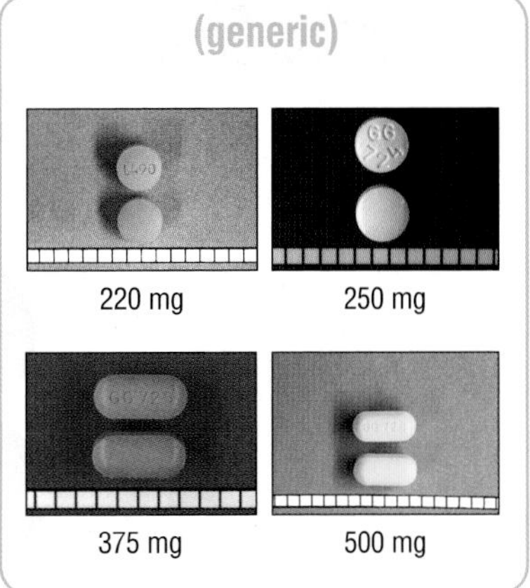
(generic)

220 mg 250 mg

375 mg 500 mg

Niacin

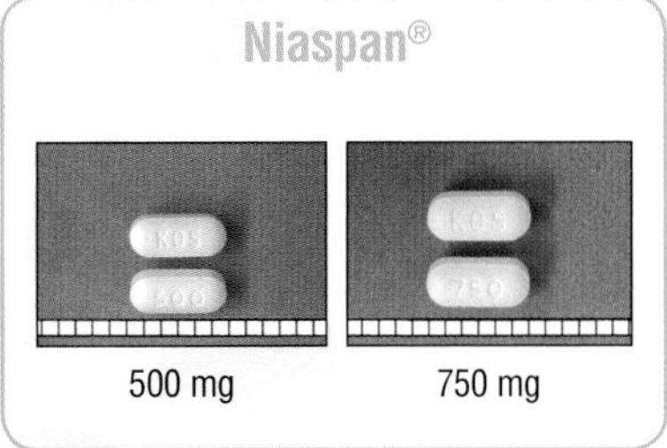
Niaspan®

500 mg 750 mg

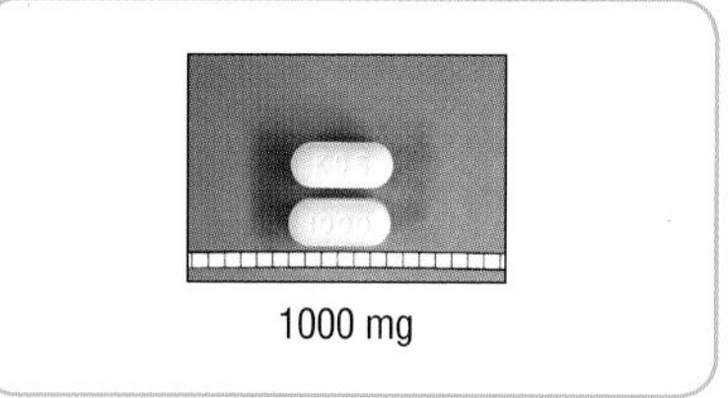

1000 mg

Nifedipine

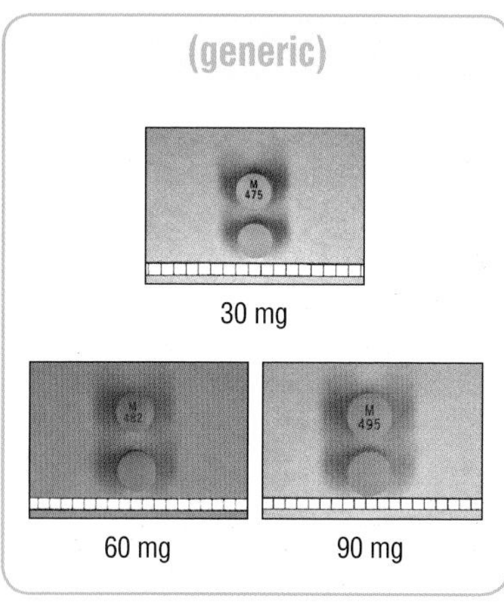

(generic)

30 mg

60 mg

90 mg

Nitrofurantoin

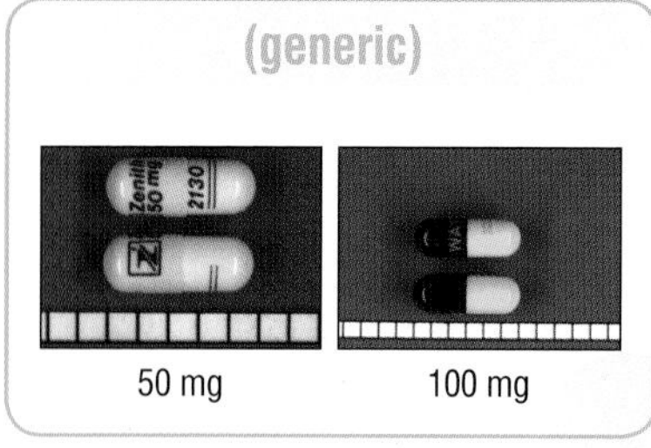

(generic)

50 mg

100 mg

Nitroglycerin

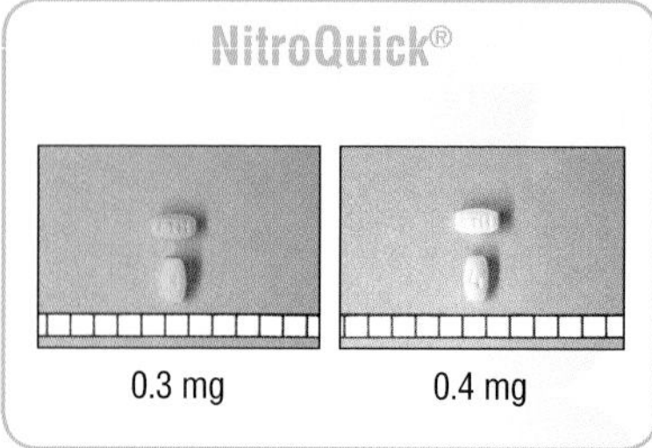

NitroQuick®

0.3 mg

0.4 mg

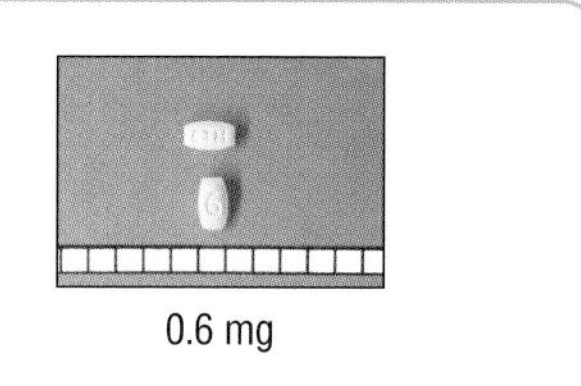

0.6 mg

Nortriptyline

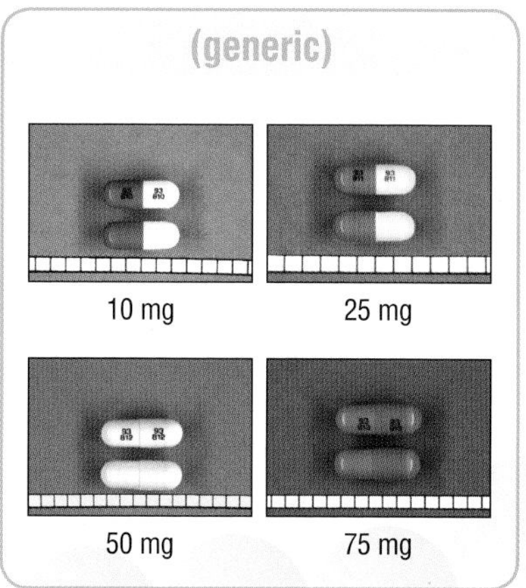

(generic)

10 mg

25 mg

50 mg

75 mg

Olanzapine

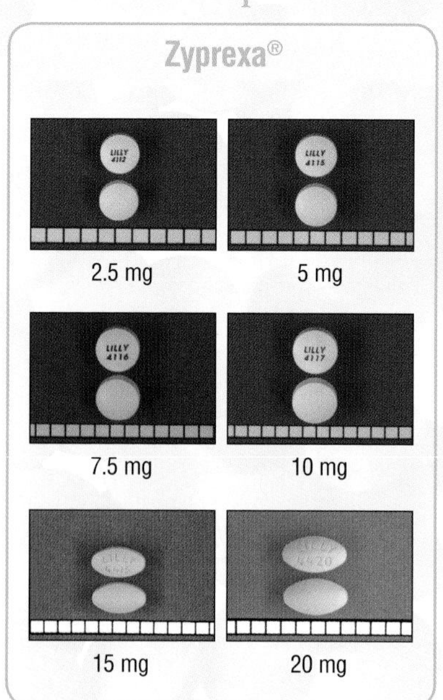

Zyprexa®

2.5 mg

5 mg

7.5 mg

10 mg

15 mg

20 mg

Olmesartan

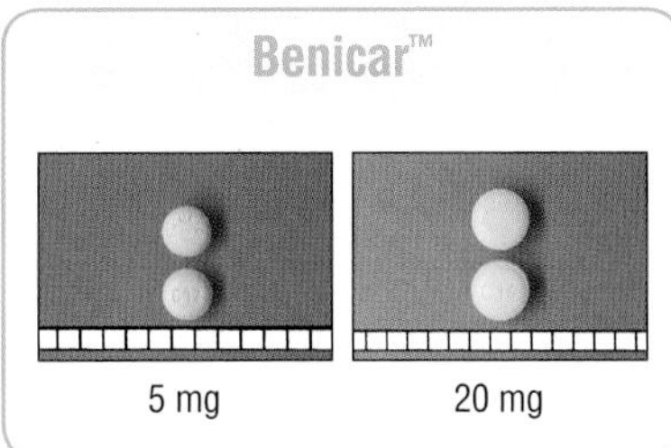

Olmesartan and Hydrochlorothiazide

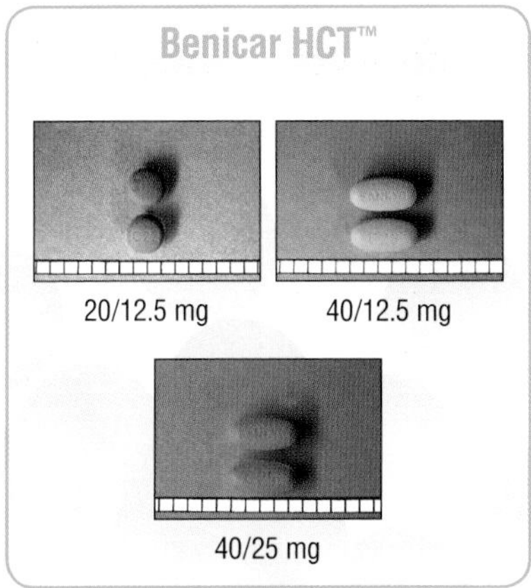

Omeprazole

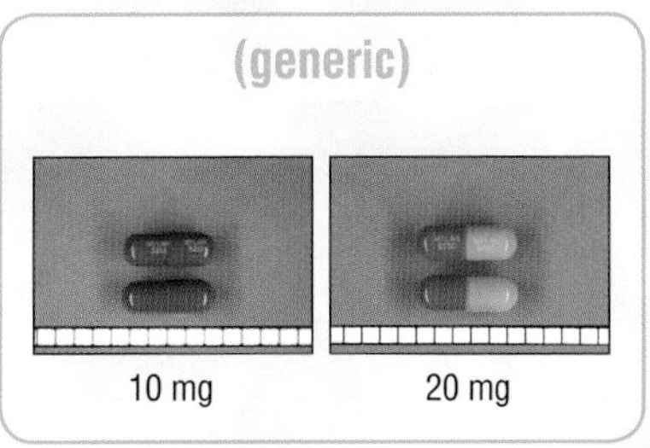

Oxycodone

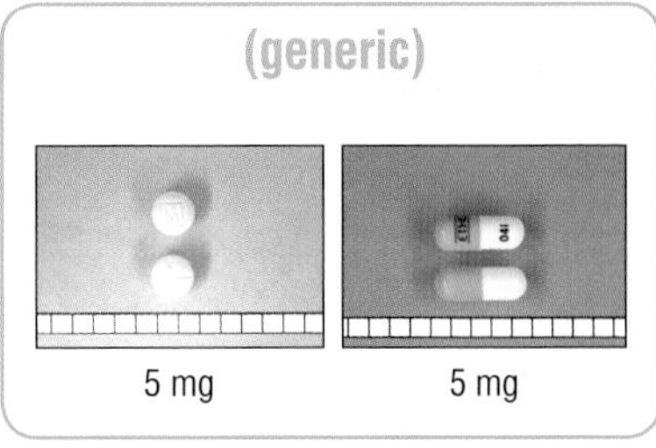

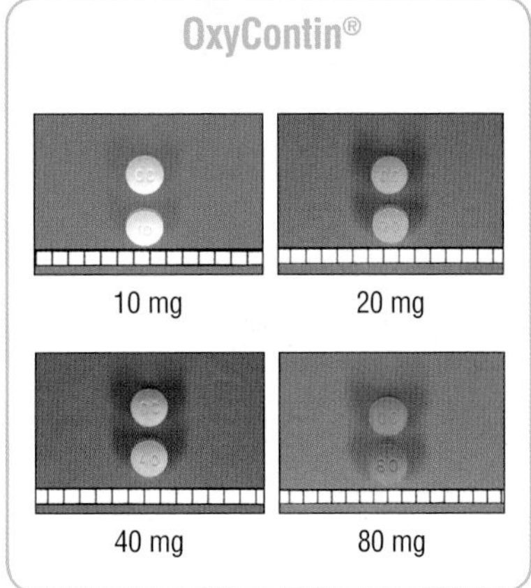

Oxycodone and Acetaminophen

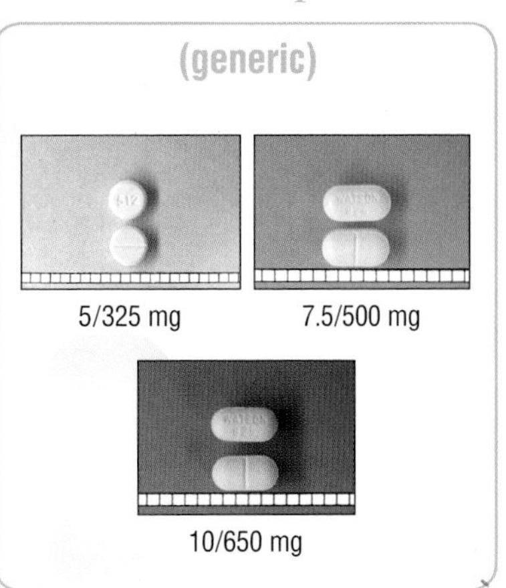

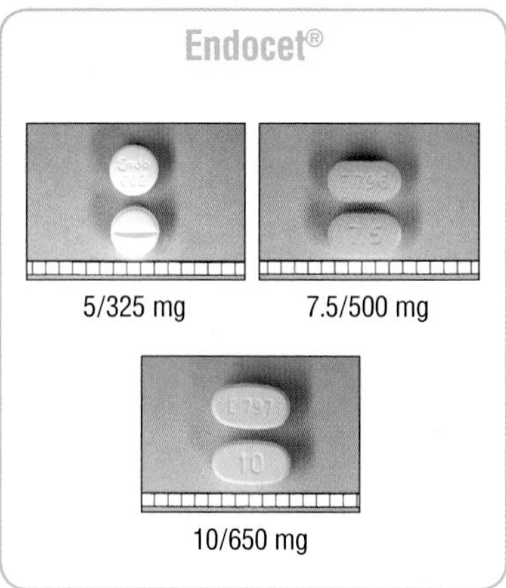

Endocet®

5/325 mg
7.5/500 mg
10/650 mg

Pantoprazole

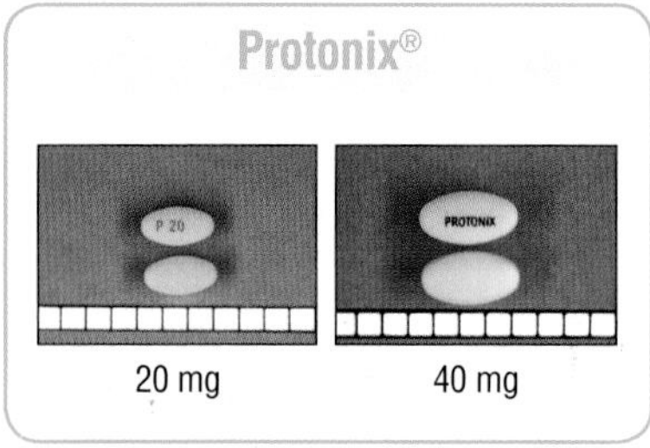

Protonix®

20 mg
40 mg

Paroxetine

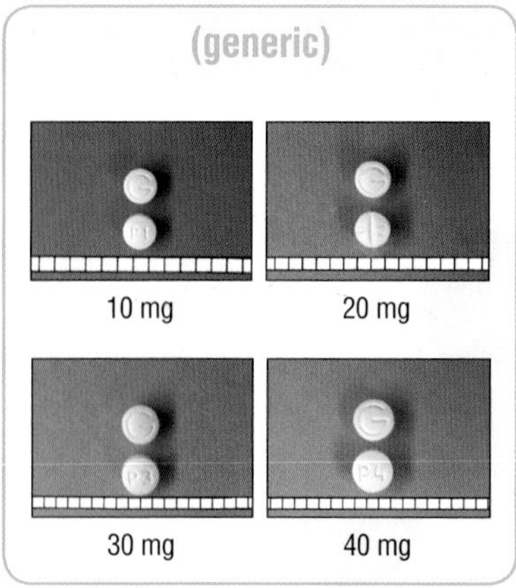

(generic)

10 mg
20 mg
30 mg
40 mg

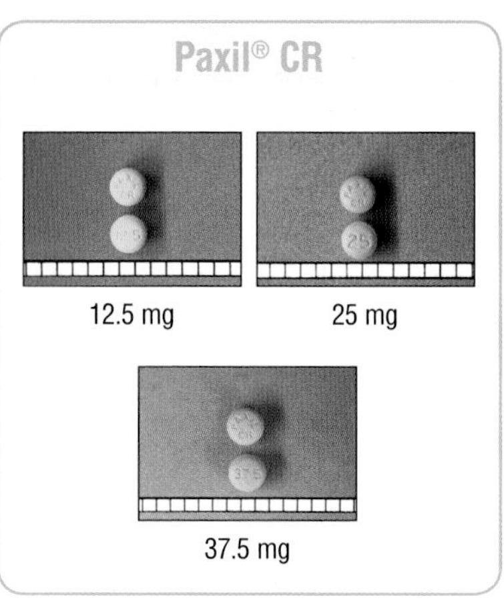

Paxil® CR

12.5 mg
25 mg
37.5 mg

Penicillin V Potassium

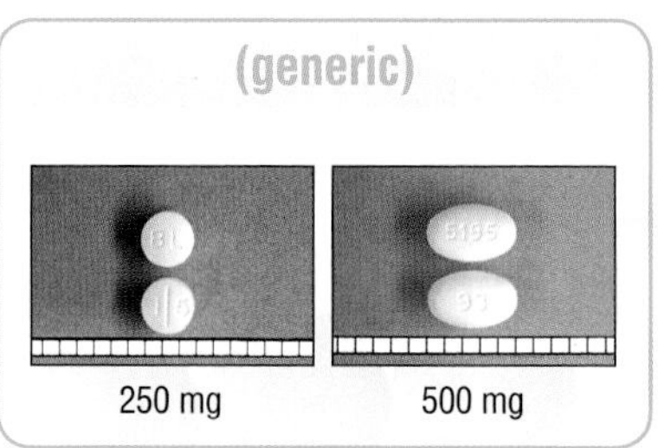

(generic)

250 mg
500 mg

Phentermine

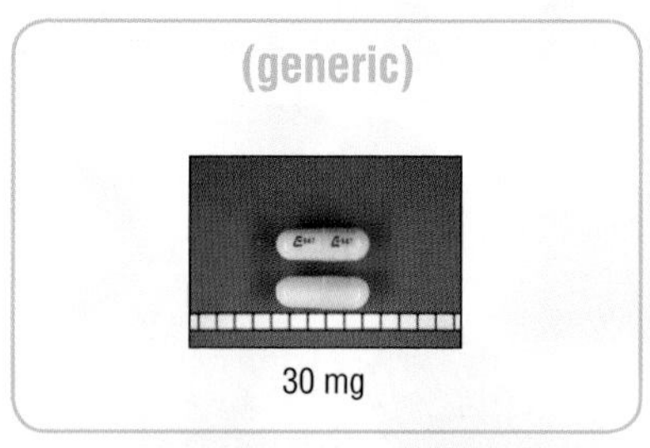

(generic)

30 mg

Pioglitazone

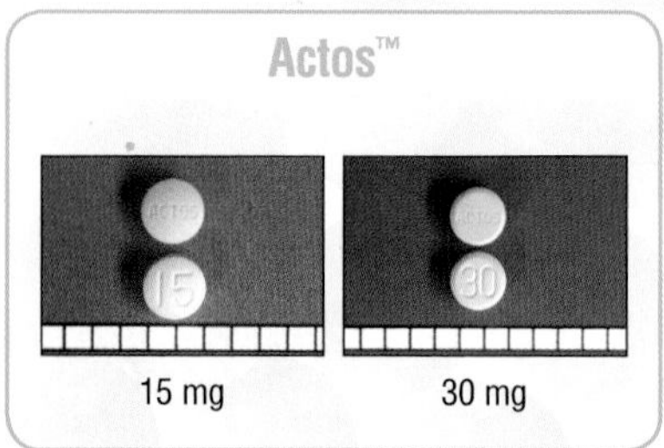

Actos™

15 mg
30 mg

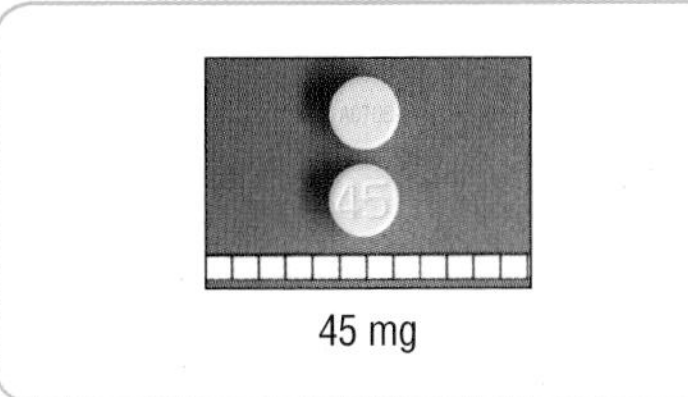

45 mg

Potassium Chloride

(generic)

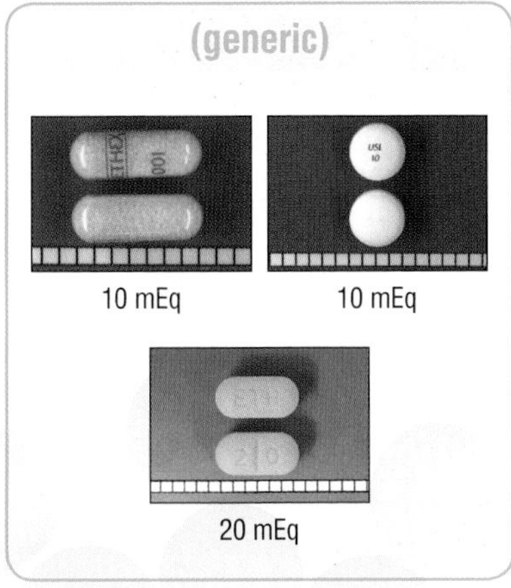

10 mEq 10 mEq

20 mEq

Klor-Con® 8

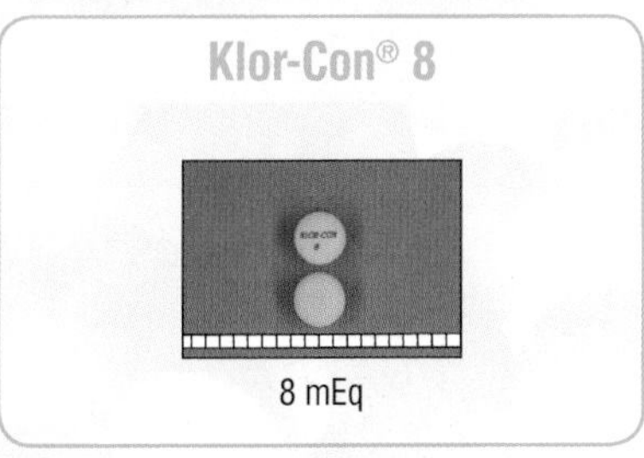

8 mEq

Klor-Con® 10

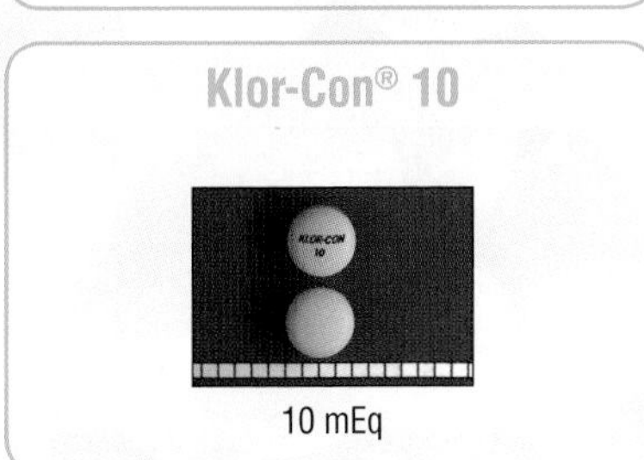

10 mEq

Pravastatin

Pravachol®

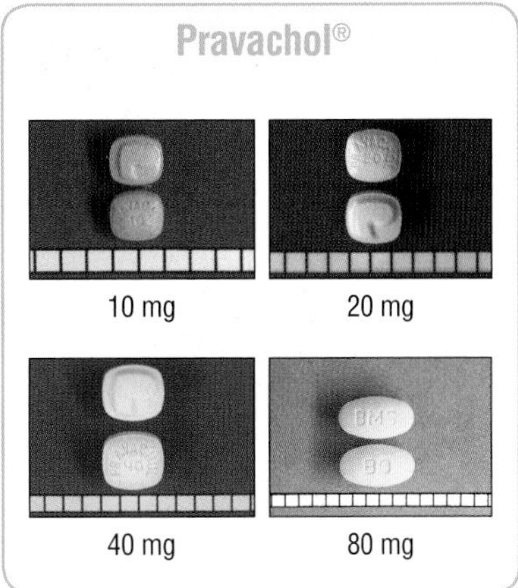

10 mg 20 mg

40 mg 80 mg

Prednisone

(generic)

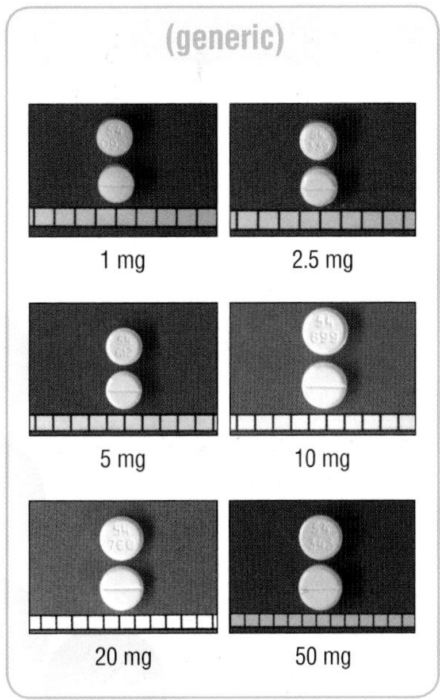

1 mg 2.5 mg

5 mg 10 mg

20 mg 50 mg

Promethazine

(generic)

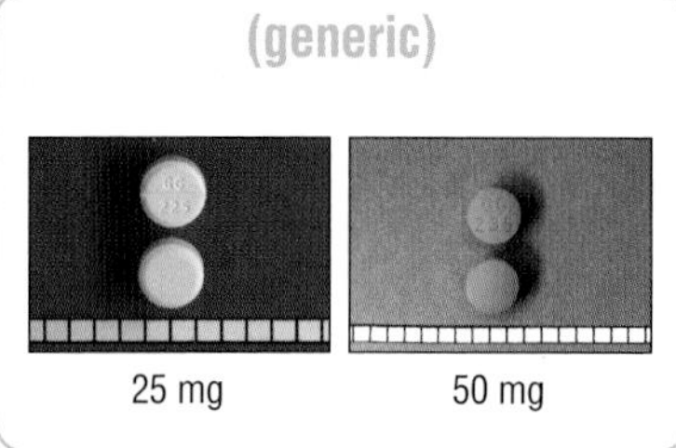

25 mg 50 mg

Propoxyphene and Acetaminophen

(generic)

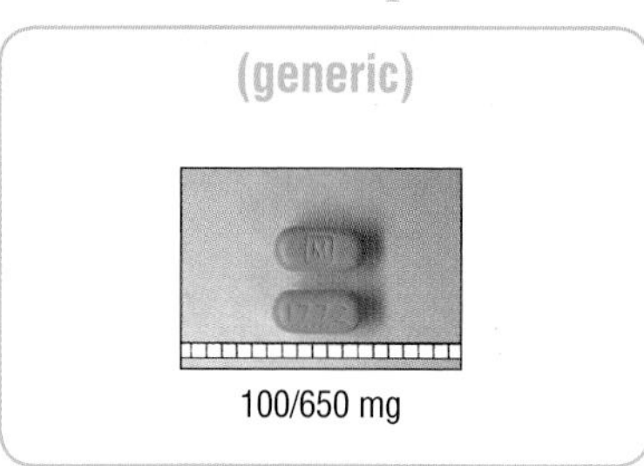

100/650 mg

Propranolol

(generic)

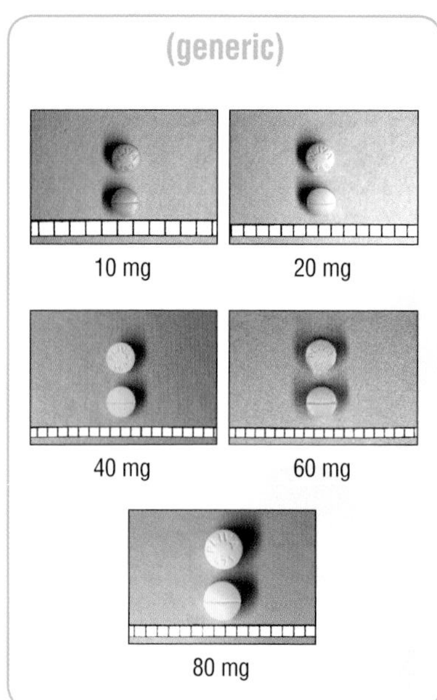

10 mg 20 mg 40 mg 60 mg 80 mg

Quetiapine

Seroquel®

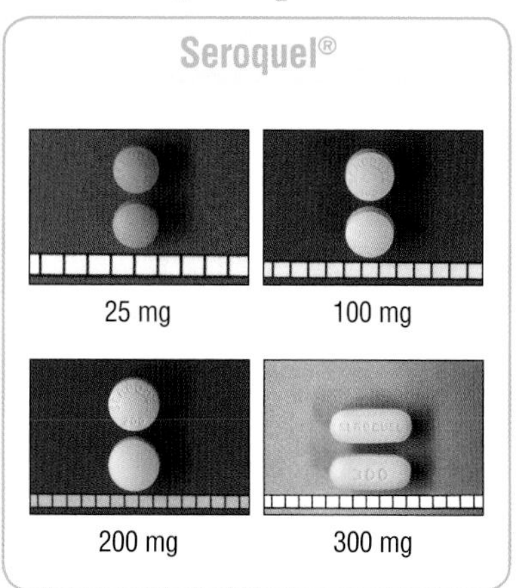

25 mg 100 mg 200 mg 300 mg

Quinapril

(generic)

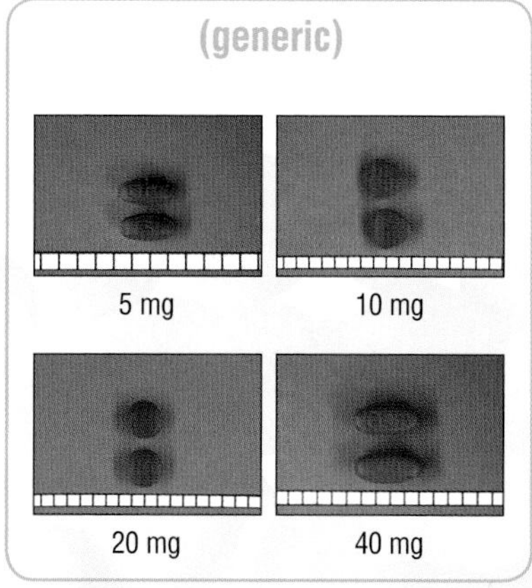

5 mg 10 mg 20 mg 40 mg

Quinine

(generic)

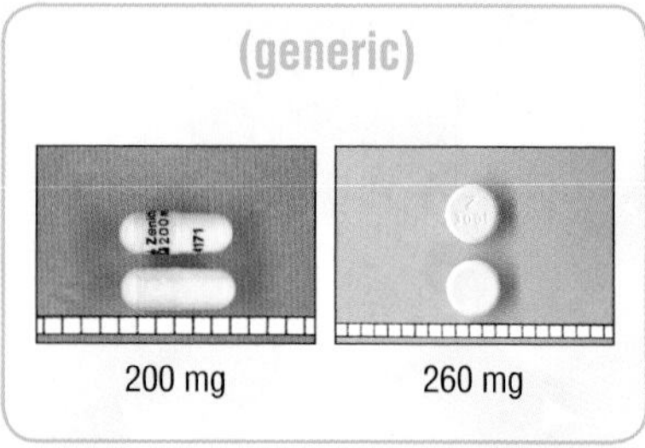

200 mg 260 mg

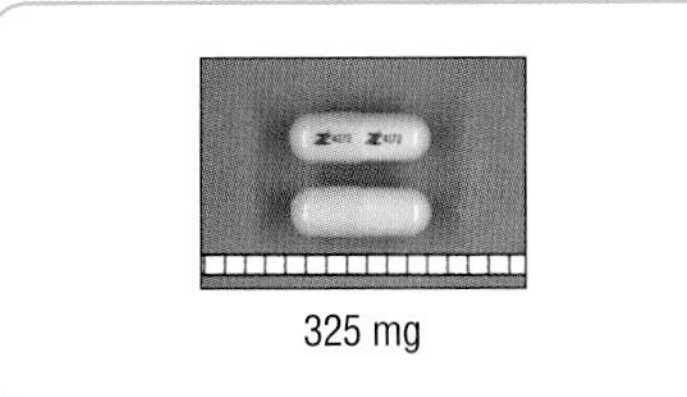
325 mg

Rabeprazole

Aciphex®

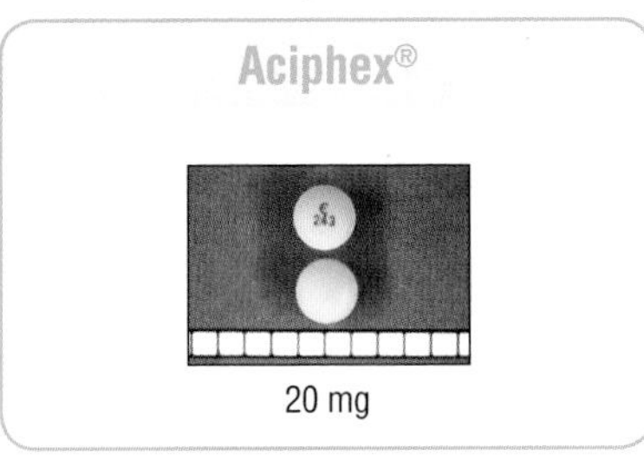
20 mg

Raloxifene

Evista®

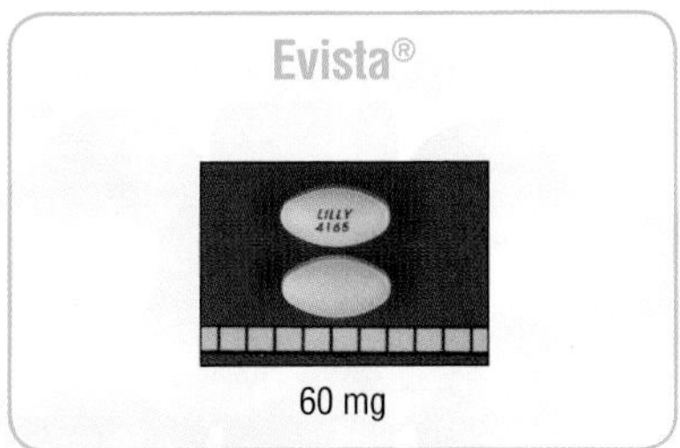
60 mg

Ramipril

Altace™

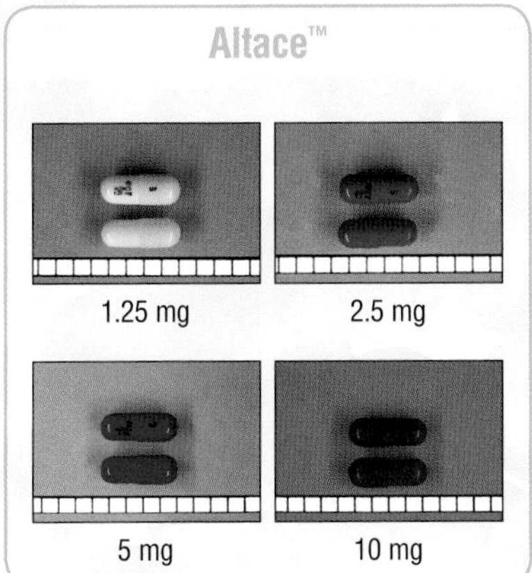
1.25 mg 2.5 mg 5 mg 10 mg

Ranitidine

(generic)

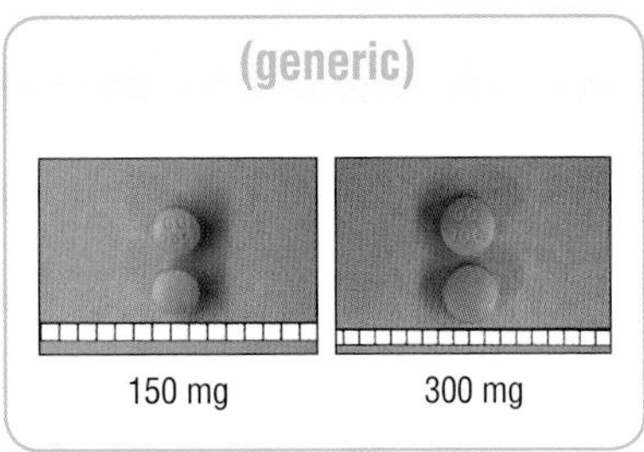
150 mg 300 mg

Risedronate

Actonel®

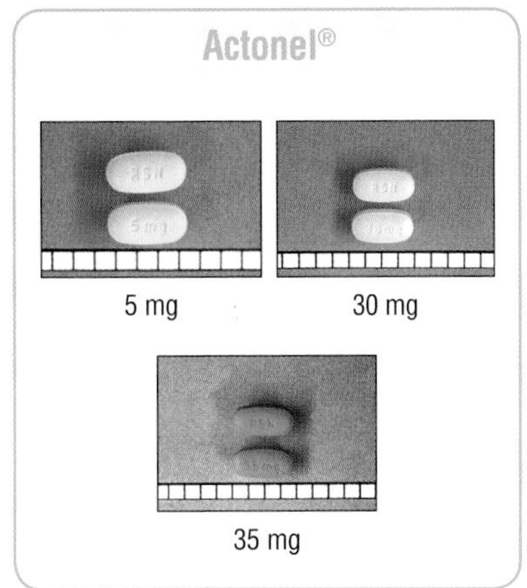
5 mg 30 mg 35 mg

Risperidone

Risperdal®

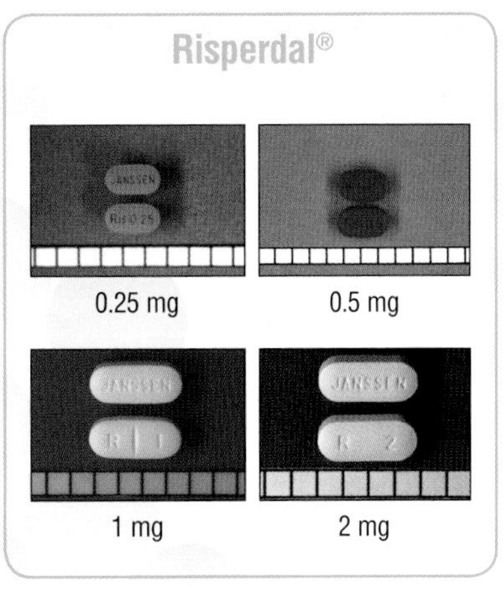
0.25 mg 0.5 mg 1 mg 2 mg

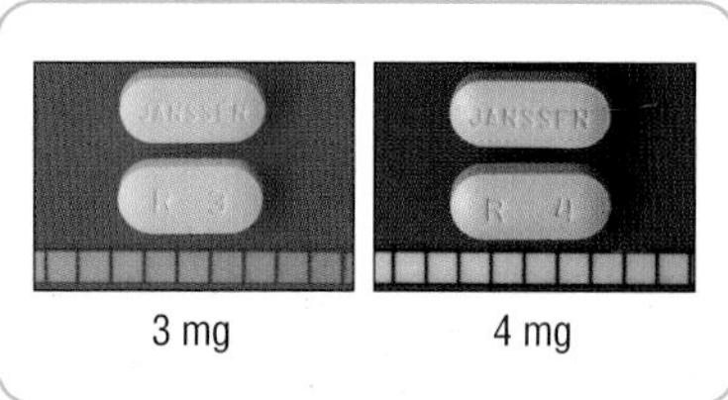

Rosiglitazone

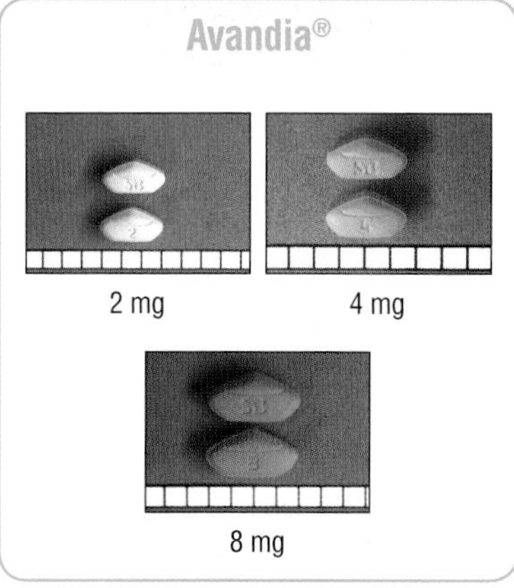

Rosuvastatin

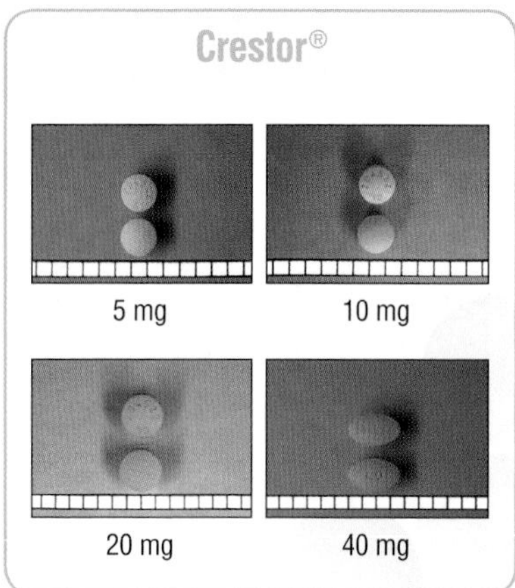

Sertraline

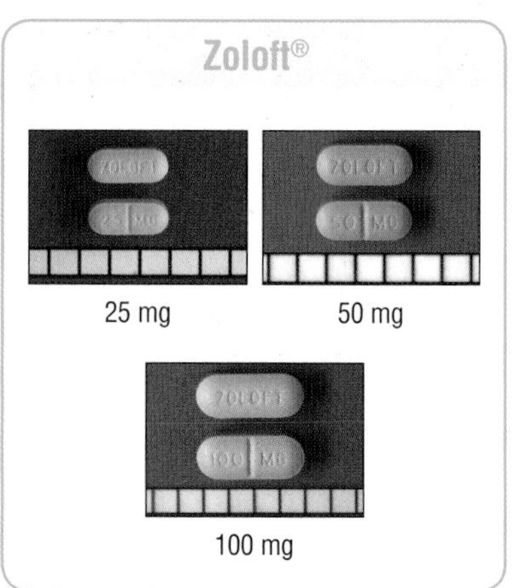

Sildenafil

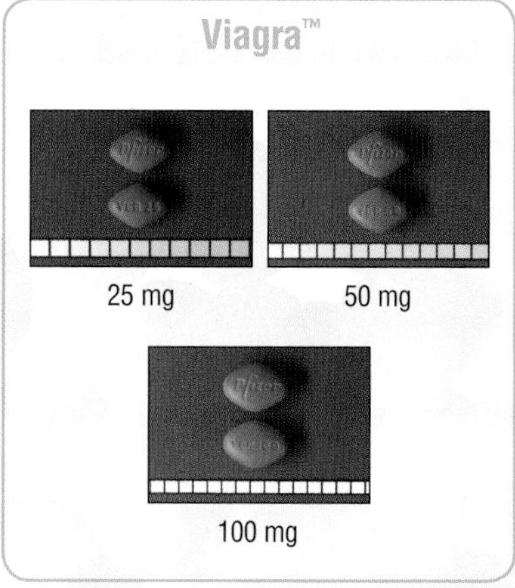

Simvastatin

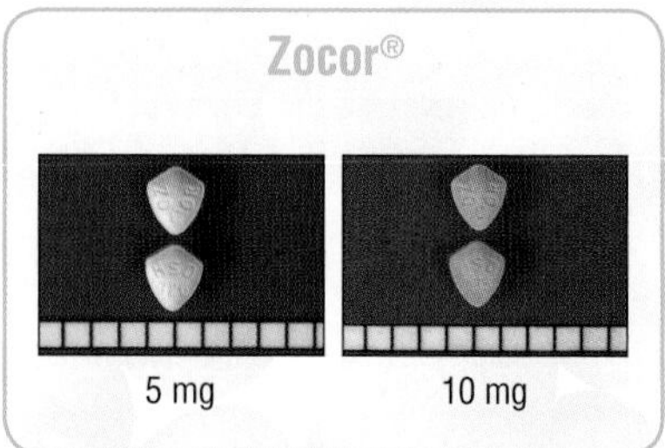

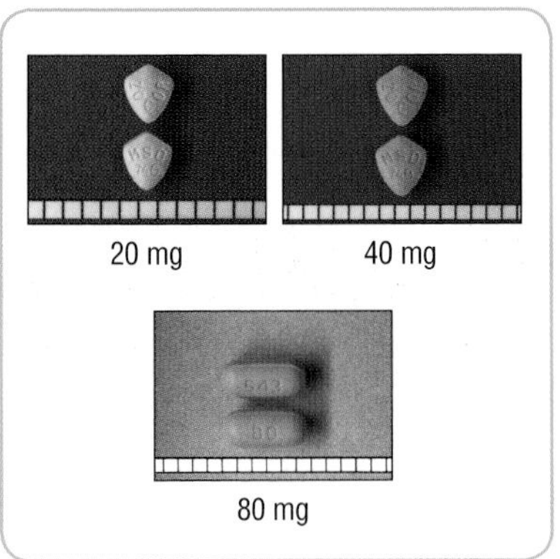

20 mg 40 mg

80 mg

Spironolactone

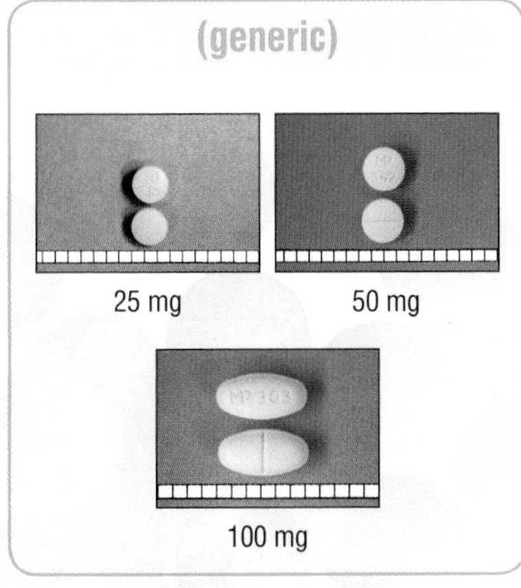

(generic)

25 mg 50 mg

100 mg

Sulfamethoxazole and Trimethoprim

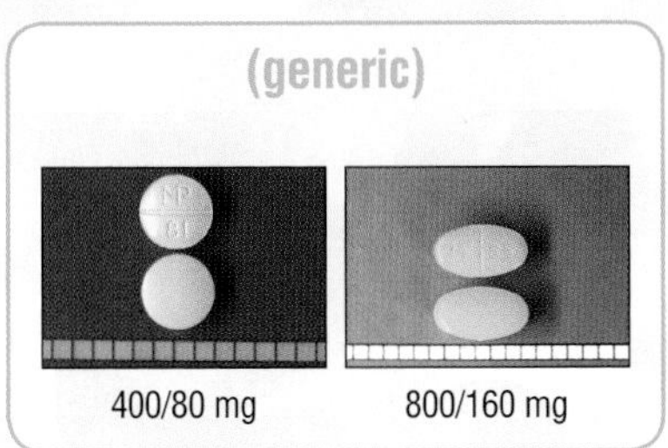

(generic)

400/80 mg 800/160 mg

Sumatriptan

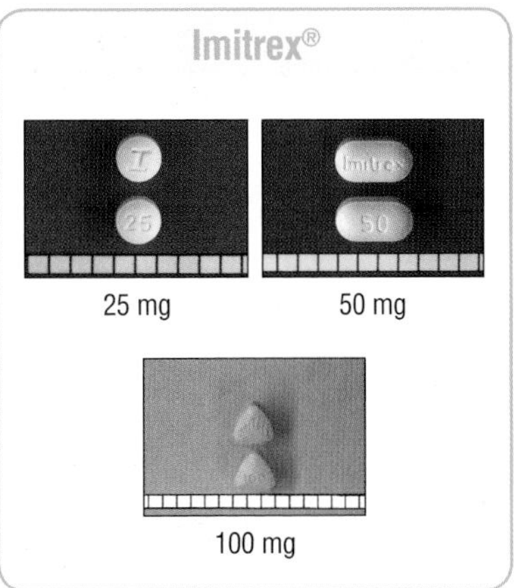

Imitrex®

25 mg 50 mg

100 mg

Tamsulosin

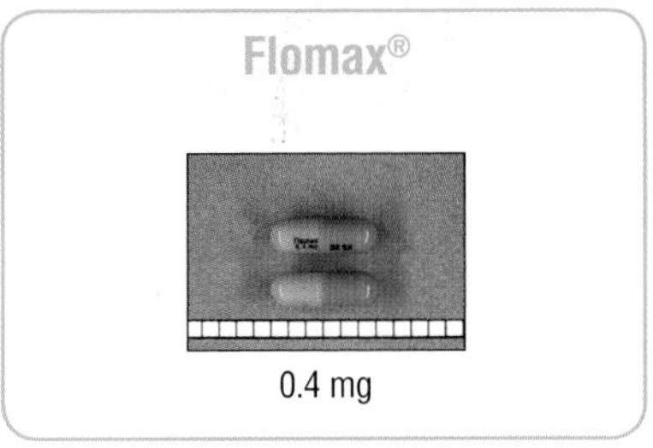

Flomax®

0.4 mg

Temazepam

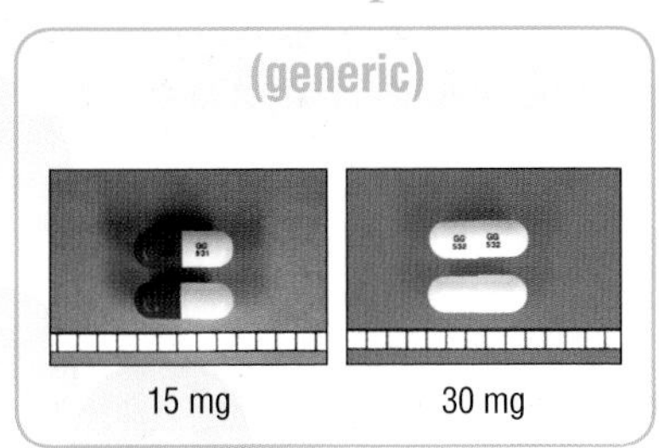

(generic)

15 mg 30 mg

Terazosin

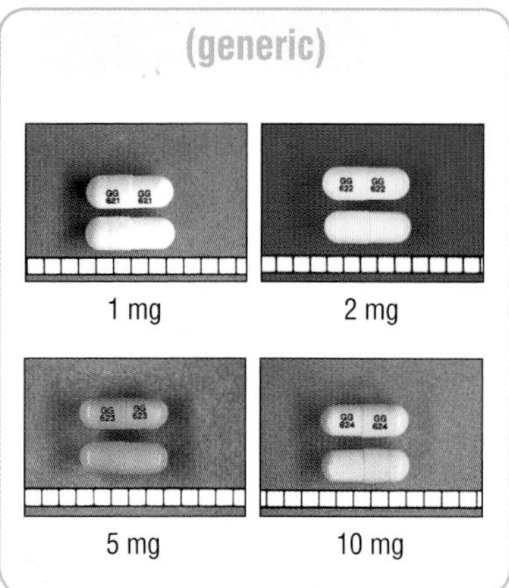

(generic)

1 mg 2 mg

5 mg 10 mg

Tolterodine

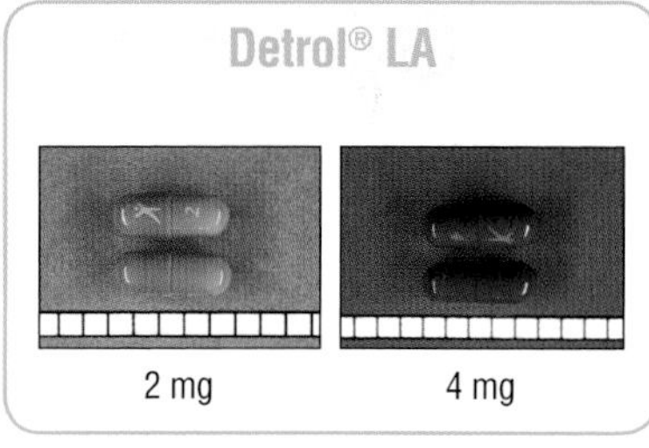

Detrol® LA

2 mg 4 mg

Topiramate

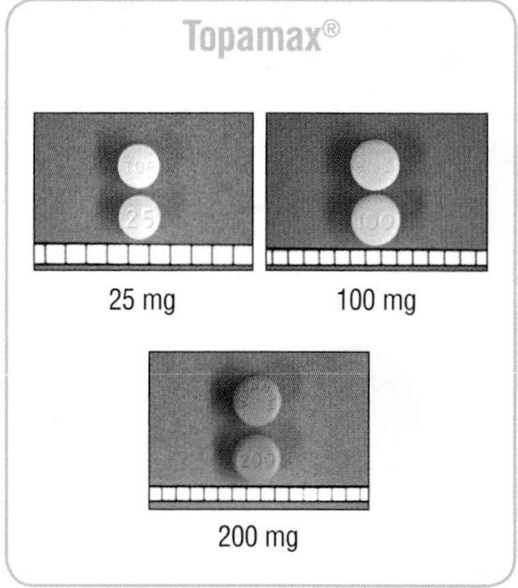

Topamax®

25 mg 100 mg

200 mg

Tramadol

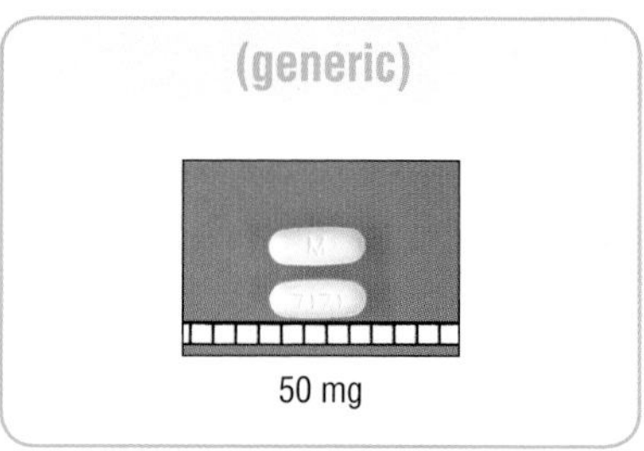

(generic)

50 mg

Trazodone

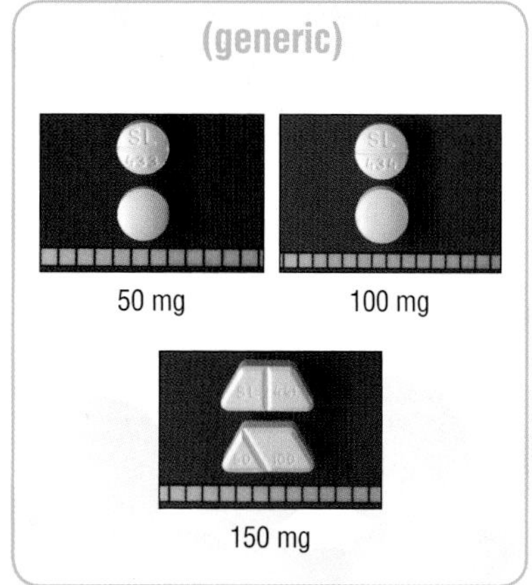

(generic)

50 mg 100 mg

150 mg

Valacyclovir

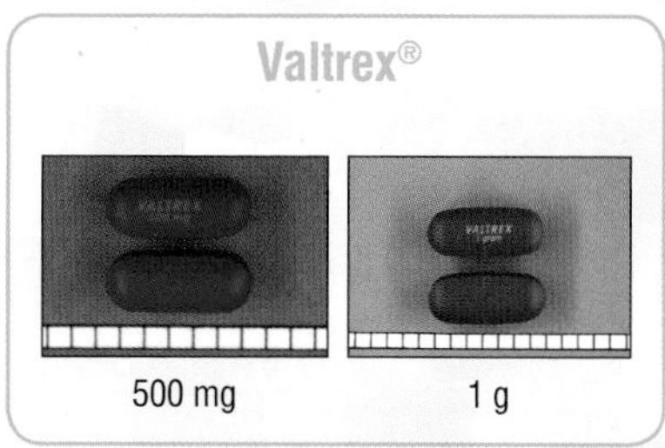

Valtrex®

500 mg 1 g